List of Nursing Procedures

Fundamentals of
NURSING

Fundamentals of NURSING

The Art & Science of Nursing Care

FOURTH EDITION

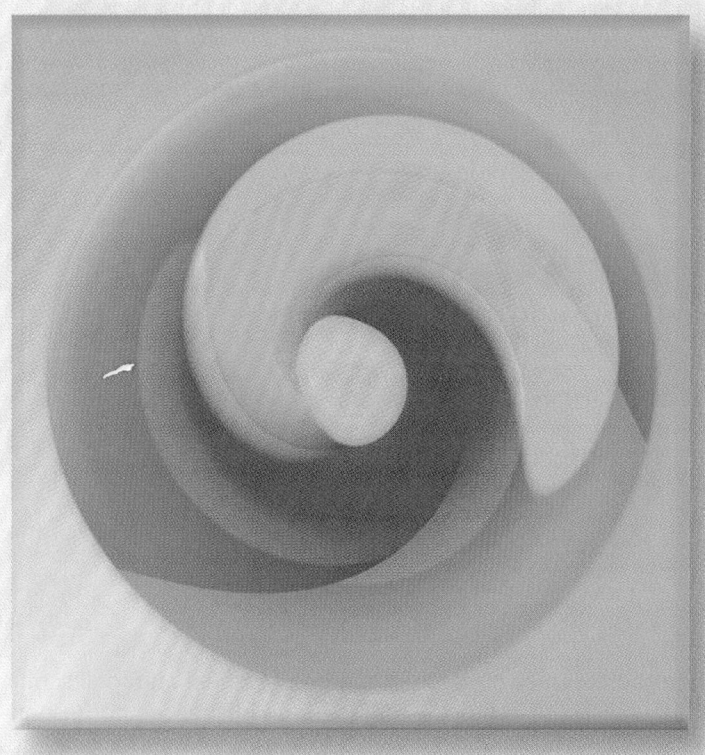

Carol Taylor • Carol Lillis • Priscilla LeMone

Carol Taylor
CSFN, RN, MSN, PhD

Director, Center for Clinical
Bioethics
Assistant Professor, Nursing
Georgetown University
Washington, DC

Carol Lillis
RN, MSN

Interim Dean, Allied Health and Nursing
Department of Nursing
Delaware County Community College
Media, Pennsylvania

Priscilla LeMone
RN, DSN, FAAN

Associate Professor and Director
Undergraduate Program
Sinclair School of Nursing
University of Missouri—Columbia
Columbia, Missouri

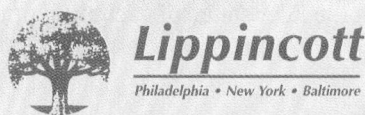

Lippincott
Philadelphia • New York • Baltimore

Acquisitions Editor: Ilze Rader
Managing Editor: Carol Loyd
Developmental Editor: Tom Lochaas
Senior Project Editor: Sandra Cherrey Scheinin
Senior Production Manager: Helen Ewan
Production Coordinator: Michael Carcel

Art Director: Doug Smock
Manufacturing Manager: William Alberti
Indexer: Maria Coughlin
Compositor: Circle Graphics
Printer: R. R. Donnelley

4th Edition

Copyright © 2001 by Lippincott Williams & Wilkins.
Copyright © 1997 by Lippincott-Raven Publishers. Copyright © 1993, 1989 by J. B. Lippincott Company.
All rights reserved. This book is protected by copyright. No part of it may be reproduced, stored in a retrieval system, or transmitted, in any form or by any means—electronic, mechanical, photocopy, recording, or otherwise—without the prior written permission of the publisher, except for brief quotations
embodied in critical articles and reviews and testing and evaluation materials provided by publisher to instructors whose schools have adopted its accompanying textbook. Printed in the United States of America.
For information write Lippincott Williams & Wilkins, 530 Walnut Street, Philadelphia, PA 19106.

Materials appearing in this book prepared by individuals as part of their official duties as U.S. Government
employees are not covered by the above-mentioned copyright.

9 8 7 6 5 4 3 2 1

Library of Congress Cataloging-in-Publication Data

Taylor, Carol, CSFN.
　Fundamentals of nursing : the art and science of nursing care / Carol Taylor, Carol Lillis, Priscilla
LeMone.—4th ed.
　　p. ; cm.
　Includes bibliographical references and index.
　ISBN 0-7817-2273-X (alk. paper)
　　1. Nursing. I. Lillis, Carol. II. LeMone, Priscilla. III. Title.
　[DNLM: 1. Nursing. 2. Health Promotion. 3. Nursing Process. WY 16 T239f 2001]
　RT41 .F882 2001
　610.73—dc21   00-057589

Care has been taken to confirm the accuracy of the information presented and to describe
generally accepted practices. However, the authors, editors, and publisher are not responsible for errors or omissions or for any consequences from application of the information
in this book and make no warranty, express or implied, with respect to the content of the
publication.

The authors, editors, and publisher have exerted every effort to ensure that drug selection and dosage set forth in this text are in accordance with the current recommendations
and practice at the time of publication. However, in view of ongoing research, changes in
government regulations, and the constant flow of information relating to drug therapy and
drug reactions, the reader is urged to check the package insert for each drug for any change
in indications and dosage and for added warnings and precautions. This is particularly important when the recommended agent is a new or infrequently employed drug.

Some drugs and medical devices presented in this publication have Food and Drug Administration (FDA) clearance for limited use in restricted research settings. It is the responsibility of the health care provider to ascertain the FDA status of each drug or device planned
for use in his or her clinical practice.

To my family and community, whose support enables me to meet each new day with love and courage.

Carol Taylor

To all my students, past and present, who are my constant inspiration.

Carol Lillis

To all my colleagues and students, who have nourished my belief in, and love for, nursing.

Priscilla LeMone

Contributors

Jane Rothrock, RN, CNOR, DNSc, FAAN Professor and Program Coordinator, Perioperative Programs, Delaware County Community College, Media, PA

Reviewers

Stasia Arcarese, RN, BS, MS, Professor, Clinton Community College, Plattsburgh, NY

Carol Braudaway, RN, MS, Assistant Professor of Nursing, Columbia Union College, Takoma Park, MD

Patricia Brien, RN, MSN, MEd, Professor of Nursing, Department Chair, ADN Program, Berkshire Community College, Pittsfield, MA

Reitha Cabaniss, RN, MSN, Nursing Faculty, Bevill State Community College, Jasper, AL

Beverly Clark, RN, MS, Associate Professor, Jefferson Community College, Watertown, NY

Patsy E. Crihfield, RN, MSN, CCRN, Assistant Professor of Nursing, Dyersburg State Community College, Dyersburg, TN

Judy Cummings, RN,C, MS, Nursing Faculty, Yavapai College, Prescott, AZ

Melanie Daniel, RN, MSN, Nursing Instructor, Bevill State Community College, Walker Campus, Sumiton, AL

Geralyn Frandsen, Nursing Faculty, Maryville University, St. Louis, MO

Wanda Gifford, St. Elizabeth School of Nursing, Lafayette, IN

Frances S. Izzo, RN, CS, MSN, Associate Professor, Nassau Community College, Garden City, NY

Jennifer Johnson, RN,C, MSN, Assistant Professor of Nursing, Kent State University, New Philadelphia, OH

Marcia Keiser, RN, CPAN, Nursing Faculty, St. Anthony Memorial Hospital, Michigan City, IN

Jo-Ann Landburg, Nursing Faculty, Western Nevada Community College, Carson City, NV

Karol Lindow, RN,C, MSN, Kent State University, Tuscarawas Campus, New Philadelphia, OH

Maureen Marthaler, RN, MS, Visiting Assistant Professor, Purdue University, Calumet, Hammond, IN

Nancye G. McAfee, RN, MSN, Program Director, Upward Mobility Nursing Program, Lamar University, Orange, Orange, TX

Donna Jo Miracle, RN, MSN, Assistant Professor, Anderson University, Anderson, IN

Connie Neuburger, RN, MN, Nursing Faculty, Kansas Wesleyan University, Salina, KS

Linda Peake, RN, MSN, Assistant Professor, St Mary's School of Nursing, Huntington, WV

Anita K. Reed, RN, MSN, Instructor of Nursing, St. Elizabeth School of Nursing, Lafayette, IN

Sharon Staib, RNCS, MS, Assistant Professor, Ohio University, Zanesville, Zanesville, OH

JoAnne Starks, BSN, MEd, Professor of Nursing, Sinclair Community College, Dayton, OH

Roselena Thorpe, RN, PhD, Department Chairperson, Nursing, Community College of Allegheny County, Allegheny Campus, Pittsburgh, PA

Cindy Warren, RN, MSN, Assistant Professor, Kent State University, Tuscarawas College of Nursing, New Philadelphia, OH,

Mary Weisel, RN, MSN, ASN Program Chair, Ivy Tech State College, South Bend, IN

Preface

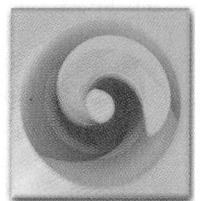

Today's competitive, market-driven healthcare environment is challenging the very nature of professional nursing practice. **Fundamentals of Nursing: The Art and Science of Nursing, fourth edition,** promotes nursing as an evolving art and science, directed to human health and well-being. It challenges students to focus on the **blended skills** they will need to serve patients and the public well. Our aim is to prepare nurses who combine the highest level of scientific knowledge and technologic skill with responsible, caring practice. We want to challenge students to identify and master the cognitive and technical skills, as well as the interpersonal and ethical/legal skills they will need to effectively nurse the patients in their care. We refuse to allow accountability and caring relationships to become relics of a bygone era.

Those new to nursing can quickly become overwhelmed by the demands placed on the nurse's knowledge, technical competence, interpersonal skills, and commitment. Therefore, much care has once again gone into the selection of both the content in this edition and the manner of its presentation. We strive to capture the unique essence of both the art and science of nursing, distilling what the person beginning the study and practice of nursing needs to know. We invite students to identify with the profession, to share in its pride, and to respond to today's challenges competently, enthusiastically, and accountably.

Those familiar with earlier editions of this text will note that we have chosen in this edition to replace the term "client" with "patient." The term *client* was initially used to highlight the active role that most individuals prefer to play in directing their healthcare. From the very first edition of this text, students were encouraged to actively partner with patients and their family caregivers in designing and implementing care. Today we have witnessed the healthcare "industry" transform patients to "customers" who buy healthcare (if they are able) as a commodity in the marketplace. We do not believe that a "customer-orientation" serves patients or nurses well. One of our students shared her belief that she owes less to a "customer" and even to a "client" than she does to a "patient." We therefore have chosen to reclaim the term *patient*—in its most positive sense—to designate the recipient of nursing care. New efforts have been made to highlight nursing strategies for actively engaging patients, family caregivers, and the public in the development of health goals and strategies to achieve these goals. Patients may be individuals, families, or communities. Care has been taken to communicate that both nurses and patients may be male or female and that they come from every racial and ethnic background and socioeconomic group. Whenever possible we have tried to avoid male/female distinctions in personal pronouns.

Organization

Fundamentals of Nursing: The Art and Science of Nursing Care is organized into eight units. Ideally, the text is followed sequentially, but every effort has been made to respect the differing needs of diverse curricula and students. Thus, each chapter stands on its own merit and may be read independently of others.

Unit I, *Foundations for Nursing Practice*, opens with a description of contemporary nursing. Successive chapters introduce content foundational to nursing practice: human needs (individual, family, and community), culture and ethnicity, health, nursing theory, ethics, and law.

Unit II, *Promoting Health Across the Life Span*, provides the basis for understanding growth and development across the life span and acknowledges nursing's differing requirements arising from the various developmental stages and abilities to meet developmental tasks.

Unit III, *Community-Based Settings for Patient Care*, introduces the multiple settings in which nursing is practiced and prepares students to ensure continuity of care in what could be a fragmented healthcare system. Chapters address the variety of community-based healthcare settings; continuity of care as the patient enters a healthcare facility, is transferred within the facility, and is discharged into another setting within the community; and care provided within the home.

Unit IV, *The Nursing Process*, offers a detailed, step-by-step guide to each component of the nursing process. Practical guidelines and examples are included in each chapter. Separate chapters address the nursing process as a whole, nursing's blended skills, assessing, diagnosing, planning, implementing, and evaluating. A chapter on documentation, reporting, and conferring highlights these nursing responsibilities.

Unit V, *Roles Basic to Nursing Care*, describes major roles in which nurses function as they interact holistically with patients. Chapters focus on the communicator, teacher and counselor, and leader, researcher, and advocate roles of the nurse as caregiver.

Unit VI, *Actions Basic to Nursing Care*, introduces the foundational skills used by nurses: measuring vital signs, assessing health, promoting safety, maintaining asepsis, administering medication, and caring for surgical patients.

Unit VII, *Promoting Healthy Psychosocial Responses*, explores the nurse's role in helping patients meet basic psychosocial needs: self-concept, stress and adaptation, loss, grief and dying, sensory stimulation, sexuality, and spirituality. In each chapter, guidelines are included for assessing and diagnosing unhealthy responses and for planning, implementing, and evaluating appropriate care strategies. Chapters conclude with a *Patient Care Study*, illustrating the use of the nursing process and nursing's blended skills to resolve selected nursing diagnoses.

Unit VIII, *Promoting Healthy Physiologic Responses*, uses the same format as Unit VII to focus on the physiologic needs of patients: hygiene, skin integrity, activity, rest and sleep, comfort, nutrition, urinary elimination, bowel elimination, oxygenation, and fluid, electrolyte, and acid–base balance.

Integrated Nursing Process

After the nursing process is introduced in Unit IV, it provides the organizational framework for successive chapters. Chapters in Units VII and VIII, which deal with psychosocial and physiologic responses, begin with a succinct background discussion of the concept, followed by an identification of factors that influence how different individuals respond to these needs. Steps in the nursing process are used to describe related nursing responsibilities.

Assessing. Common elements of both a comprehensive and problem-focused nursing assessment are presented; sample interview questions are included, and specific physical assessment techniques are described.

Diagnosing. North American Nursing Diagnosis Association (NANDA)-approved nursing diagnoses related to the human need being discussed are identified, and tables illustrate the relationship between related factors and the problem statement and provide sample defining characteristics.

Planning. Sample patient goals/expected outcomes are suggested based on patient strengths.

Implementing. Nursing interventions are clearly explained and are illustrated when this is deemed helpful. Procedures have been streamlined to facilitate mastery, and home health considerations are included. A sufficient variety of nursing interventions is provided to foster the development of a repertoire of nursing actions that makes practicing the art of nursing possible.

Evaluating. Criteria for evaluating the effectiveness of the plan of care are suggested.

Each chapter in Units VII and VIII concludes with a *Patient Care Study* that illustrates each step of the nursing process and a sample documentation of nursing assessment or intervention. Throughout these chapters, students will find numerous practical examples of how to conduct focused assessments, develop and write diagnostic statements, identify goals and outcomes, and select, implement, and evaluate appropriate nursing interventions. These examples will reinforce the student's mastery of nursing process skills. This edition incorporates the latest NANDA diagnoses as well as Nursing Interventions Classification (NIC) and Nursing Outcomes Classification (NOC) content.

Key Features

In this edition, we capitalize on the strengths of the first three editions and address new priorities. We further develop or strengthen the following features:

Nursing as an Art and Science. Nursing, as a science, is characterized by a growing body of knowledge that links technical and interpersonal interventions to desired patient outcomes; as an art, nursing demands of its practitioners sufficient competency to creatively design individualized strategies to assist patients to reach personal health goals. A unique spirit of caring always must prevail.

Health Orientation. A health rather than an illness orientation provides a framework for presentation of content. *Promoting Health* displays highlight assessment checkpoints for specific components of high-level health and include suggestions for designing a self-care prescription. These displays serve a two-fold purpose as a self-care model for the learner and an invaluable aid to the individual who is developing the role of patient healthcare educator.

The Nurse as Role Model. Nurses, because they are role models for their patients, are directed to assess their own health behaviors before attempting to help patients. Health goals for the nurse are presented in each clinical chapter.

Aims of Nursing. Learners are gradually introduced to the theory, interpersonal skills, and nursing procedures that will enable them to work successfully with patients to promote health, prevent illness, restore health, and facilitate coping with altered functioning. Early attention to these broad aims of nursing will prepare learners to meet the needs of patients in diverse healthcare settings.

Basic Human Needs. Common to all people and communities, and essential to health and survival, are basic human needs. The clinical chapters in Unit VII, *Promoting Healthy Psychosocial Responses,* and Unit VIII, *Promoting Healthy Physiologic Responses,* prepare the learner to assist patients and family members in meeting these needs. Learners are encouraged to explore human responses to health and illness as indicators of how well an individual is functioning to meet basic human needs.

Holistic Care Across the Life Span. A holistic orientation to basic human needs exists across the life span.

This orientation is emphasized through information about growth and development in Unit II, *Promoting Health Across the Life Span;* through developmental considerations and related tables and displays in Unit VII, *Promoting Healthy Psychosocial Responses;* and in Unit VIII, *Promoting Healthy Physiologic Responses,* through age consideration in many procedures, and through the diverse ages and needs of patients represented in the patient care studies in clinical chapters addressing the life span. Wherever appropriate, cultural considerations are included.

Attention to Special Needs of the Older Person. Because the age of the population is increasing, nurses encounter growing numbers of older patients in all practice settings. The section on older adults in Chapter 10, *The Aging Adult,* the *Focus on the Older Adult* displays, and general considerations for the older patient that appear within the text aim to sensitize students to the special nursing needs of this population.

Personal Accounts. Delighted with the response to the personal accounts of students in the third edition, we invited patients and family caregivers to share their experiences in the fourth edition. Displays entitled *Through the Eyes of a Student, Through the Eyes of a Patient,* and *Through the Eyes of a Family Caregiver* speak eloquently of nursing's power to "make a difference." These personal accounts will evoke smiles, pride, and empathy, and they will unite nurse caregivers in their struggles to perfect their caregiving skills as they make a difference in the lives of others.

Critical Thinking. Critical thinking is highlighted in *Chapter 14, Blended Skills and Critical Thinking Throughout the Nursing Process.* Recurring displays, *Developing Critical Thinking Skills,* help the student follow the process and develop critical thinking. New critical thinking exercises at the conclusion of each chapter challenge students to use the new knowledge they've gained to "think through" learning exercises designed to demonstrate how careful (ie, *critical*) thinking can change outcomes.

Nursing Procedures. Procedures are presented in a concise, straightforward, and simplified format that is intended to facilitate competent performance of nursing skills. Scientific rational accompany each nursing action, and many color photographs and illustrations further reinforce mastery. Special considerations, including modifications and age and home care considerations, are given where appropriate.

Broad Scope of Nursing Practice. The text is written to encompass fundamental skills in a laboratory as well as in actual clinical settings where nurses care for both well and ill patients. To acquaint students of nursing with many exciting career options in nursing, numerous examples are given to illustrate nurses interacting with patients of all ages and backgrounds and in traditional and nontraditional settings.

Research as a Strength to Practice. Updated *Research in Nursing: Making a Difference* displays, appearing throughout the book, promote the value of research and apply its relevance to nursing practice. Students are challenged to become informed participants in, or consumers of, clinical research.

Up-to-date Clinical Information. Revisions in each clinical chapter will help educators and students remain current. Sample new content includes: pain as a 5th vital sign, modified food pyramid for 70+ adults, tunneled and nontunneled percutaneous central venous catheter content, latest statistics and information on poisoning, information on the dangers of body piercing, latex allergy summary, focus on needleless equipment, information on therapeutic range, peak versus trough level of drugs, conscious sedation, AORN Perioperative Patient Focused Model, bedside bladder scanning, and MORE . . .

Revised Nursing Process Content and Presentation. This edition incorporates the latest NANDA diagnoses as well as NIC and NOC content.

New Emphasis on Partnering with Patients, Family, and Professional Caregivers. Careful attention is paid in this edition to directing students to identify, value, and develop the interpersonal skills that will allow them to effectively partner with patients, family, and professional caregivers. This will set a tone for successful practice.

Increased Community Focus and Focus on Expanded Nursing Roles. Patients today spend fewer days in the hospital, are frequently transferred both within the hospital and between healthcare institutions and home, and need to rely on rapidly proliferating community-based healthcare resources. Content, photos, and illustrations throughout the text highlight both traditional and innovative nursing roles in institutional and community-based practice settings. This text encourages students to dream about new ways nurses can serve the public by creatively responding to health needs and problems.

Self-Assessment Guides. *Fundamentals of Nursing* has always encouraged students to be independent learners. Checklists throughout the text (blended skills assessment, use of nursing process, health assessments, etc.) allow students to evaluate their personal strengths and limitations and develop related learning goals.

Student Instructional Materials within the Text

Thinking Critically about Nursing's Blended Skills. These new chapter openers offer students everyday nursing challenges and invite them to identify the cognitive, technical, interpersonal, and ethical/legal skills they would need to meet the challenge. Sample responses highlight examples of these skills. Students will begin reading each chapter understanding why the content is important and with their intellectual curiosity peaked! The emphasis on blended skills prepares nurses who combine the highest level of scientific knowledge and technologic skill with responsible, caring practice.

Learning Outcomes. By *ending* each chapter with the chapter objectives, we are offering a valuable learning checklist to assess mastery of essential content. Students can use these outcomes as a basis for learning outlines or self-testing, or the instructor may use them for evaluating student knowledge and abilities. The key terms for each chapter appear in the list of learning outcomes. When these terms are defined in the chapter, they are boldfaced for clarity. A *Glossary* appears at the back of the book for easy studying of these terms.

Nursing Process Demonstrations. *Fundamentals of Nursing* continues to set the standard for practical demonstrations of each step of the nursing process. As they read through clinical chapters, student *see* multiple examples of assessment questions and skills, diagnostic statements, plans of care, documented nursing interventions, evaluative statements, and discharge and teaching plans. For visual learners, these tools greatly facilitate mastery of the complex behaviors students must master quickly when beginning clinical experiences.

Patient Care Studies. Each clinical chapter concludes with a patient care study and related plan of care. Students will find concrete examples of each step of the nursing process (assessment, diagnosis, planning, implementation, and evaluation), as well as related examples of documentation. The diagnoses that are worked up in these studies illustrate common health problems and the wide variety of independent and collaborative interventions nurses manage in different practice settings.

Bibliography. A bibliography at the end of each chapter helps make the student aware of the variety of resources for information on nursing and gives additional reference materials for instructors or students.

Sample Test Questions. Sample test questions appear at the end of each chapter in Units VI through VIII to facilitate mastery of chapter content. These exercises will assist students who are attempting to improve their objective test-taking skills.

Summary of New Features

These features have already been discussed, but we list them here so that you can see at a glance what is new to the book. In addition to updating all of the chapters in re-

lationship to current healthcare practices, we have added the following:

- A new emphasis on the blended skills (cognitive, technical, interpersonal, and ethical/legal) nurses need to practice effectively into today's world. See the new chapter openers, Thinking Critically About Nursing's Blended Skills.
- Up-to-date Clinical Information.
- Revised Nursing Process Content and Presentation.
- New Emphasis on Partnering With Patients, Family, and Professional Caregivers.
- Increased Community Focus and Focus on Expanded Nursing Roles.
- New Critical Thinking Exercises.
- Self-Assessment Guides.

Teaching/Learning Package

To facilitate mastery of this text's foundational content, a comprehensive teaching/learning package has been developed to assist faculty and students.

- Instructor's Manual
  –Chapter objectives and learning activities encompass a range of cognitive, affective, and psychomotor domains
  –Critical thinking exercises give learning situations for further teaching (same format as those in the text, but fresh questions)
  –1000 NCLEX-style, multiple choice questions with rationale are included
- Testbank/ParTEST (CD-ROM)
  –Computerized testing program; includes 1000 NCLEX-style questions (same as in printed version), downloaded into an automatic, test-generating program; editing function allows instructors to reorganize procedures
- Image Bank CD-ROM

Carol Taylor, CSFN, RN, MSN, PHD
Carol Lillis, RN, MSN
Priscilla LeMone, RN, DSN, FAAN

How to Use
Fundamentals of Nursing

Chapter Openers. The new feature, "Thinking Critically About Nursing's Blended Skills," introduces the chapter content with a holistic approach, challenging students to consider the integration of scientific material, technical skills, and compassionate, responsible practice. By providing everyday examples, students will see the utility of relevant cognitive, technical, interpersonal, and ethical/legal skills.

The unique nature of nursing places nurses at the bedside and in groups of professionals where critical decisions are made about the best way to treat injury and illness and to solve healthcare problems. Often, the question confronting the nurse is not "How do I do this?" but rather "Should I do this?" The more that science and technology increase the options available to patients and healthcare professionals, the more frequently nurses will find themselves asking, "We can do this, but *should we*, here and now, for this patient?" The answer to this and other ethical questions is important for quality care. Nurses need to examine their intuitions, opinions, and convictions about what is ethically right and wrong and monitor how these influence their nursing care.

Ethics or morality poses questions about how we ought to act and how we should live. It is an inquiry into the justification of particular actions (eg, Are these actions right or wrong?), as well as a search for traits of moral character that promote more human flourishing

This chapter explores the influence of values on human behavior and the ethical dimensions of nursing practice. Chapter 14 describes specific ethical competencies, or skills, that are essential to nursing practice. Nurses who understand how patients' values and their own values shape nurse–patient interactions, and who continually develop sensitivity to the ethical dimensions of nursing practice, are best able to provide quality care.

Values

A **value** is a belief about the worth of som... matters, that acts as a standard to gui... you think back to how you spent yo... may observe something about your... time you devote to relationships, w... ities, leisure, and other experiences... the importance (value) you attach... ilarly, the amount of money yo... these endeavors reveals somethi...

A **value system** is an org... each value is ranked along a... value system often leads to... person's values influence... health, and illness; the p... human responses to illne... place a high value on h... often work hard to re... who value high-risk le... to life and health. N... tients are sensitive t... values influence th...

Development...

An individual i... formed over a lifetime... ment, family, and culture. As c...

Chapter 6
Values and Ethics in Nursing

Thinking Critically About Nursing's Blended Skills

Before reading this chapter, think about the types of skills you will need to practice nursing in a responsible manner, sensitive to the influence of values on human behavior and the ethical dimensions of practice.

- You are instructing a woman about lifestyle modifications (eg, diet, exercise, stress reduction) to reduce her risk for heart disease when she tells you to save your breath, "I am now any way!" I'd be better off dead than living like this. "Why should I bother about all that.
- A new nurse on your unit suggests that nurses meet on Tuesdays at lunch to discuss journal articles that recommend better ways of addressing nursing problems commonly encountered in your unit. Not everyone is enthusiastic about her suggestion.
- A woman is brought into the emergency room after an automobile collision in which her daughter was killed. The mother, who was driving, is medically unstable but keeps asking about her daughter. The emergency room attending physician tells everyone to tell the mother anything but the truth about her daughter because he believes she is too unstable to accept this news. The nurse feels uncomfortable with this deception.
- An alert woman in the intensive care unit is begging to be removed from the ventilator. She understands that it is highly likely that she will not be able to breathe on her own if this happens and she says she understands and accepts this. "If I die, I die. I can't keep living like this." The team is undecided about whether to respect her wishes.

What cognitive, technical, interpersonal, and ethical/legal skills do you think you will need to respond effectively to the ethical challenges described above?

79

COGNITIVE SKILLS

- Knowledge of how values influence behavior, specifically the behavior of the woman at risk for heart disease and the nurses who are or are not willing to meet to explore ways to improve their practice.
- Knowledge of theories of ethics, codes of professional ethics, and ethical standards for practice. When, if ever, is it justified to deceive a patient? Would the team be justified in respecting a patient's wish to be extubated even if this results in the patient's death?
- Ability to use an ethical framework and decision-making process to resolve ethical problems.

TECHNICAL SKILLS

- Ability to provide the technical nursing assistance necessary to meet the needs of the patients in the emergency room and intensive care unit.

INTERPERSONAL SKILLS

- Ability to establish trusting professional relationships with both colleagues and patients—relationships that are respectful of value differences and that enhance dignity and worth.
- Ability to advocate for patients whose preferences may be different than your own.

ETHICAL/LEGAL SKILLS

- Ability to use values clarification techniques in professional practice.
- Ability to prevent and resolve ethical conflict.
- Ability to practice nursing consistent with nursing's code of ethics.
- Ability to recognize and respond to ethical and legal issues in practice.

Self-Assessment Guides. Checklists appear throughout the book and provide an opportunity for students to evaluate their strengths and weaknesses relative to specific topics. As a teaching tool, the checklists foster independent learning.

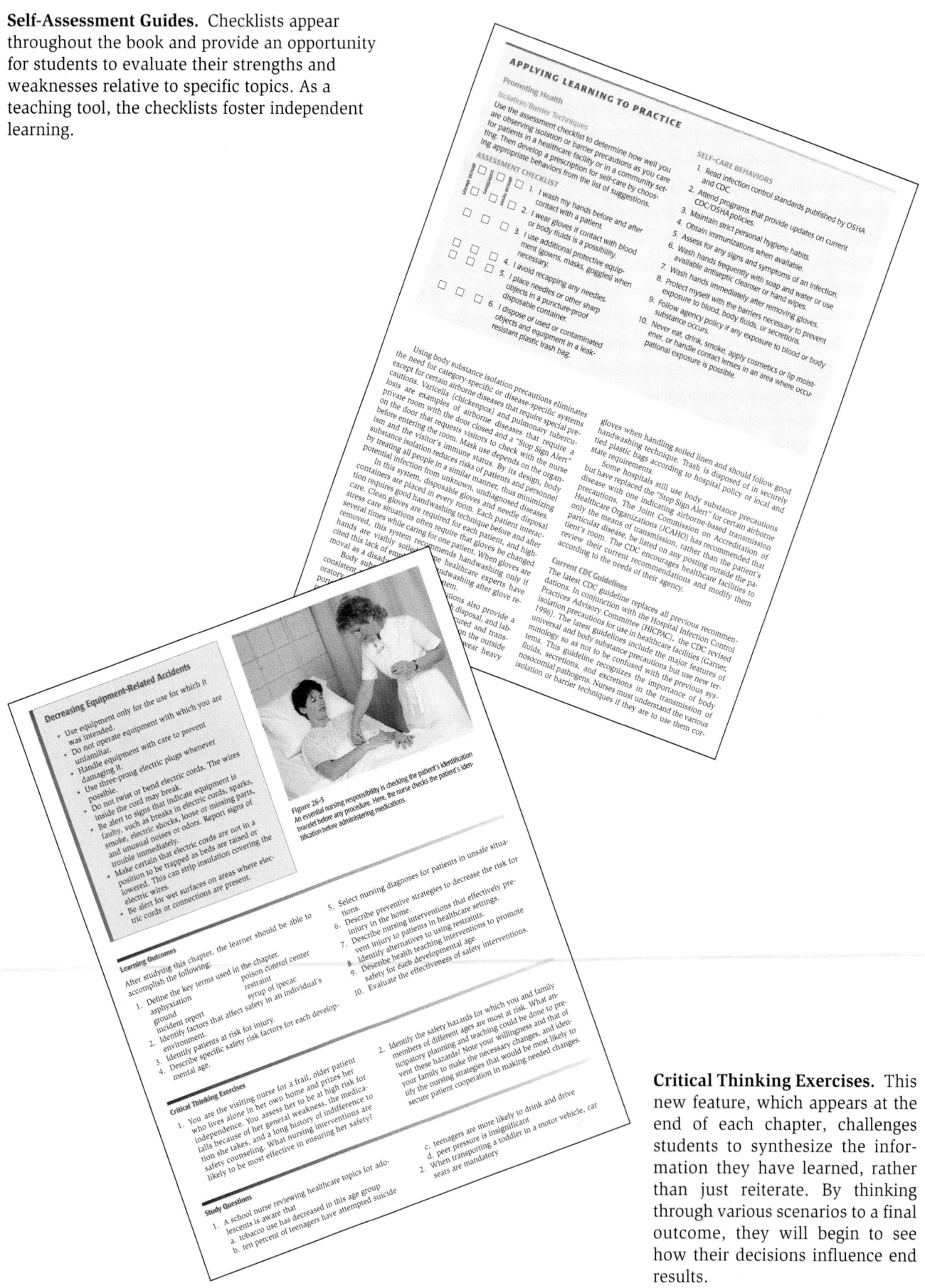

Critical Thinking Exercises. This new feature, which appears at the end of each chapter, challenges students to synthesize the information they have learned, rather than just reiterate. By thinking through various scenarios to a final outcome, they will begin to see how their decisions influence end results.

Patient Care Studies and Nursing Plans of Care. These examples, which appear at the conclusion of every chapter, represent a broad range of the health problems nurses encounter in different settings. The Care Study introduces a specific case, and the related Care Plan follows through the interventions. Each step of the nursing process is covered, and related documentation is included.

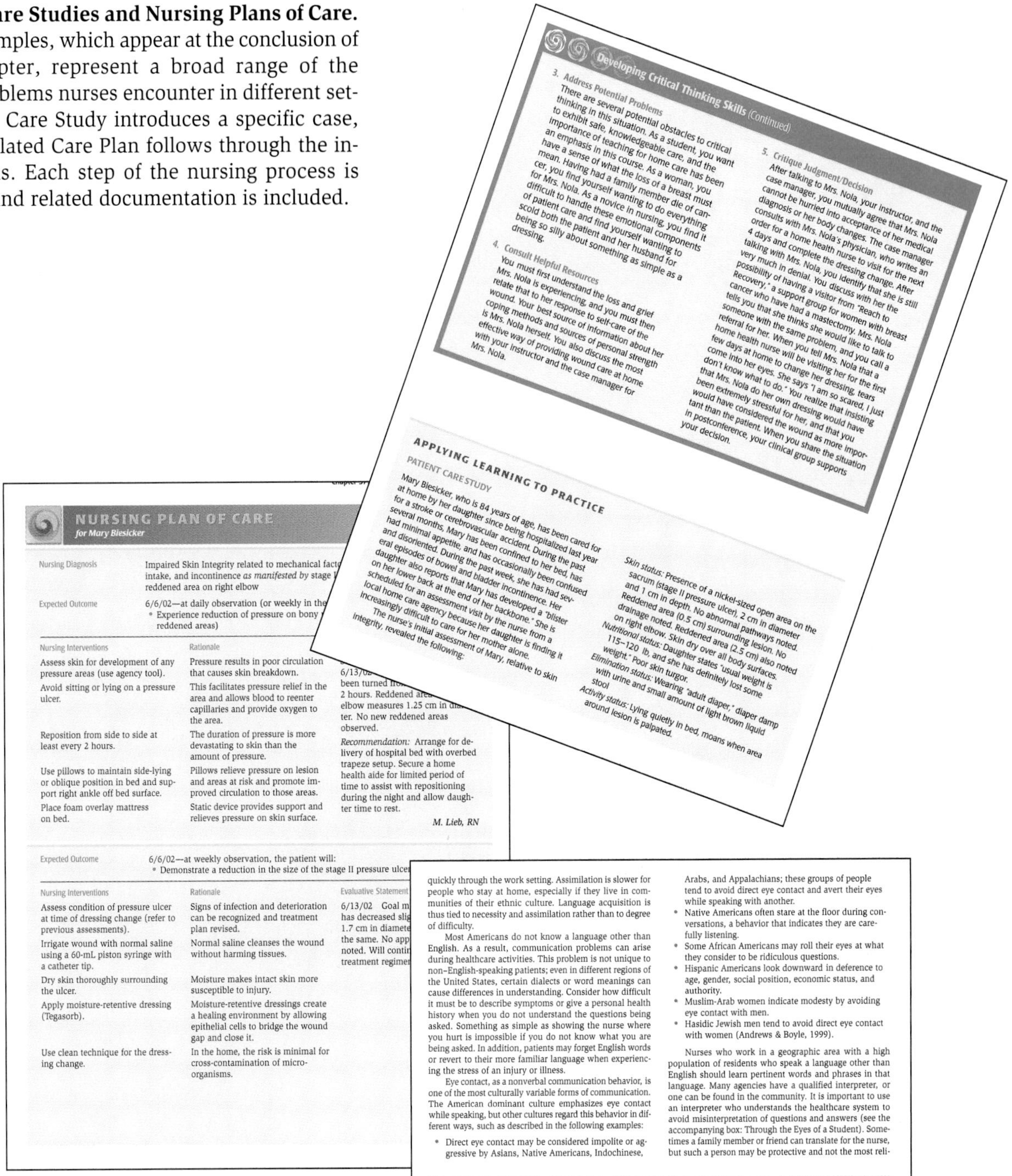

Developing Critical Thinking Skills (Continued)

3. Address Potential Problems
There are several potential obstacles to critical thinking in this situation. As a student, you want to exhibit safe, knowledgeable care, and the importance of teaching for home care has been an emphasis in this course. As a woman, you have a sense of what the loss of a breast must mean. Having had a family member die of cancer, you find yourself wanting to do everything for Mrs. Nola. As a novice in nursing, you find it difficult to handle these emotional components of patient care and find yourself wanting to scold both the patient and her husband for being so silly about something as simple as a dressing.

4. Consult Helpful Resources
You must first understand the loss and grief Mrs. Nola is experiencing, and you must then relate that to her response to self-care of the wound. Your best source of information about her coping methods and sources of personal strength is Mrs. Nola herself. You also discuss the most effective way of providing wound care at home with your instructor and the case manager for Mrs. Nola.

5. Critique Judgment/Decision
After talking to Mrs. Nola, your instructor, and the case manager, you mutually agree that Mrs. Nola cannot be hurried into acceptance of her medical diagnosis or her body changes. The case manager consults with Mrs. Nola's physician, who writes an order for a home health nurse to visit for the next 4 days and complete the dressing change. After talking with Mrs. Nola, you identify that she is still very much in denial. You discuss with her the possibility of having a visitor from "Reach to Recovery," a support group for women with breast cancer who have had a mastectomy. Mrs. Nola tells you that she thinks she would like to talk to someone with the same problem, and you call a referral for her. When you tell Mrs. Nola that a home health nurse will be visiting her for the first few days at home to change her dressing, tears come into her eyes. She says "I am so scared, I just don't know what to do." You realize that insisting that Mrs. Nola do her own dressing would have been extremely stressful for her, and that you would have considered the wound as more important than the patient. When you share the situation in postconference, your clinical group supports your decision.

APPLYING LEARNING TO PRACTICE

PATIENT CARE STUDY

Mary Biesicker, who is 84 years of age, has been cared for at home by her daughter since being hospitalized last year for a stroke or cerebrovascular accident. During the past several months, Mary has been confined to her bed, has had minimal appetite, and has occasionally been confused and disoriented. During the past week, she has had several episodes of bowel and bladder incontinence. Her daughter also reports that Mary has developed a "blister on her lower back at the end of her backbone." She is scheduled for an assessment visit by the nurse from a local home care agency because her daughter is finding it increasingly difficult to care for her mother alone.

The nurse's initial assessment of Mary, relative to skin integrity, revealed the following:

Skin status: Presence of a nickel-sized open area on the sacrum (stage II pressure ulcer), 2 cm in diameter and 1 cm in depth. No abnormal pathways noted. Reddened area (0.5 cm) surrounding lesion. No drainage noted. Reddened area (2.5 cm) also noted on right elbow. Skin dry over all body surfaces.
Nutritional status: Daughter states "usual weight is 115–120 lb, and she has definitely lost some weight." Poor skin turgor.
Elimination status: Wearing "adult diaper," diaper damp with urine and small amount of light brown liquid stool
Activity status: Lying quietly in bed, moans when area around lesion is palpated.

NURSING PLAN OF CARE
for Mary Biesicker

Nursing Diagnosis: Impaired Skin Integrity related to mechanical fact[…] intake, and incontinence *as manifested by* stage [...] reddened area on right elbow

Expected Outcome: 6/6/02—at daily observation (or weekly in the [...]
• Experience reduction of pressure on bony [...] reddened areas)

Nursing Interventions	Rationale	Evaluative Statement
Assess skin for development of any pressure areas (use agency tool).	Pressure results in poor circulation that causes skin breakdown.	6/13/0[…] been turned […] 2 hours. Reddened ar[…] elbow measures 1.25 cm in d[…]ter. No new reddened areas observed.
Avoid sitting or lying on a pressure ulcer.	This facilitates pressure relief in the area and allows blood to reenter capillaries and provide oxygen to the area.	
Reposition from side to side at least every 2 hours.	The duration of pressure is more devastating to skin than the amount of pressure.	*Recommendation:* Arrange for delivery of hospital bed with overbed trapeze setup. Secure a home health aide for limited period of time to assist with repositioning during the night and allow daughter time to rest.
Use pillows to maintain side-lying or oblique position in bed and support right ankle off bed surface.	Pillows relieve pressure on lesion and areas at risk and promote improved circulation to those areas.	
Place foam overlay mattress on bed.	Static device provides support and relieves pressure on skin surface.	M. Lieb, RN

Expected Outcome: 6/6/02—at weekly observation, the patient will:
• Demonstrate a reduction in the size of the stage II pressure ulce[r]

Nursing Interventions	Rationale	Evaluative Statement
Assess condition of pressure ulcer at time of dressing change (refer to previous assessments).	Signs of infection and deterioration can be recognized and treatment plan revised.	6/13/02 Goal m[…] has decreased sli[…] 1.7 cm in diamete[…] the same. No app[…] noted. Will conti[…] treatment regime[…]
Irrigate wound with normal saline using a 60-mL piston syringe with a catheter tip.	Normal saline cleanses the wound without harming tissues.	
Dry skin thoroughly surrounding the ulcer.	Moisture makes intact skin more susceptible to injury.	
Apply moisture-retentive dressing (Tegasorb).	Moisture-retentive dressings create a healing environment by allowing epithelial cells to bridge the wound gap and close it.	
Use clean technique for the dressing change.	In the home, the risk is minimal for cross-contamination of microorganisms.	

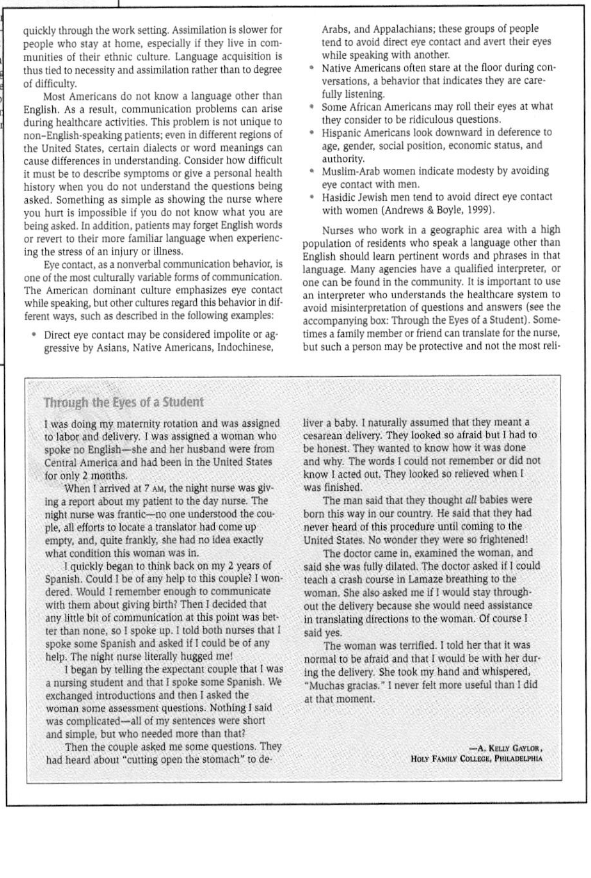

quickly through the work setting. Assimilation is slower for people who stay at home, especially if they live in communities of their ethnic culture. Language acquisition is thus tied to necessity and assimilation rather than to degree of difficulty.

Most Americans do not know a language other than English. As a result, communication problems can arise during healthcare activities. This problem is not unique to non–English-speaking patients; even in different regions of the United States, certain dialects or word meanings can cause differences in understanding. Consider how difficult it must be to describe symptoms or give a personal health history when you do not understand the questions being asked. Something as simple as showing the nurse where you hurt is impossible if you do not know what you are being asked. In addition, patients may forget English words or revert to their more familiar language when experiencing the stress of an injury or illness.

Eye contact, as a nonverbal communication behavior, is one of the most culturally variable forms of communication. The American dominant culture emphasizes eye contact while speaking, but other cultures regard this behavior in different ways, such as described in the following examples:

- Direct eye contact may be considered impolite or aggressive by Asians, Native Americans, Indochinese, Arabs, and Appalachians; these groups of people tend to avoid direct eye contact and avert their eyes while speaking with another.
- Native Americans often stare at the floor during conversations, a behavior that indicates they are carefully listening.
- Some African Americans may roll their eyes at what they consider to be ridiculous questions.
- Hispanic Americans look downward in deference to age, gender, social position, economic status, and authority.
- Muslim-Arab women indicate modesty by avoiding eye contact with men.
- Hasidic Jewish men tend to avoid direct eye contact with women (Andrews & Boyle, 1999).

Nurses who work in a geographic area with a high population of residents who speak a language other than English should learn pertinent words and phrases in that language. Many agencies have a qualified interpreter, or one can be found in the community. It is important to use an interpreter who understands the healthcare system to avoid misinterpretation of questions and answers (see the accompanying box: Through the Eyes of a Student). Sometimes a family member or friend can translate for the nurse, but such a person may be protective and not the most reli-

Through the Eyes of a Student

I was doing my maternity rotation and was assigned to labor and delivery. I was assigned a woman who spoke no English—she and her husband were from Central America and had been in the United States for only 2 months.

When I arrived at 7 AM, the night nurse was giving a report about my patient to the day nurse. The night nurse was frantic—no one understood the couple, all efforts to locate a translator had come up empty, and, quite frankly, she had no idea exactly what condition this woman was in.

I quickly began to think back on my 2 years of Spanish. Could I be of any help to this couple? I wondered. Would I remember enough to communicate with them about giving birth? Then I decided that any little bit of communication at this point was better than none, so I spoke up. I told both nurses that I spoke some Spanish and asked if I could be of any help. The night nurse literally hugged me!

I began by telling the expectant couple that I was a nursing student and that I spoke some Spanish. We exchanged introductions and then I asked the woman some assessment questions. Nothing I said was complicated—all of my sentences were short and simple, but who needed more than that?

Then the couple asked me some questions. They had heard about "cutting open the stomach" to deliver a baby. I naturally assumed that they meant a cesarean delivery. They looked so afraid but I had to be honest. They wanted to know how it was done and why. The words I could not remember or did not know I acted out. They looked so relieved when I was finished.

The man said that they thought *all* babies were born this way in our country. He said that they had never heard of this procedure until coming to the United States. No wonder they were so frightened!

The doctor came in, examined the woman, and said she was fully dilated. The doctor asked if I could teach a crash course in Lamaze breathing to the woman. She also asked me if I would stay throughout the delivery because she would need assistance in translating directions to the woman. Of course I said yes.

The woman was terrified. I told her that it was normal to be afraid and that I would be with her during the delivery. She took my hand and whispered, "Muchas gracias." I never felt more useful than I did at that moment.

—A. Kelly Gaylor,
Holy Family College, Philadelphia

Narrative Accounts. These real-life stories demonstrate how nursing can make a difference in the lives of patients and their families.

Acknowledgments

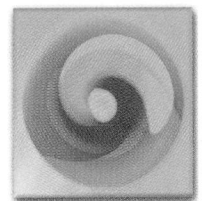

This revision is the work of many talented and committed people, and we wish to gratefully acknowledge the assistance of all who have contributed in any way to the completion of this project. Our first debt of gratitude is to all the nurse educators and students who have adopted the text and shared with us their experiences in using the teaching and learning package. We are deeply grateful for their revision suggestions and trust they will enhance the learning experiences of others.

Our special thanks to the Nursing Editorial division of Lippincott, Williams & Wilkins: Ilze Rader, Editor, and Tom Lochaas, Developmental Editor, both of whom supported our work and provided guidance throughout the project. To the members of the production department, who patiently pulled everything together to form a completed book: Sandy Cherrey Scheinin, Senior Project Editor, Mike Carcel, Senior Production Manager, and Doug Smock, Art Director.

We thank all who generously gave their time, ideas, and resources, and we gratefully acknowledge the special contributions of the following:

- Ken Kasper, Barbara Proud, Gates Rhodes, and Kathy Sloane, photographers

- Maryanne Lieb, Cheryl Meyer, Lana deRuyter, and Jane Rothrock; Delaware County Community College (DCCC) faculty, staff, and administrators; and Ed Dubin and Charity Wamae, who served as models for many of the photos.
- Patty McBride, RN, MSN, CIC coordinator of infection control at Bryn Mawr Hospital, Bryn Mawr, PA, for advising and updating us on changing infection control protocols
- Marie Clark, who developed the math problems and solutions in the "Medications" chapter

We gratefully acknowledge the influence of our mentors and teachers who have influenced our thoughts and writing; each person we have been privileged to care for as nurses; our students, who continually challenge us to find more effective means to teach nursing; our professional colleagues; and perhaps most important, our family and friends, whose love sustained us through the long hours of research and writing.

Finally, we are grateful to the reviewers of this edition and the contributors and reviewers of the previous three editions, whose expertise broadened both the scope and depth of the text.

Carol Taylor
Carol Lillis
Priscilla LeMone

Expanded Contents

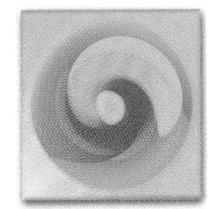

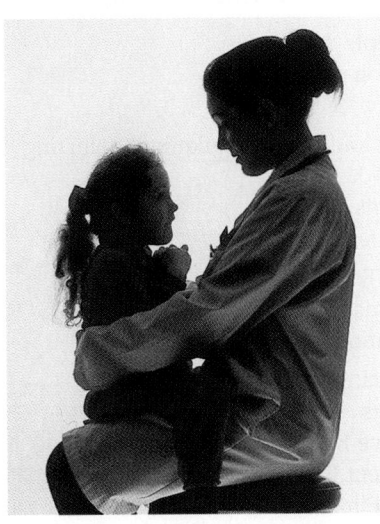

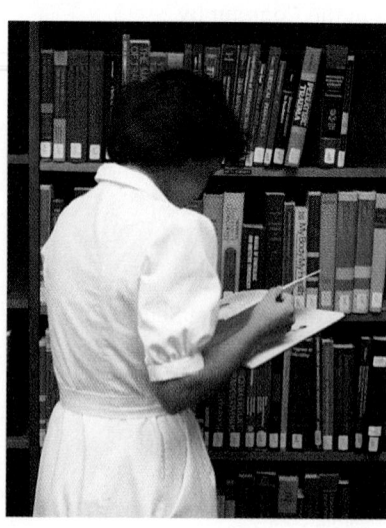

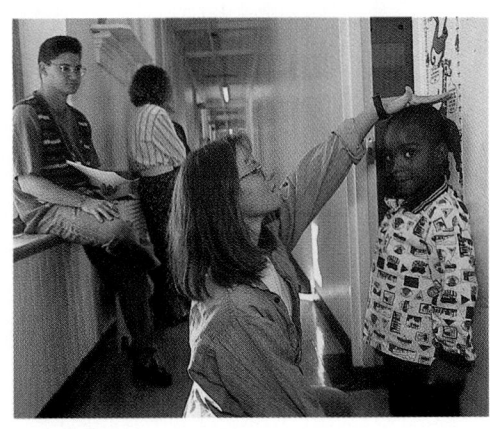

UNIT II
Promoting Health Across the Life Span   116

8 Developmental Concepts   119

9 Conception Through Young Adult   133

10 The Aging Adult   155

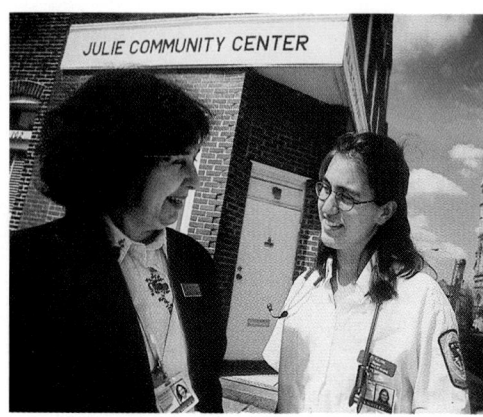

JULIE COMMUNITY CENTER

UNIT III
Community-Based Settings for Patient Care   172

11 Community-Based Healthcare   175

12 Continuity of Care   189

13 Home Healthcare   201

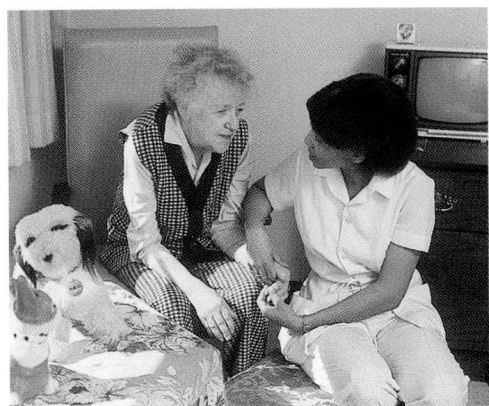

18 Implementing 289

19 Evaluating 303

20 Documenting, Reporting, and Conferring 317

UNIT V
Roles Basic to Nursing Care 344

21 Communicator 347

UNIT VI
Actions Basic to Nursing Care   414

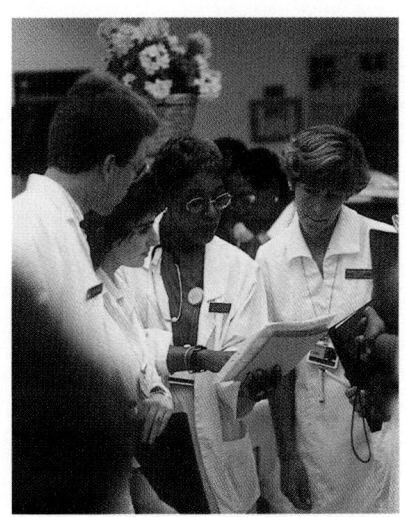

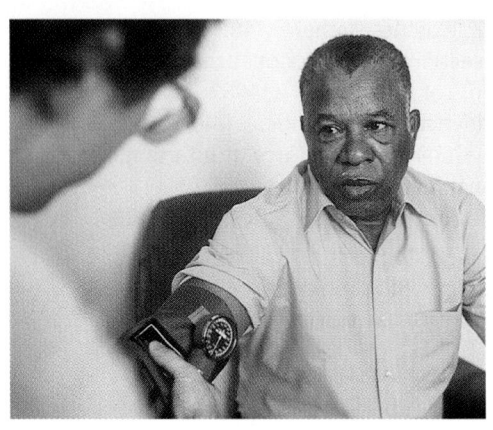

33 Sensory Stimulation 755

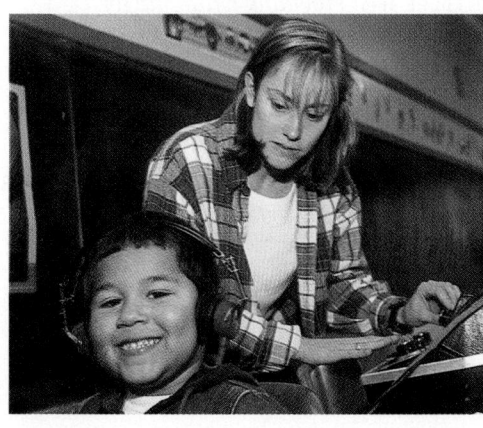

34 Sexuality 779

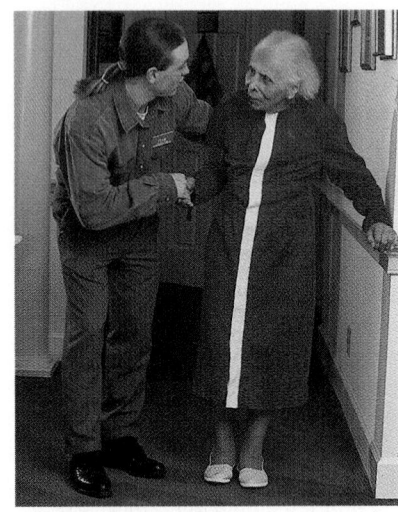

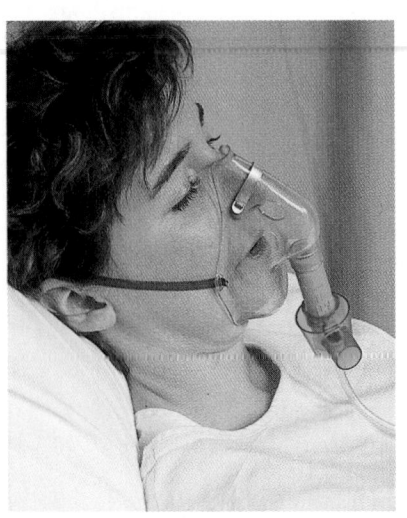

Fundamentals of
NURSING

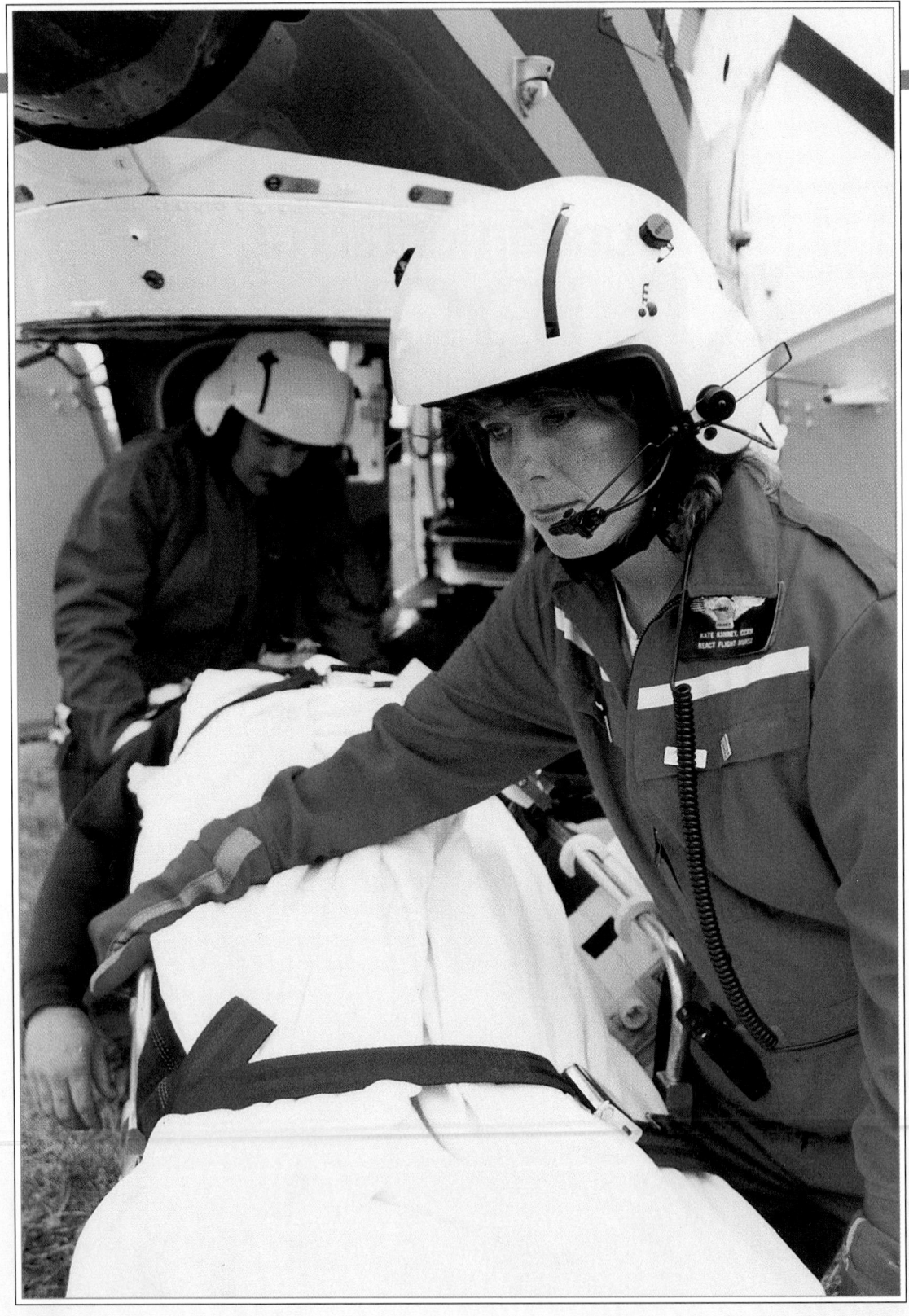

UNIT I

Foundations for Nursing Practice

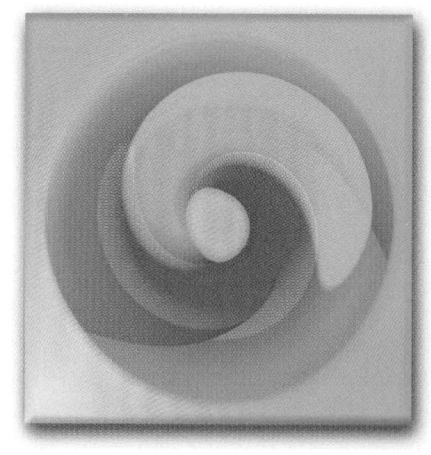

"Basic to any philosophy of nursing seems to be these three concepts: (1) reverence for the gift of life; (2) respect for the dignity, worth, autonomy, and individuality of each human being; (3) resolution to act dynamically in relation to one's beliefs."

Ernestine Wiedenbach (1900–)
a faculty member at Yale University School of Nursing, where she developed her model of nursing from years of experience in various nursing positions

Nursing is both an art and a science. It is a profession that uses specialized skills and knowledge to give care to the whole person in both health and illness and in a variety of practice settings. Unit I introduces concepts necessary to provide nurses with the foundations for nursing practice by defining nursing as a whole. Chapters in this unit introduce the profession of nursing; basic needs of individuals, their families, and the community; culture and ethnicity; promotion of wellness in both health and illness; the theoretical base for nursing; and values, with their ethical and legal implications for nursing practice.

Historic perspectives, educational preparation, professional organizations, and guidelines for professional nursing practice serve as a base for understanding what nursing is and how it is organized. An understanding of basic human needs and the individualized definitions of wellness and illness prepare the nurse to integrate the human dimensions—the physical, intellectual, emotional, sociocultural, spiritual, and environmental aspects of each person— into the care given to promote wellness, prevent illness, restore health, and facilitate coping with altered function or death. Knowledge of the varied methods of care delivery is necessary in today's complex healthcare system.

Nursing theories provide a base for nursing practice, defining the rationale for nursing actions and offering a focus for nursing care. An understanding of the influence of values on human behavior and of the ethical dimensions of nursing practice is essential to responsible and accountable patient care. Finally, sensitivity to the legal implications of professional nursing practice is imperative in today's culture.

Unit I explores the foundations for nursing practice from the perspective of the nurse and a holistic understanding of the patient. Students of nursing are introduced to a challenging and rewarding profession, and are provided with a knowledge base to ground the development of caregiving skills and professional relationships and behaviors.

Chapter 1
Introduction to Nursing

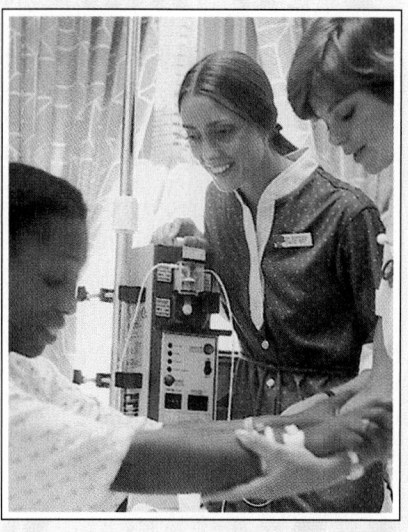

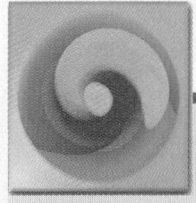

**Thinking Critically About
Nursing's Blended Skills**

Before reading this chapter, think about the types of skills you will need to master to prepare yourself for a professional nursing role.

- A young, first-time mother calls the nursery to report that her recently discharged newborn is not taking to the breast and has not had any real feeding for 24 hours.
- A colleague asks you to speak at a local meeting of oncology nurses about the education program you developed to prepare nurses to administer different types of chemotherapeutic agents.
- A group of nurses in the emergency room is becoming more and more concerned about the health needs of the increasing numbers of homeless people who appear in the emergency room with untreated medical conditions.
- You have good reason to suspect that a nurse colleague is abusing alcohol and other substances and are worried that she can no longer practice safely.

What cognitive, technical, interpersonal, and ethical/legal skills do you think you will need to meet the everyday challenges of professional nursing?

What is *nursing*? Consider the following examples of who nurses are and what they do:

- Delton Nix, RN, graduated from an associate degree nursing program 3 years ago, and is now working full-time as a staff nurse in a hospital medical unit while he attends school part-time toward a baccalaureate degree in nursing; his goal is to become a nurse anesthetist.
- Jeiping Wu, RN, MSN, FNP, specializes as an advanced practice family nurse practitioner. She has an independent practice in a rural primary health clinic.
- Samuel Cohen, LPN, decided to follow his life's dream to become a nurse after 20 years as a postal worker. After examining all his options and goals, he completed a practical nursing program and is now a member of an emergency ambulance crew in a large city.
- Amy Orlando, RN, BSN, graduated 2 years ago and recently began a new job in an urban community health service.
- Roxanne McDaniel, RN, PhD, has a doctorate in nursing and teaches and conducts research at a large university.

These examples show how difficult it is to describe nursing simply. If everyone in your class were asked to complete the sentence, "Nursing is . . . ," there would be many different responses because each person would answer based on his or her own personal experience and knowledge of nursing at that time. As you progress toward graduation and as you practice nursing after graduation, your own definition will change, reflecting changes within you as you learn about and experience nursing.

Most basically defined, **nursing** is the care of others. That care may involve any number of activities, from carrying out complicated technical procedures to something as seemingly simple as holding a hand. All nursing actions focus on the person receiving care and are a blend of the art and the science of nursing. The *science* of nursing is the knowledge base for the care that is given, and the *art* of nursing is the skilled application of that knowledge to help others reach maximum health and quality of life.

COGNITIVE SKILLS

- Knowledge of basic nutritional theory, breastfeeding, and the factors and variables that affect newborn nutrition
- Knowledge about chemotherapeutic agents and how to prepare and administer them safely
- Knowledge about how to design an effective teaching program for nurses
- Knowledge about the community resources that exist for the homeless and how to advocate for underserved populations
- Knowledge about impaired colleagues and how to work with the state board of nursing to help impaired colleagues and to ensure the safety of patients

TECHNICAL SKILLS

- Strong assessment skills to diagnose difficulties with breastfeeding and to identify the health needs of the homeless
- Competence in particular skills, such as drug preparation (chemotherapeutic agents) and intravenous therapy

INTERPERSONAL SKILLS

- Strong people skills to establish trusting relationships with the new mother, nurses interested in designing education programs, the homeless and those best able to meet their needs, and your impaired colleague
- Special interpersonal competence to mobilize your community to develop the type of resources needed to help the homeless and to needed to convince your colleague to seek help for a substance-abuse problem

ETHICAL/LEGAL SKILLS

- First and foremost, a strong sense of accountability for the health and well-being of these people, which translates into a commitment to getting them the help they need to achieve their health goals—within the scope of your nursing responsibilities and available resources
- A willingness to hold colleagues accountable for safe and high-quality practice
- Skill in working collaboratively with your colleagues and others in the community to advocate for the health needs of the homeless
- Knowledge of the ethical and legal principles that guide decision making about impaired colleagues

This chapter introduces you to nursing, including a brief history of nursing from its beginnings to the present and definitions of nursing formulated by nursing leaders and nursing organizations. Educational preparation, professional organizations, and guidelines for professional nursing practice are discussed to help you understand what nursing is and how it is organized. Because nursing is a part of an ever-changing society, current trends in nursing are also outlined.

Nursing: An Emerging Profession and Discipline

Historical Background

From the beginning, the nurse has been regarded as a caregiver. This role has traditionally been defined by groups, communities, and societies in which nursing was practiced. Healthcare and nursing as we currently know them have grown from what they were in the past.

Most early civilizations believed that illness had supernatural causes. The theory of animism attempted to understand the cause of mysterious changes in bodily functions. This theory was based on the belief that everything in nature was alive with invisible forces and endowed with power. Good spirits brought health; evil spirits brought sickness and death. The roles of the physician and the nurse were separate and distinct. The physician was the medicine man who treated disease by chanting, inspiring fear, or opening the skull to release evil spirits (Dolan, Fitzpatrick, & Herrmann, 1983). The nurse usually was the mother who cared for her family during sickness by providing physical care and herbal remedies. This nurturing and caring role of the nurse has continued to the present.

As civilizations grew, temples became the centers of medical care because of the belief that illness was caused by sin and the gods' displeasure (ie, disease literally means "dis-ease"). Priests were highly regarded as physicians, but neither human life nor women were valued by society. In some societies, the nurse was viewed as a slave, carrying out menial tasks based on the orders of the priest-physician. During the same period, the ancient Hebrews developed rules for ethical human relationships, mental health, and disease control through the Ten Commandments and the Mosaic Health Code. Nurses cared for sick people in the home and the community and also practiced as nurse-midwives (Dolan, Fitzpatrick, & Herrmann, 1983).

In the early Christian period, nursing began to have a formal and more clearly defined role. Led by the belief that love and caring for others were important, women called *deaconesses* made the first organized visits to sick people, and members of male religious orders gave nursing care and buried the dead. Both male and female nursing orders were founded during the Crusades. Hospitals were built for the enormous number of pilgrims needing healthcare, and nursing became a respected vocation. Although the early Middle Ages ended in chaos, nursing had developed purpose, direction, and leadership.

At the beginning of the 16th century, many Western societies changed from having a religious orientation to emphasizing warfare, exploration, and expansion of knowledge. Many monasteries and convents closed, leading to a tremendous shortage of people to care for the sick. To meet this need, women who had committed crimes were recruited into nursing in lieu of serving jail sentences. Along with a poor reputation, nurses received low pay and worked long hours in unfavorable conditions.

From the middle of the 18th century to the 19th century, social reforms changed the roles of nurses and of women in general. It was during this time that nursing as we now know it began, based on many of the beliefs and examples of Florence Nightingale. Florence Nightingale was born in 1820 to a wealthy family. She grew up in England and was well educated and traveled extensively. Despite strong opposition from her family, Miss Nightingale undertook nurse's training at the age of 31 years. The outbreak of the Crimean War and a request by the British to organize nursing care for a military hospital in Turkey gave Miss Nightingale an opportunity for achievement (Kalish & Kalish, 1995). As she successfully overcame enormous difficulties, Miss Nightingale challenged prejudices against women and elevated the status of all nurses. After the war, she returned to England, where she established a training school for nurses and wrote books about healthcare and nursing education.

Florence Nightingale's contributions are numerous and far-reaching:

- Identifying the personal needs of the patient and the role of the nurse in meeting those needs
- Establishing standards for hospital management
- Establishing a respected occupation for women
- Establishing nursing education
- Recognizing the two components of nursing—health and illness
- Believing that nursing is separate and distinct from medicine
- Recognizing that nutrition is important to health
- Instituting occupational and recreational therapy for sick people
- Stressing the need for continuing education for nurses
- Maintaining accurate records, recognized as the beginnings of nursing research

Florence Nightingale elevated the status of nursing to a respected occupation, improved the quality of nursing care, and founded modern nursing education. Florence Nightingale and other images of nursing care in the 19th century are shown in Figure 1-1; people important to the development of nursing are listed in Table 1-1.

Nursing in North America

The work of Florence Nightingale and the care provided for battle casualties during the Civil War focused attention on the need for educated nurses in the United States. Schools of nursing were founded in connection with hospitals. Although these schools were established on the beliefs of

Florence Nightingale, initiator of major reforms in health care and nursing training in England

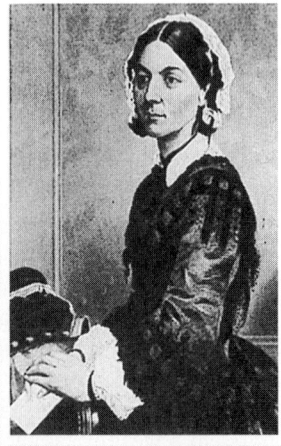

Clara Barton, founder of the American Red Cross in 1882

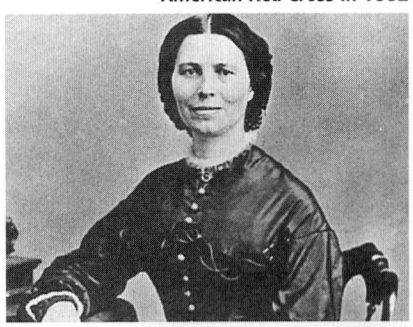

Vassar training camp classroom, 1918
Vassar training camp faculty, 1918

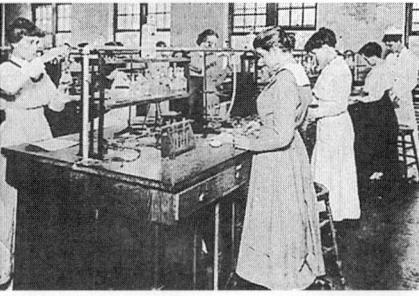

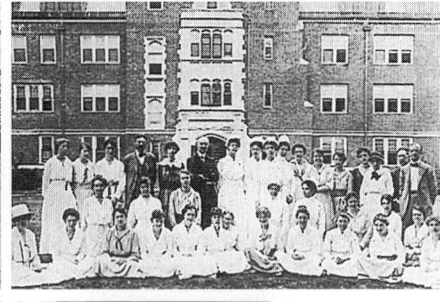

Jane Delano, an army nurse, instrumental in the organization of the Red Cross Nursing Service in the early 1900s

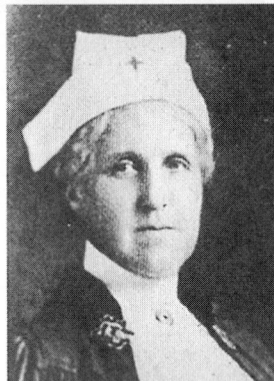

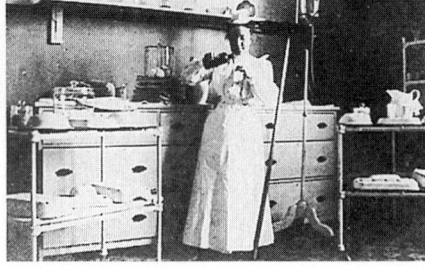

Post-WWII nursing school poster

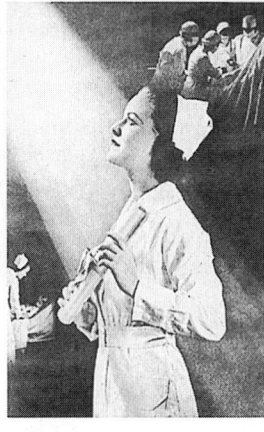

Philadelphia General Hospital nurse, late 1800s

Figure 1-1
Images of nurses spanning more than 100 years of service. (Courtesy of the Center for the Study of the History of Nursing, University of Pennsylvania.)

Nightingale, the training they provided was based more on apprenticeship than on educational principles. Hospitals saw an economic advantage in having their own school, and most hospital schools were organized to provide more easily controlled and less expensive staff for the hospital. This resulted in a lack of clear guidelines separating nursing service and nursing education. As students and as graduates, female nurses were under the control of male hospital administrators and physicians. The lack of educational standards, the male dominance in healthcare, and the pervading Victorian belief that women depended on men combined to contribute to several decades of slow progress toward professionalism in nursing (Kalish & Kalish, 1995).

World War II had an enormous effect on nursing. For the first time, large numbers of women worked outside the home. They became more independent and assertive. These changes in women and in society generally led to an increased emphasis on education. The war itself had created a need for more nurses and resulted in a knowledge explosion in medicine and technology, which broadened the role of nurses. After World War II, efforts were directed at upgrading nursing education. Schools of nursing were based on educational objectives and were increasingly developed in university and college settings, leading to degrees in nursing for both men and women.

Since the 1950s, nursing has broadened in all areas, including practice in a wide variety of healthcare settings, the development of a specific body of knowledge, the conduct and publication of nursing research, and recognition of the role of nursing in promoting health. Increased

Table 1-1
People Important to the Development of Nursing

Person	Contribution
19th Century	
Florence Nightingale	Defined nursing as both an art and a science, differentiated nursing from medicine, created freestanding nursing education; published books about nursing and healthcare; is regarded as the founder of modern nursing (see text for further information)
Clara Barton	Volunteered to care for wounds and feed Union soldiers during the Civil War; served as the supervisor of nurses for the Army of the James, organizing hospitals and nurses; established the Red Cross in the United States in 1882
Dorothea Dix	Superintendent of the Female Nurses of the Army during the Civil War; was given the authority and the responsibility for recruiting and equipping a corps of army nurses; was a pioneering crusader for the reform of the treatment of the mentally ill
Mary Ann Bickerdyke	Organized diet kitchens, laundries, and an ambulance service and supervised nursing staff during the Civil War
Louise Schuyler	A nurse during the Civil War, she returned to New York and organized the New York Charities Aid Association; this organization worked to improve care of the sick in Bellevue Hospital; one recommendation was to have standards for nursing education.
Linda Richards	The first trained nurse in the United States; a graduate of the New England Hospital for Women and Children in Boston, Massachusetts in 1873. She became the night superintendent of Bellevue Hospital in 1874 and began the practice of keeping records and writing orders.
Jane Addams	Provided social services within a neighborhood setting; a leader for women's rights; recipient of the 1931 Nobel Peace prize
Lillian Wald	Established a neighborhood nursing service for the sick poor of the lower East Side in New York City; the founder of public health nursing
Mary Elizabeth Mahoney	Graduated from the New England Hospital for Women and Children in 1879 as America's first black nurse
Harriet Tubman	A nurse and an abolitionist, she was active in the underground railroad movement before joining the Union Army during the Civil War.
Nora Gertrude Livingston	Established a training program for nurses at the Montreal General Hospital (the first 3-year program in North America)
Mary Agnes Snively	Director of the nursing school at Toronto General Hospital and one of the founders of the Canadian Nurses Association)
Sojourner Truth	A nurse who not only provided care to soldiers during the Civil War but also worked for the women's movement
Isabel Hampton Robb	A leader in nursing and nursing education, she organized the nursing school at Johns Hopkins Hospital, where she initiated policies that included limiting the number of hours in a day's work and wrote a textbook to help student learning; was the first president of the Nurses Associated Alumnae of the United States and Canada (which later became the American Nurses' Association).
20th Century	
Mary Adelaide Nutting	As a member of the faculty of Teachers' College, Columbia University, she became the first professor of nursing in the world and, with Lavinia Dock, published the four-volume *History of Nursing*.
Elizabeth Smellie	A member of the original Victorian Order of Nurses for Canada (a group who provided public health nursing); organized the Canadian Women's Army Corps during World War II.
Lavinia Dock	A nursing leader and women's right activist who was instrumental in the Constitutional amendment giving women the right to vote
Mary Breckenridge	Established the Frontier Nursing Service and one of the first midwifery schools in the United States

emphasis on nursing knowledge as the base for nursing practice has led to the growth of nursing as a profession and as a discipline. Table 1-1 summarizes the contributions of people important to the development of nursing as a profession.

Definitions of Nursing

The word *nurse* originated from the Latin word *nutrix*, meaning to nourish. Most definitions of nurse and nursing describe the nurse as a person who nourishes, fosters, and protects; a person prepared to take care of sick, injured, and aged people. With the expanding roles and functions of the nurse in today's society, however, any one definition is too limited. As stated by Ellis and Hartley (1998), one can no longer say "a nurse is a nurse is a nurse." The following sections offer several definitions that provide a broad perspective of nursing. Chapter 5 presents further definitions of nursing by specific nursing theorists.

International Council of Nurses

The following definition was written by Virginia Henderson and adopted by the International Council of Nurses (ICN) in 1973:

> The unique function of the nurse is to assist the individual, sick or well, in the performance of those activities contributing to health or its recovery (or to peaceful death) that he would perform unaided if he had the necessary strength, will, or knowledge. And to do this in such a way as to help him gain independence as rapidly as possible.

American Nurses Association

In 1965, the American Nurses Association (ANA) Committee on Education issued a position paper that broadly defined nursing as an independent profession. The statement said:

> Nursing is a helping profession and, as such, provides services which contribute to the health and well-being of people. Nursing is a vital consequence to the individual receiving services; it fills needs which cannot be met by the person, by the family, or by other persons in the community.
>
> The essential components of professional nursing are care, cure, and coordination. The care aspect is more than "to take care of"; it is "caring for" and "caring about," as well. It is dealing with human beings under stress, frequently over long periods. It is providing comfort and support in time of anxiety, loneliness, and helplessness. It is listening, evaluating, and intervening appropriately.
>
> The promotion of health and healing is the cure aspect of professional nursing. It is assisting patients to understand their health problems and helping them to cope with change. It is the administration of medication and treatments. And it is the use of critical thinking to determine, based on the patient's reactions, whether the plan for care needs to be maintained or changed. It is knowing when and how to use existing and potential resources to help patients toward recovery and adjustment by mobilizing their own resources.
>
> Professional nursing practice is this and more. It is sharing responsibility for the health and welfare of all those in the community, and participating in programs designed to prevent illness and maintain health. It is collaborating with other healthcare providers and technical services as these affect patients. It is supervising, teaching, and directing all those who provide care.

These concepts and beliefs were expanded by the ANA in 1995 in *Nursing's Social Policy Statement*, which describes the values and social responsibility of nursing, provides a definition and scope of practice for nursing, and discusses nursing's knowledge base and the methods by which nursing is regulated. Four essential features of *nursing practice* are described:

- Attention to the full range of human experiences and responses to health and illness without being restricted by a problem-focused orientation
- Integration of objective data with knowledge gained from an understanding of the patient's or group's subjective experience
- Application of scientific knowledge in the nursing process
- Provision of a caring relationship that facilitates health and healing

The central focus in all definitions of nursing is the patient (the person receiving care) and includes the physical, emotional, social, and spiritual dimensions of that person. Nursing is no longer considered to be primarily concerned with illness care. Nursing's concepts and definitions have expanded to include the prevention of illness and the promotion and maintenance of health for individuals, families, and communities.

Nursing as a Profession and a Discipline

As definitions of nursing have expanded to describe more clearly the roles and actions of nurses, increased attention has been given to nursing as a profession and as a discipline. Nursing is gaining recognition as a *profession* (ie, more than a job or occupation) based on the criteria shared by all professions:

- A well-defined body of knowledge
- A strong service orientation
- Recognized authority by a professional group
- A code of ethics
- A professional organization that sets standards
- Ongoing research
- Autonomy

A **discipline** has a specific and unique body of knowledge that uses existing and new knowledge to solve problems creatively and meet human needs within ever-changing boundaries. A discipline must meet certain criteria:

- An impressive body of lasting works
- Suitable techniques
- Concerns that are relevant to human activities

- Relevant traditions that inspire future knowledge development
- Considerable scholarly recognition and achievement

Nursing involves specialized skills and application of knowledge based on an education that has both theoretical and clinical practice components. Nurses uphold standards set forth by professional organizations and follow an established code of ethics. Nursing focuses on human responses to actual or potential health problems and is increasingly focused on wellness, an area of caring that encompasses nursing's unique knowledge and abilities. Nursing is rich in tradition. Furthermore, nursing is increasingly recognized as scholarly, with academic qualifications, research, and publications specific to nursing widely accepted and respected.

Nursing has evolved through history from a technical service to a person-centered process that allows maximizing of potential in all human dimensions. This has been an active process; the profession and the discipline of nursing have developed using lessons from the past to gain knowledge for practice in the present and in the future.

Aims of Nursing

Four broad aims of nursing practice can be identified in the definitions of nursing:

- To promote health
- To prevent illness
- To restore health
- To facilitate coping

To meet these aims, the nurse uses knowledge, skills, and critical thinking to give care in a variety of traditional and expanding nursing roles. To provide knowledgeable care, the nurse uses cognitive, technical, interpersonal, and ethical/legal competencies essential to nursing practice. The primary role of the nurse as caregiver is given shape and substance by the interrelated roles of communicator, teacher, counselor, leader, researcher, and advocate. These competencies and roles, as well as expanded educational and career roles, are described in Tables 1-2 and 1-3 and are fully discussed in Unit V. These roles are carried out by the nurse in many different settings. Examples of settings for care are listed in the accompanying box; settings for care are fully described in Chapters 11 and 12. Of these settings, care is increasingly provided out of the hospital and in the community. These activities are directed toward maximizing the functioning of the patient and his or her family.

Promoting Health

Health is a state of optimal functioning or well-being. As defined by the World Health Organization, one's health includes physical, social, and mental components and is not merely the absence of disease or infirmity. Health is often a subjective state: a person may be medically diagnosed with an illness but still consider himself or herself healthy. **Wellness** is another term with essentially the same mean-

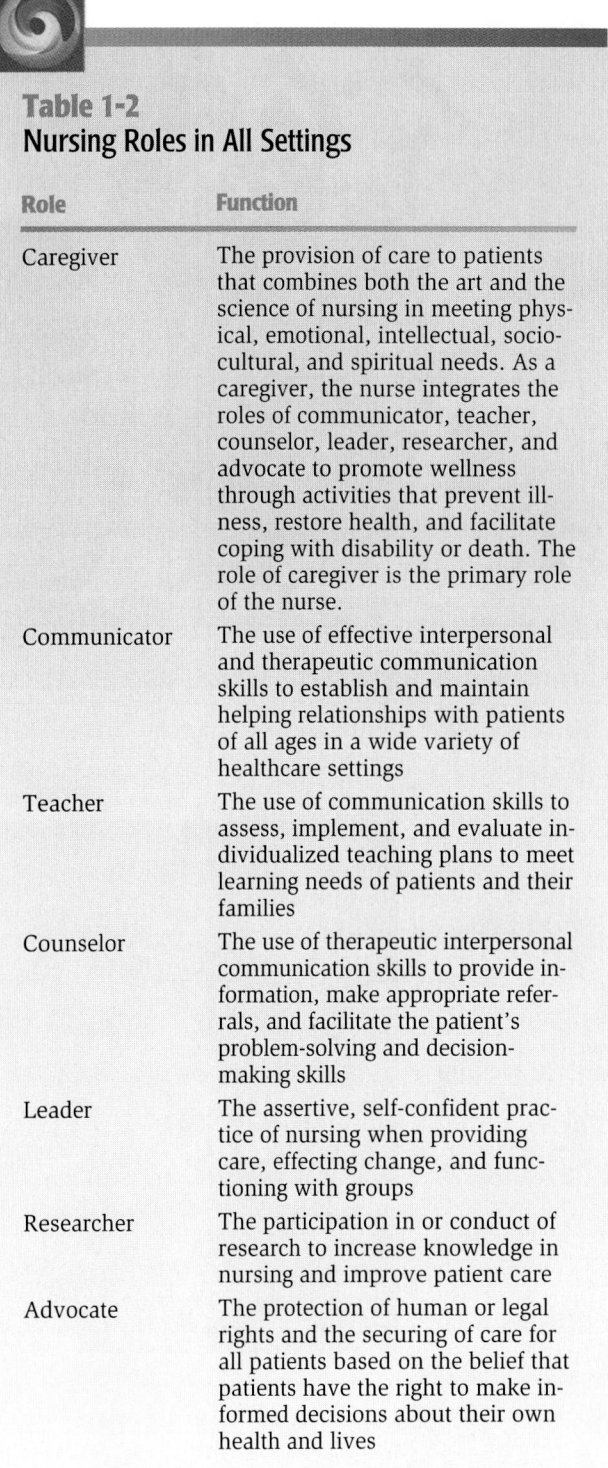

Table 1-2
Nursing Roles in All Settings

Role	Function
Caregiver	The provision of care to patients that combines both the art and the science of nursing in meeting physical, emotional, intellectual, sociocultural, and spiritual needs. As a caregiver, the nurse integrates the roles of communicator, teacher, counselor, leader, researcher, and advocate to promote wellness through activities that prevent illness, restore health, and facilitate coping with disability or death. The role of caregiver is the primary role of the nurse.
Communicator	The use of effective interpersonal and therapeutic communication skills to establish and maintain helping relationships with patients of all ages in a wide variety of healthcare settings
Teacher	The use of communication skills to assess, implement, and evaluate individualized teaching plans to meet learning needs of patients and their families
Counselor	The use of therapeutic interpersonal communication skills to provide information, make appropriate referrals, and facilitate the patient's problem-solving and decision-making skills
Leader	The assertive, self-confident practice of nursing when providing care, effecting change, and functioning with groups
Researcher	The participation in or conduct of research to increase knowledge in nursing and improve patient care
Advocate	The protection of human or legal rights and the securing of care for all patients based on the belief that patients have the right to make informed decisions about their own health and lives

ing as health. Both terms are used in this text. Models of health and wellness are described in Chapter 4.

Health promotion is motivated by the desire to increase people's well-being and health potential (Pender, 1996). A person's level of health is affected by many different interrelated factors that either promote health or increase the risk for illness. These factors include genetic inheritance, cognitive abilities, educational level, race and

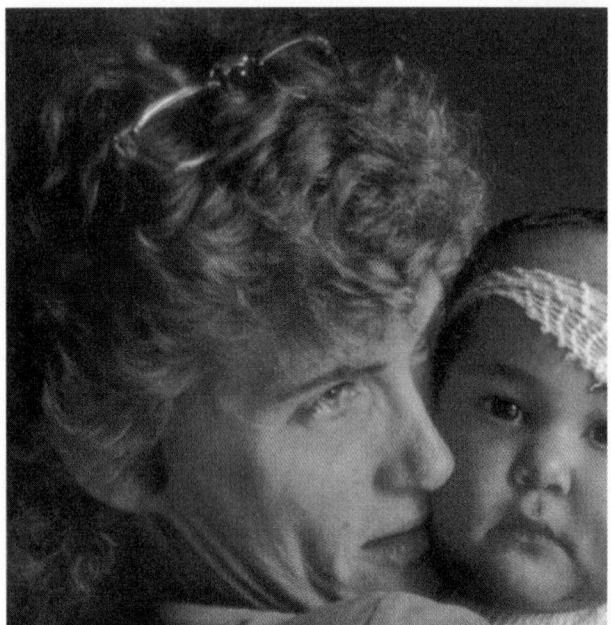

Photo © Alan Zuckerman

How can you be a nurse? How can you bear to watch children suffer?
Wait until you've rocked and soothed a suffering child into peaceful sleep, and you feel the child's relief washing over you like a blessing. Then you won't need to ask.

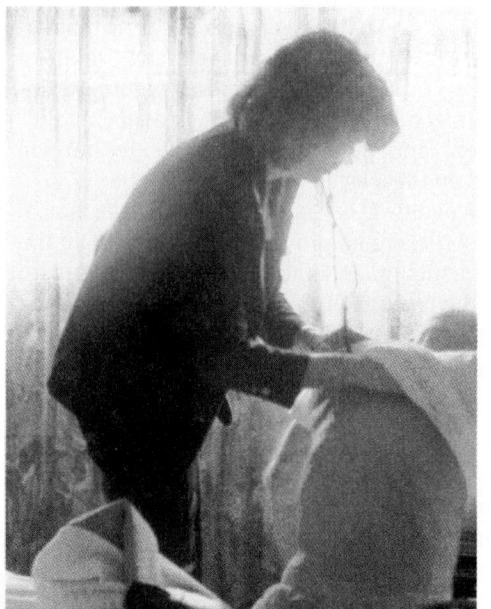

Photo © Robert Belmar

How can you be a nurse? So many of your patients are so old, so sick, these days. How can you bear the thought that, in the end, your care may make no difference?
Wait until you've used your hands and eyes and voice to dispel terror, to show a helpless person that his life is respected, that he has dignity. Your caring helps him care about himself…

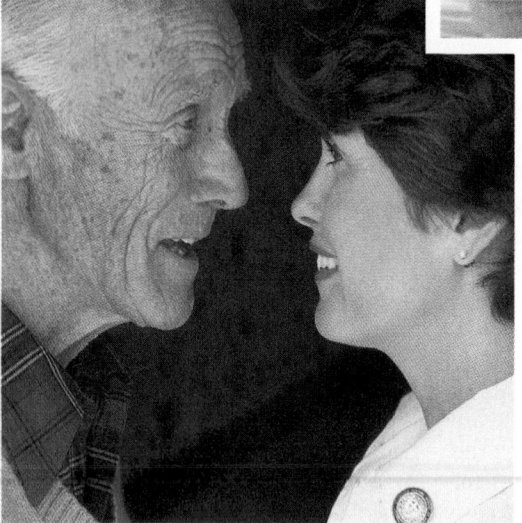

Photo © Bill Binzen

How can you be a nurse? How can you bear to care for frustrating, confused Alzheimer's patients?
Wait until you've devised a combination of strategies that provide exercise and permit safe wandering, and you see a lift, almost a spring, in a patient's shuffling gait. You'll feel the lightness of Baryshnikov in your own step that day.

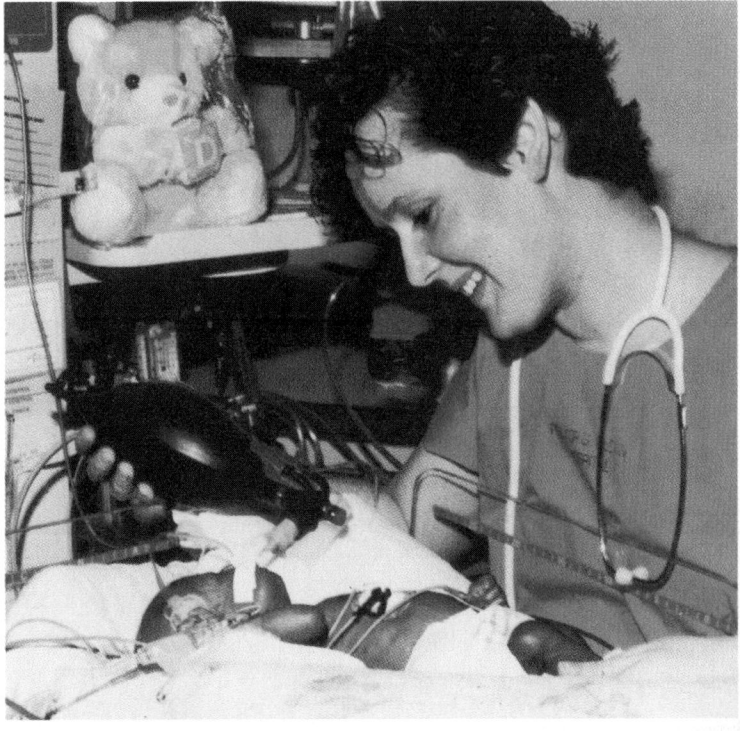

Photo © Joyce Dinello

How can you be a nurse? How can you bear the sound of babies crying?
Wait until your combination of vigilance, bulldog advocacy, and gentle handling has given a preemie's lungs the time they needed to develop, and you hear his first lusty cry. You'll laugh out loud!

Photo © Terry Wild Studios

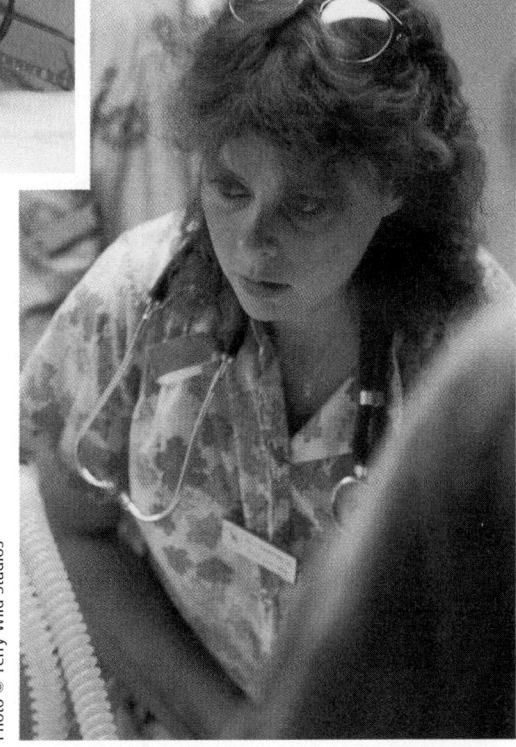

So you keep choosing to be a nurse. You have days of frustration, nights of despair, terrible angers. your highs and lows are peaks and chasms, not hills and valleys. The defeats come more than often enough to keep you humble: the problems you can't untangle, the lives that seep away too fast, the meanings that elude your understanding.

But you keep working at it, learning from it, knowing the next peak lies ahead.

Mary Mallison
Editorial, April 1987
American Journal of Nursing

Table 1-3
Expanded Educational and Career Roles of Nurses

Title	Description
Clinical nurse specialist (eg, enterostomal therapist, geriatrics, infection control, medical–surgical, maternal–child, oncology, quality assurance, nursing process)	A nurse with an advanced degree, education, or experience who is considered to be an expert in a specialized area of nursing; carries out direct patient care; consultation; teaching of patients, families, and staff; and research
Nurse practitioner	A nurse with an advanced degree, certified for a special area or age of patient care; works in a variety of health-care settings or in independent practice to make health assessments and deliver primary care
Nurse anesthetist	A nurse who completes a course of study in an anesthesia school; carries out preoperative visits and assessments, administers and monitors anesthesia during surgery, and evaluates postoperative status of patients
Nurse midwife	A nurse who completes a program in midwifery; provides prenatal and postnatal care, and delivers babies to women with uncomplicated pregnancies
Nurse educator	A nurse, usually with an advanced degree, who teaches in educational or clinical settings; teaches theoretical knowledge and clinical skills; conducts research
Nurse administrator	A nurse who functions at various levels of management in healthcare settings; is responsible for the management and administration of resources and personnel involved in giving patient care
Nurse researcher	A nurse with an advanced degree who conducts research relevant to the definition and improvement of nursing practice and education
Nurse entrepreneur	A nurse, usually with an advanced degree, who may manage a clinic or health-related business, conduct research, provide education, or serve as an adviser or consultant to institutions, political agencies, or businesses

ethnicity, culture, age and gender, developmental level, lifestyle, environment, and socioeconomic status.

Nurses promote health by maximizing the patient's own specific strengths. Health is an essential part of each of the other aims of nursing. Identification and analysis of the patient's strengths are a component of preventing illness, restoring health, and facilitating coping with disability or death. Every patient, no matter how ill, has strengths. The nurse identifies and uses these strengths to help the patient reach maximum function and quality of life or meet death with dignity.

Health promotion guidelines were established for the nation as a whole by the US Department of Health and Human Services (1990) in *Healthy People 2000*. These goals are being updated and continue to emphasize the importance of health as a national objective. Examples of national health promotion and disease prevention objectives are listed in the accompanying box.

Health promotion is the framework for nursing activities. The nurse considers the patient's self-awareness, health awareness, and use of resources while providing care. Through knowledge and skill, the nurse accomplished the following:

- Facilitates decisions about lifestyle that enhance one's quality of life and encourage acceptance of responsibility for one's own health
- Increases health awareness by assisting in the understanding that health is more than just not being ill and by teaching that certain behaviors and factors can contribute to or diminish health
- Teaches self-care activities to maximize achievement of goals that are realistic and attainable; serves as a role model
- Encourages health promotion by providing information and referrals

Examples of Settings for Nursing Care

Hospitals

Ambulatory surgery centers

Emergency helicopter services

Clinics

Homes

Educational programs

Public health offices

Doctors' offices

Industry

Long-term care facilities

Mobile healthcare units

Schools

Offices

Hospice

Mental health facilities

State health programs

Skilled-care facilities

Churches

Examples of National Health Promotion and Disease Prevention Objectives

- Increase to at least 20% the proportion of people 18 years of age and older who engage in physical activity that promotes the development and maintenance of cardiopulmonary fitness 3 or more days per week for 20 minutes or more per occasion.
- Reduce overweight to no more than 20% among people 20 years of age and older.
- Increase to at least 85% the proportion of people 18 years of age and older who use food labels to make nutritious food selection decisions.
- Reduce cigarette smoking to a prevalence of no more than 15% among people 20 years of age and older.
- Reduce deaths caused by alcohol-related motor vehicle crashes to no more than 8.5 per 100,000 people.
- Reduce drug-related deaths to no more than 3 per 100,000 people.
- Extend to 50 states laws requiring safety belt and motorcycle helmet use for all ages.
- Increase to at least 90% the proportion of all pregnant women who receive prenatal care in the first trimester of pregnancy.

From US Department of Health and Human Services. (1990). *Healthy people 2000.* Washington, DC: Author.

Preventing Illness

The objectives of illness prevention activities are to reduce the risk for illness, to promote good health habits, and to maintain optimal functioning. The motivation for illness prevention is to avoid or achieve early detection of illness or to maintain function within the constraints of an illness (Pender, 1996). Nurses primarily prevent illness by teaching and by personal example. Such activities include the following:

- Educational programs in areas such as prenatal care for pregnant women, smoking-cessation programs, and stress-reduction seminars
- Community programs and resources that encourage healthy lifestyles, such as aerobic exercise classes, "swimnastics," and physical fitness programs
- Literature and television, radio, or Internet information on diet, exercise, and the importance of good health habits
- Health assessments in institutions, clinics, and community settings that identify areas of strength and risks for illness

Restoring Health

Activities to restore health encompass those traditionally considered to be the nurse's responsibility. These focus on the individual with an illness and range from early detection of a disease to rehabilitation and teaching during recovery. Such activities include the following:

- Providing direct care of the person who is ill, by such measures as giving physical care, administer-

ing medications, and carrying out procedures and treatments
- Performing diagnostic measurements and assessments that detect an illness (eg, taking blood pressure, measuring blood sugars)
- Referring questions and abnormal findings to other healthcare providers as appropriate
- Collaborating with other healthcare providers in providing care
- Planning, teaching, and carrying out rehabilitation for illnesses such as heart attacks, arthritis, and strokes
- Working in mental health and chemical-dependency programs

Facilitating Coping

Although the major goals of healthcare are promoting, maintaining, or restoring health, these goals cannot always be met. Nurses also facilitate patient and family coping with altered function, life crisis, and death. Altered function decreases an individual's ability to carry out activities of daily living and expected roles. Nurses can facilitate an optimal level of function through maximizing the person's strengths and potentials, through teaching, and through referral to community support systems. Nurses provide care to both patients and families during terminal illness, and they do so in hospitals, long-term care facilities, and homes. Nurses are active in hospice programs, which assist patients and their families in preparing for death and in living as comfortably as possible until death occurs.

Educational Preparation for Nursing Practice

Educational preparation for nursing practice involves several different types of programs. Students may choose to enter a practical nursing program and be licensed as a licensed practical nurse (LPN), or they may enter a diploma, an associate degree, or a baccalaureate program to be licensed as a registered nurse (RN). State laws in the United States recognize both the LPN and the RN as credentials to practice nursing. Increasingly, various levels of nursing education are providing programs for educational advancement, and the LPN can complete an associate degree and become an RN, and the RN prepared at the diploma or associate degree level can attain a bachelor of science in nursing (BSN) degree. There are also programs that provide RN to master's degrees as well as BSN and master's degree to PhD. Graduate programs in nursing provide master's and doctoral degrees.

Educational preparation is a major issue in nursing. The multiple educational preparations are confusing to employers, consumers of healthcare services, and nurses themselves. Nursing organizations are working hard to answer questions such as, "What is technical nursing?" and "What is professional nursing?" as well as "Should graduates of different programs take the same licensing examination and have the same title?" These questions are likely to be resolved during your nursing career. The following sections discuss education for LPNs and RNs as well as graduate nursing education, continuing education for nurses, and in-service education.

Practical and Vocational Nursing Education

Practical nursing programs were established to teach graduates to give bedside nursing care to patients. Schools for practical nursing programs are located in varied settings, such as high schools, technical or vocational schools, community colleges, and independent agencies. Most programs are 1-year programs divided into one third classroom and two thirds clinical laboratory hours. On completion of the program, graduates can take the National Council Licensure Examination (NCLEX-PN) for licensure as a licensed practical nurse (LPN). LPNs work under the direction of a physician or RN to give direct care to patients, focusing on meeting healthcare needs in hospitals, nursing homes, and home health agencies.

Registered Nursing Education

Three primary types of educational programs lead to **licensure** as an RN: (1) diploma, (2) associate degree, and (3) baccalaureate programs. Graduates take the NCLEX-RN

examination. Although it is a national examination, it is administered by, and the nurse is licensed in, each state. It is illegal to practice nursing unless one has a license verifying completion of an accredited (by state) program in nursing and has passed the licensing examination. Nurses gain legal rights to practice nursing in another state by applying to that state's board of nursing and receiving reciprocal licensure. Table 1-4 summarizes the types of education for registered nurses.

Diploma in Nursing

Many nurses practicing in the United States received their basic nursing education in a 3-year, hospital-based diploma school of nursing (Ellis & Hartley, 1998). The first schools of nursing established to educate nurses were diploma programs, and until the 1960s, they were the major source of graduates. In recent years, the number of diploma programs has greatly decreased.

Current graduates of diploma programs have a sound foundation of the biologic and social sciences, with a strong emphasis on clinical experience in direct patient care. Graduates work in acute, long-term, and ambulatory healthcare facilities (Ellis & Hartley, 1998).

Associate Degree in Nursing

Associate degree nursing (ADN) education is based on a research project that was carried out by Dr. Mildred Montag in the 1950s. At that time, there was a shortage of nurses, and the project was created to meet the needs of society by preparing nurses in less time than was required in diploma programs. The emphasis of this type of program was education instead of service.

Currently, most associate degree programs are in community or junior colleges. These 2-year educational programs attract more men, more minorities, and more nontraditional students than do the other types of programs. Associate degree education prepares nurses to give care to patients in structured settings, including hospitals, long-term care, and home health. Graduates of these programs are technically skilled and well prepared to carry out nursing roles and functions. Competencies of the ADN on entry into practice, defined by the National League for Nursing (NLN), are encompassed into roles as provider of care, manager of care, and member of the discipline of nursing.

Baccalaureate in Nursing

The first baccalaureate nursing programs were established in the United States in the early 1900s. The number of programs and the number of enrolling students, however, did not increase markedly until the 1960s. Most graduates receive a bachelor of science in nursing (BSN) degree and often are referred to as BSN nurses.

The increase in number of these programs is the result of recommendations made by ANA, NLN, and Canadian Nurses Association that the entry level for professional practice be at the baccalaureate level. Although BSN nurses practice in a wide variety of settings, the 4-year degree is required for many administrative, managerial, and community health positions.

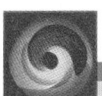

Table 1-4
Summary of Types of Educational Programs for Registered Nurses (RNs)

	Diploma	Associate Degree	Baccalaureate
Location	Hospital	Community college	Senior college or university
Length	24–36 mo	Two academic or calendar years	Four academic years
Course work	Biologic science Physical science Nursing theory Nursing practice	Basic sciences Social sciences General education Nursing theory Nursing practice	Basic sciences General education Social sciences Nursing theory Nursing practice Nursing research Community health Management
Clinical component	Both hospital and community settings	Both hospital and community settings	A variety of settings in which healthcare and nursing care are provided
Further education opportunity	If affiliated with a college, may transfer some credit toward a BSN	Credits often apply toward a bachelor of science in nursing (BSN) degree	Base for advanced education at the master's and doctoral levels
Competencies on graduation	Plans and gives direct care to patients in structured settings Works with other members of the healthcare team to plan and provide care to ill patients	Plans and gives direct care to patients in structured settings Works with other members of the healthcare team to plan and provide care to ill patients	Plans and gives direct care to individual patients, groups, and communities Directs other members of the healthcare team in planning and providing care to ill and well patients in a variety of settings; assumes beginning leadership roles; provides comprehensive healthcare, including health promotion, illness prevention, rehabilitative, and education and health counseling

In BSN programs, the major in nursing is built on a general education base with concentration on nursing at the upper level. Students acquire knowledge of theory and practice related to nursing and other disciplines, provide nursing care to individuals and groups, work with members of the healthcare team, use research to improve practice, and have a foundation for graduate study. Nurses who graduate from a diploma or associate degree program and wish to complete requirements for a BSN may choose to enroll in an RN-to-BSN program or may complete requirements through an external degree program.

Graduate Education in Nursing

The two levels of graduate education in nursing are the master's and doctoral degrees. A master's degree prepares advanced practice nurses to function in educational set-tings, in managerial roles, as clinical specialists, and as nurse midwives and nurse practitioners (Fig. 1-2). Many masters' graduates gain national certification in their specialty area, for example, as family nurse practitioners (FNPs). Nurses with doctoral degrees meet requirements for academic advancement and are prepared to carry out research necessary to advance nursing theory and practice.

Continuing Education

In its *Standards for Nursing Professional Development: Continuing Education and Staff Development*, the ANA (1994) defines **continuing education** as those professional development experiences designed to enrich the nurse's contribution to health. Formal continuing education through courses, seminars, and workshops is offered by colleges, hospitals, voluntary agencies, and private groups. In some

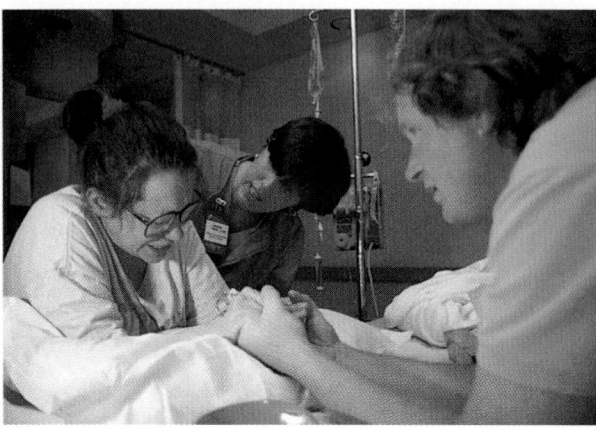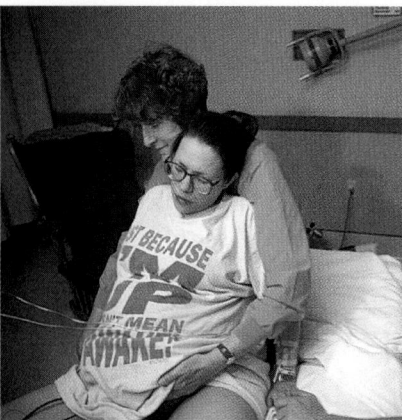

Figure 1-2
Growing numbers of women's health centers staffed with certified nurse practitioners and nurse midwives provide affordable health maintenance care. (Photo by B. A. Rupert.)

states, continuing education is required for an RN to maintain licensure.

In-Service Education

Many hospitals and healthcare agencies provide education and training for employees of their institution or organization, called **in-service education.** This is designed to increase the knowledge and skills of the nursing staff. Programs may involve learning, for example, a specific nursing skill or how to use new equipment.

Professional Nursing Organizations

One of the criteria of a profession is having a professional organization that sets standards for practice and education. Nursing's professional organizations are concerned with current issues in nursing and healthcare and influence healthcare policy and legislation. The benefits of belonging to a professional nursing organization include networking with colleagues, having a voice in legislation affecting nursing, and keeping current with trends and issues in nursing.

National Nursing Organizations

The United States has two major professional organizations for nurses: the American Nurses Association (ANA) and the National League for Nursing (NLN). The ANA is the professional organization for RNs in the United States. Founded in the late 1800s, its members are the state nurses' associations to which individual nurses belong. The ANA establishes standards of practice, encourages research to advance nursing practice, represents nursing for legislative actions, and supports the National Student Nurses' Association (NSNA).

The NLN is an organization open to all people interested in nursing, including nurses, nonnurses, and agencies. Established in 1952, its objective is to foster the development and improvement of all nursing services and

nursing education. The following are the major activities of the NLN:

- Conducts one of the largest professional testing services in the United States, including preentrance testing for potential students and achievement testing to measure student progress
- Serves as the primary source of research data about nursing education; conducts annual surveys of schools and new RNs
- Provides voluntary accreditation for educational programs in nursing

The NSNA is the national organization for student nurses. Members are students enrolled in nursing education programs. Programs and activities focus on professional development and healthcare.

International Nursing Organization

The International Council of Nurses (ICN), founded in 1899, was the first international organization of professional women. By sharing a commitment to maintaining high standards of nursing service and nursing education and by promoting ethics, the ICN provides a way for national nursing organizations to work together. The ICN's *1973 Code for Nurses* stated, "The need for nursing is universal. Inherent in nursing is respect for life, dignity and rights of man. It is unrestricted by considerations of nationality, race, creed, color, age, sex, politics, or social status."

Specialty Nursing Organizations

A wide variety of specialty nursing organizations are available to nurses. These organizations provide information on specific areas of nursing, often have publications in the specialty area, and may be involved in certification activities. Following are just a few of such organizations, illustrating their variety:

American Association of Critical Care Nurses
Association of Operating Room Nurses
American Indian Nurses' Association

National Black Nurses' Association, Inc.
Nurses' Christian Fellowship
American Public Health Association

Guidelines for Nursing Practice

As previously described, nursing continues to evolve and change to meet the needs of society. The ANA Congress for Nursing Practice (1973) stated that a profession must control its practice to guarantee the quality of its service to the public and that "a profession that does not maintain the confidence of the public will soon cease to be a social force." Nursing controls and guarantees its practice through standards of practice, nurse practice acts and licensure, and the use of the nursing process. Each of these will guide your nursing education as a student and your nursing practice after graduation.

Standards of Nursing Practice

The ANA (1998) *Standards of Clinical Nursing Practice* define the activities of nurses that are specific and unique to nursing. **Standards** allow nurses to carry out professional roles, serving as protection for the nurse, the patient, and the institution where healthcare is given. Each nurse is accountable for his or her own quality of practice and is responsible for the use of these standards to ensure knowledgeable, safe, and comprehensive nursing care. The American and Canadian Nurses Associations' standards, outlined in the accompanying boxes, apply to the practice of all RNs and lay the foundation for the practice of professional nursing in all settings.

Nurse Practice Acts and Licensure

Nurse practice acts are laws established in each state and province to regulate the practice of nursing. They are broadly worded and vary among states, but all of them have certain elements in common, such as the following:

- Are designed to protect the public by defining the legal scope of nursing practice, excluding untrained or unlicensed people from practicing nursing
- Create a state board of nursing or regulatory body having the authority to make and enforce rules and regulations concerning the nursing profession
- Define important terms and activities in nursing, including legal requirements and titles for RNs and LPNs
- Establish criteria for the education and licensure of nurses

The board of nursing for each state or province has the legal authority to allow graduates of approved schools of nursing to take the licensing examination. Those who successfully meet the requirements for licensure are then given a license to practice nursing in the state. The license, which must be renewed at specified intervals, is valid during the life of the holder and is registered in the state. The license and the right to practice nursing can be denied, revoked, or suspended for professional misconduct (eg, incompetence, negligence, chemical impairment, or criminal actions).

As nursing roles continue to expand, and as issues in nursing are resolved, new nurse practice acts will reflect those changes. All nurses must be knowledgeable about the specific nurse practice act under which they practice.

American Nurses Association: Standards of Clinical Nursing Practice

Standards of Care

Assessment: The nurse collects patient health data.

Diagnosis: The nurse analyzes the assessment data in determining diagnoses.

Outcome identification: The nurse identifies expected outcomes individualized to the patient.

Planning: The nurse develops a plan of care that prescribes interventions to attain expected outcomes.

Implementation: The nurse implements the interventions identified in the plan of care.

Evaluation: The nurse evaluates the patient's progress toward attainment of outcomes.

Standards of Professional Performance

Quality of care: The nurse systematically evaluates the quality and effectiveness of nursing practice.

Performance appraisal: The nurse evaluates her or his own nursing practice in relation to profes-

sional practice standards and relevant statutes and regulations.

Education: The nurse acquires and maintains current knowledge and competency in nursing practice.

Collegiality: The nurse interacts with and contributes to the professional development of peers and other healthcare providers as colleagues.

Ethics: The nurse's decisions and actions on behalf of patients are determined in an ethical manner.

Collaboration: The nurse collaborates with the patient, family, and other healthcare providers in providing patient care.

Research: The nurse uses research findings in practice.

Resource utilization: The nurse considers factors related to safety, effectiveness, and cost in planning and delivering patient care.

Reprinted with permission from American Nurses Association. (1998). *Standards of clinical nursing practice (2nd ed.)*. Washington, DC: American Nurses Publishing.

Canadian Nurses Association Standards for Nursing Practice

Standard I

Nursing Practice Requires That a Conceptual Model for Nursing Be the Basis of That Practice

1. Nurses are required to have a clear idea or conception of the *distinct goal of nursing.*
2. Nurses are required to have a clear idea or conception of the *client.*
3. Nurses are required to have a clear idea or conception of their *role* in response to the health needs of society.
4. Nurses are required to have a clear idea or conception of the *source of client difficulty.*
5. Nurses are required to have a clear idea or conception of the *focus and modes of nursing intervention.*
6. Nurses are required to have a clear idea or conception of the expected *consequences* of nursing activities.

Standard II

Nursing Practice Requires the Effective Use of the Nursing Process

1. Nurses are required to *collect data* in accordance with their conception of the client.
2. Nurses are required to *analyze data* collected in accordance with their conception of the goal of nursing, their role, and the source of client difficulty.
3. Nurses are required to *plan* their nursing actions based upon the identified actual and potential client problems, in accordance with their conception of the focus and modes of intervention.

4. Nurses are required to perform nursing actions which *implement* the plan.
5. Nurses are required to *evaluate* all steps of the nursing process in accordance with their conceptual model for nursing.

Standard III

Nursing Practice Requires That the Helping Relationship Be the Nature of the Client–Nurse Interaction

1. Nurses are required to initiate interaction in a way that increases the likelihood that the client will perceive the health service experience as understandable, manageable, and meaningful at the onset.
2. Nurses are required to set mutually agreed upon expectations as a means of increasing the likelihood that the client will perceive the health service experience as understandable, manageable, and meaningful.
3. Nurses are required to ensure a successful termination of the helping relationship.

Standard IV

Nursing Practice Requires Nurses to Fulfill Professional Responsibilities

1. Nurses are required to respect *statutes and policies* relevant to the profession and the practice setting.
2. Nurses are required to comply with the *Code of Ethics* of their profession.
3. Nurses are required to function as members of a *health team.*

Reprinted with permission from the Canadian Nurses Association.

Nursing Process

The nursing process, fully described in Unit IV, is one of the major guidelines for nursing practice. Nurses implement their roles through the **nursing process,** which integrates both the art and the science of nursing. That is, the nursing process is nursing made visible.

The nursing process is used by the nurse to identify the patient's healthcare needs and strengths, to establish and carry out a plan of care to meet those needs, and to evaluate the effectiveness of the plan to meet established outcomes. The nursing process allows the nurse to focus on the patient as an individual and to define those areas of care that are within the domain of nursing (Carpenito, 1997).

Trends in Nursing for the 21st Century

Nursing changes continually in response to the needs and resources of society as a whole. Nursing also changes in response to factors such as definitions of nursing, the aims

of nursing, the educational preparation for nursing, and expanded practice roles. Many trends are occurring in nursing and healthcare as we enter the 21st century:

- Healthcare is increasingly provided in community-based settings, such as clinics, outpatient settings, and homes. The impetus for this change has largely been the implementation of a system of managed care to control and monitor healthcare services to minimize costs.
- Patients who require in-hospital care are more acutely ill or injured than in the past, but their length of stay in the hospital has decreased. This trend affects nursing in several ways. Nurses employed in hospital settings must have the knowledge and skills to provide often complex care to very ill patients. In the home, nurses may find themselves providing much the same type of care as well as teaching patients and their families how to provide self-care.
- The older adult population is increasing in size more rapidly than any other age group, with the greatest

increase in those older than 75 years of age. This population trend means that patients in all healthcare settings increasingly are older and require teaching and nursing interventions designed to meet needs different from those of younger patients. Older healthcare consumers are also demanding more disease prevention interventions, new building designs to meet their housing needs, and a focus on communities of care. Nursing will increasingly need to research health issues related to the oldest old, ethnically diverse populations, quality of life, and innovative systems of care.

- Chronic health conditions, such as heart disease, cancer, respiratory diseases, and acquired immunodeficiency syndrome (AIDS), are major health problems in our society. As the population ages, it has been projected that by the year 2030, nearly 150 million people will have a chronic health condition. Meeting the healthcare needs of so many people will be more difficult for society, particularly for those who live in poverty, are homeless, are mentally ill, or are of different cultures.

- Advanced practice nurses, such as nurse practitioners and nurse midwives, are increasingly establishing independent practices in which they diagnose and treat illnesses, promote health, provide well-women care, and deliver babies (see Fig. 1-2). Depending on state certification requirements, they may practice in collaboration with a physician.

- The importance of culturally competent care and the use of alternate therapies to treat illnesses are recognized as crucial to providing holistic, individualized care. Nurses must become more culturally diverse as our society becomes increasingly global.

These trends and many others provide the background for nursing in the new century. As nurses continue to define their own practice, the special and distinctive role of nursing in caring for others will become increasingly recognized in society.

Learning Outcomes

After completing this chapter, the learner should be able to accomplish the following:

1. Define key terms used in the chapter.

continuing education	nurse practice act
discipline	nursing
health	nursing process
in-service education	standards
licensure	wellness

2. Describe the historical background of nursing, definitions of nursing, and the status of nursing as a profession and as a discipline.

3. Identify the aims of nursing as they interrelate to facilitate maximal health and quality of life for patients.

4. Describe the various levels of educational preparation in nursing.

5. Discuss the effect of nursing organizations, standards of nursing practice, nurse practice acts, and the nursing process on the practice of nursing.

6. Identify current trends in nursing.

Critical Thinking Exercises

1. Rank the roles and functions of professional nursing (see Table 1-2) in order of their importance to you. Then interview several nurses in different settings to see how much value they attach to these roles and how much time they are able to devote to them. Are their rankings the same as yours? If not, can you explain possible reasons for the differences?

2. Describe how a nurse would meet the aims of nursing as described in this chapter (promoting health, preventing illness, restoring health, and facilitating coping) when caring for the following patients. As you consider these situations, try to identify factors that either promote or inhibit the fulfilling of these aims.
   - A single mother who has just delivered her first child and is scheduled to be discharged 12 hours after delivery
   - An 82-year-old woman who wants to begin an exercise program
   - A 32-year-old man dying of AIDS at home

Bibliography

Alfaro, R. (1998). *Applying nursing diagnosis and nursing process: A step-by-step process* (3rd ed.). Philadelphia: Lippincott Williams & Wilkins.

American Nurses Association, Committee on Education. (1965). *A position paper.* New York: ANA.

American Nurses Association. (1994). *Standards for professional development: Continuing education and staff development.* Washington, DC: ANA.

American Nurses Association. (1995). *Nursing's social policy statement.* Washington, DC: ANA.

American Nurses Association. (1998). *Standards of clinical nursing practice*. Washington, DC: ANA.

Backer, B. (1993). Lillian Wald: Connecting caring with activism. *Nursing and Healthcare, 14*(3), 122–129.

Baldwin, C. (1998). Changing health outcomes for African-American children: Utilizing a self-care health promotion curriculum in urban elementary schools. *Journal of Multicultural Nursing & Health, 4*(2), 40–45.

Benson, A., & Latter, S. (1998). Implementing health promotion nursing: The integration of interpersonal skills and health promotion. *Journal of Advanced Nursing, 27*(1), 100–107.

Bulechek, G. M., & McCloskey, J. C. (1996). *Nursing interventions: Treatments for nursing diagnoses* (2nd ed.). Philadelphia: W. B. Saunders.

Burggraf, V., & Barry, R. (1998). Gerontological nursing in the 21st century. *Journal of Gerontological Nursing, 24*(6), 29–35.

Canadian Nurses Association. (1987). *A definition of nursing practice: Standards for nursing practice*. Ottawa, Canada: CNA.

Carpenito, L. J. (1997). *Nursing diagnosis: Application to clinical practice* (7th ed.). Philadelphia: Lippincott-Raven.

Deloughery, G. (1995). *Issues and trends in nursing*. St. Louis: C. V. Mosby.

Diers, D. (1990). The art and craft of nursing. *American Journal of Nursing, 90*(1), 65–66.

Dolan, J. A., Fitzpatrick, M. L., & Herrmann, E. K. (1983). *Nursing in society: A historical perspective*. Philadelphia: W. B. Saunders.

Ellis, J., & Hartley, C. (1998). *Nursing in today's world: Challenges, issues, trends* (6th ed.). Philadelphia: Lippincott Williams & Wilkins.

Floyd, J. (1999). Going global. *Reflections, 25*(1), 32–33.

Frenn, M., & Malin, S. (1998). Health promotion: Theoretical perspectives and clinical application. *Holistic Nursing Practice, 12*(2), 1–7.

International Council of Nurses. (1973). *1973 code for nurses*. Geneva: Impimeries Populaires.

Kalish, P., & Kalish, B. (1995). *The advance of American nursing* (3rd ed.). Philadelphia: J. B. Lippincott.

Keller, C., & Stevens, K. (1997). Cultural considerations in promoting wellness. *Journal of Cardiovascular Nursing, 11*(3), 15–25.

Kerfoot, K. (December 22, 1997). Role redesign: What has it accomplished? *Online Journal of Issues in Nursing*. Available: http://www.nursingworld.org/ojin/tpc5-3.htm.

Leininger, M. (1996). Culture care theory, research, and practice. *Nursing Science Quarterly, 9*(2), 71–78.

Lindberg, J., Hunter, M., & Kruszewski, A. (1998). *Introduction to nursing: Concepts, issues and opportunities* (3rd ed.). Philadelphia: Lippincott Williams & Wilkins.

McCabe, B., Walker, S., & Clark, K. (1997). Health promotion in long term care facilities. *Journal of Nursing Science, 2*(1–6), 153–167.

McCloskey, J., & Grace, H. (1994). *Current issues in nursing* (4th ed.). St. Louis: C. V. Mosby.

Nightingale, F. (1859). *Notes on nursing: What it is and what it is not*. Commemorative edition. Philadelphia: J. B. Lippincott.

Pender, N. J. (1996). *Health promotion in nursing practice*. Stamford, CT: Appleton & Lange.

Reardon, J. (1998). The history and impact of worksite wellness. *Nursing Economics, 16*(3), 117–121.

The Robert Woods Johnson Foundation. (1996). *Chronic care in America: A 21st century challenge*. Princeton, NJ: The Robert Woods Johnson Foundation.

Robinson, S., & Hill, Y. (1998). The health promoting nurse. *Journal of Clinical Nursing, 7*(3), 232–238.

Scoates, G. (1997). The burden of caregiving: What the home care nurse can do. *Home Health Focus, 4*(3), 20.

US Department of Health and Human Services. (1990). *Healthy people 2000*. Washington, DC: US Department of Health and Human Services.

Zhan, L., Cloutterbuck, J., Keshian, J., & Lombardi, L. (1998). Promoting health: Perspectives from ethnic elderly women. *Journal of Community Health Nursing, 15*(1), 31–44.

Chapter 2
Health of the Individual, Family, and Community

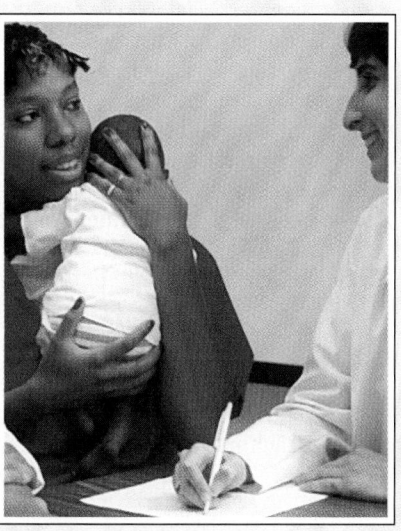

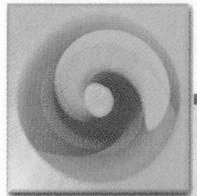

Thinking Critically About
Nursing's Blended Skills

Before reading this chapter, think about the types of skills you will need to master to prepare yourself to meet the basic human needs of those entrusted to your care.

- A sexually active 16-year-old girl wants contraceptive assistance but says her mother would "kill her" if she knew she was making this request.

- You suspect child abuse from the type of injuries you observe on a toddler brought to the emergency room by a babysitter.

- An obese 42-year-old executive says he knows he's at high risk for heart disease and seeks your help in developing a healthier lifestyle.

- The husband of a 76-year-old woman diagnosed with Alzheimer's disease 1 year ago breaks down and cries and tells you that he doesn't think he can continue to care for his wife at home but feels terrible about even considering placement in a nursing home.

What cognitive, technical, interpersonal, and ethical/legal skills do you think you will need to meet the basic human needs of those entrusted to your care?

Humans are complex organisms, influenced by and responsive to both our internal and external environments. Our behaviors, our feelings about ourselves and others, our values, and the priorities we set for ourselves all relate to our physiologic and psychosocial needs. These needs are common to all people, and meeting these needs is essential to the health and survival of all people; hence, they are labeled **basic human needs**. Basic human needs can be met or unmet in a variety of ways. A person can meet some needs independently, but most needs require relationships and interactions with other people for partial or complete fulfillment. Satisfying one's needs often depends on the social environment, especially one's family and community.

Holistic nursing care, which is based on considering all the patient's dimensions that affect how basic human needs are met in health and in illness, allows the nurse to provide person-centered and health-oriented care. Chapter 3 introduces the cultural dimension, and Chapter 4 discusses the dimensions of the whole person and the interaction of basic human needs with those dimensions. This chapter discusses how basic human needs, the family, and the community environment affect the health of the individual.

The Individual

In nursing, we consider both the physical and psychosocial needs of each individual patient. Abraham Maslow (1968) developed a **hierarchy of basic human needs** (Fig. 2-1)

that can be used to consider which needs of a person are the most important at any given time. Certain needs are more basic or essential than others and must be at least minimally met before other needs can be considered.

Levels of Needs

Maslow's hierarchy is useful for understanding the relationships of basic human needs and for establishing priorities of care. The hierarchy is based on the theory that something is a basic need if it has the following characteristics:

- Its absence results in illness.
- Its presence helps prevent illness or signals health.
- Meeting it restores health.
- It is preferred over other satisfactions when unmet.
- One feels something missing when the need is unmet.
- One feels satisfaction when the need is met.

Maslow arranged the hierarchy to show that certain needs are more basic than other needs. Although all people have all the needs all the time, people generally strive to meet certain of the needs (at least to a minimal level) before attending to other needs. The five levels of needs, with physiologic needs being the most basic, are as follows:

Level 1: Physiologic needs
Level 2: Safety and security needs

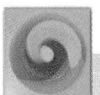

COGNITIVE SKILLS

- Knowledge of contraception and reproductive decision making
- Knowledge about child abuse and reporting responsibilities
- Knowledge about risk factors for heart disease and related prevention strategies
- Knowledge about Alzheimer's disease, associated family burdens, and community resources

TECHNICAL SKILLS

- Strong assessment skills related to sexual development and reproductive decision making, child abuse, risk prediction, and family caregiver needs.
- Competence in particular skills may be needed, such as teaching how to use contraceptive aids effectively, fitness equipment, and so on.

INTERPERSONAL SKILLS

- Strong people skills will be needed to establish trusting relationships with the new mother, nurses interested in designing education programs, the

homeless and those best able to meet their needs, and your impaired colleague.
- Special interpersonal competence will be required to mobilize your community to develop the type of resources needed to help the homeless. Special competence will also be needed to convince your colleague to seek help for a substance abuse problem.

ETHICAL/LEGAL SKILLS

- First and foremost a strong sense of accountability for the health and well-being of these individuals. This translates into a commitment to getting them the help they need to achieve their health goals—within the scope of your nursing responsibilities and available resources.
- A willingness to hold colleagues accountable for safe and good quality practice
- Skill in working collaboratively with your colleagues and others in the community to advocate for the health needs of the homeless
- A knowledge of the ethical and legal principles that guide decision making about impaired colleagues

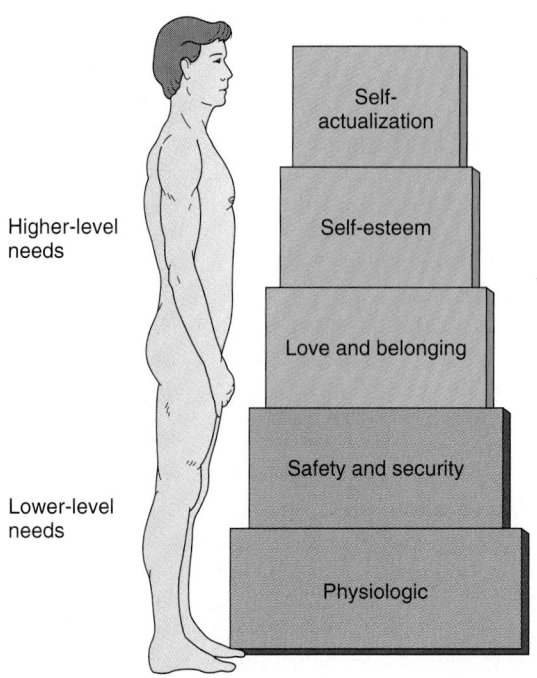

Higher-level needs

Lower-level needs

Figure 2-1
Maslow's hierarchy of basic human needs.

Level 3: Love and belonging needs
Level 4: Self-esteem needs
Level 5: Self-actualization needs

Nursing care is often directed toward meeting unmet or threatened needs. Maslow's hierarchy provides a framework for nursing assessment and for understanding the needs of patients at all levels so that interventions to meet needs become a part of the plan of care. The nursing interventions that you will learn as you progress through your education are aimed at meeting patients' basic human needs. The following sections describe each level of need in more detail.

Physiologic Needs

Physiologic needs, the most basic in the hierarchy of needs, are the most essential to life and therefore have the highest priority. **Physiologic needs**—oxygen, water, food, temperature, elimination, sexuality, physical activity, and rest—must be met at least minimally to maintain life. Most healthy children and adults meet their physiologic needs through self-care, but physiologic needs are often a major part of the nursing care plan for young, old, disabled, and ill people who require assistance in meeting them.

Oxygen is the most essential of all needs because all body cells require oxygen for survival. Oxygenation of body cells is carried out primarily by the respiratory and cardiovascular systems, and any alteration in their structure or function can result in an increased need for oxygen. This need may be acute (such as when cardiopulmonary resuscitation is needed) or chronic (requiring special positioning, treatments, and teaching). Nurses evaluate patients' oxygen needs by assessing skin color, vital signs,

anxiety levels, responses to activity, and mental responsiveness.

A balance between the intake and elimination of fluids is essential to life. Changes in the water balance of the body are evidenced by either dehydration or edema (the collection of fluid in body tissues). Dehydration occurs from conditions such as severe diarrhea or vomiting, whereas causes of edema include diseases of the cardiovascular or renal system or trauma. Water balance is assessed by measuring intake and output, testing the resiliency of the skin, checking the condition of the skin and mucous membranes, and weighing the patient.

Food is a physiologic need, with balance maintained through digestive and metabolic processes. Insufficient nutrient intake results in nutrient and electrolyte imbalances and weight loss. A component of the digestive processes that is also a physiologic need is elimination. Waste products are eliminated from the body through the skin, lungs, kidneys, and intestines. Nutritional status is assessed with a variety of indicators, including weight, muscle mass, strength, and laboratory values.

The human body functions best within a narrow range of temperatures, usually considered as plus or minus 98.6°F (37°C). This temperature is maintained by homeostatic mechanisms and adaptive responses, such as shivering. Body temperature is assessed as a vital sign by nurses.

Sexuality is an integral component of each individual and may be affected by physical and emotional illnesses. Sexual practices are dependent on a variety of factors, such as a person's age, sociocultural background, self-esteem, and level of health. There is increasing awareness in healthcare that the consideration of sexuality is a vital part of holistic care.

Physical activity and rest are also basic physiologic needs. Physical activity can be accomplished with intact and functioning neuromuscular and skeletal systems. Rest and sleep allow time for the body to rejuvenate and be free of stress. Individual requirements for rest and sleep vary widely, but the effects of deprivation have been well documented as significant. Factors that influence sleep are age, environment, exercise, stress, and drug use.

Safety and Security Needs

Safety and security needs come next in priority and involve both physical and emotional components. *Physical safety and security* means being protected from potential or actual harm. Nurses carry out a wide variety of activities to meet patients' physical safety needs, such as the following:

- Using proper handwashing and sterile techniques to prevent infection
- Using electrical equipment properly
- Administering medications knowledgeably
- Using skill when moving and ambulating patients
- Teaching parents about household chemicals that are dangerous to children

Emotional safety and security involves trusting others and being free of fear, anxiety, and apprehension. Patients entering the healthcare system often fear the unknown and may have significant emotional security needs. Nurses can help meet such needs by encouraging spiritual practices that are a source of strength and support, by allowing as much independent decision making and control as possible, and by carefully explaining new and unfamiliar procedures and treatments.

Love and Belonging Needs

All humans have a basic need for love and belonging. After physiologic and safety and security needs, this is the next priority and is often called a higher-level need. **Love and belonging needs** include the understanding and acceptance of others in both giving and receiving love, and the feeling of belonging to families, peers, friends, a neighborhood, and a community.

People who feel that their love and belonging needs are unmet often feel lonely and isolated. They may withdraw physically and emotionally, or they may become overly demanding and critical. Often, these behaviors are a signal (or cue) that the person has unmet love and belonging needs. Nurses should always consider love and belonging needs when developing a plan of care. Some nursing interventions to help meet this need are as follows:

- Including family and friends in the care of the patient (Fig. 2-2)
- Establishing a nurse–patient relationship based on mutual understanding and trust (by demonstrating caring, encouraging communication, and respecting privacy)
- Referring patients to specific support groups (such as cancer support groups or Alcoholics Anonymous)

Self-Esteem Needs

The next highest priority on the hierarchy is **self-esteem needs,** which include the need for a person to feel good about himself or herself, to feel pride and a sense of accomplishment, and to believe that others also hold one in high regard. Self-esteem gives the individual confidence and independence.

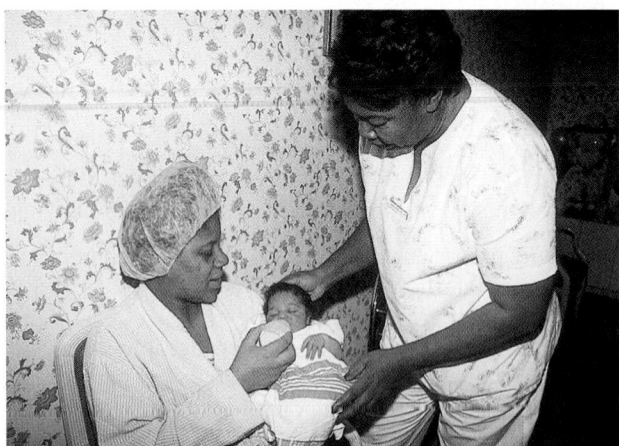

Figure 2-2
By teaching the mother to care for her infant, the nurse is helping to fulfill the need for love and belonging of both mother and child.

Many factors affect self-esteem. When a person's role changes (eg, through a job change or through the death of a spouse), self-esteem can be seriously altered because the person's responsibilities and relationships have also changed. Other changes that may affect self-esteem include a change in body image, such as the loss of a breast; an injury; or a growth spurt during puberty. Nurses must remember that the person's perception of the change—rather than the actual change itself—is what affects that individual's self-esteem.

Nurses can help meet patients' self-esteem needs by accepting their values and beliefs, encouraging patients to set attainable goals, and facilitating support from family or significant others. These actions promote a sense of worth and self-acceptance.

Self-Actualization Needs

The highest level on the hierarchy of needs is **self-actualization needs,** which include the need for individuals to reach their full potential through development of their unique capabilities. In general, each lower level of need must be met to some degree before this need can be satisfied. The process of self-actualization is one that continues throughout life. Maslow lists the following qualities that indicate achievement of one's potential:

- Acceptance of self and others as they are
- Focus of interest on problems outside oneself
- Ability to be objective
- Feelings of happiness and affection for others
- Respect for all people
- Ability to discriminate between good and evil
- Creativity as a guideline for solving problems and pursuing interests

To help meet patients' self-actualization needs, the nurse focuses on the person's strengths and possibilities rather than on problems. Nursing interventions are aimed at providing a sense of direction and hope and providing teaching that is aimed at maximizing potentials.

Applying Maslow's Theory

Nurses can apply Maslow's hierarchy of basic needs in the assessment, planning, implementation, and evaluation of patient care. The hierarchy can be used with patients at any age, in all settings where care is provided, and in both health and illness. It helps the nurse identify unmet needs as they become healthcare needs. The hierarchy of basic needs allows the nurse to locate the patient on the health–illness continuum and to incorporate health models into meeting needs (these concepts are discussed in Chap. 4).

As the nurse identifies and carries out interventions to help meet patients' needs, it is important to remember that this is only a framework or guideline and that, in actuality, each individual sets priorities for meeting needs on levels most important to that person. Additionally, basic human needs are interrelated and may require nursing actions at more than one level at a given time. For example, in caring for a person coming into the emergency department with a heart attack, the nurse's immediate concern is the patient's physiologic needs (ie, oxygen and pain relief). At the same time, however, safety needs (eg, following proper precautions with oxygen use and ensuring the person does not fall off the examining table) and love and belonging needs (eg, letting a family member stay with the person, if possible) are still major considerations. You will learn about how nurses meet basic human needs throughout the rest of this book.

The Family

Almost every person is a member of a number of groups, such as groups of friends, colleagues at work, or members of a church or school class. Each of these groups involves a specific part of the person's life and is important to the person. Only one group, however, is concerned with all parts of a person's life and with meeting his or her basic human needs to promote health. That group is the family.

What Is a Family?

A **family** can be defined simply as any group of people who live together. Families exist in all sizes and configurations and are essential to the health and survival of the individual family members as well as to society as a whole. The family is a buffer between the needs of the individual member and the demands and expectations of society. The role of the family is to help meet the basic human needs of its members while also meeting the needs of society (Friedman, 1992).

Duvall (1977) defined a family as two or more people who are related through blood, marriage, adoption, or birth. Friedman (1992) expanded that definition by including two or more people who are emotionally involved with each other and live together. The latter definition includes more of the different types of current family structures in which members may be unrelated either biologically or legally.

Family Structures

There is no single, commonly accepted form of family structure. The following sections briefly introduce many different types of family structures.

Nuclear Family

The **nuclear family,** also called the traditional family, is composed of two parents and their children. The parents are generally married, and all members of the family live in the same house until the children leave home as young adults. The traditional family may be composed of biologic parents and children, adoptive parents and children, surrogate parents and children, and stepparents and children.

In the classic nuclear family, the father was the family member who went to work, providing economic security, whereas the mother stayed at home, providing physical and emotional safety and security. This family group usually lived in close geographic proximity to relatives, such as aunts, uncles, and grandparents, who are a part of the **extended family**. Although many people still consider the nuclear family the ideal, it is no longer the dominant structure in our society.

The contemporary nuclear family still has the same basic form, but the roles of the members have changed considerably. The two major causes of this change are increased education and career opportunities for women and changes in our economy resulting in a need for additional income to maintain a desired standard of living. As a result, two-career families, in which both parents work outside the home, have become the norm instead of the exception. When both parents work, there is usually a blending of tasks, with both parents taking a more active role in housework and child care as well as economic support.

Couples without children and couples with grown children who no longer live at home are considered traditional families as well. The **blended family** is also a traditional family, formed when parents bring unrelated children from previous relationships together to form a new family.

With changes in family structure have come other influences on the basic human needs of family members. Considerations for the family, and for nursing care, include support systems (in our mobile society, family members may live hundreds or thousands of miles away), availability of child care, time for leisure and recreation, and changing role models.

Single-Parent Family

Single parents may be never married, separated, divorced, or widowed. Increasing numbers of never-married men and women are choosing to become parents. It is estimated that more than one fourth of all children in North America live in single-parent families. Most single-parent families are black and headed by women. Single parents have special problems and needs, including financial concerns and role shifts (ie, having the roles of both parents, often looking to remarriage or new relationships). These problems are important considerations when planning and implementing nursing care (Friedman, 1992). The accompanying Research in Nursing box describes a study of factors affecting low-income, single-parent women.

Other Family Structures

In addition to traditional and single-parent families are other family structures. Nurses must remember that there are no absolute "rights" or "wrongs" about what makes a family, and one person's values must not be imposed on another person. Your acceptance of all kinds of family members and relationships is essential to holistic, individualized patient care. Other family structures include cohabiting adults and single adults.

Cohabiting families are individuals who choose to live together for a variety of reasons—relationships, financial need, or changing values. Cohabiting families include unmarried adults living together and communal or group marriages.

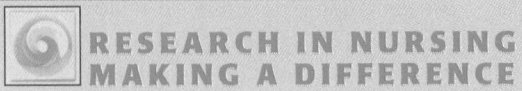

RESEARCH IN NURSING: MAKING A DIFFERENCE

Promoting Healthy Parenting in Single-Parent Families Headed by Women

Nursing care is planned and implemented with consideration of the needs of both the individual patient and the family of the patient. With changes in family structure in our society, single-parent families have become increasingly common. Most single-parent families with children younger than 18 years of age are headed by women. These women are at risk for altered parenting and abuse of their children as a result of multiple risk factors, including poor education, low income, and poor overall health.

Related Research

Lutenbacher, M., & Hall, L. (1998). The effects of maternal psychosocial factors on parenting attitudes of low-income, single mothers with young children. *Nursing Research, 47*(1), 25–34.
This study was conducted to investigate the relationships among maternal psychosocial factors in low-income, single mothers with young children (such as a history of childhood abuse, everyday stressors, self-esteem, and

depressive symptoms) and parenting attitudes of low-income single mothers with young children. Most of the mothers reported they had experienced some form of childhood abuse, had inappropriate expectations of their children, and valued corporal punishment. The findings pointed to two factors supporting at-risk parenting by the mothers: childhood physical abuse and depressive symptoms. Maternal depressive symptoms were increased by everyday stressors, which also decreased self-esteem.

Relevance to Nursing Practice

This study is an example of the importance of a family assessment to identify risk factors for child abuse, especially in low-income, single-parent families headed by women. When risk factors are identified, nurses can design interventions to provide parenting knowledge and skills and can provide information about support groups and social agencies to assist the mother with economic needs and mental health counseling.

Single adults may not be living with others, but they are part of a family of origin, usually have a social network with significant others, or may even regard a pet as family. Most single adults living alone are either young adults who achieve independence and enter the workforce or older adults who never married or are left alone after the death of a spouse.

Family Functions

Families have functions that are important for how individual family members meet their basic human needs and maintain their health. The family provides the individual with the necessary environment for development and social interactions. Families are also important to society as a whole because they provide new and socialized members for society. Five major functions of the family are as follows:

Physical: The family provides a safe, comfortable environment necessary for growth, development, and rest or recuperation.
Economic: The family provides financial aid to family members and also helps meet monetary needs of society.
Reproductive: The family raises children.
Affective and coping: The family provides emotional comfort to family members. It also helps members establish an identity and maintain that identity in times of stress.

Socialization: The family teaches; transmits beliefs, values, attitudes, and coping mechanisms; provides feedback; and guides problem solving (Friedman, 1992).

Developmental Tasks of Families

Duvall (1977) identified critical family developmental tasks and stages in the family life cycle. Duvall's theory, based on Erikson's theory of psychosocial development (described in Chap. 8), states that all families have certain basic tasks for survival and continuity and specific tasks related to the sequential stages of development throughout the life of the family.

These stages and related developmental tasks are outlined in Table 2-1. If the family does meet certain developmental tasks, societal disapproval may be lead to intervention by children's services, social services, police departments, welfare agencies, or health departments (Edelman & Mandle, 1997). The successful mastery of each developmental stage is important to the family's adaptation and growth through successive stages.

The Family in Health and Illness

Individuals learn healthcare activities, health beliefs, and health values in the family. In health and illness, as well as in other areas of life, the individual reflects behaviors learned from the family. When patients enter the healthcare

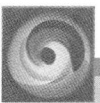

Table 2-1
Family Stages, Tasks, Health Risk Factors, and Nursing Interventions to Promote Health

Family Stage	Tasks	Risk Factors	Nursing Interventions/Referrals
Couple and family with children	Establish a mutually satisfying marriage Plan to have or not to have children Have and adjust to infant Support needs of all family members Adjust to cost of family life Adapt to needs and activity of children Cope with loss of energy and privacy Encourage and support growth and development, educational achievements	Inadequate knowledge of contraception and family Inadequate knowledge of sexual and marital roles Lack of knowledge about child safety and health Child abuse and neglect First pregnancy before age 16 Inadequate nutrition; obesity Drug and alcohol abuse Sexually transmitted diseases Rubella	Family planning clinics Prenatal classes Well-child clinics Immunization information Vision and hearing screenings Dental health information Parent support groups Communicable disease control Safety in the home, daycare, school, neighborhood, and community
Family with adolescents and young adults	Maintain open communications Support moral and ethical family values Balance teenagers' freedom with responsibility Maintain supportive home base Strengthen marital relationships	Family of origin Low socioeconomic status Family value of aggressiveness Dependence on welfare Inadequate problem-solving abilities Conflict between family members Physical or sexual abuse Use of drugs or alcohol Sexually transmitted diseases	Alcohol and drug information Accident prevention programs Sex education Nutrition support groups Mental health programs
Family with middle-aged adults	Maintain ties with younger and older generations Prepare for retirement	Diet high in fat, sugar, salt Obesity Use of drugs or alcohol Physical inactivity Depression Exposure to environmental or work-related health risks, such as sunlight, asbestos, radiation, coal dust, air or water pollution	Blood pressure screenings Screening for chronic diseases (eg, diabetes, cancer, glaucoma) Nutrition information Support groups (eg, for loss, grief, stopping smoking, alcohol or drug abuse)
Family with older adults	Adjust to retirement Adjust to loss of spouse May move from family home	Increasing age with loss of physical function Chronic illness Poor nutrition Lack of exercise Depression Death of spouse Limited income Past lifestyle	Screening for chronic diseases Nutrition information Exercise information Home safety information Retirement information Pharmacology information

Data from Duvall, E. (1977). *Marriage and family development* (5th ed.). Philadelphia: J. B. Lippincott; Aldous, J. (1975). *The developmental approach to family analysis*. Minneapolis University of Minnesota Press; *Healthy people: The Surgeon General's report on health promotion and disease prevention* (1982). Pub. No. 79-55071. Washington, DC: US Department of Health and Human Services; and *Healthy people 2000: National health promotion and disease prevention objectives* (1990). Washington, DC: American Public Health Association, US Department of Health and Human Services.

system, they bring their own personal behaviors and needs, but they also bring (in a sense) their family too. Friedman (1992) identified the importance of family-centered nursing care, based on the following rationales:

- The family is composed of interdependent members who affect one another. If some form of illness occurs in one member, all other members become a part of the illness.
- A strong relationship exists between the family and the health status of its members; therefore, the role of the family is essential in every level of nursing care.
- The level of health of the family and, in turn, each member, can be significantly improved through health promotion activities.
- Illness of one family member may suggest the possibility of the same problem in other members; through assessment and intervention, the nurse can assist in improving the health status of all family members.

Illness may precipitate a health crisis in a family. Brief changes in family tasks may occur if an illness is relatively minor, such as a viral infection in a child. If an injury or illness to a family member is serious, roles and responsibilities, as well as functions, of individual family members change. This is especially true if the illness is chronic and long-term, or results in disability. Some families find it difficult to adapt to the stress of changes in financial, social, and caregiving resources, whereas other families experience renewed family closeness and stability. Regardless of how the family adapts, members of the family must constantly adjust roles and responsibilities to manage the needs of the ill family member and the family.

Nursing interventions for the family in a health crisis include the following:

- Providing understandable information through teaching that is honest, open, and respectful
- Coordinating activities of all members of the healthcare team
- Using therapeutic communication skills, knowledge of family dynamics, and referral to community resources to support realistic hope
- Involving family members in providing physical care, if desired
- Identifying healthcare and financial resources

Family Risk Factors

Family patterns of behavior and the family environment, the environment in which the family lives, and genetic factors can place family members at risk for health problems. It is important for nurses to assess these factors before developing nursing care plans. Typical questions that should be part of a family assessment include the following:

- What is the family structure?
- What is the family's socioeconomic status?
- What are the ethnic background and religious affiliation of family members?

- Who cares for children if both parents work?
- What health practices are common (eg, types of foods eaten, meal times, immunizations, bedtime, exercise)?
- What habits are common (eg, do any family members smoke, drink to excess, or use drugs)?
- How does the family cope with stress?
- Do close friends or family members live nearby, and can they help if necessary?

When conducting a health assessment for a family, the nurse should consider the risk factors for altered health described below and listed by family developmental stage in Table 2-1.

Lifestyle Risk Factors
- Lack of knowledge about sexual and marital roles, leading to teenage marriage and pregnancy; divorce; sexually transmitted diseases; child, spouse, or elder abuse; and lack of prenatal or child care
- Alterations in nutrition—either more or less than body requirements at any age
- Chemical dependency, including the use of alcohol, drugs, and nicotine
- Inadequate dental care and hygiene
- Unsafe or unstimulating home environment

Psychosocial Risk Factors
- Inadequate child care resources when both parents work, for preschool- and school-aged children
- Inadequate income to provide safe housing, food, clothing, and healthcare
- Conflict between family members

Environmental Risk Factors
- Lack of knowledge or finances to provide safe and clean living conditions
- Work or social pressures that cause stress
- Air, water, or food pollution

Developmental Risk Factors
- Families who have new babies, especially if support systems are unavailable
- Older people, especially those living alone or on a fixed income
- Unmarried adolescent mothers who lack personal, economic, and educational resources

Biologic Risks
- Birth defects
- Mental retardation
- Genetic predisposition to certain diseases, including cardiovascular diseases and cancer

Nursing Actions to Promote Health

The role of the nurse in reducing risk factors involves activities that promote health for all family members at any level of development. Each person has his or her own definition of health, based on family beliefs and values about health and illness. Through interventions that emphasize health, the nurse assists both the individual and the family to meet their basic human needs. Examples of nursing diagnoses related to family health are listed in the accompanying Examples of NANDA Nursing Diagnoses. Examples of nursing interventions to promote health in the family are shown in Table 2-1. Nurses may carry out such activities themselves or may refer the individual or family to other healthcare providers for additional education.

The family is the primary educational and support structure for the individual. The family, as a social unit, provides the environment and relationships necessary for members to meet their basic human needs. Health beliefs and practices are learned within the family context and are influenced by the family's developmental level. Health promotion activities and nursing actions can reduce the risk for illness and facilitate healthy behaviors at any age within the family life cycle.

The Community

A person, as an individual and as a member of a family, is also a member of a community. The community environment also affects the ability of the individual to meet basic human needs. This section discusses the relationship of the community to basic human needs, including influences on health and illness.

A **community** can be defined in a variety of ways, but the most basic definition is that a community is a specific population or group of people living in the same geographic area under similar regulations and having common values, interests, and needs. Within a community, people interact and share resources.

The community has a strong influence on health promotion and illness prevention activities of individuals and families in the community (Fig. 2-3). Just as there are family risk factors for the health of individual members, so are

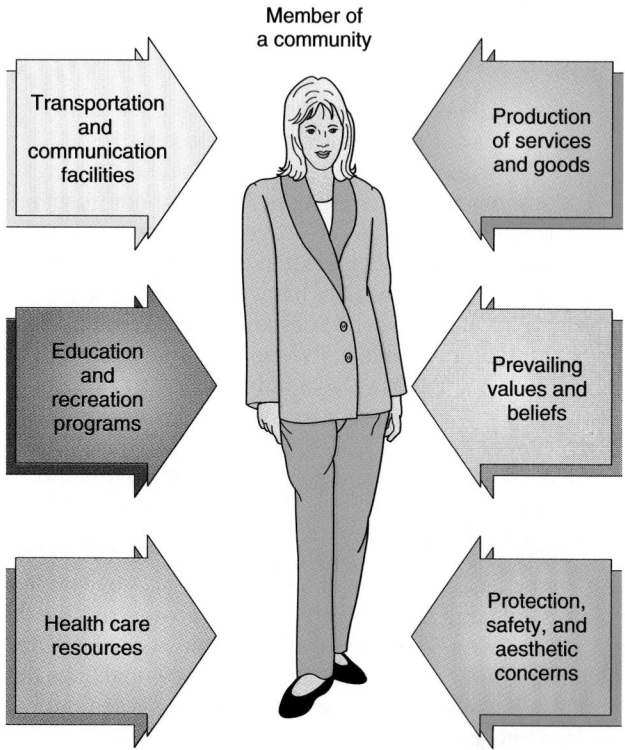

Figure 2-3
Many characteristics of a community influence the health of its members. This diagram shows six categories of characteristics that influence the health of a member of a community.

there community risk factors involving resources, economics, and services. For nursing assessments and interventions to be comprehensive and individualized, the nurse must also consider the community's influence.

Community Risk Factors

It is not within the scope of this book to discuss community health nursing as a whole. Because the community environment affects health and illness, however, it is important to discuss environmental factors influencing the health of the individuals within the community. Following are examples of community factors affecting health:

- The number and availability of healthcare institutions and services
- Housing codes and police and fire departments
- Nutritional services for low-income infants, mothers, school-aged children (eg, lunch programs), and older people
- Zoning regulations separating residential and industrial areas
- Waste disposal services and locations
- Air and water pollution
- Food sanitation
- Health education services and dissemination
- Recreational opportunities
- Violent crimes or drug use

EXAMPLES OF NANDA NURSING DIAGNOSES

The Family

The following NANDA nursing diagnoses are examples of those that might be appropriate when planning care for the patient as a member of the family.

- Risk for Infection related to presence of hepatitis C in family member
- Risk for Injury related to homeless state of family members
- Risk for Poisoning related to living in run-down urban apartment with peeling lead-based paint
- Caregiver Role Strain related to long-term home care of husband with Alzheimer's disease
- Altered Parenting related to history of child abuse by primary caretaker

To illustrate how the community can affect the individual's and family's needs, consider the following examples:

- Maria, 20 years of age, lives in an inner city, two room apartment with her 6-month-old baby girl. The apartment lacks adequate heat and plumbing. Maria has no family living nearby, and her husband has left her. Maria rarely leaves her apartment because she fears the street gangs and drug addicts. She has never taken her baby to a local clinic for checkups because she does know how to get there.
- Anne, 22 years of age, lives in a small house in a rural area with her 2-year-old son. She is a single mother and works as a secretary at an insurance agency. Anne often sees her family members, who live nearby. Anne and her son have regular health assessments.

These two different examples illustrate that the community plays a major role in the health of people who live there. Maria and her baby are at much greater risk for illness than are Anne and her son. Even if the two women had identical healthcare needs, their care plans would have different interventions because of their different community environments.

Nursing in the Community

Nurses carry out a variety of activities that involve the community, designed to promote health and prevent illness. Nurses promote health as individuals, as caregivers within institutional settings, and as community-based healthcare providers. Nurses also provide community ser-

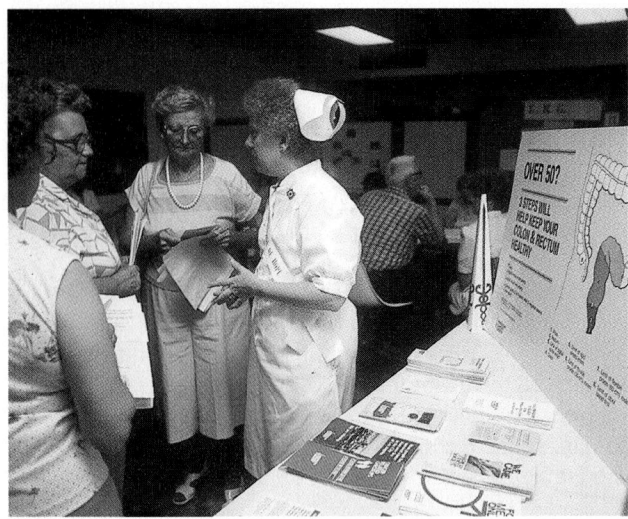

Figure 2-4
A nurse at work in an occupational (work-site) setting.

vices as volunteers in health-related activities (eg, screenings, educational programs, and blood drives) and as role models for health practices and lifestyles. Nurses working in a variety of healthcare settings consider community influences when developing individualized nursing care plans and when making referrals to community agencies and support groups. Community-based nurses are employed in many different kinds of practice settings, including home healthcare, community health centers, school nursing, occupational nursing (Fig. 2-4), and independent nursing practice. Community-based care is discussed in more detail in Chapter 11.

Learning Outcomes

After completing this chapter, the learner should be able to accomplish the following:

1. Define key terms used in the chapter.

basic human needs	love and belonging
blended family	needs
community	nuclear family
extended family	physiologic needs
family	safety and security needs
hierarchy of basic	self-actualization needs
human needs	self-esteem needs

2. Describe each level of Maslow's hierarchy of basic human needs.

3. Discuss nursing actions necessary to meet needs for each level of Maslow's hierarchy.
4. Discuss family concepts, including family roles, structures, functions, developmental stages, tasks, and health risk factors.
5. Identify aspects of the community that affect individual and family health.
6. Describe nursing interventions to promote and maintain health of the individual as a member of a family and as a member of a community.

Critical Thinking Exercises

1. Each of the following patients has tested positive for the human immunodeficiency virus (HIV) or has developed acquired immunodeficiency syndrome (AIDS). Describe how their individual needs are likely to vary.

- A woman, now in her second pregnancy. Her husband is bisexual and has also tested positive for HIV, but she did not know this before learning she is HIV-positive during a prenatal screening.

- A lesbian patient whose lover and several friends have died of AIDS.
- A child adopted from a foreign country, admitted to the hospital for treatment of pneumonia.
2. Our own family experiences often affect the way we relate to the families of our patients. Describe at least two possible responses to the families described below.
    - Suspecting child abuse, a nurse asks a mother about her child's bruises. The woman says, "In our family, we believe in spare the rod and spoil the child."
    - A single woman wants to have a child and comes to a fertility clinic for information on artificial insemination.
    - Several members of a patient's large, extended Hispanic family are in the patient's long-term facility room and are trying to do everything for the patient.

Bibliography

Ahman, E. (1998). Family matters: Examining assumptions underlying nursing practice with children and families. *Pediatric Nursing, 24*(5), 467–469.

Aldous, J. (1975). *The developmental approach to family analysis.* Minneapolis: University of Minnesota Press.

American Public Health Association. (1990). *Healthy people 2000: National health promotion and disease prevention objectives.* Washington, DC: US Department of Health and Human Services.

Bowman, K., Rose, J., & Kresevic, D. (1998). Family caregiving of hospitalized patients: Caregiver and nurse perceptions at admission and discharge. *Journal of Gerontological Nursing, 24*(8), 8–16.

Danielson, C. B., Hamel-Bissel, B. P., & Winstead-Fry, P. W. (1993). *Families, health, and illness: Perspectives on coping and interventions.* St. Louis: Mosby–Year Book.

Dowdell, E., & Sherwen, L. (1998). Grandmothers who raise grandchildren: A cross-generational challenge to caregivers. *Journal of Gerontological Nursing, 24*(5), 8–13.

Duvall, E. (1977). *Marriage and family development* (5th ed.). Philadelphia: J. B. Lippincott.

Edelman, C., & Mandle, C. (1997). *Health promotion throughout the lifespan* (4th ed.). St. Louis: Mosby–Year Book.

Friedman, M. (1992). *Family nursing: Theory and assessment* (3rd ed.). Norwalk, CT: Appleton & Lange.

Healthy people: The Surgeon General's report on health promotion and disease prevention (abridged). (1990). Washington, DC: American Public Health Association.

Hope, A., Kelleher, C., & O'Connor, M. (1998). Lifestyle practices and the health promoting environment of hospital nurses. *Journal of Advanced Nursing, 28*(2), 438–447.

Klainberg, M., Holzemer, S., Leonard, M., & Arnold, J. (1998). *Community health nursing: An alliance for health.* New York: McGraw-Hill.

Leske, J., & Jiricka, M. (1998). Impact of family demands and family strengths and capabilities on family well-being and adaptation after critical injury. *American Journal of Critical Care, 7*(5), 383–392.

Lutenbacher, M., & Hall, L. (1998). The effects of maternal psychosocial factors on parenting attitudes of low-income, single mothers with young children. *Nursing Research, 47*(1), 25–34.

Maslow, A. (1968). *Toward a psychology of being* (2nd ed.). New York: Van Nostrand–Reinhold.

O'Brien, A. (1998). Rural families as resources for family members who are mentally ill: A call for nursing involvement. *Archives of Psychiatric Nursing, 12*(4), 219–226.

Pender, N. J. (1996). *Health promotion in nursing practice* (3rd ed.). Stamford, CT: Appleton & Lange.

Shyu, Y., Archbold, P., & Imie, M. (1998). Finding a balance point: A process central to understanding family caregiving in Taiwanese families. *Research in Nursing & Health, 21*(3), 261–270.

Torres, M. (1998). Assessing health in an urban neighborhood: Community process, data results and implications for practice. *Journal of Community Health, 23*(3), 211–226.

Chapter 3
Culture and Ethnicity

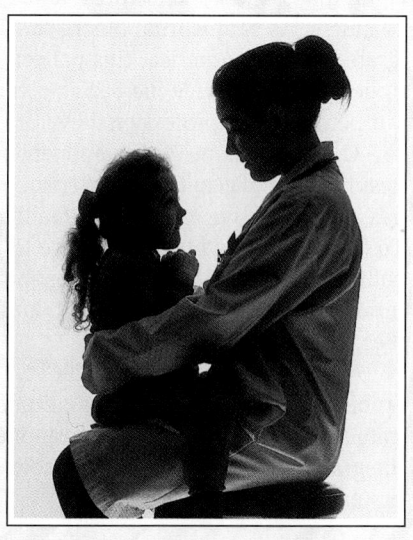

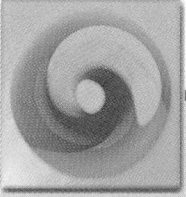

Thinking Critically About
Nursing's Blended Skills

Before reading this chapter, think about the types of skills you will need to interact effectively with colleagues, patients, and families from different cultures and ethnic groups.

- When a Haitian immigrant requests that a voodoo healer be brought into the hospital, you and your colleagues are uncomfortable with honoring her request.

- Another nurse asks you what you know about Eastern European Jews and hereditary disorders like Tay-Sachs disease. She has been dating a Jewish man she is growing to love but desperately wants children and has concerns about how her choice of a marriage partner will affect future children.

- Committed to increasing the supply of organs available for transplantation, you become frustrated when the family members of a brain-dead patient refuse organ retrieval because it violates their belief that people should enter into the next life "whole."

- A European-educated physician tells you that the family of a 70-year-old man newly diagnosed with lung cancer does not want the patient told of his diagnosis. When you protest because the patient has already started asking questions about his disease, the physician tells you that there is no need for him to hear the "bad news" that he has cancer. He further informs you that this was "common practice back home" [Italy] and that he never could understand the American ease of "dumping bad news."

What cognitive, technical, interpersonal, and ethical/legal skills do you think you will need to meet the needs of the patients described above?

Our society is made up of widely diverse groups of people. These groups include people of different racial and ethnic backgrounds, people with different sexual orientations, and people from different socio-economic backgrounds. These groups and subgroups are called *cultures*. The number of people within cultural groups other than the dominant culture continues to increase. The US Bureau of the Census (1999) estimates that the population of the United States is 272,402,000. That number is composed of the following races: 71.9% white, not Hispanic; 11.4% Hispanic; 12.1% black; 0.7% American Indian, Eskimo, and Aleut; and 4% Asian and Pacific Islanders. As people from other societies and cultures emigrate to North America, this pattern of change will continue and will provide increasing diversity and richness in our personal and professional lives.

Culture is an integral component of both health and illness because of genetic characteristics and the cultural values and beliefs we learn in our families and communities. To be able to provide holistic care to people from diverse cultural backgrounds, nurses must be sensitive to the cultural needs, characteristics, and values of individuals, families, and groups.

This chapter focuses on the concepts of culture and ethnicity and discusses various cultural characteristics that influence nursing care. It also examines the importance of integrating transcultural nursing concepts into one's daily practice of nursing.

Concepts of Culture and Ethnicity

Culture

All people have culture. Culture is apparent in the attitudes and institutions unique to particular groups. **Culture,** broadly defined, is a view of the world and a set of values, beliefs, and traditions that are handed down from generation to generation. Culture includes the beliefs, habits, likes and dislikes, and customs and rituals learned from one's family (Andrews & Boyle, 1999; Spector, 1996). As described by Leininger (1990), "culture includes all human activities taking material and nonmaterial forms and expressions . . . the political, economic, social, religious, educational, philosophical, technological, and environmental contexts in which human beings live and function" (p. 535). The characteristics of culture include the following:

- Culture guides behavior into acceptable ways for people in a specific group. It is shared by, and provides an identity for, all members of the same cultural group.
- Culture is learned by each new generation through both formal and informal life experiences. Language is the primary means of transmitting culture.
- The practices of a particular culture often arise because of the group's social and physical environment.
- Cultural practices and beliefs may evolve over time, but they mainly remain constant as long as they satisfy a group's needs.

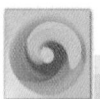

COGNITIVE SKILLS

- Knowledge of how culture and ethnicity influences a person's beliefs and values, daily living, health behaviors, decision making, and disease risk, for example, the Haitian patient's request for a voodoo healer and confidence in that healer's intervention, knowledge about Eastern European Jews and hereditary disease to facilitate decisions about marriage and childbearing, belief that the body must be intact to enter the next life, and belief that "bad news" (cancer diagnosis) is depressing and best not communicated to patients.
- Knowledge that people from different cultures and ethnic groups can think differently about what is right in any given situation.

INTERPERSONAL SKILLS

- Respect for the fact that people from different cultural and ethnic groups may believe, value, choose, and behave differently than you do.

- Ability to establish trusting relationships with colleagues, patients, family members, and others who are different from you.

ETHICAL/LEGAL SKILLS

- Commitment to securing the best possible care for patients from different cultures that is respectful of their beliefs and preferences but that does not violate your conscience or the practice of good nursing.
- Ability to advocate for the Haitian patient who has the right to be visited by a voodoo healer so long as this does not harm other patients or result in her harm while she is entrusted to the institution's care.
- Ability to advocate for the patient newly diagnosed with lung cancer if you believe that the physician's culture is interfering with good care for the patient.

- Culture influences the way people of a group view themselves, have expectations, and behave in response to certain situations. Because a culture is made up of individuals, there are differences both within cultures and among cultures.

Within most cultures are subgroups, or subcultures. A **subculture** is a large group of people who are members of a larger cultural group but have certain ethnic, occupational, or physical characteristics that are not common to the larger culture. For example, nursing is a subculture of the larger healthcare system culture, and teenagers and older adults are regarded as subcultures of the general population in North America.

Cultures include both dominant groups and minority groups. A **dominant group** is the group within a country or society that has the most authority to control values and sanctions of the society. The dominant group usually is (but does not have to be) the largest group in a society. The dominant group in the United States is currently composed of white middle-class people of European ancestry. The values of this cultural group have strongly influenced the value system of our society as a whole. Some of the dominant values include the following:

- Youth, thinness, and beauty
- Success and achievement
- Independence and self-reliance
- Use of technology
- Work
- Ownership
- Duty and conscience

A **minority group** usually has some physical or cultural characteristic (such as race, religious beliefs, or occupation) that identifies the people within it as different.

Ethnicity

Ethnicity is the sense of identification with a collective cultural group, largely based on the group's common heritage. One belongs to a specific ethnic group either through birth or through adoption of characteristics of that group. People within an ethnic group generally share unique cultural and social beliefs and behavior patterns, including language and dialect, religious practices, literature, folklore, music, political interests, food preferences, and employment patterns. Ethnicity largely develops through day-to-day life with family and friends within the community.

Race

Although the term *ethnicity* often is used interchangeably with **race,** these terms are not the same. Racial categories are typically based on specific physical characteristics, such as skin pigmentation, body stature, facial features, and hair texture. Although there has been a blending of physical characteristics through the centuries, the three major race classifications are Caucasian, Negroid, and Mongoloid.

Cultural Assimilation

When minority groups live within a dominant group, many of their members lose the cultural characteristics that once made them different. This process is called **cultural assimilation** or *acculturation.* Assimilation occurs when one's ethnic values are replaced by the values of the dominant culture. When people immigrate, their values are on one end of the spectrum and the values of the dominant culture are on the other end. As immigrants go to work, go to school, move out of the community, and learn the dominant language, they often move closer to the dominant culture. The process and the rate of assimilation are individualized. Because the degree of assimilation is so variable, nurses cannot assume characteristics based on ethnic groups.

Mutual cultural assimilation does occur, with some characteristics of both groups being traded. For example, the first Vietnamese immigrants to the United States learned to speak English, and Americans learned some dietary practices of the Vietnamese. In this way, we gain from the many cultures with which we live. Although we seldom think about it, the clothes we wear, the foods we eat, the music we enjoy, many of the words we use, and the leisure activities we practice are all characteristics in which we have become acculturated.

Factors Affecting Cultural Sensitivity

A variety of factors may negatively affect sensitivity to other cultures. When one assumes that all members of a culture or ethnic group act alike, **stereotyping** is at work. Common stereotypic beliefs are that all Italians are emotional, that all Germans are stoic, that men never cry, and that the elderly are senile. Stereotyping may be positive or negative. Negative stereotyping includes racism, ageism, and sexism. These are beliefs that certain races, an age group, or one gender is inherently superior to others, leading to discrimination against those considered inferior. Stereotyping is often done by members of the dominant group about the minority group in a culture (Fig. 3-1).

Cultural imposition is the belief that everyone should conform to the majority belief system. **Cultural blindness** occurs when one ignores differences and proceeds as though they do not exist. This has been true of the healthcare system, especially in regard to what are considered nontraditional methods of care. **Culture conflict** occurs when people become aware of cultural differences, feel threatened, and respond by ridiculing the beliefs and traditions of others to make themselves feel more secure about their own values (Andrews & Boyle, 1999).

⊚ Cultural and Ethnic Influences on Healthcare

North America is multicultural and multiethnic. As such, there is a wide diversity of people in almost every populated area. It is therefore important for nurses to be aware of and sensitive to the needs of a culturally diverse patient population (see the accompanying Research in Nursing

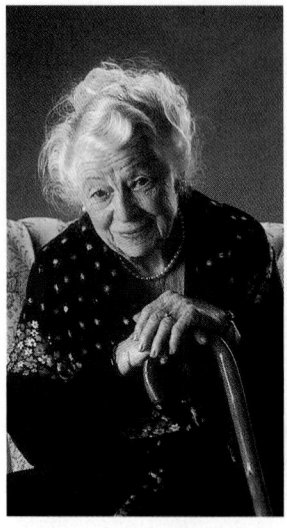

Photo © Christopher Briscoe, Science Source/Photo Researchers

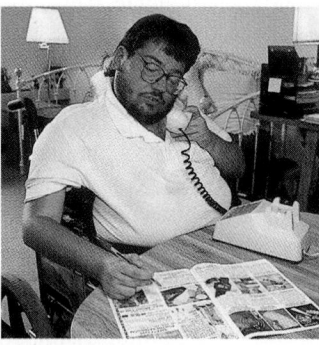

Photo © Jeff Isaac Greenberg, Science Source/Photo Researchers

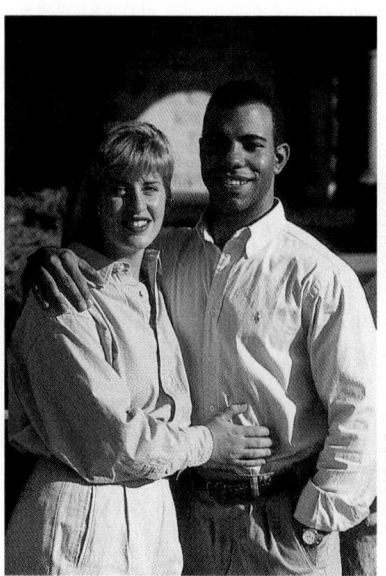

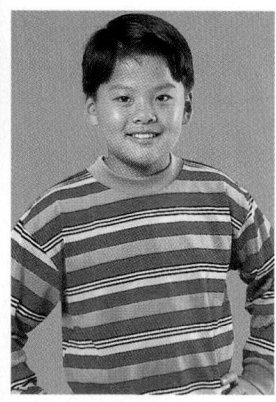

Photo © Renee Lynn, Science Source/Photo Researchers

Photo © Ken Cavanagh, Science Source/Photo Researchers

Figure 3-1
Identifying one's own prejudices is the first step toward eliminating them. Think about the assumptions you make about the people in these images.

box as an example). Table 3-1 describes selected cultural variations in the concept of health and health promotion. The following sections describe general considerations in transcultural care. (Specific values and behaviors of different groups are discussed later in the chapter.)

Gender Roles

In many cultures, the man is the dominant figure. In these cultures, men generally make decisions for other family members as well as for themselves. For example, if approval

---

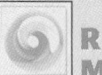 **RESEARCH IN NURSING: MAKING A DIFFERENCE**

The Meaning of Staying Healthy in Immigrant Pakistani Families

To provide culturally sensitive care, nurses need a genuine understanding of how people of other cultures view health and negotiate healthcare as well as how nurses can provide culturally sensitive care. The immigration of families from Pakistan to the United States has steadily increased in recent decades, but little has been known about how health or healthcare is experienced by these families.

Related Research
Jan, R., & Smith, C. A. (1998). Staying healthy in immigrant Pakistani families living in the United States. *Image—The Journal of Nursing Scholarship, 30*(2), 157–159.

The purpose of this study was to determine the meaning of "staying healthy" for these immigrant families. Data were collected from one member of each of four families who had lived in the United States for 14 to 15 years,

practiced the Islamic religion, conversed in English, but spoke Urdu at home. Staying healthy for these family members included the importance of feeling understood, maintaining spiritual peace, keeping family support, longing for the former way of being, and knowing how [to stay healthy].

Relevance to Nursing Practice
This study underscores the importance of sensitivity to patients' cultural values and beliefs about health. The acceptance of nursing interventions by people of other cultures depends on congruence of those interventions with what they believe is "right" and has meaning. The planning and implementing of nursing interventions must include not only physical care but also spiritual beliefs, family and community support systems, and, when appropriate, information about using the US healthcare system.

Table 3-1
Cultural Variations in Health Concept and Promotion

Cultural Group	Concept of Health	Health Promotion
Native American	Traditional health beliefs are holistic and health oriented.	Traditional health practices include physical stamina (running), relaxation (meditation), cleansing (sweats), self-sufficiency, and harmonious living. Participation in religious ceremonies and prayer promotes health of self and family.
Black/African American	Maintaining feelings of well-being, ability to fulfill role expectations, freedom from pain and excessive stress	Proper diet, proper behavior, and exercise in fresh air are prescription for maintaining health; protect against excessive cold
Cambodian	Being healthy is seen as being in equilibrium. Health needs to be individually maintained but is influenced by family and community.	Illness is seen as preventable. Nutrition is important, but not physical activity.
Chinese American	Maintaining balance between *Yin* and *Yang* influences in the body and in the environment. Harmony is important to maintain body, mind, and spirit.	One should eat a diet balanced with *Yin* and *Yang* foods and maintain harmony with friends and family.
Gypsies (Roma)	Maintaining moral purity, keeping upper and lower body separate, and practicing good behavior. Good health, prosperity, large families, and good appearance are intertwined.	Staying clean *(wuzho)* and avoiding unclean *(mahrime)*
Hmong	Being able to perform expected routines and duties.	Not a priority if considered from Western perspective
Mexican American	Feeling well and being able to maintain role function	Orientation to the present and belief that the future is in God's hands mean that health screenings and routine checkup may not be scheduled by traditional Mexican Americans.
Puerto Rican	Absence of mental, spiritual, or physical discomforts as well as *Lenities y limipios* (not being too thin and being clean) are perceived as healthy.	Eating well and drinking fruit beverages. Multivitamins are commonly used.
Samoan	Holistic approach, including aspects of body, mind, and spirit. Includes relationships with family, environment, and spiritual world.	Concept of preventive health not well established in Samoa.
Vietnamese	Principles of harmony and balance within self. Overweight a positive sign of good economic status and contentment.	Encompasses physical, spiritual, emotional, and social factors. Consuming lots of fresh vegetables, fruit, fish, and meat. Keeping clean and warm.

Data from Lipson, J., Dibble, S., & Minarik P. (Eds.). (1996). *Culture & nursing care: A pocket guide.* San Francisco: UCSF Nursing Press, pp. 21, 42, 62–63, 80–81, 136–137, 168, 219–220, 236–237, 262–263, 289.

for medical care is needed, the man gives it regardless of which family member is involved. In male-dominant cultures, women are usually passive. In many African American and white families, on the other hand, the woman is often dominant.

Knowledge of the dominant member of the family is an important consideration in planning nursing care. If the dominant member is ill and can no longer make decisions, for example, the whole family may be anxious and confused. If a nondominant family member is ill, he or she may require help in verbalizing needs, particularly if they differ from those the dominant member perceives as being important.

Language and Communication

When people from another part of the world move to North America, they may speak their own language fluently but have difficulty speaking English. This is especially true for the women or older adults in the family if they do not work outside the home and for people who live in proximity to others who speak the same language. Children usually assimilate more rapidly and learn the language of the dominant culture quickly because they leave home each day to go to school and make new friends in the dominant culture. Wage earners also tend to learn a new language more quickly through the work setting. Assimilation is slower for people who stay at home, especially if they live in communities of their ethnic culture. Language acquisition is thus tied to necessity and assimilation rather than to degree of difficulty.

Most Americans do not know a language other than English. As a result, communication problems can arise during healthcare activities. This problem is not unique to non–English-speaking patients; even in different regions of the United States, certain dialects or word meanings can cause differences in understanding. Consider how difficult it must be to describe symptoms or give a personal health history when you do not understand the questions being asked. Something as simple as showing the nurse where you hurt is impossible if you do not know what you are being asked. In addition, patients may forget English words or revert to their more familiar language when experiencing the stress of an injury or illness.

Eye contact, as a nonverbal communication behavior, is one of the most culturally variable forms of communication. The American dominant culture emphasizes eye contact while speaking, but other cultures regard this behavior in different ways, such as described in the following examples:

- Direct eye contact may be considered impolite or aggressive by Asians, Native Americans, Indochinese, Arabs, and Appalachians; these groups of people tend to avoid direct eye contact and avert their eyes while speaking with another.
- Native Americans often stare at the floor during conversations, a behavior that indicates they are carefully listening.
- Some African Americans may roll their eyes at what they consider to be ridiculous questions.
- Hispanic Americans look downward in deference to age, gender, social position, economic status, and authority.
- Muslim-Arab women indicate modesty by avoiding eye contact with men.
- Hasidic Jewish men tend to avoid direct eye contact with women (Andrews & Boyle, 1999).

Nurses who work in a geographic area with a high population of residents who speak a language other than English should learn pertinent words and phrases in that language. Many agencies have a qualified interpreter, or one can be found in the community. It is important to use an interpreter who understands the healthcare system to avoid misinterpretation of questions and answers (see the accompanying box: Through the Eyes of a Student). Sometimes a family member or friend can translate for the nurse, but such a person may be protective and not the most reli-

Through the Eyes of a Student

I was doing my maternity rotation and was assigned to labor and delivery. I was assigned a woman who spoke no English—she and her husband were from Central America and had been in the United States for only 2 months.

When I arrived at 7 AM, the night nurse was giving a report about my patient to the day nurse. The night nurse was frantic—no one understood the couple, all efforts to locate a translator had come up empty, and, quite frankly, she had no idea exactly what condition this woman was in.

I quickly began to think back on my 2 years of Spanish. Could I be of any help to this couple? I wondered. Would I remember enough to communicate with them about giving birth? Then I decided that any little bit of communication at this point was better than none, so I spoke up. I told both nurses that I spoke some Spanish and asked if I could be of any help. The night nurse literally hugged me!

I began by telling the expectant couple that I was a nursing student and that I spoke some Spanish. We exchanged introductions and then I asked the woman some assessment questions. Nothing I said was complicated—all of my sentences were short and simple, but who needed more than that?

Then the couple asked me some questions. They had heard about "cutting open the stomach" to deliver a baby. I naturally assumed that they meant a cesarean delivery. They looked so afraid but I had to be honest. They wanted to know how it was done and why. The words I could not remember or did not know I acted out. They looked so relieved when I was finished.

The man said that they thought *all* babies were born this way in our country. He said that they had never heard of this procedure until coming to the United States. No wonder they were so frightened!

The doctor came in, examined the woman, and said she was fully dilated. The doctor asked if I could teach a crash course in Lamaze breathing to the woman. She also asked me if I would stay throughout the delivery because she would need assistance in translating directions to the woman. Of course I said yes.

The woman was terrified. I told her that it was normal to be afraid and that I would be with her during the delivery. She took my hand and whispered, "Muchas gracias." I never felt more useful than I did at that moment.

—A. KELLY GAYLOR,
HOLY FAMILY COLLEGE, PHILADELPHIA

able means of transferring information. Nurses may find themselves talking in a louder tone of voice to a patient who does not understand what they are saying; remember that this is a communication problem, not a hearing problem. Following are considerations for transcultural assessment of communication, adapted from Andrews and Boyle (1999). Chapter 21 provides additional information on communicating with non–English-speaking patients.

- What language does the patient speak during usual activities of daily living?
- How well does the patient speak and write in English?
- Does the patient need an interpreter? Are family members or friends available? Are there people the patient would not want to serve as an interpreter?
- How does the patient prefer to be addressed?
- What cultural values and beliefs of the patient may change your techniques of communication and care (such as eye contact, space, or social taboos)?
- How does the patient's nonverbal behavior affect the responses of members of the healthcare team?
- How does the patient feel about healthcare providers from other cultures; would the patient prefer a healthcare provider of the same culture, gender, or age?
- What are the cultural characteristics of the patient's communications with others?

Orientation to Space and Time

Personal space is the area around a person regarded as part of the person. This area, individualized to each person and to different cultures and ethnic groups, is the area into which others should not intrude during personal interactions. When others do not consider a person's personal space, that person may become uncomfortable or even angry. When providing nursing care that involves physical contact, you should know the patient's cultural personal space preferences. For example, people of Arabic and African origin commonly sit and stand close to one another when talking, whereas people of Asian and European descent are more comfortable with some distance between themselves and others.

Many people and almost all institutions in North America value promptness and punctuality. When arriving for an appointment, doing a job, or carrying out an activity, being on time and getting the job done promptly are viewed as important. This is not true in some other cultures. For example, in some South Asian cultures, being late is considered a sign of respect. In addition, although most of middle-class North America is future oriented (including activities that promote health not only in the present but also in the future), other cultures are more concerned with the present or the past.

Food and Nutrition

Food preferences and how foods are prepared are often culturally related. Certain food groups serve as staples of the diet based on culture and remain so even when members of that culture are living in a different country. For example, rice and vegetables are the staples of Asians and Chinese, and pasta is a staple of Italians. Mexican Americans favor beans and tortillas, whereas Puerto Ricans try to eat a balance of hot, cold, and cool foods (the classification is based on type of foods, not cooking temperatures). These are only examples and should not be used to select patient foods; the nurse should always ask the patient about individual food preferences.

Patients in a hospital or long-term care setting often do not have much of a choice of foods. This means that people with cultural food preferences may not be able to select appealing foods and thus may be at risk for less than adequate nutrition. When assessing the cause of decreased appetite in patients, the nurse should determine whether the problem may be related to culture. It may be possible for family or friends to bring in foods that satisfy the patient's nutritional needs while still meeting dietary restrictions. Dietary teaching must be individualized according to cultural values about the social significance and sharing of food. Culturally sensitive assessment of nutrition includes these questions, followed by examples of differences:

1. Which foods are considered edible, and which are not?
   - In France, corn is considered an animal feed, whereas corn is a commonly eaten vegetable in the United States.
   - Religious beliefs prohibit some Jewish, Muslim, and Seventh-Day Adventist patients from eating pork.
   - Patients who follow a vegetarian diet do not eat pork, beef, or chicken.
2. What times and types of food are considered meals?
   - Anglo-Americans typically eat three meals a day, with foods such as bacon and eggs or cereal for breakfast, sandwiches and soup for lunch, and meat with potatoes and vegetables for dinner. In contrast, soup may be eaten for every meal by Vietnamese, beans are a staple for meals among Mexican people, and people from Middle Eastern countries often eat cheese and olives for breakfast.
   - Native American and Latin American people usually eat two meals a day.
   - Rural southern African Americans may eat large amounts of food on weekends and less food at meals during the week.
   - Holy days or religious holidays influence food choices for almost all cultures.
3. With whom is the food eaten?
   - Men and women eat separately in some Middle Eastern cultures; this tradition has significance for group dining in settings such as mental health institutions, schools, and long-term care facilities.

Socioeconomic Factors

Low income is a major problem in North America and is often described as having created a culture of poverty. The most recent statistics (US Bureau of the Census, 1997) noted that the number of poor—35.6 million—remained the same in 1997 as in 1996. The rate of poverty decreased, however, primarily in blacks and people of Hispanic origin. Of those defined as poor, 68.6% were white (including white, not Hispanic and Hispanic), 25.6% were black, and 5.8% were of other races. There were 7.3 million families classified as living in poverty in 1997, with more than half of those families being black. The amount of money a person or family has affects how they meet their basic needs and maintain their health. Poverty leads to other problems, such as lack of health insurance, care of infants and children, and homelessness. All these areas are of concern to nursing.

The Culture of Poverty

There has been much debate about how to define poverty. In terms of economics, a person or family whose income falls below the poverty line is considered poor. The US Bureau of the Census (1997) defines poverty by using a set of money income thresholds that vary by family size and composition. If the family's total income is less than that family's threshold, the family, as well as each member of that family, is considered poor. Others have stated that poverty is a relative term that reflects a judgment on the basis of community standards. Such standards vary at different times and in different places; what is judged poverty in one community might be regarded as wealth in another (Spector, 1996). No matter how poverty is defined, it is an increasingly devastating epidemic that has evolved into a culture of its own. At highest risk are families headed by single mothers, older people, and future generations of those now living in poverty.

The so-called feminization of poverty threatens to increase the number of people who are living at poverty level. The number of female-headed households is increasing as a result of divorce, abandonment, unmarried motherhood, and changes in abortion laws. Because it is now common in many households that two incomes are required for economic survival, a single woman supporting a household is at a financial disadvantage. The number of single-parent families headed by women is closely associated with the increasing number of children living in poverty and the number of homeless families with children.

The expanding population of older people has also raised problems associated with poverty. Many older people live on fixed incomes that often do not keep up with inflation, and many (particularly widows) are on the borderline of poverty or have already slipped into the poverty culture. Socioeconomic status often differs by the cultural group of the older adult. For example, Pacific/Asian, African American, Native American, and Hispanic elders generally have lower incomes than do elders in the Anglo-American majority population. The work history of the cultural group, especially those who have worked all their lives as agricultural workers, often means an individual has no Social Security or Medicare benefits.

In some cases, the culture of poverty is passed from generation to generation. This appears to be especially true in such groups as migrant farm workers, families living on welfare, and people who live in isolated areas of Appalachia. Poverty cultures have the following characteristics:

- Feelings of despair, resignation, and fatalism
- Day-to-day attitude toward life with no hope for the future
- Unemployment and need for financial or government aid
- Unstable family structure possibly characterized by abusiveness and abandonment
- Decline in self-respect and retreat from community involvement

Effects of Poverty on Healthcare

Poverty has long been a barrier to adequate healthcare. It prevents many people from consistently meeting their basic human needs. The lack of affordable or adequate housing is a problem frequently experienced by poor people. When low-income housing is available, it sometimes lacks such necessities as running water, heat, and electricity. To stretch their available money and to pool resources, many poor people live in crowded conditions, with several families living together in one household.

Research has demonstrated that crowded living conditions foster depersonalization, correlate with higher crime rates, and lead to psychological problems, such as schizophrenia, alienation, and feelings of worthlessness (Spector, 1996). Such conditions also contribute to an increased incidence of disease and illness because of the proximity of people, the sharing of utensils and belongings, poor sanitation, and poor health habits. The health effects of such conditions include a higher incidence and severity of illness in poor people than in people of higher income groups.

Accessing healthcare facilities frequently requires transportation, which many times is neither affordable nor available to poor people. Their access to health insurance is also frequently limited, and commonly they must choose between purchasing food and purchasing healthcare. Those in upper-income groups tend to live longer and to experience less disability than those in lower-income groups. Other barriers to healthcare include isolation, language or communication difficulties, seasonal occupations, migration patterns, depersonalization, and institutional prejudice (Spector, 1996).

Family Support

In many cultural and ethnic groups, people have large, extended families and consider the needs of any family member to be equal to or greater than their own. They may be unwilling to share private information about family members with those outside the family (including healthcare providers). Other cultural groups have great respect for the elders in the family and would never consider institutional care for them. Including the family in planning care for any patient is a major component in nursing care to meet individualized needs, especially if those needs can be met only through consideration of all members of the family.

Physical and Mental Health

Differences and similarities in both physiologic and psychological characteristics are found among various cultural and ethnic groups. These characteristics influence the individual health and illness status of group members.

Physiologic Characteristics

Researchers theorize that in the past, cultural groups slowly adapted to their environment. For example, dark-skinned people developed lighter skin as early populations moved to colder northern climates where there is less sunlight throughout the year compared with equatorial climates. Lighter skin is better able to use vitamin D from sunlight than darker skin. It also is theorized that a group's nose shape and size evolved according to the climate in which they lived (Henderson & Primeaux, 1981). From a scientific and anthropologic point of view, these adaptations were natural changes that helped improve the lives and well-being of human beings. Some of these biologic variations were effective adaptations for a particular period or for living in a certain environment.

When a person no longer is in the environment that encouraged the biologic variation, the variation might then have a detrimental effect on the person's health and well-being. Various studies have shown that certain racial groups have particular characteristics that make them more prone to developing specific diseases and conditions. These conditions may be acquired as a result of environmental factors, or they may be inherited. Some such variations are discussed in the next sections.

Keloid Formation

Keloids result from an overgrowth of connective tissue during the healing process that forms a scar after an injury, surgery, or burn. Blacks are much more likely to develop keloids. Rather than healing level with the surrounding skin tissue, the wound of a person with a tendency toward keloid formation heals with a rough, lumpy, or elevated scar.

Lactase Deficiency

Milk and many milk products contain lactose, a sugar. The enzyme lactase must be present in the body to break down lactose during digestion. Without lactase, the lactose ferments in the intestines, resulting in gas (flatus), diarrhea, and abdominal bloating and cramping. Lactase deficiency and lactose intolerance are more common in Hispanic women and in both men and women of African, Chinese, and Thai ancestry (Andrews & Boyle, 1999).

People with a lactase deficiency have to obtain their calcium and protein requirements from other sources because they are not able to tolerate regular milk products. Special lactose-free milk and milk products are available but are more expensive. Sharp cheeses (aged more than 60 days) and fermented milk products, such as yogurt, buttermilk, and sour cream, may be tolerated.

Sickle Cell Anemia

Sickle cell anemia is most common in people of African or Mediterranean origin. The sickle cell trait originally served as a protective mechanism against malaria. People with sickle cell anemia have sickle-shaped red blood cells (RBCs) that break down more rapidly than normal-shaped RBCs. The sickle shape also prevents the RBCs from moving easily through the smaller blood vessels in the body. This factor can lead to these blood vessels being clogged by the RBCs, which can cause many potentially serious problems.

Tay-Sachs Disease

People of Eastern European Jewish descent may carry a gene for a hereditary disorder called Tay-Sachs disease. A child born with this progressive disease has a short life span, usually less than 2 years. There is no cure or treatment for this devastating disease. Carriers of the disease can be identified by serum analysis.

Glucose-6-Phosphate Dehydrogenase Deficiency

Glucose-6-phosphate dehydrogenase (G6PD) is an enzyme normally found in RBCs. G6PD deficiency affects about 10% of the African American population. The deficiency is sex-linked and carried on the X female chromosome. A person with this deficiency has RBCs that cannot maintain a cell membrane. Without this protective membrane, RBCs are easily destroyed (hemolyzed) by various oxidant drugs, such as aspirin, ascorbic acid, probenecid, sulfa drugs, and vitamin K, and by fava beans (also called horse or broad beans). This destruction results in anemia, which may be severe and life-threatening, and in elevated bilirubin levels (a result of the hemolyzed RBCs), which causes jaundice (yellowing of the skin and sclerae).

Thalassemia

Thalassemia, a genetic disorder, affects the hemoglobin in the RBCs. The production of alpha or beta globin chains is defective and disrupts RBC function. This disorder is most commonly found in people of Mediterranean, Asian (especially Chinese), and African origin.

Sarcoidosis

Much more prevalent in the African American population, sarcoidosis involves the formation of multiple tubercles or nodules on various parts of the body, most commonly the lymph nodes, liver, spleen, lungs, skin, eyes, and small bones of the feet and hands. These nodules eventually form into fibrous tissue. Skeletal muscle involvement can result in muscle atrophy (wasting). If the myocardium is involved, major cardiac problems can result.

Gout

Gout is most commonly found in men, especially those of Puerto Rican or Filipino descent. Excessive quantities of uric acid are present in the blood and may be deposited in joints and cartilage. The deposits of uric acid result in swelling, inflammation, and pain in the affected area. Uric acid crystals may permanently damage the joints. These crystals also predispose the person to the formation of renal calculi (kidney stones).

Psychological Characteristics

In most situations, a person interprets the behaviors of another person in terms of her or his own familiar culture.

This process usually is multidirectional; for example, in a healthcare setting, the patient evaluates the attitudes and actions of the healthcare provider at the same time the healthcare provider interprets the behavior of the patient. Remember that what may seem reasonable and important to a patient may seem ridiculous and irrelevant to a nurse. The reverse is also true: practices a nurse perceives as logical and effective may seem senseless, incompetent, or even dangerous to a patient.

Most mental health norms are based on research and observations made of white, middle-class people. Many ethnic groups have their own norms or acceptable patterns of behavior for psychological well-being and normal psychological reactions to certain situations. For example, many Hispanic people deal with problems within the family and would view it as inappropriate to tell problems to a stranger; however, psychotherapy can be effective as long as the therapist integrates the value system of the patient into the treatment plan. Many traditional Chinese people consider mental illness a stigma; therefore, seeking psychiatric help would be a disgrace to the family. Traditionally, Chinese people prefer to avoid or minimize any type of conflict; hence, the use of any direct confrontation during psychotherapy may not work as expected. Also, Chinese people traditionally have been taught that the expression of strong emotions results in disharmony and imbalance between the body's energy forces (*yin* and *yang*) and is considered a sign of weakness. As a result of this belief, therapy involving the venting of strong feelings and emotions may be unacceptable to the patient. In situations of extreme stress or high anxiety, some Puerto Ricans may demonstrate a hyperkinetic seizure activity known as *ataques.* This behavior is a culturally accepted reaction.

Culture Shock

Culture shock, or the feelings a person experiences when placed in a different culture that the person perceives as strange, may result in psychological discomfort or disturbances. The patterns of behavior a person found acceptable and effective in his or her own culture are often not adequate in the new one. The person may then feel foolish, fearful, incompetent, inadequate, embarrassed, humiliated, or inferior. These feelings eventually can lead to frustration, anxiety, and loss of self-esteem.

Reaction to Pain

Healthcare researchers have discovered that many of the expressions and behaviors exhibited by people in pain are culturally prescribed. Some cultures allow and even encourage the open expression of emotions experienced by a person in pain, whereas other cultures frown on the open and free expression of emotions. The main issue for nurses in this area of cultural expression is their attitude toward the "ideal patient." A patient who quietly and stoically deals with pain may have pain reduction needs ignored by nurses. Nurses often assume that a patient who does not complain of pain is not experiencing any great degree of pain. Nurses should be sensitive to other signals of discomfort, such as holding or applying pressure to the painful area, self-restriction of activities that intensify the pain, and uncontrollable, spontaneous expressions of discomfort, such as facial grimacing and moaning. Nurses should not consider patients who freely express their discomfort as constant complainers whose requests for pain relief seem excessive. Pain is a warning from the body that something is wrong. Pain is what the patient says it is, and every complaint of pain should be carefully assessed.

Nursing care for the patient in pain is always individualized (see Chap. 40), but important culture-sensitive considerations include the following:

- Recognize that culture is an important component of individuality and that each person holds (and has the right to hold) various beliefs about pain.
- Respect the patient's right to respond to pain in whatever manner is culturally and individually appropriate.
- Never stereotype a patient's perceptions or responses to pain based on the person's culture.

Traditional Health Practices

People's values and beliefs about health, illness, and care for an illness develop as a direct result of cultural and ethnic influences. Many forms of folk medicine classify illnesses as natural or unnatural. Natural illnesses are caused by dangerous agents, such as cold air or impurities in the air, water, or food. Unnatural illnesses are punishments for failing to follow God's rules, resulting in evil forces or witchcraft causing physical or mental health problems.

Folk Healers

In some cultures, the power to heal is thought to be a gift from God bestowed on certain people. People in these cultures believe that these special healers know what is wrong with them through divine intervention and experience. A patient used to such healers may think of healthcare providers as incompetent because they have to ask many questions before they can treat an illness. A folk healer may prescribe boiled herbal tea as a treatment, and someone who is accustomed to this type of treatment may find it difficult to take pills that are not even steeped in hot water. Folk healers traditionally are less expensive, are usually more accessible, and are usually more understanding of the patient's cultural and personal needs, and they speak the patient's language.

Traditional Folk Medicine

Understanding traditional folk remedies used by culturally different patients greatly improves and enhances effective nursing care and facilitates a safe return of the patient to a state of health.

Herbs are a common mode of treatment in many cultures. In fact, many medications used today have a basis in herbs or other plant sources that have been used for centuries to cure illnesses. A problem may arise when a patient is being cared for by both an herbalist and a physician. The herbalist may be prescribing an herb and the physician a drug, both of which have the same action. The patient may be overmedicated or undermedicated because of the double prescription.

The nurse should not discourage the patient's use of traditional folk medicine unless it may be harmful to the patient's health and well-being or decrease the effectiveness of the nursing and medical care planned. Incorporating the patient's traditional healthcare beliefs into the care plan is an effective way to gain trust and cooperation. For example, if a patient traditionally drinks an herbal tea to alleviate symptoms of an illness, there is no reason why both the herbal tea and the prescribed medications cannot be used as long as the tea is safe to drink and the ingredients do not interfere with or exaggerate the action of the medication.

Other types of alternate therapies include the use of cutaneous stimulation, therapeutic touch, acupuncture, and acupressure. Cutaneous stimulation by massage, vibration, heat, cold, or nerve stimulation reduces the intensity of the sensation of pain. Therapeutic touch is an intentional act that involves an energy transfer from the healer to the patient to stimulate the patient's own healing potential. Acupuncture, long used in China, is a method of preventing, diagnosing, and treating pain and disease by inserting special needles into the body at specified locations. Acupressure involves a deep-pressure massage of appropriate points of the body.

Transcultural Nursing

Madeleine Leininger (1978), whose theory of transcultural care is described in Chapter 5, defines **transcultural nursing** as follows:

> Transcultural nursing is a formal area of study and practice focused on a comparative study of human cultures with respect to discovering universalities (similarities) and diversities (differences) as related to nursing phenomena of care (caring), health (wellness), or illness patterns within a cultural context and with a focus on cultural values, beliefs, and lifeways of people and institutions, and using this knowledge to provide culture-specific or universal care practices.

Providing transcultural nursing care means that care is planned and implemented in a way that is sensitive to the needs of individuals, families, and groups from diverse cultural populations within society. The nurse who recognizes and respects cultural diversity has cultural sensitivity and provides nursing care that accepts the significance of cultural factors in health and illness. Examples of nursing diagnoses for holistic transcultural care are listed in the accompanying Examples of NANDA Nursing Diagnoses. To provide culturally competent care, the nurse must be aware that the healthcare system itself is a culture and that cultural imposition and ethnocentrism (described in the following section) must be avoided.

The Culture of Healthcare

The healthcare system (described in Chap. 11) is a culture with customs, rules, values, and a language of its own. As you progress through your education, you will be acculturated into the culture of the healthcare system and will develop values related to health and healthcare. Many of the customs and rules are typical of the society in which we live; for example, cleanliness and punctuality are valued behaviors. The accompanying box outlines some common cultural norms of the healthcare system.

Nursing is the largest subculture of the healthcare system. Most nurses are members of, and have the same value systems as, the dominant middle class in North America. According to Andrews and Boyle (1999), the typical American nurse is "white, middle-class, Anglo-Saxon, Protestant,

---

EXAMPLES OF NANDA NURSING DIAGNOSES

Culture and Ethnicity

The following nursing diagnoses are examples of those that might be appropriate for providing holistic transcultural care:

- Impaired Verbal Communication related to inability to speak English and interpreter unavailable
- Impaired Social Interaction related to recent move away from neighborhood and friends of same ethnic group
- Altered Parenting related to use of culturally based discipline considered inappropriate or abusive by current country of residence

- Spiritual Distress related to inability to take part in significant culturally based rituals regularly
- Family Coping: Potential for Growth related to request for information about child care
- Ineffective Management of Therapeutic Regimen (Individual) related to mistrust of traditional healthcare personnel
- Situational Low Self-Esteem related to language difficulties and inability to secure employment
- Powerlessness related to inability to make healthcare providers understand the importance of dietary and social values and beliefs

---

Cultural Norms of the Healthcare System

Beliefs

- Standardized definitions of health and illness
- Omnipotence of technology

Practices

- Maintenance of health and prevention of illness
- Annual physical examinations and diagnostic procedures

Habits

- Documentation
- Frequent use of jargon
- Use of a systematic approach and problem-solving methodology

Likes

- Promptness
- Neatness and organization
- Compliance

Dislikes

- Tardiness
- Disorderliness and disorganization

Customs

- Professional deference and adherence to the pecking order found in autocratic and bureaucratic systems
- Use of certain procedures attending birth and death

---

female, and socialized into a subculture labeled 'healthcare professional, subdivision nurse'" (p. 37). When the nurse, with a particular set of cultural values about health, interacts with a patient who has his or her own particular set of cultural values about health, the following factors affect this interaction:

- The cultural background of each participant
- The expectations and beliefs of each about healthcare
- The cultural context of the encounter (eg, hospital, clinic, home)
- The degree of agreement between the two persons' sets of beliefs and values (Andrews & Boyle, 1999)

Cultural Imposition and Ethnocentrism in Healthcare

Cultural imposition, described by Leininger (1991) as "one of the most serious problems in the health field" (p. 36), is the tendency for health personnel to impose their beliefs, practices, and values on people of other cultures because they believe that their ideas are superior to those of another person or group. When health professionals assume that they have the right to make choices and deci-

sions for patients, patients respond in the same way that minority cultures often respond to an attitude by the dominant culture: by becoming passive, resistive, angry, or resistant to treatment.

Closely related to cultural imposition is **ethnocentrism,** the belief that one's own ideas, beliefs, and practices are the best, are superior, or are most preferred to those of others (Leininger, 1978). To avoid this practice, the nurse must carefully and critically examine his or her own values and beliefs and be willing to understand health and illness from the cultural viewpoint of the patient receiving care.

Providing Transcultural Care

A major theme of transcultural nursing care is to focus on the caring practices of various cultures. Caring is a universal phenomenon, even though the forms and manifestations may vary among cultures. Caring practices are the protecting and assisting activities related to health and performed as part of a culture.

Nursing care can become complicated when the patient and the nurse have distinctly different cultural norms. The nurse's role is to understand the patient's needs and to adapt care to meet those needs. Unless the nurse is willing to examine carefully and clarify his or her own attitudes and values and to be sensitive to others who are "different," the use of cultural concepts to provide holistic care will be unsuccessful.

Sometimes a nurse is placed in a cultural bind: the nurse's cultural upbringing influences values and beliefs, and the nurse is expected to adopt the customs of the nursing profession and at the same time accommodate the folkways and norms of individual patients. A careful merging of modern and traditional cultural beliefs is a necessary prerequisite for safe, considerate, and successful nursing care of all patients.

After a nurse attains cultural awareness and sensitivity in planning care, the nurse can more easily recognize the patient's use of traditional folk medicine and its importance. When caring for a patient who subscribes to such practices, the nurse takes this circumstance into account during assessment and planning.

Cultural Assessment

The most effective way to identify specific factors that influence a patient's behavior is to perform a cultural assessment. The primary informant should be the patient, if possible. If the patient is not able to respond to the questions, a family member or a friend can be consulted.

The nurse can anticipate a patient's values, religion, dietary practices, family lines of authority, family life patterns, and beliefs and practices related to health and illness. The nurse can obtain this anticipatory information through research before initiating contact with the patient, with the reminder that information about any culture is general and that the nurse must individualize this infor-

FOCUSED ASSESSMENT GUIDE

Transcultural Assessment: Health-Related Beliefs and Practices

1. To what cause(s) does the patient attribute illness and disease (eg, divine wrath, imbalance in hot/cold or yin/yang, punishment for moral transgressions, hex, soul loss, pathogenic organism)?
2. What are the patient's cultural beliefs about the ideal body size and shape? What is the patient's self-image compared to the ideal?
3. What name does the patient give to his or her health-related condition?
4. What does the patient believe promotes health (eating certain foods; wearing amulets to bring good luck; sleep; rest; good nutrition; reducing stress; exercise; prayer; rituals to ancestors, saints, or intermediate deities)?
5. What is the patient's religious affiliation (eg, Judaism, Islam, Pentacostalism, West African voodooism, Seventh-Day Adventism, Catholicism, Mormonism)? How actively involved in the practice of this religion is the patient?
6. Does the patient rely on cultural healers (eg, curandero, shaman, spiritualist, priest, minister,

monk)? Who determines when the patient is sick and when the patient is healthy? Who influences the choice/type of healer and treatment that should be sought?

7. In what types of cultural healing practices does the patient engage (use of herbal remedies, potions, massage; wearing of talismans, copper bracelets, or charms to discourage evil spirits; healing rituals, incantations, prayers)?
8. How are biomedical/scientific healthcare providers perceived? How does the patient and his or her family perceive nurses? What are the expectations of nurses and nursing care?
9. What comprises appropriate "sick role" behavior? Who determines what symptoms constitute disease/illness? Who decides when the patient is no longer sick? Who cares for the patient at home?
10. How does the patient's cultural group view mental disorders? Are there differences in acceptable behaviors for physical versus psychological illnesses?

From Andrews, M., & Boyle, J. (1999). *Transcultural concepts in nursing care* (3rd ed.). Philadelphia: Lippincott Williams & Wilkins, pp. 533–544, Appendix A.

---

mation for the specific patient once interaction begins. One part of the Andrews and Boyle Transcultural Nursing Assessment Guide (1999) is illustrated in the accompanying Focused Assessment Guide.

Guidelines for Transcultural Care

Table 3-2 lists cultural variations in health practices to illustrate similarities and differences among different groups in our society. It is important to remember that these are only general guidelines and that each patient must be considered as a unique individual. The following guidelines are useful in practicing transcultural nursing care:

- Become aware of the role of cultural influences in your own life. Objectively examine your own beliefs, values, practices, and family experiences. As you become more sensitive to the importance of these factors, you will also become more sensitive to cultural influences in others' lives.
- Identify biases in your own life. How do they affect your feelings about others? How could they affect your nursing care of others?
- Learn as much as possible about the belief system and practices of people in your community and of patients in the area in which you work.
- Practice techniques of observation and listening to acquire knowledge of the beliefs and values of

patients for whom you are caring. Some people, especially those of minority cultures, may have been belittled and subjected to ridicule and insults and may be hesitant to discuss their beliefs and practices. Approach this topic with patients carefully. If you are motivated by sincerity, respect, and concern, your attitude will convey this, and most patients will respond positively. On the other hand, if you are motivated by curiosity and have a condescending attitude, most patients will respond negatively.

- Incorporate factors from the patient's cultural background into healthcare whenever possible and when the practices are not considered harmful to health. To ignore or contradict the patient's background may result in the patient refusing care or failing to follow prescribed therapy.
- Keep in mind that health practices are part of the overall culture and that changing them may have widespread implications for the person. You must understand these implications accurately before attempting such a change. You also need to provide the necessary support and reinforcement for the patient if a change in a health practice with a cultural basis is considered necessary.
- Do not force the patient to participate in care that conflicts with his or her values. If the patient is

(*text continues on page 52*)

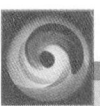

Table 3-2
Cultural Factors That Affect Nursing Care

White Middle Class

Family
- Nuclear family is highly valued.
- Elderly family members may live in a nursing home when they can no longer care for themselves.

Folk and Traditional Healthcare
- Self-diagnosis of illnesses
- Use of over-the-counter drugs (especially vitamins and analgesics)
- Dieting (especially fad diets)
- Extensive use of exercise and exercise facilities

Values and Beliefs
- Youth is valued over age
- Cleanliness
- Orderliness
- Attractiveness
- Individualism
- Achievement
- Punctuality

Common Health Problems
- Cardiovascular diseases
- Gastrointestinal diseases
- Some forms of cancer
- Motor vehicle accidents
- Suicides
- Mental illness
- Chemical abuses

Nursing Considerations
- Careful assessment of client's use of over-the-counter medications (observe for signs and symptoms of toxic medication levels, especially fat-soluble vitamins)
- Nutritional assessments of dietary habits

African American

Family
- Close and supportive extended-family relationships
- Strong kinship ties with nonblood relatives from church or organizational and social groups
- Family unity, loyalty, and cooperation are important.
- Usually matriarchal

Folk and Traditional Healthcare
- Varies extensively and may include spiritualists, herb doctors, root doctors, conjurers, skilled elder family members, voodoo, faith healing

Values and Beliefs
- Present oriented
- Members of the African American clergy are highly respected in the black community
- Frequently highly religious

Common Health Problems
- Hypertension (precise cause unknown, may be related to diet)
- Sickle cell anemia
- Skin disorders; inflammation of hair follicles, various types of dermatitis and excessive growth of scar tissue (keloids)
- Lactose enzyme deficiency resulting in poor toleration of milk products
- Higher rate of tuberculosis
- Diabetes mellitus
- Higher infant mortality rate than in the white population

Nursing Considerations
- Many African American families may still use various folk healing practices and home remedies for treating particular illnesses.
- Special care may be necessary for the hair and skin.
- Special consideration should be given to the sometimes extensive and frequently informal support networks of patients (ie, religious and community group members who offer assistance in a time of need).

(continued)

Table 3-2 (Continued)

Asian

(Beliefs and practices vary, but most Asian cultures share some characteristics.)

Family
- Welfare of the family is valued above the person.
- Extended families are common.
- A person's lineage (ancestors) is respected.
- Sharing among family members is expected.

Folk and Traditional Healthcare
- Theoretical basis is in Taoism, which seeks a balance in all things.
- Good health is achieved through the proper balance of yin (feminine, negative, dark, cold) and yang (masculine, positive, light, warm).
- An imbalance in energy is caused by an improper diet or strong emotions.
- Diseases and foods are classified as hot or cold, and a proper balance between them will promote wellness (eg, treat a cold disease with hot foods).
- Many Asian healthcare systems use herbs, diet, and the application of hot or cold therapy. Also, many Asians believe that there are points on the body that are located on the meridians or energy pathways. If the energy flow is out of balance, treatment of the pathways may be necessary to restore the energy equilibrium.

  Acumassage—Technique of manipulating points along the energy pathways

  Acupressure—Technique for compressing the energy pathway points

  Acupuncture—Technique by which fine needles are inserted into the body at energy pathway points

Values and Beliefs
- Strong sense of self-respect and self-control
- High respect for age
- Respect for authority
- Respect for hard work
- Praise of self or others is considered poor manners
- Strong emphasis on harmony and the avoidance of conflict

Common Health Problems
- Tuberculosis
- Communicable diseases
- Malnutrition
- Suicide
- Various forms of mental illness
- Lactose enzyme deficiency

Nursing Considerations
- Some members of Asian cultures may be upset by the drawing of blood for laboratory tests. They consider blood to be the body's life force, and some do not believe that it can be regenerated.
- Some members believe that it is best to die with the body intact, so they may refuse surgery except in dire circumstances.
- Members of many Asian cultures seldom complain about what is bothering them. Therefore, the nurse must carefully assess the patient for pain or discomfort by observing for nonverbal signs of discomfort, such as facial grimacing or wincing and holding of the painful area.
- Some Asians consider it polite to give a person the responses the person is expecting. Therefore, misinformation may be transmitted to the questioner in an effort, on the client's part, to be respectful.
- Some members may move from physician to physician in an attempt to be cured of an illness, but to avoid insulting or embarrassing a physician, they will not inform him or her that they are going to another physician. This can result in confusion, inaccuracies, and overmedication.
- Some Asians may refuse to have diagnostic studies done because they believe that a skilled and competent physician can diagnose an illness solely through a physical examination.
- Some members may have a difficult time understanding the importance of taking a regimen of medications because many of their folk treatments involve the ingestion of one dose of herbal mixtures.
- Dietary counseling may be necessary if the patient is on a salt-restricted diet because many Asian foods have a high salt content related to the use of soy sauce.

(continued)

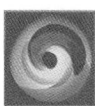

Table 3-2 (Continued)

Hispanic, Mexican American

Family
- Familial role is important.
- *Compadrazgo:* special bond between a child's parents and his or her grandparents
- Family is the primary unit of society.

Folk and Traditional Healthcare
- *Curanderas(os):* frequently folk healers who base treatments on humoral pathology—basic functions of the body are controlled by four body fluids or "humors":

  Blood—hot and wet

  Yellow bile—hot and dry

  Black bile—cold and dry

  Phlegm—cold and wet
- The secret of good health is to balance hot and cold within the body; therefore, most foods, beverages, herbs, and medications are classified as hot (*caliente*) or cold (*fresco, frio*) (a cold disease will be cured with a hot treatment).

Values and Beliefs
- Respect is given according to age (older) and sex (male).
- Roman Catholic Church may be very influential
- God gives health and allows illness for a reason; therefore, may perceive illness as a punishment from God. An illness of this type can be cured through atonement and forgiveness.

Common Health Problems
- Diabetes mellitus and its complications
- Poverty and resultant problems, such as poor nutrition, inadequate medical care, poor prenatal care
- Lactose enzyme deficiency

Nursing Considerations
- It may be difficult to convince an asymptomatic patient that he or she is ill.
- Special diet considerations are necessary if the patient believes in the hot/cold theory of treating illnesses.
- Diet counseling may be necessary at times because many members have a normal diet that is high in starch.

Hispanic, Puerto Rican

(Since the Jones Act of 1917, all Puerto Ricans are American citizens.)

Family
- *Compadrazgo*—same as in Mexican American culture

Folk and Traditional Healthcare
- Similar to that of other Spanish-speaking cultures

Common Health Problems
- Parasitic diseases, such as dysentery, malaria, filariasis, and hookworms
- Lactose enzyme deficiency

Values and Beliefs
- Place a high value on safeguarding against group pressure to violate a person's integrity (may be difficult for Puerto Ricans to accept teamwork)
- Close-mouthed about personal and family affairs (psychotherapy may be difficult to achieve at times because of this belief)
- Proper consideration should be given to cultural rituals such as shaking hands and standing up to greet and say goodbye to people.
- Time is a relative phenomenon; little attention is given to the exact time of day.
- *Ataques*—culturally acceptable reaction to situations of extreme stress, characterized by hyperkinetic seizure activity

Nursing Considerations
- It may be difficult to teach Puerto Rican patients to follow time-oriented actions (eg, taking medications, keeping appointments).

(continued)

Table 3-2 (Continued)

Native American

(Each tribe's beliefs and practices vary to some degree.)

Family
- Families are large and extended.
- Grandparents are official and symbolic leaders and decision makers.
- A child's namesake may become the same as another parent to the child.

Folk and Traditional Healthcare
- Medicine men (shaman) are heavily used.
- Heavy use of herbs and psychological treatments, ceremonies, fasting, meditation, heat, and massages

Common Health Problems
- Alcoholism
- Suicide
- Tuberculosis
- Malnutrition
- Communicable diseases
- Higher maternal and infant mortality rates than in most of the population
- Diabetes mellitus
- Hypertension
- Gallbladder disease

Values and Beliefs
- Present oriented. Taught to live in the present and not to be concerned about the future. This time consciousness emphasizes finishing current business before doing something else.
- High respect for age.
- Great value is placed on working together and sharing resources.
- Failure to achieve a personal goal frequently is believed to be the result of competition.
- High respect is given to a person who gives to others. The accumulation of money and goods often is frowned on.
- Some Native Americans practice the Peyotist religion in which the consumption of peyote, an intoxicating drug derived from mescal cacti, is part of the service. Peyote is legal if used for this purpose. It is classified as a hallucinogenic drug.

Nursing Considerations
- The family is expected to be part of the nursing care plan.
- Note taking often is taboo because it is considered an insult to the speaker because the listener is not paying full attention to the conversation. Good memory skills often are required by the nurse.
- Indirect eye contact is acceptable and sometimes preferred.
- It often is considered rude or impolite to indicate that a conversation has not been heard.
- A low tone of voice often is considered respectful.
- A Native American patient may expect the caregiver to deduce the problem through instinct and not through asking many questions and history taking. If this is the case, it may help to use declarative sentences rather than direct questioning.

Hawaiian

Family
- Familial role is important.
- Ohana, or extended families, are jointly involved in childrearing.
- Hierarchy of family structure, each gender and age have specific duties.
- Closely knit families in small, isolated communities

Folk and Traditional Healthcare
- Kahuna La'au Lapa'nu is the ancient Hawaiian medical practitioner.
- View patient's illness as part of the whole.
- Relationships between the physical, psychological, and spiritual
- Emphasis on preventative medicine
- Treatment uses more than 300 medicinal plants and minerals

Values and Beliefs
- Aloha: a deep love, respect, and affection between people and the land
- Respect given to people and land
- Christian gods replaced the myriad of Hawaiian gods.
- Lifestyle more revered than compliance with healthcare issues
- Present oriented, less initiative and drive than that of direction and achievement
- Death seen as part of life and not feared

Common Health Problems
- Diabetes mellitus and its complications
- Hypertension (unknown cause; perhaps related to diet)
- Gout (perhaps related to diet)
- Respiratory disorders: asthma, allergies, tuberculosis
- Skin disorders: bacterial, fungal, cancer
- Obesity
- Smoking, alcoholism, drug abuse

(continued)

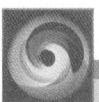

Table 3-2 (Continued)

Nursing Considerations
- Many Hawaiians may still use folk healing practices and home remedies.
- Special consideration given to the extensive family network during hospitalization
- Acceptance from healthcare practitioners of current health practices and lifestyle

Appalachian

Family
- Intense interpersonal relations
- Family is cohesive, and several generations often live close to each other.
- Elderly are respected as providers.
- Tend to live in rural, isolated areas

Folk and Traditional Healthcare
- "Granny" woman, or folk healer, provides care and may be consulted even if receiving traditional care.
- Various herbs, such as foxglove and yellow root, are used for common illnesses such as malaise, chest discomfort, heart problems, and upper respiratory infections.
- Elderly may have had only limited contact with healthcare providers and be skeptical of modern healthcare.

Values and Beliefs
- Independence and self-determination
- Isolation is accepted as a way of life.
- Person-oriented
- May be fatalistic about losses and death
- Belief in a divine existence rather than attending a particular church

Common Health Problems
- Cardiovascular disorders
- Respiratory disorders
- Nutritional disorders
- Smoking, alcoholism

Nursing Considerations
- Treat each person with regard for personal dignity.
- Allow family members to remain with patient as support system.
- Acceptance from healthcare providers of current health practices and lifestyle
- Allow patients to make decisions about care.

forced to accept it, the care may become harmful because resulting feelings of guilt and alienation from a religious or cultural group are likely to threaten the patient's well-being.
- Accommodate the cultural dietary practices of patients as much as possible. Dietary departments in many hospitals and long-term care facilities can supply patients with meals that are consistent with special dietary practices. Families may be encouraged to bring food from home for patients with particular preferences when this practice does not violate policy. Teaching patients and families about therapeutic diets can also be done within the framework of particular cultural practices.
- Take into consideration the cultural role of the family member who makes most of the important decisions. In some cultures, it is the husband or father, whereas in others, it is the grandmother or another respected elder. To disregard this fact or to proceed with nursing care that is not approved by this person can result in conflict or in disregard for what has been taught. Be careful to involve this person in the nursing care planning.
- Seek assistance of a respected family member, member of the clergy, or folk medicine practitioner as

indicated so that the patient is more likely to accept healthcare services. Acknowledging the role of the person's folk medicine practitioner can be an important way of building trust. If invited, folk medicine practitioners can work closely with professional health practitioners in the interest of the patient and family. Such efforts promote mutual understanding, respect, and cooperation.
- Modify care to include folk practices and practitioners as much as possible, and be an advocate for patients from diverse cultural groups.
- Use past transcultural experiences as a guide, but never as the answer to all transcultural solutions.
- Learn from your mistakes and do not repeat them. All nurses make mistakes at some time when caring for culturally different patients. Inadvertent mistakes are just that, but repeated mistakes are careless and disrespectful; they will adversely affect your interaction with patients and coworkers.
- Treat each person as an individual. What was true of one person will not be true of another, even if they are from the same cultural background. View each person as an individual with rights, and help the patient retain dignity.

Learning Outcomes

After completing this chapter, the learner should be able to accomplish the following:

1. Define key terms used in the chapter.

cultural assimilation	ethnocentrism
cultural imposition	minority group
cultural blindness	personal space
culture	race
culture conflict	stereotyping
culture shock	subculture
dominant group	transcultural nursing
ethnicity	

2. Discuss the concepts of culture and ethnicity.
3. Describe cultural and ethnic characteristics that influence healthcare, including gender roles, language and communication, orientation to space and time, food and nutrition, socioeconomic factors, importance of family, physical and mental characteristics, spiritual characteristics, and perceptions of health and illness.
4. Compare and contrast the culture of the healthcare system with the broad concept of culture.
5. Identify the factors that affect the interaction of the nurse and the patient in terms of culturally different healthcare values.
6. Discuss the guidelines for practicing culturally sensitive nursing care.

Critical Thinking Exercises

1. Analyze the following situations, identifying potential sources of cultural imposition.
   - A young Ethiopian woman with terminal breast cancer requests that all treatment decisions be made by her uncle, who is the family elder. Her primary nurse is an active feminist.
   - A Native American woman refuses a life-saving amputation of her leg because she believes it is essential to enter the next world "whole."

2. Interview family members or friends who have recently received healthcare, such as for a health screening, diagnostic testing, emergency care, routine checkup, or office or clinic visit or hospitalization. What aspects of the healthcare culture were most distressing to them? What factors were most helpful? Do their answers vary according to the setting for care? If so, why do you think they felt as they did?

Bibliography

Ahijevych, K., & Bernhard, L. (1994). Health-promoting behaviors of African American women. *Nursing Research, 43*(2), 86–89.

American Nurses Association. (1991). *Position statement on cultural diversity in nursing practice.* Kansas City, MO: ANA.

Andrews, M. M., & Boyle, J. S. (1999). *Transcultural concepts in nursing care* (3rd ed.). Philadelphia: Lippincott Williams & Wilkins.

Bartol, G., & Richardson, L. (1998). Clinical scholarship. Using literature to create cultural competence. *Image—The Journal of Nursing Scholarship, 30*(1), 75–79.

Campbell, J., & Campbell, D. (1996). Cultural competence in the care of abused women. *Journal of Nurse-Midwifery, 41*(6), 457–462.

Culture tips: African American/black. (1998). *Cross Cultural Connection, 3*(4), 5–6.

Dosswell, W., & Erlen, J. (1998). Multicultural issues and ethical concerns in the delivery of nursing care interventions. *Nursing Clinics of North America, 33*(2), 353–361.

Henderson, G., & Primeaux, M. (1981). *Transcultural health care.* Menlo Park, CA: Addison-Wesley.

Holland, L., & Courtney, R. (1998). Increasing cultural competence with the Latino community. *Journal of Community Health Nursing, 15*(1), 45–53.

Jan, R., & Smith, C.A. (1998). Staying healthy in immigrant Pakistani families living in the United States. *Image—The Journal of Nursing Scholarship, 30*(2), 157–159.

Juarbe, T. (1995). Access to healthcare for Hispanic women: A primary healthcare perspective. *Nursing Outlook, 43*(1), 23–28.

Leininger, M. (1978). *Transcultural nursing: Concepts, theories, and practices.* New York: John Wiley & Sons.

Leininger, M. (1990). Transcultural nursing: A worldwide necessity to advance nursing knowledge and practice. In J. McCloskey & H. Grace (Eds.), *Current issues in nursing* (3rd ed.). St. Louis: CV Mosby.

Leininger, M. (1991). Becoming aware of types of health practitioners and cultural imposition. *Journal of Transcultural Nursing, 2*(2), 32–39.

Leininger, M. (1994). Quality of life from a transcultural nursing perspective. *Nursing Science Quarterly, 7*(1), 22–28.

Lester, N. (1998). Cultural competence: A nursing dialogue. Part one. *American Journal of Nursing, 98*(8), 26–34.

Lester, N. (1998). Cultural competence: A nursing dialogue. Part two. *American Journal of Nursing, 98*(9), 36–43.

Lipson, J., Dibble, S., & Minarik, P. (Eds.). (1996). *Culture & nursing care: A pocket guide.* San Francisco: UCSF Press.

McLaughlin, L., & Braun, K. (1998). Asian and Pacific Islander cultural values: Considerations for health care decision making. *Health & Social Work, 23*(2), 116–126.

Robertson, M. (1998). Promoting cultural and racial diversity in nursing: The need for political activism. *Journal of Multicultural Nursing & Health, 4*(2), 11–15.

Rodriquez, J. (1998). Culture tips: Cuban Americans. *Cross Cultural Connection, 4*(1), 5.

Secundy, M. G. (Ed.). (1992). *Trials, tribulations, and celebrations: African-American perspectives on health, illness, aging, and loss.* Yarmouth, ME: Intercultural Press.

Sharts-Hopko, N. (1996). Health and illness concepts for cultural competence with Japanese clients. *Journal of Cultural Diversity, 3*(3), 74–79.

Smith, L. (1998). Concept analysis: Cultural competence. *Journal of Cultural Diversity, 5*(1), 4–10.

Spector, R. E. (1996). *Cultural diversity in health and illness.* (4th ed.). New York: Appleton & Lange.

Taylor, R. (1998). Check your cultural competence. *Nursing Management, 29*(8), 30–32.

US Bureau of the Census. (1999). *Resident population estimates of the US by sex, race, and Hispanic origin.* Washington, DC: Population Estimates Program, Population Division, US Government Printing Office.

US Bureau of the Census. (1997). *Poverty in the United States, 1997.* Washington, DC: US Government Printing Office.

Chapter 4
Health and Illness

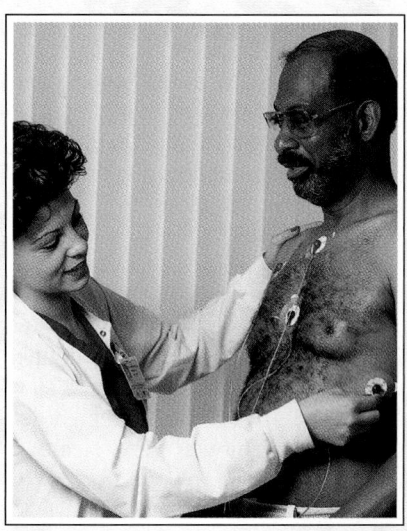

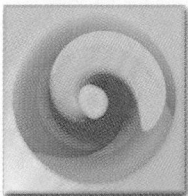

Thinking Critically About
Nursing's Blended Skills

Before reading this chapter, think about the types of skills you will need to promote and restore health and to prevent disease and illness.

- It's the end of the semester, papers are due, final examinations are right around the corner, and you can't remember when you last had a good night sleep. You watch as one friend after another gets sick and await your turn.

- You prepare to discharge a 62-year-old woman who was hospitalized after a "mini-stroke." Returned to her preevent level of functioning, she knows that she is at increased risk for a major stroke and wants to do everything possible to keep healthy.

- Six-year-old Jimmy is still in a coma after a bike accident. His family is "camped out" in the pediatric intensive care unit convinced that their love and your care will bring him "back."

- Dan is a 27-year-old man with schizophrenia who arrives in the mental health clinic demanding relief from the voices who are telling him to hurt himself. Well known to all the staff who experience him to be a difficult patient, he inspires a less than cordial welcome.

What cognitive, technical, interpersonal, and ethical/legal skills do you think you will need to meet effectively the health needs of the individuals described above?

The primary roles of the nurse as caregiver are to promote health, to prevent illness, to restore health, and to facilitate coping. These activities help maximize the health of patients of all ages, in all settings, and in both health and illness. *Health* is more than just the absence of illness; it is an active process in which an individual moves toward his or her maximum potential. One's health is influenced by a variety of factors, including the environment, how well one's basic human needs are met, and one's family and culture.

This chapter discusses how nursing care is influenced by the patient—the person receiving care. To give holistic care, the nurse must understand and respect each person's individual definition of health and responses to illness. The nurse's knowledge of health and illness, as well as a philosophy of health, is even more important because of the continuing trend toward most care being provided in the home, the increasing numbers of older adults, and the growing incidence of chronic illnesses.

Defining Health and Illness

Because *health* is individually defined by each person and is affected by so many factors, a standard definition is difficult. The most widely accepted definition of health was made in 1947 by the World Health Organization: "Health is a state of complete physical, mental, and social well being, not merely the absence of disease or infirmity" (p. 1). This definition has expanded since the 1940s, with the development of other models. On a personal level, most individuals define health according to how they feel ("I feel really sick"); the absence or presence of symptoms of illness ("I have a terrible pain in my stomach"); or their ability to carry out activities of daily living ("I felt so much better that I got up and cooked supper").

Illness is also individually defined by each person who experiences an alteration in health. It is also difficult to make a standard definition of illness, because the terms *disease* and *illness* are often used to mean the same process. **Disease** is a medical term, meaning that there is a pathologic change in the structure or function of the body or mind. A disease has specific symptoms and boundaries (see the accompanying box: Causes of Diseases). An **illness,** on the other hand, is the response of the person to a disease; it is an abnormal process in which the person's level of functioning is changed compared with a previous level. This response is unique for each person and is influenced by self-perceptions, others' perceptions, the effects of changes in body structure and function, the effects of those changes on roles and relationships, and cultural and spiritual values and beliefs. Always remember that a person may have a disease but still achieve maximum functioning and quality of life.

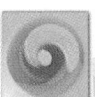

COGNITIVE SKILLS

- Knowledge of definitions of health, disease, and illness; models of health; and factors influencing health and illness
- Knowledge of risk factors and how to modify lifestyles (your own, the woman with the mini-stroke, the 6-year-old in the coma and his family, and the man with schizophrenia) to promote health and prevent disease
- Knowledge of how to implement competently a plan of nursing care for the woman with the mini-stroke, the 6-year-old in the coma and his family, and the man with schizophrenia

TECHNICAL SKILLS

- Ability to provide the technical nursing assistance necessary to meet the needs of the woman with the mini-stroke, the 6-year-old in the coma and his family, and the man with schizophrenia (eg, medication preparation and administration; assistance with feeding, hygiene, mobility; preparation for diagnostic tests; competent use of computerized documentation system)

INTERPERSONAL SKILLS

- Ability to establish caring relationships with your student colleagues, the woman with the mini-stroke, the 6-year-old in the coma and his family, and the man with schizophrenia
- Ability to work collaboratively with the interdisciplinary team
- Ability to assess health-related beliefs, goals, and practices

ETHICAL/LEGAL SKILLS

- Commitment to self-care; ability to balance responsibilities to self with care demands for others
- Advocacy skills: commitment to securing the best possible care for the patients and families assigned to your care. Ability to mobilize the mental health team's best collective efforts for the man with schizophrenia
- Knowledge of the nurse's legal responsibilities when providing care, including the need to document nursing assessment, diagnosis, planning, implementation, and evaluation

Causes of Diseases

- Inherited genetic defects
- Developmental defects resulting from exposure to such factors as virus or chemicals during pregnancy
- Biologic agents or toxins
- Physical agents such as temperature, chemicals, and radiation
- Generalized tissue responses to injury or irritation
- Physiologic and emotional reactions to stress
- Excessive or insufficient production of body secretions (hormones, enzymes, and so forth)

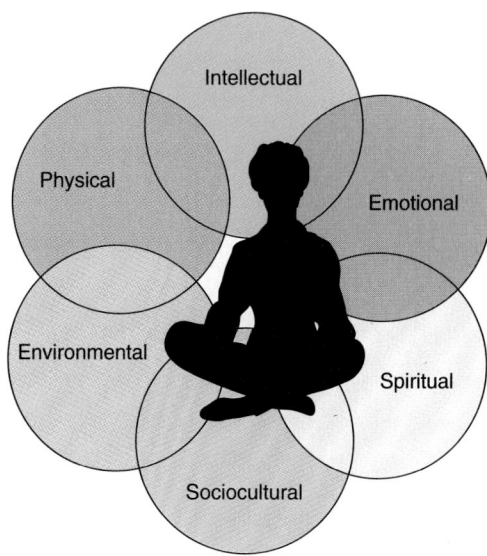

Figure 4-1
The human dimensions. All of these interdependent parts compose the whole person.

As discussed in previous chapters, every person defines health in terms of his or her own values and beliefs. A person's perception of his or her degree of health is also influenced by the family, community, and society in which the person lives. Consider the following examples:

- Meguni Kuni, 4 years of age, was born with cystic fibrosis. Although she requires ongoing treatment for this illness, she is now an active member of her preschool class, takes gymnastics lessons, and wants to be a doctor when she grows up.
- Shondra Cole is 34 years of age and married and has two school aged children. She has chronic rheumatoid arthritis and is in a wheelchair. Shondra takes care of her house and family and uses a specially designed car to get to her part-time job.
- Samuel Cohen is 67 years of age. He was diagnosed with diabetes and high blood pressure last year and takes medications for both health problems. Samuel is retired but volunteers 3 days a week in a local hospital as a transport technician.

Would you define Meguni, Shondra, and Samuel as well? Although they each have a physical condition that might lead them to define themselves as being ill, they are all productive members of their society and would say they are healthy.

Health must be defined by each person, integrating all the person's dimensions—the physical, intellectual, emotional, sociocultural, spiritual, and environmental aspects of the whole person. The nurse giving holistic nursing care must equally consider all these interrelated and interdependent dimensions of the whole person (Fig. 4-1).

⑤ Models of Health and Illness

Because health and illness cannot be given universal standard definitions, health models have been developed to help describe concepts and relationships involved in health and illness. The models described in this chapter are the health–illness continuum, the high-level wellness model, the health belief model, and the health promotion model.

Agent–Host–Environment Model

The **agent–host–environment model** of health and illness, developed by Leavell and Clark (1965) for use in community health, is useful for examining the causes of disease in an individual. The agent, host, and environment interact in ways that create risk factors, and understanding these is important for the promotion and maintenance of health. The three factors involved are defined as follows:

Agent: An environmental factor or stressor that must be present or absent for an illness to occur. For example, the factor may be bacteria or a virus, a chemical substance, or a form of radiation whose presence, excessive presence, or absence (such as in a vitamin deficiency disease) is necessary for an illness.

Host: Living beings capable of being infected or affected by an agent. The host reaction is influenced by the person's family history, age, and health habits.

Environment: All the factors external to the host that make illness more or less likely. The factors can include any that influence health, including physical, social, biologic, and cultural factors.

For example, a person who has poor nutritional habits and gets little sleep is at increased risk for infection during an outbreak of influenza. If that person also is immune deficient (as occurs in acquired immunodeficiency syndrome [AIDS]), the risk is even greater. The triangle in Figure 4-2 shows that each of the agent–host–environment factors affects and is affected by the others. These factors are constantly interacting, and a combination of factors may increase the possibility of illness. When the factors are balanced, health is maintained; when they are out of balance, disease occurs. Thus, health is an ever-changing state.

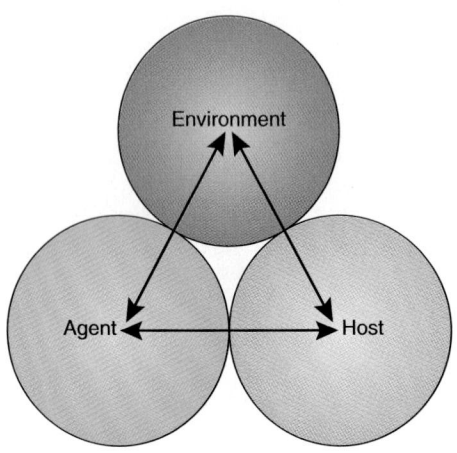

Figure 4-2
The agent–host–environment triangle.

Health–Illness Continuum

The **health–illness continuum** is one way to measure a person's level of health. This model views health as a constantly changing state, with high-level wellness and death being on opposite ends of a graduated scale, or continuum (Fig. 4-3). This continuum is a model of the dynamic state of health, as a person adapts to changes in the internal and external environments to maintain a state of well-being. A patient with a chronic illness may view himself or herself at different points on the continuum at any given time, depending on how well the patient believes he or she is functioning with the illness.

High-Level Wellness Model

Halbert Dunn (1961) described his model of **high-level wellness** as functioning to one's maximum potential while maintaining balance and a purposeful direction in the environment. Dunn differentiated "wellness" from "good health," believing that good health is a passive state wherein the person is not ill. Wellness is a more active state, oriented toward maximizing the potential of the individual, regard-

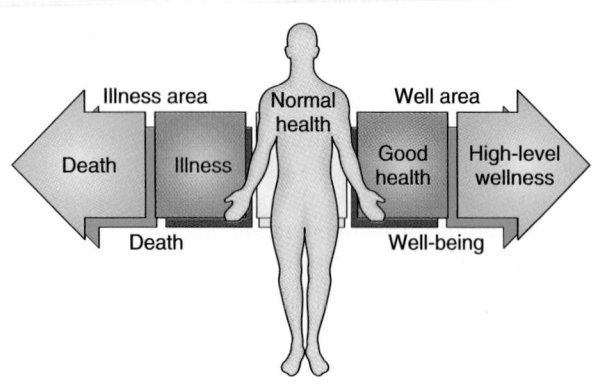

Figure 4-3
The health–illness continuum.

less of his or her state of health. Dunn also defined processes that help a person know who and what he or she is. These processes, which are a part of each individual's perception of their own wellness state, are *being* (recognizing self as separate and individual); *belonging* (being part of a whole); *becoming* (growing and developing); and *befitting* (making personal choices to befit the self for the future).

Dunn's model encourages the nurse to care for the total person with regard for all factors affecting the person's state of being while striving to reach maximum potential. For example, when planning and giving care to a young male college student paralyzed after a diving accident, the nurse would include nursing activities to meet his educational needs (intellectual dimension); incorporate friends and family (sociocultural dimension); provide or refer for counseling (emotional dimension); and ask the hospital chaplain to visit (spiritual dimension).

Health Belief Model

Free or low-cost screens and health information are available in most areas to help in the early detection of disease and to educate people about healthy living to prevent illness. Why, then, don't more people take advantage of these services or change their lifestyles? This question can be answered with the widely used health belief model, which describes health behaviors.

The **health belief model** (Rosenstock, 1974) is concerned with what people perceive, or believe, to be true about themselves in relation to their health. This model is based on three components of individual perceptions of threat of a disease: (1) perceived susceptibility to a disease, (2) perceived seriousness of a disease, and (3) perceived benefits of action.

Perceived susceptibility to a disease is the belief that one either will or will not contract a disease. Perceived susceptibility ranges from being afraid of contracting a disease to completely denying that certain behaviors will result in illness. For example, one person who smokes cigarettes may believe he or she is at danger for lung cancer and may stop smoking, while another person may believe smoking poses no serious threat and continues to smoke.

Perceived seriousness of a disease concerns the seriousness of the disease and its effect on the person's lifestyle. This component is related to how much the person knows about the disease and can result in a change in health behavior. If a person who smokes believes that lung cancer can lead to physical disability or death and would therefore affect his or her ability to work and care for the family, the person is more likely to stop smoking.

Perceived benefits of action is concerned with how effective the individual believes preventive measures will be in preventing illness. This factor is influenced by the person's conviction that carrying out a recommended action will prevent or modify the disease and by the person's perception of the cost and unpleasant effects of performing the health behavior (compared with not taking any action). For example, the person may believe that stopping smoking will prevent future breathing problems and that the initial withdrawal symptoms can be overcome; therefore, the person may stop smoking.

Modifying factors of the perceived threat of disease include demographic variables (such as age, race), sociopsychological variables (such as personality and peer group pressure), and structural variables (such as knowledge and prior contact with the disease). These factors interact to influence the perceived benefits of preventive action minus the perceived barriers to preventive action. Cues to action are also modifying factors and are provided by activities such as others' advice, mass-media campaigns, literature, appointment reminder telephone calls or postcards, and illness of a significant other. The likelihood of taking a recommended preventive health action is thus a composite of individual perceptions and modifying factors.

This model is useful when teaching individuals about health and illness. The nurse can identify the patient's health beliefs and then structure goals to help the patient realistically meet health needs. Teaching and health promotion activities are ineffective, however, unless the patient believes they are important and necessary.

Health Promotion Model

The **health promotion model** (Pender, 1996) was developed to illustrate the "multidimensional nature of persons interacting with their environment as they pursue health" (p. 53). The model incorporates individual characteristics and experiences and behavior-specific cognitions and affect, with health-promoting behavior as the outcome. The components of the model can be used to design and provide nursing interventions to promote health.

Individual characteristics and experiences include the following:

- Prior related behavior, with health-related behaviors becoming a habit, and therefore being more likely to occur
- Personal biologic, psychological, and sociocultural factors (such as age, gender, strength, self-esteem, perceived health status, definition of health, race, acculturation, and socioeconomic status) are predictive of a given health-related behavior.

Behavior-specific cognitions and affect are considered to be major motivators to engage in health-promoting behaviors. These include the following:

- The belief that there will be a positive outcome from a specific health behavior
- Barriers to action, which include perceptions of unavailability, inconvenience, expense, difficulty, or time, usually result in avoidance of a behavior.
- Perceptions of skill and competence (self-efficacy) motivate a person to engage in behaviors in which he or she excels.
- If a person feels positive about a behavior, it is likely to be repeated.

- The interpersonal influence of others, and especially of families, peers, and healthcare providers
- Situational influences (such as no-smoking policies) influence health behaviors.

The health-related behavior that is the outcome is initiated by a commitment to a plan of action, accompanied by the development of associated strategies to perform the valued behavior. Failure to sustain the behavior may result from competing demands. For example, a person may begin a low-fat diet but "give in" to the desire for fast foods. Health-related behavior is the outcome of the model and is directed toward attaining positive health outcomes and experiences throughout the life span.

Factors Affecting Health and Illness

Many factors influence a person's health status. These factors may be internal or external to the individual and may or may not be under the person's conscious control. Nonetheless, such factors do affect patient responses to nursing care. To plan and give holistic care, the nurse must understand how these factors influence behavior in both healthy and ill patients.

This section describes factors that affect health and illness, including factors in the human dimensions that influence health–illness status, beliefs, and practices; basic human needs; and self-concept.

The Human Dimensions

The factors influencing a person's health–illness status, health beliefs, and health practices relate to the person's human dimensions (see Fig. 4-1). Each person has these human dimensions, and each dimension influences the behaviors of the person receiving care. As you care for patients, consider these dimensions as an integral part of the nursing process.

Physical Dimension
Genetic makeup, age, developmental level, race, and gender are all part of an individual's physical dimension and strongly influence the person's health status and health practices. Some examples of the physical dimension are as follows:

- An adolescent boy who is prone to take risks while driving, increasing the possibility of an accident
- A young woman who has a family history of breast cancer and diabetes and therefore is at higher risk for these conditions
- A middle-aged African American man who is more prone to develop high blood pressure
- An older adult who has increased risk for one or more chronic illnesses

Emotional Dimension
How the mind affects body function and responds to body conditions also influences health. Long-term stress affects

body systems, and anxiety affects health habits; conversely, calm acceptance and relaxation can actually change body responses to illness. Consider the following examples of the emotional dimension:

- Before a test, a student always has diarrhea.
- Worried about her teenaged son, a mother chain smokes.
- An adolescent with poor self-esteem begins to experiment with drugs.
- Using relaxation techniques, a young woman reduces her pain after surgery.
- After learning biofeedback skills, a man reduces his previously elevated blood pressure.

Intellectual Dimension

The intellectual dimension encompasses cognitive abilities, educational background, and past experiences. These influence a patient's responses to teaching about health and the person's reactions to nursing care during illness. They also play a major role in health behaviors. Examples of situations involving this dimension include the following:

- An older woman who completed only the fifth grade and needs to be taught how to give herself injections
- A young college student with diabetes who follows a diabetic diet but continues to drink beer and eat pizza with friends several times a week
- A middle-aged man who quits taking his high blood pressure medication after developing unpleasant side effects

Environmental Dimension

The environment has many influences on health and illness. Housing, sanitation, climate, and pollution of air, food, and water are elements in the environmental dimension. Following are a selected few of many examples of environmental causes of illness:

- Deaths, especially among older adults, resulting from inadequate heating and cooling
- Increased incidence of asthma and respiratory problems in large cities with smog
- Increased incidence of skin cancer in people who live in hot, sunny areas of the world
- Food poisoning

Sociocultural Dimension

Health practices and beliefs are strongly influenced by a person's economic level, lifestyle, family, and culture. In general, low-income groups are less likely to seek medical care to prevent illness, and high-income groups are more prone to stress-related habits and illness. The family and the culture to which a person belongs influence the person's patterns of living and values about health and illness; such patterns are often unalterable. All of these factors are involved in personal care, patterns of eating, lifestyle habits, and emotional stability. Following are other examples of other sociocultural factors that influence health and illness:

- An adolescent who sees nothing wrong with smoking or drinking because his parents smoke and drink

- Parents of a sick infant who do not seek medical care because they have no health insurance
- A single parent, abused as a child, who in turn physically abuses her own small son
- A person of Asian descent who uses herbal remedies and acupuncture to treat an illness

Spiritual Dimension

Spiritual beliefs and values are important components of a person's health and illness behaviors. It is important that the nurse respect these values and understand their importance for the individual patient. Following are examples of the influences of the spiritual dimension:

- Roman Catholics require baptism for both live births and stillborn babies.
- Orthodox and Conservative Jews may observe kosher laws, prohibiting the intake of pork or shellfish.
- Jehovah's Witnesses are opposed to blood transfusions.

Basic Human Needs

As defined in Chapter 2, a *need* is something that is essential to the emotional and physiologic health and survival of humans. Basic human needs are essential and are common to all people. A person whose needs are met may be considered to be healthy, and a person with one or more unmet needs is at increased risk for illness.

Needs are an integral part of each person's human dimensions:

Physiologic needs (physical dimension) involve all of the body's physiologic processes, including breathing, the intake and output of food and fluids, temperature, circulation, and movement.

Safety and security needs (environmental dimension) are related to physical surroundings as they affect safety and security, including housing, the neighborhood, climate factors, and the atmosphere.

Love and belonging needs (sociocultural dimension) are related to a person's relationships and communications with family, friends, and others and a sense of belonging to a group or community and being loved by others.

Self-esteem needs (emotional dimension) involve the feelings of a person, such as fear, happiness, sadness, and loneliness, and feeling good about oneself.

Self-actualization needs (intellectual and spiritual dimension) focus on processes such as thinking, learning, problem solving, and decision making. They also encompass values and beliefs related to the experience of love, joy, peace, and fulfillment and performing activities to help others.

Self-Concept

Another variable influencing health and illness is a person's self-concept, which incorporates both how the person feels about self (*self-esteem*) and the way he or she perceives his or her physical self (*body image*). Self-concept has both physical and emotional aspects and is an important factor in the way the individual reacts to stress and illness, follows self-care health practices, and relates with others. For example, an adolescent who has anorexia nervosa and is dangerously thin may still perceive herself as being overweight and refuse to eat. In contrast, a person who is overweight may feel that nothing will change the way he or she looks and refuse to follow a diet and exercise program.

A person's self-concept results from a variety of past experiences, interpersonal interactions, physical and cultural influences, and education. It includes a person's perceptions of his or her own strengths and weaknesses. Illness can alter a person's self-concept as it affects roles, independence, and relationships with important others. Chapter 30 fully discusses self-concept.

Promoting Health and Preventing Illness

Nurses often care for patients entering the healthcare system because of an illness. Illness behaviors and the effects of illness on the family are discussed in this section, which also defines acute and chronic illness and the levels of healthcare activities carried out by nurses to promote health and prevent illness.

Risk Factors

A **risk factor** is something that increases a person's chance for illness or injury. The six general types of risk factors are described in Table 4-1. Risk factors for each developmental level across the life span are included in Unit II, and cultural influences on health are discussed in Chapter 3.

Like other components of health and illness, risk factors are often interrelated. As the number of risk factors increases, so does the possibility of disease. For example, an overweight executive, under pressure to increase sales, smokes and drinks alcohol in excess. These factors, combined with a family history of heart disease, place this person at higher risk for illness.

A health-risk appraisal is an assessment of the total person. The "picture" of the individual resulting from this assessment indicates areas of risk for disease or injury as well as areas that support health. A variety of formats are used to perform the assessment, but all of them take a broad approach to health, focusing on lifestyle and health behaviors. Such an appraisal appears in the box, Health-Style: A Self-Test, later in this chapter.

Following are examples of practices that are supportive of health:

- Sleeping regularly, 7 to 8 hours per night
- Eating breakfast
- Eating regular meals, which include recommended food groups
- Maintaining ideal body weight
- Using alcohol in moderation, if at all
- Not smoking
- Maintaining positive mental health and self-concept

Table 4-1
Major Areas of Risk Factors

Risk Factor	Examples
Age	School-aged children are at high risk for communicable diseases.
	After menopause, women are more likely to develop cardiovascular disease.
Genetic	A family history of cancer or diabetes predisposes a person to developing the disease.
Physiologic	Obesity increases the possibility of heart disease.
	Pregnancy places increased risk on both the mother and the developing fetus.
Health habits	Smoking increases the probability of lung cancer.
	Poor nutrition can lead to a variety of health problems.
Lifestyle	Multiple sexual relationships increase the risk for sexually transmitted diseases (eg, gonorrhea or acquired immunodeficiency syndrome).
	Events that increase stress (eg, divorce, retirement, work-related pressure) may precipitate accidents or illness.
Environment	Working and living environments (such as hazardous materials and poor sanitation) may contribute to disease.

Acute and Chronic Illness

Illnesses are classified as either acute or chronic. A person may have an acute illness, a chronic illness, or both at the same time; for example, an adult with diabetes (a chronic illness) may also have appendicitis (an acute illness).

Acute Illness

An **acute illness** generally has a rapid onset of symptoms and lasts only a relatively short time. Although some acute illnesses are life threatening, many do not require medical attention. If medical care is required, a specific treatment with medications (eg, antibiotics for pneumonia) or surgical procedures (eg, an appendectomy for appendicitis) usually returns the person to normal functioning. With self-treatment and use of over-the-counter medications, simple acute illnesses, such as the common cold or diarrhea, do not usually require medical treatment.

Illness Behaviors

When a person becomes acutely ill, certain illness behaviors, described by Suchman (1965), may occur in identifiable stages. These behaviors are the way people cope with alterations in function caused by the disease. Illness behaviors are unique to the individual and are influenced by age, gender, family values, economic status, culture, educational level, and mental status.

There is not a specific timetable for the stages of illness behaviors. The stages may occur rapidly or slowly. Nursing roles throughout the stages remain constant. In all stages, the nurse accepts the patient as an individual, gives nursing care based on prioritized needs, and facilitates recovery through physical care, emotional support, and health education (Fig. 4-4).

Stage 1: Experiencing Symptoms. How do people define themselves as "sick"? The first indication of an illness is usually the recognition of one or more symptoms that are incompatible with one's personal definition of health. Although pain is the most significant symptom indicating illness, other common symptoms include a rash, fever, bleeding, or a cough. If the symptoms last for a short time or are relieved by self-care, the person usually takes no further action. If the symptoms continue, however, the person enters the next stage.

Stage 2: Assuming the Sick Role. The person now defines himself or herself as being sick, seeks validation of this experience from others, gives up normal activities, and assumes a "sick role." At this stage, most people focus on their symptoms and bodily functions. Depending on his or her individual health beliefs and practices, the person may choose to do nothing, may buy over-the-counter medications to relieve symptoms, or may seek care from a healthcare provider for diagnosis and treatment. In our society,

an illness becomes legitimate when a healthcare provider diagnoses it and prescribes treatment. When help from the healthcare provider is sought, the person becomes a patient and enters the next stage.

Stage 3: Assuming a Dependent Role. This stage is characterized by the patient's decision to accept the diagnosis and follow the prescribed treatment plan. The person conforms to the opinions of others, often requires assistance in carrying out activities of daily living, and needs emotional support through acceptance, approval, physical closeness, and protection.

If the disease is serious (such as a heart attack or stroke), the patient may enter the hospital for treatment. If the symptoms can be managed by the patient or family alone or with the assistance of home care providers, however, the patient is cared for at home. To facilitate adherence to the treatment plan, the patient needs effective relationships with caregivers, knowledge about the illness, and an individualized plan of care. The patient's responses to care depend on a variety of factors, including the seriousness of the illness, the patient's degree of fear about the disease, the loss of roles, the support of others, and previous experiences with illness care. The patient is expected, by both caregivers and family, to get well and resume normal roles.

Stage 4: Achieving Recovery and Rehabilitation. Recovery and rehabilitation may begin in the hospital and conclude at home or may be totally concluded at a rehabilitation center or at home. Most patients complete this final stage of illness behavior at home. In this stage, the person gives up the dependent role and resumes normal activities and responsibilities. If the plan of care included health education, the individual may return to health at a higher level of functioning and health than before the illness.

Chronic Illness

Chronic illness is a broad term that encompasses many different physical and mental alterations in health, with one or more of the following characteristics:

- It is a permanent change.
- It causes, or is caused by, irreversible alterations in normal anatomy and physiology.
- It requires special patient education for rehabilitation.
- It requires a long period of care or support.

Chronic illnesses usually have a slow onset and commonly have periods of *remission* (when the disease is present, but the person does not experience symptoms) and *exacerbation* (the symptoms reappear). Examples of common chronic illnesses are heart problems, diabetes mellitus, lung diseases, and arthritis.

Chronic illnesses are the leading health problem in the world. Current trends resulting in an increase in chronic illnesses include increasing numbers of older adults, lifestyle choices (such as smoking and drug use), environmental factors (increasing air and water pollution), and the AIDS epidemic. Nursing care of more patients with chronic illnesses will be required in the future. Although not all people with a chronic illness require care, all people who are chronically

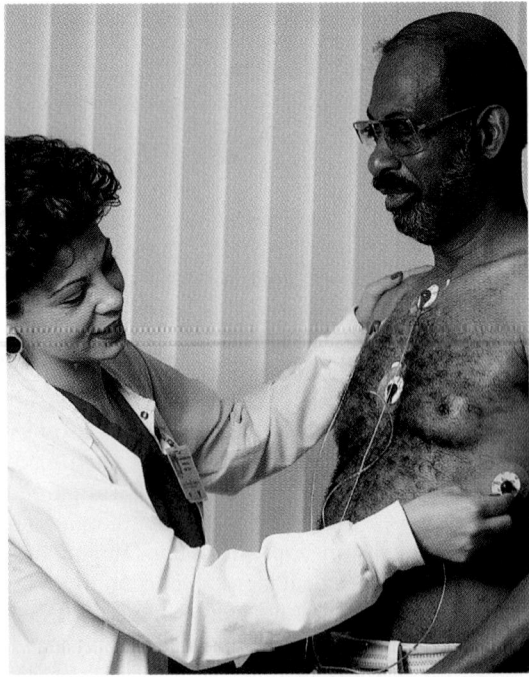

Figure 4-4
The nurse is assessing the patient as a basis for teaching healthy heart behaviors.

ill must accept certain aspects of life to be able to live with the illness on a day-to-day basis for the rest of their lives:

- Living as normally as possible, despite symptoms and treatments that make an individual feel different from others
- Learning to modify activities of daily living, relationships, and self-care activities
- Maintaining a positive self-concept and sense of hope
- Grieving over losses or changes in physical structure and function, financial income, status, role, and dignity
- Learning how to live with chronic discomfort
- Following prescribed medical therapies
- Maintaining a feeling of being in control
- Confronting the inevitability of death (Miller, 1983; Pollock, 1986)

As a nurse, you will care for individuals of all ages with chronic illnesses, and you will provide that care in all types of settings, including homes, hospitals, clinics, nursing homes, and institutions. Regardless of the age of the patient or the effects and demands of the illness or the setting, the nurse must make every effort to promote health for patients with chronic illness, with a focus of care that emphasizes what is possible rather than what can no longer be.

Effects of Illness on the Family

Most nursing care is given to patients with some form of support system, usually the family. When an illness occurs, roles change for both the patient and the family. The following are examples of family reactions to, and influences on, illness of a member.

- A chronic illness creates stress for the patient and family because it may require lifelong alterations in roles or lifestyle, frequent hospitalizations, economic problems, and decreased social interactions among members.
- Parents of a sick child often react with blame, overprotection, and severe anxiety.
- Family members of patients requiring intensive care often feel alone and frightened. They may also feel guilty and imagine the worst possible outcome.
- The reactions of family members to an illness often vary; some want to be with the patient all the time, whereas others avoid visiting.
- Family members need information about the patient's care and health status. They often rely on the nurse for answers, for emotional support, and for feeling that they are a part of the caregiving.

Nursing Care as Preventive Care

The current emphasis on health is important to nursing. In addition to providing direct care, nurses include health promotion interventions through all stages of the nursing process, as described in later chapters in this book.

Levels of Preventive Care

The current focus of healthcare is on preventive care. Leavell and Clark (1965) described the three levels of preventive care as primary, secondary, and tertiary.

Primary preventive care is directed toward health promotion and specific protections against illness. Activities at this level may focus on individuals or groups. Examples of primary-level activities are immunizations, family planning services, teaching breast self-examination, poison-control information, and accident prevention education.

Secondary preventive care focuses on early detection of disease, prompt intervention, and health maintenance for patients experiencing health problems. Examples of activities at this level are carrying out direct nursing actions (eg, providing wound care, giving medications, or exercising arms and legs); assessing children for normal growth and development; and encouraging regular medical and dental screenings and care.

Tertiary preventive care begins after an illness is diagnosed and treated and is aimed at helping rehabilitate patients and restore them to a maximum level of functioning. Nursing activities on a tertiary level include teaching a patient with diabetes how to recognize and prevent complications and referring a woman to a support group after removal of a breast because of cancer.

Nurses as Role Models for Health

Nurses must take care of their own health to be able to give effective nursing care to others. Good personal health not only enables nurses to practice more efficiently but also enables them to serve as role models for patients and families. Nurses can help patients acquire new health behaviors by modeling the very behaviors that are important to the patients' well-being.

It is difficult for nurses to be sincerely attentive to the needs of patients when their own needs are not being met. Because no one is perfectly healthy all of the time, it is important for nurses, as they prepare for professional practice, to spend time getting to know themselves. From this self-knowledge should come a commitment to pursue holistic health actively. To help you increase your self-knowledge, complete the health-style self-test in the accompanying box. As you work with patients to provide care, you can also use this self-test to help your patients learn a new health-style.

In Units VII and VIII of this text, healthcare goals for the nurse are included under the title "Applying Learning to Practice." The health promotion guides highlighted throughout the text may be useful to you as well as to your patients. Use these guides to assess and identify both strengths and risks for alterations in health. The guides can also serve as a basis for teaching self-care to patients.

Health-Style: A Self-Test

All of us want good health, but many of us do not know how to be as healthy as possible. Health experts now describe *lifestyle* as one of the most important factors affecting health. In fact, it is estimated that as many as 7 of the 10 leading causes of death could be reduced through common-sense changes in lifestyle. That's what this brief test, developed by the Public Health Service, is all about. Its purpose is simply to tell you how well you are doing to stay healthy. The behaviors covered in the test are recommended for most Americans. Some of them may not apply to people with certain chronic diseases or disabilities, or to pregnant women. Such people may require special instructions from their physicians.

Cigarette Smoking

If you <u>never smoke</u>, enter a score of 10 for this section and go the next section on *Alcohol and Drugs*.

	almost always	sometimes	almost never
1. I avoid smoking cigarettes.	2	1	0
2. I smoke only low tar and nicotine cigarettes *or* I smoke a pipe or cigars.	2	1	0

Smoking score: _____

Alcohol and Drugs

	almost always	sometimes	almost never
1. I avoid drinking alcoholic beverages *or* I drink no more than one or two drinks a day.	4	1	0
2. I avoid using alcohol or other drugs (especially illegal drugs) as a way of handling stressful situations or the problems in my life.	2	1	0
3. I am careful not to drink alcohol when taking certain medicines (eg, medicine for sleeping, pain, colds, and allergies), or when pregnant.	2	1	0
4. I read and follow the label directions when using prescribed and over-the-counter drugs.	2	1	0

Alcohol and drugs score: _____

Eating Habits

	almost always	sometimes	almost never
1. I eat a variety of foods each day, such as fruits and vegetables, whole-grain breads and cereals, lean meats, dairy products, dry peas and beans, and nuts and seeds.	4	1	0
2. I limit the amount of fat, saturated fat, and cholesterol I eat (including fat on meats, eggs, butter, cream, shortenings, and organ meats such as liver).	2	1	0
3. I limit the amount of salt I eat by cooking with only small amounts, not adding salt at the table, and avoiding salty snacks.	2	1	0
4. I avoid eating too much sugar (especially frequent snacks of sticky candy or soft drinks).	2	1	0

Eating habits score: _____

Exercise and Fitness

	almost always	sometimes	almost never
1. I maintain a desired weight, avoiding overweight and underweight.	3	1	0
2. I do vigorous exercises for 15 to 30 minutes at least three times a week (examples include running, swimming, brisk walking).	3	1	0
3. I do exercises that enhance my muscle tone for 15 to 30 minutes at least three times a week (examples include yoga and calisthenics).	2	1	0
4. I use part of my leisure time participating in individual, family, or team activities that increase my level of fitness (such as gardening, bowling, golf, and baseball).	2	1	0

Exercise/fitness score: _____

Stress Control

	almost always	sometimes	almost never
1. I have a job or do other work that I enjoy.	2	1	0
2. I find it easy to relax and express my feelings freely.	2	1	0
3. I recognize early, and prepare for, events or situations likely to be stressful for me.	2	1	0
4. I have close friends, relatives, or others whom I can talk to about personal matters and call on for help when needed.	2	1	0
5. I participate in group activities (such as church and community organizations) or hobbies that I enjoy.	2	1	0

Stress control score: _____

Safety

	almost always	sometimes	almost never
1. I wear a seat belt while riding in a car.	2	1	0
2. I avoid driving while under the influence of alcohol and other drugs.	2	1	0
3. I obey traffic rules and the speed limit when driving.	2	1	0
4. I am careful when using potentially harmful products or substances (such as household cleaners, poisons, and electrical devices).	2	1	0
5. I avoid smoking in bed.	2	1	0

Safety score: _____

(continued)

Health-Style: A Self-Test *(Continued)*

What Your Scores Mean to You

Scores of 9 and 10
Excellent! Your answers show that you are aware of the importance of this area to your health. More important, you are putting your knowledge to work for you by practicing good health habits. As long as you continue to do so, this area should not pose a serious health risk. It's likely that you are setting an example for your family and friends to follow. Because you got a very high test score on this part of the test, you may want to consider other areas where your scores indicate room for improvement.

Scores of 6 to 8
Your health practices in this area are good, but there is room for improvement. Look again at the items you answered with "Sometimes" or "Almost never." What changes can you make to improve your score? Even a small change can often help you achieve better health.

Scores of 3 to 5
Your health risks are showing! Would you like more information about the risks you are facing and about why it is important for you to change these behaviors? Perhaps you need help in deciding how to make the changes you desire. In either case, help is available.

Scores of 0 to 2
Obviously, you were concerned enough about your health to take the test, but your answers show that you may be taking serious and unnecessary risks with your health. Perhaps you are unaware of the risks and what to do about them. You can easily get the information and help you need to improve, if you wish. The next step is up to you.

Where Do You Go from Here

Start by asking yourself a few frank questions: *Am I really doing all I can to be as healthy as possible? What steps can I take to feel better? Am I willing to begin now?* If you scored low in one or more sections of the test, decide what changes you want to make for improvement. You might pick that aspect of your lifestyle where you feel you have the best chance for success and tackle that one first. Once you have improved your score there, go on to other areas.

If you already have tried to change your health habits (to stop smoking or exercise regularly, for example), don't be discouraged if you haven't yet succeeded. The difficulty you have encountered may be due to influences you've never really thought about—such as advertising—or to a lack of support and encouragement. Understanding these influences is an important step toward changing the way they affect you.

There's help available. In addition to personal actions you can take on your own, there are community programs and groups (such as the YMCA or the local chapter of the American Heart Association) that can assist you and your family to make the changes you want to make. If you want to know more about these groups or about health risks, contact your local health department or the National Health Information Clearinghouse. There's a lot you can do to stay healthy or to improve your health—and there are organizations that can help you. Start a new "health-style" today!

For assistance in locating specific information on these and other health topics, write to the National Health Information Clearinghouse:

National Health Information Clearinghouse
  P.O. Box 1133
  Washington, DC 20013

(Reprinted with permission of the National Health Information Clearinghouse.)

Learning Outcomes

After completing this chapter, the learner should be able to accomplish the following:

1. Define key terms used in the chapter.

acute illness	high-level wellness
agent–host–environment model	illness
	primary preventive care
chronic illness	risk factor
disease	secondary preventive care
health belief model	
health–illness continuum	tertiary preventive care
health promotion model	

2. Describe health and illness.
3. Identify the factors influencing health and illness, including the physical, sociocultural, intellectual, emotional, environmental, and spiritual dimensions; basic human needs; and self-concept.
4. Compare and contrast acute illness and chronic illness.
5. Summarize the role of the nurse in promoting health based on knowledge of risk factors for illness, illness behaviors, and the effects of illness on the family.
6. Describe the levels of preventive care.

Critical Thinking Exercises

1. List the six human dimensions described in this chapter, and identify your personal strengths and weaknesses in each area. For example, you may have inherited a genetic tendency toward overweight (a weakness) but have controlled your weight through nutrition and exercise (a strength). After considering your strengths and weaknesses, develop a personal plan for health promotion.

2. Identify a family in which someone has a chronic illness. Interview as many of the other family members as possible, and discuss the effect of the illness on them. What do you observe about the effects of the illness in relation to the patient's age, type of illness (eg, AIDS versus cancer), gender, and family role?

Bibliography

Bates, M., Rankin-Hill, L., & Sanchez Ayendez, M. (1997). The effects of the cultural context of health care on treatment of and response to chronic pain and illness. *Social Sciences & Medicine, 45*(9), 1433–1447.

Beckingham, C. (1995). Relinquishing the sick role: Convalescence and rehabilitation. *Australian Journal of Advance Nursing, 12*(3), 15–19.

Braden, C. (1990). A test of the self-help model: Learned response to chronic illness experience. *Nursing Research, 39*(1), 42–47.

Clemen-Stone, S., McGuire, S., & Eigsti, D. (1998). *Comprehensive community health nursing: Family, aggregate & community practice.* (5th ed.). St. Louis: Mosby.

Davidhizar, R., & Shearer, R. (1997). Helping the client with chronic disability achieve high-level wellness. *Rehabilitation Nursing, 22*(3), 131–134.

Dunn, H. (1961). *High level wellness.* Arlington, VA: Beathy.

Edelman, C., & Mandle, C. (1994). *Health promotion throughout the life span* (3rd ed.). St. Louis: Mosby.

Gallo, A., & Knafl, K. (1998). Parents' reports of "tricks of the trade" for managing childhood chronic illness. *Journal of the Society of Pediatric Nurses, 3*(3), 93–102.

Guzzettta, C. E. (1998). Reflections: Healing and wholeness in chronic illness. *Journal of Holistic Nursing, 16*(2), 197–201.

Hymovich, D., & Hagopian, G. (1992). *Chronic illness in children and adults: A psychosocial approach.* Philadelphia: W. B. Saunders.

Jensen, L., & Allen, M. (1993). Wellness: The dialectic of illness. *IMAGE—The Journal of Nursing Scholarship, 25*(3), 220–223.

Leavell, H., & Clark, E. G. (1965). *Preventive medicine for the doctor in the community* (3rd ed.). New York: McGraw Hill.

Maslow, A. (1968). *Toward a psychology of being* (2nd ed.). New York: Van Nostrand Reinhold.

Miller, J. F. (1983). *Coping with chronic illness: Overcoming powerlessness.* Philadelphia: F. A. Davis.

Murray, R. B., & Zentner, J. P. (1993). *Nursing assessment and health promotion through the lifespan* (5th ed.). Norwalk, CT: Appleton & Lange.

O'Neill, D., & Kenny, E. (1998). State of the science: Spirituality and chronic illness. *Image—The Journal of Nursing Scholarship, 30*(3), 275–280.

Pender, N.J. (1996). *Health promotion in nursing practice.* (3rd ed.). Stamford, CT: Appleton & Lange.

Pollock, S. E. (1986). Human responses to chronic illness: Physiologic and psychosocial adaptation. *Nursing Research, 35*(2), 90–95.

Robert Wood Johnson Foundation Annual Report. (1993). *Chronic health conditions.* Princeton, NJ: The Robert Wood Johnson Foundation.

Rosenstock, I. (1974). Historical origin of the health belief model. *Health Education Monographs, 2,* 334.

Suchman, E. (1965). Stages of illness and medical care. *Journal of Health and Human Behavior, 6,* 114.

Travis, J., & Ryan, R. (1988). *Wellness workbook* (2nd ed.). Berkeley, CA: Ten Speed Press.

World Health Organization. (1947). *Constitution.* Geneva: WHO.

Chapter 5
Theoretical Base for Nursing Practice

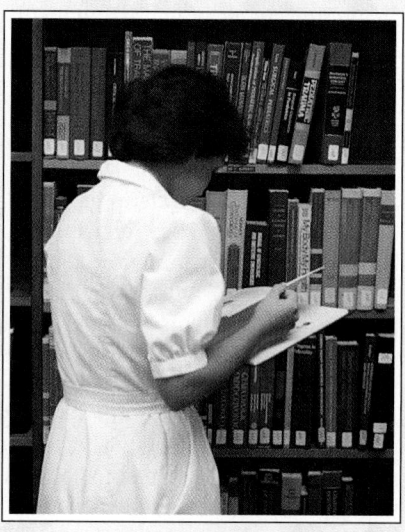

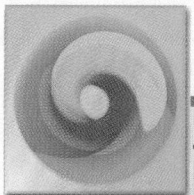

**Thinking Critically About
Nursing's Blended Skills**

Before reading this chapter, think about the types of skills you will need to practice nursing with a firm theoretical base.

- You are invited to help design an assessment tool for families caring at home for family members who are terminally ill.

- A group of nurses on your adolescent unit get together to develop care maps (plans) for some of the types of conditions that area teenagers present with often and that are most difficult for the nurses to treat (eg, eating disorders, trauma, alcohol- and substance-abuse–related problems, failed suicide attempts).

- You are the nurse member on an interdisciplinary team meeting to develop a research protocol to identify interventions to reduce the incidence of very-low-birthweight premature infants.

- The nursing home where you are employed is undergoing a $3 million renovation, and everyone's input is being solicited to ensure that the new design will facilitate healthy living for the home's aging residents and be responsive to developmental needs.

What cognitive, technical, interpersonal, and ethical/legal skills do you think you will need to meet effectively the health needs of the individuals described above?

Nursing is a unique healthcare discipline in which nurses provide others with a service based on their knowledge and skill. Nursing thus has two essential aspects: a body of knowledge and the application of that knowledge through nursing practice. This body of knowledge, called a *knowledge base*, provides the rationale for nursing actions. As you learn and practice nursing, you will come to understand rationales from many different areas, such as anatomy, physiology, chemistry, nutrition, psychology, and sociology. You will also use the knowledge base developed specifically for nursing, helping you know what nursing care is and why and how it is given. This chapter discusses how nursing theory has been developed and how it is used to give knowledgeable nursing care.

Introduction to Theory

Every individual collects, organizes, and arranges facts to build a knowledge base relevant to his or her personal reality. A similar organization and a structure of facts and events are present in large bodies of knowledge, through philosophies, concepts, theories, and processes.

Philosophy is the study of wisdom, fundamental knowledge, and the processes we use to develop and construct our perceptions of life. Philosophy provides a viewpoint and implies a system of values and beliefs. Each individual develops a personal philosophy to give meaning to experiences and to guide behavior and attitudes. We develop personal philosophies by learning from interpersonal relationships, through formal and informal educational experiences, through religion and culture, and from the environment.

Every nurse's philosophy, developed through education and practice, forms the basis for giving nursing care. Nurses have both a personal and a professional philosophy through their values and beliefs about concepts such as

goodness, health, illness, accountability, and ethics. In the same way, nursing education and nursing practice settings provide education or patient care based on philosophic beliefs about humans, health, teaching and learning, and quality patient care.

Concepts, like ideas, are abstract impressions organized into symbols of reality. Concepts describe objects, properties, and events and relationships among them. A group of concepts that follows an understandable pattern makes up a **conceptual framework or model.** Concepts can be thought of as the individual bricks and boards used to build a house, with the conceptual framework being the blueprint that specifies where each brick and board should go.

A **theory** is a group of concepts that describe a pattern of reality. A theory is a statement that explains or characterizes a process, an occurrence, or an event and is based on observed facts, but a theory cannot be proved directly or absolutely as can a fact. Theories arrange a group of related statements or concepts so that they give meaning to a series of events. Theories can be tested, changed, or used to guide research or to provide a base for evaluation. They are derived through two principal methods: (1) **deductive reasoning,** in which one examines a general idea and then considers specific actions or ideas, and (2) **inductive reasoning**, in which the reverse process is used—one builds from specific ideas or actions to conclusions about general ideas. Nursing theorists use both of these methods.

A **process** is a series of actions, changes, or functions intended to bring about a desired result. During a process, one takes systematic and continuous steps to meet a goal and uses both assessments and feedback to direct actions to meet the goal. A particular theory or conceptual framework directs how these actions are carried out. The delivery of nursing care within the nursing process (described in Unit IV) is directed by the way specific conceptual frameworks and theories define the person (patient), the environment, health, and nursing.

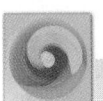

COGNITIVE SKILLS

- Knowledge of nursing models and theories
- Knowledge of how nursing models and theories dictate assessment, planning, and research design

TECHNICAL SKILLS

- Ability to access computerized literature searches to facilitate selection of appropriate nursing models and theories to direct your work

INTERPERSONAL SKILLS

- Ability to work collaboratively with nursing colleagues and the interdisciplinary team from the perspective of nursing's theoretical base. The aim

is to help others understand nursing's unique perspective and voice as healthcare is planned, implemented, and evaluated.

ETHICAL/LEGAL SKILLS

- Ability to be trusted to bring the best that nursing has to offer to the research, design, implementation, and evaluation of healthcare for different population groups.
- Knowledge of the nurse's legal responsibilities when researching, designing, implementing, and evaluating healthcare.

⑤ Basic Processes in the Development of Nursing Theories

Nursing theory, as defined by Barnum (1998), "attempts to describe or explain the phenomenon (process, occurrence, or event) called nursing." Nursing theory differentiates nursing from other disciplines and activities in that it serves the purposes of describing, explaining, predicting, and controlling desired outcomes of nursing care practices.

Nursing theories are often based on and influenced by other broadly applicable processes and theories. The ideas and principles of the theories described briefly in the following sections are basic to many nursing concepts and are a part of the nursing literature. Nurses need to understand these theories and terminologies as they develop their own knowledge base in nursing.

General Theories

General Systems Theory

General systems theory has been used in a wide range of disciplines since it emerged in the 1920s. Its primary theorist, Ludwig von Bertalanffy, developed the theory for universal application. This theory describes how to break whole things into parts and then to learn how the parts work together in "systems." It emphasizes relationships between the whole and the parts and describes how parts function and behave. These concepts may be applied to different kinds of systems, for example, to molecules in chemistry, cultures in sociology, organs in anatomy, and health in nursing.

Key points in general systems theory are as follows:

- A system is a set of interacting elements, all contributing to the overall goal of the system; the whole system is always greater than the sum of its parts.
- Systems are hierarchical in nature and are composed of interrelated subsystems that work together in such a way that a change in one element could affect other subsystems as well as the whole.
- Boundaries separate systems both from each other and from their environments.
- A system communicates with and reacts to its environment through factors that enter the system (input) or are transferred to the environment (output).
- An open system allows energy, matter, and information to move freely between systems and boundaries, whereas a closed system does not allow input from or output to the environment (no totally closed systems are known to exist in reality).
- To survive, open systems maintain balance through feedback.

Adaptation Theory

Adaptation theory defines **adaptation** as the adjustment of living matter to other living things and to environmental conditions. Adaptation is a continuously occurring process that effects change and involves interaction and response. Human adaptation occurs on three levels: the internal (self), the social (others), and the physical (biochemical reactions). Chapter 31 describes adaptation in relation to stress.

Developmental Theory

Developmental theory outlines the process of growth and development of humans as orderly and predictable, beginning with conception and ending with death. Although the pattern has definite stages, the progress and behaviors of an individual within each stage are unique. The growth and development of an individual are influenced by heredity, temperament, emotional and physical environment, life experiences, and health status.

Several theorists have made important contributions to developmental theory, but only two are mentioned here because their work is often used to develop nursing theory and to organize nursing practice. Eric Erikson based his theory of psychosocial development on the process of socialization, emphasizing how individuals learn to interact with the world. Erikson recognized the role of social, biologic, and environmental factors in development and defined specific tasks or conflicts that people accomplish or overcome during what he defined as the eight stages of life. Chapter 8 presents more information on developmental theory.

Abraham Maslow developed his theory of human needs in terms of physical and psychosocial needs considered essential to human life, rather than by chronologic age as Erikson did. As described in Chapter 2, Maslow defined five levels of need in a hierarchy, with different needs existing simultaneously.

As you continue in your nursing education and practice, you will learn how systems, adaptation, and developmental theories are used in planning and giving holistic care to patients. The following sections on specific nursing theories will help you better understand the knowledge base used to develop the concepts unique to nursing.

⑤ Nursing Theory

Nursing theory is valuable in research, education, and practice. Nursing theories identify and define interrelated concepts important in nursing and clearly state the relationships between and among these concepts. Nursing theories describe relationships that are developed logically and consistently with their basic assumptions. Nursing theories should be simple and general; simple terminology and broadly applicable concepts ensure their usefulness in a wide variety of nursing practice situations. Nursing theories should also increase the nursing profession's body of knowledge by generating research to guide and improve practice. Overall, nursing theory guides nurses by providing a knowledge base, organizing concepts, providing guidelines for practice, and identifying nursing care goals.

Common Concepts in Nursing Theories

Four concepts common in nursing theory that influence and determine nursing practice are (1) the person (patient), (2) the environment, (3) health, and (4) nursing.

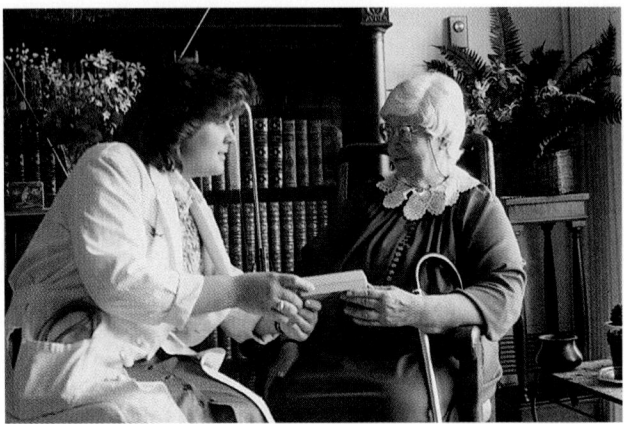

Figure 5-1
Four concepts common to all nursing theories are person, environment, health, and nursing. The most important concept, and the focus of nursing, is the person. (Photo by Gates Rhodes, courtesy of School of Nursing, University of Pennsylvania.)

Each of these concepts is usually defined and described by a nursing theorist, often uniquely; and although these concepts are common to all nursing theories, both the definitions and the relations among them may differ from one theory to another. Of the four concepts, the most important is that of the person. The focus of nursing, regardless of definition or theory, is the person (Fig. 5-1).

Nursing Theory and Nursing Practice

Historical Perspectives and Influences

Nightingale's Definition and Belief
Florence Nightingale, the nurse who established the theoretical base for nursing, developed and published a philosophy and a theory of health and nursing that has served as a solid foundation for the nursing profession (Fig. 5-2). Her contributions to nursing theory include identifying the role of the nurse in meeting the patient's personal needs, recognizing the importance of environmental influences on the care of sick people, and elevating the standards and acceptance of nursing by developing sound principles of nursing education. Nightingale also influenced nursing knowledge and practice by demonstrating efficient and knowledgeable nursing care, defining nursing practice as separate and distinct from medical practice, and differentiating between health nursing and illness nursing (Dolan, Fitzpatrick, & Herrmann, 1983).

Cultural Influences on Nursing
Certain cultural influences have affected nursing as we currently know it. Although both men and women have given comfort and assistance to sick people through history, nursing essentially was considered "women's work" until the 1970s. In the 18th and 19th centuries, in many societies, women were viewed as subservient and inferior to men. After Nightingale established an acceptable occupation for educated women and improved society's attitudes

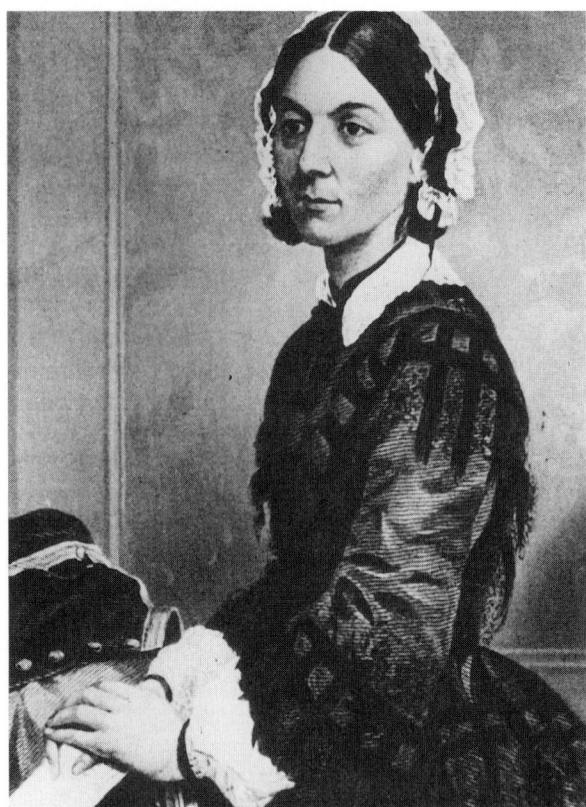

Figure 5-2
Florence Nightingale developed and published a philosophy and theory of health and nursing that has served as a solid foundation for the nursing profession. (Photo courtesy of the Center for the Study of the History of Nursing, University of Pennsylvania.)

toward nursing, the role of women as nurses became more favorably accepted.

Despite Nightingale's belief in the uniqueness of nursing, the training of nurses was initially carried out under the direction and control of the medical profession (Kalish & Kalish, 1995). Because the conceptual and theoretical basis for nursing practice came from outside the profession, nursing struggled for years to establish its own identity and to receive recognition for its significant contributions to healthcare.

Educational Influences on Nursing
Most schools of nursing established in the United States were adapted from Nightingale's model. There was no planned educational curriculum; instead, learning came from lectures by physicians and by practical experience acquired through caring for sick people in the hospital (Dolan et al., 1983). This service orientation for nursing education remained the strongest influence on nursing practice until the 1950s. Rather than developing a body of knowledge specific to nursing, nursing care was carried out under the control and direction of the hospital administration and physicians practicing in that hospital. Nursing care was based on traditional ideas about following orders as well as on common wisdom about caring for others based on either "common sense" or widely accepted scientific principles

(Chinn & Kramer, 1998). As a result, nursing knowledge remained undeveloped and fragmented.

Development of a Scientific Base for Nursing

During the first half of the 20th century, a change in the structure of society resulted in changed roles for women and, in turn, for nursing. As a result of World Wars I and II, women increasingly entered the workforce, became more independent, and sought higher education. At the same time, nursing education began to focus on true education instead of on training, and nursing research was conducted and published. As women became more assertive, nursing's need for a clearly defined identity based on unique contributions to the healthcare system emerged. In the 1950s, the idea of nursing as a science became more generally accepted, and philosophic beliefs and a knowledge base for nursing practice began to evolve.

Evolution of Nursing Theory

Research and Publishing in Nursing

Beginning in the 1950s, as great advances were made in technology and medical research, nursing leaders realized that research about the practice of nursing was necessary to meet the health needs of modern society. Increasing numbers of nurses began to conduct research and write articles telling other nurses how to conduct nursing research. Two major developments in nursing theory occurred in the 1950s: (1) the first research journal, *Nursing Research,* was published in 1950 (and continues today), and (2) as ideas were published, they served as a basis for theory development (Chinn & Kramer, 1998; Kalish & Kalish, 1995).

Educational Advances in Nursing

Beginning in the 1960s, baccalaureate programs in nursing began to increase in both number and enrollment. At the same time, master's and doctoral programs in nursing were established. This upward trend in education for nurses was reflected in the nursing literature, with more attention given to identifying knowledge specific to nursing.

Value of Nursing Theory

Even though nurses have difficulty agreeing on precise definitions of nursing, theory-based nursing directs nurses toward a common goal, with the ultimate outcome being improved patient care. Nursing theory provides rational and knowledgeable reasons for nursing actions, based on organized, written descriptions of what nursing is and what nurses do. Additionally, nursing theory gives nurses the knowledge base necessary for acting and responding appropriately in nursing care situations, provides a base for discussion, and, ideally, helps resolve current nursing issues. Furthermore, nursing theory gives nurses who know and practice theory better problem-solving skills, so that nursing actions are better organized, considered, and purposeful. Nursing theory also prepares nurses to question assumptions and values in nursing, thus further defining nursing and increasing the knowledge base.

Nursing is based on communication with others—patients, other healthcare team members, community members—as well as with nurses practicing in a variety of specialty settings. Because concepts are both abstract and highly individualized, verbal communication with others might be interpreted in different ways. As ideas are developed in nursing theory and terms precisely defined, nurses build a knowledge base and a common terminology to use in communicating with other professionals.

The term *autonomy* means independence and self-governance. As a discipline, nursing is defining its own independent functions and contributions to healthcare. The development and use of nursing theory provide autonomy in the practice of nursing in these ways:

* Having a body of knowledge specific to the discipline allows members to be viewed by others as experts; this, in turn, gives nurses authority to carry out actions.
* Actions carried out and based on sound rationales are trusted and respected.
* Nursing theory makes nursing care visible, leading to increased internal control by nurses.
* As nurses demonstrate that nursing care does indeed make a difference and that nursing services are valuable, the discipline becomes more independent.

Theoretical Frameworks for Nursing

The theories and conceptual models described in the following sections are included here because they represent different approaches to defining the reality of nursing and because they are used in a variety of educational, research, and practice settings. They are arranged alphabetically merely as a means of organization. For each theory or model, the central theme is summarized along with its basic assumptions, definitions, and applications in nursing. The terminology used in summarizing each theory or model is consistent with that used by the theorist. Table 5-1 presents the highlights of these theories. Students who find a particular framework relevant and useful are encouraged to explore the literature to learn more about the theory or model and the theorist.

Virginia Henderson: Definition of Nursing

Virginia Henderson (1966) first published her definition of nursing in 1955. She called it a definition of nursing rather than a theory because it was published before the development of concepts and theories about nursing. The purpose of her work was to identify the theoretical base for nursing practice, based on basic human needs, biophysiology, culture, and interaction-communication. Nursing is defined in functional terms, as follows:

> The unique function of the nurse is to assist the individual, sick or well, in the performance of those activities contributing to health or its recovery (or to a peaceful death that he would perform unaided if he had the necessary strength, will, or knowledge. And to do this

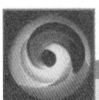

Table 5-1
Key Points of Selected Nursing Theories

Theorist	Central Theme	Emphasis of Nursing
Virginia Henderson	Definition of nursing	To assist the patient to acquire or maintain independence
Dorothy E. Johnson	Caring for the whole patient to facilitate behaviors necessary to prevent illness	Focus is on patient behaviors, assisting the patient to regain balance and health.
Imogene M. King	Individuals actively interact with others and with the environment and are changed by these experiences.	Assist the patient to identify problems and establish and achieve goals.
Madeline Leininger	Nursing is a transcultural care profession; care is the central area of concern.	Using culturally based nursing actions in culture care preservation, accommodation, and reconstruction
Myra E. Levine	The essence of nursing is human interaction	The foundation of all nursing interventions is conservation principles that maintain or restore health.
Betty Neuman	The patient's reaction to stressors in the environment	Nursing interventions can be carried out on three levels of prevention.
Dorothea E. Orem	The need for self-care to maintain life, health, and well-being	A person needs nursing when a health-related self-care deficit exists.
Hildegard E. Peplau	The nurse–patient relationship	Using a therapeutic relationship and communications to solve problems
Martha E. Rogers	Humans are the center of nursing's purpose.	To develop a science of nursing
Calista Roy	A decrease in body integrity creates a need state, followed by an act or behavior.	All nursing activity is aimed at promoting adaptation to health and illness.
Jean Watson	Caring is a human-to-human process demonstrated through therapeutic interpersonal interactions.	Caring is the mechanism by which nurses help individuals and groups reach self-actualization, maintain or attain health, or die a peaceful death.

in such a way as to help him gain independence as rapidly as possible (p.15).

The 14 components of basic nursing care encompass physiological needs (breathing, eating and drinking, eliminating, moving, sleeping and resting, selecting clothes, maintaining body temperature, keeping clean, and avoiding environmental dangers), communication and learning needs, spiritual and moral needs, and sociologic needs (working, playing). These components serve as a guide for the nurse and patient in meeting chosen goals. Henderson equated health with the individual's ability to meet these needs independently.

Henderson believed the nurse should have the knowledge to practice individualized and humane care and should be a scientific problem solver.

Dorothy E. Johnson: Behavioral Systems Model

Dorothy Johnson (1980) believes that nursing care should be directed toward caring for the patient before, during, and after an illness to facilitate effective behavioral functioning. Her behavioral systems model integrates systems,

developmental, and needs theories with a specific nursing focus. Johnson believes the four goals of nursing are to assist the person:

- Whose behavior is commensurate with social demands
- Who is able to modify his or her behavior in ways that support biologic imperatives
- Who is able to benefit, to the fullest extent during illness, from the physician's knowledge and skill
- Whose behavior does not give evidence of unnecessary trauma as a result of illness

Johnson views nursing as being separate from medicine in that medicine focuses on pathologic changes in the ill person, whereas nursing focuses on the behaviors of the person. The nursing role is complementary to the medical role. Nurses, giving care, supply functional requirements to the patient through protection, nurture, and stimulation. She views humans as individuals who act in ways that make up an individualized behavioral system. Within this behavioral system are seven interrelated subsystems. Changes in one subsystem affect all the others. The seven subsystems are as follows:

Attachment or "affiliative." This is the first behavioral subsystem to develop, initially allowing the infant to attach (bond) to a significant caregiver and continuing through life with other individuals. These attachments provide a sense of security.

Dependency. The behaviors in this subsystem precipitate nurturing by others and result in approval, attention, and physical assistance.

Ingestive. Behaviors involving the intake of food belong in this subsystem, including social and cultural factors.

Eliminative. The behaviors in this subsystem relate to the excretion of waste products from the body as well as to physical control and social situations.

Sexual. The behaviors in this subsystem are cultural and gender behaviors related to procreation and gratification.

Aggressive. In this subsystem, behaviors are concerned with protection and self-preservation.

Achievement. Behaviors that attempt to control the environment—including intellectual, physical, creative, mechanical, and social skills—belong in this subsystem.

Johnson believes that both the internal and external environments of the overall behavioral system need to be orderly and predictable to maintain balance. If subsystems are out of balance, "tension" and disequilibrium result. Nursing, as part of the external environment, can help the patient return to a state of balance.

Imogene M. King: Theory of Goal Attainment

Imogene King (1981) developed both a conceptual framework (open system) and a theory of goal attainment derived from the framework. Some assumptions basic to this framework are as follows:

- The focus of nursing is the care of humans.
- The nursing goal is the health of individuals and healthcare for groups.
- Humans are in constant interaction with their environment.

Within the framework are three interacting systems, each of which is defined and includes relevant concepts:

Personal systems. Each individual is a personal system. The concepts related to personal systems are perception, self, growth and development, body image, space, and time.

Interpersonal systems. Interpersonal systems are formed as humans interact. The concepts are interaction, communication, transaction, role, and stress.

Social systems. Social systems include families, religious groups, educational systems, work systems, and peer groups. The concepts are organization, authority, power, status, and decision making.

King developed her conceptual framework based on the belief that individuals actively interact with others and objects in the environment and are changed as a result of such experiences. King describes her theory as the interpersonal system in which two people come together in a healthcare organization to help or be helped to maintain a state of health that permits functioning in roles. A nurse (with special knowledge and skills) and a patient (with self-knowledge and personal problems) interact to identify problems and to establish and achieve goals. Based on this theory, King offers several propositions, including the following:

- If perceptual accuracy is present in nurse–patient interactions, transactions will occur.
- If nurses and patients make transactions, goals are attained.
- If goals are attained, effective nursing care will occur.
- If nurses with special knowledge and skills communicate appropriate information to patients, mutual goal setting and goal attainment will occur.

Madeline Leininger: Cultural Care Theory

Madeline Leininger's (1978) theory of nursing is based on the belief that nursing is a transcultural care profession, with care being the central area of concern for nursing. Nursing is believed to be an art and a science that provides culture-specific care to individuals and groups to promote or maintain health behaviors or recovery from illness. Within the model are the following three types of culturally based nursing actions:

Cultural care preservation (maintenance): those culturally based actions that help the individual preserve or maintain favorable health and caring lifeways

Cultural care accommodation (negotiations): those culturally based actions that reflect ways to adapt, negotiate, or adjust to the health and caring lifeways of others

Cultural care repatterning (reconstruction): those reconstructed or altered actions designed to help patients change meaningful health or life patterns

The model is based on a substantial number of propositions and assumptions, including the following:

- Culture is the blueprint for thought and action and is the dominant force in determining health–illness caring patterns and behaviors.
- Cultural values vary among all humans and groups of humans.
- Human caring is a universal phenomenon that is expressed differently in all cultures.
- Caring unifies the intellectual and practical dimensions of nursing.

Myra E. Levine: Four Conservation Principles Theory of Nursing

Myra Levine (1973) based her theory of nursing on the belief that the essence of nursing is human interaction. Assumptions that characterize this theory are as follows:

Condition. Patients entering the healthcare system are in a state of illness or altered health.

Responsibilities. The nurse is responsible for recognizing the patient's organismic response (ie, changes in behavior or level of body function) as the patient adapts or attempts to adapt to the environment (environment includes illness and nurse). The four levels of response are (1) fear, (2) stress, (3) inflammatory, and (4) sensory.

Functions. Nursing functions include interventions to promote adaptation to illness and evaluations of interventions as supportive or therapeutic. Supportive interventions help maintain the present health state and prevent further illness. Therapeutic interventions promote healing and restore health.

The foundation for all nursing interventions consists of four conservation (meaning to maintain balance) principles that support the goal of nursing, which is to maintain or restore a person to a state of health:

Conservation of energy: balancing energy intake and output to avoid excessive fatigue (rest, nutrition, exercise)

Conservation of structural integrity: maintaining or restoring the structure of the body (promoting healing)

Conservation of personal integrity: maintaining or restoring a sense of identity and self-worth (recognition of unique qualities)

Conservation of social integrity: recognizing the patient as a social being (especially with significant others)

Levine's theory is focused on one person: the patient. This theory has major implications in acute-care settings, where nursing interventions are supportive or therapeutic.

Betty Neuman: Healthcare Systems Model

Betty Neuman's (1995) model, the *total person approach,* can be used to provide an organized approach to a variety of nursing problems and to develop an understanding of humans and their environment. The model focuses on the patient's reaction to stress and the factors of reconstitution or adaptation. The person is viewed as an open system interacting with the environment. Surrounding each person are internal and external factors that are stressors. Over a lifetime, the person becomes a "normal line of defense" who uses biologic, psychological, sociocultural, and developmental skills to deal with stressors. Stressors cause the line of defense to react or respond as the total person. The stressors may be extrapersonal, interpersonal, or intrapersonal. The effect of the stressors on the system is individualized and depends on such variables as the number of stressors, how long they last, and the system's coping skills.

Nursing interventions can be carried out on three preventive levels. When the stressor is identified but no reaction has occurred, interventions can decrease the degree of reaction or increase the line of defense. This is called *primary prevention.* When the reaction has already happened, *secondary prevention* is carried out, with interventions aimed at treating symptoms and reducing reactions. After active treatment, *tertiary prevention* strengthens the lines of defense through education and uses the system's total resources to prevent further occurrences.

Dorothea E. Orem: Self-Care Deficit Theory of Nursing

Dorothea Orem's (1995) theory is based on the belief that the individual has a need for self-care actions and that nursing can assist the person in meeting that need to maintain life, health, and well-being. This is a general theory, composed of three related theories: the theory of self-care, the theory of self-care deficit, and the theory of nursing systems. The model is widely used in all areas of nursing. *Self-care,* as defined by Orem, consists of the activities that individuals carry out on their own behalf. These actions are deliberate, have pattern and sequence, and are developed from day-to-day living. The ability of the individual to perform self-care is called *self-care agency;* this is usually carried out by adults. Infants and children, as well as aged, ill, and disabled people, require help with self-care activities or complete care. Three categories of *self-care requisites* (the purposes of actions directed toward the provision of self-care) follow:

Universal self-care requisites. These are common to all humans and are associated with maintaining life, health, and well-being. They include air, water, food, elimination, activity and rest, solitude and social interaction, prevention of hazards, and promotion of human functioning.

Developmental self-care requisites. These include maintaining conditions to support life and human development.

Health deviation self-care. This is required in illness or injury or as a result of medical tests or treatments to correct a condition.

Orem suggests that a person needs nursing when the person has a health-related self-care deficit. Orem has defined three nursing systems on the premise that each nursing system depends on the self-care needs and abilities of the patient. In the first system (wholly compensatory), the nurse gives total care to meet all needs. In the second (partly compensatory), both the nurse and the patient perform care measures. In the third (supportive-educative), the patient can carry out self-care activities but requires assistance.

Hildegard E. Peplau: Psychodynamic Nursing

Hildegard Peplau (1952/1991) defines psychodynamic nursing as being able to understand one's own behavior to help others identify felt difficulties and to apply principles of human relations to the problems that arise at all levels of experience. Her model describes the phases of the nurse–patient relationship in terms of the concepts of the interpersonal process used in psychodynamic nursing. She describes the four phases that occur in sequence in mental health nursing:

Orientation, in which the person has a "felt need" and seeks professional assistance. The nurse and patient meet as strangers, and the nurse works collaboratively with the patient to identify and clarify the problem.

Identification, in which the patient identifies those who can help meet his or her needs. The nurse assists the patient in understanding illness by helping the patient explore his or her feelings. Both the patient and the nurse must clarify each other's perceptions and expectations, a process that requires a more intense therapeutic relationship. While working through this stage, the patient begins to have a feeling of belonging and capability of dealing with the problem.

Exploitation, in which the patient takes advantage of all available services, based on his or her own interests and needs, to explore problem-solving alternatives. The patient begins to feel in control of the situation and a part of the helping environment. Most patients fluctuate between being dependent on others and having independent functioning at this phase. The nurse facilitates adjustment by clarifying, listening, accepting, and interpreting during communications.

Resolution is the last phase, during which the therapeutic relationship must be terminated. This may be difficult for both the patient and the nurse, but successful resolution leads to increasing strength in both individuals.

Martha E. Rogers: A Theory of Unitary Human Beings

Martha Rogers (1970) wrote a complex theory of nursing. The goal of this theory is to develop a science of nursing to provide a growing body of theoretical knowledge applicable in nursing practice to the achievement of meaningful service to humanity. The theory is built on a knowledge base of the history of humanity and of the universe (anthropology, sociology, astronomy, religion, philosophy, history, and mythology). Based on the belief that humans are the center of nursing's purpose, Rogers' theory considers the total individual, describing the human life process and explaining and predicting the nature and direction of human development. Both systems and developmental theories are incorporated into Rogers' theory.

Rogers' basic assumptions about humans are as follows:

- Humans are unified wholes who are more than a sum of their parts.
- Humans are constantly interacting with their environment.
- Anything that occurs in life is unique because no two things in life can ever be repeated in an identical manner or under identical circumstances.
- Humans develop patterns of behaving, and their behavior becomes predictable.
- Humans are distinctive in their capacity for abstract thought, imagery, and emotion.

Nursing concepts are derived and nursing science principles are identified from these basic assumptions. Based on these assumptions, Rogers identifies four building blocks:

Energy fields. Both the human and the environment are viewed as energy fields; there is a constant exchange of energy between the two that is essential to life.

Openness. This is based on the belief that the universe consists of open systems.

Pattern and organization. These are identifying characteristics of the energy field that is undergoing continuous change.

Four-dimensionality. This is a characteristic of both human and environmental fields.

Sister Calista Roy: Adaptation Model

Sister Calista Roy (1984) developed the adaptation model of nursing. This model is widely used as a philosophic base and conceptual model in nursing education. The adaptation model is essentially a systems model. The assumptions basic to this model are as follows:

- Each person is a biophysical being and an integrated whole. All body systems are balanced to produce a functioning person with biologic, psychosocial, and social needs. Constant interaction with the changing environment of the modern world subjects the person to continual changes and stressors.
- Each person uses both innate and acquired mechanisms to cope with changes and adapt individually, with either positive or negative responses. The adaptation level reached is the result of three classes of stimuli: the primary cause of the change, other situational factors, and beliefs and past experiences shaping the response.
- Each person responds to needs (requirements within the individual stimulating a response to maintain integrity) in one or more of four modes: physiologic, self-concept, interdependent behaviors, and role-function.
- Each person's position on the health—illness continuum changes in relation to the effectiveness of coping to maintain an adaptive state.

As defined by Roy, response to a decrease in body integrity creates a need state, and the individual responds with an act or behavior. The physiologic mode involves oxygenation and circulation, fluid and electrolyte balance, nutrition, rest and activity, and regulation of temperature, hormones, and sensory function. The self-concept mode involves the perception of one's physical self and personal self, including personality, moral and ethical beliefs, and values. The interdependence mode involves social relationships, including both the need to be interdependent and the need for support by others. The role function mode involves the behaviors of a person in each role taken on in life.

In Roy's model, all nursing activity is aimed at promoting the individual's adaptation to health and illness in all four adaptive modes. This model guides the nurse to use observation and interviewing skills to make an individualized assessment of each person, and serves as a guide in planning and carrying out nursing actions.

Jean Watson: Philosophy and Science of Caring

Jean Watson's (1988) theory of caring is based on the values of kindness, concern, love of self and others, and respect for the spiritual dimension of the person. In nursing as a human science, *human caring in nursing* is defined as an art and a science in which caring is a human-to-human process demonstrated through a therapeutic interpersonal interaction. The basic assumptions of Watson's theory of nursing are as follows:

- A person's mind and emotions are windows to the soul. Although nurses give physical care and carry out procedures, the nurse's presence in the relationship transcends the physical and material world, facilitating the patient to develop a higher sense of self.
- Although a person's body is confined in time and space, the mind and soul transcend time and space and may be an indicator of the spiritual evolution of humans.
- A nurse may have access to a person's inner self, provided the physical body is not perceived and treated as separate from the mind, emotions, and sense of self.
- People need each other in a caring, loving way. Love and caring are needs that are often overlooked. We need to love, respect, and care for ourselves with dignity before we can respect, love, and care for others and treat them with dignity. (Watson, 1988, pp. 50–51)

The structure of Watson's science of caring is built on 10 "carative" factors, including forming values, instilling faith and hope, cultivating sensitivity to self and others, developing a helping–trust relationship, and promoting and accepting expression of positive and negative feelings. Other carative factors are using problem-solving for decision making; promoting interpersonal teaching and learning; providing a supportive, protective, or corrective mental, physical, sociocultural, and spiritual environment; and assisting with meeting needs.

Within the theory, optimal health is the attainment of all needs, but even when medical scientists believe that nothing can be done for a patient, the nurse can provide care by providing comfort measures and instilling hope. Caring is the mechanism by which nurses help individuals and groups reach self-actualization, maintain or attain health, or die a peaceful death. Holistic, individualized care is given through transpersonal caring, which is a human art, a human science, and the moral ideal of nursing.

Applying Conceptual and Theoretical Frameworks in Practice

As we enter a new century, it has become even more necessary and important for nurses to demonstrate efficient, cost-effective, high-quality care within organized healthcare delivery systems. By practicing theory-based nursing combined with critical thinking skills, nurses will be able not only to deliver care that meets those criteria but also to describe and document what it is they do. Kenney (1996) described how professional nurses use theories from nursing and from the behavioral sciences to accomplish the following:

- Collect, organize, and classify patient data.
- Understand, analyze, and interpret patients' health situations.
- Guide the formulation of nursing diagnoses.
- Plan, implement, and evaluate nursing care.
- Explain nursing actions and interactions with patients.
- Describe, explain, and sometimes predict patients' responses.
- Demonstrate responsibility and accountability for nursing actions.
- Achieve desired outcomes for patients (p. 9).

The major concepts of a chosen model or theory guide each step of the nursing process. The concepts serve as categories to guide the nurse in determining what information is relevant and should be collected in making assessments and formulating nursing diagnoses. The concepts also suggest the appropriate types of nursing interventions and patient outcomes to be included in the care plan. For example, if the nurse is using Orem's self-care deficit theory, data are collected about the patient's ability to meet universal and developmental self-care requisites and the presence of any health deviations. The nurse then formulates diagnoses identifying self-care deficits and determines the appropriate nursing actions for partial, compensatory, or supportive-educative nursing care.

The aims of nursing, described in Chapter 1, are the same for all nursing theorists, but the values, assumptions, and beliefs individualize each theory when it is applied to the giving of nursing care. Theoretical frameworks of nursing provide a focus for nursing care activities. The person receiving care is the central theme, but the way each theorist defines that person, the environment, health, and nursing gives a unique focus specific to a particular theory. The ultimate goal of each framework, however, is holistic patient care, individualized to meet needs, promote health, and prevent or treat illness.

Learning Outcomes

After completing this chapter, the learner should be able to accomplish the following:

1. Define key terms used in the chapter.

adaptation	general systems theory
adaptation theory	inductive reasoning
concept	nursing theory
conceptual framework or model	philosophy
deductive reasoning	process
developmental theory	theory

2. Describe the underlying processes and characteristics of nursing theory.
3. Define the four common components of nursing theory.
4. Summarize the historical background, cultural influences, and value of nursing theory.
5. Describe key concepts and beliefs in selected nursing theories.

Critical Thinking Exercises

1. Describe your own beliefs about the patient, the nurse, the environment, health, and what nursing is. Compare and contrast your answers with another student. How are they different, and how are they alike? How do you think such differences might influence nursing practice for each of you?
2. Choose one nursing theory described in the chapter and describe how it might be applied when providing care for the following patient:

Alexandar Libbus, a 17-year-old high-school senior, dove into a shallow pool of water. He fractured his neck and sustained such serious spinal cord damage that now he cannot move his arms or legs. He is angry and refuses to eat or drink.

Was the theory you chose useful? Why or why not?

Bibliography

Alligood, M., & Marriner-Tomey, A. (1999). *Nursing theory: Utilization & application.* St. Louis: C. V. Mosby.

Barnum, B. (1998). *Nursing theory: Analysis, application, evaluation* (5th ed.). Philadelphia: Lippincott Williams & Wilkins.

Chinn, P., & Kramer, M. (1998). *Theory and nursing: Integrated knowledge development* (5th ed.). St. Louis: C. V. Mosby.

Clarke, P. N. (1998). Nursing theory as a guide for inquiry in family and community health nursing. *Nursing Science Quarterly, 11*(2), 47–48.

Dolan, J. A., Fitzpatrick, M. L., & Herrmann, E. K. (1983). *Nursing in society: A historical perspective.* Philadelphia: W. B. Saunders.

George, J. (Ed.). (1995). *Nursing theories: The base for professional practice* (4th ed.). Norwalk, CT: Appleton & Lange.

Hekton, L. M. (1989). Martha E. Rogers: A life history. *Nursing Science Quarterly, 2*(2), 63–73.

Henderson, V. (1966). *The nature of nursing: A definition and its implications for practice, research, and education.* New York: Macmillan.

Johnson, D. (1980). The behavioral system model of nursing. In J. P. Riehl & C. Roy (Eds.). *Conceptual models for nursing practice.* (2nd ed.). (pp. 207-216). New York: Appleton-Century-Crofts.

Kalish, P., & Kalish, B. (1995). *The advance of American nursing.* (3rd ed.). Philadelphia: J. B. Lippincott.

King, I. (1981). *A theory for nursing.* New York: John Wiley & Sons.

Kenney, J. (1996). Relevance of theory-based nursing practice. In P. J. Christensen & J. W. Kenney (Eds.). *Nursing process: Application of conceptual models* (4th ed.). (pp. 1–23). St. Louis: C. V. Mosby.

Kenney, J. (Ed.). (1999). *Philosophical and theoretical perspectives for advanced nursing practice.* (2nd ed.). Sudbury, MA: Jones & Bartlett.

Leininger, M. M. (1978). *Transcultural nursing: Concepts, theories, and practices.* New York: John Wiley & Sons.

Levine, M. (1973). *Introduction to clinical nursing* (2nd ed.). Philadelphia: F. A. Davis.

Malenski, V. M. (1986). *Explorations on Martha Roger's science of unitary human being.* Norwalk, CT: Appleton-Century-Crofts.

Marriner-Tomey, A., & Alligood, M. (Eds.). (1997). *Nursing theorists and their work* (4th ed.). St. Louis: C. V. Mosby.

Meleis, A. I. (1997). *Theoretical nursing: Development and progress* (3rd ed.). Philadelphia: Lippincott-Raven.

Neuman, B. (1995). *The Newman systems model.* (3rd ed.). Norwalk, CT: Appleton & Lange.

Orem, D. (1995). *Nursing: Concepts of practice* (5th ed.). St. Louis: Mosby–Year Book.

Peplau, H. E. (1952/1991). *Interpersonal relations in nursing.* New York: Springer.

Raudonis, B., & Acton, G. (1997). Theory-based nursing practice. *Journal of Advanced Nursing, 26*(1), 138–145.

Rogers, M. (1970). *An introduction to the theoretical basis of nursing.* Philadelphia: F. A. Davis.

Roy, C. (1984). *Introduction to nursing: An adaptation model* (2nd ed.). Englewood Cliffs, NJ: Prentice Hall.

Roy, C., & Andrews, H. (1991). *The Roy adaptation model: The definitive statement.* Norwalk, CT: Appleton & Lange.

Watson, J. (1988). *Nursing: Human science and human care. A theory of nursing* (Pub. No. 15-2236). New York: National League for Nursing.

Weiss, M., Hastings, W., Holly, D., & Craig, D. (1994). Using Roy's adaptation model in practice: Nursing perspectives. *Nursing Science Quarterly, 7*(4), 153–157.

Woods, E. (1994). King's theory in practice with elders. *Nursing Science Quarterly, 7*(2), 65–69.

Chapter 6
Values and Ethics in Nursing

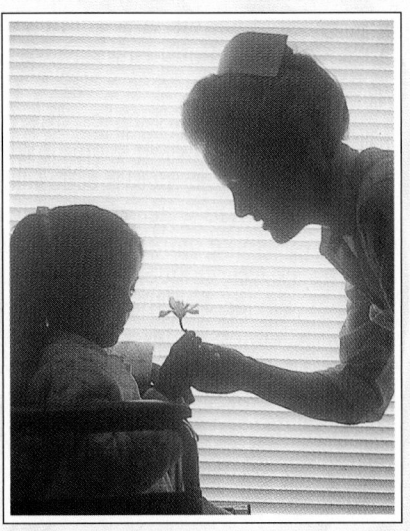

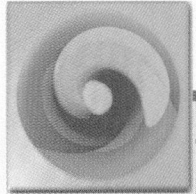

**Thinking Critically About
Nursing's Blended Skills**

Before reading this chapter, think about the types of skills you will need to practice nursing in a responsible manner, sensitive to the influence of values on human behavior and the ethical dimensions of practice.

- You are instructing a woman about lifestyle modifications (eg, diet, exercise, stress reduction) to reduce her risk for heart disease when she tells you to save your breath, "Why should I bother about all that, I'd be better off dead than living like I am now any way!"

- A new nurse on your unit suggests that nurses meet on Tuesdays at lunch to discuss journal articles that recommend better ways of addressing nursing problems commonly encountered in your unit. Not everyone is enthusiastic about her suggestion.

- A woman is brought into the emergency room after an automobile collision in which her daughter was killed. The mother, who was driving, is medically unstable but keeps asking about her daughter. The emergency room attending physician tells everyone to tell the mother anything but the truth about her daughter because he believes she is too unstable to accept this news. The nurse feels uncomfortable with this deception.

- An alert woman in the intensive care unit is begging to be removed from the ventilator. She understands that it is highly likely that she will not be able to breathe on her own if this happens and she says she understands and accepts this. "If I die, I die. I can't keep living like this." The team is undecided about whether to respect her wishes.

What cognitive, technical, interpersonal, and ethical/legal skills do you think you will need to respond effectively to the ethical challenges described above?

The unique nature of nursing places nurses at the bedside and in groups of professionals where critical decisions are made about the best way to treat injury and illness and to solve healthcare problems. Often, the question confronting the nurse is not "How do I do this?" but rather "Should I do this?" The more that science and technology increase the options available to patients and healthcare professionals, the more frequently nurses will find themselves asking, "We can do this, but *should we,* here and now, for this patient?" The answer to this and other ethical questions is important for quality care. Nurses need to examine their intuitions, opinions, and convictions about what is ethically right and wrong and monitor how these influence their nursing care.

Ethics or morality poses questions about how we ought to act and how we should live. It is an inquiry into the justification of particular actions (eg, Are these actions right or wrong?), as well as a search for traits of moral character that promote more human flourishing

This chapter explores the influence of values on human behavior and the ethical dimensions of nursing practice. Chapter 14 describes specific ethical competencies, or skills, that are essential to nursing practice. Nurses who understand how patients' values and their own values shape nurse–patient interactions, and who continually develop sensitivity to the ethical dimensions of nursing practice, are best able to provide quality care.

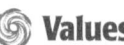 **Values**

A **value** is a belief about the worth of something, about what matters, that acts as a standard to guide one's behavior. If you think back to how you spent your last weekend, you may observe something about your values. The amount of time you devote to relationships, work, study, fitness activities, leisure, and other experiences reveals something about the importance (value) you attach to these endeavors. Similarly, the amount of money you are willing to spend on these endeavors reveals something about their value to you.

A **value system** is an organization of values in which each value is ranked along a continuum of importance; a value system often leads to a personal code of conduct. A person's values influence beliefs about human needs, health, and illness; the practice of health behaviors; and human responses to illness. For example, individuals who place a high value on health and personal responsibility often work hard to reach their fitness goals. Individuals who value high-risk leisure activities may attach less value to life and health. Nurses who work effectively with patients are sensitive to how a patient's values and their own values influence their interactions.

Development of Values

An individual is not born with values; rather, values are formed over a lifetime from information from the environment, family, and culture. As children observe the actions

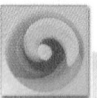

COGNITIVE SKILLS

- Knowledge of how values influence behavior, specifically the behavior of the woman at risk for heart disease and the nurses who are or are not willing to meet to explore ways to improve their practice.
- Knowledge of theories of ethics, codes of professional ethics, and ethical standards for practice. When, if ever, is it justified to deceive a patient? Would the team be justified in respecting a patient's wish to be extubated even if this results in the patient's death?
- Ability to use an ethical framework and decision-making process to resolve ethical problems.

TECHNICAL SKILLS

- Ability to provide the technical nursing assistance necessary to meet the needs of the patients in the emergency room and intensive care unit.

INTERPERSONAL SKILLS

- Ability to establish trusting professional relationships with both colleagues and patients— relationships that are respectful of value differences and that enhance dignity and worth.
- Ability to advocate for patients whose preferences may be different than your own.

ETHICAL/LEGAL SKILLS

- Ability to use values clarification techniques in professional practice.
- Ability to prevent and resolve ethical conflict.
- Ability to practice nursing consistent with nursing's code of ethics.
- Ability to recognize and respond to ethical and legal issues in practice.

of others, they quickly learn what has high and low value for family members. If the parents spend a good portion of each day cooking and the family spends a long time eating and talking at the table, the children learn to value food and the good times it represents. Similarly, children learn that helpfulness is a good and respected quality if praised when helping parents, grandparents, and siblings.

Common modes of value transmission include the following:

Modeling. Children learn what is of high or low value by observing parents, peers, and significant others. Thus, modeling may lead to socially acceptable or unacceptable behaviors.

Moralizing. Children are taught a complete value system by parents or an institution (eg, church or school) that allows little opportunity for them to weigh different values.

Laissez-faire. Children are left to explore values on their own (no one set of values is presented as best for all) and to develop a personal value system. This approach often involves little or no guidance and can lead to confusion and conflict.

Rewarding and punishing. Children are rewarded for demonstrating values held by parents and punished for demonstrating unacceptable values.

Responsible choice. Children are encouraged to explore competing values and to weigh their consequences. Support and guidance are offered as children develop a personal value system.

Values Essential to the Professional Nurse

Professional values provide the foundation for nursing practice and guide the nurse's interactions with patients, colleagues, and the public. In 1998, the American Association of Colleges of Nursing identified five values that epitomize the caring, professional nurse. The accompanying Professional Values box lists these values and sample behaviors illustrating each of these values. Every nurse should critically examine his or her personal values to see if they match these essential professional values. For example, if I value self-promotion to the extent that I am unwilling to make the sacrifices demanded by a genuine commitment to the welfare of the patients entrusted to my care, I will never be successful as a nurse. Similarly, if I attach low value to respecting people who are different from me, I may interact with patients and colleagues in a way that is demeaning and unprofessional. It is helpful to identify nurses in your practice setting who epitomize nursing's essential values and to learn from observing their behavior.

Value Neutrality

To encourage healthcare professionals to respect and accept the individuality of patients, some educators have advised that professionals be "value neutral" and "nonjudgmental" in their professional roles. Thus, the nurse has a "commitment to patients whether or not the nurse and the patients hold the same values. The nurse does not assume that personal values are right and should not judge the patient's val-ues as right or wrong depending on their congruence with the nurse's personal value system" (Steele & Harmon, 1983, p. 27). This kind of thinking encourages effective care for patients with values different from the nurse's. For example, a nurse who strongly believes that any premarital or extramarital sex is wrong can still offer competent and compassionate nursing care to a young female prostitute with active herpes lesions. On the other hand, if the same patient, after receiving education, indicates that she is unconcerned about whom she might infect in future sexual encounters, the nurse has an ethical obligation to protect the patient and others from the harm the patient's values may cause.

Values Clarification

Values clarification is a process by which people come to understand their own values and value system. "It is a process of discovery and allows the person to discover through feelings and analysis of behavior what choices to make when alternatives are presented, and to identify whether or not these choices are rationally made or are the result of previous conditioning" (Steele & Harmon, 1983, p. 13). Values clarification has a beneficial application to nursing. When nurses understand the values that motivate the decisions and behaviors of patients, they can tap these values when teaching and counseling patients. For example, a man who does not value his own health and well-being may be motivated by the value he attaches to being a good father for his children to make needed lifestyle changes.

Values theorists most often describe the process of valuing as having seven steps focusing on three main activities: (1) choosing, (2) prizing (treasuring), and (3) acting (Raths, Simon, & Harmin, 1978; Simon, 1972). When one values something, one:

Chooses
- Freely
- From alternatives
- After careful consideration of the consequences of each alternative

Prizes
- With pride and happiness
- With public affirmation

Acts
- With incorporation of the choice into one's behavior
- With consistency and regularity on the value

Example of Values Clarification by the Nurse

If respect for human dignity is a value that characterizes your nursing practice, you:

Choose
- Freely to believe in the worth and uniqueness of each individual
- To realize that you have other options (eg, you could treat with dignity only those people who are most like you)
- To believe that respecting each person's human dignity yields the best consequences for you and for all of society

Professional Values

Altruism is a concern for the welfare and well-being of others. In professional practice, altruism is reflected by the nurse's concern for the welfare of patients, other nurses, and other healthcare providers. Sample professional behaviors include the following:

- Demonstrates understanding of cultures, beliefs, and perspectives of others
- Advocates for patients, particularly the most vulnerable
- Takes risks on behalf of patients and colleagues
- Mentors other professionals

Autonomy is the right to self-determination. Professional practice reflects autonomy when the nurse respects patients' rights to make decisions about their healthcare. Sample professional behaviors include the following:

- Plans care in partnership with patients
- Honors the right of patients and families to make decisions about healthcare
- Provides information so that patients can make informed choices

Human dignity is respect for the inherent worth and uniqueness of individuals and populations. In professional practice, human dignity is reflected when the nurse values and respects all patients and colleagues. Sample professional behaviors include the following:

- Provides culturally competent and sensitive care
- Protects the patient's privacy
- Preserves the confidentiality of patients and healthcare providers
- Designs care with sensitivity to individual patient needs

Integrity is acting in accordance with an appropriate code of ethics and accepted standards of practice. Integrity is reflected in professional practice when the nurse is honest and provides care based on an ethical framework that is accepted within the profession. Sample professional behaviors include the following:

- Provides honest information to patients and the public
- Documents care accurately and honestly
- Seeks to remedy errors made by self or others
- Demonstrates accountability for own actions

Social justice is upholding moral, legal, and humanistic principles. This value is reflected in professional practice when the nurse works to assure equal treatment under the law and equal access to quality healthcare. Sample professional behaviors include the following:

- Supports fairness and nondiscrimination in the delivery of care
- Promotes universal access to healthcare
- Encourages legislation and policy consistent with the advancement of nursing care and healthcare

From American Association of Colleges of Nursing. (1998). *The essentials of baccalaureate education for professional nursing practice.* Washington, DC: American Association of Colleges of Nursing.

Prize

- Your choice (you especially enjoy when patients let you know they appreciate your care and when nursing colleagues and supervisors compliment you on interpersonal skills)
- Your ability to defend this value when someone's human dignity is being ignored

Act

- To incorporate this value into your practice
- Consistently to respect human dignity in your personal as well as professional life

As you become more conscious of this value, you will be sensitive to those of your actions that are inconsistent with it. For example, you may feel uncomfortable gossiping with other nurses during break about a patient no one likes; you realize that this behavior contradicts your basic respect for human dignity.

Clinical Applications

The accompanying box illustrates how the steps in the valuing process can be used to help a patient with high blood pressure take charge of his health and manage his medications. Other clinical examples follow here.

Patient Places Low Value on Health and Health Behaviors

You become frustrated when repeated attempts to teach or counsel a 26 year old pharmaceutical salesperson meet with failure. Although hospitalized with a serious duodenal ulcer, all he can talk about is his job and meeting his sales quota.

Values Clarification. First help this patient identify his basic life values. Ask him, "What three things are most important to you in life?" or have him rank the following behaviors in terms of how he would most likely spend an unexpected free day:

_____ Enjoy some quiet time alone (eg, thinking, reading, listening to music)
_____ Spend time with family, friends
_____ Do something active (eg, hiking, playing ball, swimming)
_____ Watch television
_____ Volunteer time and energy to help someone else
_____ Use time for my job
_____ Other

Discuss with the patient what these rankings suggest about his values. Determine whether his rankings would be different if he were asked how he *wished* he could spend the free day versus how he would *most likely* spend it.

Values of Patient and Family Members Conflict

You sense a growing tension while counseling the young parents of a child with asthma. Questioning them ("You seem uncomfortable with what I'm saying now. Is there something wrong?") reveals that the wife is a smoker and cat lover who has told her husband that even if these behaviors are hurting their child, she is unwilling to give them up.

Values Clarification. Suggest that both parents complete the following exercise, and then talk with them about their different responses.

Where do you stand on the following issues? (Indicate your responses in the following manner: SA, strongly agree; A, agree; D, disagree; SD, strongly disagree; U, undecided.)

Steps in the Valuing Process

Case: A male patient with high blood pressure

Choosing

1. *Freely.* Rehospitalized for high blood pressure after abruptly stopping his antihypertensive medication, the patient decides from now on to take his medication as prescribed.
2. *From Alternatives.* After a teaching–learning session with a nurse, the patient understands he has basically three options:
   - Comply with prescribed treatment regimen.
   - Refuse to take the medication but try harder to control his blood pressure through diet, exercise, and stress management.
   - Refuse to take the medication and assume a "we'll see" attitude.
3. *After Consideration of the Consequences.* The patient understands the *probable* consequences of these options:
   - Compliance with the treatment regimen will yield the best control of high blood pressure (but may cause some annoying side effects).
   - Diet, exercise, and stress management may reduce his blood pressure somewhat but did not yield sufficient control in the past.
   - High blood pressure may result in serious complications such as stroke, kidney disease, or impaired vision.

Prizing

4. *With Pride and Happiness.* The patient states, "Now that I understand high blood pressure better and know what I can do to control it, I feel more in charge of my life—and I like that!"
5. *With Public Affirmation.* The patient states to his wife, "I guess I was wrong to stop taking that medicine when I blamed it for how lousy I was feeling. You can bet that won't happen again. If you ever hear me complaining about my pills, remind me to see my doctor right away."

Acting

6. *With Incorporation of the Choice Into One's Behavior.* After discharge from the hospital, the patient takes the medication as prescribed.
7. *With Consistency and Regularity on the Value.* The patient seeks to understand any new medication he is prescribed (ie, reason for the medication, possible side effects, consequences of the noncompliance) and successfully manages the treatment regimen; he feels proud of his new knowledge and self-care abilities.

_____ A parent's primary obligation is to meet the needs of his or her child.

_____ Each member of a family is entitled to pursue personal pleasures, even if these are not in the best interest of all.

_____ Pleasure is more important than health.

_____ The choices one family member makes can dramatically affect other family members (positively or negatively).

This exercise will help the parents to evaluate their basic values, explore areas of conflict, and, perhaps, move toward joint choosing, prizing, and acting on several health-promoting values.

Ethics

Ethics is systematic inquiry into principles of right and wrong conduct, of virtue and vice, and of good and evil as they relate to conduct. Many people use the term *ethics* when describing the professional ethics incorporated into a code of professional conduct, such as nursing codes of ethics. The term **morals,** although similar in meaning to ethics, usually refers to personal or communal standards of right and wrong. It is important to distinguish ethics from religion, law, custom, and institutional practices. For example, the fact that an action is legal or customary does not in itself make the action ethically or morally right.

As nurses assume increasing responsibility for managing care, it is critical that we are prepared to recognize the ethical dimensions of our practice and to participate competently in ethical decision making. Common ethical issues encountered by nurses in daily practice include cost-containment issues that jeopardize patient welfare, end-of-life decisions, breaches of patient confidentiality, and incompetent, unethical, or illegal practices of colleagues.

Professional Ethical Conduct

Nurses committed to high-quality care base their practice on professional standards of ethical conduct. The study of professional ethical behavior begins in nursing school, continues in formal and informal discussions with colleagues and peers, and culminates when nurses "try on" and make their own the behaviors of role models who practice professional nursing consistent with high ethical standards. How do nurses learn the standards for professional ethical behavior? At the very least, nurses should understand the ethical theories that dictate and justify professional conduct; should be familiar with codes of professional ethics, standards of practice, and patients' bills of rights; and should be skilled in using a model of ethical decision making to resolve ethical problems. All of this entails a commitment to developing one's ability to act ethically, or one's **ethical agency.**

Ethical Agency

It is unrealistic to assume that the simple desire to be a nurse is accompanied by the natural ability to behave in an ethically professional way. This ability, ethical agency, must be cultivated in the same way that nurses cultivate the ability to do the scientifically right thing in response to a physiologic alteration. Elements of ethical agency (which are illustrated in the accompanying box) are described next.

Ethical sensibility: ability to recognize the "ethical moment" when an ethical challenge presents itself

Ethical responsiveness: ability and willingness to respond to the ethical challenge

Ethical reasoning: knowledge of and ability to use sound theoretical and practical approaches to "thinking through" ethical challenges; these approaches are used to *inform* as well as to *justify* moral behavior

Ethical accountability: ability and willingness to accept responsibility for one's ethical behavior and to learn from the experience of exercising ethical agency

Ethical character: cultivated dispositions that allow one to act as one believes one ought to act

Ethical valuing: valuing in a conscious and critical way that which squares with good ethical character and ethical integrity

Transformative ethical leadership: commitment and proven ability to create a culture that facilitates the exercise of ethical agency, a culture in which people do the right thing because it is the right thing to do

Theories of Ethics

Ethical theories are systems of thought that attempt to explain how we ought to live and why. These theories may be broadly categorized as action-guiding theories that answer the question, "What ought I to do?" or character-guiding theories that answer the question, "What kind of person ought I to be?" Action-guiding theories fall into two main categories:

Utilitarian. The rightness or wrongness of an action depends on the consequences of the action.

Deontologic. An action is right or wrong independent of its consequences.

These distinctions are important because they form the basis of many of the ethical conflicts we experience in practice. For example, one nurse may believe that abortion is ethically justified in situations in which it results in the best consequences for the woman, child, and society (utilitarian argument). Another nurse may agree that certain abortions yield better consequences than allowing an unplanned and unwanted pregnancy to continue but believe that the act of abortion is nonetheless ethically wrong because no consequences justify the taking of innocent life (deontologic argument).

Nursing ethics, which is a subset of bioethics, is the formal study of ethical issues that arise in the practice of nursing and of the analysis used by nurses to make ethical judgments. Nurse ethicists frequently use two popular theoretical and practical approaches for bioethics: the principle-based approach and the care-based approach.

Ethical Agency

Situation: A 75-year-old patient with end-stage lung cancer suffers a respiratory arrest and is coded, ventilated, and admitted to the intensive care unit (ICU). When the receiving nurse reviews his chart, she discovers that upon admission, his nurse documented that he "did not want to be resuscitated" and that he wanted to prepare an advance directive specifying "no heroics." There is no do-not-resuscitate order on the chart, and the nurse can find no advance directive.

Ethical Sensibility

The ICU nurse notes the discrepancy between the patient's documented preferences and the care that he has received. She senses personal discomfort about this disregard for his wishes.

Ethical Responsiveness

The nurse can decide to ignore her discomfort and simply provide excellent technologic care or acknowledge her discomfort and respond. She decides to talk with the attending physician about his knowledge concerning the patient's preferences and learns that the attending was unaware of the patient's documented preferences and has no personal knowledge of these. She contacts the nurse who originally admitted the patient and learns that although the patient was quite clear about his preference, no one followed up and translated this conversation into orders on his chart. She calls an ethics consult when the attending says that there is "nothing to be done now that treatment is initiated."

Ethical Reasoning

During the ethics consult, family members agree that the patient would not be happy to find himself on a ventilator and request that he be weaned—even if this results in his death. The ethicist explains that weaning him from an ineffective treatment (the ventilator will not cure his lung cancer) that is disproportionately burdensome is an ethically justified action.

Ethical Accountability

The nurse initiated the ethics consult because she believed that she could not be an advocate for this patient and merely provide good physical care. Once she knew (or suspected) that his preferences had been ignored, she felt accountable for determining how the system had failed this patient and for remedying the problem. The nurse prides herself on being responsible and accountable and therefore could not "stick her head in the sand" and pretend that this was not her problem! After the ethics consult, she participates in plans to find an optimal time and conditions to wean the patient from the ventilator and makes sure that his family is present. The patient does not survive the weaning, and although they are grieving, his family members are grateful to the nurse for her care for the patient and for them.

Ethical Character

Because she had cultivated the virtues of responsibility and fidelity, the nurse's course of action was natural.

Ethical Valuing

Because she places a high value on being an effective patient advocate, the nurse was willing to confront the attending physician and initiate an ethics consult, even though these actions caused her some discomfort and the expense of time and inconvenience.

Transformative Ethical Leadership

When her colleagues asked her where she got the "guts" to follow through with this course of action, the nurse knew that the culture within the hospital had to change so that more nurses would choose to do the same thing she did without fearing negative consequences. She asks the nurse educator on her unit to explore the possibility of pursuing this theme in a future Nursing Grand Rounds and is willing to work to make this happen.

Principle-Based Approach

The **principle-based approach** in bioethics offers specific action guides for practice. The Beauchamp/Childress principle-based approach to bioethics (1994) identifies four key principles: **autonomy, nonmaleficence, beneficence,** and **justice** (Table 6-1). Many nurses add **fidelity** to this list because it plays a central role in the tradition of nursing (and medical) ethics. The principles offer general guides to action. All things being equal, we ought to act at all times in a manner that respects the autonomy of others, does not harm and does benefit others, treats others fairly, and is faithful to the promises we make to others. Ethical dilemmas arise when attempted adherence to these principles results in two conflicting courses of action. For example, a mother demands costly, aggressive treatment for her child who is born without a brain and who will never be able to enjoy simple human pleasures. The principle of autonomy demands respect for this mother's treatment preferences, but the principle of justice dictates that public funds be used for other infants more able to benefit from aggressive treatment.

Sadly, there is no foolproof method for identifying which principle is most important when there is conflict between competing principles. Popularized versions of the principle-based approach to bioethics have too frequently resulted in a type of "quandary ethics" that diminishes in importance the everyday ethical concerns of nurses and misleadingly suggests that how ethical dilemmas are resolved is unimportant, so long as one can justify

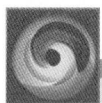

Table 6-1
Principles of Bioethics

Principle	Moral Rule	Implications for Nursing Practice
Autonomy (self-determination)	Respect the rights of patients or their surrogates to make healthcare decisions.	Provide the information and support patients and families need to make the decision that is right for them; at times, this may mean collaborating with other members of the healthcare team to advocate for the patient.
Nonmaleficence	Avoid causing harm.	Seek not to inflict harm; seek to prevent harm or risk of harm whenever possible.
Beneficence	Benefit the patient, and balance benefits against risks and harms.	Commit yourself to actively promote the patient's benefit (health and well-being). Be sensitive to the fact that individuals (patients, family members, and professional caregivers) may identify benefits and harms differently. A benefit to one may be a burden to another.
Justice	Give each his or her due; act fairly.	Always seek to distribute the benefits, risks, and costs of nursing care justly. This may involve recognizing subtle instances of bias and discrimination.
Fidelity	Keep promises.	Be faithful to the promise you made to the public to be competent and to be willing to use your competence to benefit the patients entrusted to your care. Never abandon a patient entrusted to your care without first providing for their needs.

one's recommendation with recourse to a principle. Thus, many healthcare professionals equate ethics with decisions about whether to "pull the plug" and ignore the ethical challenges involved in daily decisions about what constitutes an honest day's work, how respectful we are to others, how truthful, how compassionate.

Care-Based Approach

Dissatisfaction with the principle-based approach to bioethics led many nurses to look to care as the foundation for nursing's ethical obligations. The nurse–patient relationship is central to the **care-based approach,** which directs attention to the specific situations of individual patients viewed within the context of their life narrative. The care perspective directs that how you choose to "be" and act each time you encounter a patient or colleague is a matter of ethical significance. Ethics is not reduced to a decision to withhold or withdraw life-sustaining treatment. Characteristics of the care perspective include the following:

- Centrality of the caring relationship
- Promotion of the dignity and respect of patients as people
- Attention to the particulars of individual patients
- Cultivation of responsiveness to others and professional responsibility

- A redefinition of fundamental moral skills to include virtues like kindness, attentiveness, empathy, compassion, reliability (Taylor, 1993)

Advocacy

Nursing has traditionally held that its primary commitment is to the patient, and more recently nursing has claimed patient advocacy as a legitimate nursing role. **Advocacy,** which is discussed in Chapter 23, is the protection and support of another's rights. As a distinct ethical obligation for nurses, it finds justification in both the principle-based and care-based approaches to nursing ethics. Nurses who wish to practice in this tradition:

- Make sure that their loyalty to an employing institution or colleague does not compromise their primary commitment to the patient
- Give priority to the good of the individual patient rather than to the good of society in general
- Carefully evaluate the competing claims of the patient's autonomy (self-determination) and patient well-being

When respecting autonomy, the nurse respects and supports the patient's right to make decisions. Informed consent is described in Chapter 7. When promoting patient well-being, the nurse acts in the best interests of the patient. Ideally, both autonomy and patient well-being are promoted in every nurse–patient interaction; however, conflicts sometimes arise. For instance, if an older male patient with a serious chronic lung disease who understands well the danger of smoking asks the nurse to get him a pack of cigarettes, the nurse must decide whether to respect his autonomy and follow his wishes or to promote his medical well-being. Although there is value in the nurse refusing to perform an action that clearly compromises the *physical* well-being of a patient, one can think of situations in which a nurse might "just this one time" bend a rule because a patient's *general* well-being will be promoted. Nurses sensitive to the need to promote both patient autonomy and well-being may often experience conflict, but they are more likely than other nurses to succeed in securing the patient's genuine best interests.

Nursing Codes of Ethics

A professional code of ethics provides a framework for making ethical decisions and sets forth professional expectations. Nursing codes of ethics inform both nurses and society of the primary goals and values of the profession. These should be compatible with the nurse's personal value system and moral code. Other functions of professional nursing codes include the following:

- Indicating nursing's acceptance of the responsibility and trust with which it has been invested by society
- Providing guidance for conduct and relationships in carrying out nursing responsibilities consistent with the ethical obligations of the profession and with high-quality nursing care
- Providing a means for the exercise of professional self-regulation (American Nurses Association, 1985, pp. i–iv)

Codes are effective in accomplishing their goals only to the extent that they are upheld by members of the profession. Code requirements may exceed legal requirements. Violations of the law subject a nurse to civil or criminal liability (see Chap. 7), and violations of the code of ethics may result in reprimands, censure, suspension, and expulsion.

Codes of ethics for nursing include the International Council of Nurses (ICN) *ICN Code for Nurses* (adopted in 1953 and revised in 1965 and 1973); the ANA *Code for Nurses With Interpretive Statements* (adopted in 1950 and revised in 1968, 1976, and 1985); and the Canadian Nurses Association (CNA) *Code of Ethics for Nursing* (adopted in 1980 and revised in 1991). These are highlighted in the accompanying box: Three Codes of Ethics for Nurses.

Nursing Standards of Practice

When the American Nurses Association revised its Standards of Clinical Nursing Practice in 1991, it developed standards of professional performance as well as standards of care. The fifth standard of professional performance describes the nurse's ethical obligations:

> *Standard V: Ethics.* The nurse's decisions and actions on behalf of patients are determined in an ethical manner:

Measurement Criteria
1. The nurse's practice is guided by the *Code for Nurses*.
2. The nurse maintains patient confidentiality.
3. The nurse acts as a patient advocate.
4. The nurse delivers care in a nonjudgmental and nondiscriminatory manner that is sensitive to patient diversity.
5. The nurse delivers care in a manner that preserves or protects patient autonomy, dignity, and rights.
6. The nurse seeks available resources to help formulate ethical decisions (American Nurses Association, 1991, p. 15)

A Patient's Bill of Rights

The American Hospital Association developed *A Patient's Bill of Rights* in 1972 (revised in 1992). The bill of rights includes the rights and responsibilities of the patient while receiving care in the hospital and range from "the right to considerate and respectful care" to "the right to be informed of hospital policies and practices that relate to patient care, treatment and responsibilities." See accompanying box. With care moving increasingly from the hospital to the community, nurses must be familiar with how patient rights and responsibilities are defined by different institutions and professional groups. Other bills of rights include the Pregnant Patient's Bill of Rights, the Indian Patient's Bill of Rights, a Nursing Home Bill of Rights, and the Veterans Administration Code of Patient Concern. Each emphasizes a specific aspect of patient rights within a particular health agency and implies a code of ethics the nurse observes professionally.

Ethical Decision Making

Two types of moral and ethical problems commonly faced by nurses are moral dilemmas and moral distress. In an *ethical dilemma,* two (or more) clear moral principles apply but support mutually inconsistent courses of action. *Ethical distress* occurs when the nurse knows the right thing to do but institutional constraints make it nearly impossible to pursue the right actions (Jameton, 1993, p. 542). Nurses need sound analytic skills and the ability to engage in ethical reasoning to resolve ethical dilemmas and ethical distress. Every nurse needs to be confident in using a process of ethical decision making (see the accompanying box: Reasoning About Ethical Decisions). The accompanying patient care study illustrates a five-step model of ethical decision making that is based on the nursing process.

Examples of Ethical Problems

Ethical problems commonly arise between nurses and patients, nurses and physicians, nurses and other nurses, and nurses and their employing institutions. Moreover, nurses are often most conflicted when good practice seems to require acting against their personal moral convictions. As you read through the following mini-cases, try to determine how you would respond. The process of ethical decision making described above should prove helpful.

(*text continues on page 91*)

A Patient's Bill of Rights

Introduction

Effective health care requires collaboration between patients and physicians and other health care professionals. Open and honest communication, respect for personal and professional values, and sensitivity to differences are integral to optimal patient care. As the setting for the provision of health services, hospitals must provide a foundation for understanding and respecting the rights and responsibilities of patients, their families, physicians, and other caregivers. Hospitals must ensure a health care ethic that respects the role of patients in decision making about treatment choices and other aspects of their care. Hospitals must be sensitive to cultural, racial, linguistic, religious, age, gender, and other differences as well as the needs of persons with disabilities.

The American Hospital Association presents *A Patient's Bill of Rights* with expectation that it will contribute to more effective patient health care and be supported by the hospital on behalf of the institution, its medical staff, employees, and patients. The American Hospital Association encourages health care institutions to tailor this bill of rights to their patient community by translating and/or simplifying the language of this bill of rights as may be necessary to ensure that patients and their families understand their rights and responsibilities.

Bill of Rights*

1. The patient has the right to considerate and respectful care.
2. The patient has the right to and is encouraged to obtain from physicians and other direct caregivers relevant, current, and understandable information concerning diagnosis, treatment, and prognosis.

   Except in emergencies when the patient lacks decision-making capacity and the need for treatment is urgent, the patient is entitled to the opportunity to discuss and request information related to the specific procedures and/or treatments, the risks involved, the possible length of recuperation, and the medically reasonable alternatives and their accompanying risks and benefits.

   Patients have the right to know the identity of physicians, nurses, and others involved in their care, as well as when those involved are students, residents, or other trainees. The patient also has the right to know the immediate and long-term financial implications of treatment choices, insofar as they are known.
3. The patient has the right to make decisions about the plan of care prior to and during the course of treatment and to refuse a recommended treatment or plan of care to the extent permitted by law and hospital policy and to be informed of the medical

consequences of this action. In case of such refusal, the patient is entitled to other appropriate care and services that the hospital provides or transfer to another hospital. The hospital should notify patients of any policy that might affect patient choice within the institution.
4. The patient has the right to have an advanced directive (such as a living will, health care proxy, or durable power of attorney for health care) concerning treatment or designating a surrogate decision maker with the expectation that the hospital will honor the intent of that directive to the extent permitted by law and hospital policy.

   Health care institutions must advise patients of their rights under state law and hospital policy to make informed medical choices, ask if the patient has an advance directive, and include that information in patient records. The patient has the right to timely information about hospital policy that may limit its ability to implement fully a legally valid advance directive.
5. The patient has the right to every consideration of privacy. Case discussions, consultation, examination, and treatment should be conducted so as to protect each patient's privacy.
6. The patient has the right to expect that all communications and records pertaining to his/her care will be treated as confidential by the hospital, except in cases such as suspected abuse and public health hazards when reporting is permitted or required by law. The patient has the right to expect that the hospital will emphasize the confidentiality of this information when it releases it to any other parties entitled to review information in these records.
7. The patient has the right to review the records pertaining to his/her medical care and to have this information explained or interpreted as necessary, except when restricted by law.
8. The patient has the right to expect that, within its capacity and policies, a hospital will make reasonable response to the request of a patient for appropriate and medically indicated care and services. The hospital must provide evaluation, service, and/or referral as indicated by the urgency of the case. When medically appropriate and legally permissible, or when the patient has so requested, a patient may be transferred to another facility. The institution to which the patient is to be transferred must first have accepted the patient for transfer. The patient must also have the benefit of complete information and explanation concerning the need for, risks, benefits, and alternatives to such a transfer.
9. The patient has the right to ask and be informed of the existence of business relationships among the hospital, educational institutions, other health care providers, or payers that may influence the patient's treatment and care.

A Patient's Bill of Rights *(Continued)*

10. The patient has the right to consent to or decline to participate in proposed research studies or human experimentation affecting care and treatment or requiring direct patient involvement, and to have those studies fully explained prior to consent. A patient who declines to participate in research or experimentation is entitled to the most effective care that the hospital can otherwise provide.
11. The patient has the right to expect reasonable continuity of care when appropriate and to be informed by physicians and other caregivers of available and realistic patient care options when hospital care is no longer appropriate.
12. The patient has the right to e informed of hospital policies and practices that relate to patient care, treatment, and responsibilities. The patient has the right to be informed of available resources for resolving disputes, grievances, and conflicts, such as ethics committees, patient representatives, or other mechanisms available in the institution. The patient has the right to be informed of the hospital's charges for services and available payment methods.

The collaborative nature of health care requires that patients, or the families/surrogates, participate in their care. The effectiveness of care and patient satisfaction with the course of treatment depend, in part, on the patient fulfilling certain responsibilities. Patients are responsible for providing information about past illnesses, hospitalizations, medications, and other matters related to health status. To participate effectively in decision making, patients must be encouraged to take responsibility for requesting additional information or clarification about their health status or treatment when they do not fully understand information and instruction. Patients are also responsible for ensuring that the health care institution has a copy of their written advance directive if they have one. Patients are responsible for informing their physicians and other caregivers if they anticipate problems in following prescribed treatment.

Patients should also be aware of the hospital's obligation to be reasonably efficient and equitable in providing care to other patients and the community. The hospital's rules and regulations are designed to help the hospital meet this obligation. Patients and their families are responsible for making reasonable accommodations to the needs of the hospital, other patients, medical staff, and hospital employees. Patients are responsible for providing necessary information for insurance claims and for working with the hospital to make payment arrangements, when necessary.

A person's health depends on much more than health care services. Patients are responsible for recognizing the impact of their lifestyle on their personal health.

Conclusion

Hospitals have many functions to perform, including the enhancement of health status, health promotion, and the prevention and treatment of injury and disease; the immediate and ongoing care and rehabilitation of patients; the education of health professionals, patients, and the community; and research. All these activities must be conducted with an overriding concern for the values and dignity of patients.

*These rights can be exercised on the patient's behalf by a legally designated surrogate of proxy decision make if the patient lacks decision-making capacity, is legally incompetent, or is a minor.

Reprinted with permission of the American Hospital Association. © 1992.

Three Codes of Ethics for Nurses

International Council of Nurses Code for Nurses*

The fundamental responsibility of the nurse is fourfold—to promote health, to prevent illness, to restore health, and to alleviate suffering.

The need for nursing is universal. Inherent in nursing is respect for life, dignity, and rights of humans. It is unrestricted by considerations of nationality, race, creed, age, sex, politics, or social status.

Nurses render health services to the individual, the family, and the community and coordinate their services with those of related groups.

Nurses and People

The nurse's primary responsibility is to those people who require nursing care.

The nurse, in providing care, promotes an environment in which the values, customs, and spiritual beliefs of the individual are respected.

The nurse holds in confidence personal information and uses judgment in sharing this information.

Nurses and Practice

The nurse carries personal responsibility for nursing practice and for maintaining competence by continual learning. The nurse maintains the highest standards of

(continued)

Three Codes of Ethics for Nurses (Continued)

nursing care possible within the reality of a specific situation.

The nurse uses judgment in relation to individual competence when accepting and delegating responsibilities.

The nurse, when acting in a professional capacity, should at all times maintain standards of personal conduct that reflect credit on the profession.

Nurses and Society

The nurse shares with other citizens the responsibility for initiating and supporting action to meet the health and social needs of the public.

Nurses and Coworkers

The nurse sustains a cooperative relationship with coworkers in nursing and other fields. The nurse takes appropriate action to safeguard the individual when his or her care is endangered by a coworker or any other person.

Nurses and the Profession

The nurse plays the major role in determining and implementing desirable standards of nursing practice and nursing education.

The nurse is active in developing a core of professional knowledge.

The nurse, acting through the professional organization, participates in establishing and maintaining equitable social and economic working conditions in nursing.

American Nurses Association Code for Nurses†

1. The nurse provides services with respect for human dignity and the uniqueness of the patient unrestricted by considerations of social or economic status, personal attributes, or the nature of health problems.
2. The nurse safeguards the patient's right to privacy by judiciously protecting information of a confidential nature.
3. The nurse acts to safeguard the patient and the public when healthcare and safety are affected by the incompetent, unethical, or illegal practice of any person.
4. The nurse assumes responsibility and accountability for individual nursing judgments and actions.
5. The nurse maintains competence in nursing.
6. The nurse exercises informed judgment and uses individual competence and qualifications as criteria in seeking consultation, accepting responsibilities, and delegating nursing activities to others.

7. The nurse participates in activities that contribute to the ongoing development of the profession's body of knowledge.
8. The nurse participates in the profession's efforts to implement and improve standards of nursing.
9. The nurse participates in the profession's efforts to establish and maintain conditions of employment conducive to high-quality nursing care.
10. The nurse participates in the profession's effort to protect the public from misinformation and misrepresentation and to maintain the integrity of nursing.
11. The nurse collaborates with members of the health professions and other citizens in promoting community and national efforts to meet the health needs of the public.

Canadian Nurses Association Code of Ethics‡§

Health and Well-Being

Nurses value health and well-being and assist patients to achieve their optimal level of health in situations of normal health, illness, or injury or in the process of dying.

Choice

Nurses respect and promote the autonomy of patients and help them to express their health needs and values and to obtain appropriate information and services.

Dignity

Nurses value and advocate the dignity and self-respect of human beings.

Confidentiality

Nurses safeguard the trust of patients so that information learned in the context of a professional relationship is shared outside the healthcare team only with the patient's permission or as legally required.

Fairness

Nurses apply and promote principles of equity and fairness to assist patients in receiving unbiased treatment and a share of health services and resources proportionate to their needs.

Accountability

Nurses act in a manner consistent with their professional responsibilities and standards of practice.

Practice Environments Conducive to Safe, Competent, and Ethical Care

Nurses advocate practice environments that have the organizational and human support systems and the resource allocations necessary for safe, competent, and ethical nursing care.

---

* Adapted from International Council of Nurses. (1973). ICN Code for nurses: Ethical concepts applied to nursing. Geneva: Imprimeries Populaires.
† From American Nurses Association. (1985). Code for nurses. Kansas City, MO: ANA.
‡ This represents only one element of the code—values. Obligations, which provide more specific direction for conduct than do values by spelling out what a value requires under particular circumstances, and limitations, which describe exceptional circumstances in which a value or obligation cannot be applied, are provided with each value in the publication.
§ From the Canadian Nurses Association. (1997). Code of Ethics for Registered Nurses. Ottawa, Ontario: The Canadian Nurses Association.

Reasoning About Ethical Decisions

1. **Assess the situation (gather data)**
   Recognize and then describe the situation that gives rise to the ethical problem:
   Main people involved (their views and interests)
   Patient's overall nursing, medical, and social situation
   Relevant legal, administrative, and staff considerations
2. **Diagnose (identify) the ethical problem**
   State the problem clearly. Identify your relationship to the decision. Identify time parameters.
3. **Plan**
   Identify options and explore the probable short-term and long-term consequences of each.
   Use ethical reasoning to decide on a course of action that you can justify ethically.
   Decide on the course of action you are best able to support.
   Consultation with a respected and wise colleague or an institutional ethics committee may be helpful at this point.
4. **Implement your decision**
   Implement your decision and compare the outcome of your action with what you considered and hoped for in advance.
5. **Evaluate your decision**
   What have you learned from this process that will help you in the future? How can you improve your reasoning and decision making in the future?

Resources for ethical decision making are highlighted in the accompanying box: Ethics Resources.

Nurses and Patients

Troublesome nurse—patient situations that can result in ethical distress for nurses include **paternalism** (acting for patients without their consent to secure good or prevent harm), deception, **confidentiality,** allocation of scarce nursing resources, informed consent, and conflicts between the patient's and nurse's values and interests.

Paternalism

An alert older resident who lives in a nursing home and who is now at high risk for falls refuses to call the nurse for assistance when getting out of bed. The nurse must decide whether to obtain an order to restrain the patient. Does preventing potential harm justify violating the patient's right to autonomy and make it acceptable for the nurse to act as a "parent" and choose an action the patient does not want because the nurse believes it to be in the patient's best interest?

Deception

A postoperative patient asks the student nurse, who is about to administer an intramuscular injection for pain, "Is this your first shot?" It does happen to be the student's first injection, and the student is anxious. Would the student's intent to decrease the patient's anxiety justify telling the patient, "No, I've given several before"?

Patient Care Study Using a Five-Step Process for Resolving the Ethical

Jean W. is a labor and delivery room nurse in a small community hospital that serves both private patients and clinic patients. Jean has always felt that certain members of the obstetrics–gynecology medical staff have treated these two groups of clients differently. On this particular morning, Jean is caring for a woman who is scheduled for an elective cesarean delivery. The woman (who is a clinic patient) has made it very clear that she wants to be awake for the delivery and has requested epidural or spinal anesthesia. Jean is dismayed when the anesthesiologist enters the delivery room because the anesthesiologist's success rate with epidural anesthesia is poor. The anesthesiologist unsuccessfully attempts to perform an epidural block. After waiting 20 minutes for results, the obstetrician is growing impatient and instructs the anesthesiologist to put the patient to sleep. Jean feels the rights of this patient are being violated but is unsure of what her response should be.

Step 1: Assess the Situation (Gather Data)

The patient is in stable medical condition (elective cesarean delivery, not an emergency) and has made it very clear that she wishes to be awake for the delivery. The patient is not a private paying patient of the obstetrician. The nurse believes her role is to promote and protect the patient's interests; she knows of no

(continued)

Patient Care Study Using a Five-Step Process for Resolving the Ethical (*Continued*)

reason in this case why the patient's preferences should be disregarded.

The anesthesiologist has a poor success record with epidural anesthesia.

The obstetrician seems to want to complete delivery quickly. In the past, he has seemed to give more weight to following wishes of private patients as opposed to clinic patients. He is the head of the obstetrics–gynecology department; he believes nurses should obey physicians unquestioningly.

Nurses have in the past expressed dissatisfaction with the different levels of care being provided to private and clinic patients, but no one to date has formally addressed the concern.

Step 2: Diagnose (Identify) the Ethical

Jean W. objects to the obstetrician's intent to disregard the patient's wish to be awake for her delivery; she is aware of no good reasons justifying this course of action.

The nurse will be a participant in carrying out the decision.

The decision for this case must be made immediately; it would be helpful to plan to avoid situations like this in the future.

Step 3: Plan

a. Identify Options

The nurse can say nothing to the obstetrician and help with the delivery. If asked by the patient later why she needed to be put to sleep, the nurse can (1) tell the truth, (2) refer her to the obstetrician, (3) express sympathy that she could not be awake, or (4) say nothing. *Outcome:* The patient's wishes are disregarded; delivery occurs in record time, and the obstetrician is happy; the nurse fulfills obligation to physician and hospital but feels she has betrayed the patient's trust. *Long-term outcome:* There is a good probability the same problem will happen again.

Or

The nurse can remind the obstetrician that the patient was adamant about wanting to be awake and suggest that a different anesthesiologist be called in. If the obstetrician agrees, the patient may get her wish and everyone is satisfied with the outcome (the nurse must still decide how to prevent recurrence of this dilemma). If the obstetrician refuses and insists that the patient be put to sleep, the nurse can (1) refuse to participate (if another nurse is unavailable or unwilling to replace her, the nurse has abandoned the patient and harm may ensue); or (2) participate and proceed as above or resolve to speak to the obstetrician in a "cool moment"

after the delivery to see how to avoid this problem in the future. If the nurse does not get satisfaction with the obstetrician, then she must decide whether to move through the proper administrative channels. Depending on the institution and people involved, the nurse may be affirmed or censored for this move. *Long-term outcome:* Future patients may be helped by the nurse following through with her concerns.

Or

The nurse can say nothing and assist with this delivery, believing it to be the wisest course of action for the time being, but resolve to take the steps above to correct the perceived injustice. *Outcome:* There is no benefit for the present patient but potential benefit to future patients.

b. Think the Ethical Problem Through

Basic moral principles: The good of patients (beneficence) should be the nurse's primary concern; this strongly suggests that the nurse should act, but it does not address the nurse's obligation to do so if she feels it would jeopardize her own good (job security).

Respect for persons would suggest that the patient's autonomy (right to self-determination) should be respected unless there is strong justification for not doing so.

Justice would suggest that whether a patient pays the obstetrician privately should have no bearing on the quality of care received.

Care-based ethics would obligate Jean to serve as an effective advocate for her patient, respecting the nurse's commitment to be faithful to the nurse–patient relationship.

c. Make a Decision

Jean W. feels from past interactions with this obstetrician that her speaking up will not influence his decision to have the patient put to sleep. She decides to speak with the obstetrician after the delivery and follow up with whatever approach is necessary to avoid recurrence.

Steps 4–5: Implement and Evaluate Your Decision

Jean W. will never know if speaking up would have resulted in the patient's wishes being respected. Although she is dissatisfied with the outcome of this case, she hopes to prevent this from happening to other clinic patients in the future. In this instance, a hospital committee was formed to study the problem and make recommendations. If Jean W. had been told to "mind her own business" unless she wanted trouble, she would have to make a decision weighing patient benefit on one hand with potential personal risk or harm on the other.

Confidentiality

A nurse asks a middle-aged woman who is crying quietly, "Would you like to share what's troubling you?" The woman tells the nurse she has no idea how she will pay for this clinic visit because she entered the country illegally 2 months ago and is trying to earn enough money to help her family back home. She begs the nurse not to tell anyone. If the nurse believes this anxiety is interfering with the patient's ability to obtain needed healthcare, would it be ethical to break the woman's confidence to obtain help for her?

Allocation of Scarce Nursing Resources

A nurse has just been pulled from your unit, leaving it understaffed. Among your patients are a 33-year-old man recovering from a heart attack who is being discharged in the morning (he tells you he still has many questions); an older patient who is close to death; and a woman with cancer who has been vomiting all day and who is in severe pain. You know you cannot meet everyone's needs well. How do you "distribute" your nursing care? (You really *like* the patient who is going home in the morning.)

Advocacy in Market-Driven Environment

A hospitalized 57-year-old woman who underwent two lengthy bowel resections has just been informed by her health plan that she has exceeded her allowable length of stay and needs to be discharged immediately. She lives alone and has no family members or friends who are able to assist with her care. You believe that she would benefit immensely from extra hospital days so that she could regain her strength and learn how to provide necessary self-care. She does not have the money to pay for more days. What do you do?

Informed Consent

A resident is attempting to perform a spinal tap on an adolescent who you know dislikes the resident. After one failed attempt, the adolescent tells the resident to stop. The resident asks you to administer an antianxiety medication to the patient so the resident can get the spinal tap done quickly. Should you administer the medication knowing the patient no longer consents to the procedure?

Conflicts Between the Patient's and Nurse's Interests

Home health nurses are taking turns being assigned to care for new patients who test positive for the human immunodeficiency virus (HIV). One nurse, who is nursing her 8-month-old infant, refuses to take her turn, fearing she will transmit the disease to her baby. The other nurses tell her she must accept the assignment of this HIV-positive patient because none of them is willing to take her turn. Is a nurse ever justified in refusing to nurse a patient assigned to his or her care?

Ethics Resources

The following are ethics resources for healthcare professionals:

- American Nurses Association Center for Ethics and Human Rights
  600 Maryland Avenue, SW
  Suite 100 West
  Washington, DC 20024-2571
  202-651-7055

- National Reference Center for Bioethics Literature
  Kennedy Institute of Ethics
  Georgetown University
  Washington, DC 20057
  800-MED-ETHX

A specialized collection of library resources concerned with contemporary biomedical issues in the fields of ethics, philosophy, medicine, nursing, science, law, religion, and the social sciences. Call for bioethics information, BIOETHICSLINE searches (computerized database); search strategies; reference help; publication orders.

- The Hastings Center
  255 Elm Road
  Briarcliff Manor, NY 10510
  914-762-8500

A nonprofit, nonpartisan organization that carries out educational and research programs on ethical issues in medicine, the life sciences, and the professions. Publishes *The Hastings Center Report.*

Conflicts Concerning the Appropriate Use of Technology

An infertile woman asks you what you think about in vitro fertilization. She tells you that she is "desperate to produce a child for her husband and in-laws" but also has grave reservations about the whole process. "I've read about couples who end up with seven frozen embryos and I think that would kill me, thinking I've got seven potential kids 'on ice.'"

Nurses and Physicians

Nurse–physician situations can also result in ethical distress for nurses. Common problems include disagreements about a proposed medical regimen, conflicts regarding the scope of the nurse's role, and physician incompetence.

Disagreements About the Proposed Medical Regimen

In the nursing home where you work, any patient who loses a significant amount of weight (more than 10% of usual body weight) is automatically subjected to an exhaustive battery of tests (including a complete gastrointestinal [GI] series) to determine whether there are any physical causes for the weight loss (eg, a tumor). You strongly object to one patient being put through these tests because she has made it clear that she wants to die and will starve herself to death if that is the only way she can do it. The medical director insists that the patient undergo the diagnostic studies because there is a long history of patient family dissatisfaction with the facility's medical care. The director wants to avoid causing further dissatisfaction. Are you responsible for preparing the patient for these diagnostic studies and scheduling them? Are there grounds for refusing to participate?

Conflicts Regarding the Scope of the Nurse's Role

A young woman needing surgery that will result in a permanent colostomy tells the nurse how afraid she is and how much she dreads depending on "the thing." The nurse is certain this patient would benefit greatly from the help of the young staff enterostomal therapist (ET), who also has a colostomy. When this suggestion is mentioned to the surgeon, however, the surgeon tells the nurse that he does his own teaching and counseling for all his patients and does not "believe" in ETs. He points out that the nurse's duty here is to carry out his orders. Does it fall within the scope of nursing to recommend the ET to the woman? Is the nurse obligated to make this recommendation to the patient?

Unprofessional, Incompetent, Unethical, or Illegal Physician Practice

A nurse who works in the operating room notices that a pediatric surgeon who has been on the staff for several years and done excellent work seems suddenly not to be concentrating during surgery and to be making more mistakes than usual. Rumors have been circulating about the surgeon having a problem with cocaine abuse after his recent divorce. The parents of one pediatric patient are dissatisfied with the progress the patient is making and ask the nurse for an opinion about the surgeon. Should the nurse voice personal concerns? Is the nurse obligated to report the physician to the proper hospital authority for investigation?

Nurses and Other Nurses

Some of the most difficult ethical problems nurses encounter result from nurse–nurse interactions; these may be complicated by obligations of friendship. Problems include claims of loyalty and nurse incompetence.

Claims of Loyalty

A nurse working the 11 PM to 7 AM shift tells the other nurse on the unit, "I just made rounds and everyone is OK. Please cover for me while I catch an hour of sleep. I had an awful day." She neglects to tell the other nurse that a report mentioned that one patient needed special monitoring. This patient dies unexpectedly while the nurse sleeps. When she wakes up and discovers what happened, she begs the other nurse, her friend, never to tell anyone she was sleeping. "That patient could have died anyway between my rounds," she says.

Unprofessional, Incompetent, Unethical, or Illegal Nurse Practice

When you make your morning rounds, a patient tells you that one of the nurses fondled her body and made suggestive remarks during the previous night shift. You suspect that the patient may simply be trying to cause trouble, and because you like the nurse in question, you find it hard to believe the patient. What should you do?

Nurses and Institutional and Public Policy

As nurses assume increased responsibility for decision making at all levels of care, the institutional and public policy arenas offer unique dilemmas. Three current examples are short staffing, whistle blowing, and healthcare rationing.

Short Staffing and Whistle Blowing

Restructuring has resulted in chronic understaffing on the unit where you work. You believe that patients are now at risk because there simply are not enough nurses to provide quality care. Some nurses are talking about forming a union and going on strike. Because yours is the only major hospital in a rural area, you are unsure whether striking is a morally legitimate option. Because efforts to get management involved in addressing the issues have repeatedly failed, you are also contemplating "going public" with your concerns. Your brother works for the local newspaper, and you are pretty sure he would be willing to do a story about the situation at the hospital. What do you do?

Healthcare Rationing

In the United States, as many as 43 million people are uninsured or underinsured and have limited access to healthcare. Whether each person has a "right" (is entitled to) basic healthcare continues to be the subject of debate. There are plans for rationing healthcare that could limit the options available to the elderly, the poor, the terminally ill, and those in society whom many view as having limited "social value." What moral obligation do you have to contribute to this debate? How might you ensure that your voice and the nursing viewpoint are heard?

Nurses' Personal Moral Convictions and Institutional or Professional Ethics

Nurses sometimes experience a challenge to their personal ethical integrity because what they believe ought to be done in a particular situation is forbidden by the ethics of their place of employment or profession.

Beginning of Life Issues

You are a psychiatric mental health nurse working in a Catholic hospital whose ethical and religious directives forbid abortion and abortion counseling. You are talking with a single woman recently hospitalized with bipolar disorder who is in the first trimester of an unplanned pregnancy and who is expressing great ambivalence about continuing the pregnancy. You personally believe that your ethical obligation is to explore abortion as an option with this woman and to refer her to outside resources if she elects to abort. The charge nurse tells you that these are not appropriate options within this hospital.

End of Life Issues

You are the nurse case manager for a woman with a history of breast cancer whose cancer recurred (metastasis to the spine) after she had been cancer free for 7 years. She frequently tells you when you come to visit her at home that she is unwilling to fight anymore and wants to die with some dignity while she is still in control. She begs you to get her something that will "put me gently to sleep once and for all before my pain gets worse." You believe that this is her sincere wish, not just depression speaking, and you honestly believe that she would be better off spared the last stage of her illness. Your religious beliefs, however, tell you that assisted suicide is wrong under any circumstances. Moreover, the American Nurses Association has a position statement that claims that nurse-assisted suicide is incompatible with the ethics of nursing. How do you reconcile your desire to help this woman with your profession's ethical code and your religious conviction that what she is asking for is intrinsically wrong?

Nurses and Ethics Committees

An increasing number of healthcare institutions have developed ethics committees whose chief functions include education, policy making, case review, and consultation. Some committees focus on clinical ethics and some on organizational ethics. These committees are uniquely equipped to deal with the complexities of modern healthcare because they are multidisciplinary and provide a forum in which radically divergent views can be aired without fear of repercussion. Nurses bring an important voice to the ethics committee. When clinical issues are being reviewed, nurses can help to ensure that the technical facts are understood, that the appropriate decision makers have been identified, that the patient's medical and overall best interests have been identified, and that the course of action selected from the alternatives is justified by sound ethical principles. Nurses' strong background in interpersonal communications allow us to contribute unique knowledge about the patient and family to the discussion and to facilitate the ethics committee's group dynamics.

Nurses also play an important role in policy making. They are frequently able to identify what policies are needed to address recurring ethical concerns and to suggest needed modifications of existing policies.

Learning Outcomes

After studying this chapter, the learner should be able to accomplish the following:

1. Define key terms used in the chapter.

advocacy	morals
autonomy	nonmaleficence
beneficence	paternalism
care-based approach	principle-based approach
confidentiality	utilitarian
deontologic	value
ethical agency	value system
ethics	values certification
fidelity	
justice	

2. List five common modes of value transmission.
3. Describe seven steps in the valuing process.
4. Use values clarification strategies in clinical practice.
5. Compare and contrast the principle-based and care-based approaches to bioethics.
6. Describe three typical concerns of the nurse advocate.
7. Describe nursing practice that is consistent with the code of ethics for nursing.
8. Recognize ethical issues as they arise in nursing practice.
9. Use an ethical framework and decision-making process to resolve ethical problems.
10. Identify four functions of institutional ethics committees.

Critical Thinking Exercises

1. Students choose nursing as a career because of different values. A desire to help others, a love of money, wanting a career that allows you to work anywhere at any time, a commitment to provide for your children's well-being, a love of science and technology, and respect for your parents' wishes are

all values that may lead to choosing nursing as a career.

- Interview your classmates and identify the values that brought everyone to nursing. When a classmate lists more than one value, ask him or her to rank these in order of their importance. Compare your lists.
- Discuss which values, if any, provide the best motivation for professional nursing. Are there certain values that are incompatible with professional nursing and that ought to be grounds for rejecting candidates for professional nursing?
- Make a judgment about how well your personal values equip you for professional nursing. Are any modifications needed?

2. Make a list of all the values that might positively or negatively influence someone's ability to lose weight. Think about how you could use this knowledge when counseling obese patients.
3. Another student tells you, "Who I am outside of school is no one's business and has no effect on my nursing." Do you agree? Why or why not?
4. Take any current ethical issue (assisted suicide, human cloning, how to allocate scarce organs for transplantation, everyone's right to healthcare) and poll your class to see the range of opinions among your classmates. Reflect on what it is that causes people to reach different conclusions about what is the ethically right thing to do. How might you use this knowledge as you experience ethical conflict in your professional practice?

Bibliography

Aiken, T. D., & Catalano, J. T. (1994). *Legal, ethical, and political issues in nursing.* Philadelphia: Davis.

American Association of Colleges of Nursing. (1998). *The essentials of baccalaureate education for professional nursing practice.* Washington, DC: The Association.

American Nurses Association. (1985). *Code for nurses with interpretive statements.* Kansas City, MO: ANA.

American Nurses Association. (1988). *Ethics in nursing: Position statements and guidelines.* Kansas City, MO: ANA.

American Nurses Association. (1991). *Standards of clinical nursing practice.* Washington, DC: ANA.

Beauchamp, T. L., & Childress, J. F. (1994). *Principles of biomedical ethics* (4th ed.). New York: Oxford University Press.

Benjamin, M., & Curtis, J. (1992). *Ethics in nursing* (3rd ed.). New York: Oxford University Press.

Bishop, A. H., & Scudder, J. R. (1990). *The practical, moral, and personal sense of nursing.* Albany: State University of New York Press.

Canadian Nurses Association. (1997). *Code of ethics for nursing.* Ottawa, Ontario: CNA.

Council on Ethical and Judicial Affairs, American Medical Association. (1993). Caring for the poor. *JAMA, 269*(19), 2533–2537.

Daly, B. J. (1999). Why a new code? *American Journal of Nursing 99*(6), 64, 66.

Donley, R. (1993). Ethics in the age of health care reform. *Nursing Economics, 11*(1), 19–24, 51.

Edwards, B. S. (1993). When the physician won't give up. *American Journal of Nursing, 93*(9), 34–37.

Edwards, B. S. (1994). When the family can't let go. *American Journal of Nursing, 94*(1), 52–56.

Eriksen, J. (1993). Putting ethics into education. *Canadian Nurse, 89*(5), 18–20.

Fowler, M. (1999). Relic or resource? The Code for Nurses. *American Journal of Nursing, 99*(3), 56, 58.

Fry, S. T. (1989). The role of caring in a theory of nursing ethics. *Hypatia, 4*(2), 88–103.

Fry-Revere, S. (1994). Ethics consultations: An update on accountability issues. *Pediatric Nursing, 20*(1), 95–98.

Hughes, T. L., & Smith, L. L. (1994). Is your colleague chemically dependent? *American Journal of Nursing, 94*(9), 31–35.

Husted, G. L., & Husted, J. H. (1991). *Ethical decision making in nursing.* St. Louis: Mosby.

International Council of Nurses. (1973). *ICN code for nurses: Ethical concepts applied to nursing.* Geneva: Imprimeries Populaires.

Jameton, A. (1993). Dilemmas of moral distress: Moral responsibility and nursing practice. *AWHONN's Clinical Issues in Perinatal and Women's Health Nursing, 4*(4), 542–551.

Kirschbaum, H. (1977). *Advanced values clarification.* La Jolla, CA: University Associates.

Noddings, N. (1984). *Caring: A feminine approach to ethics and moral education.* Berkeley, CA: University of California Press.

Oddi, L. F., & Cassidy, V. R. (1990). Participation and perceptions of nurse members in the hospital ethics committee. *Western Journal of Nursing Research, 12*(3), 307–317.

Pence, T., & Cantrall, J. (Eds.). (1990). *Ethics in nursing: An anthology.* New York: National League for Nursing.

Raths, L. E., Simon, S. B., & Harmin, M. (1978). *Values and teaching* (2nd ed.). Columbus, OH: Charles E. Merrill.

Royal College of Nursing of the United Kingdom. (1980). *Guidelines on confidentiality in nursing.* London: Author.

Scanlon, C. (1994). Survey yields significant results. *American Nurses Association Center for Ethics and Human Rights Communique, 3*(3), 1–3.

Silva, M. C. (1984). The American Nurses' Association *Code for Nurses:* Purposes, content, and enforceability. *Health Matrix, 2*(2), 55–63.

Simon, S. B. (1972). *Values clarification.* New York: Hart.

Steele, S. M., & Harmon, V. M. (1983). *Values clarification in nursing* (2nd ed.). Norwalk, CT: Appleton-Century-Crofts.

Taylor, C. (1993). Nursing ethics: The role of caring. *AWHONN's Clinical Issues in Perinatal and Women's Health Nursing, 4*(4), 552–560.

Uustal, D. B. (1978). Values clarification in nursing: Application to practice. *American Journal of Nursing, 78*(12), 2058–2063.

Zink, M. R., & Titus, L. (1994). Nursing ethics committees: Where are they? *Nursing Management, 25*(6), 70–76.

Chapter 7
Legal Implications of Nursing

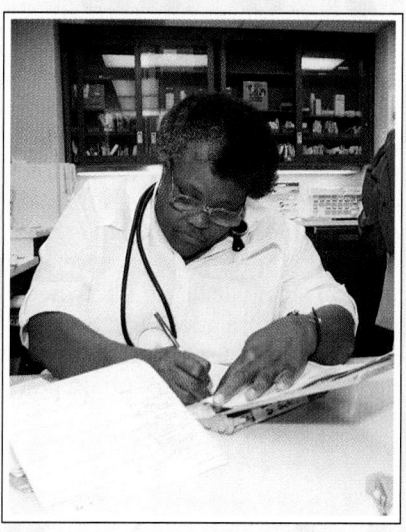

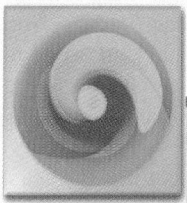

Thinking Critically About
Nursing's Blended Skills

Before reading this chapter, think about the types of skills you will need to practice nursing in a legally prudent and defensible manner.

- You realize to your horror that you just administered an intravenous antibiotic medication to the wrong patient!

- When you answer a call light, you discover an elderly patient on the floor at the side of her bed with her face bruised and her leg twisted oddly beneath her.

- A child's mother tells you in no uncertain terms that she is not happy with the care her child is receiving and she plans to see an attorney as soon as possible to press charges against the hospital.

- You arrive for practice and learn that you are responsible for 10 house calls that day. Looking at the list of patients assigned to you, you know that you will be unable to provide even the most basic assistance they require given such a heavy caseload. When you question the assignment, you are told there is no one else to help because five nurses called in sick.

What cognitive, technical, interpersonal, and ethical/legal skills do you think you will need to respond effectively to the legal challenges described above?

As the roles and duties of nurses expand, so too does their legal accountability. In the past, many nurses worked under the supervision of a physician, few carried liability insurance, and even if a nurse's actions were the direct cause of harm to a patient, the primary liability for the nursing action fell on the employing agency or physician. In modern practice, nurses assess and diagnose patients and plan, implement, and evaluate nursing care independently. Full legal responsibility and accountability for these nursing actions rest with the nurse. Nurses are increasingly the subjects of both civil and criminal negligence cases and are being brought to court to defend their practice.

Although many nurses continue to work in traditional settings like hospitals and nursing homes, more nurses are working in nontraditional community settings, such as home care agencies, clinics, day-care centers, and nurse-managed health centers. Advanced practice nurses may have independent practices. It has never been more crucial for nurses to document their actions carefully and act in ways to prevent malpractice accusations. Nurses who wish to avoid legal conflicts need to develop trusting nurse–patient relationships (satisfied patients rarely sue), practice within the scope of their competence, and identify potential liabilities in their practice and work to prevent them.

Legal Concepts

Definition of Law

A *law* is a standard or rule of conduct established and enforced by the government. Laws are intended chiefly to protect the rights of the public. *Public law* is law in which the government is directly involved. It regulates relationships between individuals and the government. Public law, for example, describes the powers of the government. Private law, also called *civil law*, regulates relationships among people. Civil law includes laws relating to contracts, ownership of property, and the practice of nursing, medicine, pharmacy, and dentistry. *Criminal law* concerns state and federal criminal statutes, which define criminal actions such as murder, manslaughter, criminal negligence, theft, and illegal possession of drugs.

Sources of Laws

Four sources of laws exist at both the federal and state level: constitutions, statutes, administrative law, and common law.

Constitutions

Federal and state constitutions indicate how the federal and state governments are created and are given authority and state the principles and provisions for establishing specific laws. Although they contain relatively few laws (called constitutional laws), constitutions serve as guides to legislative bodies.

Statutes

A **statutory law** is enacted by a legislative body. Statutory laws must be in keeping with both the federal constitution and the state constitution. Nurse practice acts are an example of statutory laws.

Nurse Practice Acts. Your state's nurse practice act is the most important law affecting your nursing practice. Each state has a nurse practice act that protects the public by broadly defining the legal scope of nursing practice. You should obtain a copy of this act from your State Board of Nursing and study it carefully. Each nurse is expected to care for patients within defined practice limits. Practicing beyond those limits (eg, performing an appendectomy) makes you vulnerable to charges of violating the state nurses practice act. Nurse practice acts list the violations that can result in disciplinary actions against a nurse and also serve to exclude untrained or unlicensed people from

COGNITIVE SKILLS

- Knowledge of how to practice nursing in a legally defensible manner
- Knowledge of how to write an incident (or variance) report
- Knowledge of how malpractice litigation works

TECHNICAL SKILLS

- Ability to provide the technical nursing assistance necessary to meet the needs of the patients entrusted to your care
- Ability to use appropriate documentation systems and tools to make a record of practice

INTERPERSONAL SKILLS

- Ability to establish trusting and respectful professional nurse–patient and nurse–colleague relationships

ETHICAL/LEGAL SKILLS

- Ability to evaluate personal areas of liability and to use appropriate legal safeguards
- Knowledge of how to challenge an unsafe patient assignment or caseload and competence in using this knowledge to effect change

practicing nursing. The accompanying box, Who Makes Nursing Practice Rules?, illustrates different sources of rules affecting nursing practice, examples of issues covered, where these rules are documented, and suggestions for initiating change.

Administrative Law

Executive officers (eg, the President of the United States, state governors, or city mayors) administer agencies that, among other functions, are responsible for law enforcement. These agencies have power to make adminis-

---

Who Makes Nursing Practice Rules?

Source of Practice Rules	Examples of Issues Covered	Where Rules Are Documented	How to Initiate Change
Federal legislation	• Medicare and Medicaid provisions related to reimbursement for nursing services	• Federal statutes	• Review documents. • Draft desired legislative changes. • Obtain support of colleagues, nursing organizations, other healthcare providers, and the public, if appropriate. • Obtain support and sponsorship from a US congressperson or senator, who will introduce the bill. • Lobby for the bill's passage.
State legislation	• Scope of practice for RNs, LPNs, advanced practice nurses • Nursing educational requirements • Composition and disciplinary authority of board of nursing	• Nurse practice act • Medical practice act • Other statutes	• Review documents. • Draft desired legislative changes. • Obtain support of colleagues, nursing organizations, other healthcare providers, and the public, if appropriate. • Obtain support and sponsorship from a state legislator, who will introduce the bill. • Lobby for the bill's passage.
Board of nursing	• Delegation • Medication administration • Unprofessional conduct • Licensing	• Rules and regulations • Position statements • Declaratory rulings (as found in meeting minutes or newsletters), which may be specific to a particular setting or institution	• Review documents. • Initiate a formal query to the licensing board. • Obtain board support for change. • The board may issue a position statement or declaratory ruling or hold a formal public hearing before voting to promulgate new rules or change existing ones.
Healthcare institution	• Clinical procedures, such as wound dressing changes • Policies specific to the institution, specialty, or practice setting • Personnel and employment policies	• Unit-based policies • Institutional policies • Institutional credentialing policies	• Review institutional policies. • Follow institutional policies or the chain of command to make inquiries or propose change.

From Laskowshi, J. L. (1998). Reaching beyond the rules: Understanding—and influencing—your scope of practice. *Nursing, 28*(9), 45.

trative rules and regulations, in conformity with enacted law, that act as laws and are enforceable. Boards of nursing are administrative agencies at the state level. The rules and regulations they adopt are administrative laws. An example of a municipal administrative agency is city board of health.

Common Law

The government provides for a judiciary system, which is responsible for reconciling controversies. It interprets legislation at the local, state, and national levels as it has been applied in specific instances and makes decisions concerning law enforcement. A body of law known as **common law** has evolved from these accumulated judiciary decisions. Common law is thus court-made law. Most law involving malpractice is court-made law.

Common law is based on the principle of *stare decisis*, or "let the decision stand." After a decision has been made in a court of law, the principle in that decision becomes the rule to follow in similar other cases. The case that first sets down the rule by decision is called a *precedent*. Court decisions can be changed but only with strong justification. Common law helps prevent one set of rules from being used to judge one person and another set to judge another person in similar circumstances.

Litigation

A lawsuit is a legal action in a court. **Litigation** is the process of bringing and trying a lawsuit. The person or government bringing suit against another is called the **plaintiff.** The one being accused of a crime or tort (defined later) is called the **defendant.** The defendant is presumed innocent until proved guilty of a crime or tort.

The two levels of courts in the United States are trial courts and appellate courts. The trial court, the first-level court, hears all the evidence in a case and makes decisions based on facts, usually through a jury. The appellate court hears only cases questioning a point of law decided by the trial court. No witnesses testify at the appellate court level. The opinions of appellate judges are published and become common law.

Professional and Legal Regulation of Nursing Practice

Nurses who practice safely respect both the voluntary and legal controls that map the boundaries of nursing practice. Both of these controls are designed to provide quality healthcare and to protect society from unsafe actions.

Standards

Voluntary standards, developed and implemented by the nursing profession itself, are not mandatory but are used as guidelines for peer review. Professional nursing organizations continually reassess the functions, standards, and qualifications of their members. These organizations are guided by their own assessment of society's need for nurs-

ing and by the public's expectations of nursing. Examples of voluntary standards include the American Nurses Association (ANA) standards of practice (see Chap. 1), professional standards for the accreditation of education programs and service organizations, and standards for the certification of individual nurses in general and specialty areas of practice.

Legal standards, on the other hand, are developed by a legislature and are implemented by authority granted by the state to determine minimum standards for the education of nurses, to set requirements for licensure or registration, and to decide when a nurse's license may be suspended or revoked. Examples of legal standards include state nurse practice acts and rules and regulations of nursing.

Credentialing

Nursing has taken several steps to ensure the competence of its practitioners, including the credentialing process. **Credentialing** refers to ways in which professional competence is ensured and maintained.

Three processes are used for credentialing in nursing. The first is **accreditation**, which is the process by which an educational program is evaluated and recognized as having met certain standards. The second is **licensure**, which is the process by which a state determines that a candidate meets certain minimum requirements to practice in the profession and grants a license to do so. The third is **certification**, which is the process by which a person who has met certain criteria established by a nongovernmental association is granted recognition in a specified practice area.

Accreditation

State constitutions give states a responsibility for the public welfare. State legislative bodies have used this principle to enact laws controlling occupational and professional groups. One function of these laws is to see that schools preparing practitioners maintain minimum standards of education. Nursing is one of the groups operating under state laws that promote the general welfare by determining minimum standards of education through accreditation of schools of nursing. State-approved, or accredited, educational programs in nursing include practical or vocational, associate degree, diploma, baccalaureate, and graduate programs in nursing.

Legal accreditation of a school preparing nursing personnel by the state board of nursing should not be confused with voluntary accreditation. The National League for Nursing Accrediting Commission (NLNAC) and the American Association of Colleges of Nursing (AACN) are voluntary agencies that accredit schools when they meet certain criteria. Most schools choose to seek this voluntary accreditation, and many prospective students prefer selecting accredited schools. Accreditation by NLNAC or AACN is not a legal requirement for a school to exist. State accreditation is a legal requirement.

Licensure

Licensure is a specialized form of credentialing based on laws passed by a state legislature. A *license* is a legal document that permits a person to offer to the public skills and knowledge in a particular jurisdiction, where such practice would otherwise be unlawful without a license. Licensure is discussed in Chapter 1.

Licensure Revocation

The State Board of Nurse Examiners in the United States may revoke or suspend a nurse's license or registration for drug or alcohol abuse, which is currently the most frequent reason. Other reasons for revocation or suspension of a license or registration include fraud, deceptive practices, criminal acts, previous disciplinary action by other state boards, gross or ordinary negligence, and physical or mental impairments, including those resulting from aging.

Once earned, a license to practice is a property right and may not be revoked without due process. This includes notice of the investigation, a fair and impartial hearing, and a proper decision based on substantial evidence. Crucial to a nurse's successful defense are early legal counsel, character and expert witnesses, and thorough preparation for all proceedings.

Certification

Many US professional organizations offer nursing certification, including two primary organizations: the American Association of Critical-Care Nurses, which represents the specialty with the largest number of certified nurses, and the ANA, which began certifying nurses in 1974. Although certification, which involves special testing, is voluntary, nurse specialists are increasingly becoming certified. Certification is one means to demonstrate advanced proficiency and a commitment to ensuring competence.

Crimes and Torts

A **crime** is a wrong against a person or his or her property, but the act is considered to be against the public as well. In a criminal case, the government, called "the people," prosecutes the offender. When a crime is committed, the factor of intent to commit wrong is present in most cases. Nonetheless, people who break certain laws are guilty of a crime regardless of whether they intended it. For example, failure to observe the Federal Food, Drug, and Cosmetic Act may constitute a crime.

In most cases, criminal law is statutory law (eg, *federal* Controlled Substance Acts and kidnapping laws or *state* criminal codes that define murder, manslaughter, criminal negligence, rape, fraud, illegal possession of drugs, theft, assault and battery) and only infrequently common law. Examples of common law are informed consent and the right to refuse treatment. Crimes are classified as felonies (rape, murder) or misdemeanors. A **misdemeanor** is a less serious crime than a felony. Misdemeanors are commonly punishable with fines, with imprisonment for less than 1 year, or with both, or with parole. A **felony** is punishable by imprisonment in a state or federal penitentiary for more than 1 year.

A **tort** is also a wrong committed by a person against another person or his or her property. A tort is subject to action in a civil court; a crime is a violation punishable by the state. In most instances, the court in a civil case settles the damages with money; rarely is imprisonment involved. Torts may be intentional or unintentional acts of wrongdoing. Some of the intentional torts for which nurses may be held liable include assault and battery, defamation of character, invasion of privacy, false imprisonment, and fraud. A person committing an intentional tort is considered to have knowledge of the permitted legal limits of his or her words or acts. Violating these limits is grounds for prosecution. For example, although there are policies that specify when a nurse may use restraints to protect an incompetent patient, restraining a competent patient to enable you to administer medications forcefully while the patient is refusing is assault and battery. Unintentional torts are referred to as **negligence.** A nurse who fails to initiate proper precautions to prevent patient harm (falls, skin breakdown) is subject to the charge of negligence.

An act that is a tort may also be a crime. For example, gross negligence that demonstrates the offender is guilty of complete disregard for another's life may be tried as both a civil and a criminal action. It is then prosecuted under both criminal and civil law. By its very nature, a wrong tried as a crime is considered a more serious offense with more legal implications than a tort.

Intentional Torts

Assault and Battery

Assault is a threat or an attempt to make bodily contact with another person without that person's consent. **Battery** is an assault that is carried out and includes every willful, angry, and violent or negligent touching of another person's body or clothes or anything attached to or held by that other person. Forcibly removing a patient's clothing, administering an injection after the patient has refused it, and pushing a patient into a chair are all examples of battery. Threatening to do any of these actions if the patient does not cooperate would be assault. When a nurse needs to defend himself or herself or others from an aggressive patient, only actions necessary for self-protection or the aid of another are permitted.

Every individual has the right to be free from invasion of his or her person, and adult patients who are alert and oriented have the right to refuse any treatment. The fact that treatment is desirable does not allow the nurse or physician to proceed without the consent of the patient or to go beyond the limits to which the patient has consented.

Informed Consent

Every person is granted freedom from bodily contact by another person unless consent is granted. In all healthcare agencies, informed and voluntary consent is needed for admission (for routine treatment), for each specialized diagnostic procedure or medical or surgical treatment, and for any experimental treatments or procedures. The consent must be written, designated for the procedure to be performed, and signed by the patient or person legally responsible for the patient. A signed consent is not needed in an emergency if there is an immediate threat to life or health, if experts would agree that it is an emergency, and if the patient is unable to consent and a legally authorized person cannot be reached. Although some value informed consent mostly as a protection against lawsuits, the central values underlying informed consent include promoting the patient's well-being and respecting the patient's self-determination (President's Commission for the Study of Ethical Problems in Medicine and Biomedical and Behavioral Research, 1982). Elements of informed consent include disclosure, comprehension, competence, and voluntariness (see the accompanying Checklist to Ensure Informed Consent).

Obtaining informed consent is the responsibility of the person who will perform the diagnostic or treatment procedure or the research study. The nurse's roles are to confirm that a signed consent form is present in the patient's chart and to answer any patient questions about the consent. In some instances, a nurse may be responsible for having a patient sign the consent form after a physician has explained to the patient the procedure, its risks and benefits, and alternative treatments.

The documentation of the consent process through the use of a printed consent form should not be confused with the actual explanation given to the patient and the informed consent itself. When documenting consent, the nurse should assess whether the patient understands what he or she is signing and report to the physician any problems. Having patients describe in their own words what they understand they are consenting to is the best way to make sure they understand. Nurses often find themselves in a position in which they question the patient's understanding of the proposed procedure and its risks or the patient's ability to consent voluntarily to the procedure. Impediments include the effects of anxiety, pain, medication, depression, and temporary or permanent states of disorientation and confusion. Unless a nurse is actually obtaining consent for a nurse-prescribed and initiated intervention, the nurse signs the consent form as a witness to having seen the patient sign the form, not as having obtained the consent (Fig. 7-1).

Consequences of not obtaining a valid consent include the possibility of charges of battery against the nurse, doctor, and healthcare agency, which has a duty to protect patients and is responsible for its employees' actions. A patient's refusal to sign a consent should be documented, and the patient should be informed of the possible consequences of the refusal. The patient should sign a release form indicating his or her refusal to consent and releasing the nurse, physician, and agency from responsibility for outcomes of this act. This statement should be witnessed.

Defamation

Defamation of character is an intentional tort in which one party makes derogatory remarks about another that diminish the other party's reputation. *Slander* is oral defamation of character; *libel* is written defamation. Defamation of character is grounds for an award of civil damages. Damages are awarded to the plaintiff based on the amount of harm done to the plaintiff. Nurses who make false or exaggerated statements about their patients or coworkers run the risk of being sued for slander or libel. A person charged with slander or libel may be found not liable if it can be proved that the statement was made not to injure another

---

Checklist to Ensure Informed Consent

Disclosure

Patient/surrogate has been informed of the (1) nature of the procedure, (2) risks (nature of the risk, magnitude, probability that the risk will materialize) and benefits, (3) alternatives (including the option of nontreatment), (4) fact that no outcomes can be guaranteed.

Comprehension

Patient/surrogate can correctly repeat in his or her own words that for which they are giving consent.

Competence

The patient understands the information needed to make *this* decision, is able to reason in accord with a relatively consistent set of values, and can communicate a preference.

The surrogate (if needed) meets the above criteria, knows the patient's wishes to the extent that this is possible, and is free from undue emotional stress and conflict of interests.

Voluntariness

The patient is voluntarily consenting or refusing. Care has been taken to avoid manipulative and coercive influences.

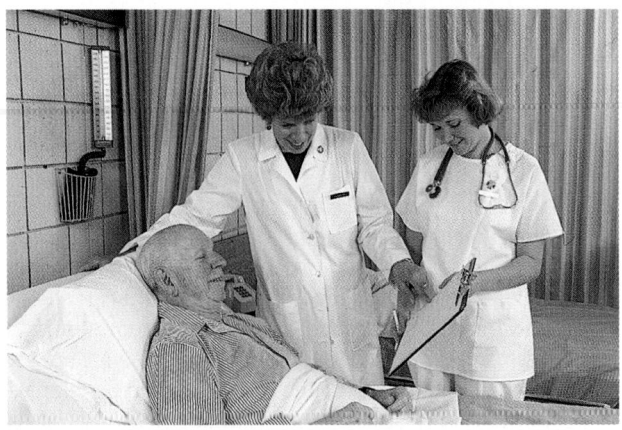

Figure 7-1
Elements of informed consent include disclosure, comprehension, competence, and voluntariness. The documentation of the consent process through the use of a printed consent form does not substitute for the actual explanation given to the patient and the informed consent itself. (Photo © B. Proud.)

but for a nonmalicious, justifiable purpose (eg, proof of consent, truth, privilege, or fair comment).

Invasion of Privacy

The US Supreme Court has interpreted the right against invasion of privacy as inherent in the US Constitution. The Fourth Amendment gives citizens the right of privacy and the right to be left alone. State courts have also been strong in protecting a patient's right to have information kept confidential. The doctrine of privileged communication specifies that individuals in a protected relationship, such as a doctor and patient, cannot be forced, even during legal proceedings, to reveal communication between them unless the person who benefits from the protection agrees to it. State laws determine which relationships are protected by the privilege doctrine, and not all states privilege nurse–patient communication. Disclosure of confidential information, such as inappropriately discussing a patient's problem with a third party, may be construed as invasion of privacy and may subject the nurse to liability. The nurse's intimate knowledge of the patient increases legal risk in this regard.

Certain acts by nurses could constitute invasion of privacy, as the following examples illustrate:

- Unnecessary exposure of patients while moving them through health agency corridors or while caring for them in rooms they share with others
- Talking with patients in rooms that are not soundproof
- Discussing patient information with people not entitled to the information (eg, with the patient's employer or the press)

- Pressing the patient for information not necessary for care planning
- Interacting with the patient's family in ways not authorized by the patient
- Using tape recorders, dictating machines, computers, and the like without taking precautions to ensure the patient's confidentiality (see accompanying box: Privacy and Confidentiality of Healthcare Records)
- Preparing written or oral class assignments about patients without concealing their identity
- Carrying out research without taking proper precautions to ensure the anonymity of patients

At times, an individual's right to privacy may conflict with other rights, such as the public's right to information. When in doubt about disclosing confidential information, the nurse should consult the nursing supervisor, ethics committee, or public relations department of the institution.

False Imprisonment

Unjustified retention or prevention of the movement of another person without proper consent can constitute false imprisonment. For example, only a reasonable amount of restraint should be used in circumstances that warrant it. The indiscriminate and thoughtless use of restraints on a patient can constitute the act of false imprisonment.

A person cannot be legally forced to remain in a health agency, such as a hospital, if he or she is of sound mind, even when health practitioners believe the person should remain for additional care. Health agencies have special forms to use when a patient insists on being discharged

---

Privacy and Confidentiality of Healthcare Records

The American Nurses Association *Code for Nurses* (1985) states. "The nurse safeguards the patient's right to privacy by judiciously protecting information of a confidential manner." It addresses the patient's right to privacy, protection of information, and access to records.

Security measures that a nurse can be aware of, particularly when using computerized healthcare records, include the following:

- Authorized users of an automated information system should have individual passwords and identification codes that are changed frequently.
- Terminals, including those at the point of care, should have key locks as an additional measure to prevent unauthorized access to data.
- The computer system should "time out" when not in use for a specific period of time. The authorized user would need to reenter the password and identification code to regain access.
- Temporary employees, such as traveling nurses, should have temporary passwords assigned.

- Employees who leave the organization should have their passwords and IDs terminated.
- The system should be able to track which users viewed, deleted, or updated patient information.
- Some information, such as results of acquired immunodeficiency syndrome testing, should not be stored on a computer.
- Computer printouts must be discarded appropriately because they may contain sensitive data about a patient.
- Your organization should have a policy regarding the use of patient data in research patient identifiers should be removed before the data are analyzed.
- Every nurse must be aware of the laws and statutes that protect the confidentiality of medical records. Most states have guidelines on the sharing of medical information. Your State Board of Nursing may revoke your license for serious breaches of patient confidentiality.

Protecting the privacy and confidentiality of healthcare records is the duty of every nurse (McMullen & Philipsen, 1996).

against medical orders. The patient signs to indicate that he or she does not hold the agency responsible for any harm that may result from leaving. People who are mentally ill may be committed to a psychiatric institution for treatment without their consent (involuntary commitment) only when it can be proved that they may be harmful to themselves or others.

Fraud

Fraud is willful and purposeful misrepresentation that could cause, or has caused, loss or harm to a person or property. Misrepresentation of a product is a common fraudulent act. A person fraudulently misrepresenting himself or herself to obtain a license to practice nursing may be prosecuted under the state's nurse practice act. Also, misrepresenting the outcome of a procedure or treatment may constitute fraud.

Unintentional Torts

Negligence and Malpractice

Negligence is defined as performing an act that a reasonably prudent person under similar circumstances would not do or, conversely, failing to perform an act that a reasonably prudent person under similar circumstances would do. As the definition implies, an act of negligence may be an act of omission or commission. **Malpractice** is the term generally used to describe negligence by professional personnel. See the example in Table 7-1.

Elements of Liability

Liability involves four elements that must be established to prove that malpractice or negligence has occurred: duty, breach of duty, causation, and damages. *Duty* refers to an obligation to use due care (what a reasonably prudent nurse would do) and is defined by the standard of care appropriate for the nurse–patient relationship. *Breach of duty* is the failure to meet the standard of care. *Causation*, the most difficult element of liability to prove, shows the failure to meet the standard of care (breach) actually caused the injury. *Damages* are the actual harm or injury resulting to the patient. Examples of these four elements are presented in Table 7-1.

Standards of Care

Whether negligence has occurred depends on a standard of care—what a reasonably prudent person would or would not have done under similar circumstances.

All nurses are responsible for following the standards of care for their particular areas of practice. For example, labor and delivery nurses must understand how standards for nursing practice differ from those for medical obstetric practice (according to the state's nurse practice act), must be familiar with specific standards for obstetric nursing (eg, Standards of the Nurses' Association of the American College of Obstetricians and Gynecologists), and must carry out the nursing responsibilities detailed in the hospital's policies and procedures and in their job description. If hospital policy dictates an assessment of each woman in the early stages of labor every 30 minutes, nurses must adhere

Table 7-1
Proof of Malpractice

An example of how a plaintiff (person bringing the lawsuit) proves that the nurse defendants are guilty of malpractice.

Element	Example
Duty	Hospital staff nurses are responsible for • Accurate assessment of patients assigned to their care • Alerting responsible healthcare professionals to changes in a patient's condition • Competent execution of safety measures for patients
Breach of duty	• Failure to note and report that an elderly patient assessed as alert on admission is exhibiting periods of confusion • Failure to execute and document use of appropriate safety measures (eg, upper and lower bedside rails, use of restraints if necessary, assisted ambulation)
Causation	• Failure to use appropriate safety measures; this failure causes the patient to fall while attempting to get out of bed, resulting in a fractured left hip
Damages	• Fractured left hip, pain and suffering, lengthened hospital stay, and need for rehabilitation

to this standard unless they document a reason for doing otherwise.

Table 7-2 lists areas of potential liability associated with each of the ANA standards of clinical nursing practice. Although any nurse can make an error, nursing errors can result in serious outcomes for the patient, as these examples show.

Malpractice Litigation

When a patient believes that he or she has been injured because of the negligence of a nurse or other healthcare professional and pursues legal action, one of three outcomes usually occurs:

• All parties work toward a fair settlement.
• The case is presented to a malpractice arbitration panel (in the United States).
• The case is brought to trial court.

The steps involved in malpractice litigation are as follows:

1. The basis for the claim is appropriate and timely; all elements of liability are present: duty, breach of duty, causation, serious damages.

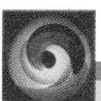

Table 7-2
Areas of Potential Liability for Nurses

Areas of Potential Liability	Examples
Standard I: Assessment The nurse collects patient health data. • Incomplete database obtained (occurs frequently when patient is too ill at admission to respond to questions) • Significant omissions or errors in recording database • Failure to note in the patient's plan of care (and to execute) need for more frequent nursing assessments • Failure to recognize and to report significant changes in the patient's condition	• Child too weak to be weighed on admission; chart contains no record of patient's weight; dosage of postoperative antibiotic therapy (which should be calculated on child's weight) too small to prevent infection; abscess develops • Nurse fails to detect and report observable signs that an older patient is at risk for abuse in her home from her granddaughter • Previously alert patient was exhibiting periods of confusion; found beating roommate with a hairbrush • Mother's labor is failing to progress, nurses unaware of signs of fetal distress; obstetrician not informed; irreversible cerebral damage to fetus • Healthy patient making slower than usual postanesthesia recovery; signs of developing cerebrovascular accident (slurred speech, difficulty moving extremities, falling to one side) present and unnoted
Standard II: Diagnosis The nurse analyzes the assessment data in determining diagnoses. • Failure to identify priority nursing diagnosis critical to the patient's care • Nursing diagnosis incorrectly developed and "labels" the patient negatively	• Nowhere in the resident's plan of care was it noted that the patient had a history of choking on food ("impaired swallowing") and that close supervision was indicated during meals; patient aspirated brussel sprout and died. • Homosexual male patient without acquired immunodeficiency syndrome (AIDS) admitted for gallbladder surgery questions the few interactions he has with staff, nursing diagnosis on cardex reads "High Risk for Violence: Directed at Others (AIDS), related to homosexuality"
Standard III and IV: Outcome Identification and Planning The nurse identifies expected outcomes individualized to the patient. • No indication in nursing care plan that nurses were aware of and sensitive to the patient's healthcare priorities	The nurse develops a plan of care that prescribes interventions to attain expected outcomes. • Obese patient with a history of impaired circulation continually refuses to ambulate after major abdominal surgery; patient dies after a massive pulmonary embolism; plan of care showed no concern or attempt to compensate for patient's lack of mobility; family states no nurse consulted them to encourage mobility
Standard V: Implementation The nurse implements the interventions identified in the plan of care. • Patient's record contains no documentation of attempts to teach appropriate self-care measures to patient and family • Nursing interventions deviate from usual standard of care (understaffing, indifference on part of nurse, inexperience of nurse, faulty or scarce equipment or resources)	• Male patient discharged from short-procedure unit on crutches; falls first day home, refracturing leg; alleges his not receiving instructions for crutch-walking caused fall; patient record contains no documentation of client education • Skin breakdown on frail, older homebound patient worsens with eventual muscle deterioration; sepsis; nurses seem confused about treatment regimen for pressure ulcers; treatment is inconsistent

(continued)

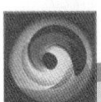

Table 7-2 (Continued)

Areas of Potential Liability	Examples
Standard VI: Evaluation	
The nurse evaluates the patient's progress toward attainment of outcomes. • No evidence in plan of care and nursing notes that nurses evaluated whether the patient achieved target goals • Patient discharged before key goals are met and without follow-up instruction	• Male patient newly started on insulin therapy discharged without understanding the relationship among food, exercise, and insulin and after giving himself the insulin only once—no referral made to visiting nurse; patient readmitted after 2 weeks with dangerously low blood sugar after overdose with insulin

Standards of care from American Nurses Association (1991). *Standards of clinical nursing practice*, Kansas City, MO: ANA.

2. All parties named as defendants (nurses, physicians, healthcare agency), as well as insurance companies and attorneys, work toward a fair settlement
3. The case is presented to a malpractice arbitration panel. The panel's decision is either accepted or rejected, in which case a complaint is filed in trial court
4. The defendants contest allegations (believe there is no basis for alleging deviation from the appropriate standard of care or for proving causation and damages).
5. Pretrial discovery activities: review of medical records and depositions of plaintiff, defendants, and witnesses
6. Trial
7. Decision or verdict reached
8. If the verdict is not accepted by both sides, it may be appealed to an appellate court.

The nurse may be involved in legal proceedings as a defendant, a fact witness, or an expert witness.

Nurse as Defendant

A nurse who is named a defendant should work closely with an attorney while preparing the defense. The attorney representing the nurse's interests is secured by either the nurse (if carrying personal liability insurance) or the employing agency. Recommendations for the nurse defendant include the following:

Do not discuss the case with anyone at your agency (with the exception of the risk manager), with the plaintiff, with the plaintiff's lawyer, with anyone testifying for the plaintiff, or with reporters.
Do not alter the patient's records. Tampering with a chart is the worst mistake you can make—you may well ruin your defense.
Cooperate fully with your attorney. Do not hide any information from your lawyer. Make sure that you are fully prepared before you go on the witness stand.
Be courteous on the witness stand. Do not volunteer any information.

Nurse as Fact Witness

A nurse who has knowledge of the actual incident prompting the legal case may be called by either attorney to testify as a **fact witness.** Fact witnesses, who are placed under oath, must base their testimony on only firsthand knowledge of the incident and not on assumptions. The nurse will be asked if the testimony is based on independent recollection of the incident or on documentation in the patient record. The nurse may testify, "I do not remember Ms. Jones but I see from review of her record that I cared for her on the evenings of June 10, 13, 14, and 17." When in doubt about facts, the nurse should simply testify, "I do not remember that." New research into memory is showing that people often remember things differently from the way they were; this challenges the value of eyewitness memory. Thus, accurate documentation remains the nurse's best defense.

Nurse as Expert Witness

A nurse may be called by either attorney to testify as an **expert witness:** to explain to the judge and jury what happened based on the patient's record and to offer an opinion about whether the nursing care met acceptable standards. Nurse expert witnesses need a solid educational background and strong clinical experience comparable with those of the nurse defendant. The expert witness also needs an understanding of the legal aspects of nursing and malpractice liability and knowledge of the state nurse practice act and the standard of nursing care where the incident occurred.

Legal Safeguards for the Nurse

Contracts

A *contract* may be defined as the exchange of promises between two parties. The agreement may be in writing or oral—although oral contracts may be more difficult to prove. The law of contracts provides a remedy for a breach of contract so that the person who suffers from a broken contract may be compensated for any resulting loss. For a contract to be legally enforceable, it must involve real consent of the parties, a valid consideration, a lawful purpose, competent parties, and the format required by law.

Practicing nurses enter into legally valid and binding contracts with both their employers and their patients. It is thus important that they understand and are able to fulfill the terms of their agreement before giving consent. Your employment contract should specify what it is reasonable for you to expect of you employer and what the employer can expect of you. An employer that repeatedly expects you to assume supervisory responsibilities without benefit or who fires you without just cause is most likely guilty of contract violations. Similarly, you may be guilty of contract violations if you refuse to accept reasonable assignments, repeatedly fail to arrive on time for work, or are habitually unable to complete reasonable work assignments. Any action by your employer that violates a federal or state law would be the basis of a grievance, even if the employment contract permits the action. Examples include a female nurse receiving less pay for performing the same work as a male nurse or a supervisor's failure to promote on the basis of race. When discrimination is suspected, complaints should be filed with the Equal Employment Opportunity Commission (EEOC). Contracts with patients are often implied. There may not be a written contract specifying what is reasonable for patients to expect of nurses, but courts will uphold that an implied contract exists obligating the nurse to be competent and to provide responsible care.

Collective Bargaining

Although individual contracts serve many nurses adequately, an increasing number of nurses have joined other groups of workers in finding their interests better protected when contracts are negotiated for them as a group. Collective bargaining is a legal process in which representatives of organized employees negotiate with employers about such matters as wages, hours, and conditions. Arbitration, strikes, and threats of strikes may be used to enhance the terms of employment and to enforce contracts. Many nurses choose their state nurses' association, versus a trade organization, as their collective bargaining representative. Other nurses question whether collective bargaining is an appropriate role for a professional organization to play. The Springhouse *Nurse's Legal Handbook* recommends asking the following questions before deciding whether to participate in collective bargaining:

- Will collective bargaining help my professional and economic status?
- Can I address my professional concerns through collective bargaining?
- Can I devote the time and effort that such organized activity demands?
- Can I change my working conditions as an individual, or do I need to organize with other nurses (Shaw, 1996, p. 261)?

Competent Practice

Competent practice remains the nurse's most important and best legal safeguard (Fig. 7-2). Each nurse is responsible for making sure that his or her educational background and clinical experience are adequate to fulfill the nursing responsibilities described in the job description. Legal safeguards include the following:

- Respecting legal boundaries of practice
- Following institutional procedures and policies
- "Owning" personal strengths and weaknesses; seeking means of growth, education, and supervised experience to ensure continued competence for new and evolving responsibilities
- Evaluating proposed assignments; refusing to accept responsibilities for which the nurse is unprepared
- Keeping current
- Respecting patient rights and developing rapport with patients
- Keeping careful documentation
- Working within the agency to develop and support management policies

Competent practice includes developing sensitivity to common sources of patient injury, such as falls, use of restraints, and malfunctioning equipment, and then taking specific measures to prevent patient injury. The accompanying box, Nursing Malpractice Prevention, lists the most frequent allegations against nurses and related prevention tips.

Patient Education

US courts affirm the patient's right to know and view patient education as the legal duty of the nurse. Standards for patient education are derived from national professional standards and from state nurse practice acts as well as the local standards described in agency policies, procedure manuals, and job descriptions. Special forms for documenting the nurse's assessment of the patient's learning needs and for subsequent teaching are available in some agencies. Failure to conduct or document the assessment of learning needs and teaching may later be construed as negligence.

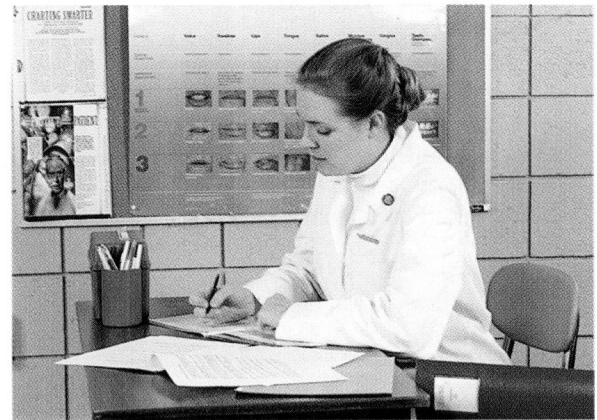

Figure 7-2
Competent practice is the nurse's most important legal safeguard. Careful documentation is the key to competent practice. (Photo © B. Proud.)

Nursing Malpractice Prevention

Most Frequent Allegations Against Nurses and Related Prevention Tips

1. **Failure to ensure patient safety**

   Monitor patients in a timely manner. Assess and document potential for injury. Incorporate safety needs into plan of care.

   Clearly define criteria for use of restrictive devices. Ensure that the use of restrictive devices is consistent with agency policy. Use the least restrictive devices that will be effective in preventing injury.

   Update knowledge on patient safety and new interventions to prevent and reduce injury.

   Evaluate whether patients at high risk for injury are routinely being identified before injury results.

2. **Improper treatment or performance of treatment**

   Question treatments you believe are improper. Know your agency's policy for questioning a problematic order.

   Use proper techniques when performing procedures, and follow agency procedures.

   Seek assistance when unsure of a new procedure. Never perform an intervention until you know what you are doing, why you are doing it, and your ongoing assessment and teaching responsibilities.

   Update your clinical skills through continuing education classes, conferences, and workshops.

3. **Failure to monitor and report**

   Follow physician orders regarding monitoring of patients unless changes in the patient's condition necessitate a change in the frequency of monitoring; report need for change to the physician.

   Report any requested information or significant changes in a patient's condition. If unsure of the significance of an observed change, consult with an experienced colleague.

   Perform appropriate and timely nursing assessments.

   Ensure that the nurse–patient ratio is adequate.

4. **Medication errors and reactions**

   Verify any questionable medical orders.

   Verify patient's name before administering medication.

   Listen to patients objections regarding medication and investigate patient's concerns *before* administering the medication.

   Refer to a drug reference for any questions about appropriate dosages, side effects, and reactions.

   Know your agency's policies on verbal and written medication orders and on medication administration.

   Update your knowledge of medications and new medication administration protocols.

5. **Failure to follow agency procedure**

   Know your agency's procedures. Ensure that your orientation to new responsibilities familiarizes you with pertinent policies and procedures.

   If you must deviate from a procedure, discuss the incident with your supervisor and decide on appropriate action.

   Advise the appropriate person of procedures that need to be revised.

6. **Documentation**

   Document significant information about your patients objectively and factually.

   Know and follow the agency's documentation policies.

   Be time specific about the information, such as when you performed actions, made observations, or performed patient assessments.

   Document legibly when writing, spell correctly, and use only agency-approved abbreviations.

   Be sensitive to privacy considerations when documenting on a computer.

   Routinely evaluate the quality of documentation and update your knowledge of new documentation methodologies.

7. **Equipment use**

   Learn how to operate equipment in a safe and appropriate manner. *Never* operate equipment with which you are unfamiliar.

   Use predetermined procedures when teaching patients how to use equipment and ensure that all the nurses involved in client education are teaching the same procedures.

   Provide home care patients with the telephone number of a 24-hour backup hospital or home care service available in case of emergency.

   Have patients demonstrate their competence with equipment before allowing them to use it.

   Attend orientations and in-services on the use of new or modified equipment.

8. **Adverse incidents**

   When adverse incidents occur, complete the appropriate documentation and report the incident to the designated individual after agency policy.

   Do not assume, voice, or record any blame for the incident.

   Know the institutional chain of command for reporting instances when patient care is at issue.

   Support agency loss prevention programs that identify potential liabilities, guard against patient injuries, and maximize the defense of the agency and its employee nurses.

(continued)

Nursing Malpractice Prevention (*Continued*)

9. **Clients with human immunodeficiency virus (HIV)**
   Be conscious of actions that could result in a lawsuit:
   Discrimination in treatment
   Nosocomial (in-hospital) transmission of virus
   Breach of confidentiality
   Participation in testing a patient for HIV without first obtaining informed consent.

Know and follow agency policies and procedures for the care of patients with infectious diseases.
Update your knowledge of HIV infection; be familiar with national standards (such as those established by the Centers for Disease Control) and pertinent state/province laws.

Adapted in part from *American Nurse,* June 1989, p. 28.

General guidelines for nurses carrying out patient education responsibilities competently include the following:

- Determine in your practice setting what specific aspects of patient education are the responsibility of nursing. Consult your job description, and be familiar with agency policies regarding patient education and its documentation.
- Remember that an important aim of nursing is to assist patients in managing their own care. Discuss the nursing plan of care with the patient and family, and identify their learning needs and learning readiness. Document the teaching plan as part of the nursing plan of care. Document all nursing efforts to educate the patient and family about healthcare management, and also document the patient's response. If a patient refuses health education or refers the nurse to a family member (eg, "Talk to my wife about my pills, she'll be giving them to me at home"), document this in the patient's record. If patient education greatly increases the patient's anxiety and the patient requests not to be given any more information, the nurse should document the patient's initial response to teaching, the patient's request that it be stopped, and, if the nurse complied, the reason for doing so.
- Because a lack of time is a frequently offered reason for failing to document patient education, nurses should assess what type of patient documentation is routinely performed. If possible, they should develop forms or checklists that will facilitate rapid documentation. For example, preoperative checklists have greatly facilitated the recording of preoperative teaching and are often introduced as evidence in court that preoperative teaching was done. Other successful models include forms for documenting diabetic patient teaching, teaching after a myocardial infarction, and teaching postpartum and baby care to mothers. The teaching role of the nurse is discussed in Chapter 22.

Executing Physician Orders

Nurses are legally responsible for carrying out the orders of the physician in charge of a patient unless an order would

lead a reasonable person to anticipate injury if it were carried out. Guidelines when executing orders follow:

1. Be familiar with the parties designated in your nurse practice act who can legally write orders for the nurse to execute (in many states, a physician's assistant cannot legally write orders for the nurse).
2. Be familiar with your institutional or agency policy regarding physician orders.
3. Attempt to get all physician's orders in writing. Verbal and telephone orders should be countersigned within 24 hours. Take the following steps to eliminate errors caused by telephone orders:
   a. Limit telephone orders to true emergency situations in which there is no alternative.
   b. Designate which nurses may take telephone orders (eg, those who have more education and experience, such as primary nurses).
   c. Repeat a telephone order back to the physician for confirmation.
   d. Document the order, its time and date, the situation necessitating the order, the physician prescribing and reconfirming the order as it is read back, and your name; indicate if the order is a VO (verbal order) or TO (telephone order).
   e. When telephone extensions make this possible, have two nurses listen to a questionable telephone order, with both nurses countersigning the order.
4. Question any physician order that is:
   a. Ambiguous
   b. Contraindicated by normal practice (eg, dose of medication that is abnormally high)
   c. Contraindicated by the patient's present condition (eg, as a patient's present condition improves, he or she may no longer need aggressive forms of treatment).

It is good practice for the nurse to double check any order a patient questions.

Documentation

Documentation is discussed in Chapter 20; this chapter addresses only the legal implications of documentation. Although most nurses prefer to spend their time interacting with patients rather than writing in a patient's record, careful documentation is a crucial legal safeguard for the nurse. Documentation must be factual, accurate, complete, and entered in a timely fashion. The presumption of the law is that if something was not documented, it was not done. This includes even routine acts, such as taking vital signs, repositioning patients, and ensuring the patient's safety.

Nurses should be sure that the nursing plan of care is part of the patient's permanent record. Agencies should have flow sheets or some type of documentation form that enables nurses to check off routine aspects of care rapidly and completely. The nurse should write a comprehensive nursing note for each patient problem the nurse addressed during his or her time of duty. The note should include the current nature of the problem, how the nurse intervened, the patient's response, and, when appropriate, future priorities for care. After a problem is noted, nursing documentation should demonstrate continuity of care until the problem is resolved.

A common problem reported by nurses is not knowing how to document an incident, for example, when the nurse believes the patient needs medical attention and intervention but the responsible physicians are not responding to calls for assistance. In this case, the best legal safeguard for the nurse is to document the facts of the incident, being careful not to make incriminatory statements, such as, "Anyone could see we were losing this patient rapidly" or "Once again, Dr. Jones was unavailable when her patient needed her." The note should document the time the physician was called, the time of response or lack of response, and the subsequent nursing response (eg, nursing supervisor notified). Such a note documents that the nurse is carefully assessing the patient, recognizing significant cues, and reporting them appropriately. The nursing supervisor should write the next note after reviewing the case and choosing a course of action. Patient noncompliance with a treatment should also be documented along with the nurse's attempts to increase compliance.

Adequate Staffing

Understaffing is a problem that results in reduced quality of nursing care and may jeopardize patient safety. Temporary management solutions to understaffing, such as floating nurses from one unit to another or asking nurses to work overtime or double (back-to-back) shifts, are ineffective because they can further jeopardize patient safety. A nurse in an understaffed agency will be held to a professional standard of judgment with respect to accepting responsibility for work and for delegating nursing responsibilities to others. Thus, if a patient claims negligent care, a nurse who claims that she was overworked that evening because of an unrealistic assignment does not have adequate grounds for a legal defense. If patient injury results, the agency and nurse employee will most likely be named as codefendants. Some state nursing associations are using "protest of assignment forms" to track employer practices of routine understaffing.

Professional Liability Insurance

Although a nurse's best legal safeguard is always competent practice, the increasing number of malpractice claims naming nurses as defendants makes it wise for nurses to carry their own liability insurance. Nurses may obtain this insurance through ANA and other nursing associations and other sources.

Reasons the ANA (1990) lists for purchasing a personal professional liability insurance policy are as follows:

Protection of the nurse's best interests. If the nurse is named defendant in a malpractice action along with the agency, a conflict of interest could arise between the nurse and the agency. Nurses have no assurance of their best interest being represented unless they have their own coverage, which provides their own attorney.

Limitations of employer's coverage. Most healthcare facilities carry "claims made" insurance, which means that if the nurse is no longer working there or the facility closes, the nurse is not covered when a claim is filed.

Care or advice given outside of work. An employer's policy only covers the nurse within the confines of the work setting.

Risk Management Programs

Hoping to reduce malpractice claims, many healthcare agencies have initiated risk management programs designed to identify, analyze, and treat risks. Elements of a comprehensive risk management program include the following:

Safety program. The aim is to provide a safe environment in which the basic safety needs of patients, employees, and visitors are met.

Products safety program. The aim is to ensure safe and adequate equipment; this involves ongoing equipment evaluation and maintenance.

Quality assurance program. The aim is to provide quality healthcare to patients; this involves ongoing evaluation of all systems used in the care of the patient.

Nurses with legal questions often find risk managers a helpful resource.

Incident, Variance, or Occurrence Reports

An incident report, also called a variance or occurrence report, is used by healthcare agencies to document the occurrence of anything out of the ordinary that results in or has the potential to result in harm to a patient, employee, or visitor. (See the Incident Report in the accompanying example.) These reports are used for quality improvement and should not be used for disciplinary action against staff members. They are a means of identifying risks. More harm than good results from ignoring mistakes. Incident reports improve the management and treatment of patients

Medication Occurrence Information Report/PI
Send completed form to Risk Management
This Document is part of a quality improvement process
CONFIDENTIAL: Do Not PHOTOCOPY
Do Not File in Patient Record
All Sections Must Be Completed

ADDRESSOGRAPH

Patient age:_____

Definition of occurrence: Any preventable event that may cause or lead to inappropriate medication use or patient harm while the medication is in the control of the healthcare professional, patient, or consumer. Such events may be related to professional practice, healthcare products, procedures and systems, including prescribing, order communication, product labeling, packaging and nomenclature; compounding; dispensing; distribution; administration; education; monitoring; and use.

Section A: Report filed by (please print): _____ Title: _____ Date/Time: _____
Location of event
Floor/Unit: _____ Date of event: _____ Time of event (24 hour): _____ ☐ Inpatient ☐ Outpatient

Error discovered: ☐ Within same shift ☐ Within 24 hours ☐ Greater than 24 hours

Staff involved in initial error: ☐ Staff RN ☐ Agency RN ☐ Pharmacist ☐ NP ☐ House staff ☐ Attending MD Name: _____
Other staff also involved (ie perpetuated the error): ☐ Staff RN ☐ Agency RN ☐ Pharmacist ☐ Physician

Staff that discovered error: ☐ Staff RN ☐ Agency RN ☐ Pharmacist ☐ Physician

Physician notified? ☐ No ☐ Yes Date: _____ Time: _____ Attending: _____

Section B: Medication type:
  ☐ IV
  ☐ Non-IV

Medication(s) involved:
A. _____
B. _____

Incident documented in medical record? ☐ Yes ☐ No
Patient/family aware of incident? ☐ Yes ☐ No
(If yes, please comment below)

TYPE OF ERROR *(See reverse for definitions)*	**BREAKDOWN POINT** *(Where in process did the initial error occur?)*	**BREAKDOWN POINT** *(Where in process did the initial error occur?)* *(continued from the previous column)*

☐ Prescribing
☐ Omission—Total #
_____ Schedule: _____
☐ Monitoring error
☐ Wrong patient
☐ Wrong time
☐ Wrong route
☐ Wrong dose/quantity/extra dose
• dose ordered _____
• dose given _____
☐ Medication D/C'd, given
• extra doses:
_____
☐ Wrong drug
• med ordered _____
• med given _____
☐ Medication not ordered
• med given _____
• dose _____
☐ Wrong drug preparation
☐ Wrong rate of administration
☐ Given to patient with known allergy
☐ Investigational protocol not followed
☐ Other _____
	☐ Prescribing
	circle:
	• illegible handwriting
	• wrong chart/order sheet
	• incorrect order
	• incomplete order
	• other, please describe below
	☐ Order processing
	circle:
	• carbon not pulled/pulled late
	• order not transcribed
	• transcribed incorrectly
	• other, please describe below
	☐ Dispensing
	circle:
	• incorrectly entered into computer by pharmacist/not entered at all
	• wrong strength sent
	• wrong med sent
	• label incorrect/unclear
	• delay in delivery of medication
	• other, please describe below
	
	(continued next column)
		☐ Administration
		circle:
		• med given, but not charted
		• med charted, but not given
		• held med given
		• incorrect medication taken from floorstock/Pyxis and given
		• incorrect dose/rate calculation
		• pump error
		  –tubing clamped
		  –incorrect rate setting
		  –pump malfunction
		  –pump turned off
		☐ Other, please describe below

ERROR SEVERITY/OUTCOME

☐ **Category A:** Circumstances or events that have the capacity to cause error
☐ **Category B:** Error occurred; medication not given
☐ **Category C:** Medication given but did not cause patient harm
☐ **Category D:** Resulted in the need for increased patient monitoring but no harm
☐ **Category E:** Resulted in the need for treatment or intervention and caused temporary patient harm
☐ **Category F:** Resulted in initial or prolonged hospitalization and caused temporary patient harm
☐ **Category G:** Resulted in permanent patient harm
☐ **Category H:** Resulted in a near-death event (eg anaphylaxis, cardiac arrest)
☐ **Category I:** Resulted in patient death

COMMENTS/DESCRIBE EVENT (include any intervention/treatment given and outcome):

_____
_____
_____

(continued on next page)

Section C: ANALYSIS/RECOMMENDATIONS/ACTION PLAN *(Manager to complete):*

<u>Possible causes:</u> ☐ abbreviation ☐ calculation error ☐ communication confusing/intimidating/lacking
☐ computer order entry ☐ decimal point/leading zero missing/trailing zero ☐ equipment design ☐ facsimile order ☐ handwriting illegible ☐ inexperienced staff ☐ staffing level ☐ labeling (GUMC) confusing/incomplete/inaccurate ☐ labeling (manufacturer) confusing/incomplete/inaccurate ☐ similar name ☐ patient identification ☐ shift change ☐ floating staff ☐ poor lighting
☐ performance deficit ☐ preparation error ☐ procedure/protocol not followed ☐ reference manual confusing/inaccurate/unclear/outdated
☐ verbal order confusing/incomplete/misunderstood ☐ written order confusing/incomplete/misunderstood ☐ other _____

_____

_____

_____

Signature of Manager: _____   Date: _____

Used with permission. Georgetown University Medical Center.

---

by identifying high-risk patterns and initiating in-service programs to prevent future problems. These forms also make all the facts about an incident available to the agency in case of litigation.

The nurse responsible for a potentially or actually harmful incident or who witnesses an injury is the one who fills in the incident form. This form should contain the complete name of the person or people involved and the names of all witnesses; a complete factual account of the incident; the date, time, and place of the incident; pertinent characteristics of the person or people involved (eg, alert, ambulatory, asleep) and of any equipment or resources being used; and any other variables believed to be important to the incident. A physician completes the incident form with documentation of the medical examination of a patient, employee, or visitor with an actual or potential injury.

In some states, incident reports may be used in court as evidence. The nurse documenting a patient incident should include a complete account of what happened in the patient's record; additionally, the nurse should prepare the incident report. Documentation in the patient record, however, should not include the fact that an incident report was filed.

Good Samaritan Laws

Good Samaritan laws are designed to protect health practitioners when they give aid to people in emergency situations. For example, a physician at the scene of an automobile accident may give emergency care without fear of legal suit if such care appears necessary, unless care is given in a grossly negligent manner.

Forty-eight states and the District of Columbia have Good Samaritan laws, although the laws vary considerably. Nurses are covered in some states but not in others.

Except in employment situations, no person has a legal obligation to help another, and a health practitioner, like any other person, may choose to help or to leave the scene of an emergency. In many situations, however, there would appear to be an ethical responsibility to assist. When health practitioners assist a person in an emergency

situation and consent for the care is impossible, they are expected to use good judgment in determining whether an emergency exists and to give care that a reasonably prudent person with a similar background and in a similar circumstance would give.

Student Liability

Student nurses are responsible for their own acts of negligence if these result in patient injury. Moreover, they are held to the same standard of care that would be used to evaluate the actions of a registered nurse. The legal responsibilities of student nurses include careful preparation for each new clinical experience and a duty to notify their clinical instructor if they feel in any way unprepared to carry out a nursing procedure. For no reason should a student attempt a clinical procedure if unsure of the correct steps involved. Student nurses are responsible for being familiar with agency policies and procedures.

A hospital may also be held liable for the negligence of a student nurse enrolled in a hospital-controlled program because the student is considered an employee of the hospital. The status of students enrolled in college and university programs is less clear, as is the liability of the educational institution in which they are enrolled and the healthcare agency offering a site for clinical practice.

Nursing instructors may share a student's responsibility for damages in the event of patient injury if the student's assignment called for clinical skills beyond the student's competency or the instructor failed to provide reasonable and prudent clinical supervision. Because the status of patients can change rapidly, especially in an acute care setting, students should notify their instructor or a staff member of any significant changes in the patient's condition, even if they are unsure of the meaning of these changes.

Most nursing programs require students to carry personal professional liability insurance. School policies provide coverage only for clinical nursing done for educational purposes. Moreover, student nurses who work as nursing assistants or in some other healthcare role are legally permitted to offer only the services contained in their job description.

Even if they feel confident with medication administration, catheter insertion, and other professional nursing acts, they risk disciplinary action when they perform these procedures outside the supervised clinical practice setting.

🌀 Laws Affecting Nursing Practice

Occupational Safety and Health

The Occupational Safety and Health Act of 1970 set legal standards in the United States in an effort to ensure safe and healthful working conditions for men and women. The act, intended to reduce work-related injuries and illnesses, has affected healthcare agencies and has increased certain responsibilities for many nurses. In December 1991, the Occupational Safety and Health Administration (OSHA) published a rule establishing safety standards for workers who may be exposed to bloodborne pathogens in the course of their employment. The following examples illustrate situations that could violate standards, if care is not taken, because of the potential threat to worker safety:

- Use of electrical equipment
- Use of isolation techniques for patients with infectious diseases and the management of contaminated equipment and supplies
- Use of radiation, such as infrared or ultraviolet radiation, sound or radio waves, and laser beams
- Use of chemicals, such as those that are toxic or flammable

The law, which continues to be updated, is specific in its applications, and fines can be severe when infractions are noted. Nurses can assist in implementing this law by promoting health and safety precautions wherever they work. Nurses employed in industrial settings have a particularly important role in conforming to the law's requirements. The US Labor Department created a new Office of Occupational Health Nursing at OSHA to underscore the major role such nurses play in striving for safe and healthful workplaces.

National Practitioner Data Bank

The Health Care Quality Improvement Act of 1986 was enacted to encourage healthcare practitioners to identify and discipline practitioners who engage in unprofessional conduct and to restrict the ability of incompetent practitioners to move from state to state without disclosure of the practitioner's previous performance. When a state licenses, certifies, or registers practitioners, they become subject to the National Practitioner Data Bank requirements. The Act contains two major provisions: (1) immunity from civil damages for peer review and (2) establishment of the National Practitioner Data Bank as an information clearinghouse. Nurses may be reported to the National Practitioner Data Bank for medical malpractice payments, adverse licensure actions, or adverse professional actions.

Reporting Obligations

The unique nature of nurse–patient interactions frequently results in the nurse's having knowledge that a state requires to be reported, such as child abuse, rape, or a communicable disease. Legislation varies in this regard, and the nurse is responsible for knowing what needs to be reported in the local area and to what authority.

Abuse

Nurses are frequently the first member of the public to detect abuse. Abuse includes physical, verbal, sexual, and emotional attack; neglect; and abandonment. Targets of abuse include infants, children, and adult men and women of all ages. Abusers are men and women of all ages, races, socioeconomic groups, and religious backgrounds. Nurses are both ethically and legally obligated to report abuse. In many states, the failure to report actual or suspected abuse is a crime in itself. The law protects individuals who erroneously file a report of suspected abuse in good faith, by suits from alleged abusers.

Controlled Substances

The United States has special laws governing the distribution and use of controlled substances (drugs with abuse potential), such as narcotics, depressants, stimulants, and hallucinogens. Drug-abuse laws are specific, and violations are considered criminal acts. Nursing responsibilities for controlled substances include their storage in special locked compartments and documentation responsibilities.

Impaired Nurses

The stresses involved in nursing and healthcare and the availability of controlled substances combine to make nurses prime candidates for alcohol- and drug-addiction problems. In earlier days, nurses with substance-abuse problems were promptly punished by firing and license suspension. Today, substance abuse is recognized as a treatable disorder, and the objective is to detect problems early and get nurses into treatment. Students are wise to recognize their level of risk and to seek help promptly if they suspect a personal problem or problem for a classmate or colleague. The public's trust and well-being and the well-being of the nurse are both at stake.

Discrimination and Sexual Harassment

Title VII of the Civil Rights Act of 1964 protects employees from discrimination based on race, color, religion, sex, or national origin and provides that pregnant women receive the same protection as other employees and applications. The EEOC, which enforces Title VII, defines sexual harassment as "unwelcome sexual advances, requests for sexual favors, and other verbal or physical conduct of a sexual nature" occurring in the following circumstances:

- Submission to sexual advances is implicitly or explicitly considered a condition of employment.

- Submission to sexual advances is used as a basis for employment decisions.
- Sexual harassment interferes with job performance even if it only creates an intimidating, offensive, or hostile atmosphere. (EEOC, 1980, sections 3950.10 to 3950.11)

People With Disabilities

Observing that there are at least 43 million Americans with physical or mental disabilities and that discrimination against such individuals persists in such crucial areas as employment, housing, public accommodations, education, transportation, communication, and health services, Congress passed the Americans With Disabilities Act (ADA) of 1990. The ADA provides a broad definition of "disability"; it covers any individual who has a physical or mental impairment that substantially limits one or more major life activities or who has a record of such impairment. In addition to covering people who have impairments that have traditionally been perceived as disabilities, the ADA also specifically protects people who have communicable diseases, such as acquired immunodeficiency syndrome or human immunodeficiency virus; people who are recovering from drug or alcohol addiction; and people who are regarded as being disabled, whether or not they are in fact disabled. The ADA imposes two requirements on businesses covered by the Act. First, it prohibits such entities from discriminating against disabled people. Second, it requires covered entities to "reasonably accommodate" individuals who are protected by the Act.

Wills

State and provincial laws regulate requirements for wills. The person who makes a will is called the *testator*. A will describes the intentions of a testator to be carried out upon his or her death. A person who receives money or property from a will is called a *beneficiary*. Nurses are occasionally asked to witness a testator's signing of his or her will and should be familiar with the following guidelines:

- The witness should feel sure that the testator is of sound mind, that is, that the testator knows what he or she is doing and is free of the influence of drugs that could likely distort his or her thinking.
- The witness should feel sure that the testator is acting voluntarily and is not being coerced in any way concerning the terms of his or her will.
- Witnesses should watch the testator sign his or her will, and they should sign in the presence of each other. State law indicates how many witnesses must acknowledge the testator's signature on a will. Two or three witnesses are most commonly required.
- Witnesses to the signature on a will do not need to read it, but they should be sure that the document being signed is a will and not some other type of document.
- In most states, a person who is a beneficiary in a will is disqualified to act as a witness to the testator's signature.

Legal Issues Related to Dying and Death

Legal responsibilities for the dying or deceased patient are discussed in Chapter 32. Legal issues include advance directives, do-not-resuscitate orders, assisted suicide, direct voluntary euthanasia, organ donation, autopsy, and inquest.

Learning Outcomes

After studying this chapter, the learner should be able to accomplish the following:

1. Define key terms used in the chapter.

accreditation	felony
assault	fraud
battery	liability
certification	licensure
common law	litigation
credentialing	malpractice
crime	misdemeanor
defamation of character	negligence
defendant	plaintiff
expert witness	statutory law
fact witness	tort

2. Define law and describe its four sources.
3. Describe the professional and legal regulation of nursing practice.
4. Identify the purpose of credentialing, using as examples accreditation, licensure or registration, and certification.
5. Identify grounds for suspending or revoking a license or registration.
6. Differentiate intentional torts (assault and battery, defamation, invasion of privacy, false imprisonment, fraud) and unintentional torts (negligence).
7. Evaluate personal areas of potential liability in nursing.
8. Describe the legal procedure once a plaintiff files a complaint against a nurse for negligence.
9. Describe the roles of the nurse as defendant, fact witness, and expert witness.
10. Use appropriate legal safeguards in nursing practice.
11. Explain the purpose of incident reports.
12. Describe laws affecting nursing practice.

Critical Thinking Exercises

1. Part of nursing's collaborative responsibilities are to help other practitioners obtain informed and voluntary consent for treatment in difficult situations. How might a nurse facilitate the process of obtaining informed consent in the following situations?
   - A 15-year-old boy with cancer who is tired of therapy needs a new course of chemotherapy.
   - Vietnamese parents who speak little English are being asked to consent to surgery for their newborn.
   - An older adult who has had pain with eating for 6 months is being offered an exploratory laparotomy. She tells the surgeon, "I don't care what you do, just get rid of this pain."
   - Rehabilitation options are being considered for an elderly man who is intermittently confused.
2. You are caring for a recently hospitalized patient who had been living in a retirement community. When his daughters, who tend to be critical, come to visit, they tell you that they hope their father's care here will be better than it is in the retirement community, which they are in the process of suing. How would you respond to the daughters and what, if anything, would you share with other nurses about this incident?
3. Recent lay-offs have reduced the number of professional nurses on your unit, and you are growing increasingly concerned about safety as well as quality issues. What would you do about your concern for your personal liability for inadequate care?
4. When you bring an antipsychotic medication to your alert nursing home resident she refuses to take it saying, "I don't like the way it makes me feel." When you report this to one of the nurses, she tells you that they always crush the medication and administer it in food so that the resident doesn't know what she is getting. How do you respond?

Bibliography

Aiken, T. D., & Catalano, J. T. (1994). *Legal, ethical and political issues in nursing.* Philadelphia: F. A. Davis.

American Nurses Association. (1990). *Liability prevention and you: What nurses and employers need to know.* Washington, DC: ANA.

American Nurses Association. (1994). *Guidelines on reporting incompetent, unethical or illegal practices.* Washington, DC: ANA.

Brent, N. J. (1997). *Nurses and the law: A guide to principles and application.* Philadelphia: W. B. Saunders.

Brown, S. M. (1999). Good Samaritan laws: Protections and limits. *RN, 62*(11), 65–68.

Calfee, B. E. (1995a). Going before the board: How to prepare yourself. *Nursing, 25*(3), 56–58.

Calfee, B. E. (1995b). Was it really wrongful termination? *Nursing, 25*(4), 65.

Calfee, B. E. (1996). Labor laws: Working to protect you. *Nursing, 26*(2); 34–40.

Creighton, H. (1986). *Law every nurse should know* (5th ed.). Philadelphia: W. B. Saunders.

Editors of *Nursing 94.* (1994). Confronting sexual harassment. *Nursing, 24*(10), 48–50.

Equal Employment Opportunity Commission. (1980). Sex discrimination guidelines. In *EEOC rules and regulations.* Chicago: Commerce Clearing House.

Eskreis, T.R. (1998). Seven common legal pitfalls in nursing. *American Journal of Nursing, 98*(4), 34–41.

Fickeissen, J. L. (1990). 56 Ways to get certified. *American Journal of Nursing, 90*(3), 50–57.

Fiesta, J. (1988). *Law and liability for nurses* (2nd ed.). Albany: Delmar Publishers.

Gallagher, R. M., Kany, K. A., Rowell, P. A., & Peterson, C. (1999). ANA's nurse staffing principles. *American Journal of Nursing 99*(4), 50–53.

Grant, A. (1994). Instructor, students and the law. *Canadian Nurse, 90*(10), 53.

Helm, A. (1998). Liability, UAPs, and you. *Nursing, 28*(11), 52–53.

Hutcherson, C., Sheets, V. R., & Williamson, S. H. (1998). What five regulatory trends mean to you. *Nursing, 28*(5), 54–57.

LaDuke, S., & Spital, J. K. (1999). What you should expect from your attorney . . . and what your attorney expects from you. *Nursing, 29*(6), 62–64.

Lammer, M. (1994). Nurses alert! Nurses and the Good Samaritan act. *Concern, 23*(2), 8–9.

Laskowshi-Jones, L. (1998). Reaching beyond the rules: Understanding—and influencing—your scope of practice. *Nursing, 28*(9), 42–48.

Mandell, M. (1986). Ten legal commandments for nurses who get sued. *Nursing Life, 6*(3), 18–21.

Martin, K., & Cepero, K. (1999). You're being deposed? Remain calm. *Nursing, 29*(3), 60–61.

McMullen, P. C., & Philipsen, N. C. (1996). Confidentiality: Computer security and data protection. In B. R. Heller, M. E. Mills, & C. A. Romano (Eds.). *Information management in nursing and health care.* Springhouse, PA: Springhouse.

Moore, G. M. (1993). Surviving a malpractice lawsuit. *Nursing, 23*(10), 55–57.

Polston, M. D. (1999). Whistleblowing: Does the law protect you? *American Journal of Nursing 99*(1), 26–32.

President's Commission for the Study of Ethical Problems in Medicine and Biomedical and Behavioral Research. (1982). *Making healthcare decisions: A report* (Vol. 1). Washington, DC: US Government Printing Office.

Shaw, M. (ed.). (1996). *Nurse's legal handbook* (3rd ed.). Springhouse, PA: Springhouse Corporation.

Smetzer, J. L. (1998). Lesson from Colorado: Beyond blaming individuals. *Nursing, 28*(5), 48–51.

Sorich, M. P. (1994). Nursing malpractice litigation: A personal journey. *MCN, 19*(5), 249–252, 254.

Wilkinson, A. D. (1998). Nursing malpractice. *Nursing 98, 28*(6), 34–39.

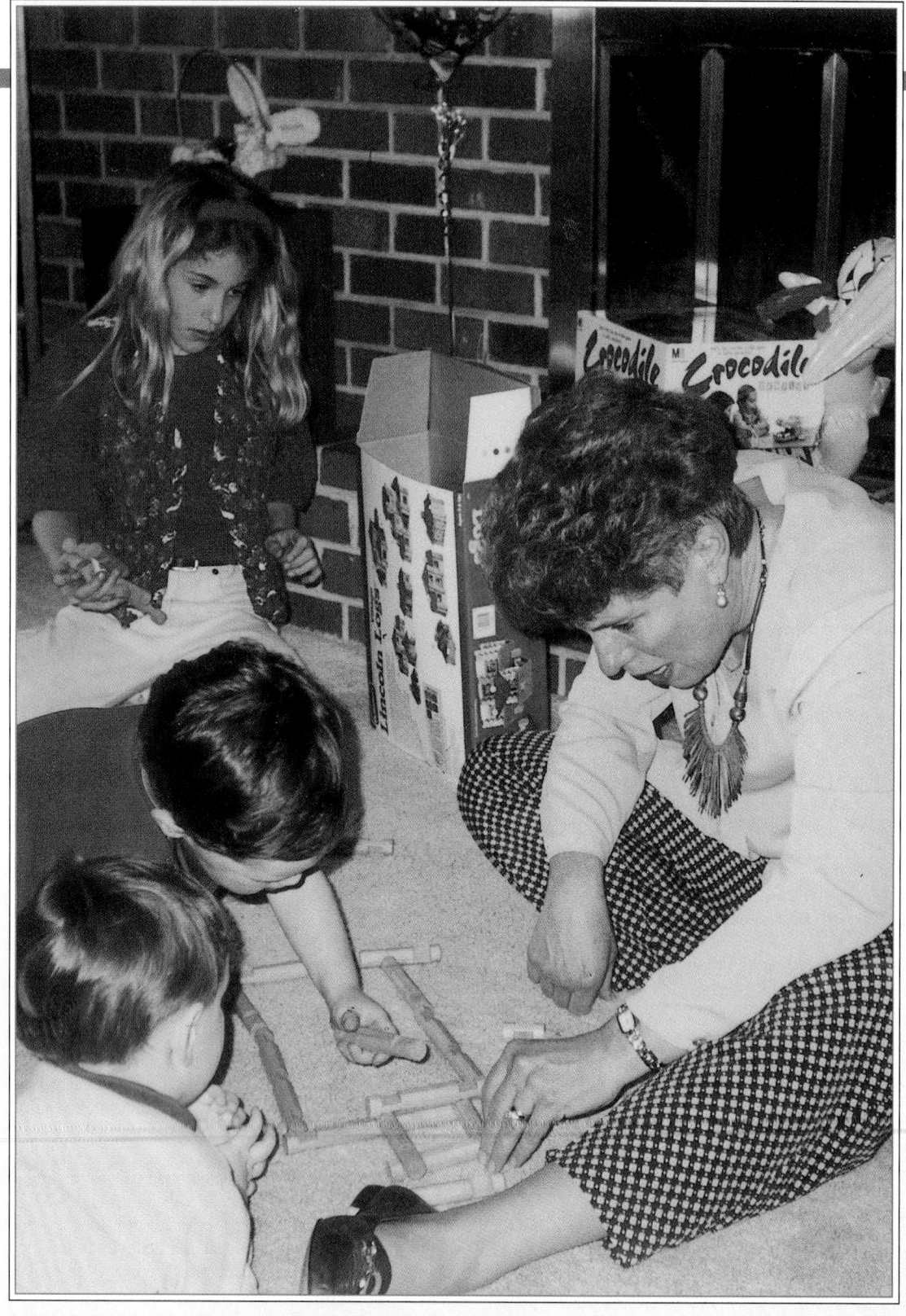

UNIT II

Promoting Health Across the Life Span

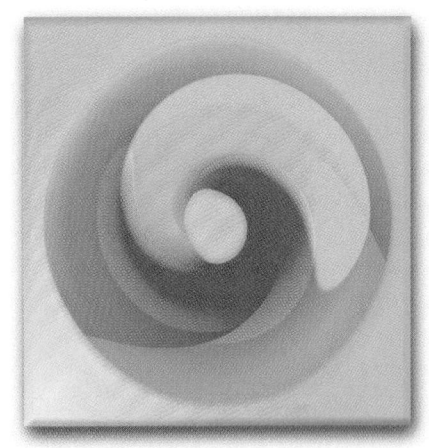

"The concern of nursing is with man in his entirety, his wholeness. Nursing's body of scientific knowledge seeks to describe, explain, and predict about human beings"

Martha Rodgers (1914–1994)
a nationally renowned nurse theoretician, author, lecturer, and consultant whose "theory of man" inspired tremendous creativity, research activity, and intellectual growth in the nursing profession.

The chapters in Unit II focus on the patient and family through the life cycle and on how the nurse provides healthcare for the individual and family. Using foundations presented in Unit I (eg, basic human needs, culture and ethnicity, values and ethics, and legal implications), this unit views the developing individual along a continuum. By considering all aspects of the individual, nurses provide healthcare oriented toward wellness and maximize the patient's strengths to reach his or her potential.

The unit begins with developmental concepts and principles necessary to understanding growth and development across the lifespan. A section on developmental theories gives an overview of major theorists and their contributions to the understanding of psychosocial, physical, cognitive, moral, and faith development. The influence of the family on the individual's growth and development are studied. The application of these concepts and theories to effective nursing is pursued.

The individual is followed through various phases of development, from conception through adolescence. Common health problems of each age group and the role of the nurse for that particular age group are considered.

The adult years are broken down into early, middle, and older-adult stages. Again developmental theories are followed as the adult continues in the life cycle. Common health problems and the nurse's role in healthcare for the adult continue through older adulthood. The unit ends with a look at the paradigm of aging and stereotypes common to the older adult. Gerontology and the healthcare system related to this field are discussed.

Chapter 8
Developmental Concepts

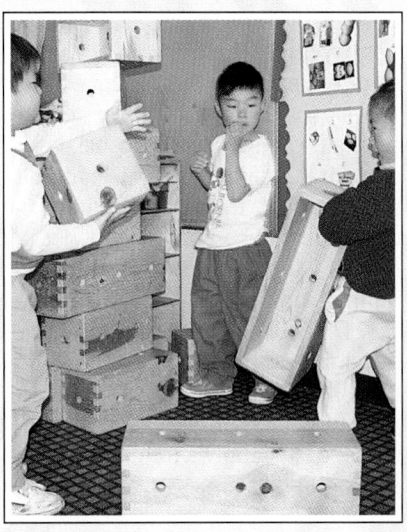

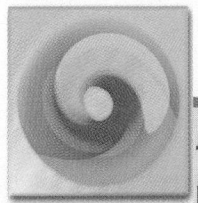

Thinking Critically About
Nursing's Blended Skills

All people, regardless of their age, have unique healthcare needs related to the physical, emotional, intellectual, social, spiritual, and cultural aspects of their developmental level. Think about the types of skills you will need to meet the developmental needs of your patients routinely.

- You have been invited to develop new diabetic instruction aids for both child and adult patients.
- Your hospital is renovating the entire pediatrics department, and it is seeking your input into its design.
- You've joined a neighborhood group committed to helping single mothers succeed.
- Moving from a pediatric rotation to a geriatric rotation, you suddenly realize that you are no longer considering developmental needs when you plan care for your older patients.
- You find yourself wondering what developmental changes an 80-year-old might face.

What cognitive, technical, interpersonal, and ethical/legal skills do you think you will need to respond effectively to the developmental challenges described above?

Nurses promote health in people from birth to death. All people, regardless of age, have unique health-care needs that result from their physical, intellectual, emotional, sociocultural, spiritual, and environmental dimensions at their developmental level. To plan and give holistic and individualized care, the nurse must understand typical growth and development characteristics, tasks, and needs of patients of all ages.

Everyone's physical development has a predetermined genetic base because of inheritance patterns carried on the person's chromosomes. Thus, an unborn child begins life with specific physical attributes. Environmental factors from birth through the early years of growth provide initial psychological and social contact through positive or negative parenting experiences. As environmental influences expand beyond the immediate caregivers or family, a broader range of psychosocial experiences affect development. Cognitive, moral, and spiritual growth are fostered through interactions within the family, school, and community. The nurse can better understand these interrelated variables at specific life stages through theories of human and family development.

This chapter presents basic principles of growth and development that help us understand human beings at various life stages. The major theories examining cognitive, psychosocial, spiritual, and moral development are discussed. The family's influence on personal development is also briefly discussed.

The Nature of Human Growth and Development

The human processes of **growth and development** result from two interrelated factors: heredity and environment. Humans simultaneously grow and develop in physical, cognitive, psychosocial, moral, and spiritual dimensions, with each dimension being an essential part of the whole person. Development is a dynamic and continuous process, characterized by a series of ascents, plateaus, and declines as one proceeds through life. Each phase of development also involves a period of disequilibrium, when adjustment to internal and external demands is more difficult, and a period of equilibrium, when adjustment to demands is more easily made (Erikson, 1963; Mussen, Conger, & Kagan, 1974). If adjustments are not made at the appropriate level of development, one may have difficulties in a later stage of life.

Principles of Growth and Development

Although growth and development occur in individual ways for different people, certain generalizations can be made about the nature of human development for everyone. These generalizations form the principles that help us understand growth and development. The broad generalizations are as follows:

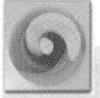

COGNITIVE SKILLS

- Knowledge of Erikson's stages of psychosocial development and related challenges that require nursing assistance, for example, the crisis of ego integrity versus despair experienced by older adults.
- Knowledge of Piaget's theory of cognitive development and its implications for nurse–patient education.
- Knowledge of Kohlberg and Gilligan's theories on moral development and how these relate to the choices a single mother makes for herself and her child.
- Ability to apply theories of growth and development to nurse care planning.

TECHNICAL SKILLS

- Ability to provide the technical nursing assistance necessary to meet the developmental needs of the patients entrusted to your care.

- Ability to use appropriate documentation systems and tools to make a record of practice

INTERPERSONAL SKILLS

- Ability to establish trusting professional relationships with patients of different ages, sensitive to their developmental needs and challenges

ETHICAL/LEGAL SKILLS

- Value for the importance of incorporating theories of growth and development when assessing and planning nursing care for individuals and families
- Ability to advocate for the unmet developmental needs of patients entrusted to your care

Growth and development are orderly and sequential as well as continuous and complex. All humans experience the same growth patterns and developmental levels. Because these patterns and levels are individualized, a wide variation in biologic and behavioral changes is considered normal. Within each developmental level, nonetheless, certain milestones can be identified, for example, the time the infant rolls over, crawls, walks, and says his or her first words.

Growth and development follow regular and predictable trends. Cephalocaudal (proceeding from head to tail) development is the first trend, with the head and brain developing first, followed by the trunk, legs, and feet. Photographs of an infant in utero show the large size of the head compared with the rest of the body (Fig. 8-1). The second trend is proximodistal development, which means that growth progresses from gross motor movements (such as learning to lift one's head) to fine motor movements (such as learning to pick up a toy with the fingers). The last trend is symmetric development of the body, with both sides of the body developing equally.

Growth and development are both differentiated and integrated. As nerve pathways develop, they become more specialized, allowing the growing child to respond to different stimuli. Throughout the life span, each new learned ability builds on previous learning and abilities, so that increasingly complex tasks can be accomplished. For example, the toddler learning to use a spoon combines motor skills, hand–eye coordination, cognitive patterning, and social imitation from watching others to repeat an act when appropriate. As children grow and develop, the task of learning to use a spoon becomes basic, forming the foundation for learning more advanced skills requiring more manual dexterity.

Different aspects of growth and development occur at different stages and at different rates and can be modified. For example, muscles and bones both grow most rapidly during the first year of life.

During the toddler and preschool years, bone growth slows, but muscle fibers increase in size and strength. The most intense period of speech development is between 3 and 5 years of age (Fig. 8-2). Sexual maturity begins during the preadolescent years and progresses into the adult years, but is based on gender and sex role identity established from birth. Many factors can modify growth and development, including nutrition, love and affection from caretakers, and illnesses.

The pace of growth and development is specific for each person. Both physical and psychological skills and maturation vary among people. For example, while learning to walk, a child may concentrate energies on the task and temporarily slow down in language development. Racial variations may also be seen; Asian children tend to be smaller than white children of the same age. In addition, one's genetic heredity places restrictions on the upper limits that can be achieved in growth and development.

Factors Influencing Growth and Development

Both growth and development are influenced by many different factors, including genetic inheritance (heredity), culture, health–illness state, nutrition, the environment, family, and community. Because of these often interrelated and interdependent factors, each person's growth and development is individualized.

Our genetic blueprint for growth is inherited from our family of origin, determining physical characteristics such as height and bone size. However, many different factors affect how growth occurs through life. Prenatal influences on fetal growth include maternal nutrition and maternal substance abuse. Factors that may alter growth from birth through adolescence include malnutrition, infection, chronic illness, lead poisoning, and poverty.

Development is influenced by prenatal, individual, environmental, and caregiver factors. Fetal development can be altered by maternal age (with risk greater in those

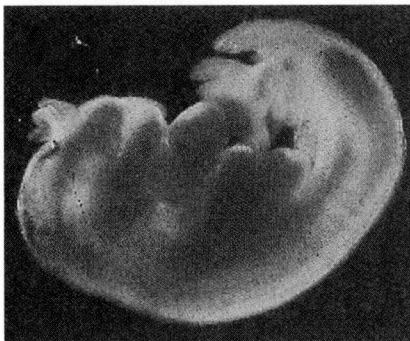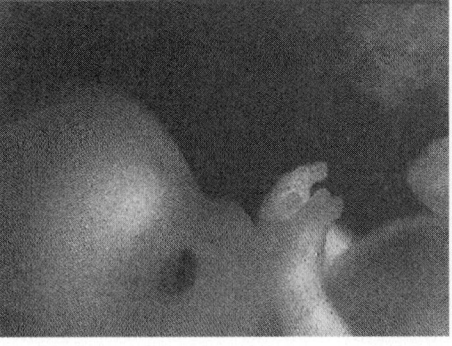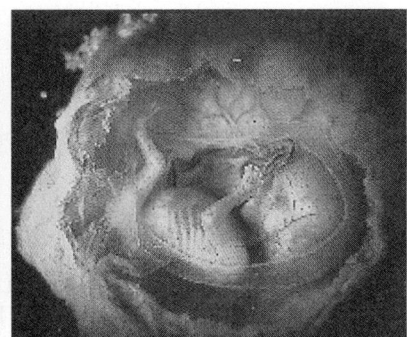

Figure 8-1
Three stages of human development in utero—at about 4, 8, and 16 weeks—showing the development first of the head and then of the trunk and limbs. (Courtesy of the Carnegie Institute, Washington, DC.)

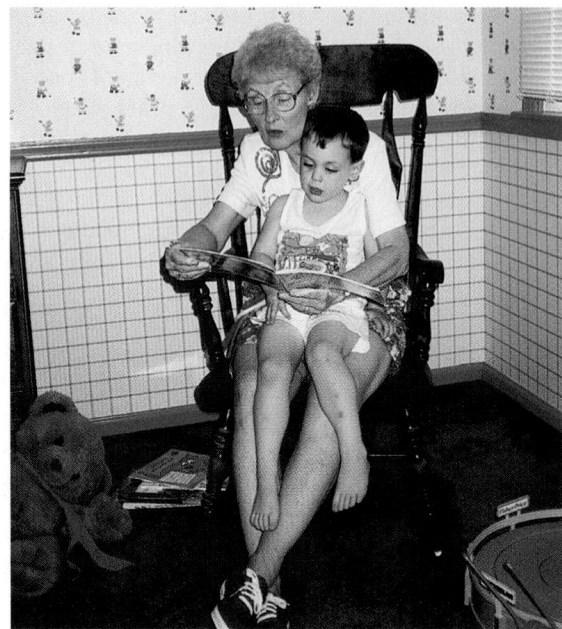

Figure 8-2
Speech development is greatest between the ages of 3 and 5 years; it is fostered by interaction and communication with caregivers.

younger than 15 years of age or older than 35 years of age), substance abuse, inadequate prenatal care, and inadequate nutrition. Individual factors that may result in altered development include congenital or genetic disorders, brain damage from accidents or abuse, vision and hearing impairments, chronic illness, inadequate nutrition, chemotherapy or radiation therapy, and substance abuse. Environmental factors that may alter development are poverty and violence. Caregiver factors that negatively affect development are neglect and abuse, mental illness, mental retardation, or a severe learning disability (North American Nursing Diagnosis Association, 1999).

Overview of Developmental Theories

Researchers have studied human development and behavior since the beginning of the 20th century and have developed theories that explain human responses expected at certain ages during life. Although a psychological approach is common to all developmental theories, each theory has a different focus. The theories discussed in the following sections examine cognitive, social, and instinctual influences on human growth and development. Key points of these are summarized in Table 8-1.

Psychoanalytic Theory: Sigmund Freud

Freud's (1923/1974) theory emphasizes the effect of instinctual human drives on behavior. The primary concepts of the theory are the unconscious mind, the id, the ego, the superego, and stages of development based on sexual motivation. Freud identified the underlying stimulus for human behavior as sexuality, which he called libido. *Li-*

bido is defined as general pleasure-seeking instincts rather than purely genital gratification. The major components of Freud's theory are as follows:

The unconscious mind: contains memories, motives, fantasies, and fears that are not accessible to recall but that directly affect behavior

The id: part of the psyche concerned with self gratification by the easiest and quickest available means

The ego: conscious part of the psyche that serves as a mediator between the desires of the id and the constraints of reality so that one may live effectively within one's social, physical, and psychological environment. The ego includes one's intelligence, memory, problem solving, separation of reality from fantasy, and incorporation of experiences and learning into future behavior. Development of the ego in the first year of life allows the infant, by 6 months of age, to view self as separate from others and to begin to alter behaviors in response to cues. Ego development continues throughout life.

The superego: part of the psyche that represents one's conscience and develops from the ego during the first year of life as the child learns praise versus punishment for actions. The superego represents the internalization of rules and values so that socially acceptable behavior is practiced.

A further contribution of Freud's theory is the description of defense mechanisms, which are means of unconscious coping when the id's impulses cannot be satisfied so as to reduce stress in the conscious mind. Defense mechanisms are discussed in Chapter 31. In addition, Freud described a series of developmental stages through which all people must pass:

Oral stage (ages 0 to 18 months). The infant's pleasures center on gratification by using the mouth for sucking and satisfying hunger.

Anal stage (ages 8 months to 4 years). This stage begins when neuromuscular control is developed to allow control of the anal sphincter. Toilet training is a crucial issue that requires delayed gratification as the child compromises between enjoyment of bowel function and limits set by social expectations.

Phallic stage (ages 3 to 7 years). The child has increased interest in gender differences, his or her own gender, and conflict and resolution of that conflict with the parent of the same sex (named the Oedipus complex in boys and the Electra complex in girls, based on feelings of intimate sexual possessiveness for the opposite-sex parent). Curiosity about the genitals and masturbation increase.

Latency stage (ages 7 to 12 years). This stage marks the transition to adult sexuality or the genital stage during adolescence. Increasing sex role identification with the parent of the same sex prepares the child for adult roles and relationships.

Table 8-1
Key Points of Developmental Theories

Theorist	Freud	Erikson	Havighurst	Piaget	Fowler	Kohlberg
Theme	Psychosexual	Psychosocial	Developmental	Cognitive	Faith	Moral
Infancy to toddlerhood	Oral stage; anal stage	Trust versus mistrust; autonomy versus shame and doubt	Learning to walk; learning to talk; learning to control body waste elimination	Basic reflexes; coordinates more than one thought at a time; begins to reason and anticipate events	Centers on relationship with primary caregiver	Oriented to obedience and punishment
Preschool to early school years	Phallic stage	Initiative versus guilt	Learning sex differences; forming concepts; getting ready to read	Increased language; increased understanding of life events and relationships	Imitates religious behaviors of others	Defines acts satisfying to self and some satisfying to others as right
School years	Latent stage	Industry versus inferiority	Learning physical skills; learning to get along with others; developing conscience and morality	Develops logical thinking; incorporates others perspectives; uses abstract thinking and deductive reasoning; tests beliefs to establish values	Accepts existence of deity; stories define religious and moral beliefs	Morality of maintaining good relations and approval of others; aware of need to respect authority
Adolescent to adult years	Genital stage	Intimacy versus generation	Achieving gender-specific social role; achieving independence; acquiring a set of values and an ethical system to guide behavior	Adopts life-guiding values or religious practices	Selects principles to follow; concern for the rights and needs of others	
Middle adult years		Generativity versus stagnation	Achieving social and civic responsibility; accepting and adjusting to physical changes	Integrates others' viewpoints into own understanding of truth		
Later adult years		Ego integrity versus despair	Adjusting to decreasing physical status and health; adjusting to retirement	Values absolute love and justice of all; believes in the existence of the future		

Genital stage (ages 12 to 20 years). At this stage, sexual interest can be expressed in overt sexual relationships. Sexual pressures and conflicts typically cause turmoil as the adolescent makes adjustments in relationships.

Psychosocial Theory: Erik Erikson

Erikson's (1963) developmental theory was based on Freud's work but was expanded to include cultural and social influences in addition to biologic processes. His **psychosocial theory** is based on four major organizing concepts: (1) stages of development, (2) developmental goals or tasks, (3) psychosocial crises, and (4) the process of coping. Erikson believed that development is a continuous process made up of distinct phases characterized by the achievement of developmental goals that are affected by the social environment and significant others.

Erikson identified eight stages that progress from birth to old age and death. Each stage is characterized by a developmental crisis to be mastered, with possible successful or unsuccessful resolution of the crisis. Unsuccessful resolution at any one stage may delay progress through the next stage, but mastery can occur later. The stages are as follows:

Trust versus mistrust (infancy). The infant learns to rely on caregivers to meet basic needs of warmth, food, and comfort, forming trust in others. Mistrust is the result of inconsistent, inadequate, or unsafe care (Fig. 8-3).

Autonomy versus shame and doubt (toddler, ages 1 to 3 years). As motor and language skills develop, the toddler learns from the environment and gains independence through encouragement from parents to feed, dress, and toilet self. If the parents are overprotective or have expectations that are too high, shame and doubt, as well as feelings of inadequacy, may develop in the child.

Initiative versus guilt (preschool, ages 4 to 6 years). Confidence gained as a toddler allows the preschooler to take the initiative in learning, so that the child actively seeks out new experiences and explores the how and why of activities. If the child experiences restrictions or reprimands for seeking new experiences and learning, guilt results, and the child becomes hesitant to attempt more challenging skills in motor or language development.

Industry versus inferiority (school-aged children). Focusing on the end result of achievements, the school-aged child gains pleasure from finishing projects and receiving recognition for accomplishments (Fig. 8-4). If the child is not accepted by peers or cannot meet parental expectations, a feeling of inferiority and lack of self-worth may develop.

Identity versus role confusion (adolescence). As many changes occur in his or her body, the adolescent is in transition from childhood to adulthood. Hormonal changes produce secondary sex characteristics and mood swings. Trying on roles and even rebellion are considered normal behaviors as the adolescent acquires a sense of who he or she is and what direction he or she will take in life. Role confusion occurs when the adolescent is unable to establish identity and a sense of direction.

Intimacy versus isolation (young adulthood). The tasks for the young adult are to unite self-identity with identities of friends and to make commitments to others. Fear of such commitments results in isolation and loneliness.

Generativity versus stagnation (middle adulthood). The middle adult years are a time of concern for the next generation as well as involvement with family, friends, and community. There is a desire to make a contribution to the world. If this task is not met,

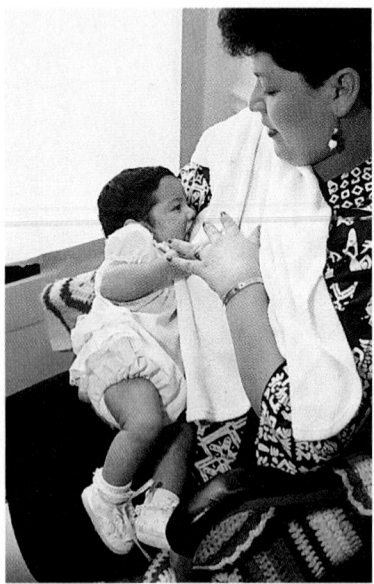

Figure 8-3
Infants develop a sense of trust and security as they learn that they can rely on their caregivers to fulfill their needs. (Photo © Kathy Sloane.)

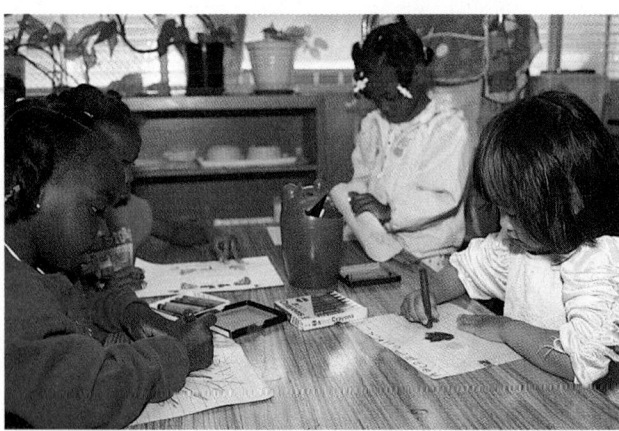

Figure 8-4
School-aged children focus on the end results of accomplishments—recognition and praise from family, teachers, and peers—in their development of a sense of competition and industry. (Photo © Kathy Sloane.)

stagnation results, and the person becomes self-absorbed and obsessed with her or his own needs or regresses to an earlier level of coping.

Ego integrity versus despair (later adulthood). As one enters the older years, reminiscence about life events provides a sense of fulfillment and purpose. If one believes that one's life has been a series of failures or missed directions, a sense of despair may prevail.

Developmental Tasks: Robert J. Havighurst

Havighurst (1972) believed that living and growing are based on learning and that a person must continuously learn to adjust to changing societal conditions. He described learned behaviors as **developmental tasks** that occur at certain periods in life. Successful achievement leads to happiness and success in later tasks, whereas unsuccessful achievement leads to unhappiness, societal disapproval, and difficulty in later tasks. The developmental tasks arise from maturation, personal motives and values that determine occupational and family choices, and civic responsibility. The developmental tasks, by age are as follows:

Infancy and Early Childhood
* Achieving physiologic stability
* Learning to eat solid foods
* Learning to walk and talk
* Forming simple concepts of social and physical reality
* Learning to relate emotionally to parents, siblings, and other people
* Learning to control the elimination of body wastes
* Learning to distinguish between right and wrong
* Learning sex differences and sexual modesty

Middle Childhood
* Learning physical skills necessary for games
* Learning to get along with age-mates
* Developing fundamental skills in reading, writing, and mathematics
* Developing a conscience, morality, and a scale of values
* Achieving personal independence

Adolescence
* Accepting one's body and using it effectively
* Achieving a masculine or feminine gender role
* Achieving emotional independence from parents and other adults
* Preparing for a career
* Preparing for marriage and family life
* Desiring and achieving socially responsible behavior
* Acquiring an ethical system as a guide to behavior

Young Adulthood
* Selecting a mate
* Learning to live with a marriage partner
* Starting a family and rearing children
* Managing a home
* Getting started in an occupation

* Taking on civic responsibility
* Finding a congenial social group

Middle Adulthood
* Accepting and adjusting to physical changes
* Attaining and maintaining a satisfactory occupational performance
* Assisting children to become responsible adults
* Relating to one's spouse as a person
* Adjusting to aging parents
* Achieving adult social and civic responsibility

Later Maturity
* Adjusting to decreasing physical strength and health
* Adjusting to retirement and reduced income
* Adjusting to death of a spouse
* Establishing an explicit affiliation with one's age group
* Adjusting and adapting social roles in a flexible way
* Establishing satisfactory physical living arrangements

Cognitive Development: Jean Piaget

Piaget (1969) developed a theory of **cognitive development** from infancy through adolescence. Piaget believed that learning occurs as a result of the internal organization of an event, which forms a mental schema and serves as a base for further schemata as one grows and develops. Intellectual growth is a continual restructuring of knowledge to progress to higher levels of problem solving and critical thinking. Two continual processes of assimilation and accommodation stimulate intellectual growth in the child. **Assimilation** is the process of integrating new experiences into existing schemata; **accommodation** is an alteration of existing thought processes to manage more complex information. Four stages of cognitive development were described by Piaget:

Sensorimotor stage (birth to 24 months). Progression through a series of developmental stages, for example:

0 to 1 month—Demonstrates basic reflexes, such as sucking

1 to 4 months—Discovers enjoyment of random behaviors (such as smiling or sucking thumb) and repeats them

4 to 8 months—Relates own behavior to a change in environment, such as shaking a rattle to hear the sound (Fig. 8-5)

8 to 12 months—Coordinates more than one thought pattern at a time to reach a goal, such as repeatedly throwing an object on the floor; only objects in sight are considered permanent

12 to 18 months—Recognizes the permanence of objects, even if out of sight; can understand simple commands

18 to 24 months—Begins to develop reasoning and can anticipate events

Preoperational stage (ages 2 to 7 years). Characterized by the beginning use of symbols, through increased language skills and pictures, to represent the preschooler's world (Fig. 8-6). This stage is

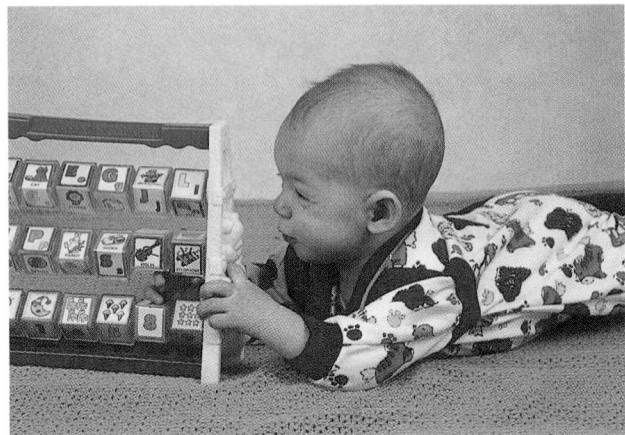

Figure 8-5
From about 4 months of age, infants can begin to relate their own behavior as causing a change in the environment, and from about 8 months of age, can integrate more than one thought pattern to obtain a purposeful goal. (Photo © B. Proud.)

divided into two parts: the preconceptual stage (ages 2 to 4 years) and the intuitive stage (ages 4 to 7 years). Play activities during this time help the child to understand life events and relationships.

Concrete operational stage (ages 7 to 11 years). Children learn by manipulating concrete or tangible objects and can classify articles according to two or more characteristics. Logical thinking is developing with an understanding of reversibility, relations between numbers, and loss of egocentricity. Also occurring is the ability to incorporate another's perspective.

Formal operational stage (age 11 years or older). The use of abstract thinking and deductive reasoning. General concepts are related to specific situations, and alternatives are considered. The world is evaluated by testing beliefs in an attempt to establish values and meaning in life (Fig. 8-7).

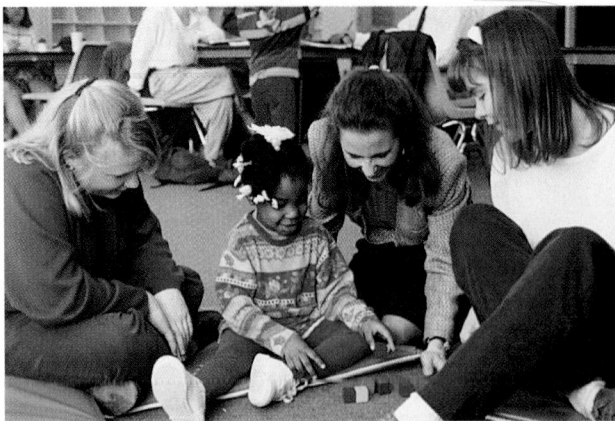

Figure 8-6
The preschool child's development is characterized by the beginning use of symbols through language and pictures, an ability to learn simple sequences, and a basic ability to categorize objects. (Photo by Gates Rhodes, courtesy of School of Nursing, University of Pennsylvania.)

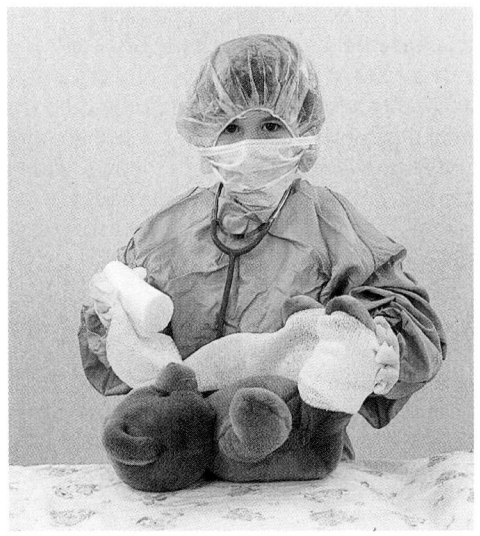

Figure 8-7
Abstract reasoning is required for children to understand that painful medical treatments given now will make them feel better later. A child who is not old enough to have reached the formal operational stage, in which abstract reasoning develops, may require special attention from the health-care staff to understand the uncomfortable experiences of the hospital stay. (Photo © B. Proud.)

Moral Development: Lawrence Kohlberg and Carol Gilligan

Lawrence Kohlberg

Kohlberg (1969) developed a theory of **moral development** in levels that closely follow Piaget's theory of cognitive development. Each level is further divided into separate stages:

The *preconventional level* is based on external control as the child learns to conform to rules imposed by authority figures. At stage 1, *punishment and obedience orientation*, the motivation for choices of action is fear of physical consequences of authority's disapproval. As a result of the consequences, a perception of goodness or badness develops. At stage 2, *instrumental relativist orientation*, the thought of receiving a reward overcomes fear of punishment, so actions that satisfy this desire are selected.

The *conventional level* involves identifying with significant others and conforming to their expectations. The person respects the values and ideals of family and friends, regardless of consequences. In stage 3, *"good boy–good girl" orientation*, the person strives for approval in an attempt to be viewed as "good." At stage 4, *"law and order" orientation*, behavior follows social or religious rules from a respect for authority. In his later work, Kohlberg maintained that many adults are at this stage because they think abstractly and view themselves as members of society (Duska & Whelan, 1975).

The *postconventional level* involves moral judgment that is rational and internalized into one's standards or values. In stage 5, *social contract, utilitarian orientation*, correct behavior is defined in terms of society's laws. Laws can be changed, however, to meet society's needs, while maintaining respect for self and others. Stage 6, *universal ethical principle orientation*, represents the person's concern for equality for all human beings, guided by personal values and standards, regardless of those set by society or laws. Justice may be internalized at an even higher level than society. Few adults ever reach this stage of development.

Kohlberg recognized that a person's moral development is influenced by cultural effects on one's perceptions of justice in interpersonal relationships. A child's beginnings of moral development result from parent and child communications during the early childhood years, as the young child tries to please his or her parents. The concept of morality emerges as a subset of a person's beliefs or values and governs choices made throughout life. Rules and regulations established by society are eventually challenged and evaluated as a person either accepts societal rules into his or her own internal set of values or rejects them.

Carol Gilligan

Gilligan (1977, 1982) originally worked with Kohlberg. As she listened to women discuss their own real-life moral conflicts, she recognized that there was a conception of morality from the female viewpoint that was not represented in Kohlberg's work. Gilligan's theory views females as developing a morality of response and care and males as developing a morality of justice.

In Gilligan's theory, males and females have different ways of looking at the world. Males are more likely to associate morality with obligations, rights, and justice. Females are more likely to see moral requirements emerging from the needs of others within the context of a relationship. This moral orientation of females is called the *ethic of care,* which develops through three levels. Each level ends with a transitional period—a time when the female considers new approaches to moral considerations and moves to a new level.

Level 1—selfishness. The focus is on one's own needs. "Should" and "would" are the same. Morality is seen in terms of sanctions by society. Relationships are often disappointing, and as a result, a woman may isolate herself to avoid getting hurt. The transition that follows this level is characterized by the move from selfishness to responsibility—a move that integrates the responsibility to care for oneself with the desire to care for others.

Level 2—goodness. Moral judgment is based on shared norms and expectations, and societal values are adopted. Acceptance by others becomes critical, and the ability to protect and care for others is seen as the defining characteristic of female goodness. This characteristic is upheld through beliefs that one is responsible for the actions of others but that others are responsible for the choices they make. As a woman examines her self-sacrifice, the second transition occurs, with the woman asking if her own needs are not also important. A shift from goodness to truth (as well as a new conception of goodness) takes place.

Level 3—nonviolence. A changed understanding of self and a redefinition of morality allow reconciliation of selfishness and responsibility. Nonviolence (the injunction against hurting) governs all moral judgments and actions. Care becomes a universal obligation toward self and others. Moral problems are usually considered within the contexts of maintaining relationships and of promoting the welfare or preventing the harm of others.

Faith Development: James Fowler

Fowler (1981) produced a developmental theory of the spiritual identity of humans, based on work by Piaget, Kohlberg, and Erikson. He describes **faith** as follows (1981, p. 4):

> Faith is not always religious in its content or context. . . . Faith is a person's or group's way of moving into the force field of life. It is our way of finding coherence in and giving meaning to the multiple forces and relations that make up our lives. Faith is a person's way of seeing him or herself in relation to others against a background of shared meaning and purpose. Faith, therefore, is not necessarily religious, but it comprises the reasons one finds life worth living.

Fowler's theory is composed of a prestage and six stages of faith development. The age when a certain stage occurs varies, but the sequence does not. Equilibrium, or a plateau in faith development, can occur at any stage from stage 2 on.

In relation to the stages of faith development, Fowler explained a triadic relationship among self, shared causes or values, and others that is the unifying factor in all stages and is based on trust. During the prestage, called *undifferentiated faith,* trust, courage, hope, and love compete with threats of abandonment and inconsistencies in the infant's environment. The strength of faith in this stage is based on the infant's relationship with the primary caregiver. The stages are as follows:

Stage 1—intuitive-projective faith: most typical of the 3- to 7-year-old child. Children imitate religious gestures and behaviors of others, primarily their parents. They take on their parents' attitudes toward religious or moral beliefs without a thorough understanding of them. Imagination in this stage leads to long-lived images and feelings that they must question and reintegrate in later stages.

Stage 2—mythical-literal faith: predominates in the school-aged child, who is having more social interaction. Stories represent religious and moral beliefs, and the child accepts the existence of a deity. The child can appreciate the perspectives of others as well as the concept of reciprocal fairness.

Stage 3—synthetic-conventional faith: the characteristic stage for many adolescents. As the person experiences increasing demands from work, school, family, and peers, the basis for identity becomes more complex. The person has an emerging ideology but has not closely examined it until now. The person begins to question life-guiding values or religious practices in an attempt to stabilize his or her own identity.

Stage 4—individuative-reflective faith: this is crucial for older adolescents and young adults because they become responsible for their own commitments, beliefs, and attitudes. Many adults do not develop to this stage, and for some people, it does not emerge until they are in their 30s or 40s. Searching for self-identity no longer defined by the faith compositions of significant others is a primary concern.

Stage 5—conjunctive faith: integrates other viewpoints about faith into one's understanding of truth. One is able to see the nature of the reality of one's own beliefs. Along with this realization, one observes the divisions of faith development among people.

Stage 6—universalizing faith: involves making tangible the values of absolute love and justice for humankind. The faith relationship is characterized by total trust in the principle of actively "being-in-relation" to others in whom we invest commitment, belief, love, risk, and hope and in the existence of the future, regardless of what religion or image of faith is involved.

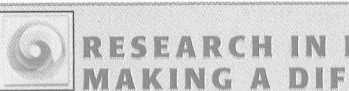 Family Influences on Growth and Development

The family is considered in this chapter because the study of growth and development would not be complete without noting the interrelationship between the individual and the family (see the accompanying Research in Nursing box). Family dynamics, a major environmental influence, begin with conception and continue throughout life. The functions, structures, and developmental tasks of the family are discussed in Chapter 2, and the establishment of a family is discussed in Chapter 9 in reference to the young adult.

The family plays a vital role in health promotion and illness prevention. Family values, along with ethnic or cultural heritage, influence how one interprets illness. A health problem or developmental crisis experienced by any one family member affects the other members. Health practices, whether positive or negative, are learned from older family members. Sometimes, the family may even cause or contribute to the cause of illness in individual members. Alterations in coping and communication patterns may predispose families to dysfunctional means of relating to one another.

Implications for Nursing

Nurses have a responsibility to assess not only the health needs of individual members of the family but also the demands on the total family in meeting every member's

---

RESEARCH IN NURSING: MAKING A DIFFERENCE

Reducing Risk Factors for Altered Growth and Development

Pregnancy and parenthood in adolescent girls continue to be a major public concern. Risk behaviors are common in adolescence, but behaviors such as unsafe sex, poor nutrition, and experimentation with tobacco, alcohol, and drugs during pregnancy place the young mother and her child at high risk for pregnancy complications and poor birth outcomes. These risks are even greater for younger adolescents, whose diet may not meet the growth needs of their fetus in addition to their own.

Related Research
Koniak-Griffin, D., Mathenge, C., Anderson, N., & Verzemnieks, I. (1999). An early intervention program for adolescent mothers: A nursing demonstration project. *Journal of Obstetric, Gynecologic, and Neonatal Nursing, 28*(1), 51–59.
This is the report of a nursing intervention research project conducted to provide comprehensive public health nursing for pregnant adolescents. The nurses included four "preparation for motherhood" classes and up to 17 home visits during pregnancy and through the first year of the infant's life. In the home visits, interventions were provided in five major areas: health, sexuality and

family planning, life skills, maternal role (including knowledge of fetal and infant growth and development), and social support systems. Telephone calls were made between visits to arrange and confirm home visits and provide follow-up information (such as referrals for healthcare). Early outcomes of this project support that home visitation by public health nurses positively affects the health of adolescent mothers and their babies.

Relevance to Nursing Practice
This study is one example of how nursing research is being used to facilitate normal growth and development—in this case, of both adolescent mothers and their infants. It supports developing and using nursing interventions to promote health in a high-risk vulnerable population and to reduce healthcare costs by preventing prematurity and reducing infant hospitalization days. Studies such as this one provide valuable information, demonstrating the effectiveness of nursing care in promoting positive health and social outcomes for pregnant adolescents. In addition, effective parenting behaviors by adolescent mothers help facilitate normal growth and development of their infants.

needs. Nurses can then function as a catalyst in planning appropriate interventions and teaching and as a collaborator with other healthcare professionals (social workers, psychologists, physicians, clergy) for achieving optimal family health.

Nurses plan and implement activities to facilitate effective family functioning to enhance growth and development. The nurse's primary role is teaching, with emphasis on the following areas (each stage of growth and development described in Chapters 9 and 10 includes nursing actions to promote health):

- Information about risk factors for individual family members, such as drinking alcohol, smoking cigarettes, or using illegal drugs
- Knowledge and skills to increase health promotion and coping behaviors
- Family strengths that foster individual and family development
- Risk factors in the home environment, such as open containers of cleaning solutions or open stairways
- Prevention of illness, injury, abuse, and neglect

These broad categories of teaching must be individualized to the needs of each family. For example, an adolescent who is a single mother requires assistance different from that of a family seeking information on child-proofing their home. Both individual developmental tasks and family developmental tasks are essential considerations for nurses providing holistic nursing care.

⑤ Applying Growth and Development Theories

The complex and interrelated elements that contribute to human development involve not only biophysical factors but also factors of personality development. The theories of Freud, Erikson, Havighurst, Piaget, Kohlberg, Gilligan, and Fowler help us understand cognitive, psychosocial, moral, and spiritual development. To understand the whole person, nurses need to evaluate all the components of development to understand certain life events or concerns.

Although these theories offer a great deal of insight into the processes of human development, they do have some limitations. When planning holistic nursing care for patients with diverse needs, backgrounds, and ages, nurses should therefore assess the patient as an individual and use interventions based on rationales from multiple developmental theories to provide comprehensive health promotion. Guidelines for incorporating the principles and theories of growth and development in nursing care are listed in the accompanying box. The following two examples demonstrate such applications:

1. While interviewing a young mother with her first child, the nurse senses a frustrated single parent when the mother talks about the task of rearing her 14-month-old child alone. Using Freud's theory, the nurse can explain to the mother the behaviors typical of the oral stage of the infants' development.

Incorporating Principles and Theories of Growth and Development

General guidelines for incorporating principles and theories of growth and development and family dynamics into daily practice of nursing care are listed below. They are provided as suggestions for working with patients of all ages.

- Be knowledgeable about the various stages of cognitive, psychosocial, moral, and spiritual development and prepared to support developmental stages typical of certain ages.
- Maintain flexibility in assessing people, and respect the uniqueness of each person. Although the literature describes development typical of a particular age, not everyone fits into an exact mold.
- Anticipate possible regression during difficult periods or times of crisis, accepting and supporting a person's return to a forward progression in development.
- Become cognizant that environmental and cultural influences have a strong effect on development, especially psychosocial development. A deprived environment can be detrimental, whereas an enriched environment enhances development.

- Assess each person with an awareness that within each stage of development, a person may retain some behaviors of a previous stage, attain goals of the current stage, and begin to exhibit behaviors of the next stage. There is a time of transition to the next stage with no definite beginning or ending to the particular stage of development.
- Remember that patients are members of families and that the family unit can have both positive and negative influences on the development of individual members. Attempt to support good family relationships and healthy environments that assist members to reach their greatest potential for growth. Provide patient teaching to individuals and their families to aid in their understanding of periods of development.
- Be ready to provide healthcare to patients who are ill or who fail to meet developmental goals. Collaborate with other members of the healthcare team in providing care to prevent or minimize disruption of development and to promote optimal health throughout life.
- Provide environments and experiences that are developmentally challenging.

Havighurst's and Erikson's theories help explain the toddler's stage of gaining independence when learning to walk. Recognizing that the mother may be limited in her support system, the nurse may need to assess further to identify the mother's potential problems with intimacy and a feeling of generativity. In planning care for this young mother, the nurse anticipates needed emotional support and health teaching about the normal toddler years. The mother's anxiety level and the child's attempts to investigate the environment through locomotion and oral exploration place the child at risk for injury from a fall or aspiration of a small object. With astute observation and knowledge of child development, the nurse has a primary role in prevention by educating the mother.

2. A 70-year-old man fell and fractured his hip while repairing the exterior of his home. Having been the traditional head of his household, he now is troubled by needing others, including his wife, to care for him. He appears withdrawn, refusing to talk and eating poorly. Reflecting on Havighurst's and Erikson's theories, the nurse understands that he may be fluctuating between feelings of nonadjustment and acceptance of his declining health and a sense of ego integrity.

These situations demonstrate how growth and development theories can be applied in the practice of nursing. Healthcare needs change quickly as a person grows and passes through life. These needs are unique for each person but include certain similarities at specific periods. The nurse must plan care based on the patient's general and unique health needs and must continually revise aspects of care as the growth process evolves or alterations in health status occur.

Learning Outcomes

After completing this chapter, the learner should be able to accomplish the following:

1. Define key terms used in the chapter.

   accommodation   faith
   assimilation   growth and development
   cognitive development   moral development
   developmental task   psychosocial theory

2. Summarize basic principles of growth and development.

3. Discuss the theories of Freud, Erikson, Havighurst, Piaget, Kohlberg, Gilligan, and Fowler.

4. Describe the importance of incorporating theories of growth and development in assessing and planning nursing care for individuals and families.

5. Describe the role of the family in growth and development.

6. List implications for nursing practice based on an understanding of growth and development.

Critical Thinking Exercises

1. Identify developmental challenges for five of your family members or friends at different ages across the life span. Explain why meeting developmental needs is an essential role of nursing.

2. Why do older adults have or not have developmental needs?

3. Using Piaget's theory of cognitive development, describe how you would explain the death of a parent to children 4, 9, and 13 years of age.

Bibliography

Coles, R. (1990). *The spiritual life of children*. Boston: Houghton & Mifflin.

Duska, R., & Whelan, M. (1975). *Moral development: A guide to Piaget and Kohlberg*. New York: Paulist.

Erikson, E. H. (1963). *Childhood and society* (2nd ed.). New York: Norton.

Flanagan, O., & Jackson, K. (1987). Justice, care, and gender: The Kohlberg–Gilligan debate revisited. *Ethics 97*, 622–637.

Fowler, J. W. (1981). *Stages of faith: The psychology of human development and the quest for meaning*. New York: Harper & Row.

Fowler, J. W. (1991). *Weaving the new creation: Stages of faith and the public church*. San Francisco: Harper Collins.

Freud, S. (1923/1974). *The ego and the id*. London: Hogarth.

Friedman, M. M. (1992). *Family nursing: Theory and assessment* (3rd ed.). Norwalk, CT: Appleton & Lange.

Garner, R. (1998). Play and its role in child development. *Assignment, 4*(1), 3–6.

Gilligan, C. (1977). In a different voice: Women's conceptions of the self and of morality. *Harvard Educational Review, 47*, 481–517.

Gilligan, C. (1982). *In a different voice*. Cambridge, MA: Harvard University Press.

Hart, D., & Schneider, D. (1997). Spiritual care for children with cancer. *Seminars in Oncology Nursing, 13*(4), 263–270.

Havighurst, R. J. (1972). *Developmental tasks and education*. New York: David McKay.

Hepler, J. (1997). Social development of children: The role of peers. *Social Work in Education, 19*(4), 242–256.

Hughes, F., & Knoppe, L. (1991). *Human development across the life span.* New York: Merrill.

Klaus, M. H., & Kennell, J. H. (1982). *Parent–infant bonding.* St. Louis: C. V. Mosby.

Kohlberg, L. (1969). Stage and sequence: The cognitive–developmental approach to socialization. In D. Gaslin (Ed.). *Handbook of socialization: Theory and research* (pp. 347–380). Chicago: Rand McNally.

Koniak-Griffin, D., Mathenge, C., Anderson, N., & Verzemnieks, I. (1999). An early intervention program for adolescent mothers: A nursing demonstration project. *Journal of Obstetric, Gynecologic, and Neonatal Nursing, 28*(1), 51–59.

Mussen, P. H., Conger, J. J., & Kagan, J. (1974). *Child development and personality* (4th ed.). New York: Harper & Row.

Newman, B. M., & Newman, P. R. (1975). *Development through life: A psychosocial approach.* Homewood, IL: Dorsey.

Nippold, M., Uhden, L., & Schwarz, I. (1997). Proverb explanation through the lifespan: A developmental study of adolescents and adults. *Journal of Speech, Language, & Hearing Research, 40*(2), 245–253.

Noppe, I., & Noppe, L. (1997). Evolving meanings of death during early, middle, and later adolescence. *Death Studies, 21*(3), 253–275.

North American Nursing Diagnosis Association (NANDA). (1999). *Nursing diagnoses: Definitions & classification 1999–2000.* Philadelphia: NANDA.

Parker, R. S. (1990). Measuring nurse's moral judgments. *Image—The Journal of Nursing Scholarship. 22*(4), 213–218.

Piaget, J., & Inhelder, B. (1969). *The psychology of the child.* New York: Basic Books.

Sherer, M. (1998). Effect of computerized simulation games on the moral development of junior and senior high-school students. *Computers in Human Behavior, 14*(2), 375–386.

Chapter 9
Conception Through Young Adult

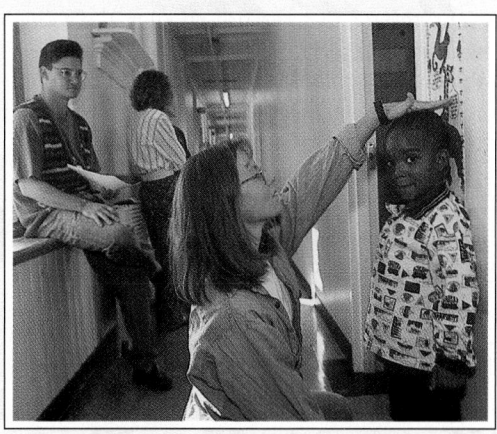

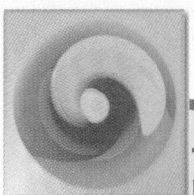

Thinking Critically About
Nursing's Blended Skills

Before reading this chapter, think about the types of skills you will need to meet effectively the developmental needs of patients in their earliest developmental stages through young adulthood.

- A 26-year-old woman in the first trimester of her pregnancy tells you that she is trying to cut back on smoking and drinking alcohol but she hasn't had much success.

- A father arrives in the emergency room with his 2-year-old daughter who is unresponsive. He says that she "took a tumble" down the stairs, but her injuries are inconsistent with this type of fall.

- Your city has a high percentage of children growing up in families that meet the federal poverty criteria, and you suspect that their nutritional and healthcare needs are grossly unmet.

- You are the school nurse in a large high school that wants to initiate a peer counseling program. You have been invited to work with the student counselors to develop their expertise in responding to student health problems.

What cognitive, technical, interpersonal, and ethical/legal skills do you think you will need to respond effectively to the developmental challenges described above?

Growth and development occur throughout the life span. The nurse's knowledge of sequential growth and developmental milestones provides a base for planning and implementing holistic, individualized nursing care for patients and their families. This chapter continues the discussion of developmental theories introduced in Chapter 8, with specific information related to the sequential stages of growth and development during conception through young adulthood.

Although divided into different stages, *childhood* encompasses the entire period before young adulthood. Included within this time span are the fetus, the neonate, the infant, the toddler, the preschooler, the school-aged child, and the adolescent. The discussion of each of these stages includes physiologic, psychosocial, and cognitive development; common health problems; and the nurse's role in meeting healthcare needs.

Although developmental milestones are summarized, the chapter focuses primarily on information necessary for the nurse to promote optimal functioning, growth, and health for patients at any age.

Environmental and Nutritional Influences

Environment and nutrition influence all stages of development. The effect of each can occur independently, but they are more likely to be interrelated, as seen in these examples:

- Infants who are malnourished in utero develop fewer brain cells than infants who have had adequate prenatal nutrition.
- Substance abuse by a pregnant woman increases the risk for congenital anomalies, low birthweight, and prematurity in her developing fetus.
- Federally sponsored school meal programs support enhanced learning with adequate nutrition.
- Failure to thrive, a condition of early infancy, has been linked to both nutritional and emotional deprivation.
- Child abuse is an extreme example of physical and emotional harm or deprivation, leading to deficits in physical or psychosocial development, or both.
- Substance abuse by adolescents and young adults is associated with an increased incidence of teenage pregnancy, violence, accidents, and suicide. Abuse of alcohol and drugs is more prevalent in teenagers who have poor family relationships, low self-esteem, and poor social skills.

Conception and Prenatal Development

Human growth and development begin at the moment the ovum is fertilized by the sperm. The fertilized ovum, or *zygote*, contains the full complement of genetic information provided by each parent that determines gender and influences personality, intellect, and physical and psychological traits. The growth and development stages of the fetus are orderly and continuous, and proceed as follows:

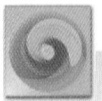

COGNITIVE SKILLS

- Knowledge of the developmental needs of fetuses and the effects of maternal behaviors, such as smoking and alcohol consumption
- Knowledge of effective strategies to help pregnant women modify behaviors that harm fetuses
- Ability to recognize potential child abuse; knowledge of your reporting obligations; knowledge of how to intervene effectively with potential abusers
- Knowledge of how to facilitate a community's responsiveness to the unmet developmental needs of vulnerable populations such as poor children
- Knowledge of the common health problems of adolescents and effective intervention strategies for peer counselors

TECHNICAL SKILLS

- Ability to provide the technical nursing assistance necessary to assess and meet the nursing needs of the pregnant woman and her fetus, the potentially abused toddler, children living in poverty, and high school adolescents

INTERPERSONAL SKILLS

- Ability to establish trusting and respectful professional relationships with patients of different ages
- Ability to mobilize groups, such as community action groups or peer counselors, to provide needed services

ETHICAL/LEGAL SKILLS

- Knowledge of the nurse's legal and ethical obligations in cases of maternal–fetal conflict, child abuse, and vulnerable populations
- Ability and willingness to advocate for vulnerable patients: fetuses, unresponsive children, children in poverty, adolescents
- Ability to practice in an ethically and legally defensible manner

1. The *preembryonic stage* lasts for about 3 weeks. The zygote, which implants in the uterine wall, has three distinct cell layers. The *endoderm,* or inner layer, becomes the respiratory system, the digestive system, the liver, and the pancreas. The *mesoderm,* or middle layer, becomes the skeleton, connective tissue, cartilage, and muscles and the circulatory, lymphoid, reproductive, and urinary systems. The *ectoderm,* or outer layer, becomes the brain, spinal cord, nervous system, and outer body parts (skin, hair, nails).

2. The *embryonic stage* occurs from the fourth through the eighth week. Rapid growth and differentiation of the cell layers take place. By the end of this stage, all basic organs have been established, the bones have begun to ossify, and some human features are recognizable. Because this is a period of such rapid growth and change, the fetus is especially vulnerable to any factor that might cause congenital anomalies (such as maternal use of alcohol, nicotine, over-the-counter medications, or drugs).

3. The *fetal stage* lasts from 9 weeks to birth. All body organs and systems continue to grow and develop. By birth, the average neonate weighs 7.5 lb (3.4 kg) and is 20 inches (50.8 cm) long.

Neonate: Birth to 28 Days

At birth, the **neonate** must adapt to extrauterine life through several significant physiologic adjustments. Although adjustments occur in all body systems, the most important occur in the respiratory and circulatory systems as the neonate begins breathing and becomes independent of the umbilical cord. The neonate is assessed immediately after birth. Of several existing measurement scales, the Apgar rating scale is the most commonly used. This scale is used to assess neonates 1 minute and 5 minutes after birth (Table 9-1).

Physiologic Development

The physical characteristics and behaviors of normal neonates include those illustrated in Figure 9-1 and the following:

- Reflexes include sucking, swallowing, blinking, sneezing, and yawning.
- Body temperature responds quickly to the environmental temperature.
- The neonate is alert to the environment, sees color and form, hears and turns toward sound, can smell and taste, and is sensitive to touch and pain.
- The neonate eliminates stool and urine.
- The neonate drinks breast milk, glucose water, and plain water.

The neonate inherits a transient immunity from infections as a result of immunoglobulins that cross the placenta. Breastfeeding provides further protection against bacterial and viral infections through antibodies, immunoglobulins, and leukocytes in breast milk. The high lactose content in breast milk, combined with limited protein, promotes an acid environment that is unsuitable for bacterial growth.

Common Health Problems

Difficulties related to the birth process, the transition to extrauterine life, or congenital anomalies (birth defects) may require intervention by healthcare personnel. Breathing difficulties may occur, especially if the neonate has been sedated by drugs given to the mother during labor

Table 9-1
Apgar Scoring Chart

Category*	0	1	2
Heart rate	Absent	Slow (less than 100 beats/min)	More than 100 beats/min
Respiratory effort	Absent	Slow, irregular	Good, crying
Muscle tone	Flaccid	Some flexion of extremities	Active motion
Reflex irritability	No response	Weak cry or grimace	Vigorous cry
Color	Blue, pale	Body pink, extremities blue	Completely pink

* Each category is rated as 0, 1, or 2. The rating for each category is then totaled to a maximum score of 10. Normal neonates score between 7 and 10. Neonates who score between 4 and 6 require special assistance; those who score below 4 are in need of immediate life-saving support.

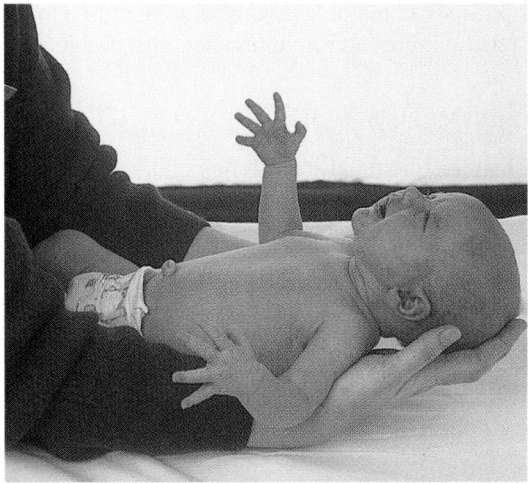

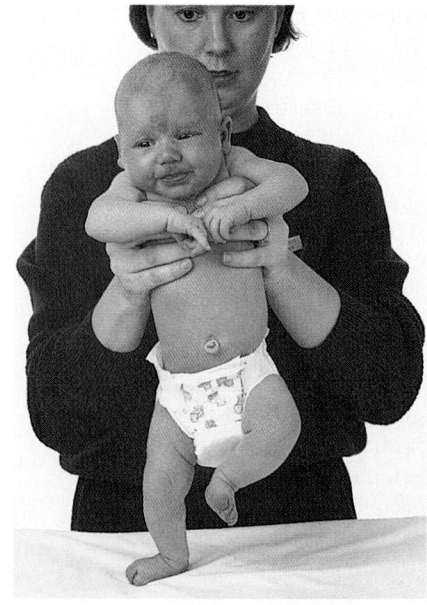

Stepping reflex (Photo © Keith Cotton)

Quiet alert state (Photo © Bob Daemmrich/Stock Boston)

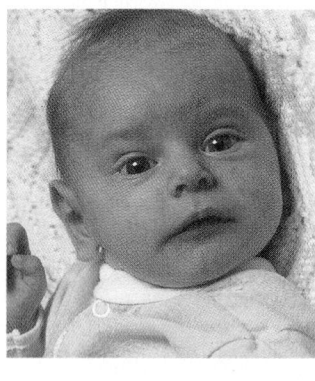

Moro reflex (Photo © Keith Cotton)

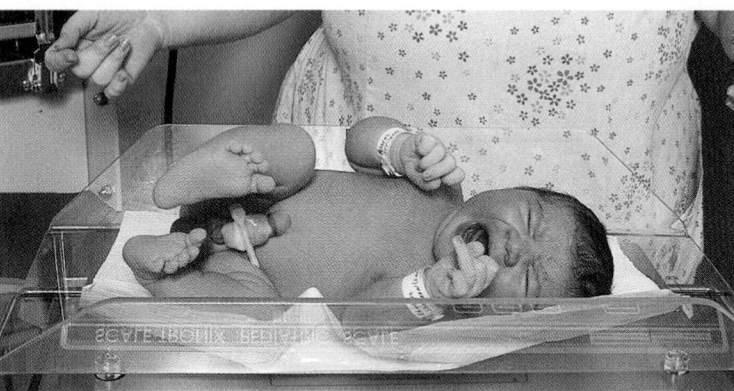

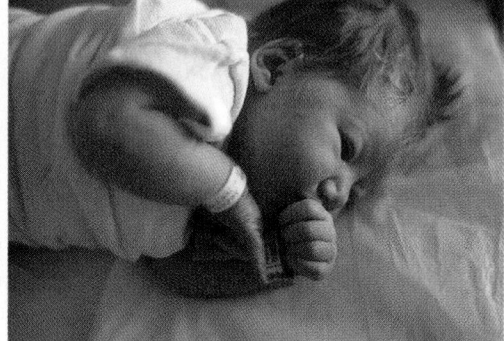

Hand to mouth and sucking activity

Active crying state

Figure 9-1
Reflexes and behaviors of the neonate.

and delivery. Premature neonates are vulnerable to respiratory distress syndrome because of the relative immature lung function. Neonates delivered by cesarean birth are at risk for respiratory difficulties because of excess mucus in the lungs, often requiring frequent suctioning.

Incompatibility between the neonate's and mother's blood groups requires prompt care at birth. Congenital malformations, such as cleft palate and cleft lip, or neural tube defects (such as spina bifida) and hydrocephalus, may result in long-term health problems. Birth traumas that cause temporary symptoms are of concern because the parents need to be reassured that the symptoms will disappear. Examples include caput succedaneum (localized edema of the scalp), molding (elongation of the skull as the baby passes through the birth canal), and subconjunctival hemorrhage. The nonthreatening nature of physiologic jaundice, which commonly occurs in the neonate's first days, should also be explained to the parents.

Neonates born to mothers who smoke cigarettes, drink alcohol, or use drugs are at risk for developmental deficits as well as complications during birth. Smoking during pregnancy may cause low birthweight. Fetal alcohol syndrome caused by maternal drinking is believed to be a leading cause of birth defects, including growth retardation, developmental delay, and impaired intellectual ability. The maternal use of cocaine, crack-cocaine, and heroin increases the probability of congenital anomalies, prematurity, low birthweight, and drug withdrawal symptoms (Wong, Wilson, Ahman, Winkelstein, Divito-Thomas, & Hockenberry-Eaton, 1998).

Cocaine use in various forms, including crack, brings about abrupt changes in the mother's blood pressure, resulting in decreased fetal blood flow and oxygenation. "Crack babies" are jittery, hypersensitive to noise or stimuli, intolerant of cuddling, and feed poorly (Wong, et al, 1998). The number of neonates born with this syndrome, which may last for 2 to 3 weeks after birth, is increasing. The long-term effects are not fully understood.

Infant: 1 Month to 1 Year

The neonate becomes an **infant** at 1 month, a period lasting until the first birthday (Fig. 9-2).

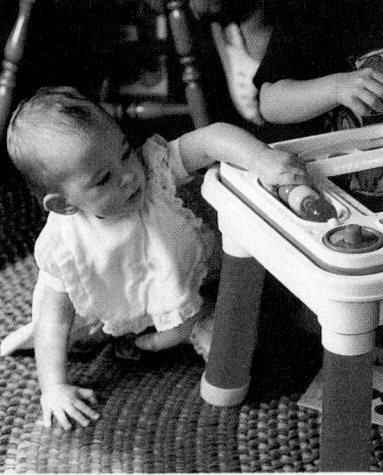

As the infant enters the second half of his first year, play will begin to involve manipulation of objects and the environment.

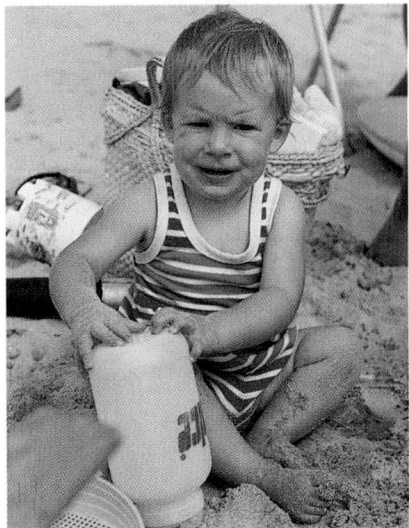

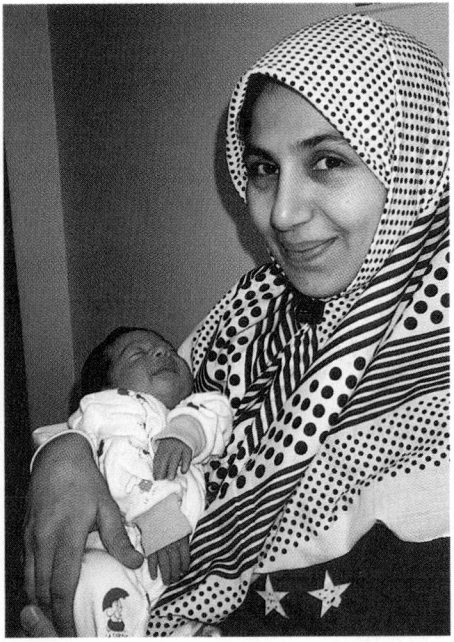

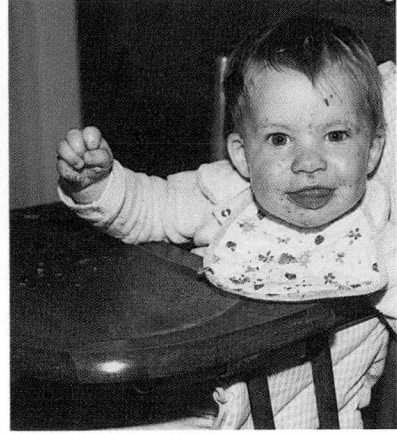

Developmental tasks of the first year include taking solid food.

Bonding may occur in the first few hours after birth or later in the first few months and is necessary for later attachment.

Figure 9-2
Development in the infant.

Physiologic Development

The physical characteristics of the infant include the following:

- Brain grows to about half the adult size.
- Body temperature stabilizes.
- Motor abilities develop, allowing using building blocks, attempts to feed self, crawling, and walking.
- Eyes begin to focus and fixate.
- Heart doubles in weight, heart rate slows, and blood pressure rises.
- Deciduous teeth begin to erupt at 4 to 6 months.
- Birthweight usually triples by 1 year, when the average male infant weighs 22 lb (10 kg) and the average female infant weighs 21 lb (9.5 kg). Length increases by 50%.

Infant and toddlers' growth rate is assessed in comparison with standardized growth charts developed for boys and girls, whose growth rates differ. Be careful when comparing an individual child's growth to standards on a chart for the following reasons:

- Every child has individual variations and short-term spurts and lags in growth.

- Atypical infants, such as those who are premature or have low birthweight, are not taken into account in such charts.
- Growth charts may be ethically and socioeconomically weighted in favor of white, middle-class children.

The Denver Developmental Screening Test (DDST) is commonly used to determine quickly and inexpensively atypical developmental patterns in infants and children. The crucial areas of development assessed in the DDST are gross motor behavior and skills, fine motor behavior and skills, language acquisition, and personal and social interaction. The test identifies problem areas that require more precise assessments. The DDST is described in more detail in most pediatric nursing texts.

Cognitive Development

Infants from birth to 1 year are in the sensorimotor stage of development described by Piaget. Language development is in the prelinguistic phase. Babies begin to coo and make pleasurable sounds soon after birth, and by 12 months of age, they can convey their wishes through a few key words.

Language development in infants has several consistent characteristics that occur with all languages:

- Use of syllable repetition (such as ma-ma, da-da, bye-bye)
- Universal early phonetic expressions (babbling sounds)
- Imitation of sounds and intonations spoken by caregivers

Psychosocial Development

In terms of the developmental theories discussed in Chapter 8, the infant has the following characteristics:

- Is in the oral stage (Freud), striving for immediate gratification of needs and having a strong sucking need
- Develops trust (Erikson) if the caregiver can be counted on to provide food when the infant is hungry; trust is also facilitated by diaper changing, warmth, and comforting
- Meets developmental tasks (Havighurst) by learning to take solid food, walk, and talk

Other components of psychosocial development in the neonate and infant include attachment, play, and temperament.

Attachment is an active, affectionate, reciprocal relationship between two people, which is somewhat different from bonding. **Bonding**, described by Klaus and Kennell (1982), occurs during a sensitive period in the first few hours after birth (although bonding also may occur later in the first few months) and is necessary for later attachment. Bonding may be considered the emotional linkage of two people, and attachment the long-term maintenance and strengthening of the linked state. Infants and children discover their environment and begin to learn how to control it through *play*. Beginning as soon as the baby is aware of sensations and the pleasure they produce, play progresses from self-pleasure to interaction with others. The two dimensions of play are social play and cognitive play. Social play, such as rolling a ball back and forth between two children, is motivated by a desire for fun, pleasure, and relationships with others. Cognitive play, as when a child puts a puzzle together, is motivated by the desire to learn.

Temperament is primarily inborn, although it is influenced by environment. A baby or child may be said to be "easy," "slow to warm," or "difficult" (Thomas, Chess, & Birch, 1968). The "easy" infant sleeps, eats, and eliminates easily; smiles spontaneously; and cries in response to significant needs. The "slow to warm" infant is more passive and distant. The "difficult" infant has volatile and labile responses, often is a restless sleeper, is highly sensitive to noises, and eats poorly. These traits often remain fairly consistent throughout the individual's life. The behavior of caregivers as they care for the baby can influence either positively and negatively the degree to which temperament dictates behavioral style.

Common Health Problems

Various health problems in infancy may require the intervention of healthcare personnel. Gastroenteritis and food allergies are common. Skin disorders, such as diaper dermatitis (diaper rash), seborrheic dermatitis (infant dandruff), prickly heat rash, and thrush (infection of the oral mucous membrane by the fungus *Candida albicans*), are also common.

Safety issues must be addressed during infancy. The inability of the infant to roll over from stomach to back makes respiratory impairment more likely if placed on the stomach to sleep. The swallowing reflex matures progressively from birth, but until it is fully developed, aspiration is a risk. Because infants put small objects in their mouths, choking is a risk. Choking may also result from small pieces of food, nuts, and popcorn. As the infant becomes more mobile, the risk for falls or for being caught in dangling cords (such as in mini-blinds) increases. Preventive measures against such safety hazards must be taught to new parents. In addition, the use of special car safety seats and restraints for infants is mandated by law. The accompanying box lists examples of nursing diagnoses for infancy through school age.

Common important health problems in infancy include infant colic, failure to thrive, sudden infant death syndrome, and child maltreatment.

Infant Colic

Colic is acute abdominal pain caused by spasmodic contractions of the intestine during the first 3 months of life. The infant cries loudly and draws the legs up to the abdomen. The exact cause of colic is not known, but several factors have been associated with this problem: swallowing excess air, feeding too rapidly or too much, improper feeding techniques, allergies, smoking, and anxiety in the primary caregiver. Despite the symptoms, the infant gains weight and thrives.

Failure to Thrive

Failure to thrive (FTT) is a condition of inadequate growth in height and weight resulting from the infant's inability to obtain or use calories needed for growth. Infants with FTT have signs of malnutrition and delayed development. Causes and contributing factors may include physiologic causes, inadequate funds to buy sufficient food, the use of a fad diet, inadequate nutritional knowledge, insufficient breast milk, and disturbances in maternal–child attachment. In most cases of FTT not caused by a physiologic problem, a team of healthcare providers (physician, nurse, dietitian, and social worker) is needed to meet the complex needs of the infant and caregivers.

Sudden Infant Death Syndrome

Sudden infant death syndrome (SIDS) is the sudden death of an infant under the age of 1 year, unexpected in light of the infant's history, in which a postmortem examination fails to reveal a cause of death. The general incidence is 2 out of every 1000 live births, with SIDS being the leading cause of death in infants ages 1 week to 1 year.

EXAMPLES OF NANDA NURSING DIAGNOSIS

Infancy Through School Age

The following are examples of nursing diagnoses that might be appropriate for the child from infancy through school age:

- Risk for Infection related to exposure to other children in childcare and at school
- Diarrhea related to milk intolerance
- Fluid Volume Deficit related to severe case of vomiting and diarrhea
- Risk for Suffocation related to parents' lack of knowledge of safety precautions

- Disorganized Infant Behavior related to environmental overstimulation
- Risk for Poisoning related to parents' lack of knowledge of proper storage of hazardous liquids
- Risk for Injury related to lack of knowledge about proper use of skates, bicycles, roller blades, and trampolines
- Self-Esteem Disturbance related to physical abuse by caregiver

---

The highest incidence occurs in the third and fourth months of life. The exact cause is still unknown, but it is believed to be associated with a brainstem abnormality in the neurologic regulation of cardiac and respiratory control. Because sleep habits have been implicated with SIDS, it is recommended that infants up to the age of 6 months sleep on their side or back (rather than the stomach) on a firm surface.

Child Maltreatment

Forms of **child maltreatment**, also called **child abuse**, include intentional physical neglect or abuse, emotional neglect or abuse, and sexual abuse. Neglect, the failure of a caregiver to provide for the child's basic needs with an adequate level of care, is the most common form. Physical abuse, often referred to as the *battered child syndrome*, refers to deliberate physical abuse and is typically inflicted by a parent. Sexual abuse includes incest, molestation, exhibitionism, child pornography, child prostitution, and pedophilia. These acts, when committed by a caregiver, such as a parent or babysitter, are considered sexual abuse. When a stranger commits such an act, it is considered sexual assault (a criminal act). Other forms of child maltreatment include violent shaking, called *shaken baby syndrome*, especially in infants younger than 6 months of age (resulting in brain trauma), and *Munchausen syndrome by proxy*, which is an illness fabricated or induced in another person. It is most often the mother who fabricates or causes an illness in a child to gain attention from healthcare providers.

Although maltreatment occurs in all ethnic groups and at all levels of society, certain factors increase the risk, including the following:

- Parents experiencing stress from unemployment, depression, poor social and marital relationships, substance abuse, or health problems.
- Children who cry frequently, have sleep difficulties, wet the bed, are hyperactive or aggressive, have difficult temperaments, or have physical, emotional, or cognitive disabilities.

- Caregivers' lack of knowledge about parenting and the normal behaviors of children.
- Lack of family and social support for caregivers.

The number of reported cases of child maltreatment has increased dramatically and is a cause of national concern. Healthcare workers are in an excellent position to recognize families at risk and offer interventions, and they have a legal obligation to report suspected maltreatment (see Chap. 7). The long-term treatment of maltreated children and their families is complex and multidisciplinary.

Role of the Nurse in Promoting Health and Preventing Illness

The most essential role of the nurse in meeting healthcare needs of the infant is promoting health and preventing illness by teaching family members. Teaching ranges from providing basic information about prevention of diaper rash to facilitating grieving in parents who have lost a baby to SIDS. Examples of specific areas of preventive teaching for parents of infants are shown in Table 9-2. Immunization against contagious diseases begins during the first year of life and should follow a regular schedule, as outlined in Table 9-3.

When an infant in late infancy is hospitalized, behaviors of separation anxiety are common. The infant may initially cry and scream in the phase of *protest*, but then stop crying and appear depressed (*despair* phase) (Wong, et al, 1998). Nurses should encourage parents to stay with the infant and provide care, or if that is not possible, consistent caregivers are important to maintain the infant's trust in others.

Toddler: 1 to 3 Years

From 1 to 3 years of age, the child is considered a **toddler** (Fig. 9-3).

Table 9-2
Promoting Health in Infancy

Areas of Concern	Teaching
Accident prevention	• Associate common accidents to developmental abilities of the infant. • Encourage relaxed, slow feeding and regular "bubbling" (burping) to prevent aspiration. • Emphasize that bottles should not be propped and left with an unattended infant. • Emphasize the use of bumper pads and keeping crib sides up at all times to prevent injury related to bumping or falling. • Teach the correct usage of infant car seats. • Emphasize never leaving an infant unattended on a table, chair, or regular bed. • Teach proper positioning of infant on back for sleeping, and discourage the use of pillows to prevent suffocation. • Keep small objects out of reach to prevent choking.
Nutrition and feeding methods	• Assist the mother with the initiation and maintenance of breastfeeding. • If bottle feeding, provide information on the preparation of formula at feeding, expulsion of air from the bottle, nipple type and hole size, and positioning for an effective feeding experience. • Emphasize the significance of emotional nurturing during feeding. • Discuss the age at which solid foods are needed. • Discuss the sequence of solid foods (ie, cereals, vegetables, fruits, meats, and protein products).
Infections	• Encourage prompt attention for infections. • Encourage completion of required immunizations of infancy.
Hygiene and skin care	• Teach proper infant bathing techniques (ie, washing eye from inner to outer canthus, washing genitals last, umbilical cord care). • Discuss the proper use of creams, oils, and powders. • Describe the nature of infant skin and its susceptibility to disturbance. • Teach diapering and hygienic practices related to the disposal of products of elimination. • Teach care related to hair, nails, and genitals (particularly circumcised boys).
Developmental norms	• Provide accurate information about development norms. This can prevent unrealistic expectations in caregivers and assist in isolating and treating developmental delays earlier.
Emotional attachment	• Encourage intimate child–caregiver contact in the crucial period immediately after birth. • Provide information about the sequence of normal attachment behaviors in infants. • Reassure concerned caregivers that attachment feelings occur at different rates for different caregivers and infants.

Physiologic Development

Physiologic development continues steadily through the toddler years, but the pace is considerably slower than that in infancy. Growth and development highlights include the following:

- Has rapid brain growth; increase in length of long bones of the arms and legs; growth of muscles
- Uses fingers to pick up small objects
- Walks forward and backward, runs, kicks, climbs stairs, and rides a tricycle
- Drinks from a cup and uses a spoon
- At 2 years of age, the toddler is typically four times the birthweight, averaging 30 to 35 lb (13.6 to 15.9 kg) and 23 to 37 inches (58.4 to 94 cm) in height.
- Has bladder control during the day and sometimes during the night (2.5 to 3 years of age)
- Turns pages in a book, and by 3 years of age, draws stick people

Cognitive Development

Toddlers are in Piaget's last two stages of sensorimotor development: beginning to understand object permanence, following simple commands, and anticipating events. Toddlers can understand self as separate from others and have a beginning perception of body image. Toddlers can identify and name several body parts and have a sense of gender identity. Language begins at about 1 year of age, with the use of single or bisyllable sounds. At about 2 years of age, children begin to use short sentences.

Psychosocial Development

In terms of psychosocial theories, the toddler has the following characteristics:

- Is in Freud's anal stage; increased muscle development and sphincter control encourage the child to focus on the pleasure of sphincter contraction and relaxation.

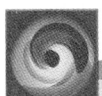

Table 9-3
Recommended Childhood Immunization Schedule United States, January–December 1999

Vaccines are listed under routinely recommended ages. Bars indicate range of recommended ages for immunization. Any dose not given at the recommended age should be given as a "catch-up" immunization at any subsequent visit when indicated and feasible. Ovals indicate vaccines to be given if previously recommended doses were missed or given earlier than the recommended minimum age.

Age ► Vaccine ▼	Birth	1 mo	2 mos	4 mos	6 mos	12 mos	15 mos	18 mos	4–6 yrs	11–12 yrs	14–16 yrs
Hepatitis B	Hep B										
			Hep B			Hep B				Hep B	
Diphtheria, tetanus, pertussis			DTaP	DTaP	DTaP		DTaP³		DTaP	Td	
Haemophilus influenzae type b			Hib	Hib	Hib	Hib					
Polio			IPV	IPV		IVP			IVP		
Rotavirus			Rv	Rv	Rv						
Measles, mumps, Rubella							MMR		MMR	MMR	
Varicella							Var			Var	

The development of new vaccines, revised recommendations on timing and dosage, and the introduction of combination vaccines have necessitated yearly revisions of the vaccine guidelines for children. For complete information about timing and specific information about immunizations, refer to recommendations from the Advisory Committee for Immunization Practices, the American Academy of Pediatrics, or the American Academy of Family Physicians.

- Enters Erikson's stage of autonomy versus shame and doubt. Autonomy is developing from independence in feeding, walking, dressing, and toileting as well as the ability to express wishes verbally. Children who do not feel autonomous may be reluctant to explore and may be fearful of activities and people.
- Has the developmental task (Havighurst) of learning to control the elimination of urine and feces; begins to learn sex differences, form concepts, learn language, and distinguish right from wrong.

Toddlers may exhibit separation anxiety, negativism, and regression. **Separation anxiety** occurs when a child is afraid of being sent away from loved ones who offer security. **Negativism** (characteristically expressed by saying no) results from the toddler's efforts at control over the environment. **Regression**, or behavior that is more characteristic of a younger age, can occur at any time in response to stressful circumstances. The most common regressive behaviors are excessive clinging to caregivers, loss of control over elimination, and the use of more infantile speech patterns.

Common Health Problems

Accidents, such as motor vehicle accidents, poisonings, burns, drowning, choking and aspiration, and falls, are the major cause of death in toddlerhood. Dental problems can occur, especially if the toddler is allowed to go to sleep while sucking on a bottle of milk or sweetened liquid. Respiratory tract and middle ear infections are common. Some surgeries, such as repair of a cleft lip and palate, may be done in the toddler years. Surgery to repair most congenital anomalies is not done until later childhood.

Role of the Nurse in Promoting Health and Preventing Illness

The role of the nurse in health promotion and illness prevention continues to be primarily teaching, as shown by the examples in Table 9-4. A significant part of teaching is in helping caregivers encourage their toddler's independence while setting firm limits.

Toddlers enter a stage of autonomy, promoting exploration.

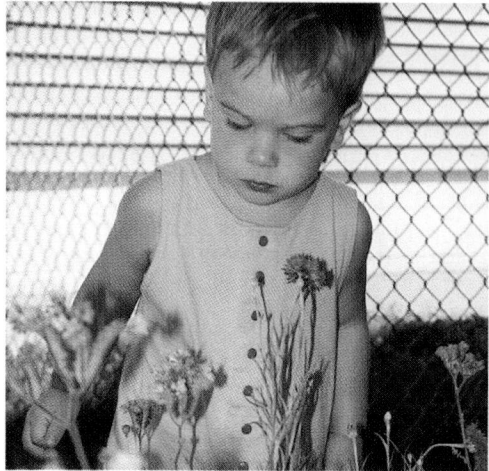

Play in toddlerhood may be solitary or parallel.

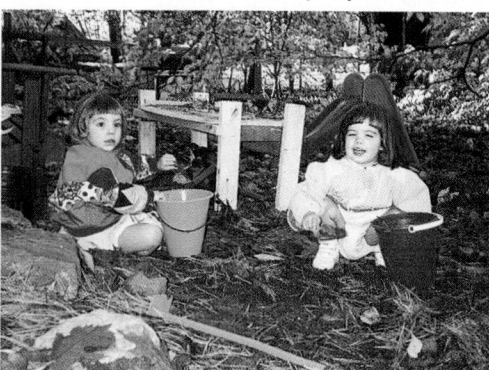

Toddlers start to see themselves as separate from others.

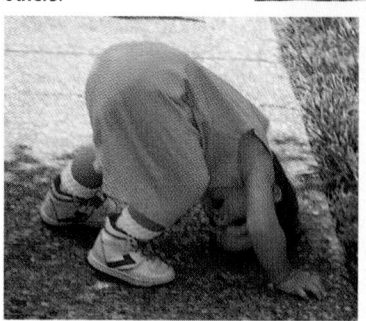

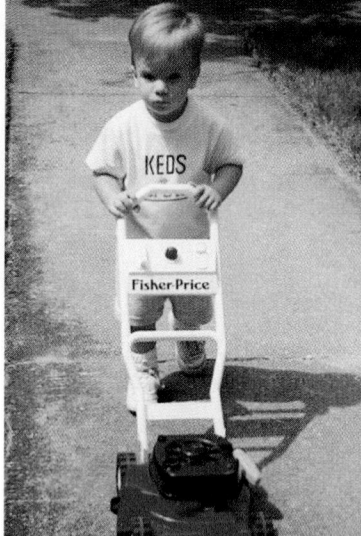

Cognitive development can be promoted by allowing the toddler the opportunity to observe and imitate.

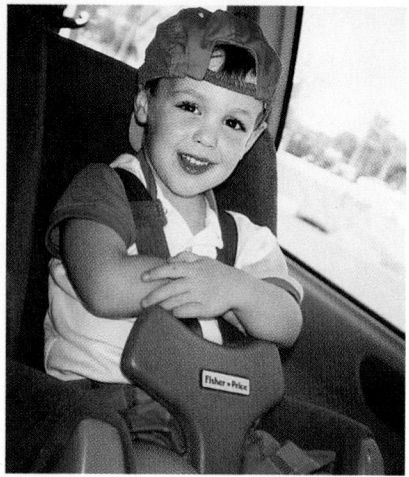

Safety becomes a common concern for caregivers.

Figure 9-3
Development in the toddler.

Toddlers who require care in the hospital setting experience stress and separation anxiety when parents are not present. To decrease stress from unfamiliar surroundings and caregivers, parents should be encouraged to provide care and remain with the toddler as much as possible. Every effort should be made to have consistency of healthcare providers and to maintain familiar routines and rituals. When they are ill or in pain, toddlers often regress to earlier behaviors, such as wanting a bottle to drink from.

Preschooler: 3 to 6 Years

At around age 3, toddlers begin to move into the next stage: **preschooler**. Although growth and development are slower than in infancy and toddlerhood, they are still steady (Fig. 9-4).

Physiologic Development

The physical characteristics of the preschooler include the following:

- Head is close to adult size by 6 years of age.
- The body is less chubby and becomes leaner and more coordinated.
- Motor abilities include skipping, throwing and catching a ball, copying figures, and printing letters and numbers.
- Full set of 20 deciduous teeth is present; baby teeth begin to fall out and are replaced by permanent teeth.
- Average weight at 5 to 6 years of age is 45 lb (20.4 kg), with boys being slightly heavier than girls.

Cognitive Development

Preschoolers are in Piaget's preoperational stage of development. Passing through the preconceptual and the intuitive phases, preschoolers demonstrate the following transitional changes:

- Egocentrism decreases as socialization with other children increases and the ability to express self verbally improves.

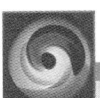

Table 9-4
Promoting Health in Toddlerhood

Areas of Concern	Teaching
Accident prevention	• Explain how the autonomy needs of the toddler need to be met while ensuring safety. • Suggest locking poisons out of child's reach. • Suggest safety plugs for electric outlets. • Advise to block stairs with a gate and then help the child learn how to maneuver stairs. • Advise not allowing toddler to have small, hard food items, such as popcorn, peanuts, raw carrots, or hard candy, or balloons, which may cause choking. • Discourage the toddler from running with food in his or her mouth. • Encourage the proper use of car seats. • Advise never to leave the child unattended near water. • Suggest teaching toddler of dangers in clear, simple terms (eg, "stove hot"). • Advise against tossing child into the air or swinging child by the arms. • Keep small objects out of reach to prevent choking.
Toilet training	• Explain developmental tasks necessary for toilet training. • Correct misconceptions about mastery of this task. • Suggest some helpful literature for caregivers.
Negativism	• Help caregivers understand the normality of negativism in toddlerhood and its meaning from the child's point of view.
Feeding and nutrition	• Suggest that food be provided in forms the toddler can manipulate independently. • Advise caregivers not to be concerned about the messiness of toddler eating habits because the independence gained by the child is more important. • Provide soft finger foods that the child can eat while playing. • Reassure caregivers that short anorexic periods are common in toddlerhood.
Hygiene and dental care	• Emphasize the teaching of good hygiene habits (eg, handwashing after toileting or before eating). • Suggest teaching the toddler how to brush teeth (with assistance). • Encourage caregivers to take the toddler with them for dental appointments as an observer.
Infections	• Encourage caregivers to attend to respiratory tract infections promptly because of the high correlation between such infections and otitis media. • Encourage the completion of initial immunization schedule and any necessary boosters.
Play habits	• Encourage the selection of toys that emphasize gross motor skills and creativity. • Advise parents that sharing is not likely to occur and that parallel play is an important precursor to interactive play.

• Play is more related to real-life events (rather than fantasy).
• Basic curiosity results in constant questions and improved reasoning ability.

Language development is seen in more elaborate and grammatically correct sentences, with 6- to 18-word sentences becoming common by 6 years of age. Incessantly asking "Why?" increases the child's knowledge, encourages further conversations, and helps develop language abilities.

Preschoolers clearly identify themselves as male or female, can understand basic body functions, and have a curiosity about sex differences. This curiosity often leads to "playing doctor," which is normal behavior at this stage. Many children in this age group want to look special or dressed up and gain increased self-esteem by receiving compliments about their appearance.

Psychosocial Development

Based on psychosocial theories of growth and development, the preschooler has the following characteristics:

• Is in Freud's phallic stage, with the biologic focus primarily genital. The child has a sexual desire for the opposite-sex parent but, as a means of defense, strongly identifies with the same-sex parent; as a result of this conflict resolution, the superego and conscience begin to develop.
• Is in Erikson's stage of initiative versus guilt. Inner turmoil occurs when natural curiosity is pitted against a constant examination of the propriety of one's actions by a rigid conscience. Realistic self-limits are learned through social interactions.
• Has four developmental tasks (Havighurst): to learn sex differences and modesty, to describe social and

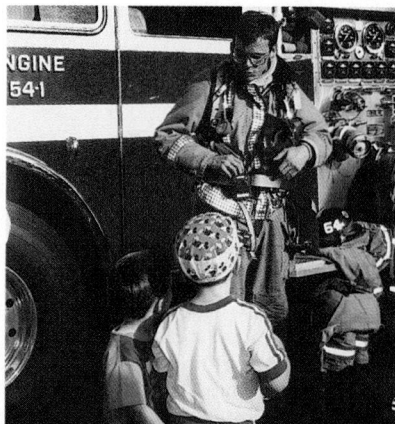

Basic curiosity results in questioning and an improved reasoning ability in the preschooler.

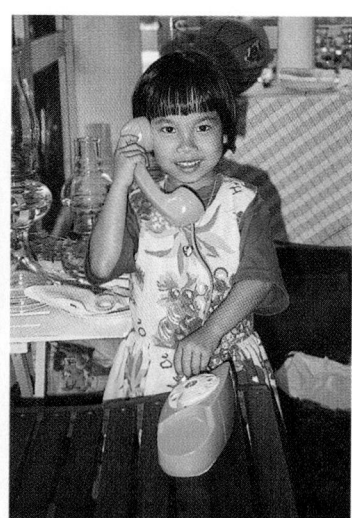

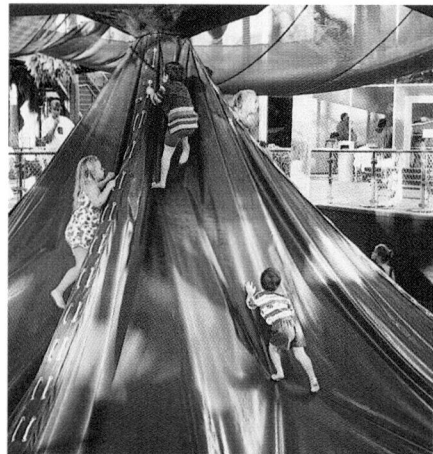

Preschooler play is associative and cooperative in its social dimension and cognitive development is demonstrated in constructive and pretend play.

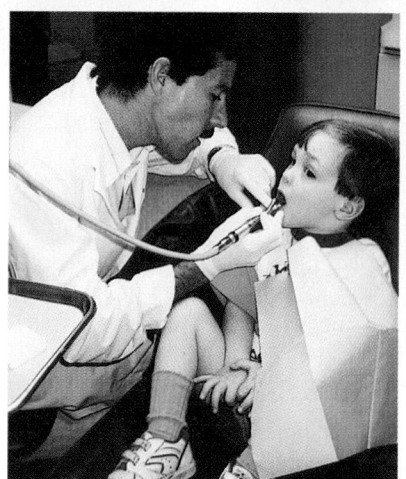

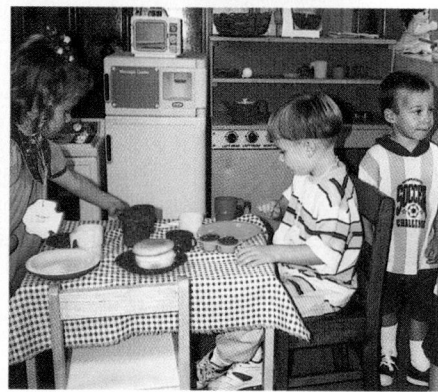

A visit to the dentist is useful for teaching dental hygiene and helps the preschooler overcome the fear of the unknown.

Symbolic play gradually becomes more related to real-life events.

Figure 9-4
Development in the preschooler.

physical reality through concept formation and language development, to get ready to read, and to learn to distinguish right from wrong.

Preschoolers often have fears—most commonly fear of new places, fear of the dark, and fear during nightmares. These fears are often made worse by the child's own fertile imagination and ability to fantasize. Support and validation of the preschooler's feelings by caregivers are essential.

Moral and Spiritual Development

Kohlberg's preconventional phase of moral reasoning dominates this age. The focus of this stage is obeying rules to avoid punishment or receive a reward.

The cognitive, psychosocial, and moral development of the preschooler provide a base for spiritual development, as described by Fowler. The preschooler may attend activities at church or synagogue with the family but does not understand religious concepts. The concept of a deity is literal, with God usually being viewed as a male human. Concepts such as heaven, hell, and holy spirits are incomprehensible and often frightening.

Common Health Problems

Preschoolers continue to have the health problems that are common in toddlerhood. Communicable diseases and respiratory tract infections are common, especially with increased interaction with other children at nursery schools and day care. Preschoolers are prone to accidents because of their increased curiosity about the world. Some congenital disorders, such as hypospadias, inguinal hernias, and cardiac anomalies, require surgery at this time. Dental caries become common if teeth are neglected. As language becomes more sophisticated, speech disorders may become apparent.

Role of the Nurse in Promoting Health and Preventing Illness

Table 9-5 provides examples of teaching for promoting health and preventing illness in preschoolers. When caring for a preschool-aged child who is scheduled for surgery or requires hospitalization, nurses must recognize the importance of the child's fear of pain as well as separation anxiety. The nurse can allay some fears by explaining procedures

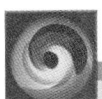

Table 9-5
Promoting Health in Preschoolers

Area of Concern	Teaching
Accident prevention and safety	• Advise that preschoolers, now out of car seats, need to learn how to use seat belts. • Advise that clear boundaries regarding where tricycles or bicycles can be ridden need to be given. • Teach simple road safety (eg, looking both ways before crossing the street). • Encourage education of children regarding strangers and block parent programs. • Encourage education about sexual abuse (ie, explaining to child what is and is not appropriate touching by an adult). • Swimming lessons can begin and basic water safety taught. • Teach the dangers of matches, and practice home fire safety drills.
Infections	• Advise that these are an inevitable result of increased socialization. • Advise teaching children sound hygiene practices such as handwashing after toileting, correct disposal of tissues after use, nonsharing of items like eating utensils. • Keep immunizations current.
Sleep disorders	• Explain to caregivers the commonality of this problem among preschoolers. • Suggest that relaxed bedtime rituals and a night light can help. • Advise that comforting and warm reassurance are needed when a child is awakened by nightmares.
Dental hygiene	• Teach that preschoolers should be brushing their teeth and flossing with caregiver assistance. • Advise that a dental visit at this time is useful for teaching dental hygiene and overcoming fear of the unknown.
Play habits	• Advise caregivers that make-believe play and imaginary friends are common and normal in the preschool years. • Encourage caregivers to promote socialization through neighborhood play groups and nursery school.
Self-esteem	• Encourage caregivers to provide opportunities to make new discoveries and gain a sense of autonomy by experiencing neighborhood and preschool activities. • Advise to avoid frequent criticism and overprotectiveness. • Teach caregivers the importance of providing opportunities for the child to plan and carry out activities and of giving appropriate praise for accomplishments.

in language the child can understand and by being honest about how much pain a procedure will cause. Many healthcare institutions and agencies have preprocedure visits so that the child having surgery becomes familiar with the setting and with the activities that will be done. Allowing the child to practice procedures on a doll and encouraging the child to express his or her feelings openly are also beneficial. Encouraging caregivers to take an active role in the child's care helps to reduce fear and separation anxiety.

School-Aged Child: 6 to 12 Years

School-aged children, from 6 to 12 years of age, are typically sturdy and strong. Physical growth during this time is relatively slow but continues steadily, with both refinement and subtle changes taking place (Fig. 9-5).

Physiologic Development

Physiologic development of school-aged children includes the following:

• The brain reaches 90% to 95% of adult size; by 12 years of age, the nervous system is almost completely matured, resulting in coordinated body movements.
• Motor abilities progress from the ability to hold a pencil and print words at 6 years of age to the ability to write in script and in sentences at 12 years of age.
• Sexual organs grow but are dormant until late in this period, when hormonal changes begin.
• All permanent teeth are present, except for the second and third molars, by 12 years of age.
• Height increases 2 to 3 inches (5.1 to 7.6 cm) and weight increases 3 to 6 lb (1.4 to 2.7 kg) a year.

Cognitive Development

The school-aged child is at Piaget's concrete operational stage of development, organizing facts about the environment to use for problem solving. In this period, the child has the following characteristics:

• Thinks logically and develops concepts of mass, volume, weight, and measurement

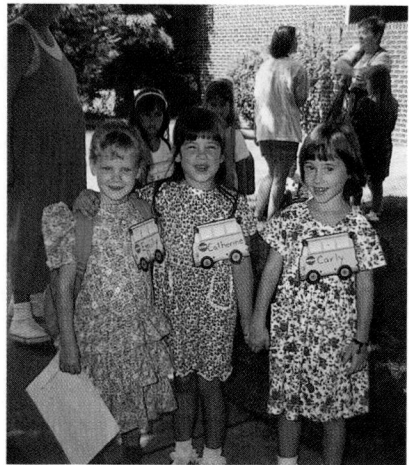
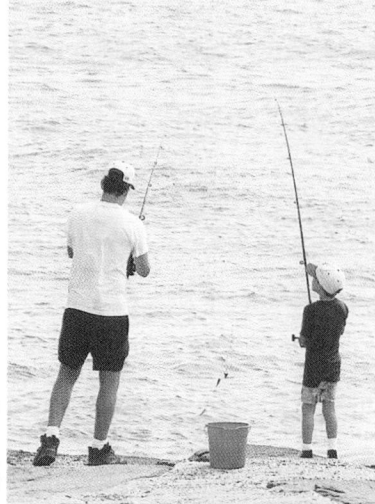
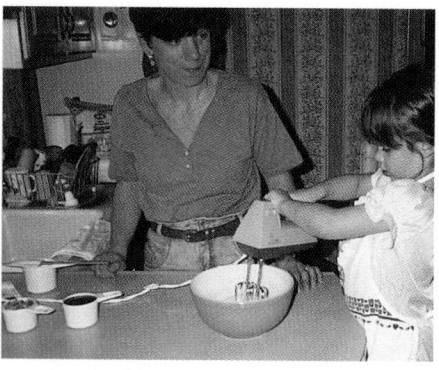

The school-aged child is aware of and understands a sequence of events.

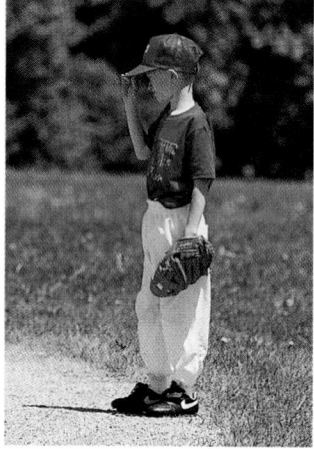

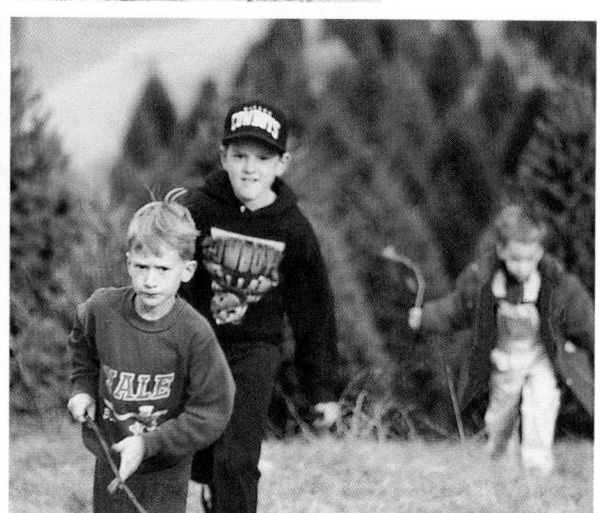

Play involves development of skill, games with rules, and competitive activities.

Figure 9-5
Development in the school-aged child.

- Deals best with actual objects and people, but can relate concepts and compare events
- Uses inductive reasoning to solve new problems
- Generalizes about people, places, and things
- Develops classification systems
- Develops an awareness and understanding of other people's feelings and points of view
- Understands reversal of events

School-aged children have well-developed language skills, using language in a more sophisticated manner. Their ability to store information in long-term memory and retrieve it in the remembering (recall) process is more efficient.

Psychosocial Development

The psychosocial development of the school-aged child is as follows:

- Is in the latency stage of Freud's theory, with psychosocial energies being channeled toward strong identification with own sex

- Is in the industry versus inferiority stage of Erikson's theory, with the child focused on learning useful skills and thereby developing positive self-esteem. A sense of identity begins to emerge, and values are integrated. The emphasis is on doing, succeeding, and accomplishing.
- Has the following developmental tasks (Havighurst):
  - Learning physical game skills
  - Learning appropriate masculine or feminine social role
  - Developing fundamental skills in reading, writing, and calculating
  - Developing concepts necessary for everyday living
  - Achieving personal independence
  - Developing conscience, morality, and a scale of values

Body image, self-concept, and sexuality are interrelated. Sexual development results in a strong need to understand body function and to have accurate information about sexuality.

Peer relationships become the major gauge for determining status, skill, and personableness. Peer groups in middle childhood help prepare the child for getting along in the larger world and teach appropriate sex role behavior. They also act as transition modes for the child as he or she leaves the total caregiver influence and heads toward adult independence.

Moral and Spiritual Development

Most of middle childhood is spent in the conventional phase of moral development. Behavior is based on familial and peer group beliefs, and conformity to the norm is common. Following school regulations, respecting teachers, and viewing justice as a means of fair play are all important.

In Fowler's theory, school-aged children view religious faith as a relationship that involves reciprocal fairness. They take part in rituals of their faith with a basic understanding of the ritual's significance. The importance of spiritual beliefs and the possibility of life after death are accepted, even if not totally understood.

Common Health Problems

Accidents continue to be common in school-aged children. With increased interactions with other children in school, communicable conditions, such as scabies, impetigo, and head lice, are more prevalent. Other common health-related problems of the school-aged child include attention deficit hyperactivity disorder (ADHD) and learning disability (LD), and enuresis (bed wetting).

ADHD is a developmentally inappropriate degree of inattention, impulsiveness, and hyperactivity. To be diagnosed with this disorder, the child must have manifested symptoms before 7 years of age and they must be present in at least two settings. LD is a group of disorders in which the child has significant difficulty in listening, speaking, reading, writing, reasoning, mathematic abilities, or social skills (Wong, et al, 1998). Both of these conditions affect all areas of the life of the child, but they are most noticeable in the classroom. Multiple approaches are used in management, including medication, environmental strategies, and classroom education. Based on the Education for All Handicapped Children's Act, children with ADHD and LD must receive free public education in the least restrictive environment.

Enuresis is diagnosed when a child is at least 5 years of age and is still having involuntary urination, usually at night. Although this problem is significant to the child and his or her parents, it is defined as a benign and self-limiting disorder, usually ending between 6 and 8 years of age.

Role of the Nurse in Health Promotion and Illness Prevention

The nurse's role in promoting health and preventing illness for the school-aged child involves individual and family teaching, such as that conducted by school nurses. Because school violence has become more common, with school-aged children involved in mass shootings, school nurses must be prepared for a potential crisis. Table 9-6 provides examples of nursing activities specific for this age group.

Because school-aged children are striving for independence and control, hospitalization may mean a loss of freedom of choice (as, for example, types of food, clothing, activities). Children of this age should be allowed to have some measure of control over allowable activities and should be encouraged to do what they can, such as making their own bed (Wong, et al, 1998).

The Adolescent and Young Adult

The adolescent and young adult years are a time of both change and stability. **Adolescence** extends from 12 to 20 years of age; the **young adult** period is considered to be the 20s and 30s. However, some people enter adolescence at age 12 and remain adolescents into the middle or late 20s; others enter adolescence at age 14 and move on into young adulthood within a year (Freiberg, 1992).

After experiencing rapid growth and development during adolescence, the young adult completes physical growth and develops internal and external controls and values acceptable to society. There are no specific measurements of maturity; each person is an individual, and a wide range of normal values and behaviors are considered healthy (Fig. 9-6).

Physiologic Development

Changes in the adolescent's body transform him or her from a child to an adult in appearance. Physiologic development includes the following:

- The feet, hands, and long bones grow rapidly, accompanied by an increase in muscle mass (especially in boys).
- Primary and secondary development occurs, with maturation of the genitalia; presence of body hair; breast development and menstruation in girls; facial hair growth, voice changes, and spermatogenesis in boys.
- Puberty (the time when the ability to reproduce begins) begins at 10 or 11 years of age in girls (with menstruation usually beginning between 11 and 14 years of age) and at 12 or 13 years of age in boys.
- Sebaceous and axillary sweat glands become active.
- Full adult size is reached, although some young men may continue to grow in their 20s.

A true assessment of adolescent development must include the profound changes in reproductive functioning. **Puberty** can be divided into the following three stages (Table 9-7):

Prepubescence: Secondary sex characteristics begin to develop, but the reproductive organs do not yet function.

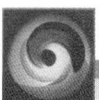

Table 9-6
Promoting Health in School-Aged Children

Area of Concern	Teaching
Accident prevention	• Emphasize traffic safety. • Encourage the use of seat belts. • Emphasize bicycle, skateboard, and scooter safety. • Teach children to take water safety programs. • Teach firearm safety. • Teach importance of bicycle helmets.
Communicable conditions	• Encourage proper hygiene habits, including not sharing personal items like combs. • Home visit may be required to discuss home health practices if a child has a communicable condition like pediculosis (head lice). • Advise of common treatment methods for conditions like scabies, impetigo, and pediculosis. • Teach about sexually transmitted diseases, including acquired immunodeficiency syndrome.
Substance abuse	• Early preventive teaching about alcohol, nicotine, and street drugs that includes guidance for families is essential.
Sexuality	• Sex education needs to begin as early as 7 or 8 years of age. • Families need encouragement to talk about sex at home. • Caregivers need encouragement to answer questions honestly and correctly. • Menstruation needs to be discussed by at least 8 years of age because some girls menstruate as young as 9 years of age.

Mental health concerns:
  School phobia
  Depression and suicide
	• Work with teachers and families so that they learn to recognize behavior that indicates mental health difficulties.
	• Provide referral for specialized assistance.

Physical fitness	• Teach good food choices that are lower in fat, salt, and sugar, but avoid strenuous dieting if child is overweight. • Emphasize the importance of physical activity: children should exercise nonstop for at least 20 to 25 minutes three times a week.
Self-esteem	• Teach caregivers to encourage independent activities and social interactions and to be sure that successes are greater in number than failures. • Provide the child with positive statements that demonstrate being valued, important, and loved.

Pubescence: Secondary sex characteristics continue to develop, and ova and sperm begin to be produced by the reproductive organs.

Postpubescence: Reproductive functioning and the development of secondary sex characteristics reach adult maturity.

Cognitive Development

According to Piaget, adolescence is the stage when the cognitive development of formal operations is developed. Deductive, reflective, and hypothetical reasoning are possible, and abstract concepts can be used. Long-term goals can be set as the concept of time, its passage, and the future become real. Challenging the decision making of adults is common. Egocentrism returns, and imaginary audiences and daydreaming are common.

Young adults, in comparison to the adolescent, are more creative in thought, are objective and realistic, and are less self-centered. Their learning is enhanced through educational and life experiences.

Psychosocial Development

In terms of developmental theories, the characteristics of the adolescent and young adult are as follows:

• Is in Freud's genital stage. The libido reemerges in a mature, adult form.
• Based on Erikson's theory, the adolescent tries out different roles, personal choices, and beliefs in the stage called *identity versus role confusion.* Self-concept is being stabilized, with the peer group acting as the greatest influence. The young adult, in the *intimacy versus isolation stage,* needs to complete tasks such as achieving independence from parents,

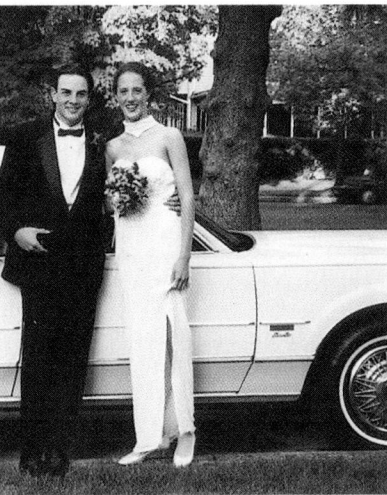

The prom is an opportunity to practice formal adult social skills among one's peers

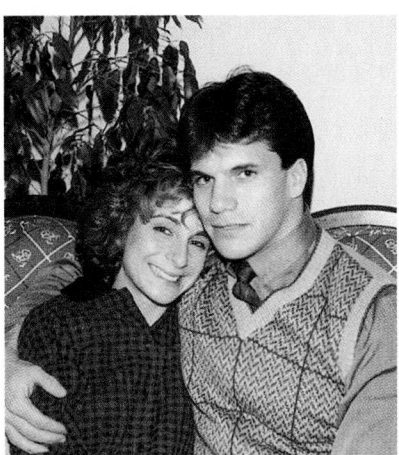

A primary developmental task of adolescence is to achieve new and more mature relationships.

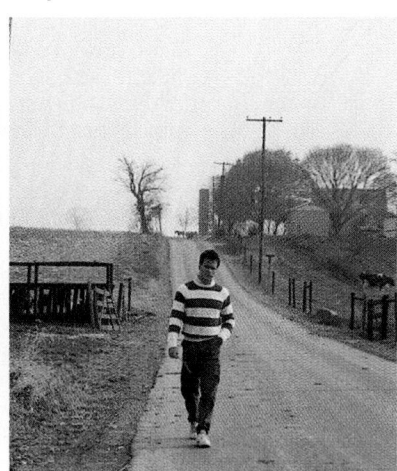

The development of self-identity in adolescence involves becoming emotionally independent.

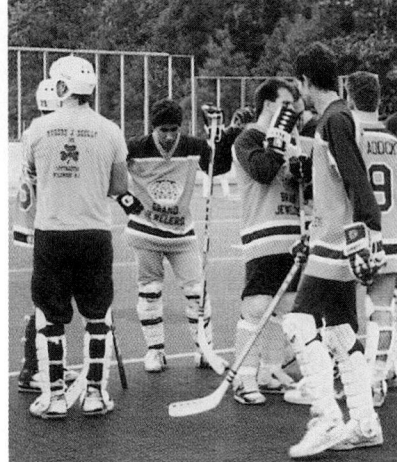

Athletic activities and skills are important in adolescence.

Figure 9-6
Development in the adolescent.

establishing intimate relationships, and choosing an occupation or career. If such developmental tasks are not accomplished, the young adult becomes isolated and self-absorbed.

- According to Havighurst, more mature relationships with both boys and girls of the same age are achieved, a masculine or feminine social role is developed, one's personal appearance is accepted, and a set of values and an ethical system as a guide to behavior are internalized.

- Based on Levinson's theory of individual life structure, the years from 18 to 22 years of age are characterized by early adult transition (Levinson, Darrow, Klein, Levinson, & McKee, 1978). This is a time of making initial career choices, establishing personal relationships, and selecting personal values and lifestyles. During the years from 22 to 28 years of age, the young adult builds on previous choices, but there may be a transient quality to occupational choices and friendships.

- Gould's (1972) theory of transformation views young adults as having established their own control as

adults separate from the family. They want to enjoy the present but also build for the future.

A major psychosocial developmental requirement for the young adult is choosing a vocation. The decision to enter the world of work is strongly influenced initially by the need to become independent of one's family and to be self-sufficient. The choice of an occupation or a career is also guided by the factors such as the desire to get married, raise a family, and become part of the community (Fig. 9-7).

Occupational and career choices are largely tied to educational choices. Many careers require a college education. Adults learn from both informal and formal experiences and are largely goal-directed learners. If the person's identified goals are to increase career opportunities, maintain financial stability, and pursue upward mobility, the adult will be motivated to learn and change. The major factor in achieving satisfaction with one's vocational choice is the belief that one is functioning to capacity and making a contribution to society.

Establishing a family involves both parents, even though the physiologic changes of pregnancy take place

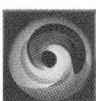

Table 9-7
Adolescent Sexual Development

Stage	Males	Females
Prepubescence	• Progressive enlargement of testicles, seminal ducts, prostate gland • Enlargement and reddening of the scrotal sac • Increase in length and circumference of penis • Appearance of downy pubic hair	• Progressive enlargement of the ovaries • Ripening of graafian follicles • Rounding of the hips • Appearance of breast buds • Enlargement of the fallopian tubes, vagina, and uterus • Appearance of downy pubic hair
Pubescence	• Increase in amount, pigmentation, and curling of pubic hair • Growth spurt involving peak pace of height and weight increase • Deepening of the voice due to growth of larynx • Enlargement of testicles • Increased pigmentation and growth of scrotum • Growth of penis in length and circumference • Beginning of spermatogenesis	• Increase in amount, pigmentation, and curling of pubic hair • Growth spurt involving peak pace of height and weight increase • Menarche • Appearance of axillary hair • Enlargement of vulva and clitoris • Development of breast tissue • Ovulation
Postpubescence	• Completion of sexual growth and development • Fertility	• Completion of sexual growth and development • Fertility

in the woman. Pregnancy may be considered a period of developmental crisis during which certain tasks must be completed for acceptance and coping by the expanding family. Completion of the tasks is influenced by the cognitive, psychosocial, cultural, and educational dimensions of the prospective parents.

The verification of pregnancy may raise conflicting emotions in the woman, influenced by such as factors as whether the pregnancy was planned or unplanned and how the baby will affect career goals. As body changes occur and fetal movement is felt, the woman begins to visualize herself as a mother and normally assumes responsibility for the health of the growing baby. As the time for delivery of the baby becomes closer, the woman centers on maternal tasks (such as preparing the baby's room and having clothing ready) and prepares herself for labor and delivery. During the pregnancy, the expectant father needs to learn the normal physiologic and psychological changes of pregnancy, accept his supportive role in meeting maternal needs, and explore his feelings about the developing infant and the birth.

Moral and Spiritual Development

The child enters adolescence with a law-and-order orientation and may never progress beyond that point. Young adults who have mastered previous levels of moral development reach the conventional level and are concerned with maintaining expectations. They also value conformity, loyalty, and social order. Some people may enter the postconventional stage, in which they make moral judgments on the basis of universal beliefs.

Adolescents and young adults can think in the abstract and may question beliefs and practices that no longer serve to stabilize their identity or purpose. The individuating-reflective period in the young adult (defined by Fowler) brings discovery of the meaning of values as they relate to the achievement of social purposes and the acceptance of the value systems of others. Often, adolescents or young adults temporarily abandon traditional religious practices.

Common Health Problems

Although adolescence and young adulthood are times of maximum physiologic development and health, a wide variety of health problems can occur. Health promotion focuses on nutrition, relationships with self and others, and safety. The accompanying box lists examples of nursing diagnoses for adolescents and young adults.

Accidents

Accidents are the leading cause of death for adolescents and young adults. Motor vehicle accidents are the most common cause of mortality, often associated with the use of alcohol or other drugs.

Substance Abuse

Smoking and the use of illegal drugs (such as marijuana and cocaine) may be a problem, and the use of alcohol is significantly related to risk-taking behavior. In addition, the use of crack-cocaine, as well as other relatively inexpensive and highly addictive drugs, has reached epidemic proportions in many areas of North America.

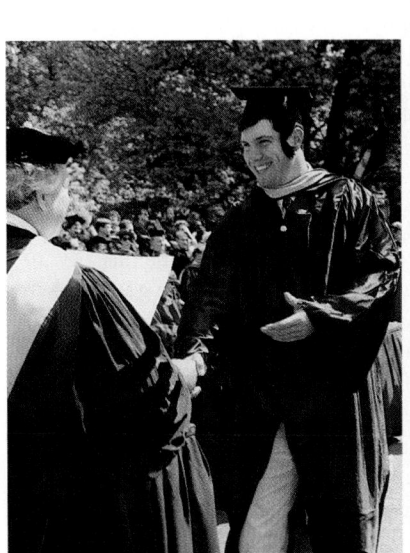
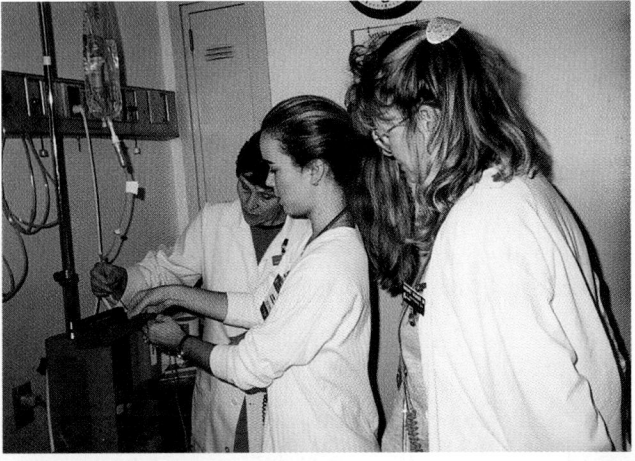
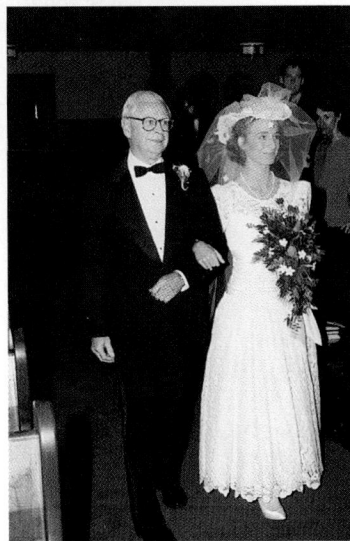
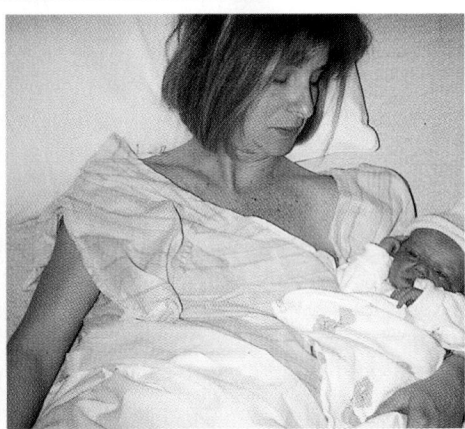

Figure 9-7
Developmental tasks of the young adult center on establishing intimate relationships and a home and on getting started in an occupation.

EXAMPLES OF NANDA NURSING DIAGNOSES

Adolescence

The following are examples of nursing diagnoses that might be appropriate for the adolescent:

- Altered Nutrition: More than body requirements related to compulsive overeating
- Altered Nutrition: Less than body requirements related to self-imposed dieting
- Risk for Fluid Volume Deficit related to extended hours of football practice in heat
- Risk for Injury related to risk-taking behavior while driving
- Risk for Trauma related to lack of knowledge about water safety

- Social Isolation related to perceived inability to be popular
- Risk for Altered Parenting related to teenage pregnancy
- Altered Family Processes related to lack of communication
- Body Image Disturbance related to obesity
- Anxiety related to fear of failure in school
- Altered Health Maintenance related to frequent use of alcohol and drugs

Suicide

The suicide rate of adolescents has increased drastically since the 1960s, with suicide being more prevalent in adolescents than in any other age group. Suicide is the third leading cause of death of adolescents and young adults. Although females attempt suicide more often than males, males are more likely to succeed. Depression is a possible contributing factor. Verbal or nonverbal indicators of suicide should not be ignored; rather, an immediate referral should be made to a professional trained in suicide intervention.

Pregnancy

The United States leads the developed countries in the number of pregnancies among adolescents 15 to 19 years old (Murray, 1996). These pregnancies are physically, psychologically, and economically costly for the adolescent mother, the infant, the family, and society. Many adolescent mothers are poor, do not complete high school, and are at high risk for complications involving the pregnancy and the infant.

Nutritional Problems

Fad dieting and habitually eating fast foods are common among adolescents and young adults. For those obsessed with body image (particularly girls and young women), severe eating disorders can result. The most common are anorexia nervosa (compulsive dieting to the point of self-starvation) and bulimia (a destructive cycle of binge eating followed by self-induced vomiting in an effort to prevent weight gain). The psychodynamics of these conditions are complex but almost always involve a negative self-concept. Although these disorders were once considered uncommon, 1 of every 100 women and girls reports symptoms of anorexia, and bulimia appears to be even more prevalent. In the young adult years, fast foods and busy lifestyles may lead to increased caloric intake with minimal exercise. As a result, obesity can become a health problem.

Sexually Transmitted Diseases

Adolescents and young adults who engage in unprotected sexual intercourse are at a higher risk for contracting **sexually transmitted diseases** (STDs) and their complications than are adults. Lack of knowledge, lack of psychosocial maturity, embarrassment, and the denial of the need to plan ahead and use condoms are the most common reasons for this increased risk. Trichomonal and monilial infections, as well as human papillomavirus, are common. Chlamydial infections occur in both genders, as do syphilis and herpes simplex type II (genital herpes). These STDs pose serious health threats.

Acquired immunodeficiency syndrome (AIDS) poses the greatest single threat to individuals and society as a whole. Although AIDS can be transmitted through means other than sexual contact, transmission is primarily through sexual intercourse. AIDS is a major cause of death in the world, and its incidence is predicted to increase still further.

Developmental and Situational Stressors

Adolescents and young adults have to deal with many stressors as a result of their choices about lifestyle, occupation, and relationships. Family-centered stressors may include both positive and negative factors: marriage, divorce, parenthood, death of a parent. Such stress may precipitate mental or physical health problems, aggravated by ineffective coping mechanisms such as substance abuse, child abuse, spouse abuse, decreased nutrition and rest, and risk-taking behavior.

Possible stressors for young adults include the following:

- An increasing number of men and women are choosing to remain single. Singlehood status has advantages and disadvantages. Being single gives one the freedom to come and go as one chooses, to have more autonomy, and to spend money and time as one wishes. On the other hand, external pressures to marry and the desire for love, to belong, and to raise a family may make a young adult question his or her decision to remain single.
- Young married couples may delay decisions to have children until their careers are established, or they may choose not to have children. If they want to have children, infertility (defined as the inability to conceive after 1 year of coitus without contraception) may add even more stress. Women who have postponed having children may realize in their middle to late 30s that their so-called biologic clock is winding down; an increasing number of women in this age group are having their first child.
- Divorce is common in our society, with rates being highest among those marrying young, having low income, and having low educational levels. It separates children from their families, has long-term emotional costs, and increases the number of single-parent families headed by women.

Role of the Nurse in Promoting Health and Preventing Illness

Preventive teaching activities for adolescents and young adults are listed in Table 9-8. Perhaps one of the more significant activities of nurses for individuals in this stage is to facilitate healthy family relationships. Mutual respect, open communications, and accurate information exchange among family members pave the road for a healthy transition from adolescence to adulthood.

Acute illness is often more of an annoyance than of serious consequence. If hospitalized, an adolescent's and young adult's motivation to recover and to resume normal activities is strong. Because independence and self-sufficiency are important to adolescents and young adults, they will not easily accept the dependent sick role. Although chronic illnesses are less common, their occurrence can lead to delayed development, loss of independence, and permanent changes in personal and career goals.

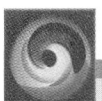

Table 9-8
Promoting Health in Adolescents and Young Adults

Area of Concern	Teaching
Substance abuse	• Advise of statistics about substance abuse. • Discuss the risks of substance abuse. • Discuss the physical consequences of substance abuse. • Discuss the psychosocial consequences of substance abuse. • Assist in preparing strategies for saying no to substance use.
Motor vehicle accidents	• Encourage driver education classes for adolescents. • Discuss the relation of alcohol consumption and motor vehicle accidents.
Suicide	• Assist teachers and caregivers to identify risk factors and data indicative of suicide risk (eg, decreased school performance, social withdrawal). • Advise those with depression where to seek help (eg, psychiatrist, community clinics, crisis centers)
Nutrition	• Discuss healthy eating habits. • Discuss dangers of excessive or nutritionally unsound dieting. • Advise those who legitimately need to lose weight to consult a physician or respected weight loss organization.
Sex education	• Provide factual information about physical and psychosexual development. • Discuss the nature and prevention of STDs. • Discuss safe-sex practices in relation to STDs, particularly AIDs. • Assist with developing strategies for saying no to sexual activity. • If is or intends to become sexually active, discuss responsible sexual behavior and birth control. • Provide assistance to pregnant adolescents by: discussing options, encouraging medical care, and encouraging psychosocial counseling.
Self-esteem	• Teach caregivers that normal behavior for adolescents includes belonging to a peer group, the desire to be like everyone else, and trying on different roles (which may include hairstyles, clothing, and jewelry). • Keep lines of communication open. • Encourage caregivers to facilitate independence while providing love and consistent rules.

Learning Outcomes

After completing this chapter, the learner should be able to accomplish the following:

1. Define key terms used in the chapter.

adolescence
attachment
bonding
child abuse
child maltreatment
colic
failure to thrive
infant

puberty
regression
school-aged child
separation anxiety
sexually transmitted
  disease
sudden infant death
  syndrome

negativism
neonate
preschooler

temperament
toddler
young adult

2. Summarize major physiologic, cognitive, psychosocial, moral, and spiritual developments from conception through the young adult.
3. List common health problems of each age period from conception through the young adult.
4. Describe nursing actions to promote health and prevent illness at each developmental level.

Critical Thinking Exercises

1. Based on the information presented in Chapters 8 and 9, describe nursing interventions to meet developmental needs for the following:

• An infant hospitalized for treatment of a serious birth defect involving the heart and lungs
• A toddler with a fracture of the left leg, treated in the emergency room and then sent home

- A school-aged child, now in rehabilitation, with burns on both arms
- A 20-year-old hospitalized for injuries resulting from an automobile accident after drinking alcohol

2. During your home visit for a 16-year-old with cancer, she says, "I don't believe in God." What would you reply? Why would you respond this way?

3. During a clinic visit, a 2-month-old appears listless and constantly cries. The mother tells you that he has colic, so she has been diluting his formula with water. What would you do now?

Bibliography

American Nurses Association. (1999). Making a difference: Immunizing infants and children. *American Nurse,* January/February, A2–A6.

Craft, N. (1997). Women's health. Life span: Conception to adolescence. *British Medical Journal, 315*(7117), 1227–1230.

Erikson, E. (1963). *Childhood and society.* New York: Norton.

Finan, S. (1997). Promoting healthy sexuality: Guidelines for the school-age child and adolescent. *Nurse Practitioner, 22*(11), 62, 65–67, 71–72.

Freiberg, K. (1992). *Human development: A lifespan approach* (4th ed.). Boston: Jones & Bartlett.

Froman, R., & Owen, S. (1999). American and Korean adolescents' physical and mental health self-efficacy. *Journal of Pediatric Nursing, 14*(1), 51–58.

Fuller, J., & Schaller-Ayers, J. (1994). *Health assessment: A nursing approach* (2nd ed.). Philadelphia: J. B. Lippincott.

Gould, R. (1972). The phases of adult life: A study in developmental psychology. *American Psychiatry, 129*, 33–43.

Grace, T. (1998). Health problems of late adolescence. *Primary Care: Clinics in Office Practice, 25*(1), 237–252.

Klaus, M. H., & Kennell, J. H. (1982). *Parent–infant bonding.* St. Louis: C. V. Mosby.

Levinson, D., Darrow, C., Klein, E., Levinson, M., & McKee, B. (1978). *The seasons of a man's life.* New York: Knopf.

Lock, S., Ferguson, S., & Wise, C. (1998). Communication of sexual risk behavior among late adolescents. *Western Journal of Nursing Research, 20*(3), 273–294.

McCaleb, A., & Edgil, A. (1994). Self-concept and self-care practices of healthy adolescents. *Journal of Pediatric Nursing: Nursing Care of Children and Families, 9*(4), 233–238.

Murray, R. (1996). *Nursing assessment and health promotion: Strategies through the life-span* (6th ed.). Norwalk, CT: Appleton & Lange.

Myers, N., & Perlmutter, M. (1978). Memory in the years from 2 to 5. In P. Ornstein (Ed.). *Memory development in children.* Hillsdale, NJ: Erlbaum.

Nelson, K. (1973). *Structure and strategy in learning to talk.* Monographs of the Society for Research in Child Development, p. 38.

Patton, G., Carlan, J., Coffey, C., Wolfe, R., Hibbert, M., & Bowes, G. (1998). Depression, anxiety, and smoking initiation: A prospective study over 3 years. *American Journal of Public Health, 88*(10), 1518–1522.

Quinn, A. (1993). Commentary on Erik Erikson: Ages, stages, and stories. *AWHONN's Women's Health Nursing Scan, 7*(6), 4.

Roth, J., Hendrickson, J., Schilling, M., & Stowell, D. (1998). The risk of teen mothers having low-birth weight babies: Implications of recent medical research for school health personnel. *Journal of School Health, 68*(7), 271–275.

Rosen, C. (1997). Sleep disorders in infancy, childhood, and adolescence. *Current Opinion in Pulmonary Medicine, 3*(6), 449–455.

Salkind, N., & Ambron, S. (1990). *Child development* (6th ed.). New York: Holt, Rinehart & Winston.

Thomas, A., Chess, S., & Birch, H. G. (1968). Temperament and behavior discussed in children. New York: New York University Press.

West, A., & Kopp, M. (1999). Making a difference: Immunizing infants and children. *American Nurse, 31*(1), A2–A6.

Wong, D. L., Wilson, D., Ahman, E. Winkelstein, M., Divito-Thomas, P., & Hockenberry-Eaton, M. (1998). *Whaley & Wong's nursing care of infants and children* (6th ed.). St. Louis: C. V. Mosby.

Zajicek-Farber, M. (1998). Promoting good health in adolescents with disabilities. *Health & Social Work, 23*(3), 203–213.

Chapter 10
The Aging Adult

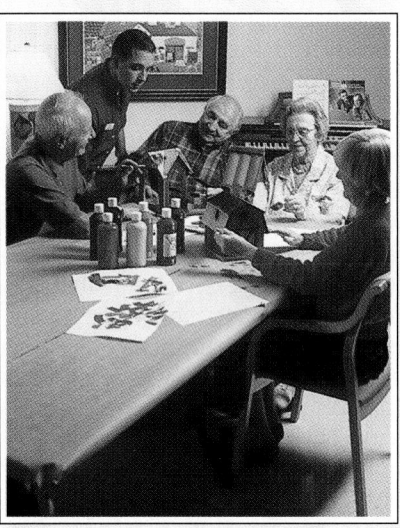

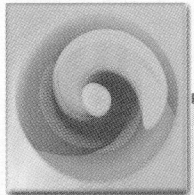

Thinking Critically About
Nursing's Blended Skills

Before reading this chapter, think about the types of skills you will need to meet effectively the developmental needs of patients in early, middle, and older adulthood.

- A woman newly diagnosed with multiple sclerosis tells you that she doesn't know how she can tell her husband. "We were just married this year, share a love of hiking and outdoor sports. It's not fair to him to be tied down to me if I can't be the life partner he thought he was getting!"

- A 59-year-old woman confides that she wishes that Viagra had never been discovered. "I was happier when we just cuddled at night. Now he wants to try all sorts of things, and I'm just not ready for this!"

- A 67-year-old man with diabetes tells you that his life has gone down hill since his retirement. "I'm bored crazy, and I've been drinking more simply because there's nothing else to do!"

- You notice that a new licensed practical nurse in your nursing home puts big bows in the older residents' hair and speaks to them as if they were children. She talks about how "cute" certain couples are who appear to enjoy one another's companionship.

What cognitive, technical, interpersonal, and ethical/legal skills do you think you will need to respond effectively to the developmental challenges described above?

Aging is a gradual process, characterized by continued development and maturation. Although the young adult years are a time of maximum physical function, the changes of aging usually begin as one enters middle adulthood. The onset and the effect of those changes throughout the middle and older adult years are influenced by numerous biologic, psychosocial, and environmental factors (described in the subsequent Theories of Aging section). The physiologic changes of aging, first beginning to be experienced in middle adulthood, become more obvious in older adults. Continued development and maturation throughout one's adult life depend to a great extent on a person's sense of self-concept and prior ability to adapt. This chapter continues the discussion of growth and development from previous chapters, focusing on the aging years.

Theories of Aging

As one ages, changes in cells, tissues, organs, and organ systems occur. Scientists do not fully understand why some people, even within the same family or environments, age much more rapidly than others. Although internal processes may in part determine aging, other factors, such as nutrition and the environment, may also play a role. Numerous theories describe how and why aging occurs, but none is universally accepted. These theories focus on a variety of factors, including genetic inheritance, cell metabolism and function, and the immune system.

The *genetic theory* of aging holds that life span depends to a great extent on genetic factors. Genes within the organism control "genetic clocks" that determine the occurrence and rate of metabolic processes, including cell division. According to the *wear-and-tear* theory, organisms wear out from increased metabolic functioning, and cells become exhausted from continual energy depletion from adapting to stressors (Sorenson & Thorson, 1995).

The *immunity theory* of aging focuses on the functions of the immune system. This system, composed primarily of the bone marrow, thymus, spleen, and lymph nodes, seeks out and destroys foreign agents (such as viruses, bacteria, and perhaps cells undergoing neoplastic changes). The immune response declines steadily after younger adulthood as the thymus loses size and function. With decreasing T-cell differentiation production by the thymus, infections, immune disorders, and cancer increase as adults age. Some authorities believe that nutrition plays an important role in maintaining the immune response, and therefore there is much interest in supplements of vitamins (such as vitamin E) to improve immune function.

Other biologic theories of aging are the *cross-linkage theory* and the *free radical theory*. Cross-linkage is a chemical reaction that produces damage to the DNA and cell death. As one ages, cross-links accumulate, leading to essential molecules in the cell binding together and interfering with normal cell function. Free radicals, formed during cellular metabolism, are molecules with separated high-energy electrons that can have adverse effects on adjacent molecules. Lipids, found in cell membranes, as well as proteins and cell organelles, are affected. Over time, irreversible damage results from the accumulated effects of this damage. The effects of vitamins (especially A, C, E, and niacin) in counteracting free radicals are being studied.

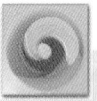

COGNITIVE SKILLS

- Knowledge of the developmental needs of early, middle, and older adults related to relationships, sexuality, family, meaningful work, and leisure
- Knowledge of how to confront a coworker who is well intentioned but insensitive to the developmental needs of older adults in a nursing home

TECHNICAL SKILLS

- Ability to provide the technical nursing assistance necessary to assess and meet the nursing needs of adults facing developmental challenges

INTERPERSONAL SKILLS

- Ability to establish trusting professional relationships with adult patients of different ages that are respectful of their developmental needs

- Ability to intervene in a way that demonstrates care and professional concern for developmental needs that may be sensitive to the individuals involved
- Ability to confront a coworker about problematic behavior and to recommend changes

ETHICAL/LEGAL SKILLS

- Ability and willingness to "get involved" with adults who present with problems related to developmental needs and a commitment to intervening in a way that "makes a difference" in their lives
- Ability to practice in an ethically and legally defensible manner

◎ The Middle Adult

The **middle adult** years are generally considered to be ages 40 to 65 years. This is a period of gradual and individualized change in both physical and psychosocial dimensions. As the average life span increases, most people in this age group still consider themselves young compared with the older population. Visible signs of aging and a heightened awareness of the time left to live, however, lead middle adults to evaluate their achievements of goals and influence their adaptation to older age.

Physiologic Development

In the early years of this period of life, physical functions are usually still effective. As time passes, gradual physiologic changes—both internal and external—occur. These are not pathologic changes but normal changes that result from aging. The person must modify his or her self-image and self-concept to adapt successfully to and accept these normal changes. Physical changes of the middle adult are outlined in the accompanying box.

The hormonal changes that take place in midlife affect men and women differently. Women undergo a change called *menopause*, a gradual decrease in ovarian function, with subsequent depletion of estrogen and progesterone. This change usually occurs between 40 and 55 years of age. With the cessation of ovulation, menstrual periods stop either gradually or abruptly, and many women experience hot flashes, mood swings, and fatigue. The loss of estrogen also increases the risk for osteoporosis and heart disease. The process can last for several years, and afterward the woman can no longer become pregnant. Men do not experience physical symptoms from the decreased levels of hormones, called *andropause*. Androgen levels diminish slowly; the man may have some loss of sexual potency but is still capable of reproduction.

Cognitive Development

Cognitive and intellectual abilities of middle adults change little from young adulthood. There is often increased motivation to learn, especially if the knowledge gained can be immediately applied and has personal relevance. Problem-solving abilities remain throughout adulthood, although response time may be slightly longer. This is due, not to any decreased ability, but rather to a longer search through more memories and to a desire to think a problem through before responding.

Psychosocial Development

The middle adult years often are a time of increased personal freedom, economic stability, and social relationships. This is also a time of increased responsibility and an awareness of one's own mortality (Fig. 10-1). One realizes that one's life may be half or more past and may feel many things are still undone. This realization can lead to a developmental crisis and situational stressors.

Developmental Tasks

In terms of adult developmental theories, the middle adult faces the following tasks:

- According to Erikson's theory (1963), the middle adult is in a period of generativity versus stagnation. The tasks are to establish and guide the next generation, accept middle-age changes, adjust to the needs of aging parents, and reevaluate one's goals and accomplishments. Adults who do not achieve these tasks tend to focus on themselves, becoming overly concerned with their own physical and emotional health needs.
- Levinson, Darrow, Klein, Levinson & McKee (1978) theorized that the middle adult may choose either to continue an established lifestyle or to reorganize one's life in a period of midlife transition.
- Gould (1972) viewed the middle years as a time when adults look inward (ages 35 to 43 years); accept their life span as having definite boundaries, and have a special interest in spouse, friends, and community (ages 43 to 50 years); and increase their feelings of self-satisfaction, value spouse as a companion, and become more concerned with health (ages 50 to 60 years).

Role Transitions

Various changes can take place during the middle years. These changes include changes in relationships with a spouse, with children who are becoming adults, and with aging parents. Midlife transition may occur in both men

---

Physical Changes in the Middle Adult

- Fatty tissue is redistributed; men tend to develop abdominal fat, women thicken through the middle
- The skin is drier
- Wrinkle lines appear on the face
- Gray hair appears, and men may lose hair on the head
- Cardiac output begins to decrease
- Muscle mass, strength, and agility gradually decrease
- There is a loss of calcium from bones, especially in perimenopausal women
- Fatigue increases
- Visual acuity diminishes, especially for near vision (presbyopia)
- Hearing acuity diminishes, especially for high-pitched sounds
- Hormone production decreases, resulting in menopause or andropause

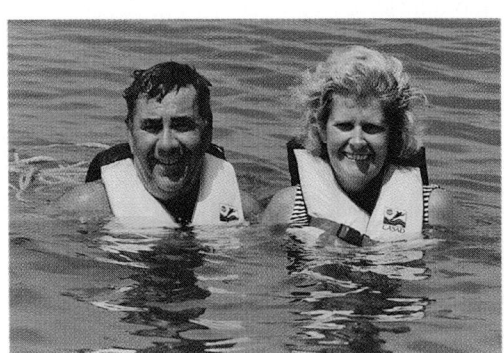
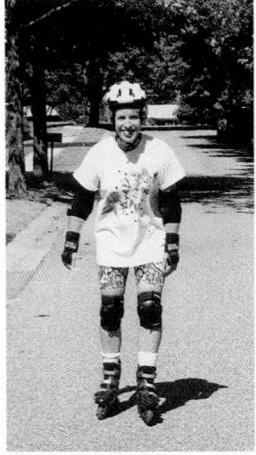
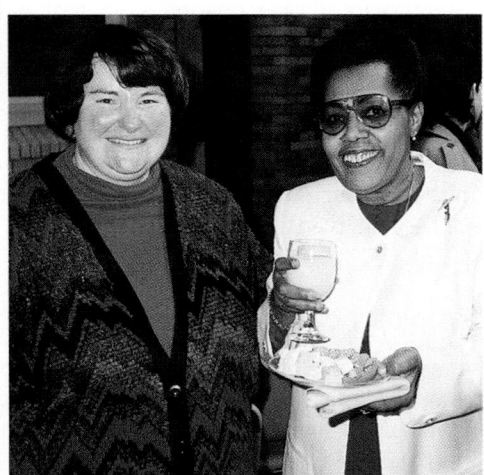
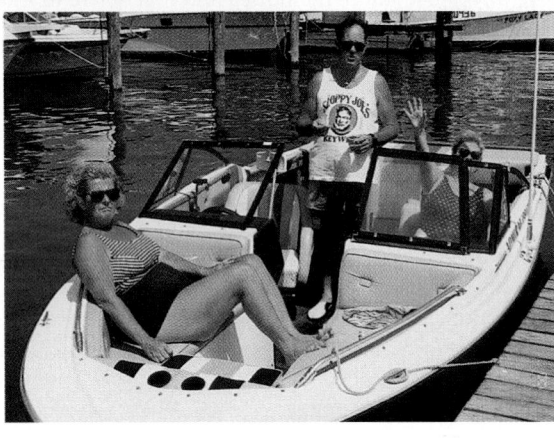

Figure 10-1
The middle adult years are characterized by greater expendable wealth, renewed relationship with one's spouse, and expanded social relationships.

and women in their 40s. The following may (but do not always) occur during this time:

- Women may choose to go to school, get a job, or change their career. Conversely, women who have been immersed in a career may decide in their early 40s to have children and not work.
- Men may become workaholics, spending little time with family or in leisure activities. Many men make career changes, often with increased emphasis on job satisfaction.
- As the 50s approach, questions about retirement and economic security become more prevalent, with an increased interest in the benefits of financial and retirement plans.
- Although one may not feel that one is aging, realizing that others consider you older can be stressful.
- Relationships with one's spouse may change. Although for many this is a time of greater security and stability with stronger emotional commitment and sharing, for some it is a time of disenchantment. A husband or wife may develop negative or

critical feelings and attitudes as a result of changes in physical appearance, energy levels, and sexual needs and abilities. Dissatisfaction with not achieving career or family goals contributes to the stresses placed on the marriage. Extramarital affairs and divorce may result.

Middle-aged adults may be caught in a "generation sandwich." Their children are often independent and married, with children of their own. Although much has been written about the *empty-nest syndrome* that occurs when the last child leaves home, most middle-aged parents welcome the increased space, time, and independence they have when active parenting ceases. As their involvement with and responsibility for children decrease, they may have an increased need to help care for aging parents and other family members. The physical aging or death of a parent makes one's own aging and inevitable death a reality.

Widowhood is more likely to occur in the middle years. The loss of a spouse is a major crisis and a threat to one's self-concept as well as a major role change. A multitude of changes may occur, including a reduced income, changes in lifestyle and social relationships, and the need for help to work through the loss and grief (see Chapter 32 on Loss, Grief, and Dying).

Moral and Spiritual Development

A middle adult may either remain at the conventional level or move to the postconventional level of moral development, especially if he or she has had sustained responsibility for the welfare of others and has consistently applied ethical principles developed in adolescence. At this level, the adult believes that the rights of others take precedence and takes steps to support those rights.

As with moral development, not all adults progress to Fowler's (1991) paradoxical-consolidative state of spiritual development. Fowler believed that only some people reach this stage, and only after 30 years of age. Most middle adults are less rigid in their beliefs and have increased faith in a supreme being as well as trust in spiritual strength.

Common Health Problems

Middle adults are subject to physical and emotional health problems associated with lifestyle behaviors, developmental or situational crises, family history, and the environment. Both acute and chronic illnesses are more likely to occur, and recovery takes longer. This is a result of slower and more prolonged responses to stressors, more pronounced reactions to an illness, and the possibility of more than one illness being present at a time.

The leading causes of death in the middle adult years are motor vehicle accidents, occupational accidents, suicide, and chronic diseases. The major health problems are cardiovascular and pulmonary diseases, cancer, rheumatoid arthritis, diabetes mellitus, obesity, alcoholism, and depression.

The risk for these common health problems often depends on a combination of lifestyle factors and aging.

As one gets older, energy requirements decrease. Middle adults tend to maintain previous eating patterns and caloric intake while being less physically active. This trend can result in obesity and atherosclerosis, with an increased risk for high blood pressure, coronary artery disease, renal failure, and diabetes. Additionally, smoking and alcohol consumption put the person at greater risk for lung cancer, chronic respiratory problems, liver disease, and peptic ulcer disease.

Chronic illness in middle adults has a major effect on self-concept and may precipitate changes in life structure. For example, after a serious heart attack, a man may face changes in his family role, his earning capacity, and his social relationships. Such changes usually cause great stress.

Middle age does not automatically result in physical or emotional health problems. Many men and women remain healthy throughout their lives, but knowing preventive healthcare practices and their special needs at this age can help middle adults have improved quality and quantity of life.

Role of the Nurse in Promoting Health and Preventing Illness

The nurse has a major role in promoting health and preventing illness in middle adults by teaching, serving as a role model, and encouraging self-care responsibilities. Examples of nursing diagnoses for the middle adult are found in the accompanying box.

The following health promotion activities are recommended:

- Have a physical and dental examination every year
- Have an eye examination every 1 to 2 years, including a test for glaucoma
- Maintain current immunizations
- Eat a diet low in fat and cholesterol, including fruits, vegetables, and fiber, and use sugar, salt, and sodium in moderation
- Make regular exercise a part of life

EXAMPLES OF NANDA NURSING DIAGNOSES

The Middle Adult

- Altered Nutrition: Potential for more than body requirements related to high calorie diet and sedentary lifestyle.
- Constipation related to diet low in fiber and lack of exercise.
- Risk for Impaired Skin Integrity related to lifetime of sun exposure.

- Sexual Dysfunction related to alcohol abuse.
- Caregiver Role Strain related to long-term care of aging parents.
- Ineffective Denial related to continued smoking despite family history of lung cancer.
- Fear related to diagnosis of breast cancer.

- For women: practice monthly breast self-examination; have a mammogram and a breast examination every year
- For men: practice testicular self-examination monthly, have testicular and prostate examination every year, and a prostate-specific antigen blood test after 50 years of age
- Have a digital rectal examination and stool blood test every year, and after 50 years of age, a sigmoidoscopy and digital examination every 3 to 5 years as recommended.

The middle adult needs to know the dangers of substance abuse. Referrals to support groups and individual counseling may be necessary to strengthen a middle adult's coping mechanisms and promote acceptance of personal and family changes. Having successfully met developmental tasks, the middle adult is ready to enjoy the rest of life. A sense of continuity and adaptability from the early 20s through the 50s is essential to meeting the developmental tasks of aging satisfactorily and to enjoying one's remaining years.

The Older Adult

The US population is growing older. Our society has arbitrarily labeled the **older adult** as one older than 65 years of age. The older adult period is often further divided into the *young-old* (ages 60 to 74 years), the *middle-old* (ages 75 to 84 years), and the *old-old* (ages 85 years and older). Currently, the average life expectancy is 72.5 years for men and 79.3 years for women (US Department of Health and Human Services, 1997). Adults older than 65 years of age comprise 12.8% of the total population, and that number is predicted to increase to 20% by the year 2030. The greatest increase is in adults older than 75 years of age. By 2050, those 85 years of age and older are expected to comprise 5% of the total population. Older women outnumber older men by a ratio of 3:2. The proportion of older people is higher in whites than in minority populations, although the number of minority older adults is increasing.

A Unique Population

The older adult population is the most unique group in today's society because its members have lived the longest and have participated in and adapted to complex societal changes. Within the life span of many older adults, society developed from a rural agricultural culture through industrialization to a service-oriented, high-technology culture. In 1900, a 20-mile trip meant an all-day undertaking in a horse-drawn wagon; today, a person can fly across the continent in less time and with considerably less effort. Lighting has progressed from kerosene and gas lamps to electricity. Information that once took weeks or months to be received now is instantaneous. Most older adults have lived through the trauma of one or two world wars. Many had parents with strong ethnic ties to another country, and many were immigrants themselves. Older adults have lived through the Great Depression of the 1930s and developed self-sufficiency.

Further adaptations become necessary with advancing age because of physical or cognitive limitations, retirement, loss of a spouse or family members, or changing income. Older adults face numerous role changes related to their age or health status. Lost roles must be replaced with new roles and activities that are acceptable and satisfying to the person.

Older people are thus living in a world that requires them to change and adapt. It is a time to reach one's potential and to satisfy long-range goals that may have been delayed because of other responsibilities. It can also be a time for older adults to turn over to others tasks such as career or community leadership. Research has shown that most older adults do adjust and adapt to new roles, and most are satisfied with their lives and with what they have. Depending on the older adult's adaptability and supportive resources, older adulthood may be a time of happiness, peace, and understanding or of sorrow, conflict, and confusion.

Ageism and Common Stereotypes

Sometimes, older adults are a victim of ageism. **Ageism** is a form of prejudice, like racism, in which older adults are stereotyped by characteristics found in only a few members of their group. Fundamental to ageism is the view that older people are different from *me* and will remain different from *me*; therefore, they do not experience the same desires, needs, and concerns. Our industrial technologic world places a high priority on productivity, and some may think that retired people have "outlived their usefulness." As well, younger generations often have lost ties to the older generation because of increased mobility of the family, and thus many young adults lack experiences with older relatives and their friends.

Older people may be *incorrectly* depicted as being rigid or narrow-minded, unable to learn, unreliable because of memory loss, too old to enjoy sexual pleasure, or childlike and dependent. Many people fear advancing age because of pervasive views that older people are poor, lonely, in frail health, and headed for institutionalization in a nursing home. These descriptors are not true for most older adults (Fig. 10-2). Common myths are compared with the realities in Table 10-1.

Most older adults are satisfied with their lives, finding retirement and old age more enjoyable than they had anticipated. Three fourths live in their own homes, and one third of these live alone. Most older adults maintain close ties with their families and have incomes above the poverty level (American Association of Retired Persons [AARP], 1998).

Older Adults and the Healthcare System

Our knowledge of aging has increased dramatically in the past 40 years. **Gerontology** is the scientific and behavioral study of all aspects of aging and its consequences.

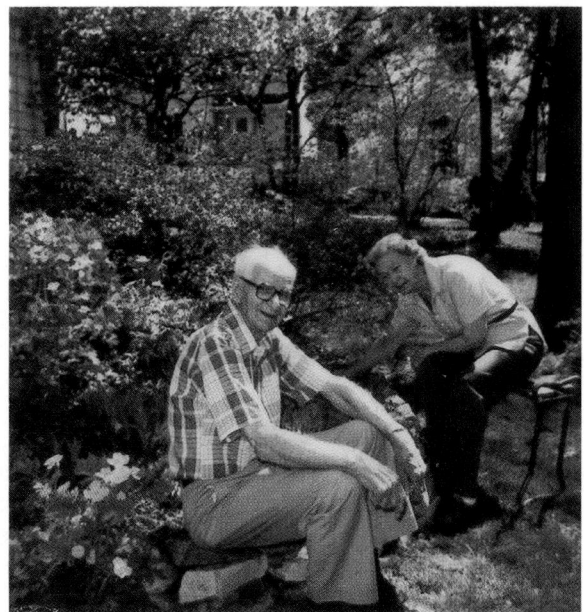

Figure 10-2
This couple, married 61 years, enjoys gardening together. They've found that they can continue most activities with only minor adjustments.

Normal changes that occur with aging are the result of complex interactions among genetics, biologic systems, and physical and social environments. Disease complicates a person's ability to adapt and maintain functional health (the ability to carry out usual and desired daily ac-

tivities). Mental or physical decline in older adults often may not be directly related to the aging process but may result from the absence of supportive care and services that could prevent disease and help maintain the older adult's ability to function.

The increasing aging population has greatly strained a healthcare system that has traditionally focused on cures and acute disease processes. For an older patient with chronic disorders, the focus of care should include the patient's and family's goals and promote functional health and independent living to the greatest extent possible. Gerontologic, or gerontic, nursing does just that. **Gerontologic nursing** combines the basic knowledge and skills of nursing with a specialized knowledge of aging in both illness and health.

Physiologic Development

In older adults, all organ systems undergo some degree of decline in overall functioning, and the body becomes less efficient. (Normal physiologic changes in structure and function of the body with aging are outlined in the accompanying box.) Body functions that require integrated activity of several organ systems are affected the most. For example, aging of the heart muscles causes fluid retention in both peripheral tissues and the lungs, causing swelling of the legs and making breathing more difficult. The most commonly encountered chronic disorders are cardiovascular diseases such as hypertension and strokes, cancers, and skeletal disorders such as arthritis and osteoporosis.

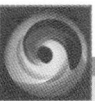

Table 10-1
Myths and Realities About Older Adults

Myth	Reality
Old age begins at 65 years of age	Defining 65 years of age as "old age" happened arbitrarily when 65 years of age was set for Social Security payments in the 1930s, based on the labor market and the economy of that time.
Most older adults live in nursing homes	Only about 5% of older adults live in nursing homes.
	Most older adults own their own homes; 31% live alone, 54% live with spouses, and the rest live with family or friends.
Most older adults are sick	Fully 71% of all older adults rate their health as good or excellent.
Old age means mental deterioration	Although response time may be prolonged from a longer processing time, neither intelligence nor personality normally decreases because of aging.
Older adults are not interested in sex	Although sexual activity may be less frequent, the ability to perform and enjoy sexual activity lasts well into the 90s in healthy older adults.
Older adults don't care how they look	Older adults want to be attractive to others.
Most older adults are isolated and lonely	Loneliness results from death of loved ones or other losses, just as it does for people of all ages. Many older adults are active in social and community activities.
Bladder problems are a problem of aging	Incontinence is not a part of aging; it requires medical attention.
Older adults do not deserve aggressive treatment for serious illnesses	Older adults deserve aggressive treatment if they want aggressive treatment.

Normal Physiologic Changes of Older Adulthood

General Status

- Progressively decreasing efficiency of physiologic processes results in a fragile balance and hinders the body's ability to maintain homeostasis.
- Physical or emotional stressors cause the older adult to be more vulnerable because of decreased physiologic reserves.
- The older adult may continue to engage in all activities of middle age but intuitively adjusts to a modified pace and more frequent rest periods.

Integumentary

- Wrinkling and sagging of skin occur with decreased skin elasticity; dryness and scaling are common.
- Balding becomes common in men and women experience thinning of hair also, hair loses pigmentation.
- Skin pigmentation and moles are common, although the skin may become pale because of loss of melanocytes.
- Nails typically thicken and become brittle and yellowed.

Musculoskeletal

- Decreases in subcutaneous tissue and weight commonly are found in the old-old.
- Muscle mass and strength decrease.
- Bone demineralization occurs, and bones become porous and brittle.
- Joints tend to stiffen and lose flexibility, and range of motion may decrease.
- Overall mobility commonly slows, and posture tends to stoop. Height decreases slightly.

Neurologic

- The central nervous system responds more slowly to multiple stimuli. Hence, the cognitive and behavioral response of the older adult may be delayed.
- Rate of reflex response decreases.
- Temperature regulation and pain perception become less efficient.
- The sense of balance declines, and fine movements may become more difficult.
- Sleep at night typically shortens, and the older adult may awaken more easily. Cat naps become common.

Special Senses

- Diminished visual acuity (*presbyopia*) occurs, with increased sensitivity to glare and decreased ability to adjust to darkness. Cataracts may further obscure vision.
- Diminished hearing acuity (*presbycusis*) occurs, particularly diminished pitch discrimination in the presence of environmental noises.
- The senses of taste and smell are decreased.

Cardiopulmonary

- Blood vessels become less elastic and often rigid and tortuous. Venous return becomes less efficient. Fatty plaque deposits continue to occur in the linings of the blood vessels. Lower-extremity edema and cooling may occur particularly with decreased mobility.
- The body is less able to increase heart rate and cardiac output with activity.
- Pulmonary elasticity and ciliary action decrease, so that clearing of the lungs becomes less efficient. Respiratory rate may increase, accompanied by diminished depth.

Gastrointestinal

- Digestive juices continue to diminish, and nutrient absorption decreases.
- Malnutrition and anemia become more common.
- With reduced muscle tone and decreased peristalsis, constipation and indigestion are common complaints.

Dentition

- Tooth decay and loss continue for most older adults.
- Eating habits may change, particularly if the older adult lacks teeth or has ill-fitting dentures.

Genitourinary

- Blood flow to the kidneys decreases with diminished cardiac output.
- The number of functioning nephron units decreases by 50%; waste products may be filtered and excreted more slowly.
- Fluids and electrolytes remain within normal ranges, but the balance is fragile.
- Bladder capacity decreases by 50%. Voiding becomes more frequent; two or three times a night is usual. A decrease in bladder and sphincter muscle control may result in stress incontinence or incomplete bladder emptying.
- About 75% of men over 65 years of age experience hypertrophy of the prostate gland; surgery may be required if urinary retention occurs.
- There is atrophy, decrease of secretions, and thinning of the older woman's genital tract.

Changes in the senses may cause alterations in many activities of daily living and increase the risk for accidents. Visual impairments result from reduced visual fields; increased sensitivity to glare; and decreased accommodation, depth perception, and color discrimination. These aging-related changes may mean that the older adult has more difficulty reading small print and driving at night, or he or she may not be able to drive at all. Hearing deficits occur from decreased hearing acuity and discrimination of pitch (so that high-pitched sounds are less well heard and understood, especially if other conversation or noise is also present) in a condition called *presbycusis*. As a result of problems with hearing, the older adult may withdraw from social events. Problems with nutrition may result from a decrease in taste buds and a reduced sensitivity to odors. There are often age-related changes in sensitivity to pain, pressure, and temperature. The older adult may also experience difficulty with balance, coordination, and spatial orientation, resulting in an increased risk for falls.

Most older adults regard themselves as healthy and deny they experience severe limitations in activities. Most are never institutionalized, nor do they suffer the effects of senility. Being healthy, however, does not necessarily mean without disease. More than four of five older adults suffer from at least one chronic illness. Like younger adults, they define their health in relation to how well they function—that is, whether they can engage in their usual and desired daily activities. This **functional health** definition includes a person's ability to remain self-reliant, to "make do," and to maintain a sense of control and independence over self and environment. There is a trend in healthcare today toward fostering increasing independence and self-care in older adults. Those who live alone are at greatest risk for loss of independence and increased need for long-term care.

There is growing evidence that aging is not synonymous with loss of function and disability. Although 90% of older adults have one or more chronic disorders, their ability to adapt determines whether they are ill or healthy. Most continue their activities from middle age and adapt intuitively to the gradual limitations of aging, although it may take longer to complete an activity or the activity may need to be modified. For examples, an older adult with arthritis may need to use an electric can opener rather than a manual one, or a person with heart disease may need 3 hours to mow the lawn, resting several times, rather than the former 1 hour.

The greatest threat to the health of older adults is loss of the physiologic reserve of the various organ systems. When illness occurs, increased physical and emotional stress places an older adult at risk for complex reactions. An older adult is more likely to develop complications and to recover more slowly (Fig. 10-3). For instance, an older patient with a hip fracture is at high risk for pneumonia and skin breakdown because of immobility, a decreased

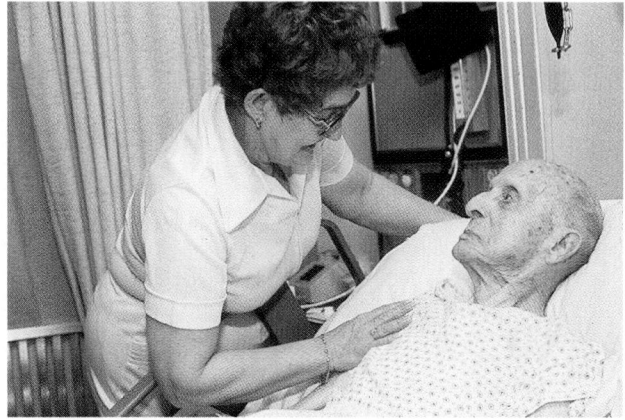

Figure 10-3
The hospitalized older adult requires nursing interventions to prevent complications. (Photo © Kathy Sloane.)

ability to expel pulmonary secretions, and thinner, more fragile skin.

Cognitive Development

The term *cognition* indicates cerebral functioning, including the ability to perceive and understand one's world. Cognition does not change appreciably with aging. In fact, intelligence increases into the 60s, and learning continues through life. It is normal for an older adult to take longer to respond and react, however, particularly in new or unfamiliar surroundings. Knowing this, the nurse should slow the pace of care and allow older patients extra time to ask questions or complete activities. Mild short-term (recent) memory loss is common but can be remedied by an older adult using notes, schedules, and calendars. Long-term memory usually remains intact.

When a serious mental impairment occurs, the effect on the patient and family can be devastating. **Dementia** refers to various organic disorders that progressively affect cognitive functioning. Of the dementias that affect older adults, **Alzheimer's disease** is the leading cause of cognitive impairment in old age, affecting about 4 million Americans. It affects brain cells and is characterized by patchy areas of the brain that degenerate. Alzheimer's disease is a progressively serious and ultimately fatal disorder. At first, forgetfulness and impaired judgment may be evident. Over a period of several years, the person becomes progressively more confused, forgetting family and becoming disoriented in familiar surroundings. When the ability to perform simple activities of daily living is lost, the person requires constant supervision and care, often in a nursing home. There is no effective medical treatment for Alzheimer's disease at this time. Comprehensive and empathetic nursing care is important (see the accompanying Research in Nursing box). Both the patient and family caregivers need emotional support and teaching and may

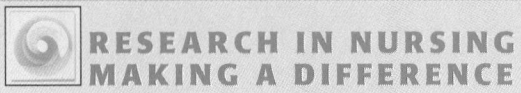

RESEARCH IN NURSING: MAKING A DIFFERENCE

Living With Dementia: The Patient's Perspective

Dementia, most often due to Alzheimer's disease, is estimated to affect nearly 10% of the population. Although research has led to better ways of caring for people with dementia and meeting the needs of caregivers, not much has been done to understand the experience of what it is like to have mild to moderate dementia.

Related Research

Phinney, A. (1998). Living with dementia from the patient's perspective. *Journal of Gerontological Nursing, 24*(6), 8–15.

To discover how patients perceive dementia, five people with Alzheimer's disease and their spouses were interviewed during home visits. Two themes were revealed: being unsure and trying to be normal. Being unsure described how people no longer take themselves for granted in how they are. They experience gaps of unawareness and memory loss that prevent them from self-trust and that lead to embarrassment. Trying to be normal is an effort to decrease the effect of changes in daily activities, roles, and relationships. Patients tried to do this through self-monitoring, keeping an active mind, staying engaged with others, and downplaying the seriousness of their diagnosis.

Relevance to Nursing Practice

This study is an example of understanding illness from the perspective of the person who experiences it. By better understanding a "hidden" illness such as Alzheimer's disease, nurses can assess not only the patient's cognitive and functional status but also his or her coping strategies used in day-to-day life. Interventions can then be individualized to meet the special needs of each patient.

---

benefit from community resources that can ease the family's burden.

Sometimes confusion and depression in an older adult are mistaken for true dementia. Drug interactions, circulatory or metabolic problems, or nutritional deficiencies are likely the real cause. An older adult may also become confused when too many changes or losses occur at one time or when moved to a different environment. A type of confusion called **sundowning syndrome** sometimes occurs, in which an older adult habitually becomes confused after dark. The nurse can help other members of the health team determine the cause of a patient's confusion and help reorient the patient. The nurse uses **reality orientation** interventions to redirect the patient's attention to what is real in the environment. Nursing interventions for reality orientation include the following:

- Calling the patient by name, and including the nurse's name, the date, and the day of the week in conversations.
- Clarifying misinformation, such as what day a family member will visit or where the patient is living.
- Using clocks and calendars.

Psychosocial Development

Most theorists agree that a person's self-concept is relatively stable throughout adult life. An older adult who has a strong sense of self-identity and has successfully met challenges earlier in life will probably continue to do so. This person substitutes new roles for old roles and perhaps continues former roles in a new context. For example, a business manager after retirement may continue to use his or her leadership talents in community or volunteer organizations. Older adults with a strong self-concept typically describe themselves as being healthier than others or "young for my years." On the other hand, events that may accompany aging can threaten a person's self-concept. Depending on the person's outlook on life and past ability to cope, events such as retirement, loss of health or income, and isolation can be devastating. For example, a retired teacher whose sense of identity was closely tied to career may suddenly find that he or she has lost friends, income, and sense of accomplishment and may consequently feel a great loss of control and self-identity.

An early psychosocial theory, called the *disengagement theory*, maintained that older adults often withdraw from usual roles and become more introspective and self-focused. This withdrawal was theorized as intrinsic and inevitable, necessary for successful aging, and beneficial for both the person and for society. Later studies have shown that isolation is not desired or acceptable and that as societal interactions decrease, healthy older adults increase their close relationships with family and friends. According to the *activity theory*, successful aging involves the ability to maintain high levels of activity and functioning. An older adult may substitute activities but does not slow down or disengage from society. The *identity-continuity theory* assumes that healthy aging is related to the older adult's ability to continue similar patterns of behavior from young and middle adulthood.

Erikson (1963) identified ego integrity versus despair and disgust as the last stage of human development, which begins at about 60 years of age. Older adults continue to look forward but now also look back and begin to reflect on their life. It is a time for realization of a "wholeness" perspective, with an inner search for meaning and order in the life cycle. Older adults search for emotional integration and acceptance of the past and present as well as acceptance of physiologic decline without fear of death. Older adults often like to tell stories of past events. This phenomenon is called **life review** or **reminiscence** and has been identified worldwide. In a sense, this is a way for an older adult to relive and restructure life experiences and is part of achieving ego integrity (Fig. 10-4). Nurses can also use reminiscence as a therapy to facilitate adaptation to present circumstances. The activities for this therapy are listed in the accompanying box: Using the Nursing Interventions Classification.

Ego integrity is facilitated when an older adult has successfully accomplished tasks earlier in life. Older adulthood can be a time for the person to look backward with pride and without regrets and forward with optimism and enthusiasm. A person who regrets the past and sees current problems as insurmountable, however, may despair. This person may view life as a series of unresolved problems and missed opportunities and feel worthless or hopeless. The despairing person may want to do things over but fears the lack of time before death.

The tasks of midlife continue or may resurface. Older adults still strive to guide the coming generations and to leave something behind (generativity versus stagnation). Their need for love and closeness continues (intimacy versus isolation), as does a strong sense of who one is in relation to family and community (identity versus role diffusion). Because of physical and social changes associated with aging, older adults are repeatedly faced with the need to adapt and to again face already completed tasks.

According to Havighurst (1972), the major tasks of old age are primarily concerned with the maintenance of social contacts and relationships. Successful aging depends on a person's ability to be flexible and adapt to new age-related roles. The person must find new and meaningful roles in

---

Using the Nursing Interventions Classification: Selected Reminiscence Therapy Activities

- Choose a comfortable setting.
- Set aside adequate time.
- Encourage verbal expression of both positive and negative feelings of past events.
- Ask open-ended questions about past events.
- Encourage writing of past events.
- Tape the reminiscence, and play it back to the patient, as appropriate.
- Ask the family to bring photo albums or scrapbooks.
- Help the patient to begin a family tree.
- Encourage the patient to write to old friends.
- Encourage writing of past events (eg, culture, traditional values, wisdom, and lessons learned).
- Inform family members about the benefits of reminiscence.
- Gauge the length of the session by the patient's attention span.
- Acknowledge previous coping skills.
- Repeat session weekly or more often over prolonged period.

From McCloskey, J., & Bulechek, G. (2000). *Nursing interventions classification (NIC)* (3rd ed.). (p. 554). St. Louis: C. V. Mosby. A full listing of nursing activities for each nursing intervention can be found in this book.

---

old age while being reasonably comfortable with the social customs of the times.

Adjusting to the Changes of Aging

Older adults use their years of experience as a guide to adjusting to the changes that come with increasing age. These changes, based on Havighurst's tasks for later life, involve many areas of life, as described in the following sections.

Physical Strength and Health

Most older adults gradually modify their lifestyle to accommodate for declining strength and health. They rest more frequently, although continued activity and exercise are important for maintaining all physiologic functions. An older adult is at high risk for accidents and falls and may need to curtail driving or use a cane or other aid to remain mobile. Diet modifications and prescribed medications may be necessary, and because of chronic illness, an older adult may need to adjust to living with some pain. With severe illness, loss of independence can occur. The loss of health is difficult to adjust to because it affects every aspect of life.

Retirement and Reduced Income

Retirement brings a change in a person's concept of time. Older adults must learn to occupy their leisure time in ways

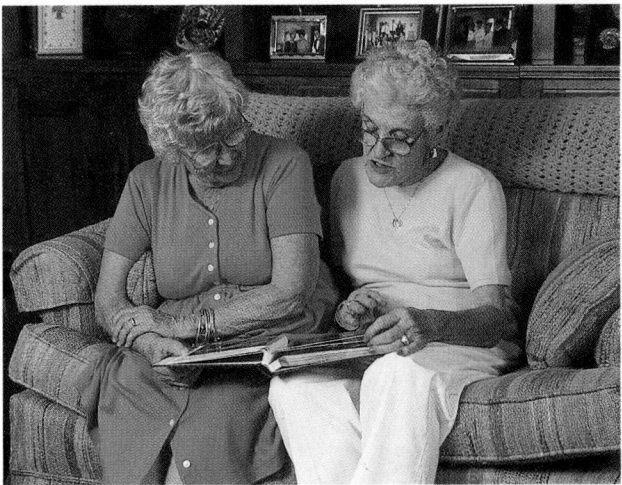

Figure 10-4
Reminiscing is a culturally universal phenomenon of aging. It is a way for the older adult to reassess life experiences and further develop a sense of accomplishment, fulfillment, and reward in life. (Photo © B. Proud.)

that maintain their self-esteem while being personally satisfying. Although increasing numbers of middle adults are retiring, retirement at 65 years of age is the hallmark of old age. Satisfaction with retirement is closely tied to income and the relationships one has outside of work. Many older adults have adequate retirement income, but a lack of adequate income can affect an older adult's ability to meet his or her needs, such as for medical care and housing or social and creative interests.

The Health of One's Spouse

When one's spouse becomes ill, numerous and difficult adjustments must be made. An older adult may face new roles for the first time. A husband may begin to cook meals; a wife may learn to handle family finances. These role changes come at a time when stress is already high. Giving physical care can be an overwhelming task if the other spouse is also frail or in poor health. Adaptations may be needed in living conditions and lifestyle, and the spouse may need to plan social and recreational events alone.

The need for love and belonging does not diminish with age and may become acute with the loss of one's spouse through illness or institutionalization. Humans are sexual beings, and sexual behavior does not necessarily stop in old age. Sexuality is part of who we are, and older adults are no exception. Like younger adults, older adults need to express their intimacy physically by touching and sexual activity and emotionally by sharing joys, sorrows, ideas, and values (Fig. 10-5).

Relating to One's Age Group

With an aging population, social organizations for older adults are becoming more numerous. For example, most communities have senior citizens' centers that offer meals, social and informational programs, and other activities for a nominal fee. Other organizations offer opportunities for travel, cultural events, and political involvement. Affiliation with others of the same age allows older adults to share common interests and concerns and to find status among their peers. It should not be assumed, however, that older adults want to associate only with others their age (Fig. 10-6).

Social Roles

Social roles change with the developmental tasks and adjustments of older adulthood, but the need to feel valued, useful, and productive continues. An older adult may develop new hobbies or increase his or her involvement in community, church, or family affairs. He or she may do volunteer work or even begin a new career. If an older adult cannot adjust and form new relationships, social isolation can become a problem. **Social isolation** is a sense of being alone and lonely as a result of having fewer meaningful relationships. It may occur because of declining health or income, transportation problems, or ageism. Whatever the cause, prolonged social isolation has been associated with declining health and higher mortality rates.

Living Arrangements

The ability to function safely and independently at home depends a great deal on one's functional health, transportation, income, and family. An older adult, for example, may need assistance with home repairs, house cleaning, or grocery shopping. Architectural barriers, such as steps, may need to be modified. Easy access to medical and recreational facilities and churches may become more important. Many older adults in poor health can

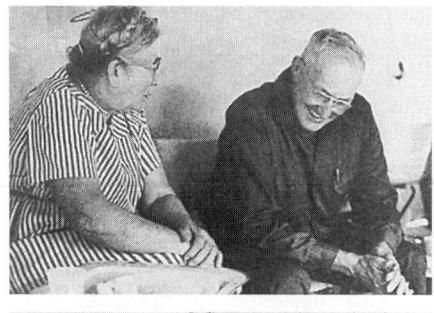
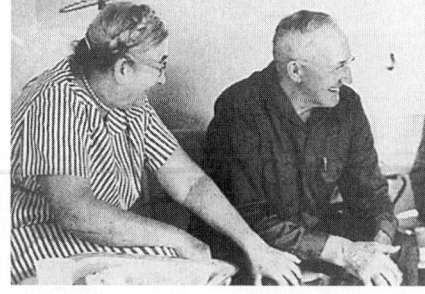
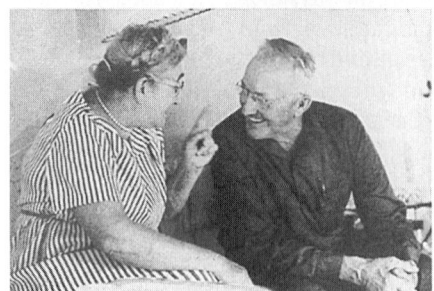
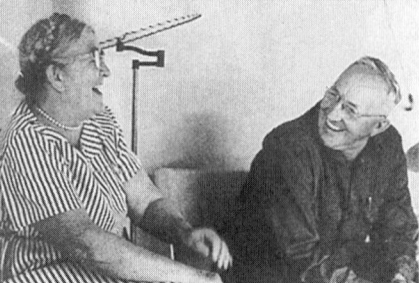

Figure 10-5
Stereotypical images of the older adult as narrow-minded, forgetful, sexless, and dependent are untrue for most of the older adult population. This couple exhibits the vitality, sensuality, joy, and playfulness of a young couple. (Photos by Karen Baldwin.)

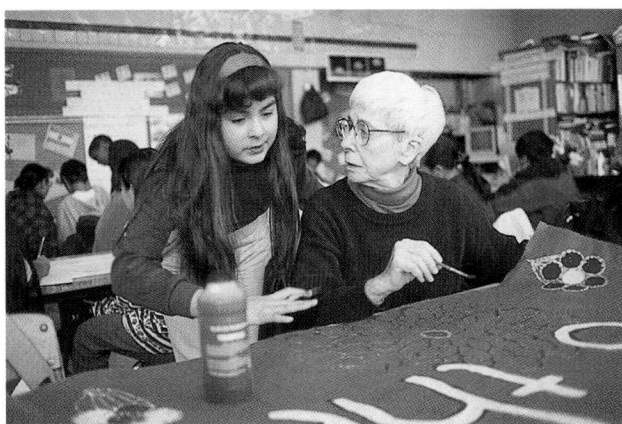

Figure 10-6
Social relationships and satisfying leisure activities remain important throughout life. This older adult volunteers in art class with 6th-grade Asian and Latina girls. (Photo © Kathy Sloane.)

continue living at home with some assistance from visiting nurses or with the aid of other services, such as home-delivered meals and senior transportation. Assisted-living housing is becoming more common, providing such requirements as meals, healthcare services, and housekeeping services.

Most older adults prefer to live in their own home and find it difficult to move. Moving in with adult children creates changes in roles and authority. If the older adult is chronically ill or cognitively impaired, the family caregivers face the need for daily caregiving, lack of freedom, and emotional stress. When one moves to an extended-care facility, such as a nursing home, the loss of one's home and possessions and the need to conform to the routines of institutional living can be traumatic for the person and family. Some people, however, choose to move for convenience, social relationships, or needed healthcare.

Retirement centers and senior citizens' housing have become common. For the family members of older adults who need healthcare, alternative methods of care have become available. Examples of alternative care are respite care facilities, which allow the family a needed rest by temporarily housing and caring for an ailing older family member, and day-care centers, which provide a safe, stimulating environment during the day when family caregivers must work. Nurses should be knowledgeable about what healthcare and social services are available in the patient's community so that the patient and family can be referred.

The old-old have special significance for nursing care because they are more likely to need help with mobility and basic activities of daily living. They may need increasing assistance to maintain a safe and comfortable living environment. The older the person, the more likely that he or she needs family and community support to maintain functional health.

Family and Role Reversal

An older adult's spouse and other family members are natural support systems who help the person maintain functional health and independence and meet the developmental tasks of old age. Supportive assistance may include the provision of transportation, food, shelter, social interactions, and even complex medical and nursing treatments. Significant others, such as close friends and neighbors, may also take on tasks formerly assumed to be the responsibilities of the traditional family.

Not all families can assist an aged member satisfactorily because of geographic distance, low income, poor health, strained marital relationships, or infringement on career or lifestyle. Adult children may feel "sandwiched" between responsibilities for their own children and careers and the needs of older parents. It can be a guilt-ridden and emotionally draining time for all involved when an older adult's physical or emotional illness reverses roles (with the child now assuming the role of parent, while the parent becomes dependent as the "child") and strains family resources.

The nurse must view the whole family as the recipient of care and assess the family for capabilities and limitations for assisting the aged member. The nurse can help ease the strain by listening to the patient's and family's concerns and by validating the importance of family needs. The nurse assists the patient and family to find workable solutions and may refer the family to community support services.

Moral and Spiritual Development

Older adults have, according to Kohlberg (1969), completed their moral development. Most are at the conventional level, following society's rules in response to others' expectations. Spiritually, an older adult may remain at an earlier level; often at the individuative-reflective level. Many older adults, however, demonstrate conjunctive faith, integrating faith and truth to see the reality of their own beliefs, or universalizing faith, in which they trust a greater power and believe in the future.

Self-transcendence is a characteristic of later life that helps one expand beyond personal limits to reach out to others and the environment and a greater awareness of others' beliefs and values. Integration of the past and future in the present facilitates acceptance of where one is in life without regretting past mistakes or fearing the future (Reed, 1996). As a person ages, spirituality and transcendence are a resource and a source of strength when faced with inevitable change and loss.

Common Health Problems

As the number of older adults increases, nurses will spend more time providing care for this population. Older adults who require care are in all types of healthcare settings, including hospitals, long-term care facilities, emergency departments, outpatient surgeries, and homes. Nursing care for older adults should be based on two principles:

- Most older people are not impaired but are functional in the community, thereby benefitting from health-oriented interventions.
- Older people are more vulnerable to physical, emotional, and socioeconomic problems than people in other age groups and may require special attention to health promotion and maintenance.

This section provides a broad introduction to the healthcare needs of the older adult in terms of chronic illness, accidental injuries, and acute illness.

Chronic Illness

The probability and incidence of a person becoming ill increase with age. The most common chronic illnesses in older adults are arthritis, hypertension, heart disease, hearing impairments, cataracts, bone disorders, sinusitis, and diabetes (AARP, 1998). Other causes of illness or disability include acute illnesses such as fractures, pneumonia, motor vehicle accidents, and falls. These acute illnesses or accidents may lead to chronic health problems. The leading causes of death in the elderly, accounting for 7 of 10 deaths, are heart disease, cancer, and stroke.

Although illness affects all dimensions of a person regardless of age, older adults have to contend with a variety of problems as they live with chronic illness. Aging is a normal process, and chronic illness is a pathologic process, but both often occur at the same time. The changes of aging and the needs imposed by chronic illness interrelate to increase the risk for problems in all areas of life, including—but not limited to—self-care, lifestyle, economics, social factors, and living arrangements. Consider the following:

- Chronic illness limits activities in about 15% of the total population, but almost half of adults older than 65 years of age have limitations as a result of one or more chronic illnesses.
- Meeting the expenses of healthcare is often difficult for older adults and their families. Medication costs related to chronic illness continue for the rest of a person's life, with multiple medications being the rule rather than the exception. Hospitalization costs continue to rise, and the price of high-quality, long-term care may well be beyond the patient's or family members' ability to pay. In addition, special diets, special equipment, and medical supplies increase economic difficulties.
- Family members must learn how to cope with the needs of the ill person. Included are personal hygiene, medication administration, special diets, elimination, activities of daily living, and recognition of symptoms that necessitate medical attention. Family members must also adapt to psychological stressors such as changes in communications, changes in roles (eg, an older mother in effect becomes dependent), and changes in their own lifestyle as they become the caregivers.

Accidents and Injuries

The older adult is at increased risk for accidental injury because of changes in vision and hearing, loss of mass and strength of muscles, slower reflexes and reaction time, and decreased sensory ability. In addition, the combined effects of chronic illness and medications may make an older adult more prone to accidents. Older adults with reduced income may live in inadequate housing in neighborhoods with heavy traffic and high crime rates. They may be isolated from family members, and many live alone. Combined with the normal changes of aging and the effects of any illness, older people not only are at increased risk but also have a more difficult time regaining health after an injury.

Role of the Nurse in Promoting Health and Preventing Illness

The nurse should teach the patient and family the following general health promotion activities. This is important because older people often believe themselves "too old" to worry about nutrition, exercise, health screenings, and immunizations.

- Eat a diet that includes all food groups; is low in fat, saturated fat, and cholesterol; balances calories with physical activity; has recommended amounts of fruits, vegetables, and grains; and uses sugar and salt in moderation.
- Make exercise a part of daily activities.
- Have annual (or as recommended) health screening examinations as recommended for the middle adult (see earlier); also include examination of the urine, thyroid, testes, mouth, skin, and lymph nodes.
- Maintain immunizations for diphtheria, tetanus, influenza, and pneumonia.

An older adult who requires surgery or medical treatment for chronic or acute illness has special, age-related needs regardless of the setting for care. Nursing care to meet age-related needs in any setting are outlined in Table 10-2.

Although nursing care adapted to the needs of older patients is described throughout this text, general principles for care are included here. Nurses must recognize physiologic and psychosocial interrelationships and view older patients holistically. Examples of nursing diagnoses for the older adult are found in the accompanying box.

Illness can severely disrupt an older adult's ability to function independently. The ill patient is under increased physical and emotional stress, which increases the risk for complications because of the lack of physiologic reserves. When a patient is hospitalized or institutionalized, family and community interactions are severely inhibited. The acute care environment itself adds new stressors, such as diagnostic tests, treatments, and surgery. In the face of new and unfamiliar routines and sensory stimulation, prior coping skills may not work, and an older patient

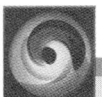

Table 10-2
Promoting Health and Preventing Illness in Older Adults

Area of Concern	Nursing Actions
Physiologic function	• Maintain physiologic reserves. Maintain ongoing assessments for early detection of problems. • Review perceptions of current health status, health problems, and prescribed or over-the-counter medications. • Include nursing care that maintains physical status, such as skin care and planned rest and activity.
Cognitive function	• Slow pace of activity and wait for responses. • Repeat teaching as often as necessary. • Be sure eyeglasses and hearing aids are used; ensure lenses are clean and batteries are strong.
Psychosocial needs	• Be aware that illness, hospitalization, or changes in living arrangements are major stressors. • Assess and support sources of strength, including cultural and spiritual values and rituals. • Encourage use of support systems: family, friends, community resources, pets. • Set mutual goals and encourage the patient's role in making decisions about care. • Encourage life review and reminiscence. • Encourage self-care. • Consider the patient's background, interests, capabilities, values, culture, and lifestyle when planning care.
Nutrition	• Assess for lost or damaged teeth; ensure dentures fit properly. Provide foods appropriate to the patient's ability to chew. • Assess height, weight, eating patterns, and food choices. If weight is being lost, assess income, storage, and transportation.
Sleep and rest	• Discourage excessive napping. • Assess normal bedtime, time for rising, bedtime rituals, effects of pain, medications, anxiety, and depression.
Elimination	• Assess frequency of bladder elimination as well as problems with incontinence. • Assess normal times for bowel movements, changes in activity, privacy, and medications. • Ensure that the floor is not cluttered, the toilet is easily accessible, lighting is adequate, and privacy is provided. • Suggest having safety bars installed in the bathroom. • Review diet for necessary fluid and fiber content.
Activity and exercise	• Assess ability to walk; ensure that assistive devices (such as a walker or cane) are available. • Consider effects of illness, surgery, medications, and changes in diet and fluid intake on strength and motor function. • Ensure an uncluttered environment with good lighting; suggest using a night light and removing throw rugs. • Slow the pace of care, allowing extra time to carry out activities.
Sexuality	• Assist as necessary with hygiene, hair care, oral care, clean clothing and bedding, makeup, and shaving. • Maintain a clean, odor-free environment. • Demonstrate genuine caring: ask preferred name, listen carefully, respect belongings, provide touch.
Meeting developmental tasks	• Promote continued development and maintenance of functional health by identifying unmet tasks, feelings of isolation, and physical or sensory limitations. • Assist in finding creative solutions to developmental tasks. • Collaborate with other healthcare providers to provide information and referral to community resources for the patient and family.

may feel less able to understand and control the new environment. An older patient is more likely than a younger patient to suffer multisystem dysfunctions, *iatrogenic* complications (caused by medications or treatments), accidents such as falls, and increasing dependence and confusion.

The focus of nursing care is to assist older patients to function as independently as possible and to support their individual strengths. The nurse collaborates with the family and other disciplines to prevent complications of illness, to secure a safe and comfortable environment, and to promote the patient's return to health.

EXAMPLES OF NANDA NURSING DIAGNOSES

Older Adult

The following are examples of nursing diagnoses that might be appropriate for the older adult:

- Risk for Infection related to dry, thin skin
- Risk for Altered Body Temperature related to very high environmental temperatures and lack of air-conditioning or fans
- Risk for Injury related to unstable gait and decreased vision from cataracts
- Risk for Loneliness related to death of spouse
- Ineffective Individual Coping related to diagnosis of chronic illness

- Impaired Physical Mobility related to severe arthritic changes in legs
- Impaired Home Maintenance Management related to recent surgery
- Impaired Memory related to cognitive impairment from onset of Alzheimer's disease
- Anxiety related to increase of crime and violence in neighborhood

Learning Outcomes

After completing this chapter, the learner should be able to accomplish the following:

1. Define key terms used in the chapter.

   ageism
   Alzheimer's disease
   dementia
   functional health
   gerontologic nursing
   gerontology
   life review

   middle adult
   older adult
   reality orientation
   reminiscence
   social isolation
   sundowning syndrome

2. Summarize major physiologic, cognitive, psychosocial, moral, and spiritual developments and tasks of middle and older adulthood.

3. Describe common health problems of middle and older adults.
4. Discuss physiologic and functional changes that occur with aging.
5. Describe common myths and stereotypes that perpetuate ageism.
6. Describe nursing actions to promote health and prevent illness for middle and older adults.
7. Identify the healthcare needs of older adults in terms of chronic illnesses, accidental injuries, and acute care needs.

Critical Thinking Exercises

1. Complete the following sentences, and then analyze the reasons for your answers:
   a. When my parents can no longer care for themselves, I will _____.
   b. If my parents were living in a nursing home, I would want the nurses to _____ _____.
   c. When I am old, I want my family to _____ _____.

2. Consider your own family. Can you identify developmental tasks for family members who are middle adults and older adults? What factors in your family facilitate or are barriers to meeting these tasks?

Bibliography

Administration on Aging. (1996). *Aging into the 21st century.* Bethesda, MD: National Aging Center, US Department of Health and Human Services.

American Association of Retired Persons (AARP). (1998). *A profile of older Americans.* Washington, DC: American Association of Retired Persons.

Blair, K., & White, N. (1998). Are older women offered adequate care? *Journal of Gerontological Nursing, 24*(10), 39–44.

Castellucci, D. (1998). Issues for nurses regarding elder autonomy. *Nursing Clinics of North America, 33*(2), 265–274.

Ebersole, P., & Hess, P. (1994). *Toward health aging: Human needs and nursing response.* (4th ed.). St. Louis: C. V. Mosby.

Eliopoulos, C. (1997). *Gerontological nursing* (4th ed.). Philadelphia: Lippincott-Raven.

Eliopoulos, C. (1995). *Manual of gerontologic nursing.* St. Louis: C. V. Mosby.

Erikson, E. (1963). *Childhood and society* (2nd ed.). New York: Norton.

Freiberg, K. L. (1992). *Human development: A lifespan approach* (4th ed.). Boston: Jones & Bartlett.

Fowler, J. W. (1991). *Weaving the new creation: Stages of faith and the public church.* San Francisco: Harper Collins.

Giger, J., Davidhizar, R., & Poole, V. (1998). Growing older is not what it used to be. *Health Care Supervisor, 16*(4), 40–47.

Gould, R. (1972). The phases of adult life: A study in developmental psychology. *American Psychiatry, 129,* 33–43.

Havighurst, R. J. (1972). *Developmental tasks and education* (3rd ed.). New York: Longman.

Hayes, J. (1999). Respite for caregivers: A community-based model in a rural setting. *Journal of Gerontological Nursing, 25*(1), 22–26.

Keister, K., & Blixen, C. (1998). Quality of life and aging. *Journal of Gerontological Nursing, 24*(5), 22–28.

Kohlberg, L. (1969). Stage and sequence: The cognitive–developmental approach to socialization. In D. Gaslin (Ed.). *Handbook of socialization: Theory and research* (pp. 347–380). Chicago: Rand McNally.

Levinson, D. J., Darrow, C. N., Klein, E. B., Levinson, M. H., & McKee, B. (1978). *The seasons of a man's life.* New York: Knopf.

Lien-Gieschen, T. (1993). Validation of social isolation related to maturational age: Elderly. *Nursing Diagnosis, 4*(1), 37–44.

Matteson, M. A., McConnell, E. S., & Linton, A. (1987). *Gerontological nursing: Concepts and practice* (2nd ed.). Philadelphia: W. B. Saunders.

McCloskey, J., & Bulechek, G. (Eds.). (2000). *Iowa intervention project: Nursing interventions classification* (3rd ed.). St. Louis: C. V. Mosby.

Miller, J. (1998). The changing face of long-term care. *Caring, 17*(8), 24–26.

Murray, R. (1996). *Nursing assessment and health promotion: Strategies through the life-span* (6th ed.). Norwalk, CT: Appleton & Lange.

Phinney, A. (1998). Living with dementia from the patient's perspective. *Journal of Gerontological Nursing, 24*(6), 8–15.

Porter, E. (1994). Older widow's experience of living alone at home. *Image—The Journal of Nursing Scholarship, 26*(1), 19–24.

Reed, P. G. (1996). Transcendence: Formulating nursing perspectives. *Nursing Science Quarterly, 9*(1), 2–4.

Ross, M., & Wright, M. (1998). Long-term care for elderly individuals and methods of financing. *Journal of Community Health Nursing, 15*(2), 77–89.

Rosseau, M. (1998). Women's midlife health: Reframing menopause. *Journal of Nurse-Midwifery, 43*(3), 145–147, 208–223.

Sheehy, G. (1998). Racing toward midlife. *Men's Health, 13*(4), 148–150, 152–153, 167.

Sorenson, H., & Thorson, J. (1995). Biological theories of aging. *Journal of Subacute Care, 1*(3), 35–39.

Stocker, S. (1996). Six tips for caring for aging parents. *American Journal of Nursing, 96*(9), 32–33.

US Census Department. (1996). *Statistical abstract of the United States.* Washington, DC: US Government Printing Office.

US Department of Health and Human Services [USDHHS]. (1997). *Administration on aging: Aging into the 21st century.* Washington, DC: Department of Health and Human Services.

Wold, G. H. (1999). *Basic geriatric nursing* (2nd ed.). St. Louis: C. V. Mosby.

Zang, S. (1998). *Nurses' guide to home care of the elderly.* Philadelphia: Lippincott Williams & Wilkins.

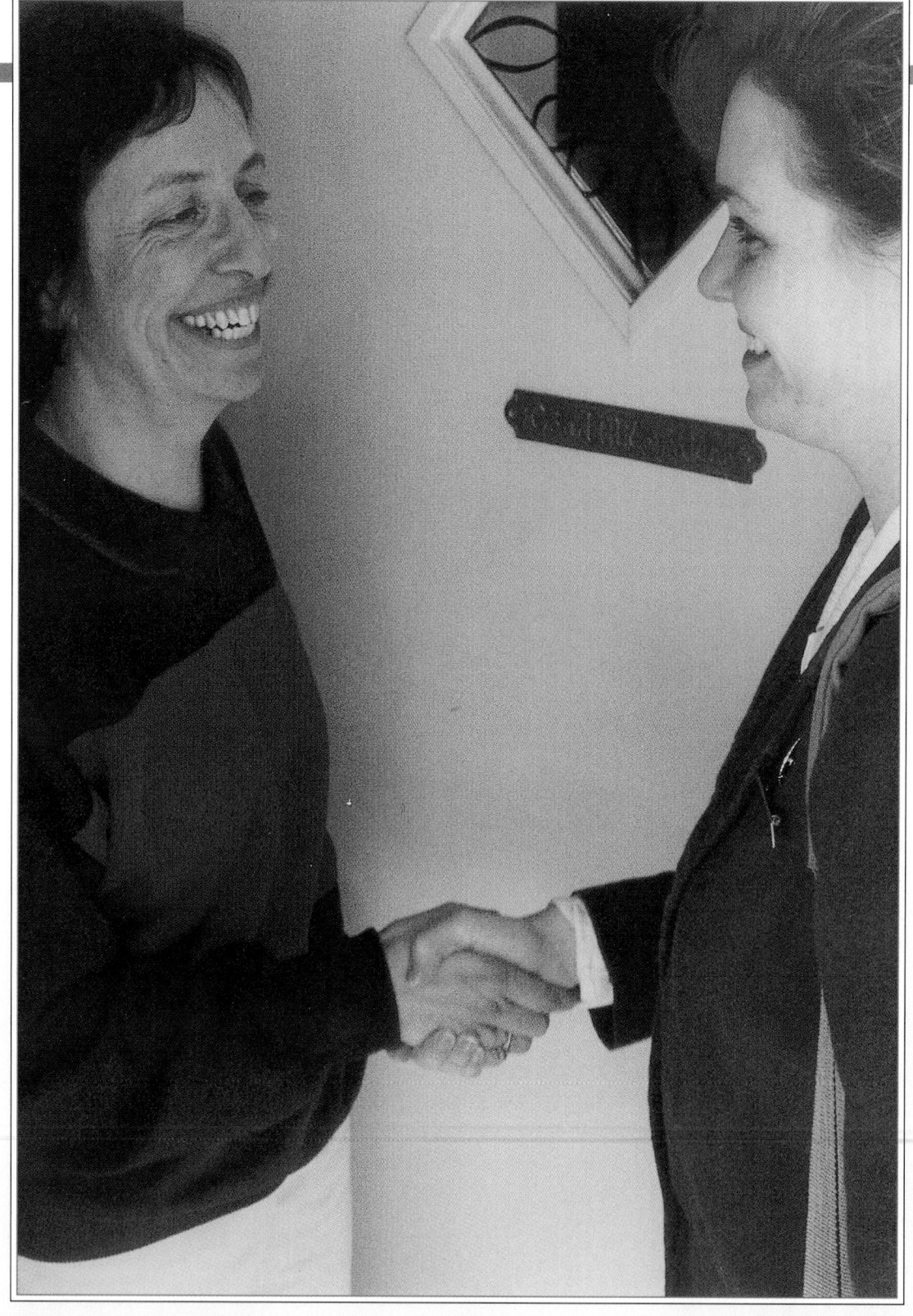

UNIT III

Community-Based Settings for Patient Care

". . . a realization that the call to the nurse is not only for the bedside care of the sick, but to help in seeking out the deep-lying basic causes of illness and misery, that in the future there may be less sickness to nurse and to cure."

Lillian Wald (1867–1940)
a visionary humanitarian who initiated child labor law revision, improved housing conditions in tenements, supported education for the mentally handicapped, originated public health nursing, and founded the Visiting Nurse Service at the Henry Street Settlement House, New York City

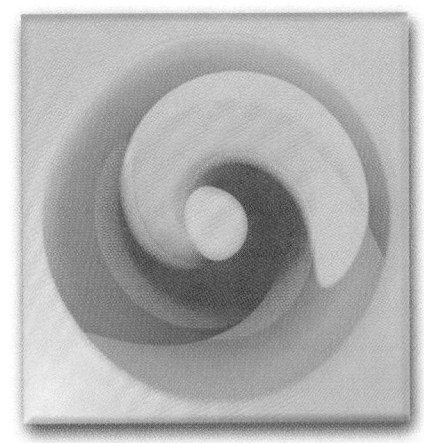

Nurses care for patients in a wide variety of settings within the community. As the healthcare environment changes, nurses increasingly provide care to promote wellness and restore health outside the traditional hospital setting. The chapters in Unit III provide information about the different community-based settings in which nursing care is provided. The chapters in this unit provide an introduction to types and methods of community-based healthcare delivery, roles of members of the healthcare team in providing collaborative interdisciplinary care, activities to provide continuity of care as patients move between and among healthcare settings, and the care provided by nurses for patients in their homes.

Community-based healthcare is provided in settings that range from very large public hospitals to one-room apartments. For example, patients may re-

ceive healthcare services as in-patients or ambulatory out-patients in a hospital, through voluntary or public health agencies, in day-care centers and schools, in offices and clinics, or through crisis intervention centers. Care is often provided by a team of healthcare providers to meet physical, psychological, sociocultural, economic, and spiritual needs. Healthcare services may be financed through federal funding, health maintenance organizations, or private insurance. All of these factors, combined with increasing concern about healthcare provision, have raised questions about cost containment, consumer rights, fragmentation of care, and changing patient populations and needs.

As patients enter, leave, and move between healthcare settings, the nurse is most often the member of the healthcare team responsible for coordinating care and teaching so that continuity of

care is maintained. Information is provided in this unit about admitting patients to hospital and ambulatory settings, transferring patients between healthcare settings, and providing discharge planning to patients and their families. Because more and more healthcare is provided to patients in their own homes, Chapter 13 provides a base for understanding what home healthcare is and what the nurse does when providing care in the patient's home. Characteristics and roles of the home health nurse are described, and components of the home visit are discussed.

Unit III provides information necessary to the provision of patient care within a variety of community-based settings. This information enables the nurse to work within the healthcare system to meet individualized patient needs and provide holistic, patient-centered care.

Chapter 11
Community-Based Healthcare

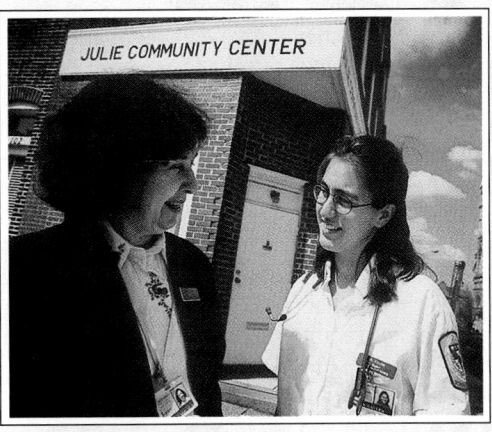

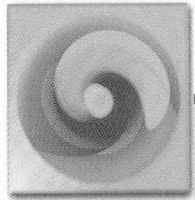

**Thinking Critically About
Nursing's Blended Skills**

Before reading this chapter, think about the types of skills you will need to nurse in community-based settings.

- You've recently become a home health nurse and are overwhelmed by the healthcare needs that families in your community are facing. Sadly, many families lack healthcare coverage for the services they need, and you often leave a family feeling terrible about your inability to provide needed care.

- You've begun volunteering as a parish nurse in your church and are excited about how the parish seems to be "pulling together" to help families with huge healthcare needs.

- Because fewer psychiatric or mental health patients can afford residential care, your hospital has opened a mental health clinic, and you have been asked to coordinate nursing services on site.

- You volunteer with a group of nurses from your hospital every year at the marathon to provide emergency first aid for runners.

What cognitive, technical, interpersonal, and ethical/legal skills do you think you will need to respond effectively to the community-based nursing challenges described above?

Community-based healthcare is care provided to people who live within a defined geographic region or have common needs. In contrast to community health nursing, which focuses on the health of the community, community-based nursing is centered on individual and family healthcare needs. Nursing care is based on the belief that it is provided for people wherever they are, including where they live, work, play, worship, and go to school (Zotti, Brown, & Stotts, 1996). The nurse practicing community-based care considers the continuity of the care the patient requires, providing direct services to manage acute or chronic illnesses and promote self-care. Community-based healthcare is designed to meet the needs of people as they move between and among different healthcare settings within the overall healthcare system. Figure 11-1 shows some of the settings for healthcare.

The healthcare system is comprised of institutions, agencies, policies, payment plans, providers, patients, families, and caregivers. This chapter introduces the healthcare system, including healthcare policy and reform; facilities and frameworks for care; collaborative care; financial aspects; and selected trends and issues affecting the healthcare system. Chapter 12 discusses the continuity of care as patients move among healthcare settings, and Chapter 13 discusses care of the patient in the home.

Healthcare Policy and Reform

Many questions have been raised about the present healthcare system. Most questions involve access to, cost of, and quality of care. These questions are debated at the local, state, and federal level as well as by healthcare providers and consumers of healthcare services. Healthcare reform plans have been proposed at both the federal and state levels, but as yet, no one plan has been accepted. Federal legislation up through the 1996 Health Insurance Portability and Accountability Act has improved access to insurance for employed persons and prohibits denial of coverage for an existing illness. Increased options for health insurance for children who do not live in poverty are available. Despite these measures, the number of people without access to private insurance continues to increase (Heinrich, 1998).

Changes taking place in healthcare give nurses the opportunity to help shape healthcare for the future. Although it is impossible to predict exactly the roles of future practitioners, projections have outlined expected competencies (listed in the accompanying box) for the year 2005 (Pew Health Professions Commission, 1991). These projections, coupled with the national health promotion and disease prevention objectives outlined in the Healthy People 2010 project (American Public Health Association, 2000), emphasize the importance of nursing's role in improving access to care, quality of care, and cost of care.

The goals of healthcare reform focus on cost containment, improved access, and increased quality of services for all citizens. Where do nurses fit into the reform movement? First, nurses are becoming a stronger voice in protesting health-related problems in our nation. Second, nurses in greater numbers are increasing their education and becoming advanced practice nurses (APNs). As such, more nurses now provide primary healthcare services in areas and to people long neglected: the elderly, women, infants, the poor, and those living in rural areas. In addition, the

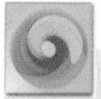

COGNITIVE SKILLS

- Knowledge of how finances and health policy affect the types of healthcare available to people in your community
- Knowledge of how to intervene politically to secure needed healthcare reform
- Knowledge of how to develop needed safe and quality community resources that are responsive to unmet healthcare needs

TECHNICAL SKILLS

- Ability to provide the technical nursing assistance necessary to meet the needs of patients and the public in community-based settings

INTERPERSONAL SKILLS

- Ability to establish trusting professional relationships with patients and colleagues in community-practice sites

- Ability to work with community groups to ensure everyone's access to safe healthcare of good quality

ETHICAL/LEGAL SKILLS

- Commitment to providing safe and quality care in any practice setting
- Commitment to healthcare reform to ensure that everyone gets at the very least a "basic decent minimum" of healthcare
- Knowledge of your legal liability when volunteering and providing professional services outside the scope of your employment, for example, as a volunteer parish nurse or first aid attendant
- Ability to practice in an ethically and legally defensible manner in community-based settings

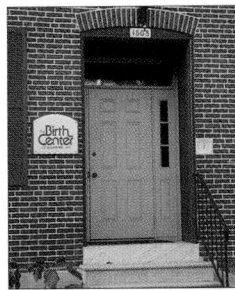
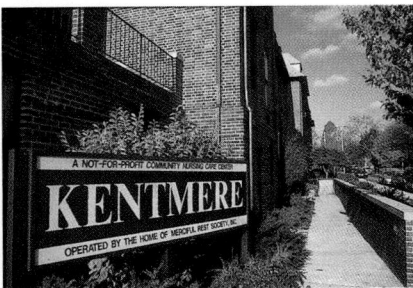
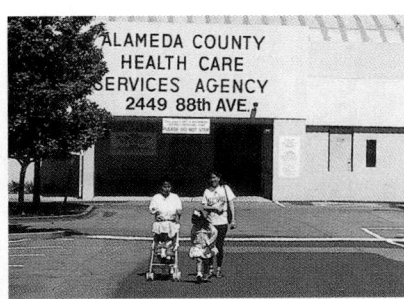
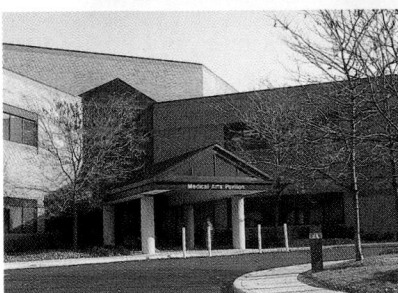
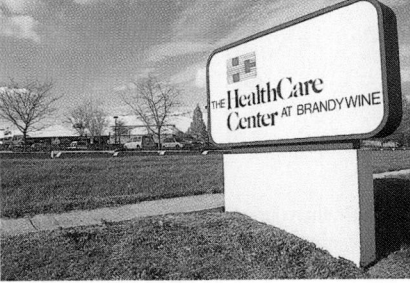
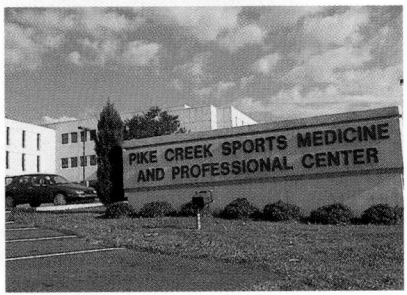

Figure 11-1
In recent years, the number and variety of healthcare settings have increased dramatically. (Photos © B. Proud.)

focus of nursing care provided by all nurses is holistic care essential to promoting health and preventing illness.

Nursing's Agenda for Healthcare Reform, published by the American Nurses Association in 1991, recommends restructuring of the healthcare system to focus on the health-care needs of consumers not only for the population in general but also in schools, homes, the community, and the workplace. The document further recommends that the focus be on health and care, not illness and cure. The document recommends restructuring the healthcare system with a standard package of essential services available to all American citizens and residents, planning for changing national demographics, and taking steps to reduce costs.

Healthcare Facilities

Community-based healthcare is provided within many different types of health-related facilities, built by and within communities to meet the needs of people. There are more than 7000 hospitals, 4000 community health agencies, and 16,000 long-term care facilities in the United States. When one considers that only patients who require complex surgery, who are acutely ill or seriously injured, or who are having babies are hospitalized—and then only for a minimum period of time—it is apparent that most healthcare services are provided in settings outside the hospital. Consideration of the patient's needs in health and in illness throughout the life span make nursing provided within a community-based healthcare framework essential. Healthcare services are provided in community-based facilities such as hospitals, clinics, homes, schools, and day-care centers for children and older people. Other facilities include crisis-intervention centers, mental health centers, drug and alcohol rehabilitation programs, storefront clinics, and churches. Some healthcare agencies provide immunizations for infants and children, screenings for sexually transmitted diseases (STDs) or tuberculosis, and verification of need and voucher distribution for milk and food for women and children with low incomes through the Women, Infants, and Children (WIC) program. Community-based healthcare

---

Competencies for Healthcare Practitioners for 2005

Practitioners for 2005 should undertake the following:

- Care for the community's health
- Expand access to effective care
- Provide contemporary clinical practice
- Emphasize primary care
- Participate in coordinated care
- Ensure cost-effective and appropriate care
- Practice prevention
- Involve patients and families in the decision-making process
- Promote healthy lifestyles
- Access and use technology appropriately
- Improve the healthcare system
- Manage information
- Understand the role of the physical environment
- Provide counseling on ethical issues
- Accommodate expanded accountability
- Participate in a racially and culturally diverse society
- Continue to learn

Pew Health Professions Commission. (1991). *Healthy America: Practitioners for 2005*. Durham, NC: The Pew Health Professions Commission.

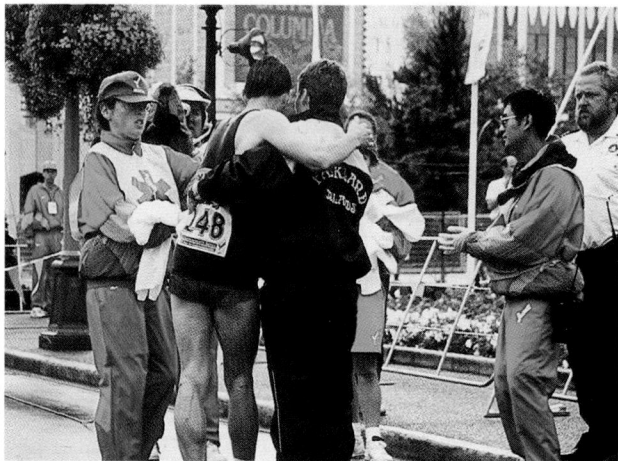

Figure 11-2
Two nurses assist a runner at the completion of the men's marathon during the Victoria Commonwealth Games, Canada. (Photo by Paul Jonson, courtesy of Sandy Gilmour.)

may also focus on special needs, such as older adults or terminally ill patients. Nurses are involved in caring for patients and families in all of these agencies and in many other settings (Fig. 11-2). The accompanying box lists examples of nursing activities in different types of community-based healthcare agencies.

People requiring care may be classified as inpatients or outpatients. People who enter a healthcare facility such as a hospital and stay for more than 24 hours are said to be **inpatients**. In addition to providing acute care, hospitals have many services for **outpatients**—those who require healthcare services but do not need to stay in the facility for those services. Individuals who do not require inpatient care can receive treatment, care, and education on an outpatient basis. Examples of outpatient services are surgical procedures, diagnostic tests, medications, physical therapy, counseling, and health education. Outpatient services are rapidly expanding and are provided not only by hospitals but also by healthcare providers' offices, ambulatory care centers, and clinics. A form of outpatient care provided by hospitals occurs in short-stay units, where patients having diagnostic tests or surgery enter the hospital, have the procedure, and then return to the hospital room for a brief (1 to 6 hours) recovery period before going home.

Home Care

Home care is one of the most rapidly growing areas of the healthcare system. (See Chap. 13 for a full discussion of this type of community-based nursing care.) Home care may be provided through community health departments, visiting nurses' associations, hospital-based case managers, and home health agencies. These agencies provide many different health-related services, including skilled nursing assessment, teaching and support of patients and family members, and direct care for patients.

The importance of home healthcare is evidenced by many factors, including the following:

Examples of Nursing Activities In Various Healthcare Settings

Home

- Assesses the home environment and the patient
- Develops the relationship based on mutual trust
- Plans, implements, and evaluates the plan of care
- Provides direct care
- Coordinates care of others
- Teaches patient and family
- Provides support for family members
- Makes referrals

Hospitals

- Serves as administrator or manager
- Assesses and monitors patient's health status
- Provides direct care
- Coordinates the care provided by others
- Teaches patients and families
- Plans, implements, and evaluates the plan of care
- Provides staff information
- Coordinates discharge planning to ensure continuity of care
- Provides specialized care
- Makes referrals

Ambulatory Care

- Makes assessments of health status of patients
- Assists (or is) the primary care provider
- Provides direct patient care
- Coordinates care provided by others
- Teaches patients and family
- Plans, implements, and evaluates the plan of care
- Serves as patient advocate

Long-Term Care

- Serves as administrator
- Coordinates the care provided by others
- Provides direct care
- Teaches patients and families
- Plans, implements, and evaluates the plan of care
- Makes referrals

- The prospective payment system of reimbursement (diagnosis-related groups, or DRGs, discussed later), which encourages early discharge from the hospital, has created a new, acutely ill population that needs skilled care at home.
- Increasing numbers of older people are living longer with multiple chronic illnesses and are not institutionalized.
- With more sophisticated technology, people can be kept alive and relatively comfortable in their own homes.

- Healthcare consumers demand that services be humane and that provisions be made for a dignified death at home.

Nurses who provide care in the home make assessments and provide physical care, administer medications, teach, and support family members. They also collaborate with other healthcare providers, such as physicians, physical therapists, occupational therapists, respiratory therapists, and social workers to plan and provide patient care.

Acute Care Providers

Hospitals have been the traditional acute care provider for people who were too ill to care for themselves at home, who were severely injured, who required surgery or complicated treatments, or who were having babies. These individuals were admitted to the hospital and were not discharged until they were fully recovered or had used all of the services available within the hospital. As a result of federal regulations and other healthcare reimbursement policies, this is no longer true. As patients are discharged earlier, hospitals now focus more often on the acute care needs of the patient.

Hospital size ranges from as few as 20 beds to large medical centers with hundreds of beds. Various services are provided, depending on the size and location of the hospital. Most hospitals provide emergency care, inpatient care, surgery, diagnostic tests, and patient education. Other hospital services might include urgent care, intensive care, obstetrical care, social services, outpatient clinics and surgery, educational programs, and long-term skilled nursing facilities. Hospitals may provide care for all types of illnesses and trauma or may specialize. Specialty hospitals, or special units in general hospitals, meet the varied needs of certain patient groups, including children, patients needing rehabilitation, patients requiring psychiatric or drug-dependency care, and patients with severe burns.

Hospitals are classified as public or private and as for-profit or nonprofit. Public hospitals, which are nonprofit institutions, are financed and operated by local, state, or national agencies. Patients admitted to a public hospital may not have health insurance, and services are provided at no cost or little cost to the patient. The cost is covered by tax revenue or public funds. Private hospitals may be for-profit or nonprofit and are operated by communities, churches, corporations, and charitable organizations. Many patients cared for in private hospitals have some type of personal health insurance or healthcare plan.

Although this trend is changing, hospitals still employ more nurses than any other type of facility. The percentage of nurses working in hospitals is declining, but it is still projected that more than half of all nurses (57.4%) will be employed in hospital jobs in the year 2005 (American Nurses Association, 1997). Nurses employed in hospitals have many roles. Although many nurses are direct care providers, other roles include manager of other members of the healthcare team providing patient care, administrator, nurse practitioner, clinical nurse specialist, patient educator, in-service educator, and researcher. The current emphasis on cost containment and restructuring has made and will continue to make changes in where and how nurses work.

Primary Care Centers

Primary healthcare services are provided by physicians and advanced practice nurses in offices and clinics offering the diagnosis and treatment of minor illnesses, minor surgical procedures, obstetrical care, well-child care, counseling, and referrals. Many offices have laboratory and radiographic facilities. Although some physicians are general practitioners who treat all types of illness, many physicians specialize in one type of illness or surgery. A nurse in a physician's office makes health assessments, performs technical procedures, assists the physician, and provides health education. Nurse practitioners or clinical nurse specialists work collaboratively with physicians to make assessments and care for patients who require health maintenance or health promotion activities. Nurse practitioners also have their own offices and clinics to provide primary care and treatment to patients and only refer complex health problems to a physician.

Ambulatory Care Centers and Clinics

Ambulatory care centers and clinics may be located in hospitals, may be a free-standing service provided by a group of healthcare providers who work together, or may be run by a nurse practitioner. Ambulatory care centers and clinics are often located in convenient areas such as shopping malls or other community agencies. Many ambulatory care centers and clinics offer walk-in services so that appointments are unnecessary, and they are also open at times other than traditional office hours. Nurses in ambulatory care centers and clinics provide technical services (such as administering medications), determine the priority of care needs, and provide teaching about all aspects of care. A special type of ambulatory care center is an urgent-care center, which provides walk-in emergency care services. Ambulatory surgical centers, discussed in Chapter 29, are another form of ambulatory care center.

Specialized Care Centers and Settings

Specialized care centers and settings provide services for a specific population or group. They are usually located in easily accessible locations within a community.

Day-Care Centers

Day-care centers have a variety of purposes. Some centers care for infants and children who are healthy but need care while parents work; some also care for children with minor illnesses. Elder-care centers and senior citizen centers provide a place for older adults to socialize and to receive care while family members work. Some day-care centers provide health-related services and care to people who do not need to be in a healthcare institution but cannot be at home alone. Such centers provide services to older people, for physical rehabilitation and special needs (eg, cerebral palsy), and for chemical dependency and mental health.

Nurses who work in day-care centers administer medications and treatments, conduct health screenings, teach, and counsel.

Respite Care

Respite care is a type of care provided to home-bound ill, disabled, or elderly patients. The primary purpose is to enable the primary caregiver some time away from the responsibilities of day-to-day care. The care may be provided in an adult day-care center or in the patient's home by either professionals or volunteers.

Mental Health Centers

Mental health centers may be associated with a hospital or may provide services as an independent agency. The services provided may be crisis centered or may involve long-term counseling. Patients receive outpatient care through a variety of interventions, including individual and group counseling, medications, and assistance with independent living. Crisis intervention centers are also mental health centers. They typically provide 24-hour services and hotlines for people who are suicidal, abusing drugs or alcohol, or in abusive situations. These centers also provide information and services for victims of rape and abuse. Nurses who work in mental health centers must have strong communication and counseling skills and must be thoroughly familiar with community resources specific to the needs of patients being served.

Rural Health Centers

Rural health centers are often located in geographically remote areas with few healthcare providers. Many rural health centers are run by nurse practitioners, who serve as the patient's primary health provider for the care of minor acute illnesses as well as chronic illnesses. Patients who are seriously ill or injured are given emergency care and then transported to the nearest large hospital. Nurses who practice independently usually do so in collaboration with a physician who approves protocols for care. Many rural hospitals, physicians, and nurse practitioners now have immediate access to information about diagnosis and treatment of illness through telecommunication and computers.

Schools

School nurses are often the major source of health assessment, health education, and emergency care for the nation's children. The role of the school nurse reflects changes in society itself: children in schools today are from many different racial and ethnic groups, have varying socioeconomic backgrounds, and have more complex disabilities requiring expert knowledge and skills for management during school hours. School nurses provide many different services, including maintaining immunization records, providing emergency care for physical and mental illnesses, administering prescribed medications, conducting routine health screenings (such as those for vision, hearing, and scoliosis), and providing health information and education.

Industry

Many large industries have their own ambulatory care clinic, staffed primarily by nurses. Occupational health nurses practicing in industrial clinics focus on preventing work-related injury and illness by conducting health assessments, teaching for health promotion (such as stopping smoking, eating sensibly, using safety equipment, and exercising regularly), caring for minor accidents and illnesses, and making referrals for more serious health problems.

Homeless Shelters

Homeless shelters are usually living units (such as an apartment building or home) that provide housing for people who do not have regular shelter. The homeless are at increased risk for illness or injury because of factors such as exposure to the elements, exposure to violence, drug and alcohol addiction, poor nutrition, poor hygiene, and overcrowding. Services provided by nurses in homeless shelters include immunizing children, teaching pregnant women, treating infections and illnesses, referring for diagnosis and treatment of sexually transmitted diseases, and providing information about maintaining health.

Rehabilitation Centers

Rehabilitation centers specialize in services for patients requiring physical or emotional rehabilitation and for treatment of chemical dependency. These centers may be either free-standing or associated with a hospital. The goal is to return patients to optimal health and to the community as independent members of society. Rehabilitation centers often use a multidisciplinary team composed of physicians, nurses, physical therapists, occupational therapists, and counselors. The role of the nurse includes direct care, teaching, and counseling. The practice of rehabilitation nursing is based on a philosophy of encouraging independent self-care within the patient's capabilities.

Long-Term Care Facilities

Long-term care facilities provide healthcare and help with the activities of daily living for people of any age who are physically or mentally unable to care for themselves independently. Long-term care may extend for periods ranging from days to years. Agencies that provide long-term care are often independent but may be associated with a hospital. Included are facilities that provide transitional subacute care, intermediate and long-term care, nursing homes; retirement centers; and residential institutions for mentally and developmentally or physically disabled patients of all ages.

One of the newest concepts in long-term care is called "aging in place." In this type of care, patients move to a living space, such as an apartment, while they are still physically able to care for themselves, and then have access to progressively more healthcare services as needed as long as they live.

Long-term care facilities have proliferated in recent years for two reasons. First, many patients discharged from the hospital earlier in their recovery period require care that is beyond the scope of home care. These patients receive transitional, subacute care in a long-term facility. Second, many older adults do not have any caregivers and are no longer be able to carry out activities of daily living independently. As the services available through home healthcare increase, however, more people are able to remain in their own homes, and the number of older adults in nursing homes has declined since the early 1990s.

Although long-term facilities—especially nursing homes—have had a negative image in the past, much has changed. Most nursing homes focus on maintaining patient function and independence, with concern for the living environment as well as the healthcare provided. Concern for the happiness of nursing home residents has led to surroundings that include plants and animals as part of the home. Many of the overall improvements in long-term care came about as a result of the 1987 Omnibus Budget Reconciliation Act (OBRA), which included legislation to maintain standards of quality assurance in the nursing home industry.

Because patients entering long-term care facilities require so many different levels of care, it is difficult to generalize about the services provided. Those entering convalescent centers remain only until they have recovered. In some instances, an older adult may choose to move into a retirement or assisted-living center that provides healthcare services only when needed. Other people who enter a nursing home may require complete care as long as they live. The nurse's roles in long-term care facilities may include being a provider of direct care, supervisor, administrator, and teacher. Because most patients are older, increasing numbers of gerontology nurse specialists are contributing their knowledge and expertise to the care of these patients. Almost all long-term care facilities require that skilled nursing care be available at all times. The care given to patients can be performed only by or under the direct supervision of a licensed nurse.

Hospice Services

Hospices are special services for terminally ill patients and their families. The hospice agency may be public or private and may provide both inpatient and home care. These agencies are committed to maintaining quality of life and dignity for the dying person by providing an environment that encourages open communication, symptom management, and comfort measures for the patient and that supports the family during and after death of the patient. Hospice agencies are usually supervised by nurses but use trained volunteers to provide emotional and physical support, assist with transportation and household care, serve as liaison between patient and healthcare providers, and provide short-term respite care for family members who are primary caregivers.

Healthcare Agencies

Many different types of agencies provide healthcare services. Discussed here are voluntary agencies, religious agencies, and government agencies.

Voluntary Agencies

Community agencies are often nonprofit **voluntary agencies.** These agencies are financed by private donations, grants, or fundraisers (although some may charge minimal fees). Examples of volunteer agencies are Meals on Wheels, which supplies meals to older and homebound people; transportation services for older and physically disabled people; hearing contact people for hearing-impaired patients; and shopping or house-cleaning services. Other nonprofit voluntary community agencies include the Heart Association and the Lung Association. Physicians and nurses are often active members of these organizations and provide health screenings and educational programs.

Voluntary agencies may also provide a setting for support groups. These groups provide an education and support system for patients who are adjusting to their health problems. Members of these support groups have experienced the same type of problem. By sharing experiences, members learn to solve problems when dealing with a stressful or crisis situation. The following are some examples of support groups:

* Alcoholics Anonymous, an international organization for recovering alcoholics. The purpose of this support group is to help individuals stop drinking and remain sober. Meetings are held in accessible community locations such as churches and hospitals.
* Cancer support groups, which focus on support and solving problems experienced by people diagnosed with cancer. Most cancer support group meetings are held at hospitals.
* Reach to Recovery is a support group for women who have had a breast removed for cancer or have had breast reconstruction surgery. Among other activities, members visit women before surgery, teach exercises to prevent muscle atrophy, and provide information about prostheses and clothing.

Religious Agencies

Parish nursing is an area of community-based nursing practice that emphasizes holistic healthcare, health promotion, and disease prevention activities. Activities are often volunteer services and are based within a church. Parish nurses function as health educators, resource and referral aids, and facilitators of lay volunteer and support groups. Parish nurses reach out to those most vulnerable—the elderly, those who have suffered a loss or change, single parents, and children.

Government Agencies

Government agencies are financed by national, state, or local taxes. City and county taxes help support hospitals and public health clinics, state taxes help support state mental health hospitals, and national taxes help finance national health and welfare programs.

Veterans Administration and Military Agencies

Veterans Administration (VA) hospitals and military hospitals all come under the umbrella of government-supported and government-operated healthcare. VA hospitals provide healthcare services to veterans, and military hospitals provide care to active members of the armed forces and their immediate families.

Public Health Service

The **Public Health Service** (PHS) is a federal health agency under the direction of the US Department of Health and Human Services. The PHS is a multifaceted program with a wide range of services. It is the medical branch of the US Coast Guard and the principal source of Native American healthcare through the Indian Health Services. The PHS supplies funds to health centers that provide care to migrant workers and to community agencies that supply healthcare to the poor and uninsured. The principal budget of the PHS goes to grant programs for poor and uninsured people.

The Centers for Disease Control and Prevention (CDC) in Atlanta and the National Institutes of Health (NIH) are both part of PHS. The CDC focuses on the epidemiology, prevention, control, and treatment of communicable diseases, such as STDs. The NIH is engaged in both funding and conducting various health research activities.

The PHS also supplies healthcare professionals (eg, nurses, physicians, dentists, and pharmacists) to the US Department of Justice to provide care in federal prisons. The service is also involved to some extent in drug and alcohol abuse and mental health programs within the state. PHS activities focus on community needs whenever possible.

Public Health Agencies

Public health agencies are those local, state, and federal agencies that provide public health services to communities of various sizes (ie, local, county, state, or federal). Public health departments are usually funded by taxes and run by elected or appointed administrators. Local agencies provide services and programs to promote health and prevent illness, such as tuberculosis screening, immunizations (Fig. 11-3), and STD screening. Public health agencies work collaboratively with state and local departments to ensure public health through activities such as inspections of restaurants and water supplies. They also provide educational programs and may provide direct care services for low-income people or people living in rural, isolated areas. Nurses who practice in public health agencies focus on prenatal care, well-child care, screening programs, education, and outreach into the community.

🌀 Frameworks for Care

Different methods are used to ensure continuity of care and cost-effective care as a patient moves through the healthcare system. These methods include managed care systems, case management, and primary healthcare.

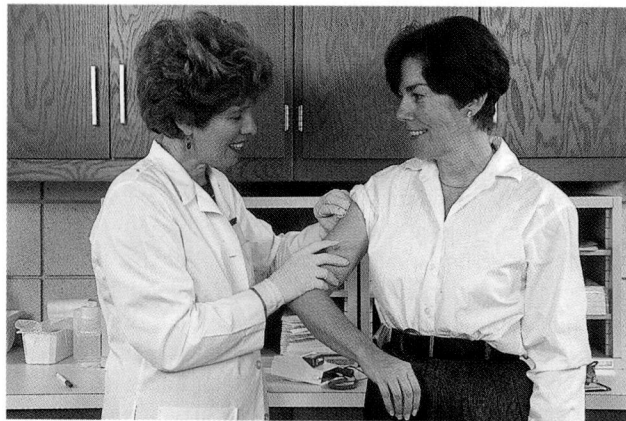

Figure 11-3
Administering an immunization at a public health clinic. (Photo © B. Proud.)

Managed Care Systems

Managed care systems are a way of providing care that are designed to control the cost of care provided while still maintaining the quality of that care. The care of the individual is carefully planned and monitored by the primary care provider, sometimes referred to as the case manager or "gatekeeper," from the initial contact to discharge from a healthcare episode. A managed care system limits the choice of care provider and requires approval for specialty care. Planning and monitoring activities are conducted to ensure that standards are followed and costs minimized. Health maintenance organizations and insurance companies are increasingly changing to managed care systems. A form of managed care has been proposed as a national healthcare plan; in general, large "umbrella" organizations would provide all aspects of care and compete for the consumer's business. Consumers would be able to choose only among managed care organizations, not among individual healthcare providers (Ellis & Hartley, 1998).

Case Management

Case management is a method used by some managed care systems to coordinate a patient's healthcare to maximize positive outcomes and contain costs (Rossi, 1999). Case managers are often nurses who maintain continuity of care across settings for patients who are seriously ill or have chronic illnesses. In this role, the nurse monitors the care provided and ensures that appropriate referrals are made and that the plan of care follows established standards (Ellis & Hartley, 1998).

Although there are different forms of case management, all focus on enhancing continuity of care and effectively using healthcare resources. The primary objective in many case management systems is to identify specific protocols and timetables for care and treatment in a format called a *critical pathway*. These written critical paths (also called *clinical pathways, care maps,* or *anticipated recovery paths*) incorporate independent and collaborative nursing interventions to reach desired patient outcomes within a specific time frame (see Chapter 20 for a further discussion of critical paths).

Nursing case management is an important method of coordinating care, controlling costs, and improving access to healthcare. The nurse case manager is responsible for these goals and may follow the patient from diagnosis of an illness to hospitalization and then back to home care. During the healthcare episode, the nurse case manager is responsible for managing the patient's interactions with the entire healthcare system. Nurses who are case managers do not give direct care; rather, they coordinate the care provided by others. In this role, nurse case managers have increased autonomy and power within the healthcare system in a variety of settings, including hospitals, long-term care facilities, and clinics.

Primary Healthcare

Primary healthcare was originally conceptualized in 1978 by the World Health Organization (WHO) and the United Nations International Children's Emergency Fund (UNICEF). The concept was developed based on decreases in illness and death in member countries that were achieved by simple, local, inexpensive solutions to health problems, especially when combined with economic and social development. Further discussion led to the Alma-Ata declaration, which focused on a global health strategy called primary healthcare. **Primary healthcare** is defined as essential healthcare based on practical, scientifically sound, and socially acceptable methods and technology, made universally accessible to individuals and families in the community through their full participation and at a cost the community can afford. It brings healthcare as close as possible to where people live and work (Barnes, Eriges, Juarbe, Nelson, Proctor, Sawyer, Shaul, & Meleis, 1995).

Primary healthcare differs from primary care. Primary care is the delivery of healthcare services, including the initial contact and ongoing care. Included in primary care is the responsibility for referral to other providers based on patient needs. Both physicians and nurse practitioners provide primary care, which focuses on the individual patient and is directed by the provider. In contrast, primary healthcare has a community-based philosophic base that emphasizes universal access and affordability of healthcare, health of the whole population, and consumer involvement. However, primary care and case management can both be practiced within a primary healthcare philosophy.

Ⓢ Collaborative Care: The Healthcare Team

In any type of agency, setting, or framework, nurses collaborate with other members of the healthcare team to plan, provide, and evaluate patient care (Fig. 11-4). For example, a nurse may request a consult with a dietitian for a patient who is not eating well or for one who needs to lose weight. After the dietitian talks with the patient and mutually determines a plan of care, the nurse can reinforce the plan and evaluate its effectiveness. The primary goal of

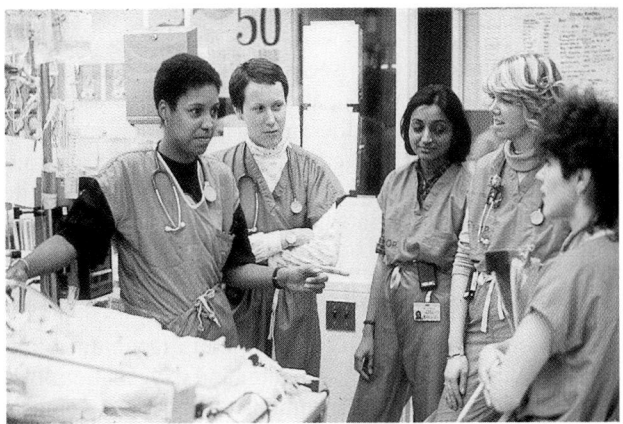

Figure 11-4
Collaboration by all members of the healthcare team facilitates quality care. (Photo by Gates Rhodes, courtesy of School of Nursing, University of Pennsylvania.)

each member of the healthcare team is to promote and restore health. The following sections describe members of the healthcare team with whom nurses work most often.

Physician

The physician is primarily responsible for the diagnosis of illness and the medical or surgical treatment of that illness. Physicians are granted the authority to admit patients to a healthcare agency by the healthcare agency or institution itself and to practice care within that setting through such actions as prescribing medications, interpreting the results of laboratory and diagnostic tests, and performing procedures and surgery. Individuals become physicians after extensive education and clinical practice and a licensing examination. Depending on the curriculum completed, a physician may graduate from a medical school and become a Doctor of Medicine (MD) or from a college of osteopathy and become a Doctor of Osteopathy (DO). MDs and DOs have similar educations and areas of practice, but osteopathic medicine emphasizes the study of mechanical changes in tissues as a cause of illness and treatment that involves manipulation of body structures. Physicians may choose to be general practitioners or to specialize in the treatment of one type of illness or body system (such as a cardiologist) or a specific type of surgery (such as an orthopedic surgeon).

Physician's Assistant

A physician's assistant (PA) has completed a specific course of study and a licensing examination in preparation for providing support to the physician. The PA's responsibilities usually depend on the supervising physician and might include conducting physical examinations and suturing lacerations. In most states, nurses are not legally bound to follow a PA's orders unless they are cosigned by a physician. This is an important aspect to investigate if PAs are employed by hospitals in your area.

Physical Therapist

A physical therapist (PT) seeks to restore function or prevent further disability in a patient after an injury or illness. PTs use various techniques to treat patients, including massage, heat, cold, water, sonar waves, exercises, and electrical stimulation. Most PTs are also educated in the use of psychological strategies to motivate patients.

Respiratory Therapist

A respiratory therapist (RT) is trained in techniques that improve pulmonary (lung) function and oxygenation. RTs may also be responsible for administering a variety of tests that measure lung function and for educating the patient about the use of various devices and machines prescribed by the physician.

Occupational Therapist

An occupational therapist (OT) assists physically challenged patients to adapt to limitations. OTs use a variety of adaptive devices and strategies to aid patients in carrying out the activities of daily living.

Speech Therapist

A speech therapist is trained to help hearing-impaired patients speak more clearly, to assist patients who have had a stroke to relearn how to speak, and to correct or modify a variety of speech disturbances in children and adults. Speech therapists also diagnose and treat swallowing problems in patients who have had a head injury or a stroke.

Dietitian

A registered dietitian (RD) manages and plans for the dietary needs of patients, based on knowledge about all aspects of nutrition. RDs can adapt specialized diets for the individual needs of patients, counsel and educate individual patients, and supervise the dietary services of an entire facility.

Pharmacist

A pharmacist is licensed to formulate and dispense medications. The pharmacist is also responsible for keeping a running file of all patient medications and for informing the physician when a potential or actual medication error in prescribing has occurred or when prescribed drugs may interact adversely. The pharmacist is an excellent resource for both patients and nurses for information related to medications.

Social Worker

A social worker counsels patients and family members and also informs them of and refers them to various community resources. Social workers are involved in many activities, such as counseling, reporting suspected drug addiction or abuse, assisting with decisions about life-sustaining treatments, placing patients in long-term care facilities, and providing support to dying patients and their family members.

Unlicensed Assistive Personnel

Unlicensed assistive personnel (UAPs) help nurses provide direct care to patients. As defined by individual state boards of nursing, UAPs may have the title of certified nursing assistants, orderlies, attendants, or technicians.

Financial Aspects of Healthcare

Healthcare is very expensive, and costs continue to increase. Few citizens can afford to pay for healthcare from their own resources. The costs of most people's healthcare are covered by federally funded programs, prepaid plans, and private insurance.

Federally Funded Healthcare Programs

The primary federally funded healthcare programs are Medicare and Medicaid.

Medicare

The 1965, **Medicare** amendments to the Social Security Act established national and state health insurance programs for the elderly under Title 18. Within a decade, almost all citizens older than 65 years of age held Medicare insurance for hospital care, extended care, and home healthcare. Medicare coverage was increased in 1972 to include permanently disabled workers and their dependents if they also qualified for Social Security benefits. In 1983, Medicare converted to a prospective payment plan based on **diagnosis-related groups** (DRGs). This plan pays the hospital a fixed amount that is predetermined by the medical diagnosis or specific procedure rather than by the actual cost of hospitalization and care. DRGs were implemented by the federal government in an effort to control rising healthcare costs. The plan pays only the amount of money preassigned to a treatment for the diagnosis (eg, an appendectomy); if the cost for hospitalization is greater than that assigned, the hospital must absorb the additional cost. If the cost is less than that assigned, the hospital makes a profit.

Medicare was again expanded in 1988 to include catastrophic care costs and expensive medications. People who receive Medicare pay both a deductible cost and a monthly premium for full insurance coverage. Part A of Medicare, which pays most inpatient hospital costs, is paid by the federal government. Part B of Medicare, which is voluntary, is paid by monthly premium; it covers most outpatient costs for physician visits, medications, and home health services. Because the full cost of some services is not covered by Medicare, a supplemental insurance policy offered by a private insurance company is recommended. Also, because

Medicare is federally funded, benefits may change annually according to decisions related to the federal budget.

Medicaid

Medicaid was also established in 1965 under Title 19 of the Social Security Act. Medicaid is a federally funded public assistance program for people with low incomes of any age; for the blind, elderly, and disabled covered by supplemental security benefits; and for beneficiaries of Aid to Families With Dependent Children. The coverage depends on individual state regulations.

Current budgetary considerations are forcing state and federal agencies to trim Medicaid expenditures. The rapid growth of an aging population and an increase in the number of poor people, many of whom are women and children, are draining the Medicaid budget. In an attempt to survive, Medicaid programs are implementing changes such as reduced benefits or placing patients into managed care programs.

Group Plans

The major group plans for financing healthcare are managed care plans, such as health maintenance organizations (HMOs), preferred provider organizations (PPOs), and private insurance. Enrollment in these plans is voluntary. An individual pays a fixed rate on a monthly or annual plan and, in turn, receives coverage for most healthcare services to maintain health and treat illness.

Because group plans such as HMOs and PPOs pay the direct costs of the healthcare services used by their subscribers, they encourage preventive healthcare to avoid the higher costs of illness and hospitalization. For the same reason, they carefully monitor the quality and quantity of the healthcare delivered to their subscribers. They also place limitations on the use of high-cost procedures and require certain guidelines to be followed when a costly procedure is recommended by a physician. Some people do not like these plans because they use a selective contracting approach that mandates subscribers use specific institutions and healthcare providers. Some consumers dislike not being able to control decisions about their own or their family's health.

Health Maintenance Organizations

Health maintenance organizations (HMOs) are prepaid, group-managed care plans that allow subscribers to receive all the medical services they require through a group of affiliated providers. There may be no additional out-of-pocket costs, or subscribers may pay only a small fee, called a *copayment*. An HMO may employ all its providers (including physicians) or may be a group of physicians in alliance who provide care as independent practitioners (an *independent practice association*). In most HMOs, the patient does not have a choice about healthcare providers but receives all services from physicians associated with or part of the HMO. HMOs are becoming popular with large employers who support the concept of managed care.

Preferred Provider Organizations

Preferred provider organizations (PPOs) allow a *third-party payer* (agencies that pay healthcare providers for services provided to individuals, such as a health insurance company) to contract with a group of healthcare providers to provide services at a lower fee in return for prompt payment and a guaranteed volume of patients and services. Although patients are encouraged to use specific providers, they may also seek care outside the panel without referral by paying additional out-of-pocket expenses. One type of PPO is called a *preferred provider arrangement*, in which a contract is made with an individual healthcare provider rather than with a group of providers. Similarly, a *point-of-service plan* encourages the use of specified physicians and services but pays a portion of expenses if referrals are made to physicians outside the organization by the patient's primary care physician.

Private Insurance

Personal healthcare can be financed by private insurance through large, nonprofit, tax-exempt organizations or through smaller, private, for-profit insurance companies. To be insured, members pay monthly premiums either by themselves or in combination with employer payments. These plans are called third-party payers because the insurance company pays all or most of the cost of care. The premiums on private insurance plans tend to be higher than those for managed care plans, but members can choose their own physician and services desired.

Long-Term Care Insurance

Increasing numbers of people are enrolling in long-term care (LTC) insurance. Most LTC insurance (about 90%) is paid for by Medicaid and out-of-pocket spending. Medicare and private insurance pays for only a minimal amount of LTC insurance. Some commercial insurance companies offer LTC benefits. Promoters of LTC insurance have developed plans that cover a variety of services, such as nursing home care and home care as well as other services that help prevent the institutionalization of older, debilitated, and chronically ill people. Adult day-care centers and respite care are also LTC services and would be covered by such benefits.

Trends and Issues in Healthcare Delivery

Some current issues and trends in healthcare are discussed in this section. In your career as a nurse, you may find that some issues are resolved, whereas other, new challenges arise. It is important for you both personally and professionally to be knowledgeable about all issues affecting the healthcare delivery system.

Focus on Self-Care and Health

Health awareness and the desire to be involved in one's own healthcare have strongly influenced the delivery of healthcare services in our society. Stress management programs,

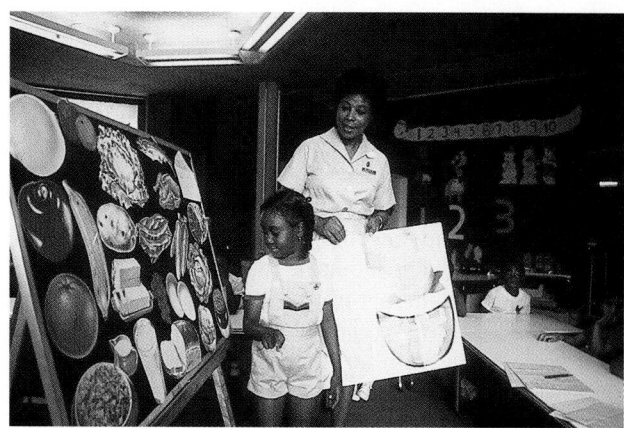

Figure 11-5
Young children in school, community centers, and other community groups can be taught the importance of eating healthful foods.

nutritional awareness, exercise and fitness programs, and antismoking and antidrug campaigns are all examples of this trend (Fig. 11-5). Equally important to health are measures such as legislating the use of seat belts, promoting automobile and airplane safety, controlling smog, controlling handguns, and eliminating hazardous wastes.

Consumer Movement

A **consumer** is someone who uses a commodity or service. Healthcare consumers are often knowledgeable about health, prefer to control and make decisions about their own health, and want to be active participants in planning and implementing their healthcare. Consumers of healthcare services have become better educated about the services they require and the services that are available. They also have become concerned about access to services and the cost of those services. Consumers have questioned escalating costs and the proliferation and duplication of services. Consumers have become actively involved in the administration of healthcare agencies and have helped develop standards for care, patient rights, and cost-containment measures as protection for patients when they enter a healthcare setting.

Cost Containment

The US healthcare system has been experiencing a financial crisis. Costs have increased dramatically, and some analysts believe that cost-containment measures were implemented too late to reverse the rise in health costs. The actual short-term and long-term results of cost-containment measures remain to be seen.

Historically, the ways healthcare was paid for encouraged the use of expensive and sometimes inappropriate or ineffective services. In the past, healthcare also focused primarily on the treatment of illnesses rather than prevention because preventive strategies were not covered by health insurance. The system of third-party reimbursement effec-

tively insulated patients, who seldom saw the bills, from knowing the actual cost of their healthcare.

Competition among hospitals has further fueled the increase in health costs. To attract patients, hospitals have invested huge sums of money in technologically advanced equipment. As new machines and more advanced procedures have been developed and used, patients' expectations of the availability and use of those resources have also tended to increase. Supporters of cost-containment measures are encouraging hospitals to cooperate and share resources rather than compete. Other efforts at cost containment include hospital restructuring and multiple hospitals joining together as one system.

Fragmentation of Care

Expanded healthcare research has led to an upward spiral of new technology and knowledge. Because many healthcare providers can no longer keep up with all of the advances being made in all areas, specialization in smaller areas has become almost the rule rather than the exception. What does this mean for patients?

A general practitioner physician diagnoses and treats a variety of common health problems; however, a patient who requires diagnosis and treatment for a more complex problem is usually referred to a specialist physician. For example, a patient with diabetes and a heart condition may be cared for by the family physician, a cardiologist, and an endocrinologist. Hospitalized patients not only come in contact with many different healthcare providers (eg, registered nurses, licensed practical nurses, nursing assistants, nurse specialists, physical therapists, dietitians, and students) but also are frequently seen by other physician specialists called in on consultation or to do surgery. No wonder that patients become confused about care and treatments. This fragmentation of care can lead to a loss of continuity of care, resulting in conflicting plans of care, too much or too little medication, and higher healthcare costs.

Healthcare: A Right or a Privilege?

Two major factors influencing the provision of healthcare in the United States are the ability to pay and the location of facilities. Poor or uninsured people, minorities, residents of rural areas, and older people often have inadequate access to healthcare services. In the United States, millions of people have inadequate insurance or none at all. Although many people assume that everyone has a right to healthcare, consider these questions that pose ethical dilemmas:

- Do uninsured people who do not take care of themselves deserve the same healthcare as employed people with insurance, even if they can't pay for it?
- Who provides funds for the healthcare needs of the homeless?
- Is someone who pays for national television coverage to ask for an organ donation for his or her child any more deserving than someone who has been waiting months for just such a transplant?

- Are you willing to pay higher insurance premiums or taxes so that drug addicts who overdose can have intensive care?
- If 20 people need a heart transplant and only one heart is available, who decides who gets another chance at life?

These are only a few of the questions being raised, and there are no easy answers. The issues of who gets healthcare and who pays the bills continue to have major importance for society in the 21st century. These issues will present both challenges and opportunities for nurses of the future.

Learning Outcomes

After completing this chapter, the learner should be able to accomplish the following:

1. Define key terms used in the chapter.

ambulatory care	managed care
case management	Medicaid
community-based healthcare	Medicare
	outpatient
consumer	preferred provider organization
day-care center	
diagnosis-related group	primary healthcare
health maintenance organization	public health agencies
	Public Health Service
inpatient	voluntary agency
long-term care	

2. Describe the role of nursing in meeting the challenges of healthcare reform.
3. Compare and contrast community-based agencies and settings in which healthcare is provided.
4. Discuss the elements of managed care, case management, and primary healthcare.
5. Describe the members of the collaborative healthcare team.
6. Discuss various methods of financing healthcare.
7. Discuss trends and issues affecting healthcare delivery.

Critical Thinking Exercises

1. Make a list of the different types of healthcare settings in which you have been provided care. How many different healthcare providers did you come in contact with? How did the structure and organization of the settings differ, and how were they alike?

2. How might prenatal and well-child care differ for two women: one without health insurance and the other with a good health insurance plan? Why do you think this happens? What can nurses do?

Bibliography

American Nurses Association. (1991). *Nursing's agenda for healthcare reform.* Washington, DC: Author.

American Nurses Association. (1997). *Supply, demand, need: Nursing's numbers revisited.* Washington, DC: Author.

American Public Health Association. (2000). *Healthy People 2010: National health promotion and disease prevention objectives.* Washington, DC: Author.

Androwich, I., & Haas, S. (1996). Ambulatory care nursing: Concerns and challenges. In J. McCloskey & H. Grace, *Current issues in nursing* (5th ed) (pp. 216–222). St. Louis: C. V. Mosby.

Armmer, F., & Humbles, P. (1995). Parish nursing: Extending health care to urban African-Americans. *Nursing & Healthcare: Perspectives on Community, 16*(2), 64–68.

Barnes, D., Eriges, C., Juarbe, T., Nelson, M., Proctor, S., Sawyer, L., Shaul, M., & Meleis, A. (1995). Primary health care and primary care: A confusion of philosophies. *Nursing Outlook, 43*(1), 7–16.

Bell, R. (1996). Promoting collaboration in community health nursing. *Nursing & Healthcare: Perspectives on Community, 17*(4), 186–188.

Chadderton, H. (1998). Thinking . . . about nursing homes. *Journal of Nursing Management, 6*(4), 191–192.

Collins, C., Butler, F., Gueldner, S., & Palmer, M. (1997). Models for community-based long-term care for the elderly in a changing health system. *Nursing Outlook, 45*(2), 59–63.

Dougherty, M., Dwyer, J., Pendergast, J., Tomlinson, B., Boyington, A., Vogel, B., Duncan, P., Coward, R., & Cox, C. (1998). Community-based nursing: Continence care for older rural women. *Nursing Outlook, 46*(5), 233–244.

Drew, J. C. (1990). Health maintenance organizations: History, evolution, & survival. *Nursing and Healthcare, 11*(3), 145–149.

Ellis, J., & Hartley, C. (1998). *Nursing in today's world: Challenges, issues, and trends.* (6th ed.). Philadelphia: Lippincott Williams & Wilkins.

Green, K., & Lydon, S. (1998). Continuing care extra: The continuum of patient care. *American Journal of Nursing, 98*(10), 16BBB–16DDD.

Health Care Financing Administration. (1997). *Managed care in Medicare and Medicaid: Fact sheet.* Washington, DC: US Department of Health and Human Services.

Heinrich, J. (1998). Incremental approaches to necessary health care reform lead to more chaos. *Nursing Outlook, 46*(3), 137–139.

Joel, L. (1997). Moving the care site from the hospital to home: Whose turf? In J. McCloskey & H. Grace, *Current issues in nursing* (5th ed.). (pp. 209–215). St. Louis: C. V. Mosby.

Klainberg, M., Holzemer, S., Leonard, M., & Arnold, J. (1998). *Community health nursing: An alliance for health.* New York: McGraw-Hill.

Miller, J. (1998). The changing face of long-term care. *Caring, 17*(8), 24–26.

Muldinger, M. (1994). Healthcare reform: Will nursing respond? *Nursing & Healthcare, 15*(1), 28–33.

National Hospice Organization. (1997). *The basics of hospice.* Arlington, VA: National Hospice Organization.

Pew Health Professions Commission. (1991). *Healthy America: Practitioners for 2005.* Durham, NC: The Pew Health Professions Commission.

Repetto, L., Granetto, C., & Venturino, A. (1997). Home care in the older person. *Clinics in Geriatric Medicine, 13*(2), 403–413.

Ross, M. E., & Wright, M. F. (1998). Long-term care for elderly individuals and methods for financing. *Journal of Community Health Nursing, 15*(2), 77–89.

Rossi, P. (1999). *Case management in health care: A practical guide.* Philadelphia: W. B. Saunders.

Shoultz, J., & Hatcher, P. (1997). Looking beyond primary care to primary health care: An approach to community-based action. *Nursing Outlook, 45*(1), 23–26.

Zotti, M., Brown, P., & Stotts, R. (1996). Community-based nursing versus community health nursing: What does it all mean? *Nursing Outlook, 44*(5), 211–217.

Chapter 12
Continuity of Care

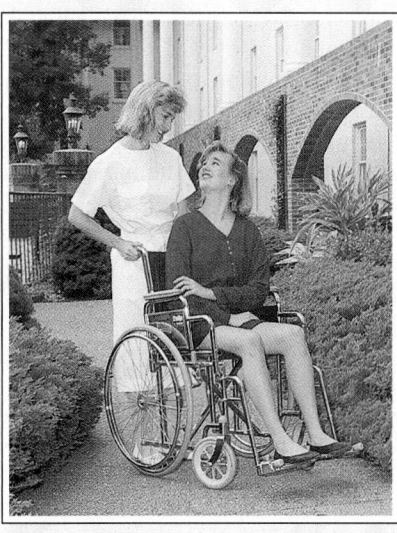

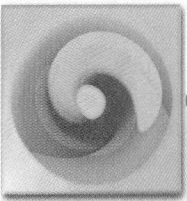

**Thinking Critically About
Nursing's Blended Skills**

Before reading this chapter, think about the types of skills you will need to ensure continuity of care in different practice settings.

- Mrs. Appleton, a 65-year-old woman who is being discharged home from same-day surgery after cataract removal appears confused about the discharge instructions she is receiving.

- Joey, a profoundly mentally retarded 7-year-old, is transferred from the state home for children to your hospital for respiratory complications.

- Jimmy is a 27-year-old homeless, schizophrenic man who frequently appears in your mental health clinic. Many of the staff dismiss his concerns and believe he comes to the clinic trying to "con" the staff for the drugs he says he needs. There is some question about whether he then sells these drugs on the street.

- Mrs. Degas was diagnosed with Alzheimer's disease 2 years ago. Her husband has been caring for her at home. She is currently in the hospital after repair of a fractured hip. Her husband wants to take her home, but both he and you are unsure of his ability to continue to provide the level of care she now needs.

What cognitive, technical, interpersonal, and ethical/legal skills do you think you will need to ensure continuity of care as the patients described above move from one place to another?

Continuity of care is a process by which healthcare providers give appropriate, uninterrupted care and facilitate the patient's transition to different settings and levels of care. Continuity of care ensures a smooth transition between ambulatory or acute care and home care or other types of community-based care. Coordination helps ensure a patient-focused and individualized continuum of healthcare so that the patient may attain maximum recovery and health.

Entering and leaving a healthcare setting, as well as receiving care at home, are experiences that produce anxiety for patients and family members. The nurse is most often the person who helps the patient make a smooth transition from one type of care setting to another. This chapter discusses admission and dismissal from a healthcare setting, transfer from one type of setting to another, and discharge planning in preparation for home care. The focus is on the patient's needs and the nurse's role in providing continuity of care.

The Nurse's Role in Providing Continuity of Care

Most people are born in a hospital and thus became consumers of healthcare from the first day of life. Most people continue to require services of some type, in a variety of healthcare settings, until they die. Although a patient's healthcare may involve many different providers and settings (see Chap. 11), the nurse is often the primary person responsible for communicating the patient's needs, teaching self-care, and, in many instances, providing care. As a result, one of the primary responsibilities of the nurse as caregiver is ensuring continuity of care.

Continuity of care is essential in the current healthcare system. The emphasis on health promotion and the prevention of illness makes teaching for individuals of all ages crucial components of patient care. To provide continuity of care, nurses must do the following:

- Include discharge planning in the care of any person admitted to any type of healthcare setting
- Collaborate with other members of the healthcare team in meeting physical, psychological, sociocultural, and spiritual needs of the patient and family in all settings and at all levels of health
- Involve the patient and family members in the planning process

The purpose of planning for continuity of care, which is more commonly referred to as *discharge planning,* is to ensure that patient and family needs are consistently met as the patient moves from one level of care to another. Discharge planning, described in detail later in the chapter, involves the following:

- Assessing the strengths and limitations of the patient, family or support person, and the environment
- Planning for continuity in healthcare from one setting to another, including the home
- Implementing and coordinating the plan of care, considering individual patient needs as well as individual, family, and community resources
- Evaluating the effectiveness of care

This chapter only introduces the different ways in which patients enter a healthcare setting and move from one type of setting to another. Discharge planning is discussed primarily in relation to the care of the patient at home; this aspect of care will be increasingly common in the future.

COGNITIVE SKILLS

- Knowledge of patient needs and the resources available to meet these needs in the patient's home and in different practice settings
- Knowledge of how to communicate effectively patient priorities and the related plan of care as a patient is transferred between home and different practice settings

TECHNICAL SKILLS

- Ability to provide the technical nursing assistance necessary to meet the needs of patients and their family and professional caregivers as patients are transferred between home and different practice settings

INTERPERSONAL SKILLS

- Ability to establish trusting professional relationships with patients, family caregivers, and healthcare professionals in different practice settings to ensure continuity of care

ETHICAL/LEGAL SKILLS

- Commitment to preparing patients and their family and professional caregivers to continue the plan of care when a patient is discharged
- Commitment to securing the best setting for care to be provided for patients and the best coordination of resources to support the level of care needed
- Knowledge of the nurse's legal and ethical obligations as patients are transferred between home and different practice settings

Admitting a Patient to a Healthcare Setting

People enter healthcare settings and become consumers of healthcare services (patients) for many different reasons. Consider the following examples:

- Joe Sol, aged 5 years, has been having increasing numbers of throat infections, and his tonsils are badly infected. Mrs. Sol takes Joe for a checkup at his pediatrician's office. Joe's pediatrician has decided that Joe must have a *tonsillectomy* (removal of tonsils) through same-day surgery at his local hospital, entering the morning of surgery and going home that afternoon.
- Jane Yee, aged 38 years, has heavy menstrual periods. After her yearly well-women check at her gynecologist's clinic, as a diagnostic procedure, her doctor schedules her for a dilation of the cervix and curettage of the uterus (*D & C*) at a community ambulatory surgery center.
- Tom Valiz, aged 28 years, injured his back while working at his construction job. After diagnostic studies as an outpatient in his local hospital, he has been going to a community health center each day for heat therapy and exercises.
- Sadie Aird, aged 78 years, has had congestive heart failure for the past 10 years. She is cared for at home by her daughter, with the help of a home health nurse and aide.
- Jim Zamba, aged 28 years, is admitted to the hospital through the emergency room, sent to surgery, and then placed in the intensive care unit for treatment of severe head injuries following a motorcycle accident. After recovery from the acute phase of care, Jim will transfer to a special rehabilitation center.

Although all of these individuals require care, they do not all have the same kind of needs, nor are they alike as patients. Some of them are admitted and discharged on the same day, some of them remain in the acute-care setting only as long as acute care is needed, and some require long-term care.

As a result of increasing costs and healthcare cost reimbursement programs that are prospective more often than retrospective, hospital admissions and lengths of hospital stay are decreasing. Increasing numbers of patients are having surgery, diagnostic tests, and emergency care in ambulatory care settings or on an outpatient basis. Even patients who are admitted may stay for less than 24 hours, may be admitted the morning of the surgery, or may go home during an interim period between diagnosis and care.

All people who enter a healthcare setting must take on a new role. They must add to their already established roles (eg, spouse, parent, sibling, student) the role of patient. They also enter an environment in which they are surrounded by strangers and in which they encounter different sounds, sights, and smells.

When meeting patients' healthcare needs during the admission process, nurses provide holistic care while establishing the base for how patients will respond to and evaluate the remainder of their stay. The accompanying box describes guidelines for establishing an effective nurse–patient relationship to ensure that each patient is considered as an individual in any setting.

During admission, the nurse acts not only as a practitioner but also as a person concerned about the welfare of the patient and family. The admission period corresponds to the orientation phase of the helping relationship described in Chapter 21. In addition, regulatory guidelines direct both the continuity and the quality of care. For example, the standards for admission and discharge from a hospital, established by the Joint Commission on Accreditation of Healthcare Organizations, include the following:

- Each patient's need for nursing care related to admission is assessed by a registered nurse.
- Each patient's assessment includes consideration of biophysical, psychosocial, environmental, self-care, educational, and discharge planning factors.

Establishing an Effective Nurse–Patient Relationship on Admission

- Recognize and take necessary steps to reduce anxiety. Anxiety is a natural reaction to the unknown. Anxiety reduction can be facilitated through therapeutic communications, teaching, and acceptance. Some common concerns that cause anxiety follow:

  Will I have pain?
  Who will take care of my family if I die?
  Will strangers be looking at my body?
  How much will this cost?
  What if I can't keep my job?

- Remember that the medical or surgical condition for which the patient is being treated is only one part of the patient's life. Although it may be the primary concern for the patient, other concerns include family needs, financial status, and the future.
- Communicate with the patient as an individual so that he or she can maintain his or her own identity. Ask patients how you should address them—some people would prefer Mr., or Mrs., Ms. [last name]; others would rather be called by their first name. Do not lump all older adults as "Grandma" or "Grandpa." Be sure that you do not refer to Mr. Jones, admitted to room 2218 for treatment of a ruptured appendix, as "the appendix in 2218."
- Take time to learn *who* the patient being admitted is, including the patient's cultural and religious background. Respect the patient's values and beliefs even though they may differ from yours.
- Provide for the patient's family participation and decision making in all aspects of care.

- The patient and family are involved in care as appropriate.
- Nursing staff members collaborate, as appropriate, with physicians and members of other clinical disciplines to make decisions regarding the patient's need for nursing care.
- In preparation for discharge, continuing care needs are assessed, and referrals for such care are documented in the patient's medical record.

Admission to an Ambulatory Care Facility

Ambulatory facilities are those in which the patient receives healthcare services but does not remain overnight. An individual may receive care in many different kinds of ambulatory facilities, including physician offices, clinics, outpatient services, emergency rooms, and same-day surgery centers. The goal of these facilities is to provide those patients who are able to provide self-care at home with assistance as necessary from healthcare providers. Individuals go to ambulatory settings for health promotion, health maintenance, or medical or surgical treatment.

In most office and clinic facilities, patients enter a reception area, where they are asked to complete a short health history unless they have already done so during a previous visit. They then go to an examination room where a physical assessment (often specific to the reason for the visit) is completed. Depending on their needs, diagnostic tests may be done, immunizations given, medications prescribed, or minor surgery performed. All patients require teaching, which should include written instructions about care at home, health promotion activities, and how to contact someone for further questions. Referrals to community agencies, support groups, or other types of healthcare settings may be necessary.

Admission to ambulatory or same-day surgery facilities is somewhat different. Screening tests, teaching, and admission procedures are usually completed before patients enter the setting. They arrive at the setting, have the procedure, and go home when recovery is satisfactory (see Chap. 29). If patients have surgery in the hospital setting, the regular admission procedures are completed on arrival; in most instances, screening tests and teaching are done before the day of surgery. It is the nurse's responsibility to assess what has been done and individualize the care plan to patients' needs.

Admission to the Hospital

In most hospitals, admission begins in the admitting office. Staff obtain information about the patient and print that information on an admission sheet. This admission sheet becomes part of the patient's permanent record. It includes the following information:

> Full name
> Address
> Date of birth
> Name of admitting physician
> Gender
> Marital status

> Nearest relative
> Occupation and employer
> Financial status for healthcare payment
> Religious preference
> Date and time of admission
> Identification number
> Admitting diagnosis

The identification number, as well as the patient's name and physician's name (and any other information required by the particular institution), is printed on the identification bracelet that is placed on the patient's wrist. This bracelet is an important safety component during the patient's treatment because it accurately identifies the individual for procedures and treatments, including medication administration, diagnostic tests, and surgery. The bracelet is essential for identifying patients who are irrational, comatose, or young.

After the necessary forms have been completed in the admitting office, the admission health history and physical assessment may be completed by a nurse who works in that area. Patients may also be taken to an assigned unit for admission procedures, but laboratory studies and radiographs, as well as the admitting office procedures, are usually completed on an outpatient basis before or on the day of admission. If the patient has an unscheduled admission or is going to have only a limited stay (eg, those who are admitted the morning of a diagnostic examination and then go home later in the day), admission procedures and assessments may be completed on the unit.

Preparing the Room for Admission

The admitting office notifies the unit before the patient's arrival so that the room can be prepared. Although the nurse may not do many of the activities listed below, it is a nursing responsibility to ensure they are done by other personnel. The following activities are carried out in anticipation of the patient's arrival:

- Position the bed (Fig. 12-1). For ambulatory patients, the bed should be in its lowest position. Place the bed in its highest position if the patient will arrive on a stretcher. Ensure that the furniture in the room is arranged to allow easy access to the bed.
- Open the bed by folding back the top bed linens.
- Assemble necessary equipment and supplies. A hospital admission pack (which contains such items as a bath basin, water pitcher, drinking glass, tissues, soap, and lotion) is placed in the room. A hospital gown or pajamas should be in the room, although the patient may choose to wear his or her own pajamas or gown. Equipment for taking vital signs (ie, stethoscope, sphygmomanometer, or thermometer) and height and weight should be in the room or readily available. If laboratory work has not been done previously, a container for a clean urine specimen should be available.
- Assemble special equipment and supplies. The patient may require oxygen therapy, cardiac monitoring, or suction equipment. The nurse ensures that

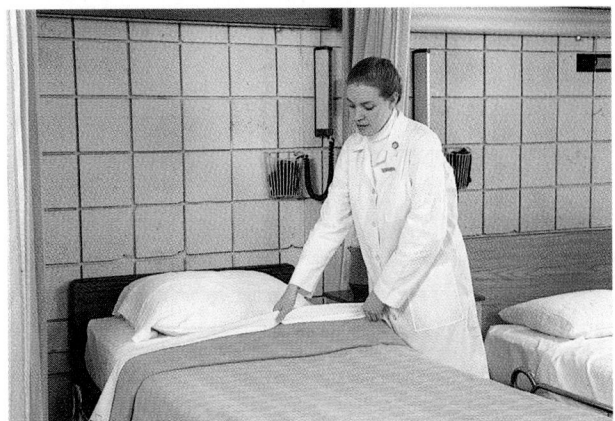
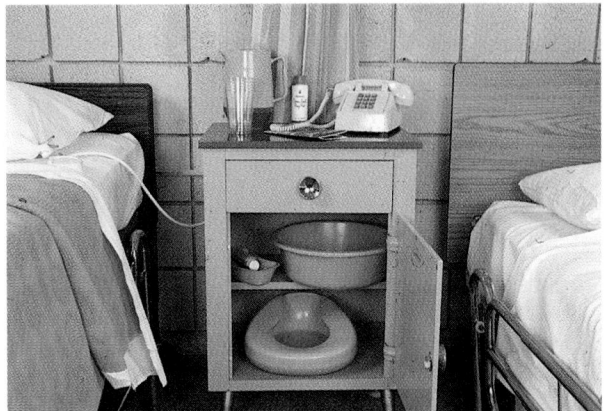

Figure 12-1
In anticipation of the patient's arrival on the hospital unit, the bed should be opened and positioned correctly, and necessary supplies and equipment should be available.

the equipment is functioning properly and is ready for the patient's use on arrival.

- Adjust the physical environment of the room. This may include turning on lights and setting the room temperature.

Welcoming the Patient to the Unit

Although other members of the healthcare team may assist in the admitting procedure, the nurse is responsible for the comfort and well-being of the patient upon arrival in the unit. The nurse completes the admission assessment and documents the information on the admission database (Fig. 12-2). The sample form (Fig. 12-3) illustrates typical information that is collected and documented. The information on the form is used to develop the nursing care plan for the patient and also is used as a database for discharge planning and home care. In addition, a patient inventory of personal belongings is often completed to ensure these are returned to the patient on discharge or transferred with the patient if a move to another unit or facility occurs.

The patient should be welcomed to the unit in the same courteous manner that would be used in welcoming a guest into one's own home. In most instances, the patient is accompanied by family members who may either remain with the patient to provide support and information or be asked to wait in the waiting room during the admission procedure. The nurse needs to assess the needs of the patient and family and mutually agree about whether family should be present during admission.

Transferring Within and Between Settings

It is common for some type of move to be made within settings as well as between settings. The following are some examples of transferring within and between settings:

- Patients often are moved within the hospital, such as from the emergency room to a hospital room, from an intensive care unit (ICU) to a hospital room (and vice versa), from one floor to another, or from one room to another room on the same floor.
- Patients are transferred to and from acute care settings and long-term settings.
- Patients are transferred from acute care settings to their homes.
- Patients are transferred from ambulatory care settings to acute care settings.

When a transfer occurs, the patient must readjust to new surroundings, new roommates, new routines, and new people providing care. If the transfer is to a higher level of care, as in a move to the ICU, the patient experiences unfamiliar sights and sounds. A transfer to a long-term facility may not be desired by the patient or family but may be necessary if family members cannot provide care at home or if no other support people are available. All of these factors cause stress and anxiety.

The nurse may not be responsible for the actual physical move but is responsible for ensuring that the comfort, safety, and knowledge needs of the patient and family are

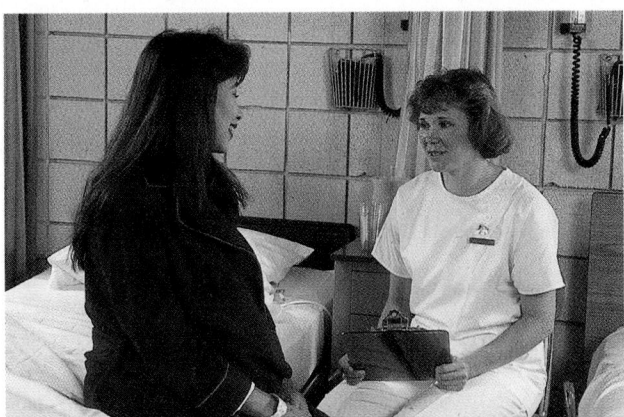

Figure 12-2
When a patient is admitted to a healthcare setting, the nurse is responsible for collecting information to complete the health history.

(*text continues on page 196*)

NURSING ADMISSION DATA

CURRENT MEDICATIONS, SUPPLEMENTS, NON-PRESCRIPTION DRUGS:

NAME	DOSE/FREQUENCY	LAST DOSE
Aspirin	2 prn	1 month
Maalox	prn	this Am

□ MEDICATION TO PHARMACY □ MEDICATION SENT HOME

ALLERGEN: (DRUGS, FOOD, TAPES, DYES, OTHERS)

ALLERGEN	SYMPTOMS
Penicillin	rash

LEGAL GUARDIAN (NAME/PHONE)_____

CONTACT PERSON (NAME/PHONE) Mrs. Solle, 335-4001

PHYSICIAN NOTIFIED ✓ TIME 0830

PRIMARY CARE PHYSICIAN Dr. Wills

DATE 1-16-00 TIME 0900

ADMISSION   □ OBSERVATION

☒ AMBULATORY □ WHEELCHAIR □ STRETCHER

□ CORRECT INDENTIFICATION BAND

ADMITTED FROM: ☒ HOME □ NURSING FACILITY
□ EMERGENCY ROOM □ OTHER_____

INFORMATION GIVEN BY: □ FAMILY MEMBER □ FRIEND ☒ PATIENT
  □ UNABLE TO TAKE HISTORY - PATIENT UNRESPONSIVE/CONFUSED/
    NOT ACCOMPANIED BY FAMILY OR FRIEND
  □ PREVIOUS MEDICAL RECORD

ORIENTATION TO ROOM

☒ VISITING HOURS ☒ CALL LIGHT IN REACH: ☒ EXPLAINED

☒ OPERATION OF BED AND SIDE RAILS ☒ USE OF PHONE

☒ VALUABLES SENT HOME □ IN SAFE □ IN POSSESSION
  SPECIFY_____

☒ PATIENT HANDBOOK   ☒ INTRODUCED TO ROOMMATE

MEDICAL HISTORY

ADMITTED MEDICAL DIAGNOSIS Peptic Ulcer

PAST HOSPITALIZATIONS AND/OR ILLNESS: (MEDICAL, SURGICAL, EMOTIONAL
PROBLEMS) 1986 - Appendectomy

WHAT IS REASON FOR ADMISSION? (PATIENT'S OWN WORDS)
"My doctor says I have An ulcer"

*SUBJECTIVE DATA:

1. HEALTH PERCEPTIONS/HEALTH MANAGEMENT PATTERN

GENERAL HEALTH Excellent

USE OF: □ TOBACCO: HOW MUCH/HOW LONG? No
  □ ALCOHOL: HOW MUCH/HOW LONG? No
  □ OTHER DRUGS TYPE(s) None

2. NUTRITIONAL/METABOLIC PATTERN

DIET/RESTRICTIONS/SUPPLEMENTS: Regular diet

□ INSTRUCTED IN DIET PREVIOUSLY BY:_____

TIME OF LAST P.O. INTAKE: 0700

FLUID INTAKE (AMOUNT/DAY) 5-6 glasses

WEIGHT: □ NO PROBLEMS

□ GAIN ☒ LOSS/HOW MUCH/HOW LONG 10 lbs / 1 month

☒ SKIN NORMAL □ HEALING PROBLEMS
  □ COLOR CHANGE OF SKIN
  □ SKIN LESIONS/RASH_____

3. RESPIRATION/CIRCULATION PATTERN

HISTORY OF: □ COUGH □ SPUTUM_____

□ SHORTNESS OF BREATH □ WITHOUT EXERCISE □ WITH EXERCISE

HISTORY OF: □ PACEMAKER □ RATE_____
  □ BLOOD CLOTS □ CHEST PAIN □ PEDAL EDEMA

☒ CHECK BOX IF DATA IS PERTINENT

*SEE NURSES NOTES FOR FURTHER NOTATIONS OR ANY CHANGES.

*OBJECTIVE DATA:

1. CLINICAL DATA

AGE 36 HEIGHT 5'6"

WEIGHT 122 ☒ BEDSCALE □ STANDING APPROXIMATE_____

TEMP: 98.4 PULSE: 118 RESPIRATIONS 16

BLOOD PRESSURE (RIGHT ARM) 120/68 (LEFT ARM) 122/70

☒ SITTING □ LYING

N.T./N.A. INITIALS O.B.

2. NUTRITIONAL/METABOLIC PATTERN

ORAL MUCOSA ☒ HEALTHY COLOR_____
  □ MOIST □ DRY □ LESIONS_____

TEETH: ☒ NO PROBLEM CONDITION:_____
  □ DENTURES □ UPPER □ LOWER □ PARTIAL
  □ MISSING TEETH □ CAPS/CROWNS

☒ WELL NOURISHED □ OBESE □ EMACIATED

SKIN: ☒ TURGOR NORMAL □ OTHER_____
  ☒ INTACT □ OTHER_____
  TEMP Warm COLOR brown □ DIAPHORESIS

□ TUBES_____

3. RESPIRATION/CIRCULATION PATTERN

BREATH SOUNDS Clear

LIP COLOR Pink _____ □ USE OF ACCESSORY MUSCLES

COUGH: □ NON-PRODUCTIVE □ PRODUCTIVE SPUTUM COLOR_____

APICAL RATE 120 RHYTHM: ☒ REGULAR □ IRREGULAR

ABNORMAL HEART SOUNDS NOTED No

NECK VEIN DISTENTION AT 45 DEGREES: □ PRESENT ☒ ABSENT

□ EDEMA: LOCATION_____

RIGHT DORSALIS PEDAL PULSE: ☒ STRONG □ WEAK □ ABSENT

LEFT DORSALIS PEDAL PULSE: ☒ STRONG □ WEAK □ ABSENT

CALF TENDERNESS ☒ NO □ YES □ N/A

EXTREMITIES COLOR brown _____

TEMP Warm

4. ELIMINATION PATTERN

ABDOMEN: ☒ SOFT   □ FIRM
  □ NON-TENDER   □ TENDER
  □ NON-DISTENDED □ DISTENDED _____ Girth

□ OSTOMIES/TUBES: TYPE_____

□ NORMAL BOWEL SOUNDS □ HYPOACTIVE ☒ HYPERACTIVE □ ABSENT

(Courtesy of Southeast Missouri Hospital, Cape Girardeau, Missouri.)

(continued)

Figure 12-3

Admission database sample.

Admission Database *(continued)*

*SUBJECTIVE DATA (Cont'd) LBM_____

4. ELIMINATION PATTERN

BOWEL HABITS: STOOLS/DAY **2** COLOR **dk. brown** ☒ SOFT/FORMED
     ☐ CONSTIPATION: ☐ LAXATIVE ☐ ENEMA
     ☐ DIARRHEA ☐ INCONTINENCE
BLADDER HABITS: URINATES/DAY **5-6** ☒ NO PROBLEM ☐ SELF-CATH
     ☐ URGENCY ☐ FREQUENCY ☐ NOCTURIA
     ☐ DYSURIA ☐ HEMATURIA ☐ INCONTINENCE

5. SEXUALITY/REPRODUCTIVE PATTERN (IF APPROPRIATE)

LAST MENSTRUAL PERIOD **1-10-00** MENSTRUAL PROBLEMS ☐ YES ☒ NO
BIRTH CONTROL MEASURES **None** # PREGNANCIES **2**
COMPLICATIONS OF PREGNANCIES **None**
HX VENEREAL DISEASE **No**
SEXUAL CONCERNS: **None**

6. ACTIVITY/EXERCISE PATTERN

ENERGY LEVEL: ☐ TIRES EASILY ☐ AVERAGE ☒ HIGH/ENERGY
ABLE TO: ☒ FEED SELF ☒ BATHE SELF
     ☐ BATHE/FEED SELF WITH ASSISTANCE
     ☒ AMBULATE ☒ CLIMB STAIRS
     ☒ CAN DO HOUSEHOLD CHORES
AIDS: ☐ CANE ☐ WALKER ☐ WHEELCHAIR ☐ OTHER _____
GAIT: ☐ STEADY ☐ UNSTEADY ☐ LIMP ☐ UNABLE TO WALK
PROTHESIS _____

7. SLEEP/REST PATTERN

DO YOU FEEL RESTED AFTER SLEEP? ☒ YES ☐ NO ☐ NO PROBLEM
SLEEP PROBLEMS: ☐ TROUBLE FALLING ASLEEP ☐ EARLY AM WAKING
     ☐ OTHER _____

8. COGNITIVE/PERCEPTUAL PATTERN

HEARING: ☒ NORMAL ☐ IMPAIRED ☐ LEFT EAR ☐ RIGHT EAR ☐ AID
VISION: ☐ NORMAL ☐ IMPAIRED ☒ GLASSES ☐ PROTHESIS
     ☐ FARSIGHTED ☐ NEARSIGHTED

OTHER PROBLEMS _____
COMMUNICATION: LANGUAGE SPOKEN **English**
UNDERSTANDS _____ UNABLE TO: ☐ READ ☐ WRITE
ABLE TO: ☒ READ ☒ WRITE ☐ LIP READ
COGNITION: ☒ NO PROBLEMS ☐ RECENT MEMORY CHANGE
     ☐ DIFFICULTY LEARNING
DISCOMFORT/PAIN: ☐ NO ☒ YES DESCRIBE **Epigastric**
HOW DO YOU MANAGE YOUR PAIN? **Bland food, Maalox**

9. COPING/STRESS TOLERANCE PATTERN

SPECIAL CONCERNS REGARDING HOSPITALIZATION? ☐ NO ☒ YES
Care of Children

10. SELF-PERCEPTION/SELF-CONCEPT PATTERN

CONCERNS ABOUT HOW YOUR ILLNESS AFFECTS YOU? ☐ NO ☒ YES
Concerned about health

11. ROLE/RELATIONSHIP PATTERN

MARITAL STATUS: ☐ MARRIED ☐ SINGLE ☐ WIDOWED ☒ DIVORCED
CHILDREN (#) **2** OTHER DEPENDENT(S) **0**
OCCUPATION **Secretary**
RESIDENCY (TYPE) **apartment**
WHO LIVES AT HOME WITH YOU? **Children**
SUPPORT SYSTEM (CLOSE FRIEND/FAMILY MEMBER) **Yes**
FAMILY CONCERNS ABOUT HOSPITALIZATION? **Yes**

12. VALUE/BELIEF PATTERN

RELIGIOUS AFFILIATION **Baptist**
RELIGIOUS RESTRICTIONS **∅**
☐ WOULD LIKE CHAPLAIN TO VISIT (IF YES, NOTIFY CHAPLAIN)

☒ WOULD LIKE FAMILY MINISTER TO VISIT
NAME **Mr. Ame** PHONE **314-6000**
RELIGIOUS ACTIVITIES IMPORTANT TO YOU **Bible**
SUBJECTIVE DATA SIGNATURE **P. LeHne RN** _____ (Nurse)

6. ACTIVITY/EXERCISE PATTERN

ROM: ☒ FULL ☐ OTHER _____
BALANCE AND GAIT: ☒ STEADY ☐ UNSTEADY ☐ LIMP _____
HAND GRASPS: ☒ EQUAL ☒ STRONG
     ☐ WEAKNESS/PARALYSIS ☐ RIGHT ☐ LEFT
LEG MUSCLES: ☒ EQUAL ☒ STRONG
     WEAKNESS/PARALYSIS ☐ RIGHT ☐ LEFT

8. COGNITIVE/PERCEPTUAL PATTERN

LEVEL OF CONSCIOUSNESS: ☒ ALERT ☒ RESPONDS TO PAIN
ORIENTED TO: ☒ TIME ☒ PLACE ☒ PERSON
MOOD: ☒ CALM ☐ SAD ☐ ANGRY
     ☐ WITHDRAWN ☐ OTHER _____
PUPILS: ☒ EQUAL ☒ REACTIVE ☐ OTHER _____
COGNITION: ☒ ABLE TO FOLLOW SIMPLE COMMANDS
     ☒ RESPONDS APPROPRIATELY TO QUESTIONS
     ☐ UNABLE TO FOLLOW COMMANDS
     ☐ OTHER _____
HEARING: ☒ NORMAL ☐ OTHER _____
VISION: ☒ NORMAL ☐ OTHER _____
MANIFESTATIONS OF PAIN _____

10. SELF-PERCEPTION/SELF-CONCEPT PATTERN

EYE CONTACT: ☒ APPROPRIATE ☐ DOWNCAST ☐ STARING
BODY POSTURE: ☒ RELAXED ☐ STOOPED ☐ RIGID
BEHAVIOR: 1 ②（2) 3 4 5 (CIRCLE)
     RELAXED   NERVOUS
     OTHER _____

11. ROLE/RELATIONSHIP PATTERN

BEHAVIOR: ①（1) 2 3 4 5 (CIRCLE)
     PASSIVE   ASSERTIVE   AGGRESSIVE
INTERACTION WITH FAMILY/SIGNIFICANT OTHER: ☐ N/A
☒ RELAXED ☐ TENSE ☐ ANGRY ☐ WITHDRAWN ☐ OTHER _____

COMMENTS: _____

Worried about effect of illness and possible surgery on care of children, job, and income. Has strong support of family.

SIGNATURE **P LeHne, RN** _____ (Nurse)

Figure 12-3 *(Continued)*

met. Although documentation and procedures differ depending on the institution and type of transfer, patient needs are always a priority in ensuring a smooth transition and continuity of care.

Transfer Within the Hospital Setting

Considerations for transfer within a hospital include the following:

- In some situations in which a patient moves from room to room on the same floor, the furniture (eg, bed or bedside table) is moved as well.
- The patient's personal belongings must be moved and put in the new room. Every effort must be made to ensure that belongings are not misplaced or lost.
- If the patient is moved to the ICU, it may be necessary for family members to take home personal belongings and flowers.
- The patient's chart, Kardex, care plan, and medications must be correctly labeled for the new room, and other hospital departments (eg, dietary, pharmacy, or physical therapy) must be notified.
- If the patient is transferred to another floor or to (or from) the ICU, the nurse in the original area gives a verbal report about the patient to the nurse in the new area. The report should include the patient's name, age, physicians, admitting diagnosis, surgical procedure (if applicable), current condition and manifestations, allergies, medications and treatments, laboratory data, and any special equipment that will be needed. Nursing care priorities are identified, and the existence of advance directives is noted. Accurate and complete communications are essential in ensuring continuity of care.

Transfer to a Long-Term Care Facility

Considerations for transfer to a long-term care facility include the following:

- All of the patient's belongings are carefully packed and sent to the facility with the patient. Prescriptions and appointment cards for return visits to the physician's office may also be sent with the patient.
- The patient is discharged from the hospital setting, but a copy of the chart may be sent to the long-term facility (depending on physician preference and agency protocol). The original chart, a legal document, remains at the hospital.
- In most instances, a detailed assessment and care plan is sent from the hospital to the long-term facility. In addition, the nurse at the hospital talks to the nurse at the long-term facility to ensure continuity of care.

Discharge From a Healthcare Setting

In meeting the needs of the patient being discharged from a healthcare setting, nurses consider that the person may be expecting a change from a dependent role to a more independent, self-care role. Patients are discharged from a healthcare facility when the expected outcomes of care are met and the patient or caregiver has the necessary knowledge and skills to provide self-care. Although discharge is almost always a welcome event, it also can be stressful.

Leaving the Hospital Against Medical Advice

A patient sometimes decides to leave the hospital *against medical advice* (AMA). Although the patient is legally free to do so, this choice carries a risk for increased illness or complications. A patient who decides to leave AMA must sign a form that releases the physician and healthcare institution from any legal responsibility for his or her health status. The patient is informed of any possible risk before signing the form. The patient's signature must be witnessed, and the form becomes part of the patient's record.

Discharge Planning

Planning for discharge actually begins on admission, when information about the patient is collected and documented. **Discharge planning** is a systematic process for preparing the patient to leave the healthcare setting and maintaining continuity of care. The key to successful discharge planning is an exchange of information among the patient, the caregivers, and those responsible for care both while the patient is in the healthcare setting and after the patient returns home. This coordination of care is usually the nurse's responsibility.

With earlier discharge, patients often are still acutely ill when they go home, and many require complicated treatment and care by family members. It is no longer unusual for family members to change sterile dressings, monitor intravenous medications, give complete physical care, and prepare special diets. If they are unprepared and unable to carry out these interventions correctly, the patient may have an exacerbation of the illness or experience complications that could require readmission or additional treatment. The nurse must ensure that family members are taught the necessary knowledge and skills (Fig. 12-4) and that referrals are made to such agencies as home healthcare or social services to provide support and assistance during the recovery period. Home care is discussed in Chapter 13.

Discharge planning anticipates and plans for the needs of a patient and family after discharge from a healthcare facility. The ultimate goal is the achievement of an optimal level of health. Effective discharge planning also helps ensure continuity of care in the least stressful manner. Discharge planning can occur in a number of ways, depending on the individual healthcare setting or provider. Discharge planning must be coordinated, interdisciplinary, initiated as early as possible, and carefully planned and should involve the patient along with family or significant others who are caregivers.

Initiating the process involves identifying patients who need discharge planning. All patients need discharge plan-

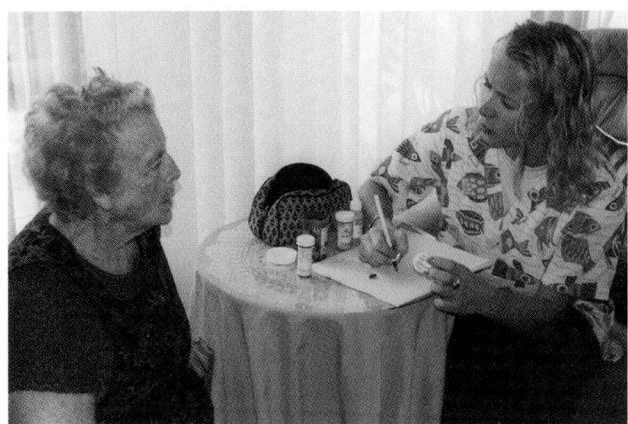

Figure 12-4
Patients or caregivers must be taught special skills, such as medication administration, diet planning, or feeding, so that they can care for themselves when nursing services are no longer provided. (Smeltzer, S. C. & Bare, B. G. [2000]. *Brunner & Suddarth's textbook of medical-surgical nursing* [9th ed., p. 42]. Philadelphia: Lippincott Williams & Wilkins.)

ning in general, but certain patients have more comprehensive needs for specific services. The nurse who conducts the initial nursing assessment is in the best position to determine these special needs. In addition to those who will be placed in a long-term care facility, patients with the following characteristics need a formal discharge plan and referral to another agency:

- Lack of knowledge of the treatment plan
- Social isolation
- Newly diagnosed chronic disease
- Major surgery
- Prolonged recuperation from major surgery or illness
- Emotional or mental instability
- Complex home care regimen
- Financial difficulties
- Lack of available or approximate referral sources
- Terminal illness

Guidelines for Discharge Planning

Discharge planning may be done over time for a patient hospitalized with a serious illness or injury, or may be completed relatively quickly for a patient treated in an ambulatory facility. A nursing case manager is often responsible for discharge planning for patients in acute care settings and may follow a plan of care or a critical path established for the patient. No matter what organizing plan is used, the nurse assesses the patient's needs and identifies problems, mutually develops goals, carries out teaching, and makes referrals (see the Discharge Planning Example later in this chapter).

Assessing and Identifying Healthcare Needs

The first step in discharge planning involves collecting and organizing data about a patient. (Assessment and inter-

viewing are covered in detail in Chaps. 15 and 25.) When assessing the patient for discharge, the nurse includes the family in the unit of care. The patient and family must both be actively involved in the discharge process if the transition from the healthcare setting to home is to be effective. Factors to assess in discharge planning are listed in the accompanying Focused Assessment Guide. Other assessment formats may be used, depending on institutional procedures, to evaluate ability to carry out activities of daily living (bathing, dressing, toileting, transfer, continence, and feeding) and instrumental activities of daily living (ability to use telephone, shop, prepare food, do housekeeping and laundry, take medications; type of transportation available). The medical record and physician orders must also be consulted for the exact medication and treatment plan before the nursing care plan is developed.

Nursing diagnoses, developed from the discharge planning assessment, recognize the needs of both the patient and the family. Examples of nursing diagnoses for a patient being discharged are listed in the accompanying box. It is important to determine whether problems are present now or are potential problems. For example, a patient with chronic respiratory problems may have assistance from a member of the family who has come to stay for 1 month, but the patient will be alone at home after that time. In this case, the problem is not an actual problem now but could become one unless planning is done to meet needs when there is no longer a family caregiver.

Mutually Setting Goals

The expected goals of the discharge plan are set mutually and must be realistic if they are to be met. When the nurse establishes goals with the patient's involvement, meeting the expected outcomes of the plan of care is more likely. Goals that are not mutually agreed on or not based on a complete assessment of the patient's needs most often result in failure of the patient to follow the plan. For example, a patient may have been taught about a special diet but does not actually follow the diet after discharge because of financial problems, lack of transportation to purchase the food items, or lack of refrigeration for food storage.

Teaching

Important teaching topics about self-care at home must be covered before discharge. These topics include the following:

Medications. The patient needs to understand the drug name, dosage, purpose, effects, times to be taken, and possible side effects. The information specific to medications should be given both verbally and in writing. It is often helpful to draw a clock face and write the names of the medications in the correct time slots.

Procedures and treatments. All steps of the procedure (eg, dressing changes) should be demonstrated, practiced, and provided in writing. The patient or caregiver should then demonstrate the procedure or treatment. Understanding the purpose of what is being done and having information about how to get supplies are important.

FOCUSED ASSESSMENT GUIDE

Discharge Planning

Factors to Assess	Questions and Approaches
Health data	Establish the following database: age; sex; height; weight; medical diagnosis; past medical history; current health problems; surgery; and functional limitations (eg, amputations, wheelchair or walker use, impaired hearing or sight).
Personal data	"How do you feel about being discharged?" (Note specifically whether patient appears anxious or frightened.) "What are your expectations for recovery?" (Unrealistic expectations require additional teaching.) "What personal coping methods do you use? Are these effective or ineffective? What language do you speak and understand?"
Caregivers	Establish who the caregivers are, and ask the following of them: "What are your expectations and fears about providing care at home? What do you believe about health and illness? Do you live with the patient?" Establish the caregivers' age, sex, relationship to the patient, past experience with this treatment or illness, and values, beliefs, and cultural practices that may affect patient care.
Environment	Assess both the home and the community: Are there barriers that will inhibit function (eg, narrow stairs if the patient requires a wheelchair)? Are there assistive devices in the bathroom? Are hot water, heat, and space needed for supplies available? Is the community rural or urban? Is healthcare accessible and readily available? Is transportation available? Are there any known hazards in the environment?
Financial and support services	Complete a financial profile, to include expenses for care after discharge (consider medications, special foods, equipment, supplies). What resources are available to assist in caring for the patient? (Consider all available resources, including Medicaid, food stamps, meal services to the home.) If the patient will be living alone, what support services are available, and how can they be obtained?

Diet. The purpose of the diet and its expected outcomes should be clearly described. Examples of written diet plans and meals are helpful. If the patient has been in the hospital, it also helpful to save menu or meal forms to use as a reference at home.

Referrals. Appointments are often made before discharge for the first visit to a physician or agency. Whether or not this is done, the patient and family members should know how to contact the providers of follow-up care and whom to call if they have questions or problems. This referral information takes into account the patient's economic situation, access to transportation, support systems, and home environment.

Health promotion. All aspects of the illness or effects of treatment should be clearly described both verbally and in written materials. Many forms of written information are available to give to patients, ranging from printed literature (eg, from the American Heart Association) to teaching materials developed by the healthcare facility. The patient should be able to talk about the anticipated physical and emotional effects of the illness and also describe what will be done to achieve the highest level of health possible.

EXAMPLES OF NANDA NURSING DIAGNOSES

Discharging From a Healthcare Setting

- Self-Care Deficit: Bathing/Hygiene related to inability to use right hand and arm secondary to right-sided weakness following a left-brain cerebrovascular accident (stroke)
- Anxiety related to uncertain outcome of treatment of cancer by chemotherapy
- Ineffective Family Coping related to lack of financial or personal support systems
- Impaired Home Maintenance Management related to limited ability to shop for food and clean the house secondary to chronic respiratory illness (emphysema)

All teaching should be documented in the patient's record and the discharge summary. Written instructions are given to the patient (Fig. 12-5). The patient's or family member's demonstrations of care procedures must be satisfactory. The patient and caregiver must have exposure to and practice with the equipment they will be using at home.

Home Care Referrals

There must be a written order by the physician for all services before a home care referral is made so that subsequent home visits are reimbursed. Patients must meet criteria for home care services to be reimbursed by Medicare and other third-party payers.

As much information as possible about the patient should be given to the home health agency. Such information includes the kind of surgery or injury, medications, the patient's physical and mental status, significant social factors (eg, frail caregiver with health problems, or no caregiver), and the family's expected needs.

Evaluating Discharge Planning Effectiveness

Evaluating the discharge plan is crucial to ensure that the discharge planning works. Planning and referrals must be scrutinized to ensure the quality and appropriateness of services. Evaluation is ongoing, and care plans may need to be changed. Further evaluation of the discharge process is usually conducted a few weeks after the patient goes home. It may be carried out by way of a telephone call, a questionnaire, or a home visit.

Discharge Planning Example

Mr. Smith is a 55-year-old married man, admitted to the hospital with a diagnosis of stroke. He now has left-side weakness and difficulty communicating verbally. He has had a history of high blood pressure for 10 years. Mr. Smith is to be discharged from the hospital in 3 days

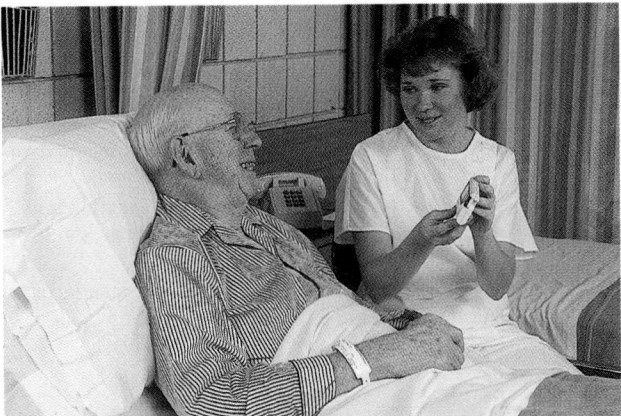

Figure 12-5
Written instructions for continuing self-care at home should be given to the patient. In addition, the nurse reviews the instructions with the patient to ensure that the patient understands. (Photo © B. Proud.)

if his blood pressure remains stable. He will be going home with four new medications and an indwelling urinary catheter.

After reviewing the medical record, the nurse interviews Mr. and Mrs. Smith. The assessment reveals that Mr. Smith is limited in his ability to transfer from bed to chair. Both Mr. and Mrs. Smith are fearful of discharge. Mr. Smith believes he will be able to return to work as an accountant in 3 weeks and hates the thought of being an invalid at his age, but Mrs. Smith thinks he'll never work again. They have never faced a life-threatening or disabling illness in the past. They have no strong cultural preferences for diet. They have two adult children who live out of state with their own families. Mrs. Smith has a younger sister who lives nearby. They are both college educated. The Smiths live in a suburban area in a two-story home with narrow stairs leading to the second floor's two baths and three bedrooms. They have adequate plumbing. Their doctor's office is about 1 mile away, and shopping is nearby.

Mrs. Smith is worried about managing care of the catheter and moving Mr. Smith in and out of bed. She needs instruction in the new medications and diet regimen. She is terrified that she may be unable to handle an emergency in the middle of the night. Financially, this two-income family has abruptly become a one-income family. Mr. Smith is not 65 years old and thus is not yet eligible for Medicare, although he does have disability insurance that will cover a portion of his salary.

How would the nurse coordinate this discharge plan? The physician must be consulted for diet, medication, other treatments, and home health orders. The dietitian needs to counsel the Smiths on a low-sodium diet and on creative ways to prepare low-salt meals. Physical therapy has already been initiated at the hospital and will continue through home health. An occupational therapist will visit to provide teaching about strengthening exercises and assistive devices, such as a walker. The social worker has been called for financial assessment to determine exactly what services the Smiths can expect to have reimbursed by their insurance plan and how they will manage their out-of-pocket expenses.

The nurse discusses Mr. and Mrs. Smith's healthcare needs with the home health agency. A teaching plan for medications and care of the urinary catheter is implemented. Mrs. Smith demonstrates how to care for the catheter. The physical therapist teaches Mrs. Smith how to transfer Mr. Smith into and out of the bed and assures her that he will help her practice at home. Written information about high blood pressure, stroke, low-salt diet, and prescribed medications are given to the Smiths, along with the telephone number of a local support group for people who have had strokes. Although Mrs. Smith still verbalizes concern about providing care at home, she says that she feels more in control now. Mr. Smith is beginning to realize that recovery may take longer than he anticipated. At the time of discharge, the nurse tells the Smiths that someone from the hospital will call them the next day and that the home health nurse will visit them that afternoon.

Learning Outcomes

After completing this chapter, the learner should be able to accomplish the following:

1. Define the key terms used in the chapter.
   ambulatory facilities   discharge planning
   continuity of care
2. Describe the role of the nurse in ensuring continuity of care between and among healthcare settings.
3. Discuss considerations for establishing an effective nurse–patient relationship when admitting a patient to a healthcare setting.

4. Compare and contrast admission of a patient to an ambulatory care setting and a hospital setting.
5. Discuss transfer of patients within and among healthcare settings.
6. Describe the components of discharge planning for providing continuity of care.

Critical Thinking Exercises

1. Interview a classmate or family member who has been admitted to a hospital. What were their concerns on admission? How did those concerns differ from those experienced on discharge?
2. Compare and contrast the needs of the following patients and their families:
   * A 2-year-old is admitted to an ambulatory surgery center to have minor surgery.

* A 34-year-old woman is discharged to her home following treatment for a fractured arm in the emergency room.
* A 50-year-old woman is returning to a clinic to learn the results of a mammogram.
* A 78-year-old man is transferred from the hospital to a nursing home.

Bibliography

Beddar, S., & Aikin, J. (1994). Continuity of care: A challenge for ambulatory oncology nursing. *Seminars in Oncology Nursing, 10*(4), 254–263.

Bulachek, G. M., & McCloskey, J. C. (1999). *Nursing interventions: Effective nursing treatments* (3rd ed.). Philadelphia: W. B. Saunders.

Carpenito, L. J. (1997). *Nursing diagnosis: Application to clinical practice* (7th ed.). Philadelphia: Lippincott-Raven.

Castro, J., Anderson, M., Hanson, K., & Helms, L. (1998). Home care referral after emergency department discharge. *Journal of Emergency Nursing, 24*(2), 127–132.

Clare, J., & Hofmeyer, A. (1998). Discharge planning and continuity of care for aged people: Indicators of satisfaction and implications for practice. *Australian Journal of Advanced Nursing, 16*(1), 7–13.

Clemen-Stone, S., McGuire, S., & Eigsti, D. (1998). *Comprehensive community health nursing: Family, aggregate & community practice.* St. Louis: C. V. Mosby.

Costello, M., & Todd-Magel, C. (1997). Bridging the gap: Hospital to home nutrition support. *MEDSURG Nursing, 6*(6), 328–337.

Green, K., & Lydon, S. (1998). The continuum of patient care. *American Journal of Nursing, 98*(10), 16BBB–16DDD.

Holzemer, S. P. (1998). Problems in providing continuity of care in a multitiered health care system. In M. Klainberg, S. Holzemer, M. Leonard, & J. Arnold. *Community health nursing: An alliance for health.* (pp. 285–298). New York: McGraw-Hill.

Joel, L. (1997). Moving the care site from hospital to home: Whose turf? In J. McCloskey & H. Grace. *Current issues in nursing* (5th ed.). (pp. 209–215). St. Louis: C. V. Mosby.

Keenan, G., & Aquilino, M. (1998). Standardized nomenclatures: Keys to continuity of care, nursing accountability and nursing effectiveness. *Outcomes Management for Nursing Practice, 2*(2), 81–86.

Mainous, A., & Gill, J. (1998). The importance of continuity of care in the likelihood of future hospitalization. *American Journal of Public Health, 88*(10), 1539–1541.

McGuire, S., Gerber, D., & Clemen-Stone, S. (1996). Meeting the diverse needs of clients in the community: Effective use of the referral process. *Nursing Outlook, 44*(5), 218–222.

McIntosh, J., & Worley, N. (1994). Beyond discharge: Telephone follow-up and aftercare. *Journal of Psychosocial Nursing & Mental Health Services, 32*(10), 21–27.

Minnid, A. (1997). Key issues in building a continuum of care. *Nursing Administration Quarterly, 21*(4), 41–46.

Ribka, J. (1998). Building systems to measure continuity of care. *Nursing Case Management, 3*(4), 151–154.

Rosswurm, M., & Sherwen, L. (1998). Discharge planning for elderly patients. *Journal of Gerontological Nursing, 24*(5), 14–21.

Welch, C., & Ludwig-Beymer, P. (1998). Shortened lengths of stay: Ensuring continuity of care for mothers and babies. *Lippincott's Primary Care Practice, 2*(3), 284–291.

Chapter 13
Home Healthcare

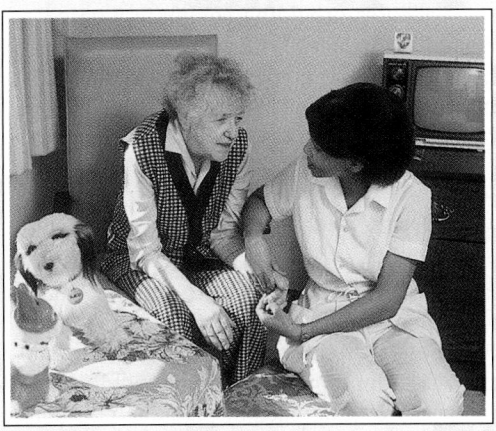

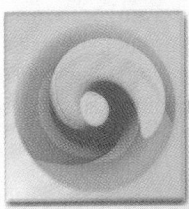

**Thinking Critically About
Nursing's Blended Skills**

Before reading this chapter, think about the types of skills you will need to meet the needs of patients and families in home healthcare settings.

- You are visiting Mrs. Cobbs to determine her need for home health nursing. She delivered twins by cesarean section last week and has been ordered to remain on bed rest for 6 weeks. One twin came home with her and the other requires surgery on his heart and is still in the neonatal intensive care unit. The Cobbs have two other children who are 2 and 3½ years of age.

- Mr. Califano, a widow who lives alone, is a patient you visit weekly. An elderly diabetic with high blood pressure and renal disease, he presents numerous nursing challenges to you.

- This is your first visit to the Flemings. Mrs. Flemings' mother has just been discharged from the hospital after treatment for a stroke, which left her unable to move on one side. Unable to return to her home, she is moving in with her daughter and family. You are to assess their need for care.

- Jane Friel is a single woman with end-stage breast cancer. She lives with a friend who provides most of her care. You are Jane's hospice nurse and visit weekly unless complications require additional visits.

What cognitive, technical, interpersonal, and ethical/legal skills do you think you will need to respond effectively to the home healthcare nursing challenges described above?

Many changes are occurring in the healthcare system and in the settings in which nurses provide care. One of these changes has been the shift from hospital-based settings to community-based home care. Home care has experienced an unprecedented rate of growth. The cost-saving methods of managed care have had a major effect on the move from hospital to home care, and this trend is expected to continue. Home care is one of the fastest growing areas of healthcare today, with the National Association for Home Care (1999) estimating that 8 million people receive home care services provided by more than 660,000 healthcare providers.

Facilities providing community-based care were discussed in Chapter 11; this chapter focuses on the care given by nurses in the home. This chapter explains what home healthcare is and how nurses provide care in the patient's home.

What is Home Healthcare?

Home healthcare is care provided in a patient's place of residence, which may include private homes, apartments, homeless shelters, boarding homes, dormitories, nursing homes, group homes, and older adult housing. It encompasses care to all ages of patients with both chronic and acute healthcare needs.

When providing home healthcare, nurses integrate community health principles focusing on environmental, socioeconomic, cultural, and personal health factors that affect the individual's and family's health. The essential components of home healthcare are the patient, the family, healthcare professionals from various disciplines, and the goals of helping the patient reach maximum independence and health status. The role of each member of the healthcare team is outlined in Table 13-1.

Care of the patient in the home is different from care of hospital patients, who conform to hospital routine and the hospital's schedule for eating, bathing, taking medications, and visiting with their families. Home care nursing is unique because when the nurse crosses the threshold of the patient's home, care must be adapted to the patient's schedules, customs, and needs. The hallmark of a home care nurse is the ability to blend clinical skills with flexibility to provide quality patient care.

The History of Home Care Nursing

The late 1800s brought a large influx of immigrants into America and a rapid population growth in most cities. Home nursing agencies emerged in New York, Boston, and Philadelphia to meet the health needs of the residents in these areas. Lillian Wald and Mary Brewster opened the Henry Street Settlement House in New York City in 1893. Visiting nurses from this agency cared for poor residents living in tenements. Eventually, these providers of home care became known as Visiting Nurse Associations (VNAs), which focused on providing personal care to the sick and health teaching to families.

Before World War II, physicians often made home care visits to treat the sick. During the war, there was a physician shift in practice from the home to the hospital and office setting. Nurses began to provide most of the home care visits during this time (Mundinger, 1983). VNAs were developed in most major urban areas throughout the country. Hospital-based home care agencies also developed as hospitals looked for ways to expand services to their communities.

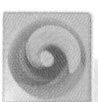

COGNITIVE SKILLS

- Knowledge of how to provide postpartal nursing care; infant care; nursing care related to diabetes, high blood pressure, and renal disease; poststroke care; and care of a terminally ill patient with breast cancer, all in the home
- Knowledge of how to coordinate the home care patients receive, drawing on family caregivers, visiting nurse assistants, and other resources
- Knowledge of the resources available within the community to meet the needs of homebound patients

TECHNICAL SKILLS

- Ability to provide the technical nursing assistance necessary to meet the nursing needs of homebound patients and their family caregivers

INTERPERSONAL SKILLS

- Ability to establish trusting professional relationships with homebound patients, their family caregivers, and others within the community
- Ability to demonstrate professional care and compassion for homebound patients and their caregivers

ETHICAL/LEGAL SKILLS

- Commitment to providing safe and quality care in home settings
- Ability to practice in an ethically and legally defensible manner in home settings
- Knowledge of the ethical and legal obligations related to caring for patients who are terminally ill

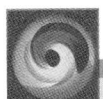

Table 13-1
Collaborative Roles of Members of the Home Healthcare Team

Member	Role
Physician	Certifies that the patient has a health problem to receive home healthcare. Prescribes and certifies a plan of care for treatment for the patient receiving home healthcare.
Nurse	Provides direct care to patients and families. Teaches patient and family self-care. Conducts research to ensure cost-effectiveness and quality of care. May be administrator of home health agency and serve as consultant to staff. Coordinates services of other healthcare providers.
Physical therapist	Provides direct care, such as muscle-strengthening exercises, gait training, and massage. Teaches patient and family to promote self-care.
Occupational therapist	Evaluates the patient's functional level and teaching activities to promote self-care in activities of daily living. Assesses the home for safety and provides adaptive equipment as necessary.
Speech pathologist	Provides direct care services to patients with speech, language, or hearing needs. Teaches patient and family to facilitate speech and language ability as well as eating and swallowing.
Social worker	Assists patient and family in dealing with the social, emotional, and environmental factors that affect their well-being. Makes referrals to appropriate community resources. Provides assistance with securing equipment and supplies, and with healthcare finances.
Home health aide	Implements the plan of care designed by the nurse. Assists patients with hygiene. May carry out light housekeeping.

Home care services expanded to include the older population in the mid-1960s. The 1965 Social Security Act provided program coverage for home healthcare to older adults participating in Medicare. Not long after, Medicaid home health benefits were initiated. The Medicare and Medicaid programs, discussed in Chapter 11, provide the structure for most home health agencies today.

There are many reasons for the increase in home care. As the American population continues to age, home care services are increasing and expanding for the growing population older than 65 years of age. The introduction of diagnosis-related groups (DRGs) in hospitals led to an earlier discharge from the hospital than in the past. Many discharged patients still need skilled professional care after they return home. Additionally, third-party payers have sought an effective way to reduce the escalating costs of healthcare through use of managed care programs that include a focus on home care.

Nursing and Home Healthcare

Before the late 1980s, home care nurses were considered generalists. Recently, many home care nurses have specialized in advanced practice skills to meet the growing demands encountered in caring for acutely ill patients at home. These specialties include enterostomal therapy, cardiac care, mental healthcare, and maternal and child healthcare (Fig. 13-1). Specialized nursing knowledge and skills, combined with sophisticated technology, means that many patients with acute and chronic healthcare needs can be treated safely and effectively in the home.

The nursing profession has its roots in home care, although in the past several decades, most nursing practice took place in hospitals. As the home care industry continues to grow, nursing practice is coming full circle and moving back to the home.

The Unique Role of the Home Care Nurse

Home care nursing is unique in that the care is provided in a setting that is unfamiliar to the nurse but familiar and comfortable to the patient. For most people, the home is a place of safety and security, having meaning and given value because of ownership, family relationships and

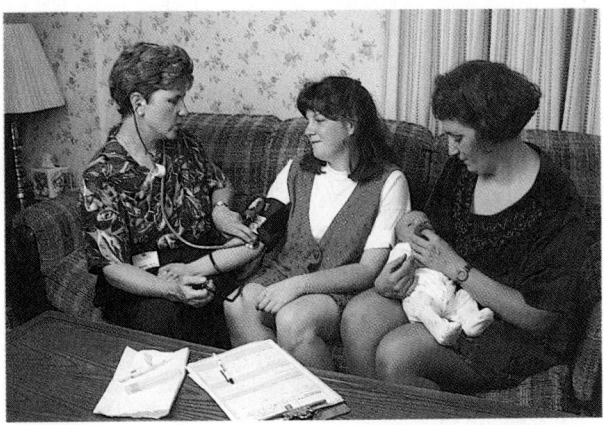

Figure 13-1
The nurse providing care in the home integrates knowledge and skills to implement family-centered specialized care.

memories, independence, and protection. Home care is provided to the patient in a setting that is controlled by the patient and family. Instead of the patient coming to the nurse, the nurse goes to the patient. Patients or their caregivers must give permission for the nurse to enter the practice setting because the nurse is a guest in their home. The nurse cannot regulate the setting where care is provided but rather must adapt to the patient's environment instead of the patient adapting to the hospital environment.

Characteristics of the Home Care Nurse

Nurses choose to practice home health nursing for various reasons. Many nurses enjoy practicing in an autonomous setting where they can use their expertise in an expanded role. Others enjoy managing their time independently and the satisfaction they derive from patients welcoming them into their home and life. Home care nurses find satisfaction in networking with other community agencies to provide individualized care. Home health nursing provides a channel through which nurses can be creative in their delivery of care.

Knowledge and Skill

Nurses who provide care in the home must be knowledgeable and skilled. Effective communication is essential, and clinical skills are important (Fig. 13-2). Physical assessment skills are necessary to identify positive and negative changes in a patient's healthcare status. Procedures such as administering intravenous fluids, changing complex wound dressings, caring for ostomies, and providing ventilator care are often required. Practicing home health nurses have identified the following areas of knowledge as most important in home care: legal regulations, physical assessment, body mechanics, nursing diagnoses, and infection control.

Independence

Nurses providing care in the home make independent decisions and assume responsibility for decision making. Home care nurses are generally alone when providing care, and consultation with other professionals is not readily available. There is no one to turn to and ask, "What does this look like to you?" Therefore, the nurse must be able to make decisions independently about the patient's care. A combination of a sound theoretical foundation, clinical skills, and creative problem solving enables the nurse to make appropriate decisions related to patient care.

Accountability

Accountability is another important characteristic of home health nurses. In a hospital, the nurse generally works a shift and reports to the next shift nurse, who then continues to care for the patient. The home care nurse generally does not have a next shift to report to but must rely on family or other caregivers to continue the care. If there is no caregiver in the home, the nurse returns to face the same issues at the next visit. The nurse is accountable to the patient, the family, and the primary healthcare provider. This increased autonomy may increase the nurse's legal risk (legal issues are discussed in Chap. 7). Home care nurses must consider such questions as the following:

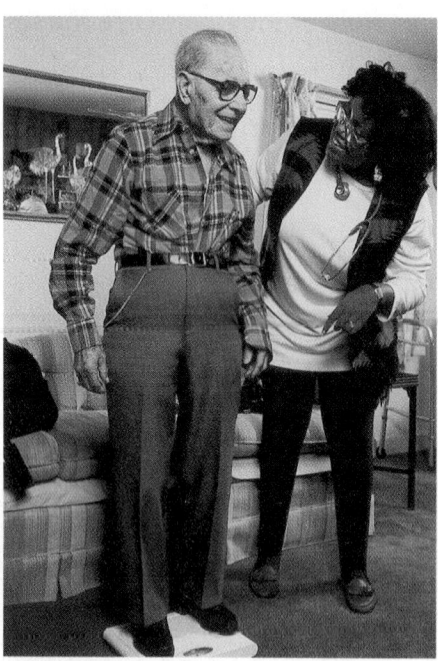
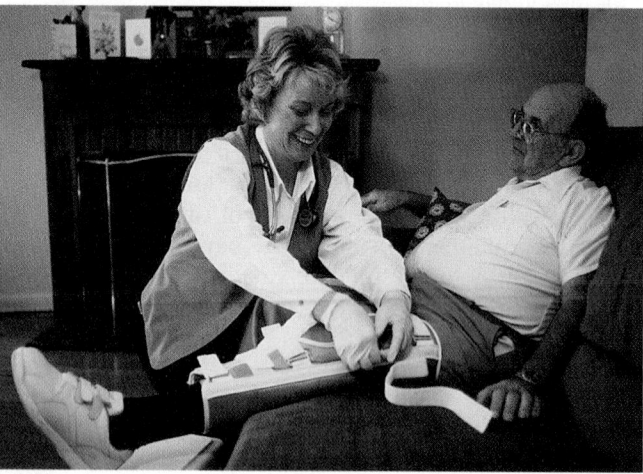

Figure 13-2
Home health nurses combine effective communication skills with a sound clinical knowledge base when caring for patients.

- Whom do I call if the patient's physician is not available?
- What should I do if a family member becomes acutely ill?
- How do I learn to perform advanced procedures?
- How do I document the patient's decisions about treatment?
- How do I ensure that other providers know about and document the plan of care?

Roles of the Home Care Nurse

In addition to having the skills necessary as a caregiver, the nurse providing care in the home is a patient advocate, coordinator of services, and patient and family educator. These roles are briefly described here; further information is found in Unit V.

Patient Advocate

Advocacy—the protection and support of another's rights—is an important role of the home health nurse. Patients may need help negotiating through the complex healthcare system or handling insurance problems or state and federal regulations affecting their care and their living environment. For example, the nurse may have to convince the patient's insurance carrier of the need for continued home health services. Patients may need help understanding complex billing issues related to their care. Home care nurses can often mobilize services needed to improve the patient's living environment. The nurse plays an advocacy role when communicating with the patient's primary healthcare provider. The physician may not be aware of the home environment and may order a treatment that cannot be accomplished in this patient's home setting. Communicating the patient's needs to the physician enables the nurse to implement appropriate treatments that fit into the patient's lifestyle.

Coordinator of Services

The home care nurse is generally the coordinator of all other healthcare providers visiting the patient, including physical therapists, occupational therapists, speech therapists, medical social workers, and home health aides. The nurse is the primary source of communication and coordination of the patient's care with the primary healthcare provider. The nurse must use effective communication skills with other healthcare providers while coordinating services for the patient. The sample forms shown in Figures 13-3 and 13-4 exemplify how the home healthcare nurse coordinates services among other healthcare providers and teaches a patient's spouse to assist in care.

The home care nurse is also responsible for coordinating community resources needed by the patient. A sound knowledge of community resources and disciplines enables the nurse to provide comprehensive services to the patient. For example, the nurse must understand the role of a social worker or physical therapist to determine a need for these services. Community resources, such as Meals on Wheels, the American Cancer Society, services for patients who are visually or hearing impaired, and local services for the aging, may be used. As the coordinator of care, the nurse directs the various services toward a common goal of improving the patient's health and promoting independence.

Educator

Nurses providing home care find that most of their time is spent teaching patients and families about the disease process, nutrition, medications, or treatment and care of wounds. The nurse identifies learning needs and, with the patient and family, mutually develops goals for teaching information necessary to promote wellness.

The nurse provides the information necessary to keep the patient safe until the next visit, using what methods work best in the home. The goal is to facilitate patients' and caregivers' ability to care for themselves. The teaching and learning process is fully described in Chapter 22.

The Home Visit

As described by Stulginsky (1993), "few families understand why people are sent home from the hospital 'still sick.' Even fewer understand what home care is. All they know is that the nurse is coming to help" (p. 477). Home care patients often feel frightened, in pain, and abandoned. Family members face the challenges of handling equipment, providing care that is totally unlike anything they have ever done for a loved one, and dealing with unfamiliar and often terrifying sounds, odors, and substances. Even family members who are themselves nurses may find providing care at home very different from providing care to others in the hospital. The accompanying box, Through the Eyes of the Family Caregiver, describes one such experience.

The Preentry Phase of the Home Visit

In the referral process, the home care agency is contacted by the physician or discharge planner of a hospital, and a brief past medical history is obtained, along with indications for home health services. The referral nurse at the home care agency collects as much information as possible about the patient's diagnoses, past surgical experience, socioeconomic status, and treatments ordered. This phase of the home care visit is called the **preentry phase**. The home health nurse is assigned the case, reviews the information, and calls the patient to make an initial contact and schedule the visit. During this conversation, the nurse can gather information to determine whether the patient's caregivers can answer questions related to their needs. It may be possible to determine the patient's cognitive abilities, orientation, and caregiver status through this conversation. All information is important to the nurse as the first visit is planned. The home care nurse must develop a trusting

HOME HEALTH CERTIFICATION AND PLAN OF TREATMENT

. Patient's HI Claim No.	2. Start Of Care Date	3. Certification Period		4. Medical Record No.	5. Provider No.
777-88-7788A	100300	From: 100300	To: 120300	S2521	78-9999

. Patient's Name and Address	7. Provider's Name, Address and Telephone Number
Smythe, Samuel A. 25952 North Hawthorne Lane Sky City, WI 50000	BHC Home Care 2001 Oak Lane Sky City, WI 50000

8. Date of Birth 021719	9. Sex ☒ M ☐ F

1. ICD-9-CM	Principal Diagnosis	Date
890.1	Open wound, left hip	100100

2. ICD-9-CM	Surgical Procedure	Date
79.35	Open reduction, left femur	092700

3. ICD-9-CM	Other Pertinent Diagnoses	Date
820.9	Fracture, left femur	092600
428.0	Congestive heart failure	090500
715.09	Osteoarthritis	030000
250.00	NIDDM	010094

10. Medications: Dose/Frequency/Route (N)ew (C)hanged

Cephradine 250 mg. Q 6 hrs. PO x 21 days
    DC p̄ 10 AM dose 102400 (N)
Tolectin 400 mg. TID (C)
Furosemide 20 mg. Q AM PO (C)
KCl 10 mEq. Q AM PO
Digoxin 0.125 mg. Q AM PO
Vitamin-mineral supplement 1 cap. QD PO
Acetaminophen tabs. 2 Q 4 hrs. PRN PO - pain

4. DME and Supplies	Wheelchair, walker

15. Safety Measures: Proper footwear, clear pathways when ambulating. O₂ precautions.

6. Nutritional Req.	1800 calorie ADA, 2 gm. Na

17. Allergies: No known allergies

8.A. Functional Limitations

1 ☐ Amputation	5 ☐ Paralysis	9 ☐ Legally Blind
2 ☐ Bowel /Bladder (Incontinence)	6 ☒ Endurance	A ☐ Dyspnea With Minimal Exertion
3 ☐ Contracture	7 ☒ Ambulation	B ☒ Other (Specify)
4 ☐ Hearing	8 ☐ Speech	Occasional orthopnea

18.B. Activities Permitted

1 ☐ Complete Bedrest	6 ☐ Partial Weight Bearing	A ☒ Wheelchair
2 ☐ Bedrest BRP	7 ☐ Independent At Home	B ☒ Walker
3 ☐ Up As Tolerated	8 ☐ Crutches	C ☐ No Restrictions
4 ☒ Transfer Bed/Chair	9 ☐ Cane	D ☐ Other (Specify)
5 ☒ Exercises Prescribed		

9. Mental Status:	1 ☒ Oriented	3 ☐ Forgetful	5 ☐ Disoriented	7 ☐ Agitated
	2 ☐ Comatose	4 ☐ Depressed	6 ☐ Lethargic	8 ☐ Other

0. Prognosis:	1 ☐ Poor	2 ☐ Guarded	3 ☒ Fair	4 ☐ Good	5 ☐ Excellent

1. Orders for Discipline and Treatments (Specify Amount/Frequency/Duration)

Wound care (L) hip daily: Irrigate with 1:1 H₂O₂/water, rinse with normal saline, pack with saline-soaked 4x4s, dress with gauze. O₂ 2L PRN HS per cannula - orthopnea.

Skilled Nursing: Daily for 62 days. Assess wound, S/S fluid retention. Perform wound care. Teach diet, O₂ precautions; new/changed medications.

Physical Therapy: One visit first week, 3 times a week for 8 weeks. Evaluation, therapeutic exercises, gait training. Teach use of walker, transfer technique. Establish home program.

Home Health Aide: 3 times a week for 9 weeks. Personal care. Assist with transfers, home exercise program.

2. Goals/Rehabilitation Potential/Discharge Plans

Anticipate daily visits to end 010301. Rehab potential good for patient to ambulate independently with walker by 120300. Will be compliant with diet, medications, therapeutic regimen. Plan discharge to care of wife when wound complications resolved.

3. Nurse's Signature and Date of Verbal SOC Where Applicable: *Jane Jayes* RN 100300	25. Date HHA Received Signed POT OCT 13 2000

4. Physician's Name and Address Albert Richard, MD 1641 Pine Circle Sky City, WI 50000	26. I certify/recertify that this patient is confined to his/her home and needs intermittent skilled nursing care, physical therapy and/or speech therapy or continues to need occupational therapy. The patient is under my care, and I have authorized the services on this plan of care and will periodically review the plan.

7. Attending Physician's Signature and Date Signed *Albert Richard* MD 10/10/00	28. Anyone who misrepresents, falsifies, or conceals essential information required for payment of Federal funds may be subject to fine, imprisonment, or civil penalty under applicable Federal laws.

Form HCFA-485 (U-4) (02-94)

(Sample data © 1995 Beacon Health Corporation, Mequon WI. Used with permission.)

Figure 13-3
Example of home health plan of care.

relationship with the patient and family during the first introductory visits.

Supplies needed for the patient are gathered in the preentry phase. The nurse organizes wound care products, dressings, and educational materials to take on the first visit. The home care nurse uses a field chart to document the assessment and care provided to the patient. This chart accompanies the nurse on subsequent visits.

The nurse should evaluate safety issues before making the first home visit. Evaluating the safety of the area

SKILLED NURSING VISIT NOTE

Patient _____ Samuel Smythe _____

DATE 061300   TIME 11:00-11:45

VISIT FREQUENCY   Daily
☐ Change   ☐ Patient informed

BP 140/86 Standing (Sitting) Lying

TEMPERATURE   98.2°

PULSE 80, regular (Apical) Radial

RESPIRATIONS 26

LUNG SOUNDS Clear

DIET/ APPETITE   1800 cal.
Taught fiber sources.

ACTIVITY LEVEL Weak. Transfers with 1.

AIDE SUPERVISION   Observed
K. Jackson

PHYSICIAN CONTACT/APPT.   Appt. 061500

CARE COORDINATION   Reviewed PT program
with aide.

CONFERENCE

☐ PROGRESS NOTE

No S/S fluid retention. Wound measures
9x5x3 cm. Small amount of purulent drainage.
Wound bed 70% slough, 30% granulation tissue.
Wound care performed: irrigated with normal
saline, packed with wet to dry 4x4s, covered
with ABD. Surrounding skin intact. Expresses
discomfort during procedure. Taught use of
pain med 1 hr. before procedure. Reports
occasional constipation. Observed aide
transfer patient. Uses safe technique.
Patient satisfied with care. Can demonstrate
exercises but reluctant to do alone. Taught
wife how to assist.

SIGNATURE *Susan Jackson RN*

SKILLED NURSING VISIT NOTE

Patient _____ Samuel Smythe _____

DATE 091900   TIME 7:30-8:20

VISIT FREQUENCY Weekly. Aide dc'd 0913
☐ Change   ☒ Patient informed

BP 132/76 Standing (Sitting) Lying

TEMPERATURE   97.6°

PULSE 70, regular (Apical) Radial

RESPIRATIONS 22

LUNG SOUNDS Clear

DIET/ APPETITE   1800 cal. ADA
"Good appetite"

ACTIVITY LEVEL Ambulates 30' - walker
No longer uses wheelchair.

AIDE SUPERVISION

PHYSICIAN CONTACT/APPT.   Appt. 092300

CARE COORDINATION

CONFERENCE

☒ PROGRESS NOTE 090500-091900

Venipuncture for FBS - (L) antecubital.
Verbalizes routine for blood, urine
testing. Still has difficult performing
finger stick. Does not get enough blood on
strip for accurate reading. Demonstrated
procedure for finger stick. Using (R) side
abdomen for all injections. Taught need to
rotate sites. Developed rotation schedule.

Change in insulin dose on 0919; blood
sugar 175-225. SN taught insulin
administration. Feeling more comfortable
about performing care.

SIGNATURE *Susan Jackson RN*

Sample data © 1995 Beacon Health Corporation.
Used with Permission.

Figure 13-4
Example of home health nursing progress note.

where the patient lives is important. The nurse may need to arrange the visit so that it is at a time when it is safe to be in that area. The nurse should always know the exact destination before arriving for the visit. In some unsafe areas, the nurse may be accompanied by police or security officers. Other guidelines for safety include using a cellular phone programmed with emergency numbers, making sure someone from the agency knows your itinerary, and being continuously alert to the environment.

The Entry Phase of the Home Visit

The second phase of the visit is the **entry phase**. In the entry phase, the nurse develops rapport with the patient and family, mutually determines desired outcomes, makes assessments, plans and implements prescribed care, and provides teaching. The nurse must remember that he or she is a guest in the patient's home and is offering services that the patient may accept or reject. Important considerations

Through the Eyes of the Family Caregiver

"I'm So Glad to Have You Home, But What Do I Do Now?" (and this is just the first day. . . .)

I am a nurse, and have been a nurse for 30 years. I have a diploma in nursing, a baccalaureate in nursing, a master's in counseling, and a doctorate in nursing. I have taught others how to be nurses for more than 25 years. Nothing in all my educational and practice experiences prepared me to care for the complex needs of my husband, Jacque, when he had surgery 2 years ago. Following diagnosis of metastatic thyroid cancer, a large lower thoracic spinal cord tumor (which put pressure on the spinal nerves, causing leg weakness and bladder malfunction) and the thyroid gland were removed surgically, and steel rods were implanted almost the entire length of the spine. After 30 days in the hospital for diagnosis, surgery, and recovery, Jacque came home—unable to do more than move from the bed to a chair, and with a catheter in his bladder that was attached to a drainage bag.

Before he came home, I got a hospital bed with electric controls, a bedside commode, and a bedside table. I cleared out the family room furniture, got a friend to put the television up on a table (so it could be seen from the hospital bed), and thought I was all ready to give my husband expert care. The first challenge came when he got up in a chair to eat his dinner—we had no chairs with a high enough seat or a straight enough back to allow use of the bedside table. I ran up and down stairs to look at chairs, and finally decided the antique arm chair in the living room would work, and it did. Now another problem— where to hang the catheter drainage bag? And how best to move so it didn't pull when he moved? And remember to empty the bag before he gets up!

I fixed a wonderful homecoming meal for this man I love, and he could only eat a few bites. Now back to bed and a new problem. He got out of the bed and into the chair just fine, but now he can't get out of the chair and into the bed because his legs are still so weak. What did I do wrong—it worked in the hospital. It took me 2 days to realize that I forgot to lower the bed height so Jacque wouldn't have to push up so hard to get his bottom on the bed.

Then, after finally literally hauling him back in bed, I realized that I did not know how to move him up in bed. The physical therapist had taught him how to get up in a chair, but not how to move himself up in bed (they always did it for him in the hospital). This is a 250-pound man we are talking about. I could turn him from side to side, but I couldn't physically move him up in bed and he couldn't stay where he was. After a lot of trials, we figured out that he could wiggle one side of his body at a time and slowly inch up in bed. Now he was exhausted and in pain, and I felt totally incompetent. Thank goodness the home health nurse is coming to visit tomorrow.

If I felt this way, how must family members feel who know nothing about caring for someone who is sick or in pain? I have such respect for all those family members who provide such wonderful care and for the nurses who provide home care that calms the fears and answers the questions.

—Priscilla LeMone

---

include negotiating and honoring visit times, establishing rapport with the patient and family, defining what nursing care will be provided, and teaching to promote independence in self-care. Examples of nursing diagnoses are found in the accompanying box.

The nurse must gain the trust of the patient and family and must recognize and respect their values. Acceptance of the patient's living conditions is necessary even when they differ from the nurse's. The nurse must ask permission before using the patient's home for activities such as handwashing. The nurse often nurse believes the furniture in the patient's home or sick room needs to be rearranged to be more accessible to equipment and to remove safety hazards. The patient should give permission before any changes are made.

Controlling Infection

The home care nurse practices infection control techniques to prevent the spread of infection from one patient's home to another's. Home care nurses carry routine equipment in a bag and use appropriate bag technique to prevent the spread of infection, including the following:

- The nurse's hands are washed each time before reaching into the bag for supplies.
- Anything that the nurse takes out of the bag is cleaned before returning it to the bag.
- The bag should be placed on a liner when it is set down in the patient's home.

Hands must be washed before and after treating the patient. Nurses use Centers for Disease Control and Prevention standard precautions during home care visits, including wearing gloves when contacting blood, body fluids, secretions, excretions, and contaminated items. Clean gloves should be put on just before touching areas of broken skin or mucous membranes.

Identifying Healthcare Needs

The ability to assess patients accurately is an important skill for home care nurses. Most of the initial assessment takes

EXAMPLES OF NANDA NURSING DIAGNOSES

Home Healthcare

The following nursing diagnoses are examples of those that might be appropriate for the patient in the home setting:

- Risk for Infection related to large draining wound and lack of clean living environment
- Constipation related to lack of bulk in diet and immobility
- Risk for Injury related to weakness and cluttered home environment
- Risk for Impaired Skin Integrity related to inability to move self in bed
- Impaired Social Interaction related to inability to take part in family and community celebrations
- Altered Family Processes related to chronic illness of head of the family

- Caregiver Role Strain related to complex health needs
- Spiritual Distress related to inaccessibility of traditional folk medicine practitioner
- Ineffective Individual Management of Therapeutic Regimen related to living alone and having limited income
- Impaired Physical Mobility related to paralysis after automobile accident
- Impaired Home Maintenance Management related to fatigue and pain
- Knowledge Deficit related to availability of community resources
- Anxiety related to care of complex medical regimen at home

place during the first home visit. Ongoing assessment occurs during subsequent visits, using various skills to collect the data needed. The nurse must be skilled not only in physical assessment but also in psychological, socioeconomic, environmental, spiritual, and cultural assessment. Providing culture-sensitive care (see Chap. 3) is even more important in the patient's home. Factors to consider include the following:

- What are the roles and responsibilities of family members? Who makes the decisions?
- What type of personal space is customary?
- How are important events celebrated?
- Are there cultural or ethnic influences on the family's usual diet?
- What cultural beliefs and taboos are followed?
- What do the patient and family believe to be the cause of this illness? The treatment of this illness?
- Are traditional medical practices followed?

The family caregivers are also considered, taking into account the various roles that each family member plays and how they contribute to the patient's health status. The nurse determines whether the patient and family understand and are agreeable with the plan of care. It is important to determine if the caregivers can understand the instructions provided and are capable of providing care. The nurse must assess the family unit overall and how the patient fits into this unit.

Home care nurses must decide whether there are any potential problems related to the family's income, lifestyle, cleanliness, or interactions. For example, the nurse may note that there is no food in the refrigerator or in the kitchen cupboards. A referral for services such as Meals on Wheels may be necessary to provide adequate nutrition for the patient. Home care nurses frequently encounter safety hazards, such as throw rugs or clutter that could easily

cause falls. Other hazards may include those related to infection control, such as an unclean home with rodent or insect infestations or a lack of running water. The nurse may determine that caregivers have an alcohol or drug problem that impairs their ability to care for the patient. Any such element is taken into consideration if it could interfere with the patient's health and safety.

Teaching the Patient and Caregivers

Because home care is meant to be short-term and intermittent, the nurse includes the family and friends in the teaching process so that they can learn how to care for the patient after the nurse's home care is no longer needed. Teaching is designed and implemented based on the following considerations:

- Teaching is geared to the patient's and caregiver's readiness to learn and is adapted to the patient's physical and emotional status.
- Major problem areas are identified, with a focus on information that is essential to keep the patient safe until the nurse's next home visit.
- Teaching is adapted to what works best in the home.
- Incentives for learning include knowing the serious consequences as well as positive benefits of carrying through with certain behaviors (Stulginsky, 1993).

Documenting Care Given in the Home

Documenting care given in the home is a critical element, mandated by regulatory and federal agencies. (Documentation is discussed in Chap. 20). Documentation may be on preprinted forms or checklists or may be by computer entry.

The documented plan of care, visit plan, and progress notes (described later) are routinely used by regulatory agencies and payer sources (such as private insurance or Medicare) to determine if various state and federal regulations are being met and if payment is warranted (Johnson,

Smith-Temple, & Carr, 1998). Figures 13-3 and 13-4 illustrate such documentation.

The initial visit is the time for assessing healthcare needs and establishing a plan of care, with schedule of visits, including all necessary information to meet agency policy, regulatory requirements, and payer source (such as Medicare) needs. The plan of care accurately reflects the condition of the patient, the need for skilled care, specific physician orders, anticipated progress, criteria for discharge, supplies needed, visit schedule for all healthcare providers, and support systems available. Other information included on the plan of care are the patient's functional limitations and safety needs. Specific measurable goals are established and a time frame for reaching the goals specified.

Progress notes are made to document each visit made by the nurse. These notes must accurately describe the patient's condition, the skilled care provided, the patient's response, the patient's progress toward discharge, and an ongoing plan for continued care. They also include the nurse's plan for the next visit. Each progress note must indicate that the care provided requires the knowledge and skills of a professional nurse.

The Needs of Caregivers in the Home

Traditionally, when a patient enters the hospital, the family plays a minor role in actual care. Families and friends visit with the patient and sometimes stay overnight, but they are generally not involved in the direct care of the patient. Hospital staff provide personal care for the patient and administer medications and treatments. After the patient is discharged, the responsibility for care is shifted to family caregivers, who may or may not be physically or mentally able to handle this responsibility. Upon discharge, the family is often given many instructions in a short time and is expected to carry them out at home.

As healthcare continues to shift to home care, families will bear the patient's healthcare needs associated with this change. Patients are discharged sooner and with a higher acuity level than in previous decades. Chronically ill patients will need continued long-term personal care at home that is not covered by the current Medicare benefit, and changes in Medicare funding may mean that fewer home visits are made. The financial burden associated with this care is more than many families can afford. In addition, the National Center for Health Statistics reports that more than 75% of all caregivers are women, and one third of those are older than 65 years of age.

The home care nurse plays an important role in facilitating patient and family access to community resources to assist the family in meeting various needs. The nurse determines when a caregiver is becoming overwhelmed with the care and attempts to provide resources to relieve the stress. The nurse also supports family decisions about complex treatments. The following questions may be used for discussion:

- What is most important to you?
- What do you want for your life and that of your family?
- How do you want to live?
- How is this technology supporting or not supporting what you want?

Hospice Nursing in the Home

Hospice nursing provides care to patients who are dying from a terminal illness. This care is most often provided in the home. Hospice care usually begins when the patient has 6 months or less to live and ends with the family 1 year after the death. This continuation of care for the family after the death is *bereavement care*. Nurses providing hospice care work with an interdisciplinary team of other health professionals, such as social workers, pastoral counselors, home health aides, and volunteers to provide comprehensive palliative care.

The American hospice movement was originally led by volunteers (many of whom were nurses) who wanted to make life better for those who were dying. These devoted volunteers promoted the dignity of dying patients and decreased their institutionalization. Dr. Elizabeth Kubler-Ross published *On Death and Dying* in 1969, which described the five stages that many terminally ill patients experience (see Chap. 32). She promoted the use of home care as a more effective means of providing support and care to dying patients and their families. In 1986, Congress passed the Medicare Hospice Benefit and also gave states the option of including hospice services in their Medicaid programs. Since then, patients who are dying of cancer or any other terminal illness may receive hospice care in the comfort of their homes with the family nearby.

The hospice nurse combines the skills of the home care nurse with the ability to provide daily emotional support to dying patients and their families. Hospice nurses are especially skilled in pain and symptom management. Their focus is on improving quality of life, as opposed to prolonging the length of it, and on preserving dignity for the patient in death. After the death, the nurse continues to care for the patient's family during the bereavement period for up to 1 year. Nurses use this time to help families work through the grief process after their loss.

Most hospice care is delivered to patients in their home. Some hospices also have an inpatient (hospital) setting where patients can receive short-term care, as a respite for caregivers, or long-term palliative care. In whatever setting, hospice care provides terminally ill patients a humane option of dying with dignity.

The Future of Home Care

The 1990s were a time of transition, growth, and specialization for the home care industry. In the 2000s, more complex services are being provided at home. Increasing numbers of surgical procedures are being performed on an outpatient or short-stay basis; thus, families and friends have more responsibility for providing care at home. Specialization will continue to expand in the areas of cardiac care, wound care, and intravenous therapy services. The role of prevention will continue to grow in home care through use of health screening, immunization, and community education programs. Keeping people healthy in the home will be a goal to prevent illness resulting in hospitalization. Home care nurses will need to expand their knowledge and skill continually to meet the challenges of providing preventive, acute, and chronic care to patients in their homes.

Learning Outcomes

After completing this chapter, the learner should be able to accomplish the following:

1. Define the key terms used in the chapter
   entry phase   hospice
   home healthcare   preentry phase
2. Outline the history of home healthcare.
3. Describe the characteristics and roles of the home health nurse.
4. Identify the essential components of the preentry and entry phases of the home visit.
5. Compare the role of the family in home care to that in hospital-based care.
6. Describe the purpose of hospice nursing.

Critical Thinking Questions

1. Interview a nurse employed in a hospital setting and a nurse employed by a home health agency. How are their roles and responsibilities alike? How do they differ?
2. Consider what you would do in the following home care situations:
   - An 85-year-old patient cannot move by himself and refuses to eat. His 83-year-old wife tries to care for him, but she begins to cry when you enter their apartment.
   - A 43-year-old woman is receiving home care after surgery to repair a herniated vertebral disk ("slipped disk"). When you arrive for the scheduled visit, you find that her speech is slurred and that she does not remember how much pain medication she took.
   - A 2-year-old has a malignant brain tumor. He is not expected to live more than 1 week and is receiving hospice care. The family's background is Native American.

Bibliography

Andrews, M., & Boyle, J. (1999). *Transcultural concepts in nursing care* (3rd ed.). Philadelphia: Lippincott Williams & Wilkins.

Askew, R., Kent, R., & McDonald, M. (1998). Assessing and responding to client needs: A framework for home care agencies. *Home Healthcare Consultant, 5*(6), 17–19.

Bennett, R. L., & Tandy, L. J. (1998). Postpartum visits: Extending the continuum of care from hospital to home. *Home Healthcare Nurse, 16*(5), 294–304.

Boland, D., & Sims, S. (1996). Family care giving at home. *Image—The Journal of Nursing Scholarship, 28*(1), 55–58.

Capone, L. (1997). Home care: A family affair. *Home Healthcare Nurse, 15*(1), 49–51.

Clemen-Stone, S., McGuire, S., & Eigsti, D. (1998). *Comprehensive community health nursing: Family, aggregate, & community practice* (5th ed.). St. Louis: C. V. Mosby.

Ellenbecker, C., & Shea, K. (1994). Documentation in home healthcare practice: Evidence of quality care. *Nursing Clinics of North America, 29*(3), 495–506.

Grossman, D. (1996). Cultural dimensions in home health nursing. *American Journal of Nursing, 96*(7), 33–36.

Holzemer, S. P. (1998). Overview of home care concepts. In M. Klainberg, S. Holzemer, M. Leonard, & J. Arnold, *Community health nursing: An alliance for health* (pp. 217–238). New York: McGraw-Hill.

Home health: 32 Tips for hospice and home health nurses. (1998). *Nursing, 28*(8), 64hh2, 64hh4.

Joel, L. (1997). Moving the care site from hospital to home. Whose turf? In J. McCloskey & H. Grace, *Current issues in nursing* (5th ed.). (pp. 209–215). St. Louis: C. V. Mosby.

Johnson, J. Y., Smith-Temple, J., & Carr, P. (1998). *Nurse's guide to home health procedures.* Philadelphia: Lippincott Williams & Wilkins.

Klebanoff, N., & Smith, N. (1977). *Lippincott's guide to behavior management in home care.* Philadelphia: J. B. Lippincott.

McCorkle, R., Robinson, L., Nuamah, I., Lev, E., & Benolil, J. (1998). The effects of home nursing care for patients during terminal illness on the bereaved's psychological distress. *Nursing Research, 47*(1), 2–10.

Mundinger, M. (1983). *Home care controversy: Too little, too late, too costly.* Rockville, MD: Aspen.

National Association for Home Care. (1999). *Basic statistics about home care.* Washington, DC: National Association for Home Care.

Pokorni, J. (1997). Promoting the overall development of infants and young children receiving home services. *Pediatric Nursing, 23*(2), 187–190.

Rice, R. (1998). Home visit safety. *Geriatric Nursing—American Journal of Care for the Aging, 19*(4), 241–242.

Stulginsky, M. (1993). Nurses' home health experience. II. The unique demands of home visits. *Nursing & Healthcare, 14*(9), 476–485.

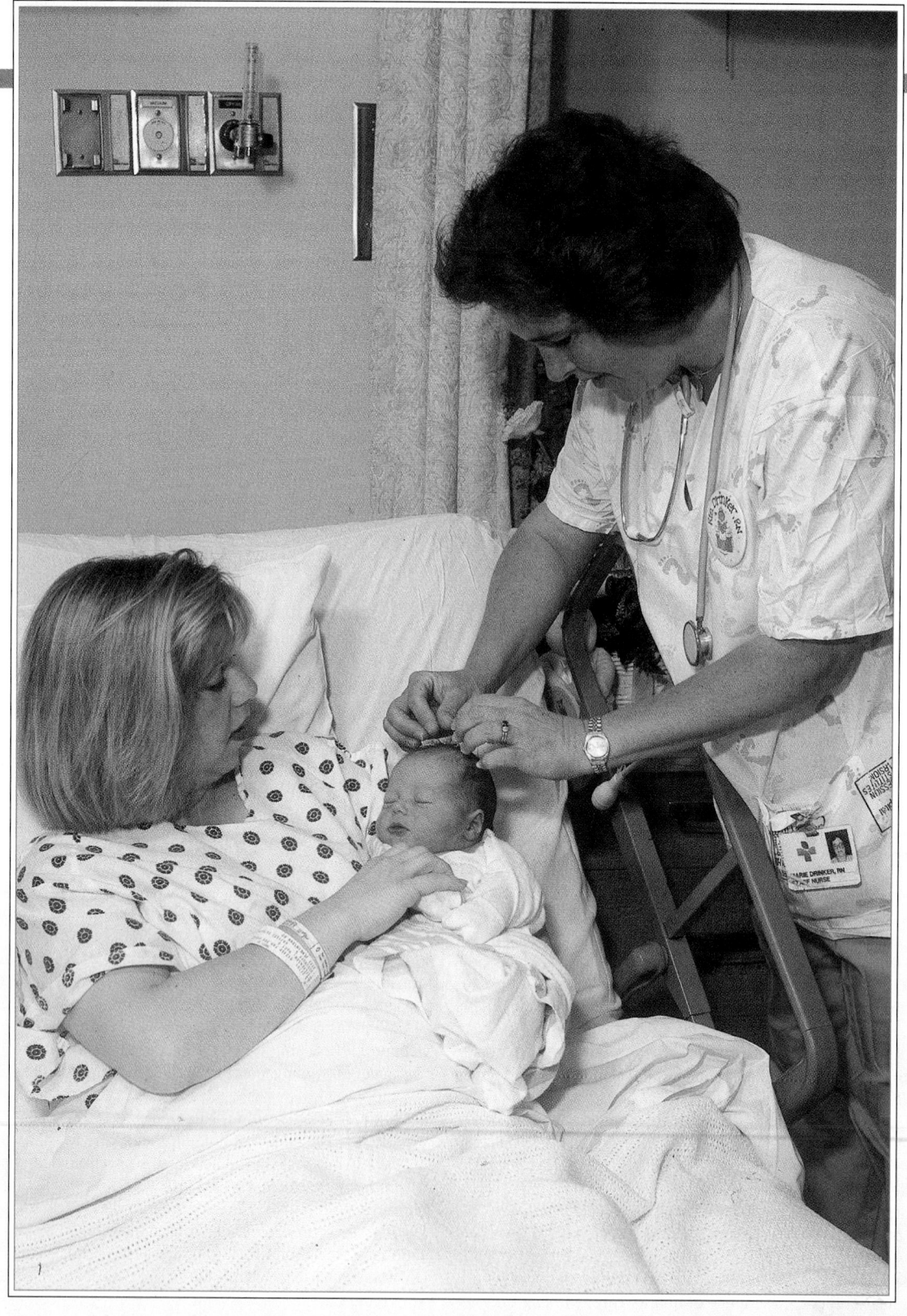

UNIT IV

The Nursing Process

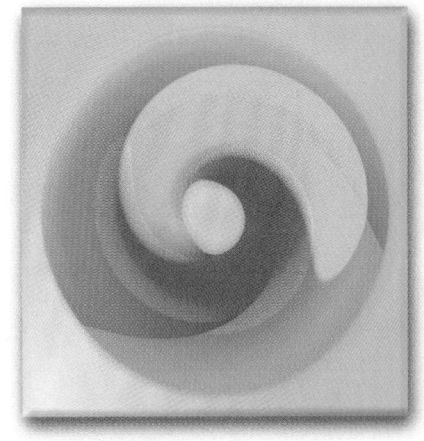

"... the nursing process is educative and therapeutic when nurse and patient can come to know and to respect each other, as persons who are alike, and yet different, as persons who share in the solution of problems."

Hildegarde Peplau (1909–)
has been an active participant in ANA and NLN and a leader in recognizing the significance of interpersonal relationships in psychiatric nursing. Her landmark book integrated theory into her model at a time when nursing theory was in its infancy.

The nursing process is a systematic, patient-centered, goal-oriented method of caring that provides a framework for nursing practice. Unit IV discusses each of the five steps of the nursing process—assessing, diagnosing, planning, implementing, and evaluating. It also describes the blended skills nurses need to use the process to promote patient well-being, and concludes with a chapter on documentation, reporting, and conferring.

The steps of the nursing process are not actually separate items but rather are parts of a whole, used to identify needs, establish priorities of care, maximize strengths, and resolve actual or potential alterations in human responses to health and illness, thereby promoting health to the highest level possible for each patient.

Assessment, the systematic and continuous collection and communication of data, allows analysis of data to identify problems and strengths of patients. During planning, the nurse and patient mutually set goals and agree on nursing interventions necessary to meet the expected outcomes. The nurse implements the plan of care, adapting it to each individual, and documents nursing actions and patient responses. After implementation, the nurse and patient evaluate the effectiveness of the plan, based on achievement of goals, and determine if the plan should be continued, modified, or terminated.

The nursing process is nursing practice in action. Unit IV provides the information necessary to begin to apply the nursing process; as blended skills are learned and practiced (both by students and by nurses), the process becomes an integral component of each nurse–patient interaction. The outcome is comprehensive and individualized nursing care.

Chapter 14
Blended Skills and Critical Thinking Throughout the Nursing Process

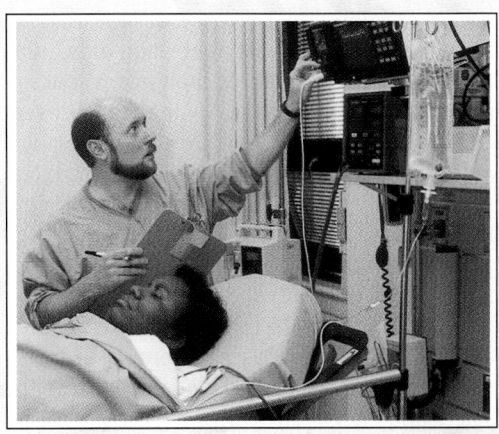

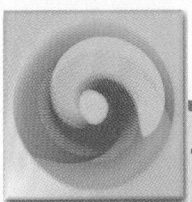

**Thinking Critically About
Nursing's Blended Skills**

Before reading this chapter, think about the types of skills you will need to use the nursing process successfully to meet the needs of the patients entrusted to your care.

- Your hospital has just started to offer cardiac transplantation services, and you are considering switching from your medical-surgical floor to the new unit.

- To discharge low-birthweight infants home earlier, your unit is thinking of providing special visiting nurse assistance to families when their infants come home.

- You have often thought about hospice nursing and decide that now is the time to make this your specialty.

- Everyone is upset with Mrs. Zuccarelli because she never follows through with the plan of care and thwarts the team's best efforts to help her. Her newly diagnosed cancer is treatable, but she continually fails to show up for appointments for both diagnostic studies and treatment.

What cognitive, technical, interpersonal, and ethical/legal skills do you think you will need to respond effectively to the nursing challenges described above?

Traditionally, nurses have prided themselves on comforting those who are ill and on executing with precision such tasks as dressing wounds, administering medications, and bathing, feeding, and ambulating patients. Many of these tasks were ordered by physicians, and few nurses in the past would have characterized their "work" as being independent, scientifically based, or creative.

The healthcare delivery system has changed, and nursing has changed with it. Nurses now work with healthy and ill patients in both private and institutional settings. In addition to their role as caregiver, nurses fill specialized roles as care managers—coordinators, teachers, counselors, advocates, and researchers. Nurses are responsible for a unique dimension of healthcare, "the diagnosis and treatment of human responses to actual or potential health problems"(American Nurses Association [ANA], 1980) and as such are knowledgeable, competent, and independent professionals who work collaboratively with other healthcare professionals to design and deliver holistic care.

As the practice of nursing became more complex, nurses began to study the *process* of nursing to both understand and improve the means nurses use to accomplish their aims. This involves paying attention to the *ever-changing mix* of blended skills needed to use the nursing process safely and effectively. One thing is certain: at no one point in your career will you ever be able to step back and say, "Now I've mastered all the cognitive, interpersonal, technical, and ethical/legal skills I need to be a good nurse!"

The Nursing Process

Historical Perspective

Since the term *nursing process* was first used by Hall in 1955, many nurses have struggled to define exactly what constitutes the "work of nursing" and what makes nurses successful. In the 1960s, nursing theorists began to describe nursing as a distinct entity among the healthcare professions and also delineated specific steps in a process approach to nursing practice. In 1967, Yura and Walsh published the first comprehensive book on nursing process, in which they described four steps in the nursing process: assessment, planning, intervention, and evaluation. They viewed the element of nursing diagnosis as the logical conclusion of the assessment phase, whereas Gebbie and Lavin (1974) made nursing diagnosis a separate step in the process. These and other studies led to the development of the five-step nursing process commonly used today: assessment, diagnosis, planning, implementation, and evaluation.

The steps of the nursing process were legitimized in 1973, when the ANA Congress for Nursing Practice developed *Standards of Practice* to guide nursing performance. These standards, which were revised in 1991, appear in Chapter 1. The standards for nursing practice were quickly reflected in revised nurse practice acts in many states.

The Joint Commission on Accreditation of Healthcare Organizations requires that care be documented according

COGNITIVE SKILLS

- Knowledge of the science of nursing care related to cardiac transplantation, low-birthweight infants, end-of-life care, and oncology.
- Knowledge of how to assess, diagnose, and then plan, implement, and evaluate nursing care for patients undergoing transplantation, couples bringing sick infants home, families caring for dying patients, and patients who are finding it difficult to exercise appropriate self-care, even in the face of serious illness.

TECHNICAL SKILLS

- Ability to provide the technical nursing assistance necessary to implement the plan of care safely and effectively for the patients described above.

INTERPERSONAL SKILLS

- Ability to establish trusting professional relationships with vulnerable patients, their family caregivers, and your colleagues.

- Ability to counsel the woman who is finding it difficult to respond to the challenge of a newly diagnosed cancer and to work with your colleagues to find a way for the team to continue to work with her.

ETHICAL/LEGAL SKILLS

- Ability and willingness to master the knowledge and skills needed to meet the nursing needs of patients and families safely and effectively in new practice areas (accountability to ensure your ongoing competence).
- Knowledge of the ethical and legal guidelines for end-of-life care.
- Ability to practice in an ethically and legally defensible manner.

to the nursing process, and the National League for Nursing has recommended that educational programs incorporate the nursing process as their intellectual process. In 1982, the state board examinations for professional nursing practice underwent major revisions and began to use the nursing process as an organizing concept. The revised examinations are structured to test the practitioner's ability to assess patients; to diagnose health problems amenable to nursing therapy; and to plan, implement, and evaluate nursing care. The examinations had previously organized content on a medical model, structured according to medical specialties—medicine, surgery, maternity, pediatrics, and psychiatry.

Description of the Nursing Process

The **nursing process** is a systematic method that directs the nurse and patient as they together accomplish the following: (1) **assess** the patient to determine the need for nursing care, (2) determine **nursing diagnoses,** (3) **plan** care, (4) **implement** the care, and (5) **evaluate** the results. The steps in this patient-centered, goal-oriented process are interrelated; each of the five steps depends on the accuracy of the steps preceding it. The process provides a framework that enables the nurse and patient to accomplish the following:

- Systematically collect patient data (assessing)
- Clearly identify patient strengths and problems (diagnosing)

- Develop a holistic plan of individualized care that specifies the desired patient goals and related outcomes and the nursing interventions most likely to assist the patient to meet those expected outcomes (planning)
- Execute the plan of care (implementing)
- Evaluate the effectiveness of the plan of care in terms of patient goal achievement (evaluating)

The five steps of the nursing process are shown in Figure 14-1 and described in Table 14-1. In each step of the process, the nurse and patient work together as partners (Fig. 14-2); the patient's health state and resources influence the patient's level of participation. When the patient is an infant or is unconscious or uncooperative, the steps of the process are worked through with the help of a family member or support person whenever possible.

Nursing Process Trends

Although experienced nurses may tell stories about lengthy handwritten plans of individualized care, the trend today is toward computerization. Nurses at centralized or bedside computer terminals have access to databases that allow them to plan and document care easily. Critical pathways (see Chap. 17), which target desired outcomes for particular illnesses, procedures, or conditions and accompanying multidisciplinary staff actions along a timeline, provide the standard guidelines for care in many institutions. Facilitating this work are national efforts to develop

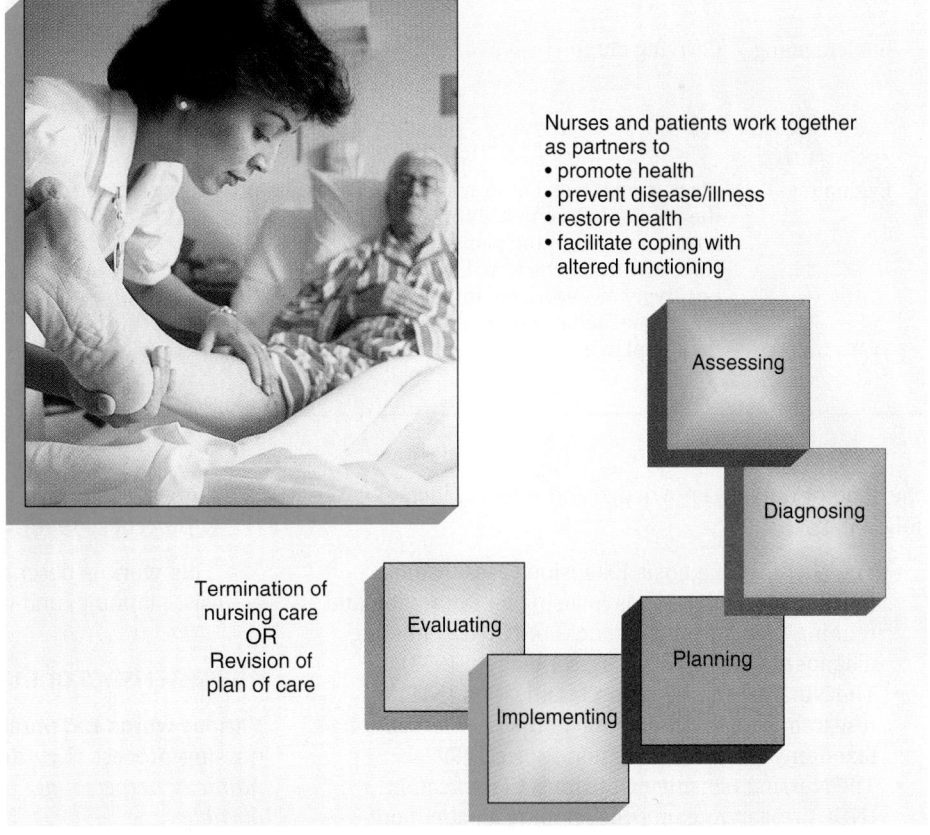

Figure 14-1
The steps in the patient-centered, goal-oriented nursing process are dynamic and interrelated. Each of the five steps depends on the accuracy of the preceding step.

Nurses and patients work together as partners to
- promote health
- prevent disease/illness
- restore health
- facilitate coping with altered functioning

Assessing

Diagnosing

Planning

Implementing

Evaluating

Termination of nursing care
OR
Revision of plan of care

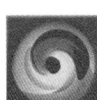

Table 14-1
Overview of the Nursing Process

Component	Description	Purpose	Activities
Assessing	Collection, validation, and communication of patient data	Make a judgment about the patient's health status, ability to manage his or her own healthcare, and need for nursing. Plan individualized holistic care that draws on patient strengths and is responsive to changes in the patient's conditions.	1. Establish the database: • Nursing history • Physical assessment • Review of patient record and nursing literature • Consultation with patient's support people and healthcare professionals 2. Continuously update the database. 3. Validate data. 4. Communicate data.
Diagnosing	Analysis of patient data to identify patient strengths and health problems that independent nursing intervention can prevent or resolve	Develop a prioritized list of nursing diagnoses.	1. Interpret and analyze patient data. 2. Identify patient strengths and health problems. 3. Formulate and validate nursing diagnoses. 4. Develop prioritized list of nursing diagnoses.
Planning	Specification of (1) patient goals/outcomes to prevent, reduce, or resolve the problems identified in the nursing diagnoses; and (2) related nursing interventions	Develop an individualized plan of nursing care.	1. Establish priorities. 2. Write goals/outcomes, and develop an evaluative strategy. 3. Select nursing interventions. 4. Communicate plan of nursing care.
Implementing	Carrying out the plan of care	Assist patients to achieve desired goals—promote wellness, prevent disease and illness, restore health, facilitate coping with altered functioning.	1. Carry out the plan of care. 2. Continue data collection, and modify the plan of care as needed. 3. Document care.
Evaluating	Measuring the extent to which the patient has achieved the goals specified in the plan of care; identifying factors that positively or negatively influenced goal achievement; revising the plan of care if necessary	Continue, modify, or terminate nursing care.	1. Measure how well the patient has achieved desired goals/outcomes. 2. Identify factors that contribute to the patient's success or failure. 3. Modify the plan of care (if indicated.)

the state of nursing knowledge and science, including the following:

- The Nursing Diagnosis Extension Classification (NDEC) research team is focusing on improving and refining the clinical usefulness of NANDA nursing diagnoses (Craft-Rosenberg & Delaney, 1997).
- The Nursing Intervention Classification (NIC) research team is developing a nursing intervention taxonomy (Iowa Intervention Project, 1997).
- The Nursing-Sensitive Outcomes Classification (NOC) research team is developing a patient out-

comes taxonomy (Johnson & Mass, 1997; McCloskey & Bulechek, 1996).

This work is described in subsequent chapters on diagnosis, planning, and implementation.

Characteristics of the Nursing Process

Various words and phrases have been used to describe the nursing process. Key descriptors include *systematic, dynamic, interpersonal, goal oriented,* and *universally applicable.*

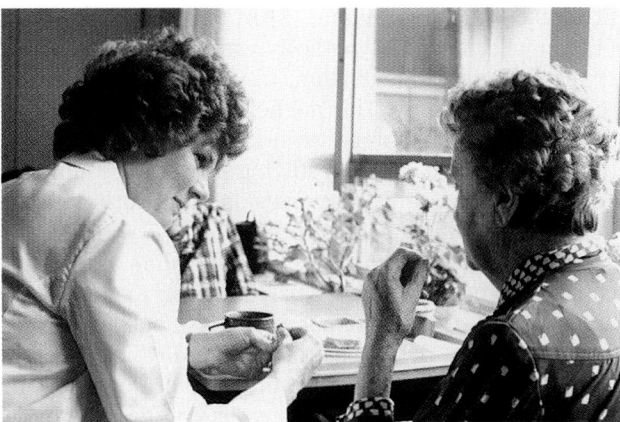

Figure 14-2
Nurses work collaboratively with patients when using the nursing process to plan and deliver care. (Photo by Gates Rhodes, courtesy of School of Nursing, University of Pennsylvania.)

Systematic

Each nursing activity is part of an ordered sequence of activities. Moreover, each activity depends on the accuracy of the activity that precedes it and influences the actions that follow it. Without a complete and accurate database, the nurse cannot identify patient strengths and problems; lacking knowledge of these, it is impossible for the nurse and patient to develop a plan of care based on realistic and valued patient goals. Unless the goals and outcomes are well written, nursing actions and evaluation lack focus and may be ineffective. The nursing process directs each step of nursing care in a sequential, ordered manner.

Dynamic

Although the nursing process is presented as an orderly progression of steps, in reality, there is great interaction and overlapping among the five steps. No one step in the nursing process is a one-time phenomenon; each step flows into the next step. In some nursing situations, all five stages occur almost simultaneously.

Interpersonal

Always at the heart of nursing is the human being. Read one student's account of this truth in the accompanying box: Through the Eyes of a Student. The nursing process ensures that nurses are patient centered rather than task centered (Fig. 14-3). Rather than simply approaching a patient to take vital signs, the nurse thinks, "How is Mrs. Barclay today? Are there any new data that indicate a need to modify her plan of care? Are our nursing actions helping her to achieve her goals? How can we better help her?"

The nursing process encourages nurses to work together to help patients use their strengths to meet all their human needs. This is different from viewing the patient as a "problem to be solved" and interacting mechanically to provide the solution. Working intimately with patients helps nurses to explore their own strengths and limitations and to develop themselves personally and professionally.

Through the Eyes of a Student

My first experience with an open wound was with a woman who had a stage IV sacral decubitus. I needed to do a dressing change with packing. I was fearful of what the wound would look like. I thought for sure I was going to be "grossed out," and I was—not by the appearance of the wound, but by the odor. The stench was awful! I started to feel queasy, and I began to sweat, and I thought I was going to pass out and fall right over on the patient. While I was packing the wound, I kept thinking that I was never going to get out of that room. I looked over at my clinical instructor and searched her face for approval of my technique, and I wondered if she also smelled anything and if it was making her feel sick too!

After the procedure was over and I left the room, I asked my instructor if all wounds smell that awful and would the smell always make me feel sick. Her response was that sometimes an odor will be really bad, and it might make me feel sick. With this kind of reassurance, I thought this is it—I never want to smell that again, and no way do I want to be a nurse. Later I realized that I had forgotten there was someone else in that room: the patient. She had to stay in there with that wound and its odor. It was for this reason I changed my mind about leaving nursing. I remembered that it was wanting to help patients to deal with their wounds that made me decide to be a nurse in the first place.

—Barbara L. Dlugosz
Holy Family College, Philadelphia, PA

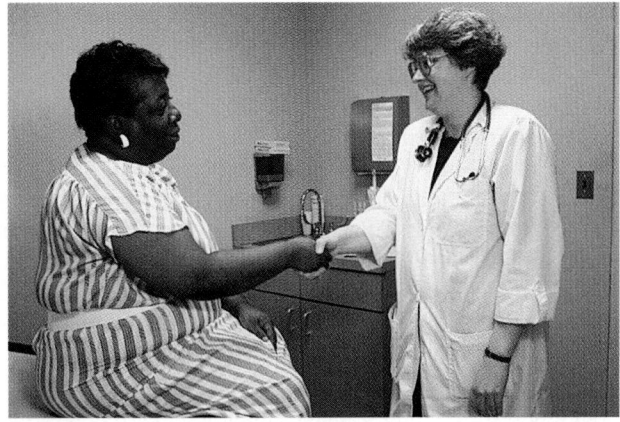

Figure 14-3
Nurses focus on people, not problems or tasks. The nursing process is patient centered, not task centered. (Photo by Gates Rhodes, courtesy of School of Nursing, University of Pennsylvania.)

Goal Oriented

The nursing process offers a means for nurses and patients to work together to identify specific goals related to health promotion, disease and illness prevention, health restoration, and coping with altered functioning; to determine which goals are most important to the patient; and to match them with the appropriate nursing actions. When these are recorded in the plan of care, each nurse can quickly determine the patient's priorities and begin nursing with a clear sense of how to proceed. The patient benefits from continuity of care, and each nurse's care moves the patient closer to goal achievement.

Universally Applicable

The one constant in healthcare is change. When nurses have a working knowledge of the nursing process, they find that they can practice nursing with well or ill people, young or old, in any type of practice setting. The student's efforts to master the nursing process result in possession of a valuable tool that can be used with ease in any nursing situation.

It should be clear from the preceding discussion that the nursing process provides a framework for all the nurse's activities. In each nurse–patient interaction, it is important to assess the patient, note any significant alterations in health status, determine whether the nursing action is helping the patient achieve his or her goals, and modify the plan of care as necessary. Thus, the nurse who feeds a child through a special tube as ordered by a physician continually assesses how the child is responding to the feeding and whether the child or family will be able to manage the feedings independently when the child is discharged. Depending on the results of the nursing assessment, new nursing diagnoses may be needed, along with related additions to the plan of care. The nursing process offers direction for *all* the activities carried out by the nurse when caring for patients.

Problem Solving and the Nursing Process

One of the strengths of the nursing process is that it is based on a methodology that is familiar to most nursing students—problem solving. Problem solving is a basic life skill; identifying a problem and then taking steps to resolve it are a matter of common sense. Different approaches to problem solving yield different results, however, some of which are more successful than others.

Trial-and-error problem solving involves testing any number of solutions until one is found that works for that particular problem. This method is not efficient for the nurse and can be dangerous to the patient; it is, therefore, not recommended as a guide for nursing practice. For example, although you may enjoy experimenting with different types of ethnic food as you discover and develop personal food preferences, you would not want to use the trial-and-error method of determining food preferences for a dehydrated and malnourished patient. You want to know, based on clinical research, exactly what food and fluid supplements are most likely to reverse his or her deficiencies.

Scientific problem solving is a systematic, seven-step problem-solving process that involves (1) problem identification, (2) data collection, (3) hypothesis formulation, (4) plan of action, (5) hypothesis testing, (6) interpretation of results, and (7) evaluation, resulting in conclusion or revision of the study. This method is used most correctly in a controlled laboratory setting but is closely related to the more general problem-solving processes commonly used by healthcare professionals as they work with patients, such as the nursing process.

For years, nurse theorists and educators argued that clinical judgments should be based on data alone (the scientific method), in an attempt to establish nursing as a science, worthy of the respect of other professions. Today, nurses acknowledge the role of **intuitive problem solving** in clinical decision making. Many veteran nurses can describe situations in which an "inner prompting" led to a quick nursing intervention that saved a patient's life. Nurses use intuitive problem solving when they directly apprehend a situation based on its similarity or dissimilarity to other situations. A recovery room nurse who realizes that a postoperative patient is "going bad" before there are measurable signs to suggest trouble is using intuitive problem solving, as is an oncology nurse who somehow senses the right moment to teach, offer encouragement, affirm or simply listen.

Advocates of intuition recommend the following:

- Welcoming flashes of intuition as additions to logical reasoning, rather than as disruptions
- Validating intuitions: when an intuition cannot be validated (eg, when the nurse senses that something is wrong with the patient, although there are no clinical signs), careful monitoring of the patient should be initiated
- Furthering nursing research to help find ways to (1) cultivate intuition and its typical results (accurate, early diagnosis; vigilant monitoring; better patient care) and (2) document the information intuition supplies (Rew, 1987)

Beginning nurses must use nursing knowledge and scientific problem solving as the basis of care they give; intuitive problem solving comes with years of practice and observation. If the beginning nurse has an intuition about a patient, that information should be discussed with the supervisor.

Documenting the Nursing Process

The ability to communicate clearly in writing is a critical nursing skill. Accurate, concise, timely, and relevant documentation provides all the members of the caregiving team with a picture of the patient. The written patient record is the chief means of communication among members of the interdisciplinary team. Legally speaking, a nursing action not documented is a nursing action not performed. If accused of negligent care, a nurse may tell the court that she faithfully assessed the patient's needs, diagnosed problems, and implemented and evaluated an effective plan of care. Unless the patient's health records contain documentation supporting her claims, however, the court has no reason to accept her word rather than that of the patient or family who are claiming that such care was not given. Each chapter in this unit offers specific documentation guidelines for nursing process activities; Chapter 20 discusses documentation in general. It is helpful to practice documentation while learning any given nursing activity; like any other nursing skill, documentation improves with practice. Examples of nursing documentation, nursing assessments, plans of care, and notes are provided throughout this text.

Benefits of the Nursing Process

When used well, the nursing process *achieves for the patient* scientifically based, holistic, individualized care; the opportunity to work collaboratively with other nurses; and continuity of the patient's care. *Nurses who use the nursing process* in a thoughtful and systematic way achieve a clear and efficient plan of action by which the entire nursing team can achieve the best results for patients; the satisfaction that they are making an important "difference" in the lives of their patients; and the opportunity to grow professionally as they evaluate the effectiveness of interventions and variables that contribute positively or negatively to the patient's goal achievement. See the accompanying box for an example of the nursing process in action.

Evaluating the Use of the Nursing Process

The chapters that follow describe each step of the nursing process in detail. Student nurses beginning to use the nursing process should evaluate their growing skill in using the

nursing process correctly. The accompanying checklist helps evaluate this personal skill in using the nursing process.

⑥ Blended Skills and Critical Thinking

The primary purpose of the nursing process is to help nurses manage each patient's care scientifically, holistically, and creatively. To do this successfully, the nurse needs many cognitive, technical, interpersonal, and ethical/legal skills along with the willingness to use them creatively and critically when working with patients to promote or restore health, to prevent disease or illness, and to facilitate coping with altered functioning.

Defining the Four Blended Skills

Before studying each step of the nursing process in more depth, it is useful to look at the skills essential to nursing practice. Understanding their importance helps the student work consciously to develop them while beginning to master the nursing process. Few nurses excel naturally in all four of these skills, and even experienced nurses continue working on becoming more proficient in the skills that lead to excellence. The remainder of this chapter discusses the blended skills that are essential to professional caregiving and successful use of the nursing process.

Cognitive Skills
Cognitively skilled nurses think about the nature of things sufficiently to "make sense" of their world and to

---

Example of the Nursing Process in Action

Assessing

You are checking on a patient who had abdominal surgery yesterday and hear that the patient has considerable pain. "It kept me up all night." The patient has been reluctant to ask for any pain medication, fearing effect of the drug. "I don't want to become a junkie." The patient's blood pressure and pulse rate are slightly elevated.

Diagnosing

You analyze the data above and write the nursing diagnosis: *Unrelieved pain related to a fear of taking pain-relieving medications.* The patient agrees that this is becoming a problem.

Planning

You decide to work with the patient to achieve the goal: *By 3:00 PM patient reports sufficient relief of pain to enable him to rest and to get out of bed to go to the bathroom.* The patient wants to accomplish the goal. You identify teaching as the primary nursing intervention.

Implementing

After asking the patient about his experiences with pain-relieving medications, you explain that although many of these drugs are addictive when abused, there is no harm if they are taken as prescribed postoperatively. You also explain that it is important for him to experience enough pain relief to be able to cough and deep breathe, ambulate, and do other things important to his recovery. You suggest that the medication will be most effective if taken before his pain peaks and becomes intense. You administer the prescribed medication for pain when the patient indicates that he is willing to give it a try.

Evaluating

After enough time has elapsed for the medication to take effect, you check back with the patient to evaluate whether he has obtained relief and met his goal. If the patient is satisfied and you both feel comfort is no longer a problem, you terminate the plan of care for this diagnosis. If the patient still feels pain or is dissatisfied with the medication, each of the preceding steps of the nursing process is reevaluated, and necessary changes are made in the plan of care.

Checklist for Evaluating Your Use of the Nursing Process

Assessing

- [ ] The initial database is obtained by means of a nursing history and nursing examination.
- [ ] Assessment data are documented:
  - [ ] Accurately—Questionable data are validated.
  - [ ] Completely—Use of a systematic guide ensures that recorded data describe (1) the patient's functional ability to meet each basic human need, and (2) responses to health and illness.
  - [ ] Concisely—Irrelevant data and meaningless generalizations are avoided.
  - [ ] Factuality—Patient behaviors are recorded rather than the nurse's interpretation of these behaviors.
- [ ] The initial database communicates a "real sense" of the patient that makes possible individualized care.
- [ ] Focused assessment data are recorded for each patient problem.
- [ ] Data collection and documentation are ongoing and responsive to changes in the patient's condition.

Diagnosing

- [ ] A prioritized list of nursing diagnoses is on the plan of care.
- [ ] Each nursing diagnosis describes an actual or potential patient health problem that independent nursing intervention can prevent or resolve. Each nursing diagnosis:
  - [ ] Is derived from an accurate and validated interpretation of a cluster of significant patient data or "cues"
  - [ ] Contains a precise problem statement describing what is unhealthy about the patient and what needs to change—suggests patient goals
  - [ ] Identifies factors that contribute to the problem (etiology)—these suggest nursing interventions
  - [ ] Uses nonjudgmental language and is written using legally advisable terms
- [ ] Old nursing diagnoses are deleted from the plan of care once resolved, and new diagnoses are added as soon as identified.

Planning

- [ ] A comprehensive, individualized, and up-to-date plan of care that specifies patient goals/outcomes and nursing orders for each nursing diagnosis is developed with the assistance of the patient and family.

- [ ] Planning is comprehensive:
  - [ ] Initial
  - [ ] Ongoing
  - [ ] Discharge
- [ ] Long-term goals alert the entire nursing team to realistic patient expectations after discharge.
- [ ] Short-term goals/outcomes:
  - [ ] When achieved, demonstrate a resolution of the problem specified in the nursing diagnosis
  - [ ] Describe a single, observable, and measurable patient behavior
  - [ ] Are valued by the patient and family
  - [ ] Are realistic in terms of the resources of the patient and the nurse
- [ ] Nursing orders:
  - [ ] Clearly and concisely describe the nursing intervention to be performed (ongoing assessment; nursing treatments and procedures; teaching, counseling, advocacy)
  - [ ] Are individualized to the patient
  - [ ] Are consistent with standards of care and supportive of other therapies
  - [ ] Are effective in accomplishing the desired patient goals/outcomes
- [ ] The plan of care encourages patient and family participation.

Implementing

- [ ] The patient record contains daily documentation of the nursing measures used to (1) assist the patient to meet basic human needs, (2) resolve health problems, and (3) implement select aspects of the medical plan of care.
- [ ] The plan of care is implemented:
  - [ ] Competently
  - [ ] Confidently
  - [ ] Caringly
  - [ ] Creatively

Evaluating

- [ ] Evaluative statements are recorded on the plan of care to document the patient's level of goal/outcome achievement at targeted times.
- [ ] Ongoing evaluation of the patient's responses to the plan of care are used to make decisions about terminating, continuing, or modifying nursing care.

grasp conceptually what is necessary to achieve valued goals. Cognitively skilled nurses are able to accomplish the following:

- Offer a scientific rationale for the patient's plan of care (prerequisite sciences include nursing and medical science as well as basic sciences, such as chemistry, microbiology, anatomy, physiology, psychology, sociology, and anthropology)
- Select those nursing interventions that are most likely to yield the desired outcomes
- Use critical thinking to solve problems creatively

Critical thinking is defined as "a systematic way to form and shape one's thinking. It functions purposefully and exactingly. It is thought that is disciplined, comprehensive, based on intellectual standards, and, as a result, well-reasoned" (Paul, 1993, p. 20). Cognitively skilled nurses are critical thinkers.

Technical Skills

Technically skilled nurses manipulate equipment skillfully to produce a desired goal. Technical competence involves everything from manual dexterity and good eye–hand coordination to an ability to troubleshoot when equipment malfunctions, based on an understanding of the technical workings of the equipment. Technically skilled nurses are able to accomplish the following:

- Use technical equipment with sufficient competence and ease to achieve goals with minimal distress to participants involved
- Creatively adapt equipment and technical procedures to the needs of particular patients in diverse circumstances

Interpersonal Skills

Interpersonally skilled nurses establish and maintain caring relationships that facilitate the achievement of valued goals while simultaneously affirming the worth of those in the relationship. Nurses skilled in interpersonal relations are able to accomplish the following:

- Use interactions with patients, their significant others, and colleagues to affirm their worth
- Elicit the personal strengths and abilities of patients and their significant others to achieve valued health goals
- Provide the healthcare team with knowledge about the patient's valued goals and expectations
- Work collaboratively with the healthcare team as a respected and credible colleague to reach valued goals

Ethical/Legal Skills

Ethically and legally skilled nurses conduct themselves in a manner consistent with their personal moral code and professional role responsibilities. Nurses skilled in ethical/legal competence are able to accomplish the following:

- Be trusted to act in ways that advance the interests of patients

- Be accountable for their practice to themselves, the patients they serve, the caregiving team, and society
- Act as effective patient advocates
- Mediate ethical conflict among the patient, significant others, healthcare team, and other interested parties
- Practice nursing faithful to the tenets of professional codes of ethics
- Use legal safeguards that reduce the risk of litigation

Cognitive and technical skills equip nurses to manage the clinical problems stemming from the patient's changing health or illness state. Interpersonal and ethical skills are essential, however, for nurses concerned about the patient's broader well-being.

Developing Cognitive Skills

The four domains of critical thinking are elements of thought (the basic building blocks of thinking), abilities (the skills essential to higher-order thinking), affective dimensions, and intellectual standards (Paul, 1993). These are illustrated in Table 14-2. The exercises below should help you to develop the ability to think critically in professional practice.

Developing the Method of Critical Thinking

Nurses who wish to develop the critical thinking skills essential to quality nursing practice will find it helpful to work methodically through a set of five types of considerations when posed with a thinking challenge. These are the purpose of thinking, adequacy of knowledge, potential problems, helpful resources, and critique of judgment/decision.

Purpose of Thinking

The first step when thinking critically about a situation is to identify the purpose or goal of your thinking. This helps to discipline your thinking by directing all thoughts to the goal. The purpose of critical thinking may be to make a judgment about a particular patient or situation or to make a decision about how best to intervene.

Adequacy of Knowledge

At the outset of critical thinking, it is important for you to judge whether the knowledge you have is accurate, complete, and relevant. If you reason with false information or a lack of important data, it is impossible to draw a sound conclusion. You also want to be sure that you understand all the details relevant to the issue. What is at stake? How much time do you have to make a decision? How much room is there for error?

Potential Problems

As you become skilled in critical thinking, you will learn to "flag" and remedy the pitfalls to sound reasoning. Common problems include working with untested or faulty assumptions, accepting an unproven claim or line of argument, allowing bias to color your thinking, and reasoning illogically, such as making a generalization on the basis of a single experience or case, or allowing emotion to rule

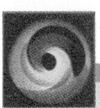

Table 14-2
The Four Domains of Critical Thinking

I. Elements of Thought: The Basic Building Blocks of Thinking

Element	Fundamental Standard	Potential Problems	Principle
Purpose	1. Clarity of purpose 2. Significance of purpose 3. Achievability of purpose 4. Consistency of purpose	1. Unclear purpose 2. Trivial purpose 3. Unrealistic purpose 4. Contradictory purposes	All reasoning has a purpose.
Question at issue or central problem	1. Clarity of question 2. Significance of question 3. Answerability 4. Relevance	1. Unclear 2. Insignificant 3. Not answerable 4. Irrelevant	To settle a question, you must understand what it requires.
Point of view	1. Flexibility in point of view 2. Fairness of point of view 3. Clarity of point of view 4. Breadth of point of view	1. Restricted 2. Biased 3. Unclear 4. Narrow	Reasoning is better when multiple, relevant points of view are sought out, articulated clearly, empathized with fairly and logically, applied consistently and dispassionately.
Empirical dimension	1. Clear evidence 2. Relevant information 3. Fairly gathered and reported evidence 4. Accurate data 5. Adequate evidence 6. Consistently applied data	1. Unclear 2. Unfairly or self-servingly gathered 3. Inaccurate 4. Insufficient	Reasoning can only be as sound as the evidence it is based on.
Concepts and ideas	1. Clarity of concepts 2. Relevance of concepts 3. Depth of concepts 4. Neutrality of concepts	1. Unclear 2. Irrelevant 3. Superficial 4. Biased	Reasoning can only be as clear, relevant, and deep as the concepts that shape it.
Assumptions	1. Clarity of assumptions 2. Justifiability of assumptions 3. Consistency of assumptions	1. Unclear 2. Unjustified 3. Contradictory	Reasoning can only be as sound as the assumptions it makes.
Implications and consequences	1. Significance of implications 2. Realistic nature of implications 3. Clarity of articulated implications 4. Precision of articulated implications 5. Completeness of articulated implications	1. Unimportant 2. Unrealistic 3. Unclear 4. Imprecise 5. Incomplete	To reason through an issue or decision, you must understand the implications and consequences that follow from it.

II. Abilities: The Skills Essential to Higher-Order Thinking	III. Affective Dimensions: The Attitudes, Dispositions, Passions, and Traits of Mind Essential to Higher-Order Thinking in Real Settings	IV. Intellectual Standards: The Standards Used to Critique Higher-Order Thinking	
• Ability to evaluate the credibility of sources of information • Ability to analyze arguments, interpretations, beliefs, or theories • Ability to clarify the meaning of words and phrases • Ability to transfer insights into new contexts • Ability to generate and assess possible solutions • Ability to develop criteria for evaluation: clarify values and standards • Ability to read, listen, write, and speak critically	• Thinking independently • Exercising fair-mindedness • Developing insight into egocentricity and sociocentricity • Developing intellectual humility and suspending judgment • Developing intellectual courage • Developing intellectual good faith and integrity • Developing intellectual perseverance • Developing confidence in reason • Developing intellectual curiosity	Clear Specific Relevant Consistent Deep Complete Adequate (for purpose)	Precise Accurate Plausible Logical Broad Significant Fair

Content from Paul, R. W. (1993). *Critical thinking: How to prepare students for a rapidly changing world.* Santa Rosa, CA: Foundation for Critical Thinking, pp. 123–132. Used with permission.

reason. The more familiar you are with these common impediments to critical thinking, the easier it is to detect them in your own thinking.

Helpful Resources

Wise professionals are quick to recognize their limits and seek help in remedying their deficiencies. Experienced clinicians know that learning is continuous and expect their practice to present challenges that demand new knowledge. Critical thinkers know what help they need to assist their reasoning and what resources to tap. Key resources include experienced clinicians, texts and journals, institutional policies and procedures, and professional groups and writings.

Critique of Judgment/Decision

Ultimately, you must identify alternative judgments or decisions, weigh the merits of each, and reach a conclusion. It is helpful to try to predict the consequences of your major options before concluding your reasoning. You will also want to evaluate the alternative you selected as your decision begins to influence your actions.

After using this method to work through an intellectually challenging situation, critique your use of the method in light of the **standards for critical thinking**: clear, precise, specific, accurate, relevant, plausible, consistent, logical, deep, broad, complete, significant, adequate (for the purpose), and fair.

The accompanying Developing Critical Thinking Skills box illustrates the use of these five considerations to facilitate critical thinking about a care dilemma experienced by a nursing student. The merits of thinking critically about which of the options is most likely to meet that patient's needs are readily apparent. Because nurses are accountable for the well-being of their patients, sloppy reasoning is both dangerous and inexcusable—even for someone new to nursing and clinical practice. Other examples of this method are found in the chapters on implementing, safety, perioperative nursing, stress and adaptation, sexuality, rest and sleep, and urinary elimination.

Developing the Attitudes and Dispositions to Think Critically

Certain habitual dispositions are needed by anyone who wants to be a critical thinker. Some of the most important of these are described below. Review this list, and assess the degree to which the dispositions characterize your thinking.

Thinking Independently

Nurses who are independent thinkers are careful not to allow the status quo or a persuasive individual to control their thinking. When confronted with an intellectual challenge, such as "Why is this patient so resistant to change?" they proceed cautiously, consulting with the patient and respected colleagues and reviewing the literature. Only then do they reach a clinical judgment. Compare this with a nurse who makes a snap judgment that a patient is "unreasonable" based on the comments of one nurse—even if this nurse is the nurse manager.

Being Fair Minded

Nurses who are fair-minded are open to different points of view and hear all sides of an argument before making a judgment. When a patient complains about another nurse or a physician, a fair-minded nurse seeks to validate the complaint and talks with the person being complained about before reaching a decision. A fair-minded thinker recognizes the limits of being egocentric ("It's right because this is what I think!") and sociocentric ("It's right because this is the way Americans—or Philadelphians—think!").

Being Intellectually Humble

One can easily differentiate nurses who are convinced that "they know it all" from those who are open and willing to learn. Intellectually humble nurses are learning all the time, often from patients and their nonprofessional caregivers, other colleagues, and the media. Never be afraid to say, "I don't know the answer to that question but I'll be happy to talk with you after I've had time to research the topic."

Being Intellectually Courageous

Nurses who are intellectually courageous are not afraid to challenge the status quo and "go against the flow." They resist the comment, "But we've always done it that way here. . ." when their experience or intuition suggests that another way may be better. They are not afraid to ask, "Is there something we might be able to do differently that would help this patient or situation?"

Demonstrating Good Faith and Integrity

Commitment to integrity helps nurses who are critical thinkers remain sensitive to discrepancies in the way one reasons in different situations and with different people. This sensitivity, for example, may result in our mind "throwing out a red flag" when it catches us reasoning unfairly.

Being Curious and Persevering

Nurses who persevere intellectually resist "easy answers." When the answer to "Why is this patient so resistant to change?" comes back, "Oh, that's just the way he is," the persevering nurse keeps questioning: "But *why* is he that way? What in his experience, values, beliefs, has made him so resistant? Until we understand these things we won't be able to help him!"

Being Disciplined

Nurses who are disciplined are thorough and take the time that is necessary to reach well-reasoned conclusions. When an initial conclusion or judgment does not "feel right," they are willing to go back to try to reason out a better judgment. They consult wise colleagues and are not afraid of doing the hard work of critical thinking.

Being Creative

Thinking critically may mean "thinking outside the box." The solution to a challenge may involve resources as yet untapped, effective and cost-saving interventions as yet undiscovered and untried. The process of brainstorm-

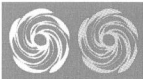 **Developing Critical Thinking Skills**

Situation

You are a nursing student. Your friend, Amy Chang, confides to you that she is very worried about her grandmother. When you meet Mrs. Chang, she demonstrates many of the assessment findings related to congestive heart failure. Although her family has entreated her to seek medical attention, Mrs. Chang insists on relying on herbal teas and traditional Chinese remedies. Now 88 years old, Mrs. Chang came to America from mainland China when she was 14. Although she raised a family that is now thoroughly "Americanized," Mrs. Chang has resisted embracing her new culture and now wants nothing to do with "American medicine." Amy, who is also a nursing student, loves her grandmother dearly and is frustrated by her stubborn refusal to see an internist. Both of you have reason to believe that she could be helped by medical attention. What do you do?

1. Identify Goal of Thinking

Clarify your thinking about alternative medicine so that you can decide how you ought to respond to Mrs. Chang's worsening physical condition.

2. Assess Adequacy of Knowledge

Pertinent circumstances: Although you have strong reason to believe that Mrs. Chang is suffering from congestive heart failure, she has not been medically diagnosed, and you lack definitive knowledge about her medical condition and the likelihood that she would respond to treatment. You do know that she places a high value on traditional Chinese culture and strongly believes that if she is to be healed, the healing will result from herbal teas and traditional Chinese remedies. She has no confidence in American medicine. Her family describe her as being extremely strong-willed and very lovable.

Prerequisite knowledge: To decide how you should respond in this situation, you need to know that traditional Western medicine is not the only beneficial system of medicine. It would be helpful for you and Mrs. Chang's family to learn more about Chinese medicine and the probability of its benefiting her (as well as the possibility of its harming her) in her present condition. You will also need to learn more about what is essential to Mrs. Chang's well-being. How much value does she place on physical health? How important is it for her to live (and possibly die) within the familiar and comforting boundaries of her culture? You will want to assess what teaching,

counseling, and support Mrs. Chang needs to reach an informed and voluntary decision that is right for her.

Room for error: Because Mrs. Chang's life may literally be at stake, there is not much room for error in the manner you and her family choose to respond. Even if her condition is not life-threatening, her sense of well-being may be severely threatened if she feels forced to pursue treatment that is alien and frightening.

Time constraints: Although you are uncertain about the seriousness of her condition, you understand that the sooner Mrs. Chang receives effective therapy, the better. Unless her condition suddenly deteriorates, this is not a decision that needs to be made within the next 24 hours.

3. Address Potential Problems

The most serious obstacle to critical thinking in this situation would be an inability to weigh the respective merits of alternative healing systems. Cultural bias may result in the untested assumption that American medicine is necessarily superior to all other systems of healing and that it would be morally wrong to support a choice of anything else. The love of Mrs. Chang's family and their desire to do everything possible to keep her well may interfere with their ability to allow her the freedom to make the choice that is right for her.

4. Consult Helpful Resources

Your first challenge will be to learn more about traditional Chinese medicine, and you will want to consult with local authorities as well as available literature. The National Institutes of Health have now established an Office of Alternative Medicine, which may provide helpful information and which is easily accessed through their web site. Your most important resource may be Mrs. Chang herself, and it will be important to try to learn from her as much as you can about what she values and what her goals are at this point in her life.

5. Critique Judgment/Decision

After getting to know Mrs. Chang better, you realize that she is firmly committed to her ways and adamant about not going to an American doctor or into a hospital at this point of her life. You (with her family) thus have only two options: to force her to see an internist against her will, possibly deceiving her to get her to the internist's

(continued)

office, or to support her choice to rely on familiar remedies, which may or may not successfully resolve her problems. The first alternative may save her life, and her family can see no other choice. You realize that by making this choice, the family is imposing its values on Mrs. Chang and violating her autonomy, her right to determine the course of her life. You decide to support her and to try to explain to her family the importance of doing this. You understand that if her condition is serious, and her traditional remedies prove ineffective her death may be hastened, but she accepts this consequence and prefers it to embracing an alien and frightening culture.

ing may bring out, along with unworkable options, one or two realistic suggestions that would not have surfaced otherwise.

Demonstrating Confidence

Nurses who routinely think critically develop confidence in their judgments and are not afraid to take and defend a position. When challenged by a patient or colleague to defend a course of action, they can reply with confidence, "I am doing it this way because research (or reason) convinced me that this is the best course of action."

Developing Technical Skills

Some people are naturally "good with their hands" and quickly master intricate procedures that involve working with technical equipment. Others have to practice procedures many times before they feel competent handling the equipment and performing clinical activities independently. Whatever your natural technical skill, you can help master the manual skills essential in the nursing process by developing the following habits.

- When a procedure demands manual dexterity, practice the necessary skill until you feel confident in its execution before attempting to perform it with a patient.
- Take time to familiarize yourself with new equipment before using it in a clinical procedure. Understand how it works and what supplies are needed to ensure optimal functioning. If possible, anticipate problems and know how to remedy them.
- Identify nurses who are technical experts, and ask them to share their secrets. Many experienced clinicians have developed quality, time-saving techniques they are willing to share.
- Never be ashamed to ask for help when feeling unsure of how to perform a procedure or manage equipment. Never forget that the patient's well-being and sometimes the patient's life depend on your technical competence.

Many nursing procedures are described in the clinical chapters in this text. Performance checklists break each procedure down into its component parts, allowing you to evaluate your performance of each step of the procedure.

This type of self-knowledge enables you to identify quickly and remedy recurrent deficiencies in technical skills.

Developing Interpersonal Skills

Characteristics of interpersonal caring that are essential to the practice of nursing include the following:

- Promotion of the dignity and respect of patients as people
- Centrality of the caring relationship
- Mutual enrichment of both participants in the nurse–patient relationship

Promoting Human Dignity and Respect

Nurses committed to respecting the human dignity of patients find it helpful to reflect on the following questions:

- What about patients obligates me to respect their human dignity? Must all patients be respected equally? Are some patients more deserving of respect? Can a patient ever forfeit the right to be respected?
- What does it mean to respect the dignity of patients? What are five concrete ways I can demonstrate respect?
- What are my strengths and deficiencies when it comes to respecting patients?
- In what ways (if any) must I change to be faithful to the duty of respecting the dignity of patients?
- What patients most challenge my ability to give care respectfully? How do I respond to this challenge? What does this teach me for the future?

Nurses often underestimate their power to help a patient heal simply through their respectful and caring presence. Each time a nurse walks into a room, he or she communicates one of two messages: (1) "You are a job to be done. You mean nothing to me," or (2) "You are a person of worth, and I care about you." Even a 60-second nurse–patient interaction can enhance or jeopardize human well-being. It is important for nurses to be sensitive to what their looks, speech, and touch communicate to patients and colleagues. The more vulnerable the patient and the more threatened the patient's sense of self, the more powerful effect the nurse's message has on the recipient's sense of worth and well-being.

The learning activity in the accompanying Applying Learning to Practice box was developed for nurses caring for older patients in a nursing home. Try these activities with a friend. Take turns being both the nurse and the older adult, and talk about how different types of nursing presence make you feel.

Establishing Caring Relationships

Increasingly, nurses are reporting that new systems of care and the demand to work "harder, faster, and smarter" to keep up in today's competitive healthcare arena are making traditional nurse–patient relationships difficult to attain. As you begin your nursing practice, ask yourself what priority you assign to caring. Nurses who accept that there can be no excellence in nursing in the absence of this relationship commit themselves to finding creative means to establish caring relationships. Obviously, many variables influence the quality of relationships that are possible, not the least of which is the acuity level of the patient and the patient's length of stay. Helpful reflection questions include the following:

- Do I know my patients well enough to promote anything more than the well-being of their body?

APPLYING LEARNING TO PRACTICE

Human Dignity: How Who I Am as a Caregiver Affects Others

Description

The purpose of this exercise is to explore the notion of "therapeutic use of self." You will be challenged to reflect on the effect your looks, speech, and touch have on other people. Role play and guided discovery will be used to enable you to experience the affirming and negating influences of different means of human relating.

Objectives

Upon conclusion of this exercise, you will be able to:

1. Demonstrate how looks, words, and touch can be used to harm or benefit others
2. Describe how the way you approach others enhances or diminishes their well-being
3. Identify one care behavior you plan to modify to improve your nursing practice

Learning Activities

Invite an experienced nurse to demonstrate how looks, words, and touch can be used to communicate two different messages to others: "You are a job to be done; you mean nothing to me"; and "You are precious, and I care about you." After the demonstration, team up with another student, and experience giving and receiving these messages. Share the feelings you both experienced. After these preliminary exercises, role play the suggested nursing situations (or others of your choosing), and once again process the experience. Talk about the relevance of this experience to human interaction in general, and conclude the exercise by writing a goal for your practice.

Worksheet

A. Practice looking at a colleague two different ways:
   1. "You are a job to be done; you mean nothing to me" look
   2. "You are precious, and I care about you" look
B. Practice speaking to a colleague in two different ways:
   1. Indifferent: "Your resident, your light."
   2. Helpful: "I think Mrs. Jones' light is on again. Do you need help?"
C. Practice touching a colleague in two different ways:
   1. Indifferent: Pick up your colleague's wrist and feel for a pulse.
   2. Using warm lotion, massage your colleague's hands.
D. Talk about how each of the above looks, words, and touches made you feel. Talk about how you think they make patients or residents feel.
E. Role play each of the situations below in two different ways, trying to incorporate looks, words, and touches that communicate:

First time: You are a job to be done; you mean nothing to me.
Second time: You are precious, and I care about you.

1. Student feels overwhelmed by patient care assignment and approaches clinical instructor to discuss her options.
2. Student walks into patient's room to begin morning care.
3. Student assists elderly patient to stand and ambulate around room.
4. Student brings medication to patient.
5. Student approaches another student and asks for help changing the bed linens of an obese patient who is on complete bed rest.

F. Name one thing you have decided to try to do differently when you take care of your patients as a result of this session.
G. Does what you experienced today have any implications for who you are when you are not nursing?

- If asked to describe a patient, would I be able to report on anything other than the patient's physical condition?
- Is the care I routinely provide *really* holistic, individualized, prioritized according to medical need *and* the patient's interests, and continuous? Do my care plans reflect this?
- What does the content of the patient report and nursing documentation communicate about nursing's priorities in my practice setting?
- What are my strengths and deficiencies in creating caring relationships?
- In what ways (if any) must I change to establish better caring relationships?

Nurses committed to caring relationships routinely use opportunities for conversation to communicate genuine interest in whom the patient is and what the patient is experiencing to provide meaningful nursing assistance. For example, rather than just "chattering" aimlessly with a talkative older adult, a nurse skilled in developing caring relationships will direct the conversation. Leading statements or questions that are often successful in eliciting useful information from older patients include the following:

- "Tell me something about your life at home. What do you miss most now that you are here?"
- "What family members and friends do you see most often? Who do you think knows you best and would you trust to be able to speak for you if you were ever unable to speak for yourself?"
- "Most of us have some goal or dream that keeps us going. It might be owning our own home, seeing some relationship patched up, or being reunited with a deceased loved one. What is your dream?"
- "When you've had troubles in the past, what did you draw on for strength? What keeps you going?"
- "Looks like you've got a lot of time for thinking these days . . . would you like to share what's been on your mind?"
- "Looks like we'll be spending some time together . . . what would you like to do with this time? How may I help you?"

Nurses who are sensitive to the well-being of their patients can find many ways to communicate caring. Happily, most caring is mutually enriching, and nurses who care find themselves reenergized for the more demanding aspects of their practice. Read one patient's account of the importance of nurse caring to her in the accompanying box: Through the Eyes of a Patient.

Enjoying the Rewards of Mutual Interchange

In any helping profession, but especially in nursing, countless opportunities exist to interact with others. Those committed to interpersonal caring enrich everyday interactions by investing them with something of themselves and, in return, receiving something of the other, as shown in Figure 14-4. Think of your last encounter with a patient. Whether you were administering a medication, checking vital signs, or preparing the patient for discharge, you had the choice of

> ### Through the Eyes of a Patient
>
> I recently spent 2 months in a university teaching hospital while doctors tried to find a way to regulate my heart beats. Many of the days were filled with tests, some of which were frightening. I was given many drugs—most of which turned out not to be helpful. I was a 2-hour car ride away from my home, family, and friends—which meant there wasn't always a familiar face at my bedside.
>
> I quickly learned I could judge what kind of day I was going to have as soon as I saw my nurse each morning.
>
> All of them brought my medicines and helped with the treatment plan. With some nurses, however, I also experienced the comfort and security of knowing that my expressed needs would be promptly and respectfully tended to. If I needed help getting up to the bathroom or asked for something for pain, I could count on help coming quickly. And finally there were those few with whom I knew I was going to have a great day because they would "make it happen" no matter how sick I was feeling. These were the nurses who offered a hug with their medicines, who had a moment to sit and listen, who teased about the "fashion statements" I was making with my nightgowns, and who "walked me through" new tests so that at least I felt better prepared to face the unknown. Most often, it wasn't what they did but how they did it.
>
> I wish all nurses understood the power they have to influence a patient's basic sense of well-being. A hospital can be a pretty scary, lonely place. Nurses can make all the difference!
>
> —MILDRED TAYLOR, PINE GROVE, PA

merely accomplishing the given task or accomplishing the task while simultaneously communicating a personal gift of support, caring, strength, and peacefulness. Frequently overlooked, these interpersonal gifts may contribute to a patient's healing as significantly as medical interventions. Rather than deplete their giver, these interpersonal gifts invite similar gifts from the recipient, which return to enrich the caregiver. Nothing causes burnout faster than a practice that is reduced to the performance of multiple tasks stripped of their human significance. When a patient is given care in a way that "makes a difference" in terms of his or her well-being, the patient's gratitude, even when unspoken, helps renew the nurse's energy. Too seldom do we stop our busy practices long enough to reflect on how who we are that day is influencing the well-being of those receiving our care. It is helpful to question:

- How conscious am I of how my mood influences the well-being of others?

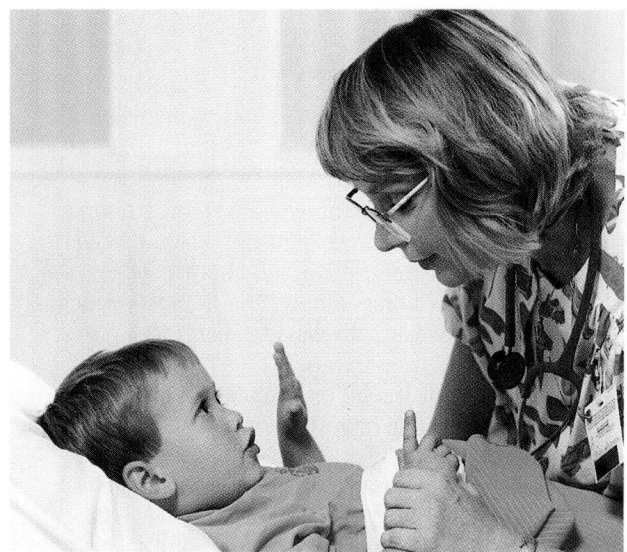

Figure 14-4
Interpersonal caring enriches the lives of everyone participating, providing a mutual exchange of giving and receiving. (Photo by Einrosia, courtesy of Shore Memorial Hospital and Nursing Spectrum.)

- Have I ever consciously tried to transmit strength, peace, support, or joy to another? What were the results?
- Am I aware of any situation in which my fatigue, anxiety, frustration, or negativity was communicated to a patient in a manner that negatively influenced his or her well-being?
- Am I conscious of ways in which patients enrich me personally or enrich my practice?
- In what ways is my practice different when I am attuned to the interpersonal dimensions of nurse–patient interactions?
- In what ways must my practice change if I am to facilitate healing by willing something of my essence to patients?

Developing Ethical/Legal Skills

Nurses who prize their role in securing patient well-being are sensitive to the ethical and legal implications of nursing practice. Chapters 6, 7, and 23 describe essential components of ethical and legal competence for nurses. Although it can take years to master effective patient advocacy skills and to become proficient in mediating ethical conflict, even beginning nurses are responsible for certain basic ethical skills. One of the greatest challenges nursing students face is balancing the competing demands of home life, school, and the hospital or practice setting. Learning to be true to oneself, to the patients for whom one is responsible, to the caregiving team, and to the profession and society is an ongoing struggle. Examining one's sense of accountability is crucial as one assumes professional responsibilities.

Developing Accountability

Nurses committed to interpersonal caring hold themselves accountable for the human well-being of patients entrusted to their care. Being accountable means being attentive and responsive to the healthcare needs of individual patients. It means that my concern for the patient transcends whatever happens during my shift, and that I ensure continuity of care when I leave a patient. In today's system of increasingly fragmented care, patients often find themselves unable to point to any one caregiver who knows their overall situation and is capable and willing to coordinate the efforts of the healthcare team. Being responsive and responsible earns a patient's trust that "all will be well" as healthcare needs are addressed. Nurses committed to responsible caring reflect on the following:

- To what extent does my commitment to securing the human well-being of those in my care dictate my work priorities?
- How comfortable am I voicing unmet patient needs to other members of the healthcare team?
- Do other caregivers listen when I present patient concerns because of my successful record of patient advocacy?
- What system variables (eg, nurse–patient ratios, skill mix, availability of resources) need to change for us to meet the human needs of our patients adequately?
- In what ways must I change for my patients to be able to count on me to respond in a responsible way to their needs?

Nurses who are sensitive to the legal dimensions of practice are careful to develop a strong sense of both ethical and legal accountability. Competent practice is a nurse's best legal safeguard. Nurses seeking to develop legal competence may find it helpful to ask the following questions:

- Do I know the legal boundaries of my practice?
- Am I familiar with pertinent institutional procedures and policies?
- Do I "own" my personal strengths and weaknesses and seek assistance as needed?
- Am I careful never to accept responsibility for an assignment for which I am unprepared?
- Am I knowledgeable about, and respectful of, patient rights?
- Does my documentation provide a legally defensible account of my practice?

When working to develop ethical and legal accountability, nurses must recognize that both deficiencies *and excesses* of responsible caring are problematic. Although it is reasonable to hold oneself accountable for promoting the human well-being of patients, nurses can err by setting for themselves unrealistic standards of responsiveness and responsibility. Prudence is always necessary to balance responsible self-care with care of others. Inexperienced nurses may feel totally responsible for effecting patient outcomes beyond their control and become frustrated and sad when unable to produce the desired outcome. Conversations about what is reasonable to hold ourselves and others accountable for are always helpful. The sample learning activity in the accompanying Applying Learning to Practice box was designed to explore such accountability issues.

APPLYING LEARNING TO PRACTICE

Accountability

Description

The purpose of this exercise is to explore the issue of accountability. You will be challenged to reflect on whether your everyday nursing practice demonstrates a commitment to ensuring the human well-being of those in your care. Individual patterns of responding to human need and responsible caring will be critiqued. Role playing and guided discovery will be used to invite you to experience the effects of both responsible caring and the indifferent provision of services.

Objectives

Upon conclusion of this session, you will be able to:

1. Describe how the way you respond (or fail to respond) to the needs of patients influences their general sense of well-being.
2. Critique the amount of responsibility you and other nurses accept for the well-being of individual patients.

3. Describe one way your practice will change in order for you to be more accountable to yourself, your patients, the nursing profession, and society.

Learning Activities

Choose another student, and work through exercises 1 to 4. Begin by describing your own positive and negative experiences of being cared for, and draw parallels to how patients feel when they believe they can count on their caregivers to recognize and respond to their needs. Then develop and discuss a list of personal, patient, and system variables that either facilitate or impede responsible caring. Finally, role play the given scenarios, and focus discussion on how different nursing responses influence patient well-being. End the discussion by developing a goal for your practice that will help you to be accountable to yourself, patients, the nursing profession, and society.

Worksheet

Objective

To critique our responsiveness to patient need and the amount of responsibility we each assume to secure patient well-being

Exercise One

Take a moment to reflect on a recent experience when you felt vulnerable (eg, new role responsibilities: first clinical rotation, new job, new spouse, new parent; car breaks down; major purchase). Share with a colleague how the conduct of the one(s) you expected to be sensitive and responsive to your need influenced your overall sense of well-being. Draw parallels to nursing.

Exercise Two

List all the *personal* variables that enable you to care for your patients responsibly (eg, coming to work rested, honestly caring about patients) and that impede your ability to do this (eg, you come to work but are mentally and emotionally back home with some other problem, such as difficulties with spouse, sick child).

Positive Personal Variables	Negative Personal Variables

Next, list all the *system* variables that enable you to care for your patients responsibly (eg, patient assignments are matched to your developing level of expertise, good team spirit among caregivers and their willingness to work together to meet complex patient needs) and that impede your doing this (eg, student assignments are unrealistic, chronic understaffing results in staff being unavailable to direct students, sense in the healthcare institution that management has "given up" and is no longer concerned about the quality; that the bottom line is always money).

Positive System Variables	Negative System Variables

Finally, list *patient* variables that positively and negatively influence your ability/willingness to care for your patients responsibly (eg, patient looks like me, patient is pleasant and makes few demands, patient has strong potential for complete recovery, or patient is homeless, has a history of self-abuse).

(continued)

APPLYING LEARNING TO PRACTICE (Continued)

Positive Patient Variables	Negative Patient Variables

Talk about how you plan to address the negative variables that interfere with your ability to care for patients responsibly. What does it mean to be accountable to yourself, your patients, the nursing profession, and society?

Exercise Three

Role play each of the scenarios below, and discuss how the nurse responds (or fails to respond) is likely to influence the patient. It would be helpful to discuss how you think nurses on your unit *would* respond to this type of situation and how you think they *should* respond. If these differ, discuss why.

1. You suspect from the blood pressure reading you just obtained that the elderly clinic patient you are examining is not taking his medication or complying with other aspects of the treatment plan. "I try to take 'em but sometimes I forgets." The clinic is understaffed, and you have many more patients to see, some of whom have waited for more than an hour.
2. You tell the resident that you don't think the pain medication one woman with metastatic cancer is receiving is adequate, and the resident tells you that it's a more than adequate dose.
3. Another nurse tells you that he's utterly frustrated because Dr. Braxton refuses to talk with a patient about advance directives because, "It might depress her." You share this nurse's belief that the patient wants to participate in decision making and that it is very possible that she will lose the ability to do this soon.
4. You are making a home visit to a 32-year-old man with end-stage AIDS. He tells you that he is tired of fighting, has no money, and no longer wants to be a bother to his friends. He asks you what he can do to end his life.

Exercise Four

Review each of the above four situations, and discuss with your colleague the legal implications of being accountable. What legal safeguards would you recommend?

Exercise Five

Name one thing about your practice that you have decided to change as a result of this session.

Reporting Incompetent, Unethical, or Illegal Practices

Each employing institution or agency providing nursing services has an obligation to establish a process for the reporting and handling of practices by individuals or by healthcare systems that jeopardize a patient's health or safety. The ANA Code for Ethics obligates nurses to report professional conduct that is incompetent, unethical, or illegal. For nurses, incompetent practice is measured by nursing standards, unethical practice is evaluated in light of professional codes of ethics, and illegal practice is identified in terms of violations of law. Parameters for evaluating each follow.

> *Parameters of competent nursing practice:* State Nurse Practice Acts and Regulations, the Scope of Practice, Professional Standards of Nursing Practice, and other practice guidelines and protocols
>
> *Parameters of ethical nursing practice:* Professional Codes of Ethics
>
> *Parameters of legal nursing practice:* Federal and State Health Regulations, Pharmacy Laws, Occupational Safety and Health Administration Standards and Regulations, Medical Records and Communicable Disease Laws, Environmental Laws, Centers for Disease Control and Prevention Guidelines, Antidiscrimination Laws, Service Facility Regulations, Clinical Improvement Act, and JCAHO regulations (ANA, 1994)

Whistle blowing refers to employees who report their employer's violation of the law to appropriate law enforcement agencies outside the employer's facilities. Citing the inadequacies of current laws to protect whistle blowers, the ANA offers the following caution: "because of the limits of current law, nurses should be advised that they may not be protected against retaliation for reporting the incompetent, unethical or illegal practices of their employers"(ANA, 1994, p. 12). Many individual nurses and nursing organizations are working to secure state and federal legislation to protect whistle blowers.

Assessing Blended Skills and Critical Thinking

Nurses who are sincerely committed to quality care learn early to make self-evaluation an integral part of their nursing practice. Self-evaluation skills promote professional development, enhance self-esteem, and help one develop self-awareness. The nurse who is just beginning to develop in the caregiver role may find it helpful to conclude each caregiving experience with a brief moment of reflection that identifies and celebrates the nursing skills used and targets skills that need to be developed. This practice can keep one from feeling overwhelmed by everything that remains to be mastered and yet strongly motivated to learn new skills.

This chapter concludes with an assessment tool you can use to assess your proficiency in the skills essential for competent use of the nursing process (see the accompanying box: Take the Challenge). After completing the exercise, share your self-evaluation with a trusted colleague or clinical instructor and see whether your assessments of your abilities agree. Celebrate your natural and developed strengths. Begin now to plan a strategy to boost those skills

in which you are deficient. This may sound trite, but it is true: your patients will be grateful you cared enough to be your best.

Identified in the patient care studies that conclude the clinical chapters in this text are the specialized knowledge and skills that the nurse needs to implement the plan of care. It is helpful when planning care to identify what nursing resources are needed to ensure you are able to meet each challenge. Nurses sensitive to mastering both the art and the science of nursing care evaluate whether they have the prerequisite skills for each nurse–patient encounter as well as the skills needed to perceive, respond to, and appreciate the uniqueness of each patient. Quality care is each nurse's responsibility.

Take the Challenge

Read the professional behaviors below, and circle the number that best reflects the proficiency you now have in each of these essential nursing competencies.

1 = no skills
2 = somewhat skilled
3 = moderately skilled
4 = well skilled
5 = excellent skills

Cognitive Competencies

1	2	3	4	5	• Offer a scientific rationale for the plan of care.
1	2	3	4	5	• Select those nursing interventions that are most likely to yield desired outcomes.
1	2	3	4	5	• Use critical thinking to problem solve creatively.

Technical Competencies

1	2	3	4	5	• Use technical equipment with sufficient competence and ease to achieve goal with a minimum of distress to involved participants.
1	2	3	4	5	• Creatively adapt equipment and technical procedures to the needs of particular patients in diverse circumstances.

Interpersonal Competencies

1	2	3	4	5	• Creative use of look, speech, and touch to communicate respect and enhance sense of worth
1	2	3	4	5	• Skilled use of presence and conversation to demonstrate empathy and to obtain sufficient knowledge about the patient to personalize care and serve as an effective advocate
1	2	3	4	5	• Responsible, competent attentiveness to the holistic needs of patients such that trust is built and patients experience comfort of security
1	2	3	4	5	• Value mutual enrichment of both participants in the nurse–patient relationship

Ethical/Legal Competencies

1	2	3	4	5	• Self-motivated to act in ways that advance the interests of patients (consistently trustworthy)
1	2	3	4	5	• Accountable for practice to self, patients served, the caregiving team, and society
1	2	3	4	5	• Consistently serve as effective patient advocate
1	2	3	4	5	• Skilled in mediating ethical conflict among the patient, significant others, healthcare team, and other interested parties
1	2	3	4	5	• Practice nursing faithful to the tenets of professional codes of ethics
1	2	3	4	5	• Use legal safeguards that reduce the risk of litigation

Learning Outcomes

After completing this chapter, the learner should be able to accomplish the following:

1. Define the key terms used in the chapter:

   assess
   cognitively skilled
   critical thinking
   ethically and legally skilled
   evaluate
   implement
   interpersonally skilled
   intuitive problem solving
   nursing diagnoses
   nursing process

   plan
   scientific problem
      solving
   standards for critical
      thinking
   technically skilled
   trial-and-error problem
      solving
   whistle blowing

2. Describe the historic evolution of the nursing process.
3. Describe the nursing process and each of its five steps.
4. List five characteristics of the nursing process.
5. List three patient and three nursing benefits of using the nursing process correctly.
6. Describe the four blended skills essential to nursing practice.
7. Use a model of critical thinking when making clinical judgments and decisions.
8. Identify four habits that assist in the development of technical skills.
9. Describe a personal plan to develop the interpersonal skills essential to quality care.
10. Explain the relationship between a nurse's sense of accountability and the patient's well-being.
11. Identify personal strengths and weaknesses in light of nursing's essential knowledge and skills.

Critical Thinking Exercises

1. A nursing student realizes that her college roommate's behavior has changed dramatically during the past month. Once outgoing and funny, she is now withdrawn and moody and rebuffs efforts to discuss the change. Compare and contrast the processes and likely outcomes of using different methods of problem solving (trial-and-error, scientific, intuitive) and the nursing process to address the roommate's needs.

2. The nursing process is an interpersonal process that is always *patient centered* rather than *task centered*. Discuss with other students the meaning of this claim. Think through (and discuss) the implications of approaching patients as "problems to be solved."

3. Describe how you would structure an assessment of the situation described below, using critical thinking considerations: purpose of thinking, adequacy of knowledge, potential problems, helpful resources, and critique of judgment/decision.

   • A 28-year-old woman is admitted to a hospital for multiple contusions and a hairline fracture of the skull. She claims that she "fell down the steps," but on examination, it appears that several of the injuries are inconsistent with a fall. The woman sticks to her story that her fall was an accident. You are her nurse.

   • Assess whether your attitudes and dispositions would help or hinder the task of critical thinking if you were the nurse in this situation. Share your self-evaluation with another student, and compare your responses.

4. Using the above scenario, identify the cognitive, technical, interpersonal, and ethical/legal skills you would need to meet the nursing needs of this woman. If possible, compare your list with that of an experienced nurse, and discuss the differences.

Bibliography

Aiken, T. D., & Catalano, J. T. (1994). *Legal, ethical, and political issues in nursing.* Philadelphia: F. A. Davis.

Alfaro, R. (1998). *Applying nursing process: A step-by-step guide* (4th ed.). Philadelphia: Lippincott Williams & Wilkins.

Alfaro-LeFevre, R. (1999). *Critical thinking in nursing: A practical approach.* Philadelphia: W. B. Saunders.

American Association of Colleges of Nursing. (1998). *Essentials of baccalaureate education for professional nursing.* Washington, DC: Author.

American Nurses Association. (1980, 1995). *Nursing: A social policy statement.* Washington, DC: Author

American Nurses Association. (1985). *Code for nurses with interpretive statements.* Kansas City, MO: Author.

American Nurses Association. (1994). *Guidelines on reporting incompetent, unethical or illegal practices.* Washington, DC: ANA.

American Nurses Association Congress for Practice. (1973; revised 1991). *Standards of practice.* Washington, DC: Author.

Aroskar, M. A. (1993). Incompetent, unethical or illegal practice—teaching students to cope. *Journal of Professional Nursing, 9*(3), 130.

Atkinson, J., & Murray, M. E. (1990). *Understanding the nursing process* (4th ed.). New York: Macmillan.

Benner, P. (1984). *From novice to expert.* Menlo Park, CA: Addison-Wesley.

Benner, P., & Wrubel, J. (1989). *The primacy of caring in health and illness.* Menlo Park, CA: Addison-Wesley.

Brooks, K. L. (1993). Critical thinking in clinical practice. *Holistic Nursing Practice, 7*(3), vi-80.

Chafree, J. (1990). *Thinking critically* (3rd ed.). Boston: Houghton Mifflin.

Christensen, P. J., & Kenney, J. W. (1994). *Nursing process: Application of conceptual models* (4th ed.). St. Louis: C. V. Mosby.

Craft-Rosenberg, M. & Delaney. (1997). Nursing diagnosis extention and classification (NDEC). In M. J. Rantz & D. LeMone (Eds.) *Classification of Nursing Diagnoses: Proceedings of the Twelfth Conference North American Nursing Diagnosis* (pp. 26–31). Glendale, CA: CINAHL Information Services.

Davies, E. (1995). Reflective practice: A focus for caring. *Journal of Nursing Education, 34*(4), 167–174.

Ennis, R. H. (1996). *Critical thinking.* Upper Saddle River, NJ: Prentice-Hall.

Fonteyn, M. E., & Cooper, L. F. (1994). The written nursing process: Is it still useful to nursing education? *Journal of Advanced Nursing, 19*(2), 315–319.

Gebbie, K., & Lavin, M. A. (1974). Classification of nursing diagnosis. *American Journal of Nursing, 74*, 250–253.

Hall, L. E. (1955). Quality of nursing care. Address given at the Department of Baccalaureate and Higher Degree Programs of the New Jersey League for Nursing. *Public Health News* (June). New Jersey: New Jersey State Department of Health.

Heinrich, K., & Killeen, M. E. (1993). The gentle art of nurturing yourself. *American Journal of Nursing, 93*(10), 41–44.

Iowa Intervention Project. (1997). Nursing interventions classification (NIC): An overview. In M. J. Rantz & P. LeMone (Eds.), *Classification of Nursing Diagnoses: Proceedings of the Twelfth Conference, North American Nursing Diagnosis* (pp. 32–39). Glendale, CA: CINAHL Information Systems.

Jacono, B. J., & Jacono, J. K. (1995). A holistic approach to teaching responsibility and accountability. *Nurse Educator, 20*(1), 20–23.

Johnson, J. (1994). A dialectical examination of the nursing art. *Advances in Nursing Science, 17*(1), 1–14.

Johnson, M., & Mass, M. L. (Eds.) (1997). *Nursing outcomes classification (NOC).* St. Louis: Mosby–Year Book.

Joint Commission on Accreditation of Healthcare Organizations. (1999). *Accreditation manual for hospitals.* Oakbrook Terrace, IL: Author.

Kataoka-Yahiro, M. (1994). A critical thinking model for nursing judgment. *Journal of Nursing Education, 33*(8), 351–356.

Kolcaba, K. Y. (1995). The art of comfort care. *Image—The Journal of Nursing Scholarship, 27*(4), 287–289.

Locsin, R. C. (1995). Machine technologies and caring in nursing. *Image—The Journal of Nursing Scholarship, 27*(3), 201–203.

McCloskey, J. C., & Bulechek, G. M. (Eds.) (1996). *Nursing intervention classification (NIC)* (2nd ed). St. Louis: Mosby–Year Book.

Miller, M. A., & Babcock, D. E. (1996). *Critical thinking applied to nursing.* St. Louis: C. V. Mosby.

Paul, R. W. (1993). *Critical thinking: How to prepare students for a rapidly changing world.* Santa Rosa, CA: Foundation for Critical Thinking.

Renz, M. C. (1993). Learning from intuition. *Nursing, 23*(7), 44–45.

Rew, L. (1987). Nursing intuition: Too powerful—and too valuable—to ignore. *Nursing, 17*(7), 43–45.

Rubenfeld, M. G., & Scheffer, B. K. (1999). *Critical thinking in nursing: An interactive approach* (2nd ed.). Philadelphia: Lippincott Williams & Wilkins.

Schraeder, B. D., & Fischer, D. K. (1986). Using knowledge to make clinical decisions. *MCN, 11*, 161–163.

Stark, J. (1995). Critical thinking: Taking the road less traveled. *Nursing, 25*(11), 53–56.

Taylor, C. (1995). Rethinking nursing's basic competencies. *Journal of Nursing Care Quality, 9*(4), 1–13.

Wilkinson, J. (1992). *Nursing process in action: A critical thinking approach.* Redwood City, CA: Addison-Wesley Nursing.

Yura, H., & Walsh, M. B. (1967, 1988). *The nursing process: Assessing, planning, implementing, evaluating* (5th ed.). Norwalk, CT: Appleton-Century-Crofts.

Chapter 15
Assessing

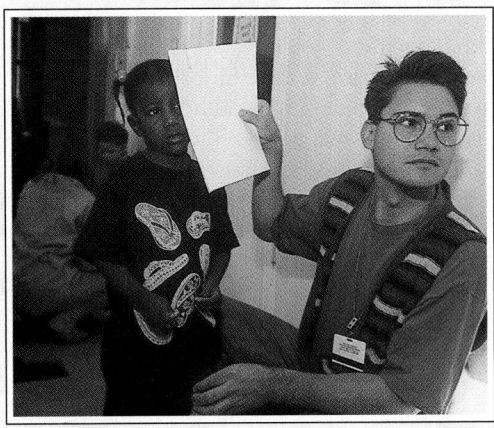

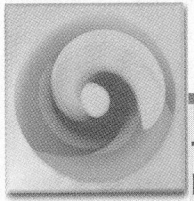

**Thinking Critically About
Nursing's Blended Skills**

Before reading this chapter, think about the types of skills you will need to develop to prepare yourself to assess patients with different types of health problems in different settings.

- You are working in a community-based well-child clinic. You become concerned when you observe negligible height and weight gains, delayed developmental milestones, and lethargy in a toddler brought to the clinic by her grandmother.

- You are working with a school nurse. Statistics reveal a pattern of teen smoking in your high school, and you are charged with developing an initiative to reverse this trend.

- You are doing a rotation on a medical floor in a hospital and learn that many of the diabetic patients being treated are repeat admissions with a history of poor self-care behavior.

- You are working in a nursing home where one alert resident with multiple chronic conditions repeatedly tells you that she has no reason to live and asks you to help her end her life.

What cognitive, technical, interpersonal, and ethical/legal skills do you think you will need to meet the everyday assessment challenges of these individuals and groups?

Assessing is the systematic and continuous collection, validation, and communication of patient data; these **data** reflect how health functioning is enhanced by health promotion or compromised by illness. A **database** includes all the pertinent patient information collected by the nurse and other healthcare professionals. The database enables a comprehensive and effective plan of care to be designed and implemented for the patient. The collection of patient data is a vital step in the nursing process because the remaining steps depend on complete, accurate, factual, and relevant data.

The initial comprehensive nursing assessment results in baseline data that enable the nurse to make a judgment about a patient's health status, ability to manage his or her own healthcare, and need for nursing; to refer the patient to a physician or other healthcare professional, if indicated; and to plan and deliver individualized, holistic nursing care that draws on the patient's strengths. In addition to an initial assessment of the patient, ongoing assessments are made by the nurse. Ongoing nursing assessment alerts the nurse to changes in the patient's responses to health and illness and suggests necessary changes in the plan of nursing care or care offered by other healthcare professionals. Ongoing nursing assessments may be problem focused, time lapsed, or emergency based.

During the assessment step of the nursing process, the nurse establishes the database by interviewing the patient to obtain a nursing history. The nurse may also perform a nursing examination to collect data. Other sources of patient information used by the nurse include the patient's support people, the patient record, the patient's healthcare professionals, and nursing and other healthcare literature. After the nurse has established the database, data about the patient are collected continuously because the patient's health status can change quickly. Questionable data are verified (validated) as part of the assessment step of the nursing process. All pertinent data are recorded and, when appropriate, communicated to other healthcare professionals so that the data can best benefit the patient (Fig. 15-1).

Unique Focus of Nursing Assessment

When nurses make nursing assessments, they do not duplicate medical assessments. Medical assessments target data pointing to pathologic conditions, whereas nursing assessments focus on the patient's responses to health problems. Is there, for example, interference with the patient's ability to meet basic human needs? Can the patient perform the activities of daily living? Although the findings from a nursing assessment may contribute to the identification of a medical diagnosis, the unique focus of nursing assessments is on the patient's responses to actual or potential health problems.

Data Collection

Types of Data

There are two types of data: subjective and objective. **Subjective data** are information perceived only by the affected person; these data cannot be perceived or verified by another person. Examples of subjective data are feeling ner-

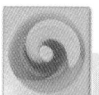

COGNITIVE SKILLS

- Knowledge of theories of growth and development, the clinical manifestations of failure to thrive, theories related to teen smoking and effective interventions, diabetic self-care and related intervention strategies, and developmental crises related to aging and end-of-life

TECHNICAL SKILLS

- Strong physical assessment skills to diagnose health problems related to failure to thrive, teen smoking, and diabetic complications
- Competence in particular skills may be needed, such as computerized documentation systems

INTERPERSONAL SKILLS

- Strong people skills to establish trusting relationships with the toddler and her grandmother, school nurse and high school

students, diabetic patients, and alert resident who wants to die

- Special interpersonal competence to mobilize the individuals involved in these scenarios to make the lifestyle changes that will result in improved levels of self-care or care for others

ETHICAL/LEGAL SKILLS

- First and foremost a strong sense of accountability for the health and well-being of these individuals. This translates into a commitment to getting them the help they need to achieve their health goals—within the scope of your nursing responsibilities and available resources
- Advocacy skills and the willingness to use them for vulnerable populations: toddler, teens, diabetics with poor history of self-care, and nursing home resident
- Knowledge of the ethical and legal principles that guide decision making about nurse-assisted suicide

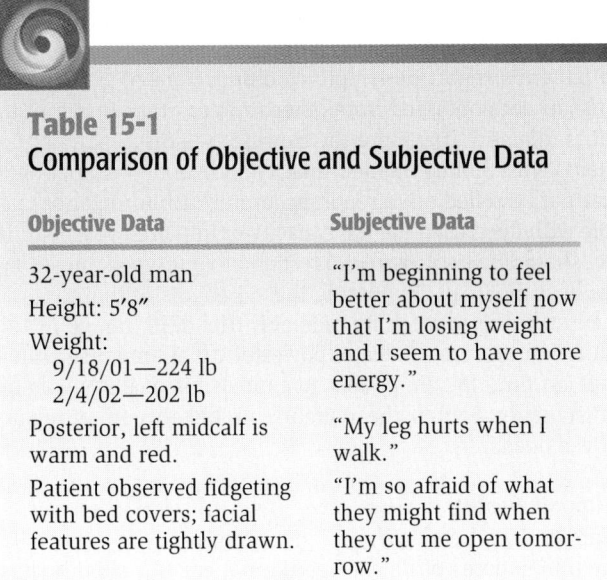

Figure 15-1
Assessing. The primary source of patient information is the patient. Resources include the patient's support people, the patient record, information from other healthcare professionals, and information from nursing and healthcare literature.

Assessing
• Identify assessment priorities determined by the purpose of the assessment and the patient's condition
• Prioritize types of data to be collected systematically
• Establish the database
  – nursing history
  – nursing examination
  – review of the patient record and nursing literature
  – consultation with the patient's support persons and healthcare professionals
• Continuously update the database
• Validate data
• Communicate data

Diagnosing

Evaluating

Planning

Implementing

vous, nauseated, or chilly and experiencing pain. Subjective data also are called symptoms or covert data.

Objective data are observable and measurable data that can be seen, heard, or felt by someone other than the person experiencing them. Objective data observed by one person can be verified by another person observing the same patient. Examples of objective data are an elevated temperature reading (eg, 101°F), skin that is moist, and refusal to look at or eat food. Objective data also are called signs or overt data (Table 15-1).

Characteristics of Data

When collecting and recording patient data, nurses should be complete, accurate, factual, and relevant.

Complete
As much as possible, all the patient data needed to understand a patient health problem and develop a plan of care to maximize health and well-being should be identified. For example, knowing that a patient has lost weight is not fully meaningful until the nurse discovers (1) if the weight loss was intentional or unintentional, (2) if it was related to a change in eating or exercise patterns or to some underlying pathological condition, and (3) how the patient views and is responding to the weight loss.

Factual and Accurate
Both the patient and the nurse may intentionally or unintentionally misrepresent or distort patient information. For

example, a patient who values being thin may describe a weight gain of several pounds as the onset of obesity. Nurses concerned with accuracy and fact continually verify what they hear with what they observe using other senses and validate all questionable data. At the outset of data collection, it is crucial to determine whether the patient or caregiver who is supplying the data is reliable. When nurses suspect that their own personal bias or

Table 15-1
Comparison of Objective and Subjective Data

Objective Data	Subjective Data
32-year-old man Height: 5'8" Weight: 9/18/01—224 lb 2/4/02—202 lb	"I'm beginning to feel better about myself now that I'm losing weight and I seem to have more energy."
Posterior, left midcalf is warm and red.	"My leg hurts when I walk."
Patient observed fidgeting with bed covers; facial features are tightly drawn.	"I'm so afraid of what they might find when they cut me open tomorrow."

stereotyping is influencing their data collection, they should consult with another nurse. It is also best to describe observed behaviors rather than an interpretation of the behavior. Such a description may read: "Patient frequently is observed lying with his face to the wall. Attempts to engage him in conversation fail. He refused lunch today and ate only soup for dinner." On the other hand, the statement "Patient is depressed" is the nurse's interpretation of the patient's behavior; it is not a factual statement. Recording the patient's behaviors factually allows other healthcare professionals to explore causes of the behavior with the patient.

Relevant

Because recording comprehensive data can become an endless task, one challenge facing nurses is to determine *what type* of data and *how much* data to collect for each patient. This chapter describes ways to do this. The aim is to record concisely all pertinent data. Often, only experience teaches nurses what data are needed in specific cases.

Learning how to collect, validate, and communicate data that are complete, accurate, factual, and relevant is the focus of the remainder of this chapter.

Sources of Data

Patient

The patient is the primary and usually the best source of information. Unless specified otherwise, it is assumed that the data recorded in the nursing history were collected from the patient. Most patients are willing to share information when they know it is helpful for planning their care. Although data collected from the patient are usually accurate, the nurse should be alert for certain difficulties. For example, a patient who is acutely ill may not be able to communicate adequately if the pain is severe or consciousness is altered in any way. An emotionally upset patient may distort information; for example, patients who are fearful because they think their illness may threaten their work or life may deny certain symptoms or deliberately give misleading facts. If the nurse becomes aware that a patient's report of symptoms differs from physical findings or data obtained from other sources, it is important to note this and to explore the cause of the discrepancy. Patients with limited mental capacity and very young patients cannot be relied on to report accurately. Children and people with decreased mental capacity or impaired verbal ability should be encouraged to respond to interview questions as best they can. Bypassing these patients and automatically turning to a family member, friend, or caregiver for information communicates powerfully that the nurse either has no time for the patient to express his or her needs or mistakenly doubts the patient's ability to communicate these needs.

Support People

Family members, friends, and caregivers are especially helpful sources of data when the patient is a child or has limited capacity to share information with the nurse. Husbands and wives can supply information concerning their spouses. Friends often accompany a patient to a health agency and can supply useful information. Care must be taken to determine that the patient does not object to data being gathered from friends and that the friends want to participate. Also, there should be a clear understanding by the patient, family, and friends of the confidentiality of the data collected. Whenever data are gathered from support people, this should be indicated in the nursing history.

Patient Record

Records prepared by different members of the healthcare team provide information essential to comprehensive nursing care. The nurse should review records early when gathering data—in some instances, before the first contact with the patient. Such a review helps to focus the nursing assessment and to confirm and amplify information obtained from other sources.

The patient's health record or chart, which lists such information as age, sex, occupation, religious preference, next of kin, and financial status, is one type of record. The health record includes information entered by various healthcare professionals, such as physicians, social workers, dietitians, physiotherapists, and laboratory technicians. Nurses who want their care to be supportive of the patient as he or she responds to changes in health status must be familiar with the many sections of the patient record in addition to the documentation of the nursing plan of care and nursing notes. The following are important sources of data for the nurse.

Medical History, Physical Examination, and Progress Notes

These sources record the findings of physicians as they assess and treat the patient; they focus on identifying pathologic conditions and their causes and on determining the medical regimen for treatment.

Consultations

The patient's physicians may invite specialists to assess and work with the patient. Their focus is on identifying findings that help establish a medical diagnosis or on planning and executing the treatment regimen.

Reports of Laboratory and Other Diagnostic Studies

Reports of laboratory studies and other diagnostic tests, such as radiographs, offer the nurse objective data that can either confirm or conflict with data collected during the nursing history or examination. Results of diagnostic studies are helpful to physicians for establishing a diagnosis and monitoring the patient's response to treatment. The results of these same studies may also be helpful to nurses in evaluating the success of nursing interventions.

Reports of Therapies by Other Healthcare Professionals

Other healthcare professionals who interact with the patient also record their findings and note any progress the patient is making in their specific areas—for example, nutrition, physical therapy, or speech therapy. These reports help the nurse to assess the patient's progress and are useful when determining the patient's ability to return home and manage care independently.

Records of previous admissions for healthcare and records from other health agencies, such as a social service agency or a home healthcare agency, are also valuable sources of data. They contain information about the patient's previous medical or surgical problems and response patterns, which may be important determinants of the current plan of care.

Other Healthcare Professionals

Nurses can learn a great deal about a patient's normal health habits and patterns and response to illness by talking with other nurses, physicians, social workers, and others on the healthcare team (Fig. 15-2). Although such communication is always important, it can be crucial when patients are transferred from home to institution or from one hospital or institution to another. The only way to ensure continuity of care is to make special efforts to share pertinent information.

Nursing and Other Healthcare Literature

To obtain a comprehensive patient database, it may be necessary to consult the nursing and related literature on specific health problems. For example, if a nurse has not cared for a patient with Paget's disease before, it is important for him or her to read about the clinical manifestations of the disease and its usual progression in order to know what to look for when assessing the patient. In addition to information concerning the medical diagnoses, treatment, and prognosis, a literature review offers nurses important information about nursing diagnoses, developmental norms, and psychosocial and spiritual practices that is helpful when assessing and caring for patients.

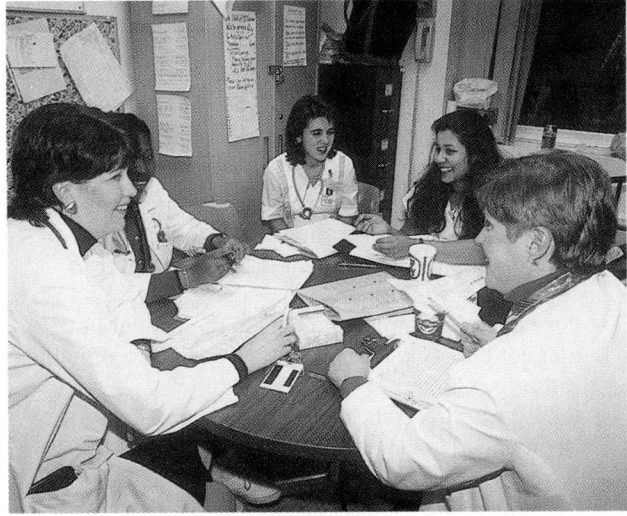

Figure 15-2
Nurses can learn a great deal about a patient's health habits and patterns and responses to illness by talking with other nurses, physicians, social workers, and other members of the healthcare team. This exchange of information is particularly important when patients transfer from one healthcare setting to another, or to home.

Data Collection Methods

Common methods used in the collection of data in nursing include observation, interview, and physical assessment.

Observation

Observation is the conscious and deliberate use of the five senses to gather data. Skilled nurses use each nurse–patient interaction to observe and interpret meaningful stimuli (data). Student nurses can develop such observation skills by training themselves to observe carefully the following each time they encounter a patient:

- What are the patient's current responses (physical and emotional) to his or her situation? Be alert to signs of distress—difficulty breathing, bleeding, pain, heightened anxiety—as well as anything out of the ordinary, such as sudden eruption of rash, changes in level of consciousness, and so forth.
- What is the patient's current ability to manage his or her care (need for additional information or nursing assistance)?
- What is the immediate environment? Consider the safety of the environment as well as the functioning of equipment (intravenous therapy, oxygen, drains). Who are the people in the room and home? What are the temperature and odor of the room?
- What is the larger environment (hospital or community)?

Interview

An **interview** is a planned communication. During the assessment step of the nursing process, the nurse interviews the patient to obtain a nursing history. Strong interviewing skills are needed to establish a successful working partnership with the patient, to communicate care and concern for the patient, and to obtain the necessary patient data. The interview can be understood in terms of its four phases, as described later.

Phases of the Interview

The four phases in the nurse–patient interview are the preparatory phase, introduction, working phase, and termination. More detailed information on interviewing techniques is provided in Chapter 21.

Preparatory Phase. Before initiating the interview, the nurse prepares to meet the patient by reading current and past records and reports, when available. During this phase, it is important not to let one's stereotypes and prejudices affect the nurse–patient relationship. Nurses who are aware of their own prejudices can deal with them constructively. Professional nurses learn to approach patients with open minds and to be sensitive to the human needs that underlie diverse behaviors.

During the preparatory phase, the nurse should ensure that the environment in which the interview is to be conducted is private and relaxed. Unless the patient wants family members or friends present during the interview, the nurse should interview the patient alone, either in the patient's room or in a quiet office.

Both the seating arrangement and the distance between nurse and patient are important (Fig. 15-3). Chairs placed at right angles to each other and about 3 to 4 feet (0.9 to 1.2 m) apart facilitate an easy exchange of information. If the patient is in bed, placing a chair at a 45-degree angle to the bed is helpful. If the nurse stands at the foot or side of the patient's bed and physically talks or looks down at the patient, a superior–inferior relationship is communicated and can negatively affect the interview. Whenever possible, it is best to communicate with patients at eye level.

The interview should be scheduled when both the nurse and the patient are free of concerns and distractions, so that they can concentrate on the task. Ten to 15 minutes may be all that is necessary in some circumstances, whereas an hour or more may be required in others. Information can be gathered in several meetings, especially if the nurse notices that the patient is tiring or is in pain.

Introduction. The interview's introduction is crucial because it sets the tone not only for the remainder of the interview but also for every following nurse–patient interaction. At the end of this phase of the interview, the patient should know the name of the primary nurse and what he or she can expect of nursing, should sense that the nurse is competent and cares about him or her, and should know what is expected of him or her in terms of developing the plan of care and participating in its execution.

The nurse initiates the interview by stating his or her name and status, identifying the purpose of the interview, and clarifying the roles of nurse and patient. A typical introduction might run like this: "Good afternoon, Miss LeBon. My name is Lisa Gray, and I'll be your student nurse. Right now I'd like to ask you a few questions about yourself so that we can plan your nursing care together. Feel free to respond only to those questions you feel comfortable answering, and know that your responses will be treated confidentially by the staff. This will take about 20 minutes.

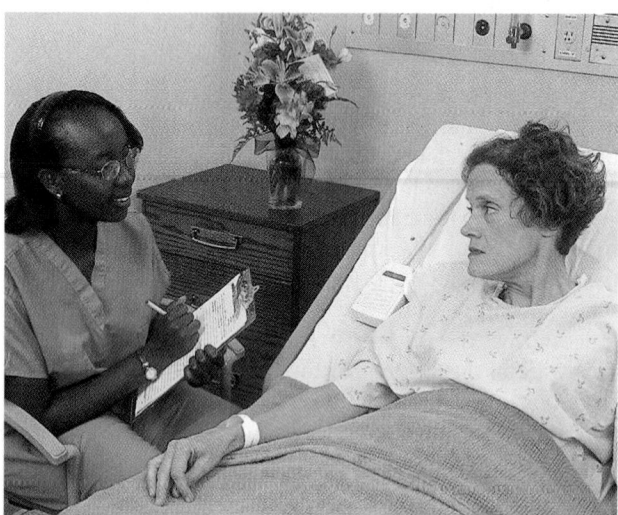

Figure 15-3
In the interview, both the seating arrangement and the distance from the patient are important in establishing a relaxed and comfortable environment for data collection. (Photo © Ken Kasper.)

Is this time convenient for you? Do you need anything before we start?"

The initial impression the nurse creates is crucial, especially with patients who are new to the healthcare environment. All nurses whom the patient encounters in the future may be judged in light of this first impression. When the nurse communicates respect and genuine concern for the patient, the patient is then encouraged to discuss health concerns and problems freely. The interpersonal qualities of a respectful presence, professionalism, and caring invite the patient's confidence and ensure the patient that help is available.

During the introduction, the nurse should assess the patient's comfort and ability to participate in the interview. It is also appropriate to assure the patient of confidentiality. The patient should know where the data being recorded are stored, how they will be used, and who has access to them. Some nurses record data on the appropriate form while with the patient, whereas other nurses take notes and complete the form later. Bedside computers are facilitating quick documentation. Documenting data should not interfere with the sharing of information during the interview, however. In unusual situations in which a contractual agreement that clearly identifies the responsibilities of both patient and nurse is indicated, terms are discussed at this time.

Working Phase. During the working phase of the interview, the nurse gathers all the information needed to form the subjective database. The accuracy, completeness, and relevance of the database depend on the nurse's use of the interviewing and basic communication techniques discussed in Chapter 21. The communication techniques highlighted below are important guidelines for a successful interview.

- Focus on the patient during the interview, demonstrating interest and concern: use the patient's name of choice, use eye contact appropriately, and avoid rushing the patient.
- Listen to the patient attentively; use reflection and paraphrase to communicate to the patient that you understand him or her.
- Ask about the patient's main problem first using terminology the patient understands; save personal or delicate questions for later when a rapport has been established. Defer less important questions until a later interview if the patient is too ill or upset to communicate easily.
- Pose questions and comments to the patient in the manner best suited to produce the desired communication (see Chap. 21):
  Closed questions elicit specific information.
  Open-ended questions allow the patient to verbalize freely.
  Reflective questions encourage the patient to elaborate on thoughts and feelings.
  Direct questioning can validate information, clarify information, or place events into a meaningful sequence.
- Avoid comments and questions that impede communication (see Chap. 21)—cliches, questions that

Through the Eyes of a Student

During my chronic medical–surgical rotation, my clinical group was placed on an oncology floor. My first thought was, "Oh no, not the cancer floor!" The word *fear* didn't even begin to describe how I felt. These patients had enough problems without some "green" nursing student aggravating them all day. I kept thinking these people are extremely ill and won't want to be bothered by my intruding questions.

Nonetheless, I knew I had to do it. Not only did I have to take care of this patient all day, I had to develop a database and plan of care. I knew I would have to do a lot more than give him his morning care and leave him alone. I would have to carry on an extended conversation with this patient to get all the information I needed.

As if all of this wasn't enough to make me throw in the white flag, when my patient assignment was given, I discovered my patient was a man only 1 year older than me. A 28-year-old man with terminal cancer—this was too scary!

Clinical day came, as I knew it would, and I was shaking. I walked in that room and together the patient and I planned his care. I explained to him the things I needed to talk about with him and I couldn't believe it—he didn't tell me to go away! We talked at length about his disease process and how it had affected his plans and goals. He opened up to me about his spirituality, his relationships with friends and family, and other personal subjects. Periodically, he would cringe, and I could tell it was time for a break. He was hurting too badly to go on at that time.

At the end of that day, my viewpoint was totally different than it had been that morning. I walked away from that room and off that floor feeling like I had made a difference for this person. We had shared a lot and he seemed so appreciative for the time I took to talk with him. The information he shared helped me to develop a better plan of care that was more responsive to his particular needs. The amazing part was that all I had to do was just be myself and allow him to do the same and our day flowed smoothly. The lesson I learned here was important for me: Keep calm and hold on to compassion, and nursing offers many rewards!

—NANCY E. DRISKILL,
SOUTHEAST MISSOURI STATE UNIVERSITY,
CAPE GIRARDEAU, MISSOURI

require a yes or no answer only, intimidating why or how questions, probing questions, giving advice, using judgmental comments, changing the subject, giving false assurance.
- Use silence and touch appropriately.

Many patient variables can positively or negatively affect the outcome of an interview. Table 15-2 identifies patient variables that can negatively influence an interview unless the nurse responds appropriately.

Termination. The successful interview is concluded carefully. A patient should be advised that the interview is coming to an end. It is helpful to recapitulate the interview, highlighting key points. Both the patient and the nurse should be satisfied that the important data are recorded. A helpful strategy is to ask the patient after the summary: "Is there anything else you would like us to know that will help us plan your care?" This gives the patient an opportunity to add data the nurse did not think to include.

Before leaving the patient, it is helpful to alert the patient as to what he or she can expect. The patient should also know when the nurse will reestablish contact, for example, "Thank you for answering these questions, Miss LeBon. Please feel free to keep us informed of anything you think we should know. I'll be leaving soon, but when I return tomorrow morning, I'll discuss your plan of care. This afternoon will be busy for you: some blood tests and a chest x-ray have been ordered. Your evening will probably be quiet. Do you have any questions? Is there anything else I can do for you before I leave?"

Techniques of Physical Assessment

Physical assessment is the examination of the patient for *objective data* that may better define the patient's condition and help the nurse in planning care. Four methods are used to collect data during a physical assessment: inspection, palpation, percussion, and auscultation. These techniques and the basic skills for physical assessment are described in Chapter 25.

Nursing History

Ideally, the nursing history captures the uniqueness of the patient and records this, so that care planning may be patterned to meet the patient's individual needs. The nursing history should therefore be obtained as soon as possible after a patient presents for care and should be followed by the nursing physical assessment. The **nursing history** should clearly identify the patient's strengths and weaknesses, health risks such as hereditary and environmental factors, and potential and existing health problems. The nursing history focuses on getting to know the *person*.

Components of a Nursing History
- Profile: name, age, sex, marital status, religion, occupation, education
- Reason for seeking healthcare
- Normal health habits and patterns and related needs for nursing assistance

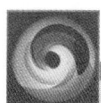

Table 15-2

Patient Variables That Can Negatively Influence an Interview and Suggested Nursing Responses

Patient Variables	Effect on Interview	Nursing Response
High anxiety	Patient may speak rapidly or incoherently and may jump from one topic to another; patient may deny or misrepresent what he or she is experiencing.	Normalize anxiety: "Many people find it difficult to talk about their health and become anxious"; approach patient gently, speak slowly and softly; underscore importance of the patient sharing what he or she is experiencing so nurses can help.
Pain	Patient offers clipped responses and "yes" or "no" answers whenever possible; overriding concern is pain relief.	Do everything possible to make patient comfortable before the interview, including obtaining an order for and administering pain medication; if pain persists, obtain only vital data and defer remainder of interview until patient is more comfortable.
Language difficulty (patient not fluent in nurse's language because patient speaks a different language, has a limited education, or fears saying the "wrong thing")	Vital patient data will not be communicated; patient may mistakenly be labeled "indifferent" or "noncommunicative."	Speak clearly (do not raise voice) using simple language; whenever possible, obtain the assistance of an interpreter (family member may help, but if patient data are confidential, a stranger may be preferable).
Previous negative experience with nurses or healthcare delivery system	Patient is aloof, unwilling to participate in interview; general attitude: "Why should I waste my time telling you anything . . . it won't do me any good."	"I know other people who have had a tough time with nurses or the system . . . life isn't perfect . . . but how about giving us a chance this time to show you what nurses can do?" Communicate respect for the patient and competence.
Unrealistic expectations of healthcare professionals	Patient expects nurses and other healthcare professionals magically to know everything about him or her and to "take care" of him or her; "surrenders" himself or herself to the system—"you know best" attitude.	Communicate clearly that no one knows or understands the patient like the patient does, and invite him or her to become involved in his or her care; "No two persons are alike, and unless you tell me a little more about yourself and how you are feeling, there is no way we'll be able to plan good care."

- Current state of health, functioning of body systems, and past medical and surgical history
- Current medications, allergies, and record of immunizations and exposure to communicable diseases
- Perception of health status and the meaning the patient attributes to health and illness and characteristic response or coping patterns
- Developmental history, family history, environmental history, and psychosocial history
- Patient's and family's expectations of nursing and of the healthcare team
- Patient's and family's ability and willingness to participate in the plan of care
- Patient's personal resources (strengths) and deficits

Nursing Physical Assessment

Physical assessment is the examination of the patient for *objective data* that may better define the patient's condition and help the nurse in planning care. The physical assess-

ment normally follows the nursing history and interview and may verify data gathered during the history or yield new data. There has been a great deal of controversy about nursing's role in the physical assessment of the patient, caused by concern that this is a duplication of medicine's role. Physicians traditionally have performed the intake physical assessment, which commonly is the mechanism of entry into the healthcare delivery system as well as the basis for medical treatment. Some nurses in advanced practice roles perform comprehensive intake physical assessments similar to their physician colleagues, which identify health and illness states, and then recommend or prescribe appropriate follow-up care. In any case, all nurses conduct selected aspects of physical assessment for nursing purposes.

Unlike the physical assessment performed by the physician to identify pathologic conditions and their causes, the nursing physical assessment focuses primarily on the patient's functional abilities. If a neurologic deficit is present, the nurse is concerned with identifying how this deficit affects the patient's reasoning and sensorimotor abilities. For example, a patient who has had a cerebrovascular accident (stroke) is examined to determine ability to comprehend and communicate information and execute the tasks of everyday life.

Purposes of the nursing physical assessment include the appraisal of health status, the identification of health problems, and the establishment of a database for nursing intervention (Fig. 15-4). See Chapter 25 for a detailed description of physical assessment skills.

Nurses practicing in different settings may use different physical assessment techniques for different purposes. Nurses in the coronary care unit use sophisticated, high-technology assessment techniques, whereas nurses in a rehabilitation center use a wide range of physical assessment skills that focus on identifying functional and nonfunctional response patterns to disabilities.

The nursing physical assessment involves the examination of all body systems in a systematic manner, commonly using a head-to-toe format. These data may be documented on a separate nursing physical assessment tool or incorporated into a combined database assessment form, as shown on pages 246–250. Nurses may also use physical assessment skills to evaluate selected body systems.

Planning Data Collection

Types of Nursing Assessments

Nursing assessments include the comprehensive initial assessment, the focused assessment, the emergency assessment, and the time-lapsed assessment.

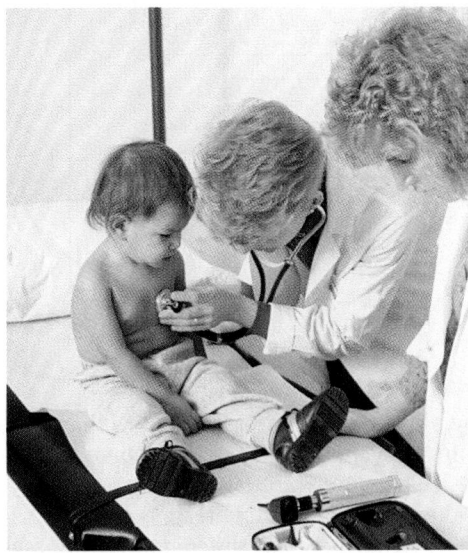

Figure 15-4
Two nurses provide a physical examination of a First Nations infant in a clinic. No matter what the setting or the age of the patient, the physical examination should include appraisal of health status, identification of health problems, and establishment of a database for nursing intervention. (Photo courtesy of Medical Services Branch, Health Canada.)

Initial Assessment

The **initial assessment** is performed shortly after the patient is admitted to a healthcare agency or service. Most institutions have policies specifying the time interval within which the assessment must be completed. The purpose of this assessment is to establish a complete database for problem identification and care planning. The nurse collects data concerning *all aspects* of the patient's health, establishing priorities for ongoing focused assessments and creating a reference for future comparison. A sample of an initial assessment structured according to Gordon's 11 functional health patterns appears in this chapter on pages 246–250.

Focused Assessment

In a **focused assessment,** the nurse gathers data about a *specific problem* that has already been identified (Alfaro, 1998, p. 41). A focused assessment may be done during the initial assessment if patient health problems surface, but it is routinely part of ongoing data collection. Another purpose of the focused assessment is to identify new or overlooked problems.

Emergency Assessment

When a physiologic or psychological crisis presents, the nurse performs an **emergency assessment** to identify life-threatening problems. A nursing home resident who begins choking in the dining room, a bleeding patient brought to the emergency room with a stab wound, an unresponsive patient in the rehabilitation unit, and a factory worker threatening violence are all candidates for an emergency assessment.

Time-Lapsed Assessment

The **time-lapsed assessment** is scheduled to compare a patient's current status to baseline data obtained earlier. Most patients in residential settings and those receiving nursing care over longer periods of time, such as homebound patients with visiting nurses, are scheduled for periodic time-lapsed assessments to reassess health status and to make necessary revisions in the plan of care.

Assessment Priorities

Before beginning to collect data on any patient, the nurse should have a good sense of the type of data needed to develop a satisfactory plan of care. Nurses spend more or less time on different components of the nursing history depending on the patient's reason for needing nursing assistance. For example, pediatric nurses are careful to establish the developmental age and milestones obtained by children admitted to a pediatric unit so that they can respect and promote these achievements. A school nurse who suspects child abuse pays careful attention to the child's statements about living conditions at home and relationships with family members and caregivers. A nurse preparing to discharge a patient from same-day surgery makes sure that the patient has the human and physical resources needed to supply appropriate postoperative care.

BRONSON METHODIST HOSPITAL
Kalamazoo, Michigan

Medical/Surgical–Critical Care Admission Assessment

A. Name: *Margaret Tembra*
Prefers to be called: *Mrs. Tembra*   Age: *72*
Date: *9/2/02*   Time of arrival to unit: *2:00 pm*
Mode of admission: *wheelchair*
I.D. bracelet on and coincides with addressograph: ☑ Yes ☐ No Information given by: *patient and her daughter Lisa*
If unable to reach next of kin/legal guardian, contact: *Barbara Tembra*   Phone: *634-5221*
Valuables (list and state disposition): *eye glasses (at bedside); purse taken home by daughter Lisa; no other valuables*
Admitted from: ☑ Home ☐ Nursing Home ☐ Assisted Living ☐ Foster Care ☐ Senior Citizens' Apartments ☐ Other
Facility Name: ____   Adm. Medical Diagnosis: *T.I.A.*

(handwritten calculations in left margin: 63.6 ×2.2 / 127.2 / 1272 / 139.92 ℔)

B. Ht: *5'2"*   Wt: *63.6* Kg
Temp: *98.2°F* ☑ Oral ☐ Ax. ☐ Rectal
Pulse: *88* ☐ Reg. ☑ Irreg.
Resp.: *18* ☑ Reg. ☐ Irreg.
BP: Left: *184/120*
   ☑ Lying ☐ Sitting ☐ Standing
   Right: *180/120*
   ☑ Lying ☐ Sitting ☐ Standing

C. (The following have been explained):

	Yes	N/A		Yes	N/A
Call system/bed-bathroom	☑		Floor restrictions	☑	
Bed operation/siderails	☑		Visitation Policy	☑	
Bathroom/bedpan-urinal	☑		Lounge	☑	
TV/CH2/telephone	☑		Newspaper/mail	☑	
Meal/cafeteria hours	☑		Siderails policy	☑	
Smoking policy	☐	☑	Chaplain services	☑	

Signature: *Margaret Tembra*

D. Health Patterns Assessment: Complete information, **including patient's words.** Indicate N/A if non-applicable. Circle, code, or check all other findings as appropriate.

1. Reason for hospitalization/chief complaint: *"I fell in the kitchen this morning and couldn't move my left leg for awhile; I've also been having headaches".*
Recent illness/exposure to communicable disease: ____

Previous hospitalizations/surgeries: *about 1970 gall bladder surgery; hospitalized for high blood pressure 1989*
What other health problems have you had? ____

Things done to manage health: *"I drink lots of water, eat fruit and avoid fried foods. I try not to worry so much."*
Statement of patient's general appearance (include condition of hair, skin, nails): *Alert, medium-built, well-nourished female; appears anxious about hospitalization: voice low, grabs daughter's hand; neat appearance; skin pale, cool and dry; gray hair—thin, scalp clean; thick nails; adequate capillary refill.*
Tobacco use: ☐ Yes ☑ No ☐ Used to smoke: ____
EtOH use: *none*

Allergies: ☐ Yes (list with reaction experienced) ☑ No
Food: ____
Medications/anesthetics: ____
Other (e.g., wool, tape, pollens): *regular soaps cause skin to be excessively dry*

FORM 102 (Revised 10/84) — Page 1

(continued)

The purpose for which the assessment is being performed offers the best guidelines about what type and how much data to collect. Assessment priorities are influenced by the patient's health orientation, developmental stage, and need for nursing.

Health Orientation

Health assessments, such as Health-Style: A Self-Test in Chapter 4, may be used by nurses to assist patients to identify potential and actual health risks and to explore their habits, behaviors, beliefs, attitudes, and values that influence levels of wellness. Hill and Smith (1990) offer nurses a variety of specialized assessment tools that focus on relationships; psychological, environmental, and physical self-care; relaxation; spirituality; humor and play; movement and exercise; sleep and dreams; nutrition; and sexuality. These assessments are different from the assessments of patients being hospitalized for disease-related treatment in terms of the type of patient data gathered.

Developmental Stage

Nursing assessments are modified according to the developmental needs of patients. For example, when assessing an infant, special attention is given to weight gain and physical

Patient's Name: _Tembra, Margaret_   Hospital No.: _4629 F_   Date: _9/2/02_

Medications: (e.g., prescript., non-prescript.) ☑Yes ☐No Did you bring? ☐Yes ☑No Taken home? ☐Yes ☐No ☐N/A

NAME	DOSE	SCHEDULE	REASON	PRESCRIBING PHYSICIAN
hydralazine	?	OD	high blood pressure	Dr. Skomar
aspirin	tt	PRN	headaches	—
metamucil	1 Tbsp	PRN	constipation	—

Have you been taking your medication(s) as prescribed? _yes_

OTHER PERTINENT DATA: _—_ | SCT | initials

NUTRITION / METABOLIC

2. Special diet? _—_   Supplements: _—_
Pattern of daily food/fluid intake: _Drinks at least 5-6 glasses H₂O daily + juices, + tea;_ _↓ fried, fatty foods; likes baked or broiled meat, vegetables + fruit "sweet tooth."_
Appetite: _"very good."_   Wt. loss/gain: _—_
Nausea/Vomiting: _—_
GI pain: _—_
Condition of oral mucous membranes: _pink, moist_
Dental condition: _dentures clean_   Dentures: ☑Upper ☑Lower ☐Partial ☐N/A
Skin: ☐Warm ☑Dry ☑Cool ☐Moist ☐Other: _pale_
Turgor: ☑Supple ☑Firm ☐Fragile ☐Dehydrated ☐Other: _—_
Color: ☐Pink ☑Pale ☐Dusky ☐Cyanotic ☐Jaundiced ☐Mottled ☐Other: _—_
Edema: _+ 1 ankles_
Wounds/drains/dressings: _—_
Skin problems (description and location): _skin on legs and upper arms dry + scaley;_ _scratch marks; reddened area under left breast – skin intact_
I.V.'s: _—_   ☐N/A
OTHER PERTINENT DATA: _—_ | SCT | initials

ELIMINATION

3. Abd. tenderness/guarding/distention: _—_
Bowel sounds: _present all 4 quadrants_   Stoma (type): _—_
Any problems with hemorrhoids/involuntary stool? _hx hemorrhoid 2° straining/constipation_
Usual bowel pattern (frequency, character, consistency, etc.): _Stools tend to be hard and dry --_
q 2-3 days   Date of last BM: _9/1/02_
If problem, describe: _occasional (1x/wk) constipation_
Use of anything to manage bowels (e.g., laxatives, enemas, suppositories, "home remedies", anti-diarrheals): _↑ fluids, ↑ fruit, metamucil; dislikes bran_
Usual urinary pattern (frequency, character, amount, incontinence, nocturia, etc.): _5-6 x per day;_ _up once at night to void_
Last void (time): _"this Am"_
If problem, describe: _—_
Perspiration/nocturnal sweats: _—_
OTHER PERTINENT DATA: _—_ | SCT | initials

FORM 102 (Revised 10/84) — Page 2

(continued)

growth, feeding and elimination problems, sleep–activity cycles, and the parenting skills of caregivers. When children are hospitalized, it is similarly important to note how independent the child is with basic care measures (toileting, hygiene, dressing, eating), what words the child uses to indicate the need to void and defecate, play preferences, and so forth.

Need for Nursing

Whether nurses will be interacting with the patient for a short or a long period (eg, same-day surgery versus surgery that necessitates a long recovery in an intensive care unit) and the nature of nursing care needed by the patient (eg, assistance with the birth of a baby versus support and home care throughout a terminal illness) both powerfully influence the type of data the nurse collects. A general guideline when assessing patients is to gather only data that are helpful when planning and delivering care. It would be inappropriate, for example, to collect a detailed sexual history on a patient admitted to the hospital overnight after a slight concussion. Conversely, a nurse should not fail to ask a pregnant woman admitted to the hospital for observation because of bleeding during her first trimester whether she has any questions about resuming sexual activity after she gets home.

4. Peripheral pulses: _palpable, strong_

☐ N/A

Neurovascular check (e.g., capillary refill) _↓ sensation (hot/cold, sharp/dull) L leg; rapid capillary refill_

Chest pain/radiation: _____

Jugular vein distention: ☐ Yes ☑ No

Hx of murmur: ☐ Yes ☑ No

Pacemaker: ☐ Yes ☑ No

Presence of A-V Shunt: _____ ☑ No

Arterio-venous bruit: _____ ☑ N/A

Monitor/rhythm: _____ ☑ N/A

Hemodynamic monitoring: _____ ☑ N/A

Tembra, M., 4269 F

CARDIO-VASCULAR STATUS

Respiratory pattern: ☑ No problem ☐ Dyspnea ☐ Nocturnal Dyspnea ☐ S.O.B. at rest

☐ S.O.B. on exertion: _____ ☐ Other: _____

Lung sounds: _clear_ Use of accessory muscles? ☐ Yes ☑ No

Cough/production: _____ O₂ supplement: _____ ☑ N/A

Resp. tubes (e.g., ET, trach, chest/describe secretions/drainage): _____ ☑ N/A

Ventilatory assistance: _____ ☑ N/A

RESPIRATORY STATUS

Use the **Activity Level Code** below to assess admission statuses:

	ADL Status		**Mobility Status**	
0–total independence	Feeding _set up tray_	Meal Preparation _—_	Bed mobility _2_	
1–assist with device	Bathing _2_	Cleaning _—_	Cart transfer _bedrest_	
2–assist with person	Dressing _0_	Shopping _—_	Chair/toilet transfer _bedrest_	
3–assist with device & person	Grooming _0_	Laundry _—_	Ambulation _bedrest_	
4–total dependence	Toileting _1_	Other _—_	R.O.M. _2_	

Handedness: ☑ Right ☐ Left

Able to use? ☑ Yes ☐ No

Reasons for ADL/Mobility limitations: _Bedrest ordered during diagnostic work-up; At present able to move all 4 extremities_ ☐ N/A

Devices used for assist: _Bed pan_ ☐ N/A

Do you need assistance with transportation? ☐ Yes ☐ No If "Yes", specify: _—_

Where do you plan to be discharged? _home_ Will you need assistance? ☐ Yes ☑ No

If "Yes", describe: _____

OTHER PERTINENT DATA: _—_

SCT initials

ACTIVITIES OF DAILY LIVING/MOBILITY STATUS

ACTIVITY / EXERCISE

5. Level of consciousness: _Alert_ Oriented to: ☑ Person ☑ Place ☐ Time

Behaviors (describe): _Face reflects concern about 's morning's paralysis + hospitalization_

Hx of epilepsy/seizures/Parkinson's, etc.: _____

Reflexes: ☑ No problem ☐ Problem (If "No problem", do not complete this section.)

Eyes: Pupil size: r _O_ l _O_ Equal? ☑ Yes ☐ No Reaction to light: r _✓_ l _✓_

Accommodation: r _✓_ l _✓_ Deviation: _____

Handgrasp: r _✓_ l _✓_ Gag: _✓_ Swallow: _✓_

Movement of extremities: _↓ strength and ↓ movement left lower extremity_

REFLEXES

Eyes/sight: ☐ No problem ☑ Deficit _"blurry vision" at times_ Aid: _eyeglasses_

Ears/hearing: ☐ No problem ☑ Deficit _"hard of hearing" Ⓛ ear_ Aid: _none_

Nose/smell: ☑ No problem ☐ Deficit _____

Tongue/taste: ☑ No problem ☐ Deficit _____

Skin/touch: ☑ No problem ☐ Deficit _____

Numbness/tingling: ☐ No problem ☑ Deficit _left leg "feels queer – pins and needles"_

Dizziness: ☐ No problem ☑ Deficit _feels "slightly dizzy – unsteady"_

SENSORIUM

COGNITIVE / PERCEPTUAL

FORM 102 (Revised 10/84) — Page 3

(continued)

Practical Considerations

Data already collected from the patient and communicated in the patient record should not be repeatedly sought from the patient unless there is a need to validate them. Repetitious questioning can be annoying to the patient and may cause the patient to wonder about the lack of communication among healthcare professionals. A careful review of the patient record before interviewing the patient helps prevent this problem.

Before meeting a new patient, it is helpful to take a minute to think carefully about the type of data needed to plan quality care. After the comprehensive nursing assessment has been completed, patient health problems dictate assessment priorities for future nurse–patient interactions.

Structuring the Assessment

Because many different types of data are collected about patients, there is a need to structure data collection systematically. Using systematic guidelines specifically developed for a nursing assessment ensures that comprehensive,

Patient's Name: _Tembra, M._ Hospital No.: _4269 F_ Date: _9/2/02_

COGNITIVE / PERCEPTUAL

PAIN

Pain: ☐ No problem ☑ Problem (If "No problem", do not complete this section.)

If "Problem", describe location, type, intensity, onset, duration: _headaches – began about 6 months ago – of increasing frequency and severity ; at present occur 1-2 x / wk, last 1-2 days_

Methods of pain management: _Asprin, other OTC extra strength pain relievers only helps "a little"_

COGNITION

Primary language: _English_ Speech deficit: _—_ Aid: _—_

Any learning difficulties? _—_

OTHER PERTINENT DATA: _—_

| | | | SCT | initials |

6. SLEEP / REST

Usual sleep/rest pattern: _11 pm – 7 am_

Adequate? ☑ Yes ☐ No Factors affecting sleep/rest: _gets up to void once during night_

Methods to promote sleep: _—_

Hx of sleep disturbances: _—_

OTHER PERTINENT DATA: _—_

| | | | SCT | initials |

7. SELF-PERCEPTION / SELF-CONCEPT

Are there any ways you feel differently about yourself since you've been ill/hospitalized? _" never questioned my health " expresses fear_

Description of non-verbal behaviors: _quiet speech, wrinkled brow, wants daughter near_

OTHER PERTINENT DATA: _daughter reports mother has been very independent, strong woman – rarely ill_

| | | | SCT | initials |

8. ROLE / RELATIONSHIP

Marital status: _Widowed_ Children: _3_

Do you live? ☐ Alone ☑ With family ☐ Other: _lives with daughter Lisa + her family_

Family feelings regarding hospitalization: _Concern_

Who are the people that will help you most at this time? _2 daughters : Lisa, Barbara_

Are you presently employed? ☐ Yes ☑ No Occupation: _____ ☐ N/A

Are you presently in school? ☐ Yes ☑ No Will illness/hospitalization interfere? _____ ☐ N/A

Upon discharge, if necessary, will you be able to afford?

Medications: ☑ Yes ☐ No Supplies: ☑ Yes ☐ No Medical Care: ☑ Yes ☐ No

OTHER PERTINENT DATA: _Husband died 8 months ago – moved in with daughter 6 months ago after selling family home – High Stress_

| | | | SCT | initials |

9. SEXUALITY / REPRODUCTIVE

Female: ☐ N/A Menopausal: ☑ Yes ☐ No Menstrual pattern: _____ ☐ N/A

Problems/changes: _—_

Date of L.N.M.P. _____ ☑ N/A Possibly pregnant? ☐ Yes ☐ No ☐ N/A

Pregnancy history: _G 3 P 3_

Use of birth control measure ☐ Yes ☐ No ☑ N/A Type: _____

Any problems with use? _____

Monthly self-breast exam? ☐ Yes ☑ No ☐ N/A

Vaginal discharge/bleeding/lesions: _____

Receiving medical attention? ☐ Yes ☑ No ☐ N/A

OTHER PERTINENT DATA: _____

| | | | SCT | initials |

Male: ☑ N/A Prostate problems? _____

Monthly self-testicular exam? ☐ Yes ☐ No ☐ N/A

Penile discharge/bleeding/lesions: _____

Receiving medical attention? ☐ Yes ☐ No ☐ N/A

OTHER PERTINENT DATA: _____

| | | | | initials |

FORM 102 (Revised 10/84) — Page 4

(continued)

holistic data are collected for each patient and lead easily to the formulation of nursing diagnoses. When the nurse internalizes such assessment guidelines, it is easier to focus on the patient during the assessment rather than worrying about what to assess next.

Most schools of nursing and healthcare institutions have developed their own structured assessment guidelines, many of which are based on a selected nursing theory. The example used in this text is based on Gordon's functional health patterns (1987), a standardized structure for delineating the basic areas of assessment applicable to all patients and compatible with all nursing theories. This framework identifies 11 functional health patterns and organizes patient data into these patterns. The North American Nursing Diagnosis Association (NANDA) uses human response patterns to organize data collection. A nonnursing model used to organize data collection with which all nurses are familiar is the body systems model or "medical model." This method organizes data collection according to organ and tissue function in various body systems. Although it is helpful in formulating diagnoses related to physiologic problems, it neglects patient problems

10. Have you experienced any recent stressful situations in addition to your illness/hospitalization? ☑Yes ☐ No

If "Yes", please describe briefly: _In past year:_
death of husband
sale of family home
relocation with daughter

Are there any ways we can be of assistance? _"can't think of any"_

How do you usually manage stresses? _talk with friends, pray_
"I used to share everything with my husband"

What do you do for relaxation? _used to crochet, watch TV_

Support groups/counselling resources used: _____

Were they helpful? _____ ☐ N/A

OTHER PERTINENT DATA: _misses husband very much_

Tembra, M. 4269F

| | SCT | initials |

COPING/STRESS

11. Will illness/hospitalization interfere with any of the following?

Spiritual or religious practices? ☐ Yes ☑No

Cultural beliefs or practices? ☐ Yes ☑No

Familial traditions? ☐ Yes ☑No

If "Yes", to any of the above, please describe briefly: _____

Would you like your clergy or hospital chaplain to be contacted? ☑Yes ☐ No ☐N/A _daughter will contact minister_

OTHER PERTINENT DATA: _____

| | SCT | initials |

VALUE/BELIEF

E. Include: a. Possible nursing diagnostic concept labels to consider for care planning.
b. Possible referral resources to consider for discharge planning needs.
c. Other pertinent information

a. _Diagnostic labels: Colonic Constipation, High Risk for Impaired Physical_
Mobility, High Risk for Altered Health Maintenance Related to
Knowledge Deficit: TIA → stroke management, disturbance in
self-concept, skin integrity impairment

b. _Social Service Referral_
referral to home minister

| | | initials |

IMPRESSIONS

DATE	TIME	INITIALS	SIGNATURES	
9/2/02	2:00 pm	SCT	S. Carol Taylor, RN	(1st Adm. R.N.)
				(2nd Adm. R.N.)
				(3rd Adm. R.N.)
				(4th Adm. R.N.)

FORM 102 (Revised 10/84) — Page 5

©1984 Bronson Methodist Hospital. All rights reserved.

(continued)

and strengths in psychosocial and spiritual dimensions of health and well-being.

Problems Related to Data Collection

Common problems encountered during data collection include inappropriate organization of the database, omission of pertinent data, inclusion of irrelevant or duplicate data, erroneous or misinterpreted data, failure to establish rapport and partnership, recording an interpretation of data rather than observed behavior, and failure to update the database. Table 15-3 describes possible causes and remedies for such problems.

Data Validation

Validation is the act of confirming or verifying. The purpose of validating is to keep data as free from error, bias, and misinterpretation as possible. Validation is an impor-

Through the Eyes of a Student

As a first-year nursing student, I often questioned myself on my technique in assessing a patient. Sure, I understood what my instructors taught me, but was I doing it right? So I find my patient has an elevated temperature, or perhaps urinary output is scanty—but what does it all mean? I often wondered if I would be able to make sense of all this information, and would I *really* be able to detect a problem should one develop. Well, it works! Keep assessing, recording, and reporting.

During my second year (first semester), I realized how an assessment can aid in saving your patient's life. A continuous assessment for 2 days saved my 91-year-old patient. I detected early signs of pulmonary edema and congestive heart failure and was able to notify appropriate medical personnel and immediately implement life-saving procedures. Sure it was scary, but how proud I felt when the nursing staff congratulated me on a job well done! I realized how significant my assessment was for my patient, when as I stood with her in the radiology department, she looked up at me from her stretcher and thanked me for taking good care of her. Knowing my patient was aware of what I had done for her meant the world to me, and at this point, I realized why I had chosen the nursing profession.

—Delores (Dee) C. Pascale,
Delaware County Community College,
Media, Pennsylvania

tant part of assessment because invalid information can lead to inappropriate nursing care.

Because validation of all data is neither possible nor necessary, nurses need to decide which items need verification. For example, data need to be verified when there are discrepancies: a patient tells the nurse he is fine and has no concerns, but the nurse notes that he demonstrates tense body musculature and seems curt in his responses. When there is a discrepancy between what the person is saying and what the nurse is observing, validation is necessary to determine accuracy. Validation in this instance may take the form of the nurse saying, "You tell me you feel fine, but right now your body and behaviors are telling me something else. Tell me more about this."

Data also need verification when they lack objectivity. For example, a nurse suspects that the patient hears from one ear but does not seem to hear well from the other. The nurse should validate the data before proceeding and

should determine whether the patient does indeed have a hearing problem. Suspicions are not objective. In this instance, the nurse needs to test the patient's hearing in both ears. Speaking toward the suspected better ear, the nurse explains, "It seems to me that you hear better out of one ear than the other. I would like to test this. I'll bring a watch slowly toward your right ear first and then toward your left. Please look straight ahead and tell me when you first hear the watch ticking." The nurse then records how far the watch was from each ear when the patient first heard it ticking.

The nurse may validate data as they are collected or at the end of the data-gathering process. When it is clear that the data are correct, the nurse is ready to analyze the data and formulate nursing diagnoses—the next step of the nursing process.

Data Communication

The patient data collected by the nurse, both initially and as patient contact continues, are of no benefit to the patient and the healthcare team unless they are appropriately communicated. Appropriate communication involves correct timing and proper documentation.

Timing

Immediate verbal communication of data is indicated whenever assessment findings reveal a critical change in the patient's health status that necessitates the involvement of other nurses or healthcare professionals. The nurse who observes an elevated temperature of 103.2°F (39.5°C) in a patient scheduled for surgery that morning must report this to the charge nurse and to the surgeon, who might then cancel surgery. Failure to communicate this finding could result in the patient's receiving preoperative sedation, being taken to the operating room, and even having the surgery performed under less than optimal conditions. Similarly, a nurse who hears a patient making suicidal remarks must communicate this information to the healthcare team, so that all are alerted to the patient's danger and so that suicide precautions may be taken immediately.

A nurse who is unsure of the significance of a particular finding is well advised to consult with another nurse. In some situations, years of experience are needed to distinguish significant from nonsignificant findings. Neither ignorance nor the fear of appearing less than competent justifies failure to report critical data.

Documentation

The initial database should be entered into the computer or recorded in ink, using the designated agency forms, the same day the patient is admitted to the agency. If, for any reason, important data cannot be obtained during the initial

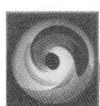

Table 15-3
Common Problems of Data Collection, Possible Causes, and Suggested Remedies

Problem	Possible Causes	Suggested Remedies
Database inappropriately organized	Failure to plan for the assessment by identifying needed data; use of inappropriate tools for data collection	Review the guidelines for specifying pertinent data. Consider modifying tool for data collection or select an alternative tool.
Pertinent data omitted	Not following up on cues during data collection; inappropriate guidelines	Identify potentially relevant factors in advance of collection. Practice interview strategies.
Irrelevant or duplicate data collected	Failure to identify specific purpose of data collection; failure to review available patient records; use of inappropriate tools for data collection	Determine specific purpose of data collection for each patient. Consider existing data before initiating collection. Consider modifying data collection tool or selecting alternative.
Erroneous or misinterpreted data collection	Failure to observe carefully or validate during data collection; interviewer prejudices or stereotypes	Sharpen observation skills by independently observing the same situation with a peer and comparing notes afterward. Role play several validation techniques.
Failure to establish rapport	Failure to establish sufficient rapport or use appropriate communication techniques with patient; failure to know what information is wanted	Review and practice communication techniques discussed in Chapter 21. Role play several explanations of purpose of data collection. Identify general data desired before collection.
Interpretation of data is recorded rather than the observed behavior	Nurse jumps to hasty conclusion about patient's behavior and deprives others of exploring with the patient possible causes of the behavior; deficient validation	Review the distinction between data and interpretation of data. Practice documenting observed patient behavior concisely.
Failure to update the database	Erroneous belief that assessment is concluded after the initial database is recorded; low priority attached to ongoing data collection	Recollect that it is impossible to give quality, individualized care without knowledge of changes in the patient's status. Ongoing data collection is critical to the deletion or modification of old problems and the identification of new problems.

assessment, this needs to be documented so that they are obtained as soon as possible. Objective and subjective patient data should be summarized and written, so that data communicate a unique sense of the patient and are comprehensive, concise, and easily retrievable. The data

Legal Alert

Nurses are responsible for alerting the appropriate healthcare professional whenever assessment data differ significantly from the patient's baseline, indicating a potentially serious problem. Interventions for which the nurse may be legally responsible include increasing the frequency of assessments and initiating necessary changes in the treatment regimen.

should be written legibly, and good grammar and only standard medical abbreviations should be used. To facilitate quick data retrieval, data should be presented under clearly marked headings.

Whenever possible, subjective data should be recorded using the patient's own words. Quotation marks should be used: "I feel tired from the moment I first get up in the morning. Any more it seems I have no energy at all." Patient reports may also be paraphrased: Patient reports feeling dyspneic, has difficulty catching breath when walking one flight of stairs.

The tendency to record data using nonspecific terms that are subject to individual definition or interpretation—words like *adequate, good, average, normal, poor, small, large*—should be avoided. One nurse's sense of what constitutes an average fluid intake may be very different from that of another nurse. It is important to be specific. Chapter 20 offers general documentation guidelines.

Learning Outcomes

After studying this chapter, the learner should be able to accomplish the following:

1. Define the key terms used in the chapter:

assessing	nursing history
data	objective data
database	observation
emergency assessment	physical assessment
focused assessment	subjective data
initial assessment	validation
interview	

2. Define and describe the purpose of four types of nursing assessments.
3. Differentiate a nursing assessment from a medical assessment.
4. Differentiate objective and subjective data.
5. Describe the purpose of nursing observation, interview, and physical assessment.
6. Obtain a nursing history using effective interviewing techniques.
7. Identify five sources of patient data useful to the nurse.
8. Plan patient assessments by identifying assessment priorities and structuring the data to be collected systematically.
9. Identify common problems encountered in data collection, noting their possible cause.
10. Explain when data need to be validated and several ways to accomplish this.
11. Describe the importance of knowing when to report significant patient data and of proper documentation.
12. Obtain and document complete, accurate, factual, and relevant patient data.

Critical Thinking Exercises

1. Working with another student, interview patients in both home and institutional settings, and record your findings separately. Make a list of the objective and subjective data you gather on each patient interviewed and compare your data lists. Explore the reasons for the differences you discover among patients, between home and residential settings, and between what you and your partner decide to record.
2. Allow another student to perform a comprehensive nursing assessment (interview and physical assessment) on you. Reflect on what you experienced. Offer the student feedback about which of her or his behaviors were helpful, comforting, distressing. Change roles and talk about what you learned from this experience.
3. Collect several different forms for recording the initial comprehensive nursing assessment (hospital, nursing home, home care, and school of nursing forms). Identify and explain the differences you see. Experiment with using the different forms, and make a list of features that help you get all the data you need in the easiest way possible.

Bibliography

Alfaro, R. (1998). *Applying the nursing process: A step-by-step guide* (4th ed.). Philadelphia: Lippincott Williams & Wilkins.

American Nurses Association (1980, 1995). *Nursing: A social policy statement*. Washington, DC: ANA.

Barkauskas, V. H., Stoltenberg-Allen, K., Ciofu-Baumann, L., & Darling-Fisher, C. (1994). *Health and physical assessment*. St. Louis: C. V. Mosby.

Bates, B. (1995). *A guide to physical examination* (6th ed.). Philadelphia: J. B. Lippincott.

Braverman, B. G. (1990). Eliciting data from the patient who is difficult to interview. *Nursing Clinics of North America, 25*(4), 743–750.

Catherman, A. (1990). Biopsychosocial nursing assessment: A way to enhance care plans. *Journal of Psychosocial Nursing, 28*(6), 31–33.

Domarad, B. R., & Buschmann, M. T. (1995). Interviewing older adults: Increasing the credibility of interview data. *Journal of Gerontological Nursing, 21*(9), 14–20.

Gordon, M. (1987). *Nursing diagnosis: Process and application* (2nd ed.). New York: McGraw-Hill.

Hill, L., & Smith, N. (1990). *Self-care nursing: Promotion of health* (2nd ed.). East Norwalk, CT: Appleton & Lange.

Laschinger, H. S. (1990). Helping students apply a nursing conceptual framework in the clinical setting. *Nurse Educator, 15*(3), 20–24.

McPhetridge, L. M. (1968). Nursing history: One means to personalize care. *American Journal of Nursing, 68*(1), 68–75.

Milholland, D. K. (1994). Privacy and confidentiality of patient information: Challenges for nursing. *JONA, 24*(2), 19–24.

Simonsen, S. M. (1996). *Telephone health assessment: Guidelines for practice*. St. Louis: C. V. Mosby.

Stewart, C. J., & Cash, W. B. (1991). *Interviewing principles and practice* (6th ed.). Dubuque, IA: Brown.

Vessey, J. A., & Richardson, B. L. (1993). A holistic approach to symptom assessment and intervention. *Holistic Nursing Practice, 7*(2), 13–21.

Chapter 16
Diagnosing

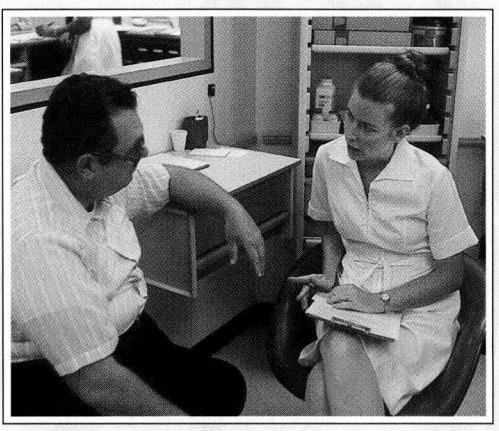

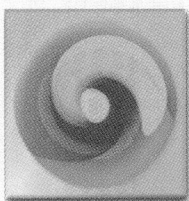

Thinking Critically About
Nursing's Blended Skills

Before reading this chapter, think about the types of skills you will need to prepare yourself to diagnose the patients you first met in the assessing chapter.

- You are working in a community-based well-child clinic. You become concerned when you observe negligible height and weight gains, delayed developmental milestones, and lethargy in a toddler brought to the clinic by her grandmother.

- You are working with a school nurse. Statistics reveal a pattern of teen smoking in your high school, and you are charged with developing an initiative to reverse this trend.

- You are doing a rotation on a medical floor in a hospital and learn that many of the diabetic patients being treated are repeat admissions with a history of poor self-care behavior.

- You are working in a nursing home where one alert resident with multiple chronic conditions repeatedly tells you that she has no reason to live and asks you to help her end her life.

What cognitive, technical, interpersonal, and ethical/legal skills do you think you will need to meet the everyday diagnostic challenges of these individuals and groups?

After the nurse has collected and recorded the patient data, the work of **diagnosing** begins—the second step in the nursing process. The purpose of diagnosing is to identify (1) actual and potential problems in the way the patient responds to health or illness, (2) factors that contribute to or cause the problems (etiologies), and (3) strengths the patient can draw on to prevent or resolve the problems.

In the diagnosing step of the nursing process, the nurse interprets and analyzes data gathered from the nursing assessment. These data help the nurse identify patient strengths and health problems. A **health problem** is a condition that necessitates intervening to prevent or resolve disease or illness or to promote coping and wellness.

When a health problem is identified, the nurse must decide which healthcare professional can best treat the problem. Actual or potential health problems that can be prevented or resolved by independent nursing intervention are termed **nursing diagnoses**. The nurse formulates, validates, and lists nursing diagnoses for each patient (Fig. 16-1).

Evolution of Nursing Diagnoses

The term *nursing diagnosis* first appeared in the literature in the 1950s. In 1976, Aspinall described nursing diagnosis as "the weak link" in nursing process. As early as 1966, Hammond wrote that nurses need to be competent in information-seeking strategies and to have a good background of theoretical knowledge with which to conduct the search for cues and evaluate evidence. These skills and knowledge result in accurate diagnosing. Key elements in the evolution of nursing diagnosis as an integral component of nursing process include the following:

- In 1972, the New York State Nurse Practice Act identified diagnosing as part of the legal domain of professional nursing; practice acts in many other states have been revised similarly since then.
- In 1973, the American Nurses Association's *Standards of Practice* included diagnosing as a function of professional nursing.
- Also in 1973, Gebbie and Lavin of St. Louis University called the First National Conference on Classification of Nursing Diagnoses, beginning a national effort to identify, standardize, and classify health problems treated by nurses. Conferences are held every 2 years, and much progress has been made in defining, classifying, and describing nursing diagnoses.

At its first meeting in 1973, the National Group, since renamed the North American Nursing Diagnosis Association (NANDA), appointed a task force to accomplish the following goals:

- Gather information and disseminate it through the Clearinghouse for Nursing Diagnosis.
- Encourage educational activities at regional and state levels to promote the implementation of nursing diagnoses. These activities include conferences to organize nurses to identify additional diagnostic labels and workshops to teach nurses about nursing diagnoses.
- Promote and organize activities to continue the development, classification, and scientific testing of nursing diagnoses. These activities include planning national conferences, identifying criteria for accept-

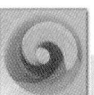

COGNITIVE SKILLS

- Ability to think critically and to engage in diagnostic reasoning
- Ability to develop nursing diagnoses that are responsive to the patient's health problems: failure to thrive, smoking, need for diabetic self-care, and loss of the will to live
- Knowledge of pertinent standards and agency or institutional policies related to diagnoses

TECHNICAL SKILLS

- Ability to research the literature to obtain the knowledge necessary for developing the list of nursing diagnoses
- Ability to use a documentation system competently to communicate the list of nursing diagnoses

INTERPERSONAL SKILLS

- Ability to establish trusting nurse–patient relationships that yield knowledge of the individual needs and strengths of patients and their family caregivers
- Ability to communicate to patients that you are concerned about their priorities and committed to their well-being

ETHICAL/LEGAL SKILLS

- Commitment to developing and communicating a list of nursing diagnoses that are responsive to the patient's individualized needs
- Knowledge of the ethical and legal principles that guide developing and documenting nursing diagnoses
- Ability to serve as a trusted and effective patient advocate

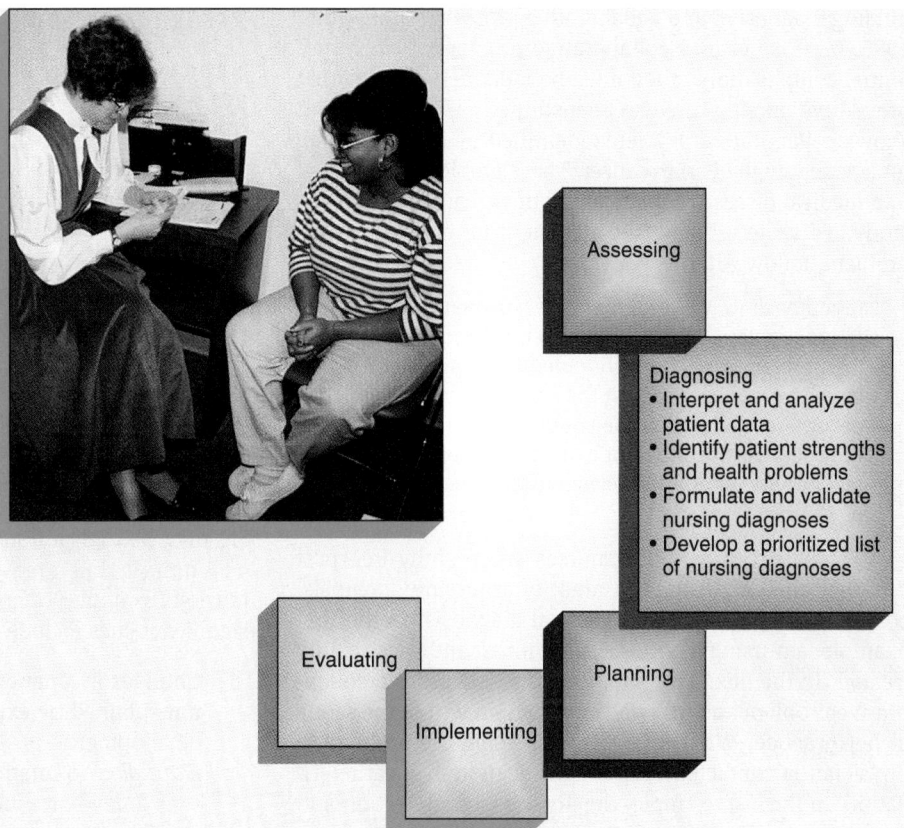

Figure 16-1
Diagnosing. Diagnosing is the interpretation and analysis of patient data to identify patient strengths and health problems that independent nursing intervention can prevent or resolve. Nursing diagnoses may change from day to day as the patient's responses to health and illness change.

ing diagnoses, surveying current research activities, and exploring varied methods for classification.

Now an accepted and essential step in the nursing process, nursing diagnosis was initially confused with medical diagnosis, and this sparked great controversy. Although this confusion has been resolved, many nurses have been slow to understand and accept the "work" of diagnosing.

Unique Focus of Nursing Diagnosis

In the diagnosing step of the nursing process, the nurse identifies nursing's unique concern for a patient (ie, what it is about the patient that gives rise to the need for nursing, as opposed to the need for medicine or for physical therapy). Nursing diagnoses are written to describe patient problems that nurses can treat independently. As nurses interpret and analyze patient data, they may identify health problems that are better treated by physicians (medical diagnoses) or by nurses working with other healthcare professionals (collaborative problems). In such a case, the nurse reports the findings to the physician or other appropriate healthcare professional and works collaboratively with him or her to resolve the problem.

Nursing Diagnosis Versus Medical Diagnosis

Medical diagnoses identify diseases, whereas nursing diagnoses focus on unhealthy responses to health and illness. Medical diagnoses describe problems for which the physician directs the primary treatment, whereas nursing diagnoses describe problems treated by nurses within the scope of independent nursing practice. A medical diagnosis remains the same for as long as the disease is present; a nursing diagnosis may change from day to day as the patient's responses change. These distinctions reflect key differences in medical and nursing practices.

Myocardial infarction (heart attack) is a medical diagnosis. Examples of nursing diagnoses for a person with myocardial infarction include Fear, Altered Health Maintenance, Knowledge Deficit, Pain, and Altered Tissue Perfusion.

Nursing Diagnosis Versus Collaborative Problems

Nursing diagnoses are also different from collaborative problems. Together, nursing diagnoses and collaborative problems constitute the range of responses that nurses treat, and as such they define the unique nature of nursing. Carpenito defines **collaborative problems** as "certain physiologic complications that nurses monitor to detect onset or changes in status. Nurses manage collaborative problems using physician-prescribed and nursing-prescribed interventions to minimize the complications of the event" (1995, p. 29).

Unlike medical diagnoses, collaborative problems are the primary responsibility of nurses. Unlike nursing diagnoses, with collaborative problems, the prescription for treatment comes from both nursing and medicine. "When the nurse writes patient outcomes that require delegated medical orders for goal achievement, the situation is not a nursing diagnosis but a collaborative problem" (Carpenito, 1995, p. 33). Because collaborative problems involve potential complications, they must be identified early so that preventive nursing care can be instituted early. Figure 16-2 shows collaborative problems identified by a nurse caring for a patient with ovarian cancer. These problems are related to a medical disease, a medical treatment, and a diagnostic study. To write a diagnostic statement for a collaborative problem, follow Alfaro's rule:

> If you need to write a diagnostic statement for a collaborative problem, focus on the *potential complications* of the problem. Use "PC" (for potential complication), followed by a colon, and list the complications that might occur. For clarity, link the potential complications and the collaborative problem by using "related to." *Example:* PC: pneumothorax related to fractured ribs. (1998, p. 115)

Table 16-1 shows how nurses successfully interpret different clusters of data to identify a nursing diagnosis, collaborative problem, and medical diagnosis. In the first example, a nursing diagnosis is identified and successfully treated. In the next example, the nurse identifies a collaborative problem and initiates intervention within the scope of her practice. When this fails to resolve the problem, a physician is contacted to order medication or a catheterization. In the last example, the nurse's early detection and reporting of the problem to the physician lead to the physician's prompt medical diagnosis of cystitis and successful antibiotic therapy.

Data Interpretation and Analysis

Most experienced nurses begin the work of interpreting and analyzing data while they are still collecting (assessing) it. The term **cue** is often used to denote significant data or data that influence this analysis. Significant data should "raise a red flag" for the nurse, who then looks for patterns or clusters of data that signal an actual, potential, or possible nursing diagnosis.

Recognizing Significant Data

Sorting out *healthy* patient responses from those that are *not healthy* is not as clearcut as it may seem. To avoid erroneously labeling selected patient health patterns as unhealthy while failing to detect an actual unhealthy behavior, nurses must be familiar with comparative standards to be used in data interpretation and analysis.

Comparing Data to Standards

A standard, or a norm, is a generally accepted rule, measure, pattern, or model to which can be compared data in the same class or category. For example, when determining the significance of a patient's blood pressure reading, appropriate standards include normative values for the patient's age group, race, and illness category. The patient's own normal range, if known, is an important standard. A pressure of $^{150}/_{90}$ mm Hg may be high for someone whose pressure normally is $^{120}/_{70}$ mm Hg, but it may be normal for a person with hypertension. Examples of how standards can be used to identify significant cues include the following (Gordon, 1994):

1. Changes in a patient's usual health patterns that are unexplained by expected norms for growth and development
   Example: An infant who took to breastfeeding easily as a newborn suddenly stops sucking when put to the breast and begins to lose weight.
2. Deviation from an appropriate population norm
   Example: A first-year college student begins to accelerate her exercise habits dramatically and starts inducing vomiting after binge eating. She rapidly loses weight.
3. Behavior that is nonproductive in the whole-person context
   Example: A college student breaks up with her boyfriend and begins to believe that she is "unfit" for any other relationship and withdraws from her friends and social activities.
4. Behavior that indicates a developmental lag or evolving dysfunctional pattern

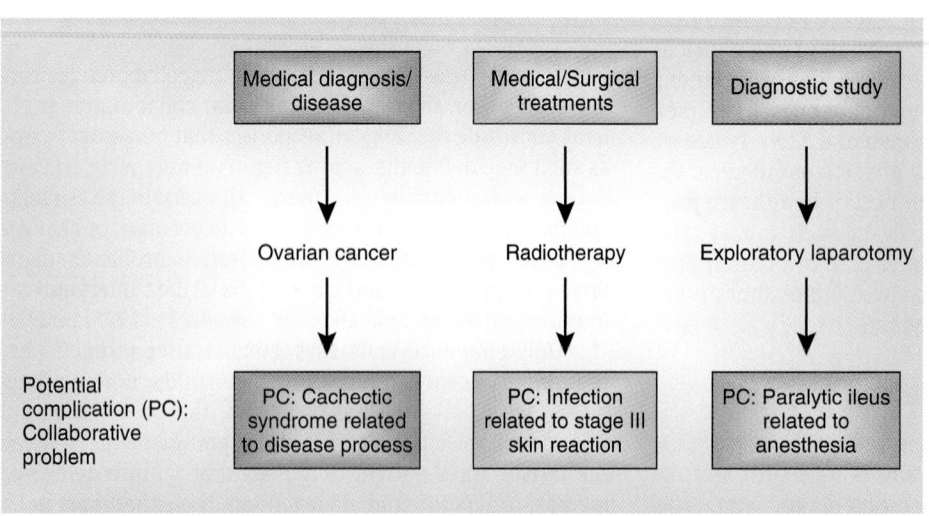

Figure 16-2
Collaborative problems.

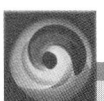

Table 16-1
A Comparison: Nursing Diagnosis, Collaborative Problem, Medical Diagnosis

	Nursing Diagnosis	Collaborative Problem	Medical Diagnosis
Definition	A nursing diagnosis is a clinical judgment about individual, family, or community responses to actual or potential health problems or life processes. Nursing diagnosis provides the basis for selection of nursing interventions to achieve outcomes for which the nurse is accountable (NANDA).	Certain physiologic complications that nurses monitor to detect onset of changes in status (Carpenito)	Traumatic or disease condition or syndrome validated by medical diagnostic studies
Focus	Monitoring human responses to actual and potential health problems	Monitoring pathophysiologic responses of body organs or systems	Correcting or preventing pathology of specific organs or body systems
Sample data cluster	56-year-old mother of seven; 5′4″, 167 lb; "Whenever I sneeze lately, I dribble urine. This is embarrassing."	42-year-old woman; 1 hour after delivery; spinal anesthesia; 1500 mL fluid infused in past 4 hours without patient voiding; unable to void	"Whenever I have to urinate it burns terribly. I also feel like I have to go all the time—real bad." Small, frequent voidings, cloudy urine; T—100.8°F
Diagnostic statement	Stress Incontinence related to degenerative changes in pelvic muscles and structural supports associated with advanced age, obesity, gravid uterus	Potential complication: Urinary Retention related to fluid overload and effects of anesthesia	Cystitis
Select nursing responses	Teach Kegel exercises to increase muscle tone; explore patient's willingness and motivation to pursue weight reduction and exercise program; evaluate need for bladder-training program.	Monitor for signs of increasing urine retention; offer bedpan, and encourage voiding with running water, warm water dripped over perineum, and so forth; if no result, administer physician-prescribed medication; if no result, perform physician-prescribed catheterization	Report signs and symptoms to physician; obtain urine culture; report results to physician; administer appropriate physician-prescribed antibiotic

Example: A 16-year-old single mother with a 6-month-old infant continues to "party hard" with her friends and hang out at the mall and shows no interest in caring for her son, who is repeatedly left with concerned family members.

Recognizing Patterns or Clusters

A **data cluster** is a grouping of patient data or cues that points to the existence of a patient health problem. Nursing diagnoses should always be derived from clusters of significant data rather than from a single cue. The danger of deriving a nursing diagnosis from a single cue is illustrated in the following example. Diagnosing a woman recovering from gallbladder surgery with ineffective coping solely on the basis of tears may misinterpret the patient's

crying, which may be a healthy release of emotion. If the same patient begins to exhibit a cluster of significant cues, such as refusing to eat, preferring bed rest to scheduled ambulation, and reporting increasing discomfort, an unhealthy pattern is emerging. Table 16-2 offers examples of how clusters of significant data lead to formulation of accurate nursing diagnoses.

Identifying Strengths and Problems

The next step in analyzing data is to determine the patient's strengths and problems.

Determining the Patient's Strengths

If a patient appears to meet a standard, the nurse concludes that the patient has a strength in that particular

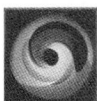

**Table 16-2
Diagnosing**

Data Interpretation and Analysis		Formulation of Tentative Nursing Diagnosis	Validation of Nursing Diagnosis
Significant Cues	**Sample Data Clusters**		
Change in a patient's usual health patterns that is unexplained by expected norms for growth and development	• "I guess I lost about 20 to 30 pounds over the last 6 months—I think I've just been too busy to eat." • Height: 5'8" • Weight: 102 lb • 35-year-old mother of 4-year-old twin boys; returned to work (executive secretary) for first time since delivery of twins 7 months ago	Altered Nutrition: Less Than Body Requirements, related to stress of new job; role conflict and demands	Accurate diagnosis: Patient validates this diagnosis, agreeing with contributing factors
Deviation from an appropriate population norm	• Teacher notices and reports frequency of bruises on third-grade boy who is repeatedly observed alone during recess periods and who is withdrawn in classroom • In conversation with the school nurse, one parent remarks: "That boy brings out the worst in me! I don't know why, but I often have to smack him hard to make him listen."	High Risk for Violence (Child Abuse) related to ? etiology (deficient parenting skills?)	Incomplete diagnosis: Additional data collection yields new information: • Father out of work for past 18 months • Father was abused as a child Diagnosis restated: High Risk For Violence (Child Abuse) related to increased family stress and father's history of being abused
Behavior that is nonproductive in the whole-person context	• Fiancé abruptly terminated relationship 3 months before established wedding date • Noticeable change in physical appearance; frequently wears same clothes; makeup, jewelry, hairstyling are absent; strong body odors present • No desire to be with others; goes home (lives alone) immediately after work • Stopped attending aerobics classes	Self-Esteem Disturbance related to feeling rejected by fiancé	Premature diagnosis resulting from incomplete data collection. Patient has a long history of major depressive states, one of which may have resulted in the breakup of this relationship. Medical diagnosis and treatment indicated. Changes in appearance are indicative of depressive state. Need to explore related nursing diagnoses.
Behavior indicating developmental lags or evolving dysfunctional patterns	• Admitted to nursing home 2 months ago • "I have nothing to live for anymore . . . why don't I die?" • Wishes to remain in room seated in chair—will only ambulate with great urging • Anything requiring movement has become "too much bother." • Decreased muscle mass, tone, and strength, reduced joint mobility	Impaired Physical Mobility related to difficult transition to nursing home	Accurate but routinized diagnosis that may result in staff's acceptance of status quo unless a more specific cause is identified

area and that this strength contributes to the patient's level of wellness. For example, a person with a history of maintaining a well-balanced diet is usually better able to cope with illness than a person who has a history of eating poorly.

Patient strengths may include healthy physiologic functioning, emotional health, cognitive abilities, coping skills, interpersonal strengths, and spiritual strengths. Resources such as the presence of support people, adequate finances, and a healthy environment may all contribute to patient strengths. Many people take their strengths for granted and may not know how to use them effectively when responding to illness. Discussing observed strengths with patients and counseling patients about ways to develop and use their strengths are important nursing measures.

Determining the Patient's Problem Areas

A person who does not meet a certain health standard probably has a limitation in this aspect of health status and may benefit from professional care. For example, a person with a long history of constipation probably needs care to help overcome this problem. As stated previously, the nurse decides whether the data represent a nursing diagnosis or a collaborative problem, or whether the data should be reported to the physician because they might lead to a medical diagnosis.

Determining Problems the Patient Is Likely to Experience

It is important for nurses to identify potential health problems. For example, a nurse notes that a patient has signs of a wound infection, but laboratory test results show that the patient's white blood cell count has not increased, as is usual when such an infection is present. The nurse concludes that the body apparently is not building up normal defenses to combat the infection. The nurse then predicts the problems this patient is likely to encounter, such as a longer than normal healing period. Potential nursing diagnoses alert other caregivers to problems the patient may experience if the certain trends in the patient's condition continue unreversed. This prediction has implications for nursing care, such as measures related to the patient's diet, fluid intake, urine output, and mobility.

When determining a patient's strengths and problems, it is helpful to determine whether the patient agrees with the nurse's identification of a problem and is motivated to work toward its resolution.

Reaching Conclusions

The nurse reaches one of four basic conclusions after interpreting and analyzing the patient data. Different nursing responses are possible for each conclusion:

No Problem
- No nursing response is indicated.
- Reinforce patient's health habits and patterns.
- Initiate health promotion activities to prevent disease or illness or to promote a higher level of wellness.
- Wellness diagnosis may be indicated.

Possible Problem
- Collect more data to confirm or disconfirm suspected problem.

Actual or Potential Nursing Diagnosis
- Nurse is unable to treat problem because patient denies problem and refuses treatment (make sure patient understands possible outcomes of this stance).
- Begin planning, implementing, and evaluating care designed to prevent, reduce, or resolve the problem.

Clinical Problem Other Than Nursing Diagnosis
- Consult with appropriate healthcare professional and work collaboratively on problem.
- Refer to medicine.

Formulating and Validating Nursing Diagnoses

Writing Nursing Diagnoses

When the nurse recognizes a cluster of significant patient data indicating a health problem that can be treated by independent nursing intervention, a nursing diagnosis should be written. Most nursing diagnoses are written either as two-part statements listing the patient's problem and its cause or as three-part statements that also include the problem's defining characteristics (Table 16-3).

Those just beginning to write nursing diagnoses may find it helpful to consult the list of health problems accepted by NANDA for testing and study (see the accompanying box). The NANDA list is a beginning list of suggested terms for health problems that may be identified and treated by nurses. Each of the diagnoses in *Nursing Diagnoses: Definitions and Classification, 1999–2000* is presented in taxonomic order and includes the basic components of a nursing diagnosis: definition, defining characteristics, and related factors or risk factors. See the example in the accompanying box. This structure has recently been simplified to facilitate the parallel development of an electronic database for nursing diagnoses. There are distinct advantages to nurses' use of common terminology when formulating nursing diagnoses. These range from communication advantages (everyone uses the same words to describe common problems) to promoting the development of nursing science by facilitating research and the dissemination of research findings.

Pocket-sized handbooks of NANDA-approved nursing diagnoses are available and help students unfamiliar with this grouping of problem statements. Nurses who encounter different health problems within the scope of their practice that they believe to be nursing diagnoses may submit these to the NANDA Diagnosis Review Committee.

Parts of Nursing Diagnoses
Problem

The purpose of the problem statement is to describe the health state or health problem of the patient as clearly and concisely as possible. Because this section of the nursing diagnosis identifies what is unhealthy about the patient and what the patient would like to change in his or her

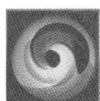

Table 16-3
Formulation of Nursing Diagnosis Statements

	Definition	Purpose	Example
Problem	Identifies what is unhealthy about the patient, indicating the need for change (clear, concise statement of the patient's health problem)	Suggests the patient goals (expectations for change)	Bathing/Hygiene Self-Care Deficit ↓ related to ↓
Etiology	Identifies the factors that are maintaining the unhealthy state or response (contributing or causative factors)	Suggests the appropriate nursing measures	Fear of falling in the tub and obesity ↓ as manifested by ↓
Defining characteristics	Identify the subjective and objective data that signal the existence of the problem (cues that reflect the existence of a problem)	Suggest evaluative criteria	Strong body and urine odor, unclean hair: "I'm afraid I'll fall in the tub and break something." (5′4″, 170 lb)

Examples:

Two-part diagnostic statement: Bathing/Hygiene Self-Care Deficit related to fear of falling in tub and obesity

Three-part diagnostic statement: Bathing/Hygiene Self-Care Deficit related to fear of falling in tub and obesity, as manifested by strong body and urine odor, unclean hair, statement of fearing fall in tub, and height and weight: 5′4″, 170 lb

---

health status, it suggests patient goals. NANDA recommends use of the following quantifiers when writing the problem statement: *altered, impaired, depleted, deficient, excessive, dysfunctional, disturbed, ineffective, decreased, increased, acute, chronic,* and *intermittent.*

Etiology

The etiology identifies the physiologic, psychological, sociologic, spiritual, and environmental factors believed to be related to the problem as either a cause or a contributing factor. Because the etiology identifies the factors that maintain the unhealthy patient state and prevent the desired change, the etiology directs nursing intervention. Unless the etiology is correctly identified, nursing actions may be inefficient and ineffective. For example, a diabetic patient who is frequently admitted to the hospital with hyperglycemia and who has a poor history of dietary and pharmacologic management is diagnosed to be noncompliant. Assuming that the noncompliance is related to a knowledge deficit and then channeling all nursing activities and energies into teaching the patient how to manage the diabetes is useless if the noncompliance is actually a result of the patient's decreased will to live, which would necessitate a different group of nursing interventions.

Defining Characteristics

The subjective and objective data that signal the existence of the actual or potential health problem are the third component of the nursing diagnosis. NANDA has identified

defining characteristics for each accepted nursing diagnosis, and familiarity with these characteristics helps nurses recognize clusters of significant data. Table 16-3 defines the three components of a nursing diagnosis statement and shows how they affect patient goals, nursing measures, and evaluation. Other examples of nursing diagnosis statements are found throughout the book.

Guidelines for Writing Nursing Diagnoses

1. Phrase the nursing diagnosis as a patient problem or alteration in health state rather than as a patient need.
2. Check to make sure that the patient problem precedes the etiology and that the two are linked by the phrase "related to."
3. Defining characteristics, when included in the nursing diagnosis, should follow the etiology and be linked by the phrase "as manifested by" or "as evidenced by."
4. Write in legally advisable terms.
5. Use nonjudgmental language.
6. Be sure the problem statement indicates what is unhealthy about the patient or what the patient wants to change (enhance).
7. Avoid using defining characteristics, medical diagnoses, or something that cannot be changed in the problem statement.
8. Reread the diagnosis to make sure the problem statement suggests patient goals and that the etiology will direct the selection of nursing measures.

(*text continues on page 265*)

NANDA-Approved Nursing Diagnoses

This list represents the NANDA-approved nursing diagnoses for clinical use and testing.

Pattern 1: Exchanging

	1.1.2.1	Altered Nutrition: More Than Body Requirements
	1.1.2.2	Altered Nutrition: Less Than Body Requirements
	1.1.2.3	Altered Nutrition: Risk for More Than Body Requirements
	1.2.1.1	Risk for Infection
	1.2.2.1	Risk for Altered Body Temperature
	1.2.2.2	Hypothermia
	1.2.2.3	Hyperthermia
	1.2.2.4	Ineffective Thermoregulation
	1.2.3.1	Dysreflexia
*	1.2.3.2	Risk for Autonomic Dysreflexia
★	1.3.1.1	Constipation
	1.3.1.1.1	Perceived Constipation
	1.3.1.1.2	Colonic Constipation (deleted in 1998)
★	1.3.1.2	Diarrhea
★	1.3.1.3	Bowel Incontinence
*	1.3.1.4	Risk for Constipation
	1.3.2	Altered Urinary Elimination
	1.3.2.1.1	Stress Incontinence
★	1.3.2.1.2	Reflex Urinary Incontinence
	1.3.2.1.3	Urge Incontinence
★	1.3.2.1.4	Functional Urinary Incontinence
	1.3.2.1.5	Total Incontinence
*	1.3.2.1.6	Risk for Urinary Urge Incontinence
	1.3.2.2	Urinary Retention
#	1.4.1.1	Altered Tissue Perfusion (Specify type: Renal, Cerebral, Cardiopulmonary, Gastrointestinal, Peripheral)
*	1.4.1.2	Risk for Fluid Volume Imbalance
	1.4.1.2.1	Fluid Volume Excess
	1.4.1.2.2.1	Fluid Volume Deficit
	1.4.1.2.2.2	Risk for Fluid Volume Deficit
	1.4.2.1	Decreased Cardiac Output
★	1.5.1.1	Impaired Gas Exchange
★	1.5.1.2	Ineffective Airway Clearance
★	1.5.1.3	Ineffective Breathing Pattern
	1.5.1.3.1	Inability to Sustain Spontaneous Ventilation
	1.5.1.3.2	Dysfunctional Ventilatory Weaning Response
	1.6.1	Risk for Injury
	1.6.1.1	Risk for Suffocation
	1.6.1.2	Risk for Poisoning
	1.6.1.3	Risk for Trauma
	1.6.1.4	Risk for Aspiration
	1.6.1.5	Risk for Disuse Syndrome
*	1.6.1.6	Latex Allergy Response
*	1.6.1.7	Risk for Latex Allergy Response
	1.6.2	Altered Protection
#	1.6.2.1	Impaired Tissue Integrity
★	1.6.2.1.1	Altered Oral Mucous Membrane
#	1.6.2.1.2.1	Impaired Skin Integrity
#	1.6.2.1.2.2	Risk for Impaired Skin Integrity
*	1.6.2.1.3	Altered Dentition
	1.7.1	Decreased Adaptive Capacity: Intracranial
	1.8	Energy Field Disturbance

Pattern 2: Communicating

#	2.1.1.1	Impaired Verbal Communication

Pattern 3: Relating

	3.1.1	Impaired Social Interaction
	3.1.2	Social Isolation
	3.1.3	Risk for Loneliness
★	3.2.1	Altered Role Performance
★	3.2.1.1.1	Altered Parenting
★	3.2.1.1.2	Risk for Altered Parenting
	3.2.1.1.2.1	Risk for Altered Parent/Infant/Child Attachment
	3.2.1.2.1	Sexual Dysfunction
★	3.2.2	Altered Family Processes
★	3.2.2.1	Caregiver Role Strain
	3.2.2.2	Risk for Caregiver Role Strain
	3.2.2.3.1	Altered Family Processes: Alcoholism
	3.2.3.1	Parental Role Conflict
	3.3	Altered Sexuality Patterns

Pattern 4: Valuing

	4.1.1	Spiritual Distress (Distress of the Human Spirit)
*	4.1.2	Risk for Spiritual Distress
	4.2	Potential for Enhanced Spiritual Well-Being

Pattern 5: Choosing

★	5.1.1.1	Ineffective Individual Coping
★	5.1.1.1.1	Impaired Adjustment

(continued)

NANDA-Approved Nursing Diagnoses (Continued)

5.1.1.1.2	Defensive Coping	
5.1.1.1.3	Ineffective Denial	
5.1.2.1.1	Ineffective Family Coping: Disabling	
5.1.2.1.2	Ineffective Family Coping: Compromised	
5.1.2.2	Family Coping: Potential for Growth	
5.1.3.1	Potential for Enhanced Community Coping	
★ 5.1.3.2	Ineffective Community Coping	
5.2.1	Ineffective Management of Therapeutic Regimen: Individuals	
5.2.1.1	Noncompliance (specify)	
5.2.2	Ineffective Management of Therapeutic Regimen: Families	
5.2.3	Ineffective Management of Therapeutic Regimen: Community	
5.2.4	Effective Management of Therapeutic Regimen: Individual	
5.3.1.1	Decisional Conflict (specify)	
5.4	Health-Seeking Behaviors (specify)	

Pattern 6: Moving

★ 6.1.1.1	Impaired Physical Mobility
6.1.1.1.1	Risk for Peripheral Neurovascular Dysfunction
6.1.1.1.2	Risk for Perioperative Positioning Injury
6.1.1.1.3	Impaired Walking
6.1.1.1.4	Impaired Wheelchair Mobility
* 6.1.1.1.5	Impaired Transfer Ability
6.1.1.1.6	Impaired Bed Mobility
6.1.1.2	Activity Intolerance
★ 6.1.1.2.1	Fatigue
6.1.1.3	Risk for Activity Intolerance
★ 6.2.1	Sleep Pattern Disturbance
6.2.1.1	Sleep Deprivation
6.3.1.1	Diversional Activity Deficit
6.4.1.1	Impaired Home Maintenance Management
6.4.2	Altered Health Maintenance
6.4.2.1	Delayed Surgical Recovery
6.4.2.2	Adult Failure to Thrive
★ 6.5.1	Feeding Self-Care Deficit
★ 6.5.1.1	Impaired Swallowing
6.5.1.2	Ineffective Breastfeeding

6.5.1.2.1	Interrupted Breastfeeding
6.5.1.3	Effective Breastfeeding
6.5.1.4	Ineffective Infant Feeding Pattern
★ 6.5.2	Bathing/Hygiene Self-Care Deficit
★ 6.5.3	Dressing/Grooming Self-Care Deficit
★ 6.5.4	Toileting Self-Care Deficit
6.6	Altered Growth and Development
6.6.1	Risk for Altered Development
6.6.2	Risk for Altered Growth
6.7	Relocation Stress Syndrome
6.8.1	Risk for Disorganized Infant Behavior
★ 6.8.2	Disorganized Infant Behavior
6.8.3	Potential for Enhanced Organized Infant Behavior

Pattern 7: Perceiving

# 7.1.1	Body Image Disturbance
7.1.2	Self-Esteem Disturbance
7.1.2.1	Chronic Low Self-Esteem
7.1.2.2	Situational Low Self-Esteem
7.1.3	Personal Identity Disturbance
# 7.2	Sensory/Perceptual Alterations (Specify: Visual, Auditory, Kinesthetic, Gustatory, Tactile, Olfactory)
7.2.1.1	Unilateral Neglect
7.3.1	Hopelessness
7.3.2	Powerlessness

Pattern 8: Knowing

8.1.1	Knowledge Deficit (Specify)
8.2.1	Impaired Environmental Interpretation Syndrome
8.2.2	Acute Confusion
8.2.3	Chronic Confusion
8.3	Altered Thought Processes
8.3.1	Impaired Memory

Pattern 9: Feeling

9.1.1	Pain
9.1.1.1	Chronic Pain
* 9.1.2	Nausea
9.2.1.1	Dysfunctional Grieving
9.2.1.2	Anticipatory Grieving
* 9.2.1.3	Chronic Sorrow
9.2.2	Risk for Violence: Directed at Others

(continued)

NANDA-Approved Nursing Diagnoses (*Continued*)

	9.2.2.1	Risk for Self-Mutilation		9.2.3.1.2	Rape-Trauma Syndrome: Silent Reaction
	9.2.2.2	Risk for Violence: Self-Directed			
★	9.2.3	Post-Trauma Syndrome	*	9.2.4	Risk for Post-Trauma Syndrome
★	9.2.3.1	Rape-Trauma Syndrome	#	9.3.1	Anxiety
	9.2.3.1.1	Rape-Trauma Syndrome: Compound Reaction	*	9.3.1.1	Death Anxiety
			#	9.3.2	Fear

*, New diagnoses accepted in 1998; ★, Revised diagnoses submitted and approved in 1998; #, Diagnoses revised by small work groups at the 1996 Biennial Conference on the Classification of Nursing Diagnoses, with changes approved and added in 1998; North American Nursing Diagnosis Association. (1999). *NANDA Nursing diagnoses: Definitions and classification, 1999–2000.* Philadelphia, PA: Author.

Common errors in writing nursing diagnoses are shown in Table 16-4, along with suggestions for correcting them.

What Is *Not* a Nursing Diagnosis

The nursing diagnosis statement is written in terms of a patient problem, alteration in health state, or patient strength *for which nursing provides the primary therapy.* Table 16-5 uses a patient with diabetes mellitus to illustrate what nursing diagnoses *are not.* For example, nursing diagnoses are not medical diagnoses or statements of patient need.

Example of a NANDA Diagnosis With Definition, Defining Characteristics, and Risk Factors or Related Factors

1.1.2.1 Altered Nutrition: More Than Body Requirements (1975)

Definition
The state in which an individual is experiencing an intake of nutrients that exceeds metabolic needs

Defining Characteristics
Triceps skin fold greater than 25 mm in women; weight 20% over ideal for height and frame; triceps skin fold greater than 15 mm in men; eating in response to external cues, such as time of day, social situation; eating in response to internal cues other than hunger (e.g., anxiety); reported or observed dysfunctional eating pattern pairing food with other activities; sedentary activity level; weight 10% over ideal for height and frame; concentrating food intake at the end of the day

Related Factors
Excessive intake in relation to metabolic need

North American Nursing Diagnosis Association. (1999). *NANDA Nursing diagnoses: Definitions and classification, 1999–2000.* Philadelphia; Author.

Actual, Potential (Risk), and Possible Nursing Diagnoses

Patient health problems may be **actual problems** (problem is present), **potential (risk) problems** (problem may occur), and **possible problems** (problem may be present). A potential nursing diagnosis is written when the health problem is likely to occur unless the nurse intervenes in a particular way. NANDA-approved diagnoses once designated as "potential" were labeled "risk" in 1992:

> A risk nursing diagnosis is a clinical judgment that an individual, family, or community is more vulnerable to develop the problem than others in the same or similar situation. Risk nursing diagnoses are supported by risk factors that guide nursing interventions to reduce or prevent the occurrence of the problem.
>
> A possible nursing diagnosis is written when the nurse suspects that a health problem exists but needs to gather more data to confirm the diagnosis. (Carpenito, 1995, p. 16)

An actual nursing diagnosis for a patient who has experienced vomiting, diarrhea, and excessive diaphoresis for 3 days is *Fluid Volume Deficit related to abnormal fluid loss.* If the diarrhea persists and weakness interferes with the patient's normal perineal hygiene, he may be at risk for skin breakdown. This is written as the potential diagnosis *Risk for Impaired Skin Integrity.* If the nurse suspects that a disturbance of self-concept is also present but lacks the necessary data (defining characteristics) to confirm this, it can be written as a possible diagnosis: *Possible Disturbance in Self-Concept.* This alerts other nurses to the need to collect more data about the patient's self-concept.

Wellness Diagnoses

A persistent critique of nursing diagnoses that focus exclusively on patient health problems is their limited applicability in nursing settings that deal primarily with healthy patients. To remedy this concern, **wellness diagnoses** were proposed and are now readily accepted. According to NANDA, a "wellness diagnosis is a clinical judgment about an individual, family, or community in

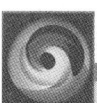

Table 16-4
Common Errors in Writing Nursing Diagnoses and Recommended Corrections

Error	Example	Correction	Example
Writing the diagnosis in terms of needs and not response	Needs assistance with bathing related to bed rest	Write the diagnosis in terms of response rather than need	Self-Care Deficit: Bathing related to immobility
Making legally inadvisable statements	Noncompliance due to hostility toward nursing staff (the words *due to* imply a direct cause-and-effect relationship)	Use "related to" rather than "due to" or "caused by" to link the etiology to the problem statement	Noncompliance related to hostility toward nursing staff (denotes a relation between the problem and etiology but not necessarily a causal relation)
	Spouse Abuse related to husband's immaturity and violent temper	Write diagnosis in legally advisable terms: statements that may be interpreted as libel or that imply nursing negligence are legally hazardous to all the nurses caring for the patient	High Risk for Violence: Spouse Abuse related to husband's reported inability to control behavior
	Impaired Skin Integrity related to patient's lying on back all night		Impaired Skin Integrity related to mobility deficit
Identifying as a problem a patient response that is not necessarily unhealthy	Mild Anxiety related to impending surgery	Include in the problem statement of the nursing diagnosis only patient responses that are unhealthy or that the patient wants to change	No need for nursing diagnosis: mild anxiety before surgery is a healthy response that motivates preoperative self-care behavior
Identifying as a problem signs and symptoms of illness	Cough related to long history of smoking	Avoid including signs and symptoms of illness in the problem statement of the nursing diagnosis	Ineffective Airway Clearance related to 20-year history of smoking
Identifying as a patient problem or etiology what cannot be changed	Alterations in Bowel Elimination: Permanent Colostomy related to cancer of bowel	Express the problem statement and etiologic factors in terms that can be changed; otherwise, nursing energies are being directed to a hopeless task	Self-Care Deficit: Care of Colostomy, related to severe anxiety about cancer and feelings of powerlessness
	Grieving related to death of spouse		Dysfunctional Grieving related to inability to accept death of spouse
Identifying environmental factors rather than patient factors as a problem	Cluttered Home related to inability to discard anything	Express the problem statement in terms of unhealthy patient responses rather than environmental conditions	High Risk for Injury related to cluttered home (inability to discard anything)
Reversing clauses	Knowledge Deficit related to alteration in parenting	Avoid reversing the problem statement and etiologic statement	Altered Parenting related to knowledge deficit: child growth and development, discipline
Having both clauses say the same thing	Alteration in Comfort related to pain (pain *is* the comfort alteration—what is contributing to the pain?)	Be sure that the *two* parts of the diagnosis do not mean the same thing	Unrelieved Incisional Pain related to fear of addiction

(continued)

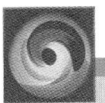

Table 16-4 (Continued)

Error	Example	Correction	Example
Including value judgments in the nursing diagnosis	Poor Home Maintenance Management related to laziness	Write the diagnosis without value judgments; avoid words such as *poor, inadequate, abnormal, unhealthy*	Impaired Home Maintenance Management related to low value ascribed to home safety and cleanliness
Including the medical diagnosis in the diagnostic statement	Impaired Home Maintenance Management related to arthritis	Do not include the medical diagnosis in the nursing diagnosis statement	Impaired Home Maintenance Management related to mobility, endurance, and comfort alterations

Common errors adapted from Mundinger, M. O., & Jauron, G. D. (1975). Developing a nursing diagnosis. *Nursing Outlook, 23*(2), 94–98. Guidelines for writing nursing diagnoses adapted from Iyer, P., Taptich, B., & Bernocchi-Losey, D. (1991). *Nursing process and nursing diagnoses* (2nd ed.). Philadelphia: W. B. Saunders.

transition from a specific level of wellness to a higher level of wellness" (1990, p. 116). The diagnostic statement for wellness diagnoses is a one-part statement that contains the label *Potential for Enhanced* followed by the desired higher-level wellness. Examples include Potential for Enhanced Family Coping, Potential for Enhanced Health Maintenance, Potential for Enhanced Parenting, and Potential for Enhanced Self-Esteem.

Validating Nursing Diagnoses

After a tentative nursing diagnosis is formulated, it should be validated. Price (1980, p. 670) indicates that an affirmative response to each of the following questions validates a tentative diagnosis:

- Is my database sufficient, accurate, and supported by nursing research?
- Does my synthesis of data (significant cues) demonstrate the existence of a pattern?
- Are the subjective and objective data I used to determine the existence of a pattern characteristic of the health problem I defined?
- Is my tentative nursing diagnosis based on scientific nursing knowledge and clinical expertise?
- Is my tentative nursing diagnosis able to be prevented, reduced, or resolved by independent nursing action?
- Is my degree of confidence above 50% that other qualified practitioners would formulate the same nursing diagnosis based on my data?

In addition, patients who are able to participate in decision making should be encouraged to validate the diagnosis. "It seems to me that bathing has become a problem now that you are afraid of falling in the tub. What's your sense of this?" Table 16-2 lists possible outcomes of validating tentative nursing diagnoses.

Documenting Nursing Diagnoses

The nurse documents validated nursing diagnoses in the patient record. Depending on the documentation system in use, nursing diagnoses may be recorded in the nursing plan of care and on the multidisciplinary problem list at the front of the patient record. Tables 16-3 and 16-4 illustrate how to document nursing diagnoses using both two- and three-part diagnostic statements.

Nursing Diagnosis: A Critique

The current nursing diagnosis literature contains many examples of nurses writing about how using nursing diagnoses has improved their clinical practice; articles also detail the many benefits nursing diagnosis brings to the profession. Conversely, other articles point out the limitations of nursing diagnosis and urge nurses to be cautious so that an uncritical use of nursing diagnosis does not restrict their practices.

The primary benefit that nursing diagnosis offers the patient is the individualization of patient care. For example, nurses may be caring simultaneously for three women who have had a modified radical mastectomy because of breast cancer. Although the postoperative nursing management of these women is similar, priorities of care may differ. A prioritized list of nursing diagnoses enables nurses to direct their energies toward these differing patient priorities:

Patient A
- Body Image Disturbance
- Ineffective Individual Coping

Patient B
- Pain
- Self-Care Deficit

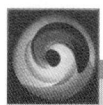

Table 16-5
What a Nursing Diagnosis Is Not, and Why

What a Nursing Diagnosis Is Not	Example	Rationale
Medical diagnosis	Diabetes mellitus	Although there is nursing care associated with medical illnesses, the illness is not primarily amenable to nursing intervention. Nursing's concern is the *person* who has the illness and the effect of the illness on human functioning.
Medical pathology	Hypoglycemia	Nurses need to understand the pathology underlying disease states to plan appropriate nursing care, but once again, nursing's focus is the person, not the pathology. The person's response to hypoglycemia, how hypoglycemia affects human functioning—these are the domain of *nursing* diagnoses.
Diagnostic tests, treatments, equipment	Fasting blood glucose Insulin therapy Insulin syringe Infusion pump	Nursing's concern is the person's response to the diagnostic study, treatment, or equipment. If the need for insulin therapy reveals a knowledge deficit or self-care deficit, this becomes the nursing diagnosis, not insulin therapy in and of itself.
Therapeutic patient needs	Needs to learn the relation among diet, exercise, and insulin	The diagnosis should be written as a patient health problem rather than a patient need. *Example:* Altered Health Maintenance (Diabetic Care) related to lack of knowledge of relation among diet, exercise, and insulin.
Therapeutic nursing goals	To develop therapeutic diabetic self-care behaviors	The diagnosis should be written from the patient perspective rather than the nursing perspective and phrased as a patient health problem. *Example:* Self-Care Deficit: Diabetic Self-Care Behaviors, related to decreased value on life and decreased motivation to learn.
A single sign or symptom	After successfully administering own insulin for 3 days, patient tells nurse, "You give me my shot today."	A nursing diagnosis is not developed until a pattern or cluster of significant cues is detected. The signs and symptoms lead to the identification of the problem statement but are not the problem statement. In this situation, no nursing diagnosis is indicated until further data collection, interpretation, and analysis take place.
An *unvalidated* nursing inference	Above incident leads to the nursing inference: Noncompliance related to depression	This is a premature nursing diagnosis that may not accurately reflect a patient problem. More data and the validation of the tentative nursing diagnosis (nursing inference) are needed before the diagnoses can be recorded.

Patient C
- Risk for Sexual Dysfunction
- Powerlessness

The use of nursing diagnosis also allows patients to be informed and willing participants in their care as they validate their diagnoses and assist in prioritizing them. The process of prioritizing nursing diagnoses is the first step in planning care and is addressed in Chapter 17.

Improved communication among nurses and other healthcare professionals is probably the most important benefit that accurate, up-to-date diagnoses—expressed in well-defined and standardized terminology—offer nurses. This communication aids in planning, charting, patient data retrieval, health team conferences, change-of-shift reports, and healthcare follow-up. It also promotes nursing accountability for the problems that nurses diagnose.

Among the other benefits of nursing diagnoses for the profession is help in defining the domain of nursing to healthcare administrators, legislators, and other healthcare providers; this is important when seeking funding for nursing and reimbursement for nursing services. Nursing diagnoses are also used to define curriculum content and to direct specialization and advancement in nursing and nursing research.

When the diagnostic process is used incorrectly, a patient may be "misdiagnosed." Common sources of error follow:

- Premature diagnoses based on an incomplete database
  Example: A diagnosis of Defensive Coping is made after the patient verbally attacks one nurse who was attempting to teach him self-care for his wound.
- Erroneous diagnoses resulting from an inaccurate database or a faulty data analysis
  Example: A diagnosis of Dysfunctional Grieving is made in a patient observed crying after learning

that her cancer had returned, before anyone had time to evaluate whether this was simply an appropriate response to bad news.

- Routinized diagnoses resulting from the nurse's failure to tailor data collection and analysis to the unique needs of the patient
  Example: A diagnosis of Knowledge Deficit is made in a diabetic patient who is frequently hospitalized with diabetes-related complications, when she actually has excellent knowledge of diabetes and related self-care demands but has lacked the motivation to care for herself appropriately.
- Errors of omission
  Failure to modify diagnoses and to identify new diagnoses as the patient's status changes may also be problems. Failures in diagnosis lead to failures in nursing care.

These are not so much limitations of nursing diagnosis as they are problems of nurses diagnosing incorrectly. More serious criticisms of nursing diagnoses are raised by nurses who claim that a classification of standardized nursing diagnoses limits nursing, curbing nurses' originality and ability to think things through.

Although some nurses believe that diagnosis offers a valued shortcut to practice, critics find this attitude offensive and respond that rather than invest nursing's energies in perfecting a shortcut, nurses need to change the working conditions that interfere with in-depth problem solving and thoughtful nursing care.

Critics of diagnostic labeling point out that instead of identifying what is unique and positive about nursing,

nursing diagnoses make a clear statement that nurses are concerned about what is deviant, wrong, or pathologic (Hagey & McDonough, 1984). The ever-changing and dynamic human person with a need for nursing care becomes objectified (Gebbie, 1984). The practice of many experienced nurses who find nursing diagnoses helpful in coordinating the care efforts of all involved in caring for unique patients with unique needs counters these concerns.

Nurses who are sensitive to transcultural issues raise important concerns about the cultural limitations of the NANDA diagnoses. Foremost among these concerns is that NANDA diagnoses and behaviors assume that the patient is "wrong" and the provider is "right" and deny the validity of cultural and healthcare beliefs and practices that are different from those of the nurse (Geissler, 1991). Examples of nursing diagnoses that often are misused in labeling such cultural deviations as abnormal include Impaired Verbal Communication, Impaired Social Interaction, and Noncompliance. Nurses who provide culturally sensitive care (see Chap. 3) and who work collaboratively with the patient as a partner avoid these problems.

In conclusion, nursing diagnosis has become a valued and essential step in the nursing process. Used correctly, it is a powerful tool for individualizing patient care and ensures that nurses' energies are being used in the most efficient way to meet patients' needs. Nurses who are as concerned about the art and spirit of nursing as they are about its science are careful to avoid labeling patients in a way that objectifies them or limits the potential range of nurse–patient interactions.

Learning Objectives

After completing this chapter, the learner should be able to accomplish the following:

1. Define the key terms used in the chapter.

actual problems	medical diagnoses
collaborative problems	nursing diagnoses
cue	possible problems
data cluster	potential (risk) problems
diagnosing	wellness diagnoses
health problem	

2. Describe the term *nursing diagnosis*, distinguishing it from a collaborative problem and a medical diagnosis.
3. Describe the four steps involved in data interpretation and analysis.
4. Use the guidelines for writing nursing diagnoses when developing diagnostic statements.
5. Describe means to validate nursing diagnoses.
6. Describe the benefits and limitations of nursing diagnoses.

Critical Thinking Exercises

1. Find a patient with a well-established medical condition. List potential medical and nursing diagnoses and collaborative problems. Explain the differing purposes of medical and nursing diagnoses and collaborative problems. What is nursing's *diagnostic contribution* to the interdisciplinary team's effort to care for this patient?
2. Interview several experienced nurses, and find at least one nurse who is strongly committed to using nursing diagnoses and another who believes they are a waste of time. Interview both until you can explain

their different experiences with nursing diagnoses. Try to identify different patient outcomes related to their use or nonuse of nursing diagnoses. List the benefits and limitations of using nursing diagnoses.
3. Interview two patients with the same medical diagnosis. Develop a prioritized list of nursing diagnoses for both, and reflect on the differences. Compare and contrast the strengths of both patients. If you can do this exercise with another student, it would be helpful to explore why there are differences in your lists of nursing diagnoses and patient strengths.

Bibliography

Alfaro, R. (1998). *Applying nursing process: A step-by-step guide* (4th ed.). Philadelphia: Lippincott Williams & Wilkins.

American Nurses' Association (1980, 1995). *Nursing: A social policy statement*. Washington, DC: Author.

Aspinall, M. J. (1976). Nursing diagnosis: the weak link. *Nursing Outlook, 24*(7), 433–436.

Atkinson, J., & Murray, M. E. (1990). *Understanding the nursing process* (4th ed.). New York: Macmillan.

Carnevali, D. L., Mitchell, P. H., Woods, N. F., & Tanner, C. A. (1984). *Diagnostic reasoning in nursing*. Philadelphia: J. B. Lippincott.

Carnevali, D. L., & Thomas, M. D. (1993). *Diagnostic reasoning and treatment decisionmaking in nursing*. Philadelphia: J. B. Lippincott.

Carpenito, L. J. (1985). Diagnostics: Actual, potential, or possible? *American Journal of Nursing, 85*(4), 485.

Carpenito, L. J. (1995). *Nursing diagnosis: Application to clinical practice* (6th ed.). Philadelphia: J. B. Lippincott.

Carroll-Johnson, R. M. (Ed.). (1991). *Classification in nursing diagnosis: Proceedings of the ninth conference*. Philadelphia: J. B. Lippincott.

Dobrzyn, J. (1995). Components of written nursing diagnostic statements. *Nursing Diagnosis, 6*(1), 29–35.

Dossey, B., & Guzzetta, C. E. (1981). Nursing diagnosis. *Nursing, 11*(6), 34–38.

Dougherty, C. M., Jankin, J. J., Lunney, M. R., & Whitley, G. G. (1993). Conceptual and research-based validation of nursing diagnoses: 1950–1993. *Nursing Diagnosis, 4*(4), 156–165.

Fitzpatrick, J. J., Kerr, M. E., Saba. V. K., Hoskins, L. M., Hurley, M. E., Milles, W. C., Rottkamp, B. C., Warren, J. J., & Carpenito, L. J. (1989). Translating nursing diagnosis into ICD code. *American Journal of Nursing, 89*(4), 493–495.

Gebbie, K. M. (Ed.). (1975). *Summary of the second national conference*. St. Louis: Clearinghouse for Nursing Diagnoses.

Gebbie, K. M. (1984). Nursing diagnosis: What is it and why does it exist? *Topics in Clinical Nursing, 5*(4), 1–9.

Gebbie, K. M., & Lavin, M. A. (1973). *Summary of the first national conference*. St. Louis: C. V. Mosby.

Geissler, E. M. (1991). Transcultural nursing and nursing and nursing diagnosis. *Nursing and Health Care, 12*(4), 190–192, 203.

Gordon, M. (1976). Nursing diagnosis and the diagnostic process. *American Journal of Nursing, 76*(8), 1298–1300.

Gordon, M. (1994). *Nursing diagnosis: Process and application* (3rd ed.). St Louis: C. V. Mosby.

Gordon, M. (1995). *Manual of nursing diagnosis: 1995–1996 edition*. St. Louis: Mosby–Year Book.

Hagey, R. S., & McDonough, P. (1984). The problem of professional labeling. *Nursing Outlook, 32*(3), 151–157.

Hammond, K. R. (1966). Clinical inference in nursing: A psychologist's view point. *Nursing Research, 15*(1), 27–38.

Hurley, M. (Ed.). (1986). *Classification of nursing diagnoses: Proceedings of the sixth conference*. St. Louis: C. V. Mosby.

Kerr, M., et al. (1993). Taxonomic validation: An overview *Nursing Diagnosis, 4*(1), 6–14.

Kim, M. J., McFarland, G. K., & McLane, A. M. (Eds.). (1984). *Classification of nursing diagnosis: Proceedings of the fifth national conference*. St. Louis: C. V. Mosby.

Kim, M. J., & Moritz, D. A. (1982). *Classification of the third and fourth national conferences*. Hightstown, NJ: McGraw-Hill.

Kritek, P. B. (1985). Nursing diagnosis in perspective: Response to a critique. *Image—The Journal of Nursing Scholarship, 16*(1), 3–8.

Lindsey, A. M. (1990). Identification and labeling of human responses. *Journal of Professional Nursing, 6*(3), 143–150.

Lunney, M. (1982). Nursing diagnosis: Refining the system. *American Journal of Nursing, 82*(3), 456–459.

Martens, K. (1986). Let's diagnose strengths, not just problems. *American Journal of Nursing, 86*(2), 192–193.

McLane, A. M. (Ed.). (1987). *Classification of nursing diagnoses: Proceedings of the seventh conference*. St. Louis: C. V. Mosby.

Mitchell, G. J. (1991). Nursing diagnosis: An ethical analysis. *Image—The Journal of Nursing Scholarship, 23*(2), 99–103.

Mundinger, M. O., & Jauron, G. D. (1975). Developing a nursing diagnosis. *Nursing Outlook, 23*, 94–98.

North American Nursing Diagnosis Association. (1990). *Taxonomy I revised with official diagnostic categories*. St. Louis: Author.

North American Nursing Diagnosis Association. (1999). *NANDA nursing diagnoses: Definitions and Classification, 1999–2000*. Philadelphia: Author.

Popkess, S. (1981). Diagnosing your patient's strengths. *Nursing, 11*(7), 34–37.

Popkess, S., & Vawter, S. (1991). Wellness nursing diagnosis: To be or not to be? *Nursing Diagnosis, 2*(1), 19–25.

Porter, E. J. (1986). Critical analysis of NANDA nursing diagnosis taxonomy I. *Image—The Journal of Nursing Scholarship, 18*(4), 136–139.

Price, M. R. (1980). Nursing diagnosis: Making a concept come alive. *American Journal of Nursing, 80*(4), 668–674.

Rasch, R. F. R. (1987). The nature of taxonomy. *Image—The Journal of Nursing Scholarship, 19*(3), 147–149.

Roberts, S. L. (1990). Achieving professional autonomy through nursing diagnosis and nursing DRGs. *Nursing Administration Quarterly, 14*(4), 54–60.

Rubenfeld, M. G., & Scheffer, B. K. (1995). *Critical thinking in nursing: An interactive approach*. Philadelphia: J. B. Lippincott.

Shamansky, S. L., & Yanni, C. R. (1983). In opposition to nursing diagnosis: A minority opinion. *Image—The Journal of Nursing Scholarship, 15*(2), 47–50.

Vincent, K. G., & Coler, M. S. (1990). A unified nursing diagnostic model. *Image—The Journal of Nursing Scholarship, 22*(2), 93–95.

Warren, J., & Hoskins, L. 1990. The development of NANDA's nursing diagnosis taxonomy. *Nursing Diagnosis, 1*(4), 162–168.

Weber, G. (1991). Making nursing diagnosis work for you and your patient: A step-by-step approach. *Nursing and Health Care, 12*(8), 424–430.

Wilkinson, J. M. (2000). Nursing diagnosis handbook with NIC interventions and NOC outcomes (7th ed.). Upper Saddle River, NJ: Prentice Hall Health.

Chapter 17
Planning

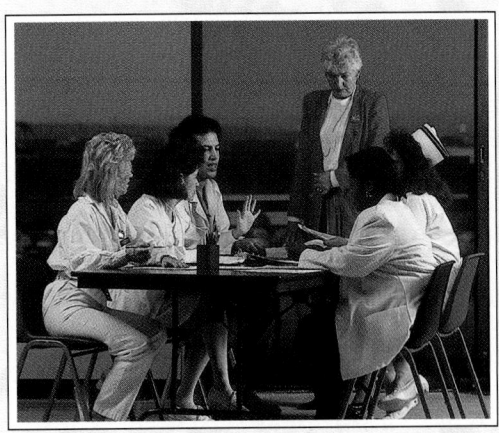

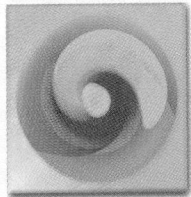

Thinking Critically About
Nursing's Blended Skills

Before reading this chapter, think about the types of skills you will need to develop a plan of care for the individuals you first met in the assessing chapter.

- You are working in a community-based well-child clinic. You become concerned when you observe negligible height and weight gains, delayed developmental milestones, and lethargy in a toddler brought to the clinic by her grandmother.

- You are working with a school nurse. Statistics reveal a pattern of teen smoking in your high school, and you are charged with developing an initiative to reverse this trend.

- You are doing a rotation on a medical floor in a hospital and learn that many of the diabetic patients being treated are repeat admissions with a history of poor self-care behavior.

- You are working in a nursing home where one alert resident with multiple chronic conditions repeatedly tells you that she has no reason to live and asks you to help her end her life.

What cognitive, technical, interpersonal, and ethical/legal skills do you think you will need to develop a plan of nursing care for these individuals and groups?

After the nurse collects and interprets patient data, identifying patient strengths and health problems, it is time to plan for nursing action. During the **planning** step of the nursing process, the nurse works in partnership with the patient and family to (1) prioritize the nursing diagnoses, (2) identify patient goals and expected outcomes that, if achieved, prevent, reduce, or eliminate the problems specified in the nursing diagnoses or secure wellness goals and design a related evaluative strategy, (3) identify the nursing interventions that are most likely to assist the patient in achieving these goals/outcomes, and (4) communicate the plan of care to all involved in its implementation.

A **goal** is an aim or an end. A **patient goal** is an expected patient outcome, an expected conclusion to a patient health problem, or in the event of a wellness diagnosis, an expected conclusion to a patient's health expectation. The words *goal, objective,* and *outcome* are often used interchangeably. In some practice settings, the term *goal* or *objective* is used to describe what is wanted, and the term *outcome* is used to describe the results achieved. In nursing, the phrase **expected outcomes** is used to refer to the more specific, measurable criteria used to evaluate the extent to which a goal has been met. This chapter uses *goal/outcome* to refer to expected patient outcomes.

Elements of planning (outlined in Fig. 17-1) include the following:

- Establishing priorities
- Writing goals/outcomes that determine the evaluative strategy
- Selecting appropriate nursing interventions
- Communicating the plan of nursing care

The nurse, patient, and family should work together as much as possible in the planning stage. If the goals/outcomes specified in the plan of care are not valued by the patient or do not contribute to the prevention, resolution, or reduction of the patient's problems or the achievement of the patient's health expectations, the plan of care may be meaningless. Goal/outcome determination is, therefore, a critical skill for successfully intervening with patients.

This chapter describes planning as a formal process, a deliberate step in the nursing process. Informal planning is often also observed by students in practice settings. This is the link between identifying a patient strength or problem and providing an appropriate nursing response. When a nurse on a busy surgical unit learns that a postoperative patient is complaining of incisional pain and quickly reshuffles priorities to allow time to assess the course and qualities of the pain and determine nursing measures to reduce discomfort, planning has occurred. When a postpartum nurse on the 3-to-11 shift realizes the evening before discharge that he or she has not seen a particular father hold his new daughter

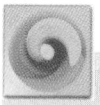

COGNITIVE SKILLS

- Knowledge of what information is needed to develop a plan of care that effectively meets the nursing needs of the toddler with failure to thrive, teens who are smoking or at risk for smoking, diabetic patients with inadequate patterns of self-care, and nursing home resident with diminished will to live (how to establish priorities, develop patient-centered goals/outcomes and related evaluative strategies, select nursing interventions, and communicate the plan of nursing care)
- Knowledge of pertinent standards of care and agency and institutional policies
- Ability to think critically about how best to respond to the patient's need for nursing

TECHNICAL SKILLS

- Ability to research the literature to obtain necessary knowledge to develop the plan of care
- Ability to use a documentation system to communicate the patient's plan of care
- Computer literacy

INTERPERSONAL SKILLS

- Ability to establish trusting nurse–patient relationships grounded in responsible caring with patients with special needs: vulnerable infant, teens, and adults who seem not to value personal health and who lack the motivation for proper self-care
- Ability to empathize with patients, sharing their struggles and celebrating their achievement of valued goals
- Ability to work collaboratively with members of the caregiving team to develop the interdisciplinary plan of care

ETHICAL/LEGAL SKILLS

- Ability to communicate respect and to promote the patient's and family caregivers' sense of worth
- Commitment to secure the patient's well-being within the bounds of your professional responsibilities
- Ability to serve as a trusted and effective patient advocate
- Consistent use of appropriate legal safeguards while developing and documenting the plan of care

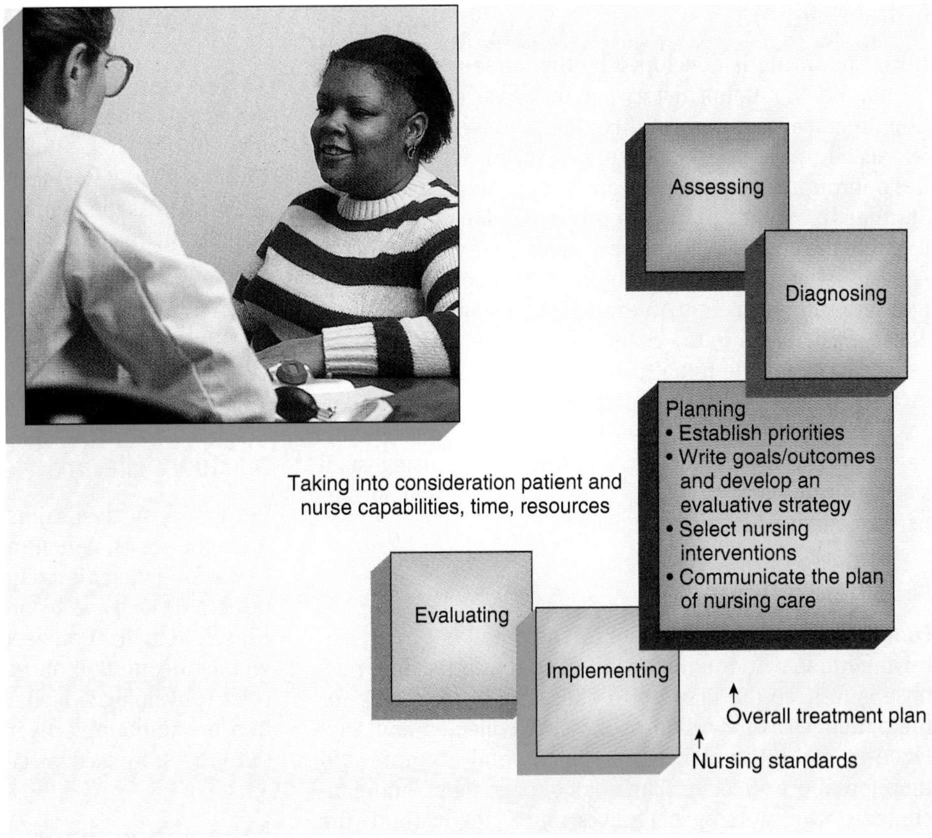

Figure 17-1
Planning. The nurse and patient work together to establish priorities, develop patient goals/outcomes, and identify the nursing interventions most likely to assist the patient to meet the goals. It is important for the plan of care to be consistent with nursing standards, congruent with other planned therapies, and realistic in terms of the patient and nurse's abilities or resources. (Photo by Gates Rhodes, courtesy of School of Nursing, University of Pennsylvania.)

and makes a mental note to observe the father–daughter interactions that evening and facilitate their bonding, planning has occurred. When a nurse in a geriatric day-care center hears a patient choking and rushes to his side to perform the Heimlich maneuver if necessary, planning has occurred. Informal planning on a more conscious level is illustrated by a hospice nurse who drives home pondering how best to support a patient with terminal cancer who is gradually relinquishing her hold on life. She may elect to initiate a more formal process of planning the next day when she consults with colleagues who have cared for patients with similar health needs. In each of the above examples, the process of informal planning allowed an individual nurse to think about how best to help a particular patient—hopefully with good results. What is lacking is a coordinated plan known by everyone caring for the patient.

A formal plan of care allows nurses to individualize care; set priorities; facilitate communication among nursing personnel and their colleagues; promote continuity of high-quality, cost-effective care; coordinate care; evaluate the patient's responses to nursing care; and promote the nurse's professional development.

Unique Focus of Nursing Planning

The primary purpose of the planning step of the nursing process is to design a plan of care for and with the patient that, once implemented, results in the prevention, reduction, or resolution of patient health problems and the attainment

of the patient's health expectations, as identified in the nursing diagnoses. A comprehensive plan of care additionally specifies any routine nursing assistance the patient needs to meet basic human needs (eg, assistance with hygiene or nutrition) and describes appropriate nursing responsibilities for fulfilling the collaborative and medical plan of care. For example, physicians may delegate to nurses caring for a surgical patient the redressing of the surgical incision, the administration of prescribed medications and intravenous therapy, and responsibility for scheduling laboratory studies. Nurses design plans of care that incorporate their independent and collaborative responsibilities. Because nursing is concerned with the patient's responses to health and illness, the plan of care is supportive of nursing's broad aims—to promote wellness, prevent disease and illness, promote recovery, and facilitate coping with altered functioning.

Comprehensive Planning

In acute care settings three basic stages of planning are critical to comprehensive nursing care—initial, ongoing problem-oriented, and discharge. In other settings such as long-term care, hospice care or a community clinic, initial and ongoing problem-oriented planning may be the primary stages used. If a nurse develops a comprehensive plan of care on the patient's first day of meeting but fails to update the plan, the plan will not be effective or efficient. Failure to update the plan of care as needed is a common problem in all healthcare settings.

Initial Planning

Initial planning is developed by the nurse who performs the admission nursing history and the physical assessment. Comprehensive in nature, this plan addresses each problem listed in the prioritized nursing diagnoses and identifies appropriate patient goals and the related nursing care. **Standardized care plans** are prepared plans of care that identify the nursing diagnoses, goals/outcomes, and related nursing interventions common to a specific population or health problem. (An example of a standardized care plan is shown later in the chapter.) They can provide an excellent basis for the initial plan *if the nurse individualizes them.* Resources for standardized plans include computerized plans, textbooks with prepared care plans, and agency-developed plans/maps/critical pathways. By using such standardized plans, the nurse is free to direct time and expertise to individualizing the plan.

Ongoing Planning

Ongoing planning is problem oriented and is carried out by any nurse who interacts with the patient. Its chief purpose is to keep the plan up to date. The nurse caring for the patient uses new data as they are collected and analyzed to make the plan more specific and accurate and therefore more effective. The work of ongoing planning includes stating nursing diagnoses more clearly (both the problem statement and the cause); developing new diagnoses; making previously developed patient goals/outcomes more realistic; developing new goals/outcomes as needed; and identifying nursing interventions that will best accomplish the patient goals.

At this stage of planning, standardized plans based on medical conditions or procedures may be useful in developing new nursing diagnoses and related nursing interventions, but the emphasis is clearly on individualizing the plan to meet unique patient needs. For example, the standard nursing order "force fluids" would be rewritten as "offer 60 mL cranberry or orange juice between meals, and keep fresh water at bedside." A preliminary order such as "explore with the patient existing supports" may be replaced with "keep daughter Barbara informed of mother's progress and coach her in effective support strategies (Barbara Clems, (h) 448-3211, (w) 654-8999)."

Discharge Planning

Discharge planning is best carried out by the nurse who has worked most closely with the patient and family, possibly in conjunction with a nurse or social worker with a broad knowledge of existing community resources. In acute care settings, comprehensive discharge planning begins when the patient is admitted for treatment. Careful planning ensures that the nurse uses teaching and counseling skills effectively to help the patient and family develop sufficient knowledge of the health problem and the therapeutic regimen to carry out necessary self-care behaviors at home competently. Discharge planning is further discussed in Chapter 11.

Establishing Priorities

To develop a prioritized list of nursing diagnoses, the nurse needs guidelines for ranking diagnoses as high, medium, or low priority. High-priority diagnoses pose the greatest threat to the patient's well-being. Non–life-threatening diagnoses are ranked as medium priorities, and diagnoses that are not specifically related to the current health problem are of low priority. In all levels, psychosocial needs must be considered as well as physiologic needs. Three helpful guides suggested by Atkinson and Murray (1990) for prioritizing patient problems are Maslow's hierarchy of human needs, patient preference, and anticipation of future problems.

Maslow's Hierarchy of Human Needs

Because basic needs must be met before a person can focus on higher ones, patient needs may be prioritized according to the following hierarchy: (1) physiologic needs, (2) safety needs, (3) love and belonging needs, (4) self-esteem needs, (5) self-actualization needs. For example, a geriatric patient who is incontinent of urine and sitting in a wet disposable brief (physiologic need) will be unable to participate fully in a music therapy diversional activity (self-esteem need) until the more basic need is met.

Patient Preference

It is best to first meet the needs the patient thinks are most important, if this order does not interfere with other vital therapies. For example, a woman is admitted to an orthopedic unit with a fractured pelvis and multiple lacerations after an automobile accident. The morning after the accident, she complains of pain and needs assistance with bathing and attention to her lacerations, but she refuses to do anything until she calls home to find out who is caring for her 15-month-old twins.

Anticipation of Future Problems

Nurses must tap their knowledge base to consider the potential effects of different nursing actions. Assigning low priority to a diagnosis that the patient wants to ignore but that can result in harmful future consequences for the patient may be nursing negligence. For example, an obese patient with multiple sclerosis and greatly decreased limb strength who spends most of her day in bed may see no value in diet modification and position changes. A nurse who is alert to the potential serious problem of pressure ulcers would assign high priority to this diagnosis, nonetheless, and incorporate weight management and position changes into the plan of care despite the patient's reluctance.

When planning nursing care for each day, it is helpful to consider the following:

- Have changes in the patient's health status influenced the priority of nursing diagnoses? For example, when a routine home visit of an older adult reveals evidence of possible elder abuse, a new set of priorities for care is needed, which may even result in a *new* diagnosis.

- Have changes in the way the patient is responding to health and illness or the plan of care affected those nursing diagnoses that can be realistically addressed? For example, a nurse may have identified ineffective individual coping as a high-priority diagnosis for the patient after the patient learned the medical diagnosis, and planned to initiate counseling. If the patient adamantly requests to be left alone for a day to think things through, however, the nurse has to modify priorities of care for that day.
- Are there relationships among diagnoses that require that one be worked on before another can be resolved?
- Can several patient problems be dealt with together?

After answering these questions, the nurse ranks diagnoses in the order in which they should be addressed. Setting priorities enables the nurse to make sure that time and energy are being directed first to the patient's most important problems.

⊚ Writing Goals/Outcomes

Deriving Goals/Outcomes From Nursing Diagnoses

Goals are derived from the problem statement of the nursing diagnosis. For each nursing diagnosis in the plan of care, at least one goal should be written that, if achieved, demonstrates a *direct resolution* of the problem statement (Table 17-1).

Other outcomes that contribute to the resolution of the problem may be written. For example, for the nursing diagnosis Nutritional Alteration: More Than Body Requirements related to excessive snacking and inactivity, in addition to the goal "within 12 weeks (12/6/02), the patient will lose 20 pounds and reach target weight: 122 lb," the following

Table 17-1
Examples of Goals to Relieve Problems

Problem Statement of the Nursing Diagnosis	Related Patient Goal/Outcome
Pain	Within 8 hours, patient will report pain is absent or diminished
Altered Nutrition: More Than Body Requirements	By 12/6/02, patient will reach target weight of 122 lb
Impaired Physical Mobility	Before discharge, patient will ambulate length of hallway independently

goals are appropriate: "within 3 days of teaching: the patient will identify 10 low-calorie snack foods he is willing to try; the patient will have 3-day diet recall consistent with nutritionally balanced 1500-calorie diet; the patient will report incorporating three ½-hour periods of walking at 5 miles per hour into each week." The difference between these goals/outcomes and the goal/outcome that the patient reach his target weight is that whereas the achievement of the former outcomes may contribute to the resolution of the problem, those outcomes may also be achieved without the problem being resolved, and the patient's plan of care may mistakenly be terminated. Remember, *at least one goal per nursing diagnosis must directly resolve the problem statement in the nursing diagnosis.*

The Nursing Outcomes Classification (NOC) developed by the Iowa Outcomes Project presents the first comprehensive standardized language used to describe the patient outcomes that are responsive to nursing intervention (Johnson & Maas, 1997). Explicit linkages between the North American Nursing Diagnosis Association (NANDA) diagnoses and the NOC facilitate a comprehensive approach to care planning.

Long-Term Versus Short-Term Goals/Outcomes

Goals/outcomes may be either long-term or short-term. Simply defined, long-term goals/outcomes require a longer period (usually more than a week) to be achieved than do short-term goals. They also may be used as discharge goals, in which case they are more broadly written and communicate to the entire nursing team the desired end results of nursing care for a particular patient. For example, two women, both 77 years of age, are on a nursing unit after undergoing similar operative procedures for fractured left hips. One woman has spent the past 2 years in bed in a nursing home; the other woman fractured her hip at the YMCA where she swims daily. Their nursing care should not be the same because it is directed to different long-term goals, even though their short-term goals may be similar (see Examples of Long-Term and Short-Term Goals).

Cognitive, Psychomotor, and Affective Goals

Goals may be categorized according to the type of change they describe for the patient. *Cognitive goals* describe increases in patient knowledge or intellectual behaviors, for example: "Within 1 day after teaching, the patient will list three benefits of continuing to apply moist compresses to leg ulcer after discharge." *Psychomotor goals* describe the patient's achievement of new skills, for example, "By 6/12/02, the patient will correctly demonstrate application of wet-to-dry dressing on leg ulcer." *Affective goals* describe changes in patient values, beliefs, and attitudes. Difficult both to write and to evaluate, affective goals may be critical to the resolution of a complex patient problem, for example, "By 6/12/02, the patient will verbalize valuing health sufficiently to practice new health behaviors to prevent recurrence of leg ulcer." In this example, even if the patient intellectually grasps the reasons for taking care of

---

Examples of Long-Term and Short-Term Goals

Patient on Bed Rest From Nursing Home

Long-Term Goal

Mrs. Goldstein returns to the nursing home pain free with her incision healed and her left leg in good alignment.

Short-Term Goals

- Whenever observed, patient will be lying in bed with legs in correct alignment (abductor pillow in place if ordered).
- Before discharge, Mrs. Goldstein's hip incision will show signs of healing (skin surfaces approximate, free from signs of infection—redness, swelling, heat, purulent drainage).
- Whenever observed, patient will report that comfort measures and medication are satisfactorily managing pain.

Active Patient from Private Home

Long-Term Goal

Mrs. Silverstein returns home to her husband pain free with incision healed, fully mobile (full weight bearing on left leg), and capable of independent activities of daily living.

Short-Term Goals

- By 1/28/02, the patient will verbalize willingness to participate in physical therapy program.
- By 2/4/02, the patient will ambulate (with nursing assistance and walker) to bathroom (full weight bearing).
- By 2/11/02, the patient will ambulate with nursing assistance only (no walker) in her room.
- Goals for incision and pain relief same as for Mrs. Goldstein.

---

her leg and can competently redress her ulcer, unless she is motivated to take care of herself, her knowledge and skills will not result in healthy outcomes.

Guidelines for Goal/Outcome Writing

One of the most important considerations in goal/outcome writing is to encourage the patient and family to be as involved in goal development as their abilities and interest permit. The more involved they are, the greater the probability that the goals will be achieved. When developing patient goals/outcomes, the nurse and patient look at the problem statement of the nursing diagnosis and ask, "What patient changes or outcomes will result in the prevention or resolution of this problem?" The answer, when carefully worded, becomes the patient goal/outcome.

Each patient goal/outcome must have a *subject*, which is the patient; a *verb*, which indicates the action the patient will perform; and **criteria**, which describe in *observable, measurable terms* the expected patient behavior or other manifestation. Verbs helpful in writing goals follow:

Define	Prepare
Identify	Design
List	Verbalize
Describe	Choose
Explain	Select
Apply	Demonstrate

The criteria must include a time criterion, which may be a realistic, actual date or other statement indicating time, such as before discharge, after viewing film, whenever observed.

Following are examples of properly constructed patient goals:

- During the next 24-hour period, the patient's fluid intake will total at least 2000 mL.
- At the next visit, 12/23/02, the patient will correctly demonstrate relaxation exercises.

It may be helpful to include special conditions when writing a goal if this information is important for other nurses (eg, "Before discharge, the patient will ambulate independently the length of hallway and back, using a Philadelphia collar to support cervical vertebrae").

Written goals/outcomes can be evaluated by seeing if they conform to the following criteria:

- Each set of goals/outcomes is derived from only one nursing diagnosis.
- At least one of the goals/outcomes shows a direct resolution of the problem statement in the nursing diagnosis.
- Each goal/outcome is brief, specific (clearly describes *one* observable, measurable patient behavior/manifestation), phrased positively, and specifies a time line.
- The patient (and family) values the goals/outcomes.
- The goals/outcomes are supportive of the total treatment plan.

Common Errors

Common errors when writing patient goals/outcomes include the following:

- Expressing the *patient* goal as a *nursing* intervention. *Incorrect:* Offer Mr. Myer 60 mL fluid every 2 hours while awake. *Correct:* Mr. Myer will drink 60 mL fluid every 2 hours while awake, beginning 2/24/02.
- Using verbs that are not *observable* and *measurable*. *Incorrect:* Mrs. Gaston will know how to bathe her newborn. *Correct:* After attending the infant care class, Mrs. Gaston will correctly demonstrate the procedure for bathing her newborn. Verbs to be avoided when writing goals include *know, understand, learn, become aware.* These verbs are too general and are unmeasurable. Verbs that are helpful when writing goals/outcomes that are observable and measurable were listed previously.
- Including more than one patient behavior/manifestation in short-term goals/outcomes. *Incorrect:* Patient will list dangers of smoking and stop smoking. *Correct:* By next meeting, 3/11/02, the patient will (1) identify three dangers of smoking and (2) describe a plan he is

willing to try to stop smoking. By 6/20/02, the patient will report that he no longer smokes.

- Writing goals/outcomes so vaguely that other nurses are unsure of the goal of nursing care. *Incorrect:* Patient will cope better. *Correct:* After teaching, 10/20/02, the patient will (1) describe two new coping strategies he is willing to try and (2) demonstrate decreased incidence of previously observed noneffective coping behaviors (chain smoking, withdrawal behavior, heavy alcohol consumption).

Developing Evaluative Strategies

Well-written goals define the evaluative strategy to be used by the nurse. Patient goals/outcomes are meaningless unless nurses evaluate the patient's progress toward their achievement. The nurse records the date the goal/outcome was written and the date it is achieved. Evaluative statements (see accompanying box) include a statement about achievement of the desired goal/outcome (met, partially met, not met) and list actual patient behavior as evidence supporting the statement. If the plan is not achieved, recommendations for revising the plan of care are included in the evaluative statement (Atkinson & Murray, 1990). Chapter 19 deals specifically with the evaluative component of the nursing process.

Identifying Nursing Interventions

A **nursing intervention** is any treatment, based on clinical judgment and knowledge, that a nurse performs to enhance patient outcomes (McCloskey & Bulechek, 1996). There are nurse-initiated, physician-initiated, and collaborative interventions.

Nurse-Initiated Interventions

A nurse-initiated intervention is an autonomous action based on scientific rationale that a nurse executes to benefit the patient in a predictable way related to the nursing diagnosis and projected outcomes. Nurse-initiated interventions do not require a physician's (or other team member's) order. Nurse-initiated interventions, like patient goals, are derived from the nursing diagnosis. But whereas the problem statement of the diagnosis suggests the patient goals, it is the cause of the problem (etiology) that suggests the nursing interventions (Fig. 17-2). Effective nurses select nursing interventions that specifically address factors that cause or contribute to the patient's problems.

For example, many factors may contribute to obesity, such as deficient nutritional knowledge, convenience of high-calorie fast foods, lifetime snacking habits, limited food budget, little exercise, and low self-esteem. The nurse working with a patient who wants to lose weight could attempt to deal with all these factors, but this approach would be inefficient. When a carefully developed nursing diagnosis identifies the specific factors that contributed to a particular patient's weight problem, nursing interventions can be selected to deal directly with these factors.

Similarly, nursing interventions for the patient with the diagnosis, Altered Nutrition: More Than Body Requirements related to lifetime snacking habits and heavy reliance on high-calorie fast foods, might include education about the fat content and calories in fast foods and an exploration of ways the patient could change eating habits to

---

Evaluative Statement

Documents that patient has met, partially met, or not met the goal/outcome

Goal/Outcome Statement

Beginning 6/8/02, the patient will ambulate half the length of hallway with assistance three times daily.

Evaluative Statement

6/8/02—Goal partially met; patient refused to ambulate in the morning but did walk to the bathroom once in the afternoon with the assistance of one nurse.

Recommendation: Review reason for progressive ambulation with patient; assess motivation to increase independence.

M. Stenulis, RN

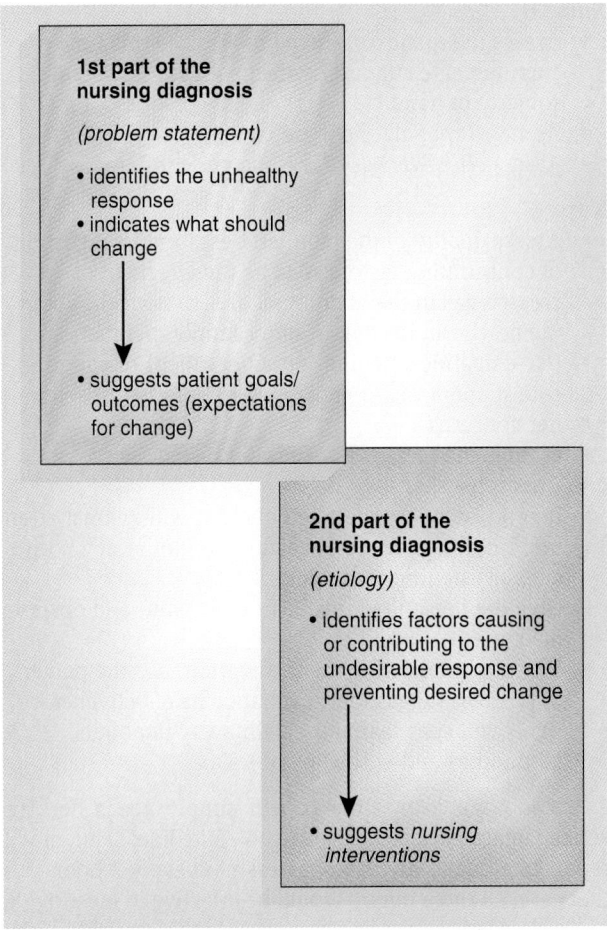

1st part of the nursing diagnosis

(problem statement)

- identifies the unhealthy response
- indicates what should change

- suggests patient goals/ outcomes (expectations for change)

2nd part of the nursing diagnosis

(etiology)

- identifies factors causing or contributing to the undesirable response and preventing desired change

- suggests *nursing interventions*

Figure 17-2

Deriving patient goals and nursing orders from nursing diagnoses.

eat more nutritionally balanced meals with fewer calories. Thus, not every patient with a weight problem is nursed the same way. The art of nursing involves the careful identification of the specific nursing interventions needed by particular patients to meet their individual needs.

Identifying and Selecting Appropriate Interventions

After the patient goals/outcomes are written, the nurse identifies various nursing interventions to help the patient achieve the goals/outcomes. The Nursing Intervention Classification System (NIC), the first comprehensive, validated list of nursing interventions applicable to all settings that can be used by nurses in multiple specialties, greatly facilitates the work of identifying appropriate interventions (McCloskey & Bulechek, 1996). Examples of using NIC to facilitate care planning for specific patient health problems may be found in each clinical chapter of this text.

The effectiveness of the nurse is directly proportional to his or her knowledge of varied nursing strategies. Consider these different nursing care options identified by three nurses when they are asked to describe nursing care for a woman 2 days after cesarean delivery who is complaining of pain in the incisional area.

Nurse A

- Check to see what type of pain medication is ordered, and give it if the time interval is sufficient.

Nurse B

- Assess the quality of the pain, and use this time to communicate support by means of expression and squeeze of hand.
- Administer analgesic if indicated.
- Assess effectiveness of the analgesic ordered.

Nurse C

- Assess quality of the pain, and explore the possibility of contributing factors such as the effects of increased gas in the abdominal area or concern about the newborn, herself, or other family members.
- Use empathic listening (possibly touch) to communicate support and to encourage the mother to share her concerns.
- Change the patient's position in bed.
- Offer a back rub.
- If appropriate, suggest activity that will distract attention from the pain (eg, watching a film of newborn care or listening to music).
- Give the prescribed medication for pain, and observe its effect.
- When administering the medication, use the power of positive suggestion to enhance its effectiveness: "This will start taking the pain away in about 10 minutes and will help you relax."

It is possible that the patient simply needs her prescribed analgesic to achieve the goal/outcome: "Patient will report minimal to no pain at assessment every 2 hours." In that case, all three nurses would be effective in meeting the patient's need for nursing care. It is highly possible, however, that the prescribed medication is not working or the

pain is compounded by the mother's fears about caring for her new baby or by her worries that the baby will ruin her relationship with her husband. Therefore, nurse C, whose knowledge level is more comprehensive, is most likely to be effective in resolving the patient's problem.

The more varied the options available to the nurse, the more effective the nursing response. In different situations, a skilled nursing procedure, an appropriate use of silence, respectful listening, humor, teaching, counseling, and touch can all be effective nursing strategies. Nurses who are merely task oriented and satisfied to meet every patient problem with a mechanical procedure are limiting their effectiveness.

When selecting nursing interventions for individual patients, use the following guidelines. Nursing interventions should be as follows:

- Appropriate in terms of the nursing diagnosis and related patient outcomes
- Consistent with research findings and standards of care
- Realistic in terms of the abilities, time, and resources available to the nurse and patient
- Compatible with the patient's values, beliefs, and psychosocial background
- Valued, whenever possible, by the patient and family
- Compatible with other planned therapies

Use of these guidelines increases the chances that the patient will successfully achieve the goal/outcome. Ongoing evaluation enables the nurse to determine the effectiveness of the selected interventions.

Nurse researchers are now attempting to establish a statistical pattern for predicting the probability of success of select nursing interventions. Competent nurses use research findings (science of nursing), experience, and knowledge of the patient (art of nursing) to aid in the selection of effective nursing interventions. Consultation with nurse colleagues and continuing education enable the nurse to develop effective nursing approaches to patient problems.

Writing Nurse-Initiated Interventions in the Plan of Care

Nursing interventions describe in writing, and thus communicate to the entire nursing staff and healthcare team, the specific nursing care to be implemented for the patient. Well-written nursing interventions accomplish the following:

- Assist the patient to meet specific goals/outcomes that are related directly to one goal/outcome
- Clearly and concisely describe the nursing action to be performed (answer the questions who? what? where? when? and how?)
- Are dated when written and when the plan of care is reviewed
- Are signed by the nurse prescribing the order or intervention
- Use only those abbreviations accepted in the institution (these are usually found in the agency's policy

manual; a list of commonly accepted abbreviations appears in Chapter 20)

- Refer the nurse to the agency's procedure manual or other literature for the steps of routine, lengthy procedures

Following are examples of well-stated nursing interventions:

- Offer patient 60 mL water or juice (prefers orange or cranberry juice) every 2 hours while awake for a total minimum P.O. intake of 500 mL.
- Teach patient the necessity of carefully monitoring fluid intake and output; remind patient each shift to mark off fluid intake on record at bedside.
- Walk with patient to bathroom for toileting every 2 hours (on even hours) while patient is awake.

The set of nursing interventions written to assist a patient to meet a goal/outcome must be comprehensive. Comprehensive nursing interventions specify what *observations* (assessments) need to be made and how often; what *nursing interventions* need to be done and when they must be done; and what *teaching, counseling, and advocacy needs* patients and families have.

Many sets of nursing interventions are inadequate because they fail to indicate the ongoing assessment priority needs for a specific problem or goal. Clearly stating assessment priorities helps all nurses to be more sensitive to important patient data. For example, when assisting a patient who wants to lose weight to reach the target weight, appropriate nursing interventions might include the following: "6/17/02—Continue to assess (1) patient's motivation to participate in weight loss program, and (2) factors that positively or negatively influence weight loss."

Similarly, it is often assumed that all patients have the same teaching needs. Nothing is farther from the truth. In fact, many patients have an excellent knowledge base (which may be greater than that of the nurse for a particular disease). Their need for nursing may be a need for counseling, instead of teaching, as they learn to live with a chronic illness. Comprehensive nursing interventions relate to individual patient needs.

Physician-Initiated Interventions

A physician-initiated intervention is an intervention initiated by a physician in response to a medical diagnosis but carried out by a nurse in response to a doctor's order. For example, a physician examining a patient brought into the emergency room after a motor vehicle accident may ask the nurse to administer a medication to relieve pain and schedule the patient for radiographs and other diagnostic tests. The nurse who performs these interventions is implementing physician-initiated interventions. Both the physician and nurse are legally responsible for these interventions, and nurses are expected to be knowledgeable about how to execute these interventions safely and effectively. Nurses who question the appropriateness of physician-initiated interventions are legally responsible to seek clarification of the order with responsible parties. Under no circumstances should a nurses implement a questionable intervention, even at the urging of a physician or other professional. Chapter 7 addresses the nurse's legal responsibility for her actions.

Collaborative Interventions

Nurses also carry out treatments initiated by other providers, such as pharmacists, respiratory therapists, or physician assistants. Nurses caring for patients in a motor vehicle accident may eventually be implementing interventions written by a physical therapist, occupational therapist, or other member of the healthcare team.

Clinical Practice Guidelines

Efforts to standardize nursing care have taken different forms. Approaches popular during different decades include: procedures (1960s), standards of care (1970s), algorithms (1980s), and clinical practice guidelines (1990s). Each of these aims to facilitate optimal care, reduce legal risks, and lower healthcare costs.

Procedure: a set of how-to action steps for performing a clinical activity or task
Standard of care: a description of an acceptable level of patient care or professional practice
Algorithm: a set of steps that approximates the decision process of an expert clinician and is used to make a decision; these clinical rules are typically embedded in a branching flow chart
Clinical practice guideline: a statement or series of statements outlining appropriate practice for a clinical condition or procedure

National guidelines such as those published by the US Agency for Health Care Policy and Research (AHCPR) are generally based on the latest, most comprehensive scientific evidence and expert analysis. They provide standards for delivering and evaluating care for patients with the same diagnosis. For free single copies of the AHCPR clinical practice guidelines, contact: AHCPR Publications Clearinghouse, P.O. Box 8547, Silver Spring, MD 20907; 1-800-358-9295; fax, 1-301-594-2800. See the accompanying box for a nationally used methodology and characteristics.

Consulting

A nurse designing the plan of care may discover that more information is needed about the nature of the problems underlying the need for nursing or about specific interventions. **Consultation**, a process in which two or more individuals with varying degrees of experience and expertise discuss a problem and its solution, often proves helpful. Nurses may consult with nurse specialists and other members of the healthcare team, including physicians, nutritionists, social workers, therapists, pastoral caregivers, and ethicists. Consultations are a valuable means for nurses to expand their nursing knowledge and repertoire of effective strategies.

Structured Care Methodology and Characteristics

Algorithm

- Useful in management of high-risk subgroups within the cohort; may be "layered" on top of a pathway to control care practices that are used to manage a specific problem
- Binary decision trees that guide stepwise assessment and intervention
- Intense specificity; no provider flexibility
- May use analytical research methods to ensure cause and effect

Critical Pathway

- Represents a sequential, interdisciplinary, minimal practice standard for a specific patient population
- Provides flexibility to alter care to meet individualized patient needs
- Abbreviated format, broad perspective
- Phase or episode driven
- Ability to measure cause-and-effect relationship between pathway and patient outcomes prohibited by lack of control; changes in patient outcomes directly attributable to the efforts of the collaborative practice team

Guideline

- Broad, research-based practice recommendations
- May or may not have been tested in clinical practice

- Practice resources helpful in construction of structured care methodologies
- No mechanism for ensuring practice implementation

Order Set

- Preprinted provider orders used to expedite the order process after a practice standard has been validated through analytical research
- Complements and increases compliance with existing practice standards
- Can be used to represent the algorithm or protocol in order format

Protocol

- Prescribes specific therapeutic interventions for a clinical problem unique to a subgroup of patients within the cohort
- Multifaceted; may be used to drive practice for more than one discipline
- Broader specificity than an algorithm; allows for minimal provider flexibility by way of treatment options
- May be "layered" on top of a pathway

Agency for Health Care Policy and Research's (AHCPR) Clinical Practice Guideline Development, AHCPR program note in Publication 93-0023, 1993.

🔁 Writing the Plan of Nursing Care

The **plan of nursing care** (patient care plan) is the written guide that directs the efforts of the nursing team as the nurses work with patients to meet health goals. It specifies nursing diagnoses, goals/outcomes, and associated nursing interventions. Well-written plans of care offer many benefits to the patient, nurse, nursing unit, nursing administration, and nursing profession. Primarily, plans of nursing care ensure that the nursing team works efficiently to deliver holistic, goal-oriented, individualized care to patients. A well-written plan of nursing care accomplishes the following:

- Represents an effective philosophy of nursing and advances nursing's four aims: promotes health, prevents disease and illness, promotes recovery, facilitates coping with altered functioning
- Is prepared by the nurse who best knows the patient and is recorded on the day the patient presents for treatment and care according to agency policy; modifications to the initial plan are signed and dated
- Is responsive to the individual characteristics and needs of the patient

- Clearly identifies the nursing assistance the patient needs and nursing's collaborative responsibilities for fulfilling the medical and interdisciplinary plan of care (clearly specifies nursing diagnoses, patient goals/outcomes, nursing interventions, and evaluative strategies)
- Directs the nurse's assessment priorities, caregiving behaviors, and teaching, counseling, and advocacy behaviors
- Is based on scientific principles and incorporates findings of nursing research
- Meets developmental, psychosocial, and spiritual needs of the patient, as well as physiologic needs
- Is updated to reflect changes in the patient's status and related needs for nursing care
- Addresses discharge needs of the patient and family
- Provides for as much patient and family participation as possible
- When appropriate, is compatible with the medical plan of care and that of the interdisciplinary team

Many suggestions for plans of care appear in the nursing literature. Each school of nursing and each healthcare institution and agency has its own format, which may reflect a particular nursing theory. Common to all formats is a minimum of three columns for documenting nursing diagnoses, patient goals/outcomes, and nursing interventions. Formats differ in the way assessment data and the nursing evaluation are addressed.

Institutional and Agency Plans of Care

The Joint Commission on Accreditation of Healthcare Organizations requires healthcare institutions and agencies to formulate, maintain, and support a patient-specific plan for care, treatment, and rehabilitation 1996. A great variety of formats are used to communicate the plan of care. In most institutions and agencies, the plans of care, regardless of their format, communicate directions for three different types of nursing care: nursing care related to basic human needs, nursing care related to nursing diagnoses, and nursing care related to the medical and interdisciplinary plan of care.

Nursing Care Related to Basic Human Needs
The plan should concisely communicate to caregivers the data about the patient's usual health habits and patterns, obtained during the nursing history, that are needed to direct daily care. For example, it is important to know whether a toddler is toilet trained and what words he or she uses to indicate the need to void or defecate. Directives about the patient's usual health habits and patterns may be modified by current treatment orders, such as an order to fast for a diagnostic procedure or to limit or increase activity. This information is useful to caregivers only if it is kept current as the patient's condition changes. Any nurse should be able to find in the plan of care the instructions needed to provide competent care.

Nursing Care Related to Nursing Diagnoses
The plan contains goals/outcomes and nursing interventions for every nursing diagnosis as well as a place to note the patient's responses to care. This section is the heart of the nursing care plan because it represents the independent component of nursing practice. If well developed, it demonstrates the nurse's clinical competence (knowledge of the science of nursing), sensitivity to the individual needs of the patient, and creativity in mobilizing the resources of the patient and the caregiving team to meet the patient's health needs.

Nursing Care Related to the Medical and Interdisciplinary Plan of Care
The plan of care also records current medical orders for diagnostic studies and treatment and specified related nursing care.

Kardex Plans of Care
Many healthcare institutions and agencies use a **Kardex care plan,** in which the plan of nursing care for each patient is concisely recorded on a folded card and placed in a central Kardex file where it is easily accessible. The plan is eventually placed in the patient's health record. The outside of the card contains basic information, such as the patient's profile, admitting diagnosis, activity levels, diet, and routine treatments, medications, and procedures. The inside of the Kardex contains the nursing care plan specifying at the very minimum nursing diagnoses or health problems and related outcomes and nursing interventions.

Computerized Plans of Care
In an increasing number of settings, nurses use **computerized plans of care**. Benefits of using computerized plans include ready access to a large knowledge base, improved record keeping with resultant improvement in audits and quality assurance, documentation by all members of the healthcare team with printouts for the patient's record and for change-of-shift reports, and reduced time spent on paperwork. One nurse researcher, however, has studied the negative impact of computerized plans on the professionalization of staff nurses. Harris (1990) cautions that computerized systems for patient care planning and the larger systems in which they are embedded contribute to the loss of autonomy, loss of individualization of care, and loss of nursing expertise. Individual nurses, as well as researchers, need to respond to this challenge from Harris: "Does a lot of nursing time spent in procedural, rule-governed, step-by-step thinking processes destroy part of the nurse's ability to care, to empathize, to intuit, to gain insight, to function in the expert mode?" (1990, p. 73).

Case Management Plans of Care
Case management is a healthcare delivery system with the objective of providing high-quality, cost-effective care for individuals, families, and groups. The emphasis is on clearly stating expected patient outcomes and the specific times within which it is reasonable to achieve these outcomes. **Clinical pathways** (**critical pathways, CareMaps**) are tools used to communicate the standardized, interdisciplinary plan of care for patients. Chapter 20 provides examples of how critical pathways are used with select documentation tools in a computerized system. The accompanying display illustrates a standardized plan of care for patients with congestive heart failure. Care guidelines and outcomes are specified for each day of the patient's stay. In this case, the patients receive a version of their own plan of care on admission, based on the rationale that knowing what to expect will result in less stress, quicker recovery, and earlier discharge.

Student Plans of Care

The care plans that students are required to develop are often more detailed than those found in practice settings. The aim is to assist students to assimilate each of the five steps of the nursing process. Although care plan formats vary among different nursing programs, most are designed so that the student systematically proceeds through the interrelated steps of the nursing process, and many use a five-column format.

The sample student care plan shown here demonstrates a plan developed for the patient whose admission assessment form is in Chapter 15. This 72-year-old woman (text continues on page 287)

Standardized Plan of Care

Chart 1
Sacred Heart—St. Mary's Hospitals, Inc.
PLAN OF CARE: CONGESTIVE HEART FAILURE
ESTIMATED LENGTH OF STAY: 4 Days
Supplies Given: Adm. Kit _PN 2-1-02_ **Urinal** _PN 2-1-02_ **Bedpan** _PN 2-1-02_ **Air Mattress** _PN 2-1-02_

FOCUS Date:	Day of Admission	Day 2	Day 3	Day 4
ACTIVITY	Activity intolerance related to dyspnea • Restrict activity 30 min before and 60 min after meals _Expected outcome_ • Activity as tolerated _PN 2-1_	• Restrict activity 30 min before and 60 min after meals • Chair 30 min t.i.d. for meals • Ambulate 60 ft in hall w/ assist • Bathroom privileges _Expected outcome_ • Able to tolerate activity without distress _PN 2-2_	• Ambulate 100 ft t.i.d. _Expected outcome_ • Able to perform ADLs and ambulation without the use of O_2 ____	• Prepare pt for discharge home _Expected outcome_ • Able to tolerate activity without distress ____
NUTRITION Needs assist _no_ Consult needed? _no_	(NAS diet or) ____ _PN 2-1_	NAS diet or ____	NAS diet or ____	NAS diet or ____
TREATMENTS Skin protocol _PN 2-1_ Fall protocol _PN 2-1_	Alteration in fluid balance related to compromised cardiac output • Vital signs q4h • I&O • Daily weight • Telemetry if ordered • Heparin lock • O_2 at _3 l/min_ • Assess lung and heart sounds q shift and p.r.n. • Assess pedal edema and pulses q shift	• Vital signs q4h • I&O • Daily weight • Telemetry if ordered • Heparin lock • O_2 at _3 l/min_ • Assess lung and heart sounds q shift and p.r.n. • Assess pedal edema and pulses q shift _Expected outcomes_ • Pt's foot edema is decreased or pt has lost weight (min 1 lb) _PN 2-2_ • Pt has improved breath sounds _PN 2-2_	• Vital signs q shift • I&O • Daily weight • Discontinue telemetry if previously ordered ____ • Heparin lock • O_2 p.r.n. (If still needed, consult cardio-pulmonary services for need for home O_2.) • Assess lung and heart sounds q shift • Assess pedal edema and pulses q shift	• Vital signs q shift • I&O • Daily weight • Discontinue heparin lock ____ • Discontinue O_2 ____ • Assess lung and heart sounds q shift • Assess pedal edema and pulses q shifts _Expected outcomes_ • Feet/ankle edema resolved • Unlabored respirations ____
TEACHING	• Review Plan of Care with pt • Explain medications to pt • Give copy of Plan of Care to pt • Give info sheet on congestive heart failure to pt • Home health referral needed _yes_ _PN 2-1-02_ • Home O_2 needed _possibly_ _PN 2-1-02_	_Expected outcomes_ • Pt can verbalize understanding of present medications _PN 2-2_	• Discharge medication sheets given ____ • Home health referral arranged if needed ____ • Home O_2 arranged if needed ____	_Expected outcomes_ • Pt can verbalize understanding of present medications ____ • Discharge medication sheet reviewed and pt can verbalize understanding ____ • Discharge instructions reviewed and pt can verbalize understanding ____ • Pt can verbalize understanding for need of follow-up visit and when to call doctor ____

OTHER FOCAL AREAS
• Durable power of attorney _yes_ _PN 2-1_
• Living will _yes_ _PN 2-1_
• Code status _full_ _PN 2-1_

Rasmussen, N., & Gengler, T. (1994). Clinical pathways of care: The route to better communication. _Nursing 94, 24_(2), 48–49. Used with permission.

Standard Plan of Care: Patient Copy

Chart 2
Sacred Heart—St. Mary's Hospitals, Inc.
PLAN OF CARE: CONGESTIVE HEART FAILURE   **PATIENT COPY**
ESTIMATED LENGTH OF STAY: 4 Days

FOCUS Date:	Day of Admission	Day 2	Day 3	Day 4
ACTIVITY	You can move around as you are able. Avoid becoming overtired or short of breath. You should remain in bed 30 minutes before and after your meals.	You should increase your activity slowly. Start by sitting up in the chair for meals and walking short distances with the help of the nurses twice a day.	You should be starting to feel better and should be able to do mild activities without your oxygen	You should be able to walk in the halls and take your own bath without trouble breathing. You'll go home today if your doctor feels you're ready.
NUTRITION	You'll be on a no-added-salt diet. The dietition will come to talk to you about this if you don't understand. A salt substitute is available if you need it. (Salt causes your body to hold in extra fluids, making your swelling worse and causing your heart to work even harder.	Low-salt diet.	Low-salt diet.	Low-salt diet. Ask your doctor or nurse if you should continue this diet at home.
TREATMENTS	The nurse will measure the amount of fluid you take in and put out. The nurse will listen to your heart and lungs to see if they are getting better. You may have to use oxygen for the first day or two to help you breathe easier. You'll be weighed daily. You'll have an intravenous needle placed in your hand or arm. This will be used to give you medication. You may have a telemetry heart monitor on. Nurses in the intensive care unit will monitor your heart's rhythm.	Treatments will remain the same.	Some treatments will remain the same. You'll use oxygen only when you feel you need it. The heart monitor will be discontinued if previously ordered.	Some treatments will remain the same. Your oxygen may be discontinued. Your needle will be removed if you're going home.
TEACHING	You'll need to understand what is going on with your body. Please ask questions if you don't understand something. You'll be given a sheet to explain what congestive heart failure is. Ask about your medications if you're unfamiliar with them.		You'll be given information sheets that explain the medication you'll take at home. You should know about the right foods to eat and what types of food you should avoid. Your doctor may order a follow-up by a home health nurse.	You'll need to follow up with your doctor. Make sure you know when your appointment is. Know what problems may require medical attention.

Rasmussen, N., & Gengler, T. (1994). Clinical pathways of care: The route to better communication. *Nursing 94, 24*(2), 48–49. Used with permission.

STUDENT CARE PLAN

Assessment/Diagnosis	*Goal/Outcome*

Subjective data: "Will I get a stroke now? I don't think I could handle that." "How can I help myself prevent it?"

Objective data: Admitting diagnosis:

TIA

BP: 184/120

Strengths: Past pattern of adhering to prescribed health behaviors.

Nursing diagnosis: High Risk for Alteration in Health Maintenance Response to TIA and Stroke Prevention related to knowledge deficit

Goal/Outcome

Before discharge, the patient will:

- Describe the terms *TIA* and *stroke,* identifying the underlying disease process, causes, symptoms, and treatment

After discussion with the physician and nurse, the patient will:

- Correctly describe the treatment plan:
  - Medications (drugs, intended effect, dose, time, route)
  - Dietary modifications
  - Exercise prescription
  - Signs and symptoms to report
  - Follow-up appointment date

Subjective data: Husband died 8 months ago; moved in with daughter 6 months ago after selling family home

Daughter reports mother has been a very independent, strong woman in the past—seemed to "crumple" after husband's death.

History of headaches

Objective data: Clutches daughter's hand

Strengths: History of handling life stressors well

Limitations: In the past, her husband was her primary support

Nursing diagnosis: Ineffective Individual Coping related to illness, recent death of husband, and relocation with daughter

Beginning 9/7/02, the patient will:

- Verbalize her feelings related to the loss of her husband, loss of family home, loss of health

- Identify coping patterns that have helped her in the past

- Identify three personal strengths and three outside supports that will help her now

Before discharge, the patient will:

- Verbalize that she feels "okay" (sufficiently in charge of her life) about returning home

STUDENT CARE PLAN (*Continued*)

Nursing Orders	*Scientific Rationale*	*Evaluation*
Assess what the patient knows about TIA and stroke (correct any misinformation). Assess learning needs, readiness to learn, and factors that will influence learning.	Each person's learning needs are different; each person learns in own unique way; learning is dependent on readiness.	9/10/02—Goal not met. Patient says her head is "too old" to learn all this stuff. Equates stroke with death. *Revision:* Reteach content in simpler terms. Reassess learning readiness. *C. Taylor, RN*
Plan teaching and learning sessions to involve family members designated by patient	The more support people knowledgeably committed to the plan of care, the greater the probability the patient will achieve goals.	9/10/02 Too early to evaluate. *C. Taylor, RN*
Include in the teaching plan a description of TIA and stroke and the underlying disease process, causes, symptoms, and treatment plan.	New self-care behaviors are dependent on knowledge.	
After the treatment plan has been developed, make sure the patient and family can restate it (teaching) and *value* the prescribed lifestyle modification (counseling).	New self-care behaviors are dependent on motivation. Unless the patient is committed to stroke prevention and values this outcome, she will not follow the treatment plan.	

Once during each shift, primary nurse should sit at patient's bedside for at least several minutes to communicate caring and to explore with the patient her current stressors and the adequacy of her coping response.
 	
• Assess factors compounding her losses.
• Reinforce her personal strengths and support systems; counsel her to tap into these now.
• Suggest local support groups if indicated.
	The nurse's unhurried, attentive, and caring presence communicates to the patient that she is important to the nurse and that the nurse values her well-being. It is an invitation to the patient to become actively involved in recovery. Also, it is logical to explore adequacy of past and current coping mechanisms before suggesting new approaches.	9/10/02 Goal partially met. Patient speaks freely about how much she misses her husband and how fearful this hospitalization makes her. When asked about living with her daughter, she becomes uncharacteristically quiet.
		
		     C. Taylor, RN
		
		9/10/02 Goal met. Patient talks about how everything seemed better in the past after she talked it over with her husband and God.
		
		     C. Taylor, RN

Primary nurse to explore with daughter, Lisa, how her mother's moving in with her has affected the family. Recommend support systems.	Adult children of aging parents frequently experience overwhelming stress as they try to deal with their own and their parents' problems. Supporting this family *is* supporting the patient indirectly.	9/10/02 Goal not met. Patient couldn't think of anything about herself that is healthy or strong. Says "maybe" her family can help her now.
		
		Revision: Counsel regarding personal strengths. Help her to experience them.
		
		     C. Taylor, RN
		
		9/11/02 Too early to evaluate.
		
		     C. Taylor, RN
		
		      (*continued*)

STUDENT CARE PLAN (*Continued*)

Assessment/Diagnosis

Subjective data: "I move my bowels every 2 or 3 days; get constipated at least once a week. Often Metamucil helps."

"I drink plenty of fluids and eat fruits and vegetables."

History of hemorrhoids secondary to straining

Objective data: No bowel movement in past 4 days

On bed rest since hospitalized

Nursing diagnosis: Constipation related to decreased physical activity and long-term laxative use (Metamucil)

Goal/Outcome

Beginning 9/7/02, the patient will:

- Pass soft, formed stool every 1 to 3 days without use of laxatives

By 9/10/02, the patient will:

- Verbalize the importance of the following natural aids to bowel elimination:
  - Daily intake of foods high in bulk
  - Daily fluid intake of 8 to 10 glasses
  - Regular time for elimination
  - Daily physical exercise: walking

Nursing Orders	*Scientific Rationale*	*Evaluation*
Monitor bowel elimination patterns; identify causative factors of constipation and successful corrective measures.	This patient's elimination problems will not be resolved until all the specific causes of her constipation and successful corrective measures are identified. Needs to be an ongoing assessment priority.	9/10/02 Goal partially met. Soft, formed stool passed every 2 to 3 days with aid of colace. *C. Taylor, RN*
Explain the importance of adhering to a regular time for defecation (patient suggests after breakfast)—adhere to this in the hospital.	This encourages positive use of circadian rhythms.	
When given medical clearance, assist patient with progressive ambulation. Recommend that she include brisk walking into daily health habits (build strength to 20- to 30-minute brisk walk daily).	Peristalsis is stimulated by physical exercise.	9/10/02 Goal met. Patient correctly related value of four natural aids to elimination. Questions whether she will be strong enough to walk. *Revision:* Encourage assisted ambulation. *C. Taylor, RN*
Explain the long-term effects of laxative abuse on the bowel, and discourage their use.	Laxative abuse leads to decreased peristaltic response to food and loss of intestinal tone	
Reinforce the patient's fluid intake and ingestion of high-bulk foods, such as fresh fruits and salad.	Commenting on these positive self-care behaviors reinforces them.	

was admitted to the hospital after experiencing a mini-stroke (transient ischemic attack) at home. Her condition is stable, and the three prioritized diagnoses written in the plan address her inability to deal with this new medical diagnosis and to prevent a major stroke (high priority), ineffective coping (medium priority), and constipation (low priority).

Assessing

The student records the assessment data that led to the determination of each diagnosis in the assessment/diagnosis column. Recording these data helps to link specific defining characteristics with diagnostic problem statements.

Diagnosing

Nursing diagnoses are recorded in the assessment/diagnosis column in a prioritized list beginning with the top-priority diagnosis. For each diagnosis, a clear and concise problem statement is followed by an etiology statement that identifies specific contributing factors.

Planning

The planning column contains the expected changes in patient health status or in patient behaviors (ie, patient goals/outcomes). If achieved, these resolve the problem statement in the nursing diagnosis.

Implementing

Sets of nursing orders that describe specific nursing interventions are written for each patient goal/outcome. These specify *what* nursing interventions are to be performed, *how* they are to be performed, *when* they are to be performed, and *who* is to perform them. In many nursing programs, students are asked to document the source of the nursing interventions they propose. Although students may be able to "pull from their head" some nursing strategies, developing the practice of consulting the nursing literature is a sure means to increase nursing knowledge. Some programs also require students to provide a scientific rationale for the interventions they propose. A succinct rationale statement demonstrates that the student is deliberately choosing the nursing intervention because of its high probability to effect the desired change.

Evaluating

Incorporating evaluative statements in the plan of care clearly communicates the message that nursing care is never complete until patient goal achievement is evaluated. Just as some say that teaching does not occur if learning does not take place, so nursing care is incomplete if the desired patient goals are not achieved.

Problems Related to Planning

Problems commonly encountered while developing plans of nursing care include insufficient data collection, nursing diagnoses developed from inaccurate or insufficient data, goals/outcomes that are stated too broadly, goals/outcomes that are derived from poorly developed nursing diagnoses, failure to write nursing orders clearly, written nursing orders that do not adequately resolve the problem, failure to involve the patient in the planning process, and failure to update the plan of care.

Learning Objectives

After studying this chapter, the learner should be able to accomplish the following:

1. Define the key terms used in the chapter.

clinical pathways (critical pathways, CareMaps)	initial planning
	Kardex care plan
computerized plans of nursing care	nursing intervention
	ongoing planning
consultation	patient goal
criteria	plan of nursing care
discharge planning	planning
expected outcome goal	standardized care plans

2. Describe the purpose and benefits of planning.
3. Identify three elements of comprehensive planning.
4. Prioritize patient health problems and nursing responses.
5. Describe how patient goals/expected outcomes and nursing orders are derived from nursing diagnoses.
6. Develop a plan of nursing care with properly constructed goals/outcomes and related nursing interventions.
7. Differentiate nurse-initiated interventions, physician-initiated interventions, and collaborative interventions.
8. Use criteria to evaluate planning skills.
9. Describe five common problems related to planning, their possible causes, and remedies.

Critical Thinking Exercises

1. Write nursing diagnoses for three obese patients, and make sure that the etiologies for the problem statement (Altered Nutrition: More Than Body Requirements) differ. Describe how these different etiologies result in different plans of care.

2. Use one of the nursing diagnoses from exercise 1 and write related cognitive, psychomotor, and affective goals. Explain the different purposes of each type of goal and why it may be necessary to include all three to resolve a patient problem successfully.

3. An alert 82-year-old widow who has a history of unsafe behaviors has recently been discharged from the hospital to her home. Caregivers attempted to secure her consent to be transferred to a nursing home, but she flatly refused. Responsible for her home care, you list High Risk for Injury as a priority nursing diagnosis. Join several students and independently list the nursing measures that are most likely to achieve the outcome of preventing injury. Compare your lists of interventions and discuss how practicing nurses can be sure they select the best nursing interventions for each expected patient outcome.

Bibliography

Alfaro, R. (1998). *Applying nursing process: A step-by-step guide* (4th ed.). Philadelphia: Lippincott Williams & Wilkins.

Alfaro-LeFevre, R. (1999). *Critical thinking in nursing: A practical approach*. Philadelphia: W. B. Saunders.

Ackley, B. J., & Ladwig, G. B. (1995). *Nursing diagnosis handbook: A guide to planning care* (2nd ed.). St. Louis: C. V. Mosby.

Atkinson, L. D., & Murray, M. E. (1990). *Understanding the nursing process* (4th ed.). New York: Pergamon.

Carpenito, L. J. (1995). *Nursing care plans and documentation* (2nd ed.). Philadelphia: J. B. Lippincott.

Carpenito, L. J. (1997). *Nursing diagnosis: Application to clinical practice* (7th ed.). Philadelphia: J. B. Lippincott.

Gage, M. (1994). The patient-driven interdisciplinary care plan. *JONA, 24*(4), 26–38.

Harris, B. L. (1990). Becoming deprofessionalized: One aspect of the staff nurse's perspective on computer-mediated nursing care plans. *Advances in Nursing Science, 13*(2), 63–74.

Iowa Intervention Project. (1997). Nursing interventions classification (NIC): An overview. In M. J. Rantz & P. LeMone (Eds.), *Classification of Nursing Diagnoses: Proceedings of the Twelfth Conference, North American Nursing Diagnosis* (pp. 32–39). Glendale, CA: CINAHL Information Systems.

Johnson, M., & Mass, M. L. (Eds.). (1997). *Nursing outcomes classification (NOC)*. St. Louis: Mosby–Year Book.

Joint Commission on Accreditation of Healthcare Organizations. (1996). *1997 Accreditation manual for hospitals*. Oakbrook Terrace, IL: JCAHO.

McCloskey, J. C., & Bulechek, G. M. (Eds.). (1996). *Nursing intervention classification (NIC)* (2nd ed.). St. Louis: Mosby–Year Book.

Raiwet, C., Halliwell, G., Andruski, L. & Wilson, D. (1997). Care maps across the continuum. *Canadian Nurse 93*(1), 26–30.

Rasmussen, N., & Gengler, T. (1994). Clinical pathways of care: The route to better communication. *Nursing, 24*(2), 47–49.

Rubenfeld, M. G., & Scheffer, B. K. (1999). *Critical thinking in nursing: An interactive approach* (2nd ed.). Philadelphia: Lippincott Williams & Wilkins.

Sparks, S. M. (1992). Computer consult: Exploring electronic support groups. *American Journal of Nursing, 92*(12), 62–65.

Ulrich, S. P., Canale, S. W., & Wendell, S. A. (1990). *Nursing care planning guides: A nursing diagnosis approach* (2nd ed.). Philadelphia: W. B. Saunders.

Vasey, E. K. (1979). Writing your patient's care plan . . . efficiently. *Nursing, 9*(4), 67–71.

Chapter 18
Implementing

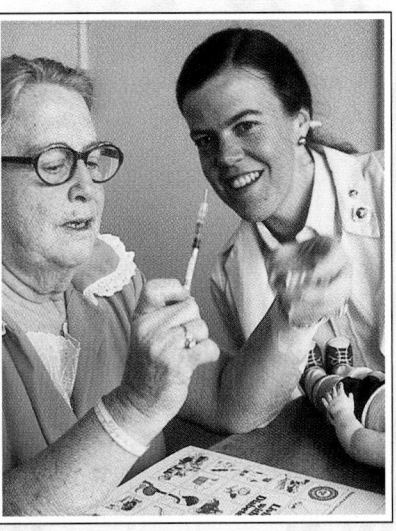

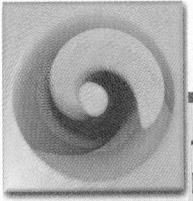

Thinking Critically About
Nursing's Blended Skills

Before reading this chapter, think about the types of skills you will need to implement a plan of care for the individuals you first met in the assessing chapter.

- You are working in a community-based well-child clinic. You become concerned when you observe negligible height and weight gains, delayed developmental milestones, and lethargy in a toddler brought to the clinic by her grandmother.

- You are working with a school nurse. Statistics reveal a pattern of teen smoking in your high school, and you are charged with developing an initiative to reverse this trend.

- You are doing a rotation on a medical floor in a hospital and learn that many of the diabetic patients being treated are repeat admissions with a history of poor self-care behaviors.

- You are working in a nursing home where one alert resident with multiple chronic conditions repeatedly tells you that she has no reason to live and asks you to help her end her life.

What cognitive, technical, interpersonal, and ethical/legal skills do you think you will need to implement a plan of nursing care for these individuals and groups?

During the **implementing** step of the nursing process, the nursing actions planned in the previous step are carried out. The purpose of implementation is to assist the patient in achieving desired health goals: promote health, prevent disease and illness, restore health, and facilitate coping with altered functioning. The plan of care is best implemented when patients who are able and willing to participate have maximum opportunities to provide self-care. Family members and other support people, as well as other healthcare professionals, may also be involved in the successful implementation of the plan of care (Table 18-1). During the implementation step, the nurse continues to collect data and to modify the plan of care as needed (Fig. 18-1). All activities are documented in the format used in the nurse's institution or agency.

Unique Focus of Nursing Implementation

In all nurse–patient interactions, the nurse is concerned with the patient's response to health and illness and ability to meet basic human needs. Whereas other healthcare professionals focus on selected aspects of the patient's treatment regimen, nurses are concerned with how the patient is responding to the plan of care in general.

Types of Nursing Interventions

When implementing the plan of care, nurses function independently, dependently, and collaboratively. These are the three types of **nursing interventions** that were described in the preceding chapter.

Nurse-initiated interventions, or independent nursing actions, involve carrying out nurse-prescribed interventions written on the nursing plan of care as well as any other actions that nurses initiate without the direction or supervision of another healthcare professional and that result from their assessment of patient needs. Nurses are legally accountable for their assessments and their nursing responses.

Physician-initiated interventions, or dependent nursing actions, involve carrying out physician-prescribed orders. State Nurse Practice Acts specify from whom nurses can receive orders. Nurses are still accountable for dependent orders they implement and are thus responsible for the clarification of any questionable order.

Collaborative interventions, or interdependent nursing actions, are those performed jointly by nurses and other members of the healthcare team. Because nurses are increasingly respected as professional colleagues with unique patient knowledge, they are increasingly involved in collaborative ventures with the healthcare team.

The three types of nursing actions can be illustrated by the example of a depressed patient whose data indicate a gastrointestinal blockage. If the physician orders a series of gastrointestinal studies, it is nursing's responsibility to prepare the patient by executing the physician's order for cleansing the bowel. This nursing action is a physician-initiated intervention. When the nurse senses that the patient seems unusually fearful of the outcome of the studies and explores the patient's fears and then follows up with appropriate teaching and counseling, the nurse is using nurse-initiated interventions. When a multidisciplinary team conference is held to discuss the patient's failure to progress, the nurse works collaboratively with the psychiatrist, gastroenterologist, social worker, and pastoral

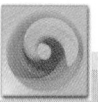

COGNITIVE SKILLS

- Knowledge of what information you need to implement the nursing interventions that effectively meet the nursing needs of the toddler with failure to thrive, teens who are smoking or at risk for smoking, diabetic patients with inadequate patterns of self-care, and nursing home resident with diminished will to live (how to carry out the plan of care, continue data collection and modify the plan as needed, and communicate care)

- Knowledge of pertinent standards of care and agency and institutional policies

- Ability to think critically about how to respond to the patient's need for nursing

TECHNICAL SKILLS

- Ability to use equipment and techniques competently that are specified by the patient's plan of care

INTERPERSONAL SKILLS

- Ability to establish a trusting nurse–patient relationship grounded in responsible caring

- Ability to communicate to the patient that you are more concerned about the patient and his or her well-being than about rote implementation of the plan of care or accomplishment of discrete tasks

- Ability to work collaboratively with members of the caregiving team to implement the interdisciplinary plan of care

ETHICAL/LEGAL SKILLS

- Commitment to implementing successfully the plan of care, within the scope of your legal practice

- Ability to be a trusted and effective patient advocate

- Consistent use of appropriate legal safeguards while implementing the plan of care

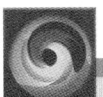

Table 18-1
Professional Nursing Relationships: Role Responsibilities and Related Competencies

Relationship	Role Responsibilities	Related Competencies
Nurse–patient	• Communicate to the patient that someone is concerned about him or her (as well as the disease) and is interested in how this change in health state will affect his or her overall well-being. • Create an environment in which the patient can commit his or her energies to health promotion or restoration or peaceful dying, confident that basic human needs are being addressed. • Challenge the patient to develop self-care abilities that promote holistic health.	• Repertoire of therapeutic interpersonal behaviors—attending, listening, interviewing, nonverbal communication, touching, facilitating, coaching • Ability to establish trusting nurse–patient–family relationships • Demonstrated competence in the nursing roles of caregiver, teacher, counselor, advocate
Nurse–patient–family	• Develop in the patient and family the knowledge, attitude, and skills that will enable them to respond to the self-care challenge of their health or illness state. • Intervene as appropriate to promote healthy family functioning. • Educate the family to be wise and assertive healthcare consumers.	
Nurse–nurse	• Support one another's efforts to deliver quality nursing care; work collaboratively with nursing administration to improve quality care. • Provide creative leadership—formally or informally—to make the nursing unit a satisfying and challenging place to work. • Supervise the nursing care given by other nursing personnel; affirm the nursing strengths of others, and constructively address the nursing deficiencies encountered. • Enhance the professional development of self and other nurses through active participation in professional organizations.	Communication Teaching/counseling/ advocacy Assertiveness Collaboration Coordination Group process Organization Leadership Delegation Change strategies Problem solving Decision making Conflict resolution
Nurse–healthcare team	• Communicate clearly nursing's perspective regarding the patient and family to the healthcare team. • Coordinate the inputs of the multidisciplinary team into a comprehensive plan of care. • Serve as a liaison between the patient and family and the healthcare team, as necessary.	

counselor to develop a comprehensive plan of care; this involves collaborative nursing interventions.

The Nursing Interventions Taxonomy Structure

In 1992, McCloskey and Bulechek published *Nursing Interventions Classification (NIC)* (Iowa Intervention Project, 1992), a report of research to construct a taxonomy of nursing interventions. Each of the 336 interventions listed has a label, a definition, a set of activities that a nurse performs to carry it out, and a short list of background readings. See the accompanying box and the NIC displays in each clinical chapter. Advantages of having a standard classification of nursing interventions include the following:

• To standardize nomenclature
• To expand nursing knowledge

• To develop information systems
• To teach decision making
• To ensure appropriate reimbursement for nursing services
• To allocate nursing resources
• To communicate nursing to nonnurses
• To link nursing content: standardized nursing diagnoses, outcomes, and interventions (Iowa Intervention Project, 1992, p. 14.)

Table 18-2 illustrates the NIC taxonomy structure designed to help clinicians to locate and select interventions most helpful for patients.

The researchers involved in the development of NICs were also committed to developing a classification of patient outcomes for nursing interventions, called *Nursing Outcomes Classifications* (NOCs). This research aimed to

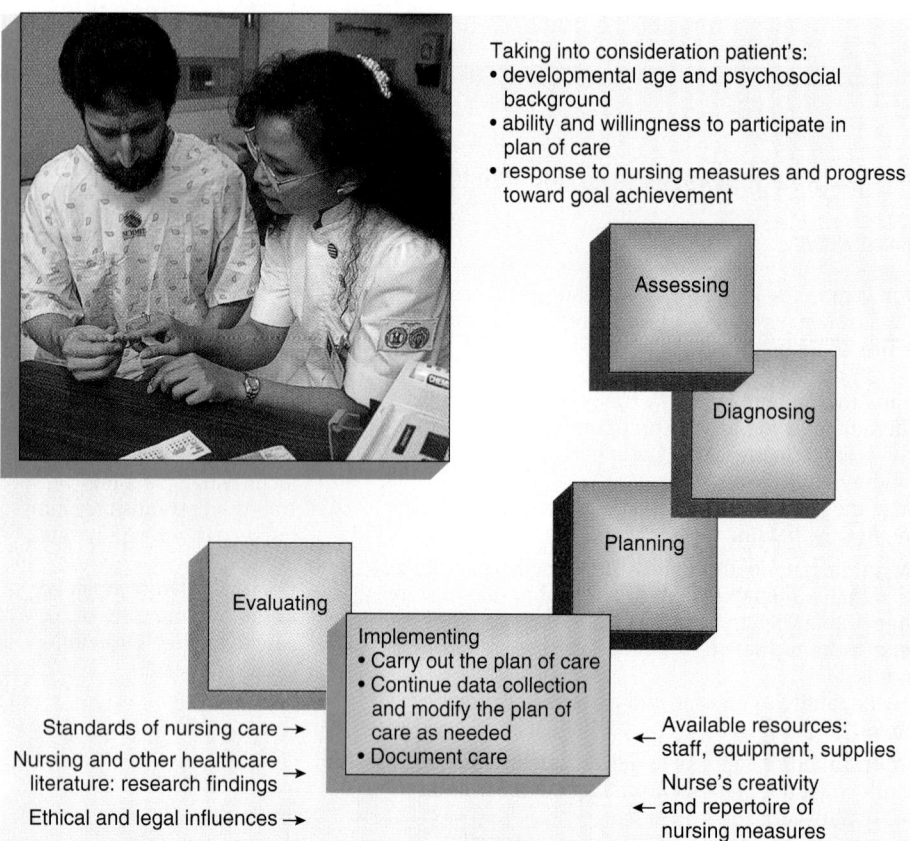

Taking into consideration patient's:
- developmental age and psychosocial background
- ability and willingness to participate in plan of care
- response to nursing measures and progress toward goal achievement

Assessing

Diagnosing

Planning

Evaluating

Implementing
- Carry out the plan of care
- Continue data collection and modify the plan of care as needed
- Document care

Standards of nursing care →

Nursing and other healthcare literature: research findings →

Ethical and legal influences →

← Available resources: staff, equipment, supplies

← Nurse's creativity and repertoire of nursing measures

Figure 18-1
Implementing. Implementing involves carrying out the plan of care, which is modified in response to patient changes. Numerous variables influence the way the plan of care is implemented (*see arrows*). (Photo © Kathy Sloane.)

(1) identify, label, validate, and classify nursing-sensitive patient outcomes and indicators; (2) evaluate the validity and usefulness of the classification in clinical field testing; and (3) define and test measurement procedures for the outcomes and indicators.

Examples of proposed NOC indicators for the outcome Caregiver Home Readiness (caregiver's preparedness to assume responsibility for the healthcare of a family member or significant other in the home) include the following:

- Willingness to assume caregiving role
- Knowledge about caregiving role
- Demonstration of positive regard for care recipient
- Participation in home care decisions
- Confidence in ability to manage care at home
- Knowledge of where to obtain needed equipment (Johnson & Mass, 1997, p. 103)

Protocols and Standing Orders

Protocols and standing orders expand the scope of nursing practice in certain clearly defined situations. **Protocols** are written plans that detail the nursing activities to be executed in specific situations. Although some protocols specify routine aspects of nursing care (eg, protocols that describe nursing responsibilities when a patient is admitted to or discharged from the institution), other protocols include **stand-**

ing orders that empower the nurse to initiate actions that ordinarily require the order or supervision of a physician. Examples include admission protocols for obstetric and gynecology patients, protocols for bowel programs that allow the nurse to select and administer necessary bowel interventions, standard orders for narcotic overdoses that specify the agents the nurse is to administer to reverse respiratory depression in an emergency, and standard orders for pain management that enable the nurse to select the strength of the medication to be given within preset ranges.

The Nurse as Coordinator

One of nursing's major contributions to the healthcare team is the role of coordinator. Care can easily become fragmented when patients are seen by numerous specialists—each interested in a different aspect of the patient. At best, patients complain that no one person really knows them and can talk with them about what is going on and how it all may affect them in the future. At worst, the orders of different specialists may conflict with one another and be counterproductive. Therefore, it is important for nurses to make rounds with other healthcare professionals and to read the results of consultations patients have had with specialists. Nurses can then interpret the specialists' findings for patients and family members, prepare patients to participate maximally in the

Using Nursing Interventions Classification to Implement Care for a Patient and Family Requiring Assistance With Home Maintenance

The Nursing Interventions Classification (NIC) can be used to implement care for a patient and family who require assistance to maintain the home as a clean, safe, and pleasant place. Based on the intervention *Home Maintenance Assistance,* representative nursing activities include the following:

- Determine patient's home maintenance requirements.
- Involve patient and family in deciding home maintenance requirements.
- Suggest necessary structural alterations to make the home accessible.
- Provide information on how to make the home environment safe and clean.
- Advise for the alleviation of all offensive odors.
- Suggest services for pest control, as needed.
- Offer solutions to financial difficulties.
- Order homemaker services, as appropriate.
- Provide information on respite care, as needed.

McCloskey, J., & Bulechek, G. (2000). *Nursing interventions classification (NIC)* (3rd ed., p. 378). St. Louis: Mosby-Year Book. (A full listing of nursing activities for each nursing intervention can be found in this book.)

plan of care before and after discharge, and serve as a liaison among the members of the healthcare team. Nurse case managers are specialists in the role of care coordinator.

Carrying Out the Plan of Care

When carrying out the plan of care, nurses use specialized abilities to (1) determine the patient's continuing need for nursing assistance, (2) promote self-care, and (3) assist the patient to achieve health goals.

Prerequisite Nursing Skills

To implement the plan of nursing care, nurses need cognitive, interpersonal, technical, and ethical/legal skills. Each nurse has a unique blend of these skills and can act effectively to the extent that her or his abilities match the patient's need for nursing care. These skills are described in Chapter 14 and illustrated in the opening of each chapter.

Determining the Need for Assistance

Although most people can independently meet their basic human needs, illness and the stress of diagnostic and therapeutic measures may interfere with a person's usual practice of self-care. The nurse assesses the patient's abil-

ities to meet his or her human needs independently. Nurses can fail patients by doing too much for them and by encouraging negative, sick-role behaviors, such as inappropriate dependence. Conversely, there is a time and a place for the "tender loving care" that says to a patient, "I know you may be able to do this for yourself, but just this once, how about if I do it and we'll talk!" Challenging a patient's best self-care effort while meeting the universal human need to feel cared for is an important component of the art of nursing.

The plan of nursing care should include specific instructions for any nursing assistance the patient needs to meet basic human needs, including the need for significant nursing encouragement to promote greater independence in functioning. When routines of self-care (or assisted self-care) are included (eg, colostomy management), instructions should include the time of the procedure, the equipment used, the process, and the level of patient involvement. Continuity of nursing care is essential to the patient's development of a comfortable routine.

Promoting Self-Care: Teaching, Counseling, and Advocacy

If patients and their families want to participate actively in seeking wellness, preventing disease and illness, recovering health, and learning to cope with altered functioning, they need to possess effective self-care behaviors. Nurses sensitive to the importance of patients learning to direct and manage their own care use nurse–patient interactions for both planned and spontaneous teaching, counseling, and advocacy. These nursing roles are described in Chapters 22 and 23. For example, while caring for a child recently diagnosed as having cystic fibrosis, the nurses work continuously with the parents and siblings, helping them to develop the knowledge and skills that will enable them to care for the child after discharge. Referring families such as this to a community support group or other resources further enhances the self-care behaviors being developed. See the accompanying box, Through the Eyes of the Family Caregiver, for a description of one wife's experiences when her husband was discharged home.

Assisting Patients to Meet Health Goals

In this phase of the implementation process, the nursing team carries out the nursing orders detailed in the nursing plan of care. If the plan of care is well constructed, carrying out its orders is the nurse's most important task and should receive top priority. The nursing actions planned to promote patient goal/outcome achievement and the resolution of health problems should be carefully executed. Implementation guidelines are listed in the accompanying box.

Because understaffing is a problem in many practice settings, nurses must learn to use their time wisely and to maximize each patient encounter. A patient bath can be simply that, or it can be an opportunity to gather additional

(*text continues on page 296*)

Table 18-2

Nursing Interventions Classification (NIC) Taxonomy

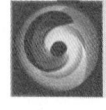

	Domain I	Domain II	Domain III	Domain IV	Domain V	Domain VI
Level 1 Domains	1. Physiologic: Basic	2. Physiologic: Complex	3. Behavioral	4. Safety	5. Family	6. Health System
	Care that supports physical functioning	Care that supports homeostatic regulation	Care that supports psychosocial functioning and facilitates lifestyle changes	Care that supports protection against harm	Care that supports the family unit	Care that supports effective use of the health-care delivery system
Level 2 Classes	A Activity and Exercise Management: Interventions to organize or assist with physical activity and energy expenditure	G Electrolyte and Acid–Base Management: Interventions to regulate electrolyte/acid–base balance and prevent complications	O Behavior Therapy: Interventions to reinforce or promote desirable behaviors or alter undesirable behaviors	U Crisis Management: Interventions to provide immediate short-term help in both psychological and physiologic crises	W Childbearing Care: Interventions to assist in understanding and coping with the psychological and physiologic changes during the childbearing period	Y Health System Mediation: Interventions to facilitate the interface between patient/family and the healthcare system
	B Elimination Management: Interventions to establish and maintain regular bowel and urinary elimination patterns and manage complications due to altered patterns	H Medication Management: Interventions to facilitate desired effects of pharmacologic agents	P Cognitive Therapy: Interventions to reinforce or promote desirable cognitive functioning or alter undesirable cognitive functioning	V Risk Management: Interventions to initiate risk reduction activities and continue monitoring risk over time	X Lifespan Care: Interventions to facilitate family unit functioning and promote the health and welfare of family members throughout the lifespan	a. Health System Management: Interventions to provide and enhance support services for the delivery of care
		I Neurologic Management: Interventions to optimize neurologic function	Q Communication Enhancement: Interventions to facilitate delivering and receiving verbal or nonverbal messages			b. Information Management: Interventions to facilitate communication among healthcare workers

C   Immobility Management: Interventions to manage restricted body movement and the sequelae

D   Nutrition Support: Interventions to modify or maintain nutritional status

E   Physical Comfort Promotion: Interventions to promote comfort using physical techniques

F   Self-Care Facilitation: Interventions to provide or assist with routine activities of daily living

J   Perioperative Care: Interventions to provide care before, during, and immediately after surgery

K   Respiratory Management: Interventions to promote airway patency and gas exchange

L   Skin/Wound Management: Interventions to maintain or restore tissue integrity

M   Thermoregulation: Interventions to maintain body temperature within a normal range

N   Tissue Perfusion Management: Interventions to optimize circulation of blood and fluids to the tissue

R   Coping Assistance: Interventions to assist another to build on own strengths, to adapt to a change in function, or to achieve a higher level of function

S   Patient Education: Interventions to facilitate learning

T   Psychological Comfort Promotion: Interventions to promote comfort using psychological techniques

McCloskey, J. C., & Bulechek, G. M. (Eds.) (2000). *Iowa Interventions Project: Nursing interventions classification* (3rd ed.). St. Louis: Mosby–Year Book. Used with permission.

Through the Eyes of the Family Caregiver

The Nurses Never Told Me There'd Be Days Like This

I wasn't prepared for a roller coaster ride when my husband became ill. My husband was admitted to the hospital in an emergency condition, became confused when his electrolytes were off balance, went into cardiac arrest and had CPR, was placed on a ventilator, and was sedated because he was too apprehensive about the ventilator. I had reached the lowest point as I sat by his bedside for days, talking to him and wondering if he heard me.

My spirits soared the day they brought him out of his sleep state and he recognized me and was hungry for real food. The next day when I went to the hospital I plummeted to the low point again when he was crumpled in bed like a confused rag doll with his hospital gown up to his chest and the sheet to his ankles. I started to cry, and the nurse came and put her arm around me. She said, "Don't think he's taken a turn for the worse. There will be good days and bad days as he recovers." No one had prepared me for that—and her arm around me and her words were so consoling.

When I brought him home after 6 weeks in the hospital, I was not prepared for his anger at being confined to the house (in a heat wave) and not being allowed to drive. His reasoning that he had to get a haircut because he hadn't had one in 2 months made sense to him. My saying no one would care about the length of his hair did not soothe his anger.

He couldn't accept the fact that he was too weak to go up and down the steps more than once a day, so he insisted on going to the basement. Going down was simple; coming up wasn't. We forgot there was no railing (which he needed to haul himself up) on the last four steps. He solved the problem by sitting on the steps and lifting himself up a step at a time. Then he got to the floor at the top and couldn't stand up. I couldn't lift him. We were stuck. Again I took a nose dive.

I thought I understood how difficult it would be for him to readjust. I knew he would be depressed and expected him to lean on me. But I was not prepared for his frustration to come out as anger at me. It would have been helpful to have someone prepare me. Or it would be nice to have a nurse put her arm around me now when my roller coaster plummets.

—ELEANOR FAVEN,
PHILADELPHIA, PENNSYLVANIA

When Implementing Nursing Care . . . Remember to Act in Partnership With the Patient/Family

- Before implementing any nursing action, reassess the patient to determine whether the action is still needed.
- Approach the patient competently. Know how to perform the nursing action, why the action is being performed, and potential adverse responses. Have all equipment and supplies ready.
- Approach the patient caringly. Explain the nursing action using language the patient understands. Communicate genuine concern for what the patient is experiencing.
- Modify nursing interventions according to the patient's (1) developmental and psychosocial background, (2) ability and willingness to participate in the plan of care, and (3) responses to previous nursing measures and progress toward goal/outcome achievement.
- Check to make sure that the nursing interventions selected are consistent with standards of care and within legal and ethical guides to practice.
- Always question that the nursing intervention selected is the best of all possible alternatives. Consult colleagues and the nursing and related literature to see if other approaches might be more successful. Evaluate the effectiveness of the intervention selected, noting any factors that positively or negatively influenced the outcome.
- Develop a repertoire of skilled nursing interventions. The more options one can choose from, the greater the likelihood of success.

focused data, to communicate concern for what the patient is experiencing and to offer support, and to teach and counsel as appropriate. How the nurse uses the 30 minutes that he or she is in the patient's room for the bath determines how effective the nurse is in helping the patient to achieve his or her goals/outcomes. See the accompanying box, Through the Eyes of a Student, for one student's account of an important bath.

Variables That Influence Goal/Outcome Achievement

When working with patients to achieve the goals/outcomes specified in the plan of care, remember that nothing about the plan of care is fixed. Some of the most important variables that influence how the plan of care is implemented follow.

Patient Variables

Ideally, the patient is primary in determining how nursing interventions are implemented. Successful nurses modify their nursing actions according to the patient's (1) changing ability and willingness to participate in the

Through the Eyes of a Student

One of my first patients was a woman with a history of Alzheimer's disease. When I was assigned this patient, I knew that I was not going to have a good day. I had been introduced to this patient the week before, when I had orientation. She was sitting in a gerry chair in the hallway, where she sang at the top of her lungs and threw tissues on the floor. Occasionally, she would curse at a person passing by.

I took a deep breath and entered her room. At her bedside I introduced myself. With a few choice words she told me to get out of her room. I tried to ignore her response and prepared her breakfast tray. She proceeded to throw her scrambled eggs around the room. After I took the tray away from her and finished cleaning up the mess, it was time for preconference. At preconference, my instructor told me were going to "tub" my patient. I had visions of a grand fiasco in the tub room, and I dreaded giving her the bath.

My instructor and I took her to the tub room by wheelchair. Once we convinced her to get in the tub, she did nothing but yell that it was cold. We started the water and she yelled even louder. I knew everyone could hear her in the hallway as she cursed and yelled, but as the bath proceeded she quieted down and stopped fighting me. We completed the bath and wheeled her back down the hall to her room. I bundled her up in blankets and put her in the gerry chair in the hallway. She was so relaxed from the bath that she let me brush her hair and put it in a ponytail. While I was brushing her hair, she fell asleep. I did my chart until her lunch arrived. When I set her up for her lunch and told her I would be leaving, she thanked me, and it made my day. All the struggling I went through all day with her and she thanked me. When I went home I felt really good about helping her. During all my worrying about the day being a fiasco and the embarrassment of having a patient yell at me, I had lost sight of the patient herself and what she needed me to do for her. By her thanking me at the end of the day, I realized that when my clinical instructor forced me to do something for my patient that the regular staff of the hospital wouldn't do, I was meeting her basic needs, and my patient recognized that.

—Jeanene C. Smith,
Delaware County Community College,
Media, Pennsylvania

plan of care and (2) previous responses to nursing interventions and progress toward goal/outcome achievement. Other important patient variables are developmental stage and psychosocial background.

Addressing the developmental needs of a patient is much more than simply identifying the patient's developmental stage on the plan of care. The developmental tasks related to this stage and their relationship to nursing care seldom need to be considered. For example, the nurse may recommend that the parents of a premature infant make a tape of their voices to stimulate their infant in the neonatal intensive care unit. Nurses must be careful not to let stereotypes about developmental stages and tasks influence patient care. For example, in nursing homes, the developmental needs of older patients are ignored when the staff select a radio station that plays rock music, make humorous comments about "romances" among the residents, embarrass some residents by calling them cute names or putting big, bright bows in their hair, or demean some patients by planning childish group activities. Perhaps the worst stereotype is the belief that all older people have to do is wait to die, that there are no developmental challenges for this age group.

To implement a comprehensive and holistic plan of care, nurses must find creative ways to meet developmental needs. This is of greatest importance when patients are separated from their families and home environments for long periods.

The same is true of the psychosocial needs of patients. Although few nurses would claim that people from all socioeconomic groups and cultures are the same, some practice nursing as if this were so. When choosing nursing interventions, the nurse should consider and respect the patient's background. Confronted with a malnourished patient on a limited income who rents a single room in a boarding home, a nurse cannot simply teach the importance of including more protein in the diet. To be effective, the nurse must explore the realistic issue of whether the patient can afford and obtain foods rich in protein. Moreover, the nurse needs to assess whether the patient values this intervention and is willing to make the necessary changes.

Nurse Variables

Nurse variables that influence the implementation of the plan of care include nurses' levels of expertise, creativity (ability to match patient needs with specific nursing strategies), willingness to provide care, and available time. The accompanying display, Developing Critical Thinking Skills, illustrates the importance of nurses' ability to think critically about intervention strategies.

Resources

The most elaborately designed plan of care cannot be fully effective in a chronically understaffed or undersupplied nursing unit. Adequate staff, equipment, and supplies are all important determinants of patient care. The financial resources of the patient and adequacy of community-based resources also influence the plan of care.

Developing Critical Thinking Skills

Situation

One of the nurses on the oncology unit where you have been working for 6 months since graduation wants to develop a "humor room" where patients, their families, and staff can "take a break" from the serious business of illness. Designed to lift the spirits, amuse, distract, and thus speed the healing process, humor rooms are gaining popularity as new therapeutic tools. Funny books, comic movies on a large-screen TV; games and puzzles; and ideally even clowns, magicians, musicians, and stand-up comedians are being envisaged (Buxman, 1991). Several nurses have vocally expressed their lack of support for the project and think the idea is "stupid" at best and potentially a great waste of money, time, and energy that could be devoted to "tried and true" methods of healing. You have been asked to support the project and must decide how to respond.

1. **Identify Goal of Thinking**
   Clarify your thinking about humor as a therapeutic measure so that you can decide whether to support this project.

2. **Assess Adequacy of Knowledge**
   Pertinent circumstances: The nurse who wants to develop the humor room is more popular with patients than she is with her colleagues. Her nurse friends are quick to point out that while it's true that she is "a bit flakey" and unorthodox, she is an efficient nurse who is well-loved by her patients and their families. The hospital is in the midst of cutting expenses and has laid off both professional and nonprofessional employees.

   Prerequisite knowledge: To decide how you should respond in this situation, you need to research the healing benefits of humor. Are there clinical studies demonstrating its effectiveness as a therapeutic measure? If studies point to humor's effectiveness, you will need to determine (1) what priority it should have among other treatment modalities and (2) the feasibility of creating a humor room in the current climate of cutting expenses. Is there a creative way to finance this venture?

   Room for error: Since life and death do not hinge on how you elect to respond to this plea

for support, there is a relatively wide margin for error. Because personal energy and finances are limited, however, you do not want to involve your unit in a futile project.

   Time constraints: There is no rush for an immediate decision on your part, which gives you adequate time to develop the knowledge base you need to make an informed decision.

3. **Address Potential Problems**
   The most serious obstacle to critical thinking in this situation would be the lack of an open mind and refusal to weigh the merits of a new treatment modality. Complicating factors include divided loyalties among the nurses and the tendency to support or refuse support for the project on the basis of whether one likes the nurse advocating the project, rather than on the merits of the project. Finally, the lowered morale caused by lay-offs may squash all creativity and willingness to "dream new dreams."

4. **Consult Helpful Resources**
   Your first challenge will be to learn more about humor as a healing measure. Ideally, you may be able to consult a local expert and invite her or him to meet with the staff. Alternately, you can research the literature looking for clinical studies and reports of the first-person experiences of others.

5. **Critical Judgment/Decision**
   After a search of the literature convinced you and some of the other nurses of the clinical benefits of humor, you decide to explore the feasibility of developing a humor room. Your options are to "play it safe" and not rock the boat during a difficult period in the hospital by trying something new, or to become an advocate for the project and commit your energies to making it happen. You decide that a creative project may be exactly what the staff needs to rediscover the "joy of nursing" and begin to explore means to fund the project. You plan to "start small" and to reassess the project every 6 months. Since your research educated you about the potential benefits *and harms* humor can create, you decide that your first objective must be to educate the staff.

Current Standards of Care

All nursing actions for implementing the plan of care must be consistent with standards for practice. All nurses are responsible for learning the standards that dictate practice in their specialty. Failure to practice according to these standards may result in a charge of negligence.

Research Findings

Nurses concerned about improving the quality of nursing care use research findings to enhance their nursing practice. Reading professional nursing journals and attending continuing education workshops and conferences are excellent ways to learn about new nursing strategies that have proved effective. Research boxes throughout this text demonstrate the difference nursing research can make in improving patient outcomes.

Ethical and Legal Guides to Practice

Nurses cannot practice good nursing if they are ignorant of the laws and regulations that affect healthcare and the ethical dimensions of clinical practice. A sincere motivation to benefit the patient and a conscientious attempt to implement nursing orders well are no longer sufficient. Each nurse is responsible for becoming sensitive to the ethical and legal dimensions of practice, and moral and legal accountability are inherent in the practice of professional nursing. Chapters 6 and 7 discuss the ethical and legal dimensions of practice. Hospital risk managers and ethics committees are increasingly available as institutional resources for nurses.

Delegating Nursing Care

Because of the pressure to reduce healthcare costs, many employers of nurses have increased their use of unlicensed assistive personnel (UAP), or "nurse extenders." In some cases, the new mix of professional and nonprofessional staff is threatening patient safety. Never has it been more important for nurses to identify critically which nursing interventions require professional nurses and which can be safely delegated. **Delegation** is the transfer of responsibility for the performance of an activity to another individual while retaining accountability for the outcome. The "five rights" of delegation are as follows:

- The *right task* (one that can be delegated)
- The *right person* (one qualified to do the job)
- The *right communication* (clear, concise description of the objective and expectations)
- The *right feedback* (evaluation in a timely manner, during and after the task is completed)
- The *right time* (Hansten & Washburn, 1992)

It is essential to understand that a nurse who delegates an intervention to a nursing assistant remains accountable for the delegated service.

Before delegating any nursing intervention, a number of factors should be considered: (1) the patient's condition, (2) the complexity of the activity, (3) the potential for harm, (4) the degree of problem-solving and innovation necessary, (5) the level of interaction required with the patient, (6) capabilities of the UAP, and (7) the availability of professional staff to accomplish the unit workload. The American Nurses Association, which is committed to monitoring the regulation, education, and use of UAP, recommends adherence to the following principles:

- It is the nursing profession that determines the scope of nursing practice.
- It is the nursing profession that defines and supervises the education, training, and use of any unlicensed assistant roles involved in providing direct nursing care.
- It is the registered nurse who is responsible and accountable for nursing practice.

- It is the registered nurse who supervises any assistant involved in providing direct patient care.
- It is the purpose of assistive personnel to work in a supportive role to the registered nurse, carrying out tasks to enable the professional nurse to concentrate on nursing care for the patient (Pennsylvania Nurses Association, 1992).

Responding to the Noncompliant Patient

When a patient fails to follow the plan of care despite the nurse's best efforts, it is time to reassess strategy. The first objective is to identify *why* the patient is not following the therapy. One possibility is that the plan of care may not be right for this patient. In this event, what is needed is not a change in the patient but rather a change in the plan of care. If the nurse determines, however, that the plan of care is adequate, he or she must identify and remedy the factors contributing to the patient's noncompliance. Common reasons for noncompliance include (1) lack of family support, (2) lack of understanding about the benefits of compliance, (3) adverse physical or emotional effects of treatment (such as pain and fatigue), (4) inability to afford treatment, and (5) limited access to treatment.

Guide for Students

Student nurses trying in advance to organize their nursing care for a particular clinical day can use the guidelines for student clinical responsibilities in the accompanying box to

---

Organizing Student Clinical Responsibilities

To organize clinical responsibilities, check:

1. Patient profile
2. Name by which patient wishes to be addressed
3. Patient's current health status
   - Note any physical or emotional changes indicating the need to modify the plan of care.
4. Routine assistance patient needs to meet basic human needs
5. Priorities for nursing care
   - Prioritized nursing diagnoses, patient goals/outcomes, and related nursing interventions
   - Medical orders that need to be implemented
   - Interdependent or collaborative nursing responsibilities
6. Special "events" of the day that may require special observation of the patient, teaching, preparation, or aftercare
   - Diagnostic tests
   - Consultations with specialists
   - New therapies (physical therapy, medications, surgery, radiotherapy, and so forth)
7. Special teaching, counseling, or advocacy needs
8. Special needs of the family

help identify nursing measures for which they will be responsible. After these have been identified, working out a time schedule may provide clear direction for the clinical day and ensure that the patient's needs are met.

Continuing Data Collection

An important nursing intervention is ongoing data collection. In every patient encounter, the nurse needs to be sensitive to both subtle and dramatic changes in the patient's condition or response to this condition. These assessment findings are used to update and revise the plan of care. Sensitivity to how the patient is responding to nursing interventions and to the patient's progress toward goal/outcome achievement allows the nurse to modify nursing interventions appropriately.

Nursing Oneself

It is difficult for nurses to be sincerely attentive to patient needs if their own human needs are not being met. Because no one is perfectly healthy or "whole" all the time, it is important that nurses preparing for professional practice spend time getting to know themselves. In an excellent chapter on psychological self-care written for nurses, Hill and Smith (1990) describe psychological self-care as a constellation of activities practiced on a regular basis to promote psychological health. These include self-awareness, communication, time management, preparation for crisis and loss, developing and maintaining support systems, and concurrent practice of self-care in all areas. The characteristics of emotional health include self-esteem, self-knowledge, satisfying interpersonal relationships, environmental mastery, stress management, a positive body image, a sense of humor, and the ability to experience pleasure.

Nurses who want to be competent practitioners learn early to nurse themselves and other nurses before attempting to nurse patients. Good personal health enables nurses not only to practice more efficiently but also to be a health model for patients and their families. Nurses can help patients to imitate health behavior and eventually integrate it into their daily life through the process of identification. Each clinical chapter contains a helpful section entitled The Nurse as Role Model.

Learning Objectives

After completing this chapter, the learner should be able to accomplish the following:

1. Define the key terms used in the chapter.
   collaborative intervention
   delegation
   implementing
   nurse-initiated
      intervention
   nursing interventions
   physician-initiated
      intervention
   protocols
   standing orders
2. Distinguish nurse-initiated, physician-initiated, and collaborative nursing interventions.
3. List advantages of having a standard classification of nursing interventions and outcomes.
4. Use cognitive, interpersonal, technical, and ethical/legal skills to implement a plan of nursing care.
5. Describe six variables that influence the way a plan of care is implemented.
6. Use seven guidelines for implementation.
7. Use ongoing data collection to direct revision of the plan of care.

Critical Thinking Exercises

1. Team up with another student and take turns role-playing a nurse visiting a homebound older man who needs his vital signs and nutritional status assessed. Discuss with each other the truth or falsity of the claim, "who the nurse is, is as important as, and sometimes more important than, what the nurse does."
2. Receive the same clinical assignment as another student, and independently outline your care priorities, specifying what you plan to accomplish during each of your clinical hours. Talk with the other student about the differences in what you both hope to accomplish and how you would do this. Try to imagine what these differences would mean to the patient.
3. Describe how you would probably respond, and how you would like to respond (if these are different), to hearing another nurse in the shift report say that one of the patients you are assigned to was a real P.I.B. ("pain in the butt") all day and "just impossible" to care for. Reflect on the importance of the language we use to report on a patient to one another.

Bibliography

Alfaro, R. (1998). *Applying nursing process: A step-by-step guide* (4th ed.). Philadelphia: Lippincott Williams & Wilkins.
Alfaro-LeFevre, R. (1999). *Critical thinking in nursing: A practical approach.* Philadelphia: W. B. Saunders.

Benner, P. (1984). *From novice to expert: Excellence and power in clinical nursing practice.* Menlo Park, CA: Addison-Wesley.
Benner, P., & Wrubel, J. (1989). *The primary of caring: Stress and coping in health and illness.* Menlo Park, CA: Addison-Wesley.

Blegen, M. A., Gardner, D. I., & McCloskey, J. C. (1992). Who helps you with your work? *American Journal of Nursing, 92*(1), 26–31.

Brider, P. (1992). The move to patient-focused care. *American Journal of Nursing, 92*(9), 26–33.

Bulechek, G. M., & McCloskey, J. C. (1987). Nursing interventions: What they are and how to choose them. *Holistic Nursing Practice, 1*(3), 36–44.

Buxman, K. (1991). Make room for laughter. *American Journal of Nursing, 91*(12), 46–51.

Dossey, B. (1991). Awakening the inner healer. *American Journal of Nursing, 91*(8), 31–34.

Eisenhauer, L. A. (1994). A typology of nursing therapeutics. *Image—The Journal of Nursing Scholarship, 26*(4), 261–264.

Ellis, J. R., & Hartley, C. L. (1995). *Managing and coordinating nursing care* (2nd ed.). Philadelphia: J. B. Lippincott.

Gibson, L. (1994). Healing with humor. *Nursing, 24*(9), 56–57.

Hansten, R., & Washburn, M. (1992a). Delegation: How to deliver care through others. *American Journal of Nursing, 92*(3), 87–90.

Hansten, R., & Washburn, M. (1992b). How to plan what to delegate. *American Journal of Nursing, 92*(4), 71–72.

Hill, L., & Smith, N. (1990). *Self-care nursing: Promotion of health* (2nd ed.). East Norwalk, CT: Appleton & Lange.

Iowa Intervention Project: McCloskey, J. C., & Bulechek, G. (Eds.) (1995). Validating and coding of the NIC taxonomy structure. *Image—The Journal of Nursing Scholarship, 27*(1), 43–49.

Iowa Intervention Project. (1993). The NIC Taxonomy Structure. *Image—The Journal of Nursing Scholarship, 25*(3), 197–192.

Iowa Intervention Project. (1997). Nursing interventions classification (NIC): An overview. In M. J. Rantz & P. LeMone (Eds.), *Classification of Nursing Diagnoses: Proceedings of the Twelfth Conference, North American Nursing Diagnosis* (pp. 32–39). Glendale, CA: CINAHL Information Systems.

Johnson, M., & Mass, M. L. (Eds.) (1997). *Nursing outcomes classification (NOC)*. St Louis: Mosby–Year Book.

Joint Commission on Accreditation of Healthcare Organizations. (1999). *1999 Accreditation manual for hospitals.* Oakbrook Terrace, IL: JCAHO.

McCloskey, J. C., & Bulechek, G. M. (Eds.) (1992). *Nursing intervention classification (NIC)*. St. Louis: Mosby–Year Book.

McCloskey, J. C., & Bulechek, G. M. (Eds.) (1996). *Nursing intervention classification (NIC)* (2nd ed.). St. Louis: Mosby–Year Book.

McCloskey, J. C., & Bulechek, G. M. (Eds.) (2000). *Nursing intervention classification (NIC)* (3rd ed.). St. Louis: Mosby–Year Book.

Neighbors, M., Eldred, E., & Sullivan, M. (1991). Nursing skills necessary for competing in the high-tech health care system. *Nursing and Health Care, 12*(2), 92–97.

Paris, L. L. (1994). Improving the process of communication at the bedside. *Journal of Nursing Care Quality, 9*(1), 10–15.

Pennsylvania Nurses Association. (1992, January). Perspectives in practice: RNs working with unlicensed assistive personnel. *Pennsylvania Nurse*, 7–8.

Prescott, P. A., Phillips, C. Y., Ryan, J. W., & Thompson, K. O. (1991). Changing how nurses spend their time. *Image—The Journal of Nursing Scholarship, 23*(1), 23–28.

Rubenfeld, M. G., & Scheffer, B. K. (1999). *Critical thinking in nursing: An interactive approach* (2nd ed.). Philadelphia: Lippincott Williams & Wilkins.

Seeger Jablonski, R. A. (1992). Remember the person attached to the ventilator. *Nursing, 92*(4), 67–70.

Sundeen, S. J., Wiscarz, S., DeSalvo-Rankin, E. A., & Cohen, S. A. (1994). *Nurse-patient interaction: Implementing the nursing process* (5th ed.). St. Louis: C. V. Mosby.

Valega, T. M. (1984). It's time for nurses to begin nursing. *Nursing and Health Care, 5*(6), 331–335.

Wichowski, H. C., & Kubsch, S. (1995). Improving your patient's compliance. *Nursing, 25*(1), 66–68.

Chapter 19
Evaluating

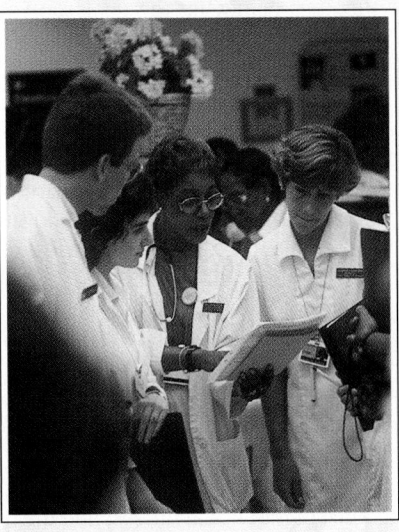

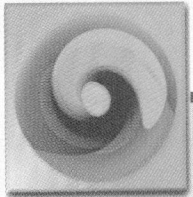

Thinking Critically About
Nursing's Blended Skills

Before reading this chapter, think about the types of skills you will need to evaluate the plan of care you designed and implemented for the individuals you first met in the assessing chapter.

- You are working in a community-based well-child clinic. You become concerned when you observe negligible height and weight gains, delayed developmental milestones, and lethargy in a toddler brought to the clinic by her grandmother.

- You are working with a school nurse. Statistics reveal a pattern of teen smoking in your high school, and you are charged with developing an initiative to reverse this trend.

- You are doing a rotation on a medical floor in a hospital and learn that many of the diabetic patients being treated are repeat admissions with a history of poor self-care behaviors.

- You are working in a nursing home where one alert resident with multiple chronic conditions repeatedly tells you that she has no reason to live and asks you to help her end her life.

What cognitive, technical, interpersonal, and ethical/legal skills do you think you will need to evaluate your nursing care for these individuals and groups?

In the fifth step of the nursing process, **evaluating**, the nurse and patient together measure how well the patient has achieved the goals/outcomes specified in the plan of care. While evaluating patient goal/outcome achievement, the nurse identifies factors that contribute to the patient's ability to achieve expected outcomes and, when necessary, modifies the plan of care (Fig. 19-1). The purpose of evaluation is to allow the patient's achievement of expected outcomes to direct future nurse–patient interactions. Based on the patient's responses to the plan of care, the nurse decides to (1) terminate the plan of care when each expected outcome is achieved, (2) modify the plan of care if there are difficulties achieving the goals/outcomes, or (3) continue the plan of care if more time is needed to achieve the goals/outcomes. When evaluation points to the need to modify nursing care, the nurse reviews each preceding step of the nursing process (assessing, diagnosing, planning, and implementing). Successful evaluation enhances the public's image of nursing and helps ensure nursing's survival by promoting continued selection and funding of nursing services in the competitive healthcare market.

Unique Focus of Nursing Evaluation

As members of the healthcare team, nurses are involved in many types of evaluation. Nurses measure patient goal/outcome achievement; how effectively nurses help targeted groups of patients to achieve their specific goals; the competence of individual nurses; and the degree to which exter-

nal factors, such as different types of healthcare services, specialized equipment or procedures, or socioeconomic factors, influence health and wellness. The patient, however, is always the nurse's primary concern. A nurse may perform a nursing procedure competently, creatively, and with care, but if this nursing action does not help the patient reach desired goals, it is not fully meaningful. Either directly or indirectly, the aim of all nursing evaluation is quality nursing care that aids patient goal/outcome achievement. Therefore, the most important act of evaluation performed by nurses is evaluating goal/outcome achievement with the patient.

Evaluation Criteria and Standards

The five classic elements of evaluation are (1) identifying evaluative criteria and standards (what you are looking for when you evaluate, eg, expected patient outcomes), (2) collecting data to determine whether these criteria and standards are met, (3) interpreting and summarizing findings, (4) documenting your judgment, and (5) terminating, continuing, or modifying the plan. In the nursing process, evaluative criteria are the patient goals/outcomes developed during the planning step. Because these reflect desired changes or outcomes in patient behavior and because nursing actions are directed toward these goals/outcomes, they are the core of evaluation. Determining whether these goals/outcomes have been or are being met and then identifying the appropriate nursing response are the functions of evaluation.

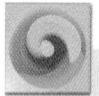

COGNITIVE SKILLS

- Knowledge of what information is needed to evaluate whether the plan of care is effectively meeting the patient's health needs (ability to measure how well the patient has achieved valued goals and to think critically about the factors contributing to patient success or failure)
- Knowledge of how to modify the plan of care, if indicated, or of how to remedy other variables interfering with the achievement of valued goals
- Knowledge of pertinent standards of care and agency and institutional policies

TECHNICAL SKILLS

- Ability to use a documentation system competently to record the patient's progress toward goal achievement

INTERPERSONAL SKILLS

- Ability to maintain a trusting nurse–patient relationship grounded in responsible caring with

the toddler with failure to thrive, teens who are smoking or at risk for smoking, diabetic patients with inadequate patterns of self-care, and nursing home resident with diminished will to live
- Ability to communicate that you are more concerned about the patient's overall well-being than the isolated task of evaluating goal achievement
- Ability to work collaboratively with the healthcare team to address factors interfering with patient's ability to meet valued goals

ETHICAL/LEGAL SKILLS

- Commitment to evaluating patient achievement of goals in a timely fashion and to addressing whatever is interfering with goal achievement
- Ability to serve as a trusted and effective patient advocate
- Ability to practice nursing with accountability to self, patient, the profession, and society

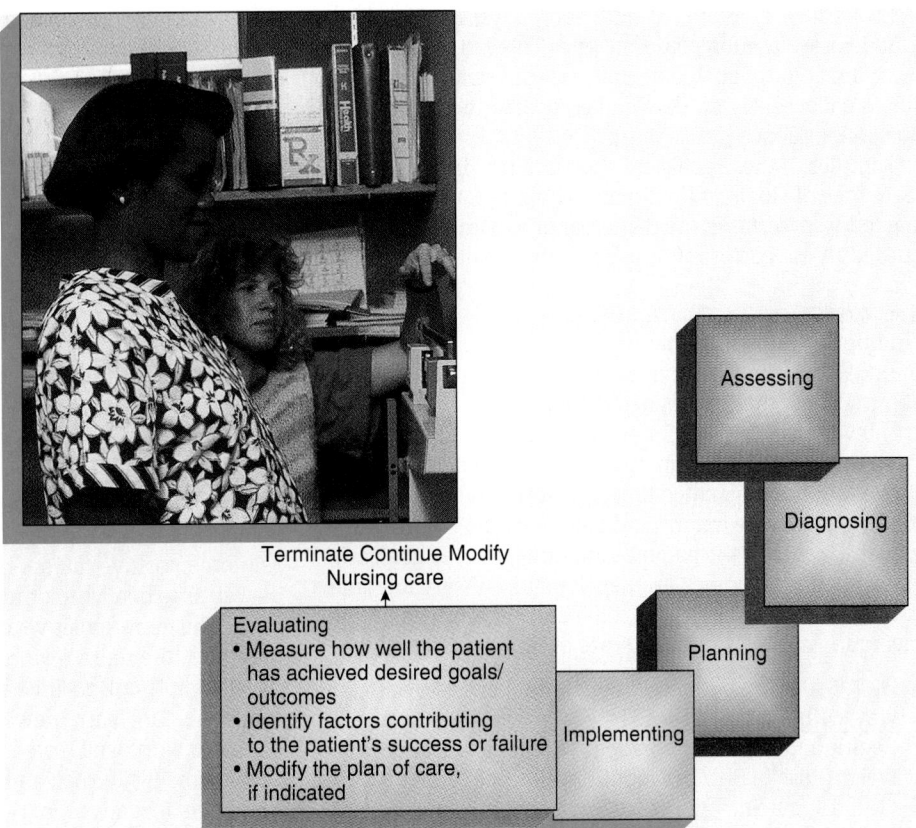

Figure 19-1
Evaluating. The nurse and patient together measure how well the patient has achieved the goals specified in the plan of care. Factors that contribute to the patient's success or failure are identified, and the plan of care is modified if necessary. Patient responses to the plan of care determine whether nursing care is to be continued as is, modified, or terminated. (Photo by David Maklem, University of Wisconsin—Milwaukee Photo Services.)

Although the terms *criteria* and *standard* are often used interchangeably in reference to the evaluation step, they have distinct definitions. **Criteria** are measurable qualities, attributes, or characteristics that specify skills, knowledge, or health states. They describe acceptable levels of performance by stating the expected behaviors of the nurse or the patient. Chapter 17 on planning describes how patient criteria are identified and formulated as patient goals or outcomes.

Standards are the levels of performance accepted and expected by the nursing staff or other health team members. They are established by authority, custom, or consent. A good example of standards is the American Nurses Association's *Standards of Nursing Practice,* which are displayed in Chapter 1.

Measuring Patient Goal/Outcome Achievement

Collecting Evaluative Data

The nurse collects evaluative data to determine whether the patient has met the desired goals/outcomes. Whereas the nurse collects data in the nursing assessment to identify patient health problems, the data collected in the evaluation step are used to determine whether the identified health problems have been or are being resolved through goal achievement. In the next paragraph and in the display, Using Four Types of Goals in the Plan of Nursing Care, which appears later in this chapter, you will find examples of the different types of data collected to evaluate the achievement of different types of patient goals/outcomes.

Types of Goals

The type of patient data collected to support the evaluation of goal achievement is determined by the nature of the goal. *Cognitive goals* involve increases in patient knowledge; these goals may be evaluated simply by asking patients to repeat information or, at a higher level of performance, by asking patients to apply the new knowledge to their everyday situations. For example, asking patients to describe new dietary restrictions is very different from asking them to plan a weekly menu compatible with these restrictions. *Psychomotor goals* describe the patient's achievement of new skills; they are evaluated by asking the patient to demonstrate the new skill. *Affective goals* pertain to changes in patient values, beliefs, and attitudes; affective goals are more complex to evaluate. Observation of patient behavior and conversation can determine whether affective goals have been achieved.

In the final type of goal statement, *physical changes* in the patient are the targeted outcome. To evaluate achievement of this type of goal, the nurse uses physical assessment skills to collect relevant data and compares these with previous patient data.

Samples of these goals are shown in the display, Using Four Types of Goals in the Plan of Nursing Care. The data collected to determine the degree of goal achievement are recorded in the corresponding evaluative statements.

Time Criteria

In addition to knowing what type of data to collect to determine goal/outcome achievement, it is important to know when to collect the data. When the patient goals/outcomes were developed, a time frame was established for when to determine whether the specified changes have been achieved. At the designated time, the nurse, in collaboration with the patient, the family, and other members of the nursing team, evaluates the patient's attainment of the goal/outcome. If goals/outcomes are developed in observable and measurable terms, the task of collecting data for evaluation is clearcut. Examples of three types of time criteria follow:

* By 7/8/02, the patient will walk the length of hallway with support of walker.
* Beginning 7/8/02, the patient will demonstrate a weight loss of 3 lb per month until target weight (135 lb) is achieved (6/8/02, weight: 151 lb).
* Before discharge, parents will correctly demonstrate chest physiotherapy procedures for patient.

It is important for nurses to evaluate patient goal/outcome achievement as early as possible. Goal attainment celebrated with the patient usually helps encourage the patient and leads to further goal achievement. When failure to meet designated goals/outcomes is detected early, the plan of care can be modified to redress the failure. The most common mistake nurses make in evaluation in acute care settings is waiting until the day the patient is to be discharged before evaluating goal/outcome achievement. At that point, it is too late to revise the plan of care.

Documenting Evaluation

After the data have been collected to determine patient goal/outcome achievement, the nurse writes an evaluative statement to summarize the findings. Atkinson and Murray (1990) suggest a two-part evaluative statement on the nursing plan of care to underscore the importance of evaluation. The evaluative statement includes a decision about how well the goal/outcome was achieved along with all patient data or behaviors that support this decision. The nurse has three decision options for how goals have been met: met, partially met, or not met.

* 1/21/02—Goal met. Patient reports 1 week of no tobacco use. C. Taylor, RN
* 1/21/02—Goal partially met. Patient reports decreasing tobacco use from one pack per day to 4 to 6 cigarettes per day. C. Taylor, RN
* 1/21/02—Goal not met. Patient reports no change in tobacco use. *Revision:* Reexplore patient's commit-

ment to try tobacco use control strategies and adequacy of personal support systems to eliminate tobacco use. C. Taylor, RN

The nurse signs and dates the evaluative statement (see the accompanying box, Using Four Types of Goals in the Plan of Nursing Care). Alternatively, the nurse follows the documentation guidelines for evaluating outcome achievement specified in the institution's computerized documentation systems.

Factors That Influence Goal/Outcome Achievement

Numerous patient, nurse, and healthcare system variables contribute positively or negatively to patient goal/outcome achievement. Identifying these variables allows the nurse to reinforce positive factors by drawing on them in the future as well as to deal with other variables that are creating problems. The more sensitive and responsive nurses are to these variables, the more rewarding their practices will be.

Examples of positive factors include a patient's strong motivation to learn new health behaviors, a nurse who comes to work well rested and with a new care idea learned from a nursing journal, and a healthcare institution or agency that offers incentives for quality nursing and has an optimal nurse-to-patient ratio.

When the nurse understands what factors are helpful to the patient who is trying to reach desired goals/outcomes, these factors can often be manipulated. For example, if a patient is learning to ambulate independently after hip surgery and you notice that he seems to make his best effort when his wife is present, mention this observation to her and plan to ambulate the patient at least once a day when she is present. Conversely, if a patient seems more fearful when his wife is present, note in the plan of care that ambulation is best attempted when the patient's wife is not on the unit. Ideally, this fear would be explored with the patient before discharge, so that he can continue to make progress when he is discharged home with his wife.

Table 19-1 presents common variables that can negatively influence patient goal achievement. Tentative nursing approaches are suggested. Nurses need to think critically about the effects of these variables and respond creatively to them.

Modifying the Plan of Care

When evaluation reveals that the patient has made little or no progress toward goal/outcome achievement and attempts to identify the contributing factors pointing to problems with the plan of care, the nurse needs to reevaluate each preceding step of the nursing process. New assessment data may need to be collected, diagnoses may be added or altered, goals/outcomes may need to be modified or rewritten, nursing orders may be changed, and evaluation may be targeted more frequently. Review the

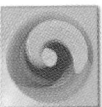

USING FOUR TYPES OF GOALS IN THE PLAN OF NURSING CARE

Nursing Diagnosis:	High Risk for Altered Parenting related to no previous experience in childrearing (fear)
Assessment Data:	*Subjective:* "My husband and I are both afraid we won't know what to do when we get the baby home."
	Objective: Both parents are single children, report no childrearing experience; healthy newborn son delivered 2/4/02; first born
Strengths:	VIB (very important baby): parents are both 38; history of infertility with one miscarriage; strong motivation to learn and use good parenting skills; strong support network

Goals (Expected Outcomes)	Nursing Interventions	Evaluative Statement (Actual Outcomes)

Psychomotor goals:
Before discharge, parents will demonstrate confidence in:
• Holding baby
• Diapering, dressing baby
• Bathing baby
• Feeding baby
	Assess both parents' knowledge of childrearing practices; identify and reinforce motivation to learn; correct any misinformation.
	
	Develop and implement at a time convenient for both parents a teaching plan to include:
	• The primary nurse role-modeling techniques for comfortably and safely holding, talking to, and dressing baby
	• Parents independently viewing videocassettes on:
	    Baby care
	    Baby bath
	    Breastfeeding
	    Followed by one-on-one discussion
	• Class for new parents: nurse to demonstrate baby bath and discuss general principles of care
	• Primary nurse observing mother and infant during initial feeding sessions and offering teaching and support as necessary
		2/6/02 Goal partially met. Both parents have correctly demonstrated safe techniques for holding, dressing, and bathing the baby. Mother is still concerned baby is not getting enough milk.
		
		Revision: Continue to spend time with mother and infant during feeding—provide positive reinforcement.
		
		F. Morales, RN

Cognitive goals: By 2/6/02, parents will report appropriate action to be taken if questions or problems arise after discharge: • Name and number of primary nurse • Name and number of pediatrician • La Leche League contact and number	Answer parents' questions and address related concerns. Assess parents' knowledge of infant problems frequently encountered by new parents. Inform parents of available community resources and describe appropriate action to take if questions or problems arise.	2/6/02 Goal met. Parents discussed some infant problems related to feeding, elimination, and illness and reported appropriate community resource to contact. *F. Morales, RN*

(continued)

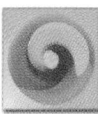

USING FOUR TYPES OF GOALS IN THE PLAN OF NURSING CARE (Continued)

Goals (Expected Outcomes)	Nursing Interventions	Evaluative Statement (Actual Outcomes)
Affective goals: Before discharge, parents will verbalize decreased anxiety in regard to caring for son.	Assess parents' level of anxiety and potential negative effects on child-rearing. Discuss this with parents. Explore adequacy of parents' coping strategies—increased knowledge, practice in supportive environment, community resources. Counsel as necessary. Compliment parents on new parenting skills. Allow for ventilation of anxiety or specific fears. Respond with teaching or emotional support as necessary.	2/6/02 Goal partially met. Except for concern about breastfeeding, *both* parents expressed feeling comfortable and eager to care for their son at home. *F. Morales, RN*
Physiologic goals: At 1-month postpartal telephone interview, 3/4/02 (by parents' report), the baby will demonstrate adequate: • Weight gain (birth weight, 7 lb 6 oz) • Sleep–wakefulness patterns • Comfort level indicating adequate parenting.	Use a 1-month postdelivery telephone interview to assess the adequacy of parenting skills. With positive report of growth and development, compliment (reinforce) the parents. With negative report, teach or counsel and refer as appropriate.	3/4/02 Goal met. Parents' report of baby's weight gain and behavior indicates good parenting skills. *F. Morales, RN*

checklist for help in evaluating your use of the nursing process in Chapter 14. Table 19-2 suggests appropriate nursing responses to common problems encountered during evaluation.

When the nurse has identified the factors contributing to the goals/outcomes not being achieved, the evaluative statement can be used to suggest the necessary revision in the plan of care: (1) delete or modify the nursing diagnosis, (2) make the goal statement more realistic, (3) increase the complexity of the goal statement, (4) adjust time criteria in goal statement, or (5) change the nursing intervention. Increasing the complexity of a goal after it has been achieved facilitates optimal function. For example, the initial goal for a patient with the diagnosis, Impaired Physical Mobility, might be "patient transfers from the bed to the chair." After this is achieved, however, the goal needs to be stepped up in complexity to "patient walks around room with support of walker."

The following evaluative statement might be noted, for example, if a patient did not meet the specified goal, "Patient will participate in a minimum of two planned social activities per week beginning 9/19/02." "9/27/02—Goal not met. Resident chose not to participate in any group activities this week." Many courses of action are then available to the nurse. Possible revisions to any plan of care include the following:

- *Delete or modify the nursing diagnosis.* This may not be a problem or concern for the resident. Evaluate and validate data pointing to the nursing diagnosis.
- *Make the goal statement more realistic.* Carefully determine the resident's need for activities and ability or desire to participate in activities.
- *Adjust time criteria in goal statement.* Reevaluate after 3 weeks; resident may need more time to adjust to being institutionalized and more encouragement.
- *Change nursing interventions.* Make a special effort to familiarize yourself with the resident's interests, and match these with available programs and activities.

Performance Improvement in Everyday Clinical Practice

It is not unusual for nurses to discover problems with how nursing care is being delivered in their practice setting. Each nurse must decide how to respond when it is perceived that patient care is being compromised. Nurses committed to

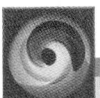

Table 19-1
Patient, Nurse, and Healthcare System Variables That May Detract From Quality Nursing Care

Variables	Possible Solution
Patient Variables	
Patient who is physically and cognitively capable of self-care gives up—refuses to cooperate with therapeutic regimen or thwarts the regimen	Identify one nurse who is able to develop a trusting relationship with the patient and determine the *reason* underlying the observed behavior: • No longer finds meaning and purpose in life • Overwhelming sense of powerlessness • Previous history of being "hurt," "exploited," "cheated" by the healthcare system • Inability to accept illness and related life-style changes Counsel appropriately. Use a team conference to develop a consistent plan of nursing care.
Patient who quietly accepts whatever is done or not done for him or her; seldom communicates needs or dissatisfaction	Note on the plan of care the need to assess this patient thoroughly because the patient will probably not advocate for himself or herself. Educate the patient to become a more assertive healthcare consumer.
Nurse Variables	
Nurse who sincerely desires to give 150% all the time and who becomes quickly frustrated when observing substandard care; may feel alienated from other staff; excellent candidate for burnout	Learn to give quality care during designated work period; leave on time; avoid the temptation to do the work of others; leave work concerns at work. After establishing a reputation for delivering quality nursing care, seek creative solutions for nursing problems (strategies to increase nursing resources, motivation, morale) and try them—hopefully with a support network. View concerns as challenges rather than overwhelming obstacles. Develop a realistic sense of how much nursing care and of what quality can be delivered with existing resources. If resources do not permit quality care, explore change strategies within the institution. If administration is not supportive, explore other practice settings.
Nurse with overwhelming outside concerns: • Preparation for marriage, childbirth, divorce • Illness (self or family members) • Role conflict (familial roles, school, work, and so forth) • New apartment, house	During periods of peak demand, may need to accept less than optimal performance at work. If this becomes the norm rather than the exception, carefully evaluate priorities. May need to cut work hours rather than "cheat" patients.
Nurse who is bored	After reflection, write down *personal* objectives related to work. Explore avenues within work setting for professional growth and development: initiate changes in nursing unit to improve patient care and to stimulate peer development; join institutional committees; participate actively in staff development programs; develop patient and family support groups. Look for new position that offers new challenges within or outside the institution. Join professional organizations and participate actively. Evaluate educational goals and explore possibilities—continuing education programs and degree work.
Healthcare System Variables	
Inadequate staffing	Develop and use a patient classification system that incorporates an identification of the kind and amount of nursing services required. Record staffing patterns and relate to needs for nursing care and patient outcomes. Clearly demonstrate and *document* that adequate staffing makes a difference. Present these data to nursing administration with the request for additional staff. If necessary, use professional bargaining unit.
Nursing administration has sold out nursing; insensitivity to nursing demands within the institution	It may be impossible to practice quality, progressive nursing in this environment. If there seems to be no hope for change after appropriate channels have been explored, look for a new practice setting. Evaluate the new setting on the basis of what experience has taught you.

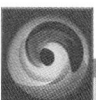

Table 19-2

Common Problems Noted During Evaluation of the Nursing Process

Problem	Nursing Response
Assessing	
1. Inaccurate database → inaccurate nursing diagnoses and a distorted plan of care	1. a. Identify the patient or nurse variables responsible for inaccuracy. b. Revise the recorded database.
2. Database does not reflect changes in patient condition.	2. Inservice the *entire* nursing staff on the importance of making assessment a priority in every patient interaction as well as the *recording* of the new data obtained.

3. Database is superficial:
• Fails to communicate uniqueness of patient
• Lacks sufficient detail on major problems or developments
	3. a. Rethink the critical relation between an adequate database and quality care.
	   b. Develop interviewing and physical assessment skills.
	   c. Begin to identify the key data that need to be collected for specific nursing diagnosis and medical diagnosis and to assess patient response to therapeutic regimen (use of a nursing diagnosis handbook may be helpful).

Diagnosing	
1. General sense that nursing diagnoses are "common sense" and therefore do not need to be put in writing → failure to address patient's real problems	1. Carefully develop and record priority nursing diagnoses for several patients and fairly evaluate whether this makes a difference in terms of the continuity of quality care.
2. General sense that nurses are too busy doing treatments, "passing meds," and doing paperwork to develop nursing diagnoses carefully → independent dimension of nursing remains underdeveloped	2. Examine practice and see whether *independent* nursing has a place; what percentage of every day is devoted to independent nursing functions? If this percentage is nonexistent or small, there understandably may be *no felt need* for nursing diagnoses—but a desperate need to revise practice priorities.

3. Nursing diagnoses are too vague to be helpful → routinized patient care	3. a. Revise the problem statement to describe more accurately what is *unhealthy* about the patient (the behavior that needs to be changed).
	   b. Revise the etiology to more accurately identify what is making the problem a problem—this should be a guide to nursing intervention.
	   c. Check NANDA lists.

4. Nursing diagnoses are not up to date → no one uses the plan of care	4. Have a process for periodically reviewing the plan of care to delete nursing diagnoses when problems have been resolved and to add a new diagnosis as needed.
Planning	
1. The plan of care contains only the standard knowledge most nurses would know without a written plan.	1. Make use of standardized (computerized) plans as a basis for care planning. Devote nursing energies to *individualizing* this plan.
2. The long-term goal is vague, standard; fails to make clear the discharge goal for this patient.	2. Practice writing specific long-term goals that clarify for all nurses the aim toward which all nursing care is directed (eg, patient returns home ambulatory with walker, right hip incision healing, able to manage activities of daily living with minimal assistance from spouse).
3. The nursing goals/outcomes, even if met, do not necessarily guarantee a resolution of the patient problem.	3. When writing goals, it often is helpful to develop outcomes related to etiologic factors. Because the stated etiology may be incomplete or inaccurate, it is essential that at least *one goal/outcome* be written so that if it is achieved, the problem in the nursing diagnosis is resolved.
4. The goals/outcomes are incorrectly developed; progress toward goal achievement is difficult to evaluate	4. After writing goals/outcomes, check them against the following criteria: • Subject is the patient or some part of the patient. • The patient behavior is stated in observable, measurable terms. • Criteria of acceptable performance are specified. • Time criteria are included in notes.

(*continued*)

Table 19-2 (Continued)

Problem	Nursing Response
Planning (continued)	
5. Nursing orders are superficial → patient receives routinized care	5. Review nursing orders to ensure that they indicate the *specific* nursing strategies most likely to result in successful goal achievement *for this patient* (eg, particular comfort measures that are successful adjuncts to analgesic administration for a particular patient. In specifying the "who, what, when, where, how, and how much" of nursing actions, be sure to list the type of equipment and supplies needed in various treatments. As new patient data are obtained, update nursing orders. Delete inappropriate or unnecessary orders.
6. The initial plan of care fails to be updated → plan of care will not be consulted by nurses—if used, it will be to patient's detriment	6. If personal accountability for updating plan fails, develop a process on the nursing unit to ensure care plan review and revision.
7. The plan of care addresses the immediate needs of the patient but fails to anticipate discharge needs → patient returns home unable to manage self-care activities	7. Work hard at developing the ability to project yourself into the patient's home after discharge. Learn to anticipate problems and concerns and prepare the patient and family for these. Use all discharge resources in the institution. Learn from patients what their needs were after previous discharge.
Implementing	
1. Nurses are not aware of patient priorities and the plan of care; lack of continuity; inefficient use of nursing resources → patient fails to achieve goals/outcomes	1. a. Use shift report to update staff on status of priority nursing diagnosis and concomitant nursing care. b. Review plan of care and nursing notes before beginning care.
2. Nursing care becomes routinized and mechanized → patient never has the sense that he or she is personally known by nurses	2. Explore creative strategies to make quality nursing care on this particular unit a *challenge* rather than a *burden;* use ongoing education, problem-solving strategies by the nursing team, gaming, and other incentives.
3. Documentation is inadequate → because there is no complete written record of nursing care, *legally* this care was never provided.	3. a. Develop the philosophy that quality nursing care *deserves* to be documented. Review legal reasons for careful documentation. b. Become familiar with the flow sheets and note format used within the work setting so that charting can be done quickly and comprehensively.
Evaluating	
1. It is not done → mastery of nursing process is stunted; severely limits accomplishment of nursing aims.	1. Develop the belief that quality nursing care does not happen automatically and that only ongoing evaluation will identify needed areas of revision. Devise an evaluative strategy and carry it out. Study its effect on quality of care after 6 months' implementation.

healthier patients, quality care, reduced costs, and the personal satisfaction of knowing that they *are actually making a difference* versus merely *wishing things were different* value **performance improvement.** The following four steps are crucial in improving performance:

- *Discover* a problem.
- *Plan* a strategy using indicators.
- *Implement* a change.
- *Assess* the change; if the goal is not met, plan a new strategy (Haase & Miller, 1999).

See the accompanying box, Steps in Performance Improvement, for an example of a performance improvement strategy.

Evaluative Programs

In addition to each nurse's evaluation of patient goal/outcome achievement and subsequent modifications to the plan of care, many formal mechanisms are used to ensure quality nursing care. In the United States, regulatory agencies, such as state boards of nursing, the Joint Commission on Accreditation of Healthcare Organizations (JCAHO), the Professional Standards Review Organization, and the National Health Planning and Resources Development Act of 1975, require nurses to document that nursing standards are being implemented and maintained. Each of these agencies is concerned with quality care and quality control. The decreased availability of resources to treat patients in hospitals and the unavailability of sufficient alternative treatment settings pose a strong challenge to the nursing profession to find ways to avoid compromising quality of care. Numerous professional organizations are working to meet this challenge (see the accompanying boxes, National Quality Initiatives and Selected Web Resources for Patients and Families).

Quality Assurance

Specially designed programs that promote excellence in nursing are called **quality-assurance programs**. These range from small programs conducted by nurses on a small nursing unit to those developed for an entire institution, state, province, or country.

Quality-assurance programs enable nursing to be accountable to society for the quality of nursing care. Such programs are also a response to the public mandate for professional accountability. They ensure survival of the profession, encourage nursing's fidelity to its moral and ethical responsibilities, and assist nursing to comply with other external pressures.

There are two different approaches to ensuring quality. *Quality by inspection* focuses on finding deficient workers and removing them. Nurses and others working in this type of setting may be afraid to admit a mistake or error and wrongly attempt to hide a problem. Such behavior is never acceptable and may result in serious harm to patients. *Quality as opportunity,* on the other hand, focuses on finding opportunities for improvement and fosters an environment that thrives on teamwork, with people sharing the skills and lessons they have learned. Mistakes are viewed not as being caused by a lack of motivation or lack of effort by a worker but rather as a result of a problem in the system. In this work environment, nurses respond with openness and a desire to learn because their integrity and self-worth are not threatened. Our goal should be to work in an environment in which quality measurements encourage our best efforts.

American Nurses Association Quality-Assurance Program

The American Nurses Association (ANA) in 1975 developed a model quality-assurance program consisting of seven steps: (1) identify values; (2) identify structure, process, and outcome standards and criteria; (3) measure the degree of attainment of criteria and standards; (4) make interpretations about strengths and weaknesses based on such measurements; (5) identify possible courses of action; (6) choose a course of action; and (7) take action. The ANA hoped the model would be used to develop and implement quality-assurance programs within institutions.

The ANA model directs attention to three essential components of quality care: structure, process, and outcome.

Steps in Performance Improvement

The following four steps are crucial in improving performance:

- **Discover a problem**
  Advance directives are a powerful legal tool for people to indicate their end-of-life care preferences. Nurses on an oncology unit are becoming frustrated because many of the patients on their unit lack advance directives. By the time decisions need to be made about ventilators, coding, dialysis, and so forth, patients are often no longer able to communicate their preferences. The hospital has a policy about advance directives, but no one seems to be taking responsibility for initiating discussions with patients when they are first admitted.
- **Plan a strategy using indicators**
  The nurses call an interdisciplinary meeting with the oncologists, social workers, and pastors, who decide that the nurse case manager will be responsible for working with patients on admission to see if they want help in preparing an advance

directive. Each case manager will be responsible for documenting within 48 hours of admission the patient's decision regarding an advance directive. Staff nurses will be able to direct patient and family requests to do advance planning to the case manager and appropriate team members. The ethics committee was asked to do an inservice on advance directives for the team.
- **Implement a change**
  Case managers begin assuming this responsibility, and one nurse volunteers to monitor progress at 3-month intervals by checking charts for advance directive content and by speaking with the staff nurses who voiced the initial frustration about decision making.
- **Assess the change;** if the goal is not met, plan a new strategy
  At the end of 6 months, everyone seems satisfied that the new plan is working, but a decision is made to a 6-month follow-up evaluation to prevent backsliding.

Four step process from Haase, R., & Miller, K. (1999). Performance improvement in everyday clinical practice. *American Journal of Nursing, 99*(5), 52, 54.

National Quality Initiatives

Organization	Initiative	Description
JCAHO (Joint Commission on Accreditation of Healthcare Organizations) Regulatory accreditation (private) < http://www.jcaho.org/ perfmeas_frm.html >	ORYX	Integrates use of outcomes and performance measures into accreditation process; requires accredited hospitals and long-term care agencies to identify two clinical measures related to at least 20% of patient population; number of measures and percentage of patient population will increase each year.
NCQA (National Committee for Quality Assurance) Accrediting body for managed care < http://www.ncqa.org >	HEDIS (Health Plan Employer Data and Information Set)	HEDIS targets these areas: effectiveness of care, access and availability of care, patient satisfaction, health plan stability, use of services, costs, and health plan descriptive information. Quality Compass reports (available on CD-ROM/electronic data file) include performance data on managed care plans.
ANA (American Nurses Association) Voluntary < http://www.nursingworld.org >	Nursing Report Card for Acute Care Settings	Indicators and measurement tools for evaluating quality of nursing care in acute care settings. The three categories of indicators are structure, process, and outcomes. Outcome indicators include nosocomial infection rate; patient injury rate; and patient satisfaction with nursing care, pain management, educational information, and care during hospitalization.
HCFA (Health Care Financing Administration) < http://www.hcfa.gov/medicare/ hsqb/oasis/oasishmp.htm >	OASIS (Outcome and Assessment Information Set)	Set of assessment questions to collect clinical, financial, and administrative data in home health agencies. Goals of OASIS: to improve quality of care delivered to home health care patients and to provide data to HCFA.
FACCT (Foundation for Accountability) Voluntary < http://www.facct.org >		Aims to improve information available to consumers when choosing health plan, provider, hospital, and treatment. Has designed outcomes-based performance measures for a number of clinical conditions, such as asthma, breast cancer, diabetes, and major depressive disorder, and for health plan satisfaction.

Oermann, M. H., & Huber, D. (1999). Patient outcomes: A measure of nursing's value. *American Journal of Nursing, 99*(9), 40–48.

Other types of quality-assurance programs may focus only on one of these components or on a mixture of components.

Structure

A **structure evaluation** or audit focuses on the environment in which care is provided. Standards describe physical facilities and equipment; organizational characteristics, policies, and procedures; fiscal resources; and personnel resources.

Process

The focus of the **process evaluation** is the nature and sequence of activities carried out by nurses implementing the nursing process. Criteria make explicit acceptable levels of performance for nursing actions related to patient assessment, diagnosis, planning, implementation, and evaluation.

Outcome

Outcome evaluation focuses on measurable changes in the health status of the patient or the end results of nursing care. Whereas the proper environment for care and the right nursing actions are important aspects of quality care, the critical element in evaluating care is demonstrable changes in patient health status.

From Quality Assurance to Quality Improvement

Concern about the spiraling costs of healthcare, coupled with the success of industrial models for quality improvement, has led to a strong commitment to quality improvement in

Selected Web Resources for Patients and Families

Organization	Internet Address	Available Information
Agency for Health Care Policy and Research (AHCPR)	< http:/www.ahcpr.gov >	Web site includes links to health information for consumers.
	< http://www.ahcpr.gov/consumer >	Healthfinder is a gateway for health information with many links. Consumer versions of clinical practice guidelines by condition available at site.
	< http://www.ahcpr.gov/consumer/hlthpln1.htm >	Consumer guide for choosing and using a health plan.
	< http://www.ahcpr.gov/consumer/qualguid.pdf >	"Your Guide to Choosing Quality Health Care" is a comprehensive consumer reference for choosing health plans, physicians, treatments, hospitals, and long-term care (PDF file).
	< http://www.ahcpr.gov/consumer/quick.htm >	"Quick Checks for Quality" is a short guide for determining quality in health care.
Foundation for Accountability (FACCT)	< http://www.facct.org >	Foundation to help the public understand healthcare quality and make informed decisions about care.
	< http://www.facct.org/measures.html >	Provides quality measures for selected clinical conditions, such as asthma, breast cancer, diabetes, and depression.
HealthCareReport Cards.com	< http://www.healthcarereportcards.com/index.cfm >	Provides data on hospital performance, such as rankings for coronary bypass surgery.
Joint Commission on Accreditation of Healthcare Organizations (JCAHO)	< http://www.jcaho.org >	General public menu includes information about reporting a complaint about a health care organization, making health care choices, and performance measurement.
	< http://www.jcaho.org/qualitycheck >	With Quality Check, consumers can retrieve information about how Joint Commission–accredited organizations have been rated in areas such as patient rights, infection control, and others.
National Committee for Quality Assurance (NCQA)	< http://www.ncqa.org/Pages/Main/consumers.htm >	NCQA Consumer Page includes links to information on healthcare organizations. Consumers can search NCQA's accreditation status list and see if their health plan has an accreditation summary report.
	< http://www.ncqa.org/pages/communications/publications/brotext.htm >	Guide for consumers in choosing a health plan.

Oermann, M. H., & Huber, D. (1999). Patient outcomes: A measure of nursing's value. *American Journal of Nursing, 99*(9), 40–48.

the 1990s. **Quality improvement** (also known as continuous quality improvement [CQI] or total quality management [TQM]) is "the commitment and approach used to continuously improve every process in every part of an organization, with the intent of meeting and exceeding customer expectations and outcomes" (Schroeder, 1994, p. 3). Unlike quality assurance, quality improvement is internally driven, focuses on patient care rather than organizational structure, focuses on processes rather than individuals, and has no end points. Its goal is *improving* quality rather than *assuring* quality. The major premises of quality improvement are as follows:

- Focus on organizational mission
- Continuous improvement
- Customer orientation
- Leadership commitment
- Empowerment
- Collaboration/crossing boundaries
- Focus on process
- Focus on data and statistical thinking (Schroeder, 1994, pp. 5–8)

From the patient's point of view, one of the most important outcomes of quality improvement is the recognition that patient satisfaction is as important as customer satisfaction in retail business. With increased competition for the healthcare dollar, providers are learning that it is important to offer services that patients value and to offer them in a way that is valued by patients. By reemphasizing the critical nature of nursing's person versus task orientation, quality improvement underscores the need for nurses to blend cognitive, technical, interpersonal, and ethical/legal skills successfully.

Nursing Audit

A **nursing audit** is a method of evaluating nursing care that involves reviewing patient records to assess the outcomes of nursing care or the process by which these outcomes were achieved. Successful nursing audits depend on careful nursing documentation.

Concurrent Versus Retrospective

Nursing care and patient outcomes may be evaluated while the patient is receiving care (ie, a concurrent evaluation) or after the patient has been discharged (ie, a retrospective evaluation). **Concurrent evaluation** is conducted by using direct observation of nursing care, patient interviews, and chart review to determine whether the specified evaluative criteria are met.

Retrospective evaluation may use postdischarge questionnaires, patient interviews (by telephone or face to face), or chart review (nursing audit) to collect data. The type of retrospective audit most familiar to nurses working in hospitals is the JCAHO retrospective chart review. This accrediting body initially required hospitals to conduct a certain number of audits per year.

Summary

The cultivation of evaluation as a critical component of the nursing process ensures nursing's continued success in achieving desired changes in patient health status. Only a firm commitment to evaluation enables nurses to answer the following questions:

- What are nursing's values?
- How can these values be formalized in standards and evaluative criteria?
- What data exist to determine whether the specified evaluative criteria are being met?
- How can these data best be collected, analyzed, and interpreted?
- To what courses of action do the findings lead?

Nursing actions are far too valuable and costly resources to be haphazardly implemented. Evaluation that is carefully planned and executed can direct and redirect these actions to maximize the patient's benefit. This is the goal and challenge of nursing evaluation. Criteria that may be helpful in determining the adequacy of the evaluation step of the nursing process include the following:

- Evaluation of the patient's achievement of desired goals/outcomes
- Review of how the process is used and revision of the plan of care if necessary
- Participation in quality-assurance programs

Learning Objectives

After studying this chapter, the learner should be able to accomplish the following:

1. Define the key terms used in the chapter:

concurrent evaluation	process evaluation
criteria	quality-assurance
evaluating	programs
nursing audit	quality improvement
outcome evaluation	retrospective evaluation
performance	standard
improvement	structure evaluation

2. Describe evaluation, its purpose, and its relation to the other steps in the nursing process.

3. Evaluate the patient's achievement of goals/outcomes specified in the plan of care.
4. Manipulate factors that contribute to the success or failure in goal/outcome achievement.
5. Use the patient's responses to the plan of care to modify the plan as needed.
6. Explain the relation between quality-assurance/quality-improvement programs and excellence in healthcare.
7. Value self-evaluation as a critical element in developing the ability to deliver quality nursing care.

Critical Thinking Exercises

1. Interview five students who have personal fitness goals. Ask them to describe what personal factors have helped or hindered their achieving their goals.

Note commonalities and differences. Reflect on how you can help patients tap their own personal strengths to achieve their goals more successfully.

2. Interview several patients and ask them what qualities in a nurse are most helpful as they try to achieve their health goals. Similarly, ask what nurse qualities are most problematic. Reflect on how you measure up in terms of both positive and negative nurse qualities.
3. Interview three or more experienced nurses in the same practice setting. Ask them what system variables (such as philosophy of care, nurse-to-patient ratio, professional and nonprofessional staff mix, nursing management, adequacy of resources) most influence their ability to deliver quality care. Identify variables you want to look for when you interview for a job.

Bibliography

Alfaro, R. (1998). *Applying nursing process: A step-by-step guide* (4th ed.). Philadelphia: Lippincott Williams & Wilkins.

Alfaro-LeFevre, R. (1999). *Critical thinking in nursing: A practical approach*. Philadelphia: W. B. Saunders.

American Nurses Association. (1975). *A plan for implementation of the standards of nursing practice*. Kansas City, MO: Author.

American Nurses Association. (1976). *ANA quality assurance workbook*. Kansas City, MO: Author.

American Nurses Association. (1991). *Standards of clinical nursing practice*. Washington, DC: Author.

American Nurses Association. (1999). *Nursing quality indicators: Guide for implementation* (2nd ed). Washington, DC: Author.

Ardabell, T. R., Turjanica, M. A., Mastorovich, J., & Hirschman, V. (1995). Business process quality improvement: A step beyond continuous quality improvement. *MEDSURG Nursing, 4*(4), 279–288.

Atkinson, L. D., & Murray, M. E. (1990). *Understanding the nursing process* (4th ed.). New York: Pergamon.

Bloch, D. (1975). Evaluation of nursing care in terms of process and outcome: Issues in research and quality assurance. *Nursing Research, 24*, 256–263.

Cassidy, C. A. (1999). Want to know how you're doing? *American Journal of Nursing, 99*(9), 51–58.

Christensen, P. J., & Griffith-Kenney, J. W. (1994). *Nursing process: Application of conceptual models* (4th ed.). St. Louis: C. V. Mosby.

Coulter, S. J., Atkins, P. M., Bailey, D., Blatt, M. E., Blashford, L., & Shumway, S. (1994). Patient satisfaction: A QI pilot project. In P. Schroeder (Ed.), *Improving quality and performance*. St. Louis: C. V. Mosby.

Donabedian, A. (1980). *The definition of quality and its approaches*. Ann Arbor, MI: Health Administration Press.

Donabedian, A. (1982). *The criteria and standards of quality: Explorations in quality assessment and monitoring*. Ann Arbor, MI: Health Administration Press.

Haase, R., & Miller, K. (1999). Performance improvement in everyday clinical practice. *American Journal of Nursing 99*(5), 52, 54.

Hughes, S. J. (1995). Point-of-care information systems: State of the art. In M. J. Ball, K. J. Hannah, S. K. Newbold, & J. V. Douglas (Eds.), *Nursing informatics: Where caring and technology meet* (2nd ed.). New York: Springer-Verlag.

Joint Commission on Accreditation of Healthcare Organizations. (1994). *1995 accreditation manual for hospitals*. Oakbrook Terrace, IL: JCAHO.

Katz, J. M., & Green, E. (1996). *Managing quality: A guide to improving performance in health care*. St. Louis: Mosby–Year Book.

Koch, M. W., & Fairly, T. M. (1993). *Integrated quality management: The key to improving nursing care quality*. St. Louis: Mosby–Year Book.

LaRochelle, D. R., & Shahinpour, N. (Eds.) (1995). Staff nurse initiated total quality management projects achieve quality nursing outcomes. *Nursing Clinics of North America, 30*(1), 1–162.

Ludwig-Beymer, P. (1993). Using patient perception to improve quality care. *Journal of Nursing Care Quality, 7*(2), 42–51.

Morin, G. D. (1995). A personal performance checklist. *Nursing Management, 26*(2), 325–326.

Oermann, M. H., & Huber, D. (1999). Patient outcomes: A measure of nursing's value. *American Journal of Nursing, 99*(9), 40–48.

Peters, D. (1991). Measuring quality: Inspection or opportunity? *Holistic Nursing Practice, 5*(3), 1–7.

Phaneuf, M. (1976). *The nursing audit: Self regulation in nursing practice*. New York: Appleton-Century-Crofts.

Phaneuf, M. (1976). Quality assurance: A nursing view. *New Zealand Nursing Journal, 69*(2), 9–11.

Rubenfeld, M. G., & Scheffer, B. K. (1995). *Critical thinking in nursing: An interactive approach*. Philadelphia: J. B. Lippincott.

Schroeder, P. (1994). *Improving quality and performance: Concepts, programs, and techniques*. St. Louis: C. V. Mosby.

Western, P. (1994). QA/QI and nursing competence: A combined model. *Nursing Management, 25*(3), 44–46.

Wright, D. (1984). An introduction to the evaluation of nursing care: A review of the literature. *Journal of Advanced Nursing, 9*(5), 457–467.

Chapter 20
Documenting, Reporting, and Conferring

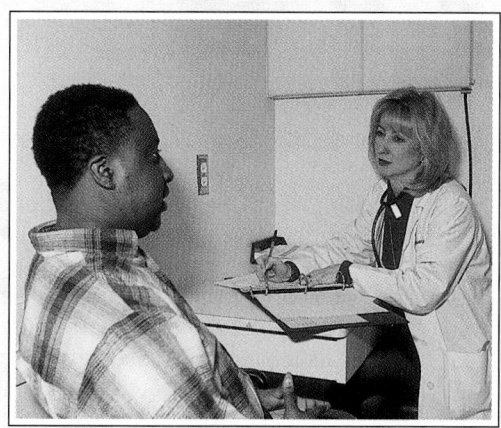

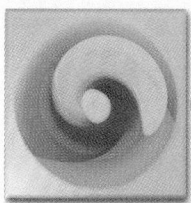

Thinking Critically About
Nursing's Blended Skills

Before reading this chapter, think about the types of skills you will need to document your plan of care for the individuals you first met in the assessing chapter and to report and confer appropriately.

- You are working in a community-based well-child clinic. You become concerned when you observe negligible height and weight gains, delayed developmental milestones, and lethargy in a toddler brought to the clinic by her grandmother.

- You are working with a school nurse. Statistics reveal a pattern of teen smoking in your high school, and you are charged with developing an initiative to reverse this trend.

- You are doing a rotation on a medical floor in a hospital and learn that many of the diabetic patients being treated are repeat admissions with a history of poor self-care behaviors.

- You are working in a nursing home where one alert resident with multiple chronic conditions repeatedly tells you that she has no reason to live and asks you to help her end her life.

What cognitive, technical, interpersonal, and ethical/legal skills do you think you will need to document a plan of nursing care for these individuals and groups and to report and confer appropriately?

Effective communication among healthcare professionals is essential to the coordination and continuity of care. Communicating effectively enables personnel to support and complement one another's services and to avoid duplications and omissions in care. This chapter describes three methods of communication central to nursing's professional role: documenting, reporting, and conferring. The first day you care for patients, you will find yourself conferring with colleagues, recording your interventions, and reporting on your patient's progress toward valued goals and outcomes. This chapter will help you assume these responsibilities with greater confidence and skill. The communication process itself and specific communication techniques are discussed in Chapter 21.

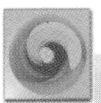 Documenting Care

Documentation is the written, legal record of all pertinent interactions with the patient—assessing, diagnosing, planning, implementing, and evaluating. Increasingly sophisticated management information systems are being designed to manage patient-specific data and information. These data are used to facilitate patient care, serve as a financial and legal record, help in clinical research, and support decision analysis. Information specialists aim to create an environment that supports timely, accurate, secure, and confidential recording and use of patient-specific information.

The **patient record** is a compilation of a patient's health information. Each healthcare institution or agency has policies that specify the nurse's documentation responsibilities. The Joint Commission for the Accreditation of Healthcare Organizations (JCAHO, 1999) specifies that nursing care data related to patient assessments, nursing diagnoses or patient needs, nursing interventions, and patient outcomes are permanently integrated into the patient record. Each nurse is expected to practice according to local policies and professional standards.

Guidelines for Effective Documentation

The patient record is the only permanent legal document that details the nurse's interactions with the patient and is the nurse's best defense if a patient or patient surrogate alleges nursing negligence. Unfortunately, there are often crucial omissions in the nursing documentation along with meaningless repetitious entries and inaccurate entries. Although these errors may go undetected and have no effect on the patient, they may also seriously affect the care the patient receives, undermine nursing's credibility as a pro-

COGNITIVE SKILLS

- Knowledge of what information you need to document the nursing interventions that effectively meet the nursing needs of the toddler with failure to thrive, teens who are smoking or at risk for smoking, diabetic patients with inadequate patterns of self-care, and nursing home resident with diminished will to live (how to carry out the plan of care, continue data collection and modify the plan as needed, and communicate care)

- Knowledge of how different documentation systems work (in a well-child clinic, public high school, hospital, and nursing home) and the purposes of documentation

- Knowledge of pertinent standards for documenting care and agency and institutional policies

- Ability to think critically about how to best respond to the patient's need for nursing and when and how to report and confer

TECHNICAL SKILLS

- Ability to use agency- and school-specified documentation systems

- Computer literacy

INTERPERSONAL SKILLS

- Ability to establish a trusting nurse–patient relationship grounded in responsible caring

- Ability to communicate to patients, their families, and professional caregivers that you are more concerned about the patient and his or her well-being than about rote documentation of the plan of care. What matters is *communicating the plan of care* so that *coordination of care* is achieved.

- Ability to establish collaborative respectful relationships with health team members to promote quality care

ETHICAL/LEGAL SKILLS

- Commitment to honesty, integrity, and accountability in professional relationships

- Respect for the confidentiality of patient information

- Ability to document nursing interventions completely, accurately, concisely, and factually—avoiding legal problems

- Ability to complete correctly an incident report to document events not consistent with the routine operation of a healthcare unit or routine patient care, which place a patient at risk of harm

fessional discipline, and cause legal problems for the nurse responsible. Adherence to the accompanying Documentation Guidelines helps to prevent errors. In brief, documentation should be consistent with professional and agency standards; complete, accurate, relevant, factual, and timely; orderly and sequential; legally prudent; and confidential.

Agency Policies

Most agencies have specific policies for patient records. Everyone who has access to the record (direct caregivers) is expected to maintain its confidentiality. At no time may a nurse let any person other than an authorized caregiver see a patient's chart. State laws differ about whether the patient has the legal right to review the chart. Most agencies grant student nurses access to patient records for purposes of education. In this instance, the student assumes responsibility to hold patient information in confidence.

Agency policies also indicate which personnel are responsible for recording on each form in the record, and such policies may also describe the order in which the forms are to appear in the record. Additional policies may concern the frequency with which entries are to be made, whether routine care is recorded, the manner in which health personnel identify themselves after making an entry, which types of abbreviations are acceptable, and the manner in which recording errors are handled (Table 20-1 provides a list of commonly used abbreviations). An issue of growing importance concerns documentation made by unlicensed personnel. Because professional nurses frequently supervise the care that unlicensed personnel give, it is essential to clarify which assessments and interventions may be charted by unlicensed personnel and which require documentation by a professional nurse.

The storage of patient records when a patient is no longer receiving treatment is a function of the health agency's record department. Many patient records are microfilmed for compact storage or are entered into a computer to expedite accessibility of information.

Purposes of Patient Records

Patient records serve many purposes.

Communication

The patient record helps healthcare professionals from different disciplines who interact with the patient at different times to communicate with one another. This is the primary purpose of the record. It is helpful to keep in mind that other healthcare professionals make judgments about nurses and nursing's contributions to the healthcare team partially on the basis of what we document in the patient record.

Care Planning

Each professional working with the patient has access to the patient's baseline and ongoing data and can see how the patient is responding to the treatment plan from day to day. Modifications of the plan of care are based on these data.

Quality Review

Charts may be reviewed to evaluate the quality of care patients have received and the competence of the nurses providing that care. For example, in a nursing audit, a committee decides in advance certain standards of care it wants to evaluate (eg, pertaining to nursing assessment, nursing documentation, or safety measures). A number of charts are then randomly selected and reviewed for evidence of the nurses' meeting the selected standards of care. If deficiencies are found, in-service training can be used to remedy the problem and improve the quality of care. Accrediting agencies, such as the JCAHO, may also use chart review to determine whether a particular agency or healthcare institution is meeting its standards.

Research

Patient records may be studied by researchers who hope to learn from the study of similar cases how best to recognize or treat identified health problems.

Decision Analysis

Information from record review often provides the data needed by strategic planners to identify needs and the means and strategies most likely to address these needs. Record review may reveal both underused and overused services, patients with prolonged stays who require special assistance, and financial information about which services generate revenue compared with those that cost the institution or agency money.

Education

Healthcare professionals and students reading a patient's chart can learn a great deal about the clinical manifestations of particular health problems, effective treatment modalities, and factors that affect patient goal achievement.

Legal Documentation

Patient records are legal documents that may be used as evidence in court proceedings, and therefore they play an important role in implicating or absolving health practitioners charged with improper care. The record can also be used in accident or injury claims made by the patient.

Reimbursement

Patient records are also used to demonstrate to payers that patients received the care for which reimbursement is being sought.

Historical Documentation

Because the dates of entries on records are specified, the record has value as a historical document. Years later, information concerning a patient's past healthcare may be pertinent.

Methods of Documentation

Source-Oriented Records

A **source-oriented record** is one in which each healthcare group keeps data on its own separate form. Sections of the

Documentation Guidelines

Content

- Enter information in a *complete, accurate, relevant* (concise), and *factual* manner.
- Record patient findings (observations of behavior) rather than your interpretation of these findings.
- Avoid words such as "good," "average," "normal," or "sufficient," which may mean different things to different readers.
- Avoid generalizations such as "seems comfortable today." A better entry would be "on a scale of 1 to 10, patient rates back pain 2 to 3 today as compared with 7 to 9 yesterday; vital signs returned to baseline."
- Note problems as they occur in an *orderly, sequential manner;* record the nursing intervention and the patient's response; update problems or delete as appropriate.
- Document all medical visits and consultations of which other nurses should be aware, either because of their impact on the patient or because of the nursing care the patient now requires.
- Document in a *legally prudent manner.* Know and adhere to professional standards and agency/institutional policy for documentation.
- Document the nursing response to questionable medical orders or treatment (or failure to treat). Factually record the date and time the physician was notified of the concern and the exact physician response. If this occurs by phone, have a second nurse listen to the conversation and cosign the note. If a nurse administrator was contacted, document this. Documentation should give legal protection to the nurse, other caregivers, the healthcare agency or institution, and the patient.
- Avoid the use of stereotypes or derogatory terms when charting.

Timing

- Chart in a *timely* manner. Follow agency policy regarding the frequency of documentation and modify this if changes in the patient's status warrant more frequent documentation.
- Indicate in each entry the date and both the time the entry was written and the time of pertinent observations and interventions. This is crucial when a case is being reconstructed for legal purposes.
- Document nursing interventions as closely as possible to the time of their execution. The more seriously ill the patient, the greater the need to keep documentation current. Never leave the unit for a break when caring for a seriously ill patient until all significant data are recorded.
- Never document interventions before carrying them out.

Format

- Chart on the proper form as designated by agency policy.
- Print or write legibly in *dark* ink to ensure permanence. Use correct grammar and spelling. Use **standard terminology,** only commonly accepted terms and abbreviations and symbols (see Table 20-1). Alternately, follow computer documentation guidelines.
- Date and time each entry.
- Chart nursing interventions chronologically on consecutive lines. Never skip lines. Draw a single line through blank spaces.

Accountability

- Sign your first initial, last name, and title to each entry. Do not sign notes describing interventions not performed by you that you have no way of verifying.
- Do not use dittos, erasures, or correcting fluids. A single line should be drawn through an incorrect entry and words "mistaken entry" or "error in charting" should be printed above or beside the entry and signed. The entry should then be rewritten correctly.
- Identify each page of the record with the patient's name and identification number.
- Recognize that the patient record is *permanent.* Follow agency policy pertaining to the color of ink and the type of pen or ink to be used. Ensure that the patient record is complete before sending it to medical records.

Confidentiality

- Patients have a moral and legal right to expect that the information contained in their patient health record will be kept private. Students should be familiar with agency policy and pertinent legislation about who has access to patient records, other than the immediate caregiving team, and the process used to obtain access.
- Most agencies allow students access to patient records for educational reasons. Students using patient records are bound professionally and ethically to keep in strict confidence all the information they learn by reading patient records. Actual patient names and other identifiers should not be used in written or oral student reports.

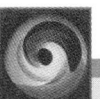

Table 20-1
Abbreviations and Symbols Commonly Used by Health Practitioners

Activities

AMB	ambulatory
BRP	bathroom privileges
CBR	complete bed rest
OOB	out of bed
up ad lib	up as desired

Assessment Data

abd	abdomen
BP	blood pressure
bx	biopsy
C	Celsius (centigrade)
cc	chief complaint
c/o	complains of
CTA	clear to auscultation
dx	diagnosis
F	Fahrenheit
FUO	fever of unknown origin
GI	gastrointestinal
GU	genitourinary
H/A	headache
h/o	history of
HPI	history of present illness
Imp	impressions
lt or Ⓛ	left
MAE	moves all extremities
NAD	no apparent distress
NKA	no known allergies
N/V	nausea and vomiting
neg	negative
P	pulse
PE	physical examination
PMH	past medical history
R	respirations
R/O	rule out
ROS	review of systems
rt or Ⓡ	right
SOB	short of breath
Sx	symptoms
T	temperature
⊕	positive
⊖	negative

Diseases

ASHD	arteriosclerotic heart disease
ASCVD	arteriosclerotic cardiovascular disease
BPH	benign prostatic hypertrophy

CA	cancer
CAD	coronary artery disease
CHF	congestive heart failure
COPD	chronic obstructive pulmonary disease
CVA	cerebrovascular accident
DM	diabetes mellitus
HTN (↑ BP)	hypertension
MI	myocardial infarction
PE	pulmonary emboli
PVD	peripheral vascular disease
STD	sexually transmitted disease
URI	upper respiratory infection

Diagnostic Studies

ABG	arterial blood gases
BE	barium enema
CBC	complete blood count
CO_2	carbon dioxide
C&S	culture and sensitivity
CXR	chest x-ray
ECG (EKG)	cardiogram
lytes	electrolytes
RBC	red blood cells
UA	urinalysis
UGI	upper GI
WBC	white blood cells

Symbols

>	greater than
<	less than
↑ ↗	increase increasing
↓ ↘	decrease decreasing
2°	secondary to
=	equal to
≠	unequal
♀	female
♂	male
°	degree
▲	change
x̄	except

Miscellaneous

ā	before
ad lib	as desired
AMA	against medical advice
ASAP	as soon as possible
BM	bowel movement
BP	blood pressure

BSD	bedside drainage
c̄ (C)	with
CABG	coronary artery bypass graft
CPR	cardiopulmonary resuscitation
dc (disc)	discontinue
Dsg	dressing
dx	diagnosis
DNR (no code)	do not resuscitate
FOB	foot of bed
Fx	fracture
GHWT	good handwashing technique
HOB	head of bed
hs	hour of sleep
Hx	history
I&O	intake and output
IV	intravenous
KVO	keep vein open
NG	nasogastric
noc	night
NPO (npo)	nothing by mouth
NS (NIS) (N/S)	normal saline
O_2	oxygen
OT	occupational therapy
p̄	after
postop	postoperative
preop	preoperative
prep	preparation
PRN (prn)	as needed
PT	physical therapy
pt	patient
q	every
QD	daily
ROM	range of motion
RX	treatment
s̄ (S)	without
SOB	side of bed
S/P	status post
STAT	immediately
TF	tube feeding
TPR	temperature, pulse, respirations
TURP	transurethral resection of prostate
TX	treatment
VS	vital signs
WA	while awake
×	times

record are designated for nurses, physicians, laboratory and x-ray personnel, and so on. Notations are entered chronologically, with the most recent entry being nearest the front of the record. An advantage of the source-oriented record is that each discipline can easily find and chart pertinent data. The main disadvantage is that data are fragmented, making it difficult to track problems chronologically with input from different groups of professionals.

Although the specifics vary among health agencies, the general characteristics of the source-oriented record have essentially remained the same. Types of forms typically used in a source-oriented patient record are presented in Table 20-2. Progress notes written by nurses in a source-oriented record are **narrative notes** that address routine care, normal findings, and the patient problems identified in the plan of care. They include a description of the status of the problem, related nursing interventions, patient responses, and needed revisions to the plan of care. Sample traditional narrative nursing notes are given in Figure 20-1. Traditional narrative nursing notes are also included in the nursing process patient care studies that conclude each clinical chapter.

Problem-Oriented Medical Records

Another type of record used in some health agencies is the **problem-oriented medical record** (POMR) or *problem-oriented record*, which was originated by Dr. Lawrence Weed in the 1960s. The POMR is organized around a patient's problems, rather than around sources of information. An example is given in Figure 20-2. All healthcare professionals record information on the same forms. The advantages of this type of record are that the entire healthcare team works together in identifying a master list of patient problems and contributes collaboratively to the plan of care. Progress notes clearly focus on patient problems. Table 20-3 and Figure 20-2 describe and illustrate the major parts of the POMR: the defined database, problem list, care plans, and progress notes.

The acronym SOAP (**S**ubjective data, **O**bjective data, **A**ssessment [the caregiver's judgment about the situation], **P**lan) is used to organize data entries in the progress notes of the POMR. Caregivers select numbered problems from the master list on the front of the patient record and then work up the problem or "SOAP it" on the progress sheet. Some nurses believe that the SOAP method of charting focuses too narrowly on problems and advocate a return to the traditional narrative format. Variants of the **SOAP format** include SOAPE, SOAPIE, and SOAPIER (**I**ntervention, **E**valuation, and **R**esponse). Figure 20-2*D* incorporates a SOAP note.

PIE—Problem, Intervention, Evaluation

The **PIE charting** system is unique in that it does not develop a separate plan of care. The plan of care is incorporated into the progress notes in which problems are identified by number. In this documentation system, a complete patient assessment is performed and documented at the beginning of each shift using preprinted fill-in-the-blank assessment forms. Patient problems identified in these assessments are numbered, worked up using the **P**roblem, **I**ntervention, **E**valuation (PIE) format, and evaluated each shift. Figure 20-3 is an example. Continuing problems are redocumented and numbered each day. One advantage of this system is that it promotes continuity of care. It also saves time because there is no separate plan of care. The disadvantage of not having a formal care plan, however, is that nurses need to read all the nursing notes to determine problems and planned interventions before initiating care.

Focus Charting

The purpose of **focus charting** is to bring the focus of care back to the patient and the patient's concerns. Instead of a problem list or list of nursing or medical diagnoses, a focus column is used that incorporates many aspects of a patient and patient care. The focus may be a patient strength, problem, or need. Topics that may appear in the focus column include patient concerns and behaviors; therapies and responses; changes of condition; and significant events, such as teaching, consultations, monitoring, management of activities of daily living, or assessment of functional health patterns. The narrative portion of focus charting uses the **D**ata, **A**ction, **R**esponse (DAR) format (Fig. 20-4). The principal advantage of focus charting is the holistic emphasis on the patient and the patient's priorities. Ease of charting is also cited as an advantage of focus charting because it is not required that each note incorporate data, action, and response. Some nurses report, however, that the DAR categories are artificial and not helpful when documenting care (Eggland, 1995).

Charting by Exception

Charting by exception is a shorthand documentation method that makes use of well-defined standards of practice; only significant findings or "exceptions" to these standards are documented in narrative notes. Benefits of this approach include decreased charting time (freeing more time for direct patient care), a greater emphasis on significant data, easy retrieval of significant data, timely bedside charting, standardized assessment, greater interdisciplinary communication, better tracking of important patient responses, and lower costs. Widely billed as "a more efficient way to document," charting by exception is rapidly gaining advocates (Murphy & Burke, 1990; Comstock & Moff, 1991). Figure 20-5 shows one example of this type of charting.

Case Management Model

Managed care's emphasis on quality, cost-effective care delivered within a limited time frame has led to the development of interdisciplinary documentation tools that clearly identify those outcomes that select groups of patients are expected to achieve on each day of care. A *collaborative pathway* (may also be called a *critical pathway* or *caremap*) for patients undergoing modified radical mastectomy is illustrated in Figures 20-6 to 20-8. In this particular documentation system, the collaborative pathway is part of a computerized documentation system that integrates the collaborative pathway and documentation flow sheets designed to match each day's expected outcomes. Developed at Vanderbilt University, this system has reduced charting (*text continues on page 326*)

Table 20-2
Examples of Forms and Information in Source-Oriented Patient Records

Form	Typical Client Information
Admission sheet	Legal name, identification number Age, birthdate, sex Marital status Occupation and employer Religious preference Next of kin and person to notify in case of emergency Date, time, reason for admission Name of the attending physician Insurance information Discharge data
Admission nursing assessment	Results of nursing history and physical assessment
Graphic sheet (see Fig. 20-9)	Daily temperatures, pulse and respiratory rates, blood pressure (vital signs), pain level Daily weight Special measurements, such as the patient's fluid intake and output
Activity flow sheet (see Fig. 20-1)	Diet and how patient has eaten Bathing and skin care Activity level, safety measures Respiratory interventions Elimination Diagnostic measures, treatments Isolation
Narrative nurse's notes (see Fig. 20-1)	Descriptions of pertinent observations of patient Statements that specify the nursing care, including teaching, received by patient and his or her responses to nursing care Statements that describe patient's condition and progress, or lack of progress, toward recovery and goal achievement Descriptions of patient's complaints and how patient is coping, or failing to cope, with them and nursing's response
Medication sheet (see Chap. 28)	Name of prescribed medications administered on a regular or p.r.n. basis Dosage of medication administered Route by which medication was administered, unless given orally Time medication was administered Name or initials of person administering the medication
Medical history and examination sheet	Results of physical examination performed by physician Current medical condition Health history, including previous illnesses Family medical history Confirmed or tentative diagnosis Plan of medical therapy
Physician's order sheet	Orders for medications Orders for treatments Other directives pertinent to a particular patient's care
Physician's progress notes	Interpretations of patient's pathology Responses of patient to medical therapy
Miscellaneous forms	Laboratory reports X-ray film reports Consultation reports Dietary requirements Results of social service consultations Types and results of physical, respiratory, and x-ray therapy

Shift	11-7:30 AM	7-3:30 PM	3-11:30 PM	Date	9/4/02 7 AM Pt. awake and
Diet or NPO	House = Soft	House = Soft	House = Soft	Time	alert. Awoke at 2 AM to void —
Nutrition		BR ☑ G ☐ F ☐ P LU ☐ G ☐ F ☐ P ☐ Feed ☑ Self	Di ☐ G ☑ F ☐ P HS Snack ☑ ☐ Feed ☑ Self		unable to fall back asleep. Refused sedative. Rested quietly. Speech clear, moving all extremities. —
Bathing Skin Care	☑ Mouth Care ☐ Skin Care *Keri lotion*	☐ S ☑ P ☐ C ☑ Mouth Care ☑ AM Care	☑ PM Care ☑ Mouth Care		L. Gray. RN
Activity	☑ CBR ☑ Pos. q2° ☐ BRP ☐ BRP c̄ Asst. ☐ OOB Chair c̄ Asst. ☐ OOB Chair s̄ Asst. ☐ AMB c̄ Asst. ☐ AMB s̄ Asst.	☑ CBR ☑ Pos. q2° ☐ BRP ☐ BRP c̄ Asst. ☐ OOB Chair c̄ Asst. ☐ OOB Chair s̄ Asst. ☐ AMB c̄ Asst. ☐ AMB s̄ Asst.	☑ CBR ☑ Pos. q2° ☐ BRP ☐ BRP c̄ Asst. ☐ OOB Chair c̄ Asst. ☐ OOB Chair s̄ Asst. ☐ AMB c̄ Asst. ☐ AMB s̄ Asst.	9/4/02 10 AM	Prune juice + cup of hot water with breakfast. resulted in soft formed BM — about 1 hour p̄ breakfast. No Straining. Keri lotion to dry skin on legs and arms. Strength seems to be increasing in left arm + leg. Performs lt. leg exercises independently. During bath talked about how much she misses her husband and her house. Explored feelings about participating in support group for widows — recommended by her friends. Feels good about babysitting her 2 grandchildren.
Resp. Assessment	☑ Cough/D. Breathe q2° ☐ Trach Care ☐ Suction Freq ___	☑ Cough/D. Breathe q2° ☐ Trach Care ☐ Suction Freq ___	☑ Cough/D. Breathe q2° ☐ Trach Care ☐ Suction Freq ___		
Treatments	Assisted ROM	P.T.	→		
Protective Precautions	☐ Full ☑ Half	— ☐ Full ☐ Half	— ☐ Full ☐ Half		C. Taylor, RN
Restraints	☐ Posey ☐ Wrist ☐ Ankle ☐ None ☑ q2° Check ☐ Other	☐ Posey ☐ Wrist ☐ Ankle ☑ None ☐ q2° Check ☐ Other	☐ Posey ☐ Wrist ☐ Ankle ☑ None ☐ q2° Check ☐ Other	2 pm	Spent 30 min. teaching patient + daughter Lisa about T.I.A. and stroke. Strong family history of PVD, CVA and MI. Reviewed importance of dietary modifications, regular exercise and taking prescribed medication. Excellent motivation for self-care — S Taylor RN
Elimination Bowel Bladder ☐ Foley	bedpan voiding q5 ☐ Commode ☐ Foley	↑BM Voiding q5 bedpan ☐ Commode ☐ Foley Care	☐ Commode ☐ Foley Care		
Diagnostic Studies +/or Specimens Obtained	—	CAT Scan	—		
Isolation Type	—	—	—	9/4/02	VS 98.8 - 78 - 18 136/92 Quiet this evening. — Napping - Not hungry at dinner: states "Busy day." Moving all extremities; alert. Daughter Barbara says her mother wants to do "too much." Still afraid TIA. automatically means stroke + death! — D. Kande RN.
Nursing Care Plan	☑ Reviewed ☐ Revised	☑ Reviewed ☐ Revised	☑ Reviewed ☐ Revised		
Comments	awake @ 2am did not fall back to sleep	"when can I go home?" napped in pm	—		
Signature	L. Gray RN	C Taylor RN	D. Kande RN		

Nazareth Hospital
Activity Flowsheet/Patient Care Notes

Figure 20-1
Sample of an activity flow sheet with narrative patient care notes. (Courtesy of Nazareth Hospital, Philadelphia.)

Summary of data base for client (20-2A)

72 year old, white, recently widowed female

brought to hospital after sudden fall caused by temporary paralysis of left leg; admitting diagnosis: transient ischemic attack (TIA), R/O cerebrovascular accident

treated for hypertension since 1990, otherwise in good health; history of headaches—once or twice a week (increasing in severity)—for last six months

ht 5'2" wt 63.6 kg   98.2 F-88-18   BP L—184/120, R—180/120
↓ strength ↓ movement left lower extremity (LLE)

Problem List (20-2B)

XXXX Medical Center   4629F

Date	No.	Problem	Identified	Resolved
9/2/02	#1	transient ischemic attack (TIA) R/O cerebro-vascular accident	J. Gleer MD	
	#1A	impaired physical mobility related to weakness in left lower extremity	D. Kande RN	
9/4/02	#2	impaired adjustment related to major life stressors and decreased supports	D. Kande RN	

Plan of Care (20-2C)

Date	Problem
9/4/02 3 pm	#2 Impaired adjustment related to major life stressors (including illness) and decreased supports Goal: Prior to discharge patient reports feeling able to go home and take one day at a time Plan: *Diagnostic*: explore adequacy of patient's usual patterns of coping and motivation to learn new strategies *Therapeutic*: 1) explain all tests/procedures to patient who wants to know and understand what is happening to her 2) create a restful environment 3) talk with patient's home minister (daughter will contact) *Educative*: Teach patient new coping skills, e.g., relaxation exercises. Refer to community support group for widows. _____ D. Kande RN

Progress Notes (20-2D)

Date	Problem-Oriented Progress Notes
9/6/02 10 am	Impaired mobility related to weakness left lower extremity (LLE) S "My left leg still feels queer, pins and needles—but I can move it alright." O Able to lift left leg off bed, positive flexion, positive extension; muscle strength in LLE 3/5 (normal movement against gravity) A recovering mobility as strength returns P *therapeutic*: consult with physician about complete bed rest order; *diagnostic*: continue to monitor muscle strength and movement at least once/shift; be alert for any signs of recurrent TIA; *educative*: instruct not to try to get out of bed without assistance until diagnostic work-up is complete; reinforce need for safety precautions. _____ D. Kande RN

Figure 20-2
Sample of a problem-oriented medical record.

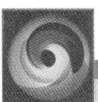

Table 20-3
Organization of the Problem-Oriented Patient Record

Part	Information
Database (see Fig. 20-2A)	The database is a compilation of all initial information about the patient and includes the following: Health state profile prepared by the nurse Medical history and the physical examination, prepared by the physician Social history Initial diagnostic test results
Problem list (see Fig. 20-2B)	The multidisciplinary problem list itemizes major aspects of the patient's life that require health attention and includes the following: Socioeconomic, demographic, psychological, and physiologic problems Each problem is labeled, numbered, and categorized as active or inactive.
Plan of care (see Fig. 20-2C)	An initial plan is formulated for each specifically numbered problem on the problem list. The nursing plan, whether *therapeutic, diagnostic,* or *educational,* is expressed through nursing orders.
Progress notes (see Fig. 20-2D) Narrative progress notes	Progress notes consist of narrative progress notes, flow sheets, and discharge notes, as follows: The narrative progress notes on the patient follow the SOAP format, as follows: S—Subjective information reported by the patient O—Objective observations made by health practitioners A—Assessments drawn from new data P—Plans or goals for action related to the patient's problems
Flow sheets	Flow sheets are used for recording information that is monitored over time. This information provides data for making comparisons of a patient's status at one time with that patient's status later.
Discharge notes	Discharge notes are the entries made at the time an episode of the patient's care is terminated and include the following information: The date of the resolution of each problem, as had been described while using the SOAP format Referrals made for the patient Recommendations for unresolved or partially resolved problems

P#1:
4/02/02
1300

Caregiver role strain related to patient's new safety needs and increased need for assistance with activities of daily living upon discharge.

I:

Sat with patient's daughter and made a list of patient's safety and basic needs upon discharge. Identified what patient already knows and feels comfortable providing and developed a teaching plan to address deficiencies. Patient is highly motivated. Explored community-based resources available to daughter and made referrals to support group for family members of persons with Alzheimer's disease. Social work will talk with daughter 4/03/02 to explore care options should it become impossible to continue providing care at home.

E:

Daughter verbalized feeling more in control and less anxious about her father's return home. ——————— *C. Taylor, RN*

Figure 20-3
Sample PIE patient care note.

time by 40% and increased staff satisfaction with the amount of paperwork from 0% to 85%. These gains were accomplished with no decrease in audited charting quality. More importantly, a time study demonstrated a directly proportional increase in time spent with the patient (Hatcher, 1995). Charting by exception is frequently used with critical pathway documentation systems.

The case management model promotes collaboration, communication, and teamwork among caregivers; makes efficient use of time; and increases quality by focusing care on carefully developed outcomes. The system works best for "typical" patients with few individualized needs. At present, there is little consensus about which documentation tools are best for recording routine aspects of care and avoiding repetition.

Variance Charting

When a patient fails to meet an expected outcome or a planned intervention is not implemented in the case man-

Date/Time	Focus	Patient Care Notes
7/11/02 9:15 am	High risk for trauma	**DATA:** *Patient crying when I entered room; confided that she is afraid to go home because her injuries are the result of husband's battery* **ACTION:** *Attending notified and discharge cancelled; Abuse network called with patient's permission and they are sending a counselor this afternoon to talk with her.* — *C. Taylor, RN*
10:00 am	Pain	**DATA:** *Patient complaining of pain in right rib area* **ACTION:** *Tylenol 3 administered as ordered.* — *C. Taylor, RN*
10:30 am	Pain	**RESPONSE:** *Patient reports relief from rib pain, still anxious about aftermath of discharge.* — *C. Taylor, RN*

Figure 20-4
Sample focus patient care notes.

agement model, this variance from the plan is documented. The usual format for **variance charting** is the unexpected event, the cause of the event, actions taken in response to the event, and discharge planning when appropriate. The variances most likely to be documented are those that affect quality, cost, or length of stay.

Computerized Records

In an increasing number of healthcare institutions, comprehensive computer systems have revolutionized nursing documentation in the patient record. Computer capacities are in operation in which the nurse (1) calls up the admission assessment tool on the computer screen and keys in patient data; (2) develops the plan of care using computerized care plans available for each North American Nursing Diagnosis Association (NANDA)-approved diagnosis; (3) adds to the patient database as new data are identified and modifies the plan of care accordingly; (4) receives a work list showing the treatments, procedures, and medications necessary for the patient throughout the shift; and (5) documents care immediately using the computer terminal at the patient's bedside. The American Nurses Association has been instrumental in developing the Computer-Based Patient Record Institute (CPRI) in response to a recommendation by the Institute of Medicine that a computer-based patient record be adopted by all healthcare providers and systems nationwide.

As healthcare reform initiatives evolve, patient outcomes will become the primary focus when evaluating the effectiveness of care. This focus will intensify as the Health Care Financing Administration and other reimbursement-management sources develop standard outcome measurements for all healthcare organizations. Outcome evaluations will be an important part of the healthcare agency's report card for consumers buying healthcare in this managed-care environment. A key component to facilitate data and outcome comparisons will be the **minimum data sets**. These specific categories of information will use uniform definitions to create a common language among multiple healthcare data users.

The nursing minimum data set is organized into three categories:

- Nursing care elements (such as nursing diagnoses and interventions)
- Patient demographic elements (such as sex, date of birth, and ethnicity)
- Service elements (such as admission and discharge dates and expected payer for services)

With **computer-based records**, these data can be distributed among many caregivers in a standardized format, allowing them to compare and uniformly evaluate patient progress easily. Besides tracking the progress of individual patients, computerized outcome information can compare the progress of groups of patients with similar diagnoses. These results will contribute to research, education, and ultimately better and more efficient nursing practice (Eggland, 1995).

The increasing use of computerized patient information systems to store and analyze patient data has necessitated the development of policies and procedures to ensure the privacy and confidentiality of patient information. Policies should specify what types of patient information can be retrieved, by whom, and for what purpose. Patient consent is necessary for the use and release of any stored information that can be linked to the patient.

The accompanying box highlights guidelines for Safe Computer Charting.

Formats for Nursing Documentation

When the nursing process is fully implemented, nursing documentation in the patient's permanent record includes information in the following areas.

Initial Nursing Assessment

A typical form used to record the initial database obtained from the nursing history and physical assessment is illustrated in Chapter 15. Accurate documentation of these data is important because they provide a baseline for later comparisons as a patient's condition changes.

(*text continues on page 333*)

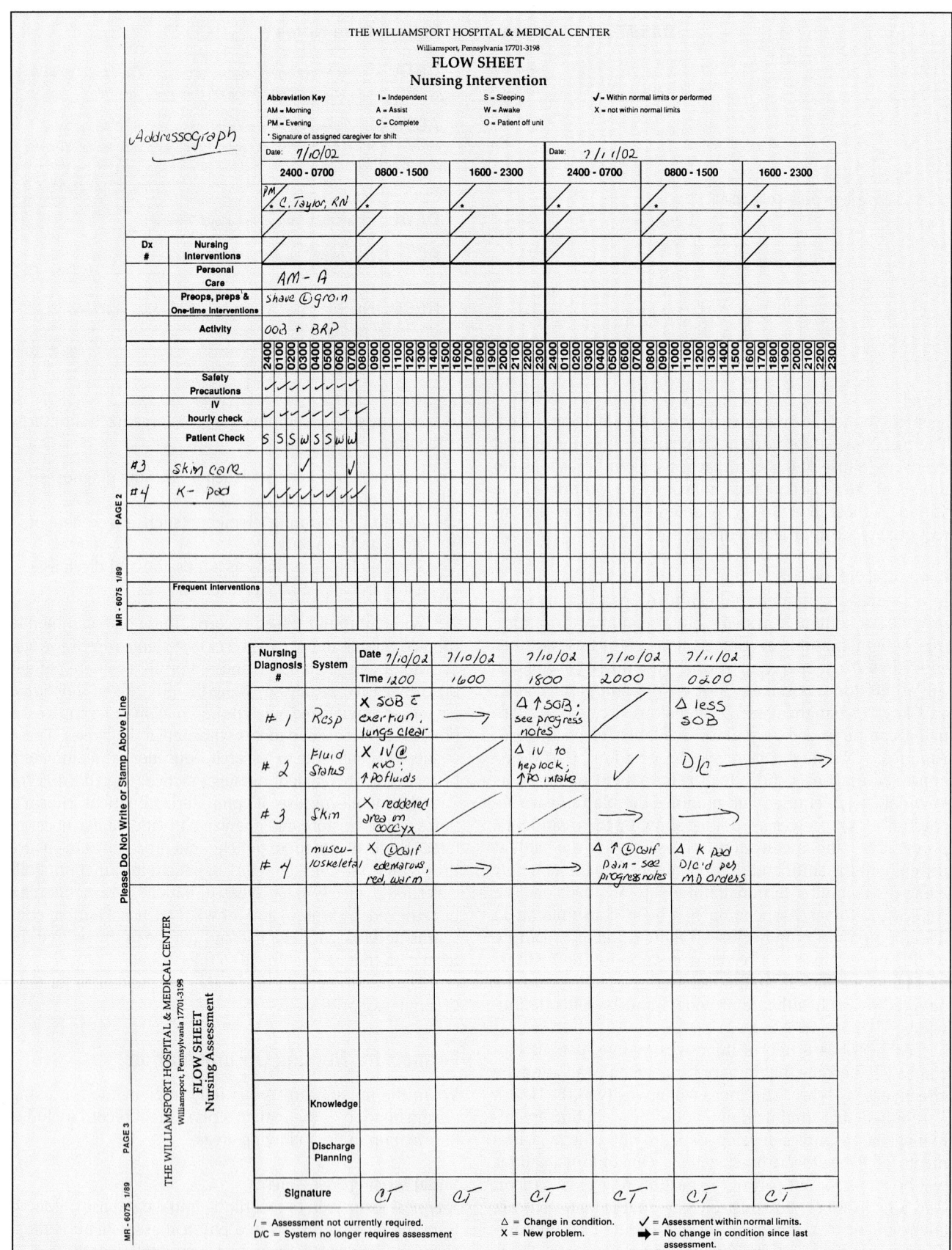

Figure 20-5
Sample documentation of nursing care using charting by exception. (Courtesy of the Department of Nursing, Williamsport Hospital and Medical Center, Williamsport, PA.)

VANDERBILT UNIVERSITY MEDICAL CENTER

Mastectomy: Modified Radical

DRG Number: _____

ELOS: _____

	Pre Op (Outpatient)	Day of Operation (Holding Room) 1 hr	Day of Operation (OR → close) 2 hr 15 min	Day of Surgery PACU (2 hr)	Day of Operation (9 S)	POD 1 (9S)	POD 2 (9S/Day of Discharge)
Goals	Pre-op testing complete and data available for review 1-4 days pre-op Pre-op testing results WNL for surgery Pt/family teaching complete Consent signed	Pre-op checklist completed Support to family Support to patient Permit signed	Pt. safety maintained → Sterile tech maintained → Pt. positioned correctly → Initial counts documented Final counts correct	Pain controlled VSS, Lung CTA Normothermia achieved SaO$_2$ ≥ 90%	Voids w/o difficulty Temp < 100°— Drsg dry & intact Incision w/o S/Sx infection — Drains patent & functioning— Tol reg diet w/o difficulty	Reach to Recovery referral made Demonstrates drain care	Home care teaching complete Drains patent and functioning till return to clinic F/U appointment scheduled
Treatments		Shave/prep	Correct position Pad extremities and bony prominence— Warm blanket— Pt. prep Bovie pad Counts x 3 if applicable	Standard PACU care Monitor drainage in hemovac Check dsg q 1 hr	No needle sticks, BP to ___ arm JP drains x 2 ———		MD remove dressing → Till RTC
Activity	Ad lib	Bedrest—	Check bony prominence	Progress as tolerated	OOB to chair in p.m.	OOB to chair Ambulate halls TID	
Diet	NPO at MN night before surg	NPO ———		Sips and chips if tolerated	Clear liquids → advance to regular as tolerated		
Labs	SMA6 SMA12 CBC with plts PT, PTT UA } → Pre-op value on charts		Specimen to Surgical Path.		PCV		
Tests	History & physical CXR EKG if > 50 yrs or indicated by history } Test results on chart						
Consults	Anesthesia—	Surgical Resident Anes. Resident Circulator for the case	Core Staff → PCM (prn) PACU Notified Pathologist	Surgeon	→	Reach to Recovery (call early w/ bra size) Assess need for HIR	
Meds/IV		IV access— Pre-op meds	Anesthesia drugs → Ancef 1 gm	Pain meds prn IV Antibotic IV (if requested) May D/C IV (if ordered)	Analgesic (IV, IM on PO)	PO analgesic	
Teaching/ D/C Plan	Procedure Plan of care VUMC orientation Consent signed	Reinforce pre-op teaching Support to family • waiting room infor. • update phone call Support to pt. • answer questions • comfort		Volurex →	TCDB Request pain med if not PCA Assess home situation/primary care giver	Drain care (empty, reactivate, record output & change dressing q d) Request pain med	Post mastectomy teaching Exercises How to take care of arm F/U Reach to Recovery Review drain care, meds, activity, reportable S/Sx, precautions Complete "patient discharge list" sheet
Patient Flow	H&P MD office Labs: Pre adm testing CXR: Radiology EKG: Heart Station	HR—	To OR suite—	→ PACU	9S		
Equipment & Supplies		IV start kit Anes. supplies X-ray folder on bed	Case cart Bovie Padded armboard OR supplies JP drains x 2 PACU stretcher	Respirator equipment	IMED		Schedule F/U 5-7 days post op to remove drains

© 1994 Vanderbilt University Medical Center. All rights reserved.

Mastectomy Modified Radical
6/3/94
General Surgery 1

Figure 20-6
Sample collaborative pathway.

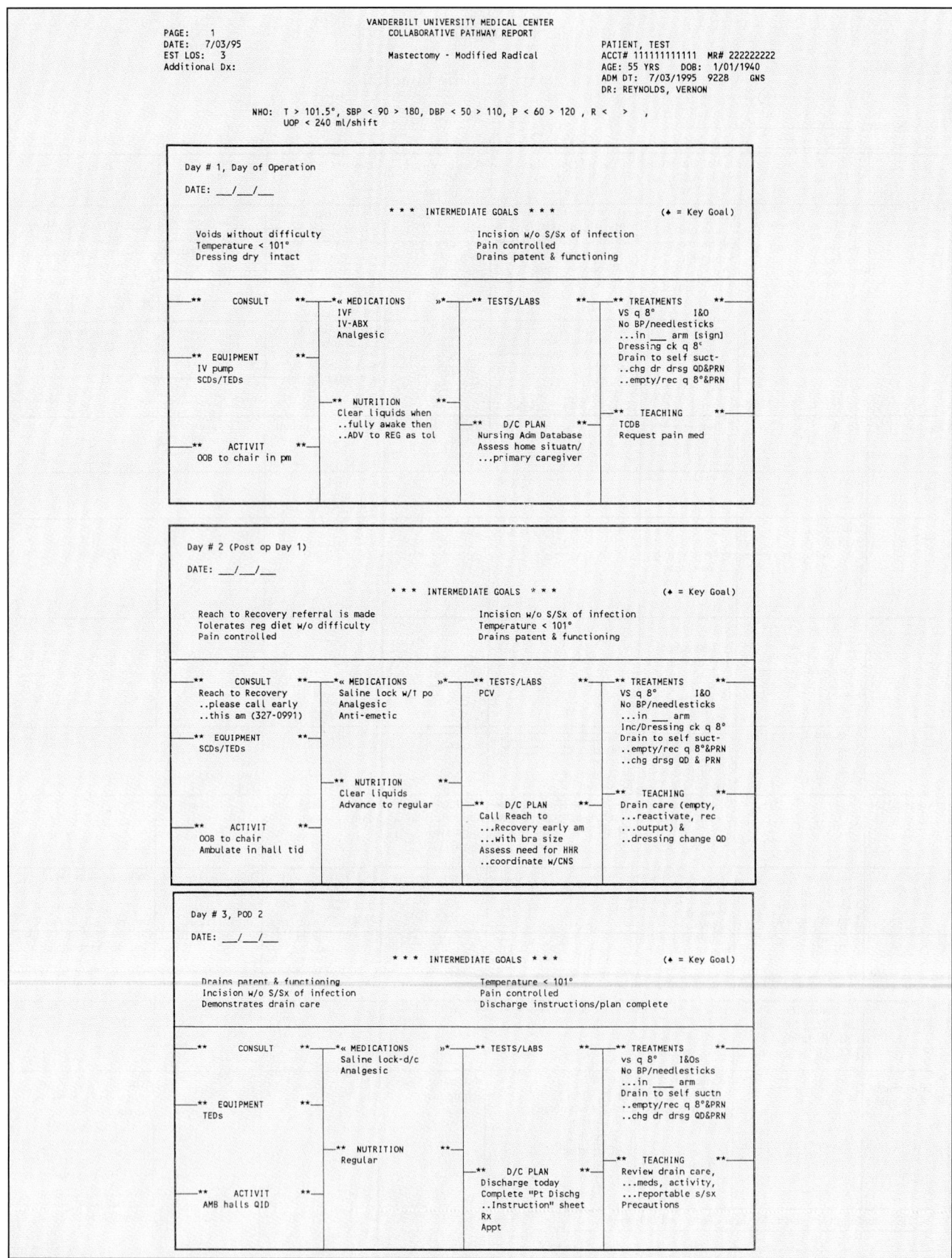

Figure 20-7

Sample collaborative pathway report. (Courtesy of Vanderbilt University Medical Center, Nashville, TN.)

VANDERBILT UNIVERSITY MEDICAL CENTER
DATE: 7/5/02

FLOWSHEET PAGE 2

PATIENT, TEST
ACCT# 111111111111   MR# 222222222
AGE: 55 YRS   DOB: 1/01/1940 9228   GNS
DR: REYNOLDS, VERNON   ADM DT: 7/03/02

COLLABORATIVE PATHWAY: Mastectomy - Modified Radical
Day # 2 (Post op Day 1)

CONSULT	Reach to Recovery					NUTRITION					
	..please call early										
	..this am (327-0991)	730 AM									
EQUIPMENT	SCDs/TEDs	✓ AB									
						NUTRITION	Clear liquids	8¹ AB			
							Advance to regular	12³⁰ AB	1730 CD		
ACTIVITY	OOB to chair	830 AB									
	Ambulate in hall tid	845 AB	1600 CD	2300 EF							
TESTS/LABS	PCV	719 AB				TREATMENTS	VS q 8° I&O				
							No BP/needlesticks	✓ AB	✓ CD	✓ EF	
							...in rt_ arm				
							Inc/Dressing ck q 8°	8 AB	1620 CD	2200 EF	
							Drain to self suct-				
							..empty/rec q 8°&PRN				
							..chg drsg QD & PRN	8⁵⁰ ✓ AB			
D/C PLAN	Call Reach to	830 AB				TEACHING	Drain care (empty,	830 AB	1135 AB	2030 CD	
	...Recovery early am						...reactivate, rec				
	...with bra size						...output) &				
	Assess need for HHR	850 AB					..dressing change QD				
	..coordinate w/CNS										

* * * * * I N C I D E N T A L   O R D E R S * * * * *

chemsticks BID

SIGNATURE	Alece Boyd RN	AB	SIGNATURE	Ellen Fisk RN	EF
SIGNATURE	Carol Davis RN	CD	SIGNATURE		

Figure 20-8
Flow sheets that accompany the collaborative pathway on day 2, mastectomy—modified radical. (Courtesy of Vanderbilt University Medical Center, Nashville, TN.)

VANDERBILT UNIVERSITY MEDICAL CENTER
DATE: 7/5/02   FLOWSHEET PAGE 3

PATIENT, TEST
ACCT# 111111111111   MR# 222222222
AGE: 55 YRS   DOB: 1/01/1940   9228   GNS
DR: REYNOLDS, VERNON   ADM DT: 7/03/02

COLLABORATIVE PATHWAY: Mastectomy - Modified Radical
Day # 2 (Post op Day 1)

ALLERGIES: penicillin

PREVIOUS DAY'S ACTIVE GOALS	Temperature < 101°

TODAY'S PATHWAY GOALS (♦ = Key Goal)	Reach to Recovery referral is made ✓AB Incision w/o S/Sx of infection ✓EF Tolerates reg diet w/o difficulty ✓EF Temperature < 101° EF Pain controlled ✓EF Drains patent & functioning ✓EF

Time		8	10	12	14	16	18	20	22	24	2	4	6
Activity		bed	ch	ch	amb	bed	amb	bed	→	→	→	→	→
Comfort	Scale												
Sal lock	flush q8												
Trach	Care												
Saline	lavage												
Suction	trach												
Tubefeed	residual												
NGT pH													
Neuro	Pupils												
	React												
	EyesOpen												
Verbal	Response												
Motor	Response												
Strength	RUE/LUE												
Strength	RLE/LLE												

Linen △ 8³⁰ BB	Bath A 8³⁰ BB	Mouth ✓BB	Skin ✓BB	Perineal ✓BB				

****** S H I F T   A S S E S S M E N T S ******

** TIME/INITIALS **	8¹⁵ AB	1510 CD	2030 EF		** TIME/INITIALS **	8¹⁵ AB	1510 CD	2030 EF	
1. NEUROLOGICAL	✓	✓	✓		8. IV SITE	✓	✓	✓	
2. CARDIOVASCULAR	✓	✓	✓		9. INCISION	✓	✓	✓	
3. PULMONARY	✓	*	*		10. DRAINS	✓	✓	✓	
4. MUSCULOSKELETAL	✓	✓	✓		11. PSYCHOSOCIAL	✓	*	→	
5. GASTROINTESTINAL	✓	✓	✓		12. SAFETY	✓	✓	✓	
6. GENITOURINARY	✓	✓	✓		13. COMFORT	✓	✓	✓	
7. INTEGUMENT	✓	✓	✓						

IV SITE: LOC/TYPE	RFA PIV				COLLABORATIVE PATH REVIEW	EF

SIGNATURE	Alece Boyd, RN	AB	SIGNATURE	Betty Brown CP	BB	✓ = No significant finding
SIGNATURE	Carol Dawn, RN	CD	SIGNATURE			* = Significant finding see note
SIGNATURE	Ellen Fisk, RN	EF	SIGNATURE			> = No change from last significant finding

Figure 20-8 (*Continued*)

Charting tips. Computer charting: Minimizing legal risks. *Nursing, 23*(5), 86.

Safe Computer Charting

The American Nurses Association, the American Medical Record Association, and the Canadian Nurses Association offer the following guidelines and strategies for safe computer charting:

- Never give your personal password or computer signature to anyone—including another nurse in the unit, a float nurse, or a doctor.
- Don't leave a computer terminal unattended after you have logged on.
- Follow the correct protocol for correcting errors. To correct an error after storage, mark the entry "mistaken entry," add the correct information, and date and initial the entry. If you record information in the wrong chart, write "mistaken entry—wrong chart" and sign off.
- Make sure that stored records have back-up files—an important safety check. If you inadvertently delete part of the permanent record, type an explanation into the computer file with the date, time, and your initials and submit an explanation in writing to your manager.
- Don't leave information about a patient displayed on a monitor where others may see it. Keep a log that accounts for every copy of a computerized file that you've generated from the system.
- Follow the agency's confidentiality procedures for documenting sensitive material, such as a diagnosis of acquired immunodeficiency syndrome or human immunodeficiency virus infection.

Kardex and Patient Care Summary

Many healthcare institutions and agencies use a **Kardex care plan** to communicate conveniently and concisely the plan of nursing care for each patient. The Kardex is recorded on a folded card and placed in a central Kardex file where it is easily accessible. The plan is eventually placed in the patient's health record. The outside of the card (activity and treatment section) contains basic information, such as the patient's profile, admitting diagnosis, and orders concerning activity levels, diet, vital signs, diagnostic tests, medications, and other treatments and procedures. The inside of the Kardex contains the nursing care plan specifying nursing diagnoses and health problems, related outcomes and nursing interventions, and special safety precautions. Some agencies now have computerized systems that are able to generate this same information in the form of a patient care summary for each shift.

Plan of Nursing Care

Patient records must communicate the patient's problems or diagnoses; related goals, outcomes, and interventions; and progress or resolution of the problems. The plan of nursing care may be written separately or incorporated into a multidisciplinary plan. In a traditional plan of nursing care, nursing diagnoses, goals and expected outcomes, and nursing interventions are written for each patient (see the sample student plan in Chapter 17 and the plans of care at the end of each clinical chapter). Standardized plans of care may also be used that identify common problems and related care for select patient cohorts. These generally incorporate standards of high-quality care, but unless such care plans are individualized, they may not sufficiently address individual patient needs. Formats for plans of care vary greatly.

Critical/Collaborative Pathways

The case management plan is a detailed, standardized plan of care that is developed for a patient population with a designated diagnosis or procedure. It includes expected outcomes, a list of interventions to be performed, and the sequence and timing of those interventions. The **critical/collaborative pathway**, illustrated in Figure 20-6 and in Chapter 17, is an abbreviated summary of key information taken from the more detailed case management plan.

Progress Notes

The purpose of **progress notes** is to inform caregivers of the progress a patient is making toward achieving expected outcomes. The method used to record the patient's progress depends on the documentation system being used. Common examples include narrative nursing notes, SOAP notes, PIE notes, focus charting, charting by exception, and flow sheets. The advantages and disadvantages of each are listed in Table 20-4.

Flow Sheets

Flow sheets are documentation tools used to record routine aspects of nursing care. Examples are shown in Figures 20-1 and 20-8.

Graphic (Clinical) Record

The **graphic sheet** is a form used to record specific patient variables, such as pulse, respiratory rate, blood pressure readings, body temperature, weight, fluid intake and output, bowel movements, and other patient characteristics (Fig. 20-9).

24-Hour Fluid Balance Record

Forms are available to document the 24-hour intake and output of fluids for patients with special needs. The forms include shift and daily fluid intake and output totals. A sample tool is shown in Chapter 45.

Medication Record

The patient's **medication record** must include documentation of all the medications administered to the patient (drug, dose, route, time), the nurse administering the drug, and, for some medications (eg, analgesics), the rea-

(*text continues on page 337*)

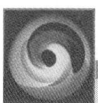

Table 20-4
Advantages and Disadvantages of Different Documentation Formats

Format	Advantages	Disadvantages
Narrative notes	Narrative notes allow nurses to describe a condition, situation, or response in their own terms, as they understand it.	It is time-consuming and difficult to read days and weeks of narrative notes to find a specific problem, its treatment, and patient response.
SOAP notes (subjective data, objective data, assessment–judgment, plan)	The location of the problem list at the front of the chart alerts all caregivers to patient priorities. Care and documentation of care is problem focused. Easy retrieval of information facilitates quality review and research. Healthcare professionals from different disciplines chart on same progress notes. SOAP format is consistent with nursing process.	The level of ability and consistency of caregivers in organizing data into the SOAP format vary. Problem focus may reduce patients to "problems to be solved." Maintaining a neat, up-to-date problem list takes constant vigilance and routine review.
PIE (problem, intervention, evaluation)	Without a formal, separate care plan, the method saves time because a nurse does not have to create or update a plan. Consistent with nursing process	Because there is no formal care plan, the nurse preparing to provide care will need to read all the nursing notes to determine problems, planned interventions, and evaluations to see if those interventions are effective.
Focus charting	Ease of charting with DAR is an advantage because categories of data, action, and response are not required for each focus cited. Components of DAR can be cited alone or out of sequence.	Many nurses have difficulty documenting information by separating the data into DAR categories. The "result" portion of the note seems to be a particularly difficult area because some nurses relate this portion to the resulting problems identified from the assessment data rather than to the patient outcome of care after nursing intervention.
Charting by exception	Abnormal status can be seen immediately, with narrative easily retrieved. The flow-sheet format shows overall trends in the patient's condition. Guidelines provide specific but concise standard information regarding "normal" assessments and expected outcomes. Documentation time is decreased because standard care is not written in narrative and duplication of charting is eliminated. This results in charting being done in a more timely manner.	Preventive and wellness-promoting functions of nursing are not documented on this format because they do not address problems. The system requires predictable, defined patient outcomes, which are more difficult to predict for some patients and in some settings than in others. More difficult to computerize
Case management model	Makes efficient use of time because each day has planned interventions and patient expected outcomes written on the plan. Increases the probability that a patient will be discharged in a timely fashion. Care is goal focused, which potentially increases quality. Promotes collaboration, communication, and teamwork among caregivers	Effective for patients with one or two diagnoses and few complications; less helpful for patients with multiple variances Space to document is limited on critical pathways, and too much writing causes illegibility. Space for individualization is limited. Separate narrative notes must be used for documentation of care. The intervention flow sheet, nursing notes, and critical path must all be reviewed to get a picture of a patient's condition.

Data for this chart were adapted in part from Eggland, E. T., & Heinemann, D. S. (1995). *Nursing documentation: Charting, recording and reporting.* Philadelphia: J. B. Lippincott.

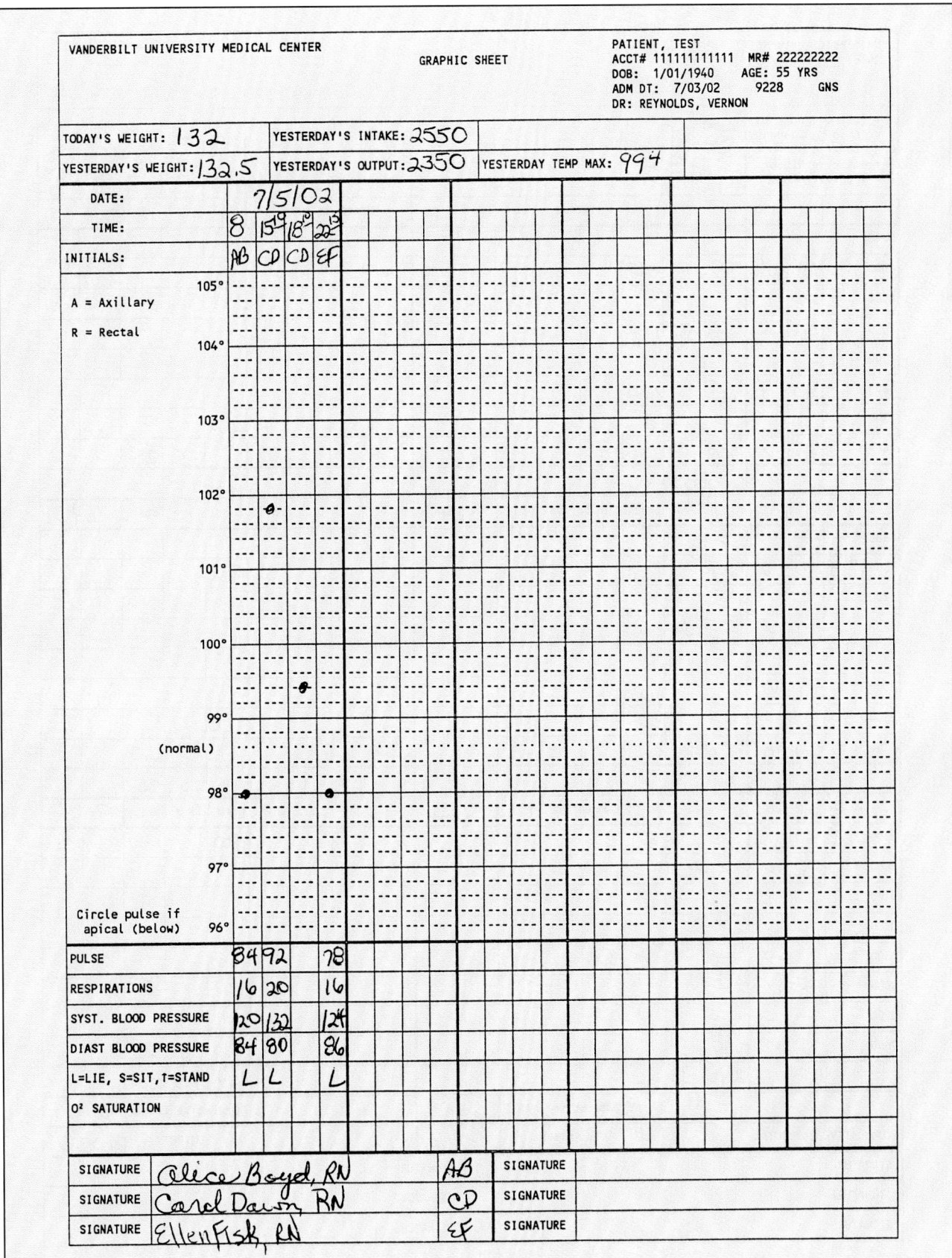

Figure 20-9
Graphic record that accompanies the collaborative pathway in Figure 20-6. (Courtesy of Vanderbilt University Medical Center, Nashville, TN.)

336   Unit IV: The Nursing Process

VANDERBILT UNIVERSITY MEDICAL CENTER
DATE: _7 / 5 /02_   I & O SHEET

PATIENT, TEST   ADM: 7/03/02
ACCT# 111111111111 MR# 222222222
DOB: 1/01/1940   AGE: 55 YRS
DR: REYNOLDS, VERNON   9228   GNS

T = Tubing Change ▲ = Dressing Change D = Diuretic + = Positive Blood - = Negative Blood			D5½NS .20K	Meds	PO										urine	JP#1	JP#2		BM
TIME	INIT	SITE✓				INTAKE						INTAKE OR OUTPUT			OUTPUT				
0700																			
0800	AB	✓	240/60		400										200				
0900																			T
1000	AB	✓	180/60	50	100														
1100																			
1200	AB	✓	120/60		400														
1300																400			
1400	AB	✓	60/60	50												15	25	
			240	100	900										600	15	25	
				Shift Cumulative Total		1240						Shift Cumulative Total				640			
1500			T															
1600	CD	✓	1000/60												400			
1700																		
1800	CD	✓	930/70	100 T	240													
1900																		
2000	CD	✓	880/50		100													
2100															500			
2200	CD	✓	810/60	50												15	30	
			240	150	340										900	15	30	
				Shift Cumulative Total		730						Shift Cumulative Total				945			
2300															400			
2400	EF	✓	770/60	50														
0100																		
0200	EF	✓	705/65															
0300																		
0400	EF	✓	650/55															
0500																		
0600	EF	✓	580/60													10	25	
			240	50											400	10	25	
				Shift Cumulative Total		290						Shift Cumulative Total				440			
CUMULATIVE 24° TOTAL					INTAKE		2260						OUTPUT		2030				
SIGNATURE									SIGNATURE									
SIGNATURE									SIGNATURE									
SIGNATURE									SIGNATURE									

Figure 20-9 (Continued)

son the drug was administered and its effectiveness. Sample medication records are shown in Chapter 28.

24-Hour Patient Care Records and Acuity Charting Forms

Flow sheets such as those illustrated in Figs. 20-1 and 20-8 are often used to document routine aspects of nursing care efficiently throughout a 24-hour period. When well designed, they enable nurses to document the routine aspects of care quickly that promote patient goal achievement, safety, and well-being.

Twenty-four hour reports are increasingly used in conjunction with acuity reports, which allow nurses to rank patients as high to low acuity in relation to both the patient's condition and need for nursing assistance or intervention. A trauma patient whose condition is changing rapidly and who requires intensive nurse monitoring and intervention will merit a higher acuity rank than a patient whose condition is stable. Acuity rankings are often used to determine staffing requirements. A nursing unit with patients with higher acuity rankings requires more professional nurses than a unit with the same number of patients but patients with lower acuity ranks.

Discharge and Transfer Summary

At the time a patient is discharged from care or transferred from one unit or institution or agency to another, a clinical resume should be written that concisely summarizes the reason for treatment, significant findings, the procedures performed and treatment rendered, the patient's condition on discharge or transfer, and any specific pertinent instructions given to the patient and family. A copy of a **discharge summary** is shown in Chapter 12.

Home Healthcare Documentation

Documentation of home care visits that reports the patient's progress serves two purposes. Sent to the attending physician with a request for signed medical orders to continue treatment, these records ensure continuity of care. Sent to third-party payers, they establish the need for continuing home care that results in continued reimbursement for necessary services. Medicare, for example, reviews progress summaries written every 60 days to determine whether a patient meets one of these Medicare requirements (Eggland, 1995, pp. 168, 172):

- The patient is homebound and still needs skilled nursing care.
- Rehabilitation potential is good (or the patient is dying).
- The patient's status is not stabilized.
- The patient is making progress in expected outcomes of care.

Chapter 13 shows a sample home health certification and a skilled nursing note.

Long-term Care Documentation

Documentation in long-term care settings is specified by the Resident Assessment Instrument (RAI), which helps staff gather definitive information on a resident's strengths and needs, which are then addressed in an individualized plan of care. The RAI helps staff track changes in a resident's status by evaluating resident goal achievement and making appropriate revisions in the plan of care. The goal is to coordinate the efforts of the multidisciplinary team to ensure that residents achieve the highest level of functioning possible (Quality of Care) and maintain their sense of individuality (Quality of Life).

The RAI consists of four basic components:

- *Minimum data set,* which is a core set of screening, clinical, and functional status elements that forms the foundation of the comprehensive assessment of all residents in long-term care facilities certified to participate in Medicare or Medicaid. The items in the minimum data set standardize communication about resident problems and condition.
- *Triggers,* which are specific resident responses for one or a combination of minimum data set elements that identify residents who either have or are at risk for developing specific functional problems and who require further evaluation using resident assessment protocols
- *Resident assessment protocols,* which are structured, problem-oriented frameworks for organizing minimum data set information and examining additional clinically relevant information about a resident. Resident assessment protocols help identify social, medical, nursing, and psychological problems and form the basis for individualized care planning.
- *Utilization guidelines,* which are specified in state operation manuals that instruct when and how to use the RAI.

Statutory law, federal regulations, and the Health Care Financing Administration specify how the RAI is implemented. An RAI must be completed for residents of Medicare skilled nursing facilities or Medicaid nursing facilities, hospice residents, and short-term stay or respite residents who are residing in a facility for longer than 14 days.

Benefits of using the RAI process include the following: (1) residents respond to individualized care, (2) staff communication becomes more effective, (3) resident and family involvement increases, and (4) documentation becomes clearer (Health Care Financing Administration, 1998).

Potential Legal Problems in Documentation

The results of one in four malpractice suits are determined on the basis of the patient's record. In the accompanying box, Potential Legal Problems in Documentation, Eggland (1995) outlines documentation content and mechanics that increase a nurse's legal risk. No nurse can afford to be ignorant or careless with respect to agency policies and professional standards for documentation.

Reporting Care

To report is to give an account of something that has been seen, heard, done, or considered. **Reporting** is the oral, written, or computer-based communication of patient data

---

Potential Legal Problems in Documentation

Documentation Content That Increases Risk for Legal Problems

- The content is not in accordance with professional or healthcare organization standards.
- The content does not reflect patient needs.
- The content does not include description(s) of situations that are out of the ordinary.
- The content overgeneralizes patient assessment or nursing interventions.
- The content is incomplete or inconsistent.
- The content does not include appropriate medical orders.
- The content implies a potential or actual risk situation.
- The content implies attitudinal bias.

Documentation Mechanics That Increase Risk for Legal Problems

- Lines between entries
- Countersigning documentation
- Tampering
- Different handwriting or obliterations
- Illegibility
- Sloppiness (some lawyers infer sloppy care from sloppy charting)
- Dates and times of entries omitted or inconsistently documented
- Improper nurse signature or unidentifiable initials
- Transcription errors (notes are made at bedside and later transcribed into patient record; problems include the amount of time that elapses between the event and when it is recorded and errors associated with recopying)

Eggland, E. T., & Heinemann, D. S. (1995). *Nursing documentation: Charting, recording and reporting.* Philadelphia: J. B. Lippincott. Used with permission.

---

to others. A laboratory report, for example, may communicate to the healthcare team that a patient's cardiac enzymes are normal or that a biopsy of breast tissue revealed malignant or atypical cells. A nurse's shift report or nursing note may communicate the progress a patient is making toward goal achievement. Common methods for reporting among health practitioners, in addition to the patient record, include face-to-face meetings, telephone conversations, messengers, written messages, audiotaped messages, and computer messages. Each of these methods has certain benefits and limitations, as detailed in Table 20-5.

Change-of-Shift Reports

A **change-of-shift report** is given by a primary nurse to the nurse replacing him or her or by the charge nurse to the nurse who assumes responsibility for continuing care of the patient. The change-of-shift report may be given in written form or orally in a meeting, or it may be audiotaped. Many charge nurses find that taped reports decrease the amount of time spent reporting and allow more time for last-minute details.

Typical information shared among nurses in a change-of-shift report includes the following:

- Basic identifying information about each patient—name, room number, bed designation, and current diagnosis
- Current appraisal of each patient's health status:
  - Changes in medical condition (results of pertinent diagnostic studies) and the patient's response to medical therapy
  - Where the patient stands in relation to identified nursing diagnoses and goal achievement
- Current orders (especially any newly changed orders):
  - Nurse-prescribed orders
  - Physician-prescribed orders (changes in medications, intravenous fluids, diet, activity level)
- Summary of each newly admitted patient, including his or her medical diagnosis, age, plan of therapy, and general condition
- Report on patients who have been transferred or discharged

It is important to avoid unprofessional comments about patients that could predispose oncoming nurses to view and respond to patients negatively.

Telephone Reports

Telephones can link healthcare professionals immediately and enable nurses to receive and give critical information about patients in a timely fashion. For example, the hematology lab may call to report a dangerously low platelet count, and the nurse may in turn notify the attending physician to obtain new medical orders. When reporting significant changes in a patient's condition to physicians and other healthcare professionals, nurses should be prepared to do the following:

- Identify themselves and the patient, and state their relationship to the patient. ("Dr. Gomez-Lobo, this is Ellen McLouglin, and I am calling about Mr. Clouser, a patient of yours who was just discharged home following a work-up for recurrent chest pain. I am his new nurse case manager.")
- Report concisely and accurately the change in the patient's condition that is of concern and what has already been done in response to this condition. ("When I first arrived in his home, he was complaining of feeling dizzy, and his blood pressure was 190/110. Yesterday morning in the hospital it was 150/90. His wife appears very flustered and says she doesn't know how she is going to take care of him. I had him rest for 30 minutes, and when I checked his pressure at that time, it was still 186/110.")
- Report the patient's current vital signs and clinical manifestations.

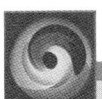

Table 20-5
Common Methods of Communication Among Healthcare Professionals

Method	Advantages	Disadvantages
Face-to-face meeting	• Message can be delivered immediately. • Nonverbal messages are readily conveyed. • Message can be clarified; receiver's questions can be raised and answered.	• Both the communicating and the receiving people must be available at the same time, in the same place. • Ordinarily there is no permanent record for later use.
Telephone conversation	• Message can be delivered immediately. • Message can be clarified; receiver's questions can be raised and answered. • Two parties need not be present in same place.	• Only the tone of voice and voice inflections can be communicated—no nonverbal messages. • Ordinarily, there is no permanent record.
Written message	• Message can be exchanged at times convenient for the people involved. • Record is available. • Time-efficient if message is understood	• Message usually cannot be validated with the sender.
Audiotaped message	• Message can be exchanged at times convenient for the people involved. • Record is available. • Time-efficient if information communicated is complete	• Message usually cannot be validated with the sender.
Computer message	• Message can be delivered immediately—even to those at a great distance. • Parties need not be present in same place. • Two-way communication is possible by e-mail. • Record is available. • Many people can participate in exchange.	• No nonverbal messages can be communicated. • Privacy concerns remain an issue.

- Have the patient's record at hand in order to make knowledgeable responses to any physician's inquiries. In this example, the physician will probably want to know all the vital signs and may ask questions about the treatment regimen both in the hospital and upon discharge.
- Concisely record the time and date of the call, what was communicated to the physician, and the physician's response.

Telephone Orders

Agency policy must be followed regarding telephone orders. Every telephone order should be repeated back to the physician to ensure that the nurse correctly understands what was ordered. If the nurse is unsure of an order given by phone, he or she asks the physician to repeat it. Telephone orders must be transcribed on an order sheet; policy usually dictates that they be cosigned by the physician within a set time. If the nurse judges a telephone order to be inappropriate, another nurse should listen to the order also. Then, agency guidelines for questioning inappropriate orders are followed.

Transfer and Discharge Reports

Nurses report a summary of a patient's condition and care when transferring patients from one unit or institution or agency to another (eg, from the postanesthesia care unit to a surgical floor) and when discharging patients. The nurse making the report should concisely summarize all the patient data that caregivers need to provide immediate care. See Chapter 12 for transfer and discharge reporting guidelines.

Reports to Family Members and Significant Others

Nurses play a crucial role in keeping the patient's family and significant others updated about the patient's condition and progress toward goal achievement. Nurses should clarify with the patient which visitors are entitled to progress reports. Similarly, nurses need to clarify what types of information they are able to communicate. The nurse is generally not the caregiver who informs family members that a patient's biopsy has revealed a malignancy. The nurse does, however, often explain what this will mean for the patient after the family has this information. Information should be shared in a manner that is honest, compassionate, and respectful of the person's ability to understand medical concepts.

Incident Reports

An *incident report,* also termed a *variance* or *occurrence report,* is a tool used by healthcare agencies to document the occurrence of anything out of the ordinary that results in or has the potential to result in harm to a patient, employee, or visitor. These reports are used for quality improvement and should not be used for disciplinary action against staff members. They are a means of identifying risks. More harm than good results from ignoring mistakes. Incident reports improve the management and treatment of patients by identifying high-risk patterns and initiating in-service programs to prevent future problems. These forms also make all the facts about an incident available to the agency in case of litigation. It is important for nurses to be familiar with agency policy about their responsibilities and obligations if they are involved personally in an incident that results in or has the potential to result in harm to a patient, employee, or visitor, or if they witness such an incident. An example of an incident report form and a fuller discussion of this topic may be found in Chapter 7.

⟳ Conferring About Care

To confer is to consult with someone to exchange ideas or to seek information, advice, or instructions. A nurse may consult with another nurse, such as when a primary care nurse consults with a nurse clinical specialist about a particular patient's care. A school nurse may confer with a child's teacher or a psychologist about a behavior problem. A community health nurse and a physician may confer about a patient's activity regimen. Health practitioners also confer with each other to validate information. Healthcare professionals increasingly use electronic support groups to consult with clinicians who share similar interests or who have expertise in other specialty areas.

Consultations and Referrals

When nurses detect problems they cannot resolve because they lie outside the scope of independent nursing practice or their expertise, they make referrals to other professionals. The process of sending or guiding someone to another source for assistance is called a **referral.** A patient may be referred by a hospital to a community health nursing service for assistance with home care. A school nurse may refer a student to a hospital emergency department. A community health nurse may refer a problem to the Department of Health.

Most health agencies have policies for referrals. An agency may have a special form that personnel are to use when making referrals. Referral policies usually indicate who may initiate a referral, how it is to be done, and so on. Referrals are especially important in providing continuity of care for people who need a variety of services. It is essential that health practitioners to whom a patient is referred receive the information that is most useful to the continuity of care. The key question is, "What would I want to know about this patient if I were the person who had to continue his or her care?" The patient must know and approve of a referral to another agency or to other health personnel.

Before making a referral, nurses should determine which profession has the needed expertise and which of its practitioners are appropriate for referral. A great disservice is done patients when referrals are poorly made. Patients and family members also appreciate a phone number and practical tips about how to reach the referred practitioner most easily.

Nursing Care Conference

Nurses and other healthcare professionals frequently confer in groups to plan and coordinate patient care. Such conferences are also used for instructing students and practitioners. A **nursing care conference** is a meeting of nurses to discuss some aspect of a patient's care. For example, several nurses who are caring for a generally uncooperative patient may initiate a conference. This would allow each nurse an opportunity to offer his or her opinion about the patient's problem and its cause, and then together they could discuss possible solutions to the problem.

Nurses may invite other healthcare practitioners to a nursing care conference concerning a patient's care. For example, a clinical psychologist may be invited in the preceding example to address the possibility that a mental disorder is influencing this patient's behavior.

Nursing Care Rounds

Nursing care rounds are procedures in which a group of nurses visit selected patients individually at each patient's bedside. The primary purposes of nursing care rounds are to gather information to help plan nursing care, to evaluate the nursing care the patient has received, and to provide the patient with an opportunity to discuss his or her care with those administering it. As each patient is visited, the nurse assigned provides a short summary of the patient's nursing diagnoses and goals and the care being given. Nursing care rounds have two principal advantages over discussions in a meeting room: nursing personnel can actually see the patient as a report of care is given, and patients can participate in discussions of their care.

Nurses should use language the patient can understand when holding discussions at the bedside. Otherwise, the patient is likely to feel excluded and cannot intelligently participate in the discussion. Nurses may also make rounds with physicians to share nursing's perspective with them.

Learning Outcomes

After completing this chapter, the learner should be able to accomplish the following:

1. Define the key terms used in the chapter:

   change-of-shift report
   charting by exception
   computer-based record
   critical/collaborative
     pathway
   discharge summary
   documentation
   flow sheet
   focus charting
   graphic sheet
   Kardex care plan
   medication record
   minimum data set

   narrative notes
   nursing care conference
   nursing care round
   patient record
   PIE charting
   problem-oriented
     medical record
   progress notes
   referral
   reporting
   SOAP format
   source-oriented record
   variance charting

2. List guidelines for effective documentation.

3. Identify abbreviations and symbols commonly used for charting.
4. Describe the purposes of patient records.
5. Compare and contrast different methods of documentation: source-oriented record; problem-oriented record; PIE—problem, intervention, evaluation; focus charting; charting by exception; case management model; computerized records.
6. Describe the purpose and correct use of each of the following formats for nursing documentation: nursing assessment, nursing care plan, critical/collaborative pathways, progress notes, flow sheets, discharge summary, and home care documentation.
7. Document nursing interventions completely, accurately, concisely, and factually—avoiding legal problems.
8. Describe nursing's role in communicating with other healthcare professionals by reporting and conferring.

Critical Thinking Exercises

1. Interview three practicing nurses and ask them to describe the documentation methods they have used in their practice. Which methods did they prefer? Which method was more effective, time efficient, and easiest to use?
2. A nurse overhears you complaining about writing narrative nursing notes and says to you, "Don't sweat it. I never worry about documentation—it's a waste of time. I'd rather spend my time doing things for patients than writing up what I did." Think about what you would like to say to this nurse and your rationale for this. Ask other students for their response, and compare your answers.
3. Imagine that you are a nurse in a nursing home and that you and the home are being sued for negligence by the family of an elderly resident who fell and fractured her hip last year. You know the resident but do not remember much about the day she fell. What data do you hope to find recorded in her health record? Which documentation system would most likely provide the type of information you think you need to reconstruct the events surrounding her fall?
4. How would you respond to each of the following requests for patient information? Compare your responses with those of another student and talk about any differences.

   • The mayor of your town who is up for reelection was just admitted to your unit after an acute myocardial infarction. You receive a phone call from his office requesting information about his condition.
   • A woman you have never seen approaches you in the hallway, identifies herself as the sexual partner of a married male patient on your unit, and requests information about his condition.
   • A case manager from a managed care organization calls you to ask about the progress an elderly surgical patient is making postoperatively. You have heard that the organization is eager to discharge her quickly, and you feel uncomfortable reporting any information over the phone.

Bibliography

Barbera, M. L. (1994). Giving report: How to sidestep common pitfalls. *Nursing, 24*(9), 41.

Buckley-Womack, C., & Gidney, B. (1987). A new dimension in documentation: The PIE method. *Journal of Neuroscience Nursing, 19*(5), 256–260.

Bulechek, G. M., McCloskey, J. C., Titler, M. G., & Denehey, J. A. (1994). Nursing interventions' use in practice. *American Journal of Nursing, 94*(10), 59–62, 64.

Burke, L., & Murphy, J. (1988). *Charting by exception: A cost effective quality approach.* Albany, NY: Delmar.

Calfee, B. (1994). 7 Things you should never chart. *Nursing, 24*(3), 43.

Capuano, T. A. (1995). Clinical pathways: Practical approaches, positive outcomes. *Nursing Management, 26*(1), 34–37.

Cohen, M. R. (1987). Play it safe: Don't use these abbreviations. *Nursing, 17*(7), 46–47.

Comstock, L. G., & Moff, T. E. (1991). Cost-effective, time-efficient charting. *Nursing Management, 22*(7), 44–48.

Cox, S. S. (1994). Taping report: Tips to record by. *Nursing, 24*(3), 64.

Eggland, E. T. (1995). Charting smarter. *Nursing, 25*(9), 35–41.

Eggland, E. T., & Heinemann, D. S. (1995). *Nursing documentation: Charting, recording and reporting.* Philadelphia: J. B. Lippincott.

Ferraro-McDuffie, A. (1993). Documenting the primary nurse's summary note: A leap toward professionalism. *Pediatric Nursing, 19*(2), 189–193.

Hatcher, I. (1995). Personal communication.

Health Care Financing Administration. (Issued 1995, updated 1998). *Long term care facility resident assessment instrument (RAI) user's manual.* Author.

House, E. (1992). Resistance to documentation: A nursing research issue. *International Journal of Nursing Studies, 29*(4), 371–381.

Iyer, P. W., & Camp, N. (1995). *Nursing documentation: A nursing process approach* (2nd ed.). St. Louis: Mosby–Year Book.

Joint Commission on Accreditation of Healthcare Organizations. (1999). *Accreditation manual for hospitals.* Oakbrook Terrace, IL: Author.

Mandell, M. (1994). Not documented, not done. *Nursing, 24*(8), 62–63.

Marr, P. B. (1993). Bedside terminals and quality of nursing documentation. Part I. *Computers in Nursing, 11*(4), 176–182.

Marrelli, T. M. (1996). *Nursing documentation handbook* (2nd ed.). St. Louis: Mosby–Year Book.

Martin, F. (1994). Documentation tips to help you stay out of court. *Nursing, 24*(6), 63–64.

Meyer, C. (1992). Bedside computer charting: Inching toward tomorrow. *American Journal of Nursing, 92*(4), 38–44.

Murphy, J., & Burke, L. J. (1990). Charting by exception: A more efficient way to document. *Nursing, 20*(5), 65–69.

North American Nursing Diagnosis Association. (1994). *NANDA nursing diagnoses: Definitions and classification, 1995–1996.* Philadelphia: Author.

Rasmussen, N. (1994). Clinical pathways of care: The route to better communication. *Nursing, 24*(2), 47–49.

Rich, P. L. (1995). Protecting patient information. *Nursing, 25*(9), 32L.

Siegrist, L., Stocks, B., & Dettor, R. (1985). The PIE system: Complete planning and documentation of nursing care. *QRB, 11*(6), 186–189.

Simpson, R. L. (1994). Ensuring patient data privacy, confidentiality, and security. *Nursing Management, 25*(7), 18–20.

Staff, E. J. (1997). Privacy, confidentiality, and security in clinical information systems. *Nursing Administration Quarterly, 21*(3), 21–28.

Sullivan, G. H. (2000) Keep your charting on course. *RN, 63*(5), 75–79.

Werley, H. H., Devine, E. C., & Zorn, C. R. (1988). Nursing needs its own minimum data set. *American Journal of Nursing, 88,* 1652.

Windle, P. E. (1994). Critical pathways: An integrated documentation tool. *Nursing Management, 25*(9), 80F–L, 80P.

Wong, C. A., & Budgell, L. (1994). Documentation redesign. *Canadian Nurse, 90*(6), 38–41.

Zolot, J. S. (1999) Computer-based patient records. *American Journal of Nursing, 99*(12), 64–69.

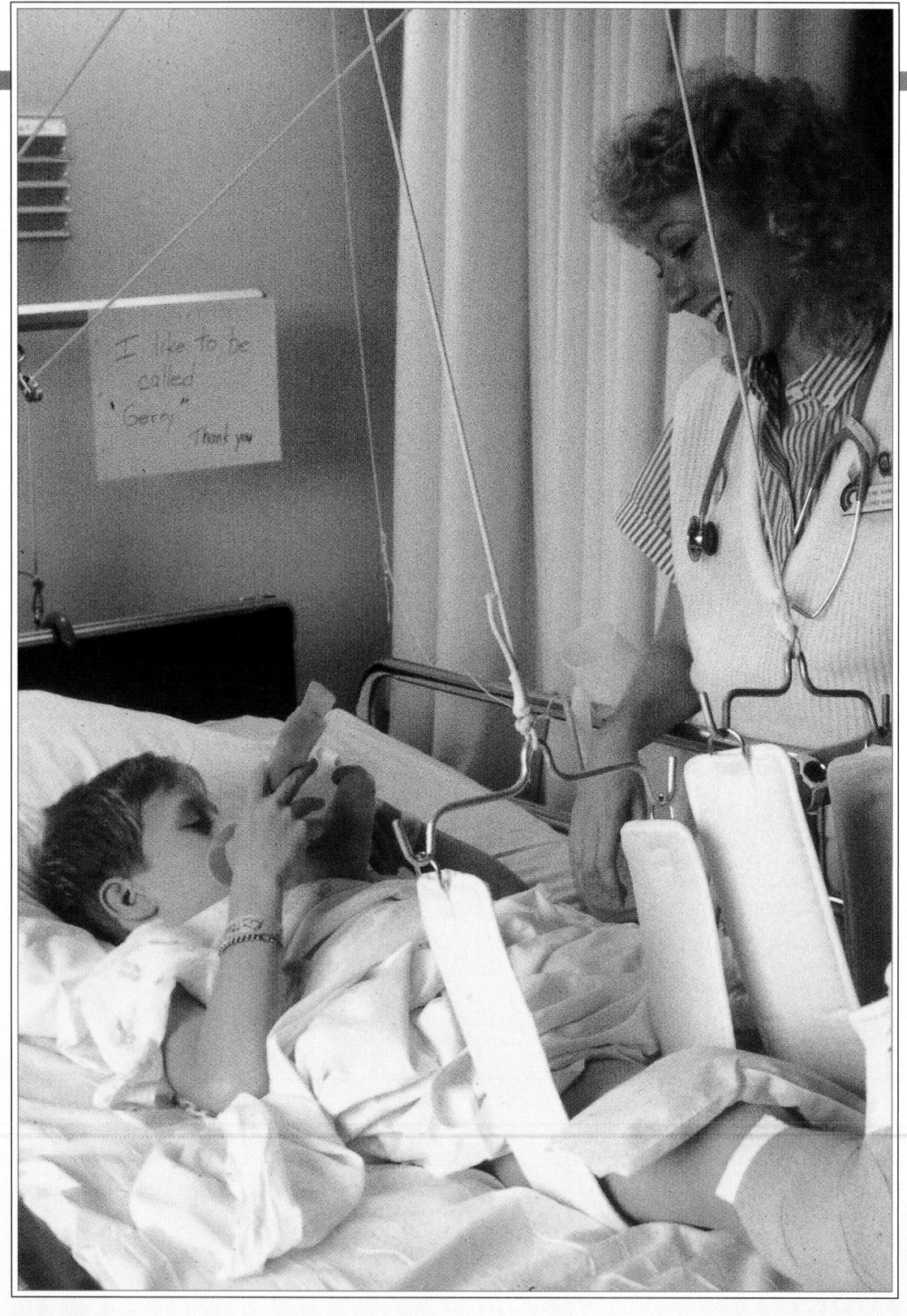

UNIT V

Roles Basic to Nursing Care

"Clinical competence . . . has three dimensions. . . . Care is the fundamental things we do to make a patient comfortable. . . . curative nursing, . . . the broader group of restorative and rehabilitative activities: to a sound knowledge of the principles on which they are based . . . counseling, . . . of emotional, intellectual, and psychological support . . ."

Frances Reiter (1904–1977)
the first chairperson of the ANA Committee on Education, she coined the term "nurse clinician" and advocated advanced preparation of nurse clinicians

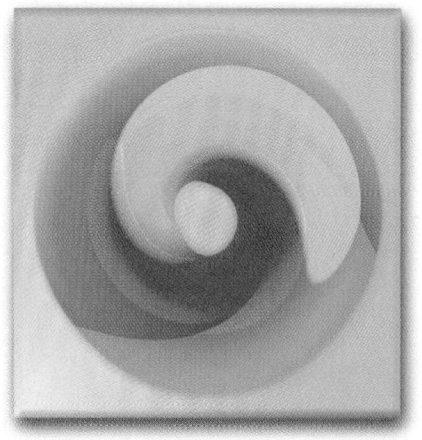

Unit V discusses the nurse's professional roles of communicator, teacher, counselor, leader, researcher, and advocate. These roles are interdependent, and each is an integral part of the broad nursing role of caregiver. The nurse in these roles helps patients of all ages to meet needs along the health continuum.

To be effective as a caregiver, the nurse must be proficient in both the art and science of nursing. Communication is essential to each professional nursing role and is the heart of caring. Nursing is a person-centered service, based on relationships with patients, peers, and other members of the healthcare team. By developing effective interpersonal skills and using therapeutic communication skills, nurses can establish and maintain helping relationships.

As teacher, the nurse uses communication skills to teach individuals and families. Teaching, implemented throughout the nursing process, is used to meet learning needs. As counselor, the nurse provides information, makes appropriate referrals, and assists the patient in developing a systematic approach to problem solving and decision making. The nurse as leader practices assertive, self-directed nursing. Abilities to lead and to bring about change begin with the student nurse and progress as the nurse develops self-confidence and skill in interpersonal relationships and experience in healthcare settings. As researcher, the nurse may conduct research, use research findings to improve patient care, or participate in research done by others. As advocate, the nurse combines all these roles to promote the right of patients to make their own decisions about health and life and to protect human and legal rights.

Unit V, therefore, enables beginning nurse caregivers to enrich their professional practice by integrating the professional nursing roles of communicator, teacher, counselor, leader, researcher, and advocate. Nursing practice, as a specialized and unique service to others, is based on the application of knowledge and skills presented in this unit.

Chapter 21
Communicator

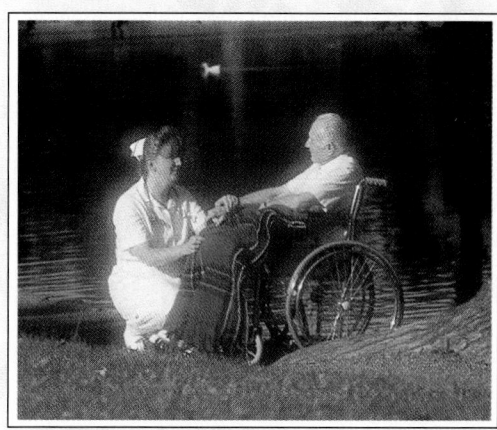

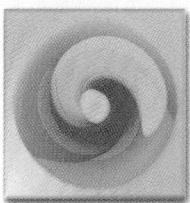

Thinking Critically About
Nursing's Blended Skills

Before reading this chapter, think about the types of interpersonal skills needed to establish effective professional relationships with patients and other team members.

- "Susie's nurse said that she seems more and more scared to be here. (Susie is a 3-year-old patient with second-degree burns on both legs.) They've started debriding her burns, and she must be in a lot of pain. I'm sure whenever she sees a doctor or nurse she is worried about what we might do to her and how much it will hurt. I wish her family could visit more often."

- Another student tells you, "The chart says that my patient, Mrs. Russell, is hard of hearing and 'pleasantly confused' at times. I have to interview her to do my nursing history—I'll probably end up shouting stupid questions at her that I don't even need to ask."

- "I've tried approaching Mr. Barnet's wife several times, but each time she screams at me and complains that no one cares about her or her husband and no one is seriously trying to help them. I'm at my wits end and can never get a word in edgewise. I don't know how I can be expected to do discharge teaching. I know Mrs. Barnet is feeling overwhelmed."

- "I've asked the staff nurse coassigned to my patient for assistance several times, and she's always 'too busy' to talk with me or help and brushes me off. I need to know what they said about my patient in report, and there are some procedures I've never done before."

What cognitive, interpersonal, and ethical/legal skills do you think you need to communicate effectively with the people described above?

Any nurse who wishes to be an effective caregiver must first learn to communicate. Good communication skills enable nurses to get to know their patients and, ultimately, to diagnose and meet their needs for nursing care. Student nurses who sit face to face with a patient for the first time to obtain a comprehensive nursing history intuitively grasp the importance of the nurse's communicator role. Communication skills are the building blocks of professional relationships between nurse and patient, nurse and nurse, and nurse and other health team members. Many experienced nurses identify the quality of their interpersonal relationships as the single most significant element in determining their helper effectiveness. Studies have shown that on nursing units where nurses freely exchange ideas and information, solve problems together when something goes wrong rather than assigning blame, compliment one another, and use humor creatively, staff morale is high, and there is a higher level of attainment of patient outcomes.

The Communication Process

Communication is the foundation of society. Without communication, it would be impossible to share family experiences, gain education, establish and maintain a government, or enjoy many forms of entertainment. By nature, humans are social, and human needs are met in collaboration with other humans. Human relationships enable us to meet not only our physical and safety needs but also our psychosocial needs for love, belonging, and self-esteem. The ability to communicate is basic to human functioning and well-being.

Communication is the process of sharing information and the process of generating and transmitting meanings. These two definitions are consistent because meaningful information is produced and transmitted in order to be shared. David K. Berlo (1960) is credited with the classic description of the communication process, which involves a source (encoder), message, channel, and receiver (decoder). This process is illustrated in Figure 21-1. The **source (encoder)** prepares and sends to the receiver a message that can be accurately decoded. The **message** is the actual product of the source or encoder. It might be a speech, interview, telephone conversation, chart, conversation, gesture, memorandum, or nursing note. The message cannot always be assumed to mean what the receiver believes it to mean or what the sender intended it to mean. The **channel** is the medium that conveys the message, which may target any of the receiver's senses. Nurses use auditory, visual, and kinesthetic (touch) channels to communicate with patients. The auditory channel involves spoken words and cues. The visual channel is sight, observation, and perception. The kinesthetic channel is experiencing sensations. The **receiver (decoder)**, upon receiving the message, translates it into its meaning and makes a decision about it. Test your knowledge of communication channels by reading the situation in the accompanying box: Communication Challenges. The nurse who is an effective communicator needs to consider the receiver at all times, seeking to send a message that appeals to the patient's interests, is phrased in words the patient understands, and requires minimal effort and time to decode. The nurse must look for verbal and nonverbal evidence—**feedback**—that the patient has received and understood the message. Noise—

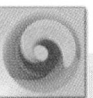

COGNITIVE SKILLS

- Knowledge of basic communication theory and factors that influence therapeutic communication.
- Knowledge of the goals and phases of helping relationships.
- Knowledge about aging, hearing disorders, and dementia as well as effective communication strategies.

INTERPERSONAL SKILLS

- Strong people skills; ability to communicate and interact effectively with frightened (Susie), confused (Mrs. Russell), hostile and probably scared (Mrs. Barnet), and indifferent (staff nurse) patients and colleagues.
- Excellent therapeutic communication skills for interacting with patients and colleagues:

conversational skills, listening skills, silence, interviewing techniques, touch, humor, assertiveness.

- Ability to establish good working relationships with colleagues—including the ability to confront colleagues who are not doing their share to make the team work.

ETHICAL/LEGAL SKILLS

- Ability to demonstrate respect, empathy, and honest caring in each professional encounter with both patients and colleagues.
- Willingness to hold colleagues accountable for contributing to the team effort essential to quality care.
- Knowledge of the ethical and legal principles that guide professional relationships and behavior.

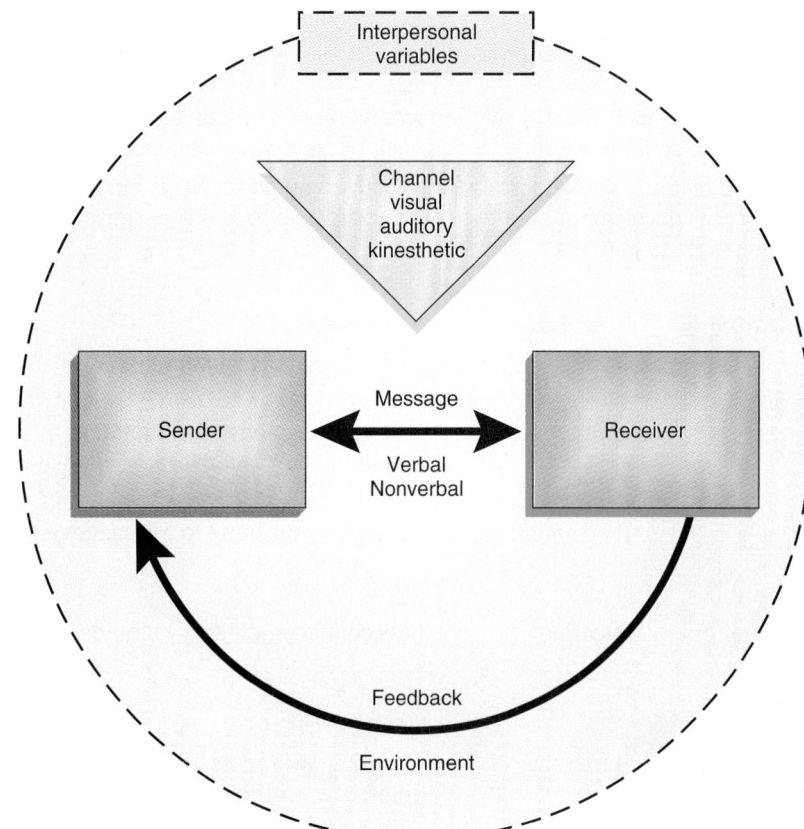

Figure 21-1
The various components in the process of communication.

any factors that distort the quality of the message—may interfere with communication at any point in the process. Examples of noise include a distracted source or receiver, a room that is uncomfortably warm, a noisy television program, and pain.

Communication is a reciprocal process in which both the sender and the receiver of messages participate simultaneously. Messages may be influenced on either end by the person's previous knowledge, past experiences, feelings, or sociocultural level.

Levels of Communication

Nurses communicate on many different levels, each of which may influence other levels. **Intrapersonal communication,** or self-talk, is the communication that happens within an individual. This communication is crucial because it affects the person's behavior. Imagine two different nursing students preparing for their first nursing experience with a critically ill patient. Both are frightened. One tells herself, "Calm down, you've been in challenging situations before and always survived. You can handle this." The other repeatedly tells herself, "There's no way you can survive this experience. The instructor will be all over you, and you may as well admit defeat before you start." Obviously, the first student's positive self-talk is more helpful than that of the second student. Understanding the importance of self-talk can help you to work with patients and families whose negative self-talk affects their health and self-care abilities.

Interpersonal communication occurs whenever two or more people interact and exchange messages. Most of the nurse's day is spent communicating with patients, family members, and other members of the team. The nurse's ability to communicate effectively at this level influences the nurse's interpersonal sharing, problem solving, goal attainment, team building, and effectiveness in critical nursing roles such as caregiver, teacher, counselor, and advocate. Interpersonal competence, described in Chapter 14 and highlighted in each clinical chapter, is essential to the practice of nursing.

Small-group communication occurs when nurses interact with two or more individuals face to face or use a medium like a conference call. To be functional, the members must communicate with one another to achieve their goal. A patient care conference, staff meeting or report, and support group are all examples of small-group communication. The more people involved in the communication process, the more complex it becomes. **Organizational communication** occurs when individuals and groups within an organization communicate to achieve established goals.

Group Dynamics

When making a determination about the effectiveness or ineffectiveness of a group, one studies the **group dynamics,** how individual group members relate to one another during the process of working toward group goals.

Although effective leadership facilitates a group's achievement of its goals, the group's success or failure is

Communication Challenges

Picture yourself walking into a patient's room to administer a pain medication by injection. What do you see yourself communicating through each of the three channels of communication?

Then read the scenario below and think about all the ways nurses might unintentionally communicate that they are not concerned about the patient or his pain. Use this exercise to guide both your verbal and nonverbal messages to patients.

Channel	Mode of Transmission	Outcome	Nursing Behavior
Visual	Sight	Receiving a visual stimulus	Patient sees nurse walking into the room holding desired medication
	Observation	Interpreting a visual stimulation by making note of nonverbal enhancement	Patient makes note of the nurse's sense of competence, confidence, and sympathetic expression
	Perception	Assigning meaning to a visual event	Patient concludes that the nurse is willing and able to help him and feels comforted
Auditory	Hearing	Receiving an auditory stimulus	Patient hears the nurse say, "I understand your hip is hurting. This injection should help you to start feeling better within 15 minutes."
	Listening	Gaining awareness of underlying messages and feelings accompanying auditory events	Patient senses that the nurse said he should start feeling better soon and really wants this to happen because she cares about him.
Kinesthetic	Procedural touch	Performing nursing procedures and techniques	Patient feels the nurse touching him while administering injection in the left buttock.
	Caring touch	Conveying emotional support	Patient feels that the nurse cares about him as a person when she touches his shoulder upon first entering the room while asking about his pain.

largely a function of its members' behaviors. Ideally, each group member uses his or her talents and interpersonal strengths to help the group accomplish its goals while maintaining sensitivity to the needs of individual group members. In effective groups, members who attempt to dominate or thwart the group process are confronted by the leader or other group members. Effective and ineffective groups are contrasted in Table 21-1. Individual group member roles can be categorized in one of three ways: (1) task-oriented roles, focusing on the work to be done; (2) group-building or maintenance roles, focusing on the well-being of people doing the work; and (3) self-serving roles, which advance the needs of individual members at the group's expense. Examples of these roles follow:

Task roles—information giver, information seeker, clarifier, coordinator, delegator, energizer, evaluator

Maintenance roles—active listener, harmonizer, trust builder, tension reliever, supporter

Self-serving roles—attention seeker, dominator, blocker, special pleader, withdrawer, aggressor

Think about groups in which you are a member and see if you can identify the roles that you and other members of your group play.

An administrative team who recognized the crucial value of staff participation in designing and implementing a hospital restructuring project used a team approach to secure needed change. Their ground rules for team members follow (Scott & Rantz, 1994, p. 13):

- I know what I have to do, and the team's goals are clear.
- Everyone takes some responsibility for leadership.
- There is active participation by everyone.
- I feel appreciated and supported by others.
- Team members listen when I speak.
- Different opinions are respected.
- We enjoy working together and have fun.
- We are aiming for excellence, not perfection.
- Everyone on the team has an equal voice.
- We are always open to more education and information.

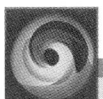

Table 21-1
Characteristics of Effective and Ineffective Groups

Variable	Effective Group	Ineffective Group
Group identity	Members value and "own" the aims of the group; aims are clearly articulated	Group's aims are not of major importance to members
Cohesiveness	Members generally trust and like one another and are loyal to the group; high commitment; high degree of cooperation	Members often feel alienated from the group and from one another; low commitment; members tend to work better alone than with the group
Patterns of interaction	Honest, direct communication flows freely; members support, praise, and critique one another	Communication is sparing; little self-disclosure; self-serving roles (ie, dominator, blocker, or aggressor) may be unchecked
Decision making	Problems are identified, appropriate method of decision making is used (ie, individual, minority, majority, consensus, or unanimous); decision is implemented and followed through; group commitment to decision is high	Problems are allowed to build without resolution; little responsibility is shown for problem solving; group commitment to decision is low
Responsibility	Members feel strong sense of responsibility for group outcomes	Little responsibility for group felt by group members
Leadership	Effective style of leadership to meet desired aims	Ineffective leadership styles
Power	Sources of power are recognized and used appropriately; needs or interests of those with little power are considered	Power is used and abused to "fix" immediate problems; little attention to needs of powerless

- Ask anything, challenge anything.
- We have a clean slate.
- We color outside the lines.
- It is OK to take a risk and fail.

Forms of Communication

Communicating people receive and send messages through verbal and nonverbal means, which can occur simultaneously.

Verbal Communication

Verbal communication is an exchange of information using words, including both the spoken and the written word. Verbal communication depends on language. **Language** is a prescribed way of using words so that people can share information effectively. Language includes a common definition of words as well as a method of arranging the words in a certain order.

Both written and spoken forms of communication reveal much about a person. The way a person pronounces certain words or uses particular phrases gives clues to such things as geographic or ethnic origin. Vocabulary, sentence structure, and spelling give indications of a person's intellectual development or educational level and may also indicate that English is a second language. Language helps nurses assess what patients know and feel. In turn, nurses must develop their own language skills to aid in reciprocal responses in the communication process.

Verbal communication is used extensively by nurses when speaking with patients, giving oral reports to other nurses, writing care plans, and recording in nursing progress notes. Other examples of verbal communication include public speaking, writing for publication, and composing signs and posters. In each of these examples, words and language are communicated to others.

Nonverbal Communication

Nonverbal communication is the transmission of information without using words; it is what is not said. Sometimes referred to as **body language**, it often helps us to understand subtle and hidden meanings in what is being said verbally. For instance, a person may respond to the question, "How are you?" by simply answering, "Fine." However, if this answer is accompanied by a rigid, tense facial expression, the true meaning of the response would need further investigation (Fig. 21-2).

Information is exchanged through nonverbal communication in various ways. It is generally accepted that nonverbal communication expresses more of the true meaning of a message than does verbal communication. Therefore, nurses must be aware of both the nonverbal messages they send and the nonverbal messages they receive from patients. The means of nonverbal communication vary considerably, depending on one's individual or cultural patterns. Nurses working with patients from diverse cultural backgrounds should attempt to understand cultural variations to avoid misunderstanding nonverbal commu-

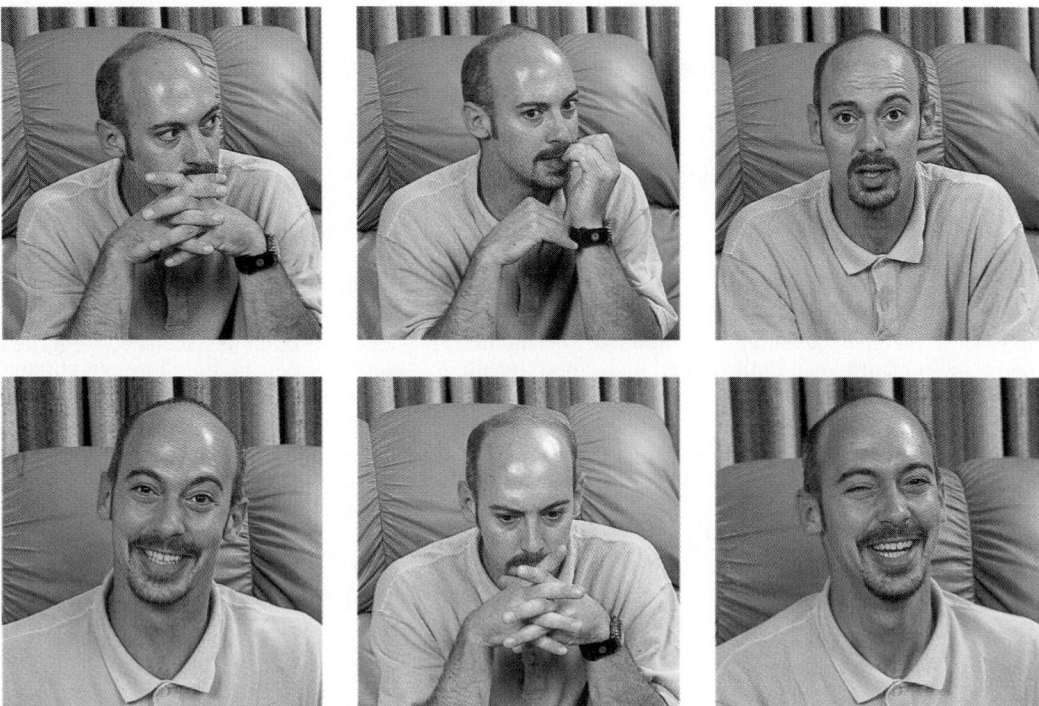

Figure 21-2
Eye contact, the lack of it, facial expression, posture, gesture, and silence send nonverbal messages to the receiver. What messages do you receive from each of these photographs?

nication. The various forms of nonverbal communication follow.

Touch

Tactile sense has been studied seriously as a form of nonverbal communication only since the 1960s. Touch is a personal behavior and means different things to different people. Investigations have shown that tactile experiences are largely shaped by familial, regional, class, and cultural influences. Such factors as age and sex also play a role in individual meanings associated with touch. Despite its individuality, touch is viewed as one of the most effective nonverbal ways to express feelings such as comfort, love, affection, security, anger, frustration, aggression, excitement, and many others.

Eye Contact

Communication often begins with eye contact. A glance, for example, is often an attention-getting method to open conversation. Eye contact also suggests respect and a willingness to listen and to keep communication open. Its absence often indicates anxiety or defenselessness, or avoidance of communication. However, young children and adolescents in some cultures are taught that it is disrespectful to look an adult in the eye. In some cultures, people are taught to avoid eye contact or, out of respect, not to make eye contact with a superior. In addition, the eyes themselves carry nonverbal messages. For example, the eyes fix in a stare during anger, tend to narrow in disgust, and ordinarily open wide in fear. A blank stare can indicate daydreaming or inattentiveness.

Facial Expressions

The face is the most expressive part of the body. Examples of the various messages facial expressions convey are anger, joy, suspicion, sadness, fear, and contempt. Some people have extremely expressive faces, whereas others mask their feelings, making it more difficult to determine what the person is really thinking. Nurses need to learn some control over their own facial expressions. For instance, a patient with extensive burns may watch the nurse's reaction when the nurse changes the burn dressings for the first time. Any sign of repulsion or disgust could have grave implications for the patient's self-image and recovery.

Posture

The way a person holds the body carries nonverbal messages. People in good health and with a positive attitude usually hold their bodies in good alignment. Depressed or tired people are more likely to slouch. Posture also often provides nonverbal clues concerning pain and physical limitations; for instance, a rigid, stiff appearance may be a good indicator of tension and pain.

Gait

A bouncy, purposeful walk usually carries a message of well-being. A less purposeful, shuffling gait often means the person is sad or discouraged. Certain gaits are associated with illness. For example, patients recovering from recent abdominal surgery usually walk slightly bent over and slowly and may need the assistance of handrails or a helping person.

Gestures

Gestures using various parts of the body can carry numerous messages; for example, thumbs up means victory, whereas thumbs down carries a negative connotation; kicking an object often expresses anger; wringing the hands or tapping a foot usually indicates anxiety or anger; a waving hand serves to beckon someone to come or, if waved in another way, signifies that someone should leave. Gestures are used extensively when two people speaking different languages attempt to communicate with each other.

General Physical Appearance

Most illnesses cause at least some alterations in general physical appearance. Observing for changes in appearance is an important nursing responsibility for detecting illness or evaluating effectiveness of care and therapy. For example, a person with an insufficient intake of fluids has dry skin that wrinkles easily, eyes that may be sunken and dull in appearance, and poor muscle tone. On the other hand, the person in good health tends to radiate his or her healthy status through general physical appearance.

Mode of Dress and Grooming

A person's clothing and grooming practices carry significant nonverbal messages. For example, healthy people with high self-esteem tend to pay attention to details of dress and grooming, whereas those with low self-esteem show much less interest in them. People feeling ill often demonstrate little interest in personal appearance, and it is often a sign of returning health when interest in mode of dress and appearance resumes.

Sounds

Crying, moaning, gasping, and sighing are oral but nonverbal forms of communication. Such sounds can be interpreted in numerous ways. For example, a person may cry because of sadness or joy. Gasping often indicates fear, pain, or surprise. A sigh may be a sign of reluctant agreement to do something or of relief.

Silence

Periods of silence during a conversation often carry important nonverbal messages. A silence between two people may indicate complete understanding of each other, or it may mean they are angry with each other. Silence and its possible uses and meanings are discussed later in this chapter.

Factors Influencing Communication

Developmental Considerations

The rate of language development varies but depends on neurologic competence and cognitive development. It is helpful for nurses to understand the process of language development as well as the stages of intellectual and psychosocial development so that they can communicate appropriately with patients of all ages. These stages are presented in Chapter 8. Knowing how each age group commonly perceives health, illness, and body functions guides nurses in their interactions with their patients. For instance, a 10-year-old child has a limited understanding of what an infection is; therefore, the nurse must explain this in simple terms so that the child cooperates with the treatment without being frightened. Because adolescents are developing abstract thinking, more detailed and accurate explanations can be given to them. Being familiar with commonly used slang usually helps nurses when communicating with adolescents. Communicating with adults can be affected by years of positive or negative health-related experiences and by inaccurate information. Nurses communicating with older patients must assess for any problems with hearing or sight (discussed later in this chapter), confusion, or depression, any of which could affect nurse–patient interactions.

Gender

Men and women have different communication styles and may give different interpretations to the same conversation. Tannen (1990) believes that this is because girls and boys grow up communicating differently. Whereas girls generally play with "best friends" and use language to seek confirmation, minimize differences, and establish or reinforce intimacy, boys use language to establish their independence and to negotiate status activities in large groups. It is important for nurses to be sensitive to the fact that men and women may use communication differently as a result of these developmental experiences. Moreover, it may be necessary for nurses working with patients of the opposite gender to validate that both the nurse and patient are accurately receiving the message the other is trying to communicate.

Sociocultural Differences

Nurses need to develop skills in recognizing the ways in which culture, economic condition, and overall lifestyle influence a patient's preferred mode of communicating. This helps the nurse understand what the patient is communicating and use language the patient understands. For example, women in some cultures may speak of personal things only to their spouses. For this reason, maternal care nurses may have to talk with the patient's husband about the woman's postdelivery care.

It is best to use lay terminology when speaking with patients unless the patient is known to be a healthcare professional. Use of medical terminology (ie, myocardial infarction for heart attack, cerebrovascular accident for stroke [brain attack], or cholecystectomy for gallbladder operation) usually alienates patients and can inhibit further communication.

Roles and Responsibilities

A person's occupation may give the nurse a general idea of his or her abilities, talents, interests, and economic status. Stereotyping a person according to occupation can be misleading, however, and should be avoided. This can be particularly dangerous when nurses assume that patients who are healthcare professionals know everything about their condition and need little nursing assistance, teaching, and counseling. The challenge for the nurse caregiver is to respect the patient's roles and responsibilities, especially because these influence their preferred manner of communicating, without denying the patient needed care. For example, a successful attorney may have a "take charge" demeanor and seem utterly self-sufficient; a skilled nurse will note this but still provide an opening for the patient to verbalize her or his needs. "You seem well prepared for this procedure and in control, but I know that patients often have questions that never get answered or fears that remain unvoiced. Is there anything I can help you with while I'm here?" Similarly, nurses should be careful not to ignore an uncomplaining lay person who never asks for anything because the power differences in the healthcare professional–patient relationship make communication intimidating.

Space and Territoriality

People are generally most comfortable in areas they claim as their own. We all generally feel relief when we come home, take our shoes and professional clothes off, and relax. This urge to maintain an exclusive right to certain spaces is termed *territoriality*. You may have already noticed that patients behave differently when being interviewed in their homes, at a health fair in the mall, or in an institutional setting. Similarly, healthcare professionals may behave differently when they are "on their own turf" in a healthcare institution from when they enter a patient's home as a guest caregiver. It is important to understand how territoriality influences the nurse–patient relationship.

The actual physical difference between the nurse and patient during an interaction is also important. Each person has a sense of how much private space is needed and of what distance between individuals is optimum; some of this is culturally dictated and some idiosyncratic. Anywhere from 18 inches to 4 feet may be the optimal distance for a nurse to sit from a patient during an intake interview. It is best to take cues from patients, noting if they are recoiling from nearness or leaning forward to draw the nurse closer. Because many nursing interventions place one in proximity to patients and entail forced intimacy, it is crucial to develop a sensitivity to how offensive this may be to certain patients who are accustomed to large areas of private space. Nurses should develop the habit of seeking the patient's permission before touching areas within a patient's private zones. Although most people consider their hands, arms, shoulders, and back within a social zone, increasing levels of privacy are accorded to (1) mouth and feet; (2) face, neck, and front of body; and (3) genitalia.

Physical, Mental, and Emotional State

The degree to which people are physically comfortable and mentally and emotionally free to engage in interactions also influences communication. A full bladder, a dull headache or crushing chest pain, anxiety about a pending diagnosis or about what is happening back home or at work, and fear can all negatively influence communica-

tion. A patient who thinks that a nurse wants to hurt him or who is thinking only about what it would be like to date the nurse will be difficult to interview. Nurses, therefore, need to develop sensitivity to the physical, mental, and emotional barriers to effective communication.

Cognitively impaired patients present nurses with special communication challenges. The accompanying box, Using the Nursing Interventions Classification, suggests helpful cognitive stimulation activities when communicating with these patients.

Values

Communication is influenced by the way people value themselves, one another, and the purpose of any human interaction. Nurses who believe that teaching is an important aspect of nursing and who value empowering patients will communicate this to patients. Conversely, a nurse who believes teaching is an unimportant chore is unlikely to be an effective teacher. Similarly, the patient's motivation (or lack of motivation) to develop new self-care behaviors cannot help but influence nurse–patient communication.

Environment

Communication happens best when the environment facilitates an easy exchange of needed information. Depending on the goals of the interaction, this may require minimizing distractions, ensuring privacy, or using music, art, and decor to place a patient at ease. A patient newly diagnosed with human immunodeficiency virus (HIV) infection will find it difficult to provide the needed sexual history or to discuss genital warts if being interviewed in a crowded hallway because no private room is available. A toddler may find it easier to communicate with a nurse if a parent, favorite stuffed animal, or blanket is nearby.

Using the Nursing Interventions Classification

Selected Cognitive Stimulation Activities

- Consult with family to establish patient's pre-injury cognitive baseline
- Inform patient of nonthreatening news events
- Offer environmental stimulation through contact with varied personnel
- Provide a calendar
- Orient to time, place, and person
- Provide planned sensory stimulation
- Use television, radio, or music as part of planned stimuli program
- Reinforce or repeat information
- Present information in small, concrete portions

McCloskey, J., & Bulechek, G. (2000). *Nursing interventions classification (NIC)* (3rd ed). (p. 220). St. Louis: Mosby–Year Book. A full listing of nursing activities for each nursing intervention can be found in this book.

Therapeutic Communication

Using Communication in the Nursing Process

The nurse's ability to communicate with patients and with other nurses is essential for effective use of the nursing process. (See the accompanying Research in Nursing box.) Knowledge of the communication process and of effective communication techniques is fundamental to all steps of the nursing process. At the same time, the nursing process provides the nurse with the guidance and direction needed to communicate with patients effectively.

Assessing

Because the major focus of the assessment step is information gathering, verbal and nonverbal communication are essential nursing tools. Nurses use the written word to obtain data concerning their patients. Nurses often read their patients' records or charts before meeting them. The spoken word is used to give and receive reports to and from other health personnel. This is a common practice

when admitting a patient to a hospital unit. Nurses use one-to-one communication with patients to obtain thorough nursing histories and physical examinations. Effective communication techniques, as well as observational skills, are used extensively during this phase. The data collected verbally and nonverbally are analyzed and then passed on to the appropriate people through oral and written communications.

Diagnosing

After a nurse formulates a nursing diagnosis, it must be communicated through the spoken and written word to other nurses as well as to the patient. The written diagnosis becomes a permanent part of the patient's record.

Planning

The planning step requires communication among the patient, nurse, and other team members as goals and outcomes are developed and interventions selected. Because a nurse is rarely able to implement all parts of a plan alone, oral and written communication is needed to inform others

 ## RESEARCH IN NURSING: MAKING A DIFFERENCE

Family Presence During Invasive Procedures and Resuscitation

Family members frequently request to be present when their loved ones undergo invasive procedures and cardiopulmonary resuscitation. Responses to these requests vary according to the preferences of professional caregivers and agency policies. Until recently, there was little research to answer the question: Is the presence of family members comforting to the patient, distressing to family members observing procedures, or uncomfortable for caregivers?

Related Research
Meyers, T. A., Eichhorn, D. J., Guzzetta, C. E., Clark, A. P., Klein, J. D., Taliaferro, E., & Calvin, A. (2000). Family presence during invasive procedures and resuscitation. *American Journal of Nursing, 100*(2), 32–43.
Meyers and colleagues (2000) designed a protocol for family presence (FP) using guidelines developed by the Emergency Nurses Association and conducted a descriptive study using quantitative and qualitative research methods at a regional level-1 trauma center. They found that families perceived visitation as a positive experience and believed that being with the patient was their right. Family members involved in FP viewed themselves as active participants in the care process, which met their needs for knowing about, providing comfort to, and connecting with the patient. Moreover, family members who visited with their loved ones during emergency care suffered no ill psychological effects.

The views of healthcare providers differed significantly: more nurses (96%) and attending physicians (79%) supported FP during resuscitation than did residents (19%). The researchers concluded that the benefits of FP justify implementing FP programs. These findings demonstrate that nurses can play an important role in meeting the needs of patients undergoing invasive procedures and resuscitation and their families by implementing FP programs and working collaboratively with physician colleagues to ensure adherence to these guidelines.

Relevance to Nursing Practice
The Emergency Nurses Association used early family presence research to establish that family members of critically ill patients have the need to be with the patient; be helpful to the patient; be informed of the patient's condition (including impending death); be comforted and supported by family; be accepted, comforted, and supported by healthcare personnel; and feel that the patient was receiving the best care possible. Family presence during invasive procedures and resuscitation efforts allows the patient and family to support each other and facilitates decision making and the grieving process. Nurses who are skilled communicators can effectively develop and implement family presence protocols.

of what needs to be done to meet the set objectives or goals. Without communication, the nurse's plan could not proceed to the implementation phase.

Implementing

Nurses assume many roles when they implement the plan of care. Verbal and nonverbal communication allows nurses to enhance basic caregiving measures and to teach, counsel, and support patients and their families during the implementation phase. Even a simple nursing order, such as "encourage to drink 100 mL of fluid every hour while awake," requires countless messages to be sent and received between the nurse and patient. The nurse explains why fluids are important, what fluids are beneficial, and how often they are needed. The patient, in turn, informs the nurse of his or her ability or inability to meet targeted objectives. The patient's verbal and nonverbal messages are assessed during each nurse–patient interaction. The implementation of the plan of care is then documented in the patient's record.

Evaluating

Nurses often rely on the verbal and nonverbal cues they receive from their patients to verify whether patient objectives or goals have been achieved. Communication also facilitates the revision of parts of the care plan through the exchange of positive and negative messages between the nurse and the patient.

Documenting Communication

Any information required for the continual assessment of the patient's needs and condition should be documented in the appropriate place, unless the information is confidential. This documentation helps promote the continuity of care given by nurses and other healthcare providers. Because one nurse cannot provide 24-hour coverage for patients, significant information must be passed on to others through nursing progress notes and care plans. Documentation is discussed in Chapter 20.

Using Communication in the Helping Relationship

Most people enter the healthcare field because they want to help people. This does not happen randomly but rather is accomplished through purposeful relationships. A **helping relationship** exists among people who provide and receive assistance in meeting human needs. In this book, that term is used to refer to helping relationships between nurses and patients (Fig. 21-3). A helping relationship sets the climate for the participants to move toward common goals to meet human needs. Therefore, need gratification occurs as the result of a successful helping relationship.

When a nurse and patient are involved in a helping relationship, the nurse assists the patient to achieve goals that allow the patient's human needs to be satisfied. The nurse is the helper, and the patient is the person being helped. The helping relationship between the nurse and patient is sometimes called the nurse–patient relationship.

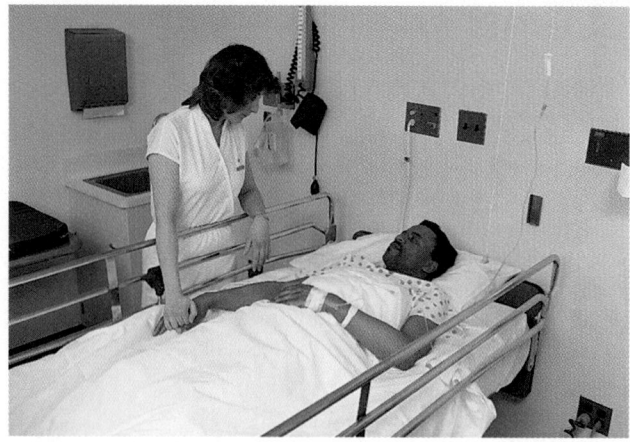

Figure 21-3
A helping relationship between the nurse and patient sets the climate for participants to move toward common goals. (Photo © B. Proud.)

The quality of one's relationship with another person is the most significant element in determining helping effectiveness. "Of all the problems that can arise in nursing care, perhaps the most common is failure to establish rapport and a helping-trust relationship with the other person" (Watson, 1985, p. 24).

A Helping Relationship Versus a Social Relationship

The difference between a helping relationship and a friendship is important. Helping relationships contain many of the qualities of a social relationship; they have in common the components of care, concern, trust, and growth. They are also very different:

- The helping relationship does not occur spontaneously, as do most social relationships. It occurs for a specific purpose with a specific person.
- The helping relationship is characterized by an unequal sharing of information. The patient shares information related to personal health problems, whereas the nurse shares information in terms of a professional role. In a friendship, information sharing is more likely to be similar in quantity and type.
- The helping relationship is built on the patient's needs, not on those of the helping person. In a friendship, needs of both participants are generally considered. A friendship may grow out of a helping relationship, but this is separate from the purposeful, time-limited interaction described as a helping relationship.

At all times, it is important for nurses to remember that their helping relationships are professional relationships. It can be helpful for those new to nursing to identify nurses who communicate a clear sense of **professionalism** in their appearance, demeanor, and behavior and to use these nurses as models. Patients and the public are more likely to trust and value nurses who appear competent and confident and who are focused on the patients entrusted to their care. Rudeness, sloppiness, inattention to person, sexually inappropriate behavior, and other breaches of professionalism undermine nursing's professional image and the effectiveness of individual nurses.

Characteristics of the Helping Relationship

The helping relationship is intangible and therefore difficult to describe. Most authorities agree, however, that it has at least the following three basic characteristics:

- It is dynamic. Both the person providing the assistance and the person being helped are active participants to the extent each is able.
- It is purposeful and time limited. This means there are specific goals that are intended to be met within a certain period.
- Although both parties in the helping relationship have responsibilities, the person providing the assistance is professionally accountable for the outcomes of the relationship and the means used to attain them. The helping person should present his or her helping abilities as honestly as possible and not promise to provide more assistance than he or she can offer.

Goals of the Helping Relationship

The goals of a helping relationship between a nurse and a patient are determined cooperatively and are defined in terms of the patient's needs. Broadly speaking, common goals might include increased independence for the patient, greater feelings of worth, and improved health and well-being. Depending on the goals/outcomes, the nurse selects nursing interventions that will help the person move toward the goal. As the patient's needs and goals change, so do the nursing care activities. The nurse may also have many needs to be met, but in the helping relationship between the nurse and the patient, the nurse's needs are temporarily set aside, and the focus is on the patient's needs.

Phases of the Helping Relationship

The helping relationship is ordinarily described as having three phases: (1) the orientation phase, (2) the working phase, and (3) the termination phase. In the helping relationship, the communication process follows the sequence of the nursing process. Both processes are continuous and reciprocal. Table 21-2 summarizes goals for patients during the three phases of an effective helping relationship. In some situations, one nurse initiates the helping relationship and works with the patient and family through to termination. More often (eg, in hospital settings), there are different nurses at different times implementing different phases of the relationship.

Orientation Phase

Ideally, the helping relationship between a nurse and a patient is initiated when the nurse starts the data-gathering part of the nursing process. It can also be initiated at other times, however. In the orientation phase, the tone and guidelines for the relationship are established. The nurse and patient meet and learn to identify each other by name. It is especially important that the nurse introduce himself or herself to the patient; it may even be helpful for the nurse to write his or her name for the patient. Failure to do so may result in the patient becoming confused and mistrustful because of the number of caregivers with whom most patients come in contact.

The following activities generally occur during the orientation phase of the helping relationship:

- The roles of both people in the relationship are clarified. A successful relationship is more likely to occur when each participant's responsibilities are known and accepted and when the nurse, by virtue of role, generally assumes leadership. Leadership does not mean control in a restrictive or manipulative sense but rather involves taking the initiative to enlist the patient's point of view. When cooperative planning occurs with consideration for the patient's needs, the

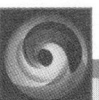

Table 21-2
Summary of Patient Goals for the Three Phases of the Helping Relationship

Orientation Phase	Working Phase	Termination
The patient will call the nurse by name.	The patient will actively participate in the relationship.	The patient will participate in identifying the goals accomplished or the progress made toward goals.
The patient will accurately describe the roles of the participants in the relationship.	The patient will cooperate in activities that work toward achieving mutually acceptable goals.	The patient will verbalize feelings about the termination of the relationship.
The patient and nurse will establish an agreement about: • Goals of the relationship • Location, frequency, and length of the contacts • Duration of the relationship	The patient will express feelings and concerns to the nurse.	

relationship between a nurse and a patient is more likely to be mutually satisfactory.

- An agreement or contract about the relationship is established. The agreement is usually a simple verbal exchange or, occasionally, a written document, especially if the relationship extends over a long period. Elements in the agreement include the goals of the relationship; location, frequency, and length of the contacts; and duration of the relationship. Depending on the purpose of the relationship, the agreement may also include the way in which personal information that the patient divulges will be handled.
- The nurse provides an orientation to the healthcare agency, its facilities and services, admission routines, and so on. The nurse identifies this orientation as one of the goals in the nurse–patient helping relationship.

It is crucial that trust is established from the outset of the relationship. Some patients may engage in testing behavior, especially if they have had negative experiences in the past in their family or with other healthcare providers. The nurse's openness to and interest in the concerns of the patient pave the way for trust to develop and communicate respect and care.

Working Phase

The working phase is usually the longest phase of the helping relationship. The nurse and the patient work together to meet the patient's needs. Interaction is the essence of the working phase. Nurse–patient interactions that occur at this time are purposeful in that they are designed to ensure achievement of health goals or objectives that were mutually agreed upon.

In the working phase, the nurse provides whatever assistance may be needed to achieve each goal. For example, if an older patient has a poor appetite and the goal is to increase food intake, the nurse discusses the idea of small, more frequent meals with the patient. With the patient's approval, the nurse makes the necessary arrangements. In another instance, a mother explains to a school nurse that she cannot afford dental care recommended for her child, although she would like to have the work done. The nurse asks if a referral to a social agency for financial assistance would be acceptable. With the mother's permission, the nurse contacts the agency.

When sentiments and feelings between people are unsatisfactory, these people often cannot work cooperatively toward achieving a common goal. When sentiments and feelings are satisfactory, they can usually work together. In the preceding examples, satisfactory sentiments and feelings between the nurse and patients may be the key aspects. The older person's relationship with the nurse may allow a positive response to the small, more frequent meals. The mother's feelings about the nurse may allow her to accept financial assistance for dental care without feeling embarrassed.

In addition, the nurse as caregiver provides the patient with whatever assistance may be needed to perform activities of daily living. For example, if a patient with impaired mobility is unable to get out of bed except to use a bedside commode, the nurse needs to help with daily hygiene.

The nursing roles of teacher and counselor (see Chap. 22) are performed primarily during this phase. These roles involve motivating the patient to learn and to implement health promotion activities, to facilitate the patient's ability to execute the plan of care, and to express feelings about health problems, nursing care, any progress or setbacks, and any other areas of concern. This is where the nurse's interpersonal skills are used to their fullest (see the discussions of interpersonal skills and effective communication techniques later in this chapter). A breakdown of the helping relationship on one of these levels could result in serious consequences. For instance, a patient begins to break clinic appointments, although he seemed to be interested in his health previously when he visited the clinic. When a community health nurse calls on the patient at home, he says, "The nurse at the clinic seems too busy; she just doesn't seem to care if I come or go. I don't like to go to that clinic." The lack of satisfactory interaction between the nurse and the patient discouraged him from continuing the relationship, even at the expense of his health. Had the nurse–patient interaction been satisfactory, the problem most likely would not have occurred.

Satisfactory interaction preserves people's integrity while promoting an atmosphere characterized by minimal fear, anxiety, distrust, and tension. People feel harmonious and contented with each other as they work cooperatively to reach common goals.

Termination Phase

The termination phase occurs when the conclusion of the initial agreement is acknowledged. This may happen at change-of-shift time, when the patient is discharged, or when a nurse leaves on vacation or for employment elsewhere. The patient and nurse examine the goals of the helping relationship for indications of their attainment or for evidence of progress toward them. If the goals/outcomes have been reached, this fact should be acknowledged. Such acknowledgment generally results in a feeling of satisfaction for both the patient and nurse. If the goals/outcomes have not been reached, the progress can be acknowledged, and either the patient or the nurse may make suggestions for future efforts.

Ordinarily, emotions are associated with the termination of a helping relationship. If the goals have been met, there is often regret about ending a satisfying relationship, even though a sense of accomplishment persists. If the goals have not been completely achieved, the patient may experience anxiety and fear about the future. Whatever the feelings, the patient should be encouraged to express his or her emotions about the termination.

The nurse can prepare for the termination of the helping relationship in various ways. The thoughtful nurse can set the stage for the patient to establish a helping relationship with another nurse, if appropriate. The nurse can assist the patient transferring from one agency to another or from one unit in an agency to another by offering explanations concerning the transfer. In some instances, the nurse may introduce the patient to personnel who will be giving care.

Occasionally, termination of the helping relationship causes a negative emotional reaction. The patient may feel angry, rejected by the nurse, or depressed and helpless, or may deny that a relationship ever really existed. If such a reaction occurs, the nurse should try to help and support the patient rather than make him or her feel bad or guilty for having such a view. Emotional reactions of this sort are less likely to occur, however, if the patient has been involved in establishing goals and has been helped to anticipate termination of the helping relationship.

Interpersonal relations in nursing are discussed more fully in the classic works of nursing theorists Orlando (1961), Paterson and Zderad (1976), Peplau (1952), Travelbee (1971), and Watson (1985).

Factors Promoting Effective Communication

Dispositional Traits

Warmth and Friendliness

The helping relationship depends on the nurse's ability to begin the orientation phase successfully. A pleasant greeting accompanied by a smile can facilitate this phase and allow the patient to relax in the nurse's presence. By maintaining qualities of warmth and friendliness throughout the helping relationship, the nurse conveys continuous acceptance of the patient and interest in discussing the patient's feelings and concerns.

Openness and Respect

A nurse who is open conveys an attitude of acceptance, frankness, respect, and lack of prejudice. A patient who feels that a nurse is being judgmental may hold back significant information. Nurses need to develop sensitivity to the unique challenges presented by each patient. Attention to patient variables that may influence the process of communicating (eg, gender, developmental level, culture, life experience) can make the difference between effective and ineffective interactions. The accompanying box highlights guidelines for relating to patients from different cultures. See also Chapter 3.

Empathy

Empathy is identifying with the way another person feels. An empathic nurse is sensitive to the patient's feelings and problems but remains objective enough to help the patient work toward positive outcomes. A nurse who retains this quality can establish successful helping relationships without becoming the cold, stern figure frequently portrayed in films and television. For example, although it is understandable for team members to become impatient with family members who never seem satisfied with the care their loved one is receiving, it is helpful if team members can empathize with the family who may be feeling frightened and helpless.

Honesty, Authenticity, and Trust

Patients should be able to trust that nurses are who they say they are (professional helpers) and that they can be trusted to do everything within their level of expertise to secure the resources and help the patient needs.

Caring

Patients quickly sense whether they are merely a "task to be performed" (task-centered caring) or a person of worth who is both cared about and cared for (relation-centered caring). Expert nurses know how to communicate genuine caring the minute they step into a patient's space by how they look at and touch the patient and by what they say and do. Patients who feel cared for feel accepted.

Competence

Competent nurses are skilled in all aspects of basic nursing and can meet their patient's healthcare needs through their technical, cognitive, interpersonal, and ethical/legal skills. Nurses are responsible for evaluating their own strengths and for strengthening any weaknesses so that all patients will receive optimal care. Consequently, patients develop trust in and respect for their nurses, facilitating helping relationships.

Rapport Builders

Good **rapport**, a feeling of mutual trust experienced by people in a satisfactory relationship (Fig. 21-4), can be achieved by paying attention to the following variables.

Specific Objectives

Having a purpose for an interaction guides the nurse toward achieving a meaningful encounter with the patient. One objective might be to do a quick head-to-toe physical assessment while greeting the patient at the beginning of a shift. Another objective might be to discuss a patient's feelings about newly diagnosed diabetes. The shortest encounter with a patient can have an objective, even if it is as simple as conveying a feeling of friendliness. Flexibility is essential at all times. The nurse should follow the patient's cues to work toward meeting all needs.

Comfortable Environment

A comfortable environment, in which both the patient and the nurse are at ease, helps to promote interactions. Suitable furniture, proper lighting, and a moderate temperature are important. Also, effective relationships are enhanced when the atmosphere is relaxed and unhurried. If the nurse seems preoccupied and on the run or if the patient is ill at ease for fear of missing visitors or because of another commitment, communication is impaired.

Privacy

It may not always be possible to carry out conversations alone with the patient in a room, but every effort should be made to provide privacy and prevent conversations from being overheard by others. Sometimes merely drawing the curtains around the bed in a hospital or nursing home or sitting in a corner of a waiting room or lounge can provide the sense of privacy that is so important in most interactions. Home visits may need to be timed to ensure the privacy the patient desires and needs.

Relating to Patients From Different Cultures

Assess your personal beliefs surrounding people from different cultures.
- Review your personal beliefs and past experiences.
- Set aside any values, biases, ideas, and attitudes that are judgmental and may negatively affect care.

Assess communication variables from a cultural perspective.
- Determine the ethnic identity of the patient, including generation in America.
- Use the patient as a source of information when possible.
- Assess cultural factors that may affect your relationship with the patient and respond appropriately.

Plan care based on the communicated needs and cultural background.
- Learn as much as possible about the patient's cultural customs and beliefs.
- Encourage the patient to reveal cultural interpretation of health, illness, and healthcare.
- Be sensitive to the uniqueness of the patient
- Identify sources of discrepancy between the patient's and your own concepts of health and illness.
- Communicate at the patient's personal level of functioning.
- Evaluate effectiveness of nursing actions and modify nursing care plan when necessary.

Modify communication approaches to meet cultural needs.
- Be attentive to signs of fear, anxiety, and confusion in the patient.
- Respond in a reassuring manner in keeping with the patient's cultural orientation.
- Be aware that in some cultural groups, discussion concerning the patient with others may be offensive and may impede the nursing process.

Understand that respect for the patient and communicated needs is central to the therapeutic relationship.
- Communicate respect by using a kind and attentive approach.
- Learn how listening is communicated in the patient's culture.

- Use appropriate active listening techniques.
- Adopt an attitude of flexibility, respect, and interest to help bridge barriers imposed by culture.

Communicate in a nonthreatening manner.
- Conduct the interview in an unhurried manner.
- Follow acceptable social and cultural amenities.
- Ask general questions during the information-gathering stage.
- Be patient with a respondent who gives information that may seem unrelated to the patient's health problem.
- Develop a trusting relationship by listening carefully, allowing time, and giving the patient your full attention.

Use validating techniques in communication.
- Be alert for feedback that the patient is not understanding.
- Do not assume meaning is interpreted without distortion.

Be considerate of reluctance to talk when the subject involves sexual matters.
- Be aware that in some cultures, sexual matters are not discussed freely with members of the opposite sex.

Adopt special approaches when the patient speaks a different language.
- Use a caring tone of voice and facial expression to help alleviate the patient's fears.
- Speak slowly and distinctly, but not loudly.
- Use gestures, pictures, and play acting to help the patient understand.
- Repeat the message in different ways if necessary.
- Be alert to words the patient seems to understand and use them frequently.
- Keep messages simple and repeat them frequently.
- Avoid using medical terms and abbreviations that the patient may not understand.
- Use an appropriate language dictionary.

Use interpreters to improve communication.
- Ask the interpreter to translate the message, not just the individual words.
- Obtain feedback to confirm understanding.
- Use an interpreter who is culturally sensitive.

Used with permission from Giger, J. N., & Davidhizar, R. E. (1995). *Transcultural nursing: Assessment and intervention* (2nd ed.) (p. 38). St. Louis: C. V. Mosby.

Confidentiality

The confidentiality with which patient information is to be treated should be established with the patient. The nurse should indicate with whom the information that the patient gives will be shared. The patient should know about the right to specify who may have access to the information. Failure to consider this factor can be considered a breach of the patient's right to privacy. See Chapter 20 for guidelines concerning patient confidentiality.

Patient Versus Task Focus

Communication in the nurse–patient relationship should focus on the patient and the patient's needs, not on the nurse or an activity in which the nurse is engaged (see

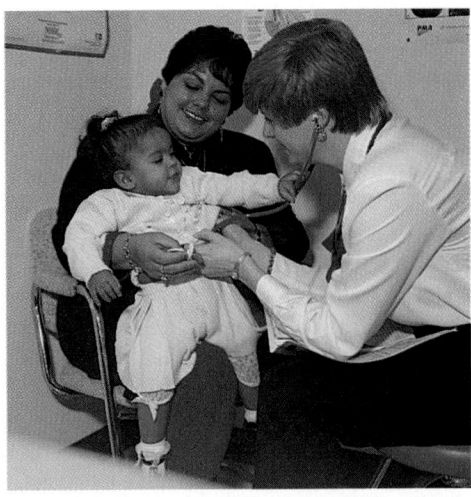 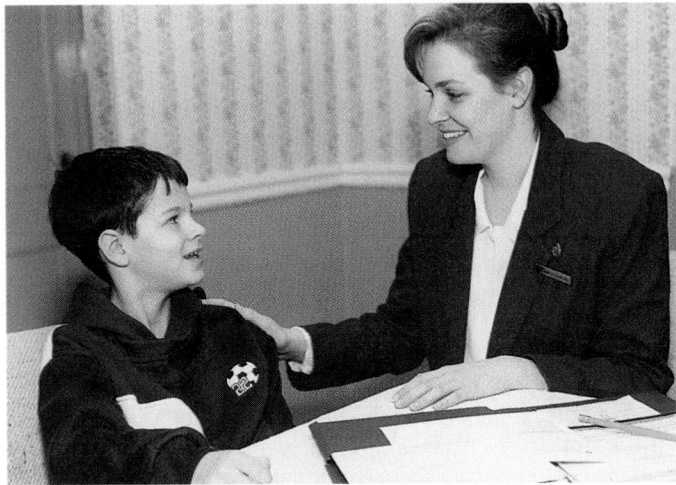

Figure 21-4
Rapport between the nurse and the patient/family is a necessary first step in planning care. (*Left*, courtesy of Nursing Spectrum; *right*, courtesy of Brett Ainsworth.)

the accompanying box: Through the Eyes of a Patient). Consider the following example, in which the nurse's comment focuses on the patient and the patient's needs:

Patient: I don't know why these injections scare me, but they do.
Nurse: You are afraid of these injections?

In contrast, consider this example, in which the nurse's comment focuses instead on the nursing activity:

Patient: I don't know why these injections scare me, but they do.
Nurse: Don't be such a baby. I've given hundreds of injections just like yours.

Use of Nursing Observations

Observation, which involves both seeing and interpreting, is especially useful for validating information. For example, a nurse suspects that a patient is afraid to hear the results of certain blood tests, but the patient insists that the tests are unimportant. The nurse then observes the patient pacing in the corridor apparently in deep thought. Observing the patient's behavior helps validate the nurse's suspicion that the patient is fearful, and the patient's assertion that he or she is unconcerned appears to be a cover-up for truer feelings.

Observation serves several important purposes:

- It helps the nurse become aware of a patient's nonverbal messages.
- It is the primary source of information when a patient is unable or unwilling to communicate verbally.
- It demonstrates the nurse's caring and interest in the patient. (Patients often recognize when a nurse is unobservant and, rightly or wrongly, usually conclude that the nurse does not care.)

Optimal Pacing

A nurse must consider the pace of any conversation or encounter with a patient. For instance, it would be in-

Through the Eyes of a Patient

I know you come to clinical every day with your head full of all the important things you need to do for me. Probably you worry about whether or not you will remember the steps to both simple and complex procedures and fear that you will never get everything done in the time allotted. I'm sure that there are many things that your clinical instructor will use as a basis for your evaluation and perhaps other things that are important to you for your self-evaluation. But I thought you might like to know what's important to me. Most of what I've listed are simple things that you can communicate each time you walk into my home or room.*

- Really listen to me.
- Ask me what I think.
- Don't dismiss my concerns.
- Don't treat me like a disease, treat me like a person.
- Talk *to* me, not *at* me.
- Respect my privacy.
- Don't keep me waiting.
- Don't tell me what to do without telling me how to do it.
- Keep me informed.
- Remember who I used to be.
- Let me know you care.

Thanks for giving me this chance to share with you what matters to me.

* The list of nursing interventions that are valued highly by patients was compiled by Roberta Messner after a review of many patient satisfaction studies. These are cited in Messner, R. L. (1993). What patients really want from their nurses. *American Journal of Nursing, 93*(8), 38–41.

effective for the nurse to rush through a list of questions when obtaining a nursing history; it is more effective to let the patient set the pace. The nurse can let the patient know at the beginning of the interaction if time is limited so that the patient does not feel that the nurse is rushing because of a lack of concern or personal interest.

Providing Personal Space

Perceptions of personal space vary. Nurses must try to determine each patient's perception of personal space because their invasion of this zone can evoke uncomfortable feelings. Nurses can assess a patient's personal space through careful observations of nonverbal communication. For example, some people like to be close to the person with whom they are speaking. They may also use touch while conversing and seem comfortable with others in close proximity. Others back away from close encounters or become nervous when their personal space is invaded. It is important for nurses to be sensitive to personal space so that patients feel comfortable during interactions.

Developing Therapeutic Communication Skills

Although humans are involved in communication in virtually all waking moments, the therapeutic use of communication requires training and practice. Students often feel awkward when first trying to develop a therapeutic relationship. Practice makes perfect, however, and you will soon feel at ease if you work on developing the following communication skills.

Conversational Skills

A good place to start is with conversation. *Conversation*, or the exchange of verbal communication, is a social interaction. As social beings, humans learn as children how to converse with others, and nursing students therefore have already had years of experience communicating verbally. However, nurses can improve their communications with patients and achieve a more effective helping relationship in the following ways:

- Control the tone of your voice so that you are conveying exactly what you mean to say and not a hidden message. The nurse's tone should indicate interest rather than boredom, patience rather than anger, acceptance rather than hostility, and so forth.
- Be knowledgeable about the topic of conversation and have accurate information. When possible, a nurse should be familiar with the subject of conversation before discussing it with the patient. If the topic is an unfamiliar one (eg, the availability of community resources for family caregivers of patients with special needs), it is best to tell the patient and family so and to direct them to other sources. Convey confidence and honesty.
- Be flexible. A nurse may want to discuss a certain subject but learns the patient wishes to discuss something else. It is better to follow the patient's lead whenever possible; in due time, the nurse can return to the subject. For example, a nurse arrives at the patient's bedside to administer a medication, but the patient begins to talk about his or her diet. It is better to take a little time to talk about the patient's interest than to insist on talking about only the procedure at hand, as long as there is enough time for the conversation.
- Be clear and concise, and make statements as simple as possible. Patients are often anxious and fail to understand the nurse's message unless the conversation is geared to a level the patient understands. Stay on one subject at a time.
- Avoid words that may be interpreted differently. The study of the meaning of words is called **semantics**. Even when two people speak the same language, some words—such as *love, hate, freedom,* and *liberty*—may have different meanings to different people.
- Be truthful. A patient who is given false information will soon distrust the nurse. If you're not sure about something, admit you don't know and seek an answer rather than make a comment that is likely to be an error.
- Keep an open mind. An attitude of "I know better than the patient" is quickly discerned by the patient. Patients can make valuable contributions to their own healthcare.
- Take advantage of available opportunities. During most caregiving situations, the nurse can facilitate conversation that makes even the most routine task meaningful. For instance, when giving a bed bath to a patient, a nurse can ask about the patient's employment. This would allow the patient to verbalize any positive or negative feelings about the job and his or her temporary absence from it, reducing the anxiety that often occurs with the loss of work. It is often comforting to know that someone understands and cares.

Listening Skills

Listening is a skill that involves both hearing and interpreting what the other says. It requires attention and concentration to sort out, evaluate, and validate clues in order to better understand the true meaning of what is being said (Fig. 21-5). The accompanying box, Through the Eyes of a Student, relates one student's experience with attentive listening. The following recommended techniques may help improve listening skills:

- Whenever possible, sit when communicating with a patient. Do not cross your arms or legs because that body language conveys a message of being closed to the patient's comments.
- Be alert but relaxed and take sufficient time so that the patient feels at ease during the conversation.
- Keep the conversation as natural as possible, and avoid sounding overly eager.
- If culturally appropriate, maintain eye contact with the patient, without staring, in a face-to-face pose.

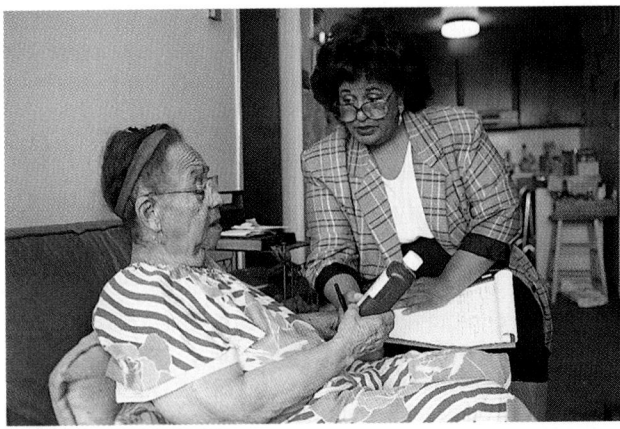

Figure 21-5
Listening attentively, with concentration and genuine concern, is key to productive communication. (Photo © Kathy Sloane.)

This technique conveys interest in the conversation and willingness to listen.

- Indicate that you are paying attention to what the patient is saying by using appropriate facial expressions and body gestures. Be attentive to both your own and the patient's verbal and nonverbal communication.
- Think before responding to the patient. Responding impulsively tends to disrupt communication and listening.
- Do not pretend to listen. Most patients are sensitive to an attitude of feigned attention or to boredom and apathy.
- Listen for themes in the patient's comments. What are the repeated themes in the person's speech and behavior? What topics does the patient tend to avoid? What subjects tend to make the patient shift the conversation to other subjects? What inconsistencies and gaps appear in the patient's conversation?

Silence

The nurse can use silence appropriately by taking the time to wait for the patient to initiate or continue speaking. During periods of silence, the nurse can reflect on what has already been shared and observe the patient without having to concentrate simultaneously on the spoken word. Periods of silence during communication can carry a variety of meanings, including the following:

- The patient may be comfortable and content in the nurse–patient relationship. Continuous talking is unnecessary.
- The patient may be trying to demonstrate stoicism and the ability to cope without help.
- The patient may be exploring his or her inner thoughts or feelings, and conversation would disrupt this. In effect, the patient is really saying, "I need some time to think."
- The patient may be fearful and use silence as an escape from a threat.

Through the Eyes of a Student

It was my first day of clinical rotation and I was assigned to Mr. Anderson, who was in his early 90s. He was in the hospital because he had a second heart attack. Mr. Anderson had lived alone for 5 years after the death of his wife. He wanted to remain independent, but his daughter, who was herself in her late 60s, and his doctor believed that he would not be able to function well on his own any longer. Mr. Anderson was distressed about this belief.

Because it was my first day and, unlike some of my classmates, I had never worked in a hospital before, I felt insecure and nervous. There really wasn't a lot of work for us to do. We weren't allowed to give medication yet, and my patient was pretty self-sufficient. Because my skills were shaky, I took my time taking vital signs, assisted Mr. Anderson with his bath and toileting, and made his bed. After checking his chart, I began my nursing interview with him. I was overjoyed to discover that he was a real talker! His memory was tremendous— either that or he was a great improvisor! He recalled stories about his childhood and his wife with great detail and emotion. He smiled and laughed when he spoke of his daughter and grandchildren. He told me about his daughter's childhood illnesses as well as his own. We talked about the Depression and world wars and about music and art and education. He asked me about my family, and I felt like I had made a friend.

The next day Mr. Anderson told me about his fears. He talked about losing his wife, about his health and body deteriorating, and about losing his independence and home. He despised having to be sent to a nursing home and having to depend on others. It hurt him a lot and made me sad. Mr. Anderson left on my second day, and as I said goodbye I wished I could do something for him.

I thought about him a lot since then and I've come to realize that in those 2 days that I knew Mr. Anderson, I did do something for him besides washing him and changing his sheets. I listened to him. Although his family had little time for him and the doctors quickly flew in and out of the room, I let him talk and heard all he said, both in words and in his eyes. He will always be a good memory for me—and I think I'll be a good memory for him.

—KRISTINA HOFMEISTER, HOLY FAMILY COLLEGE,
PHILADELPHIA, PA

In due time, the nurse may discuss the silence with the patient, especially if the nurse wishes to understand its meaning. Fear of silence sometimes leads to too much talking by the nurse. Also, excessive talking tends to place the focus on the nurse rather than on the patient.

Interviewing Techniques

The purpose of any interview is to obtain accurate and thorough information. In nursing, the interview is a major tool for collecting data during the assessment step of the nursing process (see Chap. 15). Consequently, every nurse needs to become proficient in the use of the communication techniques described previously as well as in interviewing techniques designed to gather and validate information.

All interviews should begin with an explanation of the purpose of the interview. During the interview, the nurse uses various **interviewing techniques** to obtain needed information while remaining flexible in approach. The interview itself is a therapeutic interaction and may be an essential part of the orientation phase of the helping relationship. At the end of the interview, plans for further interactions can be made. The following interviewing techniques are useful in nearly all nurse–patient interactions, especially the interview.

Open-Ended Question or Comment

When obtaining a nursing history, the nurse uses the open-ended question technique to allow the patient a wide range of possible responses. It encourages free verbalization. The greatest advantage of this technique is that it prevents the patient from answering with a simple yes or no. Consider the following example of an open-ended question and the response:

Nurse: What did your physician tell you about your
          need for this hospitalization?
Patient: He told me that my blood pressure is danger-
           ously high and that I need some special tests
           done while I am here.

This open-ended question by the nurse allows the patient to express what he or she understands to be true, yet is specific enough to prevent digressing from the issue at hand—the patient's hospital admission. The nurse could continue with an open-ended question such as the following:

Nurse: How did this news make you feel?
Patient: Well, I have to admit it shocked and scared me
           because I thought my pressure was OK and I
           know what happened to my dad as a result of
           his high pressure.

Now the nurse has even more information from the patient and can continue to seek more information. This should be done in a way that does not make the patient feel as though the nurse is prying or probing.

Closed Question or Comment

The closed question technique allows limited choices in possible responses and may often be answered by one or two words, "yes," or "no." Closed questions are used to gather specific information from a patient and allow the nurse and patient to focus on a particular area. When not used appropriately, closed questions are a barrier to effective communication. The following is an example of an appropriate use of a closed question:

Nurse: What medicines have you been taking at home?
Patient: Let me see, my doctor gave me a water pill and
           a blood pressure pill to take every day.

This technique gives the nurse the exact information that is being sought. Closed questions and comments should not be overused, however, because of their limiting effects on the patient's responses.

Validating Question or Comment

This type of question or comment serves to validate what the nurse believes he or she has heard or observed. To continue the example used in the previous technique, the nurse could validate the patient's reply as follows:

Nurse: At home you have been taking both a water pill
          and a blood pressure pill every day. Did you
          take them today?
Patient: Yes. I took one of each with my breakfast.

The nurse is able to ascertain that the patient has been taking the medication regularly, as well as the correct dosage that day. Overusing validating questions and comments, however, may lead the patient to suspect that the nurse is not listening.

Clarifying Question or Comment

With the clarifying question technique, a nurse can try to gain an understanding of a patient's comment.

Patient: I have never needed to take medicine before in
           my life.
Nurse: Is this the first health problem you have had?
Patient: Yes, I've always been healthy.

Overuse of this technique can lead the patient to believe that the nurse is not listening or is unknowledgeable. When used appropriately, however, it can avert possible misconceptions that could lead to an inappropriate nursing diagnosis. In the above example, by clarifying what the patient's health had been previously, the nurse can assess the patient's knowledge of the blood pressure problem and plan the necessary health teaching (see Chap. 22).

Reflective Question or Comment

The reflective question technique involves repeating what the person has said or describing the person's feelings. It encourages the patient to elaborate on his or her thoughts and feelings. An example of this technique follows:

Patient: I've been really upset about my blood pressure
           and having to take these pills.
Nurse: You've been upset . . .
Patient: I guess I'm worried about what could happen if
           my blood pressure gets too bad.

By saying this, the nurse has encouraged the patient to expand on this topic and express a more specific concern. Again, overusing this technique or using it mechanically may lead the patient to believe that the nurse is not listening or is uninterested.

Sequencing Question or Comment

Sequencing is used to place events in chronologic order or to investigate a possible cause-and-effect relationship between events. This technique is evident in the following example:

Patient: I don't feel like myself anymore since I've been taking my blood pressure medicine. I'm tired and don't have any energy.

Nurse: Your tiredness began after you started taking your medicine?

This type of question could lead to possible discovery of a contributing factor to the patient's problem. Nursing assessment is facilitated when events leading to a problem are placed in sequence.

Directing Question or Comment

It may become necessary at times to obtain more information about a topic brought up earlier in the interview or to introduce a new aspect of the current topic. In such an instance, the nurse can attempt to direct the patient to that topic with a technique similar to the following:

Nurse: You mentioned your dad earlier. Did he develop complications related to high blood pressure?

Patient: Yes.

Nurse: What sorts of complications?

Patient: Kidney failure. He was on dialysis for years before getting a transplant.

Nurse: And you are afraid this may happen to you?

In this way, the nurse has gained valuable information to consider in assessing the patient's health status and educational or counseling needs.

Touch

Touch is a powerful means of communication with multiple meanings. It can connect people, provide affirmation, be reassuring, decrease loneliness, share warmth, provide stimulation, and increase self-esteem. It can also communicate frustration, anger, aggression, and punishment; invade personal space and privacy; and convey a negative (eg, subservient) type of relationship with another (Giger & Davidhizar, 1995, p. 28). Because of the personal nature of touching, a nurse needs to weigh the beneficial against the detrimental use of touch for each patient. Touch can be a powerful therapeutic tool when used at the right time. Anxiety or discomfort may result, however, when a patient does not understand the meaning of a tactile gesture or when the patient simply dislikes being touched.

Touch is the most highly developed sense at birth. Tactile experiences of infants and young children appear essential for the normal development of self and awareness of others. It has also been found that many elderly people long for touch, especially when isolated from loved ones because of hospitalization or nursing home care. Many older people have no living family to provide them with the caring touch so necessary for the sense of well-being. In such an instance, a nurse can provide some special care by holding the patient's hand (Fig. 21-6).

Many situations require the nurse to touch the patient while implementing nursing care. Physical closeness between the patient and the nurse is essential and inevitable. Therefore, every nurse needs to become comfortable with the judicious use of this nonverbal communication technique so that a sense of security, rather than anxiety, results. As well, dexterity and sureness in the use of the hands help to assure the patient of the nurse's expertise when measuring blood pressure or giving an injection.

Interest has been growing in the phenomenon known as **therapeutic touch**. Therapeutic touch involves "unruffling," or unblocking, congested areas of energy in the body and redirecting this energy. After assessing a patient's "energy field," the nurse uses therapeutic touch to promote comfort, relaxation, healing, and a sense of well-being. Many nurses are studying therapeutic touch in nursing educational programs and through special courses or workshops. It is becoming a widely accepted form of therapy as well as a subject for nursing research (Hutchison, 1999).

Humor

Humor is being increasingly valued as both an interpersonal skill for the nurse and a healing strategy for patients. Nurses have a valuable tool when they can use humor effectively to maintain a balanced perspective in their work and to encourage patients to do the same. Nurses with a sense of humor are able to laugh at themselves and accept their failures, confront the absurdities of everyday practice without falling apart, and challenge patients to situate their current dilemma within the context of their larger life experiences. Laughter releases excess physical and psychological energy and reduces stress, anxiety, worry, and frustration. Humor, like other interpersonal competencies, is a learned skill.

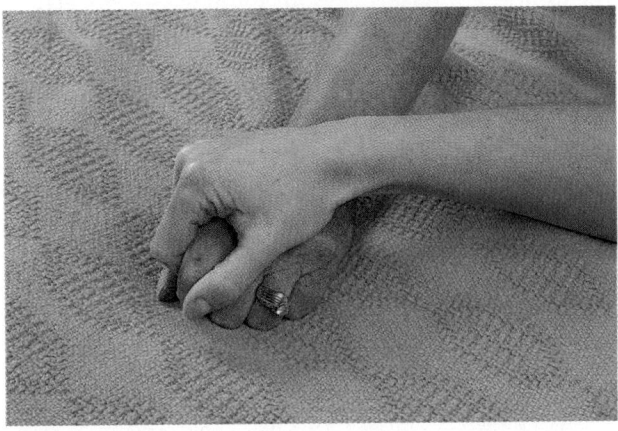

Figure 21-6
A reassuring handclasp uses touch to convey a message. Sometimes touch can be a more effective way of expressing concern and interest than verbal communication. (Photo © B. Proud.)

When used inappropriately, however, it can be destructive. Inexperienced nurses may find it helpful to identify nurses who use humor well and to "try on" behaviors they observe.

Assertive Skills

When interacting with patients, family members, nurses, physicians, and other members of the healthcare team, nurses should communicate in a way that demonstrates respect for all parties. **Assertive behaviors**, which are one hallmark of professional nursing relationships, need to be distinguished from aggressive (ie, harsh, injurious, or destructive) behaviors, which are very different from assertive behaviors, and from avoidance or acquiescent behaviors, which are the opposite of assertive behaviors. Chenevert (1994) equated learning to be assertive with learning to stand up for yourself and your patients, to trust your feelings and respect your opinions, and to like yourself. The key to assertiveness is open, honest, and direct communication. "I" statements—"I feel . . ." and "I think . . ."—play an important role in assertive statements. Table 21-3 gives examples of assertive and nonassertive speech.

Four basic components of the assertive response or approach are as follows: (1) having empathy, (2) describing one's feelings or the situation, (3) clarifying one's expectations, and (4) anticipating consequences (Angel & Petronko, 1983). For example, a student who is feeling overwhelmed by her weekly clinical assignments may communicate the following to her instructor:

Empathy: "I guess it must be hard for you to make our clinical assignments each week and to know what each one of us needs."

Description: "I have to share with you that right now I feel so overwhelmed that I go home from clinical in tears each week."

Expectation: "I am wondering if we could talk about this. I am willing to work hard, but I seem to need some help pulling everything together."

Consequences: "I expect to do well in clinical but I am afraid that if things continue the way they are right now, I may not last the semester. I would appreciate any help you can give me."

Characteristics of the assertive nurse's self-presentation include a confident, open-body posture; eye contact; use of clear, concise "I" statements; and the ability to share honestly one's thoughts, feelings, and emotions. The assertive nurse's attitude toward work is characterized by working to capacity with or without supervision, the ability to remain calm under supervision, the freedom to ask for help when necessary, the ability to give and accept compliments, and honesty in admitting mistakes and taking responsibility for them.

Blocks to Communication

Failure to Perceive the Patient as a Human Being

Patients report that nothing is more discomforting than to be treated as an object of care rather than as a patient. What distinguishes nursing from other health professions is its focus on the whole person, not simply the illness or dysfunction.

Failure to Listen

Patients may or may not feel able to speak freely to the nurse. Often, the signals indicating their readiness to talk are subtle. Nurses may miss valuable opportunities for important communication if they approach patients with

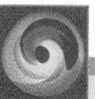

Table 21-3
Examples of Assertive and Nonassertive Speech

	Assertive	Nonassertive
Nurse to Nurse	"I know we all lose track of time occasionally but I'm finding it harder and harder to cover for you when you take extra time for lunch. I don't think it's fair for your patient and I to have to wait an extra 30 minutes every day for you to come back from lunch. Can we talk about this?"	"Huh? No, I didn't really mind. Luckily I wasn't too busy today." Thought: "What a sucker I am. Now I'll have to grab a quick bite so that I can get back to the unit in time to do 2 PM treatments."
Nurse to Physician	"I know we talked about Mr. Esposito's pain medication before but I've collected some new data. Even with the change in dosage, he is only getting 1 to 1½ hours of relief. I believe a different analgesic agent might work better for him."	"Um . . . yes I know you already changed the dosage. It's just that I thought it still wasn't working. Maybe I didn't give it enough time. Thanks for listening to me anyway. I'm sorry to bother you with this."
Student Nurse to Preceptor	"Miss Cheng has a new order to be straight cathed. I reviewed the procedure but I'd sure appreciate your talking me through this because I've never done it before and I'm terrified."	"Uh . . . I'm sorry to be such a pain again. I have to do this cath and don't know where to begin. I know you must be busy, but, uh, is there any way you might have time for me?"

closed minds or focus on their own needs rather than on the patient's needs. Nurses who lack confidence in their own ability to meet the challenges a patient presents may become defensive in response to a patient's comments. Nurse defensiveness is a huge barrier to open and trusting communication.

Inappropriate Comments and Questions

Certain types of comments and questions should be avoided in most situations because they tend to impede effective communications. A description of each type follows.

Using Cliches

A **cliche** is a stereotyped, trite, or pat answer. Most healthcare cliches suggest that there is no cause for anxiety or concern, or they offer false assurance. Their use tends to be interpreted as a lack of real interest in what has been said. For example, even though the common question, "How are you?" could start a conversation, it can cause a problem if the patient hearing this suspects that the nurse is not sincerely interested in how he or she feels. Following are some common cliches that are best not said because they tend to impede effective communications:

"Everything will be all right."
"Don't worry. You will be just fine in another day or two."
"Your doctor knows best."
"Cheer up. Tomorrow is another day."

Another type of cliche makes a sweeping generalization that does not necessarily apply to a specific patient. It also tends to cut off communications and makes the person feel as though he or she is just another insignificant being. Consider the following examples:

"Men tolerate pain poorly. That must be why you are complaining of such severe pain."
"Everybody is afraid of surgery. Why should you be any different?"
"You teenagers are all alike. You aren't being cooperative because you want to defy authority."

Such comments rarely promote communication with patients to whom they are addressed.

Using Questions Requiring Only a *Yes* or *No* Answer

Questions that can be answered by simply saying yes or no tend to cut off discussion, even when the person might wish to continue. Consider the following question:

Nurse: Did you have a good day?

The question almost begs for a noncommittal answer, which tells the nurse little. A better comment is as follows:

Nurse: Tell me about the kind of day you have had.

Another pitfall is to pose a question to which the patient can say no when that answer could present a problem. Consider the following question that a nurse asks a postoperative patient:

Nurse: Are you ready to get out of bed?

By offering the patient the chance to say no, the nurse may have created difficulties if the patient is to be out of bed.

There are times when questions that can be answered with yes or no are legitimate. Following are examples:

Nurse: Did you take your insulin before breakfast this morning?
Nurse: Do you have pain when I move your arm this way?

The problem with yes-or-no questions arises when the nurse is seeking more detailed information or when the question may create difficulty.

Using Questions Containing the Words *Why* and *How*

Questions using *why* and *how* are intimidating to many patients. Consider the following questions:

Nurse: Why were you not tired enough to sleep?
Nurse: How did you ever decide to go on a crash diet?

These two questions would be better stated as follows:

Nurse: What were you doing while you were unable to sleep?
Nurse: What things prompted you to decide to go on a crash diet?

Using Questions That Probe for Information

Questions that too obviously probe for information may cut off communication. Patients who are made to feel as though they are receiving the "third degree" become resentful and usually stop talking and try to avoid further conversation. Although the nurse may feel more information is needed, it is better to follow the patient's lead. Letting the patient take the initiative allows the nurse to delve more deeply at a time when the patient is ready. A nurse who says, "Let's get to the bottom of this" is likely to destroy conversation unless the patient is ready to face the real cause of the problem.

Using Leading Questions

A leading question suggests what response the speaker wishes to hear. Leading questions tend to produce answers that may please the nurse but are unlikely to encourage the patient to respond honestly without feeling intimidated. Consider the following examples:

Nurse: You aren't going to smoke that cigarette, are you?
Nurse: You have been well cared for by your nurses, haven't you?

These questions direct the patient to give an answer that pleases the nurse rather than to express his or her own thoughts.

Using Comments That Give Advice

Giving advice often implies that the nurse knows what is best for the patient and denies him or her the right to make decisions and have feelings. It also tends to increase the patient's dependence on caregivers. However, advice does have a rightful place when it is requested and when the person giving the advice has expert knowledge that the patient does not.

Using Judgmental Comments

Using judgmental comments tends to impose the nurse's standards on the patient. Consider the comment of a nurse who notes that a young woman is crying:

Nurse: You aren't acting very grown-up. How do you think your husband would feel if he saw you crying like this?

The nurse judges the patient as being immature, and the nurse's apparent hostility could end effective communication. A better comment in this situation might be as follows:

Nurse: I would like to help. Tell me what is making you cry.

Consider the following exchange between a nurse and a patient about to have surgery:

Patient: I think I have a right to be afraid of this operation.
Nurse: Tell me what makes you afraid.

This patient is likely to feel safe when allowed to express his or her feelings without being judged.

Changing the Subject

A quick way to stop conversation is to change the subject. The patient may be at a point of readiness to discuss something and can be expected to feel frustrated if put off by a change in the topic of conversation. The following example illustrates this:

Patient: When can I expect to be told about taking my own insulin?
Nurse: Let's discuss your diet now so that you will know what to eat when you get home. We can discuss your insulin some other time.

A nurse may also change the subject when feeling uncomfortable about the topic of conversation. For example, the patient's needs are being met when the nurse allows the patient to speak of impending death, thoughts of suicide, or a contemplated abortion. The nurse is ignoring the patient, however, when the subject is changed because the nurse feels uncomfortable talking about it.

Giving False Assurance

Because it is easier and more pleasant to deal with positive outcomes than with negative ones, the nurse may sometimes try to convince the patient that things are going to turn out well even when knowing the chances are not good. False assurance may give patients the impression that the nurse is not interested in their problems. Cliches are frequently used when a nurse gives a patient false assurance. Communication may be impeded. If the nurse inadvertently does this, explaining with an apology to the patient helps promote a return to effective communication.

Gossip and Rumor

Gossip and rumor are common forms of communication in healthcare settings. Those new to nursing are invited to explore their beneficial and negative repercussions for patients, caregivers, and the healthcare agency or institution. Gossiping may be used to inform, influence others, entertain, or ventilate. Generally occurring in small intimate groups, gossiping may be harmless, but it may also damage the reputation of others. Rumors serve similar functions as gossip but tend to be more widespread. Among their negative consequences are damage to the reputation of authority figures, coworkers, or an organization; disharmony or divisiveness; and adversarial relations (Ribeiro & Blakeley, 1995).

🌀 Impaired Verbal Communication

The ability to communicate is our most human characteristic. Human communication is essential for learning, working, and social interaction. Impaired communication can affect every aspect of a person's life. Impaired Verbal Communication is a nursing diagnosis approved by the North American Nursing Diagnosis Association (NANDA). Its definition, defining characteristics, and related factors are given here.

Definition: the state in which an individual experiences a decreased or absent ability to use or understand language in human interaction
Defining characteristics: is unable to speak dominant language; speaks or verbalizes with difficulty; does not or cannot speak; stutters; slurs; has difficulty forming words or sentences; has difficulty expressing thought verbally; uses inappropriate verbalization; has dyspnea; is disoriented
Related factors: Decrease in circulation to the brain; brain tumor; physical barrier (tracheostomy, intubation); anatomic defect, cleft palate; psychological barriers (psychosis, lack of stimuli); cultural differences; developmental or age related

The accompanying displays, Focus on the Older Adult and Communication With Patients With Special Needs, describe the speech, language, and hearing disorders that most frequently affect older people and offer guidelines for communicating with patients with special needs. The causes of hearing loss include chronic ear infections, heredity, birth defects, health problems at home, certain drugs, head injury, viral or bacterial infection, exposure to loud noise, aging, and tumors. Causes of speech and language disorders are related to hearing loss, cerebral palsy and other nerve and muscle disorders, severe head injury, stroke, viral diseases, mental retardation, certain drugs, physical impairments such as cleft lip or palate, vocal abuse or misuse, and inadequate speech and language models.

A nurse who suspects a speech, language, or hearing problem should refer the patient to a speech-language pathologist or audiologist. A speech-language pathologist is a professional educated in the study of human communication, its development, and its disorders. An audiologist is a professional educated in the study of normal and impaired hearing.

Focus on the Older Adult

What Are the Disorders of Communication That Most Frequently Affect Older People?

Our communication system, which involves speaking, hearing and understanding the speech of others, reading, and writing, is a unique human achievement. It plays a vital role in all aspects of everyday life—in our jobs, our families, and our recreation. When communication processes are damaged by disorders of speech, language, or hearing, the effects are always serious.

Disorders of speech, language, and hearing are frequently found among older adults. These individuals often find themselves at a distinct disadvantage on social, economic, and personal levels. With the number of older adults growing rapidly, and with the increased numbers of survivors of illnesses and accidents that can result in speech, language, or hearing disorders, more and more older adults with communication prob-

lems will be encountered. They require the understanding of family and friends as well as services from professionals in communication disorders.

Disorders of communication that affect older people may result from hearing impairment, stroke, cancer or other disease of the larynx, parkinsonism, or other neurologic disorders. The communication disorders vary widely and include difficulty with speaking and with understanding verbal messages. The effects of these disorders may be frustrating and bewildering and may lead to withdrawal and isolation. Participation on any social or economic level may become difficult or impossible either because of the disorder itself or the emotional consequences.

SPEECH, LANGUAGE, AND HEARING DISORDERS

APHASIA:
Aphasia is a complex problem which may result, in varying degrees, in a reduced ability to understand what others are saying, to express oneself, or to be understood. Some individuals with this disorder may have no speech, while others may have only mild difficulties recalling names or words. Others may have problems putting words in their proper order in a sentence. The ability to understand oral directions, to read, to write, and to deal with numbers may also be disturbed. Strokes are the major cause of aphasia in the older population. It has been estimated that there are over one million adults with aphasia in the United States today. Many can be helped to communicate more effectively.

DYSARTHRIA:
Dysarthria interferes with normal control of the speech mechanism. Speech may be slurred or otherwise difficult to understand due to lack of ability to produce speech sounds correctly, maintain good breath control, and coordinate the movements of the lips, tongue, palate, and larynx. Diseases such as parkinsonism, multiple sclerosis, and bulbar palsy, as well as strokes and accidents, can cause dysarthria. Many individuals with dysarthria are over 65. Their communication skills often may be improved by appropriate treatment.

HEARING PROBLEMS: It is estimated that of the approximately 27 million Americans over the age of 65, as many as 50 percent may be affected by hearing impairment. The hearing loss observed as a part of the aging process is called "presbycusis." Many of those with presbycusis describe the problem as being able to "hear" what others are saying, but being unable to understand what is being said. This condition can lead to withdrawal from personal interactions of all types. Family or friends may confuse the disorder with "forgetfulness" or "senility." A hearing aid can often improve communication for older people with hearing loss.

VOICE PROBLEMS: Laryngectomy, the surgical removal of the larynx (voice box) due to cancer, affects approximately 9,000 individuals each year, most of whom are older. They can usually learn to speak again by learning esophageal speech, by using an electronic device or by surgical implant of voice prosthesis. Other forms of disease may result in complete or partial loss of the voice. Most of these problems can be treated.

OTHER COMMUNICATION PROBLEMS: Brain diseases that result in progressive loss of mental faculties may affect memory, orientation to time, place and people, and organization of thought processes, all of which may result in reduced ability to communicate.

From *Communication Disorders and Aging.* American Speech-Language-Hearing Association, Rockville, Md. Reprinted with permission.

Communicating With Patients With Special Needs

Patients Who Are Visually Impaired

- Acknowledge your presence in the patient's room.
- Identify yourself by name.
- Remember that the visually impaired patient will be unable to pick up most nonverbal cues during communication. Speak in a normal tone of voice.
- Explain the reason for touching the patient before doing so.
- Indicate to the patient when the conversation has ended and when you are leaving the room.
- Keep a call light or bell within easy reach of the patient.
- Orient the patient to the sounds in the environment and to the arrangement of the room and its furnishings.
- Be sure eyeglasses are clean and intact or that contacts are in place.

Patients Who Are Hearing Impaired

- Orient the patient to your presence before initiating conversation. This may be done by gently touching the patient or moving so you can be seen.
- Talk directly to the patient while facing him or her. If the patient is able to lip read, use simple sentences and speak in a quiet, natural manner and pace. Be aware of nonverbal communication.
- Do not chew gum or cover your mouth when talking with the patient.
- Demonstrate or pantomime ideas you wish to express, as appropriate.
- Use sign language or finger spelling, as appropriate.
- Write any ideas that you cannot convey to the patient in another manner.
- Be sure that hearing aids are clean, functioning, and inserted properly.

Patients With a Physical Barrier
(Laryngectomy or Endotracheal Tube)

- Select one or more simple means of communication that the patient is physically able to use. Options include eye blinks or hand squeezes to communicate yes or no; writing pads or magic slates; communication boards with words, letters, or pictures; flash cards; sign language.
- Be sure that everyone communicating with the patient—family, friends, and caregivers—understands and is able to use the communication devices selected.
- Demonstrate patience with the time needed to communicate effectively, and reinforce the efforts made by the patient.

- Ensure that the patient has an effective means of signaling need for assistance, such as call bells or alarms.

Patients Who Are Cognitively Impaired

- Establish and maintain eye contact with the patient to hold attention.
- Communicate important information in a quiet environment where there is little to distract the patient's attention.
- Keep communication simple and concrete. Break down instructions into simple tasks and avoid lengthy explanations. Do not use pronouns or abstract terms. Use pictures or drawings when appropriate.
- Whenever possible, avoid open-ended questions. Ask "Would you like to wear the brown pants or the gray pants?" instead of "What would you like to wear?"
- Be patient and give the patient time to respond. If the patient does not respond after 2 minutes, repeat what you said. If there is still no response, take a break before continuing the conversation so that neither you nor the patient becomes frustrated.

An Unconscious Patient

- Be careful of what is said in the patient's presence. Hearing is believed to be the last sense lost, and therefore the unconscious patient is often likely to hear even though there is no apparent response.
- Assume the patient can hear you. Talk in a normal tone of voice about things you would ordinarily discuss.
- Speak with the patient before touching. Remember that touch can be an effective means of communication with the unconscious patient.
- Keep environment noises at as low a level as possible. This helps the patient focus on the communication.

Patients Who Do Not Speak English

- Use an interpreter whenever possible.
- Use a dictionary that translates words from one language to another so that you can speak at least some words in the patient's language.
- Speak in simple sentences and in a normal tone of voice.
- Demonstrate or pantomime ideas you wish to convey, as appropriate.
- Be aware of nonverbal communication. Remember that many nonverbal communication cues are universal.

Learning Outcomes

After studying this chapter, the learner should be able to accomplish the following:

1. Define the key terms used in the chapter:

assertiveness	message
body language	nonverbal
channel	communication
communication	organizational
empathy	communication
feedback	professionalism
group dynamics	rapport
helping relationship	receiver (decoder)
interpersonal	semantics
communication	small-group
interviewing techniques	communication
intrapersonal	source (encoder)
communication	therapeutic touch
language	verbal communication

2. Describe the communication process, identifying factors that influence communication.
3. List at least eight ways in which people communicate nonverbally.
4. Describe the interrelation between communication and the nursing process.
5. Identify patient goals for each phase of the helping relationship.
6. Use effective communication techniques when interacting with patients from different cultures.
7. Evaluate yourself in terms of the interpersonal competencies needed in nursing.
8. Describe how each type of the ineffective communication hinders communication.
9. Establish therapeutic relationships with patients assigned to your care and describe effective interventions for patients with impaired verbal communication.

Critical Thinking Exercises

1. Think about your class as a group and evaluate how effectively your class group is functioning (fair, average, good, exceptional). Identify positive and negative factors influencing your effectiveness. Talk with your classmates and see if they agree or disagree with your evaluation. Talk about how your class compares with classes of other years. What roles do you see yourself playing in your class group? Do others agree with your self-assessment?

2. Working with another student, attempt to express the following without using any form of verbal communication:
   - I am in pain.
   - I am genuinely concerned about your well-being.
   - I couldn't care less that you are my patient, and I wish I were anywhere else but here caring for you.
   - I am afraid that you will hurt me.

   Try to put into words what this exercise can teach you about the importance of nonverbal communication. Explain how this understanding will influence your nursing practice.

3. Conversation is both an art and an essential nursing tool. If you had 30 minutes to spend with each of the following patients while doing a procedure that allows you to communicate, what would you talk about (communicate) and why? Compare your answers with another student's, and explore what your conversations would communicate to the patients involved.
   - An older adult, recently admitted to a nursing home
   - A 6-year-old boy newly admitted to a hospital for asthma
   - An HIV-positive 33-year-old man who has just been given the news that he has acquired immunodeficiency syndrome (AIDS)
   - A 45-year-old amputee who has been in a rehabilitation hospital for 3 weeks after a motorcycle accident
   - A 19-year-old woman who has just had an elective abortion and is in the recovery unit
   - An unconscious patient in a critical care unit

4. An experienced nurse observes your distress after leaving the room of a patient who has just told her family that her cancer has recurred and is in an advanced state. She tells you that you better "toughen up" if you want to survive in nursing. She counsels not getting emotionally involved with patients and families: "Become a rock." How do you respond to this nurse and why? Of what value, if any, is empathy?

Bibliography

Allen, L. J., & Van Ess Coeling, H. (1995). Quality of life: Its meaning to the long term care resident. *Journal of Gerontological Nursing, 21*(2), 20–25.

Angel, G., & Petronko, D. K. (1983). *Developing the new assertive nurse: Essentials for advancement.* New York: Springer-Verlag.

Armstrong, J. (1996). Too close for comfort. *Nursing, 26*(4), 44–47.

Bergbom-Engberg, I. (1993). The communication process with ventilator patients in the ICU as perceived by the nursing staff. *Intensive Critical Care Nursing, 9*(1), 40–47.

Berlo, D. (1960). *The process of communication: An introduction to theory and practice.* New York: Holt, Rinehart, & Winston.

Bottorff, J. L., & Morse, J. M. (1994). Identifying patterns of attending: Patterns of nurse's work. *Image—The Journal of Nursing Scholarship, 26*(1), 53–60.

Chenevert, M. (1994). *STAT: Special techniques in assertiveness training for women in the health professions* (4th ed.). St. Louis: Mosby–Year Book.

Clark, C. C. (1978). *Assertive skills for nurses.* Wakefield, MA: Contemporary Publishing.

Crellin, K. (1998). 11 Easy ways to build rapport. *Nursing98, 28*(11), 48.

Deering, C. G. (1993). Working with people: Giving and taking criticism. *American Journal of Nursing, 93*(12), 56–60.

Fine, J. I., & Rouse-Bane, S. (1995). Using validation techniques to improve communication with cognitively impaired older adults. *Journal of Gerontological Nursing, 21*(6), 39–45.

Giger, J. N., & Davidhizar, R. E. (1995). *Transcultural nursing: Assessment and intervention* (2nd ed.). St. Louis: C. V. Mosby.

Grossman, D., & Taylor, R. (1995). Working with people: Cultural diversity on the unit. *American Journal of Nursing, 95*(2), 64–67.

Hagerty, B. M. K., Lynch-Sauer, J., Patusky, K. L., & Bouwsema, M. (1993). An emerging theory of human relatedness. *Image—The Journal of Nursing Scholarship, 25*(4), 291–296.

Harvey, C., Dixon, M., & Padberg, N. (1995). Support group for families of trauma patients. *Critical Care Nurse, 15*(4), 59–63.

Heidt, P. R. (1990). Openness: A qualitative analysis of nurses' and patients' experience of touch. *Image—The Journal of Nursing Research, 21*(3), 180–186.

Hermann, J. F., Cella, D. F., & Robinovitch, A. (1995). Guidelines for support group programs. *Cancer Practice, 3*(2), 111–113.

Hutchison, C. P. (1999). Healing touch: An energetic approach. *American Journal of Nursing, 99*(4), 43–48.

Laing, M. (1993). Gossip: Does it play a role in the socialization of nurses? *Image—The Journal of Nursing Scholarship, 25*(1), 37–43.

MacKay, M. (1990). *Empathy in helping relationship.* New York: Springer-Verlag.

Mackey, R. B. (1995). Discover the healing power of therapeutic touch. *American Journal of Nursing, 95*(4), 26–33.

Messner, R. L. (1993). What patients really want from their nurses. *American Journal of Nursing, 93*(8), 38–41.

Montagu, A. (1986). *Touching: The human significance of the skin* (3rd ed.). New York: Harper & Row.

Moore, J. R., & Gilbert, D. A. (1995). Elderly residents' perceptions of nurses' comforting touch. *Journal of Gerontological Nursing, 21*(1), 6–13.

Nance, T. A. (1995). Intercultural communication: Finding common ground. *Journal of Obstetric, Gynecologic, and Neonatal Nursing, 24*(3), 249–255.

Norris, R. M. (1989). Commonsense tips for working with blind patients. *American Journal of Nursing, 89*(3), 360–361.

North American Nursing Diagnosis Association. *NANDA nursing diagnoses: Definitions and classification, 1995–1996.* Philadelphia: NANDA.

Orlando, I. J. (1961). *The dynamic nurse–patient relationship.* New York: G. P. Putnam's Sons.

Paterson, J., & Zderad, L. (1976). *Humanistic nursing.* New York: Wiley.

Peplau, H. (1952). *Interpersonal relations in nursing.* New York: Putnam.

Quinn, J. F. (1988). Building a body of knowledge: Research on therapeutic touch. *Journal of Holistic Nursing, 6*(1), 37–45.

Ribeiro, V. F., & Blakeley, J. A. (1995). The proactive management of rumor and gossip. *JONA, 25*(6), 43–50.

Scott, J., & Rantz, M. (1994). Change champions at the grass roots level: Practice innovation using team process. *Nursing Administration Quarterly, 18*(3), 13.

Seldon, B. (1994). Communicating with Alzheimer's patients. *Journal of Gerontological Nursing, 20*(10), 51–53.

Sundeen, S. J., Stuart, G. W., Rankin, E. D., & Cohen, S. A. (1989). *Nurse–patient interaction* (4th ed.). St. Louis: C. V. Mosby.

Tannen, D. (1990). *You just don't understand: Women and men in conversation.* New York: Morrow.

Tennant, K. F. (1990). Laugh it off: The effect of humor on the well-being of the older adult. *Journal of Gerontological Nursing, 16*(12), 11–17.

Travelbee, J. (1971). *Interpersonal aspects of nursing* (2nd ed.). Philadelphia: F. A. Davis.

Vanore-Black, N. (1990). Maintaining healthy relationships. *Holistic Nursing Practice, 4*(4), 39–45.

Watson, J. (1985). *Nursing: The philosophy and science of caring.* Boulder: Colorado Associated University Press.

White, C., & Howse, E. (1993). Managing humor: When is it funny—and when is it not? *Nursing Management, 24*(4), 80, 84, 86–96.

Chapter 22
Teacher and Counselor

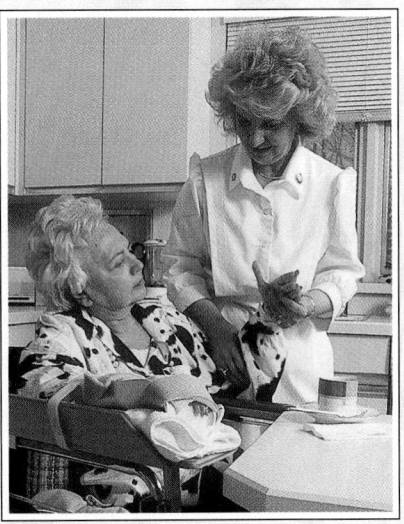

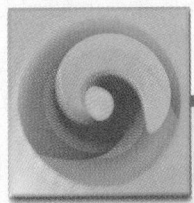

Thinking Critically About Nursing's Blended Skills

Before reading this chapter, think about the types of blended skills you will need to become an effective teacher and counselor.

- Another student asks you to help her to reach some fitness goals: weight loss, increased muscle tone, and improved cardiorespiratory capacity. She is highly motivated, but any workable plan will involve major lifestyle changes. She has numerous questions about different popular diet plans.

- Bob and Judy are expecting their first child in about 5 months and are anticipating a home birth. They characterize themselves as happy, scared, and very nervous. An intelligent couple, they ask lots of questions about childbirth and their new responsibilities as parents. They tend to lack confidence in themselves. You will be assisting with the delivery.

- Susie, a 3-year-old patient with second-degree burns on both legs, is being prepared for discharge. Her mother needs to learn how to continue to care for her burns at home but to date has missed every planned teaching session.

- Rachel asks to talk with you privately. She is the second wife of a 57-year-old patient with a serious myocardial infarction; they have been married only 1 year. She tells you that she is embarrassed to talk with the cardiologist but has lots of questions about what her husband will be able to do after he gets home, including questions about resuming sexual activity.

What cognitive, technical, interpersonal, and ethical/legal skills will you need to teach and counsel the people described above?

Many patients lack the knowledge and self-care abilities they need to achieve their health goals. To work effectively with these patients, nurses must be skilled teachers and counselors. Both roles require strong communication skills. The current trends toward shorter hospital stays and decreased time for healthcare professional–patient interactions have increased the need for effective teaching and counseling. More patients are at home in need of complex nursing assistance from their families, friends, and volunteers. Never has the demand for quality education and counseling been greater. Nurses who are skilled educators and counselors can improve patients' health and well-being and reduce the demand for professional services.

Aims of Teaching and Counseling

The basic purpose of teaching and counseling is to help patients and families develop the self-care abilities (knowledge, attitude, and skills) that enable them to maximize their functioning and quality of life (or dignified death). For example, a newly diagnosed diabetic patient must (1) acquire *knowledge* about diabetes as a disease process and related medical management and self-care, (2) value health sufficiently to make certain lifestyle modifications (*attitude*), and (3) master certain *skills*, such as insulin injection. When skillfully used by nurses, teaching and counseling are powerful tools for helping patients achieve health goals. Teaching provides the knowledge patients need to make informed healthcare decisions and to implement a plan of care. Counseling provides the resources and support patients need to participate actively in self-care.

Promoting Health

A higher level of wellness is possible for virtually everyone. Nurses can help patients to value health and develop specific health practices that promote wellness. Health teaching is varied and ranges from teaching passive exercises to a patient with left-sided paralysis to designing a safe exercise program for a young athlete.

Preventing Illness

Illness prevention, a major theme in health teaching and counseling, takes many forms. Nurses can counsel women of childbearing age about health practices that promote optimal fetal development, teach parents how to make their home safe for a toddler, or counsel individuals at high risk for heart disease, cancer, or communicable diseases.

Restoring Health

Once a patient is ill, teaching and counseling focus on developing self-care practices that facilitate recovery. Preoperative and postoperative teaching, sexual counseling for a patient recovering from a myocardial infarction, and lifestyle counseling for a patient with an ostomy are all examples of teaching and counseling directed at restoring health.

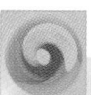

COGNITIVE SKILLS

- Knowledge of the teaching–learning and counseling processes
- Knowledge essential for designing an appropriate fitness program, nutrition program, and childbirth and parenting programs; knowledge about burn care and about sexual counseling after myocardial infarction

TECHNICAL SKILLS

- Ability to demonstrate fitness activities and fitness measurement techniques
- Ability to demonstrate childbirth and parenting psychomotor skills
- Ability to demonstrate burn dressings and treatment techniques

INTERPERSONAL SKILLS

- Strong people skills; ability to communicate and interact effectively with people and patients with complex learning and counseling needs and different levels of learning readiness and abilities to learn
- Excellent therapeutic communication skills for interacting with each of the people in these situations: the eager and highly motivated young woman, the anxious new parents, the reluctant and possibly indifferent or overwhelmed mother, and the frightened spouse—conversational skills, listening skills, silence, interviewing techniques, touch, humor, assertiveness

ETHICAL/LEGAL SKILLS

- Ability to demonstrate respect, empathy, and honest caring in each professional encounter with both patients and colleagues
- Knowledge of the ethical and legal principles that guide professional relationships and behavior in teaching and counseling situations
- Ability to document teaching and counseling interventions in a legally prudent manner

Facilitating Coping

Developmental lifestyle changes and acute, chronic, and terminal illness all place demands on patients and families that may become overwhelming. Nurses work not only with patients but also with their families and friends to help them to come to terms with illness and whatever lifestyle modifications it entails.

Nurse caregivers who are skilled teachers and counselors can effect the following outcomes:

- High-level wellness and related self-care practices
- Disease prevention or early detection
- Quick recovery from trauma or illness with minimal or no complications
- Enhanced ability to adjust to developmental life changes and acute, chronic, and terminal illness
- Family acceptance of lifestyle changes necessitated by the illness or disability of a family member

General topics for health teaching are highlighted in the accompanying box.

The Nurse as Teacher

Nurses assume the role of teacher when patients have identifiable learning needs. This teacher–learner relationship is enhanced by the helping relationship (see Chap. 21) in which mutual respect and trust are established. The nurse builds on this trust by sharing information the nurse and patient have mutually identified as important. The patient may ask for this information, or the nurse may initiate teaching after assessing and diagnosing a learning need.

Teaching–Learning Process

How the human brain stores and retrieves information is not yet fully known. People learn throughout life, although what they learn and how learning occurs change according to developmental stages. A basic understanding of the teaching–learning process aids nurses in developing their own teaching and learning skills. The accompanying box outlines each step in the teaching–learning process. This process is often condensed because of limited time or resources, but the basic principles apply each time teaching–learning occurs.

Teaching is a planned method or series of methods used to help someone learn. The person using these methods is the teacher. **Learning** is the process by which a person acquires or increases knowledge or changes behavior in a measurable way as a result of an experience.

Learning Domains

There are three ways in which people learn, called *domains:* cognitive, affective, and psychomotor (Bloom, 1956). These domains influence the teaching and evaluative strategies the nurse selects. **Cognitive learning** involves the storing and recalling of new knowledge and information in the brain (eg, the patient describes how salt intake affects blood pressure). Cognitive learning includes intellectual behaviors, such as the acquisition of knowledge, comprehension, application (using abstract ideas in concrete situations), analysis (relating ideas in an organized way), synthesis (assimilating parts of information as a whole), and evaluation (judging the worth of a body of information). Learning a physical skill involving the integration of mental and muscular activity is called **psychomotor learning** (eg, the patient demonstrates how to change

---

Topics for Health Teaching and Counseling

Promoting Health
- Developmental and maturational issues
- Normal childbearing
- Hygiene
- Nutrition
- Exercise
- Mental health
- Spiritual health

Preventing Illness
- First aid
- Safety
- Immunizations
- Screening
- Identification and management of risk factors

Restoring Health
- Orientation to treatment center and staff
- Patients' and nurses' expectations of one another

- The illness and physical condition: anatomy and physiology, etiology of problem, significance of symptoms, prognosis
- The medical and nursing regimens and how the patient can participate in care
- Self-care practices the patient and family need to manage the patient's condition independently

Facilitating Coping
- How the patient's physical and mental condition affects other areas of functioning; lifestyle counseling
- Measures that maximize independence and enhance self-concept
- Stress management
- Environmental alterations
- Community resources
- Appropriate referrals (eg, physical therapy, occupational therapy, self-help groups, psychiatric-mental health counselor)
- Grief and bereavement counseling

Steps in the Teaching–Learning Process

Assess the Client's Learning Needs

1. Use all appropriate sources of information.
2. Identify the knowledge, attitude, or skills needed by the patient and family.
3. Assess emotional and experiential readiness to learn.
4. Assess the patient's ability to learn.
5. Identify patient strengths.
6. Use anticipatory guidance.

Diagnose the Learning Needs

1. Be realistic.
2. Validate with patient or family, or both.

Develop a Teaching Plan

1. Formulate measurable learner objectives.
   - Identify short- and long-term objectives.
   - Prioritize.
   - Determine who should be included (ie, family members, significant others).
   - Include the patient in planning.
2. Create a teaching plan.
   - Match content with appropriate teaching strategies and learner activities.
   - Directly relate teaching content to the patient's interests, resources, and patterns of everyday living.
   - Schedule within limits of time constraints.
   - Decide on group versus individual teaching and formal versus informal.
   - Formulate a verbal or written contract with the patient.

Implement the Teaching Plan

1. Prepare the physical environment.
2. Gather all audiovisual materials and equipment.
3. Deliver content in organized manner using teaching strategies.
4. Be flexible.

Evaluate the Teaching–Learning

1. Evaluate completion of learner objectives.
   - Patient's comments
   - Direct questioning
   - Observational skills
   - Return demonstration
   - Postdischarge follow-ups
2. Reinforce and celebrate learning.
3. Evaluate teaching.
   - Self-evaluation
   - Patient questionnaires
4. Revise plan of learner objectives not met.
   - Alter content and teaching strategies.
   - Use motivational counseling if needed.
   - Reschedule teaching sessions.
5. Document the teaching–learning process.

---

dressings using clean technique). **Affective learning** includes changes in attitudes, values, and feelings (eg, the patient expresses renewed self-confidence after physical therapy).

Effective teaching often involves the promotion of behaviors in all three domains. In the example of a teaching plan presented later in this chapter, the nurse helps prenatal couples interested in breastfeeding master new behaviors: affective (valuing good nutrition and skin integrity, feeling confident in assuming new parenting responsibilities), cognitive (knowledge of correct feeding technique and related nipple care), and psychomotor (knowledge of nipple preparation, correct feeding technique, and aftercare).

Developmental Considerations

One of the major learning theories is Piaget's theory of intellectual development (see Chap. 8). A nurse who understands how children and adolescents develop learning abilities can use this knowledge when teaching patients at any age. For instance, if a 4-year-old girl must begin to take insulin every day, the nurses who are caring for her must recognize her limitations in understanding diabetes. Information should be simplified to only the most basic facts with concrete examples or demonstrations. A detailed discussion of the pathophysiology of diabetes would not be

appropriate. The girl could be told that she needs a shot every day to keep her from getting sick or feeling funny. She could be allowed to play with the syringes and to give shots to a doll.

A nurse who is teaching a sexually active 16-year-old girl about contraceptive methods needs to assess whether the young patient has reached the stage Piaget refers to as *formal operations* (the ability to use logical reasoning to solve hypothetical problems). If the patient's intellectual development is delayed and is still in the period of *concrete operations* (use of logical reasoning to solve concrete problems), she may be unable to think abstractly. That is, she may not perceive pregnancy as a real possibility and therefore may not understand the need for contraception. If so, the nurse can alter the teaching plan to include audiovisual (AV) teaching aids that explain the topic in concrete terms.

Some adults too have not attained the formal operations stage. Nurses must be alert to this possibility and teach or reteach material as needed. For example, an adult taking an antibiotic may not grasp the importance of taking the capsules at the prescribed times to maintain the proper blood level for the best effect. If the nurse sees that the patient is not adhering to the schedule, the effectiveness of the teaching and learning should be evaluated. Showing a simple diagram of how erratic dose scheduling affects the body may provide the concrete information the patient needs to be motivated to take the antibiotic as prescribed. In this way, the teaching is altered to meet the patient's intellectual development.

Motor development is also a concern in the teaching–learning process. The 4-year-old girl diagnosed with diabetes may not be able to learn to give her own insulin shots if she lacks the fine motor skills needed to manipulate the equipment for insulin injections. On the other hand, a 13-year-old patient could probably master the technique quickly.

Other developmental concerns related to the teaching–learning process are emotional maturity and psychosocial development. A person's age does not guarantee maturity. A 13-year-old patient may respond more maturely to health teaching than a 30-year-old patient. A great deal depends on how the patient has learned to respond to changes and stressful events in the past.

Adult Learners

Many of the developmental concerns related to teaching and learning are exacerbated by age. As people age, their personalities and their learning abilities change. Most psychologists who have studied the teaching–learning process base their work on children and adolescents because a large amount of learning occurs early in life. The science of teaching—called **pedagogy**—generally refers to the teaching of children and adolescents. In recent years, the study of teaching adults—**androgogy**—has gained more attention. The different term emphasizes that adults need to be taught differently.

Knowles (1990) lists the following four assumptions concerning adult learners:

1. As a person matures, his or her self-concept is likely to move from dependence to independence.
2. The previous experience of the adult is a rich resource for learning.
3. The readiness to learn in an adult is often related to a developmental task or a social role.
4. Most adults' orientation to learning is that material should be useful immediately, rather than at some time in the future.

These assumptions show that androgogy has a problem-centered or need-centered focus on immediate application of new material.

Most adults must believe they need to learn before they are willing to learn. Nurses often use their counseling skills (discussed later) to motivate patients to participate in the teaching–learning process. Adults may need to be shown the necessity of learning new information, health practices, or skills.

Many adults are afraid of the teaching–learning process. This may be the result of a fear of failure because many adults have not participated in formal educational programs since their school days. Older adults often express a concern over memory loss, and being required to learn new material can threaten their feelings of self-worth. Con-

sequently, the nurse's sensitivity and concern in the helping relationship are needed to build a foundation for a non-threatening learning environment.

Adults may also resist learning because of preconceived ideas about the teaching–learning process and others' expectations. Honest and open communication provides adult learners with a preview of what is involved. Many adults willingly participate once they are reassured that they are partners in the process. Retaining some control over what is taught and how it is taught gives adult learners the sense of control they are accustomed to in their daily lives.

Some older patients are especially fearful and threatened by the idea of having to learn new information. They often quote the old adage, "You can't teach an old dog new tricks," as a defensive attempt to avoid failure or change. Nurses may find that a slower approach is needed when introducing new material so that older patients do not become discouraged or overwhelmed.

Literacy

About 20% of adults are functionally illiterate (unable to read and write). Many have learned to compensate for this disability and may fool even experienced nurses. Never presume **literacy** (the ability to read and write) in a patient you are attempting to teach. By asking patients to read a sheet of printed material aloud you can assess their ability to understand printed material.

Principles of Teaching–Learning

Several basic principles of teaching–learning are guidelines for nurses in the role of teacher.

- The teaching–learning process is facilitated by a helping relationship (discussed in Chap. 21).
- Nurse-teachers need to be able to communicate effectively with individuals (Fig. 22-1), small groups, and, in some instances, large groups.
- Knowledge of the communication process is necessary to assess verbal and nonverbal feedback.
- A thorough assessment of patients and factors affecting their learning helps to diagnose their learning needs accurately.
- The teaching–learning process is more effective when the patient is included in planning learner objectives.
- Unless the patient values these objectives, little learning is likely to occur.
- The implementation of a teaching plan should include varied strategies for sensory stimulation, which promotes learning.
- Relating new learning material to patients' past life experiences helps them assimilate new knowledge.
- Proposed behavioral changes must always be realistic and explored in the context of the patient's resources and everyday lifestyle.

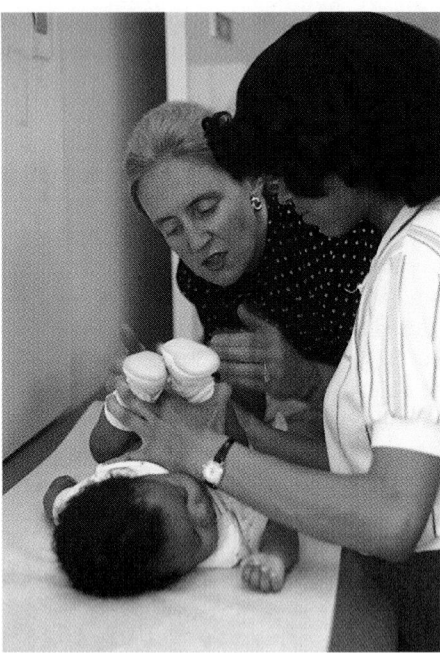

Figure 22-1
Effective communication is essential in the teaching–learning process.

- Careful attention should be paid to time constraints, scheduling, and the physical environment.
- Learner objectives are the basis for evaluating whether learning has occurred.
- When learning objectives have not been met, careful reassessment provides ideas for changing the teaching plan for subsequent implementation.

Patient teaching is approached most effectively through the steps of the nursing process. The teaching–learning process and the nursing process are interdependent.

Assessing Learning Needs

Sources of Information
Usually, patients themselves are the best source of assessment information. By using effective interviewing techniques (see Chap. 21), the nurse can obtain the data needed to identify the patient's learning needs. Relevant information can be obtained before actually meeting the patient by reviewing the patient's past and current medical records. These records provide a history of medical problems as well as documentation of nursing assessments, nursing diagnoses, nursing physical examinations, and nursing interventions that have been performed.

The patient's family and significant others are also valuable sources of assessment data. Family members or significant others are sometimes needed to provide assessment data when the patient cannot communicate with the nurse because of health problems, language barriers, or impaired sensory functions. At other times, the family members or significant others may be the most appropriate source of certain information; for example, if seeking information about how much salt is used in the family's cooking, the nurse could speak with the person who prepares the meals in the patient's home and include that person in any teaching about food preparation. The patient's permission is needed before the nurse involves family members in the teaching–learning process.

Assessment Parameters
Four elements should be considered in each assessment of patient learning needs. The nurse first identifies what new knowledge, attitudes, or skills are necessary for patients and families to manage their healthcare. Second, assessment focuses on **learning readiness**, the patient's willingness to engage in the teaching–learning process (emotional readiness) and experiential readiness to begin the challenge of learning. Readiness is distinguished from the patient's actual ability to learn, which is the third focus. The fourth focus of assessment is on patient strengths, personal resources the nurse can assist patients to tap. Many factors influence each of these elements, and all should play a role in the assessment. These factors are highlighted in the accompanying box, Assessment Parameters: Factors That Affect Nursing.

**Assessment Parameters:
Factors That Affect Learning**

Knowledge, attitudes, and skills needed for the patient and family to manage healthcare independently

Readiness to learn
- Emotional readiness
  Emotional health
  Motivation for learning
  Self-concept and body image
  Sense of responsibility for self
- Experiential readiness
  Social and economic stability
  Past experiences with learning
  Attitude toward learning
  Culture

Ability to learn
- Physical condition
- Cognitive ability to learn
- Acuity of senses
- Developmental considerations
- Level of education
- Literacy
- Communication skills
- Primary language

Learning strengths
- Successful learning in the past
- Above-average comprehension, reasoning, memory, or psychomotor skills
- High motivation
- Strong network
- Adequate financing

Diagnosing Learning Needs

When a lack of knowledge, attitude, or skill hinders a patient's self-promotion of health, the nurse diagnoses the deficit. The nurse can use diagnoses or problem statements approved by the North American Nursing Diagnosis Association (NANDA) as a guide when diagnosing learning needs (see Chap. 16). If the nurse believes that a patient's knowledge deficit is the primary problem, the nurse can write a diagnosis identifying a specific knowledge deficit as the problem, followed by its etiology and the related signs and symptoms. For example:

> Knowledge Deficit: Breastfeeding related to inexperience as manifested by anxiety and multiple questions

More often, a knowledge deficit results in an actual or potential problem; therefore, the knowledge deficit is written as the etiology (second part of the diagnostic statement):

> Infant at High Risk for Altered Nutrition: Less Than Body Requirements related to mother's lack of knowledge about infant feeding and deficient learning readiness (as manifested by mother's quick frustration when breastfeeding, refusal to engage in learning process, and infant's weight loss)

For example, if a nurse learns that a pregnant woman plans to breastfeed and knows nothing about breastfeeding, "Knowledge Deficit: Breastfeeding" is the *problem statement*. The goal is to increase the mother's knowledge. If, on the other hand, a nurse observes a newborn failing to gain weight appropriately, and it is reasonable to suspect that the mother's lack of knowledge about how to breastfeed is interfering with the infant's nutritional intake, "Knowledge Deficit: Breastfeeding" is the *etiology*. The goal is to ensure the infant's proper nutrition.

Related nursing diagnoses include the following:

Health Maintenance, Altered
Management of Therapeutic Regimen, Individuals: Ineffective
Noncompliance
Self-Care Deficit (specify)

Wellness diagnoses, such as Potential for Enhanced Parenting or Potential for Enhanced Self-Esteem, are written as one-part statements. Teaching and counseling are the primary nursing interventions used to achieve related outcome criteria.

In addition to identifying the patient's learning needs, nurses need to assess their own knowledge base and teaching skills. Nurses cannot teach information and skills to patients if they themselves lack the information and skills to be taught. Often, knowing where to find information or an appropriate resource person is the first step in correcting one's own knowledge deficits.

Planning

Planning for learning involves the development of a teaching plan. Teaching plans are similar to nursing care plans—both follow the steps of the nursing process. One type of teaching plan is presented in the accompanying display. It is directed to teaching appropriate nipple care to reduce the likelihood of nipple cracking and redness in women who are breastfeeding.

Standardized teaching plans (some computerized) are available for major topics of health teaching. When using such plans, it is imperative to individualize the plan to the patient's unique learning needs and abilities. Examples of teaching plans that are incorporated into critical path documentation systems are featured in Chapters 17 and 20.

Thoughtful planning for a patient's learning experiences maximizes the patient's learning while ensuring the most efficient use of the nurse's time and talents. Learner objectives are developed for each diagnosis of a learning need. The nursing orders become the content, teaching strategy, and learner activity columns of the written plan. This phase requires thought and creativity. The nurse's efforts are rewarded when the patient successfully meets the objectives at the end of the implementation phase.

When planning for learning, the nurse and patient together must decide who should be included in the learning sessions. When the patient is a young child, one or both parents may be the primary learners. For an adult patient, a spouse or close friend who will be giving the care that is to be learned may be included. For instance, the person who does the household cooking is usually asked to be present for nutritional teaching. Teaching plans are developed according to the needs of the individuals being taught.

One nurse or several nurses can prepare and use a teaching plan. When two or more nurses plan and coordinate the implementation of the plan, this is called *team teaching*. An advantage of team teaching is that the talents of more than one nurse are involved in promoting learning for the patient. Several factors should be considered during the formulation of any teaching plan, as discussed in the next sections.

Learner Objectives

Learner objectives are written in the same manner as the patient goals in the nursing process (see Chap. 17). When planning for the patient's learning, determine first which of the three learning domains (cognitive, psychomotor, or affective) will be the focus of teaching. The nurse can then write learner objectives that reflect what learning is to occur. A well-constructed learner objective serves as a guide for planning evaluation methods.

Choosing the verb for a learner objective is probably the most difficult part when writing objectives (see the accompanying box). Yet, when chosen carefully, it makes the planning of content, teaching strategies, learner activities, and evaluation methods easier.

The number of objectives needed for each diagnosis varies. It is better to have several specific objectives than to try to cover everything with only one or two broad objectives. Many nurses write one long-term, general objective for each diagnosis, followed by several short-term, specific objectives. For example, a long-term objective for the sample teaching plan could be as follows: "The patient will be able to breastfeed her infant as long as desired without sore nipples." This objective could be met in 2 weeks or 2 years,

Sample Teaching Plan

Diagnosis: Risk for Impaired Skin Integrity: Nipples related to knowledge and skill deficit (nipple care)

Signs and symptoms: complaints of sore nipples, redness, cracking

Long-term Objective: woman will be able to breastfeed as long as desired without nipple problems

Learner Objectives	Met	Content	Teaching Strategy	Learner Activity
Woman describes measures to prevent nipple cracking (cognitive)	8/10/02 *L.S.*	Protective measures: • Avoid soap • Avoid exposure to air and sunlight • Apply lanolin or vegetable oil • Avoid plastic liners in bra or bra pads	Lecture with discussion Audiovisual: flip chart on breastfeeding	Read handout: Nipple care
Woman begins protective measures immediately (psychomotor)	8/10/02 *L.S.*			
Woman describes the correct procedure for breastfeeding (cognitive)	8/10/02 *L.S.*	Preparation for breastfeeding • Nipple roll before the feeding	Discussion Audiovisual: flip chart on breastfeeding	Read handout: Sore nipples
Woman explains why feedings should be shorter and more frequent (cognitive)	8/10/02 *L.S.*	Breastfeeding the baby • Feed baby every 2 hours during the day • Start baby on less sore side • Get baby onto areolar area • Position properly • Change position for each feeding • Remove baby from breast	Discovery: guide through each step; assist as necessary Return demonstration	Read handout: Positioning baby for breastfeeding Borrow books on breastfeeding from reference library
Woman demonstrates correct procedure for breastfeeding (psychomotor)	8/10/02 *L.S.*			
Display increasing confidence in breastfeeding skills and self-care (affective)	8/10/02 *L.S.*			
Value good nutrition and rest at home (affective)	8/10/02 *L.S.*	After feeding • Air dry the nipples • Inspect for open or cracked areas • Apply lanolin or vegetable oil	Discovery	
List the signs of thrush (cognitive)	8/10/02 *L.S.*			
		Home considerations • Maintain "demand feedings" • Ensure good nutrition • Get adequate rest • Know the signs and symptoms of thrush	Lecture with discussion Audiovisual: poster	Refer to handouts at home as needed; call maternity department's information number for any questions

depending on how long the woman decides to breastfeed. Long-term objectives are general statements. On the other hand, the objectives written in the learner objective column of the sample teaching plan are short-term, specific behaviors to be accomplished within a specified time.

Patients and appropriate family members or significant others should be included in the planning of learner objectives. When patients value the learning objectives, learning readiness is enhanced, and goal achievement is maximized.

Content

After the learner objectives are written, the nurse must decide what information the patient needs to complete them successfully. This information is the content of the teaching plan. New nurses usually need to research the subject to be taught to determine what information exists about the topic. Books, articles, and manuals are available in many nursing units for the nurse's research. Content is often already organized and available for a variety of

Verbs That Can Be Used When Writing Learner Objectives

Cognitive Domain	Psychomotor Domain
compares	adapts
defines	arranges
describes	assembles
designs	begins
differentiates	changes
explains	constructs
gives examples	creates
identifies	demonstrates
names	manipulates
prepares	moves
plans	organizes
solves	rearranges
states	shows
summarizes	starts
	works

Affective Domain

chooses	justifies
defends	relates
displays	revises
forms	selects
gives	shares
helps	uses
initiates	values

an adult could learn similar material by discussing safety measures with the nurse.

Education experts generally agree that using a variety of teaching strategies enhances learning. In addition, some methods are better suited for certain learning objectives. The accompanying box gives suggested teaching strategies for the three learning domains. The sample teaching plan shows how teaching strategies vary according to the learner objectives and content of that particular plan. Again, the nurse can be creative in choosing the methods. However, the nurse should try to stimulate as many of the patient's senses as possible when teaching. Seeing, hearing, and touching are superior to reading or hearing alone. We reportedly remember 10% of what we read, 20% of what we hear, 30% of what we see, 50% of what we see and hear, and 80% of what we say and do. Descriptions of common teaching strategies follow.

Role Modeling

The old saying, "Actions speak louder than words," explains why role modeling is effective. Patients watch their nurses closely; the nurse can use this opportunity to influence a patient's behavior positively. For example, nurses who formerly smoked can be role models for patients who are trying to quit smoking for health reasons.

Lecture

The term *lecture* means only a presentation of information by a teacher to a learner, but to be more effective,

common health-teaching topics, thus shortening the required research time.

Nurses are often concerned about what patients should learn about topics such as illness, procedures, medications, and surgeries. "How much should they know?" is often debated. It has been found that patients benefit from explanations of the physical sensations they will experience during a procedure. They appreciate advanced knowledge of what they will feel, taste, hear, see, and smell.

Content explaining why certain treatments and medications are needed is included in a teaching plan. Information on the prevention of illness or its complications should also be covered. Patients are more likely to implement a plan that they understand and value.

Teaching Strategies

The techniques used by a teacher to promote learning are *teaching strategies*. Teaching strategies are planned before the actual teaching sessions so that every content area can be matched with an effective teaching technique. The strategies chosen depend on the teacher's familiarity with the method; the availability of computers and teaching aids, such as AV and printed materials; the facilities for using AV materials; and factors affecting the patient's learning, such as educational level and cultural background. The nurse must also consider age-appropriate methods for her patient; for example, a 10-year-old will be receptive to a comic book on personal safety, whereas

Suggested Teaching Strategies for the Three Learning Domains

Cognitive Domain

Lecture or discussion
Panel discussion
Discovery
Audiovisual materials
Printed materials
Programmed instruction
Computer-assisted instruction programs

Affective Domain

Role modeling
Discussion
Panel discussion
Audiovisual materials
Role playing
Printed materials

Psychomotor Domain

Demonstration
Discovery
Audiovisual materials
Printed materials

lectures usually include question-and-answer periods to allow for clarification. This strategy is often used to deliver information to a large group of patients. It is rarely used for individual instruction except in combination with other strategies.

Discussion

Discussion involves a two-way exchange of information, ideas, and feelings between the teacher and the learners. It is an effective method when used by a nurse who is comfortable with leading a group and knowledgeable in group process (see Chap. 21). It can also be an effective method for one-on-one instruction.

Panel Discussion

A panel discussion involves a presentation of information by two or more people. Panel discussions can be used to impart factual material but are also effective for sharing experiences and emotions. Debates are a form of panel discussion that provide exposure for multiple sides of a controversial topic.

Demonstration

Demonstration of techniques, procedures, exercises, and the use of special equipment, combined with a lecture and discussion, is an effective strategy. The patient's learning can be evaluated by a return demonstration. Practice sessions are often included for the learner. Models of body parts or practice models, such as a resuscitation model, are frequently used. When teaching breast self-examinations, the use of a breast model allows the learner to feel different types of lumps commonly found in breast tissue. Childbirth educators usually demonstrate the birth of a baby by using a pelvic model, knitted uterus, and a baby doll.

Discovery

In discovery learning, the nurse presents a problem or situation to the patient or group of patients and then guides the patients to discover the solution or approach. Discussion of other possible approaches and solutions can follow the patient's own solutions. This is a good method for teaching problem-solving techniques and independent thinking. For instance, a nurse could give a group of diabetic patients a short description of a situation that includes signs and symptoms. The group would decide whether the signs and symptoms indicate *hypoglycemia* (low blood sugar) or *hyperglycemia* (high blood sugar) and would choose what measures to take. Next, the nurse could discuss the group decision as a further learning experience. Even if the patients chose a poor solution, the nurse can turn it into an effective learning experience.

Role Playing

Role playing gives the learner a chance to experience, relive, or anticipate an event. The nurse explains the scenario and then allows the patient to play out the scene with the teacher or with one or more other learners. Role

playing can be used to work through emotional traumas or to plan for possible traumas. For example, a nurse could help a teenaged girl prepare herself to tell her mother about her pregnancy by letting the girl play herself while the nurse plays the girl's mother. This would help the patient rehearse what she wanted to say and anticipate the emotional atmosphere that she will experience. Role playing is a good strategy for adults as well as children. Puppets and dolls can help young children express negative feelings resulting from hospitalization and traumatic procedures.

Audiovisual Materials

AV materials can be effective teaching and learning tools. AV materials include films, filmstrips with or without audiotapes, slides, television programs, videotapes, overhead transparencies, flip charts, posters, and diagrams. They can be a popular and effective teaching strategy when combined with a lecture or discussion. The patient's literacy should never be assumed when using printed words. AV materials should never be the sole source of learning for a patient. It is an accepted practice to allow the patient to view AV material alone but to precede and follow it with a discussion of the material.

Printed Material

The use of printed material depends on its availability. Many nurses have written materials for distribution to patients. Writing pamphlets, instruction sheets, books, and comic books for health teaching can be rewarding as well as useful. As with AV materials, the nurse usually uses printed materials in conjunction with other strategies. Specially prepared games, which are relatively easy to make, can be a popular and fun way for patients to learn. For instance, cards with pictures of foods can be used to create a nutritional instruction game.

Print materials should be selected carefully after evaluating how well they present the needed content in a format that is attractive, understandable, and helpful. Two samples of patient education materials appear in the accompanying boxes.

Programmed Instruction

Most programmed instruction books or booklets are prepared so that learners can use them independently of a teacher. However, educators generally agree that the teacher needs to spend time with the learner before and after the completion of the program to clarify information, answer questions, and provide the personal touch necessary for a learner's motivation. Because this is a self-paced strategy, it can be beneficial for many learners.

Computer-Assisted Instruction

Computer programs for teaching are being developed, and the possibilities are unlimited. This method can even be personalized by programming the computer to address the learner by name and to give positive feedback when appropriate. Care should be taken to comple-

---

Sample Client Education Materials for Managing Cancer Pain: Pain Control Plan

Pain Control Plan

Pain control plan for

_____

At home, I will take the following medicines for pain control:

Medicine	*How to take*	*How many*	*How often*	*Comments*
_____	_____	_____	_____	_____
_____	_____	_____	_____	_____
_____	_____	_____	_____	_____

Medicines that you may take to help treat side effects:

Side effect	*Medicine*	*How to take*	*How many*	*How often*	*Comments*
_____	_____	_____	_____	_____	_____
_____	_____	_____	_____	_____	_____
_____	_____	_____	_____	_____	_____

Constipation is a very common problem when taking opioid medications. When this happens, do the following:

- Increase fluid intake (8 to 10 glasses of fluid per day).
- Exercise regularly.
- Increase fiber in the diet (bran, fresh fruits, vegetables).
- Use a mild laxative, such as milk of magnesia, if no bowel movement in 3 days.
- Take _____ every day at _____ (time) with a full glass of water.
- Use a glycerin suppository every morning (this may help make a bowel movement less painful).

Nondrug pain control methods:

_____

_____

_____

Additional instructions:

_____

_____

_____

Important phone numbers:
Your doctor _____
Your nurse _____
Your pharmacy _____
Emergencies _____
Call your doctor or nurse immediately if your pain increases or if you have new pain. Also call your doctor early for a refill of pain medicines. Do not let your medicines get below 3 or 4 days' supply.

Cancer Pain Management Guidelines Panel. (1994). *Managing cancer pain: Patient guide.* AHCPR Pub. 94-0595. Rockville, MD: Agency for Health Care Policy and Research. Public Health Service, US Department of Health and Human Services.

---

ment computer-assisted instruction with personal, human attention.

Contractual Agreements

A **contractual agreement** is a pact between two people made for the achievement of mutually set goals. Contracts between nurses and patients are becoming a common practice in many healthcare settings. The contracts are usually informal and not legally binding. When the nurse is teaching a patient, such an agreement can serve to motivate both the patient and the nurse to do what is necessary to meet the patient's learning objectives. The agreement points out the responsibilities of both the teacher and the learner, thus emphasizing the importance of the mutual commitment (see the accompanying box). Nurses can redirect "failed" teaching efforts to meet

What to Do if You Have One or More Heart Attack Warning Signs

Patient's Name: _____

Physicians now have treatments that can stop heart attacks and lessen damage to the heart. To make sure you can benefit from these treatments, you need to act promptly if you begin to experience symptoms that might signal a heart attack.

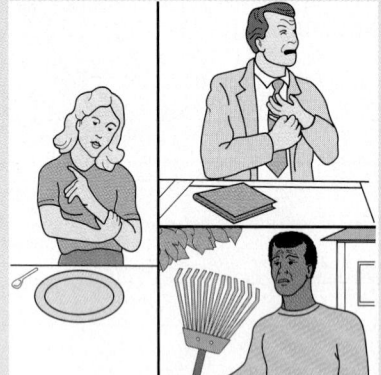

1. **This is what you may feel:**
   • Chest pain, discomfort, or pressure
   • Left arm pain or discomfort
   • Pain radiating to your neck or jaw
   • Shortness of breath
   • Sweating
   • Upset stomach
   • Discomfort in the area between your breastbone and navel
   • A sense of dread
   • Other: _____

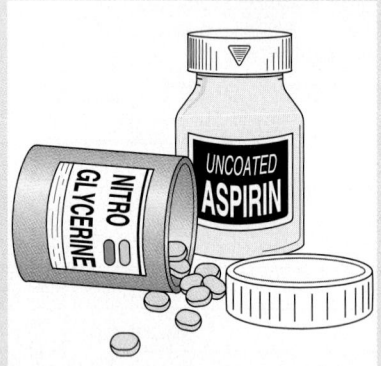

2. **Medication instructions:**
   • Chew one 325-mg tablet of uncoated adult aspirin.
   • Place one tablet of nitroglycerin under your tongue as soon as you feel discomfort. Take a second tablet if the discomfort does not go away in 5 minutes. Take a third tablet after 5 more minutes if the discomfort does not go away.
   • Other: _____

3. **If the symptoms stop, call your physician at:** _____

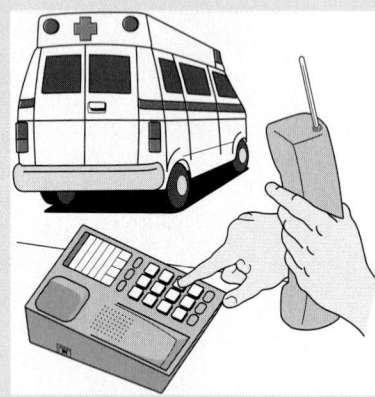

4. **If symptoms continue for more than 15 minutes, call the emergency medical services phone number below immediately. (Often this is 9-1-1, but you should check to make sure.) Never wait longer than 15 minutes.**
   At home, the emergency phone number is: _____
   At work, the emergency phone number is: _____
   At _____, the emergency phone number is: _____
   _____

(continued)

What to Do if You Have One or More Heart Attack Warning Signs (*Continued*)

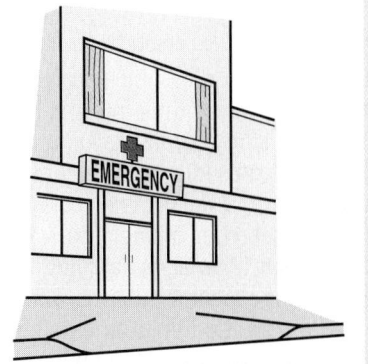

5. Know the location of the nearest 24-hour emergency department.

At home, the closest emergency department is: _____

At work, the closest emergency department is _____

At _____ , the closest emergency department is: _____

_____

Place this form next to the phone, near your other emergency numbers!

Signed: _____ MD/RN

Adapted with permission from the US Department of Health and Human Services, the Public Health Service, the National Institutes of Health, and the National Heart, Lung, and Blood Institute.

---

contracted objectives into new learning and decision-making situations and boost the patient's self-esteem by rewarding those objectives that were achieved.

Learning Activities

While planning teaching strategies, the nurse also decides what learning activities the patient is to do independently. There are many ways that the patient can preview new material or reinforce what has already been taught. Printed material, AV materials, and programmed instruction materials are often assigned in the learning activity column of the teaching plan. This column is used to guide the patient in learning activities that can be done before, between, and after planned learning sessions. The accompanying Research in Nursing display describes the success of a project to prepare older patients to become more active in their care by learning to conduct health information searches on the Internet.

Practical Considerations

Time Constraints. Time constraints must be considered when planning for the patient's learning. Nurses often have a problem finding time to meet patients' learning needs. Priorities must be set so that essential content is taught thoroughly. Less important content is taught last so that the more important learner objectives are met within the time available. If time permits, the remaining content can be addressed. Note that in the sample teaching plan, women are taught measures to use immediately.

To meet time constraints, nurses often plan together. Teamwork and cooperation allow nurses to meet deadlines. If teaching must continue beyond the hospitalization, home visit, or clinic visit, the nurse can schedule additional learning opportunities through outpatient programs or referrals to community-based programs. Home healthcare nurses often receive referrals from hospital nurses to continue teaching begun during a patient's hospitalization. Discharge planning must be started early to ensure continuity of teaching.

Scheduling. It is better to plan for shorter, more frequent teaching sessions than for one or two longer sessions. Short sessions allow patients to digest the new material and prevent them from becoming too tired or uncomfortable because of a health problem. Sessions of 15 to 30 minutes are generally well tolerated. Usually, more formal classroom programs last for more than 1 hour. In such cases, the nurse should provide breaks after every 50 minutes of class

> ### Example of a Contractual Agreement Between a Nurse and a Client
>
> I will participate in the learning activities needed to help me learn about my low-salt diet. During my hospital stay, I will attend the class on low-salt diets, read the materials given to me, and ask questions as I need to. I will work with S. Moore, RN, to plan my meals and food preparation at home. If I need help when I get home, I will contact S. Moore.
>
> *Jim Mall*
>
> I will provide Jim Mall with the experiences needed for him to follow his low-salt diet accurately.
>
> *S. Moore RN*

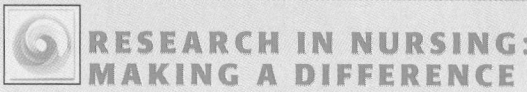

RESEARCH IN NURSING: MAKING A DIFFERENCE

Promoting Active Roles in Health Education

Advances in scientific knowledge and related health information and sharp decreases in the amount of time available for one-on-one health education are making it imperative for patients and the public to assume more independent and active roles in health education.

Related Research
Leaffer, T., & Gonda, B. (2000). The Internet: An underutilized tool in patient education. *Computers in Nursing, 18*(1), 47–52.

This two-stage pilot study involved 100 senior citizens who received instruction on how to conduct health information searches on the Internet. The

goals were to enable the seniors to assume an active role in their healthcare and to share their information with family and friends. The study results reveal a positive effect of the training on senior trainee confidence in using the computer and the Internet, conducting health information searches online, and sharing information with their physicians, families, and friends. Two thirds of the research subjects who searched for health information on the Internet talked about it with their physicians, with more than half reporting that they were more satisfied with treatment as a result of their searches and subsequent discussion with their physicians.

time. The patient should be included in planning for the time and frequency of lessons.

Group Versus Individual Teaching. The nurse must consider several factors when choosing the teaching setting for the patient. Some learner objectives are met more readily in a one-to-one encounter (Fig. 22-2), whereas others are achieved more easily in a group. For example, the objective "The patient will change the dressing using sterile tech-

nique" would be taught and evaluated during a private session with the nurse. The objective "The patient will discuss feelings about returning home after a heart attack" might be met more easily in a group discussion with other patients.

Formal Versus Informal Teaching. Most nurse–patient interactions can include **informal teaching** by the nurse. These unplanned teaching sessions are often effective because they deal with the patient's immediate learning needs and concerns. Informal teaching may also lead to additional planned, formal sessions. **Formal teaching** is the planned teaching done to fulfill learner objectives. Both forms are effective when used appropriately.

Implementing the Teaching Plan

Implementing the teaching plan requires use of interpersonal skills and effective communication techniques. Teaching the patient can be a major part of the working phase of the helping relationship (see Chap. 21). The nurse must continually observe the patient for additional assessment data that could alter the original teaching plan. This requires skill in adapting and reorganizing the teaching plan.

The nurse can facilitate patient learning by continuing a warm and accepting approach. The nurse's attitude has more effect on the patient than any other factor (Fig. 22-3). The nurse must avoid a condescending attitude. Moreover, it is always better not to use technical and medical terms unless the patient has a background in this area. A nonthreatening teaching–learning atmosphere allows learning to occur.

The physical environment is another important consideration when implementing the teaching plan. Some planning may be needed to ensure adequate space and lighting, comfortable chairs, and good ventilation. Privacy is also important, as is freedom from distractions and interruptions.

In the implementation phase, the patient as a learner has certain role functions. To avoid any misunderstandings, it is

Figure 22-2
One-to-one teaching is used in many patient–nurse situations. The nurse must be able to assess whether individual teaching is needed or whether learning can occur in a group. (Photo by Gates Rhodes, courtesy of School of Nursing, University of Pennsylvania.)

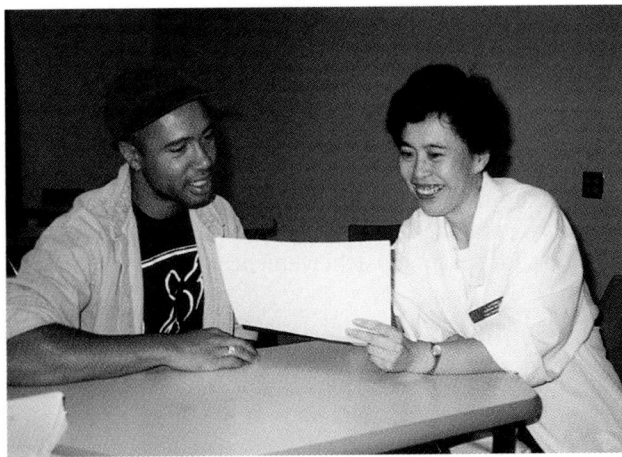

Figure 22-3
The nurse's warm approach is an important factor in interpersonal relationships.

helpful to review the contractual agreement before implementing the teaching plan. The patient is expected to listen, observe, and attempt to understand what is being taught.

Some people are uncomfortable in the role of learner; the nurse must assess this problem so that the patient can be assisted to assume the role more easily. If special techniques or procedures must be learned (eg, colostomy care, self-injections, or eye medication instillation), the nurse can assure the patient that it takes time and practice before anyone can perform new skills confidently.

The nurse must be prepared and organized before implementing the teaching plan. All teaching aids (eg, posters, films, or printed materials) should be gathered and organized before the actual teaching session. A disorganized teacher distracts the learner and has a negative effect on the learning. Also, a procedure or skill must be taught in the correct sequence so that the patient does not become confused.

An important nursing responsibility is to make each learning session interesting and enjoyable for the patient. This is facilitated by an enthusiastic and positive attitude. In addition, nurses can make learning fun through the creative use of planned teaching strategies. When nurses approach teaching positively, the patient is more likely to approach learning in a similar way.

Evaluating Teaching–Learning

Evaluating Learning

Nurses cannot assume that patients have in fact learned the content unless there is some type of proof or feedback. The key to evaluation is the learner objectives in the teaching plan, which describe what behaviors to measure. Methods for obtaining feedback about learning are discussed in the following section.

Methods of Evaluation

There are several methods of evaluation. For instance, cognitive domain learning may be evaluated through oral questioning; affective domain, through the patient's response; and psychomotor domain, by return demonstration. Consider the following learner objective in the cognitive domain: "The patient will be able to describe what a blood pressure reading represents." To evaluate this, the nurse could say to the patient, "Tell me what this blood pressure reading means to you." The patient then has a chance to talk about the current reading while the nurse evaluates the patient's understanding of it.

Sometimes, the nurse can use observational skills to determine whether the patient is using the material learned. For example, observing what the patient has ordered for lunch shows the nurse whether dietary lessons are being put into practice. The nurse depends on observation when evaluating the patient's psychomotor skills. The nurse observes the patient's demonstration of any new technique or skill to determine whether it is performed satisfactorily.

The patient's comments are also used to decide whether learner objectives have been met. Sometimes, a patient verbalizes his or her understanding of the information yet avoids further discussion of the topic. In such instances, using effective communication techniques when reintroducing the topic at a later time might provide the evaluation data needed.

Using direct questions often provides an efficient method of evaluating learner objectives. The nurse simply asks the patient a question to elicit a response that reflects the patient's level of knowledge about a topic. Direct questions can also be used to evaluate the patient's affective learning.

A return demonstration is an excellent evaluative method for learning in the psychomotor domain (Fig. 22-4). Letting the patient change his or her own dressing, for example, provides the nurse with concrete evidence of satisfactory or unsatisfactory performance of the procedure. Care must be taken to promote a nonstressful environment for the patient's return demonstration.

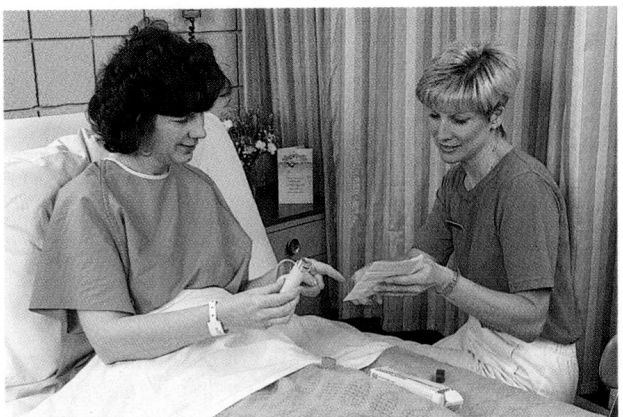

Figure 22-4
One type of evaluation is to ask the patient questions concerning what he or she has been taught. (Photo © B. Proud.)

Timing of Evaluation

Evaluation of learning is ongoing. If the nurse merely evaluates learning as soon as teaching is completed, results may be misleading. Home healthcare nurses may evaluate what the patient learned in the hospital as well as what is being taught during home visits. Hospital nurses often check with family members or significant others after discharge to evaluate whether learner objectives have been met.

Reinforcing and Celebrating Learning

Most people feel encouraged and supported when their efforts are acknowledged by another person, especially when they trust and value the other person. This is especially true in healthcare, where patients often feel overwhelmed by their illness. Nurses who recognize this dynamic can use **positive reinforcement** to affirm the efforts of patients who have mastered new knowledge, attitudes, or skills. Reinforcement may be as simple as a few words of acknowledgment—"You've mastered this diet quickly"; as spontaneous as a warm hug; or as planned as the entire staff joining to celebrate a patient's independent ambulation. **Negative reinforcement**—criticism or punishment—is generally ineffective; undesirable behavior is usually best ignored. Behavior modification programs that reward desired behaviors and ignore undesired behaviors may be designed for some patients.

Evaluating Teaching

Nurses need to evaluate their teaching to capitalize on their strengths and work on improving weaknesses. Like all nursing roles, effective teaching requires practice and experience. Even nurse educators agree that they are always learning better ways to promote learning. It is important to avoid becoming discouraged when evaluations of one's teaching are less than perfect.

It is best to evaluate one's own teaching effectiveness immediately after a teaching session. This involves a quick review of how well the nurse-teacher feels the plan was implemented. Mentally noting both the strengths and weaknesses of the teaching session helps the nurse plan better for subsequent sessions.

Nurses can also seek feedback from patients. A simple questionnaire can be used at the end of a teaching session or after discharge to gain the patient's perception of the nurse's teaching effectiveness. The questionnaire may be a standardized form used throughout the hospital or agency or one prepared by the nurse-teacher. When using an objective format that requires only circles or checkmarks as answers, space should be provided for comments.

Revising the Plan

During evaluation, nurses and patients may decide that revisions are needed in the teaching plan. A reassessment may indicate that some patient factors were not considered in the original plan. Adjustments may be made accordingly to meet the patient's needs. Often, the use of a different teaching strategy is all that is needed for a patient to achieve learner objectives. Revision is a natural part of the teaching–learning process and should not be viewed negatively.

Neither the nurse nor the patient has failed when an objective is not met. Most objectives can be met with a change in approach, although sometimes the learner objectives are unrealistic. Further assessment by the nurse may reveal that the content may be too complex or the time too short for successful achievement.

Documenting

The nurse is legally responsible to document teaching in the patient's record. Documentation of the teaching–learning process includes a summary of the learning need, the plan, the implementation of the plan, and the evaluation results. The evaluative statement is crucial and must show what concrete evidence demonstrates that learning has occurred. If the desired learning has not occurred, the nurse's notes should indicate how the problem was resolved. It is insufficient to document only what was taught. The charting has to show evidence that the patient or significant other has actually learned the material taught. See the SOAPIER note for an example of documentation.

Documentation Using a Problem-Oriented Progress Note to Meet a Learning Need

1/3/00   #2   New Problem—High Risk for Impaired Skin Integrity: Nipples

S —Patient stated that her nipples were sore during and after her newborn's first feeding

O—First day postpartum; patient is fair skinned with freckles; no reddened areas, no cracking yet; no nipple preparation before delivery

A—At high risk for cracked, open areas; patient lacks experience and knowledge of preventive measures

P—Reinforce teaching plan for nipple care

I —Teaching plan implemented

E—Patient able to meet all of the objectives satisfactorily as recorded on the teaching plan; she is currently doing protective and preparatory care for her nipples; when breastfeeding, she uses the correct feeding technique with good aftercare; she states that her nipples are no longer sore, and she is able to explain what she should do when she goes home

R—None needed, but reinforcement of content will be continued

—L. Sweeney, RN

The Nurse as Counselor

Counseling is the interpersonal process of assisting patients to make decisions that promote their overall well-being. Family members or significant others are often included in counseling sessions. Everyone participating must feel comfortable in the situation and surroundings. Like teaching, counseling may be formal or informal.

The interpersonal skills of warmth, friendliness, openness, and empathy are necessary for successful counseling. An effective counselor needs to be a caring individual. Caring is based on a humanistic philosophy (Watson, 1985), which is the core of nursing practice. A humanistic approach to counseling rooted in professional caring helps the patient strive toward the greatest health potential. Caring is important in all nursing roles but is fundamental in the counseling role.

Some advanced-practice psychiatric mental health nurses specialize in counseling, and this form of counseling has an important professional role. The focus in this chapter, however, is on the everyday counseling that is a basic component of all nurses' practice. This counseling involves listening carefully to the patient's or family's questions, concerns, demands, and complaints and then responding in an effective and facilitative manner. Appropriate responses may be difficult for the nurse at first, but practice helps develop this skill. Each nurse–patient (or nurse–family) interaction is unique. A nursing response that works well with one patient may intimidate or anger another. Sensitivity to the unique needs of each patient and a willingness to get involved and make a difference are essential for effective counseling. Table 22-1 presents typical counseling situations you might experience in your first year of nursing and analyzes both effective and ineffective nursing responses. You may want to role play these situations with a friend. Nurses who wish to succeed as a caregiver and counselor need to master the communication techniques described in Chapter 21.

In counseling situations, the nurse does not tell the patient what to do to solve the problem but instead assists and guides problem solving or decision making. Many people lack the knowledge and skills to approach a problem systematically. The nurse combines the teaching and counseling roles to help such a patient solve the dilemma successfully. The accompanying box, Promoting Lifestyle Changes, highlights the counseling steps an interdisciplinary team takes when promoting lifestyle changes in their award-winning patient education program to reduce cardiovascular risk (Chu Lai & Cohen, 1999).

The nursing process is an essential tool for the nurse when guiding and teaching the patient. Nurses are educated to approach all nursing situations in a logical, systematic way. In a crisis situation, whether minor or major, the nurse can share problem-solving abilities with the patient. The

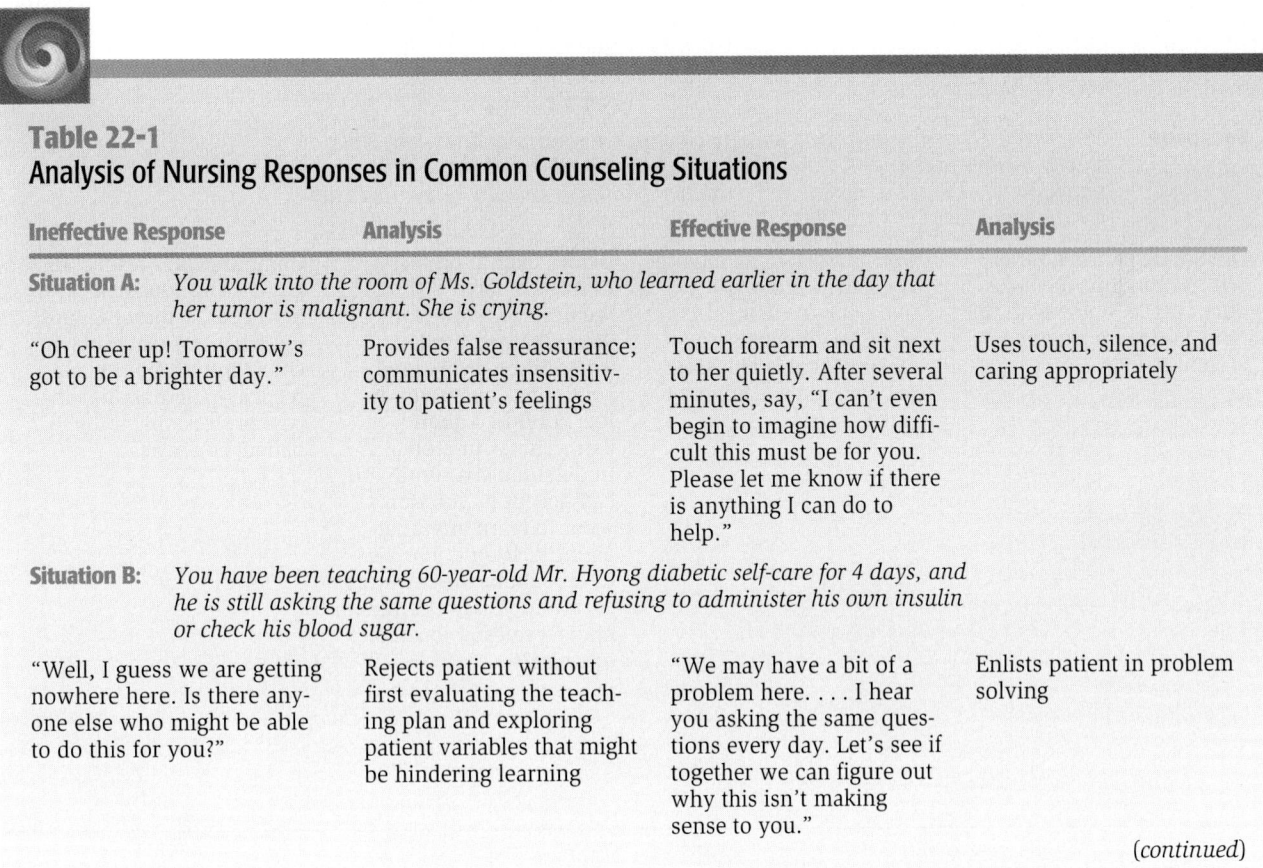

Table 22-1
Analysis of Nursing Responses in Common Counseling Situations

Ineffective Response	Analysis	Effective Response	Analysis
Situation A: You walk into the room of Ms. Goldstein, who learned earlier in the day that her tumor is malignant. She is crying.			
"Oh cheer up! Tomorrow's got to be a brighter day."	Provides false reassurance; communicates insensitivity to patient's feelings	Touch forearm and sit next to her quietly. After several minutes, say, "I can't even begin to imagine how difficult this must be for you. Please let me know if there is anything I can do to help."	Uses touch, silence, and caring appropriately
Situation B: You have been teaching 60-year-old Mr. Hyong diabetic self-care for 4 days, and he is still asking the same questions and refusing to administer his own insulin or check his blood sugar.			
"Well, I guess we are getting nowhere here. Is there anyone else who might be able to do this for you?"	Rejects patient without first evaluating the teaching plan and exploring patient variables that might be hindering learning	"We may have a bit of a problem here. . . . I hear you asking the same questions every day. Let's see if together we can figure out why this isn't making sense to you."	Enlists patient in problem solving

(continued)

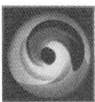

Table 22-1 (Continued)

Ineffective Response	Analysis	Effective Response	Analysis
Situation C: *One morning you walk into the room of an older resident who had withdrawn and become totally dependent on the nurses for basic care on her transfer into the nursing home. You are surprised to discover that she has washed and dressed herself—for the first time.*			
"Well, I'm happy to see that you have rejoined the ranks of the living. Did you wash off your glasses?"	Misses opportunity to celebrate the resident's achievement of an important goal	Hugs resident warmly, looks her in the eye, and exclaims, "Don't you look wonderful today? What are you celebrating?" Defers an assessment of how thorough the morning care has been until later.	Rejoices spontaneously in the resident's achievement and reinforces this behavior. Gives the resident a reason to continue to make progress. Uses touch appropriately
Situation D: *You are helping Mr. Stein, who has been on bed rest for 2 weeks because of a painful and debilitating illness, out of bed. A fiercely independent man, he is embarrassed to need your support and looks disgusted with himself when he steps on your foot.*			
"What's the problem, Honey? Haven't been eating your Wheaties?"	Uses terms of endearment, which often denote disrespect and condescension to patients, no matter in what spirit they are uttered	"No problem, Mr. Stein, my husband steps on my toes all the time when we go dancing!" After a few minutes . . . "It must be hard when you are used to doing everything for yourself to all of the sudden find yourself needing others for simple things . . . ?"	Uses humor and empathy appropriately; invites the patient to share his feelings
Situation E: *Ms. Berretta recently underwent surgery resulting in a urinary diversion. She should be able to change her own ostomy bag by this time, but she is still unwilling to look at the stoma, and participate alone in her care. The nurses are getting impatient with her "childish" refusals to learn.*			
"Really Helen, I'll do it myself but you'll be the loser once you get home with this thing and there's no one around to help."	Uses a threat in an attempt to coerce learning (negative reinforcement). Displays unwillingness to explore what is blocking Ms. Berretta's readiness to learn	Before beginning Ms. Berretta's care: "I think we need to talk before your treatment today. You will be discharged soon, and I want you to feel confident about caring for your stoma. I understand that until you can accept it, you don't want to learn anything about it. Would you like to talk about this with me, or would you prefer me to make a referral to someone else?"	Communicates respect for patient and sensitivity to her needs, without ignoring what is a real problem. Offers the possibility of a referral to another healthcare professional if the patient so wishes

Promoting Lifestyle Changes

Helping Patients Through the Stages of Change

Matching behavior-modification strategies to the stage of behavior change can facilitate patients' progress from one stage to the next and enhance long-term maintenance of new, healthier behaviors.

Stage: Precontemplation
Counseling Steps:
- Recommend lifestyle change; for example, walking 30 minutes daily as a goal.
- Provide personalized information, focusing on the patient's condition.

Stage: Contemplation
Counseling Steps:
- Identify patient willingness to change within the next 6 months.
- Discuss risks and benefits of behavior change to health. For example, patients may view possible weight gain with smoking cessation as a risk of behavior change.
- Examine barriers to change and past attempts to modify behavior.
- Explore the motivations that would keep the patient focused on changing behavior.
- Explain alternative means of achieving the behavioral goal; for example, using relaxation breathing rather than walking to help lower blood pressure.
- Provide self-help information materials, such as lists of low-fat foods.
- Refer to other resources for help, such as social support groups, psychiatric counseling, or a social worker.

Stage: Action
Counseling Steps:
- Set a date to start behavior modification.
- Outline concrete plans and develop strategies to integrate new behavior into current activities of daily living.
- Discuss potential problems and barriers based on past experiences or current obstacles.
- Investigate strategies to overcome barriers.
- Negotiate an achievable plan, allowing patients to set small intermediate goals.
- Review how to use social and professional support systems.
- Discuss potential for behavior relapse, emphasizing that it is not a personal failure, but a learning experience.

Stage: Maintenance
Counseling Steps:
- Examine parts of the plan that were helpful; identify potential and current problems.
- Revise plans and reset goals if necessary.
- Establish a schedule for periodic contact and follow-up.

Stage: Relapse
Counseling Steps:
- Identify triggers for relapse and barriers that prevented behavior maintenance.
- Discuss and reevaluate motivation to change behaviors, allowing patients to redevelop strategies to overcome barriers.
- Revisit counseling steps for precontemplation and contemplation stages, including additional referrals.

From Chu Lai, S., & Cohen, M. N. (1999). Promoting lifestyle changes. *American Journal of Nursing 99*(4), 66.

nursing process is used to organize the nurse–patient counseling situation described in the accompanying box.

Diagnosing Counseling Needs

NANDA-approved nursing diagnoses for which counseling may be indicated include the following:

Altered Parenting
Altered Role Performance
Anxiety
Body Image Disturbance
Decisional Conflict
Dysfunctional Grieving
Fear
Health Seeking Behavior (specify)
Hopelessness

Impaired Adjustment
Impaired Social Interaction
Ineffective Denial
Ineffective Family Coping
Ineffective Individual Coping
Personal Identity Disturbance
Powerlessness
Self-Esteem Disturbance
Social Isolation
Spiritual Distress

Types of Counseling

Counseling may be situational, developmental, or motivational, and short-term or long-term. *Short-term counseling* focuses on the immediate problem or concern of the patient or family. It can be a relatively minor concern or a major crisis, but in any case, it needs immediate attention (Fig. 22-5). Short-term counseling may be used during a **situational crisis**, which occurs when a patient faces an event or situation that causes a disruption in life. For example, a male patient in the hospital finds out that his spouse has been involved in a car accident; she received only a few scratches, but their only car was demolished. The nurse is in an excellent position to help the patient decide what can be done to solve this situational crisis. The nurse can guide the patient to resources to help solve the travel, financial, and emotional difficulties that arise as a result of the accident. This holistic approach is especially necessary because the crisis could adversely affect the patient's recovery.

Long-term counseling extends over a prolonged period. A patient may need the counsel of the nurse at daily, weekly, or monthly intervals. A patient experiencing a developmental crisis, for example, may need long-term counseling. A **developmental crisis** can occur when a person is going through a developmental stage or passage. For example, many women going through menopause need the assistance of a nurse when adjusting to changes they experience. Nurses may also lead support groups for group counseling.

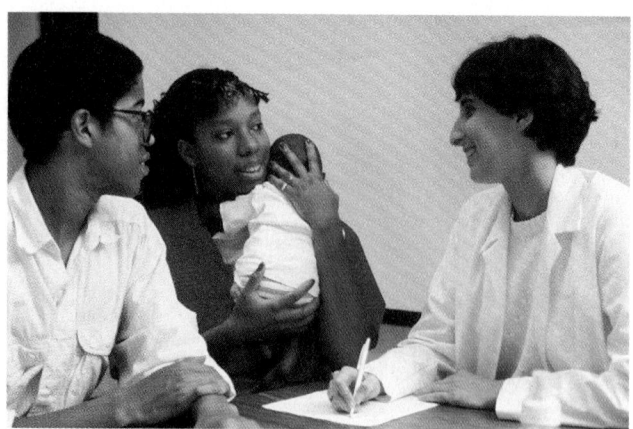

Figure 22-5
Counseling may involve a relatively minor concern that needs immediate attention. (Photo by Gates Rhodes, courtesy of School of Nursing, University of Pennsylvania.)

Motivational counseling involves discussing feelings and incentives with the patient. Nurses often become frustrated because their patients do not seem to want to get better or to learn how to care for themselves. Perhaps some

---

Short-Term Counseling

An Example of Problem Solving That Follows the Nursing Process

Situation
Monday, 7:30 PM, Amy Purcell has been admitted to the children's unit with dehydration resulting from diarrhea. Amy is responding well to intravenous (IV) fluids. Her mother is visibly distraught.

Assessing
Amy is doing well but will need 24 hours of IV therapy.

Amy and her twin sister Susan have never been separated from their parents or each other. They are 2 years old.

Ms. Purcell has no idea who will care for Susan when Mr. Purcell goes to work in the morning.

The Purcells have no regular childcare arrangements and have no family members in the area.

Ms. Purcell wants to stay with Amy during her hospitalization.

The Purcells' neighbor is home during the day. Sometimes Amy and Susan play at her house.

There is a daycare center near their home, but Susan might be upset about going there. It's also expensive.

Mr. Purcell cannot afford to take Tuesday off but will take Wednesday morning off.

Insurance does not cover a private room, which would allow Susan to come to stay in the hospital too.

Diagnosing
Anxiety related to stress of daughter's hospitalization, need for childcare for Susan, and uncertain resources.

Planning Goal
Ms. Purcell will demonstrate decreased anxiety over the care of Susan during Amy's hospitalization.

Together, Ms. Purcell and the nurse have planned the following:

- The neighbor will come to the Purcell home to care for Susan when Mr. Purcell leaves for work on Tuesday morning.
- The neighbor will bring Susan to the hospital for the afternoon visiting hours to be with Ms. Purcell and Amy.
- Mr. Purcell will come to the hospital after work to have dinner with the family.
- Mr. Purcell will take Susan home for bedtime.
- On Wednesday morning, Mr. Purcell will take off work in the morning. He and Susan will go to the hospital to pick up Ms. Purcell and Amy.

Implementing
Plan implemented by the Purcells with support of the nursing staff.

Evaluating
Ms. Purcell told the nurse that she feels that both Amy and Susan did well with the care they received from their parents. The family's stress was minimized, and she is relieved that everything went so well. The nurse decides that the goals were met.

patients do not have the inner drive or motivation to co-operate in their own healthcare. Some patients state, "I have nothing to live for." A nurse who has established a helping relationship with the patient can help him or her work through these feelings of despair. The nurse may be able to get the patient to talk about what is generating dis-interest in recovery. If a problem is identified, the nurse and patient can use the problem-solving technique to work toward an acceptable solution.

If a patient shows an unwillingness to participate in learning activities, the nurse can assess any factors from the past or present that might be negatively influencing motiva-tion for learning. Sometimes, if the nurse explains the need for certain knowledge and the consequences of not learning the material, the patient will become more receptive to the teaching–learning process. A trial learning session can be suggested to allow the patient to see what the sessions will be like. If the nurse uses the nursing process approach for counseling, the patient may become more motivated (see the accompanying box, Short-Term Counseling).

When a nurse assesses a motivational problem, con-sidering the patient's cultural values is important. Often, the way a person feels about something is strongly influenced by cultural background. For instance, if a person has grown up in a family in which illness is perceived as an inevitable result of aging, it will be difficult to motivate that person to practice preventive measures for health (see Chap. 3). These problems seem insurmountable, yet a caring nurse can work toward helping the patient become oriented to self-health. When discouraged, the nurse can confer with a col-league to help solve patient-centered problems.

Referrals

Sometimes, a patient needs specialized counseling by nurses with advanced training or by other healthcare professionals. In these cases, the best thing you can offer the patient is a referral to the appropriate professional (eg, psychiatric or mental health nurse, psychologist or psychiatrist, social worker, clergy, financial counselor, sex therapist, or occupational therapist). In other cases, a simple referral to a community resource, such as a neighborhood support group, may be all the patient needs. When making a referral, be sure to address any barriers that may prevent the patient from acting on the referral. Patients may fail to follow-up with a referral for financial reasons, because they do not understand the reason for or value the referral, because they lack trans-portation, or because the agency is not open at times when they are free.

Learning Outcomes

After completing this chapter, the learner should be able to accomplish the following:

1. Define the key terms used in the chapter:

affective learning	learning readiness
androgogy	literacy
cognitive learning	negative reinforcement
contractual agreement	pedagogy
counseling	positive reinforcement
developmental crisis	psychomotor learning
formal teaching	situational crisis
informal teaching	teaching
learning	

2. Describe the teaching–learning process, including domains, developmental concerns, and specific principles.

3. Describe what factors should be assessed in the learning process.
4. Formulate diagnoses for identified learning needs.
5. Explain how to create and implement a teaching plan for a patient.
6. Name three methods for evaluating learning.
7. Explain what should be included in the documenta-tion of the teaching–learning process.
8. Discuss the nurse's role as a counselor.
9. Summarize how the nursing process is used to assist patients in problem solving.
10. Describe how to use the counseling role to motivate a patient toward health promotion.

Critical Thinking Exercises

1. Explain what is meant by the following statement: "It is as important for patients to understand and value the **why** of the proposed treatment regimen as it is for them to understand **how** to implement the proposed regimen." What are the implications of this for teaching and counseling?
2. A patient your age has just learned that she has tested positive for the human immunodeficiency virus. Make a list of some of the learning (cognitive, psychomotor, affective) that you think should take place. What sorts of things might affect her readiness to learn? How would you tailor your nursing in response to these variables?
3. Mrs. Riley is being readmitted to your hospital unit with complications related to her diabetes. A co-worker voices her frustrations and says, "We've taught her everything she needs to know to do a better job of managing her diabetes. I don't know what more we can do." How do you respond?

Bibliography

American Nurses Association. (1994). *The scope of practice for nursing informatics.* Washington, DC: Author.

Aquilera, D. C. (1994). *Crisis intervention: Theory and methodology* (7th ed.). St. Louis: Mosby–Year Book.

Archbold, P. G., et al. (1995). The PREP system of nursing intervention: A pilot test with families caring for older members. *Research in Nursing and Health, 18*(1), 3–16.

Babcock, D. E., & Miller, M. A. (1994). *Patient education: Theory and practice.* St. Louis: C. V. Mosby.

Barnes, L. P. (1994). Useful tools in patient teaching: Interviewing skills. *MCN, 19*(5), 289.

Black, K. (1983). *Short-term counseling: A humanistic approach for the helping professions.* Menlo Park, CA: Addison-Wesley.

Bloom, B. S. (1956). *Taxonomy of educational objectives: The classification of educational goals.* New York: David McKay.

Bolwell, C. (1993). *Directory of education software for nursing* (5th ed.). New York: National League for Nursing; Athens, OH: Fuld Institute for Technology in Nursing Education.

Brazen, L., & Roth, R. A. (1995). Using learning style preferences for perioperative clinical education. *AORN Journal, 61*(1), 189, 191–195.

Canobbio, M. M. (1996). *Mosby's handbook of patient teaching.* St. Louis: C. V. Mosby.

Chu Lai, S., & Cohen, M. N. (1999). Promoting lifestyle changes. *American Journal of Nursing 99*(4), 63–67.

Cordell, B., & Smith-Blair, N. (1994). Streamlined charting for patient education. *Nursing, 24*(1), 57–59.

Dellasega, C., Clark, D., McCreary, D., Schan, P., & Helmuth, A. (1994). Nursing process: Teaching elderly patients. *Journal of Gerontological Nursing, 20*(1), 31–41.

Doak, C. C., Doak, L. G., & Root, J. H. (1995). *Teaching patients with low literacy skills.* Philadelphia: J. B. Lippincott.

Elliot, L., & Kulwicki, G. (1993). Improving patient education documentation. *Nursing Management, 24*(10), 61–62.

Farthing, M. (1994). Health education needs of a Hutterite colony. *The Canadian Nurse, 90*(7), 20–26.

Griffiths, M. (1995). Patient education needs: Opinions of oncology nurses and their patients. *Oncology Nursing Forum, 22*(1), 139–144.

Hannah, K. J., Ball, M. J., & Edwards, M. J. A. (1994). *Introduction to nursing informatics.* New York: Springer-Verlag.

Harvey, C., Dixon, M. & Padberg, N. (1995). Support group for families of trauma patients: A unique approach. *Critical Care Nurse, 15*(4), 59–63.

Hussey, L. C. (1994). Minimizing effects of low literacy on medication knowledge and compliance among the elderly. *Clinical Nursing Research, 3*(2), 132–145.

Jabeck, M. E. (1994). Teaching the elderly: A commonsense approach. *Nursing, 24*(5), 70–71.

Jacono, B., & Jacono, J. (1995). The impact of teacher characteristics on teaching. *Journal of Nursing Staff Development, 11*(3), 146–149.

Kelly, P. (1992). Counseling patients with HIV. *RN, 55*(2), 54–58.

Knowles, M. S. (1990). *The adult-learner: A neglected species* (4th ed.). Houston: Gulf Publishing.

Leaffer, T., & Gonda, B. (2000). The Internet: An underutilized tool in patient education. *Computers in Nursing, 18*(1), 47–52.

Lindberg, C. E. (1995). Perinatal transmission of HIV: How to counsel women. *MCN, 20*(4), 207–212.

Lorig, K. (1992). *Patient education: A practical approach.* St. Louis: Mosby–Year Book.

Melnyle, B. M. (1994). Coping with unplanned childhood hospitalization: Effects of informational intervention on mother and children. *Nursing Research, 43*(1), 50–55.

Miller, B. (1994). Determination of reading comprehension level for effective patient health education materials. *Nursing Research, 43*(2), 118–119.

Newbold, S. K. (1996). Maximizing technology for cost effective staff education and training. In B. R. Heller, M. E. Mills, & C. A. Romano (Eds.). *Information management in nursing and health care.* Springhouse, PA: Springhouse.

Price, J. L., & Cordell, B. (1994). Cultural diversity and patient teaching. *Journal of Continuing Education in Nursing, 25*(4), 163–166.

Rankin, S. H., & Stallings, K. D. (1990). *Patient education* (2nd ed.). Philadelphia: J. B. Lippincott.

Redman, B. K. (1992). *The process of patient education* (7th ed.). St. Louis: C. V. Mosby.

Reele, B. L. (1994). Effect of counseling on quality of life for individuals with cancer and their families. *Cancer Nursing, 17*(2), 101–112.

Ruppert, R. A. (1996). Caring for the lay caregiver. *American Journal of Nursing, 96*(3), 40–45.

Schoenly, L. (1994). Teaching in the affective domain. *Journal of Continuing Education in Nursing, 25*(5), 209–212.

Sciartelli, C. H. (1995). Using a clinical pathway approach to document patient teaching for breast cancer surgical procedures. *Oncology Nursing Forum, 22*(1), 139–144.

Seley, J. (1994). Ten strategies for successful patient teaching. *American Journal of Nursing, 94*(11), 63–65.

Sitzer, C. R. (1995). A community-based breast cancer education and screening program for elderly women. *Geriatric Nursing, 16*(4), 151–154.

Wally, B. (1994). Reading, writing and health. *Canadian Nurse, 90*(2), 29–32.

Watson, J. (1985). *Nursing: The philosophy and science of caring.* Denver: Colorado University Press.

Weaver, J. (1995). Patient education: An innovative computer approach. *Nursing Management, 26*(7), 78–83.

Weinrich, S. P., & Boyd, M. (1992). Education in the elderly: Adapting and evaluating teaching tools. *Journal of Gerontological Nursing, 18*(1), 15–20.

Wong, M. (1992). Self-care instructions: Do patients understand educational materials? *Focus on Critical Care, 19*(2), 47–49.

Chapter 23
Leader, Researcher, and Advocate

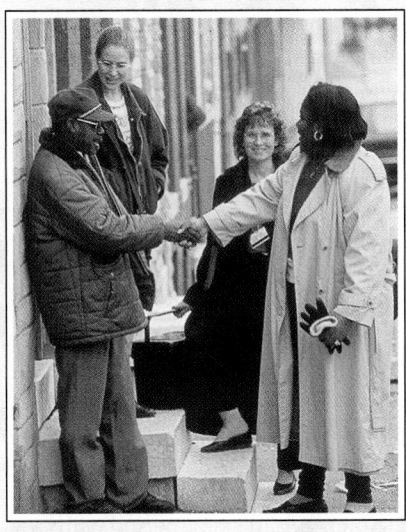

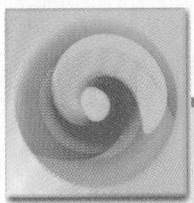

**Thinking Critically About
Nursing's Blended Skills**

Before reading this chapter, think about the types of blended skills you need to develop to become an effective leader, researcher, and advocate

- You are the newest "hire" on your orthopedic floor and have been "pulled" to other units the past three times there was a need for nurses in other areas. One of the experienced nurses tells you that it's not fair for you to be the one they always send, but there is no unit policy about who gets asked to float. You would like to be part of a solution to this problem and others like it—rather than just a "moaner-groaner"—but you aren't sure where to begin.

- A visiting nurse, you find yourself caring increasingly for couples in whom one of the spouses has advanced dementia. You are intrigued by the fact that although some family caregivers seem to cope very well with the demands on their time, energy, and good will, other spouses and families virtually fall apart—physically, mentally, and socially. You are thinking that if you could predict which families are at risk and help them to develop the resources present in the families that are coping effectively, you might help them significantly. A colleague says you have the start of a great research project.

- Emma, a woman you are caring for prenatally, tells you she wants to deliver her second child vaginally. Her first child was delivered by an emergency cesarean section. When she mentions this to the obstetrician, he tells her not to worry and that it is too early to think about this decision. You know that it is very possible that she could deliver vaginally but suspect that her obstetrician may try to convince her to have a repeat section simply because it is easier for him to avoid the risks of a vaginal delivery. You want to be an advocate for the woman.

What cognitive, interpersonal, and ethical/legal skills do you need to respond to the challenges described above?

Many changes in society and our healthcare system are jeopardizing human health and well-being and undermining nursing as a profession. Never before has there been such a need for nurses to work competently and collaboratively with other healthcare professionals to secure cost-effective quality healthcare for all. Never before has it been more important for nursing as a profession to be self-directed as it charts its future. To do all this successfully, nurses must be skilled leaders, advocates, and researchers. Nurse leaders use their abilities and skills to influence others to be their best and to achieve valued goals. Nurse advocates protect, support, and empower patients. They are committed to patient health and well-being and promote patient rights. Nurse researchers expand the body of nursing knowledge to learn improved ways to promote health and well-being.

Leadership, advocacy, and research are intertwined. Good leaders are strong advocates of patients' rights because leadership and advocacy complement each other. Research provides a knowledge base on which leaders and advocates can build. Research adds the dignity of **professionalism** to teaching, counseling, and communication—all nursing skills applied to the leadership role.

Although some nurses function as full-time leaders, researchers, or advocates, this chapter explores how the roles of leader, researcher, and advocate can enhance the basic caregiver role of nurses. It takes time and experience to develop these skills. Beginning nurses can monitor their progress by periodically reviewing the checklist provided in the accompanying box to help improve these skills.

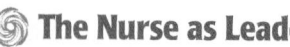

The Nurse as Leader

Leadership Dynamics

Leadership is the ability to direct or motivate an individual or group to achieve set goals. Effective leaders in groups or systems do this by encouraging others to be their best selves as they work collaboratively in the pursuit of common goals. Leaders have power, whether it is explicit or implied. For example, an elected class leader has explicit power by virtue of his or her position. A student in the class who has no designated leadership position, may, however, by force of his or her person, have more power to influence the class than designated leaders. This is implied power. Power to influence a group depends on the person's leadership style and how the person fulfills leadership responsibilities. The dynamics of leadership involve applying that power for growth or change. Nurses who use leadership skills can become proficient in effecting desired changes in many areas, including their patients' health patterns, the healthcare agency, the community, the nursing profession, and the healthcare system in general.

Leadership Qualities

Most people would agree that leaders should be dynamic, enthusiastic, and self-directed. Leaders need to be comfortable with themselves (ie, have a positive self-image) and present themselves as role models for followers. Ideally, leaders have a vision that energizes the group and brings forth the best efforts of members. Critical thinkers

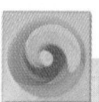

COGNITIVE SKILLS

- Basic knowledge of leadership and management theory, the research process, and advocacy responsibilities.

- Knowledge of the chain of command in hospitals, intervention strategies for the family caregivers of people with dementia, and the safety of vaginal deliveries in women who have previously delivered by cesarean section.

- Knowledge of who can help you when you first feel troubled by a workplace issue (unfair floating assignments) or clinical concerns.

INTERPERSONAL SKILLS

- Strong people skills; ability to communicate and interact effectively with nurse coworkers, patients, and family caregivers experiencing different levels

of stress, and with the obstetrician in your practice.

- Confidence in your own abilities and the willingness to get help when you need it.

ETHICAL/LEGAL SKILLS

- A strong sense of responsibility, accountability, and fair play.

- Knowledge of and respect for your rights as a worker, the pregnant woman's right to have her preferences respected when medically possible, and the rights of research subjects.

- The ability to document leadership, research, and advocacy interventions in a legally prudent and defensible manner.

Checklist for the Beginning Nurse Who Wishes to Develop Leadership, Research, and Advocacy Skills

Basic Attitudes and Skills

Read the statements on the right and circle the appropriate response: (1) rarely characterizes me, (2) sometimes characterizes me, and (3) often characterizes me.

☐ **1 2 3**   1. I am self-directed. I know what I want and take the necessary steps to get it.

☐ **1 2 3**   2. I know my strengths and limitations and feel confident with who I am and who I am becoming.

☐ **1 2 3**   3. I get an idea ("vision") and energize others to help me "make it happen."

☐ **1 2 3**   4. I coordinate or direct the activities of others, matching their abilities to the necessary task.

☐ **1 2 3**   5. I think critically about a situation without letting my feelings or those of others bias my analysis.

☐ **1 2 3**   6. Once I have identified a problem, I work at it until I resolve it—to the extent that this is within my power.

☐ **1 2 3**   7. When I need help, I know where to find it and ask for it.

☐ **1 2 3**   8. I recognize and encourage the talents of others and offer sincere compliments.

☐ **1 2 3**   9. I accept responsibility for my decisions and behavior.

☐ **1 2 3**   10. I accept compliments and enjoy my success.

☐ **1 2 3**   11. I confront individuals who are abusing my rights or those of others in my group.

☐ **1 2 3**   12. I use assertiveness techniques when defending rights.

☐ **1 2 3**   13. I am flexible and can change direction once I see the value of another course of action.

☐ **1 2 3**   14. I follow an appropriate chain of command when problem solving.

☐ **1 2 3**   15. I question how nursing interventions might be improved.

The higher your score the better. Reread the statements where you checked "1" and see how you might plan to improve in these areas.

Beginning Execution of Role Responsibilities: Leader, Researcher, Advocate

Read the list of behaviors on the right and check the appropriate box—met or not met.

Met   *Not Met*

_____ _____   1. Recognize some personal need you have been ignoring and take steps to ensure that it is met.

_____ _____   2. Think of some group you belong to (eg, school, work, church, or social) whose members' needs are not being met and plan with other members to tackle the problem.

_____ _____   3. Recognize the special advocacy needs of a patient you believe is being underserved by the healthcare system. Become an advocate for this patient.

_____ _____   4. Find a nursing research study that recommends a specific type of care for one of your patients. Implement the recommendation and compare your findings with those of the researchers.

_____ _____   5. Identify a researchable problem in your area of nursing practice. Describe what might make a good study.

_____ _____   6. Join a professional nursing organization and become an active member.

_____ _____   7. Analyze the media's portrayal of nurses in a specific television program, film, or book. Talk with a friend about how this portrayal of nursing influences your profession. Share your comments with the producer or author.

_____ _____   8. Contact your legislator to share your views about pending legislation.

_____ _____   9. Think about leaders you admire and respect; interview current nursing leaders; develop a plan for personal professional growth and development.

_____ _____   10. Develop a mentoring relationship with a nursing leader.

and responsible decision makers, they commit high energy to goal achievement and are skilled in enlisting support and cooperation.

Leaders value learning and must be knowledgeable. Because it is impossible for nurse leaders to be knowledgeable about all aspects of the profession, they develop and use resources effectively. They use one another and other healthcare workers as resources, respecting each other's expertise. Political awareness is also important for nurse leaders. Knowing how legislation at the local, state, and national levels affects healthcare helps nurses make informed decisions when voting for and supporting candidates.

Flexibility is a must for leaders. All nursing functions and roles require flexibility. The needs of patients, families, and the nursing team can change from minute to minute. A nurse coordinator may plan to involve staff in a discussion about how best to distribute new work responsibilities when three unexpected new admissions to the unit require postponing the discussion to a quieter time. Similarly, a visiting nurse may plan to dedicate more time to one dying patient and his wife when another patient on that day's caseload develops complications that require a longer visit. Flexible, responsive, and caring nurses are welcome leaders and team members.

Although aggression is never suited to the leadership role, leaders need assertiveness in nearly all leadership situations. It is very important for effecting change. **Assertiveness** is a learned quality all nurses can develop. (Assertiveness is discussed in Chap. 21.)

Leadership qualities are present in all nurses. With education and practice, these qualities can be developed to the point at which a nurse is skilled in the many behaviors necessary for leadership. A full discussion of all these qualities and skills is beyond the scope of this text, but the checklist summarizes how one might approach the role of leader.

Leadership Skills

Four basic types of skills are needed for nursing leadership:

Communication skills—the ability to establish trusting interpersonal relationships with patients, peers, subordinates, and superiors to maximize goal achievement and enhance the personal growth of all participants

Problem-solving skills—the ability to analyze all sides of a problem, to explore multiple options, and to work to a creative solution; the ability to plan, implement, and stabilize change

Management skills—the ability to direct others toward goal achievement; this ability involves the recognition and fostering of unique talents and skills of others and the ability to match these with necessary tasks; organizational skills; financial skills; and the ability to generate and use resources wisely

Self-evaluation skills—the ability to assess honestly one's effectiveness and to accept both praise and blame; the ability to direct personal professional growth and development

Leadership Styles

Different styles of leadership are present in healthcare settings, as discussed in the following sections.

Autocratic Leadership

Autocratic leadership, also called *directive leadership,* involves the leader assuming complete control over the decisions and activities of the group. A nurse with an autocratic personality can be described as "firm, insistent, self-assured, and dominating with or without intent, and keeps at the center of attention" (Douglass, 1995). An extremely autocratic leader may make all decisions for workers or followers without considering the followers' ideas or feelings.

Many nurses are used to working under autocratic leaders because this approach has been used in most hospitals until recently. It may have evolved from nursing's historical military and religious past. This style of leadership is gradually being replaced by the democratic style of leadership as nurses demand and receive more participation in decision making.

Example of Autocratic Leadership

Nurse A discovers that one of her patients is bleeding excessively from his surgical incision. She knows that he needs immediate attention, so she gives specific orders to another team member to attend to the other patients. She tells the registered nurse on her team to call the surgical resident to come as soon as possible. She implements a nursing plan of care to prevent further blood loss or complications.

Nurse A assumed the autocratic style of leadership in this situation so that all of the necessary tasks would be accomplished immediately. Although she rarely uses this style, she implemented it effectively in this emergency situation.

Democratic Leadership

Democratic leadership, also called *participative leadership,* is characterized by a sense of equality among the leader and other participants. Decisions and activities are shared. Participants are encouraged to develop their skills and strengths within the group. The group and leader work together to accomplish mutually set goals and outcomes. The leader needs skills in group dynamics to apply this type of leadership effectively.

Most nurses currently work with a democratic style of leadership. As professionals, nurses generally respond well to this style of leadership when they are the followers and feel more comfortable when they are the leaders of democratic groups. Group satisfaction and motivation are excellent benefits of this style.

Example of Democratic Leadership

Nurse B, a head nurse, observes that staff members have not been documenting patient teaching and learning in their progress notes. Nurse B is not sure why this has occurred but believes that this problem must be solved. He calls a staff meeting and leads a discussion to seek information on possible causes and planning strategies.

Nurse B has decided that staff members need to be included in the problem-solving approach. He thinks the staff will be more motivated to document their teaching and the patients' learning if they have a say in how the changes will be implemented. Nurse B has used the democratic style of leadership.

Laissez-Faire Leadership

In **laissez-faire leadership**, also called *nondirective leadership*, the leader relinquishes power to the group, such that an outsider could not identify the leader in the group. This approach encourages independent activity by group members. This style depends on the strengths of followers to direct the group activities.

This style is rarely useful in hospitals because task achievement is difficult when each nurse is working independently. However, it can be used effectively when the leader wants a problem to be solved completely by group members. It has been successful in cases in which there is resistance to a certain policy or change and the leader allows the group to work to achieve an acceptable solution.

Example of Laissez-Faire Leadership

Nurse C, a clinical coordinator, has read an interesting research study that supports a change in the current instructions being given to new mothers who are breastfeeding. She posts the article with a summary of findings in all the nurses' stations in the maternity unit.

Nurse C is using a laissez-faire leadership style in this case. She is confident that individual staff members are capable professionals who are concerned with keeping up with current research findings that they will use to improve their nursing care.

Transformational Leadership

Transformational leaders are able to create revolutionary change. Often described as charismatic, they are unique in their ability to inspire and motivate others. They create intellectually stimulating practice environments and challenge themselves and others to grow personally and professionally and to learn. Gifted in creating a common vision, they demonstrate passion for the vision and keep others similarly focused. One of the unique qualities of transformational leaders is their vulnerability. They communicate authentically and openly and are able to express emotions as well as ideas as they share themselves with others. They show concern and care for others and are willing to take risks. They pay attention to process as well as outcomes.

Example of Transformational Leadership

Nurse D, a transformational leader, is troubled by the plight of women and children in the inner city where she lives. She unites with other nurses and healthcare professionals to design and implement strategies to meet their needs; within 18 months, a nursing center is funded and running, improving maternal-child outcomes in the area. The founding group of healthcare professionals continues to meet monthly to dream about future strategies and to support each other in the work being done. They are most proud of the improved self-esteem and independence in many of the women they serve.

Situational Leadership

Generally speaking, nurses do best to use the leadership style with which they are most comfortable if that style is effective for the task at hand and those they lead. The nurse's own personality, the group's personality, and the tasks or objectives to be accomplished should be considered in each leadership situation (Fig. 23-1). **Situational leadership** theory considers the leader's style, the work group's maturity, and the situation at hand to form a comprehensive approach to management style. For example, although all nurse managers in a healthcare agency may be charged with cutting costs, both the outcomes they target and the processes they use to achieve these outcomes may vary. The unique situations in each unit influence the management style used.

Leadership and Management

All nurses—to the extent that they work with others and influence others to be their best—are leaders. Some nurses hold positions in the healthcare system that also make them managers. The role of nurse managers is to plan, organize, direct, and control available human, material, and financial resources to deliver quality care to patients and families.

> *Planning*—identifying problems and developing goals, objectives, and related strategies
> *Organizing*—mobilizing resources to meet objectives
> *Directing*—leading others in goal achievement
> *Controlling*—implementing mechanisms for ongoing evaluation

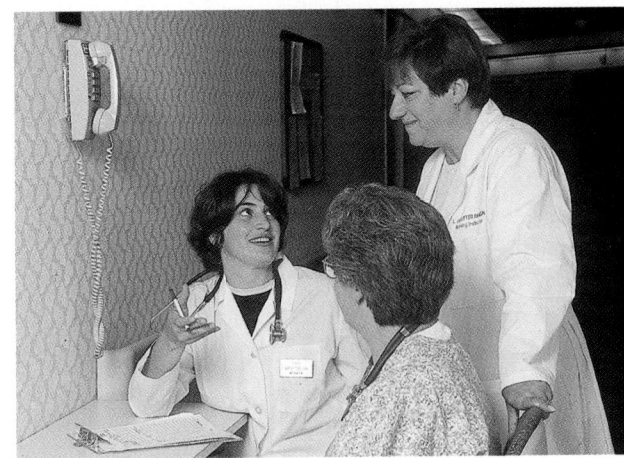

Figure 23-1
Leadership styles vary. The nurse should choose one that is comfortable and will be effective for the situation.

Hersey and Blanchard (1977) consider motivating one of the four key **management** functions, rather than directing. This is compatible with the shift in many organizations from emphasizing management (to control enterprises) to emphasizing leadership (to bring out the best in people and to respond quickly to changes). Chief nurse executives realize that nurse managers must be effective leaders to be successful. Nursing managers who cannot create a healthy group environment; who fail to resolve interpersonal issues that lower morale and result in numerous complaints from patients, nurses, and physicians; and who are unable to develop a plan to resolve detrimental interpersonal issues lack leadership skills.

Centralized and Decentralized Decision Making

In a centralized management structure, decisions are generally made by senior managers. Those at the bottom of the organization are often responsible for implementing decisions into which they had little input. In a decentralized management structure, on the other hand, decisions are made by those who are most knowledgeable about the issues being decided. Nurses are thus intimately involved in decisions concerning patient care. Nurse managers are accountable and responsible for what happens on their nursing unit, including patient census, staffing, supplies, and budget. A decentralized system invites greater accountability and responsibility because most nurses feel more responsible for decisions they have made themselves.

Nursing Care Delivery Models

Models of nursing care delivery systems are highlighted in the accompanying box. Over time, these have evolved from highly technical, industrial-based, assembly-line models to more professional, self-managed, cross-functional methods. According to Kerfoot, "As nurses have moved to accept more professional status and the responsibility of delegating and working through others, they have moved into advanced practice models in which there is less supervision, more opportunity for independent thought and creativity, and more accountability" (1995, p. 41). The evolving models of patient care delivery demonstrate that professional nurses will increasingly be expected to have significant managerial competence.

Effecting Change Through Leadership

Change is the process of transforming or modifying something. It may be planned, unplanned, or developmental. Nursing and the healthcare system are continually changing and evolving. Factors such as the increasing number of chronically ill and older people, the increasing role of government and industry in healthcare, the rising cost of healthcare, and the changing patterns of healthcare delivery have provoked a need for innovation and change in healthcare.

There are many theories of change, most based on the classic theory of change proposed by Kurt Lewin in 1951. Lewin posited the following three stages of change:

Evolving Models of Nursing Care Delivery . . . Evolving Accountability

Functional nursing	Nurses and other staff are assigned to specific tasks for a group of patients. Based on the assembly-line concept found in industry; specializing tasks increases efficiency but results in impersonal care
Team nursing	A team made up of a registered nurse and other caregivers provides care to a designated group of patients on a given shift. Modified the depersonalized approach of functional nursing and focused on individual patient care
Total care or case nursing	A nurse as caregiver provides total care to a group of patients for a designated shift. A patient-centered model; suffers from a lack of continuity between shifts and is expensive because highly paid nurses provide all aspects of care
Primary nursing	A nurse is accountable for planning, evaluating, and directing the care of a patient 24 hours a day throughout the patient's stay. A method of providing comprehensive, individualized, and consistent care; expensive
Case management	One nurse is responsible for overseeing the quality and financial outcomes of patient care; the nurse works collegially with physicians and other caregivers as well as with payers to manage patients along an agreed-on clinical pathway
Patient-centered or patient-focused care	Cross-functional teams consisting of groups of professionals and assistive personnel from nursing and other departments work together as a unit-based team to provide care to a given group of patients. Care is designed around the needs of the patients and not the needs of the departments or professionals
Collaborative practice model	Nurses and physicians work together in collaborative practice models.

Unfreezing: The need for change is recognized.

Moving: Change is initiated after a careful process of planning.

Refreezing: Change becomes operational.

Healthcare has numerous examples of using change theory to transform practice. Not so long ago, the experience of childbirth in the United States was routinely medicalized. Women who went into labor came into the hospital to deliver their babies; pain medications that interfered with the natural process of labor were routinely administered, necessitating forceps and assisted deliveries; and husbands, partners, and siblings were banished from the delivery. Nurse midwives and others recognized the need for change (*unfreezing*) and set about researching the experience of childbirth and ways to optimize infant and family outcomes. After a careful process of planning (*moving*), multiple natural childbirth options were made available to women and couples, and today they represent mainstream care (*refreezing*). Similarly, someone who takes good health for granted may fail to develop healthy lifestyle practices until illness results in recognition of the need for change (*unfreezing*). A careful process of consultation and study may lead to a well-developed fitness plan (*moving*), which ideally becomes part of the person's everyday life (*refreezing*). Effective nurses pay attention to their ability to influence thinking and behavior in each stage of change.

Planned Change

Planned change is a change agent's purposeful, systematic effort to bring about change. The eight steps in the process

of change are somewhat similar to the steps of the nursing process. These are illustrated in the accompanying box. Before planning to make a change, a nurse should consider the following:

- *What is amenable to change?* Considering this question may reveal behavior not amenable to change.
- *How does the group function as a unit?* A **change agent** may determine whether there are certain forces within a group favoring change and other forces that may resist change.
- *Is the person or group ready for change and, if so, at what rate can that change be expected to be accepted?* The pace of change must be consistent with the person's or group's readiness to assimilate change. *Readiness* involves both the ability and willingness to change.
- *Are the changes major or minor?* A series of small changes may be more easily accomplished than one large change. Also, stability in one area in which change has just occurred is often necessary before change begins in another area.

Resistance to Change

People may resist change for various reasons. The leader must decide why there is resistance and what techniques will overcome the resistance.

Threat to Self

People generally view change in terms of how they are affected personally. Personal threats may include a loss of

---

Planned Change: An Eight Step Process

Planned change is a purposeful, systematic effort to alter or bring about change through the intervention of a change agent. The same steps apply whether dealing with individuals or groups.

1. *Recognize symptoms that indicate a change is needed and collect data.*
2. *Identify a problem to be solved through change.* Analyze the symptoms and reach a conclusion. Note resistance or barriers to change and factors that promote the desired change.
3. *Determine and analyze alternative solutions to the problem.* Consider the advantages, disadvantages, and consequences of each alternative. An analysis of various proposed solutions to a problem may result in using a combination of alternatives.
4. *Select a course of action from possible alternatives.* It is best to avoid initiating too many courses of action and thereby dissipating resources and energy.
5. *Plan for making a change.* This step is crucial to effect change successfully. Start by stating specific

objectives, designing a plan for change, developing timetables, selecting people to assist with making the change, and anticipating how to stabilize change and deal with resistance to change. Unless a plan is clearly designed, effecting change is likely to be a chaotic experience.

6. *Implement the selected course of action to effect change.* The plan for change is then put into effect. During this period, flexibility is important to adapt to unforeseen problems.
7. *Evaluate the effects of change by comparing them with objectives stated in the plan for change.* Adjustments can be made in the plan as necessary after evaluation. If the results of evaluation indicate that the course of action selected to solve a problem has been unsuccessful, an adjustment should be made or another course of action selected.
8. *Stabilize the change.* When a solution has been found, take measures to make the change permanent. Continue follow-up until the change is firmly established.

self-esteem, a belief that more work will be required, or a belief that social relationships will be disrupted. For example, when hospitals began to use more unlicensed assistive personnel for routine nursing care, many nurses resisted not only because of quality concerns but also because they found themselves legally and professionally responsible for supervising the care given by these new aides. There was also concern that some professional nurses would be replaced by unlicensed assistive personnel.

Lack of Understanding

Someone who does not understand the nature of change is likely to resist. The involvement of people affected by the change is important to overcome resistance. For example, nurses who do not realize the effectiveness of using plans of care tend to resist preparing them because they believe they are not beneficial for providing patient care.

Limited Tolerance for Change

Some people simply do not like to function in a state of flux or disequilibrium. A person may understand the need for change but may be unable to cope emotionally with the change itself. For example, a nurse may resist change because of the temporary confusion the change is likely to cause.

Disagreements About the Benefits of Change

Resistance may occur when the change agent and those resisting change have different information. If the information known by the people resisting change is more accurate and relevant than the change agent's information, their resistance may be beneficial. For example, consider a plan that has been effective for implementing home healthcare in a middle-class section of a city. The supervisor of community health services proposes to implement the plan in a low-income neighborhood. The nurse in charge of the health program in the low-income area resists, believing that this plan for a middle-class section of the community cannot successfully be used in a financially and educationally disadvantaged neighborhood.

Fear of Increased Responsibility

Many people are worried about having to take on more complex responsibilities. This is especially true if they feel unprepared for the planned changes. The changes may seem overwhelming, so they naturally resist them.

Overcoming Resistance to Change

Nurses in leadership roles often find they must work to overcome resistance to change. Resistance can be subtle or distinct, gentle or aggressive. Responding to resistance is a leadership challenge for which the leader uses leadership qualities, leadership style, and knowledge of group dynamics to influence others toward a desired outcome. Nurses acting as change agents find the following guidelines helpful for overcoming resistance to change:

- Explain the proposed change to all affected people in simple, concise language.

- List the advantages of the proposed change, both for the individual and for members of the group.
- Relate the proposed change to the person's or group's existing beliefs and values.
- Help overcome resistance by providing opportunities for open communication and feedback.
- Indicate clearly how the change will be evaluated.
- Introduce change gradually. Involve everyone affected by the change in the design and implementation of the process.
- Provide incentives for commitment to change. Incentives may be money, status, time off, or a better working environment.

Power

Nurses who wish to be effective change agents are sensitive to both the uses and abuses of power. **Power**, the ability to influence others to achieve a desired effect, has many sources. Nurses in management positions within an institution (eg, director of nursing or nursing coordinator) have ascribed power associated with the role. As well, a group may attribute power to different individuals because of their expertise, leadership, or charisma. When introducing change, it is helpful to recognize and enlist the support of key power players who can then encourage others to become involved. You can probably think of people in the groups to which you belong (school, church, civic groups) who are "natural leaders" because of their demonstrated ability to influence others. These are the "key power players" whose support is essential to effecting change. Nursing leaders recognize the strengths and limitations of their own power and encourage others to develop and use power constructively.

The Nurse Caregiver's Leadership Skills

No one is born a leader. People develop leadership qualities through observation, knowledge, and experience. Nurses develop their leadership qualities in the same way, although they may enter nursing with some background in leadership experiences.

Nursing students and beginning practicing nurses have some leadership responsibilities, as described in the following sections, but they are still working at developing leadership skills and learning where and how to apply them. Fortunately, they have support systems for guidance.

Areas of Leadership

Leadership should be approached as any new role or skill is approached—slowly and carefully. Nursing students and beginning nurses should be prepared with all of the necessary tools or skills before attempting the new role. Initially, nurses develop leadership skills in well-defined situations. With each experience, growth occurs, and leadership is strengthened. It helps to remember that all nurse managers, nurse administrators, and nursing leaders also began as inexperienced nurses.

Patient Care Coordination

Even new graduate nurses have leadership responsibilities when they begin nursing. Nursing leadership begins with nursing care of the individual patient. Although patients are partners in their care planning, most do not have the knowledge base and skills to direct the plan. Through interpersonal skills and effective communication techniques, nurses lead their patients in acquiring new knowledge, solving problems, and changing behaviors. Managing care for even one patient can be an overwhelming responsibility for those new to nursing and its challenges. The student guide to organizing clinical responsibilities in Chapter 18 offers practical help. An ongoing leadership challenge for all nurses is time management. Following are helpful steps for using your time effectively:

- *Establish goals and priorities for each day.* Identify what you need to accomplish each day, differentiating "need to do" from "nice to do" tasks. Evaluate your goals in term of their ability to meet the needs of the patients entrusted to your care as well as your duties to self and your colleagues (other students and members of the team).
- *Establish a time line.* Allocate priorities to hours in your work day so that you will recognize when you are falling behind schedule in time to self-correct before the day is lost.
- *Evaluate your success or failure in managing time.* Should you fail to accomplish your goals in the time at hand, you need to determine whether your goals were overambitious, whether things happened beyond your control (eg, patient's condition worsened requiring more care, or another student required your assistance), or whether you wasted time that could have been better spent (Fig. 23-2).
- *Use the results of this evaluation to direct your next day's priorities and time line.*

Employee Responsibilities

Nurses have specific tasks or duties to perform. These tasks are determined by the plan and objective of the healthcare agency. It is important to read job descriptions carefully and to continue to evaluate how institutional factors influence one's own practice of nursing. Factors that compromise quality care should be noted and addressed in consultation with experienced nurses.

Managerial Responsibilities

New graduate nurses use leadership techniques when they cover for nurse managers or direct the work of nonprofessional staff and volunteers. Gradually, new nurses assume increased leadership responsibilities as they become primary nurses, case managers, or unit coordinators.

Nursing Department

The nursing team can also be viewed in the broader context of the entire nursing department of a healthcare institution or agency. Nurses should have an interest in the functioning of the department. Using this knowledge, nurses can seek information or change through appropriate channels. The more nurses understand how the nursing department runs, the better able they are to work constructively to meet the department's objectives.

Employing Institution or Agency

Nurses at all levels need to be knowledgeable about the administrative structure and functions of the employing institution or agency. When problems arise concerning professional, unit, departmental, or institutional or agency objectives, nurses must be able to use the proper channels of communication. For example, if a nurse believes that work assignments are routinely incompatible with basic patient safety and quality and gets no response after discussing this with her immediate nursing supervisor, she should take her complaints to the director of nursing. If the director of nursing fails to respond adequately, the nurse should determine who the director of nursing reports to and approach that individual next. Similarly, a nurse concerned about medical care should first approach the medical attending, but if he or she fails to respond, the nurse must then contact the nursing coordinator and in consult with him or her approach the medical director. The structure of these channels is shown in the agency's organization chart. The organization chart shows the relationships among the various administrative positions, departments, and job titles. Sometimes, the nurse is referred to committees that deal with specific problems or to other departments, such as public relations.

Research

Nurses should be concerned with the advancement of nursing as a profession. One of the many ways to promote nursing's development of greater autonomy and strength is nursing research. The research role of the nurse is discussed more fully later in this chapter. Nurses have always used the findings of nurse researchers to improve their efforts to deliver high-quality, cost-efficient care. Staff nurses also contribute to nursing research by doing the following:

- Observing all nursing care activities to look for any area that needs improvement

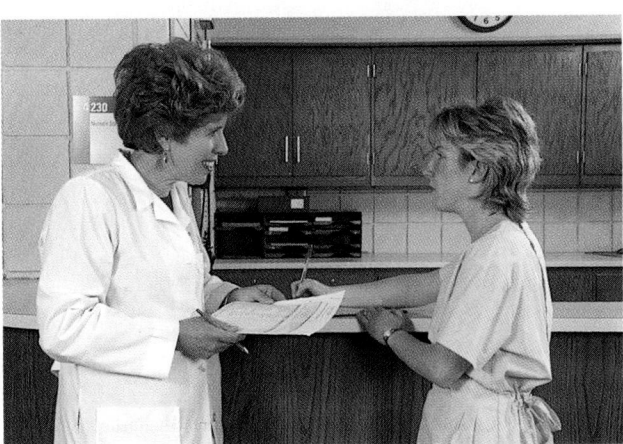

Figure 23-2
A student reviews her success in managing time with her clinical instructor.

- Questioning practices to determine whether the rationale behind caregiving activities is sound
- Participating in patient-care research done by colleagues or nurse researchers
- Making suggestions for specific topics to be researched

Legislation

Keeping informed about local, state, and national legislation allows nurses to write or call legislators before new laws are passed. Many nursing publications, newsletters, and papers give nurses specific information and guidelines on writing to elected officials concerning health-related legislation. The American and state Nurses Associations have lobbyists in Washington, DC, as well as in state capitals. The potential influence of nurses on the continued improvement of healthcare is phenomenal.

Public Image

Nurses create the public's image of nursing whenever they interact with others and are recognized as a nurse. It is crucial for beginning practitioners of nursing to understand the power they have to affect nursing's image positively or negatively. Because nurses are often portrayed negatively by the media (eg, as sex objects or as uncaring women), it is important that the public encounter nurses who are intelligent, competent, and caring to reverse this image. Nurses can change negative portrayals of nursing by organizing, monitoring and reacting to the media, and fostering an improved image. Although not all nurses are interested in joining a media watch group, all nurses can practice nursing care in a manner that promotes a positive image of nursing.

Support for Leadership Training

Mentorship

Mentorship is a relationship in which an experienced individual (the *mentor*) advises and assists a less experienced individual (*protégé*). This is an effective way of easing a new nurse into leadership responsibilities. Mentors link with protégés by common interest and provide support, information, and network links. The relationship does not include financial reward. The advantages of having an effective mentor are highlighted in the accompanying box.

Mentorship is valuable in all types of nursing positions. As a nurse climbs the ladder of leadership responsibility, a mentor who is experienced in management and administrative functions may assist. A mentor can be a critical factor in helping the less experienced nurse successfully assume added responsibilities and position changes. Many mentorship relationships also become lasting friendships.

Preceptorship

An alternative model is **preceptorship**. The *preceptor* (experienced nurse) is selected (and generally paid) to facilitate the orientee's transition to new responsibilities through teaching and guidance. The relationship is limited by the orientee's needs.

Advantages of Having an Effective Mentor

- Gives upward mobility to your career
- Boosts self-esteem by believing in you
- Shares your dreams
- Provides advice, counsel, and support
- Teaches by example
- Introduces you to the corporate structure, players, and politics
- Imparts valuable information
- Gives feedback on your progress

Heidman, M., & Cobbold, D. (1995). Mentoring and career development revisited. *Registered Nurse, 7*(1), 29–30.

Nursing Organizations

The many nursing organizations at the international, national, state, district, and local levels were discussed in Chapter 1. They are major forces for nursing leadership. These organizations have active groups throughout the United States and abroad. Membership and participation in professional organizations are important aspects of the nurse's leadership role (Fig. 23-3).

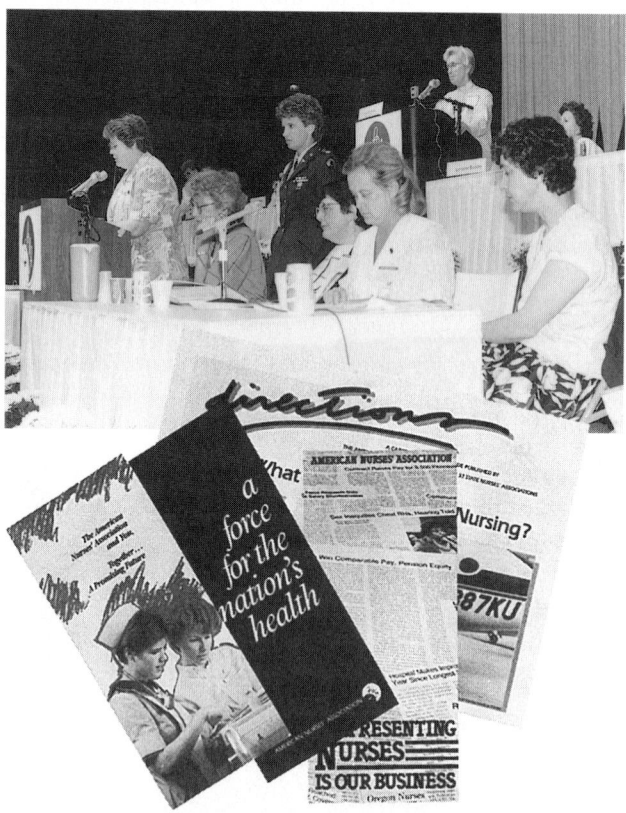

Figure 23-3
Membership and participation in professional nursing organizations help keep the individual nurse current on issues and recent developments, increase the strength of the group, and are important aspects of the nurse's leadership role. (Courtesy of the American Nurses Association.)

Continuing Education

Many programs for developing leadership, managerial, and administrative skills are available to nurses. Courses can also be taken by mail correspondence or the Internet. Periodicals and current books also provide continuing education for emerging leaders. Many continuing education programs and methods serve to prepare nurses before they assume higher levels of leadership; some are geared to nurses already in such positions. Nurses should choose a program carefully that matches their individual learning needs.

The Nurse as Researcher

While caring for victims of the Crimean War, Florence Nightingale kept careful and objective records. These records provided baseline data that she later used to determine which nursing interventions were most effective in treating her patients. Since that time, nursing research has taken many different pathways, and all nurses are involved with research either as consumers (nurses who use and evaluate research findings) or as actual investigators who design and implement research studies. The accompanying box highlights the ethical responsibilities of all involved in the conduct, dissemination, and implementation of nursing research.

Nursing research was finally recognized by the public sector when the 1985 session of the US Congress enacted legislation to establish a National Center for Nursing Research (NCNR) at the National Institutes of Health (NIH). Increasing numbers of healthcare institutions currently employ postgraduate nurses as researchers.

Research studies on nursing education, administration, and practice all affect patient care directly or indirectly. Too often, practicing nurses mistakenly think research is far removed from caring for patients at the bedside. This false impression has slowed the progress of practice-based nursing research. Yet much of what bedside nurses routinely do constitutes research. The nursing process (ie, assessing, diagnosing, planning, implementing, and evaluating) represents the basic framework of the research process. The most common impediments to nursing research include restricted access to resources, limited time to participate in research-related activities, and lack of educational preparation needed by nurses for research. Two major challenges face nursing research programs in the future:

- To continue to improve the links between research and practice
- To demonstrate nursing's unique contribution to healthcare delivery in a context of fiscal responsibility (Thurston, 1995)

Contact information for three key organizations that provide grants for nursing research is a follows:

American Nurses Foundation
    Shirley Porter, 1-202-651-7071
    http://www.nursingworld.org/anf/grants.htm
National Institute of Nursing Research
    1-301-496-0207
    E-mail: info@ninr.rih.gov
Sigma Theta Tau International
    E-mail: sandyf@stti.iupui.edu

Research and Professionalism

Nursing research is fundamental to the recognition of nursing as a profession. As an occupation, nursing has existed since the beginning of human history. Many argue,

---

Ethical Principles in the Conduct, Dissemination, and Implementation of Nursing Research

1. The investigator respects autonomous research participants' capacity to consent to participate in research and to determine the degree and duration of that participation without negative consequences.
2. The investigator prevents harm, minimizes harm, and/or promotes good to all research participants, including vulnerable groups and others affected by the research.
3. The investigator respects the personhood of research participants, their families, and significant others, valuing their diversity.
4. The investigator ensures that the benefits and burdens of research are equitably distributed in the selection of research participants.
5. The investigator protects the privacy of research participants to the maximal degree possible.
6. The investigator ensures the ethical integrity of the research process by use of appropriate checks and balances throughout the conduct, dissemination, and implementation of the research.
7. The investigator reports suspected, alleged, or known incidents of scientific misconduct in research to appropriate institutional officials for investigation.
8. The investigator maintains competency in the subject matter and methodologies of his or her research as well as in other professional and societal issues that affect nursing research and the public good.
9. The investigator involved in animal research maximizes the benefits of the research with the least possible harm or suffering to the animals.

Silva, M. (1995). *Ethical guidelines in the conduct, dissemination, and implementation of nursing research.* Washington, DC: American Nurses Association. Used with permission.

however, that the profession of nursing is still in its infancy. One of the essential elements that differentiates a profession from an occupation is the existence of a unique and distinct knowledge base. The ultimate goal of expanding nursing's body of knowledge is to learn improved ways to promote and maintain health. As healthcare and illness patterns change, nursing interventions must change. Ongoing practice-based research reflects the nursing profession's commitment to meet the ever-changing demands of healthcare consumers.

Roots of Knowledge

How does nursing expand its knowledge base to meet the healthcare needs of patients? To answer this question, one must look to the roots of knowledge. **Knowledge** comes from a variety of sources. **Traditional knowledge** is that part of nursing practice passed down from generation to generation. When questioned about the origin of such nursing practices, nurses might reply, "We've always done it this way." Changing bedclothes is an example of how traditional knowledge has affected nursing practice. It is customary in acute care settings to change a patient's bedclothes daily, whether soiled or not. There are no research data to support this, yet virtually millions of hospital beds are changed daily because this practice is accepted as a necessary component of quality patient care. Until this practice is challenged scientifically and its assumed value disproved, it will remain a traditional part of patient care.

Authoritative knowledge comes from an expert and is accepted as truth based on the person's perceived expertise, such as, for example, when a senior staff nurse teaches a new graduate nurse an easier way of doing a technical procedure such as inserting an intravenous catheter. The senior nurse has gained knowledge through experience, and the new graduate nurse accepts it as truth based on the perceived authority of the experienced nurse. Authoritative knowledge generally remains unchallenged as long as the presumed authority maintains his or her perceived expertise.

Scientific knowledge is that knowledge arrived at through the scientific method. The term *research* implies the scientific approach to acquiring new knowledge. New ideas are tested and measured systematically using objective criteria. Scientific study implies control over **variables**—factors that might affect results (outcomes). Different types of variables are involved in research studies. **Independent variables** are the factors the researcher introduces into the study and can control. **Dependent variables** are those factors already in the situation that may be affected by the independent variables. An example of scientific research that might be carried out at the bedside would be to measure the effects of two different skin emollients on a patient's opposite limbs over the course of 2 days. The dependent variable in this example are characteristics of the patient's limbs. The independent variables are the skin emollients. With careful and objective data collection, the researcher might be able to de-

termine which lotion elicited a better patient result or outcome. By testing the results of the two emollients on the same patient, the researcher maintains control over other factors that might influence outcomes within the study. Research as simple as this example could have vast implications for practice when results are shared among healthcare professionals. Scientific research relies on careful planning. If only one emollient was tested on each of two patients, instead of both emollients on each patient, the results of the research might be affected by an unknown factor, such as differing skin conditions. These factors are called **extraneous variables**. Extraneous variables (ie, those that are not being studied) can sometimes result in inaccurate research findings and therefore must be controlled.

Is one source of knowledge better than another? All sources of knowledge are useful in the collective body of knowledge that constitutes the nursing profession. Although these three sources provide nursing with important contributions, each has inherent strengths and limitations. Traditional and authoritative knowledge are practical to implement but are often based on subjective data, limiting their usefulness over a wide variety of practice settings. For this reason, nurses often focus on "evidence-based practice" or "research-based practice."

Evidence-Based Practice

Those interested in quality and cost control want evidence that the services and interventions being funded are effective in securing valued goals. Scientific research, designed to achieve high levels of objectivity, may be costly and time-consuming and can be impractical given the complexities surrounding patient care. The control and objectivity of scientific knowledge, however, allow it to be generalized, making it highly useful in a variety of care settings. Nursing's commitment to acquiring new knowledge is one reason why nurses must become more aware of and involved in the research process. Rosswurm and Larrabee (1999) designed the accompanying model to guide nurses and other healthcare professionals through a systemic process for change to evidence-based practice.

The Internet as a Source of Information

Nurses today, like others seeking health information, have access to incredible information sources through the Internet. The accompanying display highlights web sites that many nurses find helpful. If you are not sure how to access these sites, you will find it useful to spend some time with your school, hospital, or community librarian learning how to access these information sources. *Warning!* Many web sites contain data that is wrong, misleading, or inappropriate or that has not been reviewed by scientists for accuracy. Biermann and associates (1999) reviewed 400 sites for information about Ewing's sarcoma, a rare cancer. They checked the information on these sites against a preeminent oncology textbook. What they found, in addition

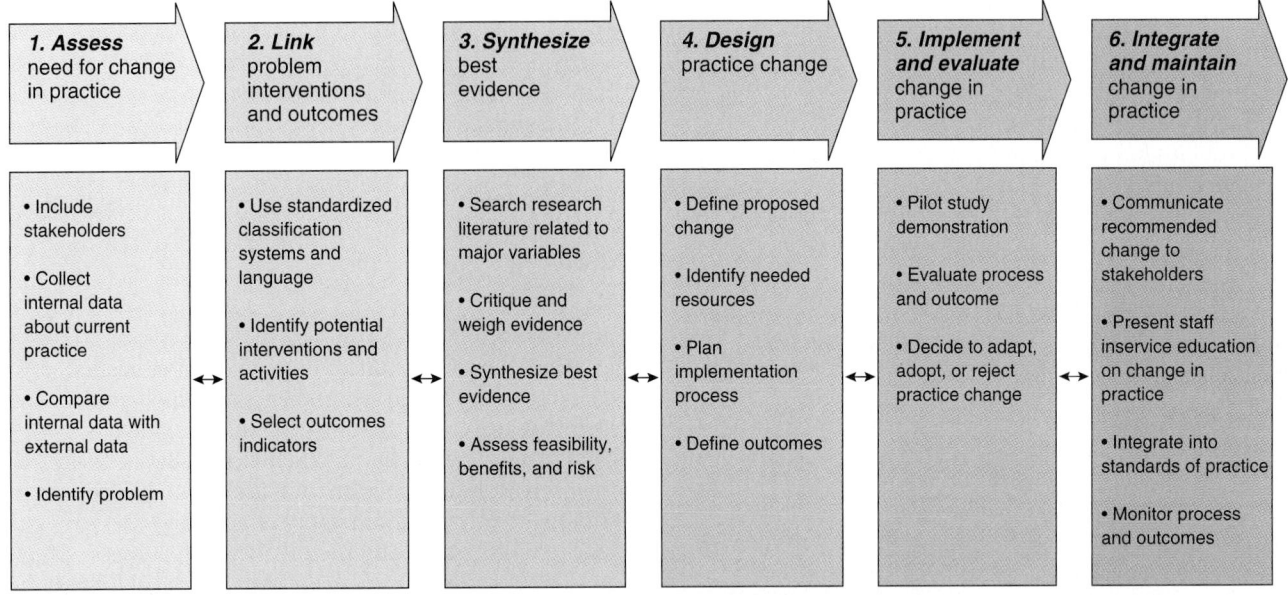

1. **Assess** need for change in practice	2. **Link** problem interventions and outcomes	3. **Synthesize** best evidence	4. **Design** practice change	5. **Implement and evaluate** change in practice	6. **Integrate and maintain** change in practice
• Include stakeholders • Collect internal data about current practice • Compare internal data with external data • Identify problem	• Use standardized classification systems and language • Identify potential interventions and activities • Select outcomes indicators	• Search research literature related to major variables • Critique and weigh evidence • Synthesize best evidence • Assess feasibility, benefits, and risk	• Define proposed change • Identify needed resources • Plan implementation process • Define outcomes	• Pilot study demonstration • Evaluate process and outcome • Decide to adapt, adopt, or reject practice change	• Communicate recommended change to stakeholders • Present staff inservice education on change in practice • Integrate into standards of practice • Monitor process and outcomes

A model for evidence-based practice. (Used with permission from Rosswurm, M. A., & Larrabee, J. H. (1999). A model for change to evidence-based practice. *Image–The Journal of Nursing Scholarship, 31*(4), 318.)

to numerous "dead ends, bad links, and pages with no medical information," was a disturbing level of inaccuracy and misinformation. It is becoming increasingly important for healthcare professionals to determine whether patients have checked their condition on the Internet so that they can dispel misinformation and refer patients to appropriate, accurate sites. Educate patients about simple ways to know whether a site is reputable, such as whether the site is provided by a professional or reputable organization, whether citations to reputable journals are provided with information, and so forth.

Consumerism

Society's attitudes about consumerism in healthcare have increased the importance of nursing research as well. The healthcare marketplace is characterized by rising concern over quality of care and cost containment. Consumers have become dissatisfied with unproved, costly treatments; they demand effective methods of treatment (evidence-based practice) at a reasonable cost. Nursing care, therefore, must focus on measurable results to assure consumers of nursing's commitment to improve patient care. Unless practice-based research is used to validate the effects of nursing interventions, consumers will not credit nursing for its important contribution.

The Nurse Caregiver's Research Skills

Relating Research to Practice
Unless the research findings of nurse researchers are used by practicing nurses to improve the quality of patient care, clinical nursing research is useless. Nursing students developing clinical skills must understand the scientific ra-

tionale that makes one course of action preferable to another. Throughout this text, Research in Nursing boxes highlight current studies that have the potential to make a positive difference in nursing practice and patient outcomes. The accompanying box lists resources nurses can explore to find research studies pertinent to their concerns. Most librarians can provide helpful introductions to these resources. As nurses develop their clinical and research skills, they are better able to critique nursing research for validity, reliability, and applicability.

Identifying Researchable Problems
Because it is the nurse as caregiver who works most immediately with patients and families, it is crucial for caregivers to approach their practice continually with the question, "Is this the best way to achieve the desired patient outcomes?" The questions, insights, and recommendations of caring, practicing nurses have assisted many nurse researchers to refine their studies in significant ways (Fig. 23-4).

Protecting the Rights of Subjects
Many nurses work in healthcare institutions in which patients are invited to participate in clinical research. With their focus on the overall well-being of the patient, nurses play an important role in ensuring that patient interests are not sacrificed to research interests. Nursing priorities on research units include determining that research studies have met appropriate scientific and ethical criteria before their implementation and protecting patient rights. Specific patient rights include **informed consent**, the patient's right to consent knowledgeably to participate in a study without coercion (knowing that this consent may be withdrawn at any time) or to refuse to participate without

Helpful Web Sites

American Diabetes Association
http://www.diabetes.org/
Provides information for patients and professionals, including up-to-date lists of conferences and educational material. Features "menu item of the week."

American Heart Association
http://www.amhrt.org/
Information on heart diseases for consumers and professionals. Includes multimedia files of normal and abnormal circulation.

American Journal of Nursing Online Services
http://www.ajn.org/
Presents online versions of *American Journal of Nursing, Nursing Research,* and *Maternal/Child Nursing* journals. A flashback feature includes quotes from archived journal volumes dating back to the early 1900s. Users can then "chat" about the relevance to today's practice.

American Nurses Association
http://www.ana.org

CarePlans
http://www.careplans.com
A free e-mail discussion group to help nurses and students share information.

Centers for Disease Control and Prevention
http://www.cdc.gov

Cybernurse
http://www.cybernurse.com

Intellihealth
http://www.intellihealth.com/IH/ihtIH

The Internet Nursing Resource
http://www.nurse.com

MEDLINE
http://igm.nlm.nih.gov
Search engine that provides abstracts of articles on a particular topic. For example, "diabetes" as a keyword retrieved 9147 articles published in the last 2 years.

MEDSCAPE
http://www.medscape.com.Default.mhtml
A free service (requires registration) for health professionals featuring full-text, peer-reviewed articles, medical news, and interactive quizzes.

National Cancer Institute CancerNet
http://cancernet.nci.nih.gov

National Institutes of Health
http://www.nih.gov

National Student Nurses Association
http://www.nsna.org

Nightingale
gopher://nightingale.con.utk.edu/00/homepage.html
An extensive gopher for nursing literature and resources on the Internet.

Nurses' Call
http://webcom.com.tsk/nrs-call/
Nursing resource list, including topics on education, conferences, research, volunteers, and employment. A unique feature of this site is a bibliographic piece called "who's who" in nursing. Selected by the users themselves, it describes an individual who has contributed to nursing. A directory enables the user to locate nurses on the Internet.

NursingNet
http://www.communique.net/ ~ nursgnt/
A forum for medical professionals and students to obtain and disseminate information about nursing and medically related subjects. Very broad areas of interest to nursing students, including nursing student help, disease links and references, nursing schools around the world, and online journals and publications (including several international journals).

The Nursing Student
http://www.csn.net/ ~ tbracket/htm.htm
An information resource for nursing students. In addition to linking to nursing web sites, it includes a math page and a "question of the day" page.

RNC Central
http://recentral.com
A place where nurses and students can enjoy themselves, support each other, and find information.

Virginia Henderson International Library
telnet://sti-suniupui.edu
A collection of databases that can search the Internet for conference proceedings, local programs, patient information pamphlets, and unpublished nursing research. A subscription is required, but a user can visit the site by typing "visitor" at the user i.d. and password prompt.

The "Virtual" Nursing Center
http://www.sci.lib.uci.edu/HSG/Nursing.html
A fascinating source of links to interactive, multimedia case studies, interactive anatomy browsers, and nursing courses and tutorials.

jeopardizing the care that he or she will receive; the right to confidentiality; and the right to be protected from harm. Nurses caring for patients who are research subjects should be familiar with the ethical directives of the American Nurses Association (1985), Silva's *Ethical Guidelines in the Conduct, Dissemination, and Implementation of Nursing Research* (1995; displayed earlier in this chapter), and *The Belmont Report* (National Commission for the Protection of Human Subjects of Biomedical and Behavioral Research, 1978).

Nursing Research Resources

Major nursing journals with a science or research focus
Advances in Nursing Science
Journal of Advanced Nursing
Canadian Journal of Nursing Research
Journal of Research in Nursing and Health
Nursing Research
International Journal of Nursing Studies
Western Journal of Nursing Studies

Indexes of journal articles
Cumulative Index to Nursing and Allied Health Literature (CINAHL)
International Nursing Index
Index Medicus

Secondary resources
Annual Review of Nursing Research
Review of Nursing Research in Nursing Education

Computerized literature searches of research
BIOETHICSLINE
Cumulative Index to Nursing and Allied Health Literature (CINAHL)
Educational Resources Information (ERIC)
Medical Literature Analysis and Retrieval System (MEDLARS)
Psychological Abstracts (PsycINFO)

Individually subscribed computer bibliographic services
Knowledge Index (available through *DIAGLOG Information Services*)
GRATEFUL MED (available through the National Library of Medicine)
BRS Colleague (available through W. B. Saunders Publishing Company)

The Nurse as Advocate

Advocacy involves combining the three roles of teacher, counselor, and leader into a new role in which the nurse protects and supports the patient's rights. Nurses have always been advocates for patients' rights. This role is increasingly important because of patients' changing expectations and demands as well as the importance the nursing profession gives to individuals' rights.

Advocacy requires that nurses inform patients and then support them in their decisions. Nurses must recognize that patients have the right to make their own decisions. Through teaching and counseling, the nurse gives patients the information they need to make educated decisions about their healthcare.

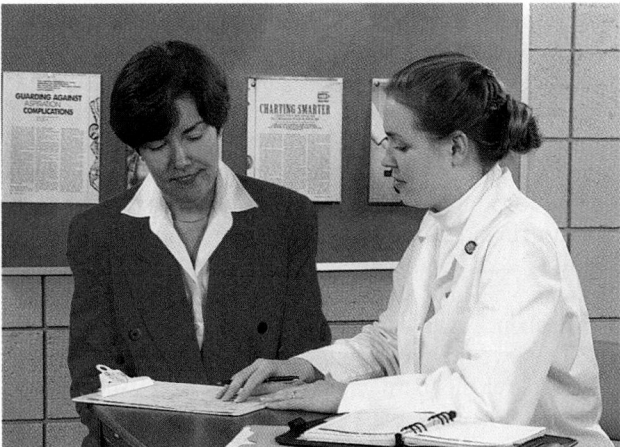

Figure 23-4
A student questions her instructor about the discrepancy between what she sees staff nurses doing to treat a wound and what her text and literature search recommend.

Some nurses view advocacy as necessary only for those who cannot defend themselves. This is not true in terms of the needs and rights of all patients. Nearly all patients need a nurse advocate to provide them with information needed for making informed decisions. Patients also need nurses to interpret what their rights are in given situations.

Patient's Bill of Rights

As holism and holistic care became popular, patients began to demand their rights as healthcare consumers. In 1972, the American Hospital Association's *A Patient's Bill of Rights* described the rights and responsibilities of patients receiving care in the hospital. This bill of rights has been widely disseminated, and in some hospitals patients receive a copy on admission. (*A Patient's Bill of Rights* is discussed and reprinted in Chap. 6.)

In the United States, the Freedom of Information Act of 1967 and the Privacy Act of 1974 were enacted primarily to open personal government records to the people described in them. Medical records were included in this enactment. Patients in health agencies operated by the US government (eg, Veteran's Administration hospitals) and patients receiving Medicare currently are entitled to see their records. Although some specifics and interpretations of the laws are still to be clarified, the trend is apparent: consumers are demanding their right to know about their healthcare and are seeking legislation to support this right.

As this text goes to press, there are new federal regulations pending on privacy that address health information and who is authorized to have access to health information. In addition, the US Congress, despite fierce lobbying and much state legislation, has yet to pass a federal Patient Protection Bill to guarantee patient rights in the new climate of managed care. Nurse advocates need to be familiar with all the ways patients and the public are at risk in today's evolving healthcare environment and continually assess the adequacy of protective mechanisms.

The Nurse Caregiver's Advocacy Skills

Representing Patients

Most nurses would agree that a great deal of nursing time is spent representing patients' interests or guiding patients in protecting their own rights. The nurse is often involved as an intermediary between the patient and the family, especially when the patient and family have conflicting ideas about the management of healthcare situations (Fig. 23-5).

For example, a patient with terminal cancer may want to go home to die. He tells this to his nurse. The patient's family, however, tells the nurse that they cannot care for him at home. As an advocate, the nurse recognizes the rights of both the patient and his family. The nurse then works to assist them in finding a solution that benefits both them and the patient. By informing the family of the availability of home care and hospice care, the nurse gives them knowledge that may help satisfy the patient's right to a dignified death. Most people on their own would be unable to get the financial help needed for such care. Nurses have the resources available to help them and can arrange referrals from other healthcare workers, such as social workers, to achieve the desired outcomes.

Nurses may also serve as intermediaries between patients and the medical profession. Patricia Murphy (1990) documented a moving account of how nurses interceded for a 43-year-old woman with amyotrophic lateral sclerosis who was on a ventilator but wished to die. The patient's primary physicians refused to help remove her from the ventilator, and more than 20 other physicians declined to accept her as a patient when they learned what she wanted to do. After unsuccessful appeals for help to the county medical society and her own attorney, the patient's visiting nurse, working with a supportive social worker, contacted her state nurses association and finally secured the assistance she needed to help the patient achieve her goal of a dignified death.

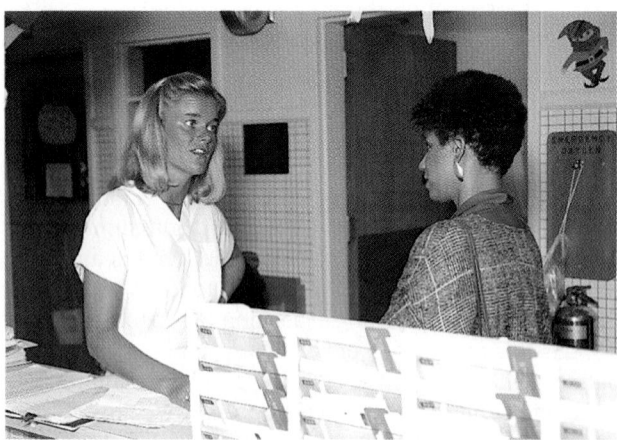

Figure 23-5
The nurse acts as a patient advocate in discussing all aspects of the patient's healthcare with family members.

Patients with special advocacy needs include those who are uninformed concerning their rights and opportunities, those with sensory impairment, those who do not speak English well or at all, the very young and the elderly, those who are seriously ill, those who are mentally or emotionally impaired, and those with physical disabilities.

Being Assertive

To help patients attain their rights, nurses need to be assertive. Occasionally, they need to teach assertive techniques to their patients. Some patient and families are intimidated in healthcare settings, and even when they disagree with a physician's treatment plan, they may feel unable to question or challenge the physician. Nurses can empower patients to claim and defend their right to knowledge, to respectful treatment, and to informed consent by legitimizing these rights and by coaching patients in the assertiveness techniques that can help them secure these rights. Basic assertiveness techniques are described in Chapter 21.

Promoting Self-Determination

Advocacy is linked to the belief that making choices about health is a fundamental human right that promotes the individual's dignity and well-being. Ethical dilemmas may arise when people are unable or unwilling to make choices or when they are not given the opportunity to do so. Faulty communication among patients, family members, and caregivers frequently contributes to these dilemmas. Nurses have an important advocacy role in educating the public about the value of written **advance directives** (described in Chap. 32).

Nurses as advocates must realize that they do not make ethical decisions for their patients. Instead, they facilitate patients' decision making. Nurses interpret findings for their patients; inform them of various aspects to be considered; help them verbalize and organize their feelings; call in those people who should be involved in the decision making (eg, family, primary nurse, physician, or clergy); and help patients assess all of their options in relation to their beliefs. In this way, nurses advocate for the right of patients to make their own decisions concerning their health. Not all individuals want to make their own treatment decisions, however, and the spirit of **autonomy** (self-determination) should not be violated by forcing it on anyone. Nurses sometimes advocate for patients by helping them to delegate decisions to a preferred decision maker whom they trust. In addition, when claiming to be a patient advocate, nurses must be careful to clarify exactly what it is they mean by advocacy because, in most instances, this is not simply supporting patients in all of their preferences. For example, if a patient in the early stages of Alzheimer's disease, with the support of her husband, asks a nurse for help in terminating her life, the nurse would have strong ethical grounds for refusing to advocate for this particular request. Ethical issues are discussed in Chapter 6.

Being Politically Active

No discussion of nursing advocacy would be complete without noting nursing's continuing voice in the political arena on behalf of those least well served by the existing healthcare system. As the government becomes more involved in the delivery and funding of healthcare services, and as those designing rationing plans speak seriously of age and other variables as criteria for limiting care, nurses must continue to advocate for the healthcare needs of those least empowered to do so for themselves, including homeless people, minorities, women, and children. Nurses are a powerful block of voters whose potential for influencing healthcare legislation is just beginning to be tapped.

Learning Outcomes

After completing this chapter, the learner should be able to accomplish the following:

1. Define the key terms used in the chapter:

   advocacy
   advance directive
   assertiveness
   autonomy
   change
     planned change
   change agent
   knowledge
     authoritative
       knowledge
     scientific knowledge
     traditional knowledge
   informed consent
   leadership
     autocratic leadership

   democratic leadership
   laissez-faire leadership
   transformational
     leadership
   situational leadership
   management
   mentorship
   power
   preceptorship
   professionalism
   variables
     independent variables
     dependent variables
     extraneous variables

2. Identify the qualities, four skills, and three styles of leaders.
3. List the four managerial functions.
4. Summarize the steps in the process of change.
5. Describe areas in which beginning nurses can develop leadership skills that enhance the caregiver role.
6. Compare the strengths and limitations of three sources of nursing knowledge.
7. Describe three ways beginning nurses can use research to enhance the caregiver role.
8. Explain different ways nurse caregivers can be advocates for patients.
9. Describe the nurse advocate's role in situations requiring ethical decision making.
10. Explain how two types of advance directives promote patient dignity and well-being.

Critical Thinking Exercises

1. Interview several experienced nurses and ask them what qualities make for the best nursing leaders. Reflect on your personal experience in groups (eg, within your family, church, school, and community). Identify the roles you characteristically assume and what qualities you personally bring to the group (eg, enthusiasm, positive thinking, vision, self-direction). Consider whether those qualities will serve you well in professional nursing groups and situations. Are there new qualities you need to develop if you want to become an effective nurse leader? Why?
2. Ask several experienced nurses for their rationale for care you observe them giving, and evaluate whether their rationale is based on traditional, authoritative, or scientific knowledge. Is the rationale they offer consistent with high-quality, cost-efficient care? Which type of knowledge supports the interventions you routinely plan for patients entrusted to your care?
3. Identify vulnerable groups in your community and describe their advocacy needs and how nursing might assist them. What in the community and the healthcare system needs to change to ensure that the healthcare needs of these groups are adequately served? What elements are likely to resist planned change? How would you address these elements?

Bibliography

Leader

Benne, K. D., & Sheats, P. (1948). Functional roles of group members. *Journal of Social Issues, 4*(2), 41.

Bennis, W. G., Benne, K. D., Chin, R., & Corey, K. E. (1976). *The planning of change* (3rd ed.). New York: Holt, Rinehart & Winston.

Bernhard, L. A., & Walsh, M. (1994). *Leadership: The key to the professionalization of nursing* (3rd ed.). St. Louis: C. V. Mosby.

Brown, B. J., & Sample, S. (Eds.). (1994). Change: The challenge for nursing. *Nursing Administration Quarterly, 18*(3), entire issue.

Chenevert, M. (1997). *Pro-nurse handbook: Designed for the nurse who wants to thrive professionally* (3rd ed.). St. Louis: C. V. Mosby.

Douglass, L. M. (1995). *The effective nurse: Leader and manager* (5th ed.). St. Louis: Mosby–Year Book.

Grensing-Pophal, L. (1998). Resolving conflicts: It's as easy as 1-2-3. *Nursing98, 28*(9), 63.

Grohar-Murray, M. E., & DiCroce, H. R. (1996). *Leadership and management in nursing.* Englewood Cliffs, NJ: Prentice-Hall.

Gurka, A. M. (1995). Transformational leadership: Qualities and strategies for the CNS. *Journal for Advanced Nursing Practice, 9*(3), 169–174.

Hagenow, N. R., & McCrea, M. A. (1994). A mentoring relationship: Two viewpoints. *Nursing Management*, 25(12), 42–43.

Heidman, M., & Cobbold, D. (1995). Mentoring and career development revisited. *Registered Nurse*, 7(1), 29–30.

Hersey, P., & Blanchard, K. (1977). *Management of organizational behavior: Utilizing human resources* (3rd ed.). Englewood Cliffs, NJ: Prentice-Hall.

Hostutler, J., Kennedy, M. S., Mason, D., & Schorr, T. M. (1999). Then and now: Nurses as leaders. *American Journal of Nursing*, 99(10), 36–38. (The first in a bimonthly series profiling nursing's ancestral, contemporary, and future leaders.)

Kerfoot, K. (1995). Models of patient care delivery. In K. W. Vestal (Ed.). *Nursing management: Concepts and issues* (2nd ed.) (pp. 37–47). Philadelphia: J. B. Lippincott.

Lewin, K. (1951). *Field theory in social science.* New York: Harper & Row.

Manfredi, C. M., & Valiga, T. M. (1994). Leadership in nursing. *Holistic Nursing Practice*, 9(1), entire issue.

Manion, J. (1995). Understanding the seven stages of change. *AJN*, 95(4), 41–43.

Marriner-Tomey, A. (1996). *Guide to nursing management and leadership.* St. Louis: Mosby–Year Book.

Tiffany, C. R., Cheatham, A. B., Doornbos, D., Loudermelt, L., & Momadi, G. G. (1994). Planned change theory: Survey of nursing periodical literature. *Nursing Management*, 25(7), 54–59.

Tiffany, C. R. (1994). Analysis of planned change theories. *Nursing Management*, 25(2), 60–62.

Trofino, J. (Ed.) (1992). Transformational leadership. *Nursing Administration Quarterly*, 17(1), entire issue.

Wolf, G. A., Boland, S., & Aukerman, M. (1994). A transformational model for the practice of professional nursing. Part I: The model. *Journal of Nursing Administration*, 23(4), 51–57.

Wolf, G. A., Boland, S., & Aukerman, M. (1994). A transformational model for the practice of professional nursing. Part II, Implementation of the model. *Journal of Nursing Administration*, 23(5), 38–46.

Wolf, P. (1998). Guide to nursing organizations. *Nursing98*, 28(12), 53–55.

Researcher

American Nurses Association, Commission on Nursing Research. (1981). *Guidelines for the investigative function of nurses.* Kansas City, MO: Author.

American Nurses Association. (1985). *Human rights guidelines for nurses in clinical and other research.* Kansas City, MO: Author.

American Nurses Association. (1987). *Research in nursing: Toward a science of nursing.* Kansas City, MO: Author.

Bierman, J. S., Golladay, G. J., Greenfield, M. & Baker, L. H. (1999). Evaluation of cancer information on the Internet. *Cancer*, 86(3), 381–390.

Lekander, B. J. (1994). Overcoming obstacles to research-based clinical practice. *AACN Clinical Issues in Critical Care Nursing*, 5(2), 115–123.

National Commission for the Protection of Human Subjects of Biomedical and Behavioral Research. (1978). *The Belmont report: Ethical principles and guidelines for the protection of human subjects of research* (DHEW Publication No. [OS] 78-0012). Washington, DC: U. S. Government Printing Office.

Pettengill, M. M., Gillies, D. A., & Clark, C. C. (1994). Factors encouraging and discouraging the use of nursing research findings. *Image—The Journal of Nursing Scholarship*, 26(2), 143–147.

Polit, D. F., & Hungler, B. P. (1996). *Essentials of nursing research: Methods, appraisal, and utilization* (4th ed.). Philadelphia: J. B. Lippincott.

Price, C. (1994). Nursing research: Everybody's business . . . here are practical steps to develop any type of nursing research program. *Journal of Maternal Child Nursing*, 19(1), 9–12, 14.

Rosswurm, M. A., & Larrabee, J. H. (1999). A model for change to evidence-based practice. *Image—The Journal of Nursing Scholarship*, 31(4), 317–322.

Roy, C. L. (1995). Developing nursing knowledge: Practice issues raised from four philosophical perspectives. *Nursing Science Quarterly*, 8(2), 79–85.

Silva, M. (1995). *Ethical guidelines in the conduct, dissemination, and implementation of nursing research.* Washington, DC: American Nurses Association.

Silva, M. (1995). *Annotated bibliography for ethical guidelines in the conduct, dissemination, and implementation of nursing research.* Washington, DC: American Nurses Association.

Taylor, D. (1998). The nurse as patient advocate. *Nursing*, 28(8), 70–71.

Thurston, D. (1995). Hospital research comes of age. *Canadian Nurse*, 91(4), 35.

Trossman, S. (1999). Nurse researchers open doors. *American Journal of Nursing*, 99(9), 68, 70.

Advocate

American Hospital Association. (1972, 1992). *A patient's bill of rights.* Chicago: Author.

Annas, G. J. (1992). *The rights of patients.* Totowa, NJ: Humana Press.

Copp, L. A. (1993). A response to, Patient advocacy—an important part of the daily work of the expert nurse. *Scholarship and Inquiry in Nursing Practice*, 7(2), 137–140.

Gadow, S. (1989). Clinical subjectivity: Advocacy with silent patients. *Nursing Clinics of North America*, 23(2), 535–541.

Kavanaugh, K. H. (1993). Transcultural nursing: Facing the challenge of advocacy and diversity/universality. *Journal of Transcultural Nursing*, 5(1), 4–13.

Kendrick, K. (1994). An advocate for whom—doctor or patient? How far can a nurse be a patient advocate? *Professional Nurse*, 9(12), 826–829.

Kenner, C. (1995). Use of professional associations for political action. The job of perinatal and neonatal nursing. *Journal of Perinatal and Neonatal Nursing*, 9(1), 78–88.

Kohnke, M. F. (1982). *Advocacy: Risk and reality.* St. Louis: C. V. Mosby.

Miller, S. H., Cohen, M. Z., & Kagan, S. H. (2000). The measure of advocacy. *American Journal of Nursing*, 100(1), 61–64.

Murphy, P. (1990). Helping Joanne die with dignity. *Nursing*, 20(9), 45–49.

Segesten, K. (1993). Patient advocacy—an important part of the daily work of the expert nurse. *Scholarship and Inquiry in Nursing Practice*, 7(2), 129–135.

Sheridan-Gonzalez, J. (2000). It's not my patient. *American Journal of Nursing*, 100(1), 13.

Teasdale, K. (1994). Advocacy and the nurse manager. *Journal of Nursing Management*, 2(2), 93–97.

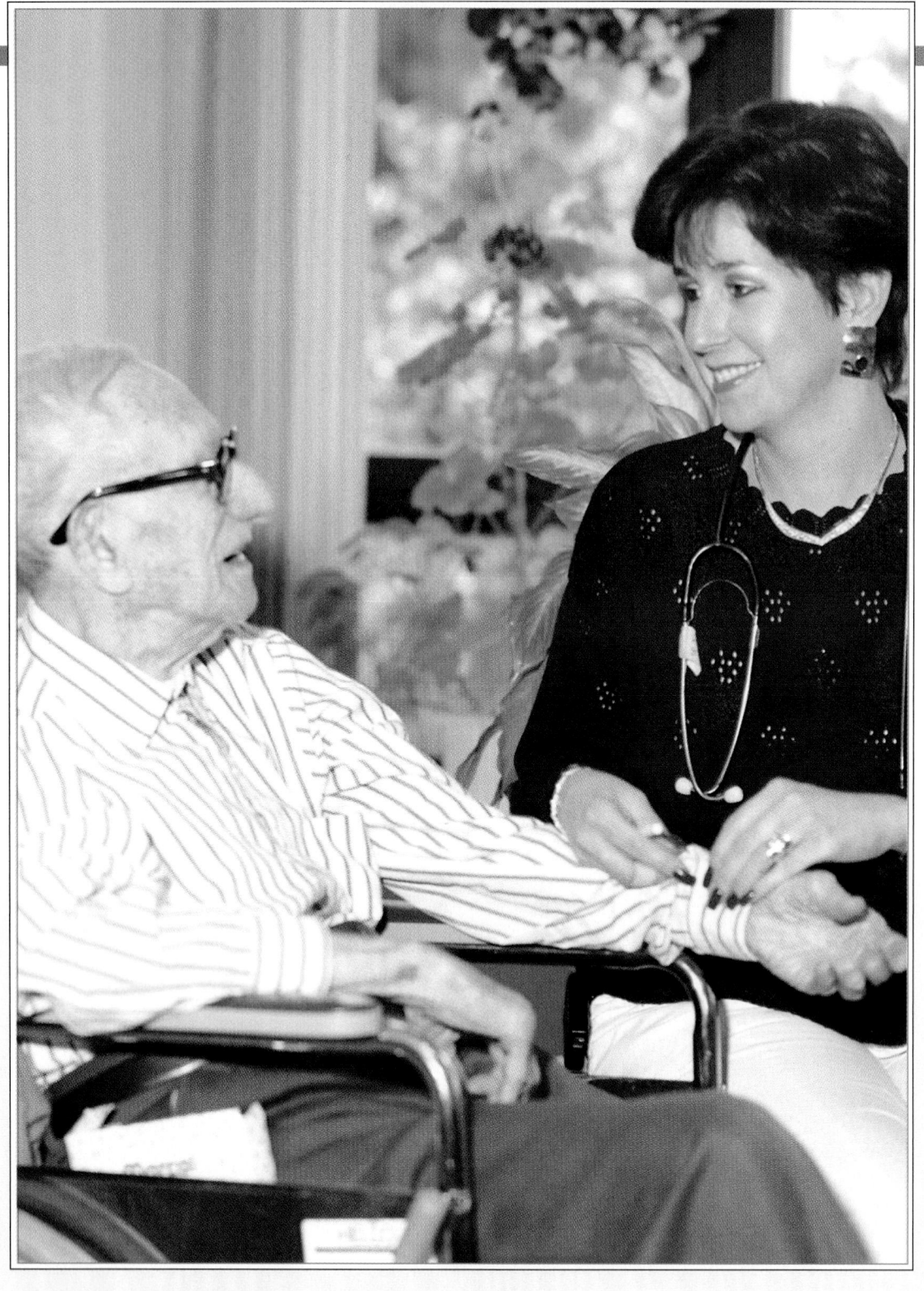

UNIT VI

Chapter 24
Vital Signs

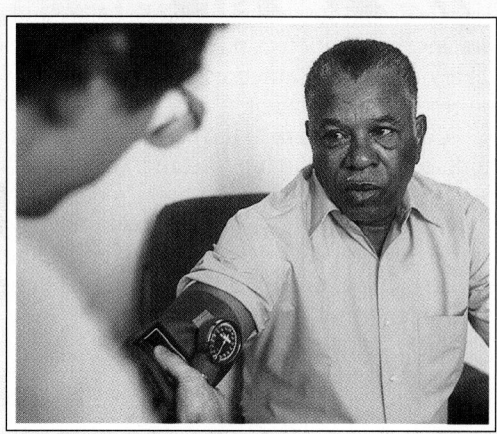

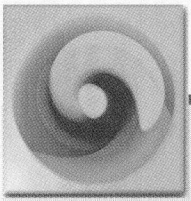

Thinking Critically About
Nursing's Blended Skills

Before reading this chapter, think about the types of blended skills you will need to develop to assess and document vital signs.

- A mother is holding her 2-year-old son in the emergency room. He screams when you attempt to obtain a tympanic membrane temperature, and his mother asks you if there is another way to get his temperature reading.

- A nursing student walks into the room of a patient who was just returned from the postanesthesia unit after surgery to assess vital signs and cannot palpate a pulse or detect respirations.

- The daughter of a 62-year-old woman being seen in your clinic for high blood pressure asks you to teach her how to monitor her mother's blood pressure. Her mother is 5 feet, 5 inches tall and weighs 287 pounds.

- When a patient is returned to your unit after vascular surgery on the femoral artery, you are instructed to check distal pulses to ensure blood flow. You are unable to palpate the posterior tibial pulse but are unsure if the reason is your lack of skill or impaired circulation.

- A record heat wave has seized your city, and you have been invited to deliver a brief statement on the local news station about hyperthermia and prevention strategies.

What cognitive, technical, interpersonal, and ethical/legal skills do you think you will need to respond to the challenges described above?

Vital signs are a person's temperature, pulse, respiration, and blood pressure. (Pain, often called the fifth vital sign, is discussed in Chap. 40). A person's physiologic status is reflected in these indicators of body function, which are normally regulated through homeostatic mechanisms and fall within certain normal ranges. A change in vital signs may indicate a change in health.

Vital signs are taken and compared with accepted normal values and the patient's usual patterns in a wide variety of instances, including screenings at health fairs and clinics, in the home, upon admission to a healthcare setting, when certain medications are given, before and after diagnostic and surgical procedures, before and after certain nursing interventions, and in emergency situations. Nurses take vital signs as often as the condition of a patient requires such assessment.

Careful attention to the details of vital sign procedures and accuracy in the interpretation of the findings are extremely important. It is the nurse's role to interpret vital sign findings. How to assess each of the vital signs, along with a discussion of normal and abnormal findings, is presented in this chapter. Additional information about health assessment can be found in Chapter 25.

Frequency of Vital Sign Assessments

Assessing vital signs is part of nursing care in any setting. Institutional and agency policies govern when and how frequently vital signs are to be routinely assessed. Vital signs are assessed at least every 4 hours in hospitalized patients with elevated temperatures, with high or low blood pressures, with changes in pulse rate or rhythm, or with respiratory difficulty as well as in patients who are taking medications that affect cardiovascular or respiratory function or who have had surgery. Severely ill patients may have vital signs taken more frequently. In critical care settings, technologically advanced devices are often used for continual monitoring of patients' vital signs. In the home and in some self-care and psychiatric units, assessments are often made as frequently as the nurse judges necessary.

Auxiliary personnel may assess vital signs in some situations, but the nurse is ultimately accountable for these assessments. If a patient has untoward symptoms (such as chest pain or dizziness) or has unexpected changes in vital signs, the nurse should double check the findings and further assess the patient. The nurse should also be familiar with normal variations in vital signs that occur at various ages (Table 24-1).

Assessing Body Temperature

Body **temperature** is the heat of the body, measured in degrees. The body temperature level reflects the difference between heat production and heat loss. The core body temperature of a healthy person is maintained within a fairly constant range by the thermoregulatory center in the hypothalamus. This center receives messages from thermal receptors located throughout the body either to pro-

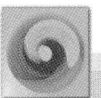

COGNITIVE SKILLS

- Basic knowledge of the anatomy and physiology underlying vital signs and the significance of normal and abnormal findings; knowledge of nursing responsibilities in assessing temperature, pulse, respirations, and blood pressure; knowledge of how to tailor vital signs technology to meet the individualized needs of patients (eg, best means to assess the temperature of a 2-year-old, the fact that a larger cuff is needed to assess with accuracy the blood pressure of the obese woman)
- Knowledge of how to respond to absent vital signs (no readily discernible pulse, respirations)
- Knowledge of how to teach patients and their family caregivers how to assess vital signs and respond to significant findings
- Knowledge about heat cramps, heat exhaustion, and heat stroke and related prevention strategies

TECHNICAL SKILLS

- Ability to use correctly the equipment necessary to assess and document vital signs

INTERPERSONAL SKILLS

- Strong people skills; ability to communicate and interact effectively with patients and their caregivers while assessing vital signs and to teach others how to assess temperature, pulse, respirations, and blood pressure accurately
- Confidence in your own abilities and the willingness to get help when you need it
- Ability to "connect" with a television audience and motivate appropriate self-care and prevention skills

ETHICAL/LEGAL SKILLS

- Commitment to safety and quality; strong sense of responsibility and accountability
- Ability to put the need to assess accurately the patient's distal pulses over your own discomfort about your questionable ability to palpate the pulse; willingness to get help when needed
- Ability to document temperature, pulse, respirations, and blood pressure findings according to agency policy

Table 24-1
Age-Related Variations in Normal Vital Signs

Age	Temperature (C)	Pulse (beats/min)	Respirations (breaths/min)	Blood Pressure (mm Hg)
Newborn	36.8 (Axillary)	80–180	30–80	73/55
1–3 yr	37.7 (Rectal)	80–140	20–40	90/55
6–8 yr	37 (Oral)	75–120	15–25	95/75
10 yr	37 (Oral)	75–110	15–25	102/62
Teens	37 (Oral)	60–100	15–20	102/80
Adults	37 (Oral)	60–100	12–20	120/80
>70 yr	36 (Oral)	60–100	15–20	120/80 (May normally be up to 160/95)

duce or conserve body heat or to increase heat loss. Under normal conditions, the thermoregulatory center's set point maintains body temperature within a range of 35.9°C (96.6°F) to 37.4°C (99.3°F). Core body temperatures reflect the temperature of the viscera and the muscles, which are insulated by the adipose tissue and skin to prevent heat loss. Heat is lost when heat from the body's inner core is transferred to the skin surface by the circulating blood (Porth, 1998).

Temperatures differ in various parts of the body, with core body temperatures being higher than surface body temperatures. Core temperatures are measured at tympanic or rectal sites, but they may also be measured in the esophagus, pulmonary artery, or bladder by invasive monitoring devices. Surface body temperatures are measured at oral (sublingual) and axillary sites.

Body Temperature Regulation

Body temperature is regulated by balancing heat production and heat loss to maintain homeostasis. Temperature regulation is influenced by various factors, including circadian rhythms, age, gender, stress, and the surrounding environment.

Heat Production
The primary source of heat in the body is metabolism, with heat produced as a byproduct of metabolic activities that generate energy for cellular functions. Various mechanisms increase body metabolism, including hormones, muscle movements, and exercise. When additional heat is required to maintain balance, epinephrine and norepinephrine (sympathetic neurotransmitters) are released and alter metabolism so that energy production decreases and heat production increases. Thyroid hormone, produced by the thyroid gland, also increases metabolism and heat production, but over a much longer time period. Shivering, a re-

sponse that increases the production of heat, is initiated by the hypothalamus and results in muscular tremors. The contraction of pilomotor muscles of the skin, causing pilo-erection, or "goose bumps," reduces the size of the surface to minimize heat loss. Exercise increases heat production through muscular activity.

Heat Loss
The skin is the primary site of heat loss. The circulating blood brings heat to the skin's surface, where small connections between the arterioles and the venules lie directly below the surface. These connections, called *arteriovenous shunts*, may remain open to allow heat to dissipate to the skin and thus to the external environment, or they may close and retain heat in the body. The sympathetic nervous system controls the opening and closing of the shunts in response to changes in core body temperature and in environmental temperature (Porth, 1998).

Other heat losses occur through evaporation of sweat, through warming and humidifying of inspired air, and through eliminating urine and feces. Heat is transferred to the external environment through the physical processes of radiation, convection, evaporation, and conduction. These processes are defined and illustrated in Table 24-2.

Factors Affecting Body Temperature

A variety of different factors affect body temperature. These factors include circadian rhythms, age, gender, stress, and environmental temperatures.

Circadian Rhythms
Many environmental and physiologic processes occur in repeated cycles of time. Some events in humans recur at 24-hour intervals, referred to as **circadian** (meaning nearly every 24 hours) **rhythm**. Predictable fluctuations

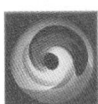

Table 24-2
Mechanisms of Heat Transfer

	Radiation	Convection	Evaporation	Conduction
Definition	The diffusion or dissemination of heat by electromagnetic waves	The dissemination of heat by motion between areas of unequal density	The conversion of a liquid to a vapor	The transfer of heat to another object during direct contact
Example	The body gives off waves of heat from uncovered surfaces.	An oscillating fan blows currents of cool air across the surface of a warm body.	Body fluid in the form of perspiration and insensible loss is vaporized from the skin.	The body transfers heat to an ice pack, causing the ice to melt.
Illustration	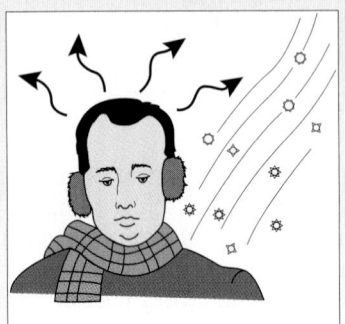	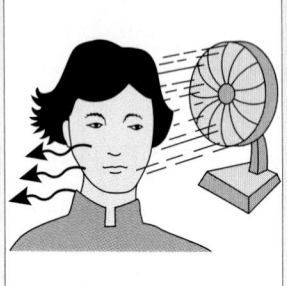	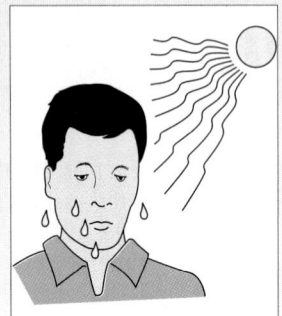	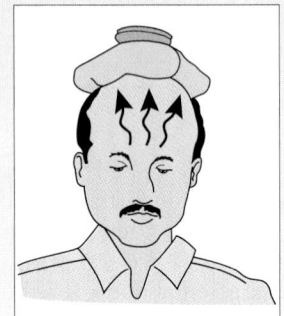

in measurements of body temperature and blood pressure are examples of functions that have a circadian rhythm. For instance, body temperature is usually about 0.6°C (1° to 2°F) lower in the early morning than in the late afternoon and early evening. This variation tends to be somewhat greater in infants and children. Research indicates that the peak elevation of a person's temperature occurs in late afternoon, between 4 and 7 PM.

Age
Both the very young and the very old are more sensitive to changes in environmental temperature. The body temperature of infants and children changes more rapidly in response to both heat and cold air temperatures. Older adults lose some thermoregulatory control and are at risk for harm from extremes of temperature.

Gender
Women tend to have more fluctuations in body temperature than men, probably the result of changes in hormones. The increase in progesterone secretion at ovulation increases body temperature as much as 0.5° to 1°F.

Stress
The body responds to both physical and emotional stress as a threat, increasing the production of epinephrine and norepinephrine. As a result, the metabolic rate increases, raising the body temperature.

Environmental Temperature
Most of us respond to changes in environmental temperature by wearing clothing that either allows increased heat loss when it is hot or retains heat when it is cold. When one is exposed to extreme cold without adequate protective clothing, however, heat loss may be increased to the point of *hypothermia* (low body temperature). Similarly, if one is exposed to extremes of heat for long periods of time, *hyperthermia* (high body temperature) may result. Both hypothermia and hyperthermia may cause serious illness or death.

Body Temperature Variations

Normal Body Temperature
Normal body temperature varies among individuals, with a range of 0.3° to 0.6°C (0.5° to 1.0°F) from the average normal temperature considered to be within normal limits. Even wider variations from the average temperature have been found to be normal for certain people.

Increased Body Temperature
Pyrexia (fever) is a body temperature above normal. A person with an increased body temperature is said to be **febrile**. A person with a normal body temperature is referred to as **afebrile**. **Hyperpyrexia** is a high fever, usually above 41°C (105.8°F), and survival is rare when the temperature reaches 44°C (110°F). Death is probably due to

damaging effects on the respiratory center but may also result from inactivation of body enzymes and destruction of
tissue proteins. Pyrexia is a common symptom of illness,
and there is evidence to indicate that an elevated temperature helps the body fight disease. In children, this response
is often seen quickly. In older adults, pyrexia may be one
of the later signs of illness, and the temperature may be elevated only 1° or 2°F above normal, even when pathologic
processes are extensive.

It is theorized that when a fever occurs, the set point
regulated by the hypothalamus is readjusted to a higher
level. As a result, heat loss is decreased or heat production
is increased, or both occur through shivering, constriction
of surface blood vessels, and absence of sweating. After the
body temperature rises to the new set point, heat loss
mechanisms again keep the body temperature from rising
to dangerous levels. Most fevers are self-limiting, and the
temperature returns to normal range after the disease
process is controlled. Relieving a moderately elevated body
temperature may reduce the body's defenses against disease. The onset of an elevated body temperature may be
sudden or gradual. Common terms used to describe types
of fever are listed in the accompanying box.

Patients with a fever usually experience loss of appetite; headache; hot, dry skin; flushed face; thirst; and
general malaise. Young children or other people with high
fevers may experience periods of delirium or seizures. Observing for other potentially dangerous manifestations of a
fever, such as dehydration, decreased urinary output, and
rapid heart rate, is an important nursing assessment. Nursing activities for the patient with a fever are outlined in the
accompanying box.

Antipyretic (fever-reducing) drugs, such as aspirin or
acetaminophen, may be administered in certain circumstances. These drugs are believed to lower the elevated set
point regulated by the hypothalamus. They do not affect
body temperature when it is within normal range. Body
temperature may also be lowered through other interventions, including cool sponge baths, cool packs, and cooling
blankets.

Terms and Definitions for Types of Fever

Intermittent: The body temperature alternates regularly between a period of fever and a period of normal or subnormal temperature.

Remittent: The body temperature fluctuates several
degrees more than 2°C (3.6°F) above normal but
does not reach normal between fluctuations.

Constant: The body temperature remains consistently elevated and fluctuates less than 2°C (3.6°F).

Relapsing: The body temperature returns to normal
for at least a day, but then the fever recurs.

Crisis: The fever returns to normal suddenly.

Lysis: The fever returns to normal gradually.

Using the Nursing Interventions Classification (NIC)

Fever Treatment

- Monitor temperature as frequently as is appropriate.
- Monitor for insensible fluid loss.
- Monitor skin color and temperature.
- Monitor blood pressure, pulse, and respiration, as appropriate.
- Monitor for decreasing levels of consciousness.
- Monitor for seizure activity.
- Monitor white blood cell count, hemoglobin, and hematocrit levels.
- Monitor intake and output.
- Monitor for electrolyte abnormalities.
- Monitor for acid–base imbalance.
- Administer antipyretic medication, as appropriate.
- Administer a tepid sponge bath, as appropriate.
- Encourage increased intake of oral fluids, as appropriate.
- Encourage or give oral hygiene, as appropriate.

McCloskey, J., & Bulechek, G. (1996). *Nursing interventions classification (NIC)* (2nd ed.). (p. 288). St. Louis: C. V. Mosby. A full listing of nursing activities for each nursing intervention can be found in this book.

Decreased Body Temperature

Hypothermia is a body temperature below the lower limit of
normal. Death may occur when the temperature falls below
about 34°C (93.2°F), but survival has been reported in isolated cases when body temperatures have fallen in the range
of severe hypothermia (28°C or 82.4°F). This may happen to
a person drowning in cold water or buried by snow.

Just as an elevated body temperature is a protective
device for the body, a lowered body temperature may be
beneficial at times. Rates of chemical reactions in the body
are slowed, thereby decreasing the metabolic demands for
oxygen. Figure 24-1 illustrates the usual ranges of human
body temperature.

Nursing Diagnoses for Altered Body Temperature

North American Nursing Diagnosis Association (NANDA)
nursing diagnoses, with definitions, for alterations in body
temperature are as follows:

- Risk for Altered Body Temperature: the state in
  which an individual is at risk for failure to maintain
  body temperature within normal range
- Hyperthermia: the state in which an individual's
  body temperature is elevated above normal range
- Hypothermia: the state in which an individual's
  body temperature is reduced below normal range

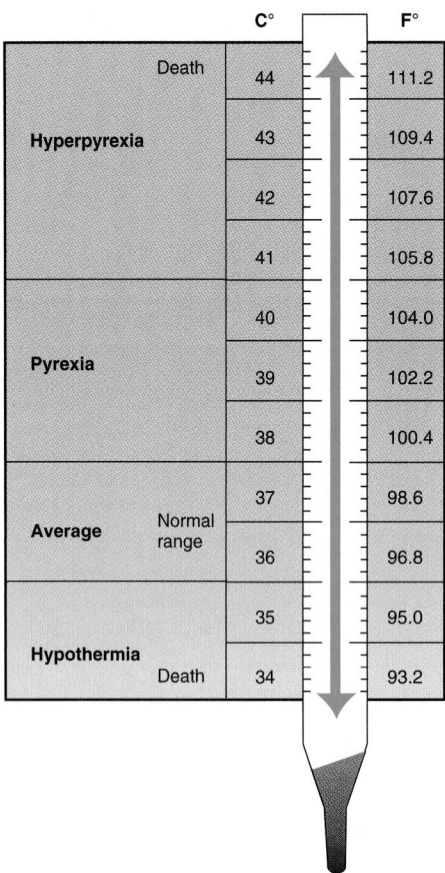

Figure 24-1
The range of human body temperature, as measured orally.

- Ineffective Thermoregulation: the state in which an individual's temperature fluctuates between hypothermia and hyperthermia

Temperature Assessment Equipment, Sites, and Methods

Equipment

Body temperature may be assessed with a variety of devices. These are electronic thermometers, tympanic membrane thermometers, glass thermometers, disposable thermometers, temperature-sensitive patches or tape, and automated monitoring devices.

Electronic Thermometer

Electronic thermometers measure body temperature in 25 to 50 seconds. Most have nonbreakable temperature probes appropriate for oral, rectal, or axillary temperature measurement. They are equipped with disposable probe covers, which minimize the risk for cross-infection. A sound indicates when the peak temperature has been recorded. Various models are available. How to assess body temperature with an electronic thermometer is described in Procedure 24-1.

Tympanic Membrane Thermometer

Tympanic membrane thermometers use infrared sensors to detect heat given off by the tympanic membrane.

The probe of the thermometer is covered with a probe cover and inserted into the ear canal tightly enough to seal the opening (see Procedure 24-1). The reading takes less than 2 seconds. Although tympanic temperatures are commonly taken in children, there is some question about the accuracy of the reading assessed with these thermometers, especially in children younger than 6 years of age (Lanham, Walker, Klocke, & Jennings, 1999).

Glass Thermometer

A glass thermometer with a mercury tip has traditionally been used to measure body temperature. This type of thermometer has a bulb at the end of a stem. The bulb contains liquid mercury, which expands when with heat and rises within the stem. Most commonly, a long, thin bulb is found on glass thermometers used to take oral temperatures, and a blunt bulb is found on glass thermometers used to take rectal temperatures.

Glass thermometers are generally calibrated in degrees of either centigrade (Celsius, C) or Fahrenheit (F) (see Fig. 24-1) in a range of about 34°C (94°) to about 42.2° (108°F). The degrees on a thermometer using the Celsius scale are subdivided into gradients of 0.1°; the subdivisions on a thermometer using the Fahrenheit scale are the equivalent of 0.2°. It is common practice to report the temperature to the nearest one tenth of a degree on a Fahrenheit thermometer when the mercury is a bit more or less from a line of calibration. Table 24-3 illustrates comparable centigrade and Fahrenheit temperatures and explains how temperatures are converted from one scale to the other. Assessing body temperature using a glass thermometer is described in Procedure 24-1.

If glass thermometers are used within a healthcare institution, each patient has his or her own thermometer for the duration of inpatient care. The thermometer is kept in the patient's room, usually in a container of liquid disinfectant. It is recommended that glass thermometers used for patients with hepatitis (an infectious disease of the liver) and acquired immune deficiency syndrome (AIDS) be discarded when the patient is discharged.

In the home, clean thermometers in lukewarm soapy water, rinse in cool water, and then store for reuse. If the thermometer is to be used by more than one person or if the person has a known or suspected infection transmitted by oral secretions, disinfect the thermometer with an appropriate solution after cleaning. Follow the manufacturer's recommendations for the care and disposal of electronic and other types of thermometers and their probe covers.

Disposable Single-Use Thermometer

Disposable single-use thermometers, such as Nex-Temp, register within seconds and are nonbreakable. Because they are used only once, they eliminate the danger of cross-infection.

Temperature-Sensitive Patch or Tape

Temperature-sensitive patches or tape, commonly applied to the abdomen or forehead, change color at different temperature ranges. These devices may be used to check

(*text continues on page 429*)

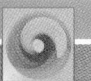

PROCEDURE 24-1

Assessing Body Temperature

Equipment

Glass thermometer or electronic
  thermometer
Probe covers for electronic
  thermometer

Lubricant (for rectal thermometers)
Disposable gloves (as appropriate or
  indicated)
Soft tissues

Pencil or pen, paper or flow sheet

Use guidelines outlined below for all sites and methods.

Guidelines for Assessing, Implementing, and Documenting Temperatures

Action	Rationale
1. Identify the patient.	Provides patient safety
2. Explain the procedure to the patient.	Reduces patient apprehension and encourages patient cooperation
3. Gather equipment.	Provides organized approach to task
4. Wash your hands and don gloves if appropriate or indicated.	Deters the spread of microorganisms
5. Select the appropriate site.	Assess the patient's age, mental, and physical condition to ensure safety and accuracy of measurement
6. Follow the steps as outlined below for the appropriate type of thermometer.	
7. Wash your hands. If gloves are worn, discard them in the proper receptacle.	Deters the spread of microorganisms
8. Record temperature on paper, flow sheet, or computerized record. Report abnormal findings to the appropriate person. Identify site of assessment if other than oral.	Provides accurate documentation and reporting

Assessing Tympanic Membrane Temperature

1. If necessary, push the "on" button and wait for the "ready" signal on the unit.
2. Attach tympanic probe cover.

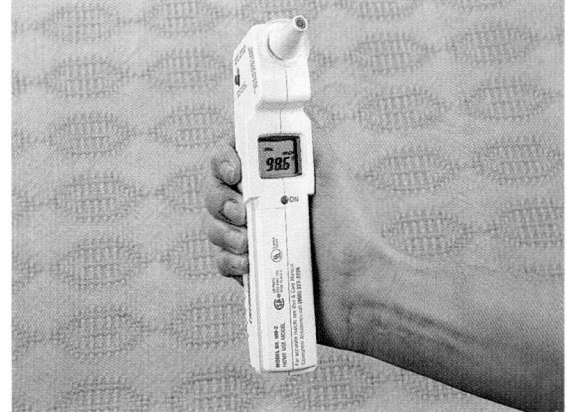

Action 1: Tympanic membrane thermometer. (Photo © B. Proud.)

3. Insert the probe snugly into the external ear, using gentle but firm pressure.

Ensures probe is positioned correctly to measure tympanic temperature

(continued)

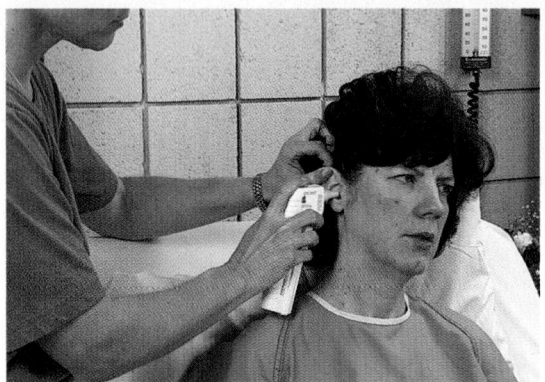

Action 3: Tympanic membrane thermometer with probe cover being placed in patient's ear. (Photo © B. Proud.)

4. Activate unit by pushing the trigger button. The reading is immediate (usually within 2 seconds).

5. Note the temperature reading, discard the probe cover, and replace the thermometer in its charger or holder.

The tympanic membrane thermometer provides a digital display of the measurement.

Assessing Oral Temperature With a Glass Thermometer

1. If stored in a chemical solution, wipe it dry with a soft tissue, using a firm twisting motion. Wipe from the bulb toward the fingers.

Chemical solutions may irritate mucous membranes and have an objectionable taste. Twisting helps cover the entire surface. Wiping from an area of few or no organisms to an area where organisms might be present minimizes spread to a cleaner area.

2. Grasp the thermometer firmly with the thumb and forefinger and, using strong wrist movements, shake it until the mercury line reaches at least 36°C (59°F).

Moves the mercury back into the bulb below the previous measurement.

3. Read thermometer by holding it horizontally at eye level, and rotate it between the fingers until the mercury line can be clearly visualized.

Facilitates reading the mercury line.

4. Place the mercury bulb of the thermometer within the back of the right or left pocket under the patient's tongue, and tell the patient to close the lips around the thermometer.

When the bulb rests deeply in the posterior sublingual pocket, it is in contact with blood vessels lying close to surface.

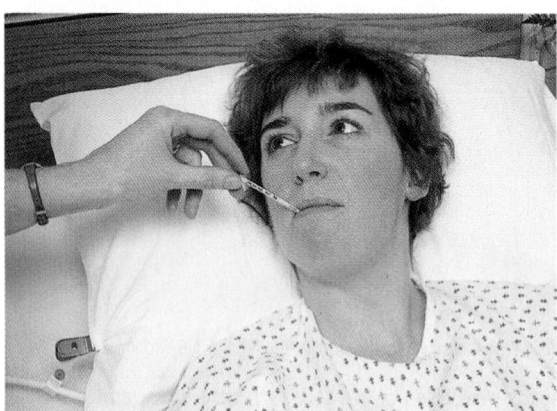

Action 4: Placing the thermometer.

(*continued*)

Assessing Body Temperature (Continued)

5. Leave the thermometer in place for 3 minutes, or according to agency protocol.	Allows time for the mercury to expand and accurately measure temperature.
6. Remove the thermometer, and wipe it once from the fingers down to the mercury bulb, using a firm, twisting motion.	Minimizes spread of organisms from an area of higher concentration to a cleaner area; friction helps loosen material from the thermometer surface.
7. Read the thermometer to the nearest tenth.	Mercury may rise a bit above or below the calibration lines.

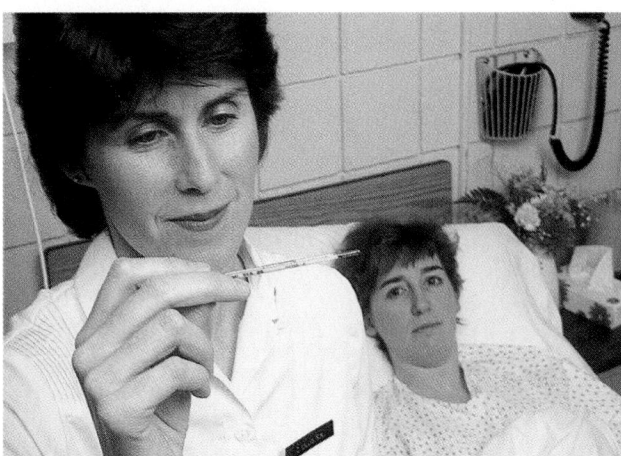

Action 7: Reading the thermometer. (Photos © Ken Kasper.)

8. Dispose of the tissues in a receptacle for contaminated items.	Confining contaminated articles helps reduce the spread of pathogens.
9. Wash thermometer in lukewarm soapy water. Rinse it in cool water. Dry and replace the thermometer in its container.	Mechanical washing action removes organic material and organisms.

Assessing Rectal Temperature Using a Glass Thermometer

1. Don gloves.	Protects nurse from microorganisms in the feces.

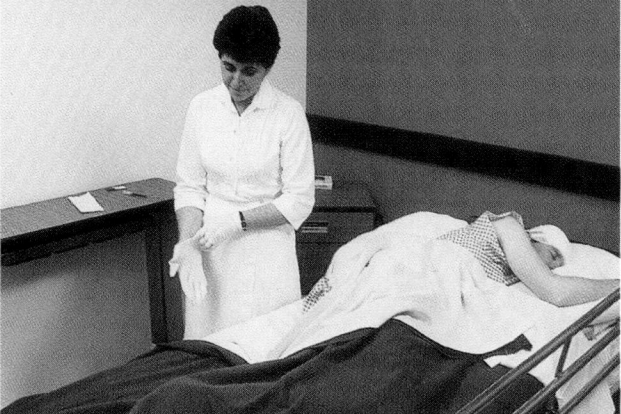

Action 1: Donning clean gloves.

2. Wipe, shake, and read the rectal thermometer.	See oral thermometer preparation.
3. Lubricate the mercury bulb up to about 2.5 cm (1 inch) up the stem.	Lubrication reduces friction and facilitates insertion, minimizing irritation or injury to the rectal mucous membranes.

(*continued*)

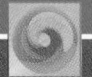
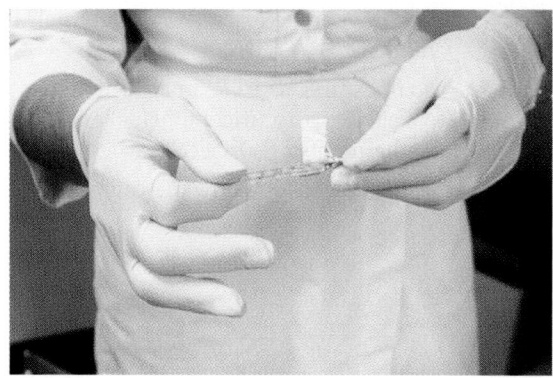

Action 3: Lubricating the mercury bulb.

4. Provide privacy. With the patient lying on the side and the buttocks exposed, separate the buttocks so the anal sphincter is seen clearly.

If not placed directly into the anal opening, the bulb of the thermometer may injure adjacent tissue or cause discomfort.

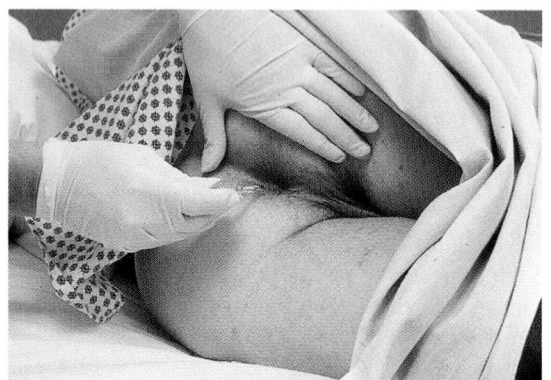

Actions 4 and 5: Separating the buttocks and inserting the thermometer.

5. Insert the thermometer about 3.8 cm (1½ inches) in an adult, 2.5 cm (1 inch) in a child, and 1.25 cm (½ inch) in an infant.

Insertion length must be adjusted to the anatomic size of the rectum based on the patient's age; rectal temperatures are not normally taken in an infant.

6. Holding the thermometer in place, let the buttocks fall into place, and continue holding the thermometer for 2 to 3 minutes.

The thermometer may be displaced internally or externally if not held.

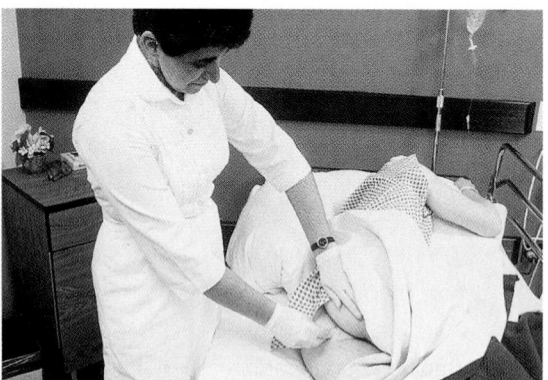

Action 6: Holding the thermometer in place.

(continued)

7. Remove the thermometer and wipe it once with soft tissue from the fingers to the mercury bulb, using a firm twisting motion.

See oral thermometer wiping.

8. Wipe the anus of any feces and the remaining lubricant.

Promotes cleanliness and comfort

9. Read the thermometer and dispose of the tissue and gloves in the proper receptacle. (Remove the gloves from the inside out.)

Avoids transmission of microorganisms

10. Wash the thermometer in lukewarm soapy water. Rinse in cool water. Dry and replace the thermometer in a container labeled "rectal thermometer."

Assessing Axillary Temperature Using a Glass Thermometer

Follow the procedure for taking an oral temperature with a glass thermometer with the following exceptions.

1. Move clothing to expose axilla.

Ensures accurate placement of the thermometer.

2. Place the bulb of the thermometer in the center of the axilla, and bring the patient's arm down close to the body.

The deepest area of the axilla provides the most accurate measurement; surrounding the bulb with skin surface ensures a more reliable measurement.

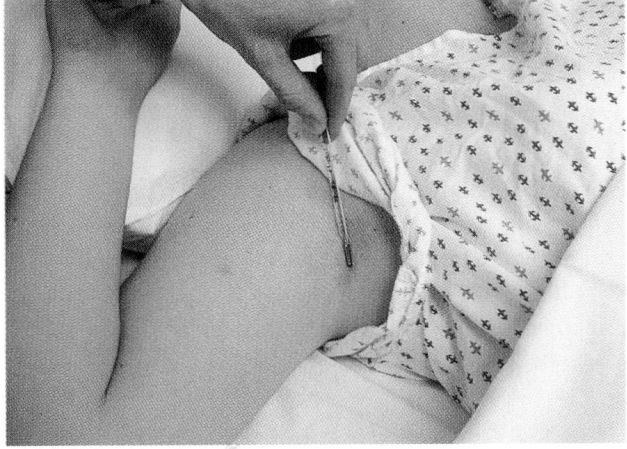

Action 2: Placing the bulb in the center of the axilla.

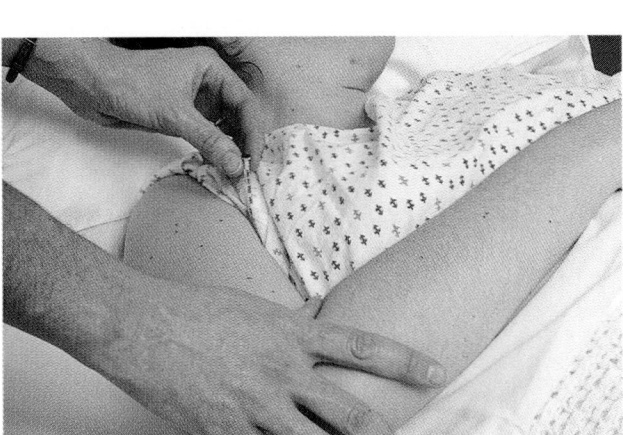

Action 2: Placing the patient's arm close to the body. (Photos © Ken Kasper.)

(continued)

PROCEDURE 24-1

Assessing Body Temperature (Continued)

3. Remain with the patient and leave the thermometer in place for 10 minutes.

Axillary measurement requires a longer time for the mercury to expand. Staying with the patient ensures that the thermometer remains in the correct position and prevents breakage.

Assessing Temperature With an Electronic Thermometer

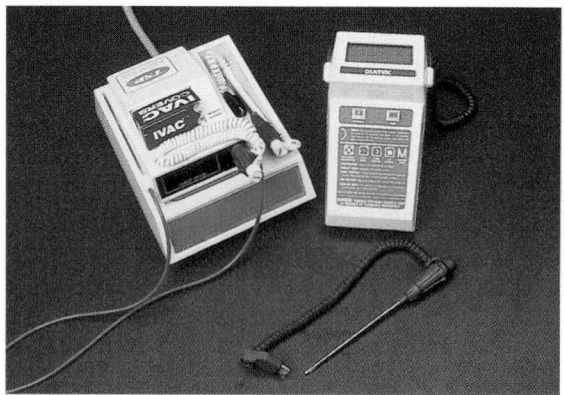

Two types of electronic thermometers and probes.

1. Release the electronic unit from the charging unit, and remove the probe from within the recording unit.

2. Cover thermometer probe with disposable probe cover, and slide it into place until it snaps into place.

Prevents contamination of the thermometer probe.

3. For rectal temperatures, lubricate probe.

See procedure for assessing rectal temperature with a glass thermometer.

4. Place probe in posterior sublingual pocket, and ask the patient to close the lips around the probe (oral); in the rectum as described when using a glass thermometer (rectal); or in the center of the axilla with arm against chest wall (axillary).

See procedures for oral, rectal, and axillary temperature assessment.

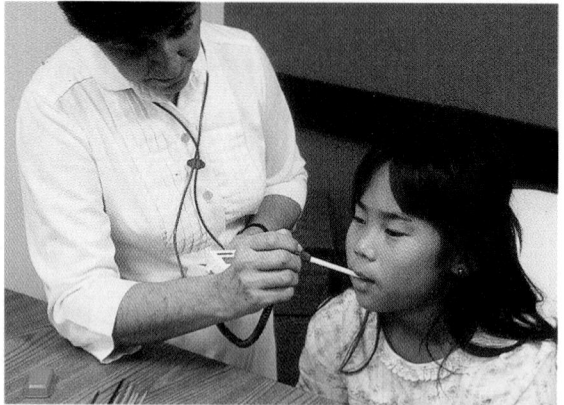

Actions 3 and 4: Placing and supporting the probe in place in the patient's mouth.

5. Hold the probe in place until an audible signal is heard.

If left unsupported, the weight of the probe tends to pull it away from the correct location. The signal indicates the measurement is completed.

(continued)

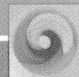

PROCEDURE 24-1

Assessing Body Temperature (Continued)

6. Note the temperature reading, and dispose of the probe cover by pressing the probe release button while holding the probe over a receptacle.

The electronic thermometer provides a digital display of the measured temperature.

7. Replace the thermometer in its charger or holder.

Recharges the thermometer for future use.

Age Considerations

The axillary, a temperature-sensitive tape, or the tympanic membrane is the preferred method of evaluating the body temperature of a child younger than 6 years of age (even though research is ongoing to determine accuracy of the measurement).

These sites should also be used for a confused, disoriented, or comatose adult.

Home Care Considerations

Reinforce differences in temperature reading depending on site used. Axillary temperatures are generally about 1° less than oral temperatures; rectal temperatures are generally about 1° higher.

---

the temperature of a toddler or young child. A thermometer should be used to reassess the temperature if the color on the tape or patch indicates that the temperature is out of the normal average range.

Automated Monitoring Devices

Automated monitoring devices are increasingly being used in various healthcare settings to measure a patient's body temperature, pulse, and blood pressure simultaneously. They require less of the nurse's time, especially when these assessments are conducted frequently.

Sites and Methods

A thermometer or electronic probe is placed under the tongue (sublingual area) of a person's mouth to assess an oral temperature, in the anal canal to assess a rectal temperature, or in an axilla (armpit) to assess an axillary temperature. A probe is placed in the ear to assess a tympanic temperature. Table 24-4 shows the average normal temperature standards for well adults at various body sites.

Health agencies specify the site to be used for assessing patients' temperatures; however, the nurse is expected to select and use alternative sites in certain situations. Factors affecting the site selection include the patient's age, state of consciousness, amount of pain, and other care being provided. It is customary to indicate the site used to assess the temperature when recording the measurement.

Assessing a Tympanic Membrane Temperature

The tympanic membrane temperature is also considered a core body temperature. Infrared sensors in the thermometer sense heat from the body as it is given off by a

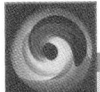

Table 24-3
Equivalent Centigrade and Fahrenheit Temperatures*

Centigrade	Fahrenheit	Centigrade	Fahrenheit
34.0	93.2	38.5	101.3
35.0	95.0	39.0	102.2
36.0	96.8	40.0	104.0
36.5	97.7	41.0	105.8
37.0	98.6	42.0	107.6
37.5	99.5	43.0	109.4
38.0	100.4	44.0	111.2

* To convert centigrade to Fahrenheit, multiply by ⁹⁄₅ and add 32. To change Fahrenheit to centigrade, subtract 32 and multiply by ⁵⁄₉.

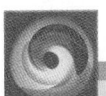

Table 24-4
Average Normal Temperatures for Healthy Adults at Various Sites

Oral	Rectal	Axillary	Tympanic	Forehead
37.0°C	37.5°C	36.5°C	37.5°C*	34.4°C†
98.6°F	99.5°F	97.6°F	99.5°F	94.0°F

* The average normal tympanic temperature depends on the calibration and mode setting of the tympanic membrane thermometer.
† The manufacturer of Digitemp forehead thermometer (Hallcrest Products, 1820 Pickwick Lane, Glenview, IL 60025) says, "Most older children and adults have normal forehead temperatures between 93 and 95 degrees F."

heat source; in the ear canal, the primary heat source is the tympanic membrane. The thermometer does not touch the tympanic membrane (see Procedure 24-1).

Assessing an Oral Temperature

One crucial criterion for selecting the oral site is that the patient must be able to close his or her mouth around the thermometer or probe. Assessing an oral temperature using a glass thermometer is contraindicated in unconscious, irrational, and seizure-prone patients and in infants and young children because of the danger of breaking the glass thermometer in the mouth. Oral temperatures are also contraindicated in people with diseases of the oral cavity and in those who have had surgery of the nose or mouth. If a patient has had either hot or cold food or fluids or has been smoking or chewing gum, it is generally recommended to wait 15 to 30 minutes to allow the oral tissues to return to normal temperature. Traditionally, oral temperatures have not been assessed in patients receiving nasal oxygen because it was believed that the oxygen causes a falsely low reading. Research is challenging this opinion. Oral temperatures should not be assessed with a glass thermometer in patients receiving oxygen by mask, however, because the time it takes to assess a reading is likely to result in a serious drop in the patient's blood oxygen level. The procedure for assessing an oral temperature is given in Procedure 24-1.

Assessing a Rectal Temperature

The rectal temperature, a core temperature, is considered to be one of the most accurate. The rectal site is a possible alternative whenever the oral site is contraindicated (see Procedure 24-1). Measuring rectal temperature is contraindicated in newborns and in patients who have undergone rectal surgery or have diarrhea or disease of the rectum. Because the insertion of the thermometer can slow the heart rate by stimulating the vagus nerve, assessing a rectal temperature may not be allowed in some institutions for people with certain heart diseases or after cardiac surgery.

Assessing an Axillary Temperature

The axillary site may be used when both oral and rectal sites are contraindicated or when these sites are inaccessible. Some hospitals assess axillary temperatures in healthy newborns to avoid the potential for perforating the wall of the rectum with the thermometer. If the axilla has just been washed, delay assessing the temperature 15 to 30 minutes. Most authorities believe that when proper procedure is used, axillary temperatures are as accurate as oral or rectal temperatures. The procedure for assessing an axillary temperature is described in Procedure 24-1.

For most clinical purposes, it would appear equally satisfactory to assess an oral, a rectal, a tympanic, or an axillary temperature provided proper technique is used and normal variations among the methods are considered. Comparing the recordings using two different sites is a method for double checking the validity of an unusual measurement.

Assessing Respirations

Respiration involves several physiologic events:

Pulmonary ventilation (or *breathing*)—movement of air in and out of the lungs; **inspiration** (or inhalation) is the act of breathing in, and **expiration** (or exhalation) is the act of breathing out

External respiration—the exchange of oxygen and carbon dioxide between the alveoli of the lungs and the circulating blood

Internal respiration—the exchange of oxygen and carbon dioxide between the circulating blood and tissue cells

Although nurses assess the manifestations of changes in all of these respiratory events, the part that is measured as a vital sign is pulmonary ventilation, called respirations. The physiology and general principles of respiration are thoroughly discussed in Chapter 44; respiratory system assessment is described further in Chapter 25.

Regulation of Respirations

The rate and depth of breathing can change in response to body demands. These changes are brought about by the inhibition or stimulation of the respiratory muscles by respiratory centers in the medulla and pons. The respiratory centers are activated by impulses from chemoreceptors located in the aortic arch and carotid arteries, from stretch and irritant receptors in the lungs, and from receptors in muscles and joints. An increase in carbon dioxide is the most powerful respiratory stimulant, causing an increase in respiratory depth and rate. The cerebral cortex of the brain allows voluntary control of breathing, such as when singing or playing a musical instrument.

Factors Affecting Respirations

Many different factors may affect respiratory rate and depth. These factors include exercise, respiratory and cardiovascular disease, alterations in fluid, electrolyte, and acid–base balances, medications, trauma, infection, pain, and anxiety.

Respiratory Rate

Under normal conditions, healthy adults breathe about 16 to 20 times each minute (**eupnea**), whereas infants and young children breath more rapidly. The relationship between the pulse rate and the respiratory rate is fairly consistent in well people: the ratio is one respiration to about four heartbeats.

In illness, the respiratory rate often varies from normal. The respiratory rate increases (**tachypnea**) in response to the increased metabolic rate during pyrexia. Cells require more oxygen at this time and have more carbon dioxide that must be removed. The rate increases as much as 4 breaths/min with every 0.6°C (1°F) that the temperature rises above normal. Any condition causing an increase in carbon dioxide and a decrease in oxygen in the blood also tends to increase the rate and depth of respirations.

Some conditions characteristically result in slow breathing (**bradypnea**). An increase in intracranial pressure depresses the respiratory center, resulting in irregular or shallow breathing, slow breathing, or both. Certain drugs, such as narcotics (eg, morphine, meperidine [Demerol]), also depress the respiratory rate.

Respiratory Depth

The depth of respirations normally varies from shallow to deep. The depth of each respiration is about the same during rest. Periodically, each person automatically inhales deeply (sighs), filling the lungs with more air than with the usual depth of respiration.

Certain terms are used to describe the nature and depth of respirations. **Apnea** refers to periods during which there is no breathing. If apnea lasts longer than 4 to 6 minutes, brain damage and death may occur. **Dyspnea** is difficult or labored breathing. A dyspneic patient usually has rapid, shallow respirations and appears anxious. Dyspneic people can often breathe more easily in an upright position, a condition known as **orthopnea**. While sitting or standing, gravity lowers organs in the abdominal cavity away from the diaphragm. This gives more room for the lungs to expand within the chest, providing intake of more air with each breath. Table 24-5 describes and illustrates various respiratory patterns.

Assessment Method

When assessing respirations, the nurse counts the patient's respiratory rate. Procedure 24-2 describes how to assess the respiratory rate.

Table 24-5
Patterns of Respiration

	Description	Pattern	Associated Features
Normal	12–20 breaths/min Regular		Normal pattern
Tachypnea	>24 breaths/min Shallow		Fever, anxiety, exercise, respiratory disorders
Bradypnea	<10 breaths/min Regular		Depression of the respiratory center by medications, brain damage
Hyperventilation	Increased rate and depth		Extreme exercise, fear, diabetic ketoacidosis (Kussmaul's respirations), overdose of aspirin
Hypoventilation	Decreased rate and depth; irregular		Overdose of narcotics or anesthetics
Cheyne-Stokes respirations	Alternating periods of deep, rapid breathing followed by periods of apnea; regular		Drug overdose, heart failure, increased intracranial pressure, renal failure
Biot's respirations	Varying depth and rate of breathing, followed by periods of apnea; irregular		Meningitis, severe brain damage

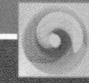

PROCEDURE 24-2

Assessing the Respiratory Rate

Equipment

Watch with second hand or digital readout

Pencil or pen, paper, or flow sheet

Action	Rationale
1. While your fingers are still in place after counting the pulse rate, observe the patient's respirations.	The patient may alter the rate of respirations if aware they are being counted.
2. Note the rise and fall of the patient's chest.	A complete cycle of an inspiration and an expiration composes one respiration.
3. Using a watch with a second hand, count the number of respirations for a minimum of 30 seconds. Multiply this number by 2 for the respiratory rate per minute.	Sufficient time is necessary to observe the rate, depth, and other characteristics.
4. If respirations are abnormal in any way, count the respirations for at least 1 full minute.	Increased time allows the detection of unequal timing between respirations.
5. Document respiratory rate on paper, the flow sheet, or the computerized record. Report any abnormal findings to the appropriate person.	Provides accurate documentation and reporting
6. Wash your hands.	Deters the spread of microorganisms

Nursing Diagnoses for Altered Respirations

NANDA nursing diagnoses, with definitions, for alterations in respirations are as follows:

- Impaired Gas Exchange: excess or deficit in oxygenation or carbon dioxide elimination at the alveolar-capillary membrane
- Ineffective Airway Clearance: inability to clear secretions or obstructions from the respiratory tract to maintain a clear airway
- Ineffective Breathing Pattern: inspiration or expiration that does not provide adequate ventilation
- Inability to Sustain Spontaneous Ventilation: a state in which the response pattern of decreased energy reserves results in an individual's inability to maintain breathing adequate to support life

Assessing Pulse and Blood Pressure

The pulse and blood pressure are indicators of cardiovascular status. Each time the left ventricle of the heart contracts to eject blood into an already full aorta, the arterial walls in the cardiovascular system expand to compensate for the increase in pressure of the blood (blood pressure). Expansion of the aorta sends a wave through the walls of the arterial system that, on palpation, can be felt as a throbbing or tapping (the pulse).

The quantity of blood forced out of the left ventricle with each contraction is called the *stroke volume*. The average amount of blood per contraction is 70 mL in an adult. The *cardiac output* is the amount of blood pumped per minute. This volume is determined by using the following formula:

$$\text{cardiac output} = \text{stroke volume} \times \text{pulse rate}$$

Thus, the cardiac output of an adult with a stroke volume of 70 mL and a pulse rate of 72 beats/min is about 5000 mL.

Many factors can affect both the heart rate and volume; however, compensatory mechanisms attempt to maintain a sufficient supply of blood to the cells at all times. For example, when the stroke volume decreases, such as when the blood volume is decreased because of hemorrhage, the contraction rate increases to try to maintain the same cardiac output. Conversely, in a physically fit athlete whose heart pumps a maximum volume of blood per stroke, the heart rate may be at the low range or below the range of normal, yet the body cells remain adequately supplied.

Nursing Diagnoses for Altered Pulse and Blood Pressure

NANDA nursing diagnoses, with definitions, for alterations in pulse and blood pressure include the following:

- Altered Tissue Perfusion (specify type—renal, cerebral, cardiopulmonary, gastrointestinal, peripheral): a decrease in oxygen resulting in the failure to nourish the tissues at the capillary level
- Risk for Fluid Volume Imbalance: risk for a decrease, increase, or rapid shift from one to the other of intravascular, interstitial, or intracellular fluid (including both a loss, an excess, or both of body fluids and replacement fluids)
- Fluid Volume Excess: the state in which an individual experiences increased isotonic fluid retention
- Fluid Volume Deficit: the state in which an individual experiences decreased intravascular, interstitial, or intracellular fluid (from water loss alone without changes in sodium)
- Decreased Cardiac Output: a state in which the blood pumped by the heart is inadequate to meet the metabolic demands of the body

Equipment Used to Assess Pulse and Blood Pressure

Stethoscope

The **stethoscope** is used to auscultate and assess body sounds, including the apical pulse and the blood pressure. The acoustical stethoscope, the most common type used, has an amplifying mechanism connected to ear pieces by tubing. The most common amplifying devices are the *diaphragm*, which is a large, flat disk, and the *bell*, which has a hollowed, upright, curved appearance. Some acoustical stethoscopes have both. The diaphragm is more useful for hearing high-frequency sounds, such as respiratory sounds, because it screens out low-frequency sounds. The bell screens out high-frequency sounds and is more useful for hearing low-frequency sounds, such as those commonly made by the heart and the blood within the vessels. Figure 24-2 illustrates the bell and diaphragm of the acoustical stethoscope.

The ear tips of the stethoscope should be selected to fit one's ear canals comfortably and snugly for the most effective auscultation. The tips should be sufficiently large to block out extraneous noises in the environment when the

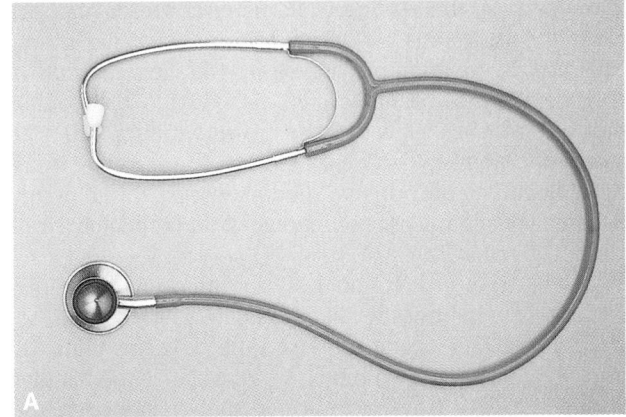

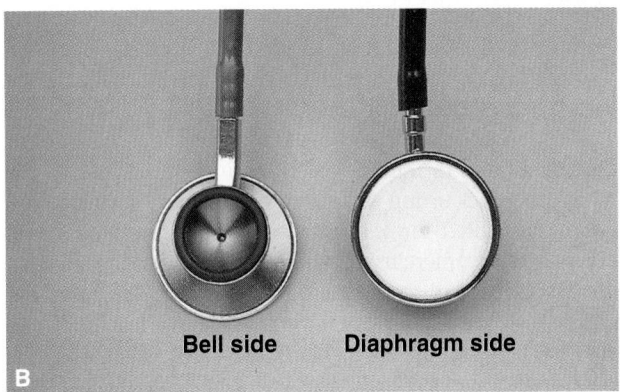

Bell side   **Diaphragm side**

Figure 24-2
(**A**) Stethoscope. (**B**) Two sides of stethoscope amplifier.
(Photo © Ken Kasper.)

stethoscope is being used. The tips should be directed into the ear canal, not against the ear itself.

Sphygmomanometer

A sphygmomanometer is used to assess blood pressure. The sphygmomanometer consists of a cuff and the manometer (Fig. 24-3). The cuff contains an airtight, flat, rubber bladder covered with cloth. A cuff of the proper width must be selected to obtain an accurate blood pressure reading. If it

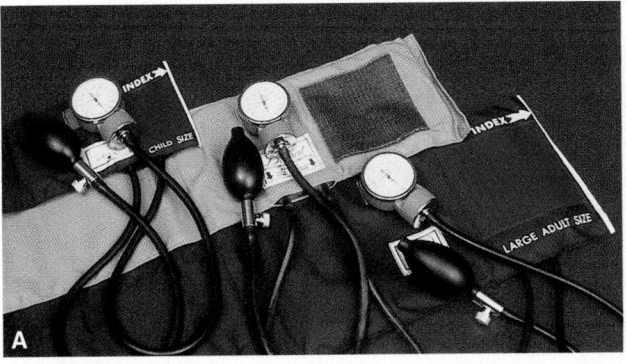

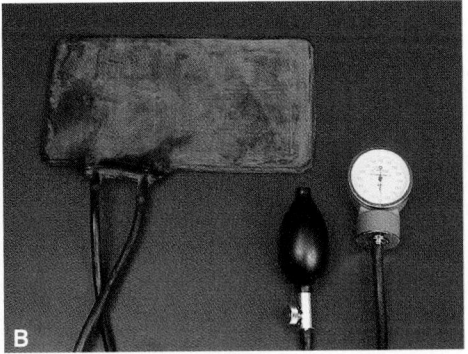

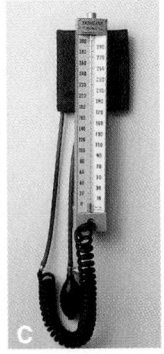

Figure 24-3
Parts of a sphygmomanometer. (**A**) Three cuff sizes: a small cuff for a child or a small or frail adult; a normal adult-sized cuff; and a large cuff, called a *leg cuff*, for measuring blood pressure on a leg or for use on an obese adult.
(**B**) An aneroid manometer. (**C**) A mercury manometer.

is too narrow, the reading could be erroneously high because the pressure is not evenly transmitted to the artery. This occurs, for example, when an average-sized cuff is used on an obese person. If a cuff is too wide, the reading may be erroneously low because pressure is dispersed over a disproportionately large surface area. For example, using an adult cuff on the arm of a child may cause this to occur. Recommendations for the selection of an appropriately sized cuff are given in Table 24-6.

Cuffs are closed around the limb with contact closures, such as nylon fabric that can be fastened to itself with Velcro or hooks. Some long cuffs are applied by encircling the arm several times. Two tubes are attached to the bladder within the cuff. One is connected to a manometer; the other is attached to a bulb used to inflate the bladder. The bladder is inflated enough to obstruct the flow of blood through the artery. A needle valve on the bulb allows the cuff to be deflated while the pressure is being read.

A mercury *manometer* has a mercury-filled cylinder or tube calibrated in millimeters. When mercury rises in the tube, the upper or top surface of the mercury forms a convex curve called the *meniscus*. When determining blood pressure with a mercury manometer, the top of the curve of the meniscus within the calibrated cylinder indicates the pressure. If the meniscus is observed above eye level, the pressure reading appears higher than it really is. If the meniscus is lower than eye level, it appears lower than it really is. The apparent change of position of an object when observed from two different angles is called *parallax*. Figure 24-4 illustrates this principle.

Another type of manometer is called the *aneroid manometer*. It too has a cuff, but it is attached to a round, calibrated dial with a needle that indicates pressure.

Equipment used to measure blood pressure must be in good repair and function properly to avoid inaccurate mea-

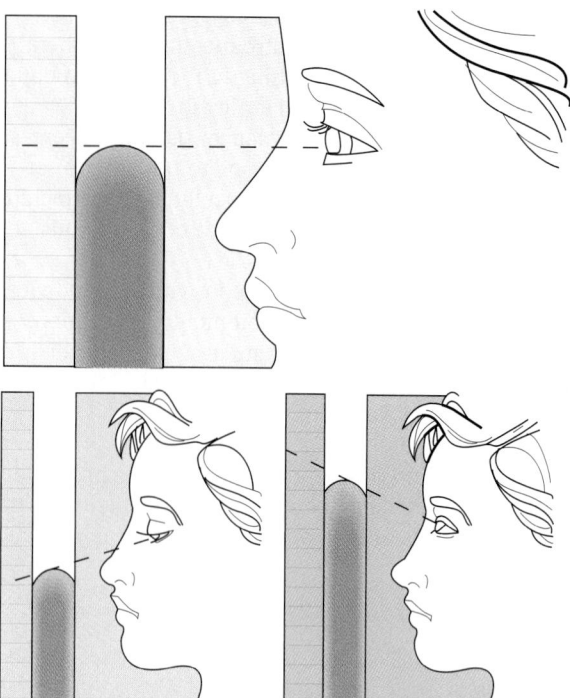

Figure 24-4
A blood pressure reading should be made with the eye at the level of the meniscus as shown in the top drawing. The two drawings at the bottom illustrate how parallax can affect the accuracy of a reading when the line of sight is not level with the meniscus.

surements. The nurse should check routinely to see that there are no air leaks in the rubber bladder, sphygmomanometer connectors, tubing, or valve. The mercury meniscus and the needle on the aneroid manometer should be checked to see that they are exactly on zero when the

Table 24-6
Recommended Bladder Sizes for a Blood Pressure Cuff

Arm Circumference at Midpoint* (cm)	Cuff Name	Bladder Width (cm)	Bladder Length (cm)
5–7.5	Newborn	3	5
7.5–13	Infant	5	8
13–20	Child	8	13
24–32	Adult	13	24
32–42	Large adult	17	32
42–50†	Thigh	20	42

* Midpoint of arm is defined as half the distance from the acromion to the olecranon. Use non-stretchable metal tape.
† In people with very large limbs, the indirect blood pressure should be measured in the leg or forearm.
(Reproduced with permission. "Recommendations for human blood pressure determination by sphygmomanometers," 1967, 1980, 1987. Copyright © American Heart Association.)

cuff is deflated. The mercury manometer should be cleaned and checked at least annually to ensure that the mercury is free of foreign matter and air. The aneroid manometer must be checked for accurate calibration against an accurate mercury manometer. Some authorities recommend weekly calibration for aneroid manometers, whereas others suggest checking it every 6 months. Any time the accuracy of the equipment is questionable, it should be checked and repaired or replaced, as indicated. If mercury leaks out of a manometer, it should be reported to the proper authorities as a hazardous waste spill.

Assessing Pulse

The **pulse** is a perceptible throbbing sensation as a wave of blood is pumped into the arteries by the contraction of the left ventricle. The pulse may be assessed at various sites of the body, described later in this section.

Regulation of Pulse
The pulse is regulated by the autonomic nervous system through the sinoatrial node (often called the *pacemaker*). Parasympathetic stimulation decreases the heart rate, and sympathetic stimulation increases the heart rate. The *pulse rate* is the number of pulsations felt over a peripheral artery or heard over the apex of the heart in 1 minute. This rate normally corresponds to the same rate at which the heart is beating. There are wide ranges for normal pulse rates. Rates change as individuals age, gradually diminishing from birth to adulthood, as shown in Table 24-7.

Factors Affecting Pulse Rate
Tachycardia
Tachycardia is a rapid heart rate. An adult has tachycardia when the pulse rate is 100 to 180 beats/min. The following factors contribute to an increase in the pulse rate:

- Pain
- Strong emotions, such as fear, anger, anxiety, and surprise
- Exercise, when the heart's compensatory ability attempts to meet the need for increased blood circulation

- Prolonged application of heat
- A decrease in blood pressure, such as occurs with blood loss, when the heart's compensatory ability attempts to meet the need for increased output of blood from the heart
- An elevated temperature, which usually causes an increase of about 7 to 10 beats/min for each 0.6°C (1°F) of elevation above normal
- Any condition resulting in poor oxygenation of blood, for example, chronic pulmonary disease or anemia
- Some medications (eg, epinephrine [Adrenalin])

Bradycardia
Bradycardia is a pulse rate below 60 beats/min in an adult. A slow pulse rate during illness is less common than a rapid pulse rate but, when present, should be reported promptly. The following factors may slow the pulse:

- The pulse rate is generally slower at rest and on awakening.
- Males have a slower pulse rate than females.
- People with thin body size tend to have slower heart rates.
- Increasing age may be associated with a slower pulse.
- Medications, such as cardiotonic glycosides, slow the pulse rate.

Pulse Rhythm
The *pulse rhythm* is the pattern of the pulsations and the pauses between them. This pattern is normally regular. An irregular pattern of heartbeats is called a **dysrhythmia**. Any irregularity in the heartbeat should be reported immediately. Common pulse rhythms are described and illustrated in Table 24-8.

Pulse Amplitude
The *pulse amplitude* describes the quality of the pulse in terms of its fullness and reflects the strength of left ventricular contraction. It is assessed by the feel of the blood flow through the vessel. The amplitude of each pulse beat is normally strong at all areas where an artery can be palpated. A strong pulse can be obliterated with relative ease by exerting pressure over the artery, but it remains perceptible with moderate pressure. Table 24-9 presents a scale often used to describe pulse amplitude; the numbers are used in documentation.

Methods of Assessing the Pulse
The pulse may be assessed by palpating (feeling) or auscultating (listening). The following methods are used:

- The middle three fingers may be used to palpate all pulse sites except the apical pulse.
- A stethoscope may be used to auscultate the apical pulse (the procedure is discussed later).
- A Doppler ultrasound may be used to assess pulses that are difficult to palpate or auscultate.
- A cardiac monitor may be used to assess the apical pulse. The monitor produces a graph or digital reading of the pulse rate and amplitude.

Table 24-7
Normal Pulse Rates per Minute at Various Ages

Age	Approximate Range	Approximate Average
Newborn to 1 mo	120–160	140
1 to 12 mo	80–140	120
12 mo to 2 yr	80–130	110
2 to 6 yr	75–120	100
6 to 12 yr	75–110	95
Adolescence to adult	60–100	80

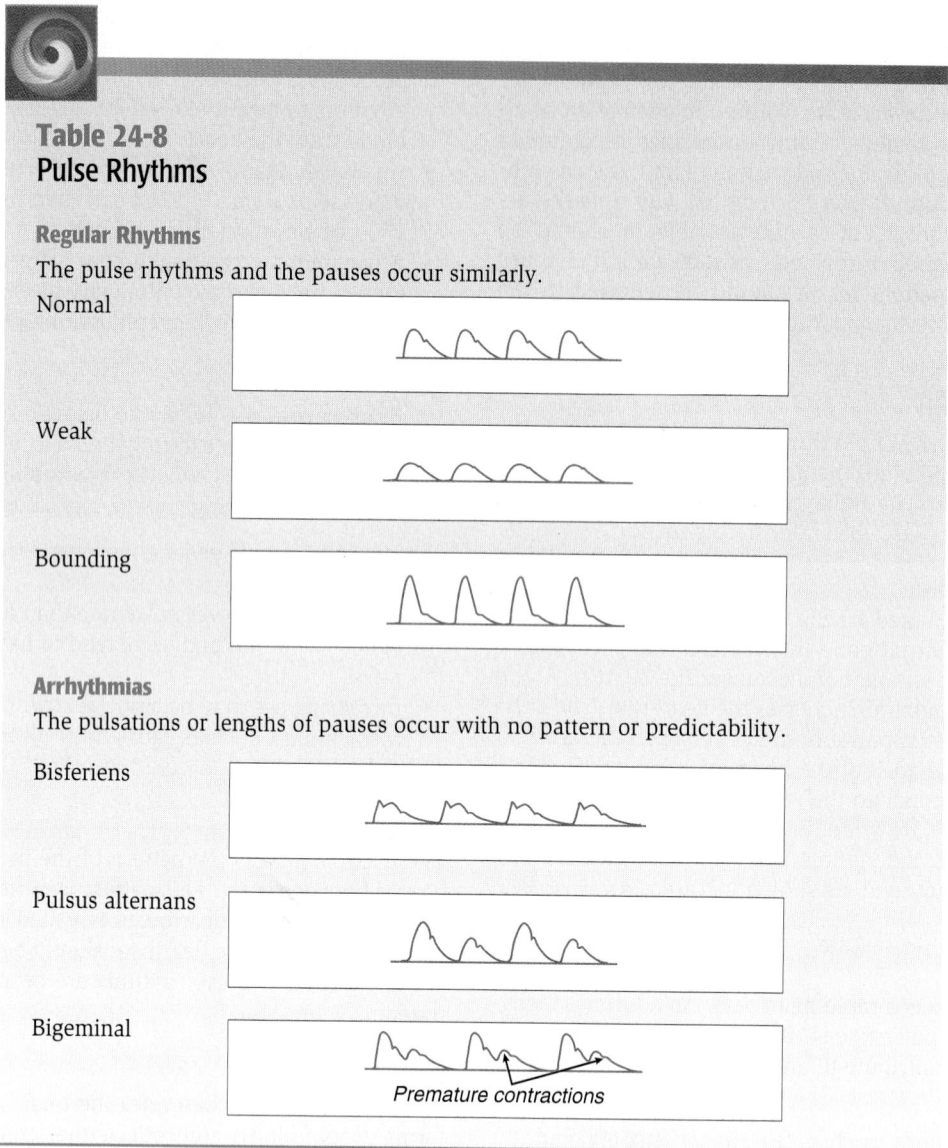

Table 24-8
Pulse Rhythms

Regular Rhythms
The pulse rhythms and the pauses occur similarly.

Normal

Weak

Bounding

Arrhythmias
The pulsations or lengths of pauses occur with no pattern or predictability.

Bisferiens

Pulsus alternans

Bigeminal

Premature contractions

Pulse Sites

Peripheral Pulses

The rate, rhythm, and amplitude of peripheral pulses may be assessed by compressing an artery against an underlying bone with the tips of the fingers. The thumb is not used to compress an artery because the thumb has its own pulse and the nurse would tend to feel his or her own pulse rather than the patient's. Arteries used for assessment of the pulse include the temporal, carotid, brachial, radial, femoral, popliteal, posterior tibial, and dorsalis pedis (Fig. 24-5).

The radial artery, located on the inner, thumb side of the wrist, is used most often for palpating the pulse because it is easily accessible. The location and the position of the fingertips for assessment are illustrated in Procedure 24-3. If this site is inaccessible, select an alternative artery that does not require exertion or cause discomfort for the person, which could alter the pulse rate. Procedure 24-3 describes how to assess the pulse rate using the radial artery site.

Apical Pulse

If a peripheral pulse is difficult to assess accurately because it is irregular, feeble, or extremely rapid, the apical rate should be assessed. An apical pulse is also assessed when giving medications that alter heart rate and rhythm, such as digoxin. In adults, the apical rate is counted for 1 full minute by listening with a stethoscope over the apex of the heart. The contraction of the heart can be heard in the space between the fifth and the sixth ribs, about 8 cm (3 inches) to the left of the median line and slightly below the nipple, as illustrated in Procedure 24-3. Nursing actions are given in Procedure 24-3. The apical rate of an infant is easily palpated with the fingertips.

Apical-Radial Pulse

When the radial pulse is irregular, the *apical-radial pulse rate* may be assessed by counting at the apex of the heart and at the radial artery simultaneously. The difference between the apical and radial pulse rates is called the **pulse deficit**. This means that all of the heartbeats are not

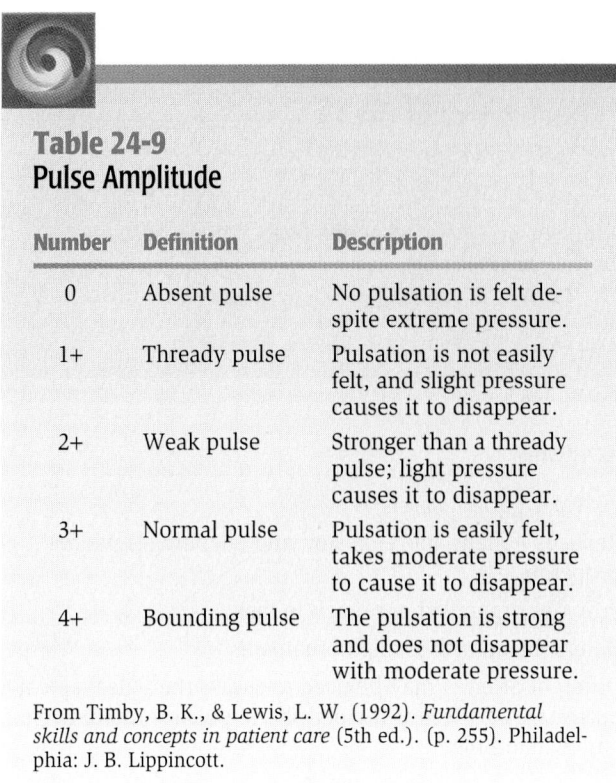

Table 24-9
Pulse Amplitude

Number	Definition	Description
0	Absent pulse	No pulsation is felt despite extreme pressure.
1+	Thready pulse	Pulsation is not easily felt, and slight pressure causes it to disappear.
2+	Weak pulse	Stronger than a thready pulse; light pressure causes it to disappear.
3+	Normal pulse	Pulsation is easily felt, takes moderate pressure to cause it to disappear.
4+	Bounding pulse	The pulsation is strong and does not disappear with moderate pressure.

From Timby, B. K., & Lewis, L. W. (1992). *Fundamental skills and concepts in patient care* (5th ed.). (p. 255). Philadelphia: J. B. Lippincott.

reaching the peripheral arteries or are too weak to be palpated. See guidelines for this procedure in the accompanying box.

Assessing Blood Pressure

Blood pressure refers to the force of the blood against arterial walls. Maximum blood pressure is exerted on the walls of arteries when the left ventricle of the heart pushes blood through the aortic valve into the aorta during systole. The highest pressure thus is called **systolic pressure**. When the heart rests between beats (*diastole*), the pressure drops. The lowest pressure present on arterial walls at this time is called **diastolic pressure**. The difference between the two is called the **pulse pressure**. Blood pressure is measured in millimeters of mercury (mm Hg) and is recorded as a fraction. The numerator is the systolic pressure; the denominator is the diastolic pressure. For example, if the blood pressure is 120/80 mm Hg, 120 is the systolic pressure and 80 is the diastolic pressure. The pulse pressure, in this case, is 40.

Regulation of Blood Pressure
The following factors are responsible for maintaining blood pressure. Deviations from normal blood pressure may result from alterations in one or more of these factors.

Peripheral Resistance
Blood leaving the heart circulates through a continuous loop of blood vessels consisting of arteries, arterioles, capillaries, venules, and veins. *Arterioles* are very small elastic

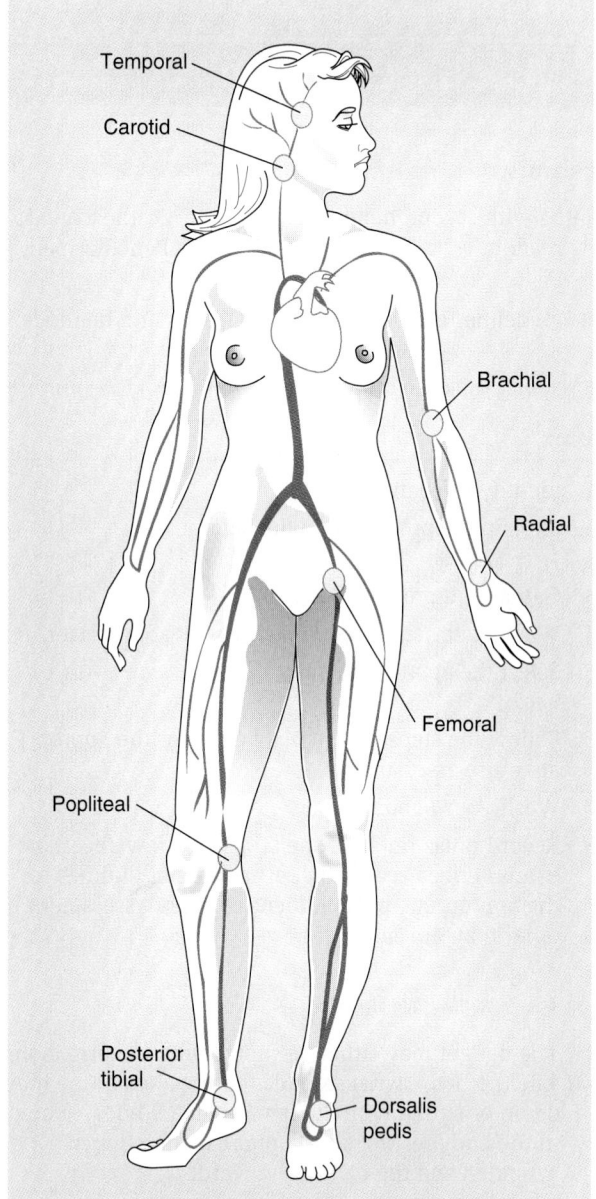

Figure 24-5
These arteries are located near the surface of the body. The pulse can be detected in any of these sites by light palpation.

tubes that can contract or dilate to regulate the distribution of blood to various organs, tissues, or cells, depending on their moment-by-moment requirements. Normally, arterioles are in a state of partial contraction, resulting in *peripheral resistance* and creating a relatively constant level of restraint to blood flow. Peripheral resistance is one of the main factors affecting blood pressure.

Pumping Action of the Heart
When cardiac output is increased, the arteries distend more, resulting in increased blood pressure. When cardiac output is decreased, blood pressure falls. Hence, a weak pumping action results in a lower blood pressure than a strong pumping action.

PROCEDURE 24-3

Assessing the Pulse

Equipment

Watch with second hand or digital readout

Stethoscope (for apical pulse)
Pencil or pen, paper, or flow sheet

Alcohol swab (for stethoscope)

Use guidelines outlined below for all sites and methods.

Guidelines for Assessing, Implementing, and Documenting Pulses

Action	Rationale
1. Identify the patient.	Provides patient safety
2. Explain the procedure to the patient.	Reduces patient apprehension and encourages patient cooperation
3. Gather equipment.	Provides organized approach to task
4. Wash your hands and don gloves as appropriate.	Deters the spread of microorganisms
5. Select the appropriate site.	Different arteries may be used to assess the pulse; apical pulses are assessed if the peripheral pulse is rapid, irregular, or inaudible.
6. Follow the steps as outlined below for the appropriate pulse assessment.	
7. Wash your hands.	Deters the spread of microorganisms
8. Record pulse rate and site on paper, flow sheet, or computerized record. Report abnormal findings to the appropriate person. Identify site of assessment if other than apical.	Provides accurate documentation and reporting

Assessing the Radial Pulse

1. The patient may either be supine with the arm alongside the body, wrist extended, and palms of the hand down or sitting with the forearm at a 90-degree angle to the body resting on a support with the wrist extended and the palm downward.	These positions are comfortable for the patient and convenient for the nurse.
2. Place your first, second, and third fingers along the patient's radial artery, and press gently against the radius. Rest your thumb on the back of the patient's wrist.	The sensitive fingertips can feel the pulsation of the artery.

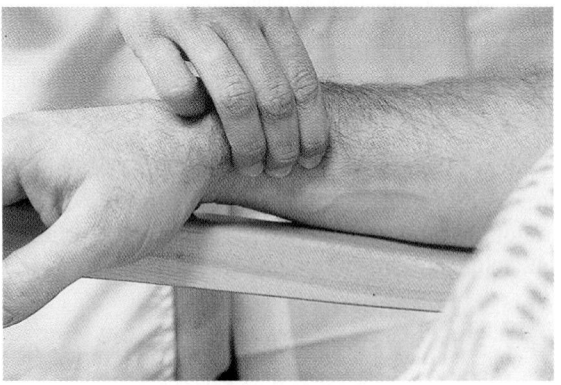

Action 2: Proper placement of the fingers along the radial artery.

(continued)

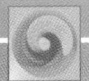

PROCEDURE 24-3

Assessing the Pulse (Continued)

3. Apply only enough pressure so that the artery can be felt distinctly.

Moderate pressure facilitates palpation of the pulsations. Too much pressure obliterates the pulse, whereas the pulse is imperceptible with too little pressure.

4. Using a watch with a second hand, count the number of pulsations felt for 30 seconds. Multiply this number by 2 to have the rate for 1 minute. If the rate, rhythm, or amplitude of the pulse are abnormal in any way, palpate and count the pulse for 1 minute or longer.

Sufficient time must be allowed to assess the rate, rhythm, and amplitude of the pulse. When pulse characteristics are abnormal, a longer time period is necessary for accurate assessment.

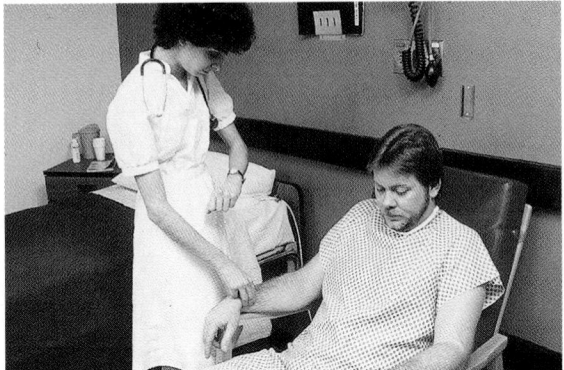

Action 4: Counting the pulsations felt for 30 seconds.

Assessing the Apical Pulse Rate

1. Use alcohol swab to clean ear pieces and diaphragm of the stethoscope.

Deters transmission of microorganisms

2. Assist patient in sitting in a chair or sitting up in bed, and expose upper chest area.

This position facilitates identification of site for stethoscope placement.

3. Hold stethoscope diaphragm against the palm of your hand for a few seconds.

Warms diaphragm, promoting patient comfort

4. Palpate fifth intercostal space, and move to the left midclavicular line. Place the diaphragm over the apex of the heart.

This is the point of maximum impulse where the heartbeat is best heard.

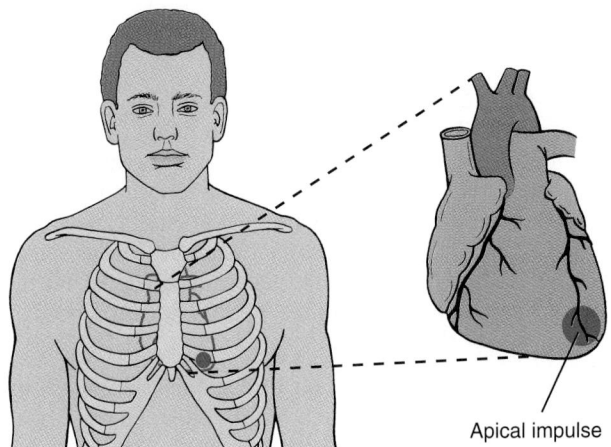

Apical impulse

Schematic depiction of the thorax showing location of apical impulse.

(continued)

PROCEDURE 24-3

Assessing the Pulse (Continued)

5. Listen for heart sounds, identified as a "lub-dub" sound.

    These sounds occur as the heart valves close.

6. Using a watch with a second hand, count the heartbeat for 1 minute.

    A longer time period increases the accuracy of assessment.

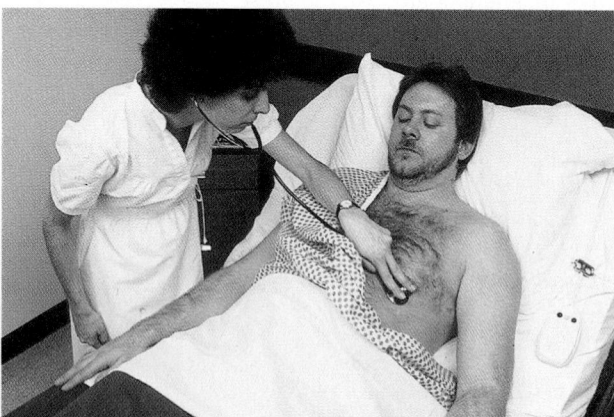

Action 6: Counting the heartbeat for 1 minute.

Age Considerations	The normal heart rate varies by age.
Home Care Considerations	Teach the patient and family how to take own pulse.
	Inform the patient and family about digital pulse monitoring devices.
	Teach family members how to locate and monitor peripheral pulse sites.

Blood Volume

When blood volume is low, as may occur with hemorrhage or dehydration, blood pressure is low because there is decreased fluid within the arteries. Increasing the quantity of blood increases the pressure because there is more fluid volume creating pressure within the arteries.

Viscosity of Blood

Viscosity is the state of being sticky or gummy. The viscosity of the blood depends on the proportion of blood cells to plasma. The more viscous the blood, the higher the blood pressure. This occurs because the heart needs to be more forceful to move the concentrated fluid throughout the circulatory system.

Elasticity of Vessel Walls

Arteries have a considerable quantity of elastic tissue that allows them to stretch and distend (called *compliance*). When the heart rests between each beat, the walls of the arteries recoil, although pressure in them does not drop to zero. The state of pressure keeps the blood entering the capillaries and veins in a continuous flow, rather than in spurts. Simultaneously, the arterioles offer resis-

tance. Therefore, the elasticity of the walls, in addition to the resistance of the arterioles, helps to maintain normal blood pressure. With age, the walls of arterioles become less elastic, which interferes with their ability to stretch and dilate. This can subsequently limit adequate blood flow and contribute to rising pressure within the vascular system.

Variations in Blood Pressure

Studies of healthy people indicate that blood pressure can be within a wide range and still be normal. Because of considerable individual differences, it is important to know the normal blood pressure of a particular person. A rise or fall of 20 to 30 mm Hg in a person's blood pressure is significant, even if it is within the generally accepted normal range. The following variations in blood pressure occur in the average healthy person:

- Readings are lowest at birth. The older adult has decreased elasticity of the arteries, which increases peripheral resistance and therefore increases blood pressure.
- Normal fluctuations occur during the day. The blood pressure is usually lowest on arising in the morning. The blood pressure has been noted to rise as much

Guidelines for Nursing Care
Taking an Apical-Radial Pulse

The following techniques are recommended to assess an apical-radial pulse rate:

- Two nurses are needed; one listens with a stethoscope over the apex of the heart for the heartbeat, and the other counts the rate at the radial artery.
- The patient's chest wall is exposed so that the stethoscope can be placed directly on the skin of the chest wall.
- One watch with a sweep second hand is placed, so that both nurses can read it simultaneously.
- The nurses determine where they can best hear and feel the pulse and decide on a time to start counting, such as when the second hand on the watch is at a specified place (such as the number 12).
- Both nurses count for 1 full minute and record their counts.

as 5 to 10 mm Hg by late afternoon, and it gradually falls again during sleep.
- Women usually have a lower blood pressure than men of the same age.
- Blood pressure increases after eating food.
- Systolic blood pressure rises during periods of exercise and strenuous activity.

- Blood pressure is usually higher in people who are obese than in those who are thin.
- Emotions, such as anger, fear, excitement, and pain, generally cause the blood pressure to rise, but the pressure falls to normal when the situation passes.
- A person's blood pressure tends to be lower in a prone or supine position than when sitting or standing.
- Race is a factor in increased blood pressure (hypertension), which is more prevalent and more severe in African American men and women.
- Oral contraceptives cause a mild increase in blood pressure in many women.

Because of the many factors that influence blood pressure, a single blood pressure measurement is not necessarily significant. The American Heart Association recommends that blood pressure readings be averaged on two or more subsequent occasions before diagnosing high blood pressure. Measurements should be taken after the patient rests for at least 5 minutes and has not consumed caffeine or smoked for 30 minutes before the measurement. Blood pressure classifications and follow-up criteria are outlined in Table 24-10.

Hypertension

Hypertension is blood pressure that is above normal for a sustained period. *Primary* or *essential* hypertension is hypertension without a known cause. When the hypertension is caused by a known pathology, it is called *secondary hypertension*. Hypertension is a major risk factor for heart disease and is the most important risk factor associated with stroke. It is often called "the silent killer" because there are few symptoms beyond the increased blood pressure.

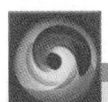

Table 24-10
Blood Pressure Classification

Stages are based on two or more readings taken on at least two separate occasions after the initial screening. The measurements, in millimeters of mercury (mm Hg), apply to adults aged 18 years and older. When systolic and diastolic readings fall into different categories, use the higher measurement to classify elevated blood pressure.

Category	Systolic	Diastolic	Follow-up
Normal	<130	<85	Recheck in 2 years
High-normal	130–139	85–89	Recheck in 1 year
Stage 1	140–159	90–99	Confirm within 2 months
Stage 2	160–179	100–109	Evaluate or refer for additional care within 1 month.
Stage 3	≥180	≥110	Evaluate or refer for additional care immediately or within 1 week.

From Joint National Committee on Prevention, Detection, Evaluation, and Treatment of High Blood Pressure. (1997). *The sixth report of the Joint National Committee on Prevention, Detection, Evaluation, and Treatment of High Blood Pressure.* Bethesda, MD: National Institutes of Health.

Hypertension is a prevalent health problem. Although hypertension can be controlled with diet and medications, many people do not follow prescribed treatment because they feel fine without it. The public and health practitioners alike are becoming increasingly aware of the importance of having regular blood pressure measurements because of the many dangers associated with hypertension. Persistent diastolic hypertension is the most serious and most common blood pressure disturbance. It is a major cause of early death and serious disability in millions of people. Although the exact reason has not been determined, hypertension is almost twice as common in African Americans as in Americans of European descent.

Hypotension

Hypotension is below-normal blood pressure. A consistently low blood pressure, for example, a systolic reading of 90 to 115 mm Hg in an adult, appears to cause no ill effects.

Orthostatic (postural) **hypotension** is a low blood pressure associated with weakness or fainting when one rises to an erect position. It is the result of peripheral vasodilation without a compensatory rise in cardiac output. This type of hypotension can usually be prevented by arising and moving about slowly, especially after a period of bed rest. Ordinarily, it can be corrected by lowering the head, which restores blood flow to the brain. Patients with postural hypotension (usually older adults) may require special monitoring.

Some drugs, such as meperidine hydrochloride (Demerol) cause hypotension. Several illnesses are also associated with hypotension. For example, the blood pressure drops when a patient is experiencing severe blood loss, burns, or severe vomiting and diarrhea, or when cardiac output is impaired after a heart attack.

Assessment Sites and Methods

The nurse assesses the blood pressure by listening for specific sounds, called Korotkoff sounds. Although various sites may be used to assess the blood pressure, the brachial artery and the popliteal artery are most commonly used. Alternate methods for assessing blood pressure include palpation and the use of mechanical devices.

Korotkoff Sounds

The series of sounds for which the nurse listens when measuring the blood pressure are called **Korotkoff sounds,** which are described in Table 24-11. In some adults, each of these sounds is distinct, whereas in others, only the beginning and ending sounds are heard. It is important to determine institutional policy for recording blood pressure sounds and to be consistent in taking and documenting the readings.

The first sound heard through the stethoscope, which is the onset of phase I, represents the systolic pressure. It is recorded as the first number in the fraction; for example, if the blood pressure reading is 120/80 mm Hg, 120 is the systolic pressure. The second number, which represents the diastolic pressure (in this case 80), notes the level at which

either a change in or cessation of the loud, distinct sounds took place. This occurs in either phase IV or phase V.

The blood pressure is most commonly recorded with two numbers written as a fraction, with the bottom number indicating either the change of the sound or the last sound heard. However, the American Heart Association recommends that in instances when both a change in the sounds and a cessation of the sounds are heard, all numbers be recorded. In this case, the blood pressure would be recorded as 120/80/64. If the sounds are heard all the way down to zero, the blood pressure recording would be 120/80/0. It is important to know the procedure for recording blood pressure at each agency or institution so that readings are consistent.

Assessing a Brachial Artery Blood Pressure

Procedure 24-4 describes how to assess the blood pressure with a mercury manometer using the brachial artery. It is important to follow the recommended techniques to avoid the common errors identified in Table 24-12.

Assessing a Popliteal Artery Blood Pressure

When the patient's brachial artery is inaccessible, the nurse can assess the blood pressure using the popliteal artery in the leg. The systolic pressure is likely to be 10 to 40 mm Hg higher at this site. A cuff of proportionately larger size should be used. The patient should be positioned on the abdomen or with the knee flexed, if in a supine position. The technique for assessment is essentially the same as when using the arm.

Palpating the Blood Pressure

Assessing the blood pressure through palpation is sometimes referred to as the *sensory detection method*. It requires only the use of the sphygmomanometer. The cuff is inflated 30 mm Hg above the point at which the pulsation in the artery disappears. As the air in the cuff is released, the nurse feels for the return of the pulse. Usually, no diastolic pressure is recorded because the artery continues to pulsate as long as blood flows through it. Some home patients assess their blood pressure this way. Instead of palpating the artery, however, the person notes the pressure on the manometer when experiencing the onset and disappearance of the throbbing sensation. The measurements using this method are fairly similar to those assessed using other, more sophisticated techniques for assessing blood pressure.

Using the Doppler Ultrasound

The blood pressure may be taken with an ultrasound or Doppler apparatus, which amplifies sounds. This is especially useful if the sounds are indistinct or are inaudible with a regular stethoscope. See guidelines for using the Doppler ultrasound to assess pulse and blood pressure in the accompanying box.

Electronic Indirect Blood Pressure Meters

Electronic blood pressure meters sense vibrations within the artery wall, record the pressure readings, and display

Table 24-11
Korotkoff Sounds

Phase	Description	Illustration
Phase I	Characterized by the first appearance of faint but clear tapping sounds that gradually increase in intensity; the first tapping sound is the systolic pressure	
Phase II	Characterized by muffled or swishing sounds; these sounds may temporarily disappear, especially in hypertensive people; the disappearance of the sound during the latter part of phase I and during phase II is called the *auscultatory gap* and may cover a range of as much as 40 mm Hg; failing to recognize this gap may cause serious errors of underestimating systolic pressure or overestimating diastolic pressure.	
Phase III	Characterized by distinct, loud sounds as the blood flows relatively freely through an increasingly open artery	
Phase IV	Characterized by a distinct, abrupt, muffling sound with a soft, blowing quality; in adults, the onset of this phase is considered to be the first diastolic figure	
Phase V	The last sound heard before a period of continuous silence; the pressure at which the last sound is heard is the second diastolic measurement	

them in digital numbers (Fig. 24-6). These devices are helpful for people who wish to measure their own blood pressure at home. They are also advantageous for people who have a hearing impairment because listening for Korotkoff sounds is unnecessary. No stethoscope is required. Because of their delicate instrumentation, however, these electronic machines should be recalibrated when readings are more than a few points different from the person's normal pattern. Patients using these devices at home should also have their blood pressure checked periodically by health personnel.

Direct Electronic Measurement

It is possible to measure blood pressure directly through the insertion of a thin catheter into an artery (an arterial line). The tip of the catheter senses the pressure and transmits this information to a machine that displays the systolic and diastolic pressure in a waveform. This technique is used primarily in intensive care areas.

(*text continues on page 449*)

PROCEDURE 24-4

Assessing the Blood Pressure

Equipment

Stethoscope
Sphygmomanometer

Blood pressure cuff of appropriate
   size

Pencil or pen, paper or flow sheet
Alcohol swab

Use guidelines outlined below.

Guidelines for Implementing and Documenting Blood Pressure

Action	Rationale
1. Identify the patient.	Provides patient safety
2. Explain the procedure to the patient.	Reduces patient apprehension and encourages patient cooperation
3. Gather equipment.	Provides organized approach to task
4. Wash your hands.	Deters the spread of microorganisms
5. Follow procedure as outlined below.	
6. Wash your hands. If gloves are worn, discard them in the proper receptacle.	Deters the spread of microorganisms
7. Record on paper, flow sheet, or computerized record. Report abnormal findings to the appropriate person. Identify site of assessment if other than brachial.	Provides accurate documentation and reporting

Guidelines for Assessing Blood Pressure

1. Delay obtaining the blood pressure if the patient is emotionally upset, is in pain, or has just exercised, unless it is urgent to obtain the blood pressure.	Factors such as emotional upset, exercise, and pain alter usual blood pressure measurements.
2. Select appropriate arm for application of cuff (no intravenous infusion, breast or axilla surgery on that side, cast, arteriovenous shunt, or injured or diseased limb).	Measurement of blood pressure may temporarily impede circulation to a diseased or compromised extremity.
3. Have the patient assume a comfortable lying or sitting position with the forearm supported at the level of the heart and the palm of the hand upward.	This position places the brachial artery on the inner aspect of the elbow, so that the bell or diaphragm of the stethoscope can rest on it easily.
4. Expose the area of the brachial artery by removing garments, or move a sleeve, if it is not too tight, above the area where the cuff will be placed.	Clothing over the artery interferes with the ability to hear sounds and may cause inaccurate blood pressure readings. Tight clothing on the arm causes congestion of blood and possibly inaccurate readings.
5. Center the bladder of the cuff over the brachial artery, about midway on the arm, so that the lower edge of the cuff is about 2.5 to 5 cm (1 to 2 inches) above the inner aspect of the elbow. The tubing should extend from the edge of the cuff nearer the patient's elbow.	Pressure in the cuff applied directly to the artery provides the most accurate readings. If the cuff gets in the way of the stethoscope, readings are likely to be inaccurate. A cuff placed upside down with the tubing toward the patient's head may give a false reading.

(continued)

PROCEDURE 24-4

Assessing the Blood Pressure (Continued)

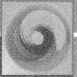

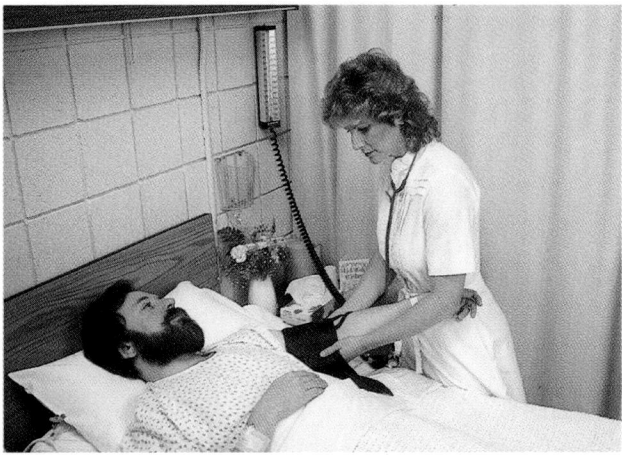

Actions 5 and 6: Centering the cuff over the brachial artery and wrapping smoothly and snugly.

6. Wrap the cuff around the arm smoothly and snugly, and fasten it securely or tuck the end of the cuff well under the preceding wrapping. Do not allow any clothing to interfere with the proper placement of the cuff.

A smooth cuff and snug wrapping produce equal pressure and help promote an accurate measurement. A cuff too loosely wrapped results in an inaccurate reading.

7. Check that a mercury manometer is in a vertical position. The mercury must be within the zero area with the gauge at eye level. If an aneroid gauge is used, the needle should be within the zero mark.

Tilting a mercury manometer, inaccurate calibration, or improper height for reading the gauge can lead to errors in determining the pressure measurements.

8. Palpate the pulse at the brachial or radial artery by pressing gently with the fingertips.

Palpation allows for measurement of the approximate systolic reading.

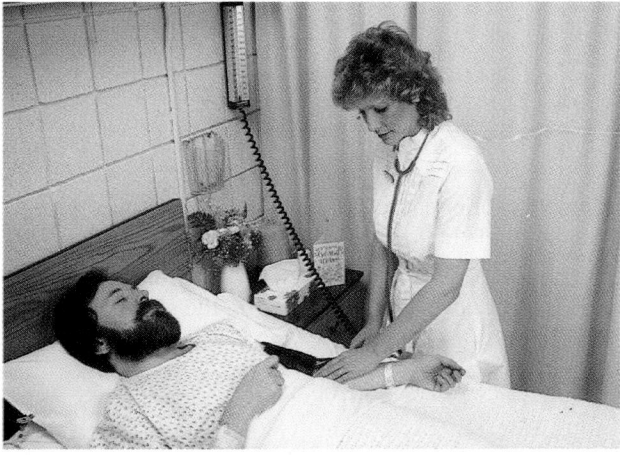

Action 8: Palpating the brachial artery.

9. Tighten the screw valve on the air pump.

The bladder within the cuff will not inflate with the valve open.

(continued)

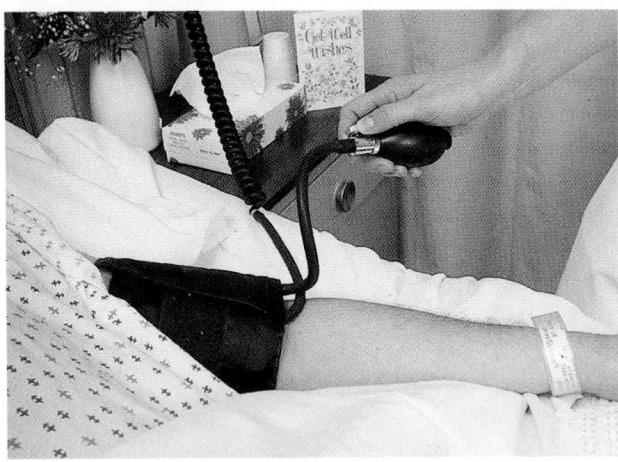

Action 9: Tightening the screw valve on air pump.

10. Inflate the cuff while continuing to palpate the artery. Note the point on the gauge where the pulse disappears.

The point where the pulse disappears provides an estimate of the systolic pressure. To identify the first Korotkoff sound accurately, the cuff must be inflated to a pressure above the point at which the pulse can no longer be felt.

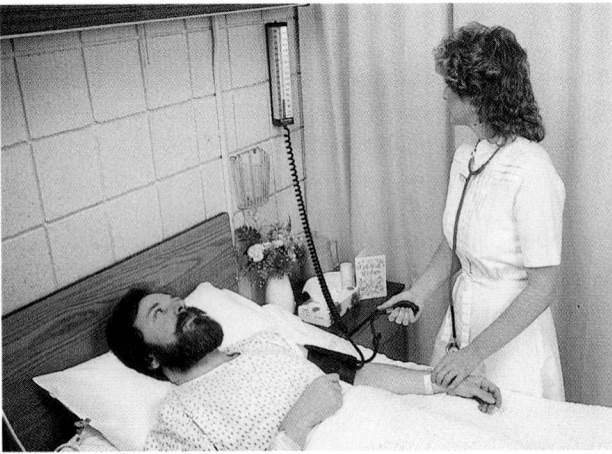

Action 10: Inflating cuff while palpating the radial artery.

11. Deflate the cuff and wait 15 seconds.

Allowing a brief pause before continuing permits the blood to refill and circulate through the arm.

12. Assume a position that is no more than 3 feet away from the gauge.

A distance of more than about 3 feet can interfere with accurate readings of the numbers on the gauge.

13. Place the stethoscope earpieces in the ears. Direct the eartips forward into the canal and not against the ear itself.

Proper placement blocks extraneous noise and allows sound to travel more clearly.

(continued)

PROCEDURE 24-4

Assessing the Blood Pressure (Continued)

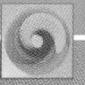

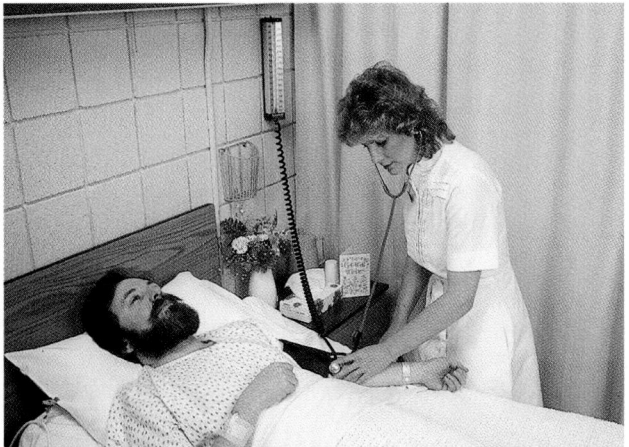

Actions 13 and 14: Placing amplifier of stethoscope over artery, reinflating cuff, and listening for disappearance of sound.

14. Place the bell or diaphragm of the stethoscope firmly but with as little pressure as possible over the brachial artery. Do not allow the stethoscope to touch clothing or the cuff.

Having the bell or diaphragm directly over the artery makes more accurate readings possible. Heavy pressure on the brachial artery distorts the shape of the artery and the sound. Placing the bell or diaphragm away from clothing and the cuff prevents noise, which will distract from the sounds made by blood flowing through the artery.

15. Pump the pressure 30 mm Hg above the point at which the systolic pressure was palpated and estimated. Open the valve on the manometer and allow air to escape slowly (allowing the gauge to drop 2 to 3 mm per heartbeat).

Increasing the pressure above where the pulse disappeared ensures a period before hearing the first sound that corresponds with the systolic pressure. It prevents misinterpreting phase II sounds as phase I.

16. Note the point on the gauge at which there is an appearance of the first faint, but clear, sound that slowly increases in intensity. Note this number as the systolic pressure.

Systolic pressure is the point at which the blood in the artery is first able to force its way through the vessel at a similar pressure exerted by the air bladder in the cuff. The first sound is phase I of Korotkoff sounds.

17. Read the pressure to the closest even number.

It is common practice to read blood pressure to the closest even number.

18. Do not reinflate the cuff once the air is being released to recheck the systolic pressure reading.

Reinflating the cuff while obtaining the blood pressure is uncomfortable for the patient and may cause an inaccurate reading. Reinflating the cuff causes congestion of blood in the lower arm, which lessens the loudness of Korotkoff sounds.

19. Note the pressure at which the sound first becomes muffled. Also, observe the point at which the sound completely disappears. These may occur separately or at the same point.

The point at which the sound changes corresponds to phase IV of Korotkoff sounds and is considered the first diastolic pressure reading. According to the American Heart Association, this is used as the diastolic pressure recording in children. The last sound heard is the beginning of phase V and is the second diastolic measurement.

(continued)

PROCEDURE 24-4

Assessing the Blood Pressure (Continued)

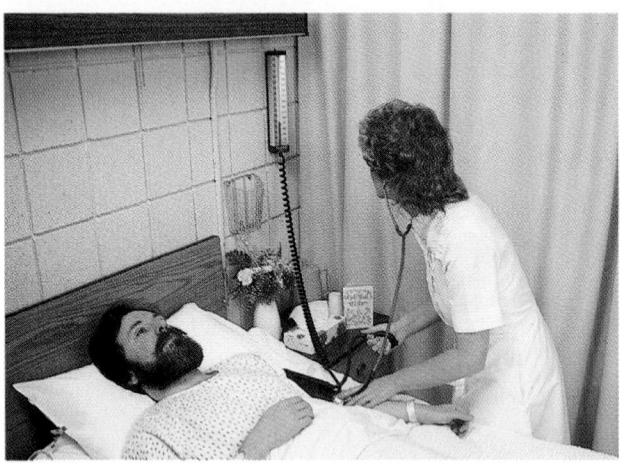

Actions 15, 16, and 18: Listening for Korotkoff sounds and noting systolic and diastolic pressure readings. (Photos © Ken Kasper.)

20. Allow the remaining air to escape quickly. Repeat any suspicious reading, but wait 30 to 60 seconds between readings to allow normal circulation to return in the limb. Be sure to deflate the cuff completely between attempts to check the blood pressure.

False readings are likely to occur if there is congestion of blood in the limb while obtaining repeated readings.

21. Remove the cuff, and clean and store the equipment.

Equipment that must be shared among personnel should be left in a manner ready for use.

Special Considerations

If this is the initial nursing assessment of a patient, take the blood pressure on both arms. It is normal to have a 5- to 10-mm Hg difference in the systolic reading between arms. Use the arm with the higher reading for subsequent pressures.

When having difficulty hearing the blood pressure sounds, the following technique is recommended:
  • Raise the patient's arm, with cuff in place, over his or her head for 15 seconds before rechecking the blood pressure.
  • Inflate the cuff while the arm is elevated, and then gently lower the arm while continuing to support it.
  • Position the stethoscope, and deflate the cuff at the usual rate while listening for Korotkoff sounds.
Raising the arm over the head helps relieve congestion of blood in the limb, increases pressure differences, and makes the sounds louder and more distinct when blood enters the lower arm.

Home Care Considerations

  • Use cuff size appropriate for limb circumference. Inform patient that cuff sizes range from a pediatric cuff to a large thigh cuff and that a poorly fitting cuff may result in an inaccurate measurement.
  • Inform patient about availability of digital blood pressure monitoring equipment. Though costly, most provide an easy-to-read recording of systolic and diastolic measurements.

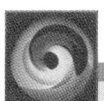

Table 24-12
Blood Pressure Assessment Errors and Contributing Causes

Error	Contributing Causes	Error	Contributing Causes
Falsely low assessments	• Hearing deficit • Noise in the environment • Viewing the meniscus from above eye level • Applying too wide a cuff • Inserting eartips of stethoscope incorrectly • Using cracked or kinked tubing • Releasing the valve rapidly • Misplacing the bell beyond the direct area of the artery • Failing to pump the cuff 20 to 30 mm Hg above the disappearance of the pulse	Falsely high assessments	• Using a manometer not calibrated at the zero mark • Assessing the blood pressure immediately after exercise • Viewing the meniscus from below eye level • Applying a cuff that is too narrow • Releasing the valve too slowly • Reinflating the bladder during auscultation

Teaching Vital Signs for Home Care

Patients at home often need to check their own temperature, pulse, or blood pressure. Guidelines for teaching self-assessment and care of equipment follow.

Taking the Temperature

• The temperature may be taken with a glass thermometer, a single-use disposable thermometer, or a temperature-sensitive tape.

• Adults who use a glass thermometer usually take an oral temperature. It is important that the temperature be taken at least 30 minutes after eating or drinking hot or cold foods or fluids or after smoking, to be sure an accurate temperature is assessed.

• Infants and small children should have their temperature taken either with a temperature-sensitive tape on the forehead or a single-use thermometer in the axilla (armpit). Infants and small children should not have rectal temperatures taken because of the risk for damage to the rectal area.

• Shake the mercury down into the bulb of the thermometer until the level of the mercury is below 98°F (36.5°C). To see the mercury level, hold the thermometer sideways at eye level and rotate it until the mercury can be seen. If the thermometer uses a Fahrenheit scale, each long mark is one degree and each short mark is two tenths of a degree; a centigrade scale uses long marks for one half of a degree and short marks for one tenth of a degree.

• Place the glass thermometer as far back as possible under the side of the tongue and close the lips. Do not talk while the thermometer is in the mouth.

• Leave the thermometer in place for 2 to 3 minutes.

• Remove the thermometer and determine the point at which the mercury is level. This is the body temperature. Call your healthcare provider if the temperature is greater than 100°F (37.7°C), or if you are concerned.

• Wash the thermometer with soap and warm water, rinse it with cold water, dry it well, and store it in a clean, dry area. Do not use the thermometer to take another person's temperature unless it has been cleaned. If several members of the household have an infection or illness, the thermometer should soak in 70% isopropyl alcohol between uses; be sure to rinse off the alcohol with cold water before using it again.

Taking the Pulse

• The pulse is often taken before taking certain medications, such as those to make the heartbeat stronger. It is also taken by people who exercise and want to monitor the effect of the exercise on heart function.

• It is necessary to be able to see a watch or a clock with a second hand when taking the pulse.

• Place one arm on a firm surface so that the palm is upward. Using the middle three fingers of the other hand, gently feel the outside of the arm just below the wrist with the fingertips. Do not press hard. When pulsations are felt, watch the second hand of the watch or clock and begin to count when the second hand reaches 12 (any number is fine, but it is often easier to remember to always begin counting when the second hand is on 12). Count each pulsation (beat) for 1 minute (when the second hand again reaches 12), and write the number down.

Guidelines for Nursing Care

Using a Doppler Ultrasound to Assess Pulse and Blood Pressure

A Doppler ultrasound may be used to assess pulses or a blood pressure that are difficult to palpate or auscultate. This device has an ultrasound transducer and an audio unit and transmits the sounds of red blood cells moving through the blood vessel. The procedure for using this device is as follows:

- Wash hands.
- Collect the Doppler ultrasound stethoscope, the transducer in the Doppler probe (the probe looks like a small transistor radio), a stethoscope headset, and transmission gel.
- Plug the headset into one of the two output jacks next to the volume control.
- Apply a small amount of transmission gel to either the probe or to the patient's skin over the selected area.
- Use the "on" button to activate the transducer.
- Hold the probe at a 90-degree angle to the skin over the pulse site while maintaining contact with the skin and the transmission gel.
- Listen for pumping sounds, indicating arterial pulse.
- Count the rate of the pulse for 1 minute; when used for blood pressure, usually the only measurement that can be assessed is the systolic reading (first sound heard).
- Remove gel from the probe and the patient's skin; do not use alcohol to clean the transducer because it may damage the transducer covering.
- Wash hands, and document pulse rate by Doppler.

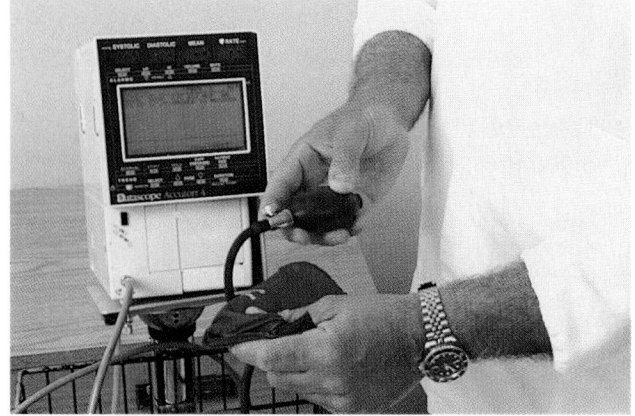

Figure 24-6
The automatic blood pressure monitor reports systolic, diastolic, and mean blood pressure. (Photo © B. Proud.)

- If the pulse is very fast, very slow, or irregular, or if you have any concerns, contact your healthcare provider.

Taking the Blood Pressure

- The blood pressure is often taken to determine how well medications are working to control high blood pressure. The blood pressure is usually checked once a week. A record of blood pressure readings over time is more important than one reading.
- The blood pressure can be measured at home with a blood pressure monitoring device or by using the mechanical devices found in many grocery or discount stores with a pharmacy. It is important to use the same device or machine each time and to write down the numbers.
- If a home device is used, be sure the cuff is the proper size and that all parts of the device are working properly. The measurement should be taken while sitting comfortably, and the arm should be supported on a firm surface.
- If the blood pressure numbers increase or decrease by more than 10, or if you have any concerns, contact your healthcare provider.

Learning Outcomes

After completing this chapter, the learner should be able to accomplish the following:

1. Define key terms used in the chapter.

afebrile	inspiration
apnea	Korotkoff sounds
blood pressure	orthopnea
bradycardia	orthostatic hypotension
bradypnea	pulse
circadian rhythm	pulse deficit
diastolic pressure	pulse pressure
dyspnea	pyrexia
dysrhythmia	respiration
eupnea	stethoscope
expiration	systolic pressure
febrile	tachycardia
hyperpyrexia	tachypnea
hypertension	temperature
hypotension	vital signs
hypothermia	

2. Discuss nursing responsibilities in assessing temperature, pulse, respirations, and blood pressure.
3. Describe the equipment necessary to assess vital signs.

4. Compare normal and abnormal vital sign assessments, including causes, effects, and implications of abnormal findings.
5. Identify sites for assessing temperature, pulse, and blood pressure.

6. Accurately assess temperature, pulse, respirations, and blood pressure.
7. Provide information to patients about taking temperature, pulse, and blood pressure at home.

Critical Thinking Questions

1. Take your own pulse several times a day, such as when you first get up, before and after meals, and before and after exercise. Write down the rate, rhythm, and quality of the pulse. What changes did you see? What are the physiologic rationale for these changes?
2. Describe differences you might expect to find in the vital signs of the following individuals, and include the physiologic reasons for these differences:

- A teenager who has his first football practice in 95°F heat
- An infant with an ear infection
- A young woman arriving at the emergency department after an attempted assault
- A middle-aged man who sustained serious trauma and bleeding in an automobile accident
- A 92-year-old woman

Study Questions

1. An elevation of the body temperature above normal is labeled
   a. pyrexia
   b. hypothermia
   c. hypertension
   d. afebrile
2. For which of the following patients would you use an oral thermometer?
   a. a 6-month-old infant
   b. a patient receiving oxygen therapy
   c. a 42-year-old healthy woman
   d. an unconscious patient
3. Insertion of a rectal thermometer may cause a potentially harmful condition. This condition is
   a. an increase in heart rate
   b. a decrease in heart rate
   c. an involuntary loss of stool
   d. an increase in respirations
4. While taking an adult patient's pulse, the nurse finds the rate to be 140 beats/min. The nurse would report and document this finding as
   a. hyperthermia
   b. bradycardia
   c. palpitations
   d. tachycardia
5. A patient complains of severe abdominal pain. When assessing the vital signs, the nurse would not be surprised to find
   a. an increase in the pulse rate
   b. a decrease in body temperature
   c. a decrease in blood pressure
   d. an increase in body temperature
6. The apical pulse is assessed by using
   a. a sphygmomanometer
   b. an electronic thermometer
   c. a stethoscope
   d. a Doppler apparatus

7. The difference between the apical and radial pulse rates is called the
   a. pulse deficit
   b. pulse amplitude
   c. ventricular rhythm
   d. heart arrhythmia
8. The normal respiratory rate in adults is considered to be
   a. 1 to 6 breaths/min
   b. 16 to 20 breaths/min
   c. 60 to 80 breaths/min
   d. 100 to 120 breaths/min
9. A patient is having dyspnea. To facilitate respirations, the nurse would
   a. remove pillows from under the head
   b. elevate the head of the bed
   c. elevate the foot of the bed
   d. take the blood pressure
10. Blood pressure is the measurement of
    a. the flow of blood through the circulation
    b. the force of blood against arterial walls
    c. the force of blood against venous walls
    d. the flow of blood through the heart
11. With aging, blood pressure is often higher due to
    a. loss of muscle mass
    b. changes in exercise and diet
    c. decreased peripheral resistance
    d. decreased elasticity in arterial walls
12. A patient has a blood pressure reading of 130/90 mm Hg when visiting a clinic. The nurse would recommend
    a. follow-up measurements of blood pressure
    b. immediate treatment by a physician
    c. nothing, because the nurse considers this reading is due to anxiety
    d. a change in diet and exercise

13. In recording a blood pressure of 120/80 mm Hg, the 120 represents
    a. the pulse rate
    b. the diastolic pressure
    c. the systolic pressure
    d. the pulse deficit
14. It is important to have the appropriate cuff size when taking the blood pressure. A cuff that is too large or too small may result in
    a. an incorrect reading
    b. injury to the patient
    c. prolonged pressure on the arm
    d. loss of Korotkoff sounds
15. A patient has intravenous fluids infusing in the right arm. When taking a blood pressure on this patient, the nurse would
    a. take the blood pressure in the right arm
    b. take the blood pressure in the left arm
    c. use the smallest possible cuff
    d. report inability to take the blood pressure

Answers With Rationale

1. The correct response is *a.* Pyrexia is an elevation of body temperature. Hypothermia is low body temperature. Hypertension is elevated blood pressure. Afebrile means that there is not an elevation of body temperature.
2. The correct response is *c.* Use of oral thermometers is contraindicated in infants, patients receiving oxygen therapy, and unconscious patients.
3. The correct response is *b.* Insertion of a rectal thermometer may stimulate the vagus nerve, which, in turn, would decrease heart rate. This may potentially be harmful for patients with cardiac problems.
4. The correct response is *d.* A pulse rate of 100 to 180 beats/min in an adult is tachycardia. Hyperthermia is high body temperature. Bradycardia is an adult pulse rate of less than 60 beats/min. The sensation one feels in being aware of the heartbeat is called palpitations.
5. The correct response is *a.* The pulse often increases when an individual is experiencing pain. Pain does not affect body temperature and may increase (not decrease) blood pressure.
6. The correct response is *c.* The apical pulse can only be assessed by listening with a stethoscope.
7. The correct response is *a.* The difference between the apical and radial pulse rate is called the pulse deficit. The other responses are names given to volume and rhythm of the pulse.
8. The correct response is *b.* The normal respiratory rate for adults is 16 to 20 breaths/min.
9. The correct response is *b.* Dyspnea is difficult respirations. Elevating the head of the bed allows the abdominal organs to descend, giving the diaphragm greater room for expansion and facilitating lung expansion. Any other intervention would not facilitate respirations.
10. The correct response is *b.* Blood pressure is the measurement of the force of blood against arterial walls. Other responses are incorrect in describing blood pressure.
11. The correct response is *d.* With aging, elasticity in arterial walls is decreased, contributing to an elevated blood pressure reading. The other responses may contribute to changes in readings, but they are not the physiologic basis for blood pressure findings in the older adult.
12. The correct response is *a.* A single blood pressure reading that is mildly elevated is not significant, but the measurement should be taken again over time to determine if hypertension is a problem. The nurse would recommend a return visit to the clinic for a recheck.
13. The correct response is *c*—120 is the systolic pressure. The diastolic pressure is 80. The other responses relate to pulse rather than blood pressure.
14. The correct response is *a.* A blood pressure cuff that is not the right size may cause an incorrect reading. It will not cause injury or loss of sounds.
15. The correct response is *b.* The blood pressure should be taken in the arm opposite the one with the infusion. Blood pressure should not be taken in the arm with an intravenous infusion because the pressure of inflating the cuff may allow the artery to clot.

Bibliography

Bayne, C. (1997). Vital signs: Are we monitoring the right parameters? *Nursing Management, 28*(5), 74–76.

Dunbar, S., & Farr, L. (1996). Temporal patterns of heart rate and blood pressure in elders. *Nursing Research, 45*(1), 43–49.

Fulbrook, P. (1997). Core body temperature: A comparison of axilla, tympanic membrane and pulmonary artery blood temperature. *Intensive & Critical Care Nursing, 13*(5), 266–272.

Grossman, D., Keen, M., Singer, M., & Asher, M. (1995). Current nursing practices in fever management. *MEDSURG Nursing, 4*(3), 193–198.

Hinojosa, R., & Beckstrand, R. (1997). Measurement of body temperature in pediatric patients. *Plastic Surgical Nursing, 17*(2), 88–90.

Holzclaw, B. (1997). Perioperative problems: Threats to thermal balance in the elderly. *Seminars in Perioperative Nursing, 6*(1), 42–48.

Holzclaw, B. (1998). New trends in thermometry for the patient in the ICU. *Critical Care Nursing Quarterly, 21*(3), 12–25.

Hurley, M. (1998). New hypertension guidelines. *RN, 61*(4), 25–28.

Joint National Committee on Prevention, Detection, Evaluation, and Treatment of High Blood Pressure. (1997). *The sixth report of the Joint National Committee on Prevention, Detection, Evaluation, and Treatment of High Blood Pressure.* Bethesda, MD: National Institutes of Health.

Jones, S., Holloman, F., & Coffin, D. (1998). Body temperature alterations in hospitalized HIV/AIDS patients. *MEDSURG Nursing, 7*(4), 217–222.

Kriesand, T., & Cohen, I. (1996). Home blood pressure monitoring. *American Family Physician, 54*(2), 537–540.

Lanham, D., Walker, B., Klocke, E., & Jennings, M. (1999). Accuracy of tympanic temperature readings in children under 6 years of age. *Pediatric Nursing, 25*(1), 39–42.

McConnell, E. A. (1995). Monitoring peripheral pulses with a Doppler ultrasound device. *Nursing, 25*(3), 18.

McConnell, E. A. (1998). Automated vital signs monitoring devices. *Nursing Management, 29*(2), 49–51.

McKenzie, N. (1998). Fever: Upping the body's thermostat. *Nursing, 28*(10), 41–45.

Pearson, J., Morrell, C., Brant, L., Landis, P., & Fleg, J. (1997). Age-associated changes in blood pressure in a longitudinal study of healthy men and women. *Journals of Gerontology, Series A, Biological Sciences & Medical Sciences, 52A*(3), M177–M183.

Porth, C. (1998). *Pathophysiology: Concepts of altered health states* (5th ed.). Philadelphia: Lippincott Williams & Wilkins.

Smith-Temple, J., & Johnson, J. (1998). *Nurses' guide to clinical procedures* (3rd ed.). Philadelphia: Lippincott Williams & Wilkins.

Watson, R. (1998). Controlling body temperature in adults. *Nursing Standard, 12*(20), 49–55.

Weber, J., & Kelley, J. (1998). *Health assessment in nursing.* Philadelphia: Lippincott Williams & Wilkins.

Chapter 25
Health Assessment

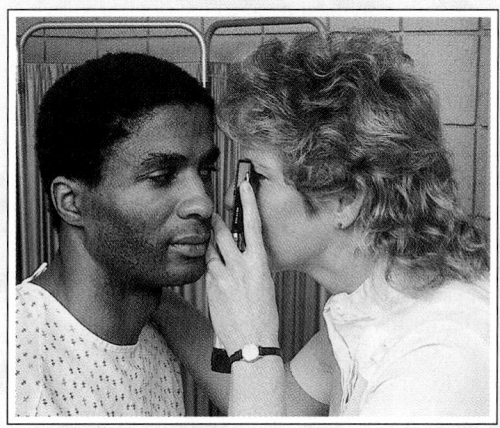

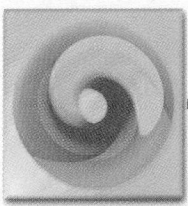

Thinking Critically About
Nursing's Blended Skills

Before reading this chapter, think about the types of blended skills you will need to develop to perform and document a health assessment competently.

- A woman in her last month of pregnancy presents in your clinic with contractions 2 minutes apart and tells you, "My baby is coming!"

- A 9-year-old child at camp runs up to you and says that he is allergic to bees and has just been stung!

- You are visiting a 76-year-old man who has been newly diagnosed with Alzheimer's disease in his home. He has just been discharged from the hospital following a motor vehicle accident–related surgery for leg fractures. Your charge is to evaluate his need for visiting nurse service. He lives with his 75-year-old wife.

- A 19-year-old female college student comes to the emergency room reporting that she was date-raped.

What cognitive, technical, interpersonal, and ethical/legal skills do you think you will need to respond to the challenges described above?

ealth assessment is an integral component of holistic nursing care and is the basis of the nursing process. Assessments are used to initiate, implement, and evaluate care in order to promote an optimal level of health through interventions to prevent illness, restore health, and facilitate coping with disabilities or death.

Health assessments may be conducted in any setting. The two components of health assessment are the health history and the physical assessment. Nurses use communication skills and interviewing techniques during the health history to gather data to determine the patient's health status. A health assessment may focus on one specific body system or may be a head-to-toe or system-by-system assessment. A head-to-toe complete physical assessment guide is outlined in the accompanying box. Both subjective and objective data are collected with the health history and the physical assessment. The health assessment helps nurses to accomplish the following:

- Establish the nurse–patient relationship.
- Gather data about the patient's general health status, including the physiologic, psychological, cognitive, sociocultural, developmental, and spiritual dimensions.
- Identify patient strengths.
- Identify actual and potential health problems.
- Establish a base for the nursing process.

Health History

A health history is a collection of subjective and objective data that provides a detailed profile of the patient's health status. Information is collected during an interview with the patient. Components of the health history and specific interviewing skills are described in Chapters 15 and 21. Each section of this chapter contains focused topics for questions to ask during the health history to identify risk factors for alterations in health. It is especially important to ask about the warning signs of cancer (listed in the accompanying box: American Cancer Society CAUTION Model) and to document and report all abnormal signs.

Guidelines for Physical Assessment

The physical assessment may be conducted in a head-to-toe sequence or a system sequence but can be adapted to meet the needs of the patient. It is often necessary to modify the sequence, positions, and specific assessments according to the patient's age, energy level, and physical state as well as time constraints. Even when modified, the physical assessment should be conducted in an organized and knowledgeable manner. Conducting an accurate physical assessment takes time and practice.

General Guidelines

The following sections discuss general guidelines for the physical assessment, including instrumentation, positioning, draping, preparation of the environment, patient preparation, and the techniques of physical assessment.

Instrumentation

The instruments (equipment) used in a physical assessment should be readily accessible, clean or sterile, in proper work-

COGNITIVE SKILLS

- Basic knowledge of how to conduct and document a health assessment in a systematic manner, identifying normal and abnormal findings.
- Knowledge of how to individualize the basic health assessment to specific populations (pregnant women, patients with Alzheimer's disease who are living at home, rape victims) and special circumstances (bee stings, fractures, date-rape).

TECHNICAL SKILLS

- Ability to use the equipment and techniques necessary to assess and document health status.
- Ability to position the patient correctly for each body system assessment.

INTERPERSONAL SKILLS

- Strong people skills; ability to communicate and interact effectively with patients and their significant

others, especially during times of stress: woman going into labor, spouse who needs to learn how to take care of her husband at home, child with bee stings, woman who was allegedly raped.

- Confidence in your own abilities and the willingness to get help when you need it.

ETHICAL/LEGAL SKILLS

- Commitment to safety and quality; strong sense of responsibility and accountability.
- Ability to document health assessment findings according to agency policy.
- Knowledge of special regulations and legislation detailing nursing responsibilities when assessing pregnancy, providing first-aid in camp situations, determining the need for home care, and caring for rape victims.

Outline of a Head-to-Toe Physical Assessment

- General survey
- Height and weight
- Vital signs
- Head
    - Skin
    - Face, skull and scalp, hair
    - Eyes
    - Ears
    - Nose and sinuses
    - Mouth and oropharynx
    - Cranial nerves
- Neck
    - Skin
    - Lymph nodes
    - Muscles
    - Thyroid
    - Trachea
    - Carotid arteries
    - Neck veins
- Chest and back
    - Skin
    - Chest size and shape
    - Heart
    - Lungs
    - Breasts and axilla
    - Spine

- Upper extremities
    - Skin, hair, and fingernails
    - Sensation
    - Muscle size, strength, and tone
    - Joint range of motion
    - Radial and brachial pulses
    - Tendon reflexes
- Abdomen
    - Skin
    - Bowel sounds
    - Vascular sounds
    - Abdominal contents
    - Specific organs, such as the liver and bladder
- Genitalia
    - Skin and hair
    - Urethra
    - Males: penis and testes
    - Females: vagina
- Anus and rectum
- Lower extremities
    - Skin, hair, and toenails
    - Gait and balance
    - Muscle size, strength, and tone
    - Joint range of motion
    - Popliteal, posterior tibial, and pedal pulses
    - Tendon and plantar reflexes

---

ing order, and organized for their sequence of use (Fig. 25-1). Equipment that will touch the patient should be warmed (by the examiner's hands or warm water) before use. Although all the instruments described below may not be needed in every assessment, they are commonly used in a total assessment. Some equipment, such as a tongue blade and penlight, may be used in the physical assessment and are not included in this discussion. Beginning students will not conduct all elements of a complete physical assessment, but the instruments and techniques are included for understanding what is being done by more advanced practitioners.

Ophthalmoscope

An *ophthalmoscope* is a lighted instrument used to visualize the interior structures of the eye. It consists of two parts: a body that contains the light source and a detachable head that contains lenses that magnify the internal eye structures. The head is secured in the body. The dial on the head, when depressed and turned, turns on the illumination. Several lenses are arranged on a wheel that controls the focus on structures in the eye. Each lens is labeled with a positive (black color) or negative (red color) number, with the units of strength called *diopters*. Red numbers are used for near-sighted (myopic) patients, and black numbers are used for far-sighted (hyperopic) patients. The zero lens is used when either the examiner or the patient has refractive errors.

Otoscope

The *otoscope* is a lighted instrument for examining the external ear canal and the tympanic membrane. The ophthalmoscope and otoscope heads are interchangeable on the same body. An attached speculum directs the light in a narrow beam for improved visualization of ear structures. The specula come in various sizes; the largest speculum that will extend into the patient's ear canal is used.

American Cancer Society CAUTION Model

Change in bowel or bladder habits

A sore that does not heal

Unusual bleeding or discharge

Thickening or lump in the breast or elsewhere

Indigestion or difficulty in swallowing

Obvious change in wart or mole

Nagging cough or hoarseness

From the American Cancer Society.

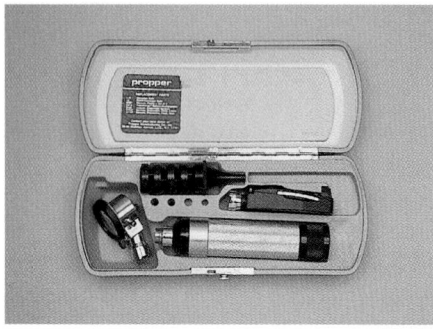

Ophthalmoscope and otoscope set

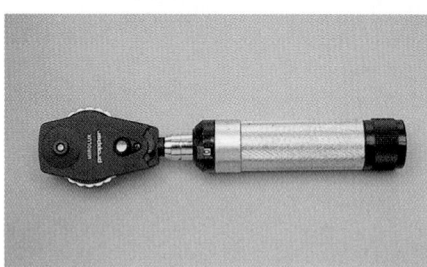

Ophthalmoscope

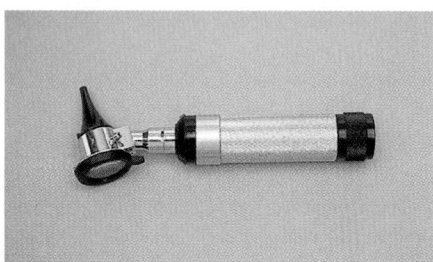

Otoscope

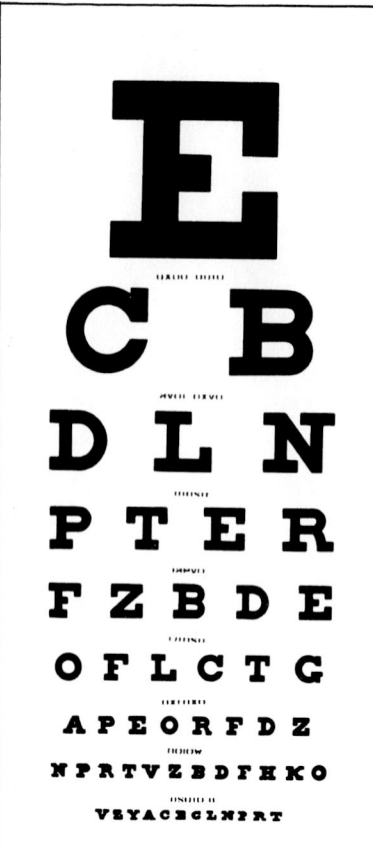

Snellen chart

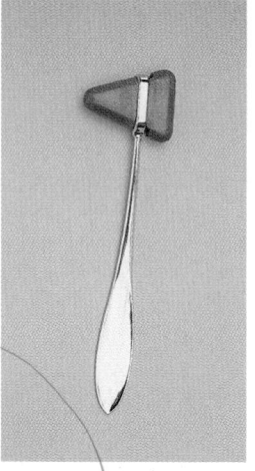

Percussion hammer

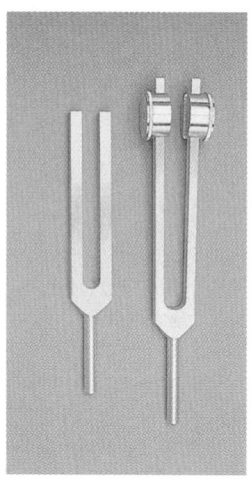

Tuning forks

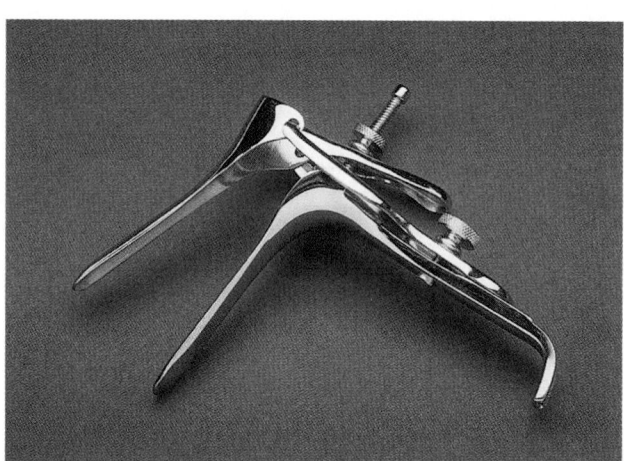

Vaginal speculum

Figure 25-1
Instruments used in the physical assessment. (Photos © Ken Kasper.)

Snellen's Chart

Snellen's chart, used as a screening test for distant vision, consists of characters in 11 lines of different-sized type, arranged with the line of largest characters at the top of the chart and the line of smallest characters at the bottom. Scores ranging from $^{20}/_{10}$ (the smallest line of characters) to $^{20}/_{200}$ (the largest line of characters) are shown in the left-hand column, and distances are in the right-hand column next to the numbers.

Nasal Speculum

The *nasal speculum* is used for visualizing the lower and middle turbinates of the nose. A penlight or flashlight is used for illumination. The blades of the speculum are inserted about $\frac{1}{2}$ inch (1 cm) into the nares and opened so that they do not press on the septum. Alternatively, the otoscope can be used to visualize the internal nares. The light is provided by the scope, and the shortest, widest speculum that will fit into the nares is used.

Vaginal Speculum

A *vaginal speculum* is a two-bladed instrument used to examine the vaginal canal and cervix. The speculum is inserted into the vagina, and the speculum blades are opened, allowing visualization and assessment of the vagina and cervix. It is essential to warm and lubricate the speculum (either with warm water or with a water-soluble agent) before insertion.

Tuning Fork

A *tuning fork* is a two-pronged metal instrument used to test auditory function and vibratory perception. The fork is activated to vibrate by gently tapping its prongs against the palm of the hand. Once vibrating, the fork is held at the base to avoid diminishing the vibration of the prongs.

Percussion Hammer

The *percussion hammer,* also called the *reflex hammer,* is an instrument with a rubber head used to test deep tendon reflexes and determine tissue density. The hammer is held between the thumb and index finger to direct a brisk tap on the selected body area. The quick, firm tap is made with a rapid downward and backward wrist action. The pointed end of the hammer is used for smaller areas.

Positioning

A variety of positions are used during a physical assessment (Fig. 25-2). During positioning, it is important to consider the patient's age, health status, mobility, physical condition, energy level, and privacy. Positioning patients who are weak may require assistance. Uncomfortable or embarrassing positions should not be maintained for long periods. The assessment should be organized so that several body systems can be assessed with the patient in one position, thus minimizing unneeded and possibly tiring movements.

Sitting Position

The patient may sit upright in a chair or on the side of an examining table or bed. A patient who is physically unable to maintain an upright position may lie supine with the head of the bed elevated. This sitting position allows visualization of the upper body and facilitates full lung expansion. It is used to take vital signs and to assess the head and neck, posterior and anterior thorax and lungs, breasts, heart, and upper extremities.

Supine Position

In the supine position, the patient lies flat on the back with legs together but extended and slightly bent at the knees. The head may be supported with a small pillow. This position allows relaxation of abdominal muscles and can be used to assess the head and neck, anterior thorax and lungs, breasts, heart, abdomen, extremities, and peripheral pulses.

Dorsal Recumbent Position

In the dorsal recumbent position, the patient lies on the back with legs separated, knees bent, and soles of the feet flat on the bed. This position may be used for patients who have difficulty maintaining the supine position but should not be used for abdominal assessment because it causes abdominal muscles to contract. Areas that can be assessed in this position are the head and neck, anterior thorax and lungs, breasts, heart, extremities, and peripheral pulses.

Sims' Position

In Sims' position, the patient lies on either the right or left side. The lower arm is behind the body, and the upper arm is bent at the shoulder and elbow. The knees are both bent, with the uppermost leg at a more acute angle. Sims' position is used to assess the rectum or vagina.

Prone Position

In the prone position, the patient lies on the abdomen, flat on the bed, with the head turned to one side. This position is difficult for many patients to assume, especially older adults. It is used to assess the hip joint and can be used to assess the posterior thorax.

Lithotomy Position

In the lithotomy position, the patient is in the dorsal recumbent position with the buttocks at the edge of the examining table and the feet supported in stirrups. This position is used for assessment of the female rectum and genitalia. It is uncomfortable for older patients and is often embarrassing; thus, it should be used only for a brief period.

Knee-Chest Position

In the knee-chest position, the patient kneels, using the knees and chest to bear the weight of the body. The body is at a 90-degree angle to the hips, with the back straight, the arms above the head, and the head turned to one side. The position is used for assessment of the rectal area. Like the lithotomy position, it should be used only briefly.

Standing Position

The standing position may be used to assess posture, gait, and balance. Patients who are unable to stand, are weak or dizzy, or are prone to fall should not be placed in the standing position.

Draping

Draping prevents unnecessary exposure, provides privacy, and keeps the patient warm during the physical assessment. Drapes may be paper, cloth, or bed linens. Only those body parts being assessed are exposed as the assessment is conducted.

Preparing the Environment

It is important to prepare the environment for conducting a physical assessment. The time for the assessment should be mutually agreed on by both the nurse and the patient.

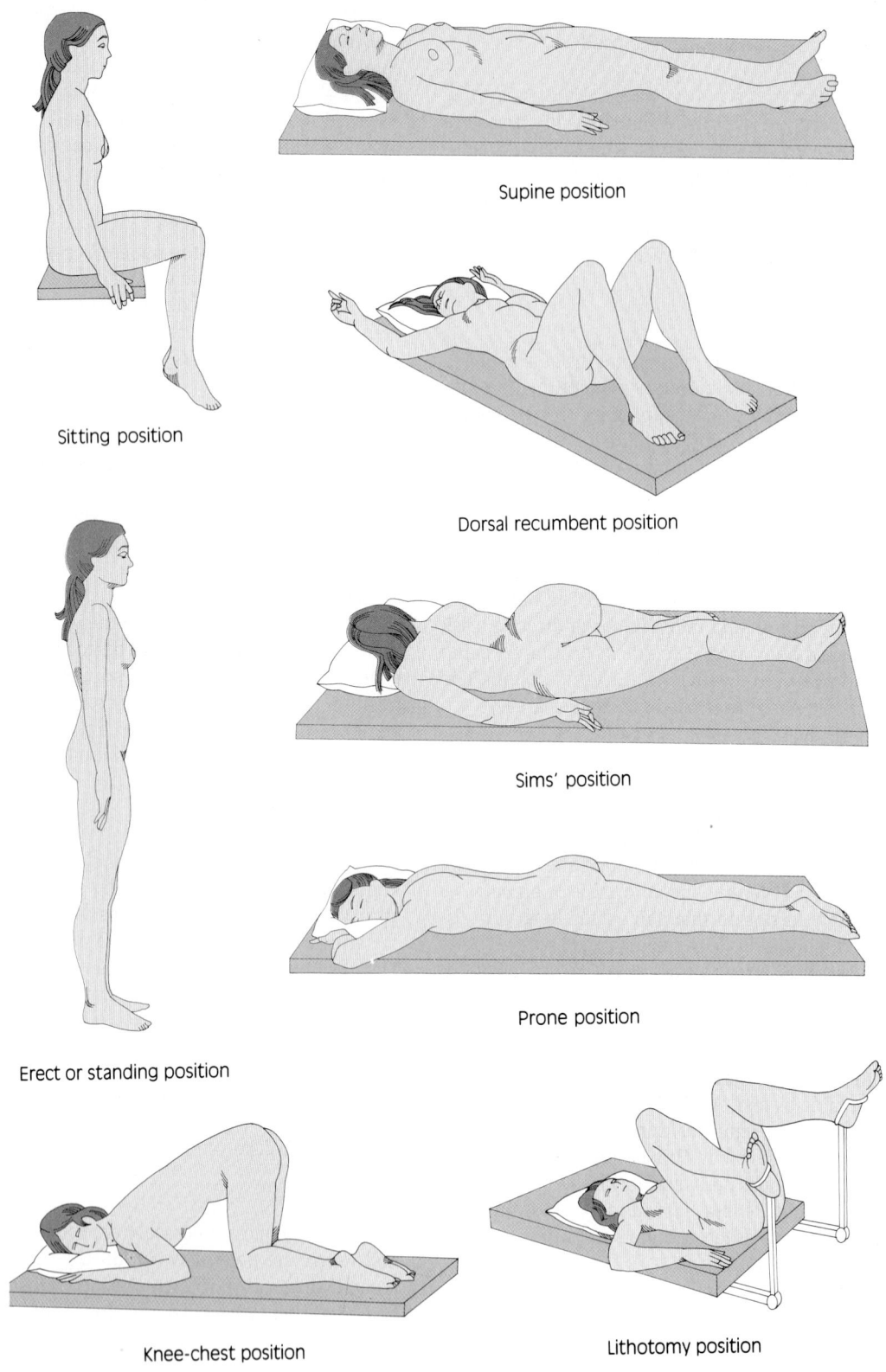

Sitting position

Supine position

Dorsal recumbent position

Sims' position

Prone position

Erect or standing position

Knee-chest position

Lithotomy position

Figure 25-2
Various patient positions used during a physical assessment.

It should not interfere with meals or daily routines for patients in the home or with treatments or visiting hours for patients in acute care settings. A time should be chosen when the patient is as free of pain as possible.

Clinics, offices, and hospitals may have a special examination room that provides a quiet, private space for assessment. If such a room is available, the examination table is prepared, a gown and drape for the patient are provided, and instruments and special supplies needed for the assessment are gathered. If the area is open to others, an enclosure with a curtain or screen is essential.

Preparing the Patient

The patient's physiologic and psychological needs should be considered before and during the physical assessment (Fig. 25-3). The nurse explains that he or she will do a physical assessment, that body structures will be examined, and that the assessments should not be painful. The patient is asked to change into a gown and directed to a private dressing area or to a comfortable area in the home. If necessary, the nurse assists the patient with undressing. The patient is asked to empty the bladder before the examination in order to be more comfortable during the assessment and to facilitate assessment of the abdomen.

The patient may be anxious for various reasons. Explaining the assessment in general terms can help decrease the patient's embarrassment, fear of possible abnormal physical findings, or fear of "failing" a test. Each assessment is then explained in greater detail as it is performed. The nurse should answer the patient's questions directly and honestly.

Techniques

The four primary assessment techniques are inspection, palpation, percussion, and auscultation. Bilateral body parts are always compared; for example, the assessment findings of one leg are compared with those of the other leg. Bilateral body parts are normally symmetric; that is, they have the same size and shape as well as the same characteristics, such as movement or pulses.

Inspection

Inspection is the process of performing deliberate, purposeful observations in a systematic manner. The nurse observes visually but also uses hearing and smelling to gather data throughout the assessment. Inspection begins with the initial patient contact and continues throughout the entire assessment. Adequate natural or artificial lighting is essential for distinguishing the color, texture, and moisture of body surfaces. A quiet environment eliminates extraneous noises and allows sounds to be heard without interference.

Inspect each area of the body for size, color, shape, position, and symmetry, noting normal findings and any deviations from normal. Inspection may be combined with the palpation phase of the assessment, with inspection preceding palpation.

Palpation

Palpation is an assessment technique that uses the sense of touch. The hands and fingers are sensitive tools and can assess temperature, turgor, texture, moisture, vibrations, and shape. The dorsum (back) surfaces of the hand and fingers are used for gross measure of temperature. The palmer (front) surfaces of the fingers and finger pads are used to assess texture, shape, fluid, size, consistency, and pulsation. Vibration is palpated best with the palm of the hand (Fig. 25-4).

For palpating, the nurse's hands should be warm and fingernails short. Any area of tenderness is palpated last. Light or deep palpation may be used, the depth being controlled by the amount of pressure applied. For light palpation, apply light pressure with the fingers together depressing the skin and underlying structures about $\frac{1}{2}$ inch (1 cm; Fig. 25-5, *top*). For deep palpation, press inward about 1 inch (2 cm; see Fig. 25-5, *bottom*). Deep palpation, which carries a risk of possible internal injury, should be used cautiously and only after considerable practice. Applying intermittent pressure to a specific area allows assessment of surface characteristics and underlying structures. Characteristics of masses, as determined by palpation, are described in Table 25-1.

Percussion

Percussion is the act of striking one object against another to produce sound. The sound waves produced by the striking action over body tissues are known as percussion tones. Percussion is used to assess the location, shape, size, and density of tissues.

Both hands are used to produce sound waves. The nondominant hand is placed directly on the area to be percussed, with the fingers slightly separated and the middle finger placed firmly on the body surface (Fig. 25-6, *left*). The other hand (dominant hand) provides the striking force, initiated by a sharp downward wrist movement with

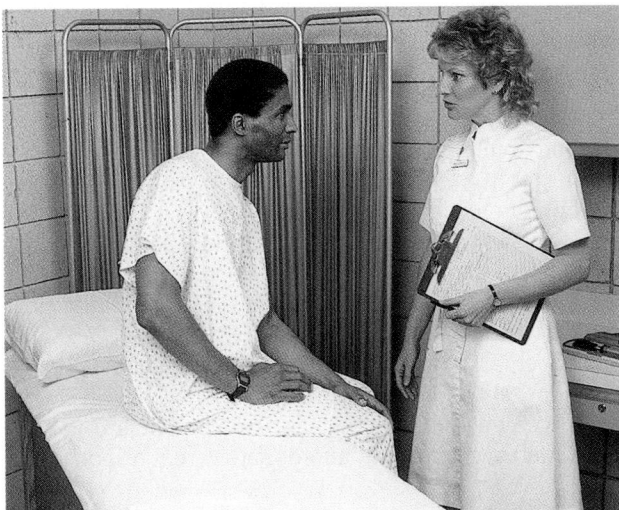

Figure 25-3
A brief explanation of the examination before beginning and just before each stage alleviates patient fear and anxiety. (Photo © Ken Kasper.)

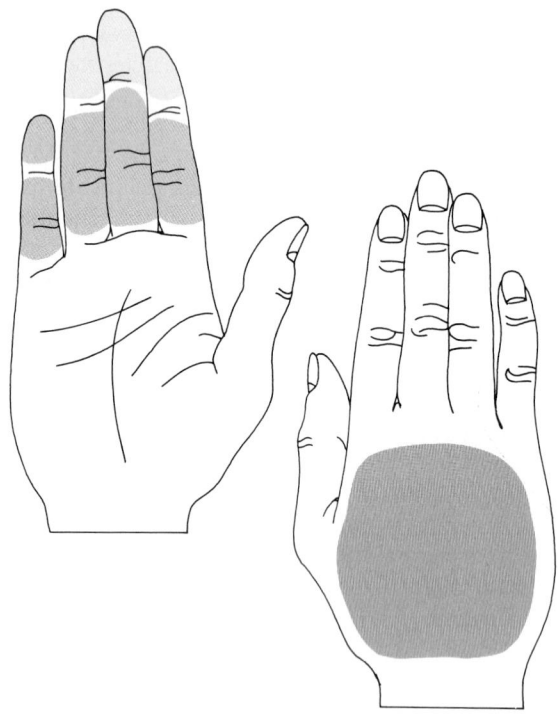

Figure 25-4
(*Top*) Palmar surfaces of the examiner's fingertips and finger pads are used for discriminatory sensation, such as texture, vibration, presence of fluid, or size and consistency of a mass. (*Bottom*) The dorsum, or back of the hand, is used to assess surface temperature.

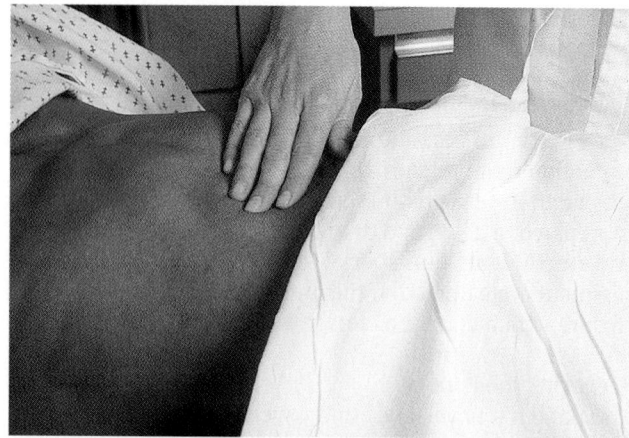

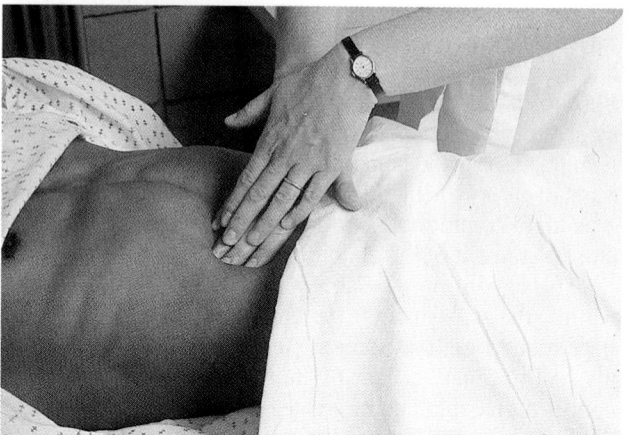

Figure 25-5
(*Top*) In light palpation, light pressure is applied by placing the fingers together and depressing the skin and underlying structures about ½ inch (1 cm). (*Bottom*) Deep palpation is used with caution. The skin and underlying structures are depressed about 1 inch (2 cm). (Photos © Ken Kasper.)

the forearm stationary and the wrist relaxed. The tip of the middle finger of the dominant hand strikes the middle finger of the opposing hand (see Fig. 25-6, *right*). This action produces a vibration that allows discrimination among five different tones, described in Table 25-2.

Auscultation

Auscultation is the act of listening with a stethoscope to sounds produced within the body. Chapter 24 discusses types of stethoscopes, their uses, and specific characteristics. Auscultation is performed by placing the stethoscope diaphragm or bell against the body part being assessed. Use firm pressure if using the diaphragm and light pressure if using the bell. The diaphragm of the stethoscope is used to detect high-pitched sounds, such as normal lung and bowel sounds. The bell of the stethoscope is used to detect low-pitched sounds, such as those produced by the heart and vascular system.

Four characteristics of sound are assessed by auscultation. They are (1) *pitch* (ranging from high to low); (2) *loudness* (ranging from soft to loud); (3) *quality* (eg, gurgling or swishing); and (4) *duration* (short, medium, or long).

General Survey

The general survey is the first component of the health assessment. Some information, such as the patient's appearance and behavior, is assessed when taking the health

history. Measuring the vital signs, height, and weight are also a part of the general survey.

General Appearance

Assessment of general appearance includes the following:

- Gender and race
- Body build, posture, and gait (note proportion of height to weight, erect or slumped posture, coordination of movements, pattern of gait)
- Hygiene, grooming (note cleanliness, body odors)
- Signs of illness (note posture, skin color, respirations, nonverbal communications of pain or distress, short attention span)
- Affect, attitude, mood (note speech, facial expressions, ability to relax, eye contact, behavior)
- Cognitive processes (note speech content and patterns, orientation, appropriate verbal responses)

Vital Signs

Vital signs are measured to establish a database and to detect actual or potential health problems. Vital signs are discussed in Chapter 24.

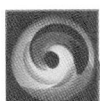

Table 25-1
Characteristics of Masses Determined by Palpation

Quality	Characteristics to Determine
Shape	Round Ovoid Tubular Irregular
Size	Measured in centimeters
Consistency	Firm Edematous Spongy Cystic
Surface	Smooth Nodular Granular
Mobility	Fixed or nonmobile Mobile
Tenderness	Amount of tenderness to touch
Pulsatile	Pulsation can or cannot be felt in the mass

Height and Weight

In adult patients, the correlation (or ratio) of height and weight is an assessment of overall health and nutrition. Height and weight should be measured using accurate scales and measuring devices. The patient should remove shoes and heavy clothing if the measurements are taken before undressing. If the patient is unable to stand erect, weight can be obtained using a chair or bed scales. The pa-

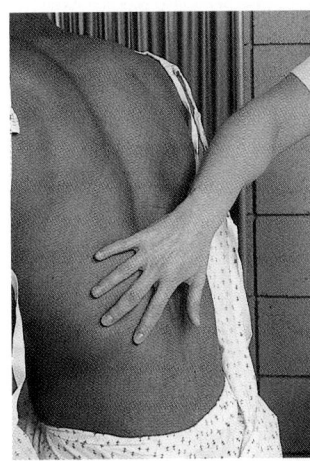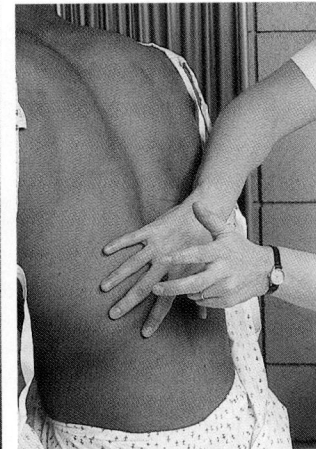

Figure 25-6
Percussion is used to access the location, shape, size, and density of tissues. (*Left*) The nondominant hand is placed directly on the area to be percussed, and the middle finger is placed firmly on the body surface. (*Right*) The tip of the middle finger of the dominant hand strikes the joint of the middle finger of the opposite hand. (Photos © Ken Kasper.)

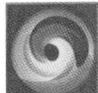

Table 25-2
Percussion Tones

Tone	Relative Intensity	Sample Location
Flat	Soft	Thigh
Dull	Medium	Liver
Resonance	Loud	Normal lung
Hyperresonance	Very loud	Emphysematous lung
Tympany	Loud	Gastric air bubble or puffed-out cheek

tient's actual height and weight can be compared with recommended average weights on a standardized chart as a general guideline for assessing nutritional status and health). The accompanying box, Guidelines for Nursing Care, describes the procedure for obtaining weight and height in adults. Table 25-3 provides a height and weight table for use as a standard reference. This table, composed by the Metropolitan Life Insurance Company, represents survey results of Americans who purchased life insurance and is adjusted according to height and frame size for adults between the ages of 25 and 59 years.

Children up to the age of 2 years should have height measured in the recumbent position with the legs fully extended. Infants should be weighed without any clothing, and children should be weighed in underwear.

Physical Assessment

The following sections discuss the physical assessment of each body system, including positions, assessment techniques, special considerations, and common normal and abnormal findings. Normal alterations in physical assessments in children and the older adult are included with each section.

Integument

The integumentary structures assessed are the skin, nails, hair, and scalp. Identify risk factors for altered health during the health history by asking about the following:

- History of rashes, lesions, change in color, or itching
- History of bruising or bleeding in the skin
- History of allergies to medications, plants, foods, or other substances
- Exposure to the sun and sunburn history
- Presence of wounds, bruises, abrasions, or burns
- Change in the color, size, or shape of a mole
- Recent treatment with chemotherapy or radiation therapy

Guidelines for Nursing Care

Obtaining Height and Weight With an Upright Balance Scale

Obtaining Height

- Ask the patient to remove shoes.
- Raise L-shaped sliding arm on the measuring device attached to the scale somewhat higher than the patient's approximate height.
- Ask the patient to step on the platform of the scale and stand erect with the back to the measuring device and the heels together.
- Lower the L-shaped sliding arm until it rests on top of the patient's head.
- Read the height in inches and record.
- Ask the patient to step down from the platform.

Obtaining Weight

- Balance the scale on zero.
- Ask the patient to remove shoes (and coat, if appropriate) and step onto the platform.
- Move the sliding indicator to the left until the scale balances.
- Read the weight in pounds and record.
- Ask the patient to step down from the platform.
- Return the scale weight indicator to zero.
- Considerations: Daily weights should be obtained at the same time each day (usually early morning), with the patient wearing the same clothing, and using the same scale.

- Exposure to chemicals that may be harmful to the skin, hair, or nails
- Degree of mobility
- Types of food eaten and liquids consumed each day

Skin

The skin is a general indicator of health status and provides information that may signify an underlying disease. The skin is assessed by inspection and palpation. The assessment begins with an overall inspection of the skin's condi-

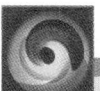

Table 25-3
Metropolitan Life Insurance Company Height and Weight Table

	Weight (lb) Men*				Weight (lb) Women†		
Height	Small Frame	Medium Frame	Large Frame	Height	Small Frame	Medium Frame	Large Frame
5′ 2″	128–134	131–141	138–150	4′ 10″	102–111	109–121	118–131
5′ 3″	130–136	133–143	140–153	4′ 11″	103–113	111–123	120–134
5′ 4″	132–138	135–145	142–156	5′ 0″	104–115	113–126	122–137
5′ 5″	134–140	137–148	144–160	5′ 1″	106–118	115–129	125–140
5′ 6″	136–142	139–151	146–164	5′ 2″	108–121	118–132	128–143
5′ 7″	138–145	142–154	149–168	5′ 3″	111–124	121–135	131–147
5′ 8″	140–148	145–157	152–172	5′ 4″	114–127	124–138	134–151
5′ 9″	142–151	148–160	155–176	5′ 5″	117–130	127–141	137–155
5′ 10″	144–154	151–163	158–180	5′ 6″	120–133	130–144	140–159
5′ 11″	146–157	154–166	161–184	5′ 7″	123–136	133–147	143–163
6′ 0″	149–160	157–170	164–188	5′ 8″	126–139	136–150	146–167
6′ 1″	152–164	160–174	168–192	5′ 9″	129–142	139–153	149–170
6′ 2″	155–168	164–178	172–197	5′ 10″	132–145	142–156	152–173
6′ 3″	158–172	167–182	176–202	5′ 11″	135–148	145–159	155–176
6′ 4″	162–176	171–187	181–207	6′ 0″	138–151	148–162	158–179

* Weights at ages 25 to 59 yr are based on lowest mortality. Weight in pounds are according to frame (in indoor clothing weighing 5 lb, shoes with 1-inch heels).
† Weights at ages 25 to 59 yr are based on lowest mortality. Weight in pounds are according to frame (in indoor clothing weighing 3 lb, shoes with 1-inch heels).
(Courtesy of Statistical Bulletin, Metropolitan Life Insurance Company.)

tion. Specific areas of the skin can be assessed during other body system assessments. Adequate lighting is essential for accurate assessments.

Inspection

The skin is inspected for color, vascularity, lesions, and body odors (Fig. 25-7).

Color. Skin color varies among races and among individuals, ranging from a pinkish white to various shades of brown. Skin areas that are normally exposed, such as the face and hands, may have a somewhat different color from areas that are usually covered by clothing, but otherwise skin color is relatively constant. Special care must be taken to detect color changes in dark-skinned people, such as African Americans, Hispanics, Native Americans, people of Mediterranean descent, and whites who are deeply suntanned. Some body areas of dark-skinned people, such as the palms of the hands and the soles of the feet, normally have less pigmentation than other areas of the body. Various terms used to describe abnormal appearance of the skin are summarized in Table 25-4.

Changes in skin color include erythema, cyanosis, jaundice, and pallor. These color changes are easier to assess in light-skinned people. **Erythema** is redness of the skin, more often seen in the face and the neck. It is associated with sunburn, inflammation, fever, trauma, and allergic reactions. **Cyanosis** is a bluish or grayish discoloration of the skin in response to inadequate oxygenation. Cyanosis is assessed as a blue tinge in patients with white skin and as a dullness in patients with dark skin. **Jaundice** is a yellow color of the skin resulting from liver and gallbladder diseases, some types of anemia, and hemolysis. It usually develops first in the sclera of the eyes and then in the skin and mucous membranes. Jaundice in dark-skinned people is more difficult to observe on the trunk of the body, but the scleral, oral mucous membranes, palms, and soles appear yellow to yellow-orange. **Pallor,** or paleness of the skin, often results from an inadequate amount of circulating blood or hemoglobin, causing inadequate oxygenation of the body tissues. Depending on severity, pallor may be visible over the entire skin surface or only in the lips, nailbeds, mucous membranes, and conjunctiva. Pallor in dark-skinned people is seen as an ashen gray or yellow-tinge.

Vascularity. The skin is inspected for vascularity, bleeding, or bruising; these signs may relate to a cardiovascular, hematologic, or liver dysfunction. **Ecchymosis** is a collection of blood in the subcutaneous tissues, causing purplish discoloration. **Petechiae** are small hemorrhagic spots caused by capillary bleeding. If present, assess their location, color, and size.

Lesions. The skin is inspected for the presence of lesions, which are areas of diseased or injured tissue (Table 25-5). Normally, the skin is smooth and intact. Bruises, scratches, cuts, insect bites, and wounds should be noted. A *wound,* a break in the continuity of the skin, is assessed for size, shape, depth, location, and presence of drainage or odor. *Scars* are healed wounds. (Wounds are discussed in Chap. 37.) A *rash* is a skin eruption. A rash should be described in terms of type, size, elevation, coloring, and presence or absence of drainage or itching. Document the exact body surface areas involved.

Palpation

The temperature, moisture, turgor, and texture of the skin are assessed by palpation.

Temperature and Moisture. The skin is normally warm and dry. An increase in skin temperature and moisture can indicate an elevated body temperature. An excessive amount of perspiration, such as when the entire skin is moist, is called *diaphoresis.* When the body is *dehydrated,* the skin is dry.

Turgor. Turgor (Fig. 25-8) is the fullness or elasticity of the skin and is usually assessed on the sternum or under the clavicle. Normal turgor results in elasticity of the skin, allowing it to be picked up in a fold and to return to its shape when released. When the patient is dehydrated, the skin's elasticity is decreased, and the skin fold returns to normal slowly. This, however, may be a normal finding in older patients. Difficulty in lifting a skin fold may indicate excess fluid in the tissues, or **edema.** Edema is characterized by swelling, with taut and shiny skin over the edematous area. If the area of edema is palpated with the fingers, an indentation may remain after the pressure is released; this is called *pitting.* Edema may be described on a scale, as follows: 0 = none, +1 = trace (2 mm), +2 = moderate (4 mm), +3 = deep (6 mm), +4 = very deep (8 mm). Edema may be the result of overhydration, heart failure, kidney failure, trauma, or peripheral vascular disease.

Texture. The texture of the skin may vary from smooth and soft to rough and dry. In the dehydrated patient, the texture is loose and wrinkled, and the mucous membranes are cracked and dry.

Nails

The nails are inspected for shape, angle, texture, and color. The shape of the nails should be somewhat convex and follow the natural curve of the finger. The angle between the nail and its base in the finger should be about 160 degrees. The texture of the nails should be smooth, and the nail base, when palpated, should be firm and nontender.

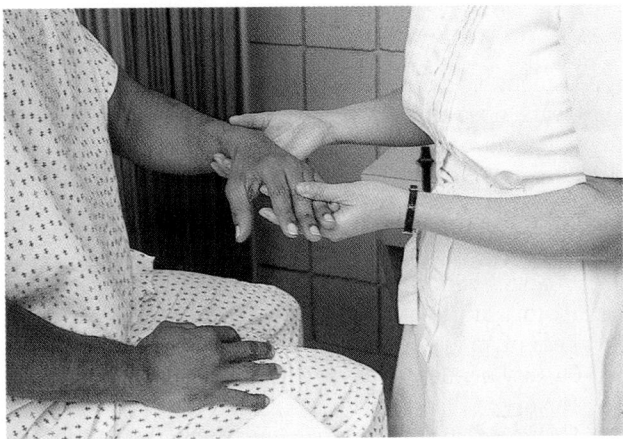

Figure 25-7
The skin is inspected for color, vascularity, and lesions.

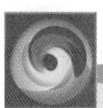

Table 25-4
Skin Color Assessment

Color Variations	Assessment Areas	Possible Causes
Redness (erythema; flushing)	Facial area, localized area of skin on the body	Blushing, alcohol intake, fever, injury trauma, infection
Bluish (cyanosis)	Exposed areas, particularly the ears, lips, inside of the mouth, hands and feet, nailbeds	Cold environment, cardiac or respiratory disease (decreased oxygenation)
Yellowish (jaundice)	Overall skin areas, mucous membranes, and sclera	Liver disease (increase in bilirubin levels)
Paleness (pallor)	Exposed areas, particularly the face and lips, conjunctivae, and mucous membranes	Anemia (decreased hemoglobin)
	Overall skin areas, lips, nailbeds, conjunctivae	Shock (decreased blood volume)
Vitiligo	Whitish patchy areas on the skin	Depigmentation (congenital or autoimmune conditions)
Tanned or brown	Sun-exposed areas	Overexposure (increased melanin production), pregnancy (brown spots?)

Abnormal findings include indentations, called *Beau's lines* (from acute illness); infection *(paronychia);* painless separation of the nail plate from the nailbed *(onycholysis)* from infection or trauma; increased brittleness or thickness and angulation (from anemia or iron-deficiency anemia); and clubbing (from long-term lack of oxygenation). Figure 25-9 illustrates nail abnormalities.

Hair and Scalp

The hair is normally resilient, evenly distributed, and neither excessively dry or oily. Hair is found on all body surfaces except the palms of the hands, the soles of the feet, and parts of the genitalia. The hair is assessed for color, texture, and distribution. Abnormal findings include unusual balding *(alopecia)* and excessive amounts of hair on the face and body *(hirsutism)*. Hair loss may be the result of chemotherapy, radiation therapy, infection, hormone disorders, or inadequate nutrition. Decreased oxygenation of peripheral tissues, especially of the lower extremities, may cause loss of hair. Excessive hair growth may occur in hormone disorders.

Separate the hair to inspect the scalp for color, dryness, scaliness, lumps, lesions, or lice. Nits, which are the white eggs of lice, can be differentiated from dandruff or lint because they are attached to the hair shaft. If any lumps or masses are palpated, note their location, size, tenderness, and mobility.

Life-Span Assessment Variations
Pediatric
- Newborns may be jaundiced and have milia (whiteheads).

- Newborns are covered with fine downy hair (lanugo) for the first 2 weeks of life.
- Skin is smooth and thin at birth.
- Pubic hair development indicates the onset of puberty.

Geriatric
- Wrinkles, dryness, scaling, decreased turgor
- Raised dark areas (senile keratosis)
- Flat brown age spots (senile lentigines)
- Small round red spots (cherry angioma)
- Fine, brittle, gray or white hair
- Hair loss
- Course facial hair in women, decreased body hair in men and women
- Thick, yellow toenails

Head and Neck

Assessment of the head and neck includes the skull, face, eyes, ears, nose and sinuses, mouth and pharynx, trachea, thyroid gland, and lymph nodes. Structures of the head and neck are assessed with inspection and palpation, with the patient sitting. Identify risk factors for altered health during the health history by asking about the following:

- Changes with aging in vision or hearing
- History of use of corrective lenses or hearing aids
- Loss of an eye with insertion of artificial eye
- History of allergies
- History of disturbances in vision or hearing
- History of chronic illnesses, such as hypertension, diabetes mellitus, or thyroid disease

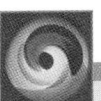

Table 25-5
Basic Types of Skin Lesions

Lesion Name	Description	Example
Primary Lesions*		
Circumscribed, Flat, Nonpalpable Change in Skin Color		
Macule	Lesion ≤1 cm	Petechiae, freckle
Patch	Lesion >1 cm	Vitiligo
Palpable, Elevated Solid Masses		
Papule	Mass ≤0.5 cm	Mole
Plaque	Mass >0.5 cm	Coalesced papules
Nodule	Mass 0.5–2 cm; firmer than a papule	Nevus (wart)
Tumor	Mass >2 cm	Lipoma
Wheal	Irregular, superficial area of localized skin edema	Hives, mosquito bite
Circumscribed, Superficial Skin Elevations Formed by Free Fluid in a Cavity Within the Skin Layers		
Vesicle	Filled with serous fluid, ≤0.5 cm	Herpes simplex
Bulla	Filled with serous fluid, >0.5 cm	2nd-degree burn
Pustule	Filled with pus	Acne, impetigo
Secondary Lesions†		
Loss of Skin Surface		
Erosion	Loss of superficial epidermis, moist, nonbleeding surface	Moist area after rupture of a vesicle, as in chickenpox
Ulcer	Loss of epidermis and dermis, may bleed and scar	Stasis ulcer
Fissure	Deep linear crack, extends into dermis	Athlete's foot
Material on the Skin Surface		
Crust	Dried residue of serum, pus, or blood	Impetigo
Scale	Thin flake of exfoliated dermis	Dandruff, dry skin
Miscellaneous Lesions		
Lichenification	Thickened and roughened epidermis, with increased visibility of skin furrows	Atrophic dermatitis
Atrophy	Thinning of the skin, loss of skin furrows, shiny appearance	Peripheral vascular disease
Excoriation	Scratch of the epidermis	
Scar	Fibrous tissue replaces tissue in the dermis or subcutaneous layer	
Keloid	Hypertrophied scar	
Other Common Skin Lesions, Not Technically Primary or Secondary		
Comedo	Plugged opening of a sebaceous gland, a hallmark of acne	Common blackhead
Telangiectasia	Small, dilated, red or bluish surface vessels; may be part of a basal cell carcinoma or skin injury from radiation	
Nevus	Flat to slightly elevated, round, evenly pigmented	Common mole

* May arise from previously normal skin.
† Result from changes in primary lesions.

- Exposure to harmful substances or loud noises
- Exposure to ultraviolet light
- History of smoking, chewing tobacco, or cocaine use
- History of eye or ear infections
- History of head trauma
- History of persistent hoarseness

Skull

The skull is assessed for size and shape by inspection and palpation. The parts of the head and face should be in proportion to each other and symmetric. Although the shape of the normal skull varies considerably, generally the shape is gently curved with prominences at the frontal and pari-

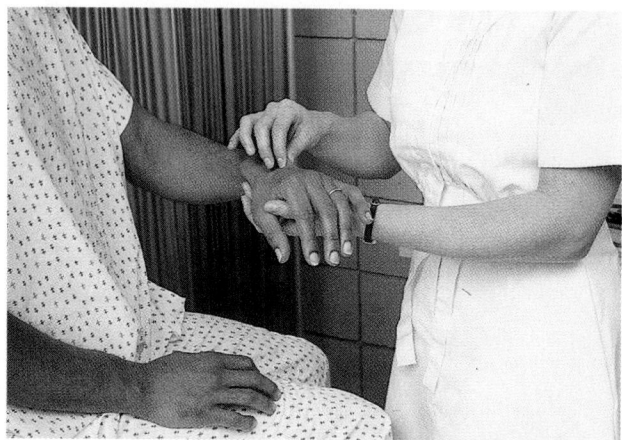

Figure 25-8
To assess skin turgor, a small fold of skin is picked up and then released to return to its normal shape. Difficulty in lifting a skin fold may indicate presence of edema. (Photo © Ken Kasper.)

etal bones. Abnormal findings include lack of symmetry or unusual size or contour of the skull (either may be the result of trauma or diseases affecting the growth of bone) and tenderness. If the skull appears disproportionately large or small, the circumference is measured. Measuring head circumference is a normal part of infant assessment up to the age of 2 years and should be conducted at each visit.

Face

The face is examined for color, symmetry, and distribution of facial hair. The facial nerve and facial muscles are assessed by asking the patient to raise the eyebrows, tightly close the eyes, puff out the cheeks, smile, and show the teeth. Edema of the face, especially around the eye *(periorbital edema)*, and involuntary facial movements (such as tics, fasciculations, and **tremors**) are abnormal findings. If abnormalities are noted, document their location, amount, and timing.

Eyes and Ears

The structures and functions of the eyes and ears are assessed using a penlight, an ophthalmoscope, an otoscope, an eye chart, a watch that ticks, and a tuning fork. The eyes and ears are assessed primarily by inspection.

Eyes

Assessments of the eye include external and internal eye structures (Fig. 25-10). Visual acuity, extraocular movements (EOMs), and peripheral vision are also assessed.

External Eye Structures. The eyes, eyebrows, eyelids, eyelashes, lacrimal gland, and pupils and iris are inspected for position and alignment (Fig. 25-11). The eyes are inspected for symmetry and parallel alignment. The eyebrows should have equal distribution, and the eyelashes should curl outward. The eyelids are inspected for color, edema, and equal coverage of the eyeball. The lacrimal glands are inspected and palpated for edema and pain.

Pupil and Iris. The pupils are normally black, equal in size, round, and smooth. The pupils may be pale and cloudy if the patient has cataracts (loss of opacity of the lens). Injury to the eye, glaucoma, and certain medications may

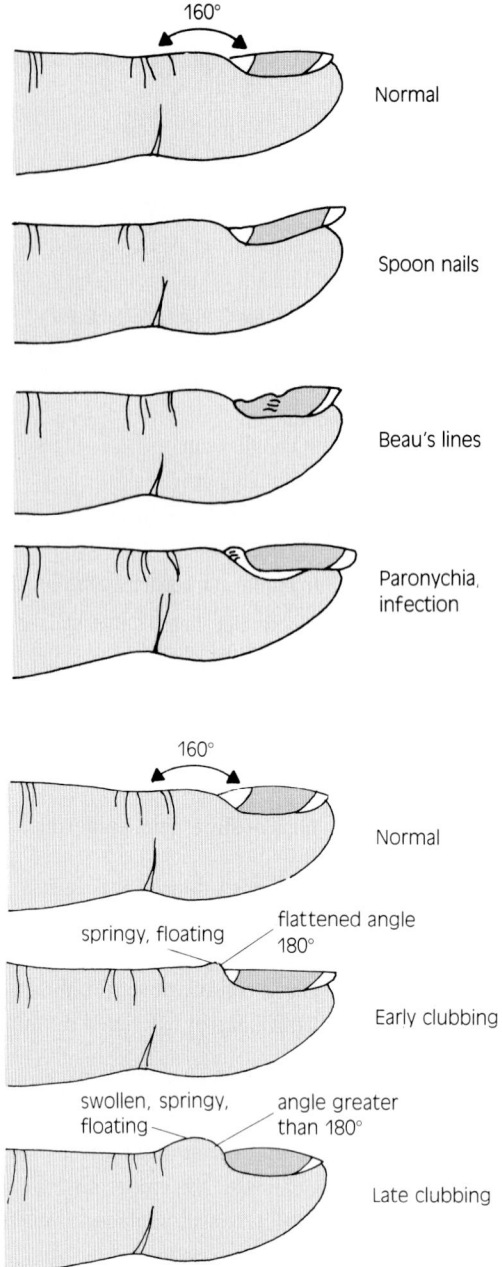

Figure 25-9
Examples of nail abnormalities.

cause the pupil to dilate *(mydriasis)*; certain drugs can cause constriction *(miosis)*; and unequal pupils may result from central nervous system injury or illness.

The pupils are assessed for their reaction to light and accommodation and for convergence. Assess pupillary *reaction to light* by following these steps (Fig. 25-12):

1. Ask the patient to look straight ahead.
2. Bring the penlight from the side of the patient's face and briefly shine the light on the pupil.
3. Observe the pupil's reaction; normally, it will rapidly constrict *(direct response)*.
4. Repeat the procedure and observe the other eye; normally, it too will constrict *(consensual reflex)*.
5. Repeat the procedure with the other eye.

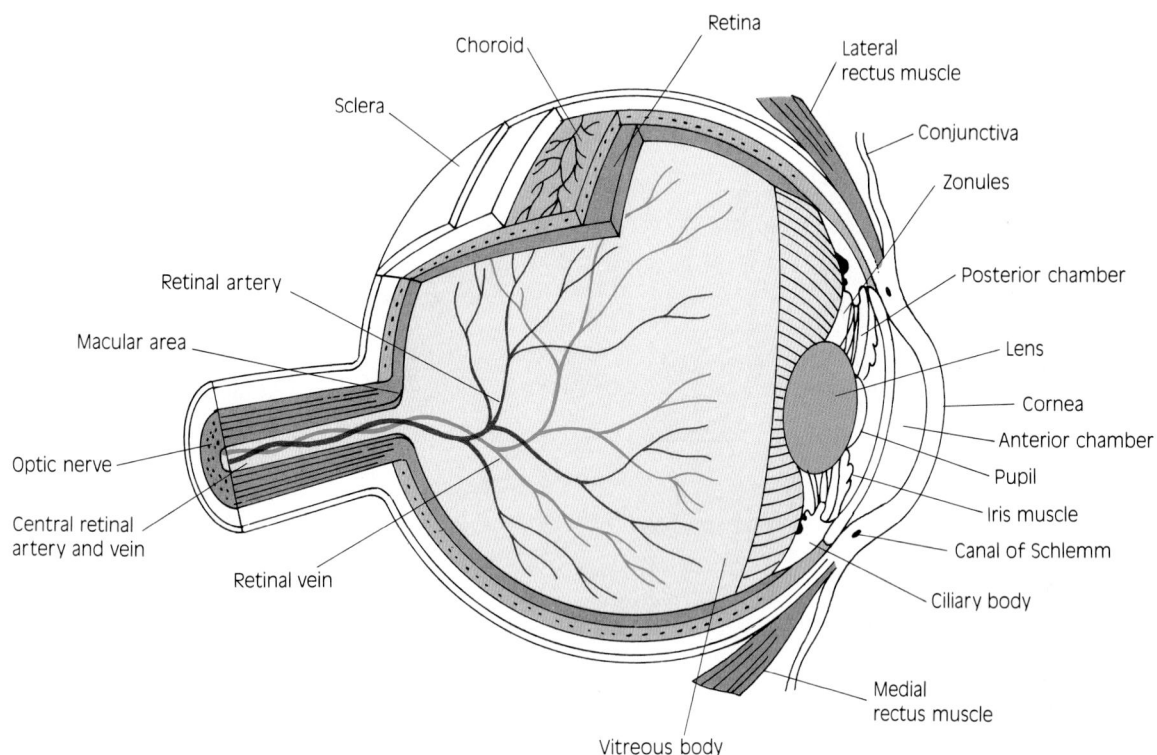

Figure 25-10
A cross-section of the eye.

Accommodation, which occurs when one moves the focus of vision from a distant point to a near point, causing the pupils to constrict, is assessed by these steps (Fig. 25-13):

1. Hold the forefinger, a pencil, or other straight object about 10 to 15 cm (4 to 6 inches) from the bridge of the patient's nose.

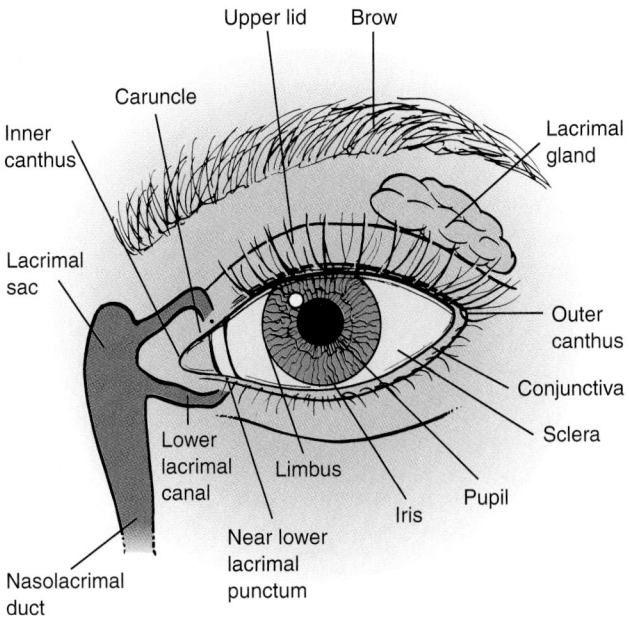

Figure 25-11
The eye and surrounding structures.

2. Ask the patient to first look at the object, then at a distant object, then back to the object being held. The pupil normally constricts when looking at a near object and dilates when looking at a distant object.

Convergence is assessed by moving your finger toward the patient's nose. The patient's eyes should normally converge (assume a cross-eyed appearance; Fig. 25-14).

Internal Eye Structures. The internal eye (Fig. 25-15) is examined with the ophthalmoscope to assess the fundus, including the retina, optic nerve disc, macula, fovea centralis, and retinal vessels. Using the ophthalmoscope takes practice. Normal findings are a uniform red reflex; clear, yellow optic nerve disc; reddish retina; and light-red arteries and dark-red veins, the veins being about $1^1/_2$ times as large as the arteries (Fig. 25-16). Guidelines for assessing the internal eye are listed in the accompanying Focused Assessment Guide. Abnormal findings include cloudiness of the lens (from cataracts), changes in the size and shape of blood vessels (which may result from hypertension or arteriosclerosis), and changes in color and surface characteristics (from such health problems as diabetes mellitus, hypertension, trauma, inflammation, or detached retina).

Vision

Visual Acuity. Visual acuity is assessed by placing the patient 20 feet from Snellen's chart and testing each eye. The patient is asked to read the smallest possible line of letters, first with both eyes and then with one eye at a time. Note where the patient's vision is being tested with or without corrective lenses. Visual acuity is measured by standardized

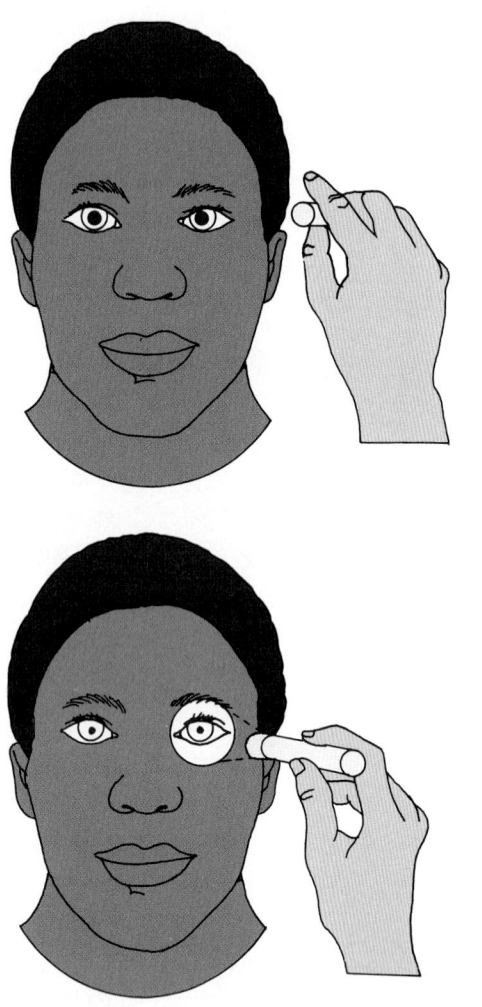

Figure 25-12
To test pupillary reaction to light, a penlight is moved from the side of the patient's face (*top*) to in front of the eye (*bottom*). The pupil should constrict when the light is present. The dilation or constriction shown is exaggerated for clarity.

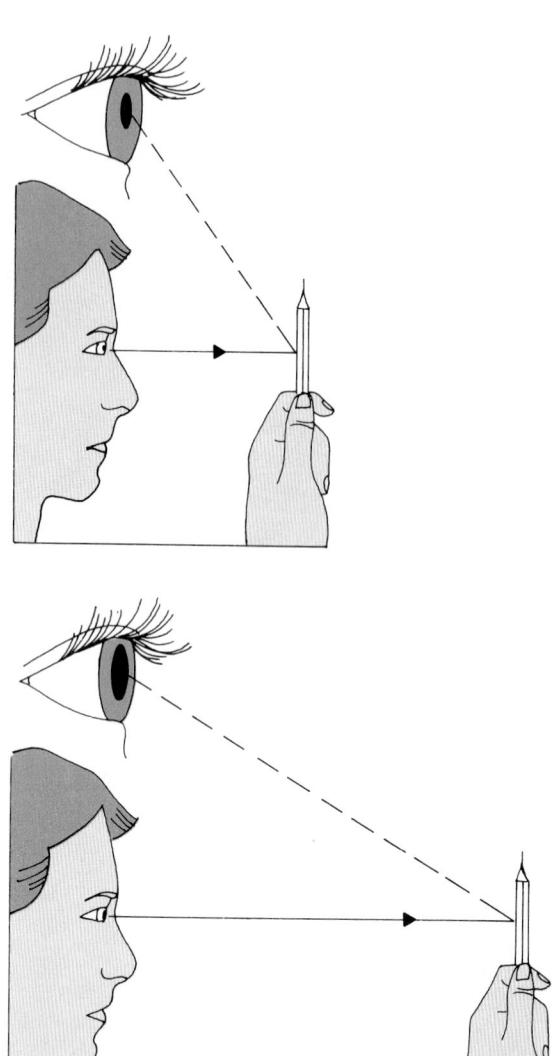

Figure 25-13
The normal pupil constricts when focused on a near object and dilates when focused on a far object. This is called *accommodation*.

numbers listed on the side of the chart. The numerator is 20, representing the distance from which a person with normal vision (recorded as $^{20}/_{20}$) can read the letters. The larger the denominator, the poorer the vision. Visual acuity is recorded as the smallest line of letters that can be read accurately with no more than two inaccurate readings (such as $^{20}/_{30-2}$ with glasses).

Extraocular Movements. EOMs are tested by assessing the cardinal fields of vision for coordination and alignment (Fig. 25-17). Normally, both eyes move together, are coordinated, and are parallel. To assess EOMs, follow these three steps:

1. Ask the patient to sit or stand about 2 feet away, facing you sitting or standing at eye level with the patient.
2. Ask the patient to hold the head still and follow the movement of your forefinger or a penlight with the eyes.
3. Keeping your finger or light about 1 foot from the patient's face, move it slowly through the cardinal

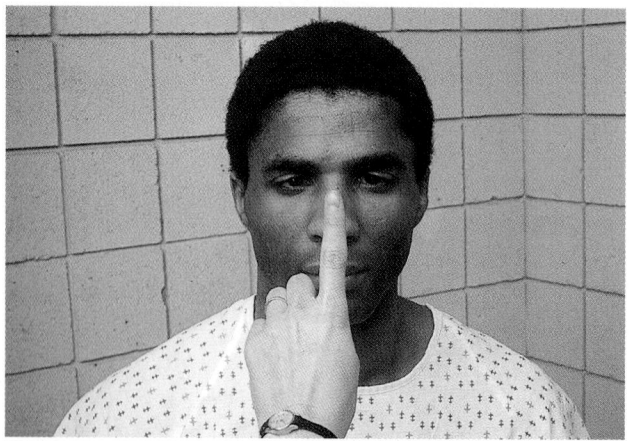

Figure 25-14
Convergence is assessed by moving the finger toward the patient's nose. (Photo © Ken Kasper.)

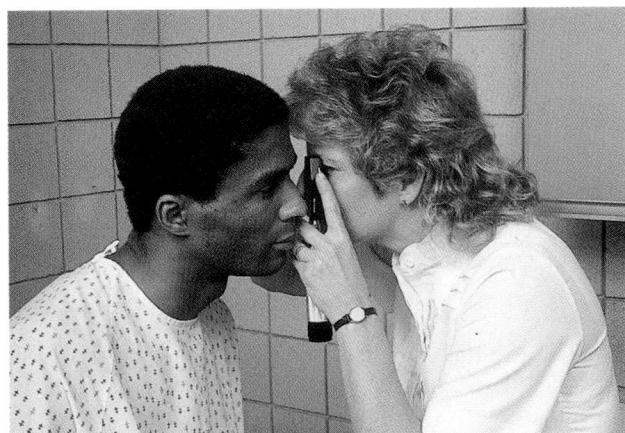

Figure 25-15
Examination of the internal structures of the eye, using an ophthalmoscope. (Photo © Ken Kasper.)

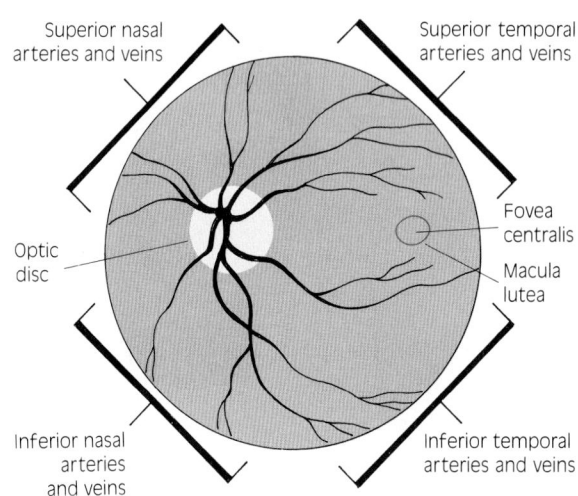

Figure 25-16
The normal fundus as seen through an ophthalmoscope.

positions—up and down, left and right, diagonally up and down to the left, diagonally up and down to the right.

Peripheral Vision. Tests for peripheral vision (or visual fields) assess retinal function and optic nerve function. Full peripheral vision is normal. Assess peripheral vision by following these steps:

1. Have the patient stand or sit about 2 feet away, facing you at eye level.
2. Ask the patient to cover one eye with a hand or an index card.
3. Ask the patient to look directly at your nose and fix his or her eyes on that spot.

4. Cover your own eye opposite the patient's closed eye.
5. Hold one arm outstretched to one side (right or left) equidistant from you and the patient, and move your fingers into the visual fields from various peripheral points.
6. Ask the patient to tell you when the fingers are first seen (both you and the patient should see the fingers at the same time).
7. Repeat the procedure for the other eye.

Abnormalities of the external eye, pupil and iris, and visual assessment include asymmetry of position and alignment (which may be due to muscle weakness or a con-

FOCUSED ASSESSMENT GUIDE

Internal Eye

General guidelines for assessment of the internal eye are as follows:

- Assemble the ophthalmoscope, beginning with the light setting at the large white light and the lens wheel at 0 setting.
- Darken the room and have the patient remove glasses. Allow time for the patient's pupils to dilate. The patient should be sitting.
- Sit facing the patient and ask him or her to look straight ahead during the examination.
- Keep both eyes open while looking through the ophthalmoscope viewer.
- Use your right hand and eye to examine the patient's right eye, and your left hand and eye for the patient's left eye.
- Shine the light on the pupil and observe the round red or orange glow (the red reflex).

- Focusing on the red reflex, slowly move the ophthalmoscope toward the patient's eye.
- Rotate the lens wheel until internal eye structures are sharp and clear.
- Follow blood vessels toward the midline to locate the optic disc; note color, size, shape, margins, and central area (physiologic cup).
- Follow blood vessels outward to each of the four quadrants, assessing color, size, and pattern.
- Ask the patient to look up, down, and from side to side, assessing the characteristics of the retina.
- Locate the macula by first locating the optic disc and then looking toward the patient's temple for a small circular structure near the disc; note color, characteristics, and area of reflected light (fovea centralis).

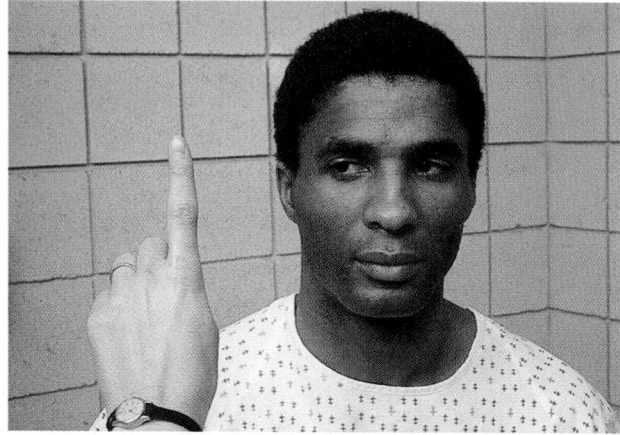

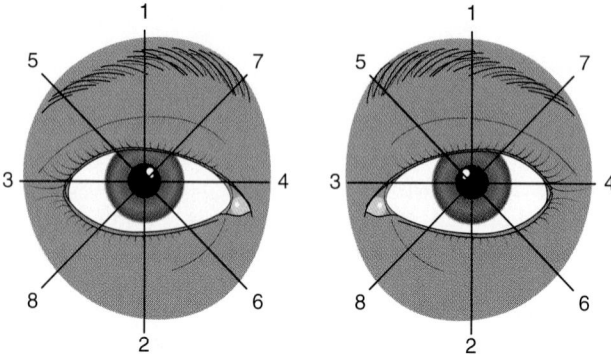

Figure 25-17
Test extraocular movement of the eye by asking the patient to hold his head still and follow the movement of your forefinger (*top*) through the cardinal positions of the eye (*bottom*). (Photo © Ken Kasper.)

genital abnormality), drooping of the upper lids (called *ptosis*; this may be the result of damage to the oculomotor nerve, myasthenia gravis, or a congenital disorder), inward turning of the lower lid *(entropion)*, outward turning of the lower lid *(ectropion)*, redness or drainage (from infection of the lid margins, conjunctivae, or hair follicles), decreased or absent pupillary response (indicating blindness or serious brain damage), inability of the eyes to accommodate or converge, and alterations in the visual fields.

Ears

The external ear, the middle ear, and the inner ear (Fig. 25-18) are assessed. The patient remains sitting while the nurse assesses the function and structure of the ears by inspection and palpation. An otoscope with the correct size of ear speculum may be used to inspect the ear canal; a tuning fork is used to assess hearing acuity.

External Ear. The external ear is inspected for shape, size, and lesions. The external surfaces of the ear should be smooth, and the shape and size of the ears should be symmetric and proportional to the head. The external ear is gently palpated for pain, edema, or presence of lesions (Fig. 25-19). Abnormal findings of the external ear include unequal height and size, uneven color, and lesions.

Ear Canal and Tympanic Membrane. The otoscope is used to examine the ear canal and the tympanic membrane with the patient sitting. The largest speculum that will fit comfortably into the patient's ear is attached to the otoscope. The otoscope speculum is inserted as the patient's head is slightly tilted away from the examiner. To achieve better visualization, the ear canal of the adult is straightened by gently pulling the pinna up and back (the ear canal is straightened in children younger than age 3 years by pulling the pinna down and back). The ear canal should be smooth and pinkish in color. It is examined for wax, discharge, and foreign bodies. The tympanic membrane should be intact,

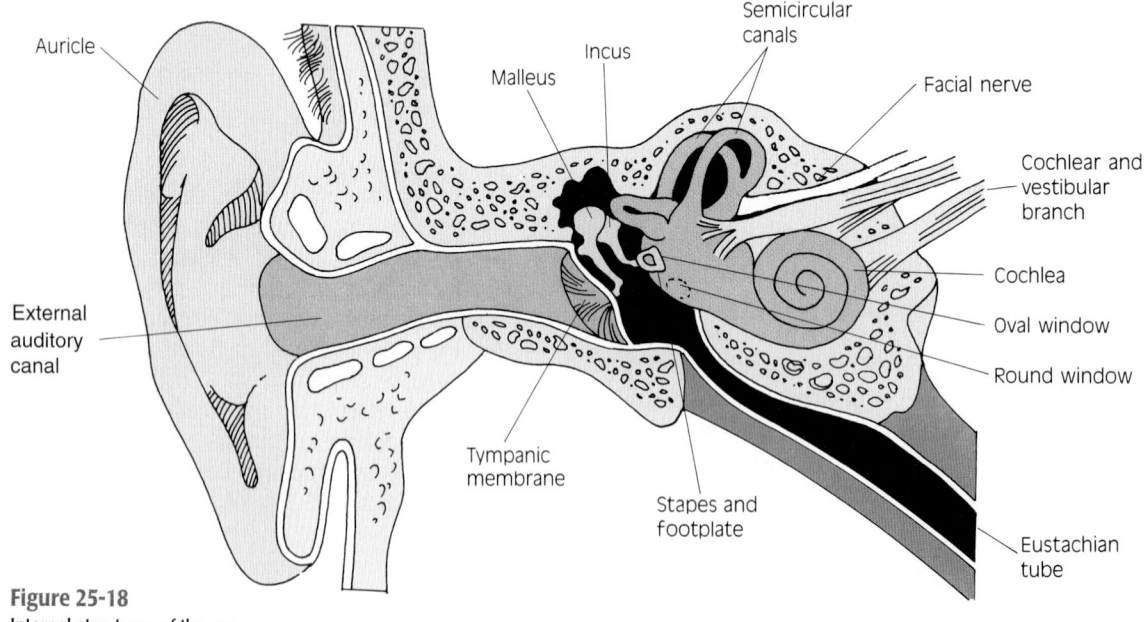

Figure 25-18
Internal structures of the ear.

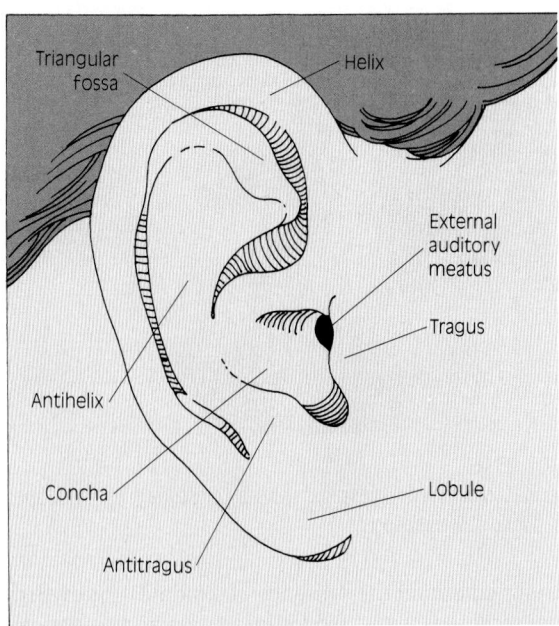

Figure 25-19
External structures of the ear.

translucent, shiny, and gray (Fig. 25-20). There should be no redness or discharge.

Abnormal findings include pain when manipulating the pinna (a symptom of an infection of the external ear), redness of the canal (from inflammation or infection), mastoid tenderness (from infection), a red and swollen eardrum (symptoms of an infection in the middle ear), a perforated eardrum (from an infection causing rupture or trauma), wax plugs in the ear canal (from an accumulation of ceru-

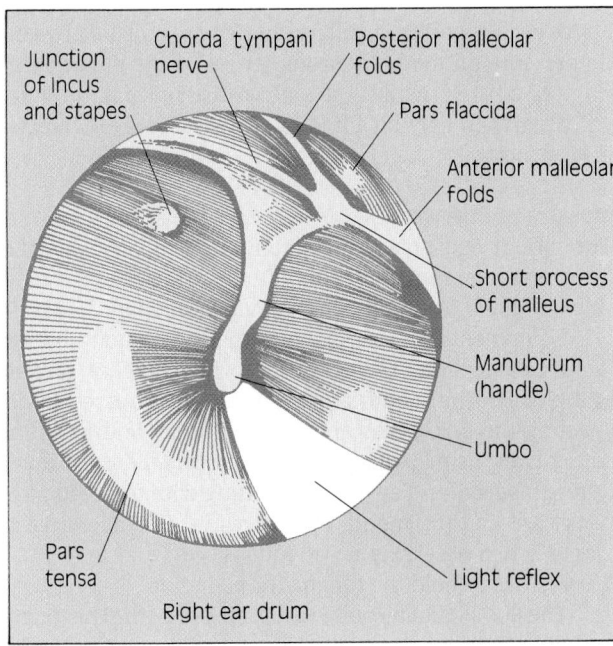

Figure 25-20
Normal tympanic membrane, as seen through an otoscope.

men), and drainage (from an infection or foreign body in the ear canal).

Hearing. Hearing is assessed, one ear at a time, by determining whether the patient can hear a whispered voice or a ticking watch from a distance of 1 to 2 feet. Assess hearing acuity out of the patient's line of vision (to prevent lip-reading), with the opposite ear covered. When a hearing loss is found, a tuning fork or audiometer may be used for more precise assessments of hearing. Audiometry is not generally used in routine physical assessment. Tuning fork tests are used to assess the type of hearing loss. Hearing loss may be *conductive* (the result of a problem with the transmission of sound waves through the outer and middle ear); *sensorineural* (from inner ear damage); or *mixed,* a combination of both.

Weber's test is used to assess bone conduction. Normally, the sound is heard in both ears or is localized at the center of the head. The three-step procedure is as follows:

1. Hold the tuning fork at its base and strike it against your other palm so that the fork vibrates.
2. Place the base of the tuning fork on the center of the top of the patient's head.
3. Ask the patient where the sound is heard best.

Patients with conductive hearing loss hear the sound better in the affected ear because bone (in this case, the ossicles) transmits the sound directly to the ear. If the sound is heard better in the ear without a problem, it indicates damage to the inner ear or a nerve disorder.

Rinne's test compares air conduction (AC) with bone conduction (BC). Air-conducted hearing is normally greater than bone-conducted hearing (documented as a positive Rinne, with AC > BC). The four-step test is as follows:

1. Strike the tuning fork.
2. Hold the base of the tuning fork against the mastoid process of the patient and ask the patient to tell you when the sound can no longer be heard.
3. Immediately place the still-vibrating tuning fork close to the external ear canal and ask whether the patient can hear the sound; the normal ear will do so.
4. Repeat the test with the other ear.

If the hearing loss is conductive, bone conduction will be the same or greater than air conduction.

Nose and Sinuses

The nose is assessed by examining the external nose, the *nares,* and the *turbinates* (Fig. 25-21). The maxillary sinuses are located in the maxillary bone; the frontal sinuses are located in the frontal bone (Fig. 25-22). The nose is assessed by inspection, and the sinuses by inspection and palpation. The patient is sitting with the head slightly tilted back.

Nose

The nose is tested for nasal patency by occluding one nostril at a time and asking the patient to inhale and exhale through the nose. Each nostril is inspected using an otoscope with a short, wide tip or using a nasal speculum and penlight (Fig. 25-23). The mucous membranes are exam-

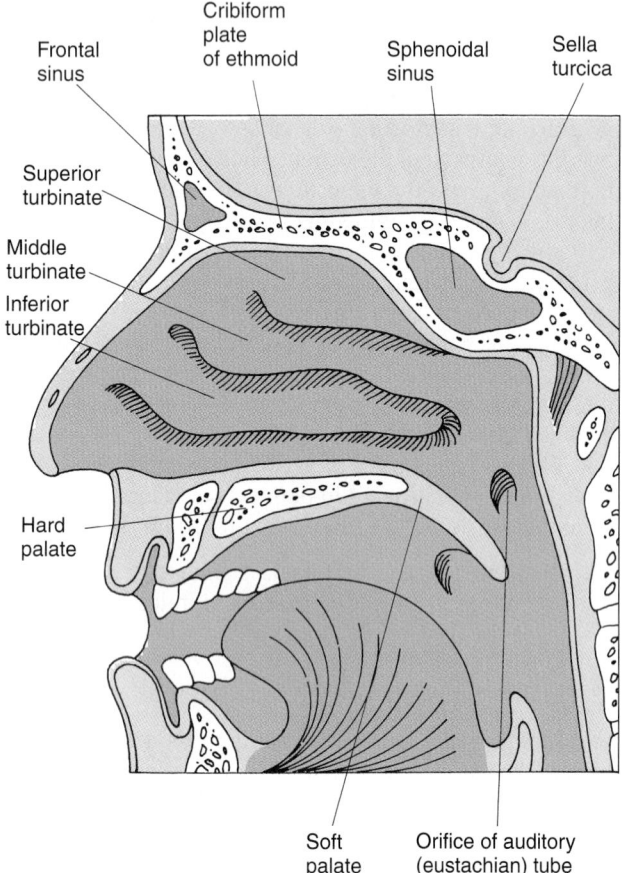

Figure 25-21
Cross-section of the nasal cavity.

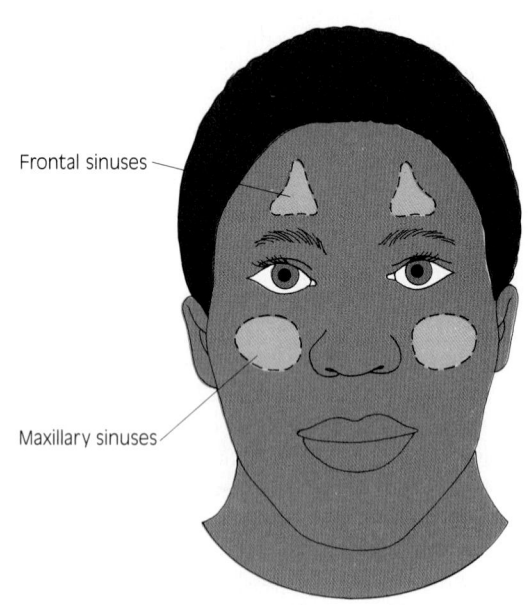

Figure 25-22
Location of the frontal and maxillary sinuses.

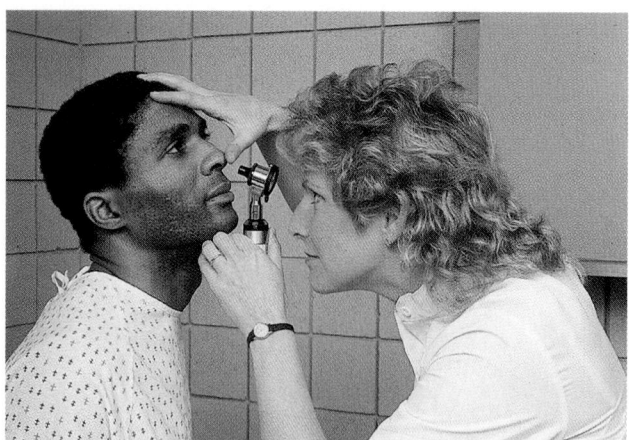

Figure 25-23
Examination of the nasal passages using an otoscope with a wide speculum. (Photo © Ken Kasper.)

ined for color and the presence of exudate or growths. The nasal septum is inspected for intactness and deviation. It is not necessary to use a nasal speculum with a child; push the tip of the nose upward with your thumb and shine a light into the nares. Normally, the nasal mucosa is moist and redder than the oral mucosa.

Abnormal findings that should be noted are swelling of the mucosa, bleeding or discharge (indicating allergies with inflammation or infection), perforation or deviation of the nasal septum (cocaine use may cause perforation; a deviated septum may be congenital or from trauma), and polyps (often seen with chronic allergies).

Sinuses

The frontal and maxillary sinuses are examined for pain and edema. The frontal sinuses are palpated by gently pressing upward on the bony prominences located above each eye. The maxillary sinuses are palpated by gentle pressure on the bony prominences of the upper cheek (Fig. 25-24). Normally, the sinuses are not painful when palpated. Pain may be a finding if the sinuses are infected or obstructed.

Mouth and Pharynx

The mouth and pharynx are composed of various structures: the lips, tongue, teeth, gums, hard and soft palate, salivary gland, tonsillar pillars, and tonsils (Fig. 25-25).

Equipment for assessment of the mouth and pharynx includes a penlight, a tongue blade, a 4 × 4 gauze sponge, and gloves. The mouth and pharynx are assessed by inspecting the lips, gums and teeth, tongue, and hard and soft palates, using palpation if any abnormalities are noted during inspection. The patient is sitting with the head tilted backward and the mouth opened wide. The nurse wears gloves when assessing a patient's mouth and may use a 4 × 4 gauze to hold the tongue for palpation.

The lips should be pink, moist, and smooth. The tongue and mucous membranes are normally pink in color, moist, and free of swelling or lesions. If the patient wears dentures, they are removed for the inspection of the gums and roof of

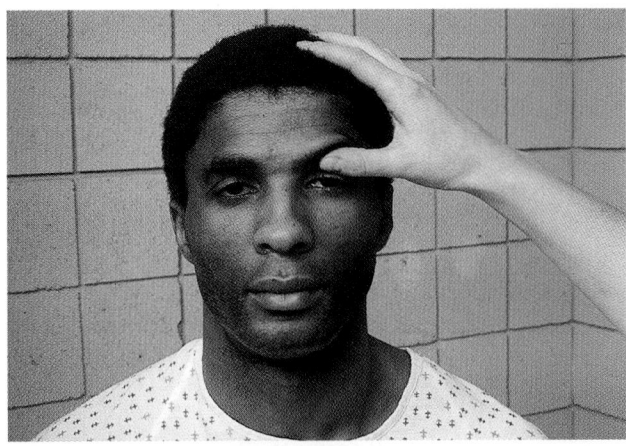

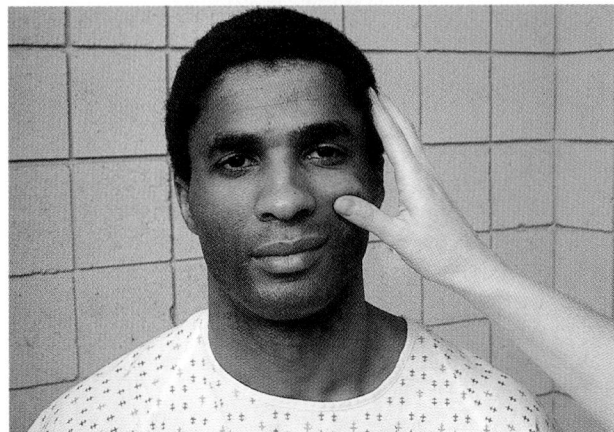

Figure 25-24
(*Top*) The frontal sinuses are palpated by gently pressing upward on the bony prominences above each eye. (*Bottom*) The maxillary sinuses are palpated by applying gentle pressure on the bony prominences of the upper cheek. (Photos © Ken Kasper.)

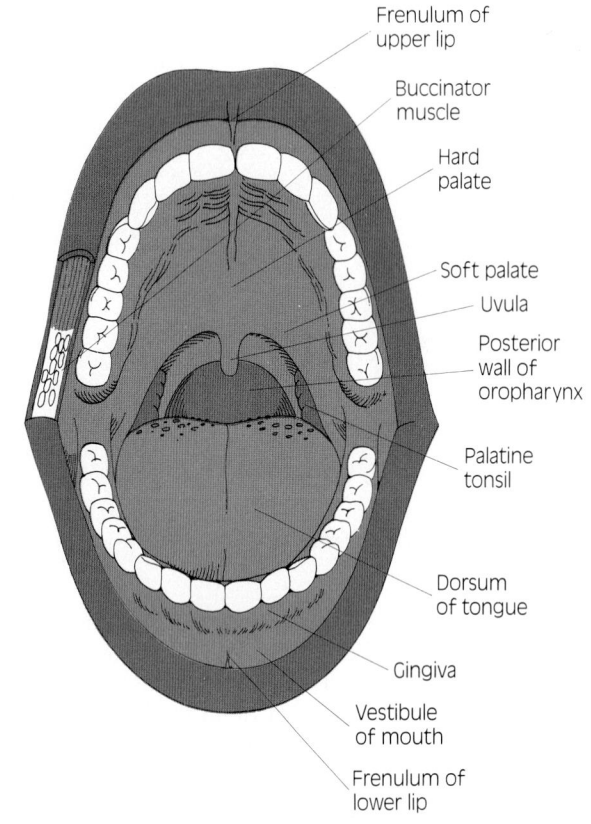

Figure 25-25
Structures of the mouth.

the mouth. The gums should be pink and smooth. With the tongue relaxed on the floor of the mouth, the mucous membrane of the oropharynx is examined while the base of the tongue is depressed with a tongue depressor. The uvula is normally centered and freely movable. The tonsils, if present, are small, pink, and symmetric in size. The teeth should be regular and free of cavities or have dental restoration.

Abnormal findings are pallor, cyanosis, or redness and swelling of the mucous membranes; lesions of the mucosa and lips; swollen, red tonsils (indicating infection); swollen, red, and bleeding gums (causes include nutritional deficits, inflammation or infection, poorly fitted dentures, or poor oral hygiene); poorly aligned, missing, or carious teeth; a white coating on the tongue (causes include poor oral hygiene, irritation, and smoking); a fissured tongue (from dehydration); a bright-red tongue (seen in deficiencies of iron, vitamin B_{12}, or niacin); or a black, hairy tongue (from antibiotic use).

Neck

With the patient sitting, the neck (Fig. 25-26) is assessed by inspection and palpation. The neck should be slightly

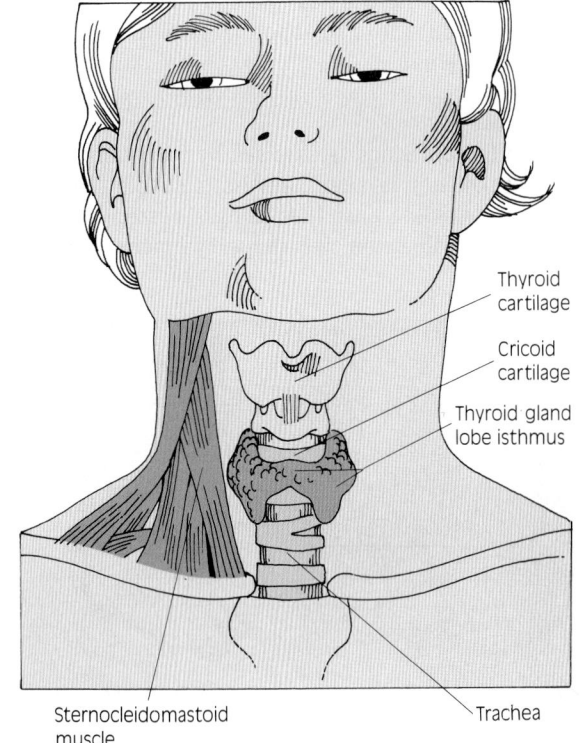

Figure 25-26
Structures of the neck.

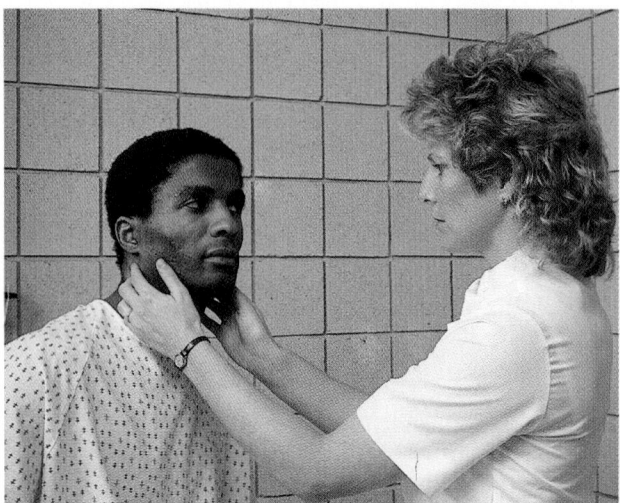

Figure 25-27
Palpating the neck. (Photo © Ken Kasper.)

hyperextended. The neck is assessed for size and position of the trachea and thyroid (Fig. 25-27), range of motion, lymph nodes, and venous distention. Range of motion is assessed by asking the patient to tilt the head backward, forward, and side to side. The neck should be symmetric with full range of motion. No neck vein distention (indicating heart problems) should be visible.

Trachea

The trachea, normally midline at the suprasternal notch, is palpated for alignment and position. An unequal space between the trachea and the sternocleidomastoid muscle on each side is an abnormal finding indicating tracheal displacement.

Thyroid

The thyroid gland is assessed by palpation, although in many patients, it is normally not palpable. The patient is sitting, with the examiner using a posterior approach (Fig. 25-28). Palpate for size, shape, symmetry, tenderness,

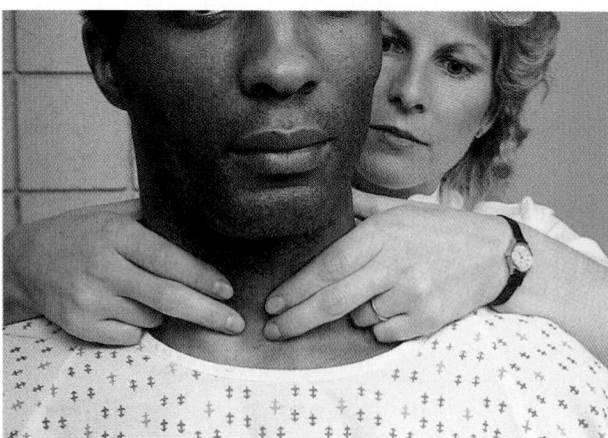

Figure 25-28
Assessing the thyroid. (Photo © Ken Kasper.)

and presence of any nodules. Follow these five steps to palpate the thyroid gland:

- Standing behind the patient, place your hands around the patient's neck, with the fingertips over the lower half of the neck and trachea.
- Ask the patient to swallow, and feel for enlargement of the gland as it rises.
- Palpate each lobe of the thyroid by having the patient turn the head slightly toward the side to be examined; then gently displace the trachea with one hand.
- Ask the patient to swallow, and palpate the thyroid with the other hand.
- Repeat for the other side.

If palpable, the thyroid gland should feel soft but elastic. It should be nontender and have no enlargement, masses, or nodules (which may indicate thyroid gland disease, infection of the thyroid, or cancer).

Lymph Nodes

The lymph nodes (Fig. 25-29) are assessed by palpating with the pads of the fingers for enlargement, tenderness, and mobility. The nodes are generally not palpable; if palpable, they should be small, mobile, smooth, and nontender. If palpable, assess location, size, consistency, mobility, and tenderness. Enlarged lymph nodes (called *lymphadenopathy*) may indicate infection, autoimmune disorders, or metastasis of cancer.

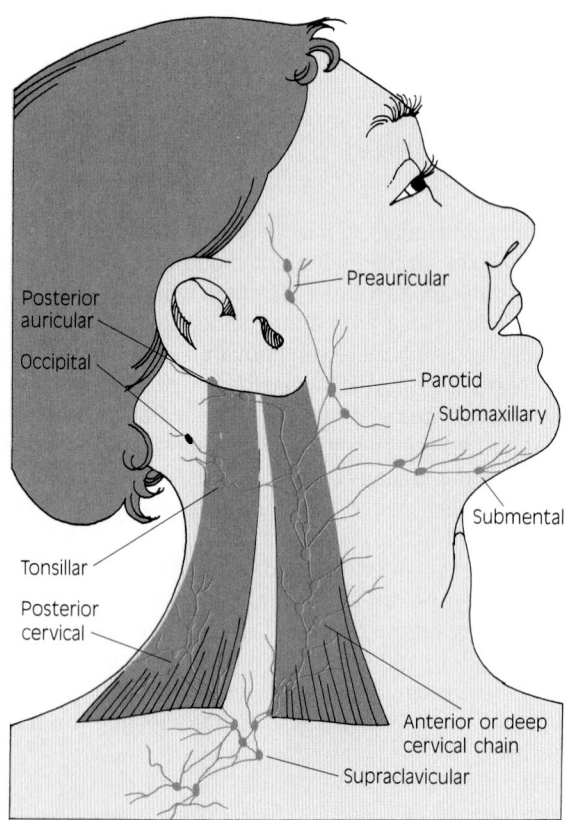

Figure 25-29
Location of the lymph nodes of the neck.

Life-Span Assessment Variations

Pediatric

- The posterior fontanel normally closes at 8 weeks of age, but the anterior fontanel remains soft until up to 18 months of age
- Ability to gaze at and follow bright objects should be present at 1 month of age
- Ability to focus with both eyes should be present at 6 months of age
- Pupils appear at the inner folds (pseudostrabismus).
- Newborns respond to loud noises with a startle reflex.

Geriatric

- Impaired near vision (presbyopia)
- Decreased color vision and peripheral vision
- Decreased adaptation to light and dark
- A white ring around the cornea (arcus senilis)
- Entropion and ectropion are common.
- Hearing loss (presbycusis)
- Impaired conductive hearing
- Elongated ear lobes
- Ear landmarks are more prominent.

- Decreased range of motion of the neck
- Thyroid gland may feel more nodular.
- Lymph glands are smaller and more easily palpated.

Thorax and Lungs

The thorax (Fig. 25-30) comprises the lungs, rib cage, cartilage, and intercostal muscles. Identify risk factors for altered health during the health history by asking about the following:

- History of trauma to the ribs or lung surgery
- Having to use several pillows to breathe when sleeping
- History of chest pain with deep breathing
- History of persistent cough with or without producing sputum
- History of allergies
- Environmental exposure to chemicals, asbestos, or smoke
- History of smoking
- History of lung disease in family members or self
- History of frequent or chronic respiratory infections

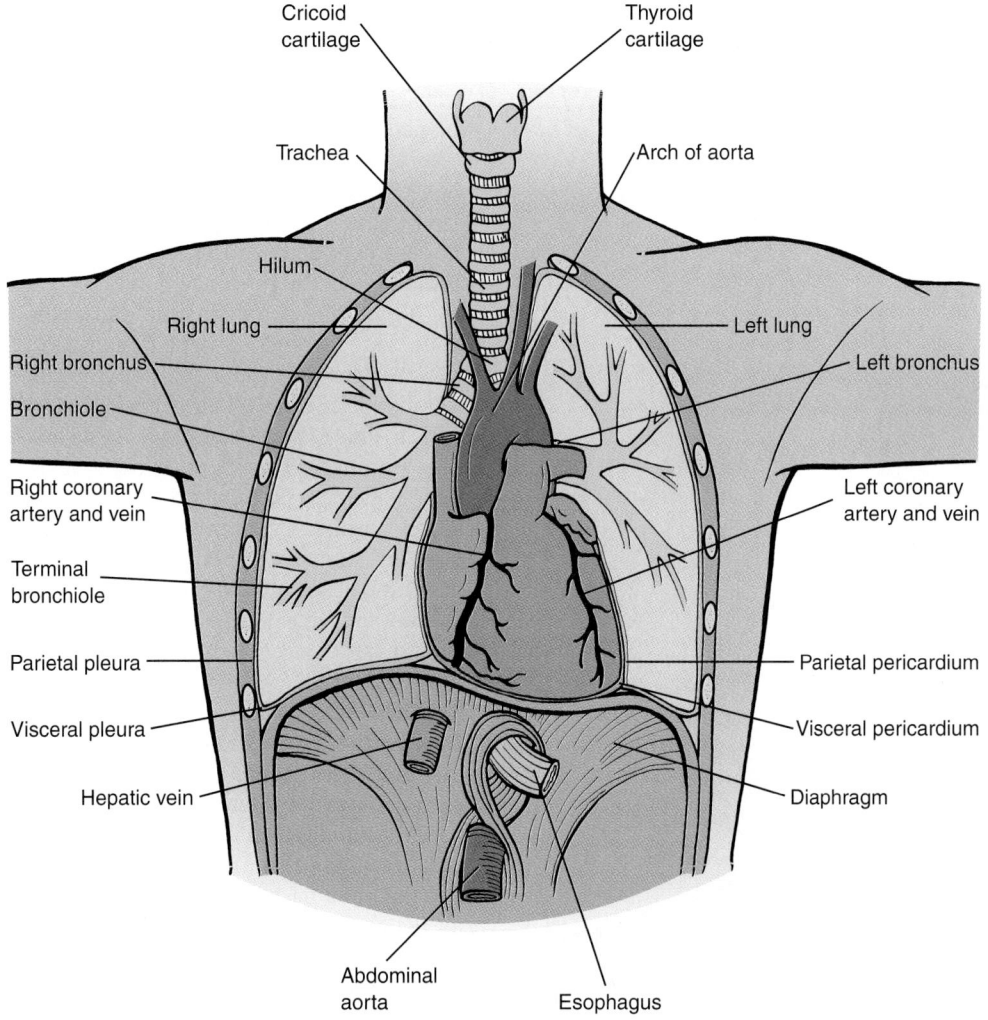

Figure 25-30
Structures of the thorax.

This assessment requires a stethoscope (warmed) and a tape measure. The environment should be warm and adequately lit. The techniques for this assessment include inspection, palpation, percussion, and auscultation. The patient is sitting during the assessment.

Inspection

Inspection begins by observing the patient's chest for color, shape or contour, breathing patterns, and muscle development. The color should be even and consistent with the color of the patient's face. The shape or contour should have a downward equal slope at the rib cage. The chest should be symmetric, with the transverse diameter greater than the anteroposterior diameter. An increased anteroposterior diameter, as seen in chronic lung diseases, is described as *barrel-chest* (Fig. 25-31). Respirations should be smooth and even, ranging from 12 to 20 breaths/min. Abnormal findings include an increase in chest size and contour, abnormal breathing patterns with use of accessory muscles (symptoms of respiratory disease, such as chronic obstructive pulmonary disease or asthma), unequal chest expansion (which may occur in chest trauma or pneumonia), and abnormal breath sounds (heard when the airways are obstructed by secretions or a foreign object).

Palpation

Palpation is used to detect areas of sensitivity, chest expansion during respirations, and vibrations *(fremitus)*. Use the palmar surface of the hands to palpate the anterior and posterior thoracic landmarks (Fig. 25-32) in a sequential pattern for temperature, moisture, muscular development, and any tenderness or masses. The same technique and sequence are used to test for tactile (vocal) fremitus, comparing bilateral sides. Normally, equal bilateral mild vibratory sensations are palpated. The skin should be warm and dry, with muscular development symmetric, and there should be no tenderness or masses.

Chest expansion is determined by placing the hands over the posterior chest wall, with the fingers at the level of T9 or T10. Ask the patient to take a deep breath, and observe the movement of your thumbs. The thorax should expand symmetrically (Fig. 25-33). Abnormal findings may be cool, excessively dry or moist skin; muscle asymmetry; tenderness; masses; increased or decreased vibratory sensation; asymmetric thoracic expansion; and abnormal breathing patterns (see Chap. 24).

Percussion

Although not used frequently in assessing the lungs, percussion may be used to determine lung position and size and to detect the presence of air, liquids, or solids within the lungs. The shoulder area and anterior and posterior thorax are percussed in a systematic pattern (see Fig. 25-32). Note the intensity, pitch, duration, and quality of sounds produced. When a normal air-filled lung is percussed, the sound is hollow, loud, low-pitched, and of long duration. This percussion tone is known as *resonance*. A *flat* tone is heard over bony or well-developed muscle tissue. *Tympany,* a hollow sound, is percussed over the stomach. Percussion sounds that are abnormal over lung tissue are *hyperresonance,* heard over emphysematous lung tissue, and *dullness,* heard over fluid or a solid mass.

Auscultation

Auscultation is used to detect air flow within the respiratory tract. The sounds of inspiration and expiration are assessed over the chest wall using the stethoscope in a pattern similar to that used with percussion. Normally, breath sounds result from the free movement of air into and out of all parts of the bronchial tree. The nurse listens for the duration, pitch, and intensity of the sounds, which normally vary over different parts of the lung. The patient should be sitting and asked to breathe slowly and deeply through the mouth. The warmed diaphragm of the stethoscope is placed over the thoracic landmarks, and breath sounds are auscultated in the same sequential pattern as

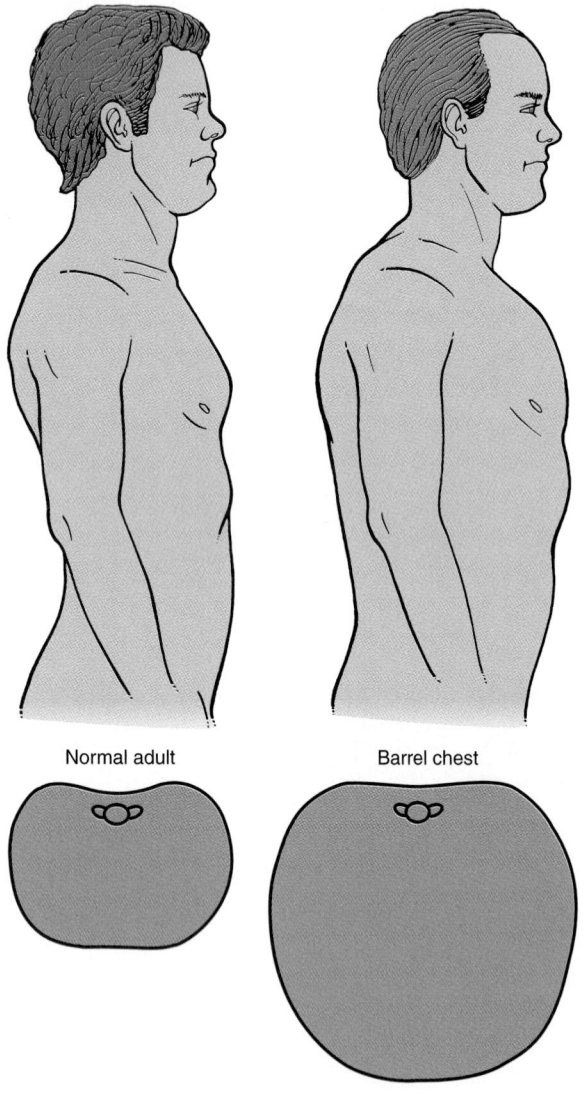

Figure 25-31
Profile and anteroposterior diameter of normal adult chest and barrel chest.

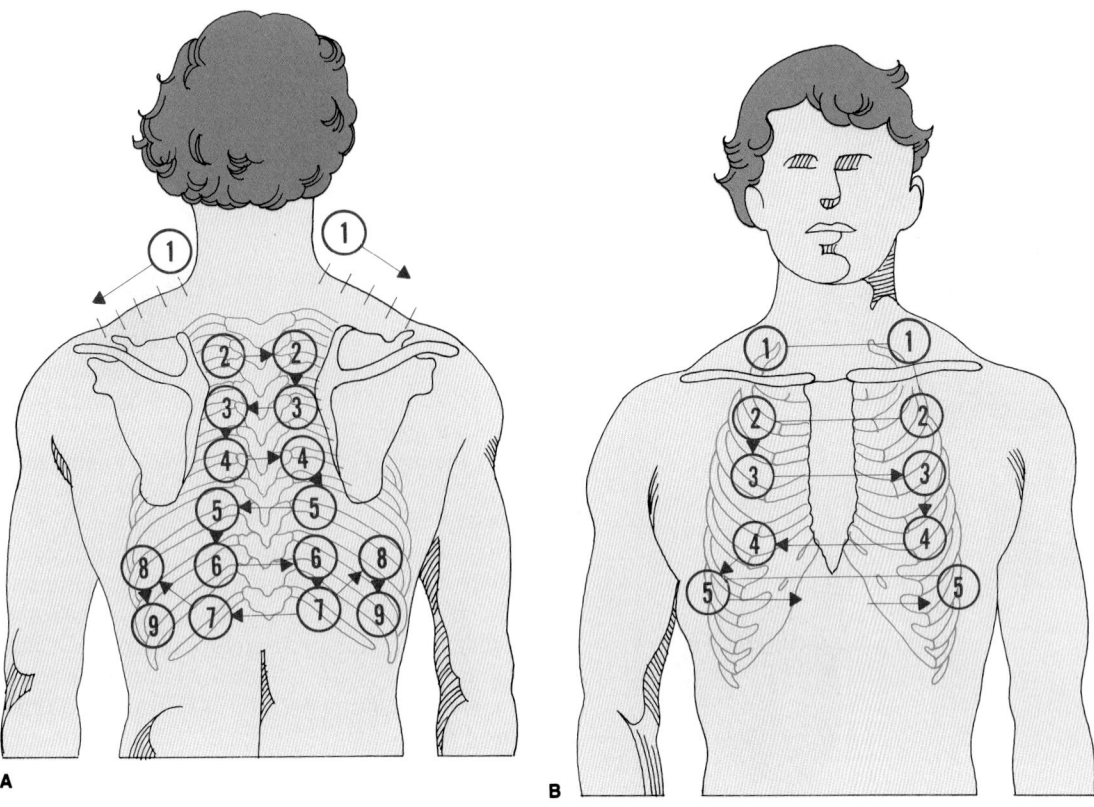

Figure 25-32
Posterior (**A**) and anterior (**B**) chest—landmarks and systematic sequence of assessment. The pattern is used for palpation, percussion, and auscultation of the chest.

used for palpation and percussion (see Fig. 25-32). Although lung sounds are not always auscultated at each site, it is important to follow a consistent pattern.

Breath Sounds

Ordinarily, respirations are not audible without auscultation. **Bronchial sounds** heard over the trachea are high-pitched, harsh sounds, with expiration being longer than inspiration. **Bronchovesicular sounds** are heard over the mainstem bronchus and are moderate "blowing" sounds, with inspiration equal to expiration. **Vesicular breath sounds** are soft, low-pitched sounds, heard best over the base of the lungs during inspiration, which is longer than expiration (Fig. 25-34).

Terms used to describe the nature of sounds that can be heard as the patient breathes are outlined and summarized in Fig. 25-35. **Adventitious breath sounds** are not normally heard in the lungs but, if present, may be auscultated along with normal breath sounds. *Stertorous* breathing is a general term used to refer to noisy, strenuous respirations. *Stridor* is a harsh, high-pitched sound heard on inspiration when there is a narrowing of the upper airway, such as the larynx or trachea. Infants or young children with croup often manifest stridor when breathing. *Crackles* are fine to course crackling sounds made as air moves through wet secretions; they are most often heard on inspiration. Crackles are described as "fine" when they are made by air passing through moisture in

small air passages and alveoli, and as "coarse" when they are made by air passing through moisture in the bronchioles, bronchi, and trachea. *Wheezes* are continuous sounds that originate in small air passages that are narrowed by secretions, swelling, or tumors. They may be inspiratory or expiratory and are high-pitched sounds. Although stertorous respirations, stridor, and wheezes can be heard without amplification, crackles and gurgles are usually heard only by auscultation with a stethoscope. A *pleural friction rub* is a grating sound, caused by an inflamed pleura rubbing against the chest wall (see Fig. 25-35). If a productive cough occurs during assessment of the thorax and lungs, the sputum should be assessed for color, consistency, and amount.

Life-Span Assessment Variations
Pediatric
- Auscultated breath sounds are louder.
- More rapid respiratory rate to age 8 to 10 years
- Abdominal muscles are used during respirations.

Geriatric
- Increased anteroposterior chest diameter
- Increase in the dorsal spinal curve (kyphosis)
- Decreased thoracic expansion
- Accessory muscles may be used to exhale.
- Decreased ciliary action increases risk for lower respiratory infections.

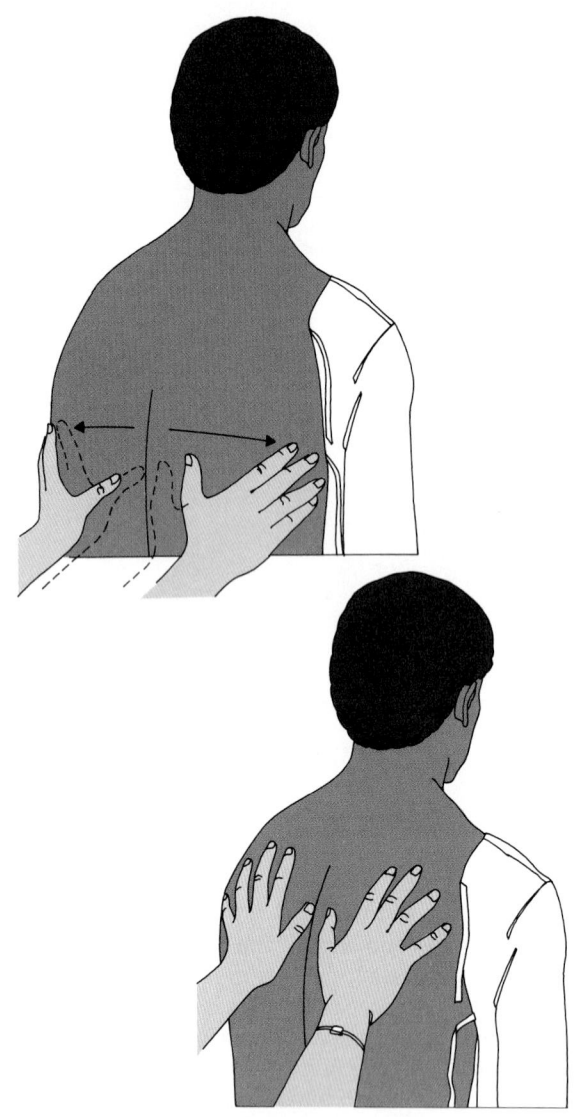

Figure 25-33
(*Top*) Palpating the posterior thorax excursion. The examiner's hands are placed symmetrically on the patient's back. As the patient inhales, the examiner's hands should move apart symmetrically. (*Bottom*) Palpation of the posterior thorax for vocal or tactile fremitus. The examiner uses the palms of the hands to detect vibrations transmitted through the lungs to the chest wall.

Cardiovascular and Peripheral Vascular Systems

Cardiovascular and peripheral vascular assessment is conducted through physical assessment of the heart and the extremities. Identify risk factors for altered health during the health history by asking about the following:

- History of chest pain, palpitations, or dizziness
- Presence of swelling in the ankles and feet
- Number of pillows used to sleep at night
- Type and amount of medications taken daily
- History of heart defect, rheumatic fever, or chest or heart surgery
- Family history of hypertension (high blood pressure), myocardial infarction (heart attack), coronary artery

disease, high blood cholesterol levels, or diabetes mellitus
- History of smoking
- History of alcohol use
- Type and amount of exercise
- Usual foods eaten each day
- Use of hormone replacement therapy (in postmenopausal women)
- Evidence of changes in color or temperature of the extremities
- History of pain in the legs when sleeping or that is worsened by walking
- History of blood clots or sores on the legs that do not heal
- History of edema of the lower extremities

Heart

The techniques used to assess the heart (Fig. 25-36) include inspection, palpation, and auscultation. (Inspection and palpation, although discussed separately here, are usually combined.) A stethoscope with a bell and diaphragm and a sphygmomanometer are used. The patient may be in a sitting position or in a supine position with the head raised about 30 degrees. Adequate lighting is essential for inspection of color and pulsations. A quiet environment is necessary for accurate auscultation of heart sounds. The nurse is usually positioned at the right side of the patient.

Inspection

The neck and **precordium** (the aortic, pulmonic, tricuspid, and apical areas; and Erb's point, illustrated in Figure 25-37) are observed for visible pulsations. Generally, there are no visible pulsations, except the apical impulse (or the point of maximal impulse [PMI]), located at about the fourth or fifth intercostal space at the left midclavicular line. Inspect the epigastric area at the tip of the sternum for pulsation of the abdominal aorta. Findings of neck vein distention (indicating heart disease) or visible pulsations in precordial areas other than the PMI (which may result from abnormalities of the ventricle) are considered abnormal.

Palpation

The precordium is palpated for the presence of pulsations. The hands, which should be warm, are used to palpate gently, using the palmar surface with the four fingers held together. Palpation proceeds in a systematic manner, with assessment of specific cardiac landmarks—the aortic, pulmonic, tricuspid, and mitral areas; and Erb's point (see Fig. 25-37). Each area is palpated to determine whether a pulsation is felt. Identify the PMI and record the apical impulse by interspace and relationship to the midsternal line or midclavicular line. Identify any precordial *thrills,* which are fine, palpable, rushing vibrations over the right or left second intercostal space, and any *lifts* or *heaves,* which involve a rise along the border of the sternum with each heartbeat. Normal findings include no pulsation palpable over the aortic and pulmonic areas, with a palpable pulsation at the PMI.

Bronchial or Tubular

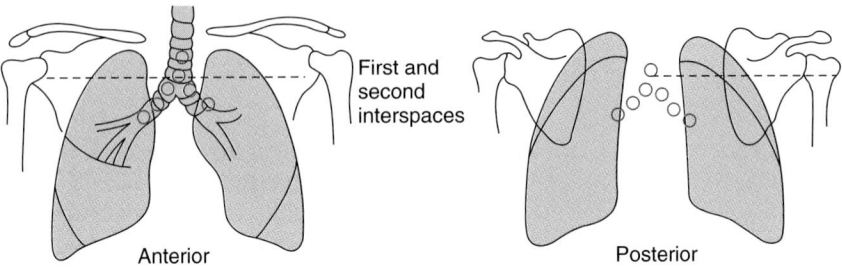

Blowing, hollow sounds auscultated over the trachea

Ratio of inspiration to expiration

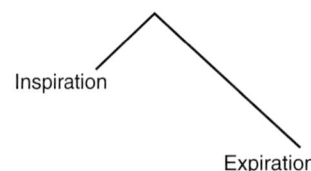

Inspiration is shorter than expiration. Expiration is longer, lower, and higher-pitched than inspiration.

Bronchovesicular

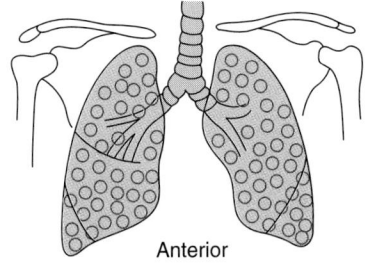

Medium-pitched, medium intensity, blowing sounds auscultated over the first and second interspaces anteriorly and the scapula posteriorly

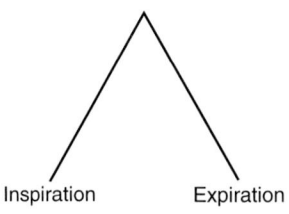

Inspiration and expiration have similar pitch.

Vesicular

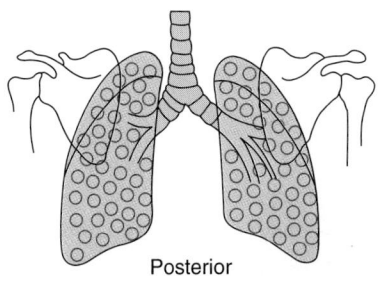

Soft, low-pitched sounds auscultated over the lung periphery

Inspiration is longer, louder, and higher-pitched than expiration.

Figure 25-34
Normal breath sounds.

Auscultation

Auscultation is used to determine the heart sounds caused by closure of the heart valves. A systematic approach is used to listen at all cardiac landmarks (Fig. 25-38): the aortic area, the pulmonic area, Erb's point, the tricuspid area, and the mitral (apical) area. Auscultation is systematic, beginning at the aortic area, moving to the pulmonic area, then to Erb's point, then to the tricuspid area, and finally to the mitral area. The patient should breathe normally. The stethoscope diaphragm is first used to listen to high-pitched sounds, followed by use of the bell to listen to low-pitched sounds. The nurse focuses on the overall rate and rhythm of the heart and the normal heart sounds (S_1 and S_2).

During auscultation, the first heart sound is heard as the "lub" of "lub-dub." This sound occurs when the mitral and tricuspid valves close and corresponds with the onset of ventricular contraction (Fig. 25-39). The sound, low-pitched and dull, is called S_1 and is heard best at the apical area. The second heart sound, S_2, occurs at the termination of systole and corresponds with the onset of ventricular diastole. It is the "dub" of "lub-dub" and represents the closure of the aortic and pulmonic valves. The sound of S_2 is higher pitched and shorter than S_1. The two sounds occur within 1 second or less, depending on the heart rate.

Normal findings include S_1 that is louder at the tricuspid and apical areas, with S_2 louder at the aortic and pulmonic areas. Abnormal findings include extra heart sounds at any of the cardiac landmarks and abnormal rate or rhythm. Extra heart sounds are often heard when the patient has anemia or heart disease. A wide variety of conditions may alter the normal heart rate or rhythm, including serious infections, diseases of the heart muscle or con-

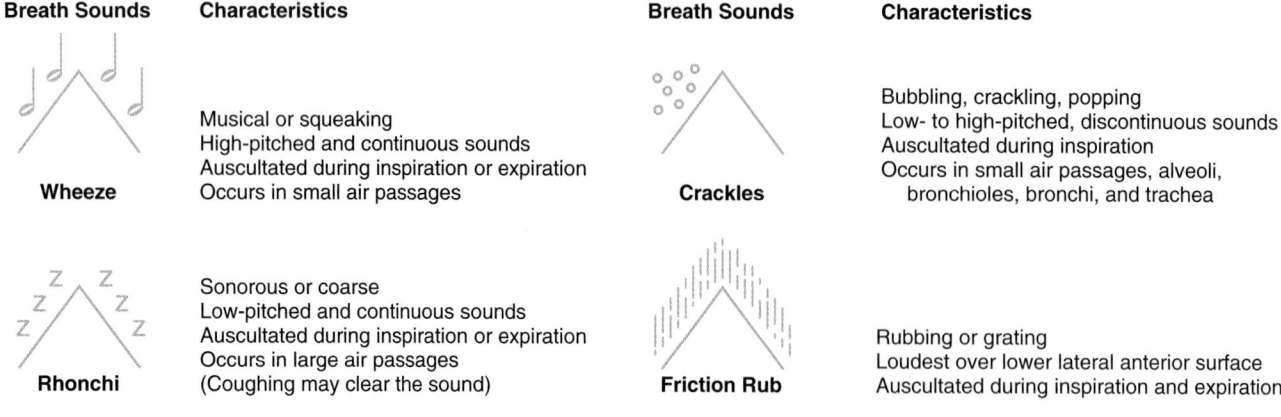

Breath Sounds	Characteristics	Breath Sounds	Characteristics
Wheeze	Musical or squeaking High-pitched and continuous sounds Auscultated during inspiration or expiration Occurs in small air passages	**Crackles**	Bubbling, crackling, popping Low- to high-pitched, discontinuous sounds Auscultated during inspiration Occurs in small air passages, alveoli, bronchioles, bronchi, and trachea
Rhonchi	Sonorous or coarse Low-pitched and continuous sounds Auscultated during inspiration or expiration Occurs in large air passages (Coughing may clear the sound)	**Friction Rub**	Rubbing or grating Loudest over lower lateral anterior surface Auscultated during inspiration and expiration

Figure 25-35
Abnormal breath sounds.

ducting system, dehydration or overhydration, endocrine disorders, respiratory disorders, and head trauma.

Extra heart sounds may be S₃, S₄, murmurs, or bruits. S_3, known as the *third heart sound,* is often represented by a "lub-dub-dee" pattern ("dee" being S_3); this sound is best heard with the stethoscope bell at the mitral area, with the patient lying on the left side. S_3 is considered normal in children and young adults and abnormal in middle-aged and older adults. S_4 is the fourth heart sound, represented by "dee-lub-dub." S_4 is considered normal in older adult pa-

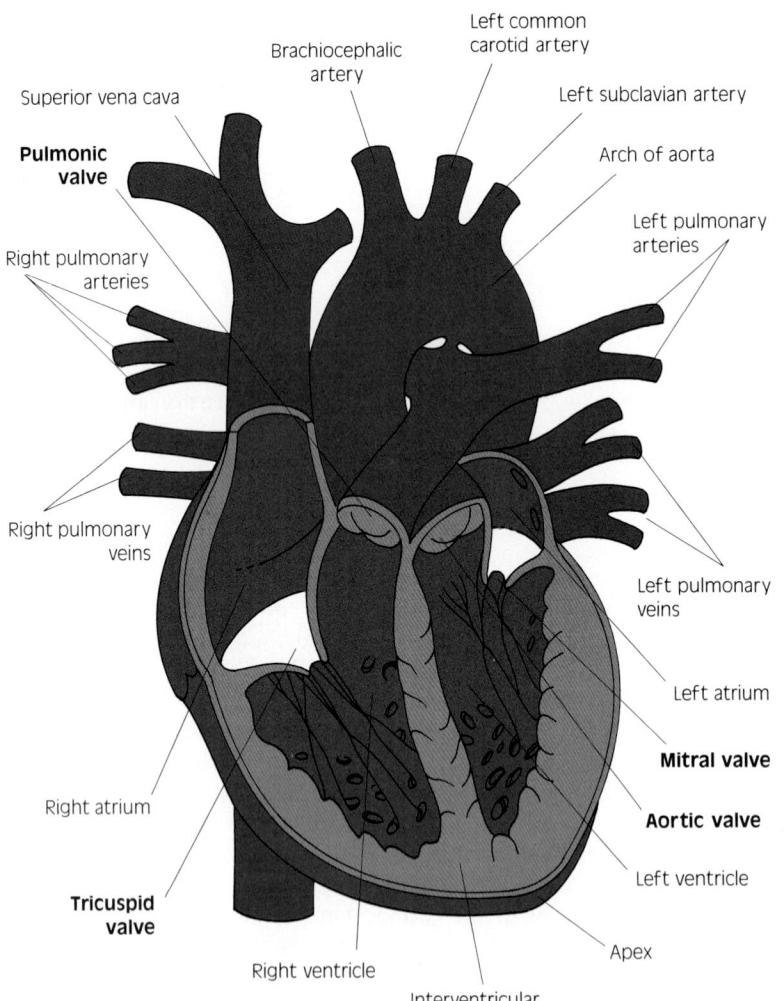

Figure 25-36
View of the interior of the heart showing the atrioventricular and semilunar valves responsible for normal heart sounds.

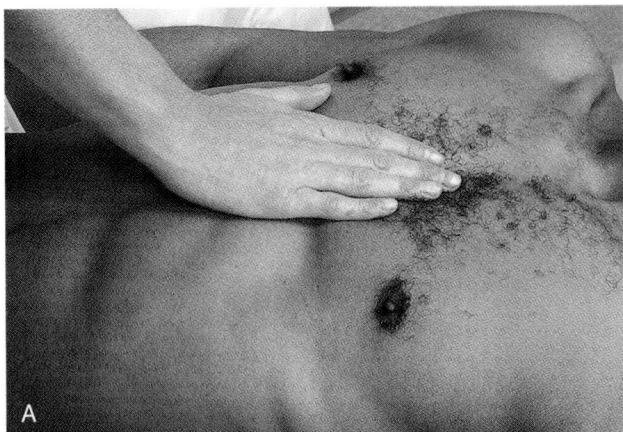

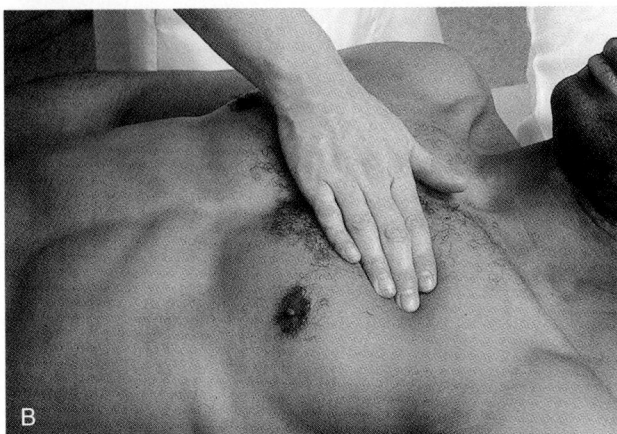

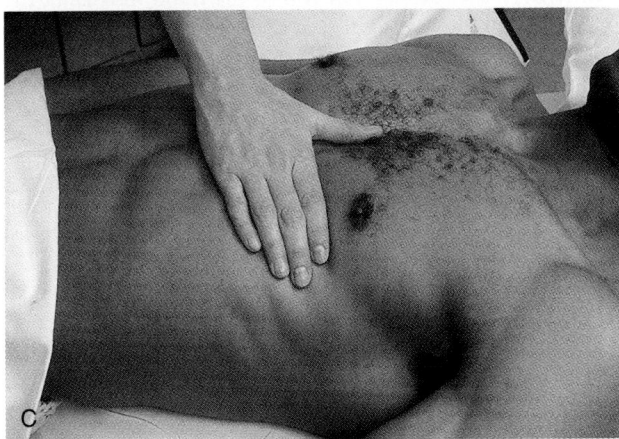

Figure 25-37
Palpating areas of the precordium: (**A**) aortic area, (**B**) pulmonic area, and (**C**) apical and tricuspic area. (Photo © Ken Kasper.)

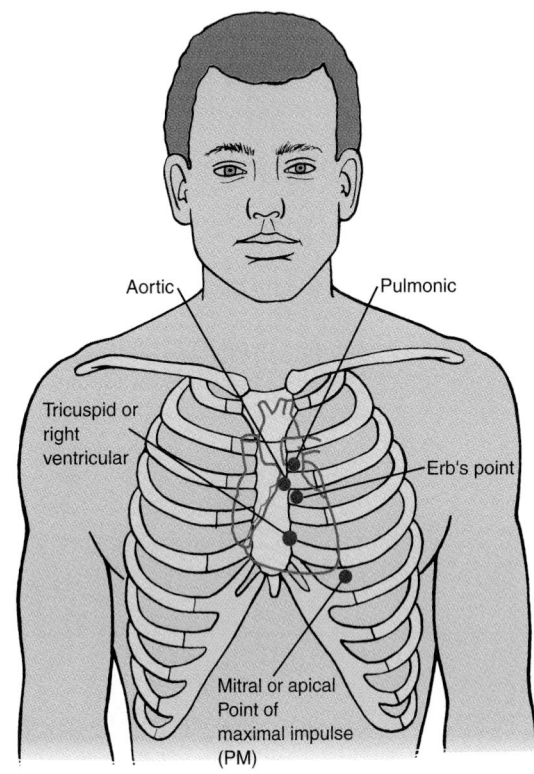

Figure 25-38
Cardiac landmarks and sequence of examination using auscultation.

swirl rather than flow normally. Bruits are most commonly heard over the carotid arteries, the abdominal aorta, and the femoral arteries.

Peripheral Vascular System

Peripheral vascular assessment includes measuring the blood pressure and assessing peripheral pulses and perfusion.

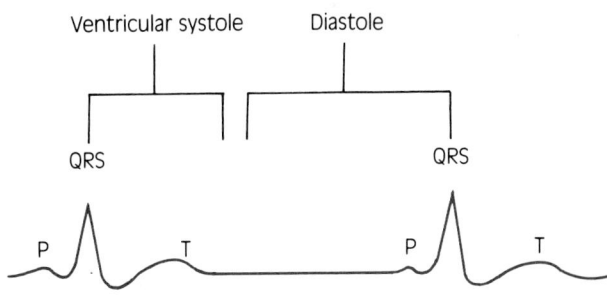

Electrocardiogram

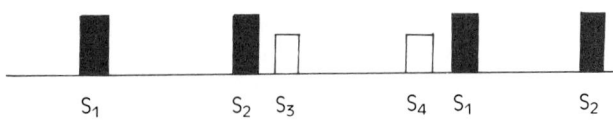

Heart sounds

Figure 25-39
Heart sounds in relation to the cardiac cycle and an electro-cardiogram.

tients but abnormal in children and adults. Heart *murmurs* are extra heart sounds caused by some disruption of blood flow through the heart. The characteristics of a murmur depend on the adequacy of valve function, rate of blood flow, and size of the valve opening. Table 25-6 illustrates the grading of heart murmurs. **Bruits**, which are abnormal sounds, are "swooshing" sounds similar to murmurs and are heard over major blood vessels. The sound indicates a partially blocked or overextended artery, causing blood to

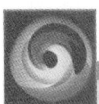

Table 25-6
Common Grading System for Heart Murmurs

Grade	Description
I	A murmur so faint that it can only be heard with great effort
II	A faint murmur but one that can be easily detected
III	A moderately loud murmur
IV	A very loud murmur that is usually associated with a thrill sound
V	An extremely loud murmur
VI	An exceptionally loud murmur that can be heard while the stethoscope is lifted off the skin

Assessments are done by inspection and palpation, with the patient sitting or supine. Peripheral vascular assessments may be combined with assessment of other body areas.

Inspection

The skin of the extremities is inspected for color, temperature, continuity, lesions (as described previously for assessment of the integument), venous patterns, and edema. There are normally no venous patterns, varicosities, rashes, ulcers, or edema on the lower extremities. The skin of the patient with peripheral vascular disease (resulting in decreased blood flow and oxygenation of tissues) is typically pale and cool, shiny with brown discolorations, and hairless. The toenails are thickened.

Palpation

To palpate peripheral pulses, use the pads of the index and middle fingers. During the peripheral vascular assessment, the peripheral pulses are palpated for amplitude and symmetry. Palpate, one at a time and with caution, the carotid brachial, radial, femoral, popliteal, dorsalis pedis, and posterior tibial pulses (see Fig. 24-5 in Chap. 24). These should be strong and equal bilaterally. The amplitude of the pulses may be documented on a scale as follows: 0 = absent, 1+ = weak, 2+ = normal, 3+ = increased, 4+ = bounding.

Abnormal findings include an absent, weak, thready pulse (which may indicate a decreased cardiac output), forceful or bounding pulse (seen in hypertension and circulatory overload), and asymmetric pulse (related to impaired circulation). *Phlebitis* (inflammation of a vein) of the lower extremity is indicated by pain, redness, and swelling of the affected calf or thigh.

Other specific assessments to determine arterial blood flow include Allen's test, Buerger's test, and capillary refill.

To conduct Allen's test, which assesses the patency of the radial and ulnar arteries, follow these three steps:

1. Ask the patient to rest his or her hand on the examining table with the palm up and to make a fist.
2. Use your thumbs to occlude the radial and ulnar arteries and ask the patient to open his or her hand (the palm will be pale).
3. Release your thumb pressure and observe the return of color to the palm (this should normally take 3 to 5 seconds).

To conduct Buerger's test, follow these three steps:

1. Ask the patient to assume a supine position and then raise one arm or one leg about 1 foot (30 cm) above the level of his or her heart.
2. Ask the patient to briskly move the leg or arm up and down for 1 minute, then to sit up and dangle the arm or leg downward.
3. Observe the time it takes for the original color of the patient's skin to return and for the veins to fill. Normally, color returns in 10 seconds, and veins fill in 15 seconds.

To assess capillary refill in adults, follow these two steps:

- Using your thumb and forefinger, squeeze the patient's fingernail or toenail until it appears white.
- Release the pressure and observe the time it takes for normal color to return. Normally, color returns immediately.

Assess capillary refill in children by pressing the skin lightly over the forehead or top of the hand, releasing the pressure, and observing the time for return of color.

Life-Span Assessment Variations
Pediatric
- A pulsation may be visible if the chest wall is thin.
- Sinus arrhythmia may occur (the rate increases with inspiration and decreases with expiration).
- S_3 may be heard in about one third of all children.
- Heart rate is more rapid until about 8 years of age.

Geriatric
- The apical pulse may be difficult to palpate.
- Distal arteries are often more difficult to palpate.
- Proximal arteries are dilated.
- Blood vessels are more prominent and tortuous, and varicosities are common.
- Systolic and diastolic blood pressure may be increased.
- Widening pulse pressure

Breasts and Axillae

The breasts and axilla are assessed in both men and women. Each breast has a lymphatic network that drains into the underlying axilla (Fig. 25-40). Although the assessments and disorders described here focus on the female breast, both male and female patients should have breast assessments. Men, as well as women, may have diseases of the breast. Identify risk factors for altered

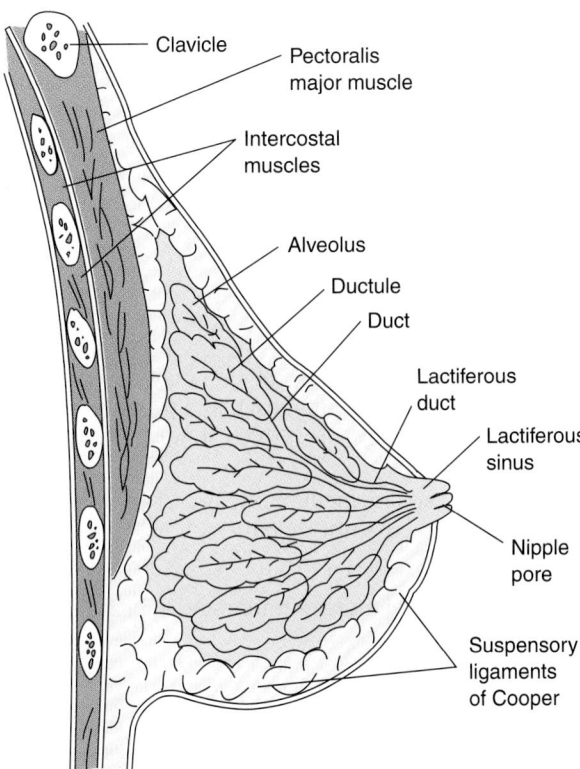

Figure 25-40
Lateral view of the female breast.

Clavicle

Pectoralis major muscle

Intercostal muscles

Alveolus

Ductule

Duct

Lactiferous duct

Lactiferous sinus

Nipple pore

Suspensory ligaments of Cooper

health during the health history by asking about the following:

- History of pain in one or both breasts, including relationship to menstrual period in women
- History of lumps or swelling, redness, change in size or dimpling in the breasts
- History of discharge from the breast
- Family history of breast cancer
- History of breast disease, biopsy, or surgery
- Menstrual and pregnancy history
- Use of hormones, oral contraceptives, or antidepressants
- Exposure to radiation, benzene, or asbestos
- Usual dietary intake and alcohol consumption
- Knowledge and practice of breast self-examination (see Chap. 34)
- Most recent breast examination by a physician and mammogram

Inspection and palpation are used in the assessment. The patient is in the sitting or supine position. When sitting, the patient should sit erect, with arms at sides or raised overhead. When supine, the patient's hand on the side being examined is placed under the head.

Inspection

The breasts and axilla are inspected for size, shape, symmetry, color, texture, and skin lesions. The breasts should be relatively symmetric, although variations are normal. The size varies among individuals. The shape of the breasts

is round and smooth, and there should be no skin depressions *(retraction)* or puckering *(dimpling)*. The color should be consistent with the rest of the skin, and the texture of the skin should be soft.

Inspect the areola and nipples for size and shape and the nipples for discharge, crusting, and inversion. The areolar and nipple areas should be equal in size, round or oval, with a smooth surface. Montgomery's tubercles (sebaceous glands on the areolae of the breasts) are a normal component of the areola. The nipples are normally everted. Lesions and discharge from the nipples are abnormal findings except in pregnancy. Leaking is normal during pregnancy.

Palpation

The primary purpose of palpation is to detect any abnormal masses or lumps. The nipple and areola are palpated, and the nipple is gently compressed between the thumb and forefinger to assess for discharge. The breast is assessed in four quadrants: the outer upper quadrant, the outer lower quadrant, the inner upper quadrant, and the inner lower quadrant (Fig. 25-41). Using the pads of the first three fingers, palpate each quadrant of each breast in a systematic method as the breast tissue is gently compressed against the chest wall (Fig. 25-42). The breast tissue should be smooth and firm with a granular consistency. If a mass is detected, its location, size, shape, consistency, and tenderness should be carefully assessed. The breasts are normally tender during the week before menstruation.

The axillary areas are palpated for lymph nodes (Fig. 25-43), which normally are nonpalpable and nontender. If

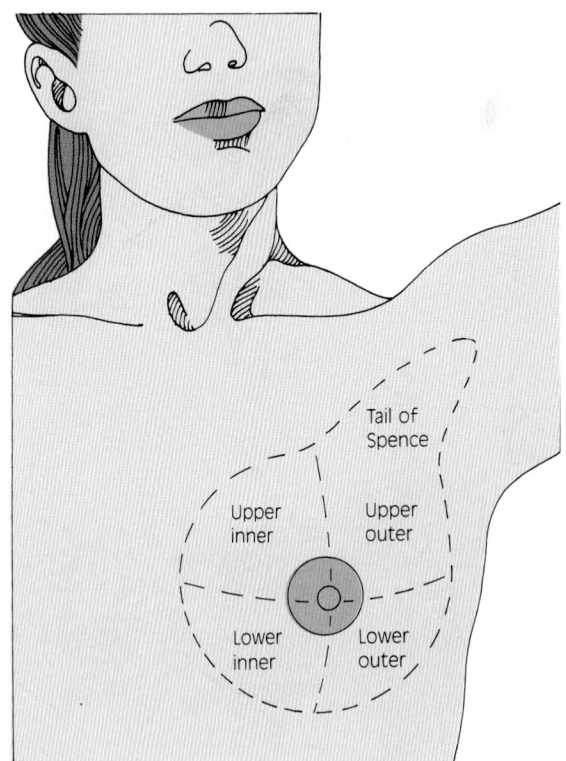

Figure 25-41
Location of assessment findings of the breast are identified by quadrant.

Tail of Spence

Upper inner

Upper outer

Lower inner

Lower outer

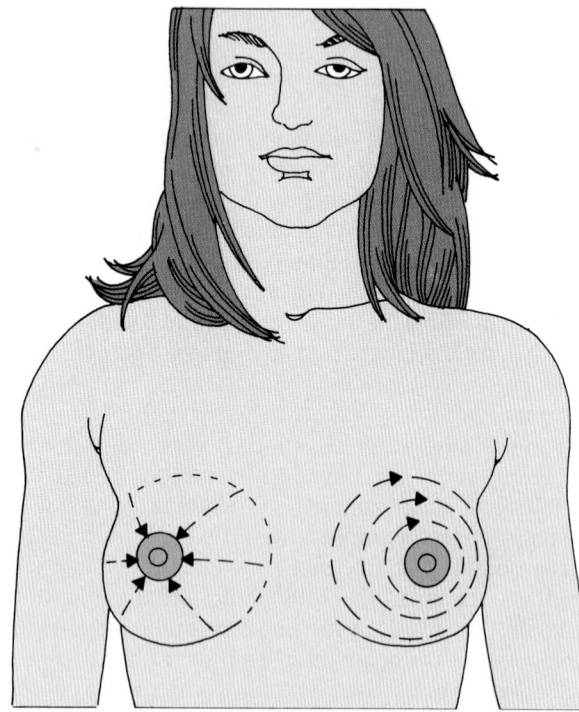

Figure 25-42
Two techniques for palpating the breast. (*Left*) Working in a clockwise direction, the examiner palpates the breast from the periphery toward the aureola at "hour" positions. (*Right*) The breast is palpated from the outer periphery in smaller and smaller circles moving toward the aureola.

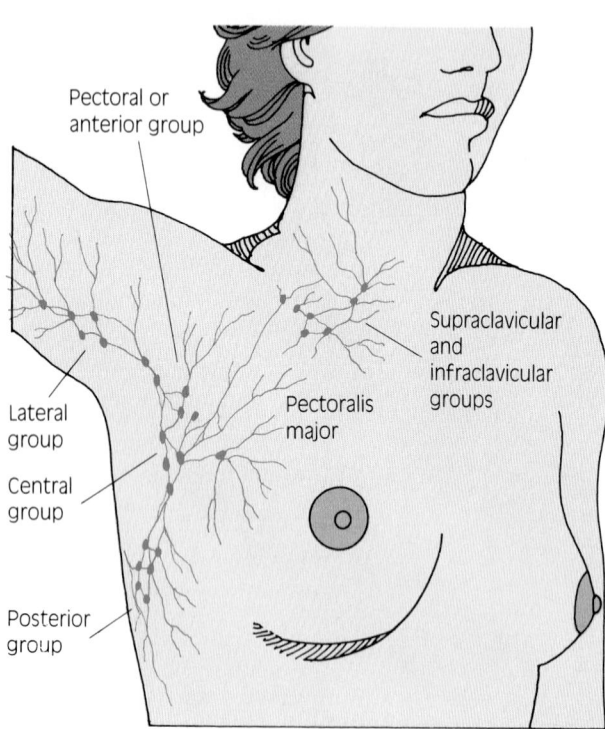

Pectoral or anterior group

Supraclavicular and infraclavicular groups

Lateral group

Pectoralis major

Central group

Posterior group

Figure 25-43
Location of the cervical, axillary, and mammary lymph nodes.

any nodes are palpable, assess their location, size, shape, consistency, tenderness, and mobility. Abnormal findings include the presence of a lump, dimpling, nipple discharge, lesions, asymmetry, and palpable lymph nodes. An increase in the nodularity and tenderness of the breasts may be associated with the menstrual period or may indicate fibrocystic disease. Discharge, lumps, lesions, dimpling, asymmetry, and palpable lymph nodes may be indicative of breast cancer.

Life-Span Assessment Variations
Pediatric
- Newborns (up to 2 weeks of age) may have breast enlargement and a white discharge from the nipples.
- Breast growth begins in girls at about 10 or 11 years of age.
- Temporary enlargement of one breast (*gynecomastia*) may occur in boys during puberty.

Geriatric
- Breasts may feel more granular and appear more pendulous.

Abdomen

The abdominal cavity (Fig. 25-44) contains several vital organs: the stomach, the small intestine, the large intestine, the liver, the gallbladder, the pancreas, the spleen, the kidneys, and the urinary bladder. Not all of these organs can be assessed. The abdominal cavity also contains the female reproductive organs, discussed in the following section. Identify risk factors for altered health during the health history by asking about the following:

- History of abdominal pain
- History of indigestion, nausea or vomiting, constipation or diarrhea
- Appetite and usual food and fluid intake
- Usual bowel and bladder elimination patterns
- History of gastrointestinal disorders, such as peptic ulcer, bowel disease, gallbladder disease, liver disease, or appendicitis
- History of urinary tract disorders, such as infections, kidney stones, or kidney disease
- History of abdominal surgery
- Type and amount of prescribed and over-the-counter medications used
- History of abdominal surgery or trauma

A warm stethoscope, adequate lighting, and warm hands with short fingernails are needed for abdominal assessment. The patient is placed supine with the head slightly elevated and arms at sides. Small pillows may be placed under the head and knees. The patient should have an empty bladder and be warm. These measures, as well as the position, help prevent contraction of the abdominal muscles, which makes palpation difficult.

To locate organs more easily and to make documentation more specific, the abdomen can be divided into four quadrants: right upper, right lower, left upper, and left lower (Fig. 25-45). The sequence of techniques used to as-

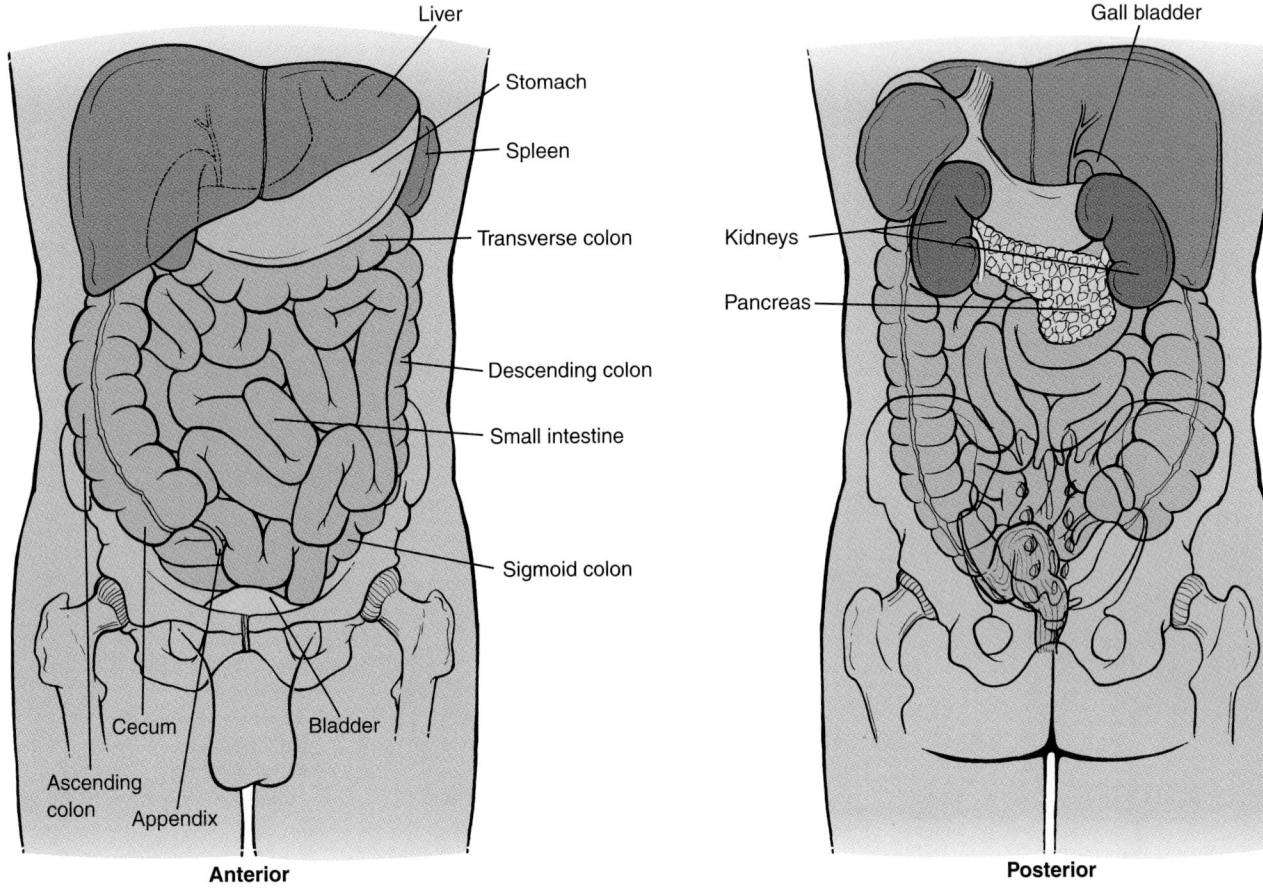

Liver
Stomach
Spleen
Transverse colon
Descending colon
Small intestine
Sigmoid colon
Cecum
Bladder
Ascending colon
Appendix

Anterior

Gall bladder
Kidneys
Pancreas

Posterior

Figure 25-44
Organs of the abdominal cavity.

sess the abdomen is as follows: inspection, auscultation, percussion, and palpation. Percussion and palpation stimulate bowel sounds and thus are done after auscultation of the abdomen.

Inspection

Inspect the abdomen while sitting at the side of the patient, using a tangential view that enhances shadows and contours. Inspect skin color and surface characteristics, including the umbilicus, contour, symmetry, peristalsis, pulsations, and masses. The skin color may be slightly lighter than exposed areas. Fine white or silver lines *(striae)* may be visible, often the result of skin stretching from weight gain or pregnancy. The umbilicus should be centrally located and normally may be flat, rounded, or concave. The abdomen should be evenly rounded or symmetric, without visible peristalsis. In thin people, an upper midline pulsation may normally be visible.

Auscultation

Auscultation is used to assess bowel sounds and vascular sounds. Auscultation is performed in a systematic manner, using the four quadrants as a guide. The stethoscope is warmed, and the flat diaphragm is placed lightly on the abdomen in one of the selected quadrants. Listen carefully for bowel sounds, and note their frequency and character.

They are heard as clicks and gurgles and usually occur every 5 to 20 seconds. Move the stethoscope in a clockwise manner, assessing all four quadrants systematically. Using the bell of the stethoscope, auscultate over the aorta, renal arteries, and iliac arteries for bruits. Abnormal findings include increased bowel sounds (often heard when the patient has diarrhea or in early bowel obstruction), decreased bowel sounds (heard after abdominal surgery or late bowel obstruction) or absent bowel sounds (indicating peritonitis or paralytic ileus). Bowel sounds of high-pitched tinkling or rushes of high-pitched sounds indicate a bowel obstruction. A *bruit* is another abnormal sound that may be heard on auscultation. Bruits are low-pitched, murmur-like sounds that occur when blood flow in an artery is obstructed. These sounds may be heard if an aneurysm or stenosis is present in an abdominal artery. Changes in bowel sounds should be reported; this is especially true if no bowel sounds are heard.

Percussion

Although abdominal percussion is not often used, it is useful in assessing a full bladder or changes in abdominal contents. All four quadrants are percussed in a systematic, clockwise manner to identify fluid, masses, or air. Note the distribution of sounds. Normal sounds are tympany over the abdomen and dullness over the liver and a full

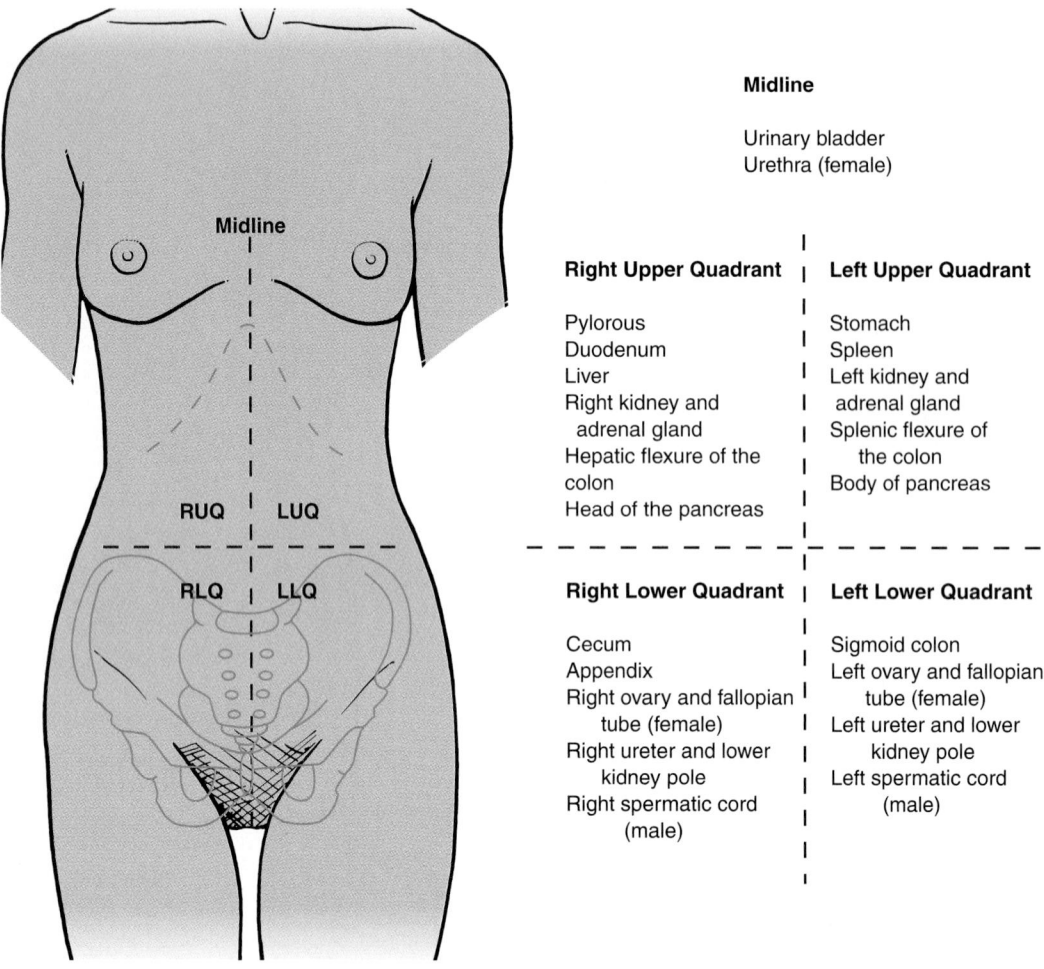

Figure 25-45
Diagram of abdominal quadrants and outline of underlying organs.

Midline

Urinary bladder
Urethra (female)

Right Upper Quadrant

Pylorous
Duodenum
Liver
Right kidney and
  adrenal gland
Hepatic flexure of the
colon
Head of the pancreas

Left Upper Quadrant

Stomach
Spleen
Left kidney and
  adrenal gland
Splenic flexure of
  the colon
Body of pancreas

Right Lower Quadrant

Cecum
Appendix
Right ovary and fallopian
  tube (female)
Right ureter and lower
  kidney pole
Right spermatic cord
  (male)

Left Lower Quadrant

Sigmoid colon
Left ovary and fallopian
  tube (female)
Left ureter and lower
  kidney pole
Left spermatic cord
  (male)

bladder. The dominant percussion note in abdominal assessment is tympany. Abnormal findings include decreased tympany and increased dullness, possibly caused by fluid or a mass.

Palpation

The pads of the fingers are used to palpate with a light, gentle, dipping motion. Watch the patient's face for nonverbal signs of pain during palpation. Palpate each quadrant in a systematic manner, noting muscular resistance, tenderness, enlargement of the organs, or masses. If the patient verbalizes abdominal pain, palpate the area of pain last. The abdomen should normally be soft, relaxed, and free of tenderness. Abnormal findings include involuntary rigidity, spasm, and pain (which may indicate trauma, peritonitis, infection, tumors, or enlarged or diseased abdominal organs).

Life-Span Assessment Variations
Pediatric
- Umbilical cord dries and falls off within the first 2 weeks of life.
- A "pot-belly" is common in children younger than 5 years of age.

- Peristaltic waves may be visible.
- The liver and spleen may be more easily palpated in young children.

Geriatric
- Decreased bowel sounds
- Decreased abdominal tone
- Liver border more easily palpated

Female and Male Genitalia

Assessment of the genitalia includes inspection and palpation. A description of an internal pelvic assessment of women is included in this chapter, although individual health agency policies vary on whether this is included as part of the health assessment. However, nurses often assist in performing vaginal examinations and need to be familiar with the procedure. Equipment required includes a vaginal speculum (for the female examination), a good light source, and disposable gloves.

Female Genitalia

The external female genitalia consist of the mons pubis, labia majora and minora, clitoris, vestibular glands, vaginal vestibule, vaginal orifice, and urethral opening (Fig. 25-46).

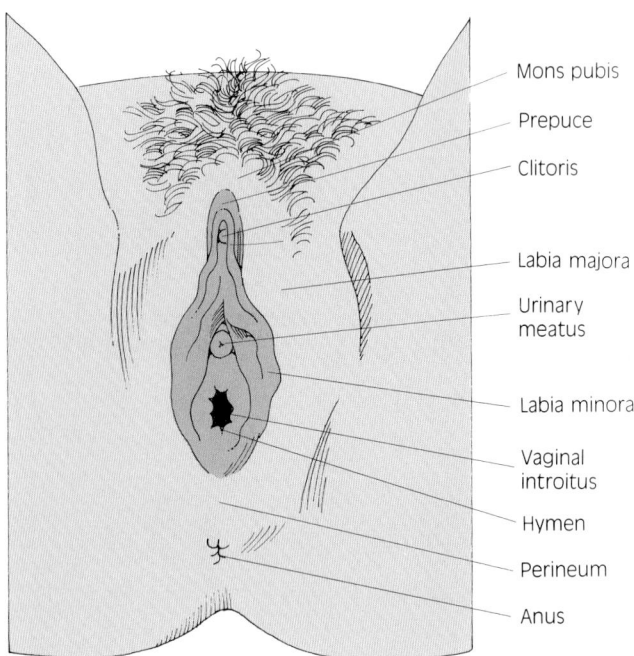

Figure 25-46
External female genitalia.

Labels: Mons pubis, Prepuce, Clitoris, Labia majora, Urinary meatus, Labia minora, Vaginal introitus, Hymen, Perineum, Anus

Identify risk factors for altered health during the health history by asking about the following:

- Menstrual history (age of first or last period, length of flow, type of flow, pain)
- Sexual history
- Number of pregnancies
- History of sexually transmitted diseases
- Use of contraceptives
- Frequency of pelvic examinations and Papanicolaou's smear
- History of vaginal discharge, itching, or pain on urination
- History of smoking
- Family history of reproductive or genital cancer

The bladder should be emptied before the examination. The woman is placed in the lithotomy position on the examination table, with the legs in stirrups, and draped so that only the genitalia are exposed. She should be told about the procedure and helped to relax as it is carried out. The nurse wears gloves during this assessment.

The external genitalia are inspected first. The pubic area is inspected for color, size, lesions, and discharge. The vulva normally has more pigmentation than other skin areas, and the mucous membranes are dark pink and moist. The skin and mucosa should be smooth, without lesions or swelling. There may normally be a small amount of clear or whitish vaginal discharge.

A speculum is used to inspect the cervix and vagina. The procedure is as follows:

1. Explain the procedure to the patient.
2. Warm the speculum under warm, running water; if cytologic specimens are to be taken, the water serves as the lubricant; if no specimens are needed, a water-soluble lubricant may be used.
3. Don gloves.
4. Using two fingers placed just inside the vagina, press down gently on the posterior vaginal wall.
5. Insert the speculum blades vertically into the vagina, the posterior portion pointed at a 45-degree angle. Ensure that no pubic hair is caught in the speculum.
6. Turn the speculum so that the handle is down and the blades are in a horizontal position.
7. Open the blades and close the screw that locks the blades open.
8. Inspect the cervix and os for size, color, shape, lesions, and discharge.
9. Obtain specimens if needed.
10. Withdraw the blades slowly, observing the vaginal walls.
11. When the speculum blades are clear of the cervix, release the screw so that the blades close, and withdraw the speculum from the vagina.
12. Provide the patient with tissues to remove the lubricating jelly (if used).

Abnormal findings include redness, swelling of glands, discharge, lesions, and pain, which may indicate infection, an abscess, a polyp, or cancer. For related assessments of the urinary tract and sexually transmitted diseases, see Chapters 42 and 34, respectively.

Male Genitalia

The male genitalia (Fig. 25-47) include the penis, testicles, epididymis, scrotum, prostate gland, and seminal vesicles. Identify risk factors for altered health during the health history by asking about the following:

- Frequency of digital rectal examinations
- Frequency of testicular self-examination
- Use of contraceptives
- Occupational exposure to chemicals (tire and rubber manufacturing, farming, mechanics)
- History of sexually transmitted disease
- History of discharge from the penis
- Difficulty with urination (hesitancy, frequency, voiding at night)
- History of incontinence
- History of erectile dysfunction

The patient may be standing or supine. Gloves are worn during this assessment. The external genitalia are inspected for size, placement, contour, appearance of the skin, redness, edema, and discharge. If uncircumcised, the foreskin is retracted for inspection of the glans penis. The location of the urinary meatus is assessed. The scrotum is inspected for symmetry; it is not unusual for the left testicle to lie lower in the scrotal sac than the right testicle. The size, shape, and consistency of the scrotal contents should be similar bilaterally.

Abnormal findings are lesions, redness, edema, pain, discharge, fluid-filled masses in the scrotum (symptoms of a hydrocele or varicocele), and displacement of the urinary meatus or difficulties with voiding. The presence of edema, redness, discharge or pain may indicate an infection. Voiding

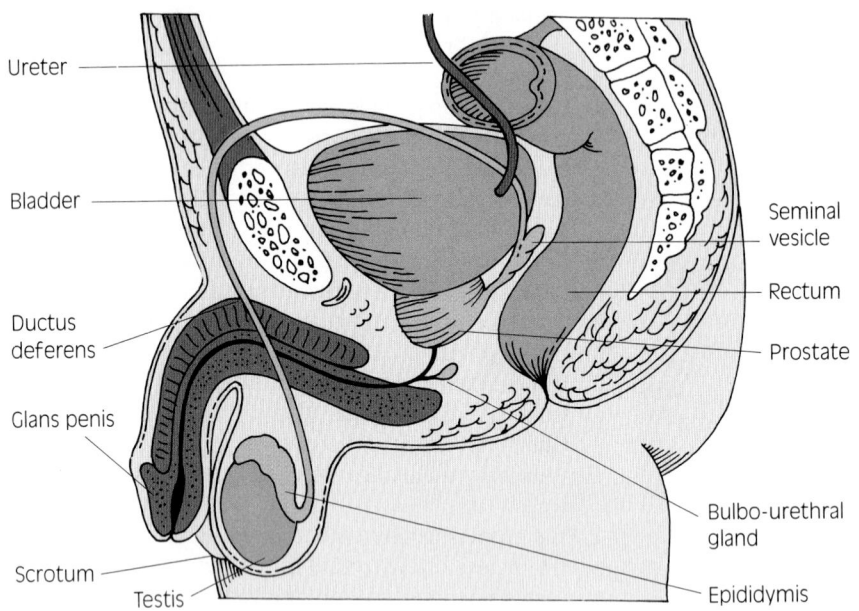

Ureter

Bladder

Ductus
deferens

Glans penis

Scrotum

Testis

Seminal
vesicle

Rectum

Prostate

Bulbo-urethral
gland

Epididymis

Figure 25-47
Organs of the male urogenital system.

difficulties may result from scarring from infections or prostate enlargement. (See Chaps. 42 and 34, respectively, for further discussion of the male urinary tract and sexually transmitted diseases.)

The rectum and anus are not assessed in all patients, but this is a part of a total health assessment. Techniques used to assess the rectum and anus are inspection and palpation. Necessary equipment includes lubricant and good lighting. Gloves are worn. The patient may be in the Sims, knee-chest, or lithotomy position or may be standing and leaning over the examination table.

Inspection is used to assess the anal area, which normally has increased pigmentation and some hair growth. Palpation is used to assess the rectum, using a well-lubricated, gloved index finger. Sphincter tone at the anus should be firm and the mucosal lining smooth. (Fecal specimens may be taken at this time, if necessary.) Abnormal findings include relaxed sphincter tone; skin cracks, nodules, or hemorrhoids at the anal sphincter; bleeding (which may indicate hemorrhoids or a colorectal cancer); and hard or abnormally colored (such as clay-colored or dark-black) stools.

If a rectal assessment is conducted, the cervix in women may be felt as a small, round mass when palpating the anterior rectal wall. Abnormal findings include changes in consistency. The prostate gland in men can be assessed for size, shape, and consistency by palpation through the anterior rectal wall; the gland is normally smooth, firm, and about 1¾ inches (4 cm) in size. Abnormal findings include enlargement or changes in consistency (which occur in benign prostatic enlargement or cancer).

Life-Span Assessment Variations
Pediatric
- The labia and clitoris may be enlarged in newborns.

Geriatric
- Decrease in the size of the labia
- Decreased vaginal secretions

- Shortened vaginal vault
- Decrease in the size of the penis
- Decreased pubic hair

Musculoskeletal System

The primary structures of the musculoskeletal system are the bones, muscles, cartilage, ligaments, tendons, and joints. Assessments are made of muscles, bones, and joints. During the assessment, the patient assumes a variety of positions, including standing, sitting, and supine. Assessments of the musculoskeletal system can be integrated into the assessment of other body systems. Identify risk factors for altered health during the health history by asking about the following:

- History of trauma, arthritis, or neurologic disorder
- History of pain or swelling in the joints
- History of pain in the bones, muscles, or joints
- Frequency and type of usual exercise
- Dietary intake of calcium
- History of smoking
- History of alcohol intake
- Use of hormone replacement therapy in women

Muscles
The muscles are examined by inspection and palpation of muscle groups and by testing muscle tone and strength. Muscle groups are observed for bilateral symmetry and palpated for tenderness. Normally, they are symmetric and nontender. Muscle *tone* (the normal condition of a muscle at rest) is evaluated by putting each joint and extremity through passive range of motion. Bilateral equal resistance should be present. Muscle strength is assessed by asking the patient to move against resistance. Observe muscle contraction and determine muscle strength exerted. An individual's dominant side is normally stronger than the nondominant side. Techniques for testing muscle strength are illustrated in Figure 25-48. Muscle strength should be bilaterally equal, with slight increase on the dominant side.

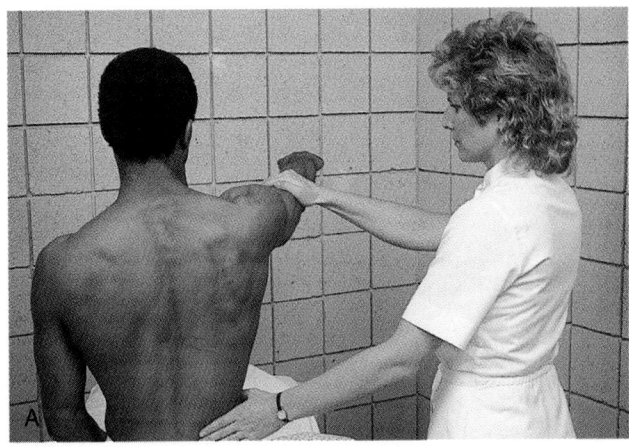

The patient flexes shoulder muscle against resistance of examiner's hand.

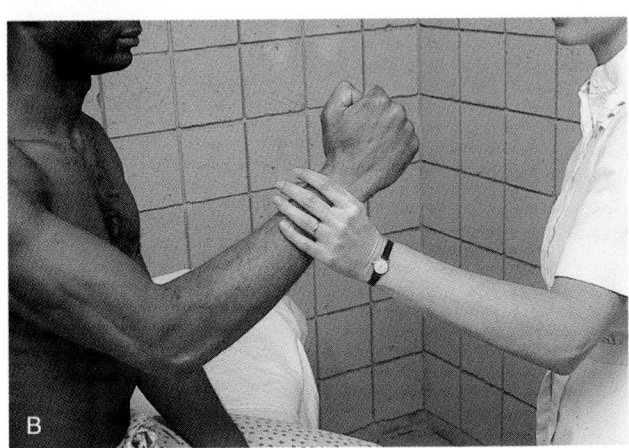

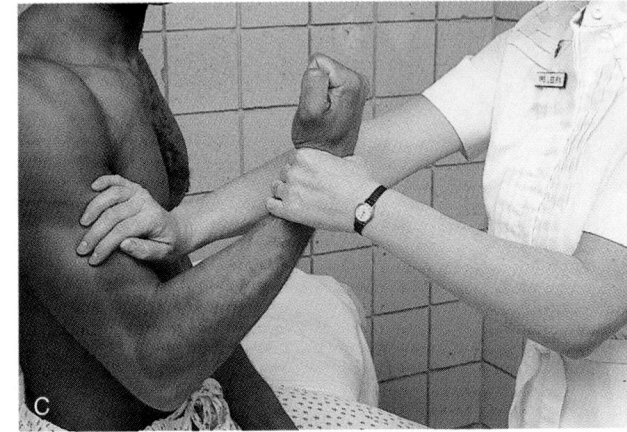

Elbow extension and flexion. The patient first extends elbow against resistance by the examiner, then flexes elbow against resistance.

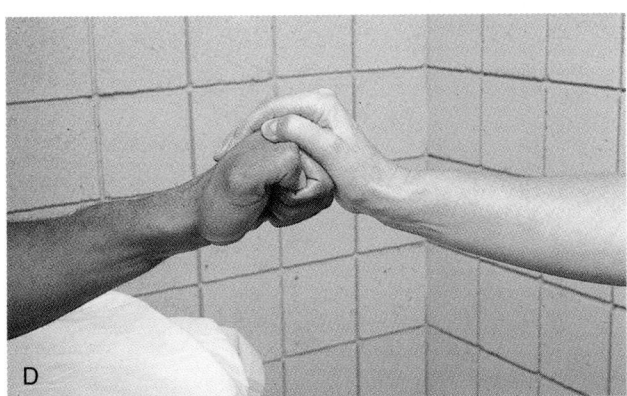

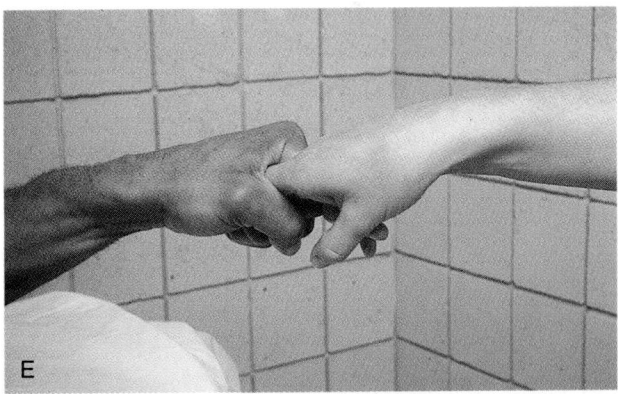

Wrist extension. The patient makes a fist and resists the examiner's attempts to pull wrist down.

Testing grip. Patient squeezes examiner's index and middle fingers.

Figure 25-48
Techniques for testing muscle strength. (Photos © Ken Kasper.)

(Continued on next page)

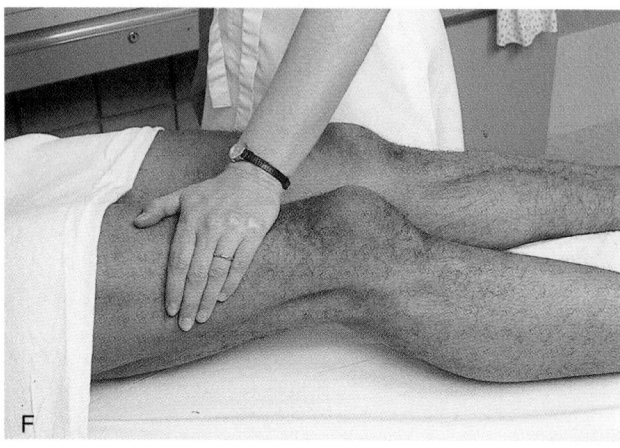

Hip flexion. Patient attempts to raise his thigh against examiner's resistance.

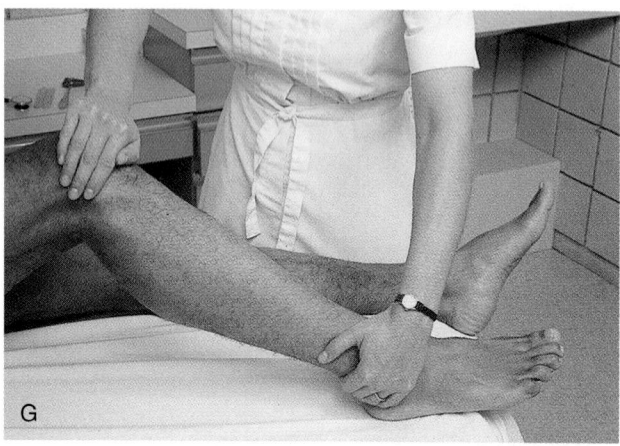

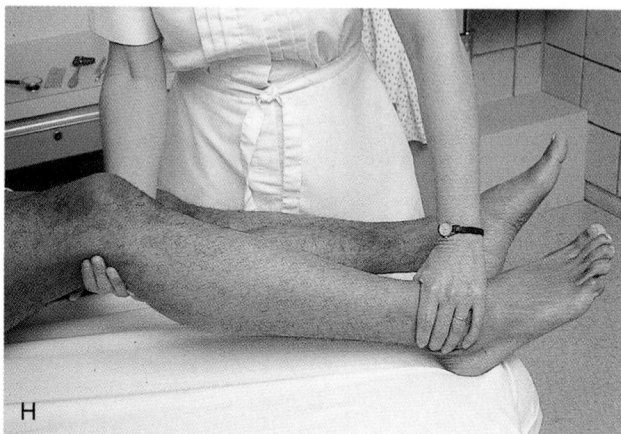

Knee flexion and extension. With the patient's knee bent and foot on the examining table, the patient attempts to keep foot down while examiner attempts to straighten the patient's leg to test flexion. To test extension, the examiner supports patient's knee, and the patient attempts to straighten his leg against examiner resistance at the ankle.

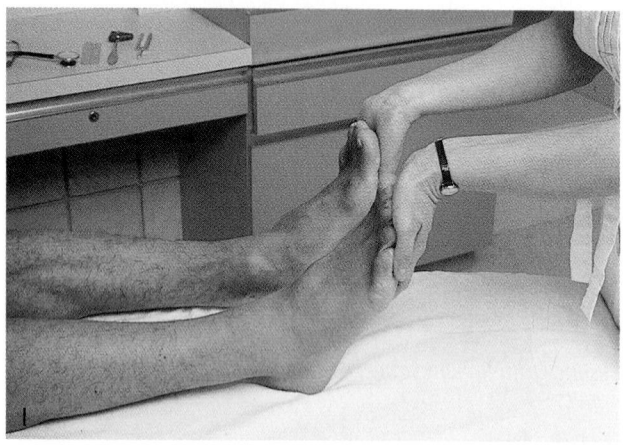

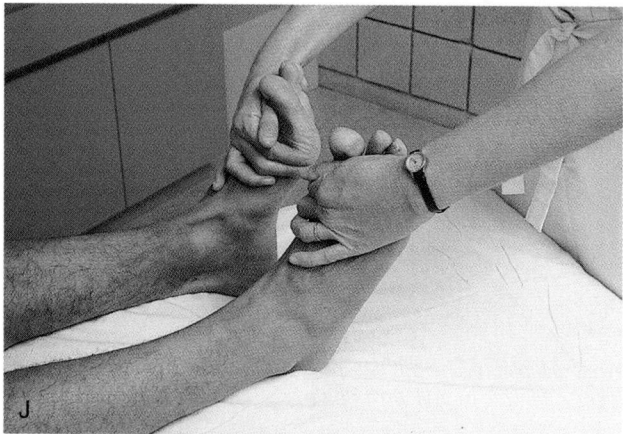

Ankle plantar flexion and dorsiflexion. The patient first pushes the balls of the feet against resistance of examiner's hands, then attempts to pull against examiner's resistance.

Figure 25-48 (*Continued*)

Muscles are normally firm, with strength and tone. Abnormal findings include *atrophy* (a decrease in size); tremors (involuntary movements) and *flaccidity* (weakness) of muscles. Other abnormal findings are loss of strength and tone, decreased range of motion, uncoordinated movements, swelling, and pain. Abnormal findings may indicate a musculoskeletal disease, trauma, or a neurologic disease.

Bones and Joints

Bones are palpated for normal contour and prominence as well as for bilateral symmetry. Abnormal findings include pain, enlargement, asymmetry, and changes in contour. Abnormal findings may indicate trauma, degenerative joint disease, musculoskeletal disease, or a neurologic disease.

Joints are assessed by inspection and palpation. Each joint is put through full range of motion, and the degree is assessed. Joint movements include flexion, extension, hyperextension, abduction, adduction, supination, and pronation. Normally, each joint has full range of motion, is nontender, and moves smoothly. Joints are palpated for the abnormal findings of pain, swelling, nodules, and *crepitation* (a grating sound heard or felt on movement). See Chapter 38 for further discussion and illustration of joint mobility.

Life-Span Assessment Variations

Pediatric
- At birth, the spine is shaped as a C curve; the anterior cervical curve develops at about 3 to 4 months of age, and the anterior lumbar curve develops between 12 and 18 months of age.
- Lordosis (an exaggerated lumbar curve) is common in young children.
- Pronation of the feet is often seen in children between 12 and 30 months of age.
- For 1 year after learning to walk, children may have genu varum (bowleg).

Geriatric
- Loss of muscle mass and strength
- Decreased range of motion
- Decreased height
- Osteoarthritic changes in joints are common.

Neurologic System

The neurologic assessment includes cerebral function, cranial nerve function, cerebellar function, motor and sensory function, and reflexes. Cerebral function is assessed by observing the patient's behavior throughout the interview and assessment and includes mental status, memory, emotional status, cognitive abilities, and behavior. Cerebellar function is evaluated by assessing fine motor skills, coordination, and balance. The sensory system is assessed by having the patient identify various sensory stimuli, and the reflexes are evaluated by contraction of specific muscles.

Identify risk factors for altered health during the health history by asking about the following:

- History of numbness, tingling, or tremors
- History of seizures
- History of headaches
- History of dizziness
- History of trauma to the head or spine
- History of infections of the brain
- History of stroke
- Changes in the ability to hear, see, taste, or smell
- Loss of ability to control bladder and bowel
- History of high blood pressure
- History of smoking
- History of chronic alcohol use
- History of diabetes mellitus or heart disease
- Use of prescription and over-the-counter medications
- Family history of high blood pressure, Alzheimer's disease, epilepsy, cancer, or Huntington's chorea
- Frequency of and level of blood cholesterol tests
- Exposure to environmental hazards (such as lead or insecticides)

Equipment includes vials of aromatic substances (eg, peppermint and vanilla); visual acuity chart; penlight; sharp object (such as a large safety pin); cotton balls; vials of solution to test taste (eg, salt or sugar); tuning fork; tongue depressor; reflex hammer; and familiar objects (eg, a key or coin). The patient should be sitting, and the environment should be quiet.

Mental Status

Mental status assessment includes orientation, level of consciousness, behavior and appearance, memory, abstract reasoning, and language. The following discussion of each of these components includes sample questions or specific assessments to use during the assessment.

Orientation

Orientation to time, place, and person are evaluated to assess level of awareness. The following questions may be used:

Time
- What is today's date?
- What day of the week is it?
- What season of the year is this?
- What was the last holiday?

Place
- Where are you now?
- What is the name of this city?
- What state are we in?

Person
- What is your name?
- How old are you?
- Who came to visit you this morning?

Although exceptions may occur, individuals who have impaired awareness first lose time orientation, followed by place orientation, and then person orientation. Remember that it is often difficult to know the exact date when one is ill, in pain, or in unfamiliar surroundings.

Level of Consciousness

Consciousness is the degree of wakefulness or the ability of a person to be aroused. This is not the same as orientation; a patient may be conscious but not oriented. Two methods to assess consciousness are (1) level of consciousness and (2) the Glasgow Coma Scale.

Level of consciousness is described as follows:

Awake and alert—is fully awake; is oriented to person, place, and time; responds to all stimuli, including verbal commands

Lethargic—appears drowsy or asleep most of the time but makes spontaneous movements; can be aroused by gentle shaking and saying patient's name

Stuporous—is unconscious most of the time; has no spontaneous movement; must be shaken or shouted at to arouse; can make verbal responses, but these are less likely to be appropriate; responds to painful stimuli with purposeful movements

Comatose—cannot be aroused, even with use of painful stimuli; may have some reflex activity (as gag reflex); if no reflexes present, is in a deep coma

The Glasgow Coma Scale is a standardized assessment tool that assesses level of consciousness. Three parameters are evaluated—eye opening, motor response, and verbal response. Scores are given in each category, and a total score is recorded, with higher scores indicating a more normal level of functioning. A score of 7 or less defines coma. This is a more accurate evaluation of mental status over time. The scale is illustrated in Table 25-7.

Memory

Memory is assessed by asking questions that call for answers demonstrating immediate recall and recall for past events. The following may be used:

Immediate

- Ask the patient to repeat a series of numbers forward or backward (eg, 3, 6, 9). Start with three numbers and gradually increase the digits until the patient

Table 25-7
Glasgow Coma Scale

Component	Response	Score
Eye opening	Spontaneous	4
	To verbal command	3
	To pain	2
	No response	1
Motor response	To verbal command	6
	To localized pain	5
	Flexes/withdraws	4
	Flexes abnormally	3
	Extends abnormally	2
	No response	1
Verbal response	Oriented/talks	5
	Disoriented/talks	4
	Inappropriate words	3
	Incomprehensible sounds	2
	No response	1

cannot respond correctly. Most adults can repeat a series of five to eight numbers forward and four to six digits backward.

- Ask, "What did you eat for breakfast this morning?"

Past

- Ask, "When is your birthday?" or "When is your wedding anniversary?"

Abstract Reasoning

Ask the patient to explain a proverb such as "The early bird catches the worm." If intellectual ability is impaired, the patient usually gives a literal explanation or repeats the phrase. Be sure that the phrase is not culture specific.

Language

The cerebral cortex controls the ability to express self through writing, words, or gestures and to understand the spoken and written word. Injury to the cortex can cause *aphasia*, which is a disorder of language ability. Aphasia may be *expressive* (the individual understands written and spoken words but cannot write or speak to communicate effectively) or *receptive* (the individual cannot understand written or spoken words). These aphasias may also be combined. Some simple methods of assessing language capabilities include the following:

- Ask the patient to name items in the room (eg, bed, flowers, gown, pajamas).
- Ask the patient to follow simple commands, such as "Point to your head."
- Ask the patient to read a short sentence aloud.
- Ask the patient to match printed and spoken words with appropriate pictures.

On initial contact, begin to evaluate the patient's orientation to person, place, and time as well as cognitive abilities and affect (eg, does the patient know who he or she is, where he or she is, and the day or month or year). Observe the patient's appearance, general behavior, and responses to questions. Any variation in responses should be noted. The nurse also assesses the patient's ability to speak clearly. The patient should have a clean, neat appearance with erect posture; be oriented to person, place, and time; have memory recall (both short-term and long-term memory); and be able to demonstrate coherent and logical thought processes. Abnormal findings include poor hygiene, inappropriate dress, disorientation, absent memory recall, and incoherent or illogical thought processes. These abnormal findings may indicate a mental health disorder, mental retardation, organic brain disease, cerebral vascular disorder, alcohol or drug intoxication, or a tumor.

Cranial Nerve Function

The function of the 12 cranial nerves is assessed primarily during the neurologic assessment, although parts of cranial nerve function are assessed with other body systems (eg, pupillary response). The cranial nerves are outlined in Table 25-8. Each nerve has a specific function and is evaluated individually.

Olfactory (I) Nerve

The olfactory nerve is a sensory nerve; its function is the sense of smell. Two or three substances with aromatic

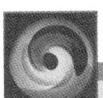

Table 25-8
Summary of Cranial Nerves

Nerve (Number)	Type	Functions	Methods for Examining Nerve
Olfactory (I)	Sensory	Sense of smell	Test each nostril for smell reception and interpretation
Optic (II)	Sensory	Sense of vision	Test vision for acuity and visual fields
Oculomotor (III)	Motor	Pupil constriction Raise eyelids	Test pupillary reaction to light and ability to open and close eyelids
Trochlear (IV)	Motor	Downward inward eye movement	Test for downward and inward movement of the eye
Trigeminal (V)	Motor	Jaw movements—chewing and mastication	Ask patient to open and clench jaws while palpating the jaw muscles
	Sensory	Sensation on the face and neck	Test face and neck for pain sensations, light touch, temperature
Abducens (VI)	Motor	Lateral movement of the eyes	Test ocular movement in all directions
Facial (VII)	Motor	Muscles of the face	Ask the patient to raise eyebrows, smile, show teeth, puff out cheeks
	Sensory	Sense of taste on the anterior two thirds of the tongue	Test for the taste sensation with various agents
Acoustic (VIII)	Sensory	Sense of hearing	Test hearing ability
Glossopharyngeal (IX)	Motor	Pharyngeal movement and swallowing	Ask the patient to say "ah," and have patient yawn to observe upward movement of the soft palate; elicit gag response; note ability to swallow
	Sensory	Sense of taste on the posterior one third of the tongue	Test for taste with various agents
Vagus (X)	Motor	Swallowing and speaking	Ask the patient to swallow and speak; note hoarseness
Accessory (XI)	Motor	Movement of shoulder muscles	Ask the patient to shrug shoulders against your resistance
Hypoglossal (XII)	Motor	Movement of the tongue; strength of the tongue	Ask the patient to protrude tongue; ask patient to push tongue against cheek

odors, such as coffee, vanilla, or peppermint, are used to assess this sense. The patient is asked to close the eyes and occlude one nostril (by pressing a finger against the side of the nose). The patient is then asked to take a breath as the vial is placed under the open nostril and to identify the odor; the process is then repeated for the opposite nostril. Normal findings are equal and bilateral sense of smell; abnormal findings are the inability to identify the odor or absence of smell.

Optic (II) Nerve

The optic nerve is a sensory nerve whose function is vision. Vision is tested for acuity and visual fields, as described in the discussion of assessment of the eye. Abnormal findings include changes in vision; blurring of vision; or inability to identify letters, numbers, or pictures.

Oculomotor (III), Trochlear (IV), and Abducens (VI) Nerves

The oculomotor, trochlear, and abducens nerves are motor nerves that control movement of the eyes through

the cardinal fields of gaze; pupil size, shape, response to light, and accommodation; and opening of the upper eyelids. These assessments are discussed in the earlier section on the assessment of the eye. Normal findings include round pupils that are equal in size, direct and consensual pupillary response, lid margin flush with the surface of the eyeball, equal and complete bilateral lid closure, and parallel movements of the eyes. Abnormal findings include asymmetric eye position, a portion of the eye not covered by the eyelid, lesions, edema, abnormal eye movements, and inability for one or both eyes to follow the cardinal fields.

Trigeminal (V) Nerve

The trigeminal nerve is a sensory and motor (sensorimotor) nerve. Motor function is assessed by observing the facial muscles for deviation of the jaw to one side and by instructing the patient to clench the jaw while palpating the tone of the muscles. Sensory status of the nerve is assessed by testing the ability to discriminate among sharp, dull, and light touch. The patient is asked to close the eyes and, as the nurse touches each side of the patient's face with a sharp object or paper clip, to report whether the sensation is sharp or dull. The same procedure is used for light touch, using a wisp of cotton and asking the patient to tell when and where on the face the sensation is felt. Normally, the patient can correctly identify sharp, dull, and soft sensation of the face and neck bilaterally. Abnormal findings are decreased or absent sensations unilaterally or bilaterally.

Facial (VII) Nerve

The facial nerve is a sensorimotor nerve that innervates the muscles of the face and functions to provide the taste sensation of the anterior two thirds of the tongue. Motor function is evaluated by observing a series of expressions the patient is asked to make, such as raising the eyebrows, smiling and showing the teeth, and puffing out the cheeks. Facial expressions should be symmetric. Abnormal findings are asymmetry and lack of expression. The taste sensation of the tongue is tested by placing a small amount of different substances (eg, sugar, salt, or lemon) on the anterior two thirds of the tongue as the patient, with eyes closed, protrudes the tongue. Various substances should be correctly identified. Abnormal findings include incorrect identification of substances or the inability to taste.

Acoustic (VIII) Nerve

The acoustic nerve is a sensory nerve that is tested by assessing hearing ability, as described in assessment of the ear. The patient should be able to hear bilaterally; abnormal findings are the inability to hear unilaterally or bilaterally.

Glossopharyngeal (IX) Nerve

The glossopharyngeal nerve is a sensorimotor nerve that allows tongue movement and swallowing as well as taste sensations of the posterior one third of the tongue. The motor function of this nerve is assessed with the vagus (X) nerve, and the taste function is assessed with the facial (VII) nerve. The patient should be able to identity various taste substances correctly, have a gag reflex, and be able to move the tongue symmetrically.

Vagus (X) Nerve

The vagus nerve is a motor nerve that is assessed by asking the patient to open the mouth and say "ah" as the upward movement of the soft palate is observed. The uvula should remain midline and rise symmetrically. The swallowing reflex can be assessed by having the patient sip and swallow water.

Accessory (XI) Nerve

The accessory nerve is a motor nerve that controls the movement of the head and shoulders. Ask the patient to shrug the shoulders upward and turn the head against the resistance of your hands (Fig. 25-49). There should be equal movement and strength of the muscles of the shoulder and head bilaterally.

Hypoglossal (XII) Nerve

The hypoglossal nerve is a motor nerve that affects the movement and strength of the tongue. Ask the patient to

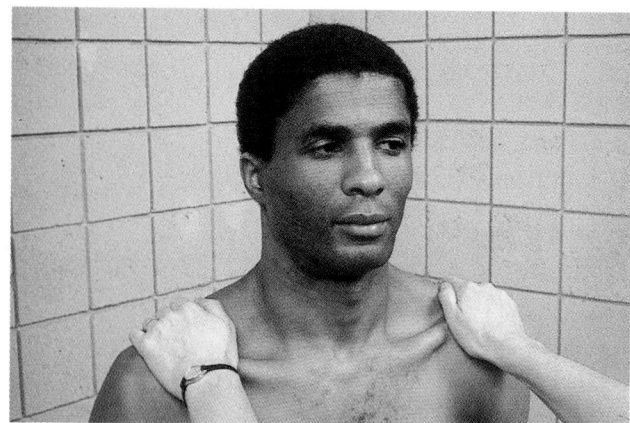

Figure 25-49
Test of the accessory nerve. The patient shrugs his shoulders against the resistance of the examiner's hands. (Photo © Ken Kasper.)

protrude the tongue forward and to push out the cheek with the tongue. The protrusion should be symmetric, and the cheek should have a puffed-out appearance. Abnormal findings include asymmetry of movements, drooping, weakness, tremors, and loss of strength.

Motor, Sensory, and Reflex Function

This part of the neurologic assessment includes the motor, sensory, and reflex abilities of the patient. Motor ability is evaluated by assessing balance, gait, and coordination; sensory function is assessed by testing sensory discrimination of pain, light touch, and vibrations; and deep tendon reflexes are evaluated to determine the functioning ability of specific spinal segment levels.

Motor Function

Balance and Gait. Balance and gait are evaluated by having the patient walk across the room on the toes, on the heels, and heel-to-toe. Observe posture, balance, and arm and leg movements. The posture should be erect, with slight swaying in the standing position, and the gait even with simultaneous arm movements. Abnormal findings include loss of balance, shuffling, wide-based gait, and abnormal patterns of gait.

Motor Function and Coordination. Motor function and coordination are evaluated by having the patient rapidly touch each finger with the thumb, rapidly pat the hand on the thigh, and tap the foot against the floor (or against your hand, if the patient is supine). Normally, the movements are coordinated.

Sensory Function

Sensory perception is tested by evaluating the patient's response to pain, light touch, and vibration. With the patient's eyes closed, a sharp object and a soft object are used randomly to touch upper and lower extremities to test sensation. This assessment proceeds from distal (ie, hands, arms, feet, or legs) to proximal (ie, trunk). The patient should be able to distinguish between sharp (pain) and soft or dull touch. The same process is repeated by using the tuning fork to test for vibratory sensation and placing the fork on bony prominences. Abnormal findings include inability to perceive pain or light touch, inability to identify the location of touch, and absence of vibratory sensation.

Reflex Function

The reflexes are assessed to evaluate the function of specific spinal segment levels. The reflex hammer is used to elicit muscle contraction and reflexes. The patient may be either sitting or supine. Selected reflexes are illustrated in Table 25-9. They are usually graded on a scale of 0 to 4, as listed in Table 25-10. A grade of 2 is considered a normal or active response.

Abdominal Reflex. Lightly stoke the abdomen on each side from above to below the umbilicus. Normally, the abdominal muscles contract, with the umbilicus deviating toward the side being stroked. This reflex may be absent in patients with lower or upper motor neuron lesions and may not be observed in patients who are obese.

Babinski's (Plantar) Reflex. Using the end of the reflex hammer, stroke the lateral aspect of the sole of the foot from the heel to the ball of the foot. Normally, the toes flex. A positive Babinski's reflex (which is abnormal) is seen in the adult when the toes fan and curl and the big toe extends, indicating lesions of the upper motor neurons, alcohol or drug intoxication, or the onset of a seizure.

Biceps Reflex. The patient's arms should be partially flexed at the elbow, with the palms down. Place your thumb or finger firmly on the patient's biceps muscle, and strike with the reflex hammer aimed directly toward the finger. Observe for flexion at the elbow, and feel for contraction of the biceps muscle.

Triceps Reflex. Flex the patient's arm at the elbow, with the palm facing the body, and position it across the chest. Strike the triceps tendon above the elbow. Observe for contraction of the triceps muscle and extension at the elbow.

Patellar or Knee Reflex. The patient is placed in a sitting or supine position with the knees in a flexed position. Briskly tap the patellar tendon just below the patella and observe for contraction of the quadriceps with knee extension.

Achilles Tendon Reflex or Ankle Reflex. The patient's leg should be slightly flexed at the knee, with dorsiflexion of the foot at the ankle joint. Strike the Achilles tendon and observe for plantar flexion at the ankle.

Life-Span Assessment Variations
Pediatric
- Positive Babinski's reflex is normal in children aged 12 to 24 months.
- Grasp reflex is present at birth.
- Motor control develops in this sequence: head, neck, trunk, extremities.

Geriatric
- Slower thought processes and verbal responses
- Decreased sensory ability (hearing, sight, smell, taste, temperature, and pain)
- Slower coordination and voluntary movements
- Decreased reflex responses
- May appear confused in unfamiliar surroundings
- Gait may be slower with a wider base and flexed hips and knees.
- Decreased deep tendon reflexes

Table 25-9
Normal Responses of Commonly Tested Reflexes

Reflex	How to Test Reflex	Normal Response
Biceps	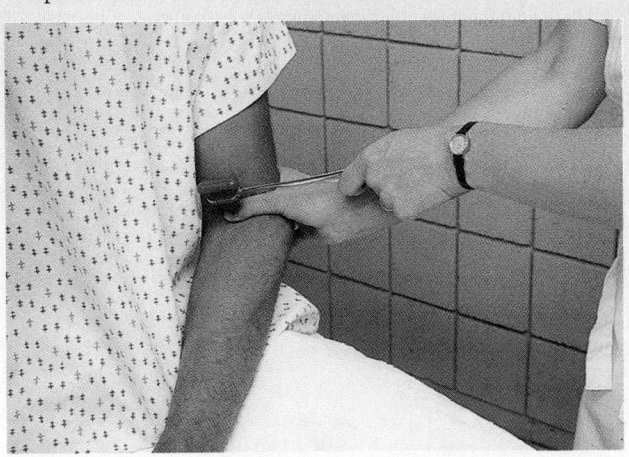	The contraction of the biceps can be seen and felt. To test the biceps reflex, the elbow is slightly bent, and the palm faces downward. The examiner's thumb is placed on the biceps tendon at the bend in the elbow. The percussion hammer strikes the examiner's thumb.

(continued)

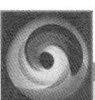

Table 25-9 (Continued)

Reflex	How to Test Reflex	Normal Response
Triceps	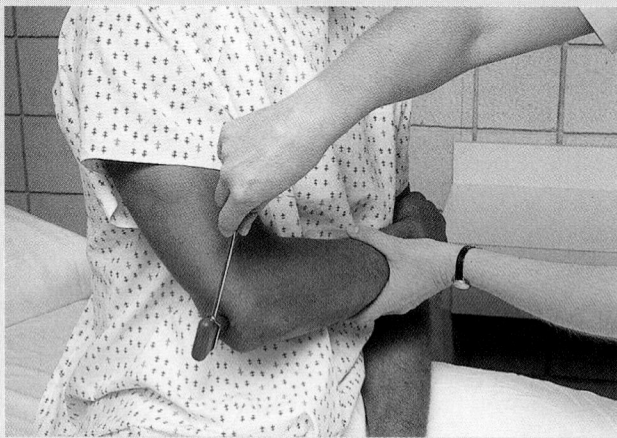	The contraction of the triceps can be seen as the elbow extends. To test the triceps reflex, the patient's elbow is sharply bent; the forearm is placed across the chest wall with the palm turned toward the body. The triceps tendon is struck with the percussion hammer just above the elbow.
Knee	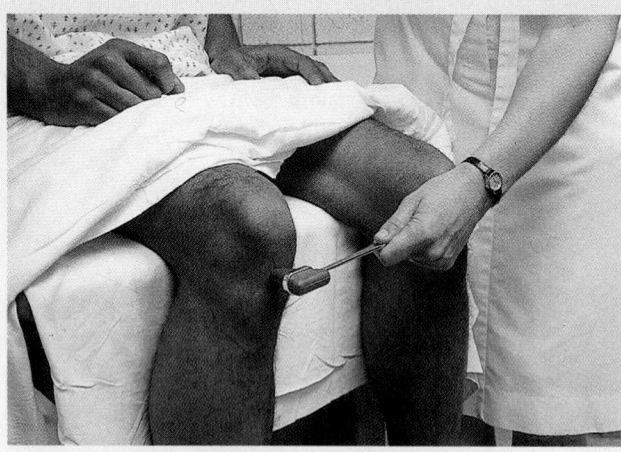	The contraction of the quadriceps causes the knee to extend. To test the knee reflex, the patient is in the sitting position. The patellar tendon just below the patella is struck with the percussion hammer. If the patient is lying down, the reflex is tested while the examiner's hands are placed under the knees to bend them.
Ankle	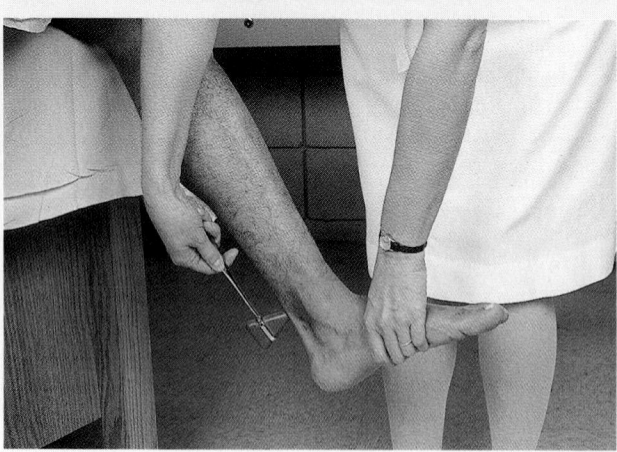	The foot jerks and moves downward. To test the ankle reflex, the leg is bent at the knee and the foot is supported in a walking position. The Achilles tendon is struck with the percussion hammer.

(continued)

Table 25-9 (Continued)

Reflex	How to Test Reflex	Normal Response
Babinski 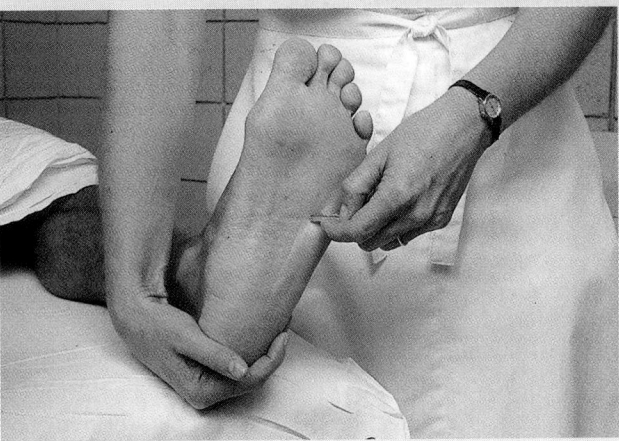		The toes bend or curl. The lateral aspect of the sole of the foot is stroked with an object, such as a key or a thumbnail, from the heel to the ball of the foot.
Abdominal 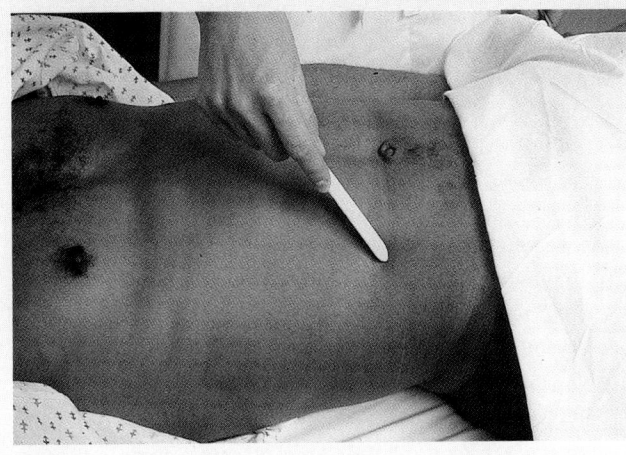		The contraction of abdominal musculature can be seen. To test the abdominal reflex, with the patient lying on the back, each side of the abdomen is stroked from the sides toward the center with a tongue blade or key.

Table 25-10
Grading of Reflexes on a 0 to 4+ Scale

Grade	Description
4+	Very brisk, hyperactive; often indicative of disease; often associated with clonus (rhythmic oscillations between flexion and extension)
3+	Brisker than average; possibly but not necessarily indicative of disease
2+	Average; normal
1+	Somewhat diminished; low normal
0	No response

Documenting the Data

After completing the nursing history and assessment, the nurse organizes all assessment data to identify actual and potential health problems, make nursing diagnoses, plan appropriate care, and evaluate the patient's responses to treatment. A pattern is often established that begins during the history and is confirmed during the physical assessment. The data are documented, with each system recorded individually. An example is illustrated in the accompanying box: Documentation of a Health Assessment.

The Nurse's Role in Diagnostic Procedures

Nurses assist before, during, and after diagnostic tests. The nurse is also responsible for other activities associated with diagnostic tests, such as witnessing the pa-

Documentation of a Health Assessment

Mrs. D. comes to a local community outpatient agency for her intolerance of eating fatty foods. She says "I just started having a lot of gas and was sick to my stomach after eating fried foods." The nurse in charge of the agency makes the following assessments.

Health History

Mrs. D. is a 52-year-old woman who lives with her 54-year-old husband on a farm in a rural midwestern area. She graduated from high school and is employed as a secretary for a local insurance agency. Mrs. D. is well-groomed, alert, and oriented. She occasionally takes over-the-counter medications for constipation and colds. She takes a prescription medication twice a day for "high blood pressure." She says she has about two mixed drinks a week and does not smoke. She has had five pregnancies, resulting in five living children. She is postmenopausal (last period, 2 years ago) and takes hormone replacement therapy in a combination of estrogen and progesterone.

Mrs. D. had her tonsils removed at 5 years of age, had an appendectomy at 22 years of age, and is allergic to penicillin (causes rash and difficulty breathing). She has had all her immunizations, but her last tetanus shot was 10 years ago. Her family history of illness is as follows:

Maternal grandfather: died of heart problems at 77 years of age

Maternal grandmother, died of diabetes complications at 69 years of age

Paternal grandfather, died of stroke at 82 years of age

Paternal grandmother, died of unknown causes at 56 years of age

Sister, 49 years of age, healthy

Brother, died at 22 years of age in a car accident

Physical Assessment

Vital signs: T = 98.8°F (orally), P = 82 beats/min, R = 16 breaths/min, BP = 150/88 mm Hg

Height/weight: 5 feet, 4 inches tall, 178 pounds

Integument: Skin warm and dry, normal turgor. Numerous freckles over face and arms. Old scar, RLQ (appendectomy). Nails convex and smooth. Hair dark brown, shiny, normal distribution.

Head and neck: Skull size and shape normal. Facial features symmetric. Can raise eyebrows, close eyes, smile, puff out cheeks. External eye structures symmetrical. Sclera white, conjunctiva pink. Wears glasses to correct near-sightedness. Vision with glasses $^{20}/_{30\text{-}2}$ on Snellen's chart. Pupils equal and react to light. Demonstrates accommodation, convergence, and peripheral vision. Lens clear. Hearing tested by use of a clock, which she heard clearly at 2 feet. External ears symmetric. Canals smooth and pink without excess cerumen. Tympanic membranes intact without redness or drainage. Right nostril clear, left nostril occluded with mucous. Left maxillary sinus slightly tender on palpation. Teeth in good repair with six fillings. Oral mucous membranes pink. Tonsils absent. Trachea midline, thyroid nonpalpable. No lymph nodes palpable.

Thorax/lungs/heart: Thorax symmetric with equal expansion. Respirations even and unlabored. Lung sounds clear. No visible pulsations noted in neck or precordium. S1 and S2 heard at pulmonic, aortic, tricuspid, and mitral areas. No extra heart sounds, murmurs, or bruits heard. Apical pulse 84 beats/min and regular.

Breasts and axilla: Skin pink. No dimpling or retraction noted. Areolae and nipples dark brown, no crusting or drainage. No masses palpated in breasts. Axillary lymph nodes are not palpable. To have mammogram at next visit.

Abdomen: Obese, rounded. Umbilicus midline. No pain on light palpation. Bowel sounds heard in all four quadrants. No bruits heard on auscultation.

Peripheral vascular: Pulses equal in both arms. Pulses equal in both legs. No edema present. Superficial varicose veins present on both lower extremities between ankle and knee. Toenails thick and yellow.

Genitalia: Will be assessed at next visit with pelvic and Papanicolaou's smear.

Rectum and anus: Inspected only. Small external hemorrhoids noted.

Musculoskeletal: Stands erect. Normal spinal curves. No joint deformities, tenderness, or crepitation. Full active range of motion in all joints. Muscle strength equal bilaterally, slightly stronger on the right (dominant side).

Neurologic: Alert and oriented to time, place, person. Facial expressions appropriate. Speech clear and appropriate. Demonstrates long-term and short-term memory. All cranial nerves tests were intact. Fine motor movements intact. Gait even. Perceives pain or light touch appropriately. All reflexes = 2.

---

tient's consent, scheduling the test, preparing the patient physically and emotionally for the test, providing care after the test, disposing of used equipment, and transporting specimens.

Diagnostic tests provide crucial information about a patient's health, and their results become a part of the total health assessment. Decisions concerning which diagnostic tests to schedule are made by nurse practitioners and physicians when problems are noted during the health history or physical assessment or because of a problem stated by the patient. Table 25-11 presents an overview of different types of diagnostic procedures.

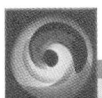

Table 25-11
A Guide to Common Laboratory and Diagnostic Procedures

Procedure	Description	Examples
Aspiration procedures	Studies in which a needle or similar instrument is inserted into a body organ or cavity. Fluid or tissue is aspirated, prepared, labeled, and sent to the laboratory for examination.	Liver biopsy Lumbar puncture Paracentesis Thoracentesis
Electrical impulse procedures	Studies that use a machine with electrodes attached to the body to monitor electric activity. Electric impulses are recorded on a graph and displayed on paper or an oscilloscope screen.	Electrocardiography (EKG) Electroencephalogram (EEG)
Endoscopic procedures	Studies that allow for direct visual examination of various body cavities and organs by means of a hollow, lighted tube, called an endoscope. The tube may be flexible or rigid. May be used to obtain tissue specimens for biopsy or microscopic examination.	Bronchoscopy Colonoscopy Gastroscopy Sigmoidoscopy Laparoscopy
Laboratory procedures	Studies in which body fluids, secretions, or tissues are sent to the laboratory for analysis.	Blood studies Urine studies Sputum studies Fecal studies Biopsies
Radiography procedures	Because of the ability of x-rays to penetrate human tissues, x-ray studies provide a picture of body structures that looks like a negative of a photograph.	Chest x-ray Dye-enhanced cardiac catheterization
Magnetic resonance imaging (MRI)	The computer-based procedure provides physiologic information and detailed views of fluid-filled soft tissues.	MRI of the brain, spine, extremities, joints, heart, pelvis, abdomen
Nuclear scanning	Studies that use the administration of a radionuclide and subsequent measurement of radiation from an organ to detect functional abnormalities.	Brain scan Heart scan Lung scan Bone scan
Ultrasonography	Studies in which a harmless, high-frequency sound wave is emitted that penetrates the organ being studied. The sound waves bounce back to the sensor and are electronically converted into a picture of the organ or the contents of the organ.	Ultrasound of the pelvis, abdomen, heart, uterus

Learning Outcomes

After completing this chapter, the learner will be able to accomplish the following:

1. Define the key terms used in the chapter.

adventitious breath sounds	inspection
auscultation	jaundice
bronchial sounds	pallor
bronchovesicular sounds	palpation
bruits	percussion
cyanosis	petechiae
ecchymosis	precordium
edema	tremor
erythema	turgor
	vesicular breath sounds

2. Identify the purposes of the health assessment.
3. Describe the techniques used during a health assessment.
4. Discuss patient preparation for a health assessment.
5. Identify equipment used in a health assessment.
6. Describe positioning used for each body system assessment.
7. Conduct a health assessment in a systematic manner, identifying normal and abnormal findings.
8. Document significant health assessment findings in a concise, descriptive manner.
9. Describe nursing responsibilities before, during, and after diagnostic procedures.

Critical Thinking Exercises

1. Describe how you would explain a cardiovascular assessment to the following patients:
   - A healthy child who is 5 years of age
   - A college student who has never been ill
   - A 50-year-old man who has never had a physical assessment
   - An 85-year-old woman with heart problems
2. When you are conducting a health history, your patient gives you strange answers. Later, during the mental status assessment, she gives you the wrong answers for the date and place. She also cannot remember what medications she takes. How would you document this information? What would you do next?
3. When you make a home visit to conduct an initial health history and physical assessment, the patient refuses to let you do more than assess vital signs. What would you do?

Study Questions

1. The internal structures of the eye can be visualized using which of the following instruments?
   a. an otoscope
   b. an ophthalmoscope
   c. a stethoscope
   d. a tuning fork
2. To make accurate assessments during inspection, the nurse must
   a. compare bilateral body parts
   b. have $^{20}/_{20}$ vision
   c. focus on selected body systems
   d. use touch judiciously
3. Palpation is a physical assessment technique that uses the sense of
   a. intuition
   b. vision
   c. hearing
   d. touch
4. When percussing over the stomach, the nurse notes the finding of a loud, drumlike sound. The term to document this percussion tone is
   a. dullness
   b. flatness
   c. tympany
   d. resonance
5. The bell of the stethoscope is used to hear
   a. tympanic sounds
   b. bowel sounds
   c. lung sounds
   d. heart sounds
6. Skin turgor may be assessed by which of the following techniques?
   a. indenting with the fingertips
   b. using special lighting
   c. touching to detect moisture
   d. lightly pinching a skin fold
7. Visual acuity may be assessed by using Snellen's chart. If a patient has acuity of $^{20}/_{40}$ in both eyes, this means
   a. the patient can see twice as well as normal
   b. the patient has double vision
   c. the patient has less than normal vision
   d. the patient has normal vision
8. When using an otoscope to assess the tympanic membrane of an adult, the ear canal is straightened by gently pulling the pinna
   a. up and back
   b. down and forward
   c. away from the examiner
   d. in any direction
9. When percussing the thorax and lungs, a dull sound indicates
   a. an air-filled structure
   b. a bony structure
   c. emphysematous tissue
   d. fluid or a solid mass
10. When auscultating the thorax and lungs, coarse gurgling sounds are heard on expiration. These sounds can be broadly labeled as
    a. adventitious breath sounds
    b. bronchovesicular breath sounds
    c. vesicular breath sounds
    d. bronchial sounds
11. Heart sounds are the result of
    a. blood flow through the heart
    b. movement of blood into the heart from the aorta
    c. closure of the heart valves
    d. contraction of the cardiac muscle
12. When palpating the breast, the assessment should be conducted by which division of areas?
    a. quadrants
    b. halves
    c. entire breast tissue
    d. bilateral comparison
13. When assessing the abdomen, which assessment technique should be conducted after inspection?
    a. percussion
    b. palpation
    c. auscultation
    d. sequence does not matter
14. Which of the following assessments of mental status is *not* an assessment of orientation?
    a. time
    b. place
    c. person
    d. consciousness
15. As part of the assessment of cranial nerves, the nurse asks the patient to raise the eyebrows, smile, and show the teeth. These actions provide information about which cranial nerve?
    a. olfactory
    b. optic
    c. facial
    d. vagus

Answers With Rationale

1. The correct response is *b*. None of the other instruments can be used to visualize the internal eye.

2. The correct response is *a*. A comparison of bilateral body parts is necessary for recognizing abnormal findings. Perfect vision is unnecessary; the nurse examines all body systems and uses touch during palpation.

3. The correct response is *d*. Palpation is the technique that uses the sense of touch. The other responses are incorrect.

4. The correct response is *c*. Tympany is a loud, drum-like sound, heard over an air-filled organ. Dullness has a thudlike quality. Flatness is a flat, high-pitched sound. Resonance is a hollow sound heard over lung tissue.

5. The correct response is *d*. The bell of the stethoscope is used to hear low-pitched sounds, such as those produced by the heart and vascular system. The diaphragm of the stethoscope is used to hear high-pitched sounds, such as normal lung and bowel sounds.

6. The correct response is *d*. Skin turgor is assessed by lightly pinching a fold of skin and allowing it to return to its shape when released. None of the other techniques would determine skin turgor.

7. The correct response is *c*. Normal vision is $^{20}/_{20}$. A finding of $^{20}/_{40}$ would mean that a patient has less than normal vision.

8. The correct response is *a*. The ear canal of an adult is straightened by gently pulling the pinna of the ear up and back. In children younger than 3 years of age, the ear canal is straightened by pulling the pinna gently down and back.

9. The correct response is *d*. A dull sound is heard when percussing over fluid or a solid mass. A flat tone is heard over a bony structure. Tympany is heard over an air-filled structure. Hyperresonance is heard over emphysematous lung tissue and is an abnormal finding.

10. The correct response is *a*. Adventitious breath sounds are sounds not normally heard in the lungs. The other responses are normal breath sounds.

11. The correct response is *c*. Heart sounds are the result of closure of the heart valves. The other responses do not result in heart sounds.

12. The correct response is *a*. The breast is divided into four quadrants—outer upper quadrant, outer lower quadrant, inner upper quadrant, and inner lower quadrant. Each quadrant is systematically palpated in a clockwise direction. Any abnormal findings are recorded by location of the involved quadrant.

13. The correct response is *c*. When assessing the abdomen, the sequence is inspection, auscultation, percussion, and palpation. Auscultation follows inspection because percussion and palpation stimulate bowel sounds.

14. The correct response is *d*. The other answers are assessments of orientation. Consciousness is the degree of wakefulness or the ability of a person to be aroused, which is not the same as orientation.

15. The correct response is *c*. Motor function of the facial nerve (cranial nerve VII) is assessed by asking the patient to raise the eyebrow, smile, and show the teeth. The other responses are also cranial nerves but have different techniques of assessment.

Bibliography

Andresen, G. (1998). Assessing the older patient. *RN, 61*(3), 46–56.

Bates, B. (1999). *Guide to physical examination and history taking* (7th ed.). Philadelphia: Lippincott Williams & Wilkins.

Cook, M. (1994). Nursing assessment for the older woman. *RN, 57*(9), 40–44.

Crigger, N., & Forbes, W. (1997). Assessing neurologic function in older adults. *American Journal of Nursing, 97*(3), 37–40.

Darovic, G. (1997). Assessing pupillary responses. *Nursing, 27*(2), 49.

Day, M. (1997). Cardiac markers: Keys to the heart. *Nursing, 27*(10 Crit Care), 1–2.

Dubin, S. (1996). Geriatric assessment. *American Journal of Nursing, 96*(5), 49–50.

Fischbach, F. (2000). *A manual of laboratory & diagnostic tests.* (6th ed.). Philadelphia: Lippincott Williams & Wilkins.

Hammond, K. (1997). Physical assessment: A nutritional perspective. *Nursing Clinics of North America, 32*(4), 779–790.

Kirton, C. (1996). Assessing breath sounds. *Nursing, 26*(6), 50–51.

Kirton, C. (1996). Assessing normal heart sounds. *Nursing, 26*(2), 56–57.

Kirton, C. (1997). Assessing a heart murmur. *Nursing, 27*(9), 51.

Kirton, C. (1997). Assessing bowel sounds. *Nursing, 27*(3), 64.

Kirton, C. (1997). Assessing S3 and S4 heart sounds. *Nursing, 27*(7), 52–53.

Ludwig, L. M. (1998). Cardiovascular assessment for home healthcare nurses. Part 1: Initial cardiovascular assessment. *Home Healthcare Nurse, 16*(7), 450–456.

Marchese, T., & Diamond, F. (1995). Primary care for women: Comprehensive assessment of the respiratory system. *Journal of Nurse-Midwifery, 40*(2), 59–64.

Neal, L. (1997). Basic musculoskeletal assessment: Tips for the home health nurse. *Home Healthcare Nurse, 15*(4), 227–235.

O'Hanlon-Nichols, T. (1998). The adult pulmonary system. *American Journal of Nursing, 98*(2), 39–45.

Pomeranz, A. (1998). Physical assessment. *Pediatric Clinics of North America, 45*(1), 1–26.

Talbot, L., & Curtis, L. (1996). The challenges of assessing skin indicators in people of color. *Home Healthcare Nurse, 14*(3), 167–173.

Weber, K., & Kelley, J. (1998). *Health assessment in nursing.* Philadelphia: Lippincott Williams & Wilkins.

Young, T. (1997). Skin assessment and usual presentations. *Community Nurse, 3*(5), 33–36.

Chapter 26
Safety

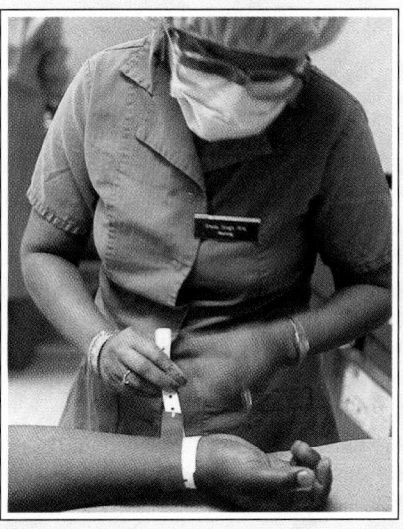

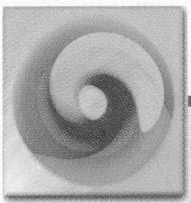

**Thinking Critically About
Nursing's Blended Skills**

Before reading this chapter, think about the types of blended skills you will need to meet the safety and security needs of patients and their families.

• You have been invited by your local Parent–Teacher Association to speak to parents on the importance of safety-proofing their homes for children of all ages.

• You work in a family health center in a poor neighborhood and are noticing an unusually high frequency of reports of suspected child abuse.

• The high school has invited your help in preparing teen peer counselors to respond to the safety challenges of high school teens.

• You are doing the initial home visit of an elderly woman recently discharged home after a stroke that has resulted in her using a walker to ambulate. You are dismayed to find so much clutter in her apartment that it will be difficult for her to navigate safely from the bedroom to the bathroom to the kitchen and sitting room.

• Two residents have been found on the floor in your nursing home unit in the past month. One fell attempting to get out of bed and the other after "escaping" from a vest restraint while seated. You have been charged with increasing safety in the home.

What cognitive, technical, interpersonal, and ethical/legal skills do you think you will need to respond to the challenges described above?

afety and security are basic human needs. Safety is a paramount concern that underlies all nursing care, and patient safety is a responsibility of *all* healthcare providers. Safety is a focus for all healthcare facilities as well as the home, workplace, and community. Many safety concerns are universal for all age groups, but there are unique safety considerations for each developmental stage.

Injuries and deaths from motor vehicle accidents, falls, fire, suffocation, and poisoning occur with alarming regularity across the life span. Violent behavior and its aftermath have also become a significant public safety concern. Many of these injuries and deaths can be prevented with appropriate safety awareness and precautions.

Ensuring that the environment is safe and secure requires an awareness of potential hazards for each developmental level. Studies have confirmed, for example, that pregnant women who use drugs, consume alcohol, or smoke expose their unborn children to substances that may adversely affect their normal growth and development. The nurse frequently is the initial healthcare provider in contact with an abused child or a battered woman. Prompt recognition of the safety problem is crucial, and the nursing assessment may play a vital role in identifying a harmful environment. As children's motor skills develop and their environment expands, the potential hazards multiply—yet many childhood accidents are preventable. Adolescents face great dangers when they abuse drugs or alcohol or engage in high-risk sexual activity. The increasing number of adolescents who become pregnant or are victims of alcohol-related motor vehicle accidents, sexually transmitted diseases, and suicide is a devastating outcome of these unsafe behaviors. Nurses have also become more aware of the growing crisis of elder abuse, which, according to Tatara (1997), may affect 1 million Americans older than 60 years of age. Nurses have firsthand experience with the specific hazards confronting each age group and situation.

This chapter provides problem-solving tools to address these safety issues. The nursing process facilitates the nurse's ability to recognize, assess, diagnose, and plan nursing interventions to ensure safety for all ages in all environments.

Factors Affecting Safety

Nursing strategies that identify potential hazards and promote wellness evolve from an awareness of factors that affect safety in the environment. Table 26-1 lists statistics for the principal causes of accidental death in the United States.

Developmental Considerations

Each developmental level has its own particular risks. Promoting safety and preventing injury are a nurse's dual responsibilities. The nurse and patient or family work together to eliminate or reduce accident risks in the home, community, or healthcare setting. Education to promote

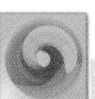

COGNITIVE SKILLS

- Basic knowledge of the safety and security needs of individuals of all ages and developmental stages and related nursing responsibilities and care
- Knowledge of how to individualize safety teaching to specific populations (parents, teenagers, older people, professional caregivers) and special circumstances (child abuse, cluttered home, restraints)
- Knowledge of available resources to meet safety and security needs

TECHNICAL SKILLS

- Ability to correctly use the equipment and techniques necessary to identify and respond to safety problems

INTERPERSONAL SKILLS

- Strong people skills; ability to communicate and interact effectively with individuals and groups to motivate safety awareness and prevention

- Ability to establish trusting relationships with patients, families, and public groups as a basis for counseling and education

ETHICAL/LEGAL SKILLS

- Commitment to safety and quality; strong sense of responsibility and accountability
- Knowledge of the fact that nurses' obligation to prevent harm may be in conflict with the obligation to respect a patient's autonomy
- Ability to initiate and participate in an ethics consult when conflict arises
- Ability to document patient harm according to agency policy (incident reports), and commitment to addressing systemic variables that contributed to the harm
- Knowledge of special regulations and laws detailing nursing responsibilities (e.g., reporting obligations) when assessing special harms, such as domestic violence

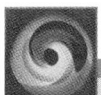

Table 26-1
Deaths and Death Rates From Accidents in the United States, 1995

Type of Accident	Total Deaths	Death Rate per 100,000 Population
Motor vehicle accidents	43,363	16.5
Falls	13,986	5.3
Poisoning (drugs and medicine)	8,000	3.0
Drowning	3,790	1.4
Fires and flames	3,761	1.4
Inhalation and ingestion of objects	3,185	1.2
Complications due to medical procedures	2,712	1.0
Firearms, handguns, and other	1,225	0.5
Air transport	851	0.3
Water transport	762	0.3
Poisoning by gas and vapors	611	0.2
Railway	569	0.2
Electric current	559	0.2
Poisoning by other solids and liquids	461	0.2

Adapted from: US Bureau of the Census (1998). *Statistical Abstract of the U.S.: 1998* (118th ed.). Washington, DC: US Bureau of Commerce).

awareness of potentially dangerous situations must begin as early as possible and continue throughout the life span. The specific risks for each developmental level, along with appropriate nursing interventions, are discussed later in this chapter.

Lifestyle

Certain occupations, recreational activities, and environments place people in more hazardous situations. A worker who frequently operates industrial machinery, works in a perilous setting, or is involved with chemical agents is at greater risk for accidental injury. Certain agents have been identified that place healthcare workers at greater risk. Nurses working in the operating room, for example, are regularly exposed to surgical smoke, a byproduct of laser and electrosurgery, that is filled with chemicals. At high concentrations, this smoke can cause visual and upper respiratory tract irritation (Sloane & Holcomb, 1997). The dramatic shift of healthcare from the hospital to community settings can lead to caregivers being in unpredictable environments that can threaten their personal safety. Reproductive haz-

ards may exist for women with long-term exposure to certain anesthetic agents, and an antiviral preparation (ribavirin) used for respiratory infections in infants and children may be harmful to a developing fetus (Eisenhauer, Nichols, Spencer, & Bergan, 1998). Exposure to excessive noise levels, such as those experienced at a construction site or when listening to extremely loud music, may eventually lead to hearing loss. The Occupational Safety and Health Administration (OSHA) is identifying risks and developing standards to prevent serious injuries and illnesses due to work-related musculoskeletal disorders resulting from repetitive motions. Back pain and carpal tunnel syndrome may occur from work-related repetitive motion.

Some people are by nature more inclined to take risks and place themselves at jeopardy. Failure to wear seat belts or follow safety precautions is common behavior for some people. Stress may precipitate an unhealthful lifestyle that involves drug or alcohol abuse. Although much has been done to identify and control environments affected by pollutants, certain areas have proved to be more hazardous and may expose residents to potentially unhealthy substances in the environment.

Living in an area where crime is prevalent often poses an additional threat to physical and emotional well-being. Security measures, such as locks and adequate exterior lighting, can provide additional safety reassurances.

Mobility

Any limitation in mobility is potentially unsafe. An older patient with an unsteady gait is more prone to falling, and an unfamiliar setting, such as a healthcare facility, may aggravate the problem. Someone with paralysis or a spinal cord injury may require assistance with even simple movements. Supportive devices, such as canes, walkers, and wheelchairs, may facilitate movement, but they require careful instruction and preparation for safe use. Recent surgery or a prolonged illness can temporarily affect a patient's mobility and necessitate special precautions to prevent falls or injuries. Nurses must assess a patient's risk for injury with a view toward maintaining independence and fostering self-esteem while providing a safe, predictable environment.

Sensory Perception

Alterations in sensory perception can have a devastating effect on safety. Any impairment in sight, hearing, smell, taste, or sense of touch can reduce one's sensitivity to the environment. Visual changes may cause a person to stumble, lose his or her balance, and fall. A hearing deficit interferes with normal communication and may result in a patient who cannot hear safety alarms, automobile horns, and sirens and who may not clearly understand instructions relating to healthcare. A reduction in one's ability to distinguish odors may lead to a failure to detect leaking gas or smoke. A loss of taste bud receptors can foster unsafe eating habits or result in eating tainted food. A patient whose tactile sense is impaired may not perceive temperature extremes that are a threat to safety.

Knowledge

An awareness of safety precautions is crucial for promoting and maintaining wellness. A patient needs instruction, for example, to adhere accurately to a medical regimen or to follow safety precautions when oxygen is in use. He or she requires a certain amount of knowledge to manage new equipment and unfamiliar procedures. Nursing assessment includes identifying and recognizing potentially threatening circumstances. Recommendations for specific safety precautions are included throughout this chapter.

Ability to Communicate

The ability to communicate with others is basic to many safety practices. The nurse must be sensitive to any factor that influences the patient's ability to receive and send messages. Fatigue, stress, medication, aphasia, and language barriers are examples of factors that can affect personal communication and prevent the patient from accurately perceiving events. A valid assessment by the nurse not only identifies the patient's level of understanding but also facilitates a positive communication experience.

Health State

Anything that affects the patient's health state potentially can affect the safety of the environment. When a person is chronically ill or in a weakened health state, the focus of healthcare includes preventing accidents as well as promoting wellness and restoring the individual to a healthy state. The nurse caring for a patient who is recovering from a stroke, for example, identifies the patient's neuromuscular impairment, pays particular attention to health teaching concerning the person's ability to maintain a sense of balance, and carefully assists the patient with ambulation to prevent falls. Many patients who fall have a primary or secondary diagnosis of cardiovascular disease, such as a stroke. Prevention of complications and return to the optimal level of functioning require attention to safety and become primary concerns in a stroke rehabilitation program. The nurse strives to maximize the patient's potential by considering safety factors in all phases of the illness and recovery experience.

Psychosocial State

Stressful situations tend to narrow a person's attention span and make him or her more prone to accidents. Stress may occur over a long period, but the effects tend to be more devastating in the person's later years when there is typically less adaptive and coping capacity. Depression may result in confusion and disorientation, accompanied by reduced awareness or concern about environmental hazards. Social isolation or lack of social contact may lead to a reduced level of concentration, errors in judgment, and a diminished awareness of external stimuli.

Assessing Safety

Environmental safety hazards result in falls, fires, poisoning, suffocation, and accidents involving motor vehicles,

equipment, and procedures. Nursing assessment includes identifying individuals at risk and unsafe situations. This requires knowledge of factors that influence safety and predispose people to accidents. Recognizing these considerations helps nurses develop an individualized plan of care and nursing interventions for protecting the patient. Assessment includes an awareness of risk factors in both the home and the healthcare agency.

As student nurses become increasingly involved in community and home care settings, they need also to assess their own environmental safety when visiting unfamiliar areas. Carroll, Morin, Hayes, & Carter (1999) suggest use of educational strategies and a questionnaire that can identify students' personal safety concerns in a community setting. Use the self-assessment checklist in the accompanying box, Promoting Wellness, to evaluate your own attention to your personal safety.

Patient

Nursing History

To help provide a safe environment, the nurse must be alert to any history of falls or accidents because a person with a history of falling is likely to fall again. Any assistive devices that the patient uses (eg, a cane or walker) should be noted. The nurse should also be alert to any history of drug or alcohol abuse. Family members and significant others are often valuable resources. Knowledge of family support systems and the home environment is crucial for the nurse to plan protective health measures.

Physical Examination

The nurse needs to assess the patient's mobility status, ability to communicate, level of awareness or orientation, and sensory perception in the physical examination. Early identification of any potential safety hazards is essential. The nurse should recognize any manifestations that suggest domestic violence or neglect. Chapters 4 and 9 discuss families experiencing violence, neglect, or abuse.

Accident-Prone Behavior

Some people seem more likely than others to have accidents. Some children, for example, are involved in multiple mishaps resulting in fractured bones or minor injuries requiring surgical repair. Adults at any age may also have this tendency. They appear unable to predict situations that may prove hazardous. Experts disagree about the cause of accident-prone behavior, but most agree that a patient with a history of accidents is likely to have another one.

Environment

Assessment of the environment requires the same attention to safety. Risks in the home, community, and healthcare agency may cause injury. Each setting must be individually assessed with the focus on the patient's developmental level and health status. Potential safety hazards in the patient's environment that require assess-

PROMOTING HEALTH

Safety in the Community

Use the following assessment checklist to determine how well you are meeting your need for maintaining personal safety as you assist with healthcare delivery in the community. Then develop a prescription for self-care by choosing appropriate behaviors from the list of suggestions.

Assessment Checklist

(almost always / sometimes / almost never)

1. I wear a badge or clothing that identifies me as a healthcare worker.
2. I dress in an unobtrusive, professional manner.
3. I keep my car in good working order.
4. I am aware of neighborhoods where personal safety and security may be a problem.
5. I confirm directions to the patient's residence before the visit.
6. I only enter patients' homes when invited in by responsible adult.

Self-Care Behaviors

1. Call patients to schedule visits for an agreeable time.
2. Carry a map of the communities you plan to visit.
3. Avoid isolated areas.
4. Request that pets be secured before your visit.
5. Do not carry money, credit cards, or handbag on your person. If necessary, lock them in your trunk.
6. Avoid wearing expensive jewelry.
7. Consider the advantages of a mobile car phone.
8. Request escort services as appropriate or make joint visits.
9. Keep your car locked when driving and when parked.
10. Make sure agency is aware of time/location of scheduled visits.

ment and intervention are described in detail later in this chapter.

Specific Risk Factors

The nurse needs to be aware of those patients who are most at risk for injury as well as specific hazards.

Falls

Falls can occur at any age but are the leading cause of accidental death in people 79 years of age or older (Hoskin, 1998). A large portion of healthcare for the elderly goes to caring for injuries resulting from falls (Rawsky, 1998). Elderly people are at risk in all settings. Falls are responsible for most hospital incidents, and about one third of those older than 65 years of age fall at home (Fortin, Yeaw, Campbell, & Jameson, 1998; Winslow & Jacobson, 1998a). Studies suggest that about half of all residents of long-term care facilities fall annually (Ray, et al., 1997; Walker, 1998). Many falls at home are unreported because they do not cause injuries requiring medical attention and because the elderly are fearful of activity restrictions, loss of independence, or placement in a nursing home. Fear of falling can also cause anxiety and panic and make an older adult more vulnerable for a fall.

Assessment of the risk for falling includes use of the nursing history and nursing examination. The nursing ex-

amination includes inspecting for factors that contribute to falls. An individual is considered at high risk for a fall if he or she has any of the following characteristics:

- Age older than 65 years
- Documented history of falls
- Impaired vision or sense of balance
- Altered gait or posture
- A medication regimen that includes diuretics, tranquilizers, sedatives, hypnotics, or analgesics
- Postural hypotension
- Slowed reaction time
- Confusion or disorientation
- Impaired mobility
- Weakness and physical frailty
- Unfamiliar environment

Surveillance must be continuous for environmental hazards in the healthcare facility and the home environment and of patients who are at risk for falls. Most healthcare agencies have fall prevention programs. Nurses have the responsibility to identify patients who are at high risk for falls, document pertinent assessments on the chart, and plan appropriate interventions to ensure their safety. A nurse whose behavior is reasonable and prudent and similar to behavior that would be expected of another nurse in similar circumstances is unlikely to be found liable if a patient falls, even if an injury results (Sullivan, 1999). Checklists for preventing falls at home and in healthcare facilities appear later in the chapter.

Fires

Many home fires are started by someone smoking in bed or falling asleep on a sofa or chair while smoking. Most fatal home fires occur while people are sleeping, and most people who die in house fires die not from burns but from smoke inhalation. Kitchen stoves, candles, and electric heaters are other causes of home fires. Faulty wiring and unsafe electrical equipment cause fires in homes and healthcare facilities. The risk for home fires can be determined by assessing the knowledge of family members.

People with limited financial resources should be questioned about how they heat their house because the electricity or gas may have been turned off and space or kerosene heaters, wood stoves, or a fireplace may be the sole source of heat. Fire safety recommendations for the home are included in the Home Safety Checklist later in this chapter.

Fire prevention and emergency response programs in healthcare facilities are sometimes viewed by staff as time-consuming or unnecessary exercises, but nurses must be prepared at all times to protect patients from injury. Hospitals are required by law to establish safety boards and to inspect the facility regularly for possible hazards. Equipment must be checked periodically, and escape routes must be kept open. Nurses, as part of their daily care procedures, must be aware of their agency's policies, review equipment and its proper functioning, and assess when and how often drills are performed.

Poisoning

Although the incidence of childhood poisoning has been reduced dramatically in the last 10 years, accidental poisoning remains a concern. According to the latest government statistics, more than 9000 deaths resulted from accidental poisoning in 1995, with many more people suffering other effects of poisons but not dying. (US Bureau of the Census, 1998). Causes of fatalities from unintentional poisoning are listed in Table 26-2. Not all poisons, however, cause death.

Consider the person's developmental stage when making a safety assessment. Younger children are more apt to

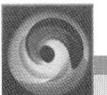

Table 26-2
Common Agents in Childhood Poisoning

Poisonous Agent	Source	Common Clinical Manifestations	Treatment
Salicylates	Products containing aspirin	Nausea, hyperpnea, dehydration, vomiting, confusion, fever, tinnitus, metabolic acidosis, respiratory alkalosis, seizures, coma	If clear history of intake is available and intake is 150–300 mg/kg,* induce emesis with syrup of ipecac. Intake > 300 mg/kg take child to ER.
Caustics	Oven cleaner Drain openers Toilet bowl cleaners Battery contents Rust removers Hair perms	Burning pain in mouth and throat, drooling, edema of lips; oral, esophageal, gastric burns; vomiting, hemoptysis	*Never induce vomiting!* Never attempt to neutralize the caustic. Dilute with milk or water. Contact physician or PCC.
Hydrocarbons	Gasoline Kerosene Furniture polish Lamp oil	Gagging, coughing, choking, dyspnea, grunting, nausea, chills, fever, lethargy	*Never induce vomiting!* Contact MD or PCC.
Iron	Vitamin preparations	Nausea, vomiting, diarrhea, abdominal pain, melena, hematemesis, lethargy, coma	If clear history of intake is available and exposure is 20–40 mg/kg,* induce vomiting with syrup of ipecac. Intake > 40 mg/kg, take child to ER.
Lead	Paint chips Paint dust	May be asymptomatic, anorexia, abdominal pain, anemia, encephalopathy, neurobehavioral deficits	Chelation therapy and monitor lead levels

*Clear history indicated knowledge of exact amount of drug ingested. Mg/Kg can be calculated by dividing the total dose ingested into the weight in kg. If unclear, visit to emergency room (ER) may be recommended by poison control center (PCC).
Adapted from: Pillitteri, A. (1999). *Maternal and Child Nursing* (3rd ed.). Philadelphia: Lippincott Williams & Wilkins; *Poison Pen Notes,* The Poison Control Center, Winter 1996 and Winter 1998.

ingest household chemicals, whereas older children may swallow medicines in a suicide attempt. Preschool-aged children are also at risk for ingestion of lead-containing substances in the home. Experimentation with drugs by adolescents and young adults may result in accidental poisoning and death. The ready availability of inhalants on store shelves and in the home may provide the opportunity for children to sniff or "huff" these dangerous substances. An older person may inadvertently take an overdose of a medication because of confusion or forgetfulness. Poor vision is also a factor in accidental poisoning in older adults.

Most exposures to toxic fumes occur in the home. Poisoning may result from improper mixing of household substances, prolonged use of strong cleaning products, or malfunctioning household appliances (gas, oil, and kerosene heaters) that can release carbon monoxide gas. Carbon monoxide gas is colorless, odorless, tasteless, and nonirritating, which makes it especially dangerous. Exposure can result in mild symptoms or progress to a life-threatening problem or long-term effects. Young children and older adults are more vulnerable to toxic fumes.

Poison control centers provide checklists for poison-proofing a home and lists of toxic household items. Such lists are helpful when assessing and teaching the family about poisonous materials. Refer to the Home Safety Checklist later in this chapter.

Suffocation and Choking

Suffocation, or **asphyxiation**, may occur at any age, but the incidence is greater in children. It results in a lack of air reaching the lungs and a stoppage of breathing.

Common causes of suffocation include drowning, choking on a foreign substance inhaled into the trachea, and gas or smoke poisoning. An infant may suffocate when a pillow or a piece of plastic inadvertently covers the nose and mouth. A young child may be accidentally strangled by the shoulder harness of a seat belt or become trapped while playing in a discarded refrigerator and suffocate.

Drowning is a form of suffocation. Nearly half of all drowning victims are children younger than 5 years of age. Most drowning deaths in young children occur because of inadequate supervision of the bathtub or pool—even a small wading pool. Older children are more likely to drown while swimming or boating.

Educating the public about the causes of suffocation can save many lives. Assessing the knowledge level of individuals—especially parents—is vitally important. Hazards that might cause a child to asphyxiate or choke are included in the Home Safety Checklist later in the chapter.

Firearm Injuries

Firearm injury prevention has become a major concern for health professionals. Some people feel that a gun in the home provides protection for family and property. Keeping a gun in the home often has dangerous consequences, however. It increases the risk for domestic homicide threefold and is responsible for many unintentional injuries and deaths. Young children are curious and like to explore their surroundings. When they encounter a loaded gun, the outcome is often tragic.

Gun ownership is a sensitive issue, and nurses need to approach this topic in a nonjudgmental manner with the focus on injury prevention. The intent is to inform families about the risks of firearm injury and discuss appropriate safety measures. Refer to the Home Safety Checklist later in the chapter.

Diagnosing

Identified unsafe situations and patients at risk are reflected in the nursing diagnosis and plan of care. The statement of the patient's actual or potential health status must be followed by the appropriate contributing or risk factors to individualize the nursing plan of care.

Samples of nursing diagnoses involving safety risks include the following:

- Risk for Injury related to lack of awareness of environmental hazards; visual or auditory sensory deficits; history of falling; unsteady gait; substance abuse; refusal to use seat belt or child safety seat; effects of medication; age greater than 65 years; generalized weakness
- Risk for Poisoning related to impaired vision; medications stored in unlocked medicine cabinet that is accessible to a child; presence of poisonous plants; excess alcohol intake; use of illicit drugs; knowledge deficit
- Risk for Suffocation related to plastic bag that is accessible to a young child; child left unattended in bathtub; smoking in bed; placing an infant prone in a water bed; lack of safety precautions (door left on discarded refrigerator); unfamiliarity with fire prevention guidelines
- Risk for Trauma related to history of previous falls; unsteady gait; presence of unsecured scatter rugs; smoking in bed; inoperable smoke detector; history of substance abuse; lack of experience operating an automobile; presence of unsecured loaded gun in the home
- Impaired Home Maintenance Management related to insufficient finances; substance abuse; physical disability
- Risk for Disuse Syndrome related to use of physical restraints

Planning: Expected Outcomes

Many accidental injuries and deaths are preventable. The nurse considers the various factors and the environment that affect the patient's safety and formulates expected outcomes uniquely suited to each situation and circumstance. Nursing interventions focus on meeting these safety needs.

Expected outcomes for patients that promote safety and prevent injury are listed next. The patient will accomplish the following:

- Identify unsafe situations in his or her environment.
- Identify potential hazards in his or her environment.
- Demonstrate safety measures to prevent falls and other accidents.
- Establish safety priorities with family members or significant others.

- Demonstrate familiarity with his or her environment.
- Identify resources for safety information.
- Remain free of injury during hospitalization.

Implementing

Integral to the nursing plan of care is the patient's safety. The nurse intervenes to control or modify the patient's environment. Safety recommendations in the following sections apply to health agency settings, the home, and the community. Nursing implementations are derived for each developmental level as well as for specific hazards in the environment. Developmentally disabled, demented, or delirious adults frequently need the same safety measures as are prescribed for children.

🌀 Teaching to Prevent Accidents

Teaching is an important intervention for accident prevention and health promotion. Many teaching opportunities concerning safety measures arise while the nurse performs regular patient care, and many resources are available to supplement health teaching (Fig. 26-1). Careful assessment, diagnosis, and planning prepare nurses to use these opportunities wisely.

Assessment data and statistical information often prove helpful to healthcare personnel who are developing a safety program for patients at risk. Safety education classes, in addition to situational health teaching, can be worthwhile for hospitalized patients and their family members. Recent studies have demonstrated that early assessment of vulnerable patients and preventive education programs can decrease the incidence of falls (Fortin et al., 1998; Shumway-Cook, Gruber, & Liao, 1997; Tideiksaar, 1996).

A school nurse has many opportunities and a ready audience for health teaching about safety, including screening programs (eg, vision and hearing), fire prevention sessions, drug and alcohol prevention programs, firearm safety, and classes on various accident prevention techniques. Managing minor accidents at school often provides an opportunity

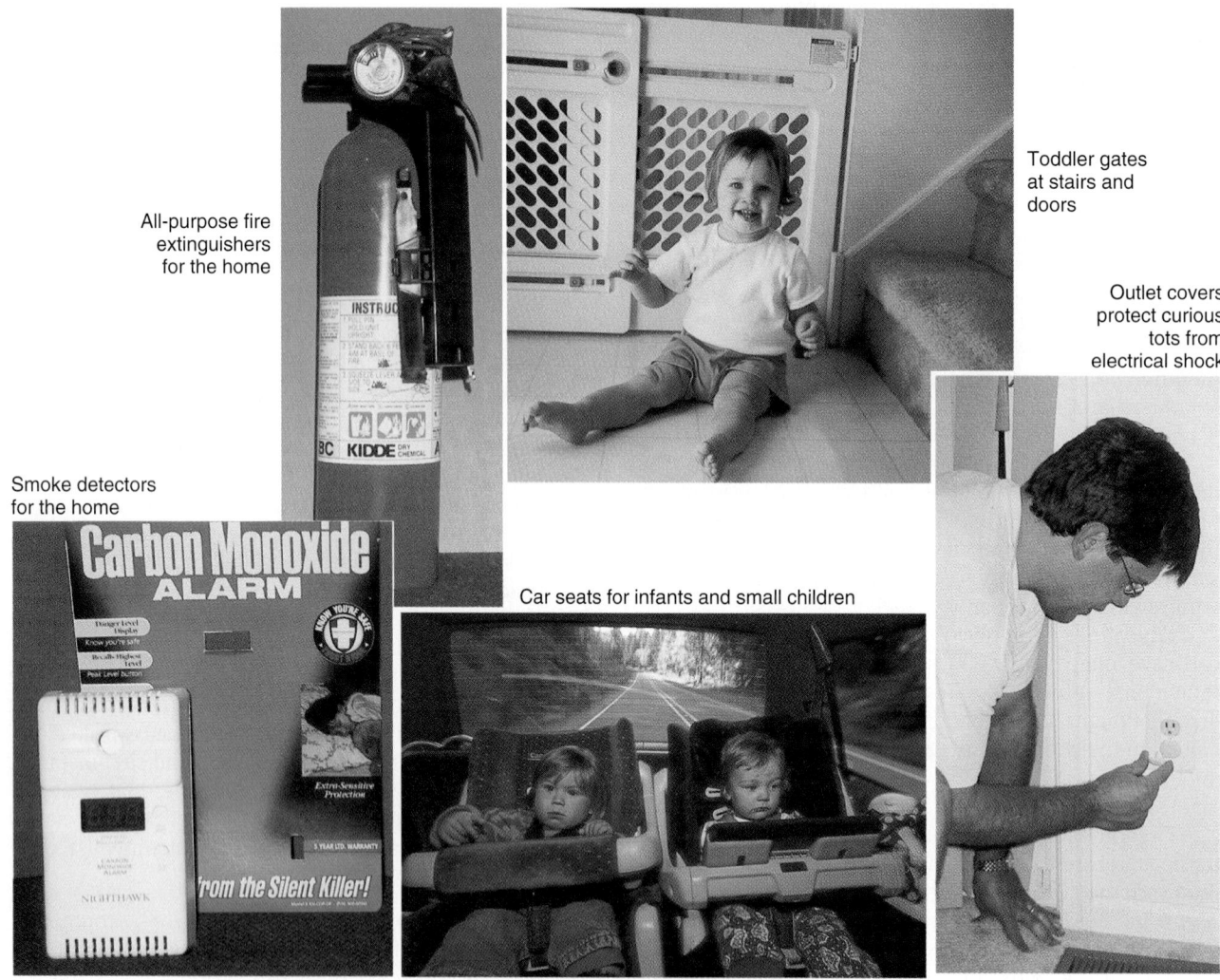

Figure 26-1
The nurse's responsibilities in home safety are primarily that of education and counseling, including providing information about home safety devices and sources for additional information. (Photos © B. Proud.)

for additional preventive teaching. School nurses also interact with the children's parents. Formal or informal health teaching can occur and should also include encouragement to do the following:

- Monitor a child's use of the Internet.
- Get involved in school activities and ask pertinent questions.
- Volunteer for safety committees that include staff and parents.

Considering Developmental Levels

Table 26-3 lists common types of accidents according to developmental age, along with safety topics that should be discussed with parents and in the school. The following discussions of developmental stages are also adaptable to teaching.

Neonate and Infant

Safety considerations begin with an awareness of behaviors that may harm the developing fetus. Newborns of mothers who smoke have a lower birthweight. Excessive alcohol consumption and use of addictive drugs may cause adverse effects that are readily apparent at birth. Nurses should reinforce a pregnant woman's knowledge of the risks associated with excess alcohol consumption, smoking, drug use, and exposure to other dangers in the environment (see Table 26-3).

The nurse has many opportunities to educate parents about safety and accident prevention for infants and young children. The lack of mobility in early infancy limits opportunities for hazardous activity, but minimal safeguards are vital to prevent accidents.

Safe care includes never leaving the infant unattended, using crib rails, and monitoring the setting for objects that the infant could place in the mouth and swallow. As the infant becomes more active, parents and caregivers must be alert to hazards that a curious, mobile infant may encounter. All items within reach must be carefully inspected and, if dangerous, secured in a safe place. Because an infant frequently climbs or pulls up on objects, scalding hot liquids must be placed out of reach.

All 50 states mandate the need for safe infant car seats and carriers when transporting a child in a motor vehicle. According to the National Highway Traffic Safety Administration, however, 40% of all children still ride without seat belts or child safety seats (Ventura, 1997). A rear-facing safety seat placed in the back seat is recommended for infants who are younger than 1 year old and weigh less than 20 lb (9.1 kg). The high force of sudden air bag inflation can cause injury to an infant in a safety seat or a child in the front seat. A recent study by the National Safe Kids Campaign found that 85% of parents use car seats incorrectly (Taft, Michalide, & Taft, 1999). Most parents do not secure the car seat tightly enough with the seat belt or fail to tighten the car seat's harness straps. These seemingly small mistakes can lead to tragic consequences. Additional

safety counseling measures that focus on health teaching for this developmental level are included in Table 26-3.

Toddler and Preschooler

To prevent accidental injury and death in the toddler and preschool years, parents need to childproof the home environment. Play areas should allow for exploration but still provide for safety. Vigilant supervision by parents and guardians should anticipate hazards in the environment and protect the child with precautionary devices. Childproofing products are available that help parents and children recognize dangerous items in the home.

Ingestion of poisons or medications is a major threat for preschoolers. Their overconfidence and initiative also make them more likely to dart into the street while chasing a ball, climb into a discarded refrigerator, or play with matches. A child who is older than 1 year of age and between 20 and 40 lb should be placed in a forward-facing safety seat in the back seat of the vehicle. An older child who must ride in the front seat should wear both shoulder and lap belts, and the seat should be moved as far back as possible to minimize danger from a deploying air bag.

Protecting a child also includes being alert to manifestations that indicate child abuse (see the accompanying box, Physical and Behavioral Manifestations of Child Abuse). In 1997, more than 3 million cases of alleged child maltreatment were reported to Child Protective Services agencies in the United States (Aggeles, 1998). Abuse can be physical, sexual, or emotional and may also be a result of neglect. All 50 states have laws that require reporting of suspected child abuse. Health teaching topics that help safeguard toddlers and preschoolers are included in Table 26-3.

School-Aged Child

As a child becomes more independent during the school years, accidents continue to be a leading cause of death. Although these children are increasingly independent, they still need help avoiding activities that are potentially dangerous. The nurse should counsel parents of school-aged children about specific interventions for safety at home, at school, and in the neighborhood.

Adolescent

Nurses and parents should collaborate to reinforce safety behaviors in adolescents. Much of the adolescent's time is spent away from home, with his or her peer group, or in automobiles. Adolescents are particularly at risk for motor vehicle accidents, and the National Center for Health Statistics lists motor vehicle accidents as the number one cause of death for school-aged children, adolescents, and young adults (see Table 26-1). Adolescent drivers are less likely to drive after drinking but are more likely to have an accident when they do. Education should focus on safe driving skills and the importance of wearing a seat belt and should include discussions about drug and alcohol use.

Tobacco is an additional health problem for teenagers. More than 3 million children smoke almost 1 billion packs of

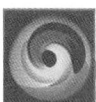

Table 26-3
Developmental Considerations and Safety Topics to Be Taught to Parents

Developmental Age	Safety Topics
Fetus	
Abnormal growth and development	Alcohol consumption
	Smoking
	Use of drugs (addicting, prescription, and over the counter)
	X-ray exposure
	Pesticides
Neonate	
Falls	Neonatal supervision
	Proper method of caring for neonate
	Environment—crib, bath, and changing area
	Infant car seats
	Use of vitamins, iron medications
	Feeding
Infant (first 6 mo)	
Falls	Many of above topics
Injuries from toys	Infant supervision
Burns	Development—rolling over and falls
	Toy safety—size, construction, lead-free paint
	Flame-retardant clothes and inflammable toys
	Smoke alarms
	Sunburns, bathwater temperature, smoking, hot beverages
	Kitchen safety
	Electrical cords and outlets
	Using medications
Infant (second 6 mo)	
Falls	Many of above topics
Injuries from toys	Close supervision for active child
Burns	Development—crawling, pulling up to stand, and pulling down objects
Suffocation or drowning	(curiosity)
Inhalation or ingestion	Safety on stairs (gates)
Foreign bodies	Teaching siblings about infant safety
	Plastic bags
	Tub and pool safety
	Child proofing entire house and any houses the infant visits
	Poisonous plants
	Child-resistant packaging of medications and all poisonous substances
Toddler	
Falls	Poison Control Center and instructions for emergencies
Cuts from sharp objects	Many of above topics
Burns	Toddler supervision
Suffocation or drowning	Development—inquisitive nature
Inhalation or ingestion	Outdoor safety—cars, driveways, parking lots
Foreign bodies	Safety glass on doors, lock doors and windows, screens
	Animal safety—pets and strange animals
	Child car seats
	Storage of hazardous substances (indoors and outdoors)
	Poisonous plants (indoors and outdoors)
	Car safety (car seats, unattended children, cars parked in sun)
	Storage of matches, use of hot liquids
	Water safety—tubs, jacuzzis, and wading and swimming pools, swimming lessons

(continued)

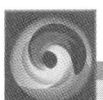

Table 26-3 (Continued)

Developmental Age	Safety Topics
Preschooler	
Falls	Many of above topics, plus use of safety equipment when riding bicycles or skateboards
Cuts	Safe play areas (equipment and supervision, streets)
Burns	Tricycles, scissors, other toys
Drowning	Guns or rifles in the house
Inhalation or ingestion	Begin to teach safety measures to child
Guns and weapons	Fire safety—prevention, emergency measures, fire drills
School-aged child	
Burns	Many of above topics
Drowning	Safety on way to school (traffic, child abuse)
Broken bones	Play equipment—bicycles, skateboards, roller skates
Inhalation or ingestion	Competitive sports
Guns and weapons	Use of machinery (farm, lawn, cooking)
Substance abuse	Teaching safety measures (bicycle, use of phone in emergencies, policeman as helper, substance abuse)
	Parental role modeling
	Drug and alcohol abuse education
	Sexuality education
Adolescent	
Drowning	Many of above topics
Vehicle accidents	Responsibilities of new freedoms of being a teenager
Guns and weapons	Driving (driver education, traffic safety, drinking and driving, motorcycles and snowmobiles)
Inhalation or ingestion	Competitive sports (proper equipment, physical examination before beginning sports or going to camp)
	Safety around water and water sports
	Emergency procedures, first-aid training
	Gun safety
	Substance abuse and role modeling for siblings
	Stress and coping
	Sexuality education and discussion of sexually transmitted diseases (including AIDS)

cigarettes each year, a figure at a 16-year high point (Shahinian & Hawke, 1998). Half of the children who experiment with cigarettes become regular smokers, and at least one third of these children will die eventually from tobacco-related diseases. Federal law mandates a minimum age of 18 years to purchase tobacco products and bans billboard advertising within 1000 feet of schools and playgrounds.

Body piercing has become increasingly popular with adolescents and young adults in recent years. Common sites include the ears, nose, eyebrows, lips, tongue, nipples, navel, and genitals. It is a quick procedure that does not require anesthesia, but the risk for infection is real. The US and Canadian Red Cross will not accept blood donations from anyone who has had a body piercing within the past year because of the risk for contracting hepatitis B virus from unsterile instruments or an unclean environment. Transmission of human immunodeficiency virus (HIV) is also possible, although less likely. Few states regulate body piercing. Meticulous postpiercing care reduces the risk for developing an infection. Nurses need to be informed about the health risks in order to be effective, informed health educators (Armstrong, 1998).

According to a recent report, almost 15% of individuals who died from gunshot wounds in 1995 were younger than 20 years of age and 65% of adolescents who committed suicide used a gun (Teret et al., 1998). Adolescents need encouragement and education about ways to solve arguments without guns and violence and guidance and direction for developing a healthful lifestyle while coping with the stresses of daily living. Providing safety information is crucial to help adolescents make mature decisions about health hazards they are likely to encounter. Refer to Table 26-3 for additional safety topics.

Adult

Young and middle-aged adults need to be reminded about the effects of stress on their lifestyle and health. Coping with the demands of raising a family and succeeding in a career may lead to unsafe health habits and a reliance on drugs or alcohol.

Domestic violence is widespread in the United States. Studies indicate that one in four women was sexually abused as a child (Winslow & Jacobson, 1998b). Many men

Physical and Behavioral Manifestations of Child Abuse

History of similar injuries

Multiple or unexplained bruises

Multiple fractures

Thermal burns in a pattern

Scars or welts

Bite marks

Multiple fractures

Vaginal discharge

Urinary tract infection

Genital pain, itching, redness, or bruising

Sexually transmitted disease

Sleeping problems (nightmares)

Psychosomatic illnesses

Excessive sexual curiosity or play

Decreased attendance and performance in school

Fear of strangers

Adapted from: Carlson, D. (1998). Uncovering the clues of child abuse. *Nursing, 28*(11), 32hn10–11.

who batter their spouses also batter their children. Recent evidence suggests a relationship between childhood sexual abuse and certain physical symptoms in adulthood, such as gastrointestinal symptoms, eating disorders, and substance abuse. The nurse may be directly involved in health education and counseling measures or may suggest other resources to the family as additional support for safety and well-being and to interrupt the cycle of violence.

Older Adult

Most accidents that involve older adults are preventable. Falls, fires, and motor vehicle accidents are significant hazards for this age group. Visual changes and slowed reaction time are realistic concerns that affect the older driver. Some become overly cautious, whereas others are prone to careless behaviors. Interventions to help older adults drive safely include maintaining the automobile in optimum driving condition, scheduling regular eye examinations, wearing corrective lenses when necessary, and keeping noise from radio and other equipment to a minimum. Some states require additional testing for older adults to renew a driving license.

Older adults are at greater risk for suffering burn injuries. Confusion, forgetfulness, and diminished visual and olfactory senses are factors. More fires occur in the home than in healthcare facilities. Additional health teaching interventions directed at helping to promote a safe environment for older patients at home are included in Table 26-3.

Accidental overdosing on medications is also a safety risk, possibly related to poor eyesight or confusion. Special devices, such as medication trays, can be prefilled and help prevent older patients from taking additional doses.

Orienting the Person to Surroundings

A person who is familiar with his or her surroundings is less likely to suffer an accidental injury. As part of the admission routine, the nurse orients the patient to the safety features and equipment in the room. An explanation and demonstration of the adjustable bed and side rails, call system, telephone, television, and bathroom area help the patient adjust to the new environment. The patient identification bracelet and a discussion of agency routine further ensure safety and assist the patient to adapt to the unfamiliar setting. Similarly, the nurse teaches the importance of orienting an older person to new surroundings when moving in with a family member or other caregiver.

Preventing Falls

Major causes of falls in the home include slippery surfaces, poor lighting, clutter, and improperly fitting clothing or slippers. Common traffic pathways in the home, the bathroom, and access areas to and from the home are the most hazardous areas for older adults (Clemson, Roland, & Cumming, 1997). Measures as simple as installing hand rails in bathrooms and on stairs, ensuring good lighting, and discarding or repairing broken equipment around the home help prevent accidents. Safety assessments by home healthcare nurses play a vital role in promoting safety in the home environment.

Safety measures recommended to reduce the number of falls in acute and extended care facilities are included in the accompanying box, Checklist: Prevention of Falls in the Healthcare Facility. Some examples are shown in Figure 26-2.

Using Side Rails

Side rails (see Fig. 26-2) provide support and aid equilibrium but can pose serious risks for a confused or agitated patient. A person of small stature has a greater risk for entrapment or injury. Patients with a history of falls from beds with elevated side rails are also seriously at risk for another serious incident (Capezuti, Talerico, Strumpt, & Evans, 1998). Between 1993 and 1996, 74 deaths from side rail use were reported to the US Consumer Product Safety Commission (Parker & Miles, 1997). Many nurses assume that side rails prevent falls, but in many cases, a comprehensive individualized assessment, along with creative alternative measures, can reduce routine reliance on side rails. In certain situations in which a patient is sedated, unconscious, or on life-support equipment, side rails may be necessary. Additional measures that promote patient safety when side rails are necessary include the following (Todd, 1997):

- Careful inspection of the hospital bed, side rails, and mattress to identify potential areas where entrapment could occur

Checklist: Prevention of Falls in the Healthcare Facility

A *no* answer to any of these questions indicates the need to take additional measures to guarantee the patient's safety.

	Yes	No
1. Has risk assessment for patient been completed?	☐	☐
2. If patient is at risk, have room and chart been clearly identified to alert all caregivers?	☐	☐
3. Are side rails up?	☐	☐
4. Is bed in low position?	☐	☐
5. Are bed wheels locked? Wheelchair brakes on?	☐	☐
6. Is call bell within patient's reach?	☐	☐
7. Does patient understand how to use the call bell?	☐	☐
8. Is the night light on?	☐	☐
9. Have physical hazards in the room been eliminated (eg, wet area on floor, clutter in pathway to bathroom)?	☐	☐
10. Does patient wear nonskid footwear?	☐	☐
11. Are patient's water, tissues, bedpan/urinal within reach?	☐	☐
12. Is patient aware of activity restrictions?	☐	☐
13. Have any changes in the patient's cognitive or sensory status been reported at change of shift?	☐	☐
14. Are alternative measures to restraints being implemented? What are they?	☐	☐
15. If necessary, are restraints being used? What type?	☐	☐
16. Is patient checked every hour and call bell answered promptly?	☐	☐
17. Are visitors aware of safety protocols?	☐	☐

- Use of a risk profile tool that identifies patients at risk for injury
- Use of padded side rail covers to protect high-risk patients
- Nursing care measures to minimize risk that the patient will try to climb out of bed (offer the bedpan frequently or help the patient out of bed to the bathroom or chair)

Using Restraints and Alternatives

Restraints are physical devices used to limit a patient's movement. Side rails, geriatric chairs with attached trays, and appliances tied at the wrist, ankle, or waist are types of physical restraints. Older patients are more likely to be restrained than younger patients. Figure 26-3 shows types of physical restraints used for adults and children.

Since 1987, the federal government and accrediting agencies have worked to reduce or eliminate using restraints. Initial guidelines formulated by the Health Care Financing Administration as part of the 1987 Omnibus Budget Reconciliation Act emphasized the limited use of restraints in long-term settings. Federal and state mandates, as well as the Joint Commission on Accreditation of Healthcare Organizations (JCAHO), have recommended that acute care agencies use restraints only as a last resort (Brenner & Duffy-Durnin,

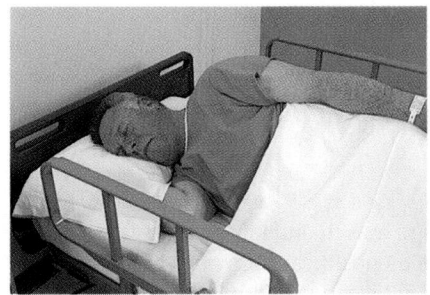
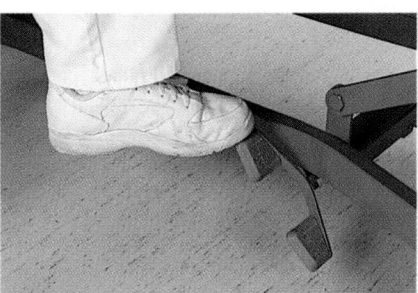
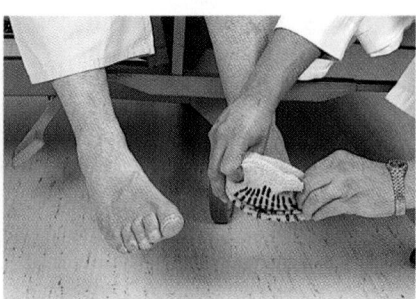

Figure 26-2
Side rails on beds, locking devices on wheeled equipment, and nonskid slippers are some of the safety devices used in healthcare agencies and in the home to prevent falls. (Photo © B. Proud.)

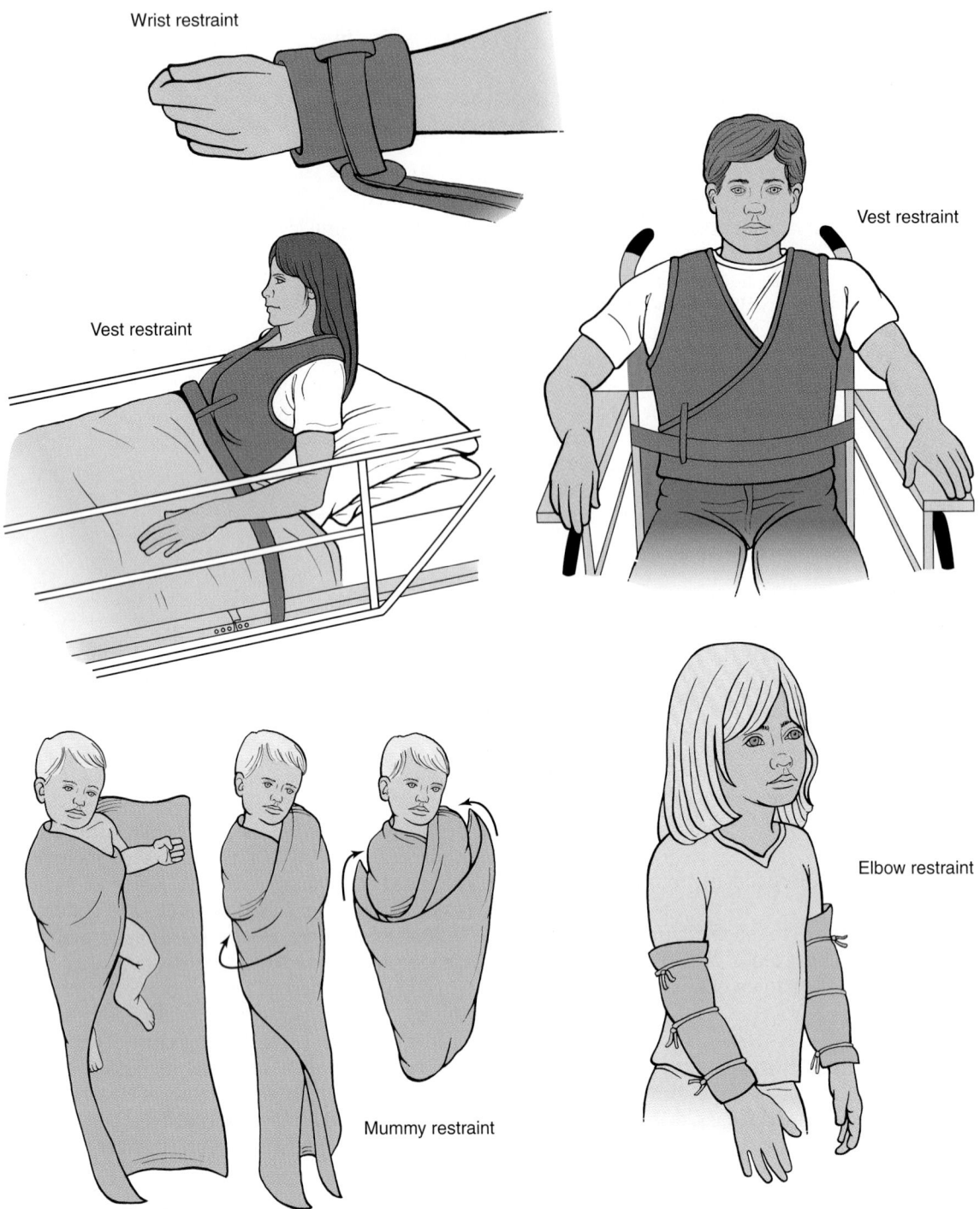

Figure 26-3
A variety of restraints used for adults and children. The purpose of restraints is to help prevent the patient from being harmed. Restraints should not interfere with physiologic functioning, such as impairing circulation, limiting muscular activity to the point of immobilization, or interfering with respiration. Restraints that can be adjusted to the desired activity limitation are most like to be accepted by the patient and family.

1998). The JCAHO, in an effort to reduce the use of restraints in all healthcare settings, stated that restraints can cause "physical and psychological harm, loss of dignity . . . and even death" (JCAHO, 1998). The US Food and Drug Administration requires that manufacturers label restraints as prescription-only devices and has issued recommendations regarding their design and manufacturing. Restraint use is definitely in decline as healthcare providers become more educated about the risks associated with restraint use and alternatives to their use (see the accompanying Research in Nursing box). Physiologic hazards associated with the use of restraints include the following:

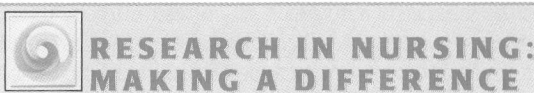

RESEARCH IN NURSING: MAKING A DIFFERENCE

Using an Educational Seminar to Alter Staff Attitudes Toward the Use of Restraints

Although the Omnibus Budget Reconciliation Act regulations have had a positive impact and lessened the use of restraints in long-term care settings, residents still suffer adverse effects from their use. Falls are a leading cause of accidental death, and some caregivers still consider restraints, both physical and pharmacologic, an effective measure to protect the patient and prevent falls. An educational program was explored as an effective measure to change the attitudes and practice of staff in long-term care.

Related Research
Middleton, H., Keene, R., Johnson, C., Elkins, A., & Lee, A. (1999). Physical and pharmacologic restraints

in long-term care facilities. *Journal of Gerontological Nursing, 25*(7), 26–33.

In addition to exploring alternative measures and identifying potential negative outcomes from the use of restraints, participants in this study reported a willingness to review the restraint policy in their agency and use less restrictive measures with elderly residents. This 8-hour educational seminar appeared to alter participants opinions significantly regarding restraint use and encouraged them to be more proactive in promoting a restraint-free environment. Implementations that promote safety while respecting a person's individualized needs can minimize the potential for falls in this population.

- Danger of suffocation from improperly applied vests
- Impaired circulation
- Altered skin integrity (eg, abrasions, skin tears, bruises)
- Pressure ulcers and contractures
- Diminished muscle and bone mass
- Fractures
- Altered nutrition and hydration
- Aspiration and breathing difficulties
- Incontinence

Research has demonstrated that restraints do not guarantee safety and in fact are associated with more lethal injuries to patients.

Careful nursing assessment is the key to identifying appropriate alternatives to restraints and finding an individualized solution (see the accompanying box, Choosing Alternatives to Restraints, and Figure 26-4 for an example of a position-sensitive electronic device [Ambularm] that is an alternative to using restraints). Nursing interventions may effectively reduce confusion or agitation and provide a safe environment. Using a restraint on an older patient who tends to wander is unjustified because a variety of alternative options can be used to keep such patients safe.

Despite all efforts, restraints may be the only solution in some situations. A patient who has threatened suicide or is attempting to remove an endotracheal tube may require a restraint as a last resort for the patient's safety, and the nurse's failure to apply a restraint in this situation may increase the liability risk. DiBartolo (1998) recommends the following R-E-S-T-R-A-I-N-T protocol, which has proved effective for confused patients in an acute care setting:

- **R**espond to the present, not the past. The patient's current condition, not his or her past history, must determine the need for restraints. This includes assessment of physical condition and mental and behavior status.

Choosing Alternatives to Restraints

- Determine whether behavior pattern exists.
- Provide pain relief.
- Involve the family in patient's care.
- Reduce noise.
- Check environment for hazards.
- Use night light.
- Identify door of room (eg, use of balloon, sign, patient's picture, ribbon).
- Use an alarm system (eg, bed or position-sensitive alarms).
- Allow restless patient to walk after ensuring that environment is safe.
- Use half rails or keep side rails in down position.
- Use a large plant or piece of furniture as a barrier to limit wandering from designated area.
- Maintain low bed position.
- Use therapeutic touch.
- Play music or video selections of the patient's choice.
- Use pillows wedged against the side of the chair to keep patient positioned safely.
- Assist with toileting at frequent intervals.
- Arrange for a bedside commode.
- Make the environment as homelike as possible.
- Provide a warm beverage.
- Provide comfortable rocking chairs.
- Allow the patient to assist the staff with simple tasks.
- Encourage daily exercise.
- Investigate possibility of discontinuing bothersome treatment devices (eg, intravenous line, catheter, feeding tube).

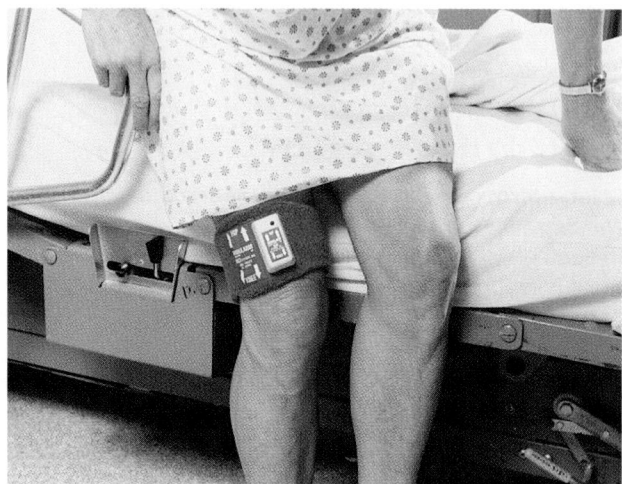

Figure 26-4
Ambularm device. (Photo courtesy of AlertCare, Inc.)

- **E**valuate the potential for injury. Determine whether the patient is at increased risk for harming self or others.
- **S**peak with family members or caregivers. Ask them for insights into the patient's behavior, and enlist their help in making a decision.
- **T**ry alternative measures first. Also, investigate the patient's medication regimen and attempt to discuss options with the patient.
- **R**eassess the patient to determine whether alternatives are successful. Agency policy dictates the frequency of assessments and documentation.
- **A**lert the physician and the patient's family if restraints are indicated. Agency policy, the JCAHO, and state and federal guidelines require an order from a physician or other healthcare professional licensed to prescribe in the state. The order should include the type of restraint, justification for the restraint, criteria for removal, and the intended duration of use.
- **I**ndividualize restraint use. Choose the least restrictive device.
- **N**ote important information on the patient's chart. Document the date and time the restraint is applied, the type of restraint, alternatives that were attempted with their results, and notification of the patient's family and physician. Include frequency of assessment, your findings, regular intervals when the restraint is removed, and nursing interventions.
- **T**ime—limit the use of restraints. Release the patient from the restraint as soon as he or she is no longer a risk to self or others. Restraints should be used no longer than 24 hours on nonpsychiatric patients. After 24 hours, a new order is required.

Clearly stated agency policies help nurses determine when to apply restraints as well as which type to use (see the accompanying Developing Critical Thinking Skills box). The policy reflects the institution's concern for patient safety as well as its respect for the quality of human life. Constant reevaluation of the need for the restraint is vital. Chapter 7

discusses the legal issues involved when restraints are used. Student nurses, from their earliest clinical experiences, need help to identify and assess the cause of a patient's behavior and not just the behavior itself. Careful patient assessment is needed to develop creative alternative strategies. Procedure 26-1 demonstrates the proper method for applying restraints.

Preventing Fires and Maintaining Fire Safety

Careless smoking, faulty electrical equipment, and combustion of anesthetic agents are the most common causes of hospital fires. Cigarettes, grease, and electrical problems are most often responsible for fires in the home.

Healthcare Agency

Orientations in healthcare agencies emphasize fire prevention information and the agency's smoking policy. Nurses are responsible for patients' safety and need to be familiar with the agency's fire safety plan, exits, the location and operation of fire extinguishers, and any special instructions for reporting a fire.

Most hospital procedures emphasize the following priorities and recommend that staff members remember the mnemonic RACE as a guide:

- **R**escue anyone in immediate danger.
- **A**ctivate the fire code system and notify the appropriate person.
- **C**onfine the fire by closing doors and windows.
- **E**vacuate patients and other people to a safe area.

Type ABC fire extinguishers, the most common kind in healthcare agencies, contain a material similar to baking soda that can be used on any type of fire.

Home

The focus of the nurse's teaching parents about home fire safety includes the family having a plan of action similar to that used in healthcare settings. Priorities and practical suggestions are included in the Home Safety Checklist (see the accompanying box).

Preventing Poisoning

Concerted efforts by individuals, communities, state governments, and the federal government have reduced the number of accidental deaths by poisoning. Childproof containers are primarily responsible for this reduction. Nursing interventions involve health education aimed at preventing accidental poisoning in the home. Every household must have the telephone number of the nearest poison control center readily available. The nurse should emphasize to parents to call the poison control center immediately—before attempting any home remedy. Parents should be instructed to keep **syrup of ipecac** on hand but not to administer it unless directed to do so by medical

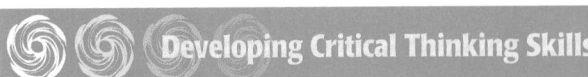

Situation

You are a nursing student caring for Mrs. Mitchell, an 82-year-old nursing home resident who was admitted to a community hospital for treatment of dehydration secondary to pneumonia. Convalescing well, she is now allowed short periods of assisted ambulation and may sit up as tolerated. On the morning you first meet her, she is awake and demanding angrily to have her vest restraint removed so that she can walk independently to the bathroom. You remove her restraint, help her to the bathroom, and wonder whether or not to reapply the restraint as you get her back into bed. She seems clear headed and tells you she has no idea why she is being tied to the bed since she knows enough to use her light to get help when she needs it. She demands you to take the restraint away and pulls back angrily when you attempt to place it over her head. You don't remember any mention of a restraint order when you read her chart the previous day and have not yet gotten report from the charge nurse. Your options are to leave her unrestrained while you clarify the need for the restraint or incur her wrath and forcibly restrain her until you can ascertain the need. You like Mrs. Mitchell and feel sorry that anyone should have to be restrained and are reluctant to wrestle with an 82-year-old woman.

1. Goal of Thinking

Short term: Reach a prudent decision about the need to restrain Mrs. Mitchell until you can clarify the need for the restraint with the charge nurse.

Long term: Evaluate the merits of restraining patients in different types of situations to facilitate future decision making.

2. Adequacy of Knowledge

Pertinent circumstances: In her weakened condition, this patient may be at high risk for falls, and should she attempt to get out of bed unassisted, a fall is a real possibility. You feel sympathetic to her plight of being tied in bed against her will and wonder whether violating patient dignity and liberty is something nurses are routinely expected to do. You are unsure of your legal risk but feel fairly certain that you are responsible for keeping her safe and that not to do so could be grounds for negligence. No other students or staff nurses are in the room, and you cannot clarify the order without leaving the patient unattended.

Prerequisite knowledge: To make a decision in this situation, you need knowledge about the patient's need to be restrained and the benefits and risks of restraining and not restraining her. Given the situation of conflicting goods—preserving her dignity and liberty versus maintaining safety—you need to know how to determine which good ought to triumph in this situation. You should be familiar with the hospital's restraint policy and understand your moral and legal obligations. For example, failure to restrain her may be construed as negligence, whereas restraining her against her will may be assault and battery.

Room for error: Given the significant risks you are incurring by choosing either option—potential fall versus assault to human dignity—there is little room for error. Until you know what her risk for fall is you should err on the side of caution.

Time constraints: You may have time to wait with the patient until another nurse comes into the room who can stay with the patient until you clarify her need to be restrained. If this is not an option, you will need to decide quickly in order to be attentive to other priorities: getting report, beginning patient care, and so forth.

3. Potential Problems

- Sincere desire to do the right thing but great anxiety about not knowing what this is
- Untested, intuitive sense that restraining an alert, uncooperative patient is wrong under any circumstances
- Fear that if you don't restrain her and she falls, you will be legally responsible
- Fear of making a wrong clinical decision that will jeopardize your clinical grade
- Hope that your good interpersonal skills may save the day and buy you the time you need to get help

4. Helpful Resources

Key resources include experienced colleagues, nursing instructor, charge nurse, hospital policy, professional literature on restraint use, hospital risk manager, patient bill of rights.

5. Critique of Judgment/Decision

There are basically two options: to restrain or not restrain Mrs. Mitchell until you can clarify the need for a restraint. If you restrain her and there is no

(continued)

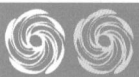

Developing Critical Thinking Skills (Continued)

need, you run the risk of increasing her agitation and violating her dignity. If you fail to restrain her and the restraint is needed, she may fall and suffer a concussion or fractured hip. You decide to reapply the restraint carefully after explaining to Mrs. Mitchell that you are a student nurse and need to check the order for the restraint before leaving it off. Given all your uncertainties, you decide that maintaining the patient's safety ought to be your first priority until you determine whether there are overriding considerations. Mrs. Mitchell is not happy with your decision but seems to understand your reasoning and does not fight you when you reapply the vest restraint. You promise to return quickly and keep your promise.

When you talk with the charge nurse she tells you that there is no need for Mrs. Mitchell to be restrained and that the night nurse tends to be overzealous about protecting elderly patients. You happily return to Mrs. Mitchell and remove the restraint. You later meet with your instructor to see what you can do to ensure that Mrs. Mitchell and other patients on the unit are not restrained for inappropriate reasons. Your instructor compliments you for reasoning well about what was in this patient's best interests. She remarks that had there been a need to restrain the patient you may have jeopardized her safety by unthinkingly following your sympathetic instinct to leave her unrestrained.

authorities to induce vomiting. Typical dosage recommendations for syrup of ipecac include the following (Eisenhauer et al., 1998):

Children
- 6 to 12 months of age—administer 10 mL orally
- Older than 1 year of age—give 15 mL orally followed by 1 to 2 glassfuls of whatever fluid the child will tolerate

Adults
- Administer 30 mL

Syrup of ipecac is effective only when given within the first 20 to 30 minutes after a poison has been ingested. Vomiting should occur within 30 minutes. Parents may be instructed to bring the child immediately to an emergency facility for treatment. The focus of emergency treatment of poisoning is to stabilize vital body functions, prevent the absorption of the poison, and encourage excretion of the toxic substance. Nursing education efforts can also change behaviors that place older adults at risk for poisoning. Suggestions for preventing poisoning in older adults are included in the accompanying box, Focus on the Older Adult.

All healthcare providers should recommend that a carbon monoxide detector be installed to alert family members to toxic levels of the gas. The gas or oil company or local health authority can help identify and remove sources of contamination. Many communities are considering legislation requiring installation of carbon monoxide detectors by homeowners and landlords.

Preventing Suffocation

Suffocation results almost immediately in unconsciousness, followed by respiratory and cardiac arrest. Emergency measures must start without delay, beginning with removal of any obstruction and administration of cardiopulmonary resuscitation. The nurse may have the opportunity to give

child care instruction emphasizing careful supervision of children and outlining specific situations that place children at risk for suffocation. Health education is a valuable preventive force. Refer to the Home Safety Checklist for specific interventions.

Preventing Injury From Firearms

Nurses are in a unique position to raise awareness and help reduce high-risk behavior that may lead to firearm injuries and deaths. In homes, schools, and other healthcare settings, nurses can provide information that may persuade parents to keep guns away from children. Parents may be unaware of how common gunshot injuries are or misinformed about the dangers when a gun is accessible to children and young adults. As a prevention partner, the nurse can begin to have an impact on this epidemic of gun injuries and death. The Home Safety Checklist recommends measures to prevent injury from firearms.

Preventing Equipment-Related Accidents

Healthcare Agency

With a marked increase in the use of highly sophisticated electrical equipment in healthcare settings, it is especially important for health practitioners to learn to use equipment properly and to recognize signs that the equipment is not functioning correctly. Using suction devices with inadequate vacuum and rate regulators or infusion equipment that delivers erratic amounts of solution has also resulted in equipment-related accidents. A failure to use protective belts or side rails on carts and to lock wheelchair wheels can also result in patient injury.

Electrical equipment can present a particular safety hazard to both patient and health practitioner when safety

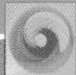

Applying Restraints

Equipment

Restraint

Padding, if necessary, for bony prominences

Action	Rationale
1. Determine the need for restraints. Assess patient's physical condition, behavior, and mental status.	Restraints should be used only as a last resort when alternative measures have failed, and the patient is at increased risk for harming himself or others.
2. Confirm agency policy for application of restraints. Secure a physician's order.	Policy protects the patient and the nurse and specifies guidelines for application as well as type of restraint and duration.
3. Explain reason for use to patient and family. Clarify how care will be given and needs will be met and that use of restraint is a temporary measure.	Explanation to patient and family may lessen confusion and anger and provide reassurance. A clearly stated agency policy on application of restraints should be available for patient and family to read. In a long-term care facility, the family must give consent before a restraint is applied.
4. Wash your hands.	Handwashing deters the spread of microorganisms.
5. Apply restraints according to manufacturer's direction:	Proper application ensures that there is no interference with patient's respiration and circulation. The US Food and Drug Administration advises manufacturers to place "front" and "back" labels on vest restraints and that correct size be used.
a. Choose the least restrictive type of device that allows the greatest possible degree of mobility.	This provides minimal restriction.
b. Pad bony prominences.	Padding prevents skin breakdown.
c. For restraint applied to extremity, ensure that two fingers can be inserted between the restraint and patient's wrist or ankle.	This prevents impaired circulation to extremity.

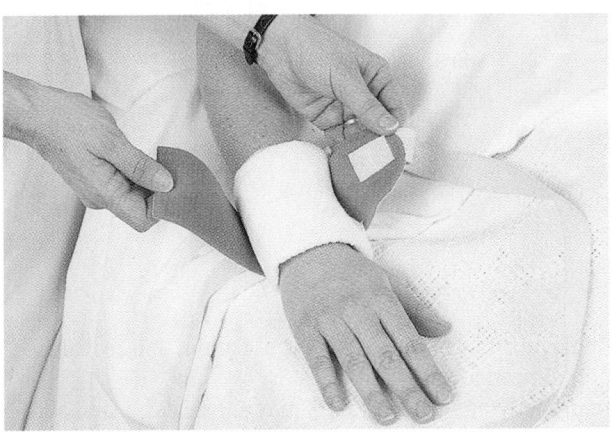

Action 5b: Applying restraint over padded bony prominences.

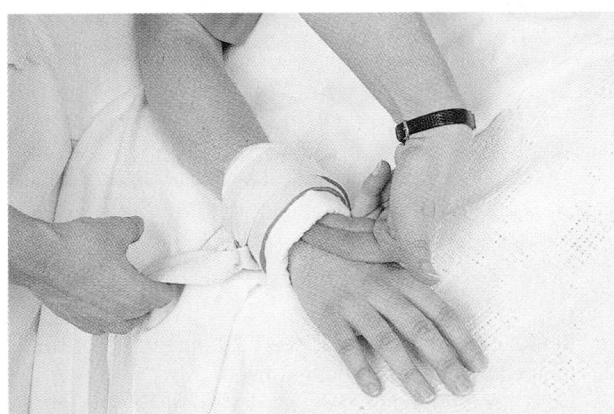

Action 5c: Ensuring that two fingers can be inserted between the restraint and the wrist.

(*continued*)

PROCEDURE 26-1

Applying Restraints (Continued)

d. Maintain restrained extremity in normal anatomic position.
e. Use appropriate tie for all restraints.

f. Fasten restraint to the bed frame and *not the side rail.* Site should not be readily accessible to the patient.

This lessens possibility of contracture or musculoskeletal injury.

A quick-release knot ensures that restraint will not tighten when pulled and can be removed quickly in an emergency. Restraint secured to a side rail may injure the patient when side rail is lowered. Tying restraint out of patient's reach promotes security.

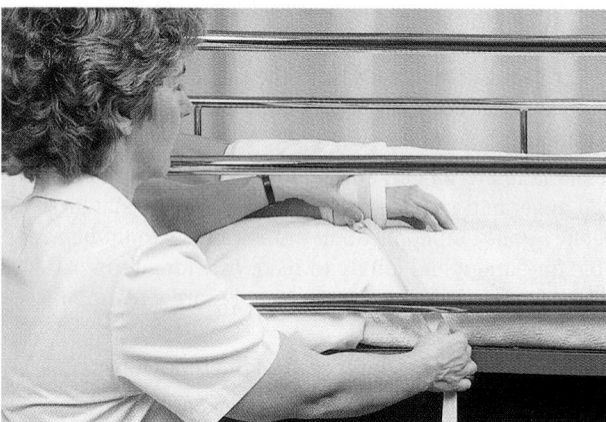

Action 5d: Keeping extremity in normal anatomic position.

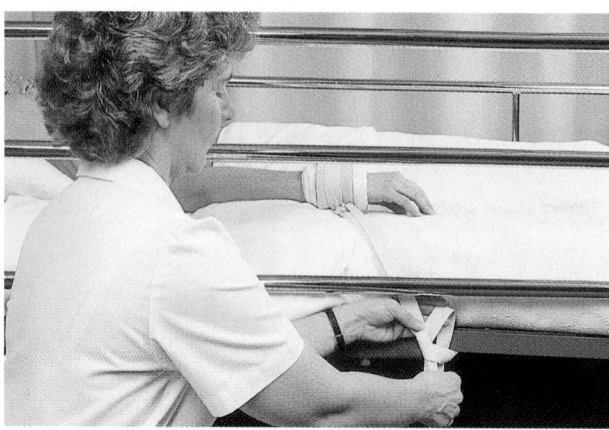

Action 5f: Fastening restraint to bed frame.

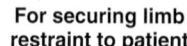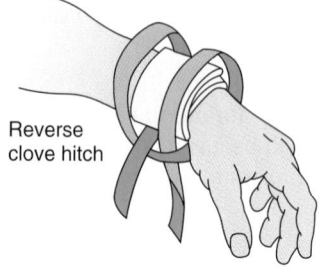

For securing limb restraint to patient

Reverse clove hitch

For securing restraint to bedframe

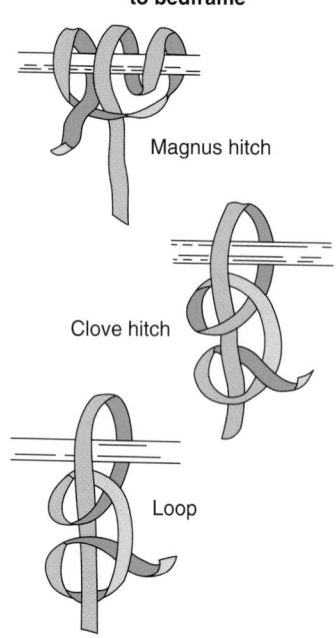

Magnus hitch

Clove hitch

Loop

Action 5e: Knots for restraints.

6. Remove restraint at least every 2 hours or according to agency policy and patient need.
   a. Check for signs of decreased circulation or impaired skin integrity.

   b. Perform range-of-motion exercises before reapplying.

Removal allows for assessment of patient and reevaluation of need for restraint.

Improperly applied restraints may cause skin tears, abrasions, or bruises. Decreased circulation may result in paleness, coolness, decreased sensation, tingling, numbness, or pain in an extremity.

Exercise increases circulation in the restrained extremity.

(continued)

PROCEDURE 26-1

Applying Restraints (Continued)
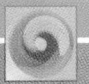

7. Reassure patient at regular intervals. Store call bell within easy reach.

8. Assess for signs of sensory deprivation, such as increased sleeping, day-dreaming, anxiety, panic, and hallucinations.

9. Wash your hands.

10. Document reason for restraining patient, alternative measures attempted before applying the restraint, date and time of application, type of restraint, times when removed, and result and frequency of nursing assessment every 2 hours. Obtain a new order after 24 hours if restraints are still necessary.

Reassurance demonstrates caring and provides opportunity for sensory stimulation as well as ongoing assessment and evaluation. Call bell can summon assistance quickly.

Use of restraints may decrease environmental stimulation and result in sensory deprivation.

Handwashing deters the spread of microorganisms.

Careful documentation supports use of restraints, alternative measures to ensure safety, and assessment data. The Joint Commission on Accreditation of Healthcare Organizations recommends a 24-hour restraint limit for all nonpsychiatric patients.

---

measures are ignored. Most electrical equipment used in hospitals is equipped with three-prong plugs. The third prong, when inserted into a properly wired wall outlet, provides a ground for the piece of equipment. A **ground** is a connection from an electricity source to the earth through which electric current leakage can be harmlessly conducted. The accompanying box lists guidelines to help reduce the number of equipment-related accidents.

Home

Accidents in the home frequently result from careless use of equipment or from malfunctioning or poorly maintained equipment. Many injuries and deaths from electric shock can be prevented. Overloaded electric circuits, faulty appliances, frayed wires, careless use of electrical equipment, and handling of electrical devices and cords when shoes and hands are wet often result in injury or death. Refer to the Home Safety Checklist for specific guidelines to prevent electrical injury.

Preventing Procedure-Related Accidents

The nurse must always be cautious and alert to prevent procedure-related accidents. Errors are possible when administering medications or intravenous solutions, transferring a patient, changing a dressing, or applying external heat to a patient's extremity. Therefore, nurses must follow correct procedures when administering care. Safeguards to prevent errors include making sure that the patient is correctly identified (Fig. 26-5). The nurse should use all available resources to answer any questions about correct procedure.

Filing an Incident Report

An accident in a healthcare agency requires filling out an **incident report,** a confidential document that objectively describes the circumstances of the accident. The report also details the patient's response and the examination and treatment of the patient after the incident. The nurse completes the incident report immediately after an accident and is responsible for recording the incident and its effect on the patient in the medical record. The incident report itself is not a part of the medical record and should not be mentioned in the documentation. Because laws vary among different states, nurses must know their own state law regarding incident reports.

All incident reports are carefully reviewed to detect any potentially threatening situation or pattern. A conference held after the incident report has been filed focuses on preventing similar occurrences in the future and continuing to deliver quality nursing care. Incident reports are discussed in more detail in Chapter 7.

Evaluating

Nurses must evaluate the effectiveness of their interventions to promote environmental safety and prevent injury. If the expected patient outcomes have been met and evaluative criteria have been satisfied, the patient should be able to accomplish the following:

• Correctly identify real and potential unsafe environmental situations
• Implement safety measures in the environment
• Use available resources for safety information
• Incorporate accident prevention practices into the activities of daily living
• Remain free of injury

Home Safety Checklist

Fire and Burn Safety

Have a list of emergency phone numbers posted near the telephone.

Install smoke detectors in each room (or at a minimum, on each floor).

Replace smoke detector batteries when you reset your clock.

Have a fire extinguisher available on each floor, and know how to use it.

Practice a fire escape plan with your family.

Teach all family members to stop, drop, and roll if clothing catches on fire.

Keep matches and lighters stored out of reach of children.

Keep lighted candles out of children's reach.

Buy flame-resistant children's clothing, particularly sleepwear.

Keep bedroom doors closed while sleeping (use monitor to listen for a child).

Have ashtrays readily available if there is a smoker in the house.

Enforce a strict "no smoking in bed" policy.

After a party, check waste baskets, ashtrays, furniture, and carpets for carelessly discarded cigarettes.

Turn off a kerosene heater when no one is in the room and at bedtime.

Operate your fireplace or wood-burning stove safely (flue open, firescreen covering the opening, annual chimney cleaning, proper disposal of ashes).

Prevent trash or paint-saturated rags from accumulating in your garage.

Store oily rags, gasoline, or other flammables away from heating sources or open flames, such as the pilot light of the water heater.

Cook on back burners, and turn pot handles toward the back of the stove.

Keep hot dishes away from the edges of tables and counters.

Set water at a safe temperature (below 120°F).

Check bath water temperature with the back of your wrist before placing a child in bath.

Use sunscreen and protective clothing to minimize exposure to the sun and prevent sunburn.

Electrical Safety

Maintain electrical cords in good condition.

Protect unused electric outlets with safety covers.

Use the proper replacement for a blown fuse.

Keep an electric space heater away from curtains and flammable material.

Turn off appliances before going to bed or leaving the house.

Hire a professional to do electrical repairs.

Never overload wall outlets or extension cords.

Unplug appliances that are not in use.

Do not permit children to use the microwave.

Preventing Poisoning

Keep the phone number for the local poison control center next to the telephone.

Keep the emergency drug, syrup of ipecac, in the home.

Store all medicines in child-resistant containers in a locked medicine cabinet.

Destroy old medicines (flush down the toilet).

Keep all poisonous plants out of a child's reach.

Avoid eating any fresh or prepared foods that look or smell spoiled.

Store cleaning products, insecticides, and corrosives safely out of a child's reach.

Avoid mixing caustic products with any other household product (dangerous chemical reactions may occur).

Keep shampoos and cosmetics stored in a safe place.

Use safety latches on cabinets.

Store alcoholic beverages out of a child's reach.

Check that paint or finish on furniture and toys is nontoxic.

Install a carbon monoxide detector in your home.

Have your furnace professionally inspected each year.

Keep vents and chimneys clear of debris, and have them checked seasonally.

Don't operate cars, motorized equipment, or charcoal or gas grills in enclosed spaces.

Preventing Falls and Other Injuries

Keep stairways clear and uncluttered.

Maintain walkways, stairs, and railings in good repair.

Keep stairs, hallways, outside walkways, and working areas well lit.

Install safety gates at tops and bottoms of stairways.

(continued)

Home Safety Checklist (*Continued*)

Apply nonslip adhesive strips to the bottom surface of the tub or shower.

Have a raised toilet seat with support arms available if necessary.

Provide grab bars next to the toilet and in the tub or shower area.

Use sturdy chairs that have armrests.

Eliminate scatter rugs, or secure them with adhesive strips on the underside.

Use a handheld device, such as pincers, when reaching for inaccessible items.

Buckle a child into an approved automobile safety seat even when making short trips.

Firearm Safety

Keep guns and ammunition stored separately and locked up.

Install trigger locks on all guns.

Make certain that the key to the locked gun storage area is not available to a child or young person.

Discuss the risk for injury from guns with your children.

Instruct your child never to touch a gun or remain in a friend's house where a gun is accessible.

Preventing Asphyxiation or Choking

Keep plastic bags out of a child's reach.

Check that crib slats are no more than $2\frac{3}{8}$ inches apart.

Ensure that the mattress fits the sides of the crib snugly.

Remove soft pillows or thick blankets from your infant's crib.

Never place an infant on a waterbed to sleep.

Cut food into small pieces before giving it to a young child.

Supervise young children when eating and drinking.

Avoid giving peanuts, hard candy, or other small treats to a young child.

Keep small objects, such as jewelry, buttons, and safety pins, out of a child's reach.

Use toys appropriate for the child's age.

Always watch a child who is in the tub.

Cover wading pools and sandboxes when not in use.

Check that nearby swimming pools are enclosed with a fence that your child cannot easily climb over.

Keep pool rescue equipment nearby.

Supervise your child closely when near water.

Know how to perform cardiopulmonary resuscitation and the Heimlich maneuver.

Focus on the Older Adult

Preventing Poisoning in the Elderly

Although poisonings happen more frequently in children, poison control centers receive many calls from adults, particularly older adults, regarding accidental poisonings. The older population uses more medications than any other age group and may also be more susceptible to the effects of various drugs. The following information includes suggestions for preventing poisonings in the older individual, as well as adults of any age:

- Do not hesitate to call the physician, nurse, or pharmacist with any questions.
- Keep the telephone numbers for your healthcare providers and the Poison Control Center in a readily accessible place.
- Develop good communication with your physician, nurse, and pharmacist.
- Report side effects from medications to healthcare provider.
- Do not stop taking any prescription drug or change the dose without first consulting the physician or nurse.
- Request large-print labels from your pharmacist.
- Use a medication calendar or diary to keep track of your dosing schedule.
- Use a pill dispenser as a medication reminder tool.
- Avoid doubling a dose if you forget a medication. Check with the physician or nurse first.
- Avoid mixing alcohol with medicines without first checking with the pharmacist.
- Do not share medications with others or take their pills.
- When a drug is discontinued, throw away any remaining medication.

Decreasing Equipment-Related Accidents

- Use equipment only for the use for which it was intended.
- Do not operate equipment with which you are unfamiliar.
- Handle equipment with care to prevent damaging it.
- Use three-prong electric plugs whenever possible.
- Do not twist or bend electric cords. The wires inside the cord may break.
- Be alert to signs that indicate equipment is faulty, such as breaks in electric cords, sparks, smoke, electric shocks, loose or missing parts, and unusual noises or odors. Report signs of trouble immediately.
- Make certain that electric cords are not in a position to be trapped as beds are raised or lowered. This can strip insulation covering the electric wires.
- Be alert for wet surfaces on areas where electric cords or connections are present.

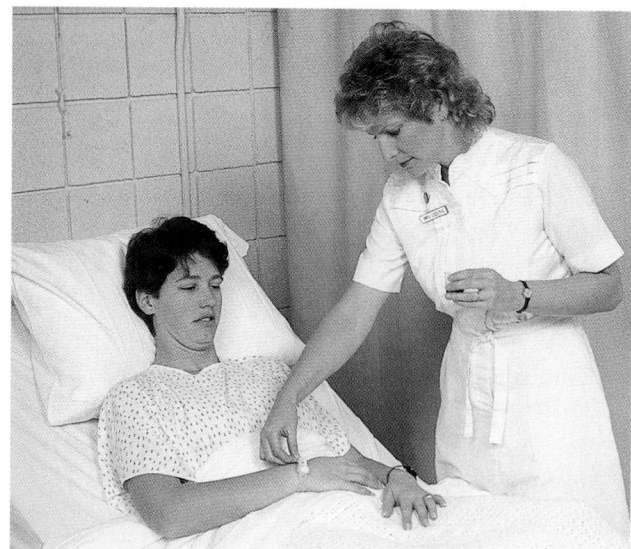

Figure 26-5
An essential nursing responsibility is checking the patient's identification bracelet before any procedure. Here, the nurse checks the patient's identification before administering medications.

Learning Outcomes

After studying this chapter, the learner should be able to accomplish the following:

1. Define the key terms used in the chapter.

    asphyxiation   poison control center
    ground   restraint
    incident report   syrup of ipecac

2. Identify factors that affect safety in an individual's environment.
3. Identify patients at risk for injury.
4. Describe specific safety risk factors for each developmental age.
5. Select nursing diagnoses for patients in unsafe situations.
6. Describe preventive strategies to decrease the risk for injury in the home.
7. Describe nursing interventions that effectively prevent injury to patients in healthcare settings.
8. Identify alternatives to using restraints.
9. Describe health teaching interventions to promote safety for each developmental age.
10. Evaluate the effectiveness of safety interventions.

Critical Thinking Exercises

1. You are the visiting nurse for a frail, older patient who lives alone in her own home and prizes her independence. You assess her to be at high risk for falls because of her general weakness, the medication she takes, and a long history of indifference to safety counseling. What nursing interventions are likely to be most effective in ensuring her safety?

2. Identify the safety hazards for which you and family members of different ages are most at risk. What anticipatory planning and teaching could be done to prevent these hazards? Note your willingness and that of your family to make the necessary changes, and identify the nursing strategies that would be most likely to secure patient cooperation in making needed changes.

Study Questions

1. A school nurse reviewing healthcare topics for adolescents is aware that
    a. tobacco use has decreased in this age group
    b. ten percent of teenagers have attempted suicide
    c. teenagers are more likely to drink and drive
    d. peer pressure is insignificant

2. When transporting a toddler in a motor vehicle, car seats are mandatory

a. in all 50 states

b. in 36 of the 50 states

c. if a seat belt is not available

d. on interstate highways

3. Which child has the greatest risk for choking and suffocating?

    a. a toddler playing with his 9-year-old brother's construction set

    b. a 4-year-old eating yogurt for lunch

    c. an infant covered with a small blanket and asleep in the crib

    d. a 3-year-old drinking a glass of juice

4. Nursing consideration regarding use of side rails for a confused patient is based on the knowledge that

    a. they prevent confused patients from wandering

    b. a history of a previous fall from a bed with raised side rails is insignificant

    c. alternative measures are ineffective to prevent wandering

    d. a person of small stature is at increased risk for injury from entrapment

5. The leading cause of accidental death for people 79 years of age and older is

    a. fires

    b. exposure to temperature extremes

    c. drug overdose

    d. falls

6. Nursing education efforts that focus on prevention of firearm injuries are important because

    a. the elder population is particularly at risk

    b. deaths among adolescents and children have increased sharply

    c. the National Safety Council recommends that every household have a gun to protect family members

    d. they have successfully contributed to a decrease in injuries and deaths from guns

7. The US and Canadian Red Cross will not accept blood donations from anyone who has had body piercing within the previous

    a. 1 year

    b. 2 years

    c. 5 years

    d. 10 years

8. Mr. Kennedy is a disoriented, older resident who likes to wander the halls of his long-term care facility. As an alternative to using restraints, the nurse might

    a. seat him in a geriatric chair

    b. use the sheets to secure him snugly in his bed

    c. keep the bed in the high position

    d. identify his door with his picture and a balloon

9. While discussing home safety with the nurse, Mrs. Fuller admits that she always smokes a cigarette in bed before falling asleep at night. An appropriate nursing diagnosis would be

a. Impaired Gas Exchange related to cigarette smoking

b. Anxiety related to inability to stop smoking

c. Risk for Suffocation related to unfamiliarity with fire prevention guidelines

d. Knowledge Deficit related to lack of follow-through of recommendation to stop smoking

10. Mr. D'Ambro has weakened knees due to arthritis. The home healthcare nurse is aware that he understands the need for safety modifications at home because he

    a. uses the towel bar for support to stand up from the commode

    b. leans on the pedestal table in his bedroom when he dresses

    c. sits only in chairs with armrests

    d. uses a small stepladder to reach an item on an upper shelf

11. When a fire occurs in a patient's room, the nurse's priority should be to

    a. rescue the patient

    b. extinguish the fire

    c. sound the alarm

    d. run for help

12. The nurse is planning a health teaching session for new parents. The topic is responding to a poisoning emergency. The initial parental response should be to

    a. use salt water to induce vomiting

    b. rush the child to the emergency department

    c. call the poison control center

    d. administer syrup of ipecac

13. JCAHO guidelines regarding use of restraints recommend that

    a. vest restraints be used because they are the least restrictive type

    b. restraints should only be used for 48 hours in nonpsychiatric patients

    c. restraints should be applied to prevent wandering behavior

    d. alternative measures must be attempted first

14. The nurse orients an older patient to the safety features in her hospital room. A vital component of this admission routine is to

    a. explain how to use the telephone

    b. introduce the patient to her roommate

    c. review the hospital policy on visiting hours

    d. explain how to operate the call bell

15. When completing an incident report, the nurse should

    a. include suggestions to prevent the accident from recurring

    b. provide minimal information about the incident

    c. discuss the details with the patient before documenting them

    d. objectively describe the incident in detail

Answers With Rationale

1. The correct response is *b.* Ten percent of teenagers attempt suicide. Tobacco use in this age group has hit a 16-year high point, with half of those who experiment with cigarettes becoming regular smokers. Teenagers are less likely to drink and drive but more likely to have an accident if they do combine both behaviors. Much of adolescents' spare time is spent away from home and with peers, and peers are most influential in their decision-making.

2. The correct response is *a.* All 50 states require safety car seats for infants and toddlers at all times.

3. The correct response is *a.* A young child may place small or loose parts in his or her mouth; a toy that is safe for a 9-year-old could kill a toddler. An infant sleeping in a crib without a pillow or large blanket and a 3- and 4-year-old drinking juice and eating yogurt are not particular safety risks.

4. The correct response is *d.* Studies of restraint-related deaths have shown that people of small stature are more likely to slip through or between the side rails. The desire to safeguard a patient from wandering is not sufficient reason to justify use of side rails. Creative use of alternative measures indicates respect for the patient's dignity and may in fact prevent more serious fall-related injuries. A history of falls from a bed with raised side rails is significant warning of a future serious incident.

5. The correct response is *d.* Falls are the leading cause of accidental death in the population 79 years of age and older. Fires, exposure to temperature extremes, and drug overdose are significant causes of accidental death, but not in this age group.

6. The correct response is *b.* Deaths among adolescents and children have increased sharply since 1990. Keeping a gun in the home can have dangerous consequences and increases the risk for domestic violence. Young children may also be unintentionally injured or killed. Recent efforts to prevent injuries from guns have become more serious because violent behavior has increased in our society.

7. The correct response is *a.* Anyone who has had a body piercing is at risk of infection from improperly sterilized instruments or an unclean environment. The greatest threat is from hepatitis B. US and Canadian blood banks restrict blood donations from these individuals for 1 year to eliminate any risk for contaminating the blood supply.

8. The correct response is *d.* Identifying his door with his picture and the balloon may work as an alternative to restraints. Using the geriatric chair and sheets are forms of physical restraint. Leaving the bed in the high position is a safety risk and would probably result in a fall.

9. The correct answer is *c.* Because Mrs. Fuller is not aware that smoking in bed is extremely dangerous, she is at risk for suffocation from fire. The other three nursing diagnoses are correctly stated but not a priority in this situation.

10. The correct response is *c.* Chairs with armrests increase the patient's leverage as he attempts to rise. Towel bars are not designed to provide support, the pedestal table is unsteady and unsafe, and standing on a stool and reaching puts the patient at risk for falling.

11. The correct response is *a.* The patient's safety is always the priority. Sounding the alarm and extinguishing the fire are important after the patient is safe. Calling for help, rather than running for assistance, allows you to remain with your patients and is more appropriate, if possible.

12. The correct response is *c.* Always call the poison control center before attempting any home remedies or administering syrup of ipecac. These responses may be dangerous for the victim. The poison control center can supply the doctor or emergency department with specific information to assist in the victim's care.

13. The correct response is *d.* Wandering behavior is not an indication for restraints. Careful assessment and attempts to find effective alternative measures must be attempted before applying a restraint. Less restrictive restraints may include side rails, a geriatric chair, or wrist restraints instead of a vest. JCAHO recommends not using restraints for more than 24 hours on nonpsychiatric patients.

14. The correct response is *d.* Knowing how to use the call bell is a safety priority, whereas knowing how to use the phone, meeting one's roommate, and an awareness of visiting hours will not necessarily prevent an accidental injury.

15. The correct response is *d.* An incident report is a legal document and must be stated as objectively and completely as possible. It is not a collaborative effort with the patient, and any suggestions to prevent this from happening again should be discussed at a postincident conference.

Bibliography

Aggeles, T. (1998). Child abuse. *The Nursing Spectrum, 7*(21), 12–13.

Allan, M. (1998). Elder abuse: A challenge for home care nurses. *Home Healthcare Nurse, 16*(2), 103–110.

Armstrong, M. (1998). A clinical look at body piercing. *RN, 61*(9), 26–30.

Benson, S. (1997). The older adult and fear of crime. *Journal of Gerontological Nursing, 23*(10), 25–31.

Brenner, Z., & Duffy-Durnin, K. (1998). Toward restraint-free care. *American Journal of Nursing, 98*(12), 16F–16I.

Carlson, D. (1998). Uncovering the clues of child abuse. *Nursing, 28*(11), 32hn10–11.

Capezuti, E., Talerico, K., Strumpt, N., & Evans, L. (1998). Individualized assessment and intervention in bilateral siderail use. *Geriatric Nursing, 19*(6), 322–330.

Carroll, M., Morin, K., Hayes, E., & Carter, S. (1999). Assessing students' perceived threats to safety in the community. *Nurse Educator, 24*(1), 31–35.

Carroll, V. (1999). Workplace violence. *American Journal of Nursing, 99*(3), 60.

Clemson, L., Roland, M., & Cumming, R. (1997). Hazards in homes for elderly people. *Occupational Therapy Journal of Research, 17*(3), 200–211.

DiBartolo, V. (1998). 9 Steps to effective restraint use. *RN, 61*(12), 23–24.

Eisenhauer, L., Nichols, L., Spencer, R., & Bergan, F. (1998). *Clinical pharmacology & nursing management* (5th ed.). Philadelphia: Lippincott Williams & Wilkins.

Fortin, J., Yeaw, E., Campbell, S., & Jameson, S. (1998). An analysis of risk assessment tolls for falls in the elderly. *Home Healthcare Nurse, 16*(9), 624–629.

Gray-Vickrey. (1999). Recognizing elder abuse. *Nursing, 29*(9), 52–53.

Hoskin, A. (1998). Fatal falls: Trends and characteristics. *Statistical Bulletin, 79*(2), 10–15.

Hunter, E. (1997). Violence prevention in the home health setting. *Home Healthcare Nurse, 15*(6), 403–408.

Joint Commission on Accreditation of Healthcare Organizations. (1998). *1998 Hospital accreditation standards*. Oakbrook Terrace, IL: Author.

Lynch, S. (1997). Elder abuse: What to look for, how to intervene. *American Journal of Nursing, 97*(1), 27–32.

Melillo, K., & Futrell, M. (1998). Wandering and technology devices. *Journal of Gerontological Nursing, 24*(8), 32–38.

Owen, B. (1999). Preventing back injuries. *American Journal of Nursing, 99*(5), 76.

Parker, K., & Miles, S. (1997). Deaths caused by bedrails. *Journal of the American Geriatrics Society, 45*(7), 797–802.

Rawsky, E. (1998). Review of literature on falls among the elderly. *Image—The Journal of Nursing Scholarship, 30*(1), 47–52.

Ray, W., Tay, J., Meador, K., Thapa, P., Brown, A., Kajihara, H., Davis, C., Gideon, P., & Griffin, M. (1997). A randomized trial of a consultation service to reduce falls in nursing homes. *Journal of the American Medical Association, 278*(7), 557–562.

Rice, R. (1998). Home visit safety. *Geriatric Nursing, 19*(4), 241–242.

Shahinian, B., & Hawke, M. (1998). The terrible truth about teens and tobacco. *The Nursing Spectrum, 7*(18), 4–5.

Shumway-Cook, A. & Gruber, W., & Liao, S. (1997). The effect of multidimensional exercises on balance, mobility, and fall risk in community-dwelling older adults. *Physical Therapy, 77*(1), 46–57.

Sloane, M., & Holcomb, C. (1997). Where there's smoke. . . . *The Nursing Spectrum, 6*, 4–5.

Sullivan, G. (1999). Minimizing your risk in patient falls. *RN, 62*(4), 69–72.

Taft, C., Michalide, A., & Taft, A. *Child passengers at risk in America: A national study of car seat misuse*. Washington, DC: National SAFE KIDS Campaign, February 1999.

Tatara, T. (1997). *Summaries of the statistical data on elder abuse in domestic settings for FY 95 and FY 96*. Washington, DC: National Center on Elder Abuse.

Teret, S., et al. (1998). Making guns safer. *Issues in Science and Technology, 14*(4), 37–40.

Tideiksaar, R. (1996). Preventing falls: Home hazard checklists to help older patients protect themselves. *Geriatrics, 41*, 26–28.

Todd, J. (1997). Hospital bed side rails. *Nursing, 27*(5), 67.

US Bureau of the Census (1998). *Statistical Abstract of the US: 1998* (118th ed.). Washington, DC: Author.

Ventura, M. (1997). Air bag safety alert. *RN, 60*(4), 43–44.

Walker, B. (1998). Preventing falls. *RN, 61*(5), 40–42.

Winslow, E., & Jacobson, A. (1998a). Reducing falls in older patients. *American Journal of Nursing, 98*(10), 22.

Winslow, E., & Jacobson, A. (1998b). The effects of childhood sexual abuse on women. *American Journal of Nursing, 98*(8), 67–70.

Chapter 27
Asepsis

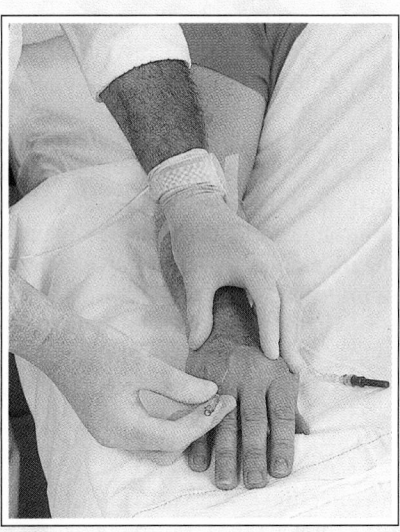

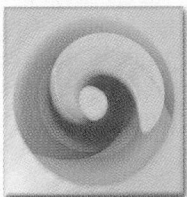

Thinking Critically About
Nursing's Blended Skills

Before reading this chapter, think about the types of blended skills you will need to break the chain of infection effectively by using the appropriate medical and surgical asepsis techniques.

- You are working on a medical floor in a hospital where some nurses are rarely seen with gloves while others are rarely seen without gloves. You are asked to lead a noon conference about when to glove.

- You are scrubbing in for a surgical procedure and notice a colleague "going through the motions" of a scrub but not really "working up a lather." When questioned, she replies that her hands have been very dry and she's trying to "give them a break" until they heal.

- A woman undergoing chemotherapy treatment for leukemia tells you that she understands she is at high risk for infection because of her compromised immune status. Her concern is how to respond to the 20 to 30 children in her Church who know and love her and who are used to greeting her with a big hug Sunday morning. I want to "play it safe" but I know that I need these hugs too!

- Family members of a teenager with varicella see the isolation sign and setup and ask for your help before they enter the room.

What cognitive, technical, interpersonal, and ethical/legal skills do you think you will need to respond to the challenges described above?

A major concern for health practitioners is the danger of spreading microorganisms from person to person and from place to place. Microorganisms are naturally present in almost all environments. Some are beneficial, but some are not. Some are harmless to most people, and others are harmful to many people. Still others are harmless except in certain circumstances.

The efforts of many groups are directed toward a microorganism-safe environment: government agencies at the international, national, state, and local levels; health personnel; and individuals. Such efforts include mass immunization programs, laws concerning safe sewage disposal, regulations for the control of communicable diseases, and hospital infection-surveillance programs. Medical science continues to grapple with increasingly virulent organisms that have become drug resistant and with problems related to immunologically compromised patients. Prevention of infection is a major focus for nurses. As primary caregivers, nurses are involved in identifying, preventing, controlling, and teaching the patient about infection. Use of the nursing process can prove critical in breaking the chain of infection.

Infection Prevention and Control

Infection Cycle

An **infection** is a disease state that results from the presence of pathogens in or on the body. A **pathogen** is a disease-producing microorganism. An infection occurs as a result of a cyclic process, as shown in Figure 27-1. The six components in the infection cycle are as follows:

- Infectious agent
- Reservoir
- Portal of exit
- Means of transmission
- Portal of entry
- Susceptible host

Infectious Agent

Some of the more prevalent agents that cause infection are bacteria, viruses, and fungi. **Bacteria** are the most significant and most commonly observed infection-causing agents in healthcare institutions. Bacteria can be categorized in various ways. According to shape, they are classified as spherical (cocci), rod shaped (bacilli), or corkscrew shaped (spirochetes). Based on their reaction to the Gram stain, bacteria are either gram positive or gram negative. *Gram-positive bacteria* have a thick cell wall that resists decolorization (loss of color) and are stained violet. *Gram-negative bacteria* have chemically more complex cell walls and can be decolorized by alcohol. This difference is vital for the physician selecting an antibiotic to prevent or treat an infection. Antibiotics are classified as specifically effective against only gram-positive organisms or as broad spectrum and effective against several groups of microorganisms.

Another distinguishing characteristic of bacteria is their need for oxygen. Most bacteria require oxygen to live and grow and are therefore referred to as **aerobic**. Those that can live without oxygen are **anaerobic** bacteria.

A **virus** is the smallest of all microorganisms and can be seen only with an electron microscope. Many infections are caused by viruses, including the common cold and the

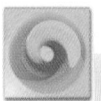

COGNITIVE SKILLS

- Basic knowledge of the infection cycle and nursing interventions to break the chain of infection
- Knowledge of factors that reduce the incidence of nosocomial infection
- Knowledge of Centers for Disease Control and Prevention guidelines for standard and transmission-based precautions and isolation systems

TECHNICAL SKILLS

- Ability to implement techniques correctly for medical and surgical asepsis
- Ability to use isolation and barrier techniques for infection prevention and control

INTERPERSONAL SKILLS

- Strong people skills; ability to communicate and interact effectively with individuals and groups.

Ability to communicate care and compassion to patients placed on isolation precautions

- Ability to establish trusting relationships with patients, families, public groups, and colleagues as a basis for teaching, counseling, and securing compliance with infection control programs

ETHICAL/LEGAL SKILLS

- Commitment to safety and quality; strong sense of responsibility, accountability; strong advocacy abilities
- Ability to confront colleagues who fail to observe proper asepsis and isolation procedures
- Knowledge of special regulations, legislation, and policy detailing nursing responsibilities related to asepsis and infection control

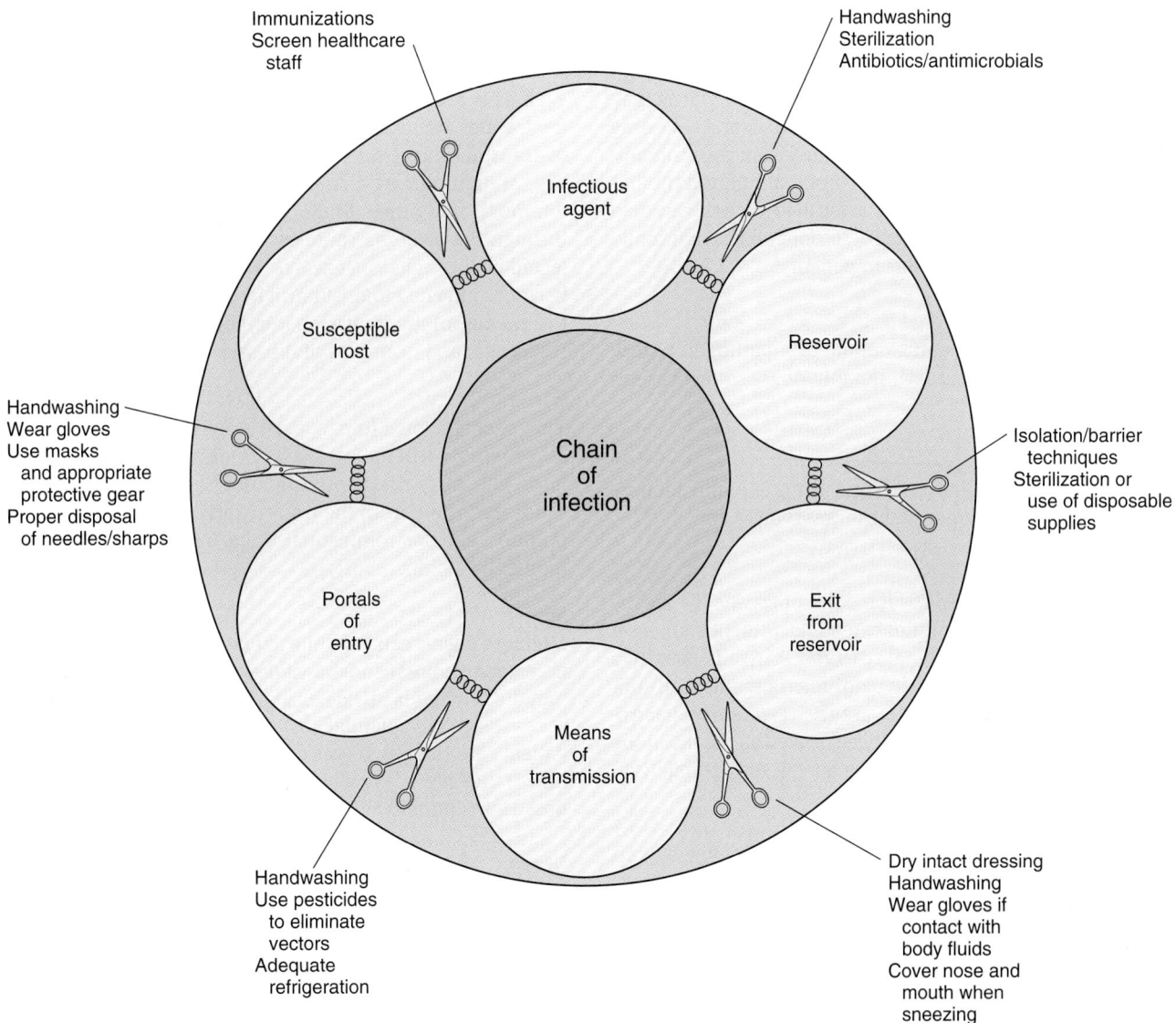

Figure 27-1
The cyclic process through which an infection occurs. (Adapted from Murphy, Q. [1998]. Infectious microbes and disease: General principles. *Nursing Spectrum, 7* (2), 12–14.)

deadly disease, acquired immunodeficiency syndrome (AIDS).

Fungi are plantlike organisms (molds and yeasts) that also can cause infection. They are present in the air, soil, and water, and many are resistant to treatment.

An organism's potential to produce disease in a person depends on a variety of factors, including the following:

- Number of organisms
- *Virulence* of the organism, or its ability to cause disease
- Competence of the person's immune system
- Length and intimacy of the contact between the person and the microorganism

Under normal conditions, some organisms may not produce disease. Microorganisms that commonly inhabit various body sites and are part of the body's natural defense system are referred to as *normal flora*. Other factors may intervene and cause this relatively harmless organism to cause an infection. Bacteria that may potentially be harmful are referred to as *opportunists*. For example, *Escherichia coli*, which normally resides in the intestinal tract, may produce infection when it migrates into the urinary tract.

Reservoir

The **reservoir** for growth and multiplication of microorganisms is the natural habitat of the organism. Possible reservoirs that support organisms pathogenic to humans include other humans, animals, food, water, milk, and inanimate objects.

Other Humans

Some humans are reservoirs who experience symptoms of disease, whereas others are *carriers* of the disease but do not have any symptoms. For example, a person who has tested positive on a human immunodeficiency virus (HIV) antibody test is probably infected with HIV. Even though symptoms of AIDS may not occur for years, the virus may be transmitted to others by intimate sexual contact, sharing a contaminated needle and syringe, transfusion with contaminated blood or blood products, or from an infected mother to her child during pregnancy or birth. Humans can also serve as reservoirs for nosocomial infections and inadvertently transfer pathogenic organisms to patients.

Animals

The rabies virus is an example of a pathogen whose reservoir is various animals, notably dogs, squirrels, and raccoons.

Soil

The organisms that cause gas gangrene and tetanus are examples of pathogens whose reservoir is soil.

Portal of Exit

The *exit from the reservoir* is the point of escape for the organism. The organism cannot extend its influence unless it moves away from its original reservoir. There is usually a primary exit route for each type of microorganism. In humans, common escape routes are the respiratory, gastrointestinal, and genitourinary tracts, as well as breaks in the skin. Blood and tissue can also be an exit for pathogens.

Means of Transmission

An organism may be transmitted from its reservoir by various means or routes. Some organisms can be transmitted by more than one route. Organisms can enter the body by way of the *contact* route, either directly or indirectly. Direct contact involves proximity between the susceptible host and an infected person or a carrier, such as occurs in touching, kissing, and sexual intercourse. The indirect contact route involves personal contact with an inanimate object, such as a contaminated instrument. Contaminated blood, food, water, or inanimate objects (fomites) are *vehicle* routes of transmission. *Vectors*, such as mosquitoes, ticks, and lice, are nonhuman carriers that transmit organisms from one host to another. Microorganisms can also be spread through the *airborne* route by droplet nuclei when an infected host coughs, sneezes, or talks or when the organism becomes attached to dust particles. Table 27-1 summarizes the means of transmission for several organisms, their reservoirs, and examples of diseases they transmit.

Portal of Entry

The organism must find a portal of entry to a host. The *portal of entry* is the point at which organisms enter a new host. The entry route into the new host often is the same as the exit route from the prior reservoir. The urinary, respiratory, and gastrointestinal tracts and the skin are common entry points.

Susceptible Host

Microorganisms can continue to exist only in a source that is acceptable (a **host**) and only if they overcome any resistance mounted by the host's defenses. *Susceptibility* is the degree of resistance the potential host has to the pathogen. Hospital patients are often in a weakened state of health because of illness and have less resistance. Many factors influence a host's susceptibility; these are discussed later in the chapter.

Stages of Infection

Nurses need to understand the stages in the development of an infection in order to intervene and disrupt the infection cycle. An infection progresses through the following phases:

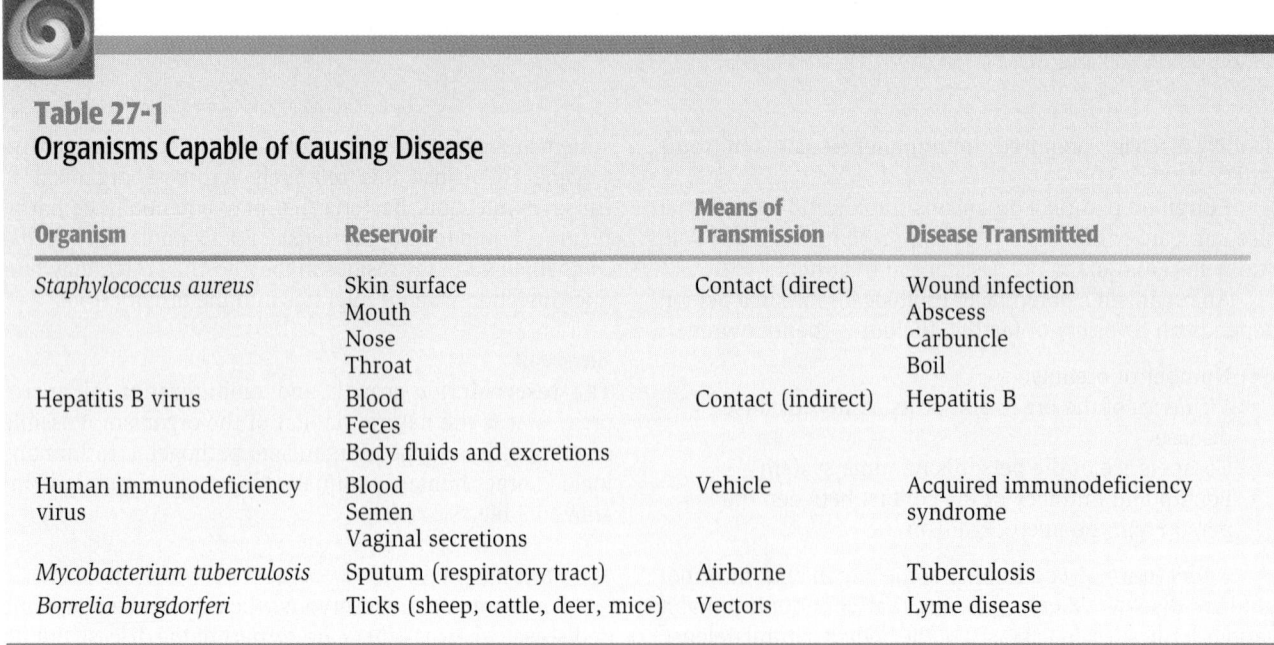

Table 27-1
Organisms Capable of Causing Disease

Organism	Reservoir	Means of Transmission	Disease Transmitted
Staphylococcus aureus	Skin surface Mouth Nose Throat	Contact (direct)	Wound infection Abscess Carbuncle Boil
Hepatitis B virus	Blood Feces Body fluids and excretions	Contact (indirect)	Hepatitis B
Human immunodeficiency virus	Blood Semen Vaginal secretions	Vehicle	Acquired immunodeficiency syndrome
Mycobacterium tuberculosis	Sputum (respiratory tract)	Airborne	Tuberculosis
Borrelia burgdorferi	Ticks (sheep, cattle, deer, mice)	Vectors	Lyme disease

- Incubation period
- Prodromal stage
- Full stage of illness
- Convalescent period

The course and severity of the infection, as well as the patient's response, influence the type and extent of nursing care provided.

Incubation Period

The *incubation period* is the interval between the invasion of the body by the pathogen and the appearance of symptoms of infection. During this stage, the organisms are growing and multiplying. The length of incubation may vary. The common cold develops in 1 to 2 days, whereas tetanus has an incubation period ranging from 2 to 21 days.

Prodromal Stage

A person is most infectious during the *prodromal stage.* Early signs and symptoms of disease are present but are often vague and nonspecific, ranging from fatigue and malaise to a low-grade fever. This period lasts from several hours to several days.

Full Stage of Illness

The presence of specific signs and symptoms indicates the *full stage of illness.* The type of infection determines the length of the illness and the severity of the manifestations. Symptoms that are limited or occur in only one body area are referred to as *localized symptoms*, whereas *systemic symptoms* are manifested throughout the entire body.

Convalescent Period

The *convalescent period* is the recovery from the infection. The signs and symptoms disappear, and the person returns to a healthy state. Convalescence may vary according to the severity of the infection and the patient's general condition.

The Body's Defense Against Infection

In addition to the normal flora that inhabit various body sites, other defense systems help a person combat infection.

The *inflammatory response* is a protective mechanism that eliminates the invading pathogen and allows for tissue repair to occur.

The *immune response* involves specific reactions in the body as it responds to an invading foreign protein, such as bacteria, or in some cases, to the body's own proteins. The complex mechanisms that constitute the immune response occur as the body attempts to protect and defend itself. The foreign material is called an *antigen*, and the body commonly responds to the antigen by producing an *antibody*. This antigen–antibody reaction, also known as *humoral immunity,* is one component of the overall immune response. The cell-mediated defense, or *cellular immunity,* involves an increase in the number of lymphocytes (white blood cells) that destroy or react with cells the body recognizes as harmful. Although these complicated chemical and mechanical responses are not completely understood, it is known that they help to defend the body specifically against bacterial, viral, and fungal infections as well as malignant cells.

Factors Affecting the Risk for Infection

The susceptibility of the host depends on various factors, including the following:

- Intact skin and mucous membranes protect the body against microbial invasion.
- The normal pH levels in the gastrointestinal and genitourinary tracts help to ward off microbial invasion.
- The body's white blood cells provide resistance to certain pathogens.
- Age, sex, race, and hereditary factors influence susceptibility. Neonates and older adults appear to be more vulnerable to infection. (The accompanying box discusses older adults' predisposition to infection.)
- Immunization, natural or acquired, acts to resist infection.
- Fatigue, climate, nutritional and general health status, the presence of preexisting illnesses, previous or current treatments, and some kinds of medications may play a part in the susceptibility of a potential host.
- Stress may adversely affect the body's normal defense mechanisms.
- The increasing use of invasive or indwelling medical devices provides more potential sources of disease-producing organisms, particularly in a patient whose defenses are already weakened by disease.

Health habits that promote wellness positively influence the susceptibility of a host. Sensible nutrition, adequate rest and exercise, stress-reduction techniques, and good personal hygiene habits can help maintain optimum bodily function and immune response. Unsafe sex practices and sharing intravenous needles are potentially dangerous and can introduce pathogens that cause infection.

The Nursing Process

ASSESSING

The nurse's critical role in controlling infection begins with early detection and surveillance techniques. The extent of nursing interventions depends on the susceptibility of the host, the virulence of the organism, and the patient's signs and symptoms.

The nurse should inquire about the patient's immunization status and previous or recurring infections, observe nonverbal cues, and gather information about the history of the current disease. Nursing assessments include observation for signs and symptoms of a local or systemic infection. A localized infection can result in redness, swelling, warmth in the involved area, pain or tenderness, and loss of function of the affected part. Manifestations of

Focus on the Older Adult
Predisposition for Infection

There are specific *physiologic alterations* that predispose an older adult to infection. Common infections seen in the elderly are pneumonia, tuberculosis, and urinary tract and skin infections. Morbidity and mortality are increased in this age group, and the signs and symptoms may be atypical. In addition to a *reduced inflammatory response* and a *decrease in immune function,* specific physiologic alterations in each body system that are associated with the development of these common infections include the following:

Pulmonary Infections (Pneumonia and Tuberculosis)

Decreased cough reflex

Decreased elastic recoil of the lungs

Decreased activity of the cilia

Abnormal swallowing reflexes

Urinary Tract Infections

Incomplete emptying of the bladder

Decreased sphincter control

Bladder outlet obstruction due to an enlarged prostate gland

Pelvic floor relaxation due to estrogen depletion

Reduced renal blood flow

Skin Infections

Loss of elasticity

Increased dryness

Thinning of epidermis

Slowing of cell replacement

Decreased vascular supply

Atypical clinical manifestations of infection in an older adult include confusion, disorientation, lethargy, anorexia, delayed fever response, falls, incontinence, and failure to thrive.

a systemic infection include fever, often accompanied by an increase in pulse and respiratory rate, lethargy, anorexia, and tenderness and enlargement of lymph nodes that drain the area when an infection is present. Laboratory data can provide further insight into the presence of an infectious process. Any of the laboratory test results outlined in the accompanying box may indicate the presence of an infection.

This compilation of assessment data constitutes a unique nursing database that suggests nursing interventions for patients at risk for infection or those in whom an infection is already present.

DIAGNOSING

The potential for infection or the presence of an infection in a patient suggests possible nursing diagnoses. The focus of nursing care depends on a nursing diagnosis that accurately reflects the patient's condition. The following are examples of nursing diagnoses related to an infectious process:

Risk for Infection related to presence of chronic disease; altered immune response; effects of medication; altered skin integrity; malnutrition; presence of invasive or indwelling medical device; lack of proper immunization

Social Isolation related to presence of communicable disease (AIDS)

Altered Oral Mucous Membrane related to ineffective dental hygiene; trauma; side effect of medication

Diversional Activity Deficit related to lack of visitors; restrictions imposed by airborne isolation precautions

Risk for Altered Body Temperature related to infectious process, dehydration

Anxiety related to high risk for infection

Risk for latex allergy response related to occupational exposure; history of multiple surgical procedures

PLANNING: EXPECTED OUTCOMES

Effective nursing interventions can control or prevent infection. The nurse reviews the assessment data, considers the cycle of events that results in the development of an infection, and incorporates principles of infection control while formulating patient outcomes. Planning outcomes that prevent infection or interfere with the infection cycle is an exciting challenge and an opportunity to see positive results from one's efforts. The following expected patient outcomes are appropriate for preventing infection and using infection control techniques. The patient will accomplish the following:

- Demonstrate effective handwashing
- Identify the signs of an infection
- Maintain adequate nutritional intake
- Demonstrate proper disposal of soiled articles
- Use appropriate cleansing and disinfecting techniques
- Demonstrate an awareness of the necessity of proper immunizations
- Demonstrate stress-reduction techniques
- Verbalize an understanding of health risks associated with a latex allergy

IMPLEMENTING

The nurse uses aseptic technique to halt the spread of microorganisms and minimize the threat of infection. To control the number of organisms, medical and surgical asepsis is vital. The practice of **asepsis** includes all activities to prevent infection or break the chain of infection. **Medical asepsis**, or clean technique, involves procedures and practices

Laboratory Data Indicating an Infection

- Elevated white blood cell (leukocyte) count—normal value is 5000 to 10,000/mm³
- Increase in specific types of white blood cells (differential count or percentage of each cell type)

Neutrophils	Normal = 60% to 70%	Increased in acute infections that produce pus; may be decreased in acute bacterial infection
Lymphocytes	Normal = 20% to 40%	Increased in chronic bacterial and viral infections
Monocytes	Normal = 2% to 8%	Increased in severe infections and function as a scavenger or phagocyte
Eosinophil	Normal = 1% to 4%	May be increased in allergic reaction and parasitic infection
Basophil	Normal = 0.5% to 1%	Usually unaffected by infections

- Elevated erythrocyte sedimentation rate—red blood cells settle more rapidly to the bottom of a tube of whole blood when an inflammation is present
- Presence of pathogen in urine, blood, sputum, or other draining cultures

that reduce the number and transfers of pathogens. **Surgical asepsis,** or sterile technique, includes practices used to render and keep objects and areas free from microorganisms.

Teaching About Infection Control

Teaching about medical asepsis and infection control is a challenging nursing responsibility. Patients need to be aware of techniques that prevent the spread of infection. Use of the nursing process in infection control protects both the patient and the nurse.

In the home, medical asepsis techniques are appropriate for most procedures, except for self-injection technique, which requires surgical asepsis. The patient must frequently make adjustments and improvise with the resources and supplies available for his or her use. The nurse emphasizes effective handwashing and hygiene practices that interrupt the infection chain. To satisfy Occupational Safety and Health Administration (OSHA) requirements, many home care agencies have either a full-time or part-time infection control practitioner.

Patients should be taught to use basic principles of asepsis at home and in public facilities. These involve the activities of daily living (see Chap. 36 for a discussion of personal hygiene). Following are examples of medical asepsis practices recommended in the home:

- Wash hands before preparing food and before eating.
- Prepare foods at temperatures high enough to ensure that they are safe to eat, the most common example being the preparation of fresh pork.
- Use care with cutting boards and utensils, and wash hands before and after handling raw meat.
- Keep foods refrigerated, especially those containing mayonnaise.
- Wash raw fruits and vegetables before serving them.
- Use pasteurized milk.
- Wash hands after using the bathroom.
- Use individual personal care items, such as washcloths, towels, and toothbrushes, rather than sharing.

Prevent infection in public facilities by following these guidelines:

- Wash hands after using any public bathroom.
- Use paper towels or hot-air dryers in restrooms.
- Use individually wrapped drinking straws.
- Use tongs to lift food from common service trays in cafeterias, food stores, and salad bars.

The community reinforces medical asepsis practices in various ways, including the following:

- Use of sterilized combs and brushes in barber and beauty shops.
- Examination of food handlers for evidence of disease.
- Enforcement of frequent handwashing by food handlers.

Using Medical Asepsis

Medical asepsis techniques are used continuously both within and outside health agencies because it is always assumed that pathogens are likely to be present. For example, public drinking cups are unsanitary because pathogens may be present on the cup after being used by someone who may harbor them. In a healthcare facility, if a specific pathogen is known to be present, special methods of medical asepsis are used to prevent further spread of the organism. Nearly every nursing activity includes practices of medical asepsis. Breaking the chain of infection is the nurse's responsibility. It involves giving safe patient care and protecting the patient as well as oneself from microorganisms that may cause disease. See the accompanying box for basic practices of medical asepsis that nurses should use when giving care to patients.

Preventing Nosocomial Infections

For various reasons and sometimes despite our best efforts, certain patients in health agencies develop infections that were not noted to be present on admission. The term

Practicing Basic Principles of Medical Asepsis in Patient Care

- Wash hands frequently but especially before handling foods, before eating, after using a handkerchief, after going to the toilet, before and after each patient contact, and after removing gloves.
- Keep soiled items and equipment from touching the clothing. Carry soiled linens or other used articles so that they do not touch the uniform.
- Do not place soiled bed linen or any other items on the floor, which is grossly contaminated. It increases contamination of both surfaces.
- Avoid having patient cough, sneeze, or breathe directly on others. Provide them with disposable tissues, and instruct them, as indicated, to cover their mouth and nose to prevent spread by airborne droplets.
- Move equipment away from you when brushing, dusting, or scrubbing articles. This helps prevent contaminated particles from settling on the hair, face, and uniform.
- Avoid raising dust. Use a specially treated cloth or a dampened cloth. Do not shake linens. Dust and lint particles constitute a vehicle by which organisms may be transported from one area to another.

- Clean the least soiled areas first and then the more soiled ones. This helps prevent having the cleaner areas soiled by the dirtier areas.
- Dispose of soiled or used items directly into appropriate containers. Wrap items that are moist from body discharge or drainage in waterproof containers, such as plastic bags, before discarding into the refuse holder so that handlers will not come in contact with them.
- Pour liquids that are to be discarded, such as bath water, mouth rinse, and the like, directly into the drain to avoid splattering in the sink and onto you.
- Sterilize items that are suspected of containing pathogens. After sterilization, they can be managed as clean items, if appropriate.
- Use practices of personal grooming that help prevent spreading microorganisms. Examples include shampooing the hair regularly, keeping it short or pinned up to limit the possibility of carrying microorganisms on hair shafts, keeping the fingernails short and free of broken cuticles and ragged nail edges, and avoiding wearing rings with grooves and stones that may harbor microorganisms.
- Follow guidelines conscientiously for isolation or barrier techniques as prescribed by agency.

nosocomial infection is used to describe a hospital-acquired infection. In its broad meaning, nosocomial means that the infection results while the patient is receiving healthcare, and the source may be either exogenous or endogenous. An infection is referred to as **exogenous** when the causative organism is acquired from other people. An **endogenous** infection occurs when the causative organism comes from microbial life harbored in the person. An infection is referred to as **iatrogenic** when it results from a treatment or diagnostic procedure. Not all nosocomial infections are iatrogenic.

Prevention of nosocomial infections is a major challenge for healthcare providers. At least 5% of all people admitted to a hospital contract a nosocomial infection, and these hospital-acquired infections are the 11th leading cause of death in the United States, costing an estimated $4.65 billion yearly (Crow, 1998). The cost of the additional hospital care days necessary to treat a nosocomial infection is staggering, particularly in light of the efforts to control spiraling healthcare expenses.

Invasive Medical Devices

Most hospital-acquired infections are caused by bacteria. *E. coli, Staphylococcus aureus, Streptococcus faecalis, Pseudomonas aeruginosa,* and *Klebsiella* species are common causative organisms. Urinary tract infections account for 40% of all nosocomial infections, and most of these infections are related to catheterization (Burke &

Riley, 1996; Ritter, 1998). Surgical wounds are a common site for infections to develop. Nosocomial pneumonia is the most difficult infection to prevent; its mortality rate ranges from 13% to 55% (Carroll, 1998). The increasing use of biomedical equipment is often cited as a causative factor. In addition to indwelling urinary catheters, other devices causing infection include hemodynamic monitoring lines, hemodialysis equipment, and respiratory equipment. Patients on mechanical ventilation are especially at risk for nosocomial pneumonia. Often, the hands of the healthcare worker using the instruments or equipment are the most significant means for the transmission of the pathogens.

Antibiotic-Resistant Organisms

A significant and disturbing trend continues to be the development of hospital-acquired pathogens resistant to antibiotics. The indiscriminate use of broad-spectrum antibiotics has allowed once-susceptible bacteria to develop defenses against antibiotics. This has been the major factor in the emergence of resistant organisms such as methicillin-resistant *S. aureus* (MRSA). When *S. aureus*, a common cause of nosocomial wound and skin infections postoperatively, developed resistance to methicillin, vancomycin became the drug of choice. Most recently, vancomycin intermediate-resistant *S. aureus* (VISA) has emerged, suggesting to epidemiologists that a *S. aureus* fully resistant to vancomycin (VRSA) is a distinct possibility in the near future.

This will present a formidable challenge because other antibiotics that are able to treat this organism are limited. Vancomycin-resistant enterococcus (VRE) is another serious pathogen in hospitals. More than 40 states have reported this pathogen, and the incidence has increased from 0.3% in 1989 to 7.9% in 1993 (Turco, et al, 1998). Enterococci, a species of streptococcus often found in normal intestinal and female genital tracts, can cause nosocomial infections with a high mortality rate if the organism is vancomycin resistant. When resistance to penicillin, ampicillin, and gentamycin first appeared, physicians again prescribed vancomycin as the drug of choice. Several new drugs are being investigated that may become alternatives for treating drug-resistant bacteria. The US Food and Drug Administration (FDA) recently approved a new antibiotic, quinupristin/dalfopristin (Synercid), that is effective against the deadliest enterococcal germs and provides another option if the organism is resistant to vancomycin. Quinupristin/dalfopristin is administered intravenously, is more expensive than vancomycin, and should not be used if other antibiotics are effective against a particular organism. A culture of a wound or of blood or other body fluids can identify the specific organism present, and a sensitivity test determines which antibiotic is most effective against the organism.

Strategies to Protect the Patient

Nurses are in a unique position to prevent the transmission of nosocomial infections. MRSA and VRE are most often transmitted by the hands of healthcare providers, but VRE lives much longer in the environment and can also be spread through patient contact with a contaminated surface, such as side rails or an overbed table. Careful assessment and evaluation of high-risk patients and situations, coupled with strict observance of medical and surgical asepsis techniques, minimize infection and reduce the unnecessary suffering imposed on patients. Using nursing diagnoses to generate appropriate nursing interventions makes a significant difference. Specific barrier precautions are discussed later in this section.

Healthcare agencies have found the following measures to be successful in reducing the incidence of nosocomial infections:

- Instituting constant surveillance by infection-control committees and nurse epidemiologists. Their work can reduce infections significantly when aggressive control measures are initiated based on their findings.
- Having written infection-prevention practices for all agency personnel. Adherence to thorough handwashing and barrier precautions or isolation techniques can prevent many nosocomial infections. Typical guidelines are described later in this chapter.
- Using practices to promote and keep patients in the best possible physical condition. Measures include meeting the patient's needs for nutrition, fluids, rest, oxygen, and physical and psychological comfort and security.

Outbreaks of nosocomial infection in acute care hospitals and long-term care facilities are costly, frequently difficult to control, and debilitating for patients. Infection-control measures save lives and reduce the risk for transmission of pathogens to patients as well as personnel.

Handwashing

Handwashing is the most effective way to help prevent the spread of organisms. There are differences of opinion about proper cleaning agents, the minimum length of time for washing, and ideal frequency of adequate handwashing, but everyone agrees that handwashing is the most important procedure for preventing nosocomial infections. Nurses need to focus on this simple procedure that can interrupt the chain of infection.

Bacterial Flora on Hands

Two types of bacterial flora are normally found on the hands: transient bacteria and resident bacteria. *Transient bacteria*, normally picked up by the hands in the usual activities of daily living, are relatively few on clean and exposed areas of the skin. They are attached loosely on the skin, usually in grease, fats, and dirt, and are found in greater numbers under the fingernails. Transient bacteria, pathogenic as well as nonpathogenic, can be removed with relative ease by washing the hands thoroughly and frequently. *Resident bacteria*, normally found in creases in the skin, are relatively stable in number and type. They cling tenaciously to the skin by adhesion and adsorption, and considerable friction with a brush is required to remove them. They are less susceptible to antiseptics than transient bacteria. It is not possible to clean the skin completely of all bacteria.

Transient bacteria may adjust to the environment of the skin when they are present in large numbers over a long enough time. They then become resident bacteria. If pathogenic organisms become resident bacteria on the skin, the hands then become carriers of the particular organism. Therefore, it is important to clean the hands promptly when they are visibly soiled, after each contact with contaminated materials, and after removing gloves to help prevent transient bacteria from becoming resident bacteria.

Cleansing Agents

Various products are available for handwashing. Soaps and detergents, also referred to as *nonantimicrobial* agents, are considered adequate for routine mechanical cleansing of the hands and removal of most transient microorganisms. They help remove soil because they lower surface tension and act as emulsifying agents. Bar, liquid, leaflet, and powdered soap are all effective. Use of a particular type in a healthcare agency often depends on personnel or agency preference.

Using handwashing products that contain an *antimicrobial* or antibacterial ingredient is recommended in any setting in which there is a high risk for infection. When present in certain concentrations, these agents can kill bacteria or suppress their growth. Antimicrobial soaps are suggested for intensive care units, emergency departments, and any patient care setting in which exposure to blood and body fluids is likely or patients are immunosuppressed. Handwashing with antimicrobial soap is also recommended to prevent nosocomial spread of disease. Some soaps containing antimicrobial agents have reportedly caused skin dryness and cracking. Usually, this irritation can be traced to the detergent base of the soap rather than to the antiseptic. These irritations defeat the purpose of decreasing the number of surface organisms because damaged skin harbors organisms and is more difficult to clean adequately. Some products are available that contain an emollient or softening agent, but lotions may also be used to comfort damaged skin. They are best applied after patient care is completed. Small, nonrefillable containers for personal use are recommended. Check with infection control personnel to determine whether a particular lotion interferes with the action of soaps used in that agency.

Recommended Techniques

Recommended handwashing techniques for medical asepsis are listed in Procedure 27-1. Handwashing before assisting with a surgical procedure involves a more lengthy scrub and reduces resident and transient flora from the forearms and hands. This procedure, known as surgical handwashing, incorporates surgical asepsis and is described in texts that deal with operating and delivery room procedures. Effective handwashing requires at least a 10- to 15-second scrub with plain soap or disinfectant and water. Hands that are visibly soiled need a longer scrub. Many studies have established the merits of handwashing, and several agencies have published directions and recommendations. The Association for Professionals in Infection Control and Epidemiology (APIC) has published guidelines for handwashing in various settings and reviewed the variety of products available for handwashing.

Most guidelines recommend removing all jewelry except wedding bands and paying particular attention to the area beneath the fingernails, where bacteria tend to accumulate. Rings also increase the likelihood that gloves may tear when donned over the jewelry. Nails should be kept short because most organisms are found under and around the nails. Nail polish does not appear to increase the number of microorganisms, but a clear polish is preferable to color because the area under the nails is more visible. Artificial nails are not recommended because they harbor more bacteria than natural nails, place the wearer at risk for developing a fungal infection in the nail bed, and are associated with less vigorous scrubbing in the nail area. A recent study suggests that two nurses' long or artificial nails may have been a factor in exposing neonates in a neonatal intensive care unit to an infection caused by *Pseudomonas aeruginosa* (Moore et al., 2000).

Even though healthcare personnel know the importance of handwashing, most studies report that compliance with this simple preventive measure is difficult to achieve. Despite intensive educational efforts, handwashing is infrequently practiced. Wearing gloves does not eliminate the need for proper handwashing. In reality, the warmth and moisture inside gloves create an ideal environment for bacteria to multiply, making it even more important to wash hands before and after using gloves. Research also indicates that gloving does not guarantee complete protection from infectious organisms. Gloves provide a barrier but are not impenetrable. One study of latex and vinyl gloves found that 20% to 34% allowed penetration of bacteria even though only 4% had visible defects (Beaumont, 1997). Often, the healthcare worker is unaware that a leak has occurred. Routine handwashing should be done after each patient contact, whether or not gloves were worn.

Controlling Infectious Agents by Sterilization and Disinfection

Cleansing, disinfection, and sterilization help to break the chain of infection and prevent nosocomial disease. Most health agencies provide patient care items that are sterile when purchased and disposed of after use. Some items, such as pitchers, water glasses, and thermometers, may be used repeatedly but by one patient only; they are then discarded or sent home with the patient on discharge.

Health agencies usually maintain a central supply unit where most reusable equipment is cleaned, kept in good working order, and sterilized as indicated. In the home and in some small health agencies, the nurse sometimes must make decisions about how to prepare equipment and supplies that are safe for patient use. Although nurses may not be directly involved in the actual process, they must be aware of the critical role they play in preventing infection.

Several processes are used to destroy microorganisms. *Disinfection* destroys all pathogenic organisms except spores; *sterilization* is the process by which all microorganisms, including spores, are destroyed. Disinfection and sterilization of contaminated or infected objects and good handwashing diminish and often eliminate microorganisms as potential sources of infection.

Factors in Selecting Method

Various factors influence the choice of sterilization and disinfection methods, including the following:

Nature of organisms present: The **Centers for Disease Control and Prevention** (CDC), the government agency responsible for investigating, preventing, and controlling disease, recommends that all supplies, linens, and equipment in a healthcare setting should be treated as if the patient were infectious. Some organisms are easily destroyed, whereas others can withstand certain common sterilization and disinfection methods.

Number of organisms present: The more organisms present on an item, the longer it takes to destroy them.

Type of equipment: Equipment with small lumens, crevices, or joints requires special care. Certain articles that may be damaged by various sterilization and disinfection methods require special handling.

Intended use of equipment: The need for medical or surgical asepsis influences the preparation and cleaning of equipment. In the home, it may be safe to use equipment and supplies that are clean, but most health agencies prefer to use sterilized articles for patient care.

Available means for sterilization and disinfection: The choice of chemical or physical means of sterilization and disinfection depends on the nature and

PROCEDURE 27-1

Handwashing

Equipment

Liquid, bar soap, granules, or leaflet   Paper towels   Oil-free lotion (optional)

Action	Rationale
1. Stand in front of the sink. Do not allow your uniform to touch the sink during the washing procedure.	The sink is considered contaminated. Uniforms may carry organisms from place to place.
2. Remove jewelry, if possible, and secure in a safe place or allow plain wedding band to remain in place.	Removal of jewelry facilitates proper cleansing. Micro-organisms may accumulate in settings of jewelry. If jewelry was worn during care, it should be left on during handwashing.
3. Turn on water and adjust force. Regulate the temperature until the water is warm.	Water splashed from the contaminated sink will contaminate your uniform. Warm water is more comfortable and has less tendency to open pores and remove oils from the skin. Organisms can lodge in roughened and broken areas of chapped skin.
4. Wet the hands and wrist area. Keep hands lower than elbows to allow water to flow toward fingertips.	Water should flow from the cleaner toward the more contaminated area. Hands are more contaminated than forearms.
5. Use about 1 teaspoon liquid soap (3–5 mL) from dispenser or rinse bar of soap and lather thoroughly. Cover all areas of hands with the soap product. Rinse soap bar again and return to soap dish.	Rinsing the soap before and after use removes the lather that may contain microorganisms.
6. With firm rubbing and circular motions, wash the palms and backs of the hands, each finger, the areas between the fingers, the knuckles, wrists, and forearms. Wash at least one inch above area of contamination. If hands are not visibly soiled, wash to one inch above the wrists.	Friction caused by firm rubbing and circular motions helps to loosen dirt and organisms that can lodge between the fingers, in skin crevices of knuckles, on palms and backs of the hands, and on the wrists and forearms. Cleaning less contaminated areas (forearms and wrists) after hands are clean prevents spreading organisms from the hands to the forearms and wrists.

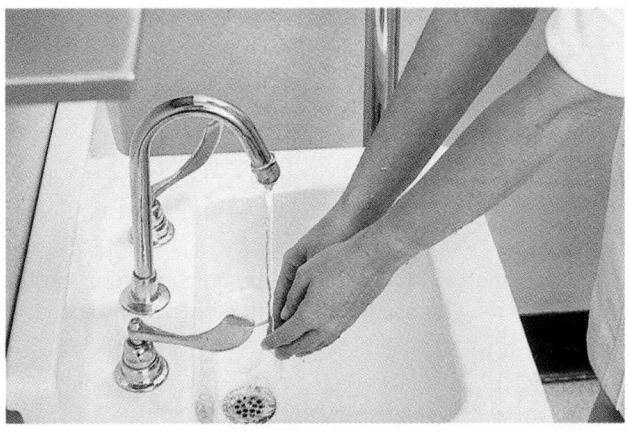

Action 4: Wetting hands and wrists.

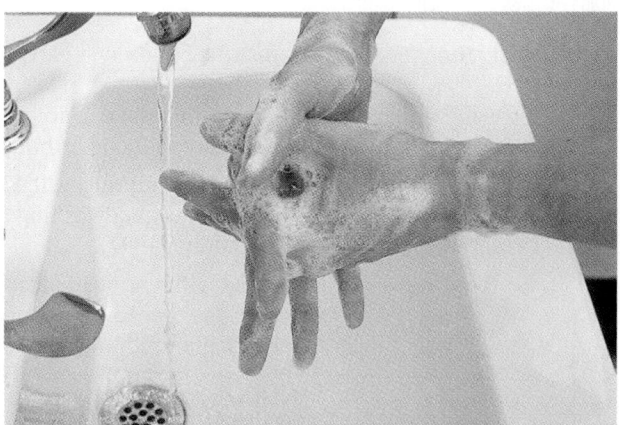

Action 6: Washing hands and forearms with firm rubbing and circular motions.

(continued)

PROCEDURE 27-1

Handwashing (Continued)

7. Continue this friction motion for 10 to 15 seconds.

Length of handwashing is determined by degree of contamination.

8. Use fingernails of the other hand or a clean orange-wood stick to clean under fingernails.

Area under nails has a high microorganism count, and organisms may remain under the nails where they can grow and be spread to others.

9. Rinse thoroughly.

Running water rinses organisms and dirt into the sink.

10. Dry hands, beginning with the fingers and moving upward toward forearms, with a paper towel and discard it immediately. Use another clean towel to turn off the faucet. Discard towel immediately without touching other clean hand.

Drying the skin well prevents chapping. Dry hands first because they are the cleanest and least contaminated area. Turning the faucet off with a clean paper towel protects the clean hands from contact with a soiled surface.

11. Use lotion on hands if desired.

Oil-free lotion helps to keep the skin soft and prevents chapping. It is best applied after patient care is complete and from small, personal containers. Oil-based lotions should be avoided when wearing gloves because they can cause deterioration.

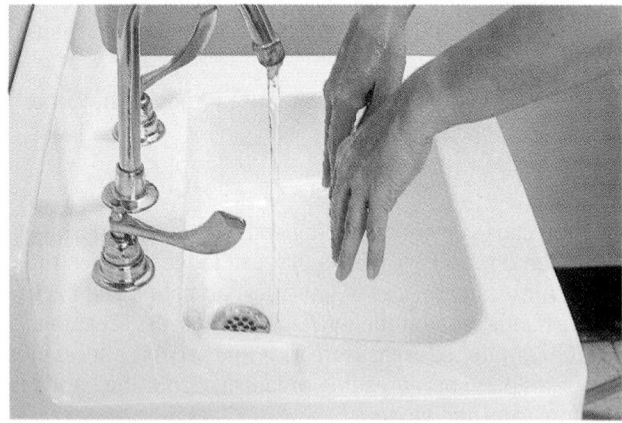

Action 9: Rinsing thoroughly.

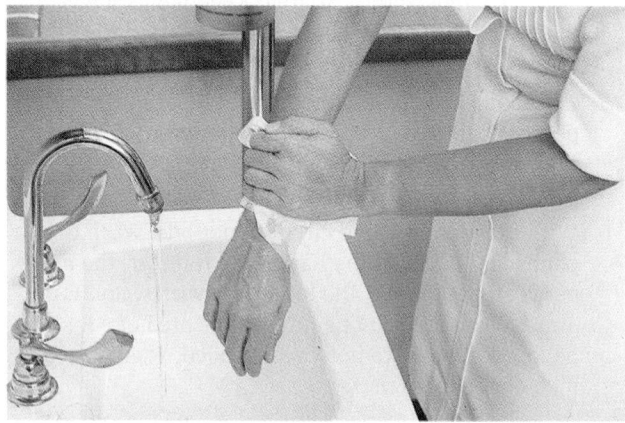

Action 10: Finishing drying with a paper towel.

Age Considerations

Instruct children at early age in proper handwashing techniques.

Special Considerations

An antimicrobial soap product is recommended before an invasive procedure and after exposure to blood or body fluids. The length of the scrub will vary based on need.

A recent study suggested that healthcare workers who wear rings have a higher bacteria count after handwashing than those who wore no rings (Salisbury, Hutfilz, Treen, Bollin, & Gautam, 1997).

Sinks with various faucet controls are available. In addition to the more common hand faucets, knee- and foot-operated controls may be used. Sinks with elbow controls are generally used in a surgical setting.

number of organisms, the type and intended use of the equipment, and the availability and practicality of the means.

Time: Time is a key factor when sterilizing or disinfecting articles. Failure to follow the recommended time periods is grossly negligent.

Cleaning Supplies and Equipment

Proper cleaning of items used in healthcare before they are sterilized or disinfected is essential to reduce the number of organisms and to dislodge them from crevices and from under layers of contaminating substances. The following techniques are recommended for cleaning equipment:

- Wear waterproof gloves at all times.
- Rinse the articles first with cold running water to remove organic material. Heat coagulates certain organic material, which makes removal more difficult.
- Wash the articles, after rinsing them, in warm water that contains detergent or soap. The combination of warm water and soap facilitates emulsification and removal of dirt and debris.
- Use a brush with stiff bristles as indicated to clean the articles thoroughly. Friction aids in the removal of organisms and debris from difficult-to-reach areas.
- Rinse and dry the article thoroughly.
- Prepare the cleaned equipment for sterilization or disinfection.
- Consider the brush, gloves, and the sink or basin in which the articles were cleaned as highly contaminated, and treat or discard them accordingly.

See Table 27-2 for an explanation of physical and chemical means of sterilization and disinfection.

Home Care Considerations

The increasing number of individuals who are ill or immunocompromised, coupled with increasingly virulent organisms, poses sterilization and disinfection concerns for home environments. After thorough cleaning, contaminated items may be disinfected by placing them in boiling water for 10 minutes or using common disinfectants such as bleach, isopropyl alcohol (70%), acetic acid (white vinegar), or a phenol agent such as Lysol (Rice, 1998).

Using Surgical Asepsis

Surgical asepsis techniques, used regularly in the operating room, labor and delivery areas, and certain diagnostic testing areas, are also used by the nurse at the patient's bedside. Procedures that involve the insertion of a urinary catheter, sterile dressing changes, or preparing an injectable medication are examples of surgical asepsis techniques. An object is considered sterile when all microorganisms, including pathogens and spores, have been destroyed. For example, the needle for an injection must be handled so that it is sterile when inserted into a patient. A sterile forceps or sterile gloves are used to handle sterile dressings to protect against contamination. The basic principles of surgical asepsis are listed in the accompanying box.

When observing medical asepsis, areas are considered contaminated if they bear or are suspected of bearing pathogens. When following surgical asepsis, areas are con-

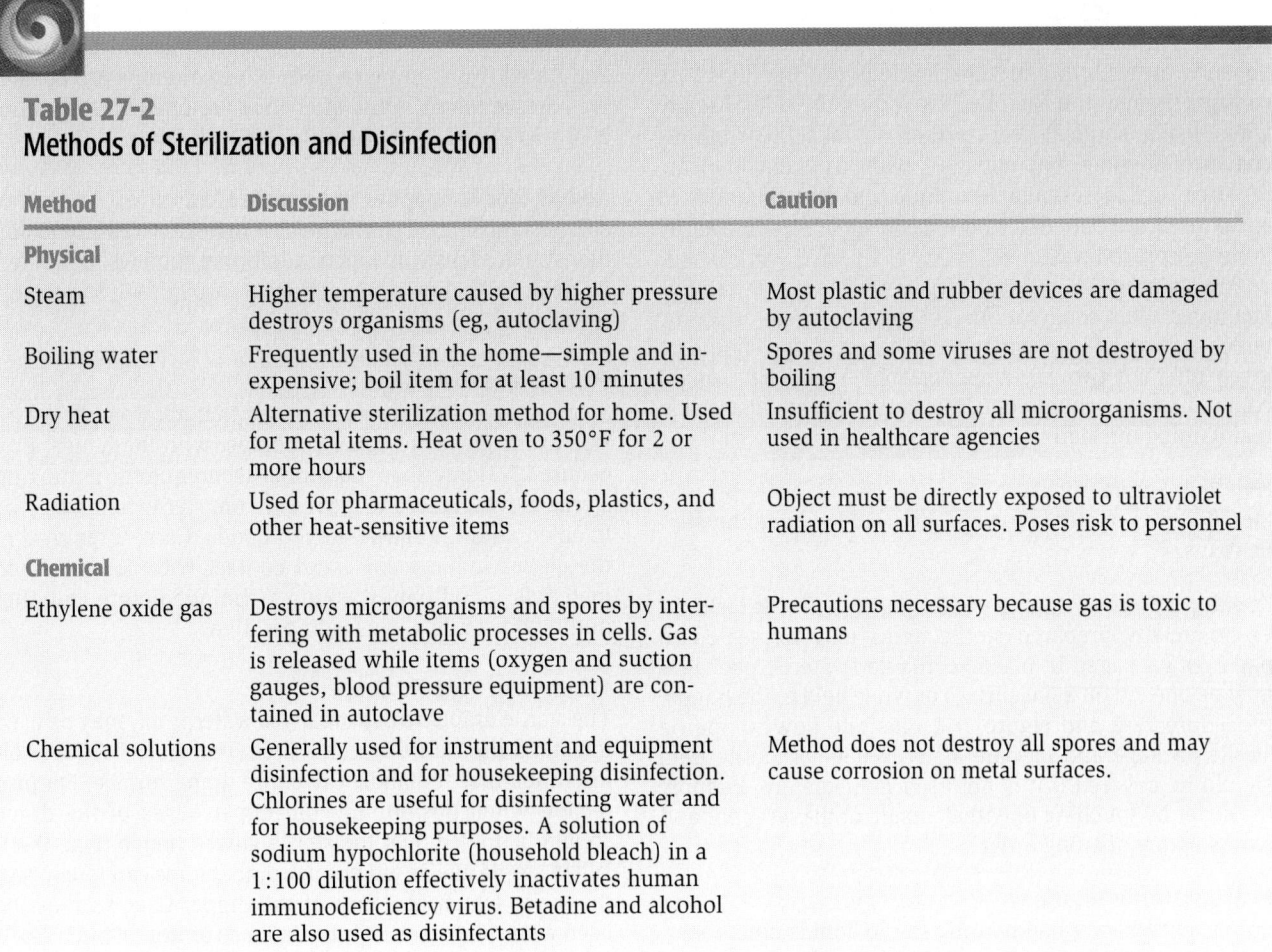

Table 27-2
Methods of Sterilization and Disinfection

Method	Discussion	Caution
Physical		
Steam	Higher temperature caused by higher pressure destroys organisms (eg, autoclaving)	Most plastic and rubber devices are damaged by autoclaving
Boiling water	Frequently used in the home—simple and inexpensive; boil item for at least 10 minutes	Spores and some viruses are not destroyed by boiling
Dry heat	Alternative sterilization method for home. Used for metal items. Heat oven to 350°F for 2 or more hours	Insufficient to destroy all microorganisms. Not used in healthcare agencies
Radiation	Used for pharmaceuticals, foods, plastics, and other heat-sensitive items	Object must be directly exposed to ultraviolet radiation on all surfaces. Poses risk to personnel
Chemical		
Ethylene oxide gas	Destroys microorganisms and spores by interfering with metabolic processes in cells. Gas is released while items (oxygen and suction gauges, blood pressure equipment) are contained in autoclave	Precautions necessary because gas is toxic to humans
Chemical solutions	Generally used for instrument and equipment disinfection and for housekeeping disinfection. Chlorines are useful for disinfecting water and for housekeeping purposes. A solution of sodium hypochlorite (household bleach) in a 1:100 dilution effectively inactivates human immunodeficiency virus. Betadine and alcohol are also used as disinfectants	Method does not destroy all spores and may cause corrosion on metal surfaces.

Practicing Basic Principles of Surgical Asepsis

- Only a sterile object can touch another sterile object. Unsterile touching sterile means contamination has occurred.
- Open sterile packages so that the first edge of the wrapper is directed away from the worker to avoid the possibility of a sterile surface touching unsterile clothing. The outside of the sterile package is considered contaminated. Opening a sterile package is shown and described in Figure 27-2.
- Avoid spilling any solution on a cloth or paper used as a field for a sterile setup. The moisture penetrates through the sterile cloth or paper and carries organisms by capillary action to contaminate the field. A wet field is considered contaminated if the surface immediately below it is not sterile.
- Hold sterile objects above the level of the waist. This will ensure keeping the object within sight and preventing accidental contamination.
- Avoid talking, coughing, sneezing, or reaching over a sterile field or object. This helps to prevent contamination by droplets from the nose and the mouth or by particles dropping from the worker's arm.
- Never walk away from or turn your back on a sterile field. This prevents possible contamination while the field is out of the worker's view.
- All items brought into contact with broken skin, or used to penetrate the skin in order to inject substances into the body, or to enter normally sterile body cavities, should be sterile. These items include dressings used to cover wounds and incisions, needles for injection, and tubes (catheters) used to drain urine from the bladder.
- Use dry, sterile forceps when necessary. Forceps soaked in disinfectant are not considered sterile.
- Consider the edge (outer 1 inch) of a sterile field to be contaminated.
- Consider an object contaminated if you have any doubt as to its sterility.

sidered contaminated if they are touched by any object that is not also sterile. One of the most important aspects of surgical and medical asepsis is that the effectiveness of both depends on faithful and conscientious practice by those carrying them out. It is far better to err on the side of safety when using surgical asepsis than to take the slightest chance of possible contamination. Being a patient advocate requires vigilant aseptic technique and a willingness to speak up if the patient's safety has been compromised by improper procedures.

Explaining the surgical asepsis procedure to patients facilitates their cooperation. The patient needs to know which objects and areas may not be touched and should be given directions to avoid sudden movements that might contaminate the equipment. This helps the patient assist in maintaining the sterility of the procedure.

Handling Sterile Objects
Sterile gloves or sterile forceps are used for handling sterile items.

Opening a Sterile Package and Preparing a Sterile Field
Commercially prepared sterile items may be sealed in paper or packaged in plastic containers. Sterile packages may be opened on a flat surface or while held in the hands. Procedure 27-2 and Figure 27-2 illustrate how to open a sterile package and prepare a sterile field. A sterile item should be covered if it is not used immediately. Reapply the cover by touching only the outside of the wrapper and reversing the opening order.

Pouring Sterile Solutions
Care is necessary when pouring sterile liquids onto a sterile dressing or into a sterile basin. The outer surfaces of the bottle and cap are considered unsterile, whereas the inside areas and the solution are considered sterile. After a solution has been opened, the outer bottle should be labeled and dated if it is to be reused. Most solutions are considered sterile for 24 hours after they are opened. Procedure 27-2 and Figure 27-3 illustrate this technique.

Adding Sterile Supplies to a Sterile Field
After establishing a sterile field, it may be necessary to add items such as instruments or additional supplies to the sterile field. Procedure 27-2, actions 8 through 10, shows this technique.

Putting on Sterile Gloves
Sterile gloves are donned in a way that allows only the inside of the gloves to come in contact with the hands. Procedure 27-3 describes the proper technique for putting on sterile gloves. After the gloves are on, sterile items may be handled with the sterile-gloved hands. Careful removal of the gloves reduces any hand contact with contaminated materials. Good handwashing technique before and after putting on sterile gloves is imperative.

Positioning a Sterile Drape
The sterile drape, which ideally is waterproof, may be used to extend the sterile working area. Using sterile gloves allows the nurse to handle the entire drape surface. For protection when positioning, the upper edges of the drape should be folded over the sterile-gloved hands (Fig. 27-4). When sterile gloves are not worn, the nurse can touch only the outer 1 inch (2.5 cm) of the drape. Caution must be used when shaking the drape open so as not to touch one's uniform or an unsterile object. Holding the drape by the

PROCEDURE 27-2

Preparing a Sterile Field

Equipment

Sterile wrapped drape or commercially prepared sterile package

Additional sterile supplies as needed (dressings, container, solution)

Action	Rationale
Initially Preparing the Field	
1. Explain procedure to patient.	An explanation encourages patient cooperation and reduces apprehension.
2. Gather equipment.	Preparation provides for an organized approach to task.
3. Wash your hands.	Handwashing deters the spread of microorganisms.
4. Check that sterile wrapped drape or package is dry and unopened. Also note expiration date.	Moisture contaminates a sterile package. Expiration date indicates period that package remains sterile.
5. Select a work area that is waist level or higher.	Work area is within sight. Bacteria tend to settle, so there is less contamination above waist level.
6. Open sterile wrapped drape or commercially prepared sterile package.	
a. For *sterile wrapped drape,* open outer covering. Remove sterile drape, lifting it carefully by its corners. Shake open, hold away from your body, and lay drape on selected work area.	Outer 1 inch (2.5 cm) of drape is considered contaminated. Any item touching this area is also considered contaminated.
b. Place *commercially prepared package* in center of work area. Touching outer surface only, carefully reach around item and fold topmost flap of wrapper away from you. Open right and left flap before grasping the nearest flap and opening toward you.	Proper placement prevents contamination by reaching across sterile field. Touching outer side of wrapper maintains sterile field.
7. Place additional sterile items on field as needed.	Sterile field is maintained.
Adding a Sterile Item to a Sterile Field	
8. Open agency-prepared item or commercially packaged item:	
a. Hold *agency-wrapped item* in one hand with top flap opening away from you. With other hand, unfold top flap and both sides. Keeping a secure hold on item, grasp the corners of the wrapper and pull back toward wrist, covering hand and wrist.	Only sterile surface and item are exposed before dropping onto sterile field.
b. If *commercially packaged item* has an unsealed corner, hold package in one hand and pull back on top cover with the other hand. If edge is partially sealed, use both hands to carefully peel apart.	Contents remain uncontaminated by hands.
9. Drop sterile item onto sterile field from a 6-inch (15 cm) height or add item to field from the side. Be careful to avoid 1-inch border.	Wrapper does not contaminate sterile field. Any items landing on 1-inch border are considered contaminated.
10. Discard wrapper.	A neat work area promotes proper technique.

(continued)

PROCEDURE 27-2

Preparing a Sterile Field (Continued)

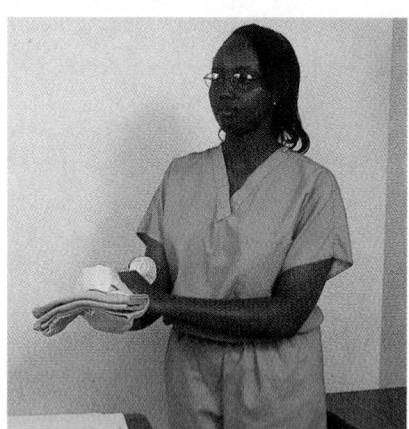

Action 8a: Preparing to drop sterile towel onto the sterile field.

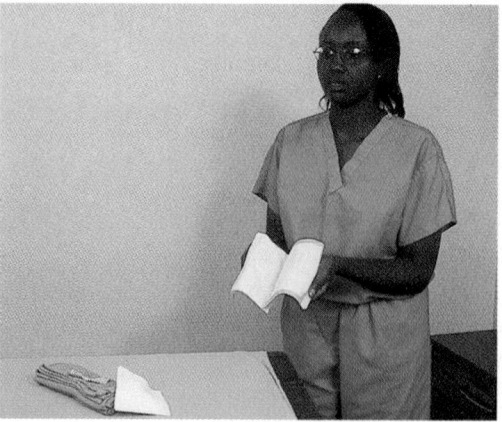

Action 8b: Using both hands to peel apart edges of a commercially packaged item.

Pouring a Sterile Solution

11. Obtain appropriate solution and check expiration date.

Once opened, a bottle should be labeled with date and time. Solution remains sterile for 24 hours.

12. Open solution container according to directions and place cap on table with edges up.

Sterility of inside cap is maintained.

13. If bottle has previously been opened, "lip" it by pouring a small amount of solution into waste container.

This cleanses the lip of the bottle.

14. Hold bottle outside the edge of the sterile field with the label side uppermost and prepare to pour from a height of 4 to 6 inches (10 to 15 cm). The tip of the bottle should never touch a sterile container or dressing.

Label remains dry, and solution may be poured without reaching across sterile field. Minimal splashing occurs from that height. Accidentally touching the tip of the bottle to a container or dressing contaminates both items.

15. Pour required amount of solution steadily into sterile container positioned at side of sterile field. Avoid splashing any liquid.

Moisture contaminates sterile field.

16. Touch only the outside of the lid when recapping.

Solution remains uncontaminated.

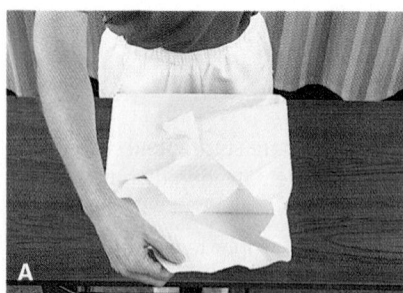

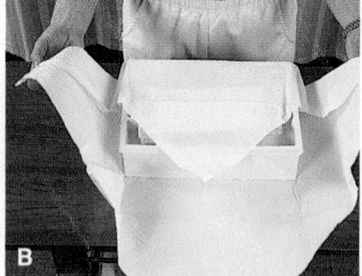

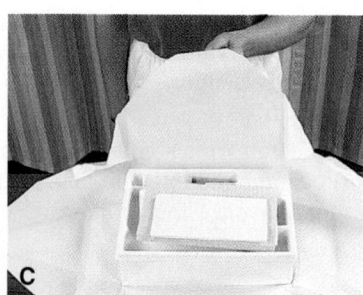

Figure 27-2
Opening a sterile package. (**A**) The nurse folds the topmost part of the covering wrapper away from the nurse. (**B**) Then he or she opens the next layer of the wrapper to the sides. (**C**) The last layer of the wrapper is opened toward the nurse to prevent any reaching over the sterile field. (Photos © B. Proud.)

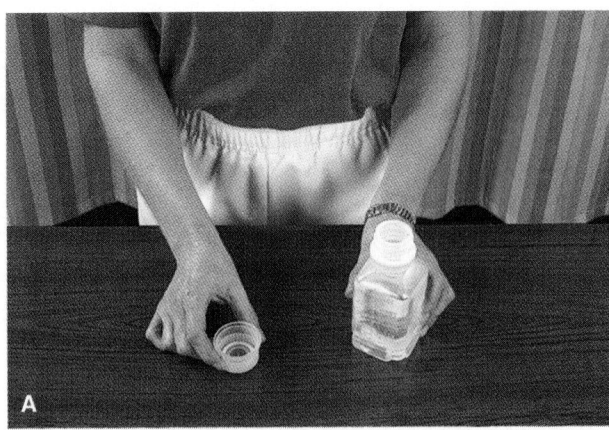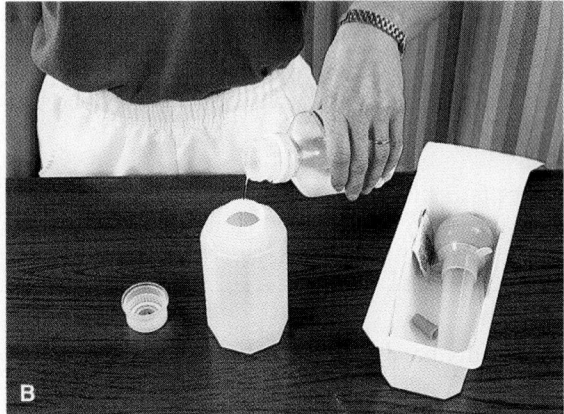

Figure 27-3

Pouring sterile liquids. (**A**) The nurse opens the sterile liquid container while touching only the outside of the cap. The cap is then placed aside with the open side up. (**B**) The nurse pours the sterile liquid into a sterile container without reaching over the sterile container. (Photo © B. Proud.)

1-inch upper edge, the nurse positions the drape over the desired area. The nurse must not reach over the drape because this would contaminate a sterile area.

Using Isolation and Barrier Techniques for Infection Prevention and Control

Isolation is a protective procedure that limits the spread of infectious diseases among hospitalized patients, hospital personnel, and visitors. The transfer of pathogens from person to person can be decreased by limiting dissemination of pathogens. The most practical way to accomplish this is barriers that prevent common vehicles from transmitting the pathogens. Figure 27-5 shows how barriers break the infection cycle. The next section provides background on the development of the current CDC isolation precautions.

Historical Perspective

Early isolation practices involved quarantining infected patients together in a separate facility where few, if any, aseptic techniques were employed. At the beginning of the 20th century, efforts at isolation moved toward placing infected individuals together in one hospital or a hospital ward where caregivers used gowns and antiseptic solutions for handwashing as barriers to transmitting a disease. Eventually, infectious disease hospitals closed, including those set aside for people with tuberculosis, and infected patients were routinely placed on general hospital units in separate rooms or in multiple-patient rooms.

Early CDC Guidelines

By 1970, the CDC was actively involved in developing and recommending infection-control practices and procedures for hospitals. Initial guidelines from the CDC included procedures for *category-specific isolation*, in which all infectious diseases that required similar infection-control techniques were grouped together in categories. The CDC recommended that hospitals use the specific isolation techniques to prevent transmission of all the diseases in each category. The seven

categories were strict isolation, contact isolation, respiratory isolation, protective isolation, enteric precautions, drainage and secretion precautions, and blood and body fluid precautions. The specific precautions for each category were outlined on color-coded cards placed outside the patient's room.

In 1983, rather than group similar infectious diseases together, the CDC initiated *disease-specific isolation*, which listed each infectious disease separately along with the individual interventions and barriers necessary to prevent transmission of that specific pathogenic organism. This system eliminated unnecessary isolation practices because caregivers responded to specific directions for that disease and thus individualized care for each patient based on the specific pathogenic organism. Because of the many diseases and modes of transmission, this isolation method required knowledgeable practitioners and accurate medical diagnoses and laboratory reports in order to choose the correct isolation category (see the accompanying box, Promoting Health).

Universal Precautions

Concern about the transmission of bloodborne diseases (eg, AIDS, hepatitis B virus [HBV]) and the increasing incidence of nosocomial infections caused a shift in the focus of infection-control programs. In 1987, in an effort to protect healthcare workers, the CDC issued recommendations for *universal precautions*. The CDC recommended that healthcare workers use gloves, gowns, masks, and protective eyewear when exposure to blood or body fluids was likely and that all patients should be considered potentially infected. A later update from the CDC clarified the specific body fluids affected by universal precautions. Epidemiologic evidence suggested that only blood, semen, vaginal secretions, and possibly breast milk could transmit an infection. Although the risk was unknown, universal precautions also applied to cerebrospinal, synovial, pleural, peritoneal, pericardial, and amniotic fluids. Universal precautions did not include feces, nasal secretions, sputum, sweat, tears, urine, and vomitus, unless they contained visible blood. The risk
(*text continues on page 552*)

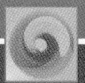

PROCEDURE 27-3

Donning and Removing Sterile Gloves

Equipment
Sterile gloves (size of gloves is indicated on outer wrapping; select appropriate size)

Action	Rationale
To Apply Gloves	
1. Wash and dry hands carefully.	Handwashing deters the spread of microorganisms. Gloves are easier to don when hands are dry.
2. Place sterile glove package on clean, dry surface above your waist.	Moisture could contaminate the sterile gloves. Any sterile object held below the waist is considered contaminated.
3. Open the outside wrapper by carefully peeling the top layer back. Remove inner package, handling only the outside of it.	This maintains sterility of gloves in inner packet.
4. Carefully open the inner package and expose the sterile gloves with the cuff end closest to you.	The inner surface of the package is considered sterile.

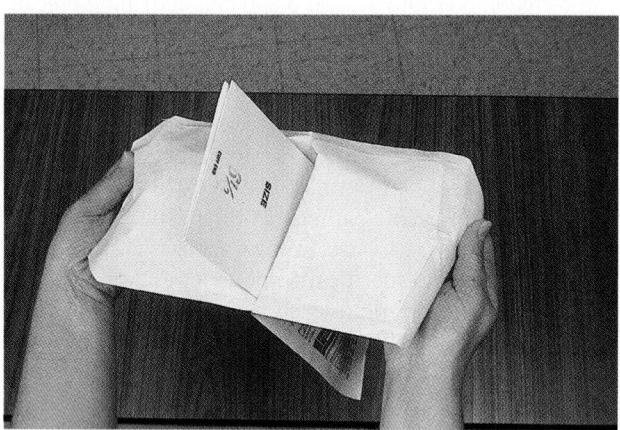

Action 3: Peeling back top layer of outer package.

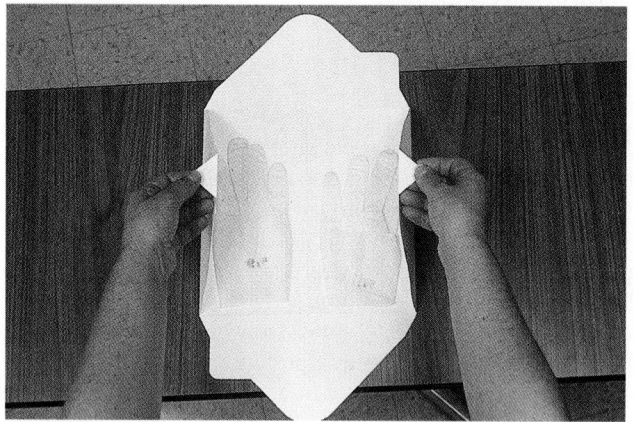

Action 4: Opening inner package.

Action	Rationale
5. With the thumb and forefinger of nondominant hand, grasp the folded cuff of the sterile glove for dominant hand.	Unsterile hand only touches inside of glove. Outside remains sterile.
6. Lift and hold glove with fingers down. Be careful it does not touch any unsterile object.	Glove is contaminated if it touches unsterile objects.
7. Carefully insert the dominant hand into glove and pull glove on. Leave cuff folded down until other hand is gloved.	Attempts to turn upward with unsterile hand may result in contamination of sterile glove.
8. Holding thumb outward, slide fingers of gloved hand under cuff of remaining glove and lift glove upward.	Thumb is less likely to become contaminated if held outward.
9. Carefully insert nondominant hand into glove. Adjust gloves on both hands touching only sterile areas.	Sterile surface touching sterile surface prevents contamination.

(continued)

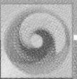

PROCEDURE 27-3
Donning and Removing Sterile Gloves (Continued)

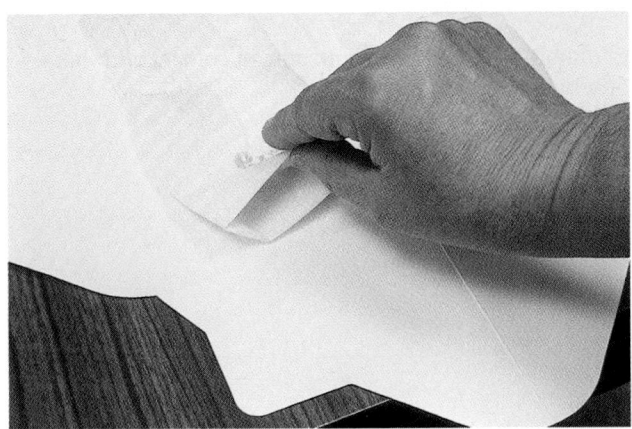

Action 5: Grasping edge of folded cuff.

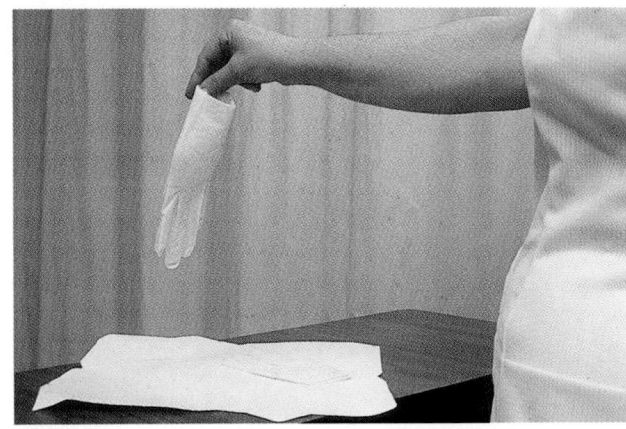

Action 6: Lifting and holding glove with fingers down.

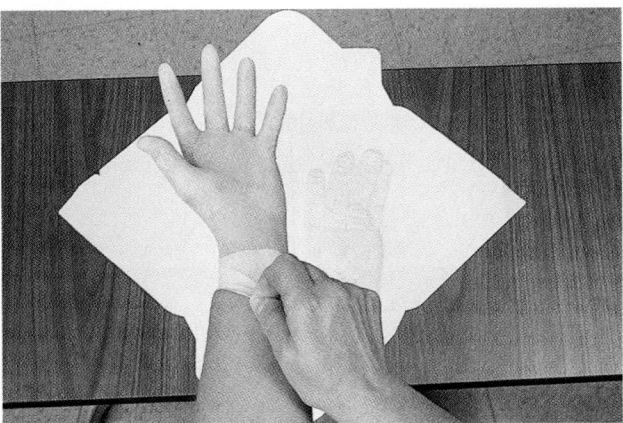

Action 7: Pulling first glove on with cuff folded.

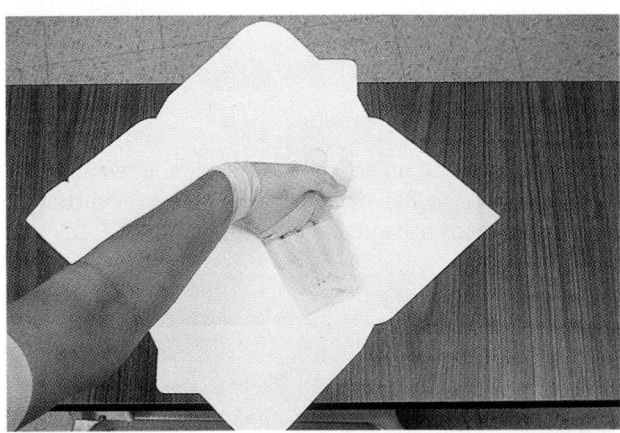

Action 8: Sliding fingers of gloved hand under cuff of second glove.

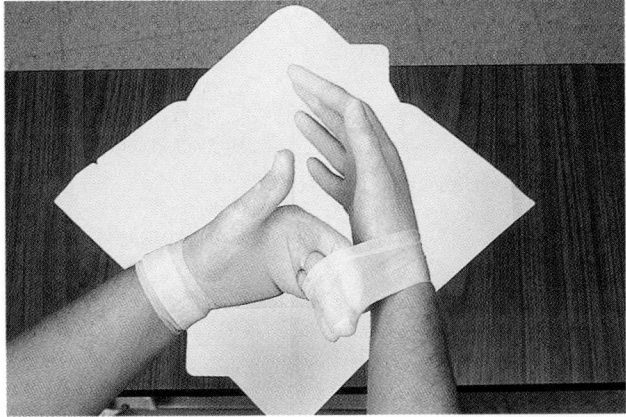

Action 9: Inserting hand with cuff folded.

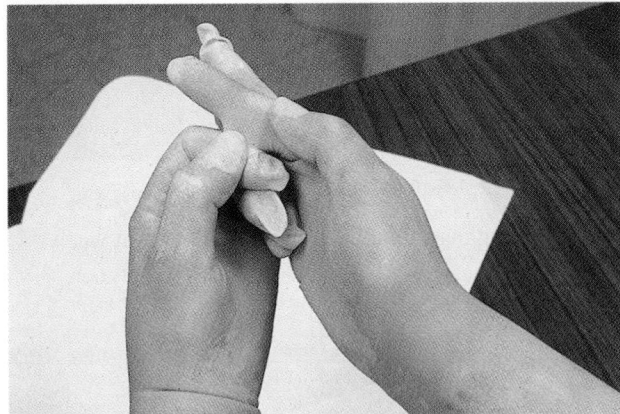

Action 9: Adjusting gloves on both hands.

(continued)

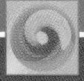

PROCEDURE 27-3

Donning and Removing Sterile Gloves (Continued)

To Remove Gloves

1. Using dominant gloved hand, grasp other glove near cuff end and remove by inverting it, keeping the contaminated area on the inside. Continue to hold on to glove.

Contaminated area does not come in contact with hands or wrists.

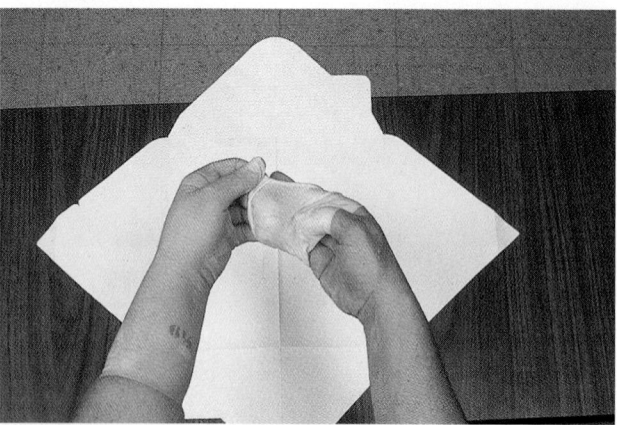

Action 1: Inverting glove as it is removed.

2. Slide fingers of ungloved hand inside the remaining glove. Grasp glove on inside and remove by turning inside out over hand *and other* glove.

Contaminated area does not come in contact with hands or wrists.

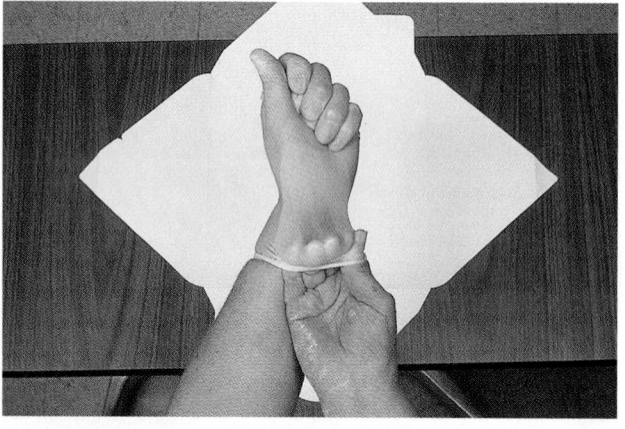

Action 2: Sliding ungloved fingers inside second glove.

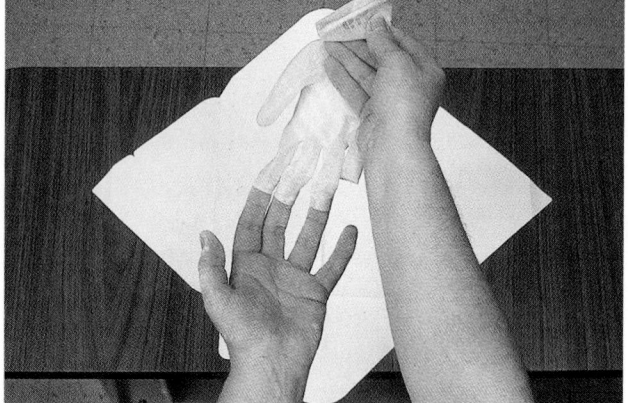

Action 2: Removing second glove inside out.

3. Discard gloves in appropriate container and wash hands.

Handwashing reduces the spread of microorganisms.

---

of HIV or HBV being transmitted through these materials was thought to be very low or nonexistent.

Universal precautions also recommended the use of puncture-resistant containers for disposing of all needles and sharps. Needles were not to be recapped because most needlestick injuries occur during recapping. The use of universal precaution strategies was not meant to replace other isolation system safeguards. The CDC recommended using universal precautions along with category-specific or disease-specific isolation systems.

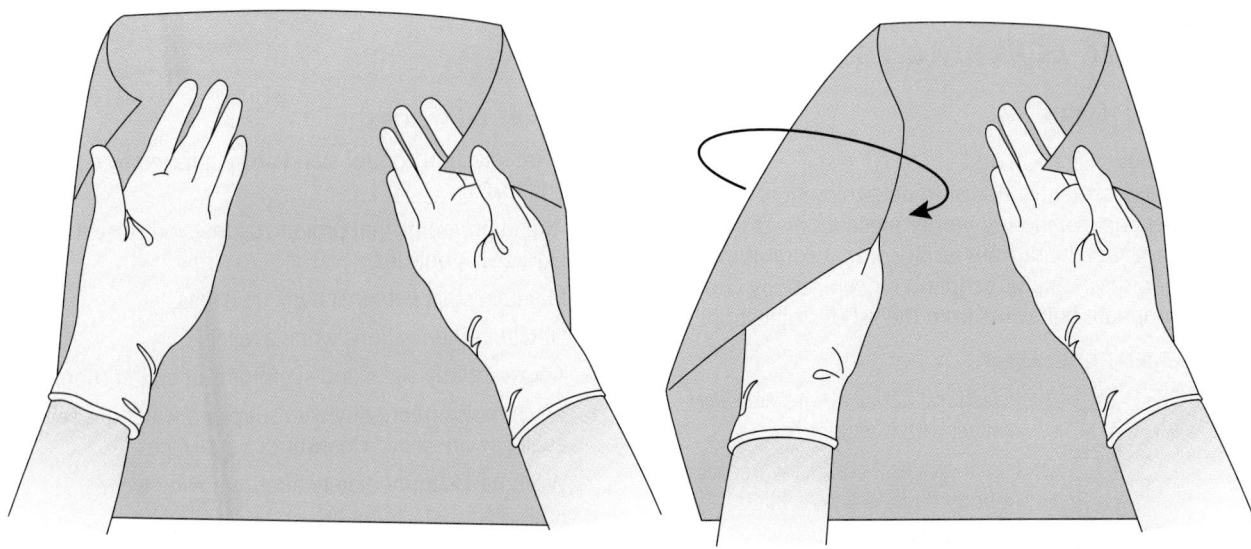

Figure 27-4
Techniques of cuffing a sterile drape over gloved hands.

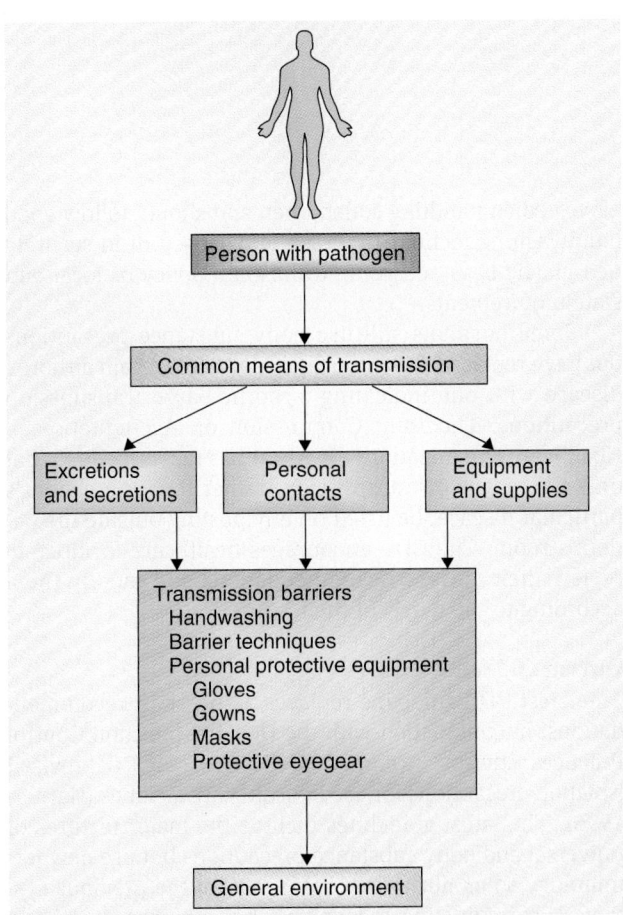

Figure 27-5
Transmission barriers prevent common means of transmission from transporting pathogens from the infected person to the general environment.

OSHA Regulations

OSHA is a government agency that administers the Occupational Safety and Health Act of 1970 and establishes minimum health and safety standards for workers. In 1991, OSHA issued regulations for use of universal precautions in all situations and settings in which occupational exposures to blood and other potentially infectious materials were possible. This ruling reinforced CDC guidelines for universal precautions and made violations punishable with severe fines. Recognizing that HBV poses the greatest bloodborne risk to healthcare workers, OSHA also required that employers offer HBV vaccine free of charge to employees to prevent its transmission. The American Nurses Association is urging OSHA to extend this directive to provide immunization and mandate protection against bloodborne diseases for nursing students who practice in these healthcare facilities.

OSHA has also fined hospitals that fail to use equipment or devices that reduce the risk for needlestick injuries for employees.

Body Substance Precautions

Body substance precautions (or body substance isolation) are an extension of universal precautions. First implemented at Harborview Medical Center in Seattle in 1985, they were designed to reduce the risk for cross-transmission of organisms between patients and minimize the risk for infection in healthcare personnel. Body substance isolation precautions consider *all* body substances potentially infective, regardless of a person's diagnosis, and advocate consistent use of barriers whenever healthcare personnel have contact with moist body substances, mucous membranes, and nonintact skin. The more inclusive term "body substance" includes not only blood and blood-tinged fluids but also feces, urine, wound drainage, oral secretions, vomitus, and any other body substance. Advocates of body substance isolation consider it a simple, straightforward approach to infection control.

APPLYING LEARNING TO PRACTICE

Promoting Health

Isolation/Barrier Techniques

Use the assessment checklist to determine how well you are observing isolation or barrier precautions as you care for patients in a healthcare facility or in a community setting. Then develop a prescription for self-care by choosing appropriate behaviors from the list of suggestions.

ASSESSMENT CHECKLIST

almost always | sometimes | almost never

☐	☐	☐	1. I wash my hands before and after contact with a patient.
☐	☐	☐	2. I wear gloves if contact with blood or body fluids is a possibility.
☐	☐	☐	3. I use additional protective equipment (gowns, masks, goggles) when necessary.
☐	☐	☐	4. I avoid recapping any needles.
☐	☐	☐	5. I place needles or other sharp objects in a puncture-proof disposable container.
☐	☐	☐	6. I dispose of used or contaminated objects and equipment in a leak-resistant plastic trash bag.

SELF-CARE BEHAVIORS

1. Read infection control standards published by OSHA and CDC.
2. Attend programs that provide updates on current CDC/OSHA policies.
3. Maintain strict personal hygiene habits.
4. Obtain immunizations when available.
5. Assess for any signs and symptoms of an infection.
6. Wash hands frequently with soap and water or use available antiseptic cleanser or hand wipes.
7. Wash hands immediately after removing gloves.
8. Protect myself with the barriers necessary to prevent exposure to blood, body fluids, or secretions.
9. Follow agency policy if any exposure to blood or body substance occurs.
10. Never eat, drink, smoke, apply cosmetics or lip moistener, or handle contact lenses in an area where occupational exposure is possible.

Using body substance isolation precautions eliminates the need for category-specific or disease-specific systems except for certain airborne diseases that require special precautions. Varicella (chickenpox) and pulmonary tuberculosis are examples of airborne diseases that require a private room with the door closed and a "Stop Sign Alert" on the door that requests visitors to check with the nurse before entering the room. Mask use depends on the organism and the visitor's immune status. By its design, body substance isolation reduces risks of patients and personnel by treating all people in a similar manner, thus minimizing potential infection from unknown, undiagnosed diseases.

In this system, disposable gloves and needle disposal containers are placed in every room. Each patient interaction requires good handwashing technique before and after care. Clean gloves are required for each patient, and high-stress care situations often require that gloves be changed several times while caring for one patient. When gloves are removed, this system recommends handwashing only if hands are visibly soiled. Some healthcare experts have cited this lack of emphasis on handwashing after glove removal as a disadvantage of this system.

Body substance isolation precautions also provide a consistent approach to soiled linen, trash disposal, and laboratory specimens. Laundry bags are secured and transported in the usual manner. Visible soiling on the outside requires double bagging. Laundry workers wear heavy gloves when handling soiled linen and should follow good handwashing technique. Trash is disposed of in securely tied plastic bags according to hospital policy or local and state requirements.

Some hospitals still use body substance precautions but have replaced the "Stop Sign Alert" for certain airborne disease with one indicating airborne-based transmission precautions. The Joint Commission on Accreditation of Healthcare Organizations (JCAHO) has recommended that only the means of transmission, rather than the patient's particular disease, be listed on any posting outside the patient's room. The CDC encourages healthcare facilities to review their current recommendations and modify them according to the needs of their agency.

Current CDC Guidelines

The latest CDC guideline replaces all previous recommendations. In conjunction with the Hospital Infection Control Practices Advisory Committee (HICPAC), the CDC revised isolation precautions for use in healthcare facilities (Garner, 1996). The latest guidelines include the major features of universal and body substance precautions but use new terminology so as not to be confused with the previous systems. This guideline recognizes the importance of body fluids, secretions, and excretions in the transmission of nosocomial pathogens. Nurses must understand the various isolation or barrier techniques if they are to use them correctly and minimize infection risks to patients as well as themselves.

The revised guideline designates two tiers of precautions:

Standard precautions: precautions used in the care of all hospitalized individuals regardless of their diagnosis or possible infection status. These precautions apply to blood, all body fluids, secretions, and excretions *except sweat* (whether or not blood is present or visible), nonintact skin, and mucous membranes.

Transmission-based precautions: precautions used in addition to standard precautions for patients in hospitals with suspected infection with pathogens that can be transmitted by *airborne, droplet,* or *contact* routes. These precautions encompass all the diseases or conditions previously listed in the disease-specific or category-specific classifications. These categories recognize that a disease may have multiple routes of transmission.

The three types of transmission-based precautions (airborne, droplet, or contact) may be used alone or in combination but always in addition to standard precautions. The accompanying box summarizes the CDC guidelines along with specific recommendations for both tiers of precautions. Hospitals are encouraged to modify these recommendations as needed for implementation of their infection-control strategy (see the accompanying box).

The CDC continues to recommend the use of puncture-resistant containers for disposal of all needles and sharps. Needles should never be recapped because most needlestick injuries occur during recapping. Since the 1980s, when the universal precautions first emphasized prevention of needlestick injuries, needlestick injuries caused by recapping have declined from 25% to 4% (Jagger & Perry, 1999). The most serious risk with this injury is exposure to bloodborne pathogens such as HBV, hepatitis C virus (HCV), and HIV. According to some estimates, healthcare workers have a 1 in 300 chance of acquiring AIDS from a needlestick and a 1 in 6 chance of acquiring HBV (Peterson, 1997). Most hospitals now purchase needleless or protected or recessed intravenous systems. Although more expensive, studies have determined that higher costs for the newer equipment may be almost totally offset by lower costs of treatment and follow-up of needlestick injuries to employees. Although alternative equipment is available, nurses must still be accountable for their own safe work practices. In certain situations, as when access to a needle disposal unit is not immediately possible, it may be necessary to recap a needle. See Figure 27-6 for an example of how to recap a needle to prevent needlestick injuries.

Special Situations

When caring for a patient with MRSA or VRE, the nurse has responsibility to help contain the infection. The CDC guideline for standard precautions applies to all patients, and the second level of transmission-based precautions, particularly contact isolation precautions (see box in

previous section summarizing CDC guidelines), should be implemented when MRSA or VRE has been identified. To help prevent the spread of these organisms, the following additional measures are effective (Sheff, 1998):

- After gloves or gown are removed, avoid touching the bed or overbed table because these areas may be contaminated. This is more likely with VRE.
- Remember to change gloves after caring for a patient who is incontinent or has diarrhea before moving to a "clean" area.
- Instruct family members or visitors about the need for protective equipment. Demonstrate how to put it on, remove and dispose of it, and wash hands thoroughly when leaving the room.
- Clean any additional equipment with a disinfectant before removing it from the room. Avoid placing any such item on the bed or overbed table.
- Use aseptic technique when performing procedures such as suctioning, inserting an intravenous line, or catheterization. Any breach in technique may further compromise the patient.

Occasionally, nurses need to use *neutropenic precautions* for an immunocompromised patient (eg, one recovering from transplantation surgery). Those who are immunosuppressed more often than not become infected by organisms harbored in their own bodies rather than by pathogens present in the environment or transmitted from other people. As with all patients, standard precautions are required, but some additional measures are helpful when a patient's ability to withstand any bacterial invasion is compromised. Recommendations in this situation include the following (Dikon, 1998):

- A healthy caregiver
- Restricting visits from friends and family members who have colds or contagious illnesses
- No standing collection of water in the room (eg, with flowers or in humidifiers) to avoid bacteria typically found in this water

Personal Protective Equipment and Supplies

According to the 1992 OSHA ruling, healthcare agencies must provide employees with the equipment and supplies necessary to minimize or prevent exposure to infectious material. This personal protective equipment includes gloves, gowns, masks, and protective eye gear. Procedure 27-4 summarizes proper use of this equipment.

Gloves

Wearing gloves is not a substitute for good handwashing. Gloves are worn only once and discarded appropriately according to agency policy, and then hands should be thoroughly washed. Each patient interaction requires a clean pair of gloves, and some care activities for an individual patient may necessitate changing gloves more than once. Gloves are not necessary when care activities do not not involve the possibility of soilage of hands with body fluids. Activities such as turning a patient, feeding a patient, taking vital signs, and changing intravenous fluid bags

---

Summary of CDC Recommended Practices for Standard and Transmission-Based Precautions

Standard Precautions (Tier 1)

- *Wash hands* after touching blood, body fluids, secretions, excretions, and contaminated items, regardless of whether gloves are worn. Wash hands immediately after gloves are removed, between patient contacts, and whenever indicated to prevent transfer of microorganisms to other patients or environments. Use plain soap for routine handwashing and an antimicrobial or waterless antiseptic agent for specific circumstances.
- *Wear clean nonsterile gloves* when touching blood, body fluids, excretions of secretions, contaminated items, mucous membranes, and nonintact skin. Change gloves between tasks on the same patient as necessary and remove gloves promptly after use.
- *Wear personal protective equipment* such as mask, eye protection, face shield, or fluid-repellant gown during procedures and care activities that are likely to generate splashes or sprays of blood or body fluids. Use gown to protect skin and prevent soiling of clothing.
- *Avoid recapping used needles.* If you must recap, never use two hands. Use a needle-recapping device or the one-handed scoop technique (see Fig. 28-??). Place needles, sharps, and scalpels in appropriate puncture-resistant containers after use.
- *Handle used patient care equipment that is soiled with blood or identified body fluids, secretions, and excretions carefully* to prevent transfer of microorganisms. Clean and reprocess items appropriately if used for another patient.
- *Use adequate environmental controls* to ensure that routine care, cleaning, and disinfection procedures are followed.
- *Review room assignments carefully.* Place patients who may contaminate the environment in private rooms (such as an incontinent patient).

Transmission-Based Precautions (Tier 2)

The following precautions are recommended in addition to standard precautions:

Airborne Precautions
- Use these for patients who have infections that spread through the air, such as tuberculosis, varicella (chicken pox) and rubeola (measles).

- Place patient in private room that has monitored negative air pressure in relation to surrounding areas, 6 to 12 air changes per hour, and appropriate discharge of air outside or monitored filtration if air is recirculated. Keep door closed and patient in room.
- Use respiratory protection when entering room of patient with known or suspected tuberculosis. If patient has known or suspected rubeola (measles) or varicella (chicken pox), respiratory protection should be worn unless person entering room is immune to these diseases.
- Transport patient out of room only when necessary and place a surgical mask on the patient if possible.
- Consult CDC Guidelines for additional prevention strategies for tuberculosis.

Droplet Precautions
- Use these for patients with an infection that is spread by large particle droplets, such as rubella, mumps, diphtheria, and the adenovirus infection in infants and young children.
- Use a private room, if available. Door may remain open.
- Wear a mask when working within 3 feet of patient.
- Transport patient out of room only when necessary and place a surgical mask on the patient if possible.
- Keep visitors 3 feet from the infected person.

Contact Precautions
- Use these for patients who are infected or colonized by a microorganism that spreads by direct or indirect contact, such as MRSA, VRE, or VISA.
- Place the patient in a private room if available.
- Wear gloves whenever you enter the room. Change gloves after having contact with infective material. Remove gloves before leaving the patient environment, and wash hands with an antimicrobial or waterless antiseptic agent.
- Wear a gown if contact with infectious agent is likely or patient has diarrhea, an ileostomy, colostomy, or wound drainage not contained by a dressing.
- Limit movement of the patient out of the room.
- Avoid sharing patient care equipment.

Adapted from Garner, J. 1996. Guideline for Isolation Precautions in Hospitals. *Infection Control and Hospital Epidemiology, 17*(1), 53–80.

---

do not require gloving so long as body fluids are not present. The nurse should never do the following while wearing gloves: leave the patient's room (unless transporting a contaminated item or a patient under isolation precautions), write in the patient's chart, or use the computer keyboard or telephone in the nurses' station (Crow, 1997; Borton, 1998).

As mentioned earlier, gloves are not always an impenetrable barrier. In high-risk settings such as the operating room, glove failure is common. Reports indicate that during surgery, particularly operative procedures longer than three hours, gloves fail almost 50% of the time (Korniewicz & Rabussay, 1997). Being exposed to body fluids and blood and handling many surgical instruments are both factors in

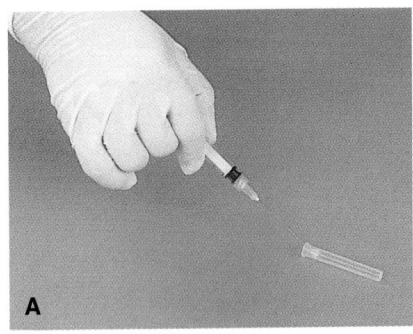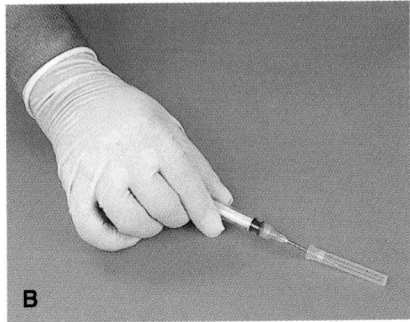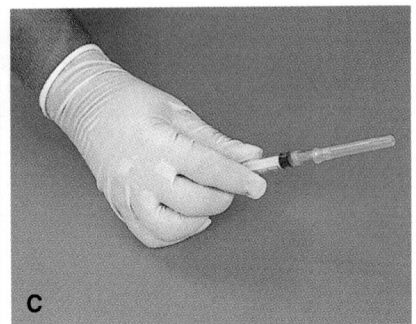

Figure 27-6
If it is necessary to a recap a needle, use a one-handed scoop technique or a needle-recapping device. (**A**) Preparing to slide needle into cap. (**B**) Lifting cap onto needle. (**C**) Covering needle with cap.

glove destruction. Tiny tears or cuts that occur in the gloves are often not observed until the gloves are removed after surgery and blood is visible on the hands. Electronic glove-monitoring devices combined with ongoing education about safe gloving technique and injury prevention help provide a safer work environment.

Latex Allergy. Latex allergy is recognized as an occupational hazard for healthcare workers. Reports reveal that 8% to 17% of healthcare workers may be allergic to latex, compared with 1% to 6% of the general population who do not use these products regularly. The FDA reported 27 latex-related deaths as of June 1996 (Burt, 1998). Reactions have ranged from local skin reactions to urticaria (hives) to systemic anaphylaxis, an exaggerated allergic reaction that can result in death. The initial CDC recommendation for universal precautions contributed to an increased use of latex gloves for patient care activities. Changes in the manufacturing process to meet supply demands may also have been a factor. The cornstarch powder or talc used to make gloves easier to put on is a major causative factor in any latex allergy. The powder binds with the latex protein and becomes airborne, where it can remain for 5 to 12 hours after healthcare workers don or remove gloves. These particles may be inhaled, be absorbed into skin or mucous membranes, or enter the bloodstream.

The National Institute for Occupational Safety and Health (NIOSH) recommends that nonlatex gloves or powder-free, low-allergen latex gloves (if latex gloves are used) be available for employees (Gritter, 1998). Nitrile gloves that are made of a synthetic material that resembles latex are now also available (Carroll, 1999). For patients with a latex allergy, a "latex-safe" healthcare environment is essential. A 1998 FDA ruling required all products or packaging containing natural rubber latex to carry a warning that these products may cause allergic responses in sensitive individuals. All healthcare facilities should have a written policy dealing with latex-sensitive employees and patients. Before admission, the room for a patient with known or suspected latex allergy should be cleaned to remove any trace of residual glove powders. A latex-safe environment involves removal or covering of any natural latex rubber items. Items such as wall-mounted blood pressure

cuffs, sharps containers, injection port caps on intravenous tubing, and urinary catheters are examples of medical products that could elicit an allergic response. Awareness of an allergy to latex is also important for safe home care. Nurses should ask whether patients have experienced any unusual signs or symptoms when blowing up balloons, using latex condoms, or wearing rubber gloves for dish washing or cleaning. The accompanying box summarizes information on latex allergy for healthcare personnel and patients.

Gowns

Gowns are usually worn to prevent soiling of the healthcare worker's clothing by the patient's blood and body fluids. They provide barrier protection and should be donned immediately before entering the patient's room. Individual gown technique is recommended; this means that a gown is worn only once and is then discarded appropriately according to agency policy. If a gown becomes heavily soiled or moistened with blood or body fluids when caring for a patient, it should be removed, the hands should be thoroughly washed, and a clean gown should be donned. There is no one special technique for applying a gown used as a barrier, but recommended practices for removing a soiled gown are included in Procedure 27-4.

Masks

Masks help prevent the wearer from inhaling large-particle aerosols, which usually travel short distances (about 3 feet), and small-particle droplet nuclei, which can remain suspended in the air and travel longer distances. Masks also discourage the wearer from touching the eyes, nose, and mouth, thus limiting contact of organisms with mucous membranes.

Various mask practices are used. In some instances, all personnel and all the patient's visitors wear masks; in other situations, a patient on respiratory precautions wears the mask when transported outside his or her room to protect healthcare personnel and other patients from any exposure to pathogens. A mask should be worn only once and should *never* be lowered around the neck and then brought back over the mouth and nose for reuse. How long one can wear one mask while caring for one patient is debated. It should (*text continues on page 560*)

PROCEDURE 27-4

Using Personal Protective Equipment

Equipment (may vary)

Gloves
Gown

Mask (surgical or particulate
    respirator)

Protective eyewear

Action	Rationale
1. Check physician's order for type of isolation and review precautions in Infection-Control Manual.	Mode of transmission or organism determines type and degree of precautions.
2. Plan nursing activities and gather necessary equipment before entering patient's room.	Organization facilitates performance of task and adherence to isolation precautions.
3. Provide instruction about isolation precautions to patient, family members, and visitors.	An explanation encourages cooperation of patient and family and reduces apprehension about isolation procedures.
4. Wash your hands.	Handwashing deters the spread of microorganisms.
5. Put on gown, gloves, mask, and protective eyewear, if recommended as isolation precaution:	Interrupts chain of infection. Protects patient and nurse.
a. Tie gown securely at neck and waist.	Gown should protect entire uniform.
b. Use clean disposable gloves. If worn with gown, draw glove cuffs over gown sleeves.	Protect hands and wrists from microorganisms.
c. Mask must be securely tied and fitted to face.	Protects nurse from droplet nuclei and large-particle aerosols.
d. Eyewear must have protection on side of face or side shields.	Protects mucous membranes in the eye from splashes.
6. When patient care is completed, remove gloves first.	Gloves have been involved in patient care and are most soiled.
a. Untie waist strings of gown first. Grasp outside of one glove and turn inside out to remove. Continue to hold on to glove.	Ungloved hand is clean and should not touch contaminated areas. Waist strings of gown are considered contaminated.
b. Insert fingers of ungloved hand inside the cuff of the remaining glove. Grasp glove on inside and remove by turning inside out. Drop in appropriate container.	

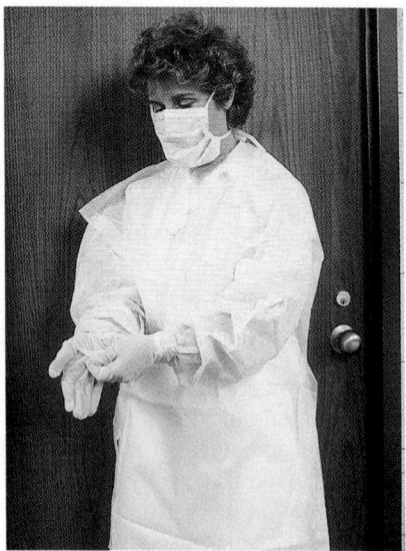

Action 6a: Grasping outside of first glove and pulling it off inside out.

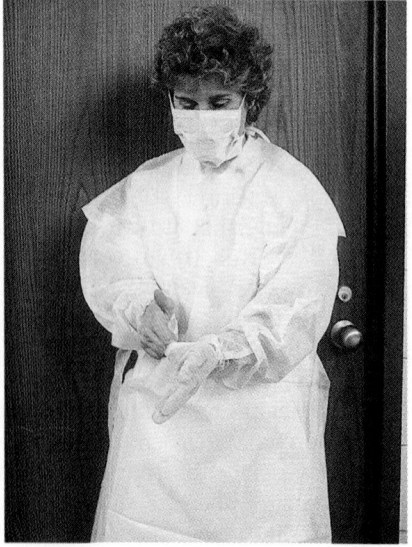

Action 6b: Placing fingers of ungloved hand inside cuff of the remaining glove.

(*continued*)

PROCEDURE 27-4

Using Personal Protective Equipment (Continued)

7. After gloves are removed, remove mask:

   Surgical mask
   a. Untie mask and drop by strings into waste container.

   Center of mask is contaminated. Strings are considered clean.

   Particulate respirator
   b. Use hand to hold respirator in place.
   c. Pull bottom strap up and over head.
   d. Pull top strap over head.
   e. Remove respirator from face and save for future use or discard according to manufacturer's directions.

   Prevents respirator from falling off face onto floor.

8. Remove gown:
   a. Gown that is not visibly soiled requires no particular technique for removal

   For gown that is visibly soiled:
   b. Untie neck strings of gown. Remove gown without touching outside of gown by keeping one hand up and under the gown cuff and using this protected hand to pull the opposite sleeve down and off.

   Neck strings are considered clean. Outside of gown is contaminated.

   c. Use ungowned arm and hand to grasp the gown from the inside and remove from the remaining arm. Remove gown and turn inside out and drop in appropriate container.

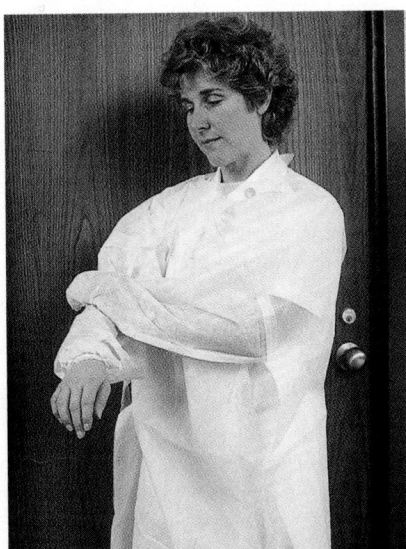

Action 8b: Using protected hand to pull the opposite sleeve down and off.

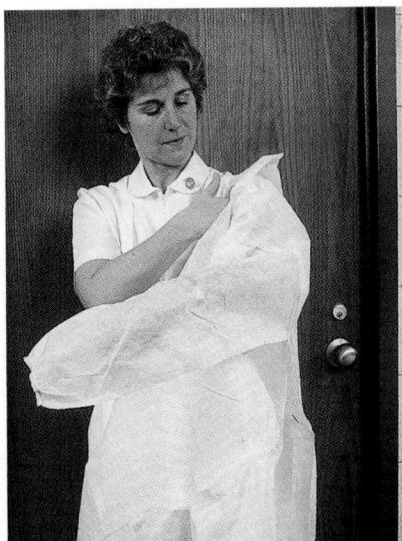

Action 8c: Using ungowned hand to grasp gown from the inside.

9. Remove eyewear last and clean according to agency policy.

   Eyewear is reusable.

10. Wash hands thoroughly.

   Prevents spread of microorganisms.

Latex Allergy Summary

Those at Risk

- Healthcare personnel who wear latex gloves
- Anyone who had frequent surgical procedures at an early age necessitating contact with latex products, such as a child with spina bifida
- Workers in plants manufacturing latex items
- People with a history of allergies
- Anyone with a food allergy to bananas, kiwifruit, avocados, chestnuts, and pineapples

Types of Reactions

- Irritant contact dermatitis—red and itchy skin found on hands after latex glove use
- Delayed hypersensitivity—(the most common reaction) redness, itching, localized swelling, running eyes and nose, and coughing
- Immediate hypersensitivity—(immediate response that has the potential to be life-threatening) may include hives, generalized edema, itching, rash, wheezing, bronchospasm with progression to respiratory or cardiac arrest

Diagnosis of Those at Risk

- A detailed history indicating allergic responses to latex exposures
- Skin prick test—a drop of dilute latex allergen extract is placed on the skin before making a small prick. This test may cause an allergic response in a highly sensitive person, and treatment must be immediately available.
- RAST test (radioallergosorbent testing)—a blood test that measures the quantity of a latex-specific immune globulin in serum
- Challenge or patch test—small pieces of glove are taped to a person's back for 48–96 hours. Inflamed skin under the patch indicates latex sensitivity.

For the Healthcare Worker

- Avoid latex products. Wear synthetic gloves.
- Become aware of medical and household products that contain latex.
- Inform all healthcare providers (eg, dentist, doctor) of latex allergy.
- Carry a quick-acting oral antihistamine and an epinephrine autoinjector at all times.
- Wear a MedicAlert bracelet stating "latex allergy"
- Join a latex allergy support group.
- Investigate employer's policy for latex-sensitive employees.

For Latex-Sensitive Patients

- Provide a latex-safe environment using the following measures:
  - Before surgery, document any reactions to latex products. Indicate "latex allergy" on the front of the chart.
  - A private room is advisable during the hospital stay. Indicate "latex allergy" on the door, over the bed, and on patient's identification bracelet.
  - Avoid contact with any latex product (eg, gloves, tourniquets, blood pressure devices).
  - Keep a latex-safe equipment cart in the room.
  - Use latex-free medication procedures (eg, remove rubber stoppers from vial before withdrawing medication, use syringes with latex-free plungers.

Adapted from McGann, S., O'Boyle, E., & Brochard, B. (1997). Latex allergy alert. *Nursing Spectrum, 6*(15), 12–13; Burt, S. (1998). What you need to know about latex allergy. *Nursing, 28*(10), 33–39; and Gritter, M. (1998), The latex threat. *American Journal of Nursing, 98*(9), 26–32.

certainly be changed before it becomes damp from the wearer's exhalations. Recommended practices for masks are summarized in Procedure 27-4.

The serious increase in the number of multidrug-resistant tuberculosis cases prompted new guidelines to prevent the transmission of this disease. According to CDC guidelines for airborne precautions, either a high-efficiency particulate air (HEPA) filter respirator or N95 respirator certified by NIOSH must be worn when entering the room of a patient with known or suspected tuberculosis. These respirators filter inspired air, whereas surgical masks filter only expired air (Borton, 1997; Jones & Hannum, 1998). Caregivers have expressed difficulty wearing the HEPA-style respirator for extended periods of time, but the N95 respirator, which is designed to filter out particles as small as 1 μm with 95% efficiency, fits more comfortably against the face (Fig. 27-7). It also costs considerably less than the HEPA filter respirators. The elastic straps on these respirators provide more protection and a better fit than the ties on regular surgical masks.

Protective Eyewear

Protective eyewear, such as goggles or a face shield, should be available whenever there is a risk of contaminating the mucous membranes of the eyes. Suctioning a tracheostomy or assisting with an invasive procedure that may result in splattering of blood or other body fluids requires protection for the caregiver. Plain glasses are unacceptable because side shields are required.

Other Isolation Supplies and Procedures

Used equipment may be disposed of after use or, if reusable, bagged according to agency policy, sent to a central cleaning area, and sterilized or disinfected. Double bagging may be required if the single bag is not secure or is soiled on the outside. A contaminated item should never be used for another patient.

Double bagging of trash and linen is usually needed only if the outside of the bag is visibly soiled. Some linen bags are water soluble and dissolve in hot water, making it unnecessary for workers to handle the contaminated linen. The use of paper trays and plastic eating utensils does not prevent transmission of organisms and is no longer recommended. The combined hot water and detergent used in commercial dishwashers sufficiently decontaminates dishes, glasses, and utensils. All spills of body fluids or substances must be immediately cleaned with the appropriate chemical germicide or disinfectant.

When a specimen is collected, care must be taken to prevent the outside of the container from becoming contaminated with any secretions or bodily fluids. All laboratory specimens are placed in plastic bags and sealed to prevent leakage during transportation. No special labels are applied to specimen containers or bags.

Meeting Needs of Patients in Isolation

The psychological implications of isolation precautions are usually great, whether the patient is strictly separated from others or needs only to observe relatively simple precautions (see the accompanying box, Through the Eyes of a Student).

The current standard precautions of the CDC treat all people in a similar manner and greatly minimize the psychological trauma of feeling unclean and undesirable that

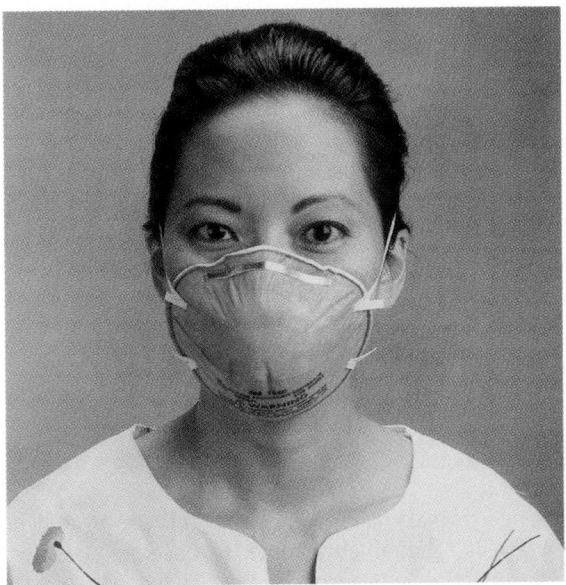

Figure 27-7
The Type N95 healthcare particulate respirator is NIOSH approved. It meets CDC guidelines for tuberculosis exposure control and is designed specifically for use in a healthcare setting. (Courtesy of 3M Health Care.)

Through the Eyes of a Student

She was the cutest little girl I have ever known. She was infected with the HIV from birth. Her mother was an IV drug user and engaged in unprotected sex with multiple partners. This little girl, who came in to the world with an innocent, fresh, new face full of unconditional love, could not walk, could not talk, could not chew, could not control her urine or bowel movements—but boy could she smile! In the beginning I was so terrified of contracting AIDS that I couldn't walk into her room without a mask, gown, gloves, protective eyewear, and basically a full protective body spacesuit. At the end I wanted to take her into my home and give her all the love, support, and care she needed. I am not saying that I didn't wear gloves when I changed her diapers or when I flushed her heparin lock because I did . . . I was very careful. But I realized that she is a person, a person full of feelings, a person who needed me and from whom I could learn. People with the AIDS virus are just that—people. We need to learn to treat them as such.

I also learned not to fear the person who is diagnosed with HIV infection or AIDS. I know that I will take the proper safety precautions with this person. The person I need to fear is the cute little old man who would never have AIDS because "he's not the type." If I don't use precautions, it is possible that one day I'll become infected through contact with someone who is "not the type." If that should ever happen, I hope everyone who cares for me will treat me as a real person and not be afraid.

—Karmi N. Soder, Georgetown University Washington, DC

often occurred with earlier isolation measures. Sensory deprivation and loss of self-esteem may occur, however, with transmission-based precautions. Friends and relatives, as well as healthcare personnel, may be inclined to spend less time with the patient because they are afraid that they will contract the disease or because of the inconvenience of coping with specific transmission precaution procedures. Nursing measures to help prevent sensory deprivation and loss of self-esteem are discussed in Chapters 30 and 33.

Health teaching about transmission-based precautions can ease the fears of patients and family members. Both must understand the pertinent epidemiologic facts and how to carry out the specific precautions. It is helpful to emphasize the following (Marx, 1998):

- Isolation is temporary.
- The precautions and protective equipment worn by the staff protect the patient, the caregiver, and other patients.
- Handwashing before and after visiting the patient is the most effective measure to prevent spread of the disease.

Nurses must document their health teaching about barrier precautions in the patient's care plan. A well-informed nurse who understands how to protect both self and patients and a well-informed patient who is cooperating in his or her care represent superior communicable disease precautions.

Raising Ethical Concerns About Infection Risks

Isolation and barrier precautions minimize infection risks for patients as well as healthcare workers. The increasing numbers of people infected with HIV, HBV, and HCV have led to serious ethical concerns and controversy related to the risk for transmitting these diseases. At issue are the rights of the patient versus the rights of the healthcare worker and the healthcare agency. Questions such as these are being debated:

- Should all hospital patients be routinely tested for HIV infections?
- Should HIV testing be mandatory for all healthcare workers?
- Should healthcare workers infected with HIV be permitted to perform exposure-prone invasive procedures?
- What procedures should be considered exposure prone?
- Will healthcare facilities be liable if they allow HIV-positive staff to care for patients?
- Should pregnant healthcare providers be expected to care for patients with infectious diseases?

The CDC and various medical and nursing groups are seeking consensus on these issues based on scientific information and valid statistical evidence. All agree, however, that healthcare workers who conscientiously adhere to isolation or barrier precautions seriously reduce the risk for infection for patients and themselves.

Reporting an Accidental Exposure

Nurses are accountable for their own safety. Any needlestick injury or accidental exposure to blood or body fluids must be reported immediately so that appropriate interventions can be used. Failure to notify an employer of an exposure may result in personal jeopardy as well as loss of compensation if an infection develops. An agency's plan for this type of exposure typically includes the following:

- Wash the exposed area immediately with warm water and soap.
- Report the incident to the appropriate person and complete an incident or injury report if required by the agency.
- Inform the agency of the source (patient's name) and nature of the exposure.
- Consent to an initial baseline blood test, if agreeable, to determine personal HIV and HBV status. Repeat blood test 6 weeks after exposure and at 3-month, 6-month, and 1-year intervals.
- Consent to postexposure prophylaxis, if recommended, at the appropriate time.
- Await blood test results of the involved patient (with his or her consent) to determine HIV and HBV status. State laws may vary concerning this practice.
- Attend counseling session regarding safe practices to protect self and others.

Using the Infection-Control Nurse

In the hospital, the infection-control nurse is responsible for educating patients and staff about effective infection-control techniques and for collecting statistics about infections. Many hospitals rely on this specialized practitioner to survey laboratory reports and review records for patients at risk as well as suggest approaches to potentially dangerous situations. Intensive investigative strategies create a positive environment that significantly reduces the incidence of nosocomial infections in healthcare facilities. The infection-control nurse knows the devastating effects of infection and is intent on promoting health and fostering a systematic approach to infection control.

In the home, the infection control nurse's duties include surveillance for agency-associated infections, education, consultation, epidemiologic investigation, quality-improvement activities, and policy and procedure development. OSHA regulations state that home care agencies must have an infection-control program and that OSHA infection-control standards and policies must be available to all staff for reference.

EVALUATING

Nurses as primary caregivers can intervene in and positively affect a patient's outcome. By assessing the person at risk, selecting appropriate nursing diagnoses, planning, and intervening to maintain a safe environment, the nurse can reduce a patient's potential for developing an infection. Evaluation of the plan of care determines whether the individual's need for safety is being effectively met. Ongoing systematic evaluation is crucial for nurses who strive to maintain a secure environment for their patients as well as themselves. If patient goals have been met and evaluative criteria have been satisfied, the patient will accomplish the following:

- Correctly use techniques of medical asepsis
- Identify health habits and lifestyle patterns that promote health
- State the signs and symptoms of an infection
- Identify unsafe situations in the home environment

Learning Outcomes

After studying this chapter, the learner should be able to accomplish the following:

1. Define the key terms used in the chapter.

aerobic	iatrogenic
anaerobic	infection
asepsis	isolation
bacteria	medical asepsis
Centers for Disease	nosocomial infection
Control and Prevention	pathogen
endogenous	reservoir
exogenous	surgical asepsis
fungi	virus
host	

2. Explain the infection cycle.
3. Describe nursing interventions used to break the chain of infection.
4. List the stages of an infection.
5. Identify patients at risk for developing an infection.
6. Identify factors that reduce the incidence of nosocomial infection.
7. Identify situations in which handwashing is indicated.
8. Identify nursing diagnoses for a patient who has an infection or is at risk for infection.
9. Describe strategies for implementing CDC guidelines for standard and transmission-based precautions when caring for patients.
10. Implement recommended techniques for medical and surgical asepsis.

Critical Thinking Exercises

1. A nurse cannot help but notice that whenever a particular surgeon makes rounds, he ignores basic principles of asepsis. He will move from one patient to another, touching dressings without washing his hands between patients. He is also inconsistent in his practice of sterile technique. You suspect that there is a higher rate of post-operative infection among his patients. What do you do?

2. A friend who is a nursing student always wears gloves when doing anything for ill patients. You are more selective in your use of gloves. She tells you that you are a fool for "taking chances" because you never know what you may pick up and bring home. Should this be a matter of personal preference? Is one position more consistent with good nursing? Are your instructors consistent in how they would respond to the above question?

Study Questions

1. The smallest infectious agents capable of causing an infection are
   a. bacteria
   b. viruses
   c. molds
   d. yeasts
2. Your patient has developed a low-grade fever and states that she has felt very tired lately. This phase of an infection is known as the
   a. incubation period
   b. prodromal stage
   c. full stage of illness
   d. convalescent period
3. The highest mortality rate is associated with nosocomial infections that involve the
   a. respiratory tract
   b. integumentary system
   c. urinary tract
   d. intestines
4. A patient develops a urinary tract infection after an indwelling urinary catheter has been inserted. This would most accurately be termed
   a. a viral infection
   b. a chronic infection
   c. an iatrogenic infection
   d. an opportunistic infection
5. The nurse has opened the sterile supplies and donned two sterile gloves to complete a sterile dressing change. Maintaining surgical asepsis requires that the nurse
   a. keep splashes on the sterile field to a minimum
   b. cover the nose and mouth with gloved hands if a sneeze is imminent

c. use the dominant hand to cleanse the incision with a moist saline sponge and then apply the dry dressing

d. consider the outer 1 inch of the sterile field as contaminated

6. The CDC standard precaution recommendations apply to
    a. only patients with diagnosed infections
    b. only blood and body fluids with visible blood
    c. all body fluids including sweat
    d. all patients receiving care in hospitals

7. In addition to standard precautions, the nurse caring for a patient with rubella would plan to implement
    a. droplet precautions
    b. airborne precautions
    c. contact precautions
    d. universal precautions

8. When caring for a patient with latex allergy, the nurse creates a latex-safe environment by
    a. carefully cleaning the wall-mounted blood pressure device before using it
    b. donning latex gloves outside the room to limit powder dispersal
    c. using a latex-free pharmacy protocol
    d. placing the patient in a semi-private room

9. The guidelines for minimum protection standards for infection prevention and control were initially developed by
    a. OSHA
    b. individual healthcare facilities
    c. the state governing body
    d. the CDC

10. The recommended sequence when the nurse removes soiled personal protective equipment when preparing to leave the patient's room is
    a. remove gown, goggles, mask, gloves, and exit the room
    b. remove gloves, wash hands, remove gown, mask, and goggles
    c. remove gloves, mask, gown, goggles, and wash hands

d. remove goggles, mask, gloves, gown, and wash hands

11. For a nurse under normal conditions with unsoiled hands, effective handwashing between patients requires
    a. at least a 10- to 15-second scrub
    b. at least a 23-minute scrub
    c. use of an antimicrobial product
    d. that a mask be worn when scrubbing

12. Which hospitalized patient is most at risk for developing a nosocomial infection?
    a. Mr. Y, a 60-year-old patient who smokes two packs of cigarettes daily
    b. Mrs. J, a 40-year-old patient who has a white blood cell count of $6000/mm^3$
    c. Mr. L, a 65-year-old patient who has an indwelling urinary catheter in place
    d. Mrs. M, a 60-year-old patient who is a vegetarian and slightly underweight

13. A patient develops food poisoning from contaminated potato salad. The means of transmission for the infecting organism is
    a. direct contact
    b. vector
    c. vehicle
    d. airborne

14. A nurse is caring for an obese 62-year-old patient with arthritis who has developed an open reddened area over his sacrum. A priority nursing diagnosis is
    a. Altered Nutrition: More Than Body Requirements related to immobility
    b. Impaired Physical Mobility related to pain and discomfort
    c. Chronic Pain related to immobility
    d. Risk for Infection related to altered skin integrity

15. The nurse teaches a patient at home to use clean technique when changing a wound dressing. This is
    a. the nurse's preference
    b. safe for the home setting
    c. unethical behavior
    d. grossly negligent

Answers With Rationale

1. The correct response is *b*. A virus is the smallest of all microorganisms and can only be seen with a special microscope. Molds and yeasts (fungi) and bacteria are larger infectious agents.

2. The correct response is *b*. During the prodromal stage, the person has vague signs and symptoms, such as fatigue and a low-grade fever. There are no obvious symptoms of infection during the incubation period, and they are more specific during the full stage of illness before disappearing by the convalescent period.

3. The correct response is *a*. Urinary tract infections and surgical wounds are common sites for nosocomial infections to develop, but the highest mortality

rate is associated with those infections that involve the respiratory tract. The intestine is not particularly prone to nosocomial infections.

4. The correct response is *c*. An infection that develops as a result of the insertion of an indwelling catheter is termed iatrogenic. Because this infection just developed, it is not chronic, nor did it occur because of any altered physiology that may give an opportunistic organism a chance to cause infection. Urinary infections are bacterial, not viral.

5. The correct response is *d*. Considering the outer inch of a sterile field as contaminated is a principle of surgical asepsis. Moisture contaminates the sterile field, and sneezing would contaminate the sterile gloves.

The sterile hand that cleaned a wound should not be used or should be regloved before applying a sterile dressing.

6. The correct response is *d*. Standard precautions apply to all patients receiving care in hospitals regardless of their diagnosis or possible infection status. These recommendations include blood, all body fluids, secretions, and excretions except sweat, nonintact skin, and mucous membranes.

7. The correct response is *a*. Rubella is an illness transmitted by large-particle droplets and requires droplet precautions in addition to standard precautions. Universal precautions and body substance isolation are incorporated into the new CDC standard precautions recommendations.

8. The correct response is *c*. Wall-mounted blood pressure devices have latex tubing and should not be touched or used on the patient. Latex gloves could cause a serious allergic response; only synthetic gloves are allowed in a latex-free environment. A private room is best to minimize the possibility of latex exposure from something used for the other patient. A latex-free pharmacy protocol is a vital component when creating a safe environment for this patient.

9. The correct response is *d*. The CDC established the initial minimum requirements for infection prevention and control. OSHA has issued and monitors regulations for use of universal precautions in situations and settings in which exposure to blood and other infectious materials is possible.

10. The correct response is *c*. Gloves are always removed first because they are most likely to be contaminated, and hands should be washed thoroughly after the equipment has been removed and before leaving the room.

11. The correct response is *a*. Hands that are not visibly soiled can be effectively cleaned with a 10- to 15-second scrub. Neither a mask nor an antimicrobial product is required in this situation or setting. Hands that are visibly soiled require a longer scrub.

12. The correct response is *c*. Indwelling urinary catheters have been implicated in most nosocomial infections. Cigarette smoking, a normal white blood cell count, and a vegetarian diet have not been implicated as risk factors for infection.

13. The correct response is *c*. Contaminated food is a vehicle for transmitting an infection. Direct contact requires proximity between the susceptible host and an infected person. A vector is a nonhuman carrier, such as an insect, and the airborne means of transmission carries the organism in droplet nuclei or with dust.

14. The correct response is *d*. The priority diagnosis in this situation is the possibility of an infection developing in the open skin area. The others may be potential or probable diagnoses for this patient and may also require nursing interventions after the first diagnosis is addressed.

15. The correct response is *b*. In the home setting, where the patient's environment is more controlled, medical asepsis is usually recommended, with the exception of self-injection. This is the appropriate procedure for the home and is neither unethical nor grossly negligent.

Bibliography

Ames, A. (1999). Accidental needlesticks. *RN, 62*(3), 62–65.

Beaumont, E. (1997). Technology scorecard: Focus on infection control. *American Journal of Nursing, 97*(12), 51–54.

Borton, D. (1997). Isolation precautions: Clearing up the confusion. *Nursing, 27*(1), 49–51.

Borton, D. (1998). Taking a commonsense approach to infection control. *Nursing, 28*(5), 32hn1–32hn4.

Burke, J., & Riley, D. (1996). Nosocomial urinary tract infections. In *Hospital infections. Hospital epidemiology and infection control* (pp. 141–153). Baltimore: Williams & Wilkins.

Burt, S. (1998). What you need to know about latex allergy. *Nursing, 28*(10), 33–39.

Carroll, P. (1998). Preventing nosocomial pneumonia. *RN, 61*(6), 44–47.

Carroll, P. (1999). Latex allergy: What you need to know. *RN, 62*(9), 41–45.

Casey, K., Curry, J., & Douglas, S. (1998). Infection control: HIV/AIDS and other bloodborne pathogens. *Nursing Spectrum, 7*(1), 12–14.

Centers for Disease Control and Prevention. (1997). *Staphylococcus aureus* with reduced susceptibility to vancomycin—United States. *Morbidity and Mortality Weekly Report, 46,* 765–766.

Crow, S. (1997). Your guide to gloves. *Nursing, 27*(3), 26–27.

Crow, S. (1998). Asepsis: Back to the basics. *Urologic Nursing, 18*(1), 42–46.

Dikon, A. (1998). Ways to prevent infection in patients with special needs. *Nursing, 28*(5), 32hn17–32hn19.

Edmond, M., Wenzel, R., & Pasculle, A. (1996). Vancomycin-resistant *Staphylococcus aureus:* Perspectives on measures needed for control. *Annals of Internal Medicine, 124,* 329–334.

Finkelstein, L. (1998). Exposure to bloodborne pathogens. *American Journal of Nursing, 98*(3), 67–68.

Fraser, D. (1997). Assessing the elderly for infections. *Journal of Gerontological Nursing, 23*(11), 5–10.

Garner, J. (1996). Guideline for isolation precautions in hospitals. *Infection Control Hospital Epidemiology, 17,* 53–80.

Gritter, M. (1998). The latex threat. *American Journal of Nursing, 98*(9), 26–32.

Hawke, M. (1997). Infection control practice: Much more than handwashing. *Nursing Spectrum, 6*(21), 4–6.

Jagger, J., & Perry, J. (1999). Power in numbers: Reducing your risk of bloodborne exposures. *Nursing, 29*(1), 51–52.

Jones, L., & Hannum, D. (1998). Playing it safe with a particulate respirator. *Nursing, 28*(1), 50–51.

Korniewicz, D., & Rabussay, D. (1997). Surgical glove failures in clinical practice settings. *AORN Journal, 66*(4), 660–667.

Marx, J. (1998). Teaching your patient about isolation precautions. *Nursing, 28*(5), 32hn20–32hn21.

McConnell, E. (1998). How to choose and use needle-stick prevention devices. *Nursing, 28*(5), 32hn6–32hn8.

McConnell, E. (1999). Proper handwashing technique. *Nursing, 29*(4), 26.

McGann, S., O'Boyle, E., & Brochard, B. (1997). Latex allergy alert. *Nursing Spectrum, 6*(15), 12–13.

Moolenar, R., Crutcher, M., SanJoaquin, V., Sewell, L., Hutwagner, L., Carson, L., Robinson, D., Smithee, L., & Jarvis, W. (2000). A prolonged outbreak of *Pseudomonas aeruginosa* in a neonatal intensive care unit: Did staff fingernails play a role in disease transmission? *Infection Control and Hospital Epidemiology, 21*(2), 80–85.

Murphy, D. (1998). Infectious microbes and disease: General principles. *Nursing Spectrum, 7*(2), 12–14.

North American Nursing Diagnosis Association (1999). *Nursing Diagnoses: Definitions and Classification 1999–2000,* Philadelphia: Author.

Peterson, C. (1997). ANA applauds safer needle device bill. *American Journal of Nursing, 97*(12), 16.

Povolny, K. (1997). Needle sticks: The ugly truth. *RN, 60*(6), 41–43.

Rice, R. (1998). Infection control in the home: 1998 Update. *Geriatric Nursing, 19*(5), 297–300.

Ritter, J. (1998). Using invasive medical devices safely. *Nursing, 28*(5), 32hn12–32hn16.

Salisbury, D., Hutfilz, P., Treen, L., Bollin, G., & Gautam, S. (1997). The effect of rings on microbial load of health care workers' hands. *American Journal of Infection Control, 25*(1), 24–27.

Sarver-Steffenson, J. (1999). When MRSA reaches into long-term care. *RN, 62*(3), 39–41.

Scott, A. (1999). Latex allergies: Mild or severe, allergies to latex products require attention. *Advance for Nurses, 1*(8), 32.

Sheff, B. (1998). VRE & MRSA: Putting bad bugs out of business. *Nursing, 28*(3), 40–44.

Turco, T., et al. (1998). Press release, American Academy of Orthopedic Surgeons. *Annals of Pharmacotherapy, 32,* 758–760.

Chapter 28
Medications

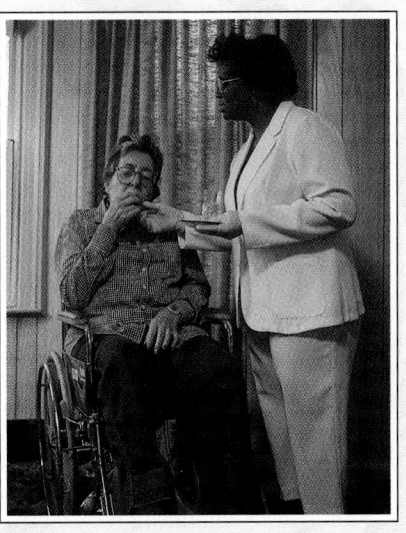

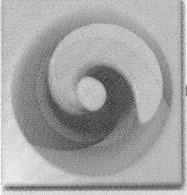

Thinking Critically About
Nursing's Blended Skills

Before reading this chapter, think about the types of blended skills you will need to administer medications safely.

- You are "pulled" to pediatrics and realize that you are unfamiliar with pediatric dosages of the medications ordered for the children assigned to your care.

- You realize to your horror that you just gave one nursing home resident another resident's morning medications.

- You discover as a school nurse that more and more doctors seem to be prescribing stimulants such as Ritalin and antidepressants such as Prozac for preschoolers. Alarmed about pharmacologic "fixes" to behavior problems, you are uncertain of how to respond but know that you do not want to participate in inappropriately medicating children.

- A family member with arthritis who frequently complains about joint pain asks your advice about a new medication he saw advertised on television. Another family member asks what you think about Viagra and whether there are any reasons why he should not try it.

What cognitive, technical, interpersonal, and ethical/legal skills do you think you will need to respond to the challenges described above?

edication administration is a basic nursing function that involves skillful technique and consideration of the patient's development and safety. The nurse administering medications needs a knowledge base about drugs, including drug names, preparations, classifications, adverse effects, and physiologic factors that affect drug action (see the accompanying box, Through the Eyes of a Student).

The nursing process can be applied to the fundamental nursing skill of medication administration. Assessment includes a comprehensive medication history as well as ongoing assessments of the patient's response during and after drug therapy. Nursing diagnoses are developed from the assessment data. Patient-centered outcomes are evaluated after implementation of the plan of care, tailored to the patient's needs.

A *drug* or *medication* is any substance that modifies body functions when taken into the body. The study that deals with chemicals that affect the body's functioning is called *pharmacology*. A *pharmacist* is a person licensed to prepare and dispense drugs. The physician is legally responsible for prescribing medications, although in some states, nurse practitioners have this privilege also. The physician or nurse practitioner conveys the medication plans to others by an order called a *prescription*. After the medication is prepared by the pharmacist, the nurse administers the medication to the patient.

Some medications are given frequently, and the nurse becomes familiar with the facts about these drugs. With other medications not given often, the nurse needs information before administering the drugs. Information about specific drugs is available in pharmacology texts. Many drug references are available to nurses to increase one's knowledge of medications.

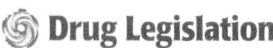

Drug Legislation

In 1906, the Pure Food and Drug Act designated the United States Pharmacopeia (USP) and the National Formulary (NF) as official standards of drugs and empowered the federal government to enforce these standards. This legislation was updated in 1938 by the Federal Food, Drug and Cosmetic Act. The Food and Drug Administration (FDA) enforces this law. Extensive testing of new drugs is required before they may be marketed for use. An amendment to the Federal Food, Drug and Cosmetic Act in 1952 distinguished prescription drugs from nonprescription (over-the-counter) drugs and provided directions for dispensing prescription drugs.

The Comprehensive Drug Abuse Prevention and Control Act, also known as the Controlled Substances Act, was passed in 1970. This law regulates the distribution of narcotics and other drugs of abuse. Such drugs have been categorized according to their therapeutic usefulness and potential for abuse. Government programs for the prevention and treatment of drug abuse were established.

Introduction to Pharmacology

Drug Preparations

Nomenclature

Drugs have several names. The **chemical name** is a precise description of the drug's chemical composition; it identifies the drug's atomic and molecular structure. This name is of significance to the pharmacist. The **generic name** is

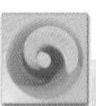

COGNITIVE SKILLS

• Basic knowledge of pharmacology; drug names, types of preparations, types of orders; drug classifications and actions; adverse effects; drug dose calculations

• Knowledge of how to prepare and administer medications safely by the oral, parenteral, topical, and inhalation routes

• Knowledge of how to develop teaching plans to meet patient needs specific to medication administration

• Knowledge of resources to contact when encountering questions about medications or dosing parameters with which you are unfamiliar

TECHNICAL SKILLS

• Ability to use equipment correctly and implement techniques for safe and effective preparation and administration of medications

INTERPERSONAL SKILLS

• Strong people skills; ability to communicate and interact effectively with individuals and groups

• Ability to establish trusting relationships with patients, families, public groups, and colleagues as a basis for teaching and counseling with respect to medication regimens

ETHICAL/LEGAL SKILLS

• Commitment to safety and quality; strong sense of responsibility, accountability; strong advocacy abilities

• Knowledge of pertinent drug legislation and policy

• Commitment to report medication errors and to follow agency policy for working to prevent their recurrence

Through the Eyes of a Student

I entered my patient's room, knowing that she had had surgery less than 12 hours before my arrival, and introduced myself. I asked how she was feeling, to which she immediately responded, "I need pain medication—*now!*" I told her that I would check the medication orders and be back as soon as possible. I walked quickly to the medication Kardex, and there it was glaring at me in neatly printed black and white: "Demerol, 100 mg IM q 3–4 hr p.r.n." My mind raced as I thought, "I have never given an IM injection. There has to be something else ordered for pain." I knew there wasn't. I found my clinical instructor and announced, "My patient needs an IM injection." Given the anxiety I was feeling, everything went surprisingly well as we prepared the medication. I went over the procedure one last time before entering the patient's room.

We approached the patient just in time for her to look at us in sheer terror and cry, "I hope that shot isn't for me; I hate them," which did nothing for my already shaking hands. I explained that she couldn't take a pill because she could not have anything by mouth because of the nature of her surgery. My instructor and I positioned the patient on her side—a feat in itself—so that I could give her the shot in the dorsogluteal area. I marked the landmarks at least half a dozen times, wiped the area with alcohol, and asked her if she was ready for the injection. *Big mistake!* She swiftly replied, "No, but get it over with."

A little voice in my head repeated the words my technologies professor had said a million times, "Darting action is the key to a successful injection." So I aimed at the bull's-eye that appeared in front of my eyes. My hand, which seemed to be moving in slow motion, propelled downward at a 90-degree angle. Secretly I prayed that I would not hit my own hand. I must have closed my eyes because the next thing I remember was the loudest scream I had ever heard! I looked down and it was a bull's-eye, thank God, but the needle had not penetrated the muscle! The patient successfully tensed her muscle tight enough to intercept the needle midflight. At that moment she relaxed, probably because she thought the worst was over, and I pushed the needle into place. I slowly drew back the plunger to make sure no blood appeared in the syringe. I began injecting the Demerol slowly, watching my hands shake. Then I withdrew the needle and gently applied pressure over the site. It was over and I wanted to scream, "I did it!" but I kept my composure to feign the experience I lacked. Giving my first IM injection was not as bad as I thought it would be!

—Alison L. Moriarty, Georgetown University, Washington, DC

the name assigned by the manufacturer that first develops the drug. Often, the generic name is derived from the chemical name. The **official name** is the name by which the drug is identified in the official publication, *United States Pharmacopeia and National Formulary* (USP and NF). The **trade name**, also referred to as the *brand name* or *proprietary name*, is selected by the drug company that sells the drug and is copyrighted. A drug can have several trade names when produced by different manufacturers.

Nurses should be familiar with a drug's generic and trade names. For example, acetaminophen (generic name) has trade names such as Tylenol, Tempra, and Liquiprin.

Types of Preparations

Drugs are available in many forms, or preparations. The form in which the drug is prepared may determine the route of administration. Some drugs may be prepared in only one form to be administered by a certain route. Others may be supplied in several preparations, which allow them to be given through various routes. One type of preparation may be desirable in a given situation. For example, a liquid preparation of a medication would be indicated for young children who are not able to swallow solid preparations such as tablets. Drug preparations are available for oral, topical, and injectable administration. Table 28-1 describes drug preparations commonly used by the nurse.

Classifications

How do nurses organize the vast amount of information about medications? Where do nurses begin their study of medications? Nurses should begin with a focus on drug classifications.

Drugs are classified from different perspectives. For example, drugs may be classified by body systems (eg, drugs that affect the respiratory system, drugs that affect the cardiovascular system), by the symptom relieved by the drug, or by the clinical indication for the drug (eg, analgesic, antibiotic).

Mechanisms of Drug Action

Pharmacodynamics

Drugs act at the cellular level to achieve the desired effects. The process by which drugs alter cell physiology is called *pharmacodynamics* (Abrams, 1998). One mechanism of drug action is a drug–receptor interaction in which the drug interacts with one or more cellular structures to alter cell function. These specialized structures are called *receptor*

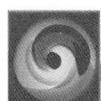

Table 28-1
Common Types of Drug Preparations

Preparation	Description
Capsule	Powder or gel form of an active drug enclosed in a gelatinous container
Elixir	Medication in a clear liquid containing water, alcohol, sweeteners, and flavor
Extended release	Preparation of a medication that allows for slow and continuous release over a predetermined period; may also be referred to as CR or CRT (controlled release), SR (sustained or slow release), SA (sustained action), LA (long acting), or TR (timed release)
Liniment	Medication mixed with alcohol, oil, or soap, which is rubbed on the skin
Lotion	Drug particles in a solution for topical use
Lozenge	Small oval, round, or oblong preparation containing a drug in a flavored or sweetened base, which dissolves in the mouth and releases the medication; also called *troche*
Ointment	Semisolid preparation containing a drug to be applied externally; also called an *unction*
Pill	Mixture of a powdered drug with a cohesive material; may be round or oval
Powder	Single or mixture of finely ground drugs
Solution	A drug dissolved in another substance (eg, in an aqueous solution)
Suppository	An easily melted medication preparation in a firm base such as gelatin that is inserted into the body (rectum, vagina, urethra)
Suspension	Finely divided, undissolved particles in a liquid medium; should be shaken before use
Syrup	Medication combined in a water and sugar solution
Tablet	Small, solid dose of medication, compressed or molded; may be any color, size, or shape; *enteric-coated tablets* are coated with a substance that is insoluble in gastric acids to reduce gastric irritation by the drug
Transdermal patch	Unit dose of medication applied directly to skin for diffusion through skin and absorption into the bloodstream

sites. The drug fits the receptor as a key fits a lock. Drugs may also combine with enzymes to achieve the desired effect, which is referred to as a *drug–enzyme interaction.* Some drugs act on the cell membrane or alter the cellular environment.

Pharmacokinetics

Pharmacokinetics is the study of the movement of drug molecules in the body in relation to the drug's absorption, distribution, metabolism, and excretion.

Absorption

Absorption is the process by which a drug is transferred from its site of entry into the body to the bloodstream. Absorption of a drug is influenced by several factors:

Route of administration: Injected medications are usually absorbed more rapidly than oral medications.

Drug solubility: Liquid medications are absorbed more rapidly than solid preparations. Liquid preparations do not have to be dissolved in the gastrointestinal fluids. Most drugs are weak acids and bases. When in solution, drugs are a mixture of ionized and unionized forms. The *unionized form* is lipid soluble and more readily absorbed, whereas the *ionized form* is not easily absorbed and is lipid insoluble. This factor is important because cell membranes have a fatty acid layer and a drug that is more lipid soluble can be more readily absorbed and pass through the cell membrane (McKenry & Salerno, 1998).

pH: The form in which the drug is found depends on the pH of the environment. Acidic drugs are well absorbed in the stomach. Drugs that are basic remain ionized or insoluble in an acid environment. These drugs are not absorbed before reaching the small intestine. The concept of acid–base balance is further discussed in Chapter 45.

Local conditions at the site of administration: The more extensive the absorbing surface, the greater the absorption of the drug and the more rapid the effect. A patient with burns would have poor absorption from an intramuscular injection. Food in the stomach can delay the absorption of some medications or enhance the rate of absorption of other drugs. Drug absorption can be manipulated with sustained-release preparations or enteric-coated preparations. Enteric-coated preparations are resistant to the digestive action of the stomach.

Drug dosage: A loading dose, or a larger than normal dose, is usually given when a patient is in acute distress and it is necessary to achieve the maximum therapeutic effect as quickly as possible. If drug toxicity occurs, it can quickly be detected and treated in the controlled hospital environment. A maintenance dose is a lower dosage that becomes the usual or daily dosage. Patients who receive digoxin or phenobarbital may receive loading doses when therapy is initiated.

After a drug has been absorbed, its serum level can be monitored by drawing a blood specimen and measuring the drug's peak and trough levels. This is recommended for certain medications (eg, aminoglycoside antibiotics, digoxin, and theophylline) to ensure that a therapeutic range is maintained. A drug's *therapeutic range* is that concentration of drug in the blood serum that produces the desired effect without causing toxicity. The *peak level,* or highest plasma concentration, of the drug should be measured when absorption is complete. The peak level may be affected by factors that affect drug absorption as well as the route of administration. The *trough level* is the point when the drug is at its lowest concentration, and this specimen is usually drawn in the 30-minute interval before the next dose. The dosage schedule, as well as the half-life of the drug, can modify the trough level. Simply stated, a drug's *half-life* is the amount of time it takes for half a dose of a drug to be eliminated from the body (Chase, 1997). Monitoring these levels ensures the effectiveness and safety of certain drugs (Shirrell, Gibbar-Clements, Dooley, & Free 1999).

Distribution

After a drug has been absorbed into the bloodstream, it is distributed throughout the body. The drug accumulates in specific tissues for its action. **Distribution** depends on the rate of perfusion and capillary permeability to the drug. Certain other factors may also influence distribution. The drug may bind to plasma proteins, which causes unequal distribution and may prevent the drug from reaching its intended site of action. The blood-brain barrier is poorly permeable to water-soluble drugs. Some drugs fail to penetrate the tissues of the central nervous system as readily as others. The placenta, on the other hand, is not a selective barrier to the distribution of drugs. Drugs move across the placenta readily, and many produce harmful effects in the fetus.

Metabolism

Metabolism, or biotransformation, is the breakdown of the drug to an inactive form. The liver is the primary site for drug metabolism. Various processes and enzymes are involved in metabolism. Physiologic changes associated with aging or the presence of liver disease may complicate the process. Pharmacology texts provide more detailed explanations of metabolism.

Excretion

After the drug is broken down to an inactive form, **excretion** of the drug from the body occurs. Most drugs are excreted by the kidneys. The lungs are the primary route for the excretion of gaseous substances, such as inhalation anesthetics. Many drugs are excreted through the intestines. The sweat, salivary, and mammary glands are also routes of drug excretion.

Some medications may be contraindicated, or dosages may need to be adjusted downward if renal excretion is affected by age or disease. A recent FDA directive orders drug manufacturers to include specific information regarding implications for geriatric patients on the package inserts of certain drugs. Of particular concern are details concerning the excretion of these drugs in older adults whose renal function has declined. This ruling affects psychotropic drugs, nonsteroidal antiinflammatory agents, oral hypoglycemic agents, anticoagulants, certain broad-spectrum antibiotics, and cardiac drugs (Skolnick, 1997).

Factors Affecting Drug Action

Certain variables influence the action or effect of a medication.

Developmental Considerations

During pregnancy, most drugs are contraindicated because of their possible adverse effects on the fetus, and certain drugs, referred to as *teratogenic drugs,* are known to have potential to cause developmental defects in the embryo or fetus. Examples of teratogenic drugs include cocaine, alcohol, phenytoin (Dilantin; an anticonvulsant), and isotretinoin (Accutane; a medication used to treat severe acne). Breastfed infants are also at risk for adverse effects from drugs in the mother's circulation. A child's dose for medication is smaller than an adult's dose. Infants are especially responsive to medications because of the immaturity of their organs. Older people are responsive to medications because their bodies have experienced physiologic changes associated with the aging process, including decreased gastric motility, acid production, and blood flow, which affect drug absorption. Small body size, reduced weight, and reduced body water also alter distribution, as do decreases in cardiac output and organ perfusion. Decreased plasma binding increases the possibility of drug toxicity. Liver function declines with advancing age and changes in hepatic enzymes involved in drug metabolism. Blood flow to the liver decreases secondary to a decrease in cardiac output. Drugs are excreted more slowly from the body as a result of changes in kidney function. Receptor sensitivity is altered in older people, and their sensitivity to certain drugs increases. The physiologic changes in older people that increase drug susceptibility are summarized in the accompanying box, Focus on Older Adults.

Weight

Expected responses to drugs are based largely on those reactions that occur when the drugs are given to healthy adults (18 to 65 years of age, 150 lb [68 kg]). Nurses should know the usual dose for a particular medication. Drug doses for children are calculated by weight or body surface area.

Focus on the Older Adult

Altered Drug Response in Older People

Physiologic Basis	Adverse Reaction	Nursing Action
Decreased gastric emptying time and increased pH of gastric juices	Stomach irritation and ulceration	Assess for symptoms of stomach discomfort. Test stools for blood.
Increased adipose tissue and decreased total body fluid in proportion to the total body mass	Increased possibility of drug toxicity	Assess for early signs of drug interactions or toxicity. Monitor blood levels of drugs. Monitor laboratory values.
Decreased number of protein-binding sites		
Decline in liver function and enzyme production needed for drug metabolism		
Decreased kidney function, resulting in diminished filtration and excretion		
Altered peripheral venous tone	More pronounced hypotensive effects from medications (particularly antihypertensives and diuretics)	Monitor vital signs. Caution patient to change position slowly.
Changes in blood-brain barrier allowing for easier penetration of fat-soluble drugs	Increased risk for dizziness and confusion, particularly with beta blockers	Assess for dizziness and light-headedness. Be aware of safety precautions.

Sex

The difference in the distribution of body fat and fluids in men and women is a minor factor affecting the action of some drugs. To date, most research on drugs and their actions and effects has been conducted on men. Future clinical drug trials are expected to include more women in order to document the effects of hormonal fluctuations (see the accompanying Research in Nursing box).

Genetic and Cultural Factors

Differences in the responses of patients receiving the same medication may result from genetic and cultural differences. *Pharmacoanthropology*, a relatively new field of study, investigates differences in drug response in various ethnic or racial groups (Abrams, 1998). Enzyme deficiencies or metabolic disturbances can alter the way the body handles medication or metabolizes a drug. For example, Asian patients may require smaller doses of a drug because they metabolize it at a slower rate. A drug dose that is normal for a white patient may cause unexpected side effects in an Asian; differences in body heights and weights do not appear to be a factor in this response. African Americans appear to require larger doses of some medications that are used to lower blood pressure. Culturally related health beliefs can also affect compliance and response to a medication regimen. Herbal treatments that are popular in some

cultures may interfere with or counteract the action of prescribed medication. Nurses who are aware of the specific needs and beliefs of culturally diverse patients are better able to communicate effectively with them. The accompanying box gives guidelines for effective communication about medication with culturally diverse patients.

Psychological Factors

The patient's expectations of the medication affect the response to the medication, as, for instance, in studies of drug effects in which some patients receive a placebo. A *placebo* is a pharmacologically inactive substance. In clinical drug trials, one group of patients receives the active drug, whereas another group receives a placebo to study the drug's effects. Some patients appear to have the same response with the placebo as with the active drug.

Pathology

The presence of disease can affect drug action. The liver is the primary organ for drug breakdown. Pathologic conditions that involve the liver may slow down metabolism.

Environment

The patient's environment may influence the response to medications. Sensory deprivation and overload may affect drug responses. The relative oxygen deprivation at high

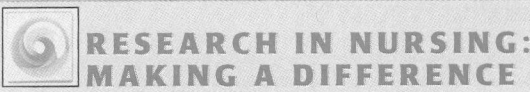
RESEARCH IN NURSING: MAKING A DIFFERENCE

Enhancing Medication Compliance in Elderly People Living in the Community

Noncompliance with a medical regimen places an individual at risk for complications from disease. Many previous studies have documented that elderly individuals living at home who require medication for chronic diseases are particularly at risk for noncompliance with their medication schedules. Managed care and the accompanying cuts in home care reimbursement limit the nurse's ability to improve compliance, yet simple measures that serve as reminders for this population can have a positive effect on management of symptoms and overall well-being.

Related Research
Fulmer, T., Feldman, P., Kim, T., Carty, B., Beers, M., Molina, M., & Putnam, M. (1999). An intervention study to enhance medication compliance in community-dwelling elderly individuals. *Journal of Gerontological Nursing, 25*(6), 6–14.
Individuals, 65 years of age and older, who had a primary or secondary diagnosis of congestive heart failure (CHF) and were living at home were recruited to participate in this study to improve medication compliance. The participants were randomly placed in three groups. The control group received the usual care, which included prepoured medications prepared

by the home care nurse during a weekly visit. The second group received a daily telephone call, and the third group received a daily videotelephone call. Over the course of the study, the two groups receiving daily telephone or videotelephone reminders demonstrated improved medication compliance. Electronic prescription bottlecaps measured the pill-taking of the participants. This study reinforced the effectiveness of a simple strategy, such as a telephone call, in improving compliance with a medication regimen and demonstrated the potential impact that technologic advances can have on patient care.

Relevance to Nursing Practice
Interventions that enable the nurse to monitor medication compliance of a high-risk group in a community setting can have a significant impact on preventing the rehospitalization that is common with a chronic disease such as CHF. The increased contact offered by a simple daily telephone call provided additional reminders to take prescribed medications. The nurse can play an essential role in helping elderly people to maintain their independence, avoid complications, and remain in their home setting.

altitudes may increase sensitivity to some drugs. The patient who receives pain medication or a sedative in an active, noisy environment may not be able to benefit fully from the medication's effects. Nutritional state can also affect the body's reaction to certain drugs.

Timing of Administration
The presence of food in the stomach delays the absorption of orally administered medications. Some medications should be given with food to prevent gastric irritation, and the nurse should consider this when establishing a patient's

Communicating Effectively About Medication With Culturally Diverse Patients

- Acquire basic information about health beliefs and practices of various cultural groups in your healthcare setting.
- Be alert to atypical drug responses or unexpected side effects that may occur in certain ethnic groups.
- Ask specifically about the use of folk or home remedies prescribed by a nontraditional healer.
- Utilize printed or audiovisual information that is in the language spoken by your patients.
- Encourage cultural sensitivity in healthcare workers in your particular setting.

- Recognize that diversity exists within cultural groups. For example, the Hispanic population includes Mexicans, Cubans, Puerto Ricans, and other Latino groups.
- Emphasize threads or messages in health teaching that are common to all cultures (eg, concern about family, faith, and home).
- Include culturally sensitive information in all basic health teaching.
- Help culturally diverse patients to value and understand the importance of communicating concerns and asking questions about prescribed medications.

Adapted from Eisenhauer, L., Nichols, L., Spencer, R. & Bergan, F. (1998). *Clinical pharmacology and nursing management* (5th ed.). Philadelphia: Lippincott Willliams & Wilkins.

medication schedule. Human rhythms and cycles may also influence drug action.

Adverse Drug Effects

Although therapeutic effect is the desired effect in medication administration, sometimes adverse effects or side effects may occur. Those secondary effects that are often predictable and can usually be tolerated are referred to as side effects, whereas adverse effects are more severe and may require discontinuation of the drug. Not all side effects are necessarily adverse. Thirty percent of hospitalized patients experience an adverse drug effect. Most often, analgesics, sedatives, antibiotics, or antipsychotics are involved (Edwards, 1997).

An *iatrogenic disease* is caused unintentionally by drug therapy. *Drug allergy* occurs in a person who has been previously exposed to the drug and has developed antibodies. Drug allergies can be manifested in a variety of symptoms ranging from minor to serious. The reaction can occur immediately after the patient receives the medication or be delayed for hours to days. Some of the signs and symptoms of a drug allergy are rash, urticaria, fever, diarrhea, nausea, and vomiting. A life-threatening immediate reaction is called an **anaphylactic reaction** and results in respiratory distress, sudden severe bronchospasm, and cardiovascular collapse. This reaction is treated with epinephrine, bronchodilators, and antihistamines. Serious adverse drug reactions must be documented according to agency policy and reported to the FDA MEDWATCH program. According to FDA criteria, a serious drug event is defined as an action that is life-threatening, requires intervention to prevent death or permanent impairment, and leads to death, hospitalization, disability, or congenital anomaly. Nurses and healthcare professionals are encouraged to complete a one-page form that provides information on a medication or medical product that they suspect either has caused harm or has the potential to cause harm. The facility risk manager can provide this form (McKenry & Salerno, 1998).

Drug tolerance occurs when the body becomes accustomed to a particular drug over a period of time. Larger doses of the drug must be taken to produce the same effects. A **cumulative effect** occurs when the body cannot metabolize one dose of a drug before another dose is administered. The drug is taken in more frequently than it is excreted, and each new dose increases the total quantity in the body. An **idiosyncratic effect** is any abnormal or peculiar response to a drug that may manifest itself by overresponse, underresponse, or response different from the expected outcome. Older patients often have unpredictable or erratic responses to medications. Idiosyncratic effects are thought to be the result of genetic enzyme deficiencies that lead to an abnormal mechanism of drug breakdown.

In a *drug interaction*, the combined effect of two or more drugs acting simultaneously produces an effect either less than that of each drug alone (**antagonist effect**) or greater than that of each drug alone (**synergistic effect**). Alcohol and barbiturates, for example, when taken together create a synergistic effect. Nurses must be knowledgeable and alert for drug interactions and the effects of drug therapy.

The Nursing Process

ASSESSING THE MEDICATION HISTORY

Assessment of the patient receiving medications begins during a nursing history, one component of which is the medication history. During the interview, the nurse can adapt questions to meet the patient's needs and level of understanding. The nurse should avoid using medical jargon that the patient may not understand but instead should use familiar terms. For instance, the patient may refer to a diuretic as the "water pill" or to an anticoagulant as a "blood thinner."

Areas to be included in the medication history are listed in the accompanying Focused Assessment Guide.

The nurse not only assesses the patient with regard to medications during the nursing history but also continues the assessment during and after medication administration.

The accompanying box, Applying Learning to Practice: Promoting Health, describes medication self-care behaviors for healthcare workers.

DIAGNOSING

Data that the nurse collects may lead to the development of several nursing diagnoses related to medication administration. The following are examples of appropriate nursing diagnoses:

Altered Health Maintenance related to lack of knowledge about anticoagulant medication regimen
Altered Sexuality Patterns related to adverse effects of antihypertensive drug
Anxiety related to daily self-injection of insulin
Body Image Disturbance related to effects of chemotherapy
Risk for Aspiration related to impaired swallowing of oral medications
Risk for Poisoning related to confusion about medication dosages
Knowledge Deficit related to lack of interest in learning about medication regimen
Noncompliance With Medication Regimen related to adverse drug effects, cost of medications, confusion, lack of motivation, visual impairment, complexity of regimen
Sleep Pattern Disturbance related to consistent use of sedative-hypnotics

PLANNING: EXPECTED OUTCOMES

Medication Orders

No medication may be given to a patient without a *medication order* from a physician or, in some states, a nurse practitioner. Each health agency has a policy specifying the manner in which a physician writes an order. In most instances, orders are written on a form specifically designed

FOCUSED ASSESSMENT GUIDE

Medications

Factors to Assess	Questions and Approaches
Previous and current drug use	What medications are you taking that the doctor prescribed for you?
	What over-the-counter medications are you taking on a regular basis?
	Do you use nonmedicinal drugs (eg, alcohol, caffeine, home remedies)?
	How often do you use them?
	What is the reason for taking the medication?
	What medications have you taken during the past year and for what reasons?
	Is there anything else you have tried to alleviate your symptoms?
Medication schedule	At what times do you take your medications?
	Is there any special way your medication has to be prepared (eg, crushing and mixing with applesauce)?
	Do you have any special method for remembering to take your medications?
Response to medications	Have the medications had the expected effects?
	Have you ever experienced any adverse or unexpected reactions to the medications?
	Is there a family history of this type of reaction to medication?
	Do you have any allergies to medications?
	What happens when you take this medication?
Attitude toward drugs and use of drugs	How do you feel about taking medications?
	Why do you take the medications?
Compliance with regimen	Can you tell me your understanding of the reason for taking the medications?
	Can you describe how you follow the medication schedule?
	Are there any problems that prevent you from following the medication regimen?
Storage	Where are your medications stored at home?
	How long do you keep medications in the home?
	Can you show me any medications you have on hand?

for a physician's order. This becomes part of a patient's permanent record. Many healthcare facilities use a computer-generated pharmacy order system and can receive a medication order by fax from the physician.

Safe practice dictates that a nurse follow only a written order. A written order by a physician is least likely to result in error or misunderstanding. Under certain circumstances, such as in an emergency, a verbal order from the physician may be given to a registered nurse or a pharmacist. In most

settings, a student nurse is not permitted to accept a verbal order from a physician. The legal implications for dispensing and administering an agent without a written order vary, and nurses must be familiar with the exact agency policy whenever called on to administer therapeutic agents. The legal implications of verbal orders are discussed in Chapter 7.

Usual hospital policy dictates that when a patient is admitted, unless specific orders to the contrary are written, all drugs that the physician may have ordered while

APPLYING LEARNING TO PRACTICE

Promoting Health

Medications

Use the following assessment checklist to determine how well you are meeting your own need for safe medication practices. Then develop a prescription for self-care by choosing appropriate behaviors from the list of suggestions.

ASSESSMENT CHECKLIST

almost always | sometimes | almost never

☐ ☐ ☐ 1. I store medications in a safe place (eg, a cool, dry place, away from direct sunlight, out of the reach of children).

☐ ☐ ☐ 2. I discard medications that have passed their expiration date.

☐ ☐ ☐ 3. I wear a Medic-Alert tag or carry information that identifies a drug allergy or required medication.

☐ ☐ ☐ 4. I am cautious about combining prescribed medication with OTC drugs, alcohol, or foods that can interact with the drug.

SELF-CARE BEHAVIORS

1. Finish all prescriptions as ordered by physician or nurse practitioner.
2. Avoid foods, alcohol, or over-the-counter drugs that may interact with a prescribed drug.
3. Use available resources (textbooks, pharmacist, physician) to verify the potential for drug interactions or possible side effects of a medication.
4. Use a reminder system to maintain medication schedule.
5. Avoid sharing medications or taking someone else's prescribed pills.
6. Complete any laboratory tests necessary for maintenance or adjustment of a medication regimen.
7. Practice safe behaviors when storing medications.
8. Purchase drugs from the same pharmacy as an additional safeguard with multiple medication regimens.

the patient was at home are discontinued. This can be a problem when a patient brings medications from home to the hospital. To avoid the possibility of having the patient continue taking the home medications while receiving the same ones or others under new orders, all medications should be sent home with the family or removed from the patient's unit and placed in safekeeping. This requires an explanation to the patient and the family of how the patient's drug plan is to be implemented.

In some inpatient facilities, patients keep their medications at their bedside and learn or continue to administer them as they would at home. It is believed that this approach helps to promote patients' independence. The nurse should be aware when patients are allowed to take their own medications while hospitalized and should know each agent's purpose and possible adverse effects. Also, a notation should be made on the patient's plan of care so that everyone knows the patient has medications at the bedside.

When a patient has had surgery or is transferred to another clinical service or another health agency, it is general practice that all orders related to drugs are discontinued and that new orders are written. To keep physicians aware of orders in effect, some hospitals specify a day of the week when orders are to be rewritten, or they automatically are discontinued.

Types of Orders

There are several types of orders that a physician may write.

A *standing order* is carried out as specified until it is canceled by another order. Many physicians whose practices are limited to a particular clinical area have a specified set of written orders for all their hospitalized patients. These are also referred to as standing orders. Occasionally, a physician writes a standing order and its cancellation simultaneously; that is, the physician specifies that a certain order is to be carried out for a stated number of days or times. After the stated period has passed, the order is canceled automatically.

The physician may write an *"as needed" (p.r.n.) order* for medication. The patient receives medication when it is requested or needed. A p.r.n. order commonly is written for postoperative pain medication.

Another type of order is called a *single order*; that is, the directive is carried out only once, at a time specified by the physician. Medication to be administered immediately before surgery is an example of a single order.

A *stat order* also is a single order but one that is carried out at once. A stat order for epinephrine or an antihistamine would be carried out immediately for a patient who is experiencing an anaphylactic drug reaction.

Parts of the Medication Order

The medication order consists of seven parts:

- Patient's name
- Date and time the order is written
- Name of drug to be administered

- Dosage of the drug
- Route by which the drug is to be administered
- Frequency of administration of the drug
- Signature of person writing the order

Patient's Name

The patient's full name is used. The middle name or initial should be included to avoid confusion with other patients. In most agencies, the patient's full name and identification number and the physician's name are mechanically imprinted on all sheets on the patient's chart, including the physician's order sheet.

Date and Time the Order Is Written

The date the order is written is given, sometimes including the time as well. Because the nursing staffs in inpatient agencies change several times during each 24-hour period, the date and time help to prevent errors of oversight as different nurses take charge of a unit. When an order is to be followed for a specified number of days, the date and time are important so that the discontinuation date and time can be determined accurately. The length of time an order for a narcotic remains valid is determined by law. Therefore, the date and time the order is written are essential for determining when the order for a narcotic becomes invalid.

Name of Drug to Be Administered

The name of the drug is stated in the order, either by the brand name or by the generic name. Certain brand names are well known, but the practice of using the generic name is considered safest and is required by some healthcare agencies.

A nurse unfamiliar with a drug has several sources for obtaining information. The USP and NF are the official sources in the United States. Most other countries have similar references that describe official therapeutic agents. Many agencies also provide their own book listing the official drugs commonly used by the agency. The *Physician's Desk Reference* (PDR) is another source of information based on that supplied by pharmaceutical companies. In addition, the nurse may obtain information about drugs from the hospital pharmacist, the physician, and any of several texts written specifically for the nursing role in the management of drug therapy.

Dosage of the Drug

The dosage of a drug can be stated in either the apothecary or the metric system. The metric system has been adopted internationally. These systems are described in a following section.

Apothecary measurements are used less frequently. A medication error may occur if nurses are unfamiliar with the apothecary system, if the doctor's handwriting is illegible, or if administration equipment, such as syringes, cups, or reference sources, use only metric measurement. Self-administered drugs are commonly labeled in household measurements to facilitate administration. Most agencies post a table of common equivalent dosages for people who have learned to use one system and find

that the agency for which they work uses the other system. Although these tables are convenient and useful, the nurse should be prepared to convert from one system to the other because such tables are not available in every situation. The nurse should also be familiar with common equivalent measurements when using household equipment, such as teaspoons and tablespoons, because the home is usually not equipped with special measuring devices. The most common equivalents can be found in Appendix A.

Certain standard abbreviations are used to indicate drug amounts, and the nurse should know the common abbreviations before administering drugs. See Table 20-1 in Chapter 20 for common abbreviations used in drug orders.

Route by Which the Drug Is to Be Administered

The route to be used when administering a medication is stated clearly because some drugs can be given in more than one way and some may be used safely only through one route. Table 28-2 describes common routes by which medications are administered.

Frequency of Administration of the Drug

The time and frequency with which a drug is to be administered are usually stated in standard abbreviations in the medication order. Common abbreviations used in writing prescriptions, including time and frequency, are listed in Chapter 20, Table 20-1.

The nursing service department of inpatient facilities usually determines the hours at which routine drugs are given. For example, if certain drugs are to be given every 4 hours, the nursing service policy indicates the times. Every 4-hour administration may be at the times of 12 noon, 4 PM, 8 PM, 12 midnight, 4 AM, and 8 AM. Another agency may use the hours 1 PM, 5 PM, 9 PM, 1 AM, 5 AM, and 9 AM. To lessen the risk for error, some healthcare facilities use the 24-hour clock (or military time), which designates midnight as 0000 hours and runs until 2400 hours. If a drug is ordered to be given before or after meals, time of administration depends on the hours at which meals are served. It is a nursing responsibility to check that times for medication administration correspond to safe practice for that drug.

If a drug is to be given only once or twice a day, the decision about which hours to use depends on the nature of the drug and the patient's plan of care. Whenever possible, the patient's choice of time should be considered.

Drugs should be administered punctually as ordered. A nurse administering drugs to several patients, however, cannot give all of the drugs exactly on the hour indicated. Agency policies vary, but a common one is that drugs should be administered within a half hour before or after the indicated hour. Thus, a drug to be administered at 9 AM can be administered any time between 8:30 AM and 9:30 AM using this policy. This policy does not apply to all drugs. A preoperative medication ordered to be given at 7:30 AM should be administered at that hour because the time was planned in relation to the time surgery is to begin. Preoperative medications may also be given when the nursing unit receives a call from the operating room to premedicate the surgical

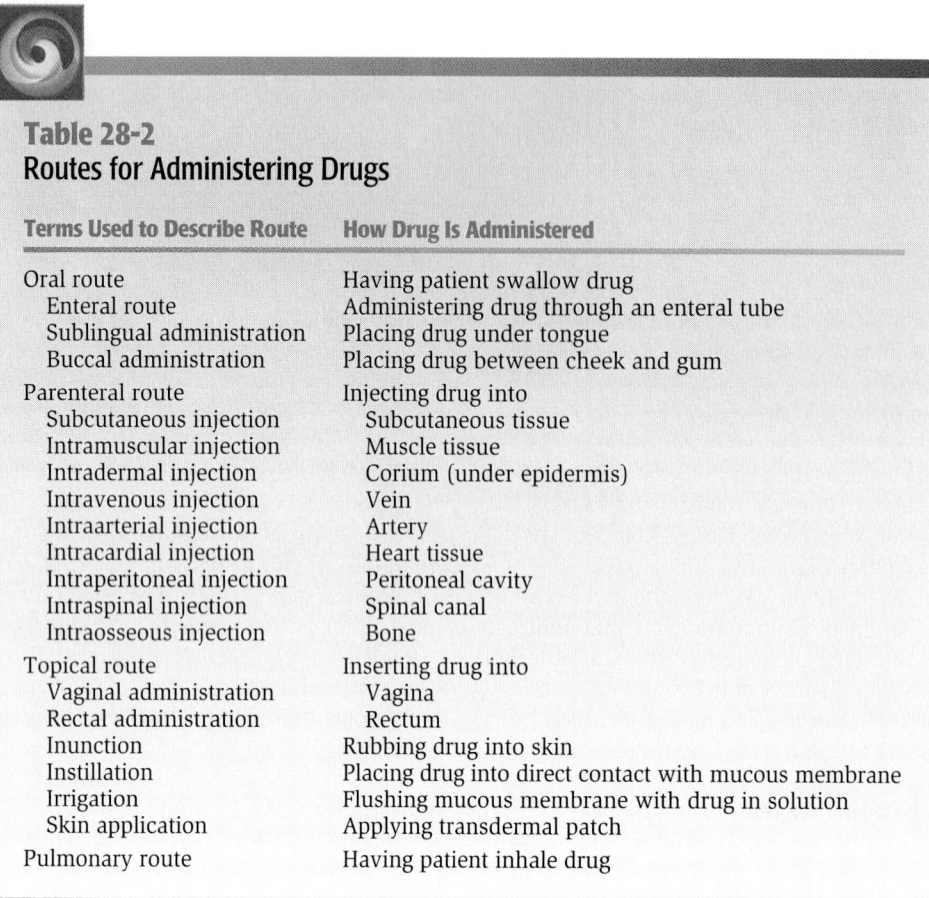

Table 28-2
Routes for Administering Drugs

Terms Used to Describe Route	How Drug Is Administered
Oral route	Having patient swallow drug
Enteral route	Administering drug through an enteral tube
Sublingual administration	Placing drug under tongue
Buccal administration	Placing drug between cheek and gum
Parenteral route	Injecting drug into
Subcutaneous injection	Subcutaneous tissue
Intramuscular injection	Muscle tissue
Intradermal injection	Corium (under epidermis)
Intravenous injection	Vein
Intraarterial injection	Artery
Intracardial injection	Heart tissue
Intraperitoneal injection	Peritoneal cavity
Intraspinal injection	Spinal canal
Intraosseous injection	Bone
Topical route	Inserting drug into
Vaginal administration	Vagina
Rectal administration	Rectum
Inunction	Rubbing drug into skin
Instillation	Placing drug into direct contact with mucous membrane
Irrigation	Flushing mucous membrane with drug in solution
Skin application	Applying transdermal patch
Pulmonary route	Having patient inhale drug

patient. This also holds true when patients are given drugs before certain diagnostic procedures and with stat orders.

Signature of Person Writing the Order

The signature of the person writing the order follows the order. The signature is of importance for legal reasons because the authority to prescribe drugs is defined by state laws. Also, if there is a question about the order, the signature indicates who should be contacted.

Checking the Medication Order

Agency policy specifies the manner in which the medication order is checked. Various systems are used. Nurses should be familiar with the system used in the agency where they care for patients and should implement it correctly to minimize errors.

In many institutions, the order is copied onto the patient's medication record, often called a *Kardex* or MAR (medication administration record). Increasing numbers of healthcare facilities are computerizing patient records, including medication records. The nurse is responsible for checking that the transcription of the medication order is correct by comparing it with the original order.

Questioning the Medication Order

The nurse is legally responsible for drugs administered. Any drug order suspected to be in error should be questioned.

The suspected error may be in any part of the order. The legal implications are serious in a situation in which there is an error in a drug order and the nurse could be expected, based on knowledge and experience, to have noted and reported the error.

On occasion, the nurse may not think that there is an error in the order but may not understand why the medication has been prescribed. In such instances, the nurse should ask how the order relates to the patient's plan of care.

Confusion over the placement of a decimal point can lead to a medication error. A zero should always precede a decimal point (eg, 0.1 mg) for clarity, but there is no need to use a zero after a decimal point (eg, 1.0 mg) because this can cause confusion if the decimal point is unclear or missed completely (Lilley & Guanci, 1997).

A drug to which the patient is allergic may be inadvertently prescribed. The patient may describe past adverse reactions with the drug. It is general practice to indicate any drug allergies clearly on the patient's chart. The drug should not be given, and the order should be questioned when, in the nurse's judgment, the patient is allergic to a drug. In many healthcare facilities, the patient may also wear a wrist band that indicates specific allergies. An allergic reaction can be life-threatening to the patient.

A nurse may have difficulty reading an order. Guessing is gross carelessness. Rechecking with the person who wrote the order is the only safe procedure.

The nurse has the right to refuse to administer any medication that, based on knowledge and experience, may be harmful to the patient. Although this situation seldom occurs, the nurse needs to understand that the patient's safety is a primary objective in the administration of medications.

Medication Supply Systems

Medications are supplied in a number of ways. With a *stock supply* system, large quantities of medications are kept on the nursing unit. With an *individual supply* system, each patient is supplied with the medication needed for a period of time. The nurse is responsible for accurately measuring the dosage from the medication containers. In the *unit dose* system, the pharmacist simplifies medication preparation by packaging and labeling each dosage for a 24-hour period.

Most nursing units use a medication cart for the administration of medications. The standard cart contains individual drawers into which the medications for each patient are placed. The drawer is labeled with the patient's name. The nurse moves the cart from room to room when dispensing medications. A computerized medication cart usually remains in a central area, has drawers stocked with approved medications, and provides access to the medications ordered for each patient. A computerized medication dispensing system and the traditional medication cart are shown in Figure 28-1.

Dosage Calculations

Systems of Measurement

Nurses need to be proficient in the use of weights and measures as well as systems of measurement to calculate drug dosages and prepare medications for administration. Three systems of measurement are used for administering medications: the metric system, the apothecary system, and the household system.

Metric System
The metric system is the most widely accepted and convenient system. The basic units of measurement are the meter (linear), the liter (volume), and the gram (weight). The metric system is a decimal system, in which each unit can be divided into multiples of 10 (10, 100, 1000). Calculations in the metric system often involve moving the decimal point to the right or left. In the preparation of medications, the nurse usually uses the following metric units:

Weight
    1 kilogram = 1000 grams
    1 gram = 1000 milligrams
    1 milligram = 1000 micrograms

Volume
    1 liter = 1000 milliliters or cubic centimeters

Converting Dosages
It may be necessary to convert drug dosages to a different unit in the metric system. To convert a larger unit into a

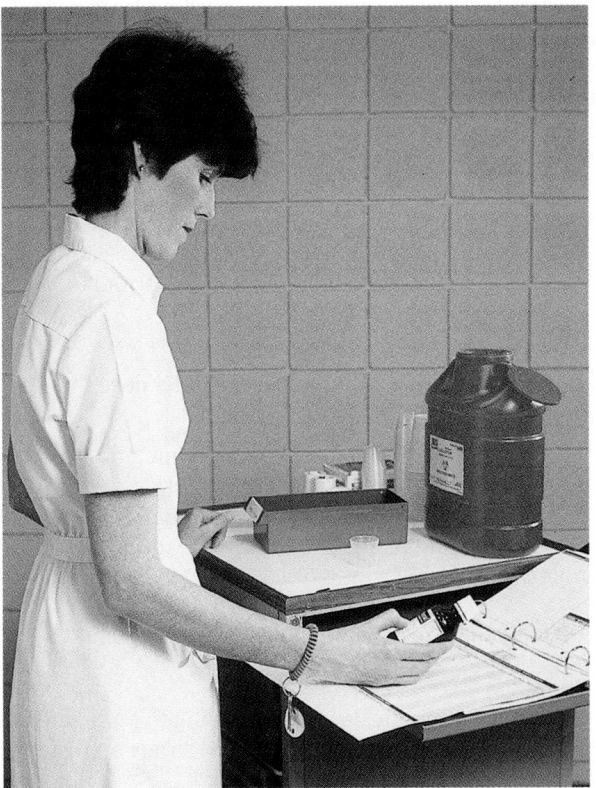

Figure 28-1
Traditional medication cart.

smaller unit, move the decimal point to the right (the new number is larger than the original). To convert a smaller unit into a larger unit, move the decimal point to the left (the new number is smaller than the original).

Example

0.5 g = ? mg
Move decimal point three places to right.
Answer = 500 mg
900 mg = ? g
Move decimal point three places to the left.
Answer = 0.9 g

Apothecary System

The apothecary system is less convenient and precise than the metric system and infrequently used. The basic unit of weight is the grain. The minim, dram, ounce, pint, and quart are used for volume. In the apothecary system, Roman numerals are used to express numbers (grains X) and quantities less than 1 are written in fraction form (grains $\frac{1}{4}$).

Household System

The household system is the least accurate system of measurement. It is not widely used except in home settings. Teaspoon, tablespoon, teacup, and glass are commonly used household measures.

Equivalents of Measurement

All three systems of measurement are in use in the United States. The nurse may be called on to convert dosages from one system to another. It is then extremely important that the nurse know and be able to calculate commonly used equivalents, as listed in Appendix A.

Formulas for Computing Drug Dosages

Drugs are sometimes prepared and supplied in the amount ordered by the physician, and the nurse can see when checking the medication label that no calculation is necessary. At other times, drugs are not prepared and supplied in the exact quantities called for in the medication order, and the nurse must do a dosage calculation to determine what quantity of medication the patient is to receive.

Several formulas can be used to calculate drug dosages. One such formula consists of ratios to set up a proportion and can be used to calculate dosages for both solid and liquid preparations. A ratio shows the relation between numbers. A proportion contains two ratios. The nurse is usually seeking the quantity of on-hand medication that is equal to the desired dosage (the dosage ordered). The formula is as follows:

$$\frac{\text{dose on hand}}{\text{quantity on hand}} = \frac{\text{dose desired}}{X \,(\text{quantity desired})}$$

The dosage must be in the same unit of measurement. This applies to the quantity as well. Dosages are on the top line of the proportion, and quantities are on the bottom line. After the numbers are placed in the proportion, the nurse cross-multiplies to find the desired quantity.

Example: Amoxicillin, 625 mg PO, is ordered. It is supplied as a liquid preparation containing 250 mg in 5 mL. How much does the nurse administer?

$$\frac{250 \text{ mg}}{5 \text{ mL}} = \frac{625 \text{ mg}}{X \text{ mL}}$$

cross-multiply:

$$3125 = 250X$$
$$X = 12.5 \text{ mL}$$

Example: Phenobarbital, gr i PO, is ordered. It is available in 30-mg tablets. How many tablets does the nurse administer?

There are two systems of measurement in this problem. The nurse checks the list of equivalents to learn that 60 mg is equivalent to grains i.

$$\frac{30 \text{ mg}}{1 \text{ tablet}} = \frac{60 \text{ mg}}{X \text{ tablets}}$$
$$60 = 30X$$
$$X = 2 \text{ tablets}$$

Another formula that can be used to calculate drug dosages is as follows:

$$\frac{\text{dose desired}}{\text{dose on hand}} \times \text{quantity on hand} = \frac{\text{desired}}{\text{quantity}}$$

This formula can be used for both liquid dosages and fractions of tablets.

Pediatric Calculations

Pediatric dosages are calculated according to the child's weight or *body surface area* (BSA).

The *BSA formula* provides the most accuracy in calculating pediatric dosages because it considers weight and height. To find a child's BSA, the West nomogram is used (Fig. 28-2). The child's height is located at a point in the left-hand column, and the weight is located at a point in the right-hand column. The two points are connected with a straight line. The point at which the line crosses the surface area column is the child's BSA. The formula for calculating the child's dosage is as follows:

$$\frac{\text{BSA (child)}}{\text{BSA (adult)}} \times \text{adult dose} = \text{child's dose}$$

The average adult BSA is 1.7 square meters.

A less commonly used formula is *Clark's rule* for children aged 2 years or younger. This formula assumes that the average adult weighs 150 lb (68 kg) and is calculated as follows:

$$\frac{\text{usual adult}}{\text{dose}} \times \frac{\text{weight of child in pounds}}{150} = \frac{\text{child's}}{\text{dose}}$$

Accepted pediatric dosages according to milligram per kilogram weight per 24 hours for many drugs are listed in medication references.

Nomogram for Estimating the Surface Area of Infants and Young Children				
Height		Surface Area	Weight	
feet	centimeters	in square meters	pounds	kilograms

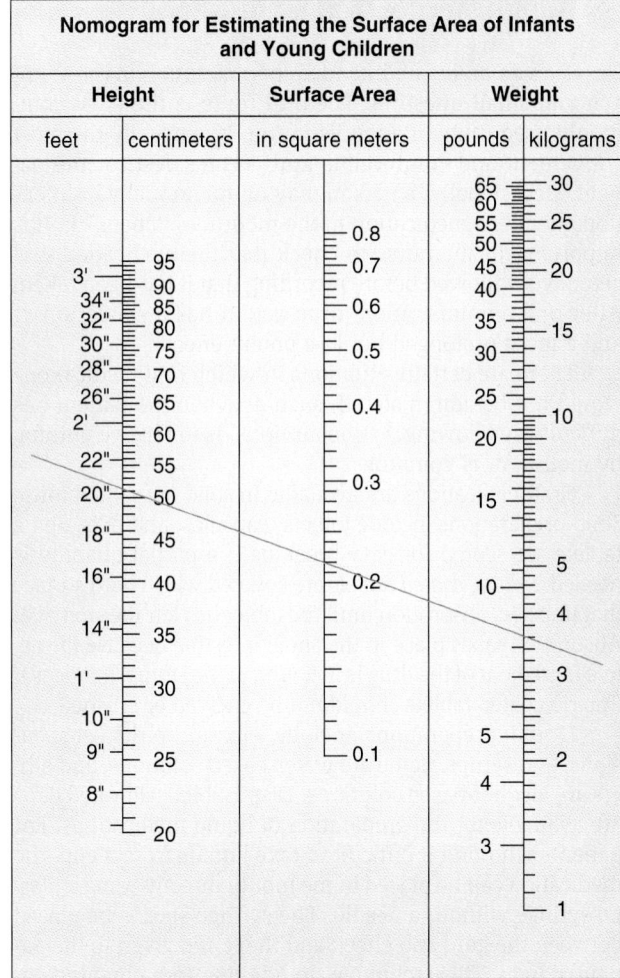

Figure 28-2

Body-surface area nomogram. To determine the surface area of the child, draw a straight line between the point representing his or her height on the left vertical scale to the point representing weight on the right vertical scale. The point at which this line intersects the middle vertical scale represents the child's surface area in square meters. (Courtesy of Abbott Laboratories.)

⑤ Using Safety Measures While Preparing Drugs

Three Checks and Five Rights

Safety is of the utmost importance in preparing and implementing drug administration. The nurse observes the *three checks* and the *five rights* when administering medications.

The label on the medication container should be checked three times during medication preparation. The label should be read (1) when the nurse reaches for the container or unit dose package, (2) immediately before pouring or opening the medication, and (3) when replacing the container to the drawer or shelf or before giving the unit dose medication to the patient.

The *five rights* help to ensure accuracy when administering medications. The nurse gives the (1) *right medica-* tion to the (2) *right patient* in the (3) *right dosage* through the (4) *right route* at the (5) *right time.*

The importance of the three checks and the five rights cannot be overemphasized. The safe nurse does not allow automatic habits of preparing medications to replace constant thinking, purposeful action, and repeated checking for accuracy.

Maintaining a Safe Environment

An environment that promotes safety and good working habits contributes to accuracy in the preparation of drugs for administration. Good lighting must be present when preparing drugs. Also, the nurse who is preparing drugs should work alone. This practice helps to avoid distractions and interruptions, which may lead to errors.

After the nurse begins to prepare drugs for administration, they should not be left unattended. If it is imperative to leave for a short time, the drugs that have been prepared should be placed in a locked area. The nurse who prepares the medication also administers the drug and records the drug administration. When the nurse is not working at the medication cart, it should be locked.

Caring for Controlled Substances Safely

Controlled substances are kept in a locked drawer or container as a safety measure. Narcotics or controlled substances may be ordered only by physicians who are registered with the Department of Justice, Bureau of Narcotics and Dangerous Drugs. According to federal law, a record must be kept for each narcotic that is administered. Healthcare agencies provide forms for keeping such records, and these forms are kept with the narcotics. Although the forms differ, the following information is usually required: the name of the patient receiving the narcotic, the amount of the narcotic used, the hour the narcotic was given, the name of the physician who prescribed the narcotic, and the name of the nurse who administered the narcotic. It is common practice to check narcotics daily at specified intervals. In hospitals, checking is usually performed at each shift change. The amount of narcotics on hand is counted, and each used narcotic must be accounted for on the narcotic record. Some agencies use a computerized system for dispensing narcotics. The nurse has a secure identification code that provides access into the system, identifies the patient by name or identification number, and verifies the count for each drug as it is removed. Unless the number is incorrect, this eliminates the need to check the narcotic count at specific intervals each day. A narcotic count that does not check properly must be reported immediately. The law requires these special precautions to aid in the control of drug abuse. The nurse administering narcotics has an important responsibility to see that the federal law is observed. If for any reason a narcotic prepared for administration has to be discarded, a second person should act as a witness and that person should also sign the narcotic sheet.

Identifying the Patient

The nurse prepares medications, considering safety at all times, as discussed in the previous sections. *Positive identification of the patient is essential to safe drug administration.* Before administering the drug, the nurse must check carefully to see that the right drug is given to the right patient. Patients in inpatient healthcare agencies usually wear identification bracelets. The nurse identifies the patient by checking the identification bracelet, as shown in Figure 26-5 in Chapter 26. Also, the patient should be asked to state his or her name if possible. It is considered unsafe to call the patient by name because the patient may respond even if the nurse uses the wrong name. In some long-term care facilities, a current photograph of the resident can also be used as a form of identification.

IMPLEMENTING: ADMINISTERING A MEDICATION

The nurse should remain with the patient and see that the medication is taken. If the patient receives several drugs, offer them separately so that if one is refused or dropped, positive identification can be made and the drug recorded or replaced. Never leave medications at the bedside for the patient to take later. This is unsafe practice because the patient may forget to take the medication or someone else may take the medication. The nurse records medication administration as soon as possible after the patient takes the medication. Some agencies allow patients to self-administer certain drugs to promote the patient's independence. The nurse should be familiar with agency policy on this matter. Nursing responsibilities for administering drugs are listed in the accompanying box.

Nursing Responsibilities for Administering Drugs

- Assessment of the patient and clear understanding of why the patient is receiving a particular medication
- Preparing the medication to be administered (ie, checking labels, preparing injections, observing proper asepsis techniques with needles and syringes)
- Accurate dosage calculations
- Administration of the medication (proper injection techniques, aids to help swallowing, topical methods)
- Documentation of medications given
- Monitoring the patient's reaction and evaluating the patient's response
- Educating the patient regarding his or her medications and medication regimen

---

Administering Oral Medications

Drugs given orally are intended for absorption in the stomach and small intestine. The oral route is the most commonly used route of administration. It is usually the most convenient and comfortable and is the safest for the patient. Occasionally, a person may unintentionally or intentionally hide a medication in the mouth, or "cheek" it. It is important for the nurse to check that the medication was actually swallowed before recording that it has been taken. After oral administration, drug action has a slower onset and a more prolonged but less potent effect.

There are certain situations in which oral medications would not be administered, such as when the patient has difficulty swallowing, is unconscious, is to receive nothing by mouth, or is vomiting.

Oral medications are available in solid and liquid form. Solid preparations include tablets, capsules, and pills. Some tablets are scored for easy breaking if a partial quantity is needed. *Enteric-coated tablets* are covered with a hard surface that impedes absorption until the tablet has left the stomach. Absorption takes place in the small intestine because the active ingredient of the drug is irritating to the stomach mucosa. Enteric-coated tablets should not be chewed or crushed.

Liquid preparations include elixirs, spirits, suspensions, and syrups. Some are water-based solutions, and others are alcohol-based solutions. Disposable, calibrated cups are available for the preparation of liquid medications. For patients who find it difficult to take liquids from a cup, the medication can be placed in the mouth directly using a plastic syringe without a needle. The syringe should be placed between the gum and cheek and the liquid given to the patient slowly. This technique, in addition to having the patient in an upright or side-lying position, helps prevent the patient from choking and aspirating the medication.

Certain narcotics that were previously administered parenterally can now also be administered in a lollipop or oral-transmucosal form.

If a label becomes difficult to read or accidentally comes off the container, the container should be returned to the pharmacy. A medication should never be given from a bottle without a label or with a label that cannot be read with accuracy. Because of the danger of error, unused medications should not be returned to their bottles. Care should be exercised in pouring, to prevent unnecessary loss. Medications should not be transferred from one pharmacy container to another. Many medication bottles now have an identification code number on them. If similar medications were mixed and a patient had a reaction, it would be difficult to identify which drug was responsible. A medication with an unexpected precipitate should not be used, nor should one that has changed color.

Procedure 28-1 describes the techniques for preparing and administering oral medications.

Special Techniques

Certain drugs that are given orally discolor the teeth or damage the enamel. Such medications are mixed well with water or some other liquid; the patient takes it through a

(*text continues on page 586*)

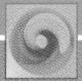

PROCEDURE 28-1

Administering Oral Medications

Equipment

Medication Kardex or computer-
    generated MAR

Medication cart or tray
Medication cups (disposable)

Straws
Water or juice

Action	Rationale
1. Gather equipment. Check each medication order against the original physician's order according to agency policy. Clarify any inconsistencies. Check the patient's chart for allergies.	This comparison helps to identify errors that may have occurred when orders were transcribed. The physician's order is the legal record of medication orders for each agency.
2. Know the actions, special nursing considerations, safe-dose ranges, purpose of administration, and adverse effects of medications to be administered.	This knowledge aids the nurse in evaluating the therapeutic effect of the medication in relation to the patient's disorder and can also be used to educate the patient about their medications.
3. Wash your hands.	Handwashing prevents the spread of microorganisms.
4. Move the medication cart to the outside of the patient's room or prepare for administration in the medication area.	Organization facilitates error-free administration and saves time.
5. Unlock the medication cart or drawer.	Locking of the cart or drawer safeguards each patient's medication supply.
6. Prepare medications for one patient at a time.	This prevents errors in medication administration.
7. Select the proper medication from the drawer or stock and compare with the Kardex or order. Check expiration dates and perform calculations if necessary.	Comparison of medication to physician's order reduces errors in medication administration. Verify calculations with another nurse if necessary. This is the *first* safety check.
a. Place unit dose–packaged medications in a disposable cup. *Do not open wrapper* until at bedside. Keep narcotics and medications that require special nursing assessments in a separate container.	The label is needed for an additional safety check. Prerequisites to giving certain medications may include monitoring of certain vital signs.
b. When removing tablets or capsules from a bottle, pour the necessary number into the bottle cap and then place the tablets in a medication cup. Break only scored tablets, if necessary, to obtain the proper dose.	Pouring medication into the cap allows for easy return of excess medication to bottle. Pouring tablets or capsules into the nurse's hand is unsanitary.
c. Hold liquid medication bottles with the label against the palm. Use the appropriate measuring device when pouring liquids, and read the amount of medication at the bottom of the meniscus at eye level. Wipe the lip of the bottle with a paper towel.	Accuracy is possible when the appropriate measuring device is used and then read accurately. Liquid that may drip onto the label makes the label difficult to read.
8. Recheck each medication package or preparation with the order as it is poured.	This is a *second* check to guard against a medication error.
9. When all medications for one client have been prepared, recheck once again with the medication order before taking them to the client.	This is a *third* check to ensure accuracy and to prevent errors.

(*continued*)

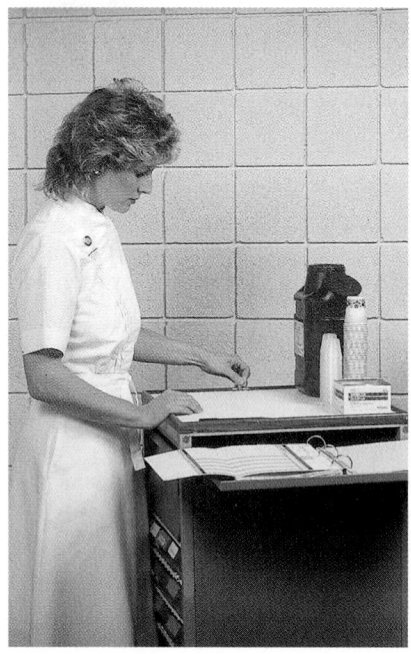

Action 5: Unlocking medication cart.

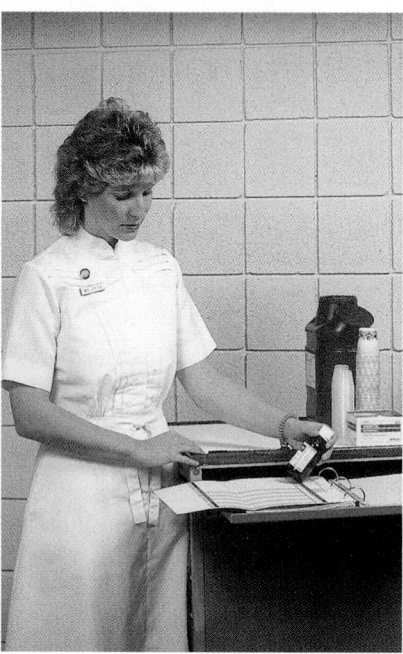

Action 7: Comparing medication with Kardex or order.

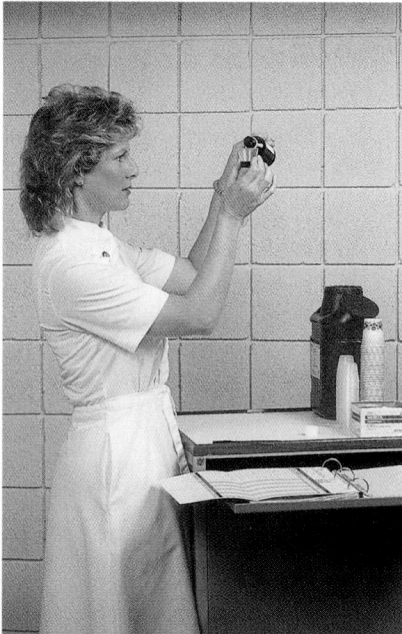

Action 7c: Measuring at eye level.

10. Transport medications to the patient's bedside carefully, and keep the medications in sight at all times.

Careful handling and close observation prevent accidental or deliberate disarrangement of medications.

11. See that the patient receives medications at the correct time.

Check agency policy, which may allow for administration within a period of 30 minutes before or 30 minutes after designated time.

12. Identify the patient carefully. There are three correct ways to do this:
    a. Check the name on the patient's identification band.
    b. Ask the patient his or her name.

    c. Verify the patient's identification with a staff member who knows the patient.

Identifying the patient is the nurse's responsibility to guard against error.
This is the most reliable method. Replace the identification band if it is missing or inaccurate in any way.
This requires a response from the patient, but illness and strange surroundings often cause patients to be confused.
This is another way to double check identity. Do not use the name on the door or over the bed because these may be inaccurate.

13. Complete necessary assessments before administration of medications. Check allergy bracelet or ask patient about allergies. Explain the purpose and action of each medication to the patient.

Assessment is a prerequisite to administration of medications.

14. Assist the patient to an upright or lateral position.

Swallowing is facilitated by proper positioning. An upright or side-lying position protects the patient from aspiration.

(continued)

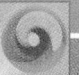

PROCEDURE 28-1

Administering Oral Medications (Continued)

15. Administer medications:
    a. Offer water or other permitted fluids with pills, capsules, tablets, and some liquid medications.

    b. Ask the patient's preference regarding medications to be taken by hand or in a cup and one at a time or all at once.
    c. If the capsule or tablet falls to the floor, it must be discarded and a new one administered.
    d. Record any fluid intake if intake and output measurement is ordered.
16. Remain with the patient until each medication is swallowed. Unless the nurse has seen the patient swallow the drug, it cannot be recorded that the drug was administered.

Liquids facilitate swallowing of solid drugs. Some liquid drugs are intended to adhere to the pharyngeal area, in which case liquid is not offered with the medication. This encourages the patient's participation in taking the medications.

This prevents contamination.

This provides for accurate documentation.

The patient's chart is a legal record. Only with a physician's order can medications be left at the bedside.

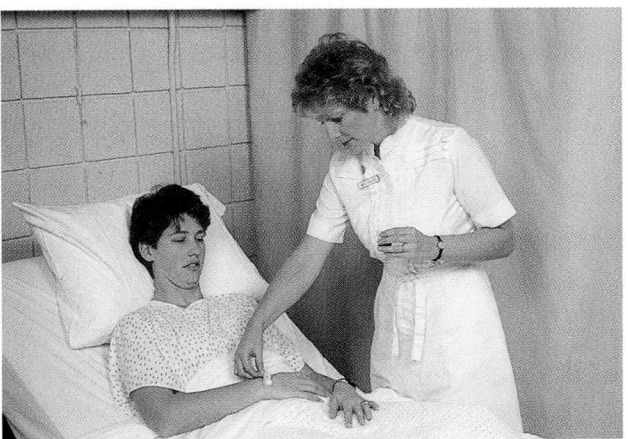

Action 12a: Checking patient identity.

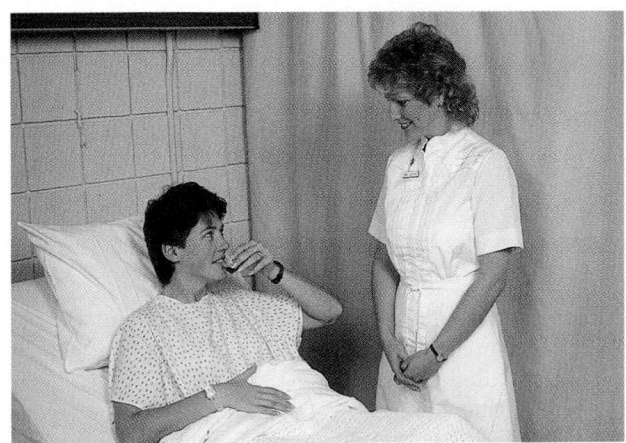

Action 16: Observing patient swallowing medication. (PHOTOS © KEN KASPER.)

17. Wash your hands.
18. Record each medication given on the medication chart or record using the required format.
    a. If the drug was refused or omitted, record this in the appropriate area on the medication record.
    b. Recording of administration of a narcotic requires additional documentation on a narcotic record stating drug count and other specific information.
19. Check on the patient within 30 minutes to verify response to medication.

Handwashing prevents the spread of microorganisms.
Prompt recording avoids the possibility of accidentally repeating the administration of the drug.
This verifies the reason medication was omitted.

Controlled substance laws necessitate careful recording of narcotic use.

This provides opportunity for further documentation and additional assessment of effectiveness of pain relief and adverse effects of medications.

(continued)

PROCEDURE 28-1

Administering Oral Medications (Continued)

Age Considerations

Special devices are available in a pharmacy to ensure accurate dose calculations for young children and infants.

Elderly patients with arthritis may have difficulty opening childproof caps. On request, the pharmacist can substitute a cap that is easier to open. A rubber band twisted around the cap may provide a more secure grip for older patients.

The FDA has received reports of infants choking on the plastic caps that fit on the end of syringes used to administer oral medication. They recommend: removal and disposal of caps before giving syringes to patients or families, caution family caregivers to dispose of caps on syringes they buy over the counter, and report any problems with syringe caps to the FDA.

Home Care Considerations

Encourage the patient to discard outdated prescription medications.

Discuss safe storage of medications when there are children and pets in the environment.

Special Considerations

If the patient questions a medication order or states the medication is different from the usual dose, *always* recheck and clarify with the original order before giving medication

If the patient's level of consciousness is altered or his or her swallowing is impaired, check with the physician to clarify the route of administration or alternative forms of medication.

Patients with poor vision can request labels printed with larger type on medication containers. A magnifying lens also may prove helpful.

---

drinking straw, and water is taken after administration. This practice reduces the strength of the drug that comes in contact with the teeth.

Some patients object to the taste of certain medications. The following techniques help disguise or mask the objectionable taste:

- It is sometimes necessary to crush a medication or add it to food so that the patient can swallow it. Some drugs cannot be crushed (eg, enteric-coated and sustained-release capsules). Check with the pharmacist or a pharmacology reference when uncertain about crushing a medication.
- Allow the patient to suck on a small piece of ice for a few minutes before taking the medication. The ice numbs the taste buds, and the objectionable taste is less discernible.
- Store oily medications in the refrigerator. Cold oil is less aromatic than oil at room temperature.
- Place the medication in a syringe, and place the syringe well back on the tongue, being careful not to trigger the patient's gag reflex. This places the medication on the part of the tongue where there are few taste buds.
- Offer oral hygiene immediately after giving the medication.
- Give the medication with generous amounts of water or other liquids, if permitted, to dilute the taste.

Children

Nurses find administration of medications to infants and children challenging as well as frustrating at times. Children younger than 5 years of age have difficulty swallowing tablets and capsules. Most medications are available in liquid form. Nursing responsibility also includes teaching and preparing family members to administer medications to a child at home. In addition to understanding the medication order and the reason for the medication, the caregiver should be able to demonstrate any special techniques involved in administering the prescribed drugs. Helpful strategies for administering medications to children include the following:

- Use a dropper to give infants or very young children liquid medications while holding them in a sitting or semi-sitting position. Place the medication between the gum and cheek to prevent possible aspiration.
- Crush uncoated tablets or empty a soft capsule and mix the medication with soft foods, such as potatoes or cooked or hot cereal, for patients who are likely to aspirate liquids. Proper absorption may not occur if coated tablets or hard capsules are added to food.
- Explain to the child when a medication has an objectionable taste if the child is old enough to understand. Failing to warn the child is likely to decrease the child's trust in the nurse.
- Care should be taken when selecting the food to be mixed with the medication. The item should not be

an essential part of the child's diet, such as formula or the child's favorite food. The child may refuse a food associated with medications.

- Offer the child a flavored ice pop or frozen fruit bar immediately before taking the medication. It numbs the tongue, making the taste of the medication less evident.
- Praise the child for a job well done after he or she swallows the medication.

Older Adults

Techniques for administering medications to older people include the following:

- Allow extra time to administer medications to older patients because their reflexes may be slowed and their understanding of the treatment decreased.
- Older patients may experience some difficulty swallowing medications and may find it easier to take their medications when crushed or given in liquid form. Swallowing can be initiated by massaging the laryngeal prominence or the area just below the chin prominence. The pressure from the gentle massage creates the desire to swallow. A speech therapist may offer additional suggestions for patients who have difficulty swallowing.
- Reevaluation of the drug dosage is necessary with the older patient. Weight and age should be used as criteria for determining the dosage.
- The nurse should assist the older patient to set up a home medication schedule as a reminder to take medications as scheduled.
- Monitor carefully for adverse effects that may result from the drug regimen. These may be magnified in older individuals.
- Teach patients the names of drugs rather than distinguishing them by color. Manufacturers may vary the colors of generic drugs, and the visual changes associated with aging may make it more difficult to identify medications by their color.

Administering Medications Through an Enteral Feeding Tube

Patients with a gastrointestinal tube (nasogastric, nasointestinal, percutaneous endoscopic gastrostomy [PEG] tube, or J tube) often receive medication through the tube. The insertion of the tube and care of the patient with an enteral feeding tube are described in Chapter 41. The following are suggestions for giving medications through the tube:

- Use liquid medications or medications that can be crushed and combined with liquid.
- Bring the liquid medication to room temperature. Cold liquids may cause patient discomfort.
- Remove the clamp from the tube and use the recommended procedure for checking tube placement in the stomach or intestine *before* administering the drug.
- Flush the tube with 15 to 30 mL of water (5 to 10 mL for children) before giving the medication and imme-

diately after giving the medication. Flushing before may warn you if the tube is clogged and helps to maintain tube patency.

- It is best to give medications separately and flush with water between each drug. Some medications may interact with each other or become less effective if mixed with other drugs.
- If the tube is connected to suction, keep it disconnected from the suction and clamped for 20 to 30 minutes after administration of the medication to allow for absorption.
- Disconnect a continuous tube feeding before giving medications, and leave the tube clamped for a short period of time after medication has been given according to agency protocol.
- Document the water intake and liquid medication by tube on the intake and output record. Adjust the amount of water used if the patient is on restricted fluid intake.

Administering Sublingual Medications

Certain drugs, such as sublingual nitroglycerin, are administered *sublingually*; that is, a tablet is placed under the patient's tongue. This area is rich in superficial blood vessels, which allows the drug to be absorbed relatively rapidly into the bloodstream for quick systemic effects. Sublingual medications should not be swallowed but rather are held under the tongue so that complete absorption can occur.

Administering Parenteral Medications

The term *enteral* means within the intestines; parenteral means outside the intestines or alimentary canal. Many people use the term **parenteral** to refer to injection routes only, although technically, the term includes routes for administering agents given by inhalation, those placed on the skin, and most of those placed on the mucous membrane.

Table 28-2 defines terms used to describe various types of *injections*. Medications may be injected into an artery, the peritoneum, heart tissues, the spinal canal, and bones. Techniques for injecting medications into these areas are discussed in clinical texts. In most instances, physicians are responsible for these procedures, and nurses assist.

Absorption occurs more rapidly with injection than when other routes are used. It is also more nearly complete; therefore, the results are more predictable, and the desired dosage can be determined with greater accuracy. Giving drugs by injection is necessary if the drug is available in no other form. Injections are particularly desirable for patients who are irrational, unconscious, or having gastrointestinal disturbances. The injection of drugs is also used in emergencies because absorption and desired results occur rapidly.

Needles and Syringes

Needles are available in various lengths and gauges with different sizes of bevels. Figure 28-3 shows the parts of a needle. The most commonly used needle lengths vary from

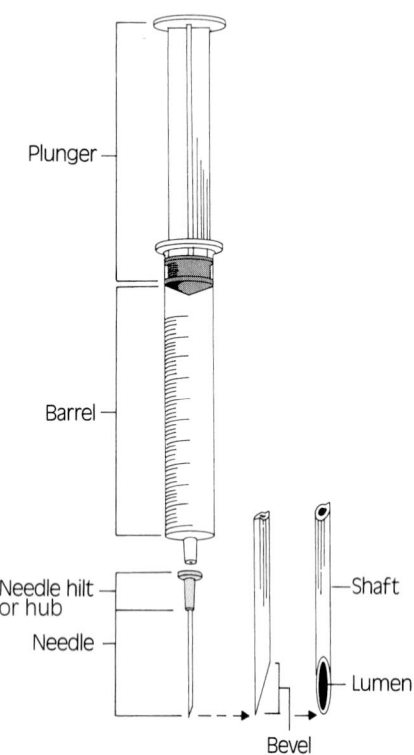

Plunger

Barrel

Needle hilt
or hub

Needle

Shaft

Lumen

Bevel

Figure 28-3
Parts of a needle and syringe.

$5/16$ inch to 2 inches (0.8 to 5.1 cm). The length of the needle chosen is determined by the route of administration. The gauge is determined by the diameter of the needle. Needle gauges are numbered 18 through 30. As the diameter of the needle increases, the gauge number decreases. An 18-gauge needle is larger than a 30-gauge needle. The bevel of the needle is its sloped edge, designed to make a narrow, slitlike opening that closes quickly.

Syringes are supplied in various sizes. Most syringes are plastic and disposable. Some syringes are supplied with the needle attached, whereas others are not, in which case the nurse selects an appropriate needle. The parts of a needle and syringe are shown in Figure 28-3.

The nurse chooses the equipment needed for an injection based on the following criteria:

Route of administration: A longer needle is required for an intramuscular injection than for an intradermal or a subcutaneous injection.
Viscosity of the solution: Some medications are more viscous than others and require a large-lumen needle to inject the drug.
Quantity to be administered: The larger the amount of medication to be injected, the greater the capacity of the syringe.
Body size: An obese person requires a longer needle to reach muscle tissue than a thin person.
Type of medication: There are special syringes for certain uses. An example is the insulin syringe used to inject insulin. Some medications, such as iron dextran injection (Imferon), are irritating to subcutaneous tissue. Therefore, a longer needle

should be used to ensure proper placement of the medication in the muscle tissue.

After use, the needles and syringes are placed in puncture-resistant containers without being recapped. Most needle-stick injuries occur during recapping. The one-handed technique is used when a needle must be recapped. This technique and additional measures to protect healthcare workers from accidental transmission of infectious diseases are discussed in Chapter 27.

Techniques of surgical asepsis must be strictly followed for parenteral injections to help avoid introducing organisms into the body. The parts of the syringe and needle that must be kept sterile during the procedure of preparing and administering an injection are the inside of the barrel, the part of the plunger that enters the barrel, the tip of the barrel, and the needle, except for the needle's hub.

Surgical asepsis applies to cleaning the skin for an injection. The skin is cleaned with alcohol or povidone-iodine (Betadine) in a circular motion, working from the center of the designated site outward.

Needleless Systems

The risk for accidental needlestick and possible exposure to bloodborne pathogens is reduced significantly with the use of needleless devices or protected needles. Chapter 27 describes the rationale for these systems of protection for healthcare workers. These devices prevent needlestick injuries in a variety of ways. Examples include needles that can be sheathed in a plastic guard after the needle is withdrawn from the skin and syringes that have a retractable needle that locks and seals inside the syringe barrel. Needleless systems are also available for intravenous use, including recessed and shielded intravenous needle connectors as well as blunt cannulas that are inserted into special receptor sites on tubing or lock setups. All needleless devices or blunt cannulas are discarded in special containers that are puncture proof, leak proof, clearly labeled, and available at various locations on each healthcare unit. Figure 28-4 shows an example of a needleless device.

Preparing Medications for Administration by Injection

Drugs for administration by injection are packaged in several ways. Those that deteriorate in solution are usually dispensed as powders and are reconstituted immediately before injection. If drugs remain stable in solution, they are usually dispensed in ampules, bottles, or vials in an aqueous or oily solution or suspension.

Drugs may be dispensed in single-dose glass ampules, single-dose rubber-capped vials, multidose rubber-capped vials, and prefilled cartridges. Figure 28-5 shows several types of ampules and vials as well as prefilled cartridges.

Ampules

An **ampule** is a glass flask that contains a single dose of medication for parenteral administration. There is no way to prevent airborne contamination of any unused portion of medication after the ampule is opened. If all the med-

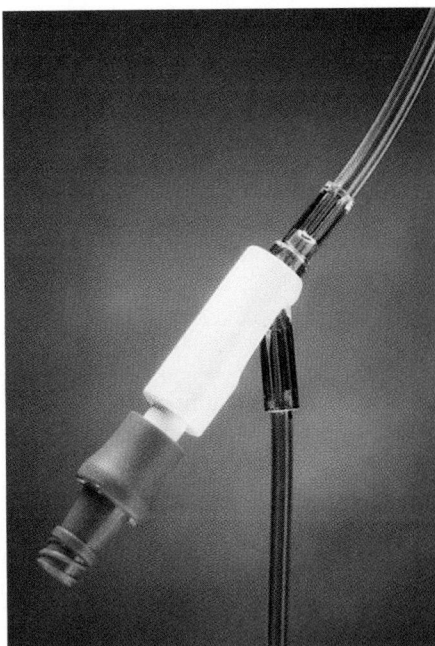

Figure 28-4
Example of a needleless system. (Courtesy of ICU Medical, Inc., San Clemente, CA.)

ication is not used, the remainder must be discarded. Medication is removed from an ampule after its thin neck is broken. The ampule can be inverted or placed on a flat surface to draw the solution into the syringe. Care must be taken not to contaminate the needle by touching the rim of the ampule. Procedure 28-2 shows how to remove medication from an ampule.

Vials

As Figure 28-5 shows, a **vial** is a glass bottle with a self-sealing stopper through which medication is removed. For safety in transporting and storing, the single-dose rubber-capped vial is usually covered with a soft metal cap that can be easily removed. The rubber stopper that is then exposed is the means of entrance into the vial.

Some drugs are dispensed in vials that contain several doses. This means that the nurse can remove several doses from the same container. To facilitate removal of medica-

tion, the nurse injects air into the vial. The amount of air is the same as the desired quantity of solution. Procedure 28-3 details how to remove medication from a vial.

Prefilled Cartridges

Prefilled cartridges provide a single dose of medication. The nurse inserts the cartridge into a reusable holder. Before giving the injection, the nurse checks the dosage in the cartridge and clears the cartridge of excess air. Most prefilled cartridges are overfilled, and the nurse should eject any excess medication to give an exact dose and avoid a medication error. Tubex and Carpuject are two types of prefilled cartridges.

Mixing Medications in One Syringe

Preparation of medications in one syringe depends on how the medication is supplied. When using a single-dose vial and a multidose vial, air is injected into both vials, and the medication in the multidose vial is drawn into the syringe first. This prevents the contents of the multidose vial from being contaminated with the medication in the single-dose vial. The nurse must first ensure that the two drugs are compatible.

The steps to follow when preparing medications from two multidose vials in one syringe are illustrated in Figure 28-6 and Procedure 28-4.

When preparing medications from an ampule and a vial, the medication in the vial is prepared first. The medication in the ampule is drawn up after the medication in the vial.

Nurses must be aware of drug incompatibilities when preparing medications in one syringe. Certain medications, such as diazepam (Valium), are incompatible with other drugs in the same syringe. Other drugs have limited compatibility and should be administered within 15 minutes of preparation. Incompatible drugs may become cloudy or form a precipitate in the syringe. Such medications are discarded and reprepared in separate syringes. Mixing more than two drugs in one syringe is not recommended (McConnell, 1998b). If it must be done, the pharmacist should be contacted to determine the compatibility of the three drugs as well as the compatibility of their pH values and the preservatives that may be present in each drug. A drug compatibility table should be available to nurses who are preparing medications.

Mixing Insulins in One Syringe

Insulin, a naturally occurring hormone produced by the islets of Langerhans in the pancreas, enables cells to use carbohydrates. Patients with diabetes mellitus produce no insulin or produce insulin in insufficient amounts. Several types of insulin are available for use by patients with diabetes mellitus. Insulins vary in their onset and duration of action and are classified as short acting, intermediate acting, and long acting. Some insulins have a modifying protein that slows absorption. The modifying proteins are globin and protamine (NPH, globin zinc, protamine zinc).

Insulin dosages are calculated in units. The scale commonly used is U100, which is based on 100 units of insulin
(*text continues on page 594*)

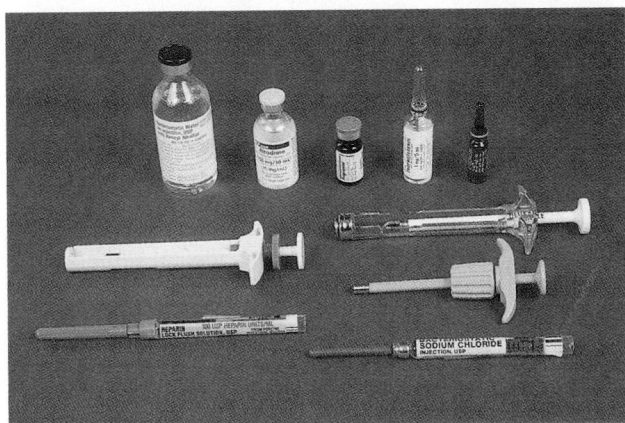

Figure 28-5
Vials, ampules, prefilled cartridges, and holders.

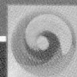

PROCEDURE 28-2

Removing Medication From an Ampule

Equipment

Sterile syringe and needle (size depends on medication being administered and patient)

Ampule of medication
Medication Kardex or computer-generated MAR

Alcohol swab or gauze pad
Filter needle (optional)

Action	Rationale
1. Gather equipment. Check the medication order against the original physician's order according to agency policy.	This comparison helps to identify errors that may have occurred when orders were transcribed.
2. Wash your hands.	Handwashing deters the spread of microorganisms.
3. Tap the stem of the ampule or twist your wrist quickly while holding the ampule vertically.	This facilitates movement of medication in the stem to the body of the ampule.
4. Wrap a small gauze pad or dry alcohol swab around the neck of the ampule.	This protects the nurse's fingers from the glass as the ampule is broken.
5. Use a snapping motion to break off the top of the ampule along the prescored line at its neck. Always break away from your body.	This protects the nurse's face and fingers from any shattered glass fragments.

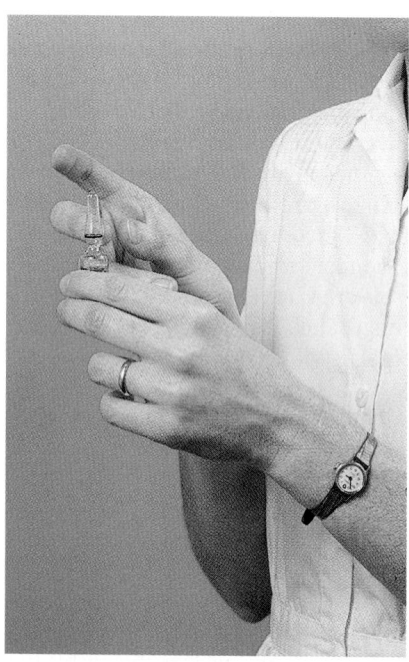

Action 3: Tapping stem of ampule.

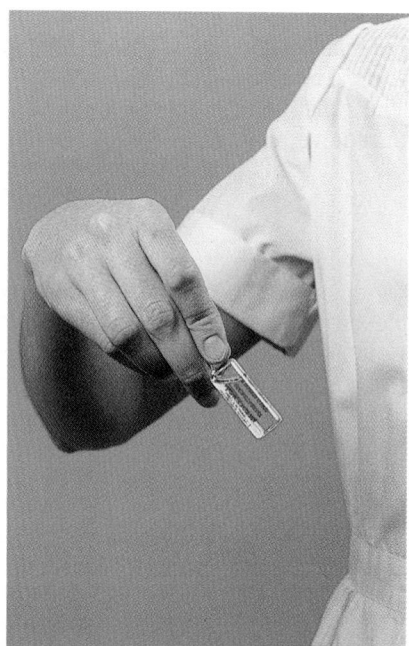

Action 3: Twisting motion of wrist while holding ampule.

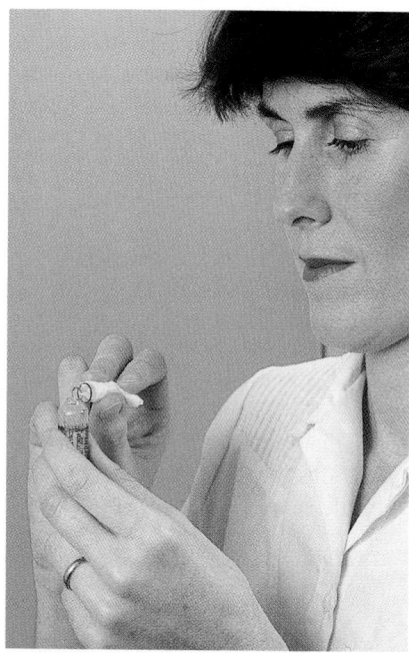

Action 5: Snapping off top of ampule.

6. Remove the cap from the needle by pulling it straight off. Insert the needle into the ampule, being careful not to touch the rim. (Some agencies recommend use of a filter needle when withdrawing solution from an ampule.)

The rim of the ampule is considered contaminated. (Use of a filter needle prevents the accidental withdrawing of small glass particles with the medication.)

(continued)

PROCEDURE 28-2

Removing Medication From an Ampule (Continued)

7. Withdraw medication in the amount ordered. Do not inject air into solutions. Use either of the following methods:

   a. Insert the tip of the needle into the ampule, which is *upright* on a flat surface, and withdraw fluid into the syringe. Touch plunger at knob only.

   b. Insert the tip of the needle into the ampule and *invert* the ampule. Keep the needle centered and not touching the sides of the ampule. Remove the prescribed amount of medication. Touch plunger at knob only.

The contents of the ampule are not under pressure; therefore, air is unnecessary and will cause the contents to overflow. Handling plunger at knob only will keep shaft of plunger sterile.

Surface tension holds the fluid in the ampule when inverted. If the needle touches the sides or is removed and then reinserted into the ampule, surface tension is broken, and fluid runs out. Handling plunger at knob only will keep shaft of plunger sterile.

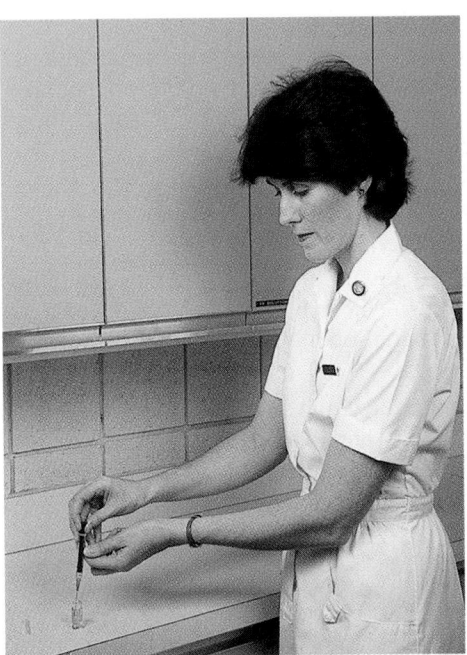

Action 7a: Withdrawing medication from upright ampule.

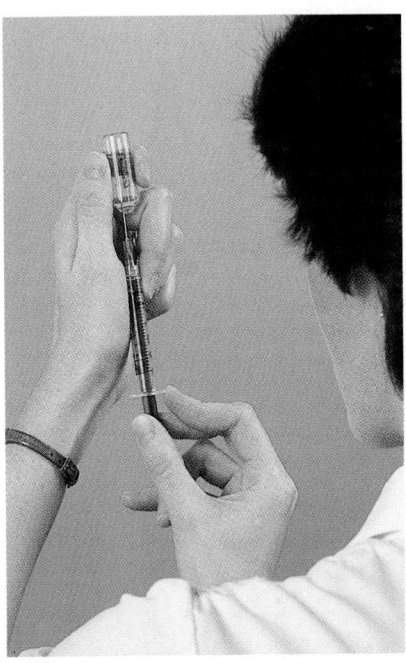

Action 7b: Withdrawing medication from inverted ampule. (PHOTOS © KEN KASPER.)

8. Do not expel any air bubbles that may form in the solution. Wait until the needle has been withdrawn to tap the syringe and expel the air carefully. Check the amount of medication in the syringe and discard any surplus.

9. Discard the ampule in a suitable container after comparing with the medication Kardex.

10. Replace the cap carefully over the needle on the syringe.

11. Wash your hands.

Ejecting air into the solution increases pressure in the ampule and can force the medication to spill out over the ampule. Ampules may have overfill. Careful measurement ensures that correct dose is withdrawn.

If all of the medication has been removed from the ampule, it must be discarded because there is no way to maintain sterility of contents in an unopened ampule.

This prevents contamination of the needle and protects the nurse against inadvertent needlesticks. A one-handed recap method may be used.

Handwashing deters the spread of microorganisms.

PROCEDURE 28-3

Removing Medication From a Vial

Equipment

Sterile syringe and needle (size
   depends on medication being
   administered and patient)

Vial of medication
Medication Kardex or computer-
   generated MAR

Alcohol swab
Filter needle (optional)

Action	Rationale
1. Gather equipment. Check medication order against the original physician's order according to agency policy.	This comparison helps to identify errors that may have occurred when orders were transcribed.
2. Wash your hands.	Handwashing deters the spread of microorganisms.
3. Remove the metal or plastic cap on the vial that protects the rubber stopper.	The metal or plastic cap prevents contamination of the rubber top.
4. Swab the rubber top with the alcohol swab.	Alcohol removes surface bacteria contamination. This is not necessary the first time the rubber stopper is entered, but subsequent reentries into the vial require the use of alcohol cleansing.
5. Remove the cap from the needle by pulling it straight off. (Some agencies recommend use of a filter needle when withdrawing premixed medication from multi-dose vials.) Draw back an amount of air into the syringe that is equal to the specific dose of medication to be withdrawn.	Before fluid is removed, injection of an equal amount of air is required to prevent the formation of a partial vacuum because a vial is a sealed container. If not enough air is injected, the negative pressure makes it difficult to withdraw the medication. (Use of a filter needle prevents any solid material from being withdrawn through the needle.)
6. Pierce the rubber stopper in the center with the needle tip and inject the measured air into the space above the solution. (Do not inject air into the solution.) The vial may be positioned upright on a flat surface or inverted.	Air bubbled through the solution could result in withdrawal of an inaccurate amount of medication.

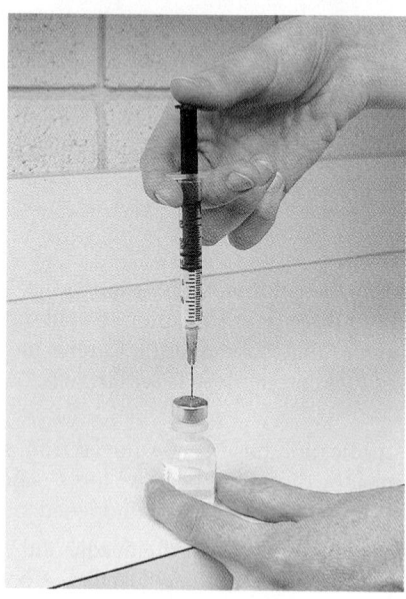

Action 6: Injecting air with vial upright.

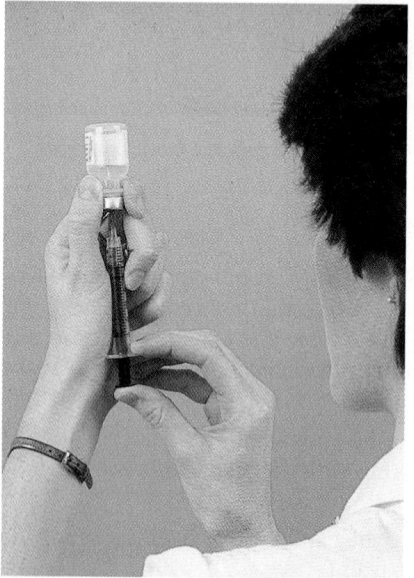

Action 6: Injecting air with vial inverted and needle above solution.

(continued)

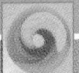

PROCEDURE 28-3

Removing Medication From a Vial (Continued)

7. Invert the vial and withdraw the needle tip slightly so that it is below the fluid level.

This prevents air from being aspirated into the syringe.

8. Draw up the prescribed amount of medication while holding the syringe at eye level and vertically. Be careful to touch the plunger at knob only.

Holding the syringe at eye level facilitates accurate reading, and the vertical position makes removal of air bubbles from the syringe easy. Handling plunger at knob only will keep shaft of plunger sterile.

9. If any air bubbles accumulate in the syringe, tap the barrel of the syringe sharply and move the needle past the fluid into the air space to reinject the air bubble into the vial. Return the needle tip to the solution and continue withdrawal of the medication.

Removal of air bubbles is necessary to ensure accurate dose of medication.

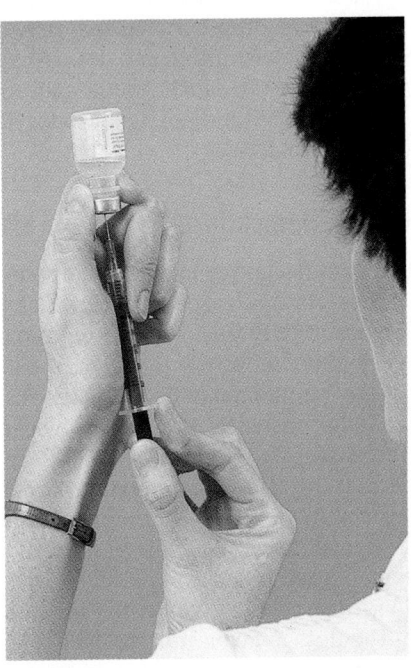

Action 8: Withdrawing medication at eye level.

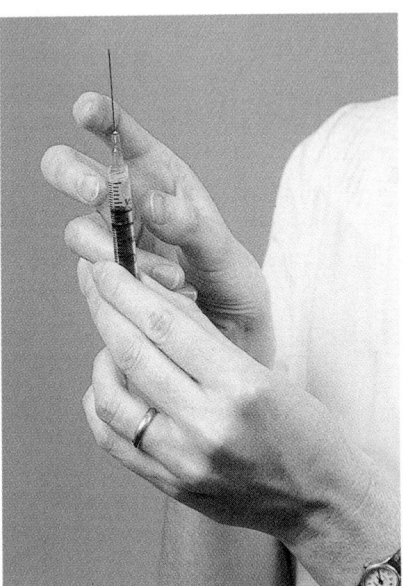

Action 9: Tapping to remove air bubbles. (PHOTOS © KEN KASPER.)

10. After the correct dose is withdrawn, remove the needle from the vial and carefully replace the cap over the needle.

This prevents contamination of the needle and protects the nurse against accidental needlesticks. A one-handed recap method may be used.

11. If a multidose vial is being used, store the vial containing the remaining medication according to agency policy.

Because the vial is sealed, the medication inside remains sterile and can be used for future injections. Some agencies require labeling opened vials with a date and limiting its use after a specific time period.

12. Wash your hands.

Handwashing deters the spread of microorganisms.

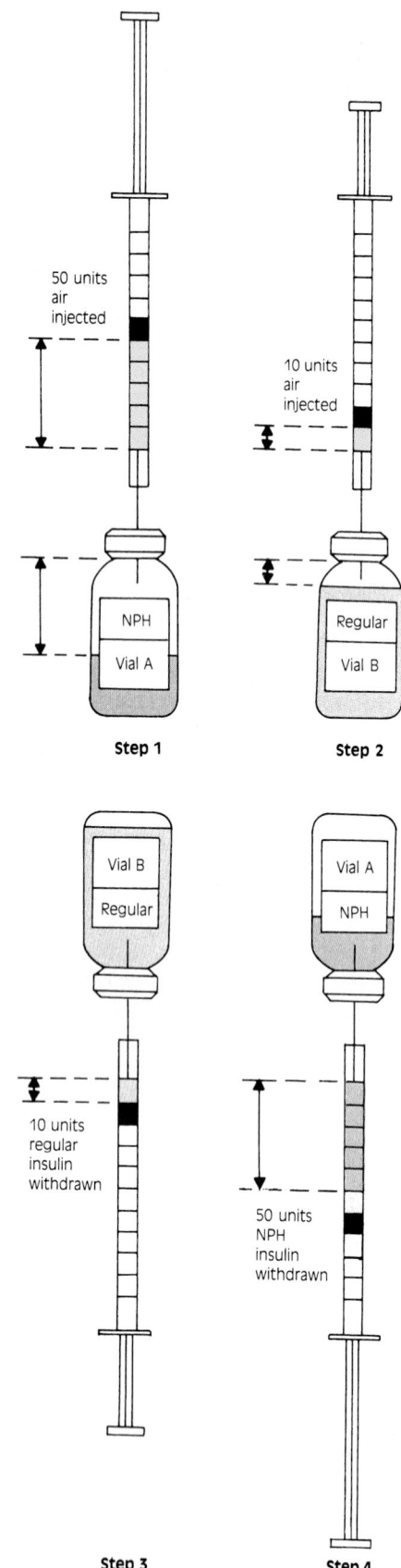

50 units
air
injected

10 units
air
injected

NPH

Vial A

Regular

Vial B

Step 1

Step 2

Vial B

Regular

Vial A

NPH

10 units
regular
insulin
withdrawn

50 units
NPH
insulin
withdrawn

Step 3

Step 4

Figure 28-6
Mixing medications in one syringe.

contained in 1 mL of solution. An insulin syringe is calibrated in units also. Before administering insulin, the nurse should check the dosage with the physician's orders. Many cases of diabetes mellitus are regulated with a combination of two insulins (eg, regular and NPH insulins). Procedure 28-4 gives the steps for mixing two types of insulins in the same syringe.

The importance of rotating injection sites for insulin administration cannot be overemphasized. Injection sites are discussed in the later section, Administering Medications Subcutaneously. A 10-mL vial of unrefrigerated insulin may be safely used for 1 month if stored in a cool place (Fleming, 1999).

Reconstituting Powdered Medications

Occasionally, a drug may be supplied as a powder in a vial. A liquid, or *diluent*, must be added to the powder before it is administered as a solution. The technique of adding a diluent to a powdered drug is called *reconstitution*. Information needed for reconstitution and dosage calculation is usually located on the vial label. Additional sources of information about reconstitution of medications are package inserts and the pharmacist.

Administering Medications Intradermally

The intradermal route has the longest absorption time of all parenteral routes. For this reason, intradermal injections are used for diagnostic purposes, such as the tuberculin test and tests to determine sensitivity to various substances. The advantage of the intradermal route for these tests is that the body's reaction to substances is easily visible, and degrees of reaction are discernible by comparative study.

Intradermal injections are placed just below the epidermis. Sites commonly used are the inner surface of the forearm, the dorsal aspect of the upper arm, and the upper back. Equipment used for an intradermal injection include a tuberculin syringe calibrated in tenths and hundredths of a milliliter. The dosage given intradermally is small, usually less than 0.5 mL. A ¼- to ½-inch (0.6 to 1.3 cm), 26- or 27-gauge needle is used. Procedure 28-5 shows how to administer an intradermal injection.

Administering Medications Subcutaneously

Subcutaneous tissue lies between the epidermis and the muscle. Because there is subcutaneous tissue all over the body, various sites are used for **subcutaneous injections**. These sites are the outer aspect of the upper arm, the abdomen (from below the costal margin to the iliac crests), anterior aspects of the thigh, upper back, and the upper ventral or dorsogluteal area. Figure 28-7 includes the sites on the body where subcutaneous injections can be given. This route is used to administer insulin, heparin, and certain immunizations.

Equipment used for a subcutaneous injection depends on the medication to be given. For instance, insulin is prepared with an insulin syringe. Heparin is prepared with a tuberculin syringe or supplied in a prefilled cartridge.

PROCEDURE 28-4

Mixing Insulins in One Syringe

Equipment

Two vials of insulin
Medication Kardex or computer-
   generated MAR

Sterile insulin syringe with 25-gauge
   or 27-gauge needle
Alcohol swabs

Action	Rationale
1. Gather equipment. Check medication order against the original physician's order according to agency policy.	This comparison helps to identify errors that may have occurred when orders were transcribed.
2. Wash your hands.	Handwashing deters the spread of microorganisms.
3. If necessary, remove the metal cap that protects the rubber stopper on each vial.	The metal cap prevents contamination of the rubber top.
4. If insulin is a suspension (NPH, Lente), shake the vial vigorously.	Rolling a vial does not adequately mix NPH or LENTE insulin and may result in an inconsistent dose. Regular insulin or clear insulin does not need to be mixed before withdrawal.
5. Cleanse the rubber tops with alcohol swabs.	It is questionable whether cleaning with alcohol actually disinfects or, instead, transfers resident bacteria from the hands to another surface. Because it is difficult in a healthcare facility to keep an insulin vial in its original box as recommended, cleansing with alcohol will most likely continue.
6. Remove cap from needle. Inject air into the modified insulin preparation (eg, NPH insulin). Touch plunger at knob only. Use an amount of air equal to the amount of medication to be withdrawn. Do not allow the needle to touch the medication in the vial. Remove the needle.	Regular, or short-acting, insulin should never be contaminated with NPH or any insulin modified with added protein. Placing air in the NPH insulin first without allowing the needle to contact the insulin ensures that regular insulin is not contaminated with the additional protein in the NPH. Handling the plunger by the knob only assures sterility of shaft of plunger.
7. Inject air into the clear insulin without additional protein (eg, regular insulin). Use an amount of air equal to the amount of medication to be withdrawn.	An equal amount of air must be injected into the vacuum to allow easy withdrawal of medication.

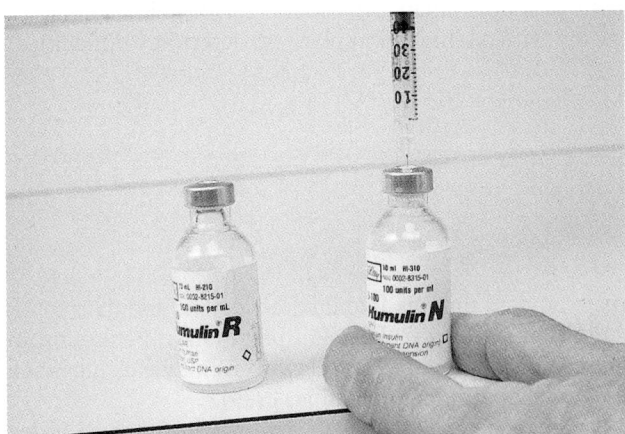

Action 6: Injecting air into modified insulin preparation.

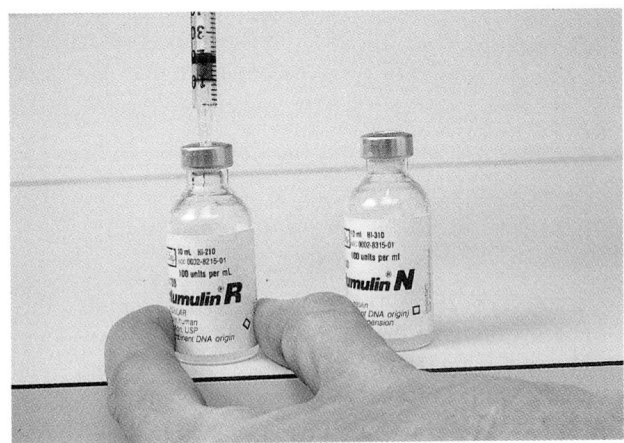

Action 7: Injecting air into clear insulin.

(continued)

PROCEDURE 28-4

Mixing Insulins in One Syringe (Continued)

8. Invert the vial of clear insulin and aspirate the amount prescribed. Remove the needle from the vial.

Regular insulin that contains no additional protein is not contaminated by insulin that contains globulin or protamine.

9. Cleanse the rubber top of the modified insulin vial. Insert the needle into this vial, invert it, and withdraw the medication. Carefully replace the cap over the needle.

Previous addition of air eliminates need to create positive pressure. Capping the needle prevents contamination and protects the nurse against accidental needlesticks. A one-handed recap method may be used.

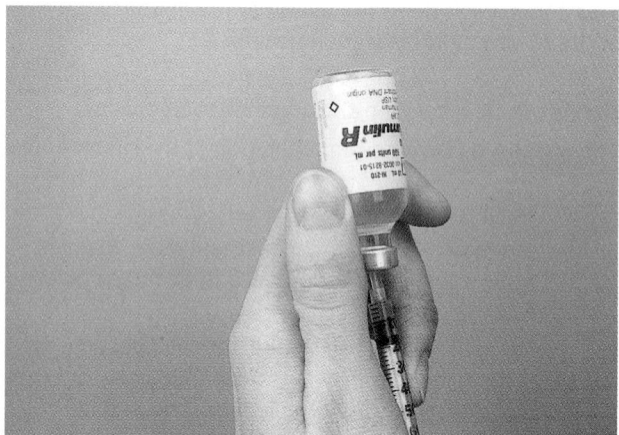

Action 8: Withdrawing clear insulin.

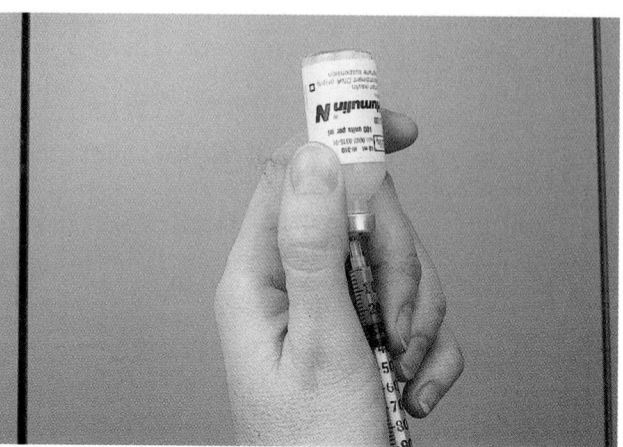

Action 9: Withdrawing modified insulin. (PHOTOS © KEN KASPER.)

10. Store the vials according to agency recommendations.

Insulin need not be refrigerated but must be protected from temperature extremes.

11. Wash your hands.

Handwashing deters the spread of microorganisms.

Special Considerations   An insulin-dependent diabetic patient who is visually impaired may find it helpful to use a magnifying apparatus that fits around the syringe.

An insulin-cartridge pen (the Novalin Pen) is available that allows the patient to dial the correct dose of insulin and press a button to release the dose quickly through a short, fine, 27-gauge needle.

Before attempting to explain or demonstrate devices that aid low-vision diabetic patients to prepare their medication, the nurse should attempt to use the device under similar circumstances. Practice using the aid with a blindfold in place, to detect any difficulties the patient may experience.

A $5/16$- to 1-inch, 25- to 30-gauge needle is used for this route. Ordinarily, no more than 1 mL of solution is given subcutaneously. Giving larger amounts adds to the patient's discomfort and may predispose to poor absorption.

The skin is cleaned for a subcutaneous injection in the same manner as for an intradermal injection. Recent research has questioned the need to clean the skin with an alcohol prep before an insulin injection. The combination of a small-gauge needle that limits the number of bacteria

that can pass through it and bacteriostatic additives in insulin preparations makes skin preparation before an insulin injection unnecessary. However, this cleansing is still commonly performed (Fleming, 1999).

The nurse chooses the angle of needle insertion based on the amount of subcutaneous tissue present and the length of the needle. In most cases, a $5/8$-inch needle is inserted at a 45-degree angle and a $1/2$-inch needle is inserted at a 90-degree angle. The patient's size may also determine

PROCEDURE 28-5

Administering an Intradermal Injection

Equipment

Medication
Medication Kardex or computer-
   generated MAR
Disposable gloves

Sterile syringe and needle (size
   depends on medication being
   administered and patient)

Alcohol swab
Acetone and 2 × 2 sterile gauze
   square (optional)

Action	Rationale
1. Assemble equipment and check the physician's order.	This ensures that the patient receives the right medication at the right time by the proper route. Many intradermal drugs are potent allergens and may cause a significant reaction if given in an incorrect dose.
2. Explain the procedure to the patient.	Explanation encourages cooperation and reduces apprehension.
3. Wash your hands. Don disposable gloves.	Handwashing deters the spread of microorganisms. Gloves act as a barrier and protect the nurse's hands from accidental exposure to blood during the injection procedure.
4. If necessary, withdraw medication from an ampule or vial as described in Procedures 28-2 and 28-3.	
5. Select an area on the inner aspect of the forearm that is not heavily pigmented or covered with hair. The upper chest or upper back beneath the scapulae also are sites for intradermal injections.	The forearm is a convenient and easy location for introducing an agent intradermally. Hair or lesions at the injection site may interfere with assessments of skin changes at the site.
6. Cleanse the area with an alcohol swab while wiping with a firm, circular motion and moving outward from the injection site. Allow the skin to dry. If the skin is oily, clean the area with a pledget moistened with acetone.	Pathogens on the skin can be forced into the tissues by the needle. Introducing alcohol into tissues irritates the tissues and is uncomfortable for the patient. Acetone is effective for removing oily substances from the skin.
7. Use the nondominant hand to spread the skin taut over the injection site.	Taut skin provides an easy entrance into intradermal tissue.
8. Remove the needle cap with the nondominant hand by pulling it straight off.	The cap protects the needle from contact with microorganisms. This technique lessens the risk of an accidental needlestick.
9. Place the needle almost flat against the patient's skin, bevel side up, and insert the needle into the skin so that the point of the needle can be seen through the skin. Insert the needle only about ⅛ inch.	Intradermal tissue is entered when the needle is held as nearly parallel to the skin as possible and is inserted about ⅛ inch.
10. Slowly inject the agent while watching for a small wheal or blister to appear. If none appears, withdraw the needle slightly.	If a small wheal or blister appears, the agent is in intradermal tissue.
11. Withdraw the needle quickly at the same angle that it was inserted.	Withdrawing the needle quickly and at the angle at which it entered the skin minimizes tissue damage and discomfort for the patient.

(continued)

PROCEDURE 28-5

Administering an Intradermal Injection (Continued)

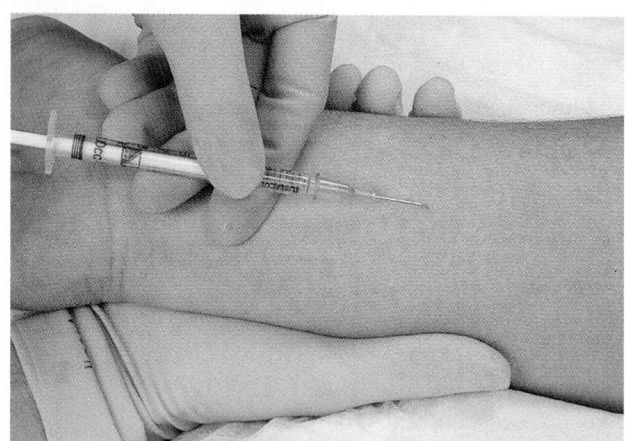

Action 9: Inserting the needle almost level with the skin.

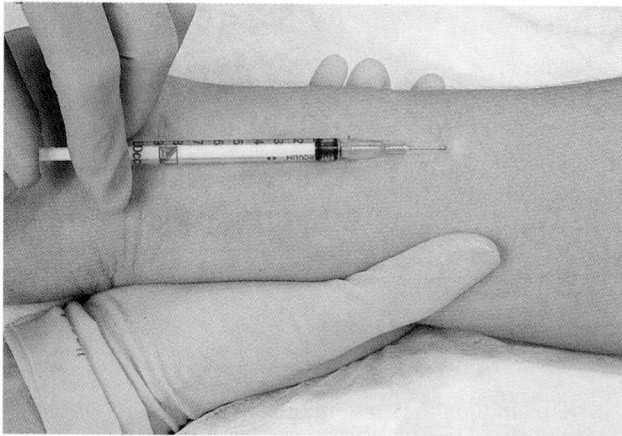

Action 10: Observing for wheal while injecting medication.

12. Do not massage the area after removing the needle.

Massaging the area where an intradermal injection is given may interfere with test results by spreading medication to underlying subcutaneous tissue.

13. Do not recap the used needle. Discard the needle and syringe in the appropriate receptacle.

Proper disposal of the needle protects the nurse from accidental injection. Most accidental puncture wounds occur when recapping needles.

14. Assist the patient to a position of comfort.

This provides for the well-being of the patient.

15. Remove gloves and dispose of them properly. Wash your hands.

Handwashing deters the spread of microorganisms.

16. Chart the administration of the medication.

Accurate documentation is necessary to prevent medication error.

17. Observe the area for signs of a reaction at ordered intervals, usually at 24- to 72-hour periods. Inform the patient of this inspection. In some agencies, a circle may be drawn on the skin around the injection site.

This easily identifies the site of the intradermal injection and allows for careful observation of the exact area.

Special Considerations   Recent research has indicated that a bevel-down technique may be preferable when performing skin testing (Howard et al., 1997).

the angle of needle insertion. For a thin patient, it is best to bunch the skin to create a skin fold and insert the needle at a 45-degree angle. The risk for injecting a medication intramuscularly is lower for a heavier person, and a 90-degree angle may be used. Because the needle frequently used now for insulin injections is thinner (30 gauge) and shorter ($^5/_{16}$ inch), the angle of needle insertion is less important. It is unlikely, even in a thin person, that this smaller needle will reach muscle tissue.

Heparin is also administered subcutaneously; the abdomen is the most commonly used site. The area two inches

around the umbilicus and the belt line must be avoided. Manufacturer's directions for subcutaneous administration of low-molecular-weight heparin preparations (eg, Lovenox) include specific instructions to pinch the tissue gently and insert the needle at a 90-degree angle into a fat pad on either side of the abdomen. Aspiration or pulling back on the plunger is not recommended with administration of heparin because this action can result in hematoma formation. Aspiration after an insulin injection is also unnecessary and has not proved a reliable indicator of needle placement. For a subcutaneous injection, the site is gently massaged after

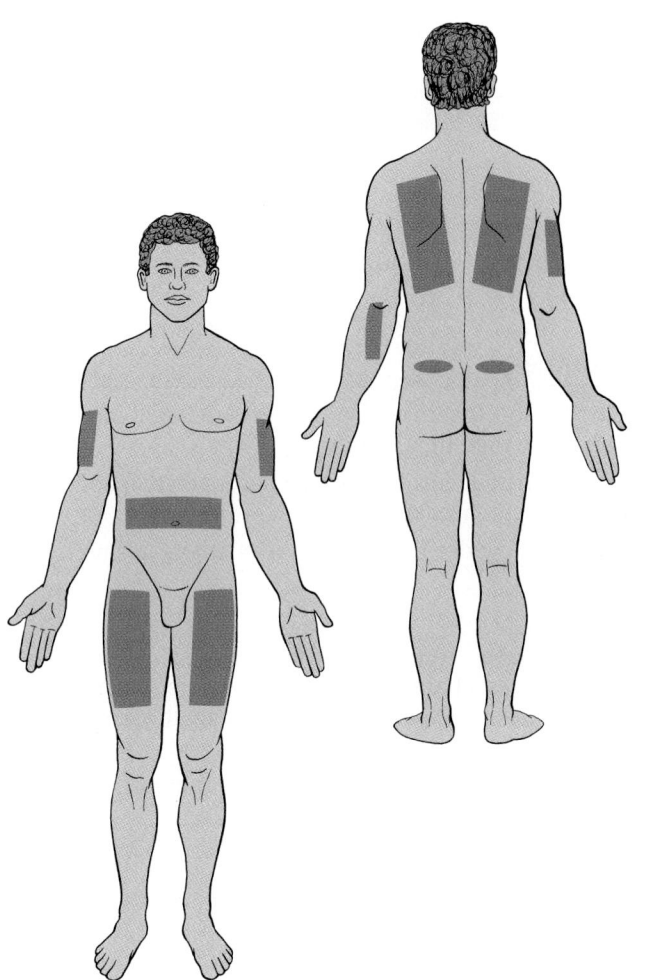

Figure 28-7
Sites on the body where subcutaneous injections can be given.

the medication has been given, except in the case of heparin and insulin because massaging the site can increase the rate of absorption of these agents.

It is necessary to rotate sites or areas for injection if the patient is to receive frequent injections. This helps to prevent buildup of fibrous tissue and permits complete absorption of the medication. It is recommended that patients administering their own insulin use the same area of the body at the same time every day to ensure more consistent absorption (Fleming, 1999). Insulin is absorbed most quickly in the abdomen, followed by the arms, thighs, and buttocks. For instance, every morning the patient uses the abdomen for insulin injection and every evening before dinner, the patient injects the insulin into the arms or thighs. In each case, the injections should be given an inch away from the previous injection site so that the same area will not be used again in the same month. A small spot bandage or piece of tape can be used to mark the first injection site, with subsequent injections rotated in a circle around that site. After this area has been used, an adjacent site, an inch away, can be selected, using the same rotation format. A marked diagram incorporated into the patient's plan of care is also helpful for noting alternative sites. It is futile to rely on mem-

ory. Not even the patient can always recall the site of the previous injection. The site of administration is recorded in the patient's record. Procedure 28-6 shows the procedure for administering medications subcutaneously. Techniques for reducing discomfort in subcutaneous administrations are listed after the discussion Administering Medications Intramuscularly.

Administering Medications Intramuscularly

The intramuscular route is often used for drugs that are irritating because there are few nerve endings in deep muscle tissue. If a sore or inflamed muscle is entered, however, the muscle may act as a trigger area, and severe referred pain often results. It is best to palpate a muscle before injection. A site should be selected that does not feel tender to the patient and where the tissue does not contract and become firm and tense.

Absorption occurs as in subcutaneous administration but more rapidly because of the greater vascularity of muscle tissue. The amount of 4 mL is considered the maximum to be given in one site for an adult with well-developed muscles, although the patient's size and the site used (eg, deltoid muscle) may necessitate that a smaller amount is injected (Beyea & Nicoll, 1996).

Intramuscular Injection Sites

An important point in the administration of an **intramuscular injection** is the selection of a safe site away from large nerves, bones, and blood vessels (Fig. 28-8). When care is not taken, common complications include abscesses, necrosis and skin slough, nerve injuries, lingering pain, and periostitis (inflammation of the membrane covering a bone).

The sites for injecting intramuscular medications should be rotated when therapy requires repeated injections. The sites described in this chapter may all be used on a rotating basis. Whatever pattern of rotating sites is used, a description of it should appear in the patient's plan of nursing care.

Ventrogluteal Site

The ventrogluteal site (see Fig. 28-8A) involves the gluteus medius and gluteus minimus muscles in the hip area. The ventrogluteal site is recommended for both adults and children older than 7 months of age as a safe site for most intramuscular injections. There are no large nerves or blood vessels in the injection area, the site is removed from bone tissue, the area is clean because fecal contamination is rare at this site, and the patient can be on the back, abdomen, or side for the injection. To relax the gluteal muscle, the patient may flex the knees while lying on the back, point the toes inward while lying in the prone position, and flex the upper leg in front of the lower leg in the side-lying position. Although any of the three positions just described may be used when injecting the ventrogluteal site, nurses increasingly prefer the side-lying position.

To locate the ventrogluteal site, the nurse places the palm over the greater trochanter, with the fingers facing the patient's head. The right hand is used for the patient's
(*text continues on page 602*)

PROCEDURE 28-6

Administering a Subcutaneous Injection

Equipment

Medication
Medication Kardex or computer-
generated MAR

A sterile syringe and needle (size
depends on medication being
administered and patient)

Alcohol swabs
Disposable gloves

Action	Rationale
1. Assemble equipment and check the physician's order.	This ensures that the patient receives the right medication at the right time by the proper route.
2. Explain the procedure to the patient.	An explanation encourages patient cooperation and reduces apprehension.
3. Wash your hands.	Handwashing deters the spread of microorganisms.
4. If necessary, withdraw medication from an ampule or vial as described in Procedures 28-2 and 28-3.	
5. Identify the patient carefully. See Procedure 28-1, action 12. Close the curtain to provide privacy. Don disposable gloves.	It is the nurse's responsibility to guard against error. Gloves act as a barrier and protect the nurse's hands from accidental exposure to blood during the injection procedure.

6. Have the patient assume a position appropriate for the most commonly used sites:
    a. Outer aspect of upper arm—the patient's arm should be relaxed and at the side of the body.
    b. Anterior thighs—the patient may sit or lie with the leg relaxed.
    c. Abdomen—the patient may lie in a semi-recumbent position.
	Injection into a tense muscle causes discomfort.

7. Locate the site of choice according to directions given in this chapter. Ensure that the area is not tender and is free of lumps or nodules.	Good visualization is necessary to establish the correct location of the site and avoid damage to tissues. Nodules or lumps may indicate a previous injection site where absorption was inadequate.
8. Clean the area around the injection site with an alcohol swab. Use a firm, circular motion while moving outward from the injection site. Allow the antiseptic to dry. Leave the alcohol swab in a clean area for reuse when withdrawing the needle.	Friction helps to clean the skin. A clean area is contaminated when a soiled object is rubbed over its surface.
9. Remove the needle cap with the nondominant hand, pulling it straight off.	The cap protects the needle from contact with microorganisms. This technique lessens the risk of an accidental needlestick.
10. Grasp and bunch the area surrounding the injection site or spread the skin at the site.	This provides for easy, less painful entry into the subcutaneous tissue. The decision to pinch or spread tissue at the injection site depends on the size of the patient. If the patient is thin, skin needs to be bunched to create a skinfold.
11. Hold the syringe in the dominant hand between the thumb and forefinger. Inject the needle quickly at an angle at 45 to 90 degrees, depending on the amount and turgor of the tissue and the length of the needle, as shown.	Subcutaneous tissue is abundant in well-nourished, well-hydrated people and spare in emaciated, dehydrated, or very thin persons. For a thin person, it is best to insert the needle at a 45-degree angle.

(continued)

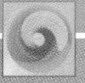

PROCEDURE 28-6

Administering a Subcutaneous Injection (Continued)

12. After the needle is in place, release the tissue and immediately move your nondominant hand to steady the lower end of the syringe. Slide your dominant hand to the tip of the barrel.

Injecting the solution into compressed tissues results in pressure against nerve fibers and creates discomfort. The nondominant hand secures the syringe and allows for smooth aspiration.

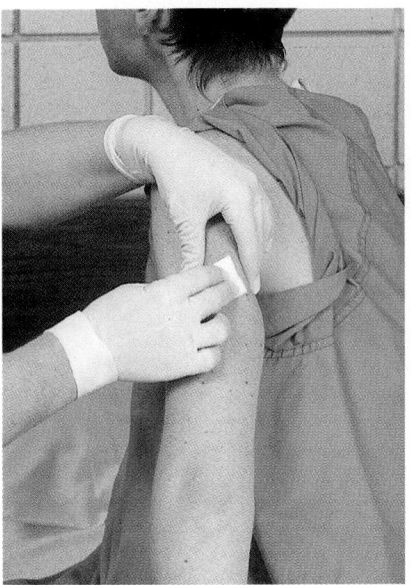

Action 8: Cleaning injection site.

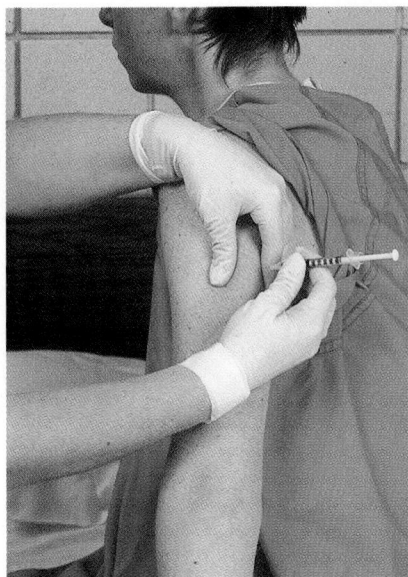

Action 10: Bunching tissue around injection site.

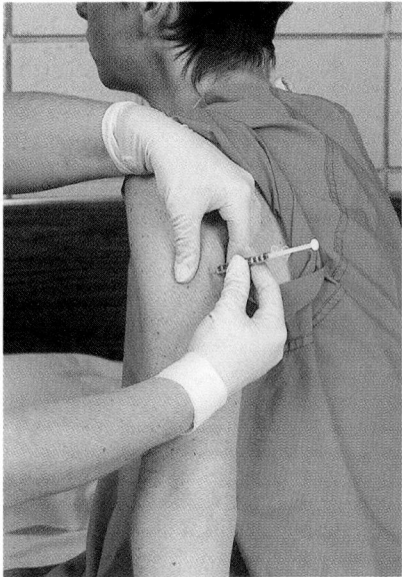

Action 11: Inserting needle.

13. Aspirate, if recommended, by pulling back gently on the plunger of the syringe to determine whether the needle is in a blood vessel. If blood appears, the needle should be withdrawn, the medication syringe and needle discarded, and a new syringe with new medication prepared. *Do not aspirate when giving insulin or heparin.*

14. If no blood appears, inject the solution slowly.

15. Withdraw the needle quickly at the same angle at which it was inserted, as shown.

16. Massage the area gently with the alcohol swab. (Do not massage a subcutaneous heparin or insulin injection site.)

Discomfort and possibly a serious reaction may occur if a drug intended for subcutaneous use is injected into a vein. Heparin is an anticoagulant and may cause bruising if aspirated. Because the insulin needle is so small, aspiration after insulin has proved unreliable in predicting needle placement.

Rapid injection of the solution creates pressure in the tissues, resulting in discomfort.

Slow withdrawal of the needle pulls the tissues and causes discomfort. Applying countertraction around the injection site helps to prevent pulling on the tissue as the needle is withdrawn. Removing the needle at the same angle at which it was inserted minimizes tissue damage and discomfort for the patient.

Massaging helps to distribute the solution and hastens its absorption. Massaging the site of a heparin injection causes additional bruising. Massaging after an insulin injection may contribute to unpredictable absorption of the medication.

(continued)

PROCEDURE 28-6

Administering a Subcutaneous Injection (Continued)

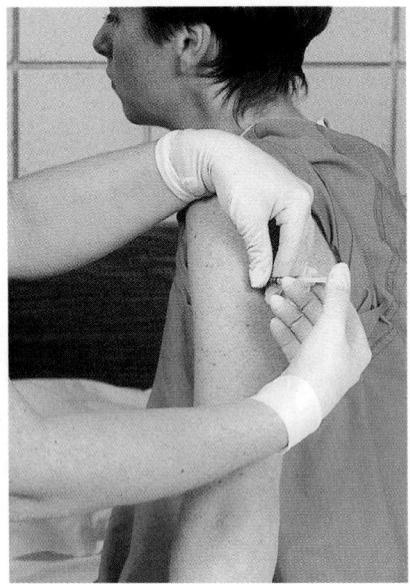

Action 14: Injecting medication.

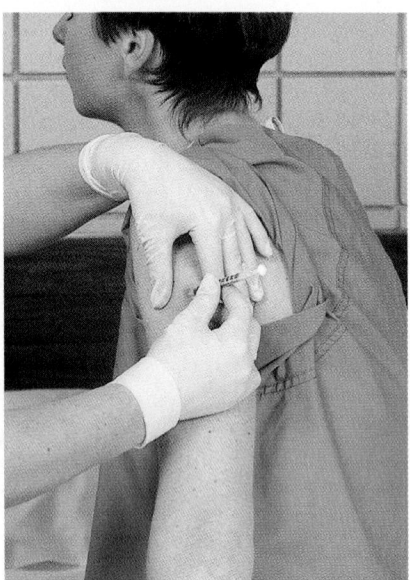

Action 15: Withdrawing needle. (PHOTOS © B. PROUD.)

17. Do not recap the used needle. Discard the needle and syringe in the appropriate receptacle.

Proper disposal of the needle protects the nurse from accidental injection. Most accidental puncture wounds occur when recapping needles.

18. Assist the patient to a position of comfort.

This provides for the well-being of the patient.

19. Remove gloves and dispose of them properly. Wash your hands.

Handwashing deters the spread of microorganisms.

20. Chart the administration of the medication.

Accurate documentation is necessary to prevent medication error.

21. Evaluate the response of the patient to medication within an appropriate time frame.

Reaction to medication given by the parenteral route may occur within 15 to 30 minutes after injection.

Home Care Considerations   According to the American Diabetes Association, reuse of insulin syringes in this setting appears safe. Once the needle is dull, it should be discarded (usually after 2 to 10 uses). Only in this situation and setting, can the needle be recapped between uses (Fleming, 1999).

left hip, or the left hand for the right hip, to identify landmarks. The index finger is placed on the anterosuperior iliac spine, and the middle finger extends dorsally, palpating the crest of the ileum. A triangle is formed. The injection is made in the center of the triangle.

Vastus Lateralis Site

The vastus lateralis muscle is recommended frequently for the injection of medications if the ventrogluteal site cannot be used (see Fig. 28-8B). It is a thick muscle,

and there is little or no danger of serious injury. There are no large nerves or vessels in proximity, and it does not cover a joint. The muscle covers the anterolateral aspect of the thigh. It is bounded by the midanterior thigh on the front of the leg and the midlateral thigh on the side. The thigh is divided into thirds horizontally and vertically. The injection is given in the *outer middle* third. This space provides a large number of injection sites. The vastus lateralis site is particularly desirable for infants and children, whose gluteal muscles are poorly developed.

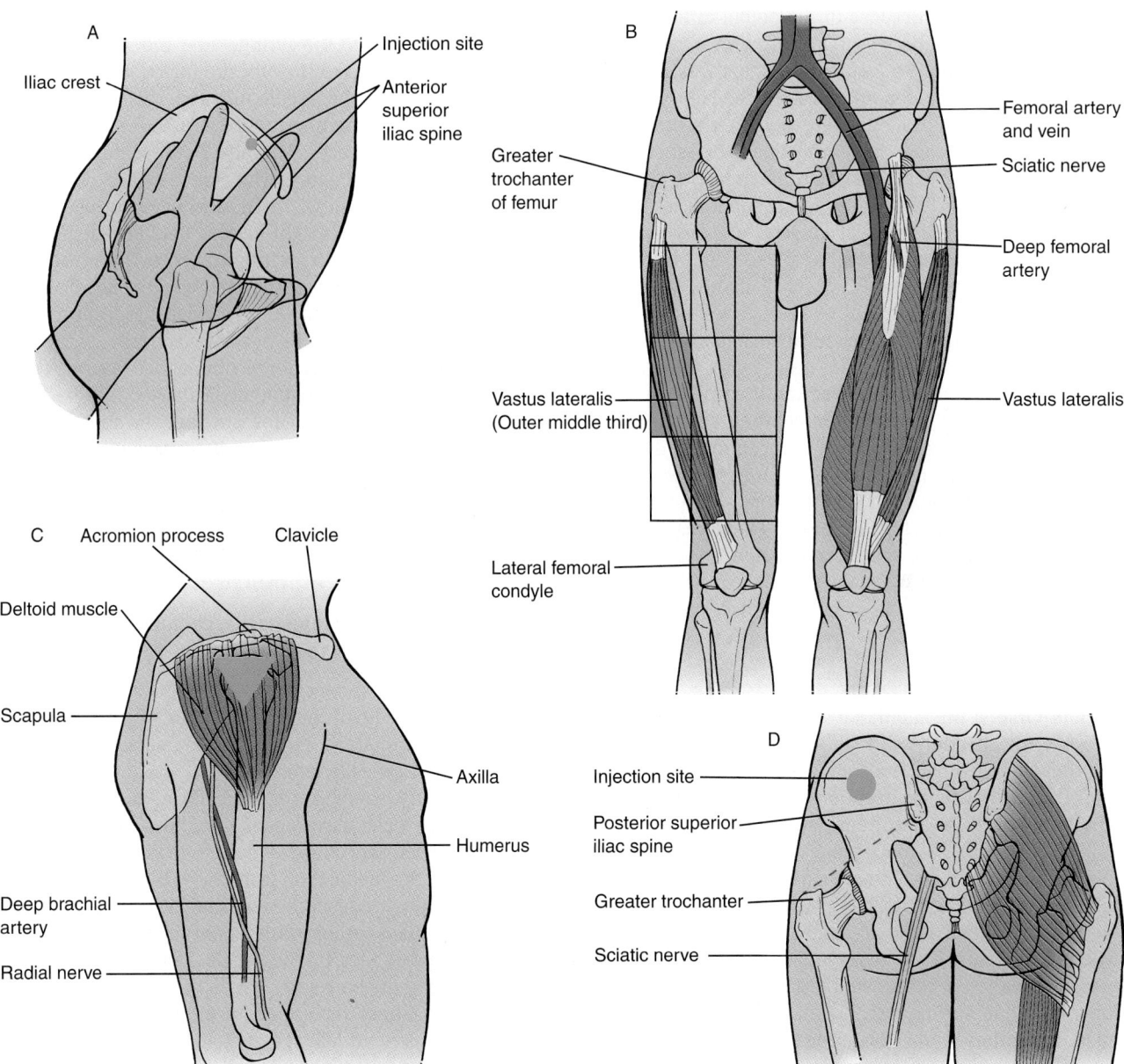

Figure 28-8
Sites for intramuscular injections. Descriptions for locating the sites are given in the text. (**A**) The *ventrogluteal site* is located by placing the palm on the greater trochanter and the index finger toward the anterosuperior iliac spine. (**B**) The *vastus lateralis site* is identified by dividing the thigh into thirds, horizontally and vertically. (**C**) The *deltoid muscle site* is located by palpating the lower edge of the acromion process. (**D**) The *dorsogluteal site* is lateral and slightly superior to the midpoint of a line drawn from the trochanter to the posterior superior iliac spine.

Deltoid Muscle Site

The deltoid muscle is located in the lateral aspect of the upper arm (see Fig. 28-8C). It is not often used because it is a small muscle and is not capable of absorbing large amounts of solution. Damage to the radial nerve and artery is a risk of the deltoid site. Intramuscular injections into the deltoid muscle should be limited to 1 mL of solution and used only for adults. The deltoid muscle is not developed enough in infants and children to absorb medication adequately.

The deltoid muscle can be located by palpating the lower edge of the acromion process. A triangle is formed at the midpoint in line with the axilla on the lateral aspect of the upper arm. Hepatitis B virus vaccine is one medication that should be given in the deltoid muscle in adults to induce adequate levels of the antibody.

Dorsogluteal Site

The dorsogluteal site (see Fig. 28-8D), located in the buttock, has been a common site for administering intramuscular injections. Because of the potential for accidental injury to the sciatic nerve and the presence of major blood vessels and bone mass near the site, the dorsogluteal muscle is not considered an optimal site. The posterosuperior iliac spine and the greater trochanter represent the anatomic landmarks. An imaginary line is drawn between the posterosuperior iliac spine and the greater trochanter. The injection site is lateral and slightly superior to the midpoint of the line. The gluteal muscles are developed by walking; therefore, the dorsogluteal site is not to be used for children younger than 3 years of age because their gluteal muscles are too small.

Good visualization of the entire area and careful mapping are necessary to locate the proper site. This necessitates adequate exposure by lowering the undergarments. Merely raising one side of underclothing permits only a partial visualization of the area. It is recommended that the patient be in a prone position with the toes pointed inward, or in the side-lying position with the upper knee flexed and the upper leg in front of the lower leg. These positions help to promote maximum muscle relaxation and, therefore, minimum discomfort. When the patient is in a standing position, the gluteus muscle usually is tense, and then this site should not be used.

Intramuscular Injection Procedure

No more than 4 mL should be injected into a single injection site for an adult with well-developed muscles. The less developed muscles of children and elderly people limit the intramuscular injection to 1 to 2 mL. Equipment commonly used for an intramuscular injection includes a 1½-inch (3.8 cm), 21- to 23-gauge needle. The length of the needle should be selected with care for any intramuscular injection. Prepackaged, loaded syringes usually have a needle that is 1 inch long. If there is any question about whether the belly of the target muscle can be reached, the medication should be transferred to another syringe with the appropriate needle size. A short needle does not minimize discomfort, and a longer one does not increase discomfort. The characteristics of the patient's anatomy should dictate the needle length chosen. The most important consideration is to use a needle with a tip that will reach deep into the muscle.

The addition of an air bubble to the syringe is unnecessary and a potentially dangerous procedure that could result in an overdose of medication. Disposable syringes are calibrated to deliver a correct dose without the use of an air bubble (Beyea & Nicoll, 1996). The technique for administering an intramuscular injection is outlined in Procedure 28-7. Figure 28-9 compares the angles for needle insertion for different forms of injections.

Z-Track Technique

Any intramuscular injection may be given using the **Z-track** technique. Beyea & Nicoll (1996) state that Z-track is the safest and most comfortable technique for giving any intramuscular injection. This prevents seepage of the medication into the needle track and reduces the pain and discomfort, particularly for patients receiving injections

over an extended period. In the Z-track technique, a clean needle is attached to the syringe after the syringe is filled with the medication to prevent the injection of any residual medication on the needle into superficial tissues. The needle should be a minimum of 1½ inches (3.8 cm) long. The ventrogluteal, vastus lateralis, or dorsogluteal site can be used for this procedure. The skin is pulled down or to one side about 1 inch (2.5 cm), and held in this position with the left hand for a right-handed person. The needle is inserted and aspirated carefully to detect the presence of blood. The medication is injected slowly, the needle is then steadily withdrawn, and the displaced tissue is released and allowed to return to its normal position.

Massage of the site is not recommended because it may cause irritation by forcing the medication to leak back into the needle track, but gentle pressure may be applied with a dry sponge. The procedure for administering a Z-track injection is outlined in Figure 28-10.

Reducing Discomfort in Subcutaneous and Intramuscular Administrations

The following are recommended techniques to help reduce discomfort when injecting medications subcutaneously or intramuscularly:

- Select a needle of the smallest gauge that is appropriate for the site and solution to be injected, and select the correct needle length.
- Be sure the needle is free of medication that may irritate superficial tissues as the needle is inserted. Recommended procedure is to use two needles—one to remove the medication from the vial or ampule and a second one to inject the medication. If medication is in a prefilled syringe with a nonremovable needle and has dripped back on the needle during preparation, gently tap the barrel to remove the excess solution.
- Use the Z-track technique for intramuscular injections to prevent leakage of medication into the needle track, thus minimizing the patient's discomfort.
- Inject the medication into relaxed muscles. There is more pressure and discomfort when the medication is injected into a contracted muscle.
- Do not inject areas that feel hard on palpation or tender to the patient.
- Insert the needle with a dartlike motion without hesitation, and remove it quickly at the same angle at which it was inserted. These techniques help to reduce discomfort and tissue irritation.
- Do not administer more solution in one injection than is recommended for the site. Injecting more solution creates excess pressure in the area and increases discomfort.
- Inject the solution slowly so that it may be dispersed more easily into the surrounding tissue (10 seconds per 1 mL).
- Apply gentle pressure after injection, unless this technique is contraindicated.

(text continues on page 607)

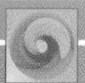

PROCEDURE 28-7

Administering an Intramuscular Injection

Equipment

Medication
Medication Kardex or computer-
 generated MAR

Sterile syringe and needle (size
 depends on medication being
 administered and patient)

Alcohol swab
Dry sponge
Disposable gloves

Action	Rationale
1. Assemble equipment and check the physician's order.	This ensures that the patient receives the right medication at the right time by the proper route.
2. Explain the procedure to the patient.	Explanation encourages cooperation and alleviates apprehension.
3. Wash your hands.	Handwashing deters the spread of microorganisms.
4. If necessary, withdraw medication from an ampule or vial as described in Procedures 28-2 and 28-3.	
5. Do not add air to the syringe.	The addition of air to the syringe is potentially dangerous and may result in an overdose of medication.

6. Provide for privacy. Have the patient assume a position appropriate for the site selected.
  a. Ventrogluteal—the patient may lie on the back or side with the hip and knee flexed.
  b. Vastus lateralis—the patient may lie on the back or may assume a sitting position.
  c. Deltoid—the patient may sit or lie with arm relaxed.
  d. Dorsogluteal—the patient may lie prone with toes pointing inward or on the side with the upper leg flexed and placed in front of the lower leg.
	Injection into a tense muscle causes discomfort.

7. Locate the site of choice according to directions given in this chapter and ensure that the area is nontender and free of lumps or nodules. Don disposable gloves.	Good visualization is necessary to establish the correct location of the site and avoid damage to tissues. Nodules or lumps may indicate a previous injection site where absorption was inadequate. Gloves act as a barrier and protect the nurse's hands from accidental exposure to blood during the injection procedure.
8. Clean the area thoroughly with an alcohol swab, using friction. Allow alcohol to dry.	Pathogens present on the skin and alcohol can be forced into the tissues by the needle.
9. Remove the needle cap by pulling it straight off.	The cap protects the needle from contact with micro-organisms. This technique lessens the risk of an accidental needlestick and also prevents inadvertently unscrewing the needle from the barrel of the syringe.
10. Displace the skin in a Z-track manner or spread the skin at the site using your nondominant hand.	This makes the tissue taut and minimizes discomfort. Z-track prevents seepage of the medication into the needle track and is less painful.
11. Hold the syringe in your dominant hand between the thumb and forefinger. Quickly dart the needle into the tissue at a 90-degree angle.	A quick injection is less painful. Inserting the needle at a 90-degree angle facilitates entry into muscle tissue.

(continued)

Administering an Intramuscular Injection (Continued)

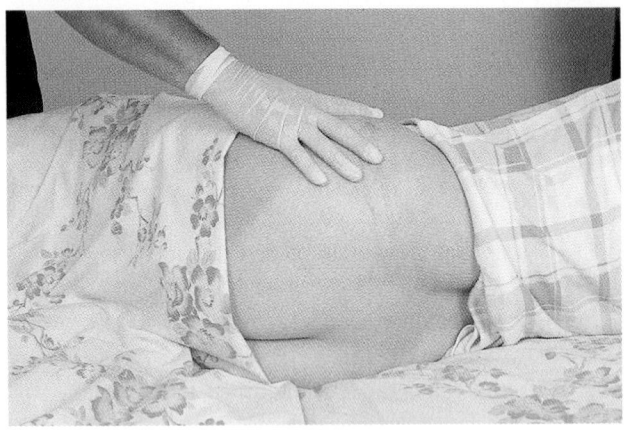

Action 7: Identifying landmarks for ventrogluteal injection site.

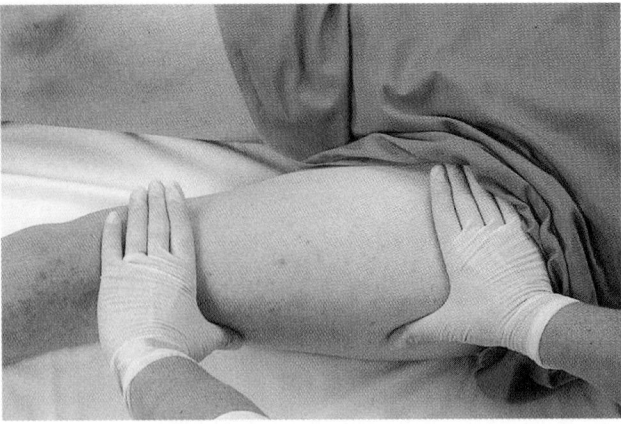

Action 7: Identifying vastus lateralis injection site.

12. As soon as the needle is in place, use your nondominant hand to hold the lower end of the syringe. Slide your dominant hand to the tip of the barrel.

13. Aspirate by slowly (for at least 5 seconds) pulling back on the plunger to determine whether the needle is in a blood vessel. If blood is aspirated, discard the needle, syringe, and medication, prepare a new sterile setup, and inject another site.

14. If no blood is aspirated, inject the solution slowly (10 seconds per mL of medication).

This acts to steady the syringe and allows for smooth aspiration.

Discomfort and possibly a serious reaction may occur if a drug intended for intramuscular use is injected into a vein. Allowing slow aspiration facilitates back-flow of blood even if needle is in a small, low-flow blood vessel.

Injecting slowly helps to reduce discomfort by allowing time for the solution to disperse in the tissues.

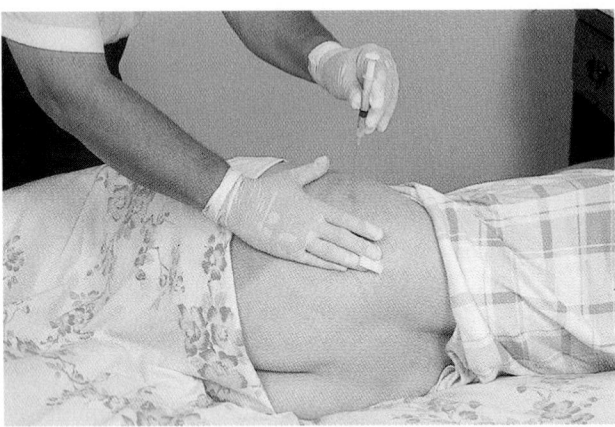

Actions 10 and 11: Displacing tissue in a Z-track manner and darting needle into tissue.

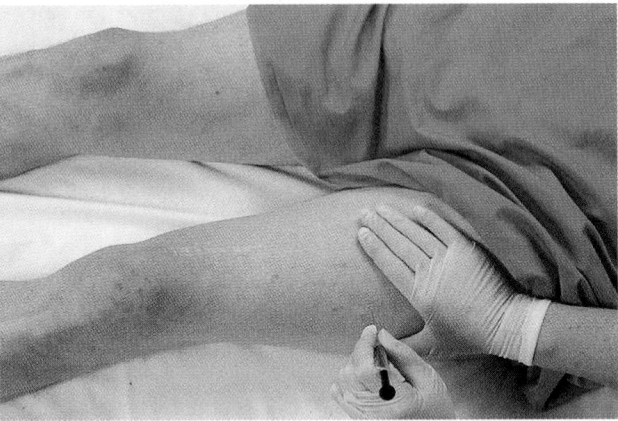

Actions 10 and 11: Spreading the skin at vastus lateralis site and darting needle into the tissue. (PHOTOS © B. PROUD.)

(continued)

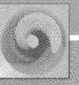

PROCEDURE 28-7

Administering an Intramuscular Injection (Continued)

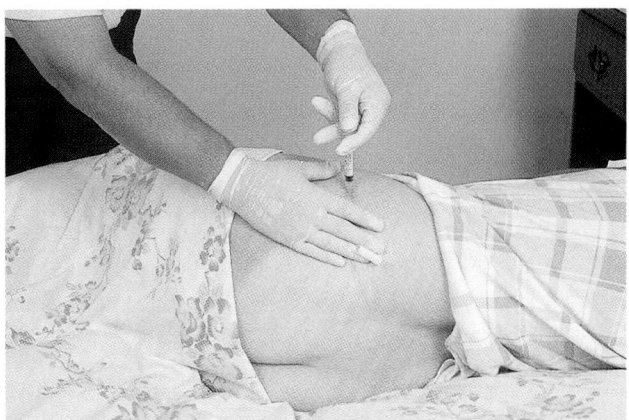

Action 13: Aspirating.

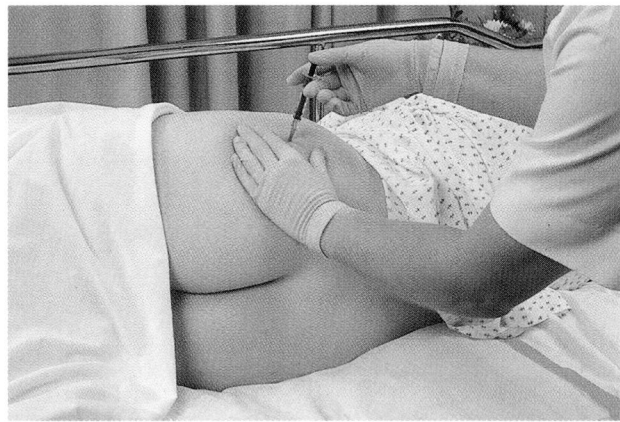

Action 14: Injecting.

15. Remove the needle slowly and steadily. Release displaced tissue if Z-track technique was used.	Slow withdrawal allows the medication to begin to be diffused through the muscle.
16. Apply gentle pressure at the site with a small, dry sponge.	Light pressure causes less trauma and irritation to the tissues.
17. Do not recap the used needle. Discard the needle and syringe in the appropriate receptacle.	Proper disposal of the needle protects the nurse from accidental injection. Most accidental puncture wounds occur when recapping needles.
18. Assist the patient to a position of comfort. Encourage patient to exercise leg if possible.	Exercise promotes absorption of the medication.
19. Remove gloves and dispose of them properly. Wash your hands.	Handwashing deters the spread of microorganisms.
20. Chart the administration of the medication.	Accurate documentation is necessary to prevent medication error.
21. Evaluate the response of the patient to the medication within an appropriate time frame. Assess site, if possible, within 2–4 hours after administration.	Reaction to medication given by the parenteral route is a possibility. Assessment also allows for visualization of the site for any untoward effects.

Age Considerations   Safe administration of an intramuscular injection into an infant's vastus lateralis muscle may require use of a 1-inch needle rather than the commonly used ⅝-inch needle. A 1-inch needle consistently allows penetration into the muscle and safe administration of the medication.

- Allow the patient who is fearful of injections to talk about his or her fears. Answer the patient's questions truthfully, and explain the nature and purpose of the injection. Taking the time to offer support often allays fears that ordinarily add to the discomfort of the procedure for the patient.
- Rotate the sites when the patient is to receive repeated injections. Injections in the same site may cause undue discomfort, irritation, or abscesses in tissues.

Administering Medications Intravenously

Medications administered intravenously have an immediate effect. The **intravenous route** is the most dangerous route of administration. Because the drug is placed directly into the bloodstream, it cannot be recalled, nor can its actions be slowed. Intravenous administration is the route used in most emergency situations when immediate absorption is required. There also are many nonemergency clinical situations

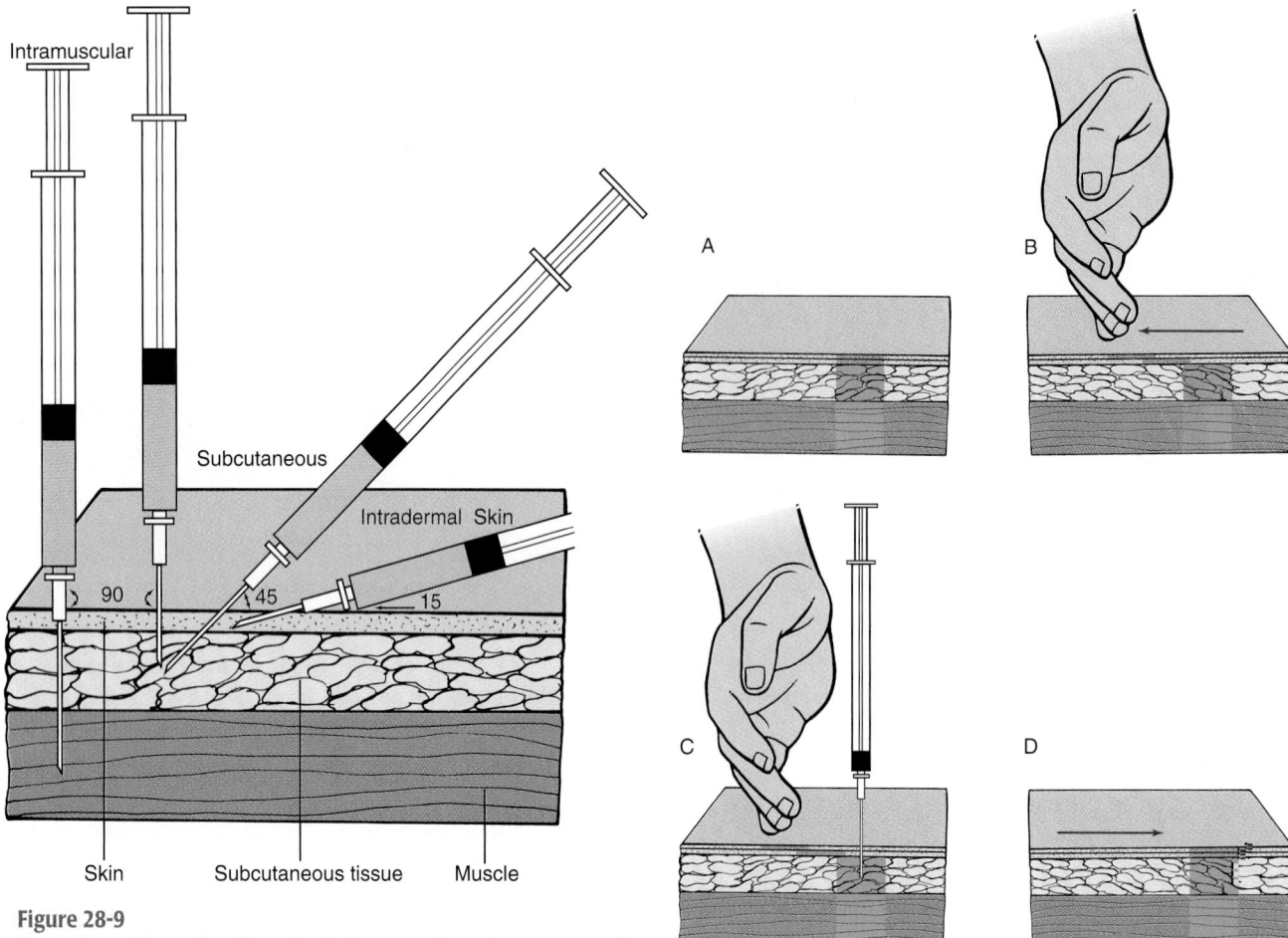

Figure 28-9
Comparison of the angles of insertion for intramuscular, subcutaneous, and intradermal injections.

Figure 28-10
The Z-track or zigzag technique is recommended for intramuscular injections. (**A**) Normal skin and tissues. (**B**) Moving the skin to one side. (**C**) Needle is inserted at a 90-degree angle, and needle is aspirated for blood. (**D**) Once the needle is withdrawn, displaced tissue is allowed to return to its normal position, preventing the solution from escaping from the muscle tissue.

in which drugs are administered intravenously. Patient-controlled analgesia allows the patient to control administration of an intravenous analgesic for pain management (see Chap. 40). Procedure 45-1 in Chapter 45 describes the basic technique for administering an intravenous infusion.

There are several ways to administer medications intravenously. Medications may be added to the patient's infusion solution. The recommended procedure is for the pharmacist to add the prescribed drug to a large volume of intravenous solution, but sometimes the drug is added in the nursing unit, in which case sterile technique must be maintained. Steps for adding medications to intravenous solutions are given in Procedure 28-8.

When medication is administered by *continuous infusion*, the patient receives it slowly and over a long period. Although sometimes this can be an advantage when it is desirable to give the medication slowly, it is a disadvantage when the patient needs to receive the drug more quickly. Also, if for some reason all of the solution cannot be infused, the patient will not receive the prescribed amount of the medication. The patient receiving medication by a continuous intravenous infusion should be checked for possible adverse effects at least every hour.

A medication can be administered as an intravenous *bolus* or push. This involves a single injection of a concen-trated solution administered directly into an intravenous line (Procedure 28-9).

Medications can be administered by *intermittent intravenous infusion*. The drug is mixed with a small amount of the intravenous solution, such as 50 to 100 mL, and administered over a short period at the prescribed interval, for example, every 4 hours. As mentioned earlier, needleless devices are recommended by the Centers for Disease Control and Prevention and the Occupational Safety and Health Administration, and they effectively prevent needlesticks and provide access to the primary venous line. Either blunt-ended cannulas or recessed connection ports may be used. A patient with an intravenous line in place can receive the solution containing the medication by way of a piggyback setup, a volume-control administration set (eg, Pediatrol or Volutrol), or a miniinfusion pump. The intravenous *piggy-*
(*text continues on page 612*)

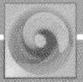

PROCEDURE 28-8

Adding Medications to an IV Solution Container

Equipment

Medication prepared in a syringe
   with a 19- to 21-gauge needle
   (or needleless device)

Alcohol swab
IV fluid container (bag or bottle)

Label to be attached to the IV
   container

Action	Rationale
1. Gather all equipment and bring to the patient's bedside. Check the medication order with the physician's order.	Having equipment available saves time and facilitates performance of the task. Checking the orders ensures that the patient receives the correct medication at the correct time and in the right manner.
2. Explain the procedure to the patient.	Explanation allays the patient's anxiety.
3. Wash your hands.	Handwashing deters the spread of microorganisms.
4. Identify the patient by checking the band on the patient's wrist and asking the patient his or her name.	This ensures that medication is given to the right person.
5. Add the medication to the IV solution that is infusing:	
a. Check that the volume in the bag or bottle is adequate.	The volume should be sufficient to dilute the drug.
b. Close the IV clamp.	This prevents back-flow directly to the patient of improperly diluted medication.
c. Clean the medication port with an alcohol swab.	This deters entry of microorganisms when the needle punctures the port.
d. Steady the container and uncap the needle or needleless device and insert it into the port. Inject the medication.	This ensures that the needle or needleless device enters the container and medication can be dispersed into the solution.
e. Remove the container from the IV pole and gently rotate the solutions.	This mixes the medication with the solution.

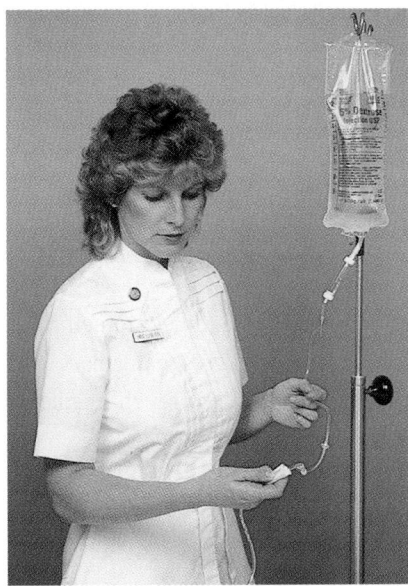

Action 5b: Closing the IV clamp.

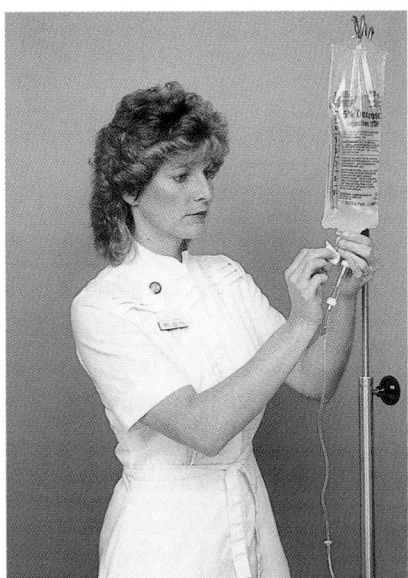

Action 5c: Cleaning the medication port.

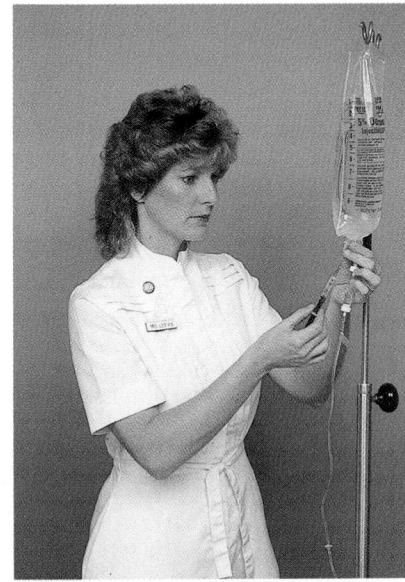

Action 5d: Inserting the needle or needleless device into the port.

(*continued*)

Adding Medications to an IV Solution Container (Continued)

f. Rehang the container, open the clamp, and readjust the flow rate.

This ensures the infusion of the IV with medication at the prescribed rate.

g. Attach the label to the container so that the dose of medication that has been added is apparent.

This confirms that the prescribed dose of medication has been added to the IV solution.

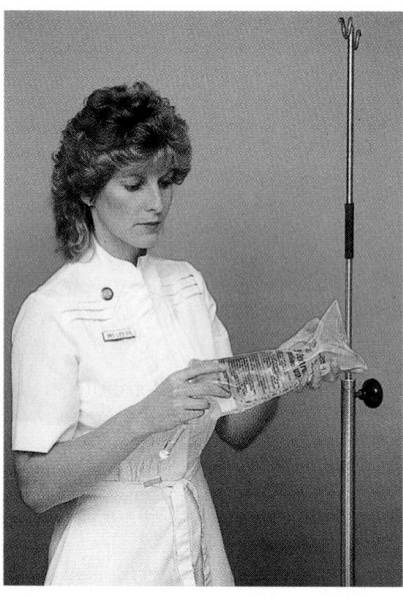

Action 5e: Rotating solution to distribute medication.

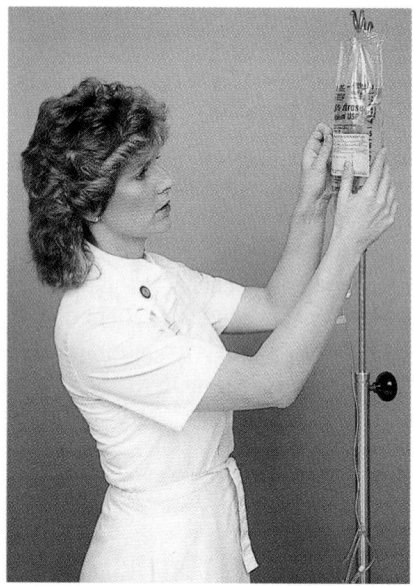

Action 5g: Labeling container to show medication.
(PHOTOS © KEN KASPER.)

6. Add the medication to the IV solution before infusion:
   a. Carefully remove any protective cover and locate the injection port. Clean with an alcohol swab.
   b. Uncap the needle or needleless device and insert into the port. Inject the medication.
   c. Withdraw and insert the spike into the proper entry site on the bag or bottle.
   d. With tubing clamped, gently rotate the IV solution in the bag or bottle. Hang the IV.
   e. Attach the label to the container so that the dose of medication that has been added is apparent.
7. Dispose of equipment according to agency policy.
8. Wash your hands.
9. Chart the addition of medication to the IV solution.

10. Evaluate the patient's response to medication within the appropriate time frame.

This deters entry of microorganisms when the needle punctures the port.

This ensures that the needle enters the container and that medication can be dispersed into the solution.

This punctures the seal in the IV bag or bottle.

This mixes medication with the solution.

This confirms that the prescribed dose of medication has been added to the IV solution.

This prevents inadvertent injury from the equipment.

Handwashing deters the spread of microorganisms.

Accurate documentation is necessary to prevent medication errors.

Patients require careful observation because medications given by the IV route may have a rapid effect.

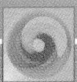

PROCEDURE 28-9

Adding a Bolus IV Medication to an Existing IV

Equipment

Medication prepared in a syringe
   with needleless device or 23- to
   25-gauge, 1-inch needle

Alcohol swab
Watch with second hand
Disposable gloves

Action	Rationale
1. Gather the equipment and bring to the patient's bedside. Check the medication order with the physician's order. Check a drug resource to clarify if medication needs to be diluted before administration.	Having equipment available saves time and facilitates performance of the task. Checking the orders ensures that the patient receives the correct medication at the correct time and in the right manner.
2. Explain the procedure to the patient.	Explanation allays the patient's anxiety.
3. Wash your hands. Don clean gloves.	Handwashing deters the spread of microorganisms. Gloves protect the nurse from exposure to blood-borne pathogens.
4. Identify the patient by checking the band on the patient's wrist and asking the patient his or her name.	This ensures that medication is given to the right person.
5. Assess the IV site for the presence of inflammation or infiltration.	IV medication must be given directly into a vein for safe administration.
6. Select the injection port on the tubing that is closest to the venipuncture site. Clean the port with an alcohol swab.	Using the port closest to the needle insertion site minimizes dilution of the medication. Cleaning with alcohol deters entry of microorganisms when the needle punctures the port.
7. Uncap the syringe. Steady the port with your nondominant hand while inserting the needleless device or needle into the center of the port.	This supports the injection port and lessens the risk for accidentally dislodging the IV or entering the port incorrectly.
8. Move your nondominant hand to the section of IV tubing just beyond the injection port. Fold the tubing between your fingers to temporarily stop the flow of the IV solution.	This minimizes the dilution of the IV medication with IV solution.
9. Pull back slightly on the plunger just until blood appears in the tubing.	This ensures injection of medication into a vein.

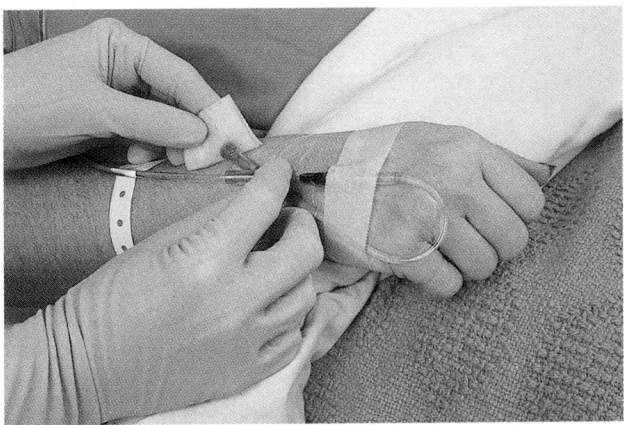

Action 6: Cleaning injection port.

(continued)

PROCEDURE 28-9

Adding a Bolus IV Medication to an Existing IV (Continued)

10. Inject the medication at the prescribed rate. (see Special Considerations, below).

This delivers the correct amount of medication at the proper interval according to manufacturer's directions.

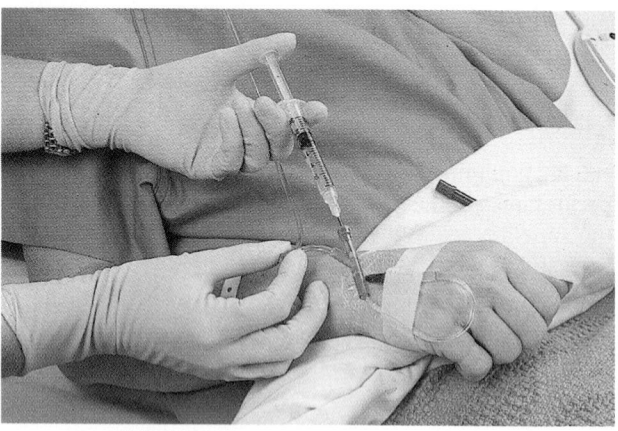

Action 10: Injecting medication while interrupting IV flow. (PHOTO © B. PROUD)

11. Remove the needle. Do not cap it. Release the tubing and allow the IV to flow at the proper rate.

This prevents accidental needlestick.

12. Dispose of the syringe in the proper receptacle.

Proper disposal prevents accidental injury and spread of microorganisms.

13. Remove gloves and wash your hands.

Handwashing deters the spread of microorganisms.

14. Chart the administration of the medication.

Accurate documentation is necessary to prevent medication errors.

15. Evaluate the patient's response to medication within the appropriate time frame.

The patient requires careful observation because medications given by an IV bolus injection may have a rapid effect.

Special Considerations

Agency policy may recommend the following variations when injecting a bolus IV medication:
- Release the folded tubing after a portion of the drug has been administered at the prescribed rate to facilitate delivery of the medication.
- Use a syringe with 1 mL normal saline to flush the tubing after an IV bolus is delivered to ensure that residual medication in the tubing is not delivered too rapidly.

back delivery system requires the intermittent or additive solution to be placed higher than the primary solution container. An extension hook provided by the manufacturer provides for easy lowering of the main intravenous container. The port on the primary intravenous line has a back-check valve that automatically stops the flow of the primary solution, allowing the secondary or piggyback solution to flow when connected. A *tandem* delivery setup is similar, except that both solutions remain at the same height and there is no back-check valve at the secondary port on the primary line. This type of setup is used infre-

quently because the solution from the primary intravenous line will back up into the tandem line if this intermittent infusion is not clamped immediately after it is infused. Because manufacturer's designs vary, nurses are advised to check the directions carefully for the systems used in their agency. The nurse is responsible for calculating and manually adjusting the flow rate of the intravenous intermittent infusion or regulating the infusion with an infusion pump or controller. Intravenous administration of medications using additive sets is explained in Procedure 28-10.

(*text continues on page 616*)

Administering IV Medications by Piggyback, Volume-Control Administration Set, or Miniinfusion Pump

Equipment

For Piggyback or Miniinfusion Pump

Gloves (optional)
Medication prepared in labeled
    piggyback set or syringe
    (5 to 100 mL)
Secondary infusion tubing (microdrip
    or macrodrip)
Needleless device, stopcock, or sterile
    needle (21- to 23-gauge)
Alcohol swab
Tape
Metal or plastic hook
Miniinfusion pump
Date label for tubing

For Volume Control Set

Gloves (optional)
Volume-control set (eg, Volutrol,
    Buretrol)
Medication (in vial or ampule)
Syringe with needleless device
    attached or a 20- or 21-gauge
    needle
Alcohol swab
Medication label

Action	Rationale
1. Gather all equipment and bring to the patient's bedside. Check the medication order against the original physician's order according to agency policy.	Having equipment available saves time and facilitates performance of the task. Checking the orders ensures that the patient receives the correct medication at the correct time and in the right manner.
2. Identify the patient by checking the identification band on the patient's wrist and asking the patient his or her name.	This ensures that the medication is given to the right person.
3. Explain the procedure to the patient.	Explanation allays the patient's anxiety.
4. Wash your hands and don gloves.	Handwashing deters the spread of microorganisms. Gloves protect the nurse when connecting setup to an existing IV.
5. Assess the IV site for the presence of inflammation or infiltration.	The medication must be administered directly into the vein that is not inflamed to avoid injuring surrounding tissue.

For Piggyback Infusion

6. Attach the infusion tubing to the piggyback set containing diluted medication. Place label on tubing with appropriate date and attach needle or needleless device to end of tubing according to manufacturer's directions. Open the clamp and prime the tubing (see action 4, Procedure 45-1). Close the clamp.	This removes air from the tubing and preserves the sterility of the setup. Tubing for piggyback setup may be used for 48 to 72 hours, depending on agency policy.
7. Hang the piggyback container on the IV pole, positioning it higher than the primary IV according to the manufacturer's recommendations. Use metal or plastic hook to lower primary IV.	The position of the container influences the flow of the IV fluid into the primary setup.
8. Use an alcohol swab to clean the appropriate port.	This deters entry of microorganisms when the piggyback setup is connected to the port.

(continued)

PROCEDURE 28-10

Administering IV Medications by Piggyback, Volume-Control Administration Set, or Miniinfusion Pump (Continued)

9. Connect the piggyback setup to either:
   a. Needleless port
   b. Stopcock: turn stopcock to open position

   c. Primary IV line: uncap needle and insert into secondary IV port closest to the top of the primary tubing. Use a strip of tape to secure the secondary set tubing to the primary infusion tubing. Primary line is left unclamped if port has a back-flow valve.

Needleless systems and stopcock setup eliminate the need for a needle and are recommended by the Centers for Disease Control and Prevention.
The tape stabilizes the needle in the infusion port and prevents it from slipping out. Back-flow valve in primary line secondary port stops flow of primary infusion while piggyback solution is infusing. Once completed, the back-flow valve opens, and flow of primary solution resumes.

10. Open the clamp on the piggyback set and regulate the flow at the prescribed delivery rate or set rate for secondary infusion on infusion pump. Monitor the medication infusion at periodic intervals.

Delivery over a 30- to 60-minute interval is usually a safe method of administering IV medication. It is important to verify safe administration rate for each drug to prevent adverse effects.

11. Clamp the tubing on the piggyback set when the solution is infused. Follow agency policy regarding disposal of equipment.

This reduces the risk for contaminating the primary IV setup.

12. Readjust the flow rate of the primary IV.

Piggyback medication administration may interrupt the normal flow rate of the primary IV. Readjustment of the rate may be necessary.

Using a Miniinfusion Pump

13. Connect prepared syringe to miniinfusion tubing.

Special tubing connects prepared medication to primary IV line.

14. Fill tubing with medication by applying gentle pressure to syringe plunger.

This removes air from the tubing.

15. Insert syringe into miniinfusion pump according to manufacturer's directions.

Syringe must fit securely in pump apparatus for proper operation.

16. Connect miniinfusion tubing to appropriate connector as in action 9.

Proper connection allows IV medication to flow into primary IV line.

17. Program pump to begin infusion. Set alarm if recommended by manufacturer.

Pump delivers medication at controlled rate. Alarm is recommended for use with IV lock apparatus.

18. Recheck flow rate of primary IV once pump has completed delivery of medication.

Normal flow rate of the primary IV may have been altered by the miniinfusion pump.

Using a Volume-Control Administration Set

19. Withdraw medication from the vial or ampule into the prepared syringe. See Procedure 28-2 or 28-3.

The correct dose is prepared for dilution in the IV solution.

20. Open the clamp between the IV solution and the volume-control administration set or secondary setup. Follow the manufacturer's instructions and fill with the desired amount of IV solution. Close the clamp.

This dilutes the medication in the minimal amount of solution. Reclamping prevents the continued addition of fluid to the volume to be mixed with the medication.

21. Use an alcohol swab to clean the injection port on the secondary setup.

This deters entry of microorganisms when the needle punctures the port.

(continued)

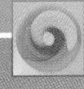

PROCEDURE 28-10

Administering IV Medications by Piggyback, Volume-Control Administration Set, or Miniinfusion Pump (Continued)

22. Remove the cap and insert the needle or blunt needle-less device into the port while holding the syringe steady. Inject the medication. Mix gently with IV solution.

This ensures that the medication is evenly mixed with solution.

23. Open the clamp below the secondary setup and regulate at the prescribed delivery rate. Monitor the medication infusion at periodic intervals.

Delivery over a 30- to 60-minute interval is a safe method of administering IV medication.

24. Attach the label to the volume-control device.

This prevents medication error.

25. Place the syringe with the uncapped needle in the designated container.

Proper disposal of the needle prevents inadvertent needlestick.

26. Wash your hands.

Handwashing deters the spread of microorganisms.

27. Chart the administration of medication after it has been infused.

Accurate documentation is necessary to prevent medication errors.

28. Evaluate the patient's response to medication within the appropriate time frame.

The patient requires careful observation because medications given by the IV route may have a rapid effect.

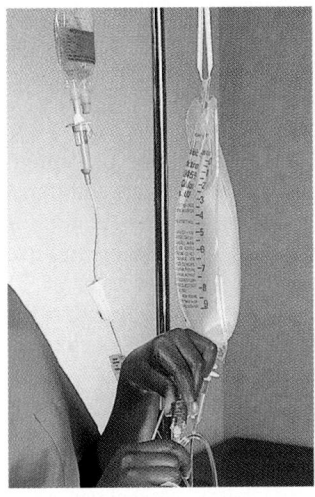

Action 6: Attaching tubing to piggyback set.

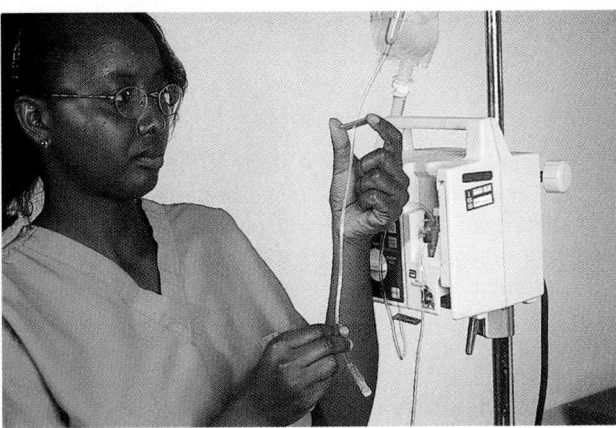
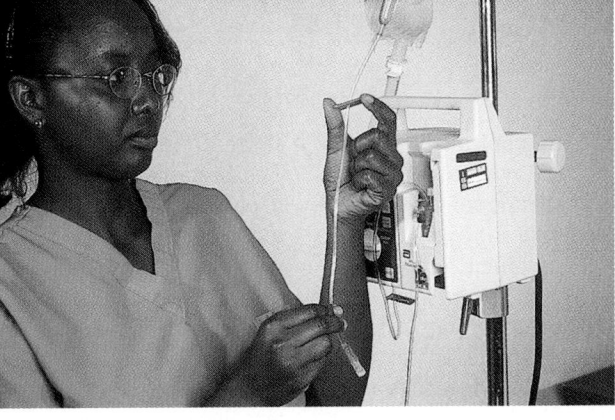

Action 6: Opening clamp and priming the tube.

Action 9a: Connecting piggyback setup to needleless port.

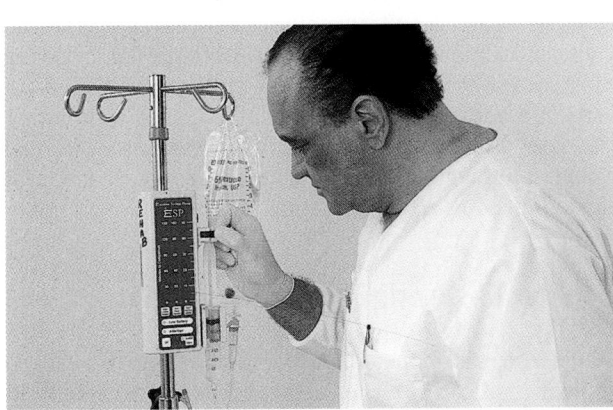

Action 15: Inserting syringe into mini-infusion pump.

(continued)

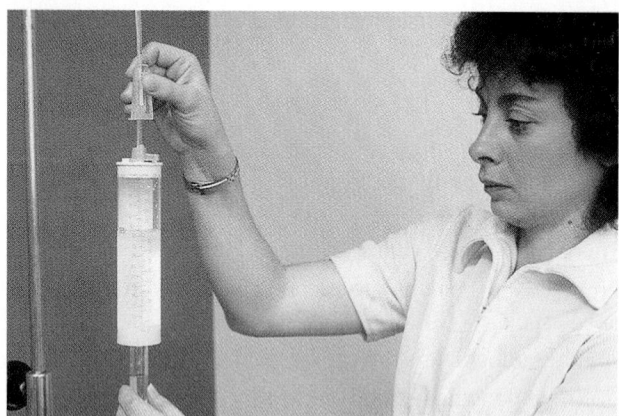

Action 20: Filling volume-control set.

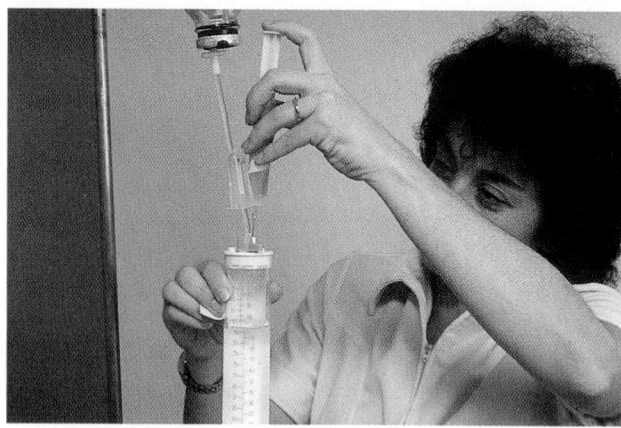

Action 22: Injecting medication.

Medications can also be placed in a controlled-volume administration set for intermittent intravenous infusion. The medication is diluted with a small amount of solution and administered through the patient's intravenous line (see Procedure 28-10). This type of equipment is also used for infusing solutions into children and older patients when the volume of fluid infused must be carefully monitored.

The minisyringe pump for intermittent infusion is battery operated and allows medication mixed in a syringe to be connected to the primary line and delivered by mechanical pressure applied to the syringe plunger (see Procedure 28-10).

A *heparin or saline lock*, or intermittent venous access device, is used for patients who require intermittent intravenous medication but not a continuous intravenous infusion. This device consists of a needle or catheter connected to a short length of tubing capped with a sealed injection port. An intravenous lock is shown in Procedure 28-11. After the needle is in place in the patient's vein, the needle and tubing are anchored to the patient's arm so that the needle remains in place until the patient no longer requires the repeated medication intravenously.

An intravenous lock allows the patient more freedom than a continuous intravenous infusion. The patient is connected to the intravenous line when it is time to receive the medication and disconnected when the medication is completed. A saline flush rather than a heparin flush is used in many agencies to maintain patency of the heparin lock. Using saline eliminates any possible systemic effects on coagulation or drug incompatibility that may occur when a heparin solution is used. The intermittent infusion is not

started until the nurse confirms intravenous placement. The heparin lock is flushed after the infusion is completed to clear the vein of any medication and to prevent clot formation in the needle. The procedure for flushing an intravenous lock with saline is discussed in Procedure 28-11. The intravenous site is assessed for complications discussed in Chapter 45. If infiltration or phlebitis occurs, the lock is removed and replaced in a new site.

In addition to a peripheral intravenous line, intermittent intravenous medication may be administered through a centrally placed line into the subclavian or internal jugular veins or through peripherally inserted central catheters. These venous access devices are discussed in more detail in Chapter 45. Medications are prepared under laminar flow in a sterile environment if they are to be administered through a central intravenous line, such as a Hickman catheter. Laminar flow is a special technique that helps regulate air flow to prevent bacterial contamination and collection of hazardous chemical fumes. Aseptic technique is observed when the nurse administers medications through a central intravenous line. All connections are cleaned with povidone-iodine or an antiseptic agent.

Administering Topical Medications

When a drug is applied directly to a body site, it is called a **topical application**. Topical applications are usually intended for direct action at a particular site, although some

(*text continues on page 619*)

PROCEDURE 28-11

Introducing Drugs Through a Heparin or Intravenous Lock Using the Saline Flush

Equipment

Medication
Medication Kardex or computer-
    generated MAR
Saline vial
Sterile syringe (2) with needleless
    device or 25-gauge needle
Alcohol swabs
Watch with second hand or digital
    readout
Gloves

For Bolus Injection

Sterile syringe (2) with needleless
    device or 25-gauge needle

For Intermittent IV Delivery

IV setup with needleless device
    attached to tubing or a 25-gauge
    needle
Adhesive tape (optional)
IV pump or controller (optional)

Action	Rationale
1. Assemble the equipment and check the physician's order.	This ensures that the patient receives the right medication at the right time by the proper route.
2. Explain the procedure to the patient.	Explanation alleviates the patient's apprehension about IV drug administration.
3. Wash your hands.	Handwashing deters the spread of microorganisms.
4. Withdraw 1 to 2 mL of sterile saline from the vial into the syringe as described in Procedure 28-3.	Using saline eliminates concern about drug incompatibilities and effect on systemic circulation that exists with heparin flush.
5. Don the clean gloves.	Gloves protect the nurse's hands from contact with the patient's blood.
6. Administer the medication. *For bolus IV injection:*	
a. Check the drug package for the correct injection rate for the IV push route.	Using the correct injection rate prevents speed shock from occurring.
b. Clean the port of the lock with an alcohol swab.	Cleaning removes surface bacteria at the heparin lock entry site.
c. Stabilize the port with your nondominant hand and insert the needleless device or needle of syringe of normal saline into the port.	This allows for careful insertion into the center circle of the lock.
d. Aspirate gently and check for blood return (blood return does not always occur even though lock is patent).	Blood return usually indicates that the catheter is in vein.
e. Gently flush with 1 mL of normal saline. Remove the syringe.	Saline flush ensures that the IV line is patent. A patient's complaint of pain or resistance to the flush detected by the nurse may indicate that the IV line is not patent.
f. Insert blunt needleless device or needle of syringe with medication into port and gently inject the medication, using a watch to verify correct injection rate. Do not force the injection if resistance is felt. If the lock is clogged, it has to be changed. Remove the medication syringe and needle when administration is completed.	Easy instillation of the medication usually indicates that the lock is still patent and in the vein. If force is used against resistance, a clot may break away and cause a blockage somewhere else in the body.

(continued)

PROCEDURE 28-11

Introducing Drugs Through a Heparin or Intravenous Lock
Using the Saline Flush (Continued)

For administration of a drug by way of an intermittent delivery system:

a. Use a drug resource book to check for the correct flow rate of the medication. (The usual rate is 30 to 60 minutes.)

Using the correct injection rate prevents speed shock from occurring.

b. Connect the infusion tubing to the medication setup according to the manufacturer's directions. Hang the IV setup on a pole. Open clamp and allow solution to clear IV tubing of air. Reclamp tubing.

This removes air from the tubing and preserves the sterility of the setup.

c. Attach needleless connector or sterile 25-gauge needle to the end of the infusion tubing.

A small-gauge needle prevents damage to the lock.

d. Clean the port of the lock with an alcohol swab.

Cleaning removes surface bacteria at the lock entry site. This allows for careful insertion into the port.

e. Stabilize the port with your nondominant hand and insert the needleless device or needle of syringe of normal saline into the port.

f. Aspirate gently and check for blood return (blood return does not always occur even though lock is patent).

Blood return usually indicates that the catheter is in vein.

g. Gently flush with 1 mL of normal saline. Remove the syringe.

Saline flush ensures that the IV line is patent.

h. Insert blunt needleless device or needle attached to tubing into port. If necessary, secure with tape.

Tape secures the needle in the lock port.

i. Open the clamp and regulate the flow rate or attach to IV pump or controller according to manufacturer's directions. Close clamp when infusion is complete.

This ensures that the patient receives the medication at the correct rate.

j. Remove the needleless connector or needle from lock. Carefully replace uncapped, used needle or needleless device with a new sterile one. Allow the medication setup to hang on the pole for future use according to agency policy. Stabilize the port with your nondominant hand and insert the needleless device or needle of syringe of normal saline into the port. Flush the reservoir with 1 to 2 mL of sterile saline. Remove the syringe and discard uncapped needles and syringes in the appropriate receptacle. Remove gloves and discard appropriately.

This prevents possible needlestick with contaminated needle. Agency policy specifies length of time for safe use of IV infusion tubing.

Saline clears the line of medication with less of the systemic effects of the heparin flush.

7. Wash your hands.

Handwashing deters the spread of microorganisms.

8. The injection site and IV lock should be checked at least every 8 hours and a small amount of saline administered if medication is not given at least that often.

This ensures the patency of the system for continuing injections.

9. The heparin lock should be changed at least every 48 hours or according to agency policy. A clogged lock should be changed immediately.

Changing a heparin lock regularly and having it free of clotted blood reduces dangers of infection and emboli in the circulating blood.

10. Chart the administration of the medication or saline flush.

Accurate documentation is necessary to prevent medication error.

(continued)

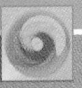

PROCEDURE 28-11

Introducing Drugs Through a Heparin or Intravenous Lock Using the Saline Flush (Continued)

Safety Considerations Some agencies recommend the use of single-dose saline vials without preservatives in the solution. Preservatives may be linked to an increased incidence of phlebitis with heparin locks.

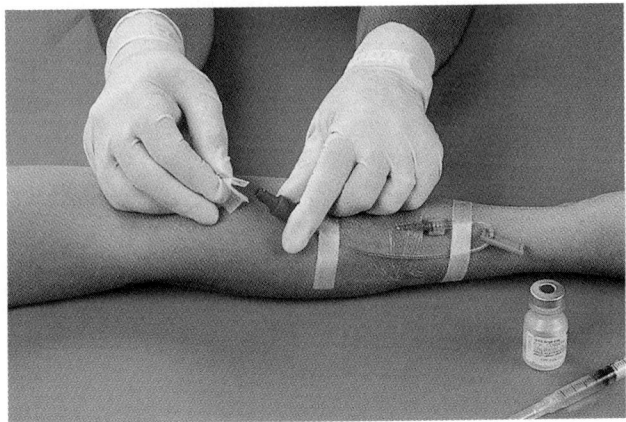

Action 6b: Cleaning the port with an alcohol swab.

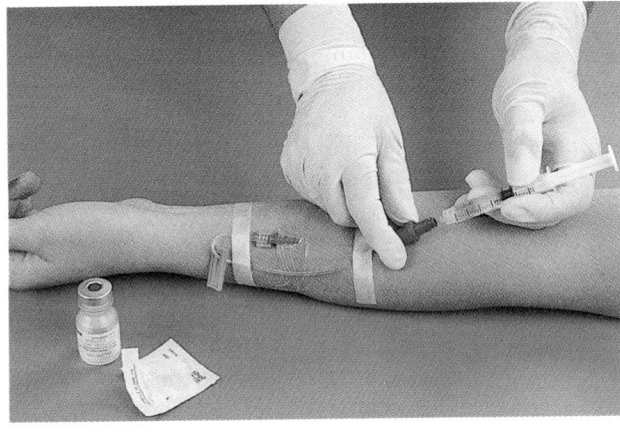

Action 6c: Inserting syringe with blunt needle into port.

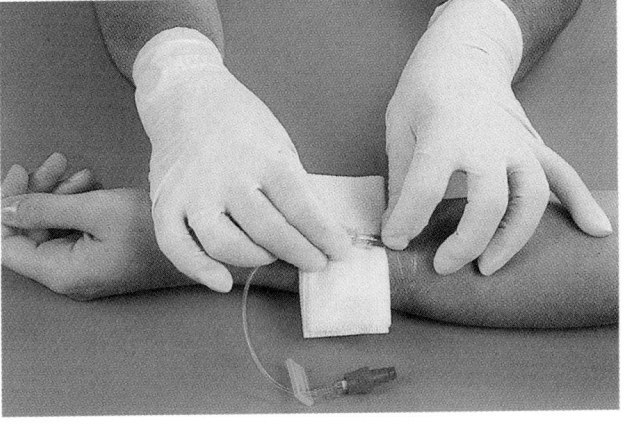

Action 6d: Aspirating for a blood return.

---

systemic effect may also occur. The action depends on the type of tissue and the nature of the agent.

If the site of application is readily accessible, such as the skin, an agent can easily be placed on it. If it is a cavity, such as the nose, or is enclosed, such as the eye, it is necessary to use a mechanical applicator for introducing the drug.

Skin Applications

The skin is a mechanical and chemical barrier that protects the underlying tissues. It is a sense organ, having receptors that respond to touch, pain, pressure, and temperature. The skin helps in excretion, in regulating body tempera-

ture, and in storing essentials to the body, such as water, salts, and glucose.

When a drug is incorporated in an agent, such as an ointment, and rubbed into the skin for absorption, the procedure is referred to as an *inunction*. On normal skin, drugs are absorbed into the lining of the sebaceous glands. Absorption is hindered because of the protective outer layer of the skin, which makes penetration difficult, and because of the fatty substances that protect the lining of the glands. Absorption can be enhanced by cleaning the skin well with soap or detergent and water before administration and then rubbing the medicated preparation into the skin. Absorption can also be improved by using a drug mixed in an ointment or added to a liniment that will mix with the fat in the gland lining. When indicated, local heat applied to the application area can improve blood circulation and promote absorption. The following are typical preparations applied to skin areas:

Powders are used to promote drying of the skin and prevent friction on the skin. Use caution when applying to prevent inhalation of the powder.

Ointments provide prolonged contact of a medication with the skin and soften the skin. They are usually thoroughly massaged into intact skin.

Creams and oils lubricate and soften the skin and prevent drying of the skin. The preparation should be warmed in the hands or fingers if a large part of the body is to be covered, to prevent chilling.

Lotions protect and soothe the skin. Shake lotions thoroughly before using and apply with cotton balls or gauze.

The *transdermal* route is being used more frequently to deliver medication. This involves application of a disk or patch to the skin that contains medication intended for daily use or for longer intervals. Despite a slow onset of action, transdermal drug patches maintain consistent serum drug levels (see the accompanying Guidelines for Nursing Care: Applying Transdermal Patches).

Eye Instillations and Irrigations

The receptors for the sense of sight are located in the eye. The outer layer of the eyeball is called the *sclera*. The cornea is the transparent part of the sclera in front of the eyeball. The sclera is fibrous and tough, but the cornea is easily injured by trauma. For this reason, applications to the eye seldom are placed directly onto the eyeball.

Because direct application cannot be made onto the sensitive cornea, applications intended to act on the eye or the lids are placed onto, or instilled or irrigated into, the lower conjunctival sac.

The eye is a delicate organ, highly susceptible to infection and injury. Although the eye is never free of microorganisms, the secretions of the conjunctiva have a protective action against many pathogens. For maximum safety for the patient, the equipment, solutions, and ointments introduced into the conjunctival sac should be sterile. If this is not possible, the most careful guidelines for medical asepsis should be followed.

Eyedrops

Instillation of eyedrops is performed for their local effects, such as for pupil dilation or constriction when examining the eye, for treating an infection, or to aid in controlling intraocular pressure for patients with glaucoma. The type and amount of solution depend on the purpose of the instillation. See the accompanying box, Guidelines for Nursing Care: Instilling Eyedrops, for a description of techniques to expose the lower conjunctival sac and instill eyedrops.

Ointments

Various types of medication in an ointment form may be prescribed for the eye. These ointments are usually used

---

Guidelines for Nursing Care
Applying Transdermal Patches

- Wear gloves when applying or removing patches. Handwashing is also a necessity.
- Remove the old patch before applying the new one. The physician may order a specific time for removal of the patch that may not coincide with the application time.
- Dispose of old patches carefully. Keep out of the reach of children and away from pets.
- Follow directions and use the patch as prescribed. Remove the patch from its protective covering and then remove the clear plastic covering without touching the adhesive. Apply the patch and use the palm to press firmly for about 10 seconds.
- Rotate application sites.
- Apply the patch at the same time of the day and write the date and time on the patch. Document application on the MAR.
- Monitor the patient's response carefully. Be alert for adverse effects specific to the medication applied.
- Check for dislodgment of the patch if the patient is active. Read information about the patch or consult with the pharmacist to determine reapplication schedule and procedure.
- Assess for any skin irritation. If necessary, remove the patch, wash the area carefully with soap and water, and allow skin to air dry.
- Aluminum backing on a patch necessitates precautions if defibrillation is required. Burns and smoke may result.

Adapted from McConnell, E. (1997). Using transdermal medication patches. *Nursing, 27*(7), 18.

---

for a local infection or irritation. Eye ointments are dispensed in a tube. A small amount of ointment is distributed along the exposed lower conjunctival sac after the eyelids and eyelashes have been cleansed. About $1/2$ inch of ointment is squeezed from the tube along the exposed sac. After the application, the eyes should be closed. The warmth helps to liquefy the ointment. Also, the patient should be instructed to move the eye because this helps to spread ointment under the lids and over the surface of the eyeball.

Eye Irrigation

An eye *irrigation* is performed to remove secretions or foreign bodies or to cleanse and soothe the eye. In an emergency, eye irrigation can be used to remove chemicals that may burn the eye. Copious amounts of tap water should be

Guidelines for Nursing Care

Instilling Eyedrops

- Offer the patient paper tissues to remove solution and tears that may spill from the eye during the procedure.
- Wash hands before putting on gloves.
- Clean the eyelids and eyelashes of any drainage with cotton balls or gauze pledgets moistened with normal saline solution because debris can be carried into the eye when the conjunctival sac is exposed. Use each cotton ball for only one stroke, moving from the inner toward the outer canthus to prevent carrying debris to the lacrimal ducts.
- Tilt the patient's head back slightly if sitting, or place the patient's head over a pillow if lying down. The head may be turned slightly to the affected side to prevent solution or tears from flowing toward the opposite eye.
- Invert the monodrip plastic container that is commonly used to instill eyedrops.
- Have the patient look up while focusing on something on the ceiling.
- Place the thumb or two fingers near the margin of the lower eyelid immediately below the eye-lashes, and exert pressure downward over the bony prominence of the cheek. The lower conjunctival sac is exposed as the lower lid is pulled down.
- Hold the dropper close to the eye, but avoid touching the eyelids or lashes, which may startle the patient and cause blinking. Also, avoid touching the eyeball with the dropper because this could easily injure the eye.
- Squeeze the container and allow the prescribed number of drops to fall in the lower conjunctival sac. Do not allow drops to fall onto the cornea because of the danger of injuring it and the unpleasant sensation it causes the patient.
- Release the lower lid after the eyedrops are instilled. Ask the patient to close the eyes gently.
- Apply gentle pressure over the inner canthus to prevent the eyedrops from flowing into the tear duct. This minimizes the risk of systemic effects from the medication.
- Instruct patient not to rub the affected eye.

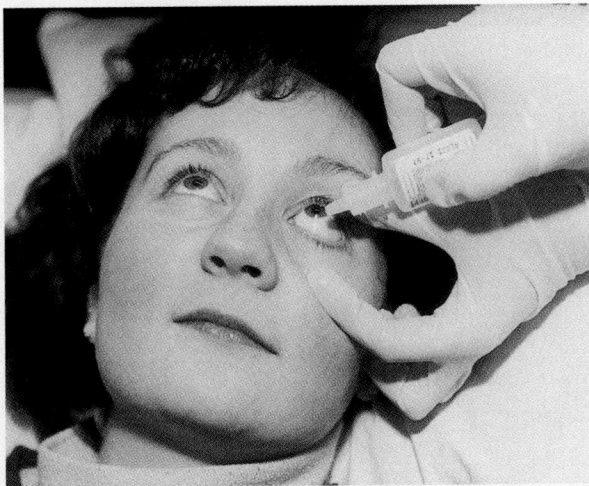

With the lower lid pulled down, the nurse prepares to administer the eyedrops on the lower conjunctival sac.

used to remove chemicals such as acid. The irrigation should continue for at least 15 minutes, and then professional help should be sought.

The techniques for administering an eye irrigation are described in Procedure 28-12.

Eye Medication Disks

An eye medication disk is flexible, resembles a contact lens, and contains medication that is gradually released into the conjunctival sac. It can remain in place for up to a week before being removed and discarded. When properly placed, the disk is completely covered by the lower eyelid, allowing the patient to wear contact lenses, swim, and sleep with the disk in place. Gloves should be worn when applying and removing the disk. Additional nursing guidelines for inserting and removing an intraocular disk include the following:

- Position the disk with the convex side adhering to your fingertip.

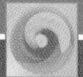

PROCEDURE 28-12

Administering an Eye Irrigation

Equipment

Sterile irrigating solution (warmed to 37°C [98.6°F])
Sterile irrigation set (sterile container and irrigating or bulb syringe)

Cotton balls
Emesis basin or irrigation basin
Disposable gloves

Waterproof pad
Towel

Action	Rationale
1. Explain procedure to patient.	Explanation facilitates cooperation and reassures the patient.
2. Assemble equipment.	This provides for an organized approach to the task.
3. Wash your hands.	Handwashing deters the spread of microorganisms.
4. Have the patient sit or lie with the head tilted toward the side of the affected eye. Protect the patient and the bed with a waterproof pad.	Gravity aids the flow of solution away from the unaffected eye and from the inner canthus of the affected eye toward the outer canthus.
5. Don disposable gloves. Clean the lids and the lashes with a cotton ball moistened with normal saline or the solution ordered for the irrigation. Wipe from the inner to the outer canthus. Discard the cotton ball after each wipe.	Materials lodged on the lids or in the lashes may be washed into the eye. This cleaning motion protects the nasolacrimal duct and the other eye.
6. Place the curved basin at the cheek on the side of the affected eye to receive the irrigating solution. If the patient is sitting up, ask him or her to support the basin.	Gravity aids the flow of solution.
7. Expose the lower conjunctival sac and hold the upper lid open with your nondominant hand.	The solution is directed onto the lower conjunctival sac because the cornea is sensitive and easily injured. This also prevents reflex blinking.

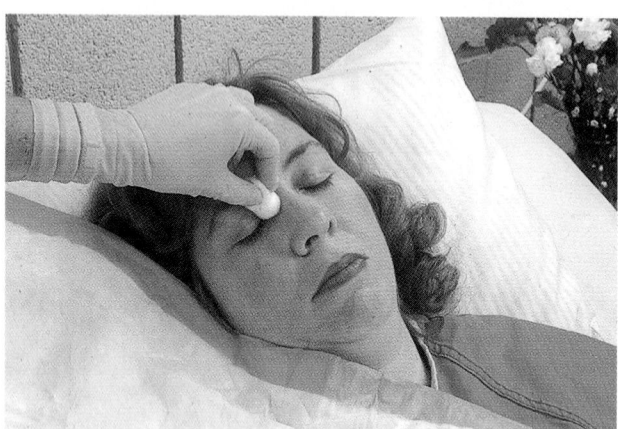

Action 5: Cleaning lids and lashes from inside of eye to outside.

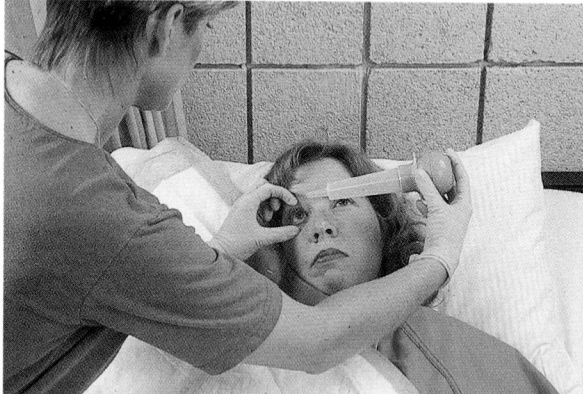

Action 7: Preparing to irrigate the eye. (PHOTOS © B. PROUD.)

8. Hold the irrigator about 2.5 cm (1 inch) from the eye. Direct the flow of the solution from the inner to the outer canthus along the conjunctival sac.

This minimizes the risk for injury to the cornea. Solution directed toward the outer canthus helps to prevent the spread of contamination from the eye to the lacrimal sac, the lacrimal duct, and the nose.

(continued)

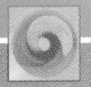

PROCEDURE 28-12

Administering an Eye Irrigation (Continued)

9. Irrigate until the solution is clear or all of the solution has been used. Use only sufficient force to remove secretions gently from the conjunctiva. Avoid touching any part of the eye with the irrigating tip.

Directing solutions with force may cause injury to the tissues of the eye as well as to the conjunctiva. Touching the eye is uncomfortable for the patient.

10. Have the patient close the eye periodically during the procedure.

Movement of the eye when the lids are closed helps to move secretions from the upper to the lower conjunctival sac.

11. Dry the area after the irrigation with cotton balls or a gauze sponge. Offer a towel to the patient if the face and neck are wet.

Leaving the skin moist after an irrigation is uncomfortable for the patient.

12. Remove gloves and wash your hands.

Handwashing deters the spread of microorganisms.

13. Chart the irrigation, appearance of the eye, drainage, and the patient's response.

This provides accurate documentation.

- Ask the patient to look up, and use the other hand to pull the patient's lower eyelid down gently.
- Place the disk in the conjunctival sac and lift the lower eyelid up and over the disk. *If properly positioned, the disk should not be visible at this time.*
- For removal, expose the disk by pulling down on the patient's lower eyelid.
- Use the forefinger and thumb of the other hand to gently pinch the disk and lift it out of the patient's eye.

These medication disks are usually applied at bedtime because they initially cause blurring of vision.

Ear Instillations and Irrigations

The ear contains the receptors for hearing and for equilibrium. It consists of the external ear, the middle ear, and the inner ear. The external ear consists of the auricle or pinna and the exterior auditory canal. The auditory canal serves as a passageway for sound waves. Drugs or irrigations are instilled into the auditory canal for their local effect. They are used to soften wax, relieve pain, apply local anesthesia, destroy organisms, or destroy an insect lodged in the canal, which can cause almost intolerable discomfort.

The tympanic membrane separates the external ear from the middle ear. Normally, it is intact and closes the entrance to the middle ear completely. If it is ruptured or has been opened by surgical intervention, the middle ear and the inner ear have a direct passage to the external ear. When this occurs, instillations and irrigations should be performed with the greatest of care to prevent forcing materials from the outer ear into the middle ear and the inner ear. Sterile technique is used to prevent infection.

Ear Drops
The techniques listed in the accompanying box, Guidelines for Nursing Care: Instilling Ear Drops, are recommended to place drops in the external auditory canal.

Ear Irrigations
Irrigations of the external auditory canal are ordinarily for cleaning purposes or for applying heat to the area. Typically, normal saline solution is used, although an antiseptic solution may be indicated for local action. An irrigation syringe is used in most instances. An irrigating container with tubing and an ear tip may also be used, especially if the purpose of the irrigation is to apply heat to the area. The techniques for administering an irrigation of the external auditory canal are described in Procedure 28-13.

Nasal Instillations

Besides serving as the olfactory organ, the nose functions as an airway to the lower respiratory tract and protects the tract by cleaning and warming the air taken in by inspiration. Cilia project on most of the surfaces of the nasal mucous membrane and help remove particles of dirt and dust from the inspired air. The nose also serves as a resonator when speaking and singing.

Nasal instillations are used to treat sinus infections and nasal congestion. Medications with a systemic effect, such as vasopressin, may also be prepared as a nasal instillation. The nose is normally not a sterile cavity, but because of its connection with the sinuses, medical asepsis should be carefully observed when using nasal instillations. See the accompanying box, Guidelines for Nursing Care: Instilling Nose Drops, for recommended techniques to instill nose drops.

Guidelines for Nursing Care

Instilling Ear Drops

- Warm the solution to be instilled to body temperature to minimize discomfort for the patient.
- Clean the external ear of drainage with cotton balls moistened with normal saline solution, as necessary. (Disposable gloves should be worn if drainage is present.)
- Place the patient on the unaffected side in bed, or if ambulatory, have the patient sit with the head well tilted to the side so that the affected ear is uppermost. This positioning prevents the drops from escaping from the ear.
- Draw up the amount of solution needed in the dropper. Excess medication should not be returned to a stock bottle. A monodrip plastic container may also be used.
- Straighten the auditory canal by pulling the cartilaginous portion of the pinna up and back in an adult and down and back in an infant or a child under age 3 years, and straight back for a school-aged child. Pulling on the pinna as

described helps to straighten the canal properly for ear instillation.
- Hold the dropper in the ear with its tip above the auditory canal. For an infant or an irrational or restless patient, protect the dropper with a piece of soft tubing to help prevent injury to the ear.
- Allow the drops to fall on the side of the canal. It is uncomfortable for the patient if drops fall directly onto the tympanic membrane.
- Release the pinna after instilling the drops, and have the patient maintain the position to prevent the escape of the medication.
- Gently press on the tragus a few times to help move the medication from the canal toward the tympanic membrane.
- If ordered, loosely insert a cotton ball to prevent medication from leaking out.
- Wait 5 minutes before instilling drops in the second ear, if ordered.

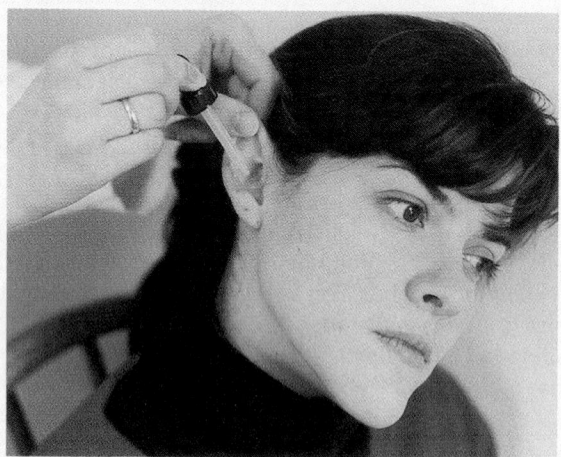

Adult

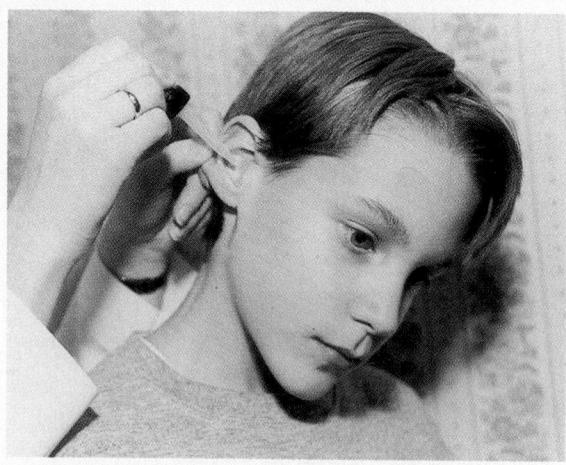

School-aged child

Solutions that are instilled by drops may also be applied to the nasal mucous membrane in a spray. A small atomizer is used. The end of the nose is held up, and the tip of the nozzle is placed just inside the nares and directed backward. Only sufficient force is used to bring the spray into contact with the membrane. Too much force may drive the solution and contamination into the sinuses and eustachian tubes.

Vaginal Applications

A healthy vagina contains few pathogens but many nonpathogenic organisms. The nonpathogens are important because they protect the vagina from the invasion of pathogens. The normal secretions in the vagina are acidic

and further serve to protect the vagina from microbial invasion. Therefore, the normal mucous membrane is its own best protection.

Creams can be applied intravaginally, using a narrow, tubular applicator with an attached plunger. Suppositories that melt when exposed to body heat are also administered by vaginal insertion. Suppositories should be refrigerated for storage.

The patient should be asked to void before inserting the medication. The patient is positioned lying on her back with the knees flexed. Privacy should be maintained with draping. Adequate light should be available to visualize the vaginal opening (see the accompanying box, Guidelines for Nursing Care: Inserting Vaginal Suppository or Cream).

PROCEDURE 28-13

Administering an Ear Irrigation

Equipment

Prescribed irrigating solution
    (warmed to 37°C [98.6°F])
Irrigation set (container and
    irrigating or bulb syringe)

Emesis basin
Cotton-tipped applicators
Disposable gloves (optional)

Cotton balls
Waterproof pad

Action	Rationale
1. Explain procedure to patient.	Explanation facilitates cooperation and provides reassurance for the patient.
2. Assemble the equipment. Protect the patient and bed linens with a moisture-proof pad.	This provides for an organized approach to the task.
3. Wash your hands.	Handwashing deters the spread of microorganisms.
4. Have the patient sit up or lie with the head tilted toward the side of the affected ear. Have the patient support a basin under the ear to receive the irrigating solution.	Gravity causes the irrigating solution to flow from the ear to the basin.
5. Clean the pinna and the meatus at the auditory canal as necessary with the applicators dipped in normal saline or the irrigating solution.	Materials lodged on the pinna and at the meatus may be washed into the ear.
6. Fill the bulb syringe with solution. If an irrigating container is used, allow air to escape from the tubing.	Air forced into the ear canal is noisy and therefore unpleasant for the patient.
7. Straighten the auditory canal by pulling the pinna down and back for an infant and up and back for an adult.	Straightening the ear canal aids in allowing solution to reach all areas of the canal easily.
8. Direct a steady, slow stream of solution against the roof of the auditory canal, using only sufficient force to remove secretions. Do not occlude the auditory canal with the irrigating nozzle. Allow solution to flow out unimpeded.	Solution directed at the roof of the canal aids in preventing injury to the tympanic membrane. Continuous in-and-out flow of the irrigating solution helps to prevent pressure in the canal.

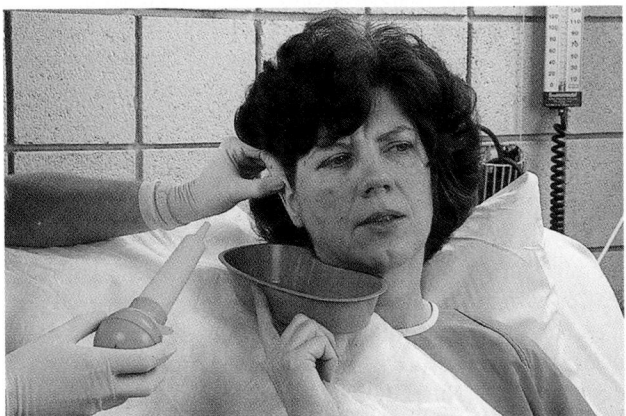

Action 7: Straightening the auditory canal.

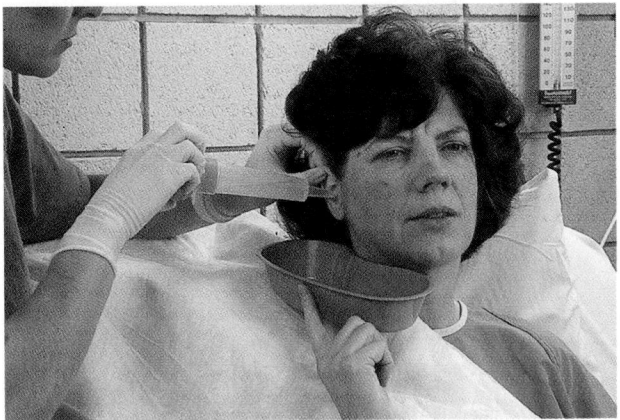

Action 8: Instilling irrigation fluid. (PHOTOS © KEN KASPER.)

(continued)

PROCEDURE 28-13

Administering an Ear Irrigation (Continued)

9. When the irrigation is completed, place a cotton ball loosely in the auditory meatus and have the patient lie on the side of the affected ear on a towel or an absorbent pad.

The cotton ball absorbs excess fluid, and gravity allows the remaining solution in the canal to escape from the ear.

10. Wash your hands.

Handwashing deters the spread of microorganisms.

11. Chart the irrigation, the appearance of the drainage, and the patient's response.

This provides accurate documentation.

12. Return in 10 to 15 minutes and remove the cotton ball and assess drainage.

Drainage or pain may indicate injury to the tympanic membrane.

Rectal Instillations

Rectal suppositories are used primarily for their local action, such as laxatives and fecal softeners. Systemic effects are also achieved with rectal suppositories. Acetaminophen suppositories are used for an antipyretic effect, and many antiemetics are available in suppository form to relieve nausea and vomiting.

Clean disposable gloves should be used to prevent contamination with feces and microorganisms. See the Nursing Guidelines for Inserting a Rectal Suppository in Chapter 43. After the suppository is inserted, the patient should remain in that position for 5 minutes. If the suppository is for laxative purposes, it must remain in position for 35 to 45 minutes or until the patient feels the urge to defecate.

Administering Medications by Inhalation

The lungs are richly supplied with blood and have a large surface area. These characteristics allow drugs to be absorbed easily from the lower respiratory tract. The smaller the particles of inhaled medication, the lower in the respiratory tract the medication tends to travel. A disadvantage of using this route is that the drug dosage is difficult to establish.

Drugs classified as bronchodilators and decongestants commonly are administered by **inhalation**. They act to decrease resistance to air flow by enlarging air passageways. Decongestants are local vasoconstrictors. Bronchodilators promote relaxation of musculature in the tracheobronchial tree. The relaxed passages produce less resistance to air flow and provide an opened respiratory passageway. Bronchodilators are further discussed in Chapter 44.

Drugs for inhalation may be administered by a hand atomizer or a nebulizer. These devices break up the medication into a mist for more efficient inhalation.

The hand-held, metered-dose inhaler (MDI) is often used incorrectly, and the correct dose of medication is not delivered. See Nursing Guidelines for using an inhaler in Chapter 44.

Nebulization may also result from the force of an oxygen stream or compressed air passed through the fluid in a nebulizer or an atomizer. This method is valuable for patients who require inhalation of a drug several times a day when the hand atomizer or nebulizer is fatiguing. The oxygen stream is also useful in the production of vapors when

Guidelines for Nursing Care

Instilling Nose Drops

- Provide the patient with paper tissues and ask that the patient blow his or her nose before instilling the nose drops.
- Have the patient sit up with head tilted well back. Or, if the patient is lying down, tilt the head back over a pillow. These positions allow the solution to flow well back into the nares.
- Draw sufficient solution into the dropper for both nares. Excess solution should not be returned to a stock bottle.
- Hold up the tip of the nose and place the dropper just inside the nares about one third of an inch. Instill the prescribed number of drops in one naris and then into the other. Protect the dropper with a piece of soft tubing when the patient is an infant or young child.
- Avoid touching the nares with the dropper because it may cause the patient to sneeze.
- Have the patient remain in position with the head tilted back for a few minutes to prevent the escape of the solution.

Guidelines for Nursing Care

Inserting Vaginal Suppository or Cream

- Fill a vaginal applicator with the prescribed amount of cream, or have a suppository ready.
- Lubricate the applicator with water, as necessary. A suppository may be lubricated with a water-soluble gel. Ordinarily, lubrication is unnecessary but may be used to reduce friction while inserting the applicator or suppository.
- Wear disposable gloves.
- Use clean aseptic technique to administer the medication.
- Spread the labia well with the fingers, and clean the area at the vaginal orifice with cotton balls and warm water to remove discharge, as necessary. With each cotton ball, use a single stroke moving from above the orifice downward toward the sacrum. These techniques prevent contamination of the vaginal orifice with debris surrounding the anus.
- Introduce the applicator gently in a rolling manner while directing it downward and backward to follow the normal contour of the vagina for its full length. Push the plunger to its full length, and then gently remove the applicator with the plunger depressed. After the applicator is properly positioned, the labia may be allowed to fall in place to free the nurse's hand for manipulating the plunger. Insert a suppository with gloved fingers well into the vagina.

- Ask the patient to remain in the supine position for 5 to 10 minutes after insertion.
- Offer the patient a perineal pad to collect excess drainage.
- Teach proper techniques to the patient who wants to administer vaginal suppositories and creams herself.

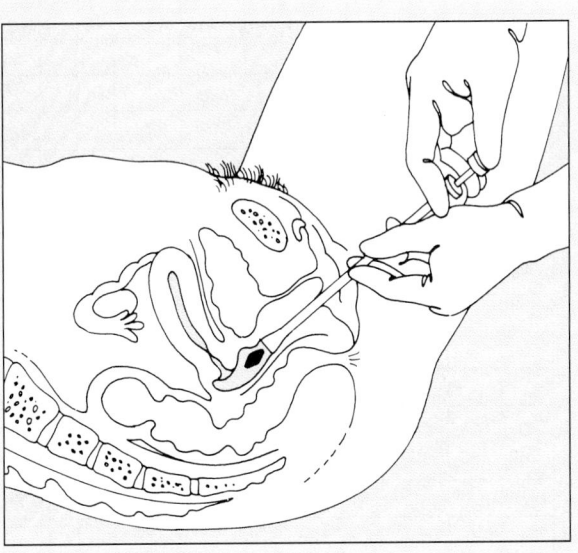

high humidity is needed continuously for long periods. One of the most common means of administering a nebulized drug using air pressure is the intermittent positive-pressure breathing machine (see Chap. 44).

Documenting Medication Administration

The medication record is a legal document. Recording each dose of medication as soon as possible after it is given provides a documented record that can be consulted if there are any questions about whether the patient received the medication. The nurse should not record medications before they are given: if the medication is then not given, the medication record would falsely show that the patient received the medication. Different forms are used for recording medications. An example is given in Figure 28-11. The name of the medication, dosage, route of administration, time given, and nurse's initials are noted on the form. The site used for an injection should be recorded. The nurse's full signature must appear on the form for initial identification. Other specific patient information may be required. For instance, the pulse rate may be recorded when administering some car-

diac drugs, or a description of the effects on the patient's pain when administering analgesics may be recorded.

Omitted Drugs

Drugs may be omitted intentionally or inadvertently. The omission and the reason for it are documented on the patient's record. Drugs may be omitted intentionally for the following reasons:

- The patient is to have a diagnostic test and is to fast before the test. Oral drugs are usually omitted, or their administration is delayed, depending on the physician's orders.
- The problem for which the medication is intended no longer exists. For example, a laxative has been ordered for a patient. The patient has had a bowel movement and no longer needs the laxative. The laxative is then omitted.
- The patient is suspected of having an allergy to the medication. Any suspected allergy should be reported to the physician.

To reduce the incidence of medication errors, many healthcare facilities are using computerized medication

CROZER-CHESTER MEDICAL CENTER
MEDICATION ADMINISTRATION + PARENTERAL THERAPY RECORD

FORM NS-MAR-1

Allergies:

Operative Date:
Procedure:

Penicillin

Legend for Injection Sites

RA- Right Arm   RT- Right Thigh
LA- Left Arm   LT- Left Thigh
RB- Right Buttock R.Abd.- Right Abdomen
LB- Left Buttock   L.Abd.- Left Abdomen

STANDING ORDERS (MEDICATION ORDERED PER ROUTINE SCHEDULE OR WITH SPECIFIC NUMBER OF DOSES)

ORDER DATE & RN INIT.	EXP. DATE & TIME	MEDICATION, DOSAGE, FREQUENCY, ROUTE	HOURS	11/29 INJ. SITE	11/29 INIT.	11/30 INJ. SITE	11/30 INIT.	12/1 INJ. SITE	12/1 INIT.	12/2 INJ. SITE	12/2 INIT.	12/3 INJ. SITE	12/3 INIT.	12/4 INJ. SITE	12/4 INIT.	12/5 INJ. SITE	12/5 INIT.	12/6 INJ. SITE	12/6 INIT.	12/7 INJ. SITE	12/7 INIT.	12/8 INJ. SITE	12/8 INIT.
11/29/01 sm		Digoxin 0.25 mg po QD	10A		AC		AC		CL														
					AR =88		AR =92		AR =86														
11/29/01 sm		Lasix 20 mg QD po	10A		AC		AC		CL														
11/29/01 sm		Trental 400 mg TIO Po	10A		AC		AC		CL														
			2P		AC		AC		CL														
			6P		PR		PR		PR														
11/29/01 sm		Slow Ktt po QD	10A		AC		AC		(CL)														
11/29/01 sm		Serax 15 mg Po q. 8°	6A		SP		SP		MS														
			2P		AC		AC		CL														
			10P		PR		PR		PR														
11/29/01 sm		Procardia 20 mg po TIO	10A		AC		AC		CL														
			2P		AC		AC		CL														
			6P		PR		PR		PR														

SINGLE ORDERS (STAT, PRE-OP, ONE TIME DOSE, ON CALL, DIAGNOSTIC PREP)

ORDER DATE & RN INIT.	MEDICATION, DOSAGE, ROUTE	TO BE GIVEN DATE	TO BE GIVEN TIME	INJ. SITE	RN INIT.	ORDER DATE & RN INIT.	MEDICATION, DOSAGE, ROUTE	TO BE GIVEN DATE	TO BE GIVEN TIME	INJ. SITE	RN INIT.
11/29 PR	Dalmane 15 mg po now	11/29	11P	–	PR						
11/30	Dulcolax tab. iii po at 6 pm	11/30	6P		PR						

Figure 28-11
Example of a medication record.

PRN MEDICATIONS (ENTER DATE, TIME GIVEN, INJECTION SITE AND RN INITIALS)																
ORDER DATE & RN INIT.	EXP. DATE & TIME	MEDICATION, DOSES, FREQUENCY, ROUTE		DOSES GIVEN												
11/29/01 SM		Tylox tab ii po q 3° prn	DATE	11/29	11/30											
			TIME	1q	3A											
			INJ.SITE													
			RN INIT.	AC	SP											
11/29/01 SM		Maalox 30 cc po q 6° prn	DATE													
			TIME													
			INJ.SITE													
			RN INIT.													
			DATE													
			TIME													
			INJ.SITE													
			RN INIT.													

PARENTERAL THERAPY			DOCUMENTATION FOR MEDICATION WITHHELD			
ORDER DATE & RN INIT.	I.V. SOLUTIONS	SCHEDULE	DATE	TIME	MEDICATION	REASON FOR WITHHOLDING
11/29/01 SM	1000 cc D5W	q.8°	12/1	10A	Slow K tab ii	patient refused

RN IDENTIFICATION						
INIT.	SIGNATURE	INIT.	SIGNATURE	INIT.	SIGNATURE
AC	a. Christopher RN				
PR	P Rogers RN				
SP	S. Pointer RN				
CL	C. Lewis RN				

Figure 28-11 (*Continued*)

administration record systems. These automated records give the pharmacy the capability to track statistical information, maintain inventory control of drugs, and integrate this information with the central billing system (see the accompanying box, Developing Critical Thinking Skills).

Refused Drugs

If the patient refuses a drug that is considered essential to the therapeutic regimen, the nurse should report this promptly. The nurse can often play an important role in determining the reason for the refusal and can help the patient accept needed drugs. If the patient is not persuaded by reasonable efforts and adamantly refuses a medication, it is unwise to continue urging the patient. Patients have the right to refuse therapy, and the nurse should recognize and respect that right. The refusal to take prescribed drugs and the manner in which the situation was managed should be described on the patient's record and reported according to agency policy.

Medication Errors

Nurses should take every precaution to avoid errors when administering therapeutic agents. Common types of medication errors include the following:

- Inappropriate prescribing of the drug (eg, incorrect dose, quantity, or route, or inadequate instruction)
- Extra, omitted, or wrong doses
- Administration of a medication to a patient that was not ordered for him or her
- Administration of a drug by an incorrect route or rate
- Failure to give a medication within the prescribed time interval
- Incorrect preparation of a drug before giving it
- Improper technique when administering a drug
- Giving a drug that has deteriorated

Prompt acknowledgment of errors may minimize their possible detrimental effect. The immediate priority is the safety of the patient. The following steps are recommended when a medication error occurs:

1. Check the patient's condition immediately when the error is noted. Observe for the development of adverse effects related to the error.
2. Notify the nurse manager and the physician to discuss possible courses of action depending on the patient's condition.
3. Write a description of the error on the patient's medical record, including remedial steps that are taken.

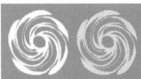 **Developing Critical Thinking Skills**

Situation

You are caring for two residents in a long-term care facility. One of your residents is scheduled to receive a B_{12} injection, and because it will be your first intramuscular injection, it has you more than a little apprehensive. You are eagerly awaiting the moment when your instructor will be free to supervise your injection. Meanwhile, she has cleared you to administer the 10:00 AM meds, and you bring a multivitamin, a diuretic, and an antiinflammatory agent to one of your assigned residents. When you go to record the medications you administered you suddenly realize to your horror that you brought them to the wrong resident. When you grab your buddy and confide your error, she says, "Whatever you do, don't tell Miss McMullen [the clinical instructor]. She gets spastic about med errors and has a reputation for gleefully failing students!" You remember that the resident who received the wrong medications has no known drug allergies and think that she probably wouldn't suffer any adverse effects from the meds she received. What should you do?

1. **Identify Goal of Thinking**

   Determine how you ought to respond to the realization that you administered medications to the wrong resident.

2. **Assess Adequacy of Knowledge**

   Pertinent circumstances: A resident has received three medications which were not ordered for her. You are a nursing student in your first clinical rotation and fear your clinical instructor's response should you inform her about your error. You are unsure of the harm that might result from the resident receiving the wrong medication.

   Prerequisite knowledge: In order to decide how you should respond in this situation you need to understand your professional obligations, which include your moral and legal accountability for having committed a medication error. You will need knowledge of the pharmacologic action of each of the medications you administered and their potential adverse effects for the resident who received them (possible interactions with other medications she is receiving, contraindications with related adverse effects, etc.). You recognize that there is no way for you to get the knowledge you need to make a morally and legally defensible response unless you admit your error to a responsible party.

   Room for error/Time constraints: Because you do not know the effects of these medications, you

are not in a position to judge how much room there is for error, nor are you able to make a prudent decision about how much time you have to act. The only defensible response is to seek help to clarify your position immediately because a resident's well-being is potentially at stake. No imagined personal costs would justify a delay in your admission of your error.

3. **Address Potential Problems**

   The most serious obstacle to critical thinking in this situation would be an inability to think rationally about your obligation to report the error because of your fear of being censured by your clinical instructor. You will want to examine critically your friend's claim that your instructor will respond harshly because this may, in fact, not be the case. You will also want to test your friend's unstated assumption that your primary obligation in this sort of situation is to take care of yourself—even if this course of action results in harm to a patient. It would be helpful to think through the consequences of every healthcare professional behaving in this manner.

4. **Consult Helpful Resources**

   Given that you are new to medication administration and are unable to assess the potential harm caused to the resident who received the wrong medications, you will find that your most helpful resource is your instructor and you will need to enlist her or his assistance immediately. She or he will probably want to contact the resident's physician to determine whether there are any contraindications to this resident's receiving the medications you administered or possible interactions with other medications. A pharmacist may also need to be consulted. You will want to be familiar with the institution's policy on medication errors and will need to know how to complete an incident report. If the nursing home has a risk manager you may want to consult with him or her.

5. **Critique Judgment/Decision**

   You have two options here: admit your error and initiate appropriate follow-up, or attempt to cover-up your error and "hope for the best." Your decision will basically be decided on the strength of your moral conviction that your primary obligation is to safeguard patient well-being, even should this involve some self-sacrifice. Once you recognize the potential disastrous consequences of patients not being able to trust healthcare professionals to act in

(continued)

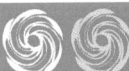 **Developing Critical Thinking Skills (Continued)**

their best interests, you decide that there really is only one professionally acceptable response in this situation, and you inform your instructor. It turns out that the resident who received the wrong medications suffered no adverse reactions. You, on the other hand, spend an awful morning following up on your error, and even have to delegate your B$_{12}$ injection to another student while you are admitting

your error to the resident, her attending, and the charge nurse and completing the incident report. At the end of the day, your instructor compliments you for your honesty and sense of responsibility and cautions you not to repeat the mistake. You are grateful that your worst fears (*failing*) weren't confirmed and leave the unit having learned a powerful lesson about the costs of being accountable.

4. Complete a special form for reporting errors, as dictated by agency policy. These forms, called *accident, incident,* or *unusual occurrence reports,* require an objective, complete account of the medication errors. Include the steps taken after the error was recognized. For legal reasons, it is essential that an error be described fully and accurately. Medication errors are a common allegation in nursing liability cases.

Although incident reports have a negative connotation for many nurses, they can provide vital information that can be used to prevent the error from being repeated in the future. The emphasis should be on the collaborative efforts necessary to provide safe patient care and decrease the incidence of errors. Peer review committees have proved effective in some healthcare settings.

Teaching About Medications and Abuse

Teaching about medications is an ongoing process and should begin as soon as the patient is admitted to the healthcare facility. In many cases, patients continue a prescribed medication regimen at home after discharge from the hospital. A factor that affects the patient's compliance to the medication regimen at home is education about the prescribed medications. Teaching should be tailored to the patient's level of understanding. Written instructions can be used as a reference for the patient and should include the following:

- The drug name and its intended effects
- Special instructions about taking the medication
- What to do when adverse effects occur
- Foods, beverages, and other medications that should be avoided while taking a medication
- Proper storage of the drug
- What to do if a dose is missed

Techniques of medication administration should be explained to the patient and family. Before discharge from a healthcare facility, the patient should practice the necessary techniques under the supervision of a nurse to acquire sufficient skill for safe administration. Many patients have learned to give themselves injections, as well as many other medications, when the teaching was planned well and the patient able and willing to learn.

The nurse should emphasize the importance of taking medications as prescribed and for as long as prescribed. A common error made by patients is simply omitting a drug, either through carelessness or because they believe that missing a dose is not important. Various aids are available to help nurses identify patients who are noncompliant and remind the patient to take his or her medication on schedule. Medication containers that beep when a dose is due to be taken, scratch-off dots on a medication label, and an electronic cap that signals dosage time and records each time the cap is removed are available as compliance aids. Patients should be advised to keep their medications with them when they travel. If luggage is lost or misplaced, refilling the prescription may be difficult.

The patient should be instructed not to alter the dosage without consulting the physician. Medications should not be discontinued when symptoms disappear. Drugs used to maintain health, such as those to control high blood pressure, need to be continued as ordered to avoid recurrence of symptoms.

Caution the patient not to share prescribed medications with other family members or with friends and neighbors. Inappropriate use of another person's drugs can have serious consequences.

Nurses have a teaching responsibility in relation to the abuse of any drug. Teaching may take place on an individual basis or on a family or community level. Drug abuse is a major public health concern worldwide, especially among teenagers and young adults. Not only is continued public and individual education indicated, but nurses are also expected to teach by setting high standards for their own behavior and the use of drugs. Because drug abuse is increasingly common and impairs healthcare providers, it is imperative that nurses observe, document, and intervene for the patient's safety, if drug abuse by a professional caregiver is suspected.

EVALUATING THE PATIENT'S RESPONSE TO MEDICATIONS

Drug effectiveness can be assessed in several ways. Clinical observation is the first method. Subjective data from the patient (eg, "My pain has disappeared") can be collected. Objective data (eg, the patient's vital signs) help the nurse evaluate medication effectiveness. The alert nurse assesses the patient for adverse drug effects.

Measurement of drug levels in body fluids provides data about the patient's response to a particular medication. For many drugs, including digoxin, theophylline, anticonvulsants, and aminoglycoside antibiotics, monitoring blood levels is an important component of therapy.

The patient is tested to determine whether the drug level in the blood is within the therapeutic range. Drug dosages may be adjusted as a result of the serum drug level.

Monitoring systems can also assist the nurse in evaluating drug effectiveness. For the patient with an arrhythmia, for example, a cardiac monitor can show a change in heart rhythm.

Learning Outcomes

After studying this chapter, the learner should be able to accomplish the following:

1. Define the key terms used in the chapter.

absorption	intramuscular injection
ampule	intravenous route
anaphylactic reaction	metabolism
antagonist effect	official name
chemical name	parenteral
cumulative effect	subcutaneous injection
distribution	synergistic effect
excretion	topical application
generic name	trade name
idiosyncratic effect	vial
inhalation	Z-track
intradermal injection	

2. Discuss drug legislation in the United States.
3. Describe drug names, types of preparations, and types of drug orders.
4. Identify drug classifications and actions.
5. Discuss adverse effects of drugs, including allergy, tolerance, cumulative effect, idiosyncratic effect, and interactions.
6. Obtain patient information necessary to establish a medication history.
7. Calculate drug dosages, using the various systems of equivalents.
8. Describe principles used to prepare and administer medications safely by the oral, parenteral, topical, and inhalation routes.
9. Develop teaching plans to meet patient needs specific to medication administration.

Critical Thinking Exercises

1. You are scheduled to give an intramuscular injection in the ventrogluteal site and remember learning that it should be administered using the Z-track technique. When you mention this to the nurse in the hospital who has been taking care of your resident, she tells you to be sure to remember the air lock. You remember your instructor telling you not to use an air lock. What do you do?
2. You are caring for two residents and have just completed giving medications to the first when you realize that you gave her the medications ordered for your other resident. How do you respond?

Study Questions

1. The name of a drug that is selected by the pharmaceutical company selling the drug and copyrighted by it is the drug's
   a. chemical name
   b. generic name
   c. official name
   d. trade name
2. The process by which a drug is transferred from its site of entry into the body to the bloodstream is known as
   a. absorption
   b. distribution
   c. metabolism
   d. excretion
3. A patient has an abnormal, unexpected response to a drug. This is defined as
   a. drug tolerance
   b. a cumulative effect
   c. an idiosyncratic effect
   d. an anaphylactic reaction
4. A medication order reads: "Digoxin, 0.125 mg PO qod." The nurse correctly gives this drug
   a. daily before bedtime
   b. by mouth every other day
   c. twice a day by way of the oral route
   d. once a week after recording an apical rate
5. In addition to checking a patient's identification bracelet, the nurse can correctly verify his identity by
   a. asking Mr. Brown his name
   b. reading his name on the sign over the bed
   c. asking his roommate to verify his name
   d. asking, "Are you Mr. Brown?"
6. Medication needs to be administered by way of a nasogastric tube. Before giving the medication, it is important for the nurse to

a. crush the enteric-coated pill for mixing in a liquid

b. flush open the tube with 60 mL of very warm water

c. check for proper placement of the nasogastric tube

d. take the patient's vital signs

7. The medication order reads: "Meperidine, 50 mg IM stat." The prefilled cartridge is available with a label reading 50 mg/1 mL. The cartridge contains 1.2 mL of meperidine. The nurse should

a. give all the medication in the cartridge because it expanded when it was mixed

b. call the pharmacy and request the proper dose

c. refuse to give the medication

d. dispose of 0.2 mL correctly before administering the drug

8. A patient requires 40 units of NPH insulin and 10 units of regular insulin daily subcutaneously. The correct sequence when mixing insulins is

a. inject air into the regular insulin vial and withdraw 10 units; then, using the same syringe, inject air into the NPH vial and withdraw 40 units of NPH insulin

b. inject air into the NPH insulin vial, being careful not to allow the solution to touch the needle; next, inject air into the regular insulin vial and withdraw 10 units; then, withdraw 40 units of NLH insulin

c. inject air into the regular insulin vial, being careful not to allow the solution to touch the needle; next, inject air into the NPH insulin vial and withdraw 40 units; then, withdraw 10 units of regular insulin

d. inject air into the NPH insulin vial and withdraw 40 units; then, using the same syringe, inject air into the regular insulin vial and withdraw 10 units of regular insulin

9. Ms. Hall has an order for meperidine, 100 mg q 4 h p.r.n. The nurse notes that according to Ms. Hall's chart, Ms. Hall is allergic to Demerol. The order for medication was signed by Dr. Long. Which of the following would be the correct procedure for this situation?

a. Administer the medication; the doctor knows best.

b. Call Dr. Long and ask that she change the medication.

c. Ask the supervisor to administer the medication.

d. Ask the pharmacist to provide a medication to take the place of Demerol.

10. The nurse manager on your unit prepared medications for Mr. Giles. She is called to the phone and asks you to give the patient his medications. Which is the best response to this request?

a. Give Mr. Giles the medication and record it in his chart.

b. Tell the nurse manager that you do not have time and ask her to get someone else.

c. Tell the nurse manager that because you did not pour the medication, you cannot administer it.

d. Give the medication to Mr. Giles but have the nurse manager chart it.

11. Which of the following is the reason the intravenous method of medication administration is called the "most dangerous route of administration"?

a. The vein can take only a small amount of fluid at a time.

b. The vein may harden and become nonfunctional.

c. Blood clots may become a serious problem.

d. The drug is placed directly into the bloodstream, and its action is immediate.

12. Mr. King is receiving heparin subcutaneously. Which of the following demonstrates correct technique for this procedure?

a. Aspirate before giving and gently massage after the injection.

b. Do not aspirate; massage the site for 1 minute.

c. Do not aspirate before or massage after the injection.

d. Massage the site of the injection; aspiration is not necessary but will do no harm.

13. A patient refuses to take her noon medication, saying that she does not need it. Which of the following would be the best response?

a. Tell her that she must take the medication because the doctor ordered it.

b. Tell her that you went through a lot of preparation to get her medications ready, and it's the least she can do.

c. Tell her that you don't care whether she takes the medications or not.

d. Tell her that you will return the medications to the cart but would like to discuss her reasons for refusing the medications.

14. The nurse discovers that she has made a medication error. Which of the following would be the first response?

a. Record the error on the medication sheet.

b. Notify the physician regarding course of action.

c. Check the patient's condition to note any possible effect of the error.

d. Complete an incident report, explaining how the mistake was made.

15. The nurse takes an 8 AM medication to the patient and properly identifies her. The patient asks the nurse to leave the medication on the bedside table and states that she will take it with breakfast when it comes. What is the best response to this request?

a. Leave the medication and return later to make sure that it was taken.

b. Tell her that it is against the rules and take the medication with you.

c. Tell her that you cannot leave the medication but will return with it when breakfast arrives.

d. Take the drug from the room and record it as refused.

Answers With Rationale

1. The correct response is *d*. The chemical name identifies the drug's chemical composition and molecular structure. The generic name is assigned by the manufacturer who develops the drug, and the official name is the name that identifies the drug in the official publication.
2. The correct response is *a*. Distribution, metabolism, and excretion occur after the drug has been absorbed.
3. The correct response is *c*. Drug tolerance results when the body becomes accustomed to the drug over time. A cumulative effect occurs when the body cannot metabolize one dose of a drug before another one is given. An anaphylactic reaction is a life-threatening, immediate response to a drug that can result in respiratory distress and cardiovascular response.
4. The correct response is *b*. The abbreviation qod refers to every-other-day administration.
5. The correct response is *a*. A sign over the patient's bed may not always be current and updated. The roommate is an unsafe source of information, and the patient may not even hear his name and reply in the affirmative (eg, a person with a hearing deficit).
6. The correct response is *c*. Tube placement should always be checked before administering any medication to prevent the possibility of aspiration if the tube is not in the stomach. Enteric-coated pills should never be crushed, and very warm water may injure stomach mucosa. Taking the vital signs is not necessary unless a particular medication requires it before administration.
7. The correct response is *d*. Many cartridges are overfilled, and some of the medication needs to be discarded. Giving the excess medication in the cartridge may result in adverse effects for the patient. For this dose, it is not necessary to call the pharmacy or refuse to give the medication, provided the order is written correctly.
8. The correct response is *b*. Regular or short-acting insulin should never be contaminated with NPH or any insulin modified with added protein. Placing air in the NPH vial first without allowing the needle to contact the solution ensures that the regular insulin will not be contaminated.
9. The correct response is *b*. The nurse is responsible for any medications he or she gives and must contact the doctor to inform her of the patient's allergy to the drug. The nurse should not give the medication and might speak with the supervisor only if he or she is uncomfortable with the physician's response once she is notified. The nurse is legally unable to order a replacement medication, as is the pharmacist.
10. The correct response is *c*. The nurse should never give medications prepared by someone else because she is responsible for what she administers.
11. The correct response is *d*. The intravenous route is a direct access to the bloodstream, and medications act quickly when given intravenously. The condition of the veins is not as important as the rapid effect of the medication administered by way of the intravenous route.
12. The correct response is *c*. Heparin that is given subcutaneously should not be aspirated or massaged, so as not to cause trauma or bleeding in the tissues.
13. The correct response is *d*. The patient has the right to refuse medications, but the nurse should assess the patient's reasons for refusal, document them, and report them to the physician.
14. The correct response is *c*. The nurse's first responsibility is the patient, and careful observation is necessary to assess for any effect of the medication error. The other nursing actions are pertinent but only after checking the patient's welfare.
15. The correct response is *c*. Safe nursing practice requires that a medication never be left at the patient's bedside. It is not correct to say that the patient has refused medication in this situation.

Medication Calculation Problems

1. Metoprolol (Lopressor), 25 mg PO, is ordered. Metoprolol is available as 50-mg tablets. How many tablets would the nurse administer?
2. Phenytoin (Dilantin), 100 mg PO, is ordered to be given through a nasogastric tube. Phenytoin is available as 30 mg/5 mL. How much would the nurse administer?
3. Captopril (Capoten), 12.5 mg PO, is ordered. Captopril is available as 25 mg tablets. How many tablets would the nurse administer?
4. Potassium chloride (MicroK), 20 mEq, is ordered. Potassium chloride is available as 10 mEq per tablet. How many tablets would the nurse administer?
5. Digoxin (Lanoxin), 0.0625 mg PO, is ordered. Digoxin is available as 0.125-mg tablets. How many tablets would the nurse administer?
6. Propantheline bromide (ProBanthine), 15 mg, is ordered. Propantheline bromide is available as 7.5-mg tablets. How many tablets would the nurse administer?
7. Ciprofloxacin (Cipro), 500 mg PO, is ordered. Ciprofloxacin is available as 250-mg tablets. How many tablets would the nurse administer?
8. Furosemide (Lasix), 20 mg PO, is ordered. Furosemide is available as 40-mg tablets. How many tablets would the nurse administer?
9. Theophylline elixir, 100 mg PO, is ordered by way of a percutaneous endoscopic gastrostomy tube. Theophylline elixir is available as 8 mg/15 mL. How much would the nurse administer?

10. Clonidine (Catapres), 0.1 mg PO, is ordered. Clonidine is available as 0.2-mg tablets. How many tablets would the nurse administer?
11. Vitamin K, 10 mg IM, is ordered. Vitamin K is available as 5 mg/mL. How much would the nurse administer?
12. Meperidine (Demerol), 35 mg IM, is ordered. Meperidine is available as 50 mg/mL. How much would the nurse administer?
13. Midazolam (Versed), 3 mg IM, is ordered. Midazolam is available as 5 mg/mL. How much would the nurse administer?
14. Hydroxyzine (Vistaril), 50 mg IM, is ordered. Hydroxyzine is available as 25 mg/mL. How much would the nurse administer?
15. Epoetin alfa (Epogen), 2000 units SC, is ordered. Epoetin alfa is available as 4000 units/mL. How much would the nurse administer?

16. Nalbuphine (Nubain), 1.5 mg IM, is ordered. Nalbuphine is available as 1 mg/mL. How much would the nurse administer?
17. Octreotide acetate (Sandostatin), 50 µg SC, is ordered. Octreotide is available as 100 µg/mL. How much would the nurse administer?
18. Morphine sulfate, 4 mg SC, is ordered. Morphine sulfate is available as 8 mg/mL. How much would the nurse administer?
19. Prochlorperazine (Compazine), 7.5 mg IM, is ordered. Prochlorperazine is available as 5 mg/mL. How much would the nurse administer?
20. Glycopyrrolate (Robinul), 0.4 mg IM, is ordered. Glycopyrrolate is available as 0.2 mg/mL. How much would the nurse administer?

Answers to Medication Calculation Problems

1. $\dfrac{\text{dose on hand}}{\text{quantity on hand}} = \dfrac{\text{dose required}}{X \text{ (quantity desired)}}$

$$\dfrac{50 \text{ mg}}{1 \text{ tablet}} = \dfrac{25 \text{ mg}}{X}$$

cross-multiply:

$$50X = 25$$
$$X = 0.5 \text{ or } \tfrac{1}{2} \text{ tablet}$$

2. $\dfrac{\text{dose on hand}}{\text{quantity on hand}} = \dfrac{\text{dose desired}}{X \text{ (quantity desired)}}$

$$\dfrac{30 \text{ mg}}{5 \text{ ml}} = \dfrac{100 \text{ mg}}{X}$$

cross-multiply:

$$30X = 500$$
$$X = 16.66 \text{ or } 17 \text{ ml}$$

3. $\dfrac{\text{dose on hand}}{\text{quantity on hand}} = \dfrac{\text{dose desired}}{X \text{ (quantity desired)}}$

$$\dfrac{25 \text{ mg}}{1 \text{ tablet}} = \dfrac{12.5 \text{ mg}}{X}$$

cross-multiply:

$$25X = 12.5$$
$$X = 0.5 \text{ or } \tfrac{1}{2} \text{ tablet}$$

4. $\dfrac{\text{dose on hand}}{\text{quantity on hand}} = \dfrac{\text{dose desired}}{X \text{ (quantity desired)}}$

$$\dfrac{10 \text{ mEq}}{1 \text{ tablet}} = \dfrac{20 \text{ mEq}}{X}$$

cross-multiply:

$$10X = 20$$
$$X = 2 \text{ tablets}$$

5. $\dfrac{\text{dose on hand}}{\text{quantity on hand}} = \dfrac{\text{dose desired}}{X \text{ (quantity desired)}}$

$$\dfrac{0.125 \text{ mg}}{1 \text{ tablet}} = \dfrac{0.0625 \text{ mg}}{X}$$

cross-multiply:

$$0.125X = 0.0625$$
$$X = 0.5 \text{ or } \tfrac{1}{2} \text{ tablet}$$

6. $\dfrac{\text{dose desired}}{\text{dose on hand}} \times \dfrac{\text{quantity}}{\text{on hand}} = X \text{ (desired quantity)}$

$$\dfrac{15 \text{ mg}}{7.5 \text{ mg}} \times 1 \text{ tablet} = X$$
$$2 \times 1 = 2 \text{ tablets}$$

7. $\dfrac{\text{dose desired}}{\text{dose on hand}} \times \dfrac{\text{quantity}}{\text{on hand}} = X \text{ (desired quantity)}$

$$\dfrac{500 \text{ mg}}{250 \text{ mg}} \times 1 \text{ tablet} = X$$
$$2 \times 1 = 2 \text{ tablets}$$

8. $\dfrac{\text{dose desired}}{\text{dose on hand}} \times \dfrac{\text{quantity}}{\text{on hand}} = X \text{ (desired quantity)}$

$$\dfrac{20 \text{ mg}}{40 \text{ mg}} \times 1 \text{ tablet} = X$$
$$\tfrac{1}{2} \times 1 = X$$
$$X = \tfrac{1}{2} \text{ tablet}$$

9. $\dfrac{\text{dose desired}}{\text{dose on hand}} \times \dfrac{\text{quantity}}{\text{on hand}} = X \text{ (desired quantity)}$

$$\dfrac{100 \text{ mg}}{80 \text{ mg}} \times 15 \text{ ml} = X$$
$$\dfrac{1500}{80} = X$$
$$X = 18.75 = 19 \text{ ml}$$

10. $\dfrac{\text{dose desired}}{\text{dose on hand}} \times \dfrac{\text{quantity}}{\text{on hand}} = X \text{ (desired quantity)}$

$$\dfrac{0.1 \text{ mg}}{0.2 \text{ mg}} \times 1 \text{ tablet} = X$$

$$\tfrac{1}{2} \times 1 = X$$
$$X = \tfrac{1}{2} \text{ tablet}$$

11. $\dfrac{\text{dose on hand}}{\text{quantity on hand}} = \dfrac{\text{dose desired}}{X \text{ (quantity desired)}}$

$$\dfrac{5 \text{ mg}}{1 \text{ mL}} = \dfrac{10 \text{ mg}}{X}$$

cross-multiply:

$$5X = 10$$
$$X = 2 \text{ mL}$$

12. $\dfrac{\text{dose on hand}}{\text{quantity on hand}} = \dfrac{\text{dose desired}}{X \text{ (quantity desired)}}$

$$\dfrac{50 \text{ mg}}{1 \text{ mL}} = \dfrac{35 \text{ mg}}{X}$$

cross-multiply:

$$50X = 35$$
$$X = 0.7 \text{ mL}$$

13. $\dfrac{\text{dose on hand}}{\text{quantity on hand}} = \dfrac{\text{dose desired}}{X \text{ (quantity desired)}}$

$$\dfrac{5 \text{ mg}}{1 \text{ mL}} = \dfrac{3 \text{ mg}}{X}$$

cross-multiply:

$$5X = 3$$
$$X = 0.6 \text{ mL}$$

14. $\dfrac{\text{dose on hand}}{\text{quantity on hand}} = \dfrac{\text{dose desired}}{X \text{ (quantity desired)}}$

$$\dfrac{25 \text{ mg}}{1 \text{ mL}} = \dfrac{50 \text{ mg}}{X}$$

cross-multiply:

$$25X = 50$$
$$X = 2 \text{ mL}$$

15. $\dfrac{\text{dose on hand}}{\text{quantity on hand}} = \dfrac{\text{dose desired}}{X \text{ (quantity desired)}}$

$$\dfrac{4000 \text{ U}}{1 \text{ mL}} = \dfrac{2000 \text{ U}}{X}$$

cross-multiply:

$$4000X = 2000$$
$$X = \tfrac{1}{2} \text{ mL}$$

16. $\dfrac{\text{dose desired}}{\text{dose on hand}} \times \dfrac{\text{quantity}}{\text{on hand}} = X \text{ (desired quantity)}$

$$\dfrac{1.5 \text{ mg}}{1 \text{ mg}} \times 1 \text{ mL} = X$$

$$1.5 \times 1 = X$$
$$X = 1.5 \text{ mL}$$

17. $\dfrac{\text{dose desired}}{\text{dose on hand}} \times \dfrac{\text{quantity}}{\text{on hand}} = X \text{ (desired quantity)}$

$$\dfrac{50 \text{ μg}}{100 \text{ μg}} \times 1 \text{ mL} = X$$

$$\tfrac{1}{2} \times 1 = X$$
$$X = \tfrac{1}{2} \text{ mL}$$

18. $\dfrac{\text{dose desired}}{\text{dose on hand}} \times \dfrac{\text{quantity}}{\text{on hand}} = X \text{ (desired quantity)}$

$$\dfrac{4 \text{ mg}}{8 \text{ mg}} \times 1 \text{ mL} = X$$

$$\tfrac{1}{2} \times 1 = X$$
$$X = \tfrac{1}{2} \text{ mL}$$

19. $\dfrac{\text{dose desired}}{\text{dose on hand}} \times \dfrac{\text{quantity}}{\text{on hand}} = X \text{ (desired quantity)}$

$$\dfrac{7.5 \text{ mg}}{5 \text{ mg}} \times 1 \text{ mL} = X$$

$$1.5 \times 1 = X$$
$$X = 1.5 \text{ mL}$$

20. $\dfrac{\text{dose desired}}{\text{dose on hand}} \times \dfrac{\text{quantity}}{\text{on hand}} = X \text{ (desired quantity)}$

$$\dfrac{0.4 \text{ mg}}{0.2 \text{ mg}} \times 1 \text{ mL} = X$$

$$2 \times 1 = X$$
$$X = 2 \text{ mL}$$

Bibliography

Abrams, A. (1998). *Clinical Drug Therapy* (5th ed.). Philadelphia: Lippincott Williams & Wilkins.

Beyea, S., & Nicoll, L. (1996). Back to basics: Administering IM injections the right way. *American Journal of Nursing, 96*(1), 34–35.

Chase, S. (1997). Pharmacology in practice: Back to basics. *RN, 60*(3), 24–26.

Covington, T., & Trattler, M. (1997). Bull's eye: Finding the right target for IM injections. *Nursing, 27*(1), 62–63.

DeBrew, J., Barba, B., & Tesh, A. (1998). Assessing medication knowledge and practices of older adults. *Home Healthcare Nurse, 16*(10), 686–691.

Edwards, J. (1997). Guarding against adverse drug events. *American Journal of Nursing, 97*(5), 26–31.

Eisenhauer, L., Nichols, L., Spencer, R., & Bergan, F. (1998). *Clinical Pharmacology and Nursing Management* (5th ed.). Philadelphia: Lippincott Williams & Wilkins.

Fleming, D. (1999). Challenging traditional insulin injection practices. *American Journal of Nursing, 99*(2), 72–74.

Gever, M. (1998). Transdermal patches: What's in a brand name? *Nursing, 28*(5), 58–59.

Guttadore, D. (1999). A quick way to identify compatible drugs. *RN, 62*(9), 53–55.

Chapter 29
Perioperative Nursing

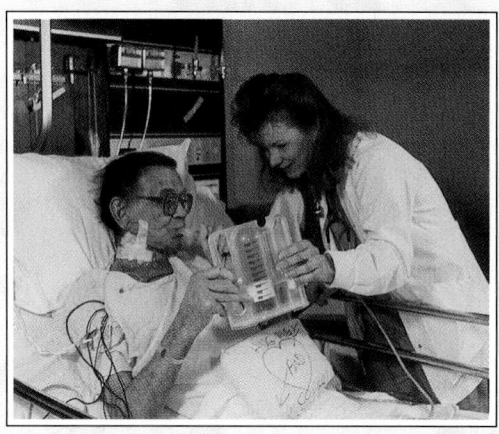

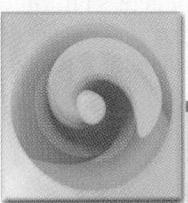

Thinking Critically About
Nursing's Blended Skills

Before reading this chapter, think about the types of blended skills you will need to care for patients undergoing surgical experiences.

- Molly is a 38-year-old woman who arrives in same-day surgery at 6:30 AM for a breast biopsy. As you begin her admission history, you quickly see how frightened she is.

- Jim is a 22-year-old man being discharged home from same-day surgery. He underwent a surgical procedure to crush kidney stones. You are doing the postoperative teaching.

- You have been assigned to scrub in for a vaginal hysterectomy.

- Mr. Peters had a total hip replacement and is in the postanesthesia care unit (PACU). You are responsible for monitoring his vital signs, keeping him comfortable, and preventing complications. He has an intravenous line, a Foley catheter, and a drain.

What cognitive, technical, interpersonal, and ethical/legal skills do you think you will need to respond to the challenges described above?

The treatment of a wide variety of illnesses and injuries includes some type of surgical intervention. Surgery may be planned or unplanned, major or minor, and invasive or noninvasive and may involve any body part or system. A surgical procedure of any extent is a stressor for both the patient and the family that requires physical and psychosocial adaptations. The patient's recovery from a surgical procedure requires skillful and knowledgeable nursing care whether the surgery is done on an outpatient basis or in the hospital. All phases of the nursing process are used to make assessments and provide interventions to promote the recovery of health, prevent further injury or illness, and facilitate coping with alterations in physical structure and function.

This chapter discusses nursing care for preparing the patient for surgery, supporting the patient during surgery, and assisting with recovery after surgery. The nurse's role in each stage is described for the stages of the nursing process. Selected nursing diagnoses and expected outcomes are included for each phase of care of the surgical patient.

The Surgical Experience

Regardless of the surgical intervention required or the setting in which the surgery is performed, all patients progress through specific perioperative phases, require some type of anesthesia, and give their consent for surgery. The following sections describe those components of the surgical experience.

Phases of the Perioperative Period

The patient who is having surgery progresses through several distinct phases. The entire time frame is called the **perioperative period**. **Perioperative nursing** is the name for the wide variety of nursing activities carried out before, during, and after surgery. The three phases of perioperative patient care are the **preoperative phase**, beginning with the decision that surgical intervention is necessary and lasting until the patient is transferred to the operating room bed; the **intraoperative phase**, extending from admission to the surgical department (or operating room) to transfer to the recovery area; and the **postoperative phase**, lasting from admission to the recovery area to the complete recovery from surgery. The postoperative phase itself can further be broken down to phase I (providing patient care from a totally anesthetized state to one requiring less acute nursing interventions), phase II (preparing the patient for self or family care or for care in a phase III extended care environment), and phase III (providing ongoing care for those patients requiring extended observation or intervention after transfer or discharge from phase I or II) (American Society of PeriAnesthesia Nurses [ASPAN], 1998).

With the increasing trend toward short-stay or same-day surgical treatment, the nursing interventions in each phase of perioperative or postanesthesia nursing care may vary somewhat but remain basically the same. The nursing process is used during each phase to meet physical and psychosocial needs and to facilitate the patient's return to health. Each of these phases, with related patient needs and nursing activities, is described in detail in this chapter.

COGNITIVE SKILLS

- Basic knowledge of the surgical experience, including perioperative phases, categories of surgery, types of anesthesia, informed consent, and related nursing care
- Ability to use the nursing process to develop an individualized plan of care for patients undergoing surgery during each phase of the surgical experience
- Knowledge of wound care
- Knowledge of resources to contact when encountering questions about the surgical experience or care with which you are unfamiliar

TECHNICAL SKILLS

- Ability to use equipment correctly and implement techniques for safe and effective nursing care of patients in each perioperative phase.

INTERPERSONAL SKILLS

- Strong people skills; ability to communicate and interact effectively with surgical patients, their families, and other members of the professional caregiving team.
- Ability to establish trusting relationships with patients, families, and colleagues as a basis for quality perioperative care.

ETHICAL/LEGAL SKILLS

- Commitment to safety and quality; strong sense of responsibility, accountability; strong advocacy abilities.
- Knowledge of pertinent agency policy for perioperative nursing responsibilities.

Classification of Surgical Procedures

Surgical procedures are usually categorized according to urgency, risk, and purpose. Table 29–1 lists each classification, with purposes and selected examples for each.

Based on Urgency

Surgery may be classified as **elective surgery**, meaning that it is preplanned and based on the patient's choice; *urgent surgery*, in which the surgery is necessary for the patient's health but not an emergency; and **emergency surgery**, which must be done immediately to preserve the patient's life, body part, or body function.

Based on Degree of Risk

Surgery is classified as *minor* or *major* based on the degree of risk for the patient. Minor surgery is almost always performed in settings such as a physician's office, an outpatient clinic, or a same-day, ambulatory surgery setting. This classification means that the surgical procedure is usually brief, carries a low risk, and results in few complications. In contrast, major surgery may require hospitalization, is

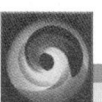

Table 29-1
Classification of Surgical Procedures

Classification	Purpose	Examples
Based on Urgency		
Elective: Delay of surgery has no ill effects; can be scheduled in advance based on patient's choice	• To remove or repair a body part • To restore function • To improve health • To improve self-concept	Tonsillectomy, hernia repair, cataract extraction and lens implantation, hemorrhoidectomy, hip prosthesis, scar revision, facelift, mammoplasty
Urgent: Usually done within 24–48 hours	• To remove or repair a body part • To preserve or restore health • To restore function • To prevent further tissue damage	Removal of gallbladder, coronary artery bypass, surgical removal of a malignant tumor, colon resection, amputation
Emergency: Done immediately	• To preserve life (plus purposes listed above)	Control of hemorrhage; repair of trauma, perforated ulcer, intestinal obstruction; tracheostomy
Based on Degree of Risk		
Major: may be elective, urgent, or emergency	• To preserve life • To remove or repair a body part • To restore function • To improve or maintain health	Carotid endarterectomy, cholecystectomy, nephrectomy, colostomy, hysterectomy, radical mastectomy, amputation, trauma repair
Minor: Primarily elective	• To restore function • To remove skin lesions • To correct deformities	Teeth extraction, removal of warts, skin biopsy, dilation and curettage, laparoscopy, cataract extraction, arthroscopy
Based on Purpose		
Diagnostic	• To make or confirm a diagnosis	Breast biopsy, laparoscopy, bronchoscopy, exploratory laparotomy
Ablative	• To remove a diseased body part	Appendectomy, subtotal thyroidectomy, partial gastrectomy, colon resection, amputation
Palliative	• To relieve or reduce intensity of an illness; is not curative	Colostomy, nerve root resection, débridement of necrotic tissue, balloon angioplasties, arthroscopy
Reconstructive	• To restore function to traumatized or malfunctioning tissue • To improve self-concept	Scar revision, plastic surgery, skin graft, internal fixation of a fracture, breast reconstruction
Transplantation	• To replace organs or structures that are diseased or malfunctioning	Kidney, liver, cornea, heart, joints
Constructive	• To restore function in congenital anomalies	Cleft palate repair, closure of atrial–septal defect

usually prolonged, has a higher degree of risk, involves major body organs or life-threatening situations, and has more potential for postoperative complications. Advances in the use of laser techniques and minimally invasive approaches involving very small incisions have made major surgery less traumatic, requiring shortened hospital stays. New surgical approaches using minimally invasive techniques continue to evolve. Many surgical procedures, even though they are classified as major, may now be performed on an ambulatory basis or as a 23-hour stay.

Based on Purpose

Some descriptors used to classify surgical procedures based on purpose include *diagnostic*, *ablative*, *palliative*, *reconstructive*, *transplantation*, and *constructive* (see Table 29-1).

Combinations

Surgical procedures may combine several classifications and labels (eg, a patient who has been in an automobile accident and has severe trauma and bleeding may require major, reconstructive, emergency surgery). No matter the defined degree of risk, any surgical procedure imposes physical and psychological stress and is seldom considered minor by the patient.

Anesthesia

Anesthesia, depending on its classification as *general* or *regional*, produces such states as narcosis (loss of consciousness), analgesia, relaxation, and loss of reflexes. General anesthesia produces all of these responses, whereas regional anesthesia does not cause narcosis but results in analgesia and reflex loss. Anesthetic agents are administered by a physician, an anesthesiologist (medical doctor), or a nurse anesthetist.

General Anesthesia

When a patient is given drugs by the inhalation, intravenous, rectal, or oral route to produce central nervous system depression, this is termed **general anesthesia**. The desired actions of general anesthesia are loss of consciousness, analgesia, relaxation of skeletal muscles, and depression of reflexes. The choices of route and type of anesthesia are made primarily by the anesthesia provider after discussion with the patient. Many factors influence these choices, including the type and length of surgery and the physical and psychological status of the patient (Meeker & Rothrock, 1999). Inhalation anesthesia is often used because it has the advantage of rapid excretion and reversal of effects.

The three phases of general anesthesia are induction, maintenance, and emergence. Induction begins with administration of the anesthetic agent and continues until the patient is ready for the incision. Maintenance continues from this point until near the completion of the procedure. Emergence starts as the patient begins to emerge from the anesthesia and usually ends when the patient is ready to leave the operating room; the length of time depends on the depth and length of anesthesia (Meeker & Rothrock,

1999). New anesthetic agents enable patients to emerge from anesthesia and "wake up" in a fraction of the time required in the past. As these agents become more commonly used, patients will frequently bypass the PACU; such agents also enable more surgical procedures to be safely done in doctors' offices.

The advantages of general anesthesia are that it can be used for patients of any age and for any surgical procedure, with the patient unaware of the physical trauma of the surgery. There are, however, major associated risks for circulatory and respiratory depression, postoperative nausea and vomiting, and alterations in thermoregulation.

Regional Anesthesia

Regional anesthesia occurs when an anesthetic agent is injected near a nerve or nerve pathway in or around the operative site, inhibiting the transmission of sensory stimuli to central nervous system receptors. The patient receiving regional anesthesia remains awake but loses sensation in a specific area or region of the body. In some instances, reflexes may also be lost. Regional anesthesia may be accomplished through major nerve blocks or through spinal (subarachnoid block), caudal, or epidural blocks, defined as follows:

- *Nerve blocks* are accomplished by injecting a local anesthetic around a nerve trunk supplying the area of surgery, such as the jaw, face, and extremities. Onset and duration of the block depend on the anesthetic drug, its concentration, the amount injected, and the addition of epinephrine, which prolongs the block.
- *Spinal anesthesia* is achieved by the injection of a local anesthetic into the subarachnoid space through a lumbar puncture, causing sensory, motor, and autonomic blockage. This type of anesthesia is used for surgery of the lower abdomen, perineum, and legs. Adverse effects of spinal anesthesia may include hypotension, postdural headache, and urine retention.
- *Caudal anesthesia* is the injection of the local anesthetic into the epidural space through the caudal canal in the sacrum; it may be used for procedures on the lower extremities or perineum.
- *Epidural anesthesia* involves the injection of the anesthetic through the intervertebral spaces, usually in the lumbar region (although it may also be used in the thoracic or cervical regions).

Although regional anesthesia may be selected for numerous types of surgery and patients, research indicates that it is especially useful in reducing postsurgical pain, bowel dysfunction, and length of hospital stay for elderly patients (Goodwin, 1999).

Conscious Sedation/Analgesia

Conscious sedation/analgesia is used for short-term procedures; the patient maintains cardiorespiratory function and can respond to verbal commands while the intravenous administration of sedatives and analgesics raises the pain threshold and produces an altered mood and some degree of amnesia. This type of anesthesia is often administered by a perioperative nurse with specialized training and competence in administering the medications and monitoring the patient's cardiac rate and rhythm, respiratory rate, oxygen saturation, level of consciousness, blood pressure, and skin condition.

> *Topical anesthesia* is used on mucous membranes, open skin surfaces, wounds, and burns. Cocaine in 4% to 10% solution is the most commonly used agent; others are lidocaine (Xylocaine) and benzocaine.
>
> *Local anesthesia* is the injection of an anesthetic agent such as lidocaine, bupivacaine or, tetracaine to a specific area of the body. It is administered by the surgeon in minor, short-term surgical or diagnostic procedures such as tissue biopsy.

Informed Consent

Informed consent is the patient's voluntary agreement to undergo a particular procedure or treatment (such as surgery) after having received the following information, which should be provided in understandable words (layman's terms) by the physician:

- Description of the procedure or treatment along with potential alternative therapies
- The underlying disease process and its natural course
- Name and qualifications of the person performing the procedure or treatment
- Explanation of the risks involved, including potential for damage, disfigurement, or death, and how often they occur
- Explanation that the patient has the right to refuse treatment and that consent can be withdrawn

Informed consent protects the patient, the physician, and the healthcare institution. The signed form is a legal document as well as an ethical imperative. The responsibility for securing informed consent from the patient lies with the person who will perform the procedure; this is usually the physician. The nurse may sign as a witness, signifying that the patient signed the consent form without coercion and was alert and aware of the act. The patient always has the right to refuse treatment.

Consent forms are not legal if the patient is confused, unconscious, sedated, mentally incompetent, or a minor (as determined by state laws). Consent may be given in those instances by a parent, spouse, next of kin, or legal guardian. In emergency situations, the physician may obtain consent over the telephone or by court order. More detailed information about informed consent is included in Chapter 7.

Advance Directives

Advance directives are another form of legal document that allows the patient to specify instructions for his or her healthcare treatment should they be unable to communicate these wishes postoperatively. This allows the patient to discuss his or her wishes with family members in advance of the surgery. If the patient should experience a serious, life-threatening complication, such as intraoperative cardiac arrest, the family has previous knowledge of the patient's wishes regarding cessation of treatment, resuscitative efforts, or end-of-life decisions. Two common forms of advanced directive include *living wills* and *durable power of attorney* for healthcare. The risk management or legal department of the facility should be consulted if there are questions about the validity of the document or its contents (Gillanders & Moley, 1997).

Ambulatory Surgery

Surgical procedures performed in ambulatory (also referred to as *outpatient* or *same-day*) surgical settings have become common as the healthcare system has reduced length of hospital stay to lower costs of healthcare. These surgical settings may be found as free-standing units, in hospitals, and in physicians' offices. Some free-standing ambulatory surgery centers specialize in selected types of surgery, such as orthopedics or hernia repair. Others perform a wide variety of surgical interventions, including major surgical procedures that formerly required a 3-week stay in a hospital (Pessagno, 1999).

By allowing the patient to spend the night before surgery at home and to return to his or her own home to convalesce, much of the stress associated with surgery is eliminated. Patients who are older or chronically ill or who do not have support systems or access to resources to provide the care needed after surgery may require additional teaching and referral for home care services.

Preoperative nursing assessments and teaching are key processes of care for ambulatory surgical patients (Fig. 29–1). Preoperative teaching can often can be combined with preoperative screening tests, which are usually done 2 to 5 days before the scheduled surgery. Preoperative teaching for ambulatory surgery includes the following instructions to the patient and family:

- List medications routinely taken and ask the physician which should be taken or omitted the morning of surgery.
- Notify the surgeon's office if a cold or infection develops before surgery.
- List allergies and be sure the operating staff is aware of these.
- Remove nail polish and do not wear makeup for the procedure.
- Leave all jewelry and valuables at home.
- Wear clothing that buttons in front; short-sleeved garments are better for surgery on the hands.
- Have someone available for transportation home after recovery from anesthesia.

Teaching should also include written instructions covering the following:

- Limitations on eating or drinking before surgery, with a specific time to begin the limitations

PREADMISSION TEACHING/TESTING PERIOPERATIVE ASSESSMENT

Planned Surgery And Date: _Arthroscopy, debridement_
foreign body (L) knee   8/7/00

Date Of Visit: _7/14/00_
Surgical History: _(L) Knee arthroscopy x3_
(1997 = most recent with little improvement.) (R) inguinal hernia repair 10
years ago.

Anesthesia History: _No problems_

Systems Review: _____   Allergy: _NKA_
_____   Dental: _N/A - no bridges or crowns_
Contact Lens/IOL: _N/A_
Hearing Aid: _N/A_

Cardiovascular
Angina: _____   Stroke: _____
Rheumatic Fever: _____ Murmur: _____
Hypertension: _____   Infarction: _____
Date Last EKG: _1997_   Pacemaker: _____

Respiratory
Pneumonia: _____   Smoke: _____
Asthma: _____   Recent URI: _____
Date Last CXR: _1997_

Hematology
Bleeding Tendency: _On ASA - to D/C 8 days pre-op._

GI
Recent Vomiting: _____   Diarrhea: _____
Jaundice: _____   Hepatitis: _____

GYN
L.M.P.: _N/A_   Para: _____
                       Gravida: _____

GU
UTI/Problems: _____

Neuropsych
Syncope: _____   Epilepsy: _____

Musculoskeletal
                          Neck Or
Arthritis: _(L) Knee_   Back Inj.: _____
R.O.M.: _Limit = (L) Knee only_ Prothesis: _____
Skin Integrity: _No problems noted_

Metabolic
Diabetes: _____
Thyroid: _____

Medications (including over-the-counter, herbal):
ASA daily
Lipitor 40 mg (each evening)

B/P _130/82_ T. _98²_ P. _86_ R. _20_ Wt. _185_
                                           Ht. _6'1"_
Advance Directive: _Done_
Escort Name/Phone: _Wife (207) 143-4444_

Lab Ordered:
H & H — results WNL

Abnormal Lab work called to

Dr. _____ on _____ Initials _____

X-ray _Chest xray — Normal_
AP/Lat (L) knee — Medial joint line spurs, lateral compartment well preserved

Abnormal X-ray called to

Dr. _____ on _____ Initials _____

EKG
NSR — WNL

Abnormal EKG work called to

Dr. _____ on _____ Initials _____

Pre-op Teaching Guidelines
✓ Pre-Op Medications   ✓ Skin Prep
✓ Transported to Holding Room ✓ Awake in Postanesthesia
                                 Care Unit
✓ Visitors to Waiting Room   ✓ Oxygen Delivery
✓ I.V. Fluids   ✓ Deep Breaths and Cough
__ Sequential Compressive   ✓ Frequent Check BP & P
   Device (Appr. Surg.)   ✓ Fluid and Food Restrictions
__ Leggings (Cysto or GYN)   ✓ Cannot Drive Self Home
✓ Taken to O.R.   ✓ Jewelry, Make-up Left Home
✓ Safety Belt   ✓ Wear Loose Clothing
✓ BP Cuff, Monitor Pads, Pulse __ Video _____
   Oximeter   ✓ Hand-out Packet _____
✓ Electrosurgical Pad
✓ Use of Pain Scale

Notes: _____
Scheduled for knee classes

Postanesthesia Care Unit Follow Up: _Has voided, Using ice bag_
on (L) knee. Pain 2 on scale 1 → 10. Has post-op appt made. Reviewed signs
and symptoms that should be called to MD.

Post-Op Follow Up: _____
Will do knee rehab unless contradicted by physician

Phone: _(207) 143-4444_

Figure 29-1
Example of an ambulatory surgery assessment record.

- When and where to arrive for the procedure as well as the estimated time when the procedure will be performed

Preoperative Nursing Care

Patients who require surgical intervention and nursing care enter the healthcare setting in a wide variety of situations, ranging from essentially healthy people who have planned elective procedures to emergency admissions for treatment of trauma. Surgical patients may be any age and at any point on the health–illness continuum. It is the nurse's responsibility to identify factors that affect the risk of a surgical procedure. This includes assessing the physical and psychosocial needs of the patient and family and establishing a plan of care, based on appropriate nursing diagnoses. Also included are interventions to meet needs and facilitate recovery as the patient progresses through the perioperative period. Some of the desired outcomes of the plan of care for the surgical patient, outlined by the Association of peri-Operative Registered Nurses (AORN, 1999), are that the patient will meet the following goals:

- Be free from injury and adverse effects related to positioning; retained foreign objects; or chemical, physical, or electrical hazards
- Be free from infection
- Maintain fluid and electrolyte balance; skin integrity
- Demonstrate an understanding of the physiologic and psychological responses to the planned surgery
- Participate in a rehabilitation process following surgery

The Nursing Process

ASSESSING

The importance of preoperative assessment cannot be overemphasized. Surgery is a major trauma to the body, and preoperative assessments identify factors that may place the patient at greater risk for complications during and after surgery. Assessment of the surgical patient includes a nursing history and physical assessment to establish baseline data, identify risk factors, and determine teaching and psychosocial needs of the patient and the patient's family. The assessment is often conducted several days before surgery as part of preoperative laboratory screening and teaching; this is referred to as *preadmission testing*. It may be conducted in the hospital, a surgical clinic, office, or even in the patient's own home.

Nursing History

The nursing history identifies risk factors and strengths in the patient's physical and psychosocial status. Information significant to the surgical experience includes a health history, lifestyle habits, cultural and ethnic beliefs, functional status, coping strategies and support systems, including patient perceptions of self, and surgery and learning needs.

Health History

Health history data that identify risk factors and individualize assessments include the patient's developmental level, medical history, medications, previous surgeries, and perceptions and knowledge of the surgery to be done.

Developmental Considerations

Infants and older adults are at a greater risk from surgery than are children and young or middle-aged adults. The infant has a lower total blood volume, making even a small loss of blood a serious consideration because of the risk for dehydration and the inability to respond to the need for increased oxygen during surgery. The infant also has difficulty maintaining stable body temperature during surgery because the shivering reflex is not well developed, making potential hypothermia or hyperthermia more likely. The renal system has a lower glomerular filtration rate and creatinine clearance, leading to a slower metabolism of drugs that require renal biotransformation. Because the liver is immature until after the first year of life, the effects of muscle relaxants and narcotics may be prolonged.

Physiologic changes associated with aging (described in Chap. 10) increase the surgical risk for older patients (AORN, 1997). These changes, summarized in the accompanying box, Focus on the Older Adult, decrease older adults' ability to respond to the stress of surgery, alter the response to preoperative and postoperative medications and anesthesia, and prolong or alter wound healing processes. With an increasing older adult population, assessment of physiologic changes is crucial to providing knowledgeable, safe, holistic nursing care to older surgical patients. Chronic illnesses, more common in the older population, also increase surgical risk and may require adaptations of usual perioperative procedures. For example, a patient with congestive heart failure may be more easily fatigued and thus unable to be up and about as rapidly after surgery.

Medical History

The medical history provides information about past and current illnesses. Pathologic changes associated with past and current illnesses increase surgical risk as well as the potential for postoperative complications. Preoperative assessments and documentation are necessary to provide a database for individualized assessments and interventions in the intraoperative and postoperative phases of care. Following are selected examples and associated risks:

Cardiovascular diseases, such as thrombocytopenia, hemophilia, recent myocardial infarction or cardiac surgery, congestive heart failure, and dysrhythmias, increase the risk for hemorrhage and hypovolemic shock, hypotension, venous stasis, thrombophlebitis, and overhydration with intravenous fluids.
Pulmonary disorders, such as pneumonia, bronchitis, asthma, emphysema, and chronic obstructive

Focus on the Older Adult

Physiologic Changes With Aging That Increase Surgical Risk

System	Change	Preoperative Nursing Interventions
Cardiovascular	• Decreased cardiac output, stroke volume, and cardiac reserve • Decreased peripheral circulation • Increased vascular rigidity	• Obtain and record baseline vital signs. • Assess peripheral pulses. • Teach leg exercises, turning, and ambulating. • Document normal activity levels and tolerance of fatigue. • Monitor fluid administration. • Allow sufficient time for medication effects to occur.
Respiratory	• Reduced vital capacity • Diminished cough reflex • Decreased oxygenation of blood • Decreased chest expansion (arthritic changes in ribs) • Decreased muscle strength of diaphragm and intercostals	• Obtain and record baseline respiratory depth and rate. • Teach coughing and deep-breathing exercises. • Assess color of skin. • Explain use of pulse oximeter for monitoring postoperative oxygenation.
Central Nervous System	• Sensory deficit • Decreased reaction time, coordination • Reduced short-term memory • Reduced thermoregulation ability	• Orient to surroundings. • Institute safety measures (eg, elevate side rails, use night light). • Allow additional time for questions and teaching. • Use appropriate thermoregulation measures to conserve body heat.
Renal	• Decreased renal blood flow • Reduced bladder capacity	• Assess amount and times of voiding. • Monitor fluid and electrolyte status. • Record intake and output.
Integument	• Decreased vascularity • Dry, inelastic skin • Decreased subcutaneous fat	• Assess skin status. • Monitor fluid status. • Use minimal amounts of tape on intravenous sites. • Pad and protect bony prominences, pressure sites.
Gastrointestinal	• Increased gastric pH • Prolonged gastric-emptying time • Decreased hepatic blood flow, liver mass, and enzyme function	• Monitor nutritional status. • Observe for prolonged medication effects.

pulmonary diseases, increase the risk for respiratory depression from anesthesia as well as postoperative pneumonia, atelectasis, and alterations in acid–base balance.

Kidney and liver function alterations influence the patient's response to anesthesia, affect fluid and electrolyte as well as acid–base balance, alter the metabolism and excretion of drugs, and impair wound healing.

Metabolic disorders, especially diabetes mellitus, increase the potential for hypoglycemia or acidosis and slow wound healing and present an increased risk for postoperative cardiovascular complications.

Medications

The use of either prescribed or over-the-counter drugs can affect the patient's reaction to and increase the risk from the stress of surgery and the effects of the anesthetic agent. Many medications are cancelled before the surgery, but the nurse should know the purposes and actions of the patient's drugs as well as the physician's orders. Specific medications may be given even when the patient is going to surgery (eg, patients with heart or cardiovascular problems or diabetes mellitus).

Surgical risk is increased by drugs in the following categories:

Anticoagulants: may precipitate hemorrhage.
Diuretics: may cause electrolyte imbalances, with resulting respiratory depression from anesthesia.
Tranquilizers: may increase the hypotensive effect of anesthetic agents.
Adrenal steroids: abrupt withdrawal may cause cardiovascular collapse in long-term users.
Antibiotics: those in the mycin group, when combined with certain muscle relaxants used during surgery, can cause respiratory paralysis.

Previous Surgery

Data about previous surgeries are important for meeting the patient's physical and psychological needs throughout the perioperative period. Physical implications of previous surgeries are important to the intraoperative and postoperative phases (eg, previous heart or lung surgery may necessitate adaptations in anesthesia and in positioning during surgery). Complications during or after prior surgery, such as malignant hyperthermia, latex sensitivity, pneumonia, thrombophlebitis, or surgical site infection, may necessitate careful postoperative monitoring or alter intraoperative care.

The patient's past experiences with surgery also affect the plan of care established in the preoperative phase, especially if a past experience was negative. When the interview elicits negative feelings about the surgical experience, pain management, or nursing interventions carried out to prevent complications during previous surgeries, teaching and mutual goal setting are even more important.

Perceptions and Knowledge of Surgery

Included in the medical history review are the patient's perceptions and knowledge of the surgical procedure to be performed. The patient's questions or statements are important for meeting psychological and family needs when preparing the patient for surgery and planning for patient and family teaching and preparation for discharge.

Lifestyle

The nursing history data about the patient's lifestyle and cultural and ethnic background provide valuable information related to surgical risk and postoperative recovery and rehabilitation. Areas especially important are nutrition; the use of alcohol, illicit drugs, or nicotine; activities of daily living; and occupation.

Nutrition

Both malnutrition and obesity increase surgical risk. Surgery increases the body's need for nutrients that are necessary for normal tissue healing and resistance to infection. A patient who is malnourished is at higher risk for alterations in fluid and electrolyte balance, delay in wound healing, and wound infection. Obese patients are increased risk for pulmonary, cardiovascular, and gastrointestinal problems. Fatty tissue has a poor blood supply and therefore has less resistance to infection; postoperative complications of delayed wound healing, wound infection, and disruption in the integrity of the wound are more common (Smeltzer & Bare, 2000).

Use of Alcohol, Illicit Drugs, or Nicotine

Patients with a large habitual alcohol intake require larger doses of anesthetic agents and postoperative analgesics, increasing the risk for drug-related complications. Patients who use illicit drugs are at risk for potential interactions with anesthetic agents. These are specific to the illicit drug used and should be noted on the medical record for safe anesthetic management. Patients who smoke are at higher risk for respiratory complications after surgery. Pulmonary secretions are retained by all patients during anesthesia, but smokers, who already have increased mucous secretions and decreased ciliary action in the tracheobronchial tree, have more difficulty clearing the respiratory passages after surgery. In addition, the tracheobronchial mucosa is chronically irritated in people who smoke; anesthesia further increases this irritation.

Activities of Daily Living

Exercise and rest and sleep habits are important for preventing postoperative complications and facilitating recovery. A patient with a well-established exercise program has improved cardiovascular, respiratory, metabolic, and musculoskeletal function, thereby lowering the risks of surgery. Rest and sleep are essential to physical and emotional adaptation and recovery from the stress of surgery. Information from the nursing history allows the nurse to individualize interventions to promote rest and sleep.

Occupation

Many surgical procedures require a delay in returning to a career or occupation or may affect how the patient earns a living. Knowledge of a patient's usual work and concerns about returning to work help the nurse plan necessary teaching and referrals.

Coping Patterns and Support Systems

Assessment of the patient's psychological, sociocultural, and spiritual dimensions is as important as the physical history and examination. Surgery is a major psychological stressor and affects coping patterns, support systems, and individual human needs.

Coping Patterns

A surgical procedure, no matter whether planned or unexpected, major or minor, causes anxiety and fear. While obtaining the nursing history, the nurse can use cues from the patient's and family's verbal and nonverbal communication to identify fears and concerns and to plan nursing interventions to provide information and emotional support necessary to successful recovery from surgery.

Surgery is an unfamiliar experience over which a person has no control; the resulting anxiety may be expressed in many ways, such as anger, withdrawal, apathy, confrontation, or questioning. Therapeutic communication skills are essential for establishing the trusting nurse–patient relationship that is necessary to identify and resolve fear. The causes of fear in the preoperative phase include the following:

Fear of the unknown: The patient has fears about the surgery itself, the anesthesia, the diagnosis, the future, financial and family responsibilities, response to pain, or possible disfigurement or disability.

Fear of pain or death: Common fears are that the anesthesia will not "put me to sleep," that death will occur during surgery, or that the patient will not be able to handle postoperative pain.

Fear of changes in body image and self-concept: Surgical procedures often leave the patient with permanent changes in body structure, function, or appearance. Patients commonly fear alterations in physical attractiveness, social relationships, lifestyle, and sexuality.

The nurse should encourage the patient to identify and verbalize fears; often simply talking about fears helps to diminish their magnitude. At the same time, incorrect knowledge can be identified and corrected, strengths can be identified, and teaching can be done. The reduction of fear is of major importance in preoperative preparation; emotional stress added to the physical stress of surgery increases the surgical risk.

Support Systems

Coping with stress can be facilitated through support systems identified in the assessment phase of preoperative nursing care. As much as possible, family members or significant others should be part of the initial interview and should be included in discussions of fears and concerns. Family members should be encouraged to provide support before and after surgery.

By identifying spiritual beliefs in the nursing history, the nurse can support the patient's spiritual needs through acceptance, participation in prayer or other rituals, or referral to a spiritual leader. Faith in a higher being provides support and helps to reduce fears.

The need for other support systems can also be identified in the initial interview. For example, a patient having a colostomy, heart transplantation, or mastectomy may have many questions answered and anxieties reduced by a preoperative visit from a person who has had the same operation and adapted successfully.

The nursing history should elicit those ways in which a patient provides self-support to reduce stress. These are discussed in Chapter 31 and range from listening to music to practicing active relaxation techniques.

Sociocultural Needs

A person's perceptions of and reactions to the surgical experience are influenced by individual factors, including family health beliefs and practices, economic factors, and cultural/ethnic background.

As discussed in Chapter 4, each person is influenced by family health beliefs and practices. A patient who requires surgery but has grown up in a family that believes that surgical intervention is the last possible option for treating illness may be hesitant about the surgery or may be convinced that death will result. The resulting anxiety may make this patient even more susceptible to surgical risk. Reactions to teaching, physical care, and pain are also influenced by family values and cultural/ethnic identity. For example, a male patient reared with the belief that it is unmanly to acknowledge pain may demonstrate a stoic acceptance of pain and refuse needed medications postoperatively.

Cultural and ethnic influences also affect the patient's responses to and perceptions of the surgical experience. The patient's cultural background may require that nursing interventions be individualized to meet needs in such areas as language, food preferences, family interactions and participation, personal space, and health beliefs and practices. For example, a patient from a culture that believes that bed rest is the most important treatment for illness or injury may have difficulty accepting the need for postoperative exercises and early ambulation.

Physical Assessment

Assessing the patient's current physical status provides data for interventions to decrease surgical risk and potential postoperative complications. Depending on the situation, the physical assessment is conducted as described in Chapter 25. The accompanying box summarizes key Preoperative Physical Assessment areas for surgical patients.

Presurgical Screening Tests

Various presurgical screening tests provide objective data of normal body function. In cases of abnormalities, such tests provide data for medical interventions to improve the patient's physical status and thus decrease the risks for potential surgical complications. The nurse's role is to ensure that the tests are explained to the patient, that the results are recorded in the patient's record before surgery, and that abnormal findings are reported. Additionally, abnormal results are data for determining additional nursing diagnoses and collaborative problems. Usual presurgical screening tests include chest x-ray, electrocardiography, complete blood count, measurement of electrolyte levels, and urinalysis. Normal findings for laboratory tests are found in Appendix B. Significant abnormal findings include an elevated white blood cell count (presence of infection), decreased hematocrit and hemoglobin level (presence of bleeding, anemia), hyperkalemia or hypokalemia (increased risk for cardiac problems), elevated blood urea nitrogen or

Preoperative Physical Assessment

General survey: Note the patient's general state of health, body posture, and stature. Record height, weight (assists in determining nutritional problems and medication calculation), and vital signs (pulse rate and rhythm, respiratory rate and rhythm, blood pressure, and temperature (note route used), which will be used as a baseline for future comparisons).

Skin: Inspect skin for color and characteristics. Note in nursing record any lesions and their location and character. Check skin turgor and condition of skin over bony prominences and pressure areas. These results are important in determining outcomes regarding the prevention of injury.

Chest and lungs: Palpate for any tenderness. Auscultate breath sounds. Evaluate chest excursion and diameter and shape of thorax.

Cardiovascular system: Determine apical rate, rhythm, and character. Auscultate heart sounds and note any jugular venous pulsations. Locate and palpate peripheral pulses; if the patient is undergoing vascular surgery, these may need to be marked for intraoperative and postoperative assessment. Note and record any peripheral edema.

Abdomen: Inspect the contour of the abdomen. Note any areas of asymmetry. Auscultate bowel sounds.

Musculoskeletal system: Inspect and note range of motion in joints. Record any limitations in range of motion to assist in surgical and postoperative patient positioning to prevent injury.

Neurologic status: Note the patient's level of consciousness, awareness, and speech. Watch facial expression and note manner, affect, and any asymmetry. Determine whether there are any motor or sensory deficits. These assessments assist in evaluating the patient's recovery from anesthesia and other potential postoperative complications such as stroke, injury related to surgical position or surgical intervention in the area of the head and neck.

creatinine levels (possible renal failure), and abnormal urine constituents (indicating infection, fluid imbalances, renal failure).

DIAGNOSING

Nursing diagnoses for patients in the preoperative phase may be identified for various problems that exist or for which a patient is at risk. These are derived from the analysis of subjective and objective data obtained from the nursing history and physical examination as well as information from other health team members and screening tests. Many diagnoses reflect assessment of risk and are made to guide

interventions for patient needs in the intraoperative and postoperative phases. Nursing care throughout the perioperative period must be consistent and documented; the preoperative nursing diagnoses are the bases for consistent, holistic care from admission through recovery.

Examples of North American Nursing Diagnosis Association (NANDA) nursing diagnoses appropriate to the preoperative period are as follows:

Anticipatory Grieving related to perceived loss of normal body image resulting from scheduled amputation of left leg

Anxiety related to the effects of surgical procedure on ability to function as primary wage earner and head of the family

Fear related to surgery for treatment of cancer of the breast and unknown future

Risk for Infection related to age (77 years), obesity, and abdominal incision to remove intestinal tumor

Ineffective Airway Clearance related to 25-year history of smoking and administration of anesthesia during surgery

Ineffective Individual Coping related to conflict between need for surgery and religious belief (member of Christian Scientist faith)

PLANNING: EXPECTED OUTCOMES

Preoperative nursing care is affected by the length of the preoperative phase. Patients who enter the hospital through the emergency department with the need for immediate surgery and those who have ambulatory surgery may not have time for comprehensive assessments and teaching. There has been a tremendous increase in the number of ambulatory and short-stay surgeries, in which patients are admitted early the morning of surgery. In such cases, the nurse must use standardized preoperative plans and individualize the plans for the particular patient and family. Outcome criteria are standard for all patients having surgery, but nursing interventions are designed to meet the priority needs of individual patients and situations.

Planning for the entire perioperative period is done in the preoperative phase and includes expected outcomes that are discussed and agreed on by the nurse, the patient, and the family. Specific appropriate outcomes are as follows. The patient will meet the following goals:

- Be physically and emotionally prepared for surgery
- Demonstrate turning, coughing, and deep-breathing exercises
- Verbalize understanding of postoperative pain management
- Maintain fluid intake and nutritional balance to meet needs

To help the patient meet these goals during the preoperative phase, the nurse must accomplish the following:

- Establish a database and plan of care to meet patient needs throughout the perioperative period

- Identify and meet patient and family learning needs
- Identify physical and psychosocial risk factors
- Provide interventions to maximize physical and emotional safety and security

IMPLEMENTING

Preoperative nursing interventions provide the patient with the necessary physical and psychological preparation for surgery and the postoperative phase. This section discusses implementing the plan of care to meet established patient goals; Procedure 29-1 outlines the actions and rationale for preoperative patient care.

Preparing the Patient Psychologically

Surgery is almost always viewed as a life crisis and evokes anxiety and fear. Anxiety can be reduced and recovery facilitated by nursing actions that focus on therapeutic communications and patient and family teaching.

Communicating

The nurse uses therapeutic communication skills and techniques, as described in Chapter 21, to establish a supportive and trusting nurse–patient relationship and to facilitate psychological safety and security. Guidelines for the nurse to meet psychological needs of the surgical patient are as follows:

- Establish and maintain a therapeutic relationship, allowing the patient to verbalize fears and concerns.
- Use active listening skills to identify and validate verbal and nonverbal responses revealing anxiety and fear.
- Use touch, as appropriate, to demonstrate genuine empathy and caring.
- Be prepared to respond to common patient questions about surgery:
    - Will I lose control of body functions while I'm having surgery?
    - How long will I be in the operating room and PACU?
    - Where will my family be?
    - Will I have pain when I wake up?
    - Will the anesthetic make me sick?
    - Will I need a blood transfusion?
    - How long will it be before I can eat?
    - What kind of scar will I have?
    - When will I be able to be sexually active?
    - When can I go back to work?

Remember that each patient is a unique individual and responds to the surgical experience in a unique way. One note of caution: false reassurance must be avoided. In an attempt to allay anxiety and fear, the nurse may be tempted to reassure the patient that he or she will be fine. Such a response denies the patient's emotional needs, shuts off therapeutic communications and trust, and may not be true.

Teaching

Teaching about postoperative activities is implemented in the preoperative phase and is the nurse's responsibility. Patients and families need to know about surgical events and sensations, how to manage pain, and how to perform the physical activities necessary to decrease postoperative complications and facilitate recovery. The teaching–learning process (see Chap. 22) is individualized to meet common and individual patient needs.

The timing of teaching is a significant consideration; teaching too far in advance of surgery or when the patient is anxious is less effective. In today's healthcare system, patients often enter the hospital the day before or the day of surgery, and teaching must be adapted to this schedule. Many institutions provide teaching sessions before admission to prepare the patient for surgery. Whether done before or after admission, a preoperative teaching checklist gives nurses organized and comprehensive guidelines for instruction (see the accompanying Sample Preoperative Teaching box).

Nursing research has indicated that the success of preoperative teaching varies with the timing of the teaching, the individual patient and his or her support systems, the type of surgery, and group versus individual sessions. Preoperative teaching has proved beneficial in decreasing postoperative complications and length of stay as well as positively influencing recovery.

Surgical Events and Sensations

Patients and their families need to know when surgery is scheduled; about how long the surgery and postanesthesia care will last; and what will be done before, during, and after surgery (procedures, medications, equipment). If the surgery is elective, a tour of the operating room suite may be helpful in reducing anxiety and fear of the unknown; although especially helpful for children, this is also useful in preparing adult patients. An explanation of surgical events includes a description of the various members of the healthcare team. An outline of surgical events is found in the preoperative teaching checklist box.

Patients also need to know what sensations they will experience during the perioperative period. Although the sensations differ depending on the type of surgery, teaching should include the following:

- Feelings experienced from preoperative medications, such as a dry mouth and drowsiness
- Sensations that normally occur after surgery and anesthesia, such as a sore throat from an endotracheal tube, a gradual return of feeling and movement after spinal anesthesia, and a lower tolerance of activity with increased fatigue
- Sensations experienced after surgery, such as incisional pain, intravenous lines and fluids, tight dressings, dry mouth, and drowsiness

Pain Management

Pain is a normal part of the surgical experience and a major concern for the patient and family. Guidelines for the management of acute surgical pain have been established by

PROCEDURE 29-1

Preoperative Patient Care: Hospitalized Patient

Action	Rationale

General

1. Identify patients for whom surgery is a greater risk:
   a. Very young and elderly patients
   b. Obese or malnourished patients
   c. Patients with fluid and electrolyte imbalances
   d. Patients in poor general health from chronic diseases and infectious processes
   e. Patients taking certain medications (ie, anti-coagulants, antibiotics, diuretics, depressants, steroids)
   f. Patients who are extremely anxious

This allows for recognition of patients who may be prone to complications after surgery.

2. Review nursing database, history, and physical examination. Check that baseline data are recorded; report those that are abnormal.

Review identifies patients who are surgical risks.

3. Check that diagnostic testing has been completed and results are available; identify and report abnormal results.

This check may influence type of surgery and anesthetic as well as timing of surgery or need for additional consultation.

4. Promote optimal nutrition and hydration status.

This promotes wound healing.

5. Identify learning needs of patient and family. Conduct preoperative teaching regarding the following:
   a. Coughing and deep-breathing exercises; respiratory therapy regimens
   b. Management of pain after surgery
   c. Leg exercises and early ambulation
   d. Postoperative equipment and monitoring devices
   e. Home care requirements

This enhances surgical recovery and allays anxiety by preparing patients for postoperative convalescence, discharge plans, and self-care.

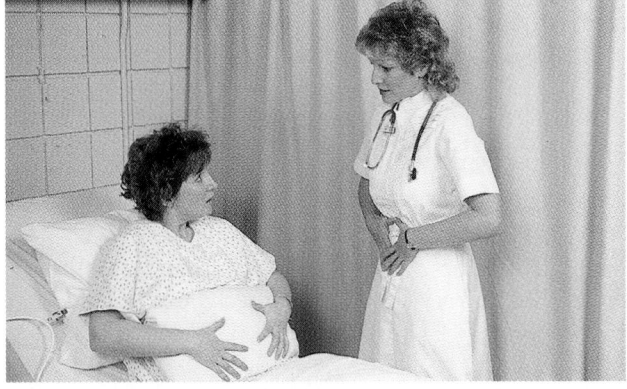

Action 5a: Teaching patient to splint incision before coughing. (PHOTO © KEN KASPER.)

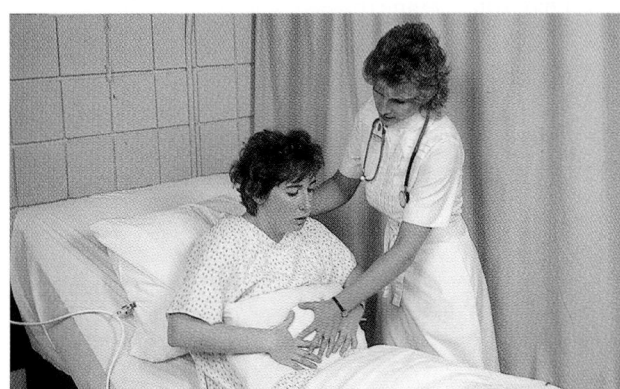

Action 5a: Teaching patient to cough. (PHOTO © KEN KASPER.)

Day Before Surgery

6. Provide emotional support. Answer questions realistically. Provide spiritual assistance if requested. Include family when possible.

This allays family and patient misconceptions and fears.

(continued)

PROCEDURE 29-1

Preoperative Patient Care: Hospitalized Patient (Continued)

7. Follow preoperative fluid and food restrictions.	This reduces risk for vomiting and aspiration during surgery. Anesthetic agents temporarily depress gastro-intestinal function and processes.
8. Prepare for elimination needs during and after surgery.	Anesthetic agents and abdominal surgery interfere with normal elimination function. A urinary catheter inserted preoperatively minimizes risk for inadvertent trauma to bladder during surgery.
9. Attend to patient's special hygiene needs (ie, use of antiseptic cleaning agents to prepare surgical site).	This decreases risk for infection.
10. Provide for adequate rest.	Rest minimizes stress before surgery.

Day Before Surgery

11. Check that proper identification band is on patient.	Double-checking ensures identity of patient.
12. Check that preoperative consent forms are signed, witnessed, and correct, that advance directives are in medical record (as applicable), and that medical record is in order.	This fulfills legal requirement related to informed consent and educates patients regarding advance directives.
13. Check vital signs. Notify physician of any pertinent changes (ie, rise or drop in blood pressure, elevated temperature, cough, symptoms of infection).	This provides baseline data for comparison.
14. Provide hygiene and oral care. Remind patient of food and fluid restrictions and time when NPO for surgery.	This promotes comfort and prevents intraoperative complications during anesthesia induction.
15. Continue nutritional and hydration preparation.	This prepares patient for operative procedure.
16. Remove cosmetics and prostheses (eg, contact lenses, false eyelashes, dentures, and so forth). Assess for loose teeth.	These interfere with assessment during surgery.
17. Have patient empty bladder and bowel before surgery.	An empty bladder and bowel minimize risk for injury or complications during and after surgery.
18. Place valuables in appropriate area. Hospital safe is most appropriate place for valuables. They should not be placed in narcotics drawer.	This ensures safety of valuables and personal possessions.
19. Attend to any special preoperative orders.	This prepares patient for operative procedure.
20. Complete preoperative checklist and record of patient's preoperative preparation.	This ensures accurate documentation and communication with perioperative nurse caring for patient.
21. Administer preoperative medication as prescribed by physician/anesthesia provider.	Medication reduces anxiety, provides sedation, and diminishes salivary and bronchial secretions.

the Agency for Health Care Policy and Research (1992). The guidelines are based on these principles: (1) the pain reported by the patient is the determining factor of pain control, (2) pain must be assessed as often as every 2 hours after major surgery, and (3) the older patient is at risk for both undertreatment and overtreatment of pain. Following are guidelines for teaching the patient about pain control:

- Medications to relieve pain will be ordered by the physician and administered by the nurse.
- Pain medications may be ordered to be given on a regular basis or on an as-needed (p.r.n.) basis. If medication is ordered p.r.n., there is a time restriction between doses (eg, every 2 to 4 hours). The patient needs to ask for the medication and should do so

Sample Preoperative Teaching: Activities and Events for In-Hospital Surgery

Preoperative Phase

- ☐ Exercises and physical activities
  - ☐ Deep-breathing exercises
  - ☐ Coughing
  - ☐ Incentive spirometry
  - ☐ Coughing
  - ☐ Turning
  - ☐ Leg exercises
- ☐ Pain management
  - ☐ Meaning of PRN orders for medications
  - ☐ Timing for best effect of medications
  - ☐ Splinting incision
  - ☐ Nonpharmacologic pain management options
- ☐ Visit by anesthesiologist
- ☐ Physical preparation
  - ☐ NPO
  - ☐ Sleeping medication the night before
  - ☐ Preoperative checklist (review items)
- ☐ Visitors and waiting room
- ☐ Transported to operating room by stretcher

Intraoperative Phase

- ☐ Holding area
  - ☐ Skin preparation
  - ☐ Intravenous lines and fluids
  - ☐ Medications
- ☐ Operating room
  - ☐ Operating room bed

- ☐ Lights and common equipment (eg, cardiac monitor, pulse oximeter, warming device, etc.).
- ☐ Safety belt
- ☐ Sensations
- ☐ Staff

Postoperative Phase

- ☐ Postanesthesia care unit
  - ☐ Frequent vital signs, assessments (eg, orientation, movement or extremities, strength of grasp)
  - ☐ Dressings/drains/tubes/catheters
  - ☐ Intravenous lines
  - ☐ Pain medications/comfort measures
  - ☐ Family notification
  - ☐ Sensations
  - ☐ Airway/oxygen therapy/pulse oximetry
  - ☐ Staff
- ☐ Transfer to unit (on stretcher)
  - ☐ Frequent vital signs
  - ☐ Sensations
  - ☐ Pain medications/nonpharmacologic strategies
  - ☐ NPO, diet progression
  - ☐ Exercises
  - ☐ Early ambulation
  - ☐ Family visits

---

before the pain becomes severe. If the medication does not control the pain, a different one can be ordered.

- Medications for pain are usually given by injection or intravenously for the first few days (and as long as the patient is NPO). With food intake and decreasing pain levels, oral medications can be used.
- There is little danger of addiction to pain medications used in the postoperative management of pain.
- The use of relaxation techniques (such as deep breathing, music, and guided imagery) enhances the effects of pain medications.
- Pain medications facilitate the management of pain and increase the patient's ability to carry out activities and exercises necessary for recovery.

Alternative methods of pain control, including *transcutaneous electrical nerve stimulation* (TENS) and *patient-controlled analgesia* (PCA), may be used after surgery. TENS is a nonpharmacologic technique that affects nerve fiber activity; it is also believed to stimulate the release of endorphins, which are chemicals produced in the body that mediate pain perception. The TENS unit electrodes are placed on the skin along each side of the surgical incision. The patient controls the electric current by pushing a button when feeling pain. A PCA pump allows the patient to administer his or her own analgesic. When the patient pushes the control button on the pump, a preset dose of analgesic medication is administered automatically. The time intervals between doses and the amount of medication that can be used within a given period are programmed into the device. The patient must be taught before surgery how to use these methods of pain control, and the nurse is responsible for assessing the effectiveness of the pain relief. Pain management is further discussed in Chapter 40.

Physical Activities

The most common causes of postoperative complications are cardiovascular and pulmonary alterations, including atelectasis, pneumonia, thrombophlebitis, and emboli. Physical activities to reduce the potential for these complications are taught in the preoperative period. The following sections describe deep (diaphragmatic) breathing, coughing, incentive spirometry, leg exercises, and turning in bed. The patient should be able to state the purpose and demonstrate the activities before going to surgery. (This section gives the rationale for the activities; postoperative complications are discussed later in the chapter.)

Deep Breathing. During surgery, the cough reflex is suppressed, mucus accumulates in the tracheobronchial passageways, and the lungs do not ventilate fully. After surgery, respirations often are less effective as a result of the anesthesia, pain medications, and pain from the incision (eg, patients who have thoracic or high abdominal incisions are especially prone to shallow breathing because of incisional pain with deeper respirations). As a result, alveoli do not inflate and may collapse, and secretions are retained, increasing the potential for atelectasis and pulmonary infection. Deep-breathing exercises hyperventilate the alveoli and prevent their recollapse, improve lung expansion and volume, help to expel anesthetic gases and mucus, and facilitate oxygenation of tissues.

Following are guidelines for teaching effective deep-breathing exercises:

- Place the patient in semi-Fowler's position, with the neck and shoulders supported.
- Ask the patient to place the hands over the rib cage, so he or she can feel the chest rise as the lungs expand.
- Ask the patient to:
  - Exhale gently and completely.
  - Inhale through the nose gently and completely.
  - Hold his or her breath for 3 to 5 seconds and mentally count "one, one thousand, two, one thousand," and so forth.
  - Inhale as completely as possible through the mouth with lips pursed (as if whistling).
  - Repeat three times.
  - This exercise should be done every 1 to 2 hours while the patient is awake for the first 24 to 48 hours after surgery and as necessary thereafter, depending on risk factors and pulmonary status.

Coughing. Coughing facilitates the removal of retained mucus from the respiratory tract and is usually is taught in conjunction with deep breathing. Coughing is especially important in patients with an increased risk for pulmonary complications. Because coughing is often painful, the patient should be taught how to splint the incision (ie, to support the incision with a pillow or folded bath blanket, as shown in Procedure 29-1) and to use the period after pain medication has been administered to best advantage. Following are guidelines for teaching effective coughing:

- Place the patient in a semi-Fowler's position, leaning forward.
- Provide a pillow or folded bath blanket to use in splinting the incision.
- Ask the patient to:
  - Inhale and exhale deeply and slowly through the nose three times.
  - Take a deep breath and hold it for 3 seconds.
  - "Hack" out for three short breaths.
  - With mouth open, take a quick breath.
  - Cough deeply once or twice.
  - Take another deep breath.
  - Repeat the exercise every 2 hours while awake.

Incentive Spirometry. An incentive spirometer is often ordered for patients having surgery, and the proper tech-

nique for using it should be practiced preoperatively. This device helps to increase lung volume and inflation of alveoli and facilitates venous return. A gauge on the incentive spirometry device allows the patient to measure his or her progress and provides immediate positive reinforcement for the breathing efforts (refer to Chap. 44 for additional discussion of incentive spirometry). The following points should be included in patient teaching:

- Sit upright or elevate the head of the bed 45 degrees.
- Take two or three normal breaths and then insert the spirometer's mouthpiece into the mouth.
- Inhale through the mouth and hold the breath for 3 to 5 seconds.
- Exhale slowly and fully.
- Repeat the sequence 10 times during each waking hour for the first 5 days after surgery (except immediately before or after meals).

Leg Exercises. During surgery, venous blood return from the legs slows; some surgical positions also decrease venous return. With circulatory stasis of the legs, thrombophlebitis and resultant emboli are potential complications. Leg exercises increase venous return through flexion and contraction of the quadriceps and gastrocnemius muscles. Guidelines for teaching the patient leg exercises are shown in Figure 29-2.

Leg exercises must be individualized to patient needs, physical condition, physician preference, and agency protocol.

Turning in Bed. Turning in bed improves venous return, respiratory function, and gastrointestinal peristalsis and prevents unrelieved pressure if the patient were to remain in one position only. Although turning in bed sounds like a simple procedure, incisional pain makes it difficult, and it should be practiced before surgery. To turn in bed, the patient should raise one knee, reach across to grasp the side rail on the side toward which he or she is turning, and roll over while pushing with the bent leg and pulling on the side rail. A small pillow is useful for splinting the incision while turning. The patient should turn and change positions in bed every 2 hours.

Preparing the Patient Physically

The physical preparation of the patient for surgery varies, depending on the patient's physical status and special needs, type of surgery, and physician's orders. Certain nursing interventions are appropriate for all surgical patients in the areas of hygiene and skin preparation, elimination, nutrition and fluids, and rest and sleep. The nurse is also responsible for the preparation and safety of the patient on the day of surgery.

Hygiene and Skin Preparation

Intact skin is the body's first line of defense against microorganisms, and an alteration in skin integrity (such as the surgical incision) provides a potential source of infection. Therefore, the skin is prepared to minimize skin contamination and decrease the risk for postoperative surgical site infection.

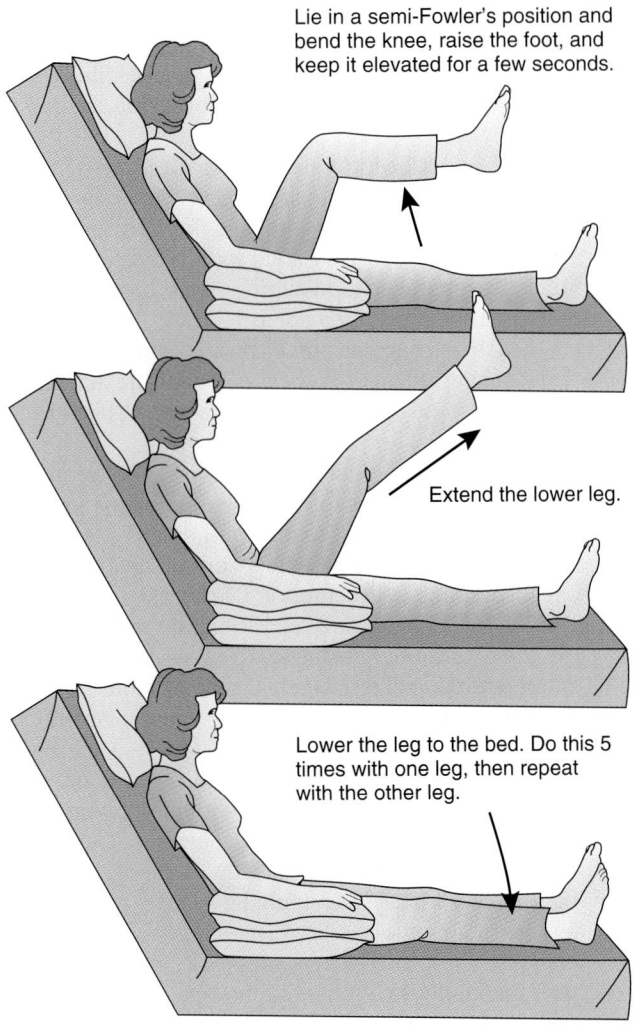

Lie in a semi-Fowler's position and bend the knee, raise the foot, and keep it elevated for a few seconds.

Extend the lower leg.

Lower the leg to the bed. Do this 5 times with one leg, then repeat with the other leg.

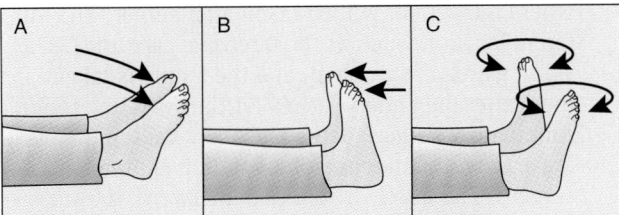

A. Point the toes of both feet toward the foot of the bed. Relax both feet.
B. Pull toes toward the chin. Relax both feet.
C. Make circles with both ankles. First circle to the right, then to the left. Repeat 3 times. Relax feet.

Figure 29-2
Leg exercises to increase venous return.

The skin is cleaned at the operative site with an antibacterial soap or solution to remove bacteria. The patient can do this while taking a bath or shower. Ideally, a shower is taken the evening before or the morning of surgery. Shampooing the hair and cleaning the fingernails also help to reduce the number of organisms present.

The incisional area may require removal of hair before surgery. The need for hair removal depends on the amount of hair, the location of the incision, and the type of surgical procedure being performed. This may be done on the unit or in the surgical suite immediately before the operation, usually in the surgical holding area. If hair must be removed, depilatory creams or hair clippers are recommended by the Centers for Disease Control and Prevention, rather than shaving the surgical site as done in the past. If the surgeon requires a shave prep, it should be done as close to the time of surgery as possible. Agency protocol should be followed for the timing, people responsible, and documentation of the condition of the skin and method of preparation.

Elimination

Emptying the bowel of feces is no longer a routine procedure before surgery, but the nurse should use preoperative assessments to determine the need for an order for bowel elimination. If the patient has not had a bowel movement for several days or has had preoperative barium diagnostic tests, an enema helps to prevent postoperative constipation.

If the patient is scheduled for surgery of the gastrointestinal tract, a cleansing enema is usually ordered. Peristalsis does not return for 24 to 48 hours after the bowel is handled, so preoperative cleansing helps to decrease postoperative constipation. An empty bowel also prevents contamination of the surgical area during surgery.

Insertion of an indwelling urinary catheter may be ordered before surgery, especially in patients having pelvic surgery, to prevent bladder distention or accidental injury. If an indwelling catheter is not in place, the patient should void immediately before receiving preoperative medications to ensure an empty bladder during surgery.

Nutrition and Fluids

The diet order for a patient having surgery depends on the type of surgery and type of anesthesia to be used. In the past, most surgical patients could not eat or drink anything for 8 to 12 hours before the surgery. More current practice is to allow patients to drink clear liquids up to 2 hours before surgery with the permission of the physician. Clear liquids must be carefully defined for the patient: water, fruit juices without pulp, carbonated beverages, clear tea, and black coffee. According to the American Society of Anesthesiologists, patients, especially children, may be less anxious, better hydrated, and have fewer headaches and nausea after surgery with these revised practice guidelines for preoperative fasting (Goodwin, 1999). The nurse explains the reason for being NPO to the patient and, at the appropriate time, removes all food and fluids from the bedside and places a sign over the bed so that all health team members and visitors know about the restriction. If the patient eats or drinks, the physician should be notified at once.

Patients need to be well nourished and hydrated before surgery to counterbalance fluid, blood, and electrolyte loss during surgery and to facilitate tissue healing after surgery. Preoperative assessments provide a base for physical preparation for surgery, including the need for supplemental nutrition, fluids, or electrolytes. A patient who is undernourished may require parenteral nutrition (see Chap. 41) and intravenous electrolyte replacements. If the patient's screening tests show a hemoglobin level of less than 10 g/dL and a hematocrit of less than 33%, blood or blood component therapy may be given preoperatively to maintain volume and increase oxygenation of tissue during surgery.

Rest and Sleep

Rest and sleep are important components for reducing stress before surgery and for healing and recovery after surgery. The nurse can facilitate rest and sleep in the immediate preoperative period by meeting psychological needs, carrying out teaching, providing a quiet environment, encouraging relaxation or comfort measures that are personally effective for the individual patient, or administering the prescribed bedtime sedative medication for hospitalized surgical patients.

Preparing the Patient on the Day of Surgery

The preoperative checklist outlines the nurse's responsibilities on the day of surgery; these activities must be completed before the patient is transported to surgery. Some of these activities have already been described (NPO, preoperative teaching, informed consent, skin preparation, screening tests, bladder elimination). Other nursing responsibilities include the following:

- Obtain and record vital signs to serve as baseline data for the intraoperative phase, and assess for and report any abnormal findings (such as an elevated temperature).
- Prepare the patient physically for the intraoperative phase.
- Have the patient remove all personal clothing and put on an operating room gown.
- Remove all hairpins or hairpieces. This prevents injury to the patient during surgery and possible loss of hairpieces.
- Remove makeup and fingernail polish to allow intraoperative and postoperative assessment of skin and nailbeds for circulation and oxygenation of tissues.
- Remove all prostheses, such as dentures or partial plates, eyeglasses, contact lenses, and artificial limbs. Dentures may cause respiratory obstruction during anesthesia; other prostheses may be damaged or lost. Be sure items are stored safely while the patient is in surgery.
- Remove jewelry, including body-piercing jewelry, to prevent loss or injury (such as swelling or getting caught on a piece of equipment during or after surgery); if the patient prefers not to remove a wedding band, it can be securely taped to the finger (in some types of surgery, leaving jewelry on is not allowed). When jewelry is removed, it should be given to a family member or locked in a safe place and its disposition noted.
- Leave on a hearing aid, and be certain that perioperative and PACU nurses know the patient has one.
- Be sure that the patient's identification bracelet is in place to ensure accurate identity.
- Note allergies according to institutional policy (eg, on the front of the patient's record or on an allergy bracelet).

- Carry out any special procedures ordered, such as securing previous records, inserting a nasogastric tube, starting an intravenous line, applying antiembolic stockings or compression devices, or giving medications.
- Give the prescribed preoperative medications at either the scheduled time or "on call" (the operating room calls to tell the nurse to give the medication). With ambulatory surgery and rapid recovery tracks, much less premedication is prescribed. Medications that might be prescribed are as follows:
  - Sedatives, such as diazepam (Valium), midazolam (Versed), or lorazepam (Ativan) to alleviate anxiety and decrease recall of events related to surgery
  - Anticholinergics, such as atropine and glycopyrrolate (Robinul), to decrease pulmonary and oral secretions and to prevent laryngospasm
  - Narcotic analgesics, such as morphine and meperidine hydrochloride (Demerol), to facilitate patient sedation and relaxation and to decrease the amount of anesthetic agent needed
  - Neuroleptanalgesic agents, such as fentanyl citrate-droperidol (Innovar), to cause a general state of calmness and sleepiness
  - Histamine receptor antihistaminics, such as cimetidine (Tagamet) and ranitidine (Zantac), to decrease gastric acidity and volume
- Maintain patient safety by elevating side rails, lowering the bed (if possible), applying a safety restraint, and instructing the patient to stay in bed or on the stretcher.
- Meet the family's (or other support person's) needs. The family of the hospitalized surgical patient is told where the patient will be taken after surgery (if a different location, such as the intensive care unit). The waiting area is described, and the family is taken there after the patient leaves for the operating room. Ambulatory surgery patients usually wait in the waiting area with family members until it is time for surgery. The family is told that afterward, the surgeon will come to the waiting area to tell them what happened in surgery.
- Document, through checklists and narrative charting, the nursing interventions carried out.
- Assist in moving the patient from the bed to the operating room stretcher when it is time to transport the patient to surgery, ensuring accurate identification.
- Prepare the hospitalized patient's bed (make a surgical bed) and room for postoperative care.
- Have necessary equipment and supplies in the room for postoperative care (equipment to measure vital signs, hang intravenous fluids, and so forth).

EVALUATING

Evaluating the plan of care for the preoperative phase is based on the expected outcomes. The plan is effective if the patient is physically and emotionally prepared for surgery, can verbalize events and sensations of the perioperative period, and can demonstrate postoperative exercises and activities.

Intraoperative Nursing Care

The intraoperative phase of surgery begins with admission of the patient to the surgical area and lasts until the patient is transferred to the PACU. Although the surgeon has a dominant role during this phase, the perioperative nurse has critical responsibilities and roles in collaboratively meeting patient needs. The nursing process uses the preoperative data and plan as a basis for the intraoperative plan of care. A conceptual model for perioperative nursing care is shown in Figure 29–3. In this model, the patient is at the center of all care activities. The three critical domains for patient care include safety, physiologic responses, and the patient and family behavioral responses. For each of these domains, there are desired outcomes. These, rather than the usual progression of the nursing process, which begins with assessment, are identified first in the model because perioperative nursing is preventive in nature. Therefore, perioperative

nurses base plans of care on already known and recognized desired outcomes. The patient is assessed for the relevance of the outcome, nursing diagnoses are then identified, and interventions are planned. The domain in the model that relates to the health system is intended to represent the structure elements and other system activities that must be present to support safe, effective, quality patient care.

The type of surgery scheduled influences the desired outcomes, nursing diagnoses, assessments, and interventions carried out by the nurse. For example, the nurse's role when caring for the patient having ambulatory surgery may be that of providing patient care from admission through discharge. The nurse's role for hospital-based surgery is usually specific to one phase. This section of the chapter discusses the role of the nurse specific to intraoperative care.

The Nursing Process

ASSESSING

The first room the patient enters when transferred to the surgical area is usually the holding area. Nurses in surgical

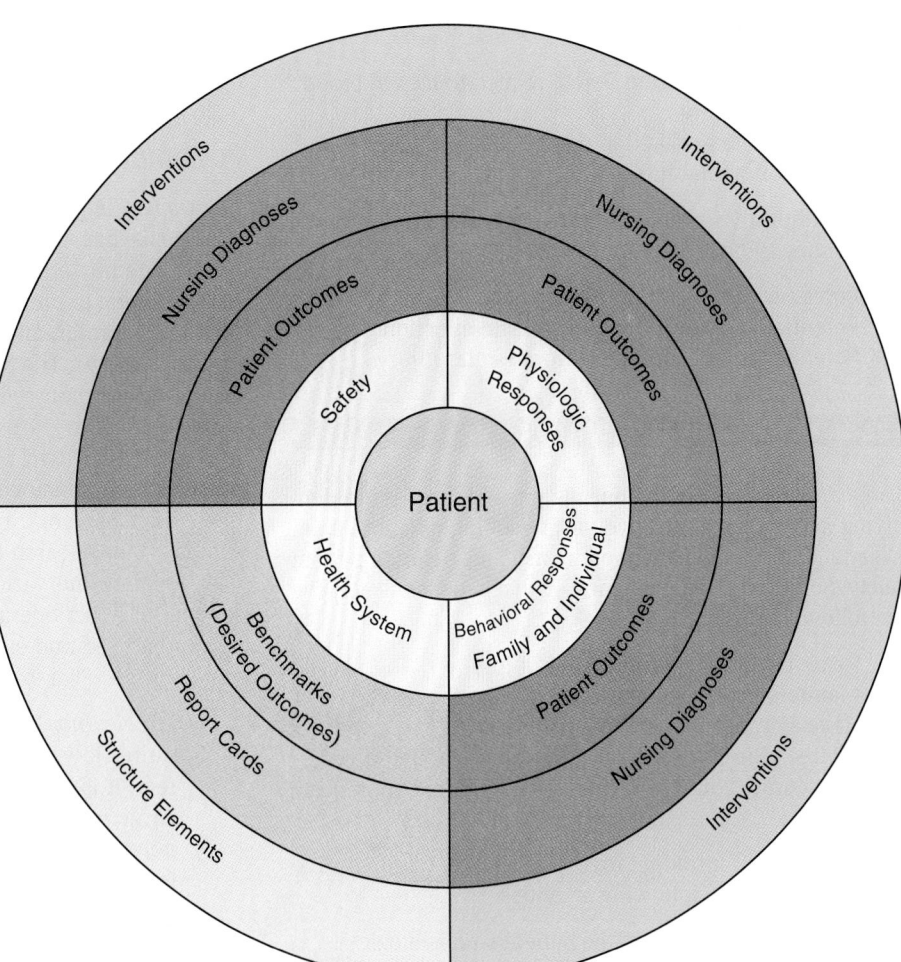

Figure 29-3
Association of Operating Room Nurses perioperative patient-focused model. Reproduced with permission, *AORN Perioperative Patient Focused Model.* Copyright © AORN, Inc., 2170 S. Parker Road, Suite 300, Denver, CO 80231.

scrub attire identify the surgical patient, assess the patient's emotional and physical status, and verify the information on the preoperative checklist. They may also carry out required immediate preoperative care, including performing skin preparation, starting intravenous fluids, and giving preoperative medications. The patient's response to procedures is assessed, and the events of surgery are explained. When the operating room is prepared, a perioperative nurse helps transport the patient to the operating room.

In the operating room, the patient is positioned on the operating bed, anesthetized, and draped. The perioperative nurse assesses the patient and reviews preoperative data, paying particular attention to factors that increase surgical risk. The nurse also assesses the patient during positioning and monitors supplies used to maintain safety for the patient.

DIAGNOSING

Patient problems in the intraoperative period may occur in relation to the position of the patient during the procedure, the effects of the anesthesia, equipment used and potential hazards, disruption of tissues during surgery, and the incision. Appropriate nursing diagnoses include the following:

> Impaired Skin Integrity related to 4-inch midline abdominal incision
>
> Risk for Fluid Volume Deficit related to loss of blood during surgery
>
> Risk for Injury related to positioning, anesthesia, and environmental hazards

Collaborative problems might include the following (Carpenito, 1999):

> Potential complication: Hemorrhage
> Potential complication: Surgical site infection
> Potential complication: Neuromuscular injury

PLANNING: EXPECTED OUTCOMES

The planning phase of the nursing process focuses on identifying actions most effective for preventing potential complications, resolving patient problems, and ensuring patient safety. Some expected outcomes are that patient will achieve the following goals:

* Remain free of neuromuscular injury
* Maintain intact skin surfaces
* Have symmetric breathing patterns
* Be free of injury from burns, retained foreign objects (inaccurate count of supplies), and wound contamination

During the intraoperative phase, the perioperative nurse performs the following activities:

* Assesses and monitors the patient's physiologic response

* Positions the patient to prevent injury or alterations in skin, respiratory, or neuromuscular function
* Maintains the patient's physical safety
* Maintains aseptic technique

IMPLEMENTING

During surgery, nurses function as scrub nurses, circulating nurses, in an expanded role as **registered nurse first assistants** (RNFAs), or in an advanced practice role as acute care nurse practitioners (APNs). *Scrub nurses* are members of the sterile team who maintain surgical asepsis while draping and handling instruments and supplies. The **circulating nurse** assesses the patient on admission to the operating room, collaborates in safely positioning the patient on the operating bed, assists with monitoring the patient during surgery, provides additional supplies, maintains environmental safety, and, throughout the surgical procedure, counts the number of instruments, needles, and sponges used during the surgery to prevent the accidental loss of an item in the wound. The RNFA actively assists the surgeon by providing exposure, hemostasis, and wound closure. The APN coordinates care activities, collaborates with physicians and nurses in all phases of perioperative and postanesthesia care, and integrates case management, critical paths, and research into care of the surgical patient (Hodson, 1998). Additional educational preparation is required for both roles of the RNFA and the APN.

Positioning

The patient is placed in a specific operative position after anesthesia has produced loss of consciousness and reflexes. The nurse must ensure patient safety and comfort in positioning to prevent alterations in integumentary, respiratory, vascular, and neuromuscular function (Meeker & Rothrock, 1999). The potential for skin injury is avoided by lifting, rather than rolling or pulling, the patient into the surgical position. Rolling or pulling can cause a shearing force, in which two or more tissue layers slide on each other, stretching subcutaneous blood vessels, obstructing blood flow, and contributing to pressure ulcers (see the accompanying Research in Nursing box).

Although the various operative positions are not described here, perioperative nurses need to know the position to be used and significant nursing considerations for that position. Two examples are as follows:

> *Trendelenburg's position:* This surgical position requires lowering the upper torso and raising the feet. It is commonly used in minimally invasive surgery (laparoscopy) of the lower abdomen or pelvis. The displacement of the abdominal viscera toward the head decreases diaphragm movement and respiratory exchange; blood pools in the upper torso, and blood pressure increases; hypotension can result with return to the supine

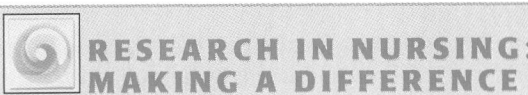

RESEARCH IN NURSING: MAKING A DIFFERENCE

Protecting the Skin Integrity of Patients in the Operating Room

Studies have determined that 12% to 66% of patients develop tissue damage to the sacral, heel, or elbow area as a result of the pressure and sheer experienced during surgery. The combination of the positions used during surgery and the typical operating room (OR) mattress subject a patient's vulnerable areas to uneven pressure that can progress to a pressure ulcer. Nursing assessments that identify patients at risk and individualized interventions that minimize or prevent pressure ulcers present a challenge for the nurse.

Related Research

Schultz, A., Bien, M., Dumond, K., Brown, K., & Myers, A. (1999). Etiology and incidence of pressure ulcers in surgical patients. *AORN, 70*(3), 434–449.

This study was designed to identify the etiology and incidence of pressure ulcer development in a large sample of surgical patients. Participants in the study either received the standardized care or used a special mattress overlay as well as heel and elbow pro-

tectors as a preventive measure while in the OR. Results of the study indicated that patients who developed pressure ulcers (primarily stage I) were older, had a smaller body mass, and had a secondary diagnosis of diabetes mellitus. Evaluation of the mattress overlay, however, confirmed that it was not effective in preventing the development of pressure ulcers during the OR experience. Standard procedure proved as effective in reducing postoperative skin changes.

Relevance to Nursing Practice

Nurses are actively involved in identifying patient needs and solving problems in patient care during the perioperative period. Continued attention to variables, particularly the peripheral vascular changes that often accompany diabetes mellitus, is imperative as nurses attempt to predict alterations in skin integrity. Nursing research in these areas will continue to expand the knowledge base for interventions that improve patient outcomes during and after surgery.

---

position. Shearing is also a significant risk in this position.

Lithotomy position: This surgical position is used for gynecologic, rectal, and urologic procedures. The placement of legs in stirrups causes pooling of blood in the legs, increasing the potential of thrombophlebitis. Pressure can also damage the peroneal nerve, with resultant footdrop.

Draping

Drapes are used to create and maintain a sterile field around the operative site, preventing the passage of microorganisms, particulate matter, and fluids between sterile and nonsterile areas. The only area left exposed is the incision site. Plastic adhesive drapes may be used to form a complete seal over the skin; with these drapes, skin color is visible, and the incision is made through the impermeable adhesive drape.

Documenting

Throughout surgery, the perioperative nurse documents ongoing patient assessment, item counts (sponges, sharps, instruments), monitoring data (such as vital signs, urine output, blood loss, pulse oximetry results), positioning, medications, dressings and drains, and so forth on the intraoperative record. This documentation includes planning and implementation of perioperative nursing activities and evaluation of the achievement of patient outcomes.

Transferring to the Postanesthesia Care Unit

After the surgery, the patient is carefully moved from the operating bed to a stretcher. This is an especially critical time; sudden or rough handling can cause severe hypotension or potentially lethal cardiac or respiratory arrest. The patient is then transported to the PACU room, and relevant preoperative and postoperative assessments and interventions are communicated to the PACU nurses.

EVALUATING

Evaluation of the effectiveness of the plan of care for the intraoperative phase is based on the expected outcomes. If met, the plan was effective.

Postoperative Nursing Care

The postoperative phase can be divided into two stages: immediate care (usually provided in the PACU in both inhospital and ambulatory surgery centers) and ongoing postoperative care, lasting from return to the unit through convalescence. Nursing assessments and interventions are consistent with those in the preoperative and intraoperative phases and are carried out to maintain function, promote recovery, and facilitate coping with alterations in structure or function (see the accompanying box: Through the Eyes of a Student).

Assessments and nursing interventions are combined here in discussing immediate postoperative care; the phases

Through the Eyes of a Student

The first time I took care of a patient with "multiple tubes," I was horrified at the thought of actually touching the patient. I hadn't really been exposed to that many critically ill patients until my last semester as a student nurse. I remember being assigned a patient in the cardiothoracic intensive care unit in the hospital where I trained. The patient was a "fresh heart"—a cardiopulmonary bypass graft patient who had just been operated on that morning.

I remember walking into the room and thinking, "What do I do with all of these tubes?" and then with horror thinking, "What if one of them falls out?" Needless to say, I was overwhelmed and frightened but at the same time excited at the challenge that faced me. I asked my preceptor what each tube was for and where it was hooked up and whether it would fall out if I touched it. She answered all my questions with patience and understanding and asked me if I wanted to handle the lines. I looked at her as if she were insane, but went ahead and did it. Would you believe that nothing fell out! I must admit that the experience taught me a lot, but it also got me over the fear of tubes.

I now chuckle every time I see a nursing student's face with that same look of horror as I had, and I try to answer every question with the same degree of patience and understanding that my preceptor had for me.

—LYNDA L. ULLMER, R.N.
GAITHERSBURG, MD

of the nursing process are used to describe ongoing postoperative care.

Immediate Postoperative Care

Postanesthesia care in the PACU involves assessment of postoperative patients, with emphasis on preventing complications from anesthesia or the surgery. Assessments are continuous and ongoing, using preoperative and intraoperative data as bases for comparison. The assessments made in the PACU include respiratory status, cardiovascular status, central nervous system status, fluid status, wound status, and general condition. These assessments are made every 10 to 15 minutes initially. Some institutions use a head-to-toe assessment to organize data; others use a body systems approach. The average PACU stay is about 2 hours but will vary depending on the type of surgery, length of anesthesia, and patient response.

Respiratory Status

Assessments of respiratory function are made by monitoring respiratory rate, rhythm, and depth; by auscultating breath sounds; and by noting oxygen-saturation level. During a surgical procedure with general anesthesia, an artificial airway (endotracheal tube) may be inserted to administer the anesthetic gases and maintain patent air passages. The airway is not removed until the laryngeal and pharyngeal reflexes return, allowing the patient to control the tongue, cough, and swallow. The airway is assessed for patency, humidified oxygen applied, and pulse oximetry initiated. Cardiovascular and mental status assessments provide additional data about oxygenation. The following assessments indicate ineffective ventilation:

- Restlessness, apprehension
- Unequal chest expansion with use of accessory muscles
- Shallow, noisy respirations
- Cyanosis
- Rapid pulse rate

Respiratory obstruction is the most common PACU emergency. It may occur as a result of secretion accumulation, obstruction by the tongue, laryngospasm (a sudden, violent contraction of the vocal cords), or laryngeal edema. Assessments of respiratory obstruction include those outlined previously plus observation for wheezing or crowing sounds with respiratory effort.

Positioning, administering humidified oxygen, encouraging the patient to take deep breaths, and suctioning may be used to maintain a patent airway and tissue oxygenation.

Cardiovascular Status

Evaluation of cardiovascular function includes assessing blood pressure and pulses, electrocardiogram rate and rhythm, skin color and condition, respirations, temperature, and the wound.

Blood pressure findings are compared with baseline data from the preoperative period; hypotension may be the result of varied factors, including anesthetic agents, preoperative medications, position changes, blood loss, respiratory alterations, and peripheral blood pooling. Transient hypertension can also occur as a result of anesthetic effects, respiratory insufficiency, the surgical procedure, or the excitement phase of recovery from anesthesia. Low blood pressure can be increased by oxygen administration, deep breathing, leg exercises, verbal stimulation (to help expel anesthetic gases and facilitate increasing level of consciousness), and maintaining accurate intravenous flow rates.

All pulses are assessed for bilateral equality, rhythm, rate, and character. Of special significance are assessments of abnormal function—an irregular rhythm, absence of pulses, or tachycardia. Tachycardia, an early symptom of shock, must be carefully evaluated. Other related assessments are cyanosis, edema, a cool skin temperature, and a decrease in urine output.

Patients are at risk for altered body temperature related to the surgical procedure, its length, anesthetic agents, a cool surgical environment, age, and use of cool irrigating or infusion fluids. Inadvertent hypothermia (temperature below 35.5°C [96°F]) can lead to potential complications of poor wound healing, hemodynamic stress, cardiac disturbances, coagulopathy, delayed emergence from anesthesia, and shivering and its associated discomfort (Sessler, 1997). The patient's body temperature is measured, usually by the oral or tympanic route, and measures are initiated if the patient complains of being cold or is hypothermic. Warmed blankets are placed on the patient's body and head, and forced warm-air devices are used for rewarming.

Central Nervous System Status

Anesthetics cause loss of consciousness and reflexes; the return of central nervous system function is assessed through response to stimuli and orientation. Consciousness returns in reverse order, with the usual pattern being (1) unconsciousness, (2) response to touch and sounds, (3) drowsiness, (4) awake but not oriented, and (5) awake and oriented. Nurses in the PACU verbally reorient the patient by touching and calling him or her by name.

Fluid Status

Fluid imbalance may result from factors such as preoperative fluid restriction, fluid loss during surgery, wound drainage, or the surgical stress response (with retention of sodium and water). Fluid volume deficit or excess is a risk for all surgical patients but is especially so in children and older adults. Assessment of fluid status includes skin turgor, vital signs, urine output, wound drainage, and intravenous fluid intake. Assessment of intravenous fluid administration includes the type of fluid infused, the rate, location of lines, condition of intravenous insertion site, and the security and patency of the tubing.

Wound Status

The nurse in the PACU assesses the wound dressing for amount, consistency, and color of drainage as well as for any tubes or drains and the amount and type of drainage by that route. The area underneath the patient is also assessed for drainage.

Large amounts of bright red drainage, combined with other abnormal physical status assessments (restlessness, pallor, cold moist skin, decreasing blood pressure, increasing pulse and respiratory rates), may indicate hemorrhage and hypovolemic shock. These symptoms should be reported immediately.

Pain Management

Pain is both a subjective (what the patient feels) and an objective (what the nurse observes, such as grimacing, moaning, reluctance to move a body part, crying) experience. Clinical practice guidelines developed by the Agency for Health Care Policy and Research recommend the assessment of pain using a rating scale. These may be verbal (ranging from no pain to worst possible pain), numeric (with 10 on a scale of 0 to 10 being the worst possible pain), or a "faces" rating scale, ranging from a smiley face indicating no pain to a face that has frowns and tears for worst possible pain (see Fig. 40-6 in Chap. 40). Early administration of analgesia,

using nonsteroidal antiinflammatory drugs and opiates, occurs in the PACU. Opiates may be delivered by PCA, allowing the patient to control the analgesic administration. Other nonpharmacologic methods to decrease pain and improve comfort include positioning, verbal reassurance, touch, applications of heat or cold, massage, music therapy, humor therapy (see box in Chap. 40, Using Humor to Help Patients Cope With Pain), meditation, and guided imagery. Preoperative assessments, noting personally effective methods for the patient, assist in effective implementation in the PACU. These should supplement, not substitute for, pharmacologic pain relief.

General Condition

Other assessments and interventions are made to ensure physical and emotional comfort and safety. Constant reorientation and reassurance that the surgery is completed provide psychological comfort. Careful assessments, proper positioning, and use of side rails and restraints maintain physical safety.

The patient is discharged from the PACU when physical status and level of consciousness are considered stable. The family is notified that the patient is being transferred back to his or her room, and the PACU nurse gives a verbal report to the unit nurse about the assessments and interventions during the intraoperative and immediate postoperative phases.

Ongoing Postoperative Care

Ongoing postoperative care is planned to facilitate recovery from surgery and coping with alterations. The plan of care is based on individualized nursing diagnoses and includes promoting physical and psychological health, preventing complications, and teaching self-care when the patient returns home. Procedure 29-2 outlines postoperative patient care.

The Nursing Process

ASSESSING

The nurse on the unit assists PACU personnel in transferring the patient to the bed in the unit room and makes an initial assessment using data from the preoperative and intraoperative phases. A postoperative checklist or flow sheet (Fig. 29-4) may be used. The initial assessment is often combined with the implementation of postoperative physician orders and includes the following:

Vital signs: Assess temperature, blood pressure, and pulse and respiratory rates. Note deviations from preoperative and PACU data as well as symptoms of complications.
Color and temperature of skin: Assess for warmth, pallor, cyanosis, and diaphoresis.
Level of consciousness: Assess orientation to time, place, and person as well as reaction to stimuli and ability to move extremities.

(*text continues on page 664*)

PROCEDURE 29-2

Postoperative Care When Patient Returns to Room

Action	**Rationale**

Immediate

1. Place patient in safe position (high Fowler's or side-lying). Note level of consciousness.

A sitting position facilitates deep breathing; side-lying with neck slightly extended prevents aspiration and airway obstruction.

2. Monitor and record vital signs frequently. Assessment order may vary, but usual frequency includes taking vital signs every 15 minutes the first hour, every 30 minutes the next 2 hours, every hour for 4 hours, and finally, every 4 hours.

Comparison with baseline preoperative vital signs may indicate impending shock or hemorrhage.

3. Provide for warmth. Assess skin color and condition.

Hypothermia is uncomfortable and may lead to cardiac dysrhythmias and impaired wound healing.

4. Check dressings for color, odor, and amount of drainage, and feel under patient for bleeding.

Hemorrhage and shock are life-threatening complications of surgery.

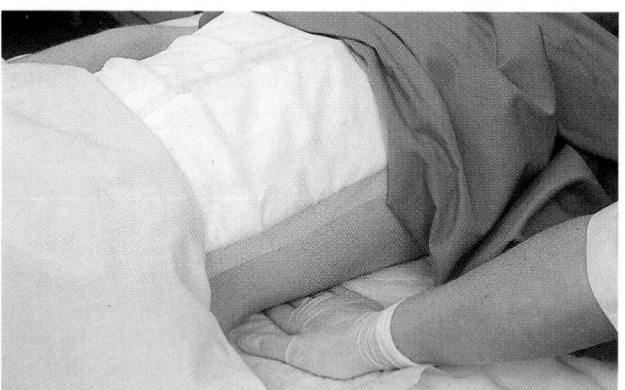

5. Verify that all tubes and drains are patent and equipment is operative; note amount of drainage in collection device.

This ensures maintenance of vital functions.

6. Maintain intravenous infusion at correct rate.

This prevents dehydration and electrolyte imbalances.

7. Provide for a safe environment. Keep bed in low position with side rails up. Have call bell within patient's reach.

This prevents accidental injury.

8. Relieve pain by administering medications ordered by physician. Check record to verify if analgesic medication was administered in the postanesthesia care unit.

Analgesics are used for relief of postoperative pain.

9. Record assessments and interventions on chart.

This provides for accurate documentation.

General

10. Promote optimal respiratory function:
    a. Coughing and deep breathing
    b. Incentive spirometry
    c. Early ambulation
    d. Frequent position change
    e. Administration of oxygen as ordered

Anesthetic agents may depress respiratory function: patients who have existing respiratory or cardiovascular disease or abdominal or chest incisions or who are obese or elderly or in a poor state of nutrition are at greater risk for respiratory complications.

(*continued*)

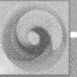

PROCEDURE 29-2

Postoperative Care When Patient Returns to Room (Continued)

11. Maintain adequate circulation:
    a. Frequent position changes
    b. Early ambulation
    c. Application of antiembolic stockings or pneumatic compression devices, if ordered by physician
    d. Leg and range-of-motion exercises if not contra-indicated

Preventive measures can improve venous return and circulatory status.

12. Assess urinary elimination status:
    a. Promote voiding by offering bedpan at regular intervals
    b. Monitor catheter drainage if present
    c. Measure intake and output

Anesthetic agents may temporarily depress bladder tone and response.

13. Promote optimal nutrition status and return of gastro-intestinal function:
    a. Assess for return of peristalsis
    b. Assist with diet progression
    c. Encourage fluid intake
    d. Monitor intake
    e. Medicate for nausea and vomiting as ordered by physician

Anesthetic agents and narcotics depress peristalsis and normal functioning of gastrointestinal tract.

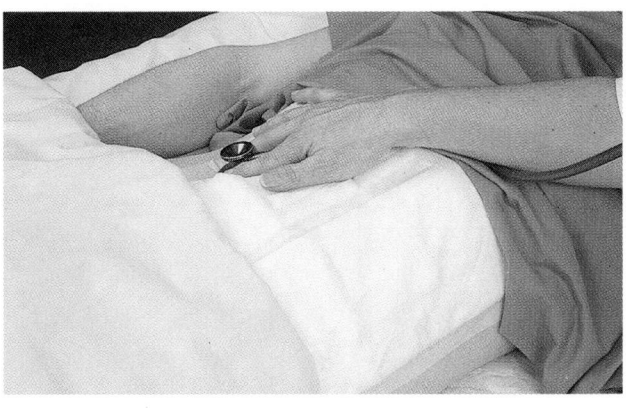

14. Promote wound healing:
    a. Use surgical asepsis
    b. Assess condition of wound
    c. Assess any drainage

Alterations in nutrition, circulatory, and metabolic status may predispose patients to infection and delayed healing.

15. Provide for rest and comfort.

This shortens recovery period and facilitates return to normal function.

16. Provide emotional and spiritual support

This facilitates individualized care and patient's return to normal health.

Name _Dale Courtney_

M.R. # _302-59910_

POSTOP
PROGRESS FLOW RECORD

Date	8/7/00									
Time	10	10^{15}	10^{30}	11	11^{15}	11^{30}	12	12^{30}		
BP	120/80	126/82	128/80	130/80	130/82	130/80	130/82	128/80		
Pulse	90	88	88	90	88	86	86	86		
Respirations	22	24	22	20	20	22	20	20		
Temperature	98^8	98^8	98^8	98^8	98^8	98^8	98^8	98^8		
I.V.	Dc'd	———————————————————————→							Discharged to home with wife	
Wound	DD&I	———————————————————→								
Drain(s)	N/A									
LOC	AAA x3	———————————————————————→							Reviewed D/C instructions	
Pain	SPA	————————————→		+4 (Iced)	+3	+3	+2		Immobilizer on for D/C	
Nausea	No	———————————————————————→								
Foley/Other Cath or Voiding	No				Voided 45cc				Voided	
Turn, Cough Deep Breathe	C & DB	———————————————————→							Ambulated	
Moves All Extremities	+4	———————————————————→							Returned to baseline	
Initials	JCR	JCR	JCR	JCR	JCR	JCR	JCR			

Key _____   _____

_____

Figure 29-4
Example of a postoperative progress record.

Intravenous fluids: Assess type and amount of solution, flow rate, security and patency of tubing, and infusion site.

Surgical site: Assess dressing and dependent areas for drainage (color, amount, and consistency). Assess drains and tubes and be sure they are intact, patent, and properly connected to drainage systems.

Other tubes: Assess indwelling urinary catheter, gastrointestinal suction, and so forth, for drainage, patency, and amount of output. Be sure dependent drainage bags are hanging properly and suction

drainage is attached and functioning. If oxygen is ordered, ensure placement of ordered application and flow rate.

Comfort level: Assess for pain (location, duration, and intensity) and determine whether analgesics were given in the PACU. Assess for nausea and vomiting.

Position and safety: Place the patient in an ordered position (eg, after spinal anesthesia, patient may have to remain flat for a specified period), or if the patient is not fully conscious, place him or her in the side-lying position. Elevate the side rails and place the bed in low position.

Comfort: Cover the patient with a blanket, reorient him or her to the room as necessary, and allow family members to remain with the patient after the initial assessment is completed.

After assessment, document the time of arrival and all assessment data obtained. Follow agency protocol for assessment routines: common time frames are every 15 minutes until stable, changing to every 1 to 2 hours for the first 24 hours, and to every 4 hours thereafter. Although agency protocols are used for guidelines in the immediate postoperative period, the nurse is responsible for adjusting the frequency and priorities of assessment to the specific needs of each patient.

DIAGNOSING

Nursing diagnoses in the postoperative phase may represent actual problems or those for which the patient is at risk for altered responses. Collaborative problems are identified to implement nursing actions necessary for monitoring and preventing postoperative complications. When making nursing diagnoses, the nurse uses assessment data and plans of care established before and during surgery and includes the family. Examples of postoperative nursing diagnoses and their etiology might include the following:

Risk for Surgical Site Infection related to traumatic wound of right arm in farm vehicle accident

Pain related to right flank incision

Altered Family Processes related to loss of economic stability after surgical treatment for bone malignancy

Impaired Verbal Communication related to repair and wiring of fractured jaw

Impaired Skin Integrity related to incision on left anterior thorax

Impaired Physical Mobility related to inability to be independent in movement secondary to surgical repair of fractured right hip

Appropriate collaborative problems for the patient in the postoperative period include the following (Carpenito, 1999):

Potential complication: Hemorrhage
Potential complication: Evisceration
Potential complication: Dehiscence
Potential complication: Urinary retention
Potential complication: Thrombophlebitis
Potential complication: Paralytic ileus

PLANNING: EXPECTED OUTCOMES

The plan of care in the postoperative phase begins in the preoperative phase, when nursing activities to reduce stress and teach postoperative activities are carried out. From admission, the patient and family are prepared for uneventful recovery and self-care after discharge. Specific expected outcomes are individualized, based on risk fac-

tors, the surgical procedure, and the patient's unique needs. Examples of desired postoperative outcomes for a patient after major surgery are as follows. The patient will achieve the following goals:

*   Carry out leg exercises every 2 to 4 hours
*   Deep breathe and cough effectively every 2 hours
*   Verbalize decreasing levels of pain
*   Have a balanced intake and output
*   Regain normal bowel and bladder elimination
*   Have a well-healed surgical incision
*   Remain free of infection
*   Verbalize any concerns about appearance of wound
*   Verbalize and demonstrate wound self-care
    The aims of nursing are as follows:
*   Assess and monitor the patient's physical and emotional status
*   Promote physical and psychological comfort and safety
*   Prevent complications
*   Facilitate coping with alterations in structure or function
*   Promote a return to health and maximize wellness

IMPLEMENTING

Many nursing activities implemented in the postoperative phase have already been discussed in this chapter or are fully discussed in other chapters; therefore, this section focuses on the nursing interventions implemented to meet the expected outcomes of the plan of care. Nursing care to prevent complications, promote a return to health, and facilitate coping with alterations are discussed.

Preventing Postoperative Complications

A wide variety of factors increase the risk of postoperative complications. These have been described in the preoperative and intraoperative sections of this chapter and include age, health habits, physical condition, medical history, psychological status, and surgical intervention (anesthesia, positioning, wound). Ongoing postoperative assessments and teaching are implemented to decrease the risk for postoperative complications, as discussed in the following sections.

Preventing Cardiovascular Complications

Nursing interventions to prevent or monitor for cardiovascular complications are as follows:

*   Assess and document vital signs as ordered and as the patient's status dictates, using preoperative assessments as a baseline.
*   Provide covers, forced warm air, or other warming device or techniques as necessary to prevent shivering and hypothermia.
*   Maintain fluid balance.
    *   Maintain accurate intake and output.
    *   Monitor rate, type, access site of intravenous fluids.

- Assess skin turgor and hydration of mucous membranes.
- Monitor amount, color, and consistency of wound drainage (dressings and drains or tubes).
- Implement leg exercises and turning in bed every 2 hours.
- Assist with ambulation. Ambulation usually begins the evening of surgery and increases as tolerated; blood pressure and pulse and respiratory rates monitor tolerance.
- Apply and follow protocols for antiembolic stockings or compression devices, if ordered.
- Administer prescribed anticoagulant medications.
- Measure bilateral calf and thigh circumference daily. This is a more accurate assessment of thrombophlebitis than Homans' sign (pain in the calf when the foot is dorsiflexed).
- Avoid positioning that impedes venous return (eg, do not mechanically raise the knee portion of the bed or place pillows under the knees).

Specific cardiovascular complications include shock, hemorrhage, thrombophlebitis, and pulmonary embolus.

Shock

Shock is the body's reaction to acute peripheral circulatory failure as the result of an alteration in circulatory control or as a response to a loss of circulating fluid. The type of shock most commonly seen in postoperative patients is *hypovolemic shock*, which occurs from a decrease in blood volume. Common indications of shock are hypotension; cold, clammy skin; a weak, thready, and rapid pulse; cool, mottled extremities; deep, rapid respirations; decreased urine output; thirst; apprehension; and restlessness. The primary purpose of care for a patient in shock is to improve and maintain tissue perfusion by eliminating the cause of the shock. Following are recommended interventions when caring for a patient in shock:

- Establish and maintain airway.
- Place the patient in a flat position with the legs elevated 45 degrees. (The Trendelenburg, or "shock," position is no longer recommended because it causes the diaphragm to ascend, reducing total lung volume and ventilation.)
- Be prepared to assist with the insertion of intravenous lines (cutdowns in the long saphenous vein at the ankle or in the basilic vein in the antecubital space to monitor central venous pressure may be initiated) and fluid administration as well as administration of whole blood or its components.
- Administer oxygen therapy as indicated.
- Place extra covering on the patient to maintain warmth.
- Administer medications as prescribed.
- Monitor vital signs, urine output, hematocrit, blood gas results, and general condition.
- Provide psychological support to the patient and family.

Hemorrhage

Hemorrhage is an excessive blood loss, either internally or externally. Hemorrhage may lead to hypovolemic shock. It may occur from a slipped suture, a dislodged clot in the wound, or stress on the surgical site; it may also be the result of pathophysiologic conditions or certain medications. Common indications of hemorrhage are restlessness, anxiety, and frank bleeding as well as the symptoms listed previously for shock. The primary purposes of care for the patient having a hemorrhage include stopping the bleeding and replacing blood volume. The following interventions are recommended when caring for the patient who is hemorrhaging:

- Apply a pressure dressing to the bleeding site.
- Be prepared to have the patient return to the operating room if bleeding cannot be stopped or is massive.
- Provide nursing care as outlined for the patient in shock.

Thrombophlebitis

Thrombophlebitis is an inflammation of a vein associated with thrombus (blood clot) formation. Thrombophlebitis from venous stasis is most commonly seen in the legs of postoperative patients, especially in varicose veins (Minkes & Baumann, 1997). Common indications of thrombophlebitis are pain and cramping in the calf or thigh of the involved extremity, redness and swelling in the affected area, elevated temperature, and an increase in the diameter of the involved extremity. Care for the patient with thrombophlebitis includes preventing a clot from breaking loose and becoming an embolus that travels to the lungs, heart, or brain and preventing further clot formation. Interventions in caring for the patient with thrombophlebitis are as follows:

- Administer antiinflammatory medications as prescribed; anticoagulants are usually ordered for deep-vein thrombosis.
- Maintain bed rest (sometimes with limb elevation) as ordered.
- Use high antiembolic stockings or sequential pneumatic compression devices (see the accompanying box), and follow protocols for care.
- Do not massage or rub the legs.
- Give analgesics and use external heat applications as ordered.
- Measure bilateral calf or thigh circumference every shift.
- Provide emotional support to the patient and family.

Pulmonary Embolus

An *embolus* is a blood clot or other foreign substance that is dislodged and travels through the bloodstream until it lodges in another smaller vessel. In postoperative patients, the embolus is often part of a thrombus that breaks free from a vein wall. If the embolus lodges in the pulmonary vessels, it is called a *pulmonary embolus*. Common indications of a pulmonary embolus include dyspnea, chest pain, cough, cyanosis, rapid respirations, tachycardia, and anxiety. The primary goals of care are to stabilize cardiovascular and respiratory function and to prevent further

Pneumatic Compression Devices

Pneumatic compression devices are composed of an air pump, connecting tubes, and an extremity sleeve. The sleeve may cover the entire leg or may extend from the foot to the knee. A variety of types are available; the accompanying figure provides one example. The devices apply brief pressure to the legs to enhance blood flow and venous return, thereby decreasing the risk for thrombophlebitis after surgery. The devices may apply either intermittent or sequential pressure. Intermittent pneumatic compression devices fit over the entire leg, with inflation and deflation of the sleeve covering the leg alternating from one leg to the other by a preset timer. Sequential pneumatic compression devices are designed so that pressure moves up the leg in increments. They may inflate and deflate by alternating from one leg to the other, or they may do so for both legs at once.

Nursing Care

- Explain the purpose of the device to the patient.
- Apply the device so that two fingers fit between the leg and the sleeve.

- Position the tubing so the patient can move about without interrupting the air flow.
- Remove the sleeves at least once a day for skin care and assessment.
- Assess the extremities for peripheral pulses, edema, changes in sensation, and movement on a regular schedule.
- Ensure that all chambers are inflating in proper sequence once per shift.

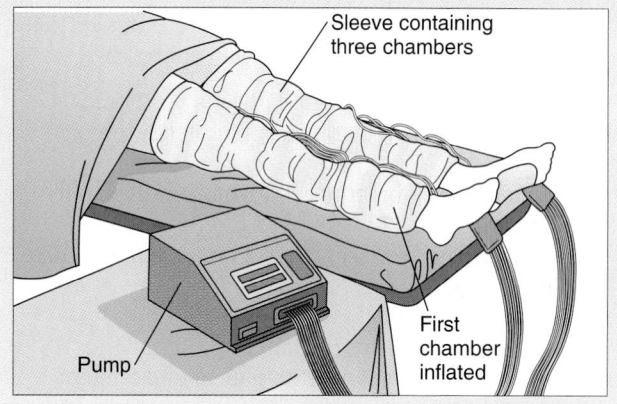

Sleeve containing three chambers

Pump

First chamber inflated

---

emboli. Following are recommended interventions for the patient with a pulmonary embolus:

- Contact the physician immediately if symptoms occur; pulmonary embolus is a life-threatening complication, and immediate treatment is necessary.
- Maintain bed rest with the patient in the semi-Fowler's position.
- Maintain fluid balance; avoid overhydration with intravenous fluids.
- Administer oxygen therapy as appropriate.
- Administer anticoagulant medications as ordered.
- Administer prescribed analgesic medications for pain; use caution with narcotic analgesics, which depress respirations.
- Assess vital signs and general status frequently.
- Instruct the patient to avoid Valsalva's maneuver (forced exhalation against a closed glottis, such as straining to have a bowel movement) to prevent increased intrathoracic pressure and, possibly, increased emboli.
- Provide emotional support for the patient and family.

Preventing Respiratory Complications

Nursing interventions to prevent or monitor for respiratory complications are as follows:

- Assess and monitor vital signs, using preoperative assessments as a baseline.
- Implement deep breathing, coughing, incentive spirometry, and turning in bed every 2 hours.

- Ambulate as ordered.
- Maintain hydration.
- Avoid positioning that decreases ventilation.
- Carefully monitor responses to narcotic analgesics.

Specific respiratory complications include pneumonia and atelectasis.

Pneumonia

Pneumonia is an inflammation of the alveoli as the result of an infectious process or presence of foreign material. Pneumonia may occur postoperatively as a result of aspiration, infection, depressed cough reflex, increased secretions from anesthesia, dehydration, and immobilization. Indications of pneumonia are an elevated temperature, chills, a cough that produces rusty or purulent sputum, crackles and wheezes, dyspnea, and chest pain. The goals of care are to treat the underlying infection, maintain respiratory status, and prevent spread of microorganisms. Following are recommended interventions in caring for the patient with pneumonia:

- Promote full aeration of the lungs by positioning the patient in semi-Fowler's or Fowler's position.
- Administer oxygen therapy as indicated or prescribed.
- Maintain fluid and nutritional status.
- Administer antibiotics as prescribed.
- Administer expectorants and analgesics as prescribed.
- Implement deep-breathing and coughing exercises every 2 hours.

- Provide frequent oral hygiene.
- Teach proper disposal of tissues and sputum.
- Ensure rest and comfort.
- Provide emotional support to patient and family.

Atelectasis

Atelectasis is the incomplete expansion or collapse of alveoli with retained mucus, involving a portion of lung and resulting in poor gas exchange. Indications of atelectasis include decreased lung sounds over the affected area, dyspnea, cyanosis, crackles, restlessness, and apprehension. The primary goals of care for patients with atelectasis are to ensure oxygenation of tissues, prevent further atelectasis, and expand involved lung tissues. Following are recommended interventions in caring for the patient with atelectasis:

- Position the patient in semi-Fowler's position.
- Administer oxygen therapy as indicated or prescribed.
- Implement deep breathing, coughing, and incentive spirometry every 2 hours.
- Implement leg exercises every 2 hours and ambulate as prescribed.
- Maintain hydration.
- Administer analgesics for pain as prescribed.
- Provide emotional support to patient and family.

Preventing Surgical Site Complications

The nurse assesses and cares for the surgical site to promote healing and prevent complications. Wound care is discussed in Chapter 37. Specific nursing interventions to prevent and monitor for complications at the surgical site are as follows:

- Assess vital signs, especially temperature elevation.
- Maintain hydration.
- Maintain nutritional status; encourage diet high in proteins, carbohydrates, calories, and vitamins
- Use proper handwashing techniques.
- Maintain aseptic technique when changing dressings at the surgical site and exit sites for tubes and drains. Follow standard precautions for disposing of soiled gloves, dressings, and so forth.

Promoting a Return to Health

Nurses provide interventions during postoperative recovery to promote the return of the patient's physical and psychological functioning to as near a normal state as possible. The plan of care to achieve this goal includes activities to meet elimination, fluid and electrolyte, nutrition, and rest and comfort needs.

Meeting Elimination Needs

Both urinary and bowel elimination can be altered by anesthesia, manipulation of organs during the surgical intervention, inactivity, and altered fluid and food intake during the perioperative period. The following nursing assessments and interventions promote the return of normal bowel elimination:

- Assess for the return of peristalsis by auscultating bowel sounds every 4 hours when the patient is awake.
  - Assess abdominal distention, especially if bowel sounds are not audible or are high pitched (indicative of possible paralytic ileus, which is an absence of intestinal peristalsis).
  - Assess the patient's ability to pass flatus and stool.
- Assist with movement in bed and ambulation to relieve gas pains, a common postoperative discomfort.
- Encourage food and fluid intake when ordered, especially fruit juices and high-fiber foods.
- Maintain privacy when patient is using the bedpan, commode, or bathroom.
- Administer suppositories, enemas, or medications, such as stool softeners, as prescribed.

The following nursing assessments and interventions promote the return of normal urinary elimination:

- Monitor intake and output.
- Assist the patient in assuming normal position to void by using an upright position when on a bedpan and using a bedside commode or bathroom when able, or by assisting the male patient to stand upright to void with a urinal.
- Assess for bladder distention by palpating above the symphysis pubis if the patient has not voided within 8 hours after surgery or if the patient has been voiding frequently in amounts of less than 50 mL; notify the physician with assessment results.
- Maintain prescribed intravenous fluid infusion rates.
- Encourage oral fluid intake when prescribed.
- Provide privacy when the patient is using bedpan, bedside commode, urinal, or bathroom.
- Initiate urinary catheterization if prescribed.

Meeting Fluid and Nutrition Needs

Fluid and nutrition needs can be met by implementing the following nursing assessments and interventions:

- Monitor intake and output.
- Maintain prescribed intravenous fluid infusion rates.
- Assess for dehydration and weight loss.
- Provide oral hygiene before meals and as needed.
- Monitor tolerance of postoperative dietary progression (often from clear to full liquids, then from soft to regular diet).
- Maintain an environment conducive to appetite (clean and neat, with elimination of odors).
- Encourage the patient to sit up in bed or a chair for meals.
- Encourage family participation in meals.

Meeting Comfort and Rest Needs

After surgery, comfort needs are a priority. Factors that interfere with the surgical patient's comfort include nausea, vomiting, thirst, hiccups, and pain at the surgical site. Following are suggested nursing interventions that promote rest and comfort by providing relief for these potential problems.

Nausea and Vomiting

- Avoid large intake of fluids or food at one time, especially after being NPO.
- Administer prescribed medications.
- Provide oral hygiene as needed.
- Maintain clean environment.
- Avoid use of a straw.
- Avoid strong-smelling food.
- Assess for possible allergic response to medications, such as antibiotics or analgesics.
- Maintain bowel elimination.

Thirst

- Offer sips of water or ice chips when NPO (if permitted).
- Maintain oral hygiene.

Hiccups

- Have the patient do the following:
  - Take several swallows of water while holding the breath (if not NPO).
  - Rebreathe into a paper bag.
  - Eat a teaspoon of granulated sugar.

Surgical Pain

- Assess pain frequently; administer prescribed analgesics every 2 to 4 hours on a regular schedule during the first 24 to 36 hours after surgery.
- Reinforce preoperative teaching for pain management.
- Offer nonpharmacologic measures to supplement medications: massage, position changes, relaxation, guided imagery, meditation, music.

Comfort and rest are also promoted by providing personal hygiene, keeping bed linens clean, providing quiet rest periods, and allowing family members to remain with the patient.

Helping the Patient Cope

Surgery may alter physical appearance as well as normal physiologic function, leading to the risk for or actual alterations in self-concept and body image. Changes in a person's self-perception can influence all of the human dimensions and areas of human functioning, including self-esteem, relationships with others, sexual identity, spiritual beliefs, sociocultural values, and independent and fulfilling engagement in activities of daily living.

Many surgical patients have the same reaction to loss of a body part as to a death (see Chap. 31 for a discussion of crisis; loss and grief are more fully discussed in Chap. 32). The response and adaptation to it are influenced by multiple factors, including age, cultural values and beliefs, sociocultural background, significance of the body part, visibility of the body part, time to prepare for the change, and support people available. A surgical patient's grief is a normal, appropriate response. It is unique to the person experiencing it, and although there are stages and phases of grief, there is no timetable for it. The nurse must be aware and accepting of the patient's needs and must establish interventions to meet needs in coping with change. The nursing process is used to implement interventions, beginning with the patient's decision to have surgery and continuing through convalescence. Nursing activities to facilitate coping are as follows:

- Accept each patient as a unique individual.
- Identify through verbal and nonverbal cues those patients who are at risk for alteration in self-concept (risk is increased if the patient has little support from others, a visible alteration, or an alteration that will seriously affect functional ability).
- Allow time for patients and families to verbalize their feelings about the alteration, and do not assume that all patients will have problems.
- Identify and support strengths and effective coping mechanisms.
- Encourage the patient and family to be part of goal setting and decision making throughout the surgical experience.
- Provide teaching and honest information to the patient and family about all aspects of care.
- Work collaboratively with other members of the health team to provide referrals and resources as necessary to meet physical, psychological, and spiritual needs.

Providing Ambulatory Surgery Postoperative Care

Evaluating the patient's postoperative status after ambulatory surgery focuses on ensuring that the patient can be safely cared for at home. After surgery and recovery from the anesthetic, the patient is asked to sit up and drink liquids. A patient who is no longer drowsy or dizzy, has stable vital signs, and has voided is allowed to go home accompanied by a responsible adult. The patient is not allowed to drive a car to go home. The usual length of time from completion of surgery to discharge is 1 to 3 hours, provided that established criteria have been met. Written and verbal instructions for home care are given to the patient and family.

EVALUATING

Evaluating the patient's achievement of desired outcomes for postoperative recovery and rehabilitation may be accomplished in a number of ways. Because the final resolution of some desired outcomes may not be apparent or measurable at the time of discharge, many institutions use follow-up telephone calls or written surveys that are mailed to patients. It may also be possible to work with the physician's office to have a patient complete a survey on the first postoperative visit. Whatever mechanism is selected, important outcomes, such as the absence of surgical site infection, the patient's satisfaction with pain management measures, return to former levels of mobility and activity, and the absence of postoperative complications for which the patient was at risk, should be included as part of evaluative criteria.

Learning Outcomes

After studying this chapter, the learner should be able to accomplish the following:

1. Define the key terms used in the chapter.

   advance directives
   circulating nurse
   conscious sedation/
     analgesia
   elective surgery
   emergency surgery
   general anesthesia
   informed consent
   intraoperative phase

   perioperative nursing
   perioperative period
   postanesthesia care
   postoperative phase
   preoperative phase
   registered nurse first
     assistant
   regional anesthesia

2. Describe the surgical experience, including perioperative phases, postanesthesia phases, categories of surgery, types of anesthesia, informed consent, and advance directives.

3. Conduct a preoperative nursing history and physical assessment to identify patient strengths as well as factors that increase the risks for surgical and postoperative complications.
4. Teach preoperative exercises: deep breathing, coughing, and leg exercises.
5. Prepare a patient physically and psychologically for surgery.
6. Identify assessments specific to the prevention of complications in the immediate postoperative phase.
7. Use the nursing process to develop knowledgeably an individualized plan of care for the surgical patient during each phase of the perioperative period.
8. Provide information to patients and caregivers for self-care at home.

Critical Thinking Exercises

1. You are providing the immediate preoperative care for a woman scheduled for surgery to debulk a brain tumor. She tells you that she does not want the surgery because she knows she is dying and just wants to go home to be with her husband and children. She also knows that her husband cannot accept the fact that she is dying and wants the surgery. What do you do?

2. You are assigned to discharge a woman from your same-day surgery unit to her home. You strongly believe that she is not ready to go home, and there is no caretaker in her home. When you voice your concern to the surgeon, you are told that this is not your problem, and that there is nothing anyone can do about the situation because her insurer will not approve hospitalization. How do you respond?

Study Questions

1. Mrs. Ogg requires surgery for treatment of a ruptured spleen as the result of an automobile accident. This type of surgery belongs in which of the following categories?
   a. minor, diagnostic
   b. minor, elective
   c. major, emergency
   d. major, palliative
2. A general anesthetic is given for specific purposes during a surgical procedure. Which one of the following purposes is not included?
   a. loss of consciousness
   b. relaxation of skeletal muscles
   c. reduction of reflex action
   d. localized loss of sensation
3. You have been asked to witness a patient signature on an informed consent form for surgery. You recognize that the document is valid for which one of these patients?
   a. a 92-year-old patient who is severely confused
   b. a 45-year-old patient who is oriented and alert
   c. a 10-year-old patient who is oriented and alert
   d. a 36-year-old patient who has had a narcotic premedication

4. Although surgical patients may be taking any number of medications before surgery, which of the following categories of drugs would be most likely to increase surgical risk?
   a. anticoagulants
   b. antacids
   c. laxatives
   d. sedatives
5. An obese patient who has surgery is at risk for which of the following postoperative complications?
   a. hunger
   b. impaired wound healing
   c. hemorrhage
   d. gas pains
6. Which of these teaching methods would be most effective in preoperative teaching for ambulatory surgery?
   a. lecture with video
   b. discussion
   c. audiovisuals
   d. written instructions
7. Mr. Ying is scheduled for surgery. He says to you, "I am so frightened—what if I don't wake up?" What would be your best response?

a. "You have a wonderful doctor."
b. "Let's talk about how you are feeling."
c. "Everyone wakes up from surgery!"
d. "Don't worry, you will be just fine."

8. A PCA pump allows postoperative patients to
   a. be totally pain free
   b. take unlimited amounts of medication
   c. choose the type of pain medication
   d. administer his or her own analgesic

9. Mr. Moreno has had a surgical procedure that necessitated a thoracic incision. You anticipate that he will have a higher risk for postoperative complications involving which body system?
   a. respiratory system
   b. circulatory system
   c. digestive system
   d. nervous system

10. While assessing a patient in the PACU, the perianesthesia nurse notes increased wound drainage, restlessness, a decreasing blood pressure, and an increase in the pulse rate. The most probable cause for these findings is
    a. thrombophlebitis
    b. atelectasis
    c. infection
    d. hemorrhage

11. Your patient tells you she is having pain in her right lower leg. You assess the presence of thrombophlebitis by
    a. palpating the skin over the tibia and fibula
    b. measuring and documenting calf circumference daily

c. taking and recording vital signs four times a day
d. noting difficulty with ambulation

12. Gas pains are a common postoperative discomfort. Which of the following nursing actions implemented in the plan of care would be most likely to relieve gas pains?
    a. cough and deep breathe every 2 hours
    b. maintain NPO status for 48 hours
    c. encourage frequent ambulation
    d. take vital signs every 4 hours

13. Which of the following surgical patients is at a greater risk for alterations in body image?
    a. female, aged 19 years, large facial laceration
    b. female, aged 42 years, gallbladder surgery
    c. male, aged 14 years, fractured clavicle
    d. male, aged 52 years, hernia repair

14. Older adults often have reduced vital capacity as a normal physiologic change. Which nursing action would be most important for the postoperative care of an older surgical patient specific to this change?
    a. Take and record vital signs every shift.
    b. Turn, cough, and deep breathe every 4 hours.
    c. Encourage increased intake of oral fluids.
    d. Assess bowel sounds daily.

15. The rationale for the use of leg exercises after surgery is that leg exercises
    a. promote respiratory function
    b. maintain functional abilities
    c. provide diversional activities
    d. increase venous return

Answers With Rationale

1. The correct response is c. This surgery would involve a major body organ, has the potential for postoperative complications, requires hospitalization, and must be done immediately to preserve the patient's life.

2. The correct response is d. Whereas a, b, and c are all purposes of a general anesthetic, a localized loss of sensation occurs with a regional anesthetic.

3. The correct response is b. A consent form is not legal if the patient signing the form is confused, sedated, or a minor.

4. The correct response is a. Anticoagulant drug therapy would increase the risk for hemorrhage during surgery. The other categories of drugs normally would not increase surgical risk.

5. The correct response is b. Fatty tissue is less vascular and therefore less resistant to infection and more prone to delayed wound healing.

6. The correct response is d. Although all of the responses might be useful in teaching patients and families before ambulatory surgery, written instructions are most effective in providing information.

7. The correct response is b. This response allows the patient to talk about feelings and fears and is

therapeutic. The other responses give false reassurance.

8. The correct response is d. A PCA pump allows the patient to administer his or her own analgesic. Use of this device does not allow the patient to take unlimited amounts of medication, choose the type of pain medication, or be totally pain free.

9. The correct response is a. A thoracic incision makes it more painful for the patient to take deep breaths or cough. Shallow respirations and ineffective coughing increase the risk for respiratory complications.

10. The correct response is d. Increased wound drainage, restlessness, decreasing blood pressure, and increasing pulse rate are assessment findings that indicate hemorrhage.

11. The correct response is b. Inflammation from thrombophlebitis increases the size of the affected extremity and can be assessed by measuring circumference on a regular basis.

12. The correct response is c. Frequent ambulation stimulates peristalsis and relieves gas pains. The other responses are incorrect in this situation.

13. The correct response is a. The reaction of the patient to an accidental or intentional incision is influenced by age, time to prepare for the change, and visibility of the trauma. Large facial wounds increase the risk for an alteration in body image.

14. The correct response is b. Reduced vital capacity in older adults increases the risk for respiratory complications, including pneumonia and atelectasis. Having the patient turn, cough, and deep breathe every 4 hours maintains respiratory function and helps to prevent complications.

15. The correct response is d. Leg exercises in the postoperative period do increase venous return. As a result, the patient has decreased risk for thrombophlebitis and emboli.

Bibliography

Agency for Health Care Policy and Research. (1992). *Acute pain management: Operative or medical procedures and trauma. Clinical practice guidelines.* DHHS Pub. No. (AHCPR) 920032. Silver Spring, MD: Author.

American Society of PeriAnesthesia Nurses. (1998). *Standards of perianesthesia nursing practice.* Thorofare, NJ: Author.

Association of Operating Room Nurses. (1997). *AORN's Age-Specific Competency Series.* Denver, CO: Author.

Association of Operating Room Nurses. (1999). *AORN standards, recommended practices and guidelines.* Denver, CO: Author.

Berg, M. (1998). An introduction to anesthesia-related medications. *Journal of Perianesthesia Nursing, 13*(4), 239–242.

Borchardt, M. (1999). Review of the clinical pharmacology and use of the benzodiazepines. *Journal of Perianesthesia Nursing,14*(2), 65–72.

Carpenito, L. J. (1999). *Nursing care plans and documentation: Nursing diagnoses and collaborative problems* (3rd ed.). Philadelphia: Lippincott Williams & Wilkins.

Christie, F. (1998). Pulmonary embolism. *American Journal of Nursing, 98*(11), 36–37.

Crenshaw, J. (1999). Research for practice: New guidelines for preoperative fasting. *American Journal of Nursing, 99*(4), 49.

Faries, J. (1998). Easing your patient's postoperative pain. *Nursing, 28*(6), 58–60.

Gillanders, W. E., & Moley, J. F. (1997). *The Washington manual of surgery.* Boston, MA: Little, Brown.

Goodwin, S. A. (1999). Notes from the American Society of Anesthesiologists meeting. *Journal of Perianesthesia Nursing, 14*(2), 102–105.

Haynor, P. M. (1998). Meeting the challenges of advanced directives. *American Journal of Nursing, 98*(3), 27–33.

Heiser, R. M., Chiles, K., Fudge, M., & Gray, S. E. (1997). The use of music during the immediate postoperative recovery period. *AORN Journal, 65*(4), 777–784.

Hodson, D. M. (1998). The evolving role of advanced practice nurses in surgery. *AORN Journal, 67*(5), 998–1009.

Hoshowsky, V. M. (1998). Surgical positioning. *Orthopaedic Nursing, 17*(5), 55–65.

Janikowski, D. L., & Rockefeller, C. A. (1998). Awake and talking: Ambulatory surgery and conscious sedation. *Nursing Economics, 16*(1), 37–42.

Kost, M. (1999). Conscious sedation: Guarding your patient against complications. *Nursing, 29*(4), 34–39.

Meeker, M. H., & Rothrock, J. C. (1999). *Alexander's care of the patient in surgery* (11th ed.). St. Louis: C. V. Mosby.

Minkes, R. K., & Baumann, D. S. (1997). *The Washington manual of surgery.* Boston, MA: Little, Brown.

Noble, K. (1999). PACU: Ensuring a safe experience. *Advance for Nurses, 1*(5), 11–13.

Patton, C. M. (1999). Preoperative nursing assessment of the adult patient. *Seminars in Perioperative Nursing, 8*(1), 42–47.

Pessagno, J. J. (1999). Ambulatory care: Adjusting to the evolution of a changing health care system. *Advances for Nurses, 1*(8), 20–21.

Ramnarine-Singh, S. (1999). The surgical significance of therapeutic touch. *AORN Journal, 69*(2), 358–369.

Sessler, D. I. (1997). Mild perioperative hypothermia. *New England Journal of Medicine, 336,* 1730–1737.

Smeltzer, S. C. & Bare, B. G (2000). *Brunner & Suddarth's textbook of medical-surgical nursing* (9th ed.). Philadelphia: Lippincott Williams & Wilkins.

Stoller, J. K., & Kester, L. (1998). Respiratory care protocols in postanesthesia care. *Journal of Perianesthesia Nursing, 13*(6), 349–357.

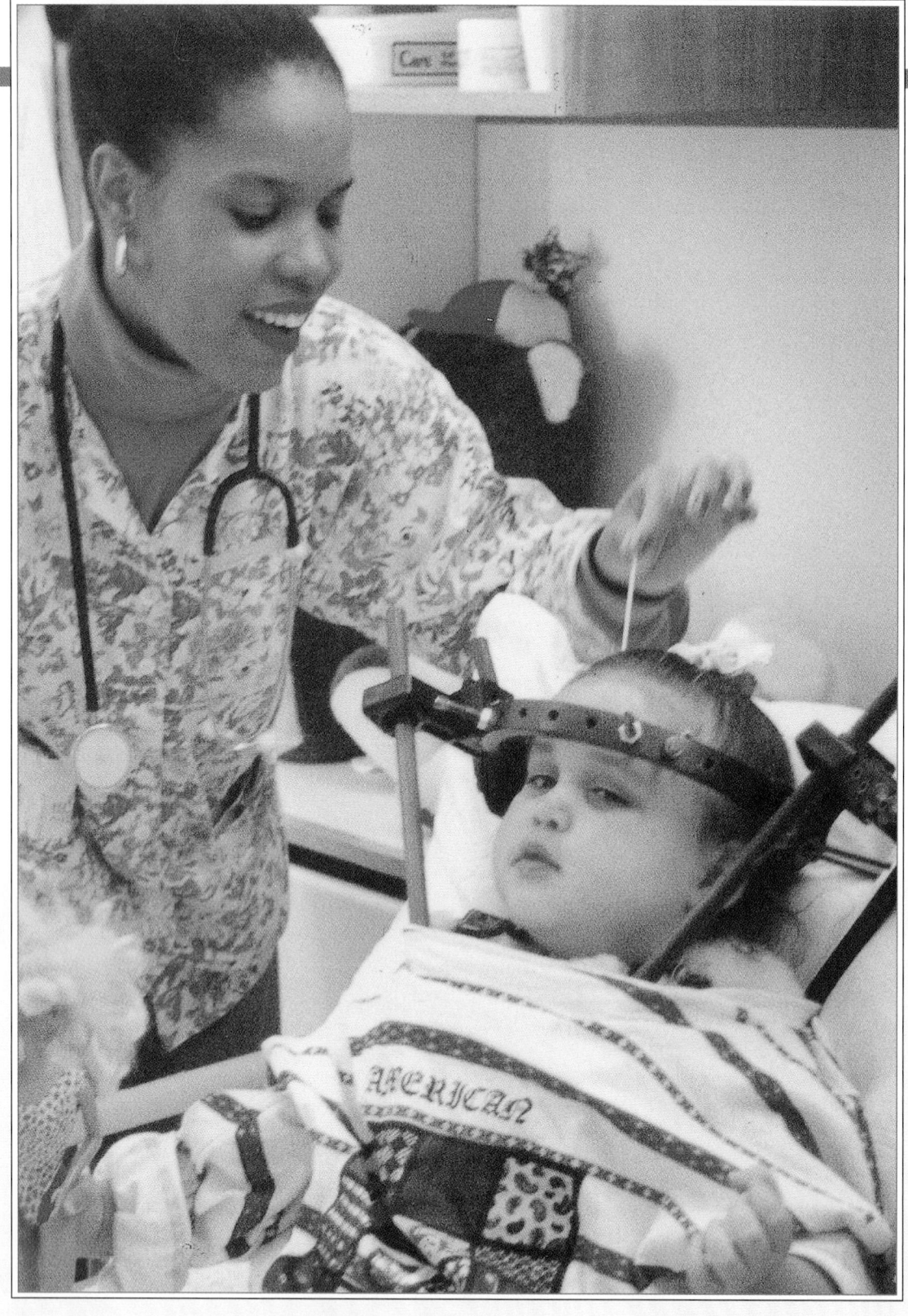

UNIT VII

Promoting Healthy Psychosocial Responses

"The unique function of the nurse is to assist the individual . . . in the performance of those activities contributing to health or its recovery (or to peaceful death) that he would perform unaided if he had the necessary strength, will or knowledge . . . in such a way as to help him gain independence as rapidly as possible."

Virginia Henderson (1897–   )
the "first lady of nursing," whose career spanned almost 70 years as both author and researcher; her works on nursing principles are research based and have been translated into 25 languages

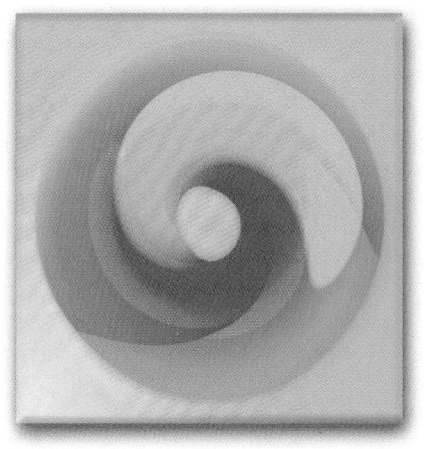

Each individual is a composite of interrelated physiologic and psychosocial dimensions; alterations in one dimension affect all of the others. Unit VII discusses psychosocial considerations in holistic patient care, focusing on self-concept; stress and adaptation; loss, grief, and dying; sensory stimulation; sexuality; and spirituality.

One's sense of self may contribute positively or negatively to health and self-care abilities. Similarly, stress can motivate or thwart growth and self-actualization. Nursing interventions to maintain, strengthen, or change self-concept and to promote healthy adaptation are basic to all aspects of patient care.

Loss, grief, and dying are universal human experiences that most nurses encounter in some form on a daily basis. Effective nurses are competent and willing to assist people struggling with loss, grief, and dying.

Intact and functioning senses are necessary for life, normal growth and development, and pleasurable experiences. Alterations in any of the senses require caring, knowledgeable, and individualized nursing interventions to meet needs and prevent further overload or deprivation.

Sexuality and spirituality are important components of human functioning. These dimensions are an integral part of each person's identity and are critical elements in holistic patient care. To facilitate sexual and spiritual wellness, nurses must develop self-awareness in these areas and become aware of values and practices different than their own. Nursing interventions and therapeutic interpersonal skills are used to elicit concerns, identify needs, implement teaching, make referrals, and demonstrate empathic acceptance and caring.

Unit VII provides the knowledge base for promoting healthy psychosocial responses in patients. Using the nursing process, interventions can be planned and implemented to meet needs and support strengths in both health and illness.

Chapter 30
Self-Concept

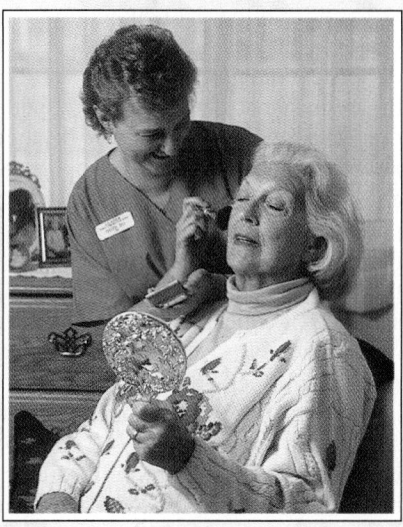

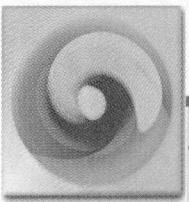

**Thinking Critically About
Nursing's Blended Skills**

Before reading this chapter, think about the types of skills you will need to enhance the self-concepts of patients, family caregivers, and colleagues.

- Lourie, a 16-year-old single teenager, confides to you, the school nurse, that she is pregnant, wants to keep the baby, and knows her life is over. "My mother told me I'd never amount to anything."

- A colleague invites you to speak at a local nursing home to the nursing assistants about meeting the self-esteem needs of the residents.

- Chad is 12 years of age and has cancer. He is refusing his chemotherapy medications because he is tired of being sick and says that losing his hair will be the last straw. "I can't go to school bald!"

- Raul is 22 years of age and has just learned that he has herpes simplex, a sexually transmitted disease. He does not know how this will affect his ability to be intimate with sexual partners. "I sort of feel like 'damaged goods' now."

What cognitive, interpersonal, and ethical/legal skills do you think you will need to meet the everyday challenges of professional nursing?

As people move through the hierarchy of human needs to higher levels, needs for self-esteem and self-actualization arise, as discussed in Chapter 2. The need for **self-esteem** is the need to feel good about oneself and to believe that others hold one in high regard. The need for **self-actualization** is the need to reach one's potential through full development of one's unique capability. A critical component of both these needs is self-concept. One's self-image or **self-concept** has the power to either encourage or thwart personal growth.

People with deficient self-concept may lack the motivation to learn self-care behaviors in response to illness, injury, and trauma. Nursing efforts aimed at teaching new health behaviors may fail until the patient values himself or herself enough to want to invest energy in self-care. On the other hand, patients may desperately want to modify their self-concept and self-care behaviors and have no idea how to do it. The experience of illness, diagnostic testing, and treatment can severely threaten the self-concept of a patient. Nurses sensitive to the self-concept needs of patients can use each nurse–patient interaction to enhance the patient's sense of self and to assist the patient in resolving self-concept disturbances.

Study of this chapter provides knowledge of the dimensions of self-concept, formation of self-concept, and key factors affecting self-concept. Practical interview guides are offered for assessing self-concept (personal identity, body image, self-esteem, role performance). Strategies for enhancing the self-esteem of the nurse are provided. Numerous examples of nursing diagnoses are given, and specific nursing strategies for assisting patients to meet self-concept goals/outcomes are described. These guides and the concluding patient care study illustrate how the nurse's knowledge of self-concept may be combined with skilled nursing interventions and caring to resolve successfully disturbances in self-concept.

Overview of Self-Concept

Dimensions of Self-Concept

Self-concept is the mental image or picture of self. All the feelings, beliefs, and values associated with "I" or "me" compose self-concept. Included in the notion of self-concept are personal identity, body image, self-esteem, and role performance.

The dimensions of self-knowledge, self-expectations, and self-evaluation describe self-concept. People with a positive self-concept have broad and diversified knowledge of the self, realistic expectations, and high self-esteem.

Self-Knowledge: "Who Am I?"
A person's self-knowledge includes basic facts (age, race, occupation), which place that person in social groups, and a listing of qualities or traits, which describe typical behaviors, feelings, moods, and other characteristics (generous, hot-headed, ambitious, intelligent, sexy). Although some labels cannot be changed (eg, sex, age, and race), most are unstable and subjective. **Global self** is the term used to describe the composite of all the basic facts, qualities, traits, and images one holds about oneself.

Self-Expectations: "Who or What Do I Want to Be?"
Expectations for the self flow from the **ideal self,** the self one wants to be or thinks one should be. These expectations often develop early in childhood and are based on the image of a role model. These expectations may be healthy or unhealthy. Many contemporary thinkers are expressing

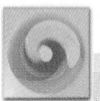

COGNITIVE SKILLS

- Knowledge of basic self-concept theory and variables that influence the development of self-concept and its relationship to health and health behaviors
- Knowledge of how to use the nursing process to identify, diagnose, and resolve self-concept disturbances
- Knowledge of how to teach others to use self therapeutically to meet the needs of nursing home residents

INTERPERSONAL SKILLS

- Strong people skills to establish trusting relationships with the new mother, nursing assistants, preteen with cancer, and young adult with herpes simplex

- Ability to use self therapeutically to enhance the self-concept of patients, family caregivers, and colleagues
- Ability to help patients find the motivation to develop new health and coping behaviors

ETHICAL/LEGAL SKILLS

- First and foremost, a strong sense of accountability for the health and well-being of these individuals; a commitment to getting them the help they need to achieve their health goals—within the scope of your nursing responsibilities and available resources
- Knowledge of the nurse's legal responsibilities when providing care, including the need to document nursing assessment, diagnosis, planning, implementation, and evaluation concerning disturbances in self-concept

concern that many children identify rock stars or pimps, prostitutes, and drug dealers as their heroes, rather than parents, government leaders, or other professional people.

Self-Evaluation: "How Well Do I Like Myself?"

Self-esteem is the evaluative and affective component of the self-concept, sometimes termed self-respect, self-approval, or self-worth. According to Maslow (1954), all people "have a need or desire for a stable, firmly based, usually high evaluation of themselves, for self-respect or self-esteem, and for the esteem of others." (p. 90) Accordingly, he identified two subsets of esteem needs: (1) self-esteem needs (strength, achievement, mastery and competence, confidence in the face of the world, independence, and freedom) and (2) respect needs or the need for esteem from others (status, dominance, recognition, attention, importance, and appreciation). Self-esteem comes from two major sources: how competent children think they are in various aspects of life and how much social support they receive from other people. One's self-esteem, like the various self-images that make up one's self-concept, varies considerably depending on a specific relationship or situation.

Coopersmith (1967) identified the four bases of self-esteem as (1) significance—the way a person feels he or she is loved and approved of by the people important to that person; (2) competence—the way tasks that are considered important are performed; (3) virtue—the attainment of moral–ethical standards; and (4) power—the extent to which a person influences his or her own and others' lives. According to Coopersmith, people with high, medium, and low self-esteem differ in their expectations of the future, in their affective reactions, and in their basic styles of adapting to environmental demands. People with high self-esteem are accustomed to being well received and successful. They are able to approach people, tasks, and new situations freely, with confidence in their ability to interact and to get along with people and to respond successfully to life's challenges.

Formation of Self-Concept

A person is not born with a self-concept. Rather, it is a social creation that develops as a result of interactions with others (Fig. 30-1). Steps in the formation of self-concept include the following:

1. An infant learns that the physical self is different from the environment. If basic needs are met and warmth and affection are experienced, the child begins life with positive feelings about self.
2. The child next internalizes (incorporates into self) other people's attitudes toward self. Parents play the most influential role; peers play the second most influential role.
3. The child or adult internalizes the standards of society.

Stages in the development of the self include self-awareness (infancy); self-recognition (18 months); self-definition (3 years); and self-concept (6 to 7 years).

Coleman, Morris, and Glaros (1990) identified the following psychological conditions that foster healthy development of the self in children:

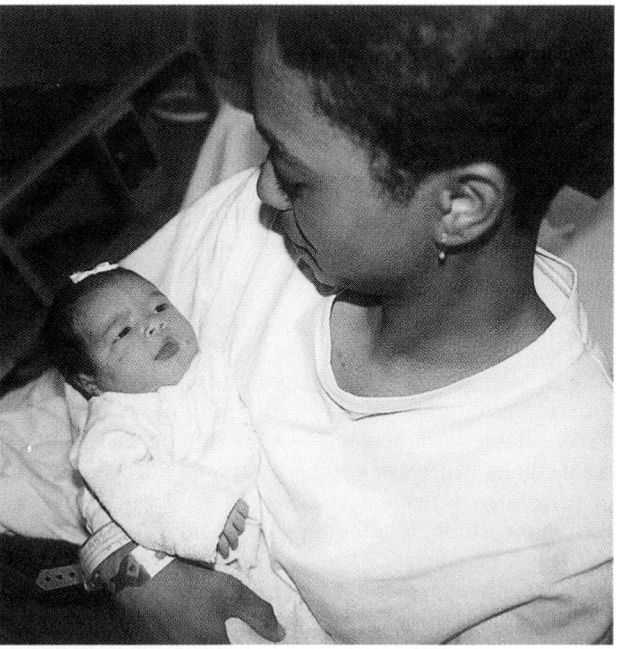

Figure 30-1
Interaction between parents and the infant are important to the child's development. Feeding, holding, cuddling, and cooing are forms of interaction.

- Emotional warmth and acceptance
- Effective structure and discipline
- Clearly defined standards and limits, so that children understand what goals, procedures, and conduct are approved
- Adequately defined roles for both older and younger members of the family
- Established methods of handling children that produce the desired behavior, discourage misbehavior, and deal with infractions when they occur
- Encouragement of competence and self-confidence
- Helping children meet challenges
- Appropriate role models
- A stimulating and responsive environment

Formation of self-concept is further described in developmental theories, especially in Erikson's stages of development, Piaget's cognitive developmental stages, and Havighurst's developmental tasks (see Chaps. 8 and 9).

Threats to Self-Concept

Anxiety is a threat to self-concept. According to psychoanalysts, the ego uses many different methods to protect itself from anxiety. Among these methods are coping and defense mechanisms. Anxiety, coping, and defense mechanisms are discussed in Chapter 31.

Factors Affecting Self-Concept

Almost any life experience can influence a person's self-concept. Key factors include developmental considerations, culture, internal and external resources, history of success and failure, stressors, and illness or trauma.

Developmental Considerations

As a person matures, the criteria that mark the experiences necessary for a positive self-concept change. Although the infant needs a supportive environment in which all human needs are met, the growing child needs the freedom to explore and develop the ability to meet increasing personal needs. Table 30-1 highlights developmental changes affecting self-concept, related implications for nursing, and potential causes of self-concept disturbances.

Culture

As a child internalizes the values of parents and peers, culture begins to influence a sense of self. If the culture is relatively stable, little tension may be experienced between what culture expects of the child and what the child expects of self. When parents, peers, and the adult world confront the child with different cultural expectations, the sense of self may be confused. For example, an adolescent may realize his or her parents live by the work ethic and believe it is necessary to rise early every day and put in a full day's work. The adolescent's peer group has few demands placed on it and encourages the adolescent to hang out with the group. The adolescent's vocational aptitudes, meanwhile, are leading him or her to consider a music career in a rock group, which will keep the adolescent out late many nights doing something the parents do not classify as work.

Internal and External Resources

The personal strengths an individual recognizes, develops, and uses are powerful but subjective determinants of self-concept. One person may use humor as both an effective coping mechanism and a successful interpersonal tool. Another person may use humor to avoid facing conflict and may feel bad about being known as a joker or clown. External resources such as a network of support people (see accompanying Research in Nursing box), adequate finances, and organizational supports are also subjective determinants of self-concept. Generally, the more resources a person has and uses wisely, the better the feelings about self.

History of Success and Failure

People with a history of repeated failure (in school, friendships, work, or marriage) may perceive themselves as failures and actually perpetuate this image by unconsciously instructing others to treat them this way. They may come to fear success and actually find it easier to fail even though they do not like themselves that way. Thus, failure influences an individual's self-concept negatively, and his or her self-concept instructs the person to continue to fail. On the other hand, one successful experience conditions a person to strive for the next success, and a positive self-concept is forged that expects success and makes it happen.

Stressors

Life stressors (marriage, divorce, an exam, a new job, a gray hair, a fire) may call forth a personal response and mobilize an individual's talents, resulting in good feelings about oneself. Stressors may also evoke maladaptive responses that di-minish the self-concept. Examples of these include withdrawal, depression, extreme anxiety, and substance abuse. How the person perceives the stressor (threat, challenge, defeat) and his or her ability to mobilize personal strengths and other resources are determined largely by that person's self-concept, which in turn is influenced by the response the person chooses.

Aging, Illness, or Trauma

Because most people take a healthy body for granted, the diminishment of physical attractiveness or functioning, the suggestion of disease, or sudden impact of trauma may pose serious threats to the self (Fig. 30-2). People vary greatly in their response to aging, illness, and trauma.

The Nursing Process

Before reading this section, review the box, Applying Learning to Practice: The Nurse as Role Model (p. 683).

ASSESSING

The nurse assessing self-concept focuses on the patient's personal identity, body image, self-esteem, and role performance. A general assessment of self-concept should be included in every comprehensive nursing assessment. It is as important to identify and label a patient's positive self-concept as it is to note problems. The following self-concept assessment was recorded on the nursing history of a 17-year-old single mother of a healthy newborn:

> Describes herself as a strong, healthy, fun-loving person who is "going to make it." Is unafraid of new parenting responsibilities. Identifies the following as strengths: experience with younger brothers and sisters; program for single parents in her high school; strong motivation to make something of herself (plans on getting an associate degree in x-ray technology); support of family and friends; and belief that "God will help me." Expresses concern about always being able to make the right decisions about going out with friends, dating, and so forth. Views motherhood as an achievement about which she is proud. Basically has positive self-concept with high self-esteem.
>
> M. LeBon, RN

Patients experiencing illness or trauma resulting in body disfigurement, altered functioning, or life crises that arrest development and thwart the achievement of life goals are at high risk for problems related to self-concept and should be assessed more carefully. If problems surface during the interview, a more thorough assessment should be carried out. The accompanying Focused Assessment Guide highlights elements common to any self-concept assessment and high-risk factors.

It is important for the nurse conducting this assessment to realize the limitations of self-reporting. A patient may give what he or she believes are the desired or socially acceptable responses to interview questions. "Why, of course I like myself. I'm a pretty good person. Yes, I have friends." For this reason, the nurse must evaluate the pa-

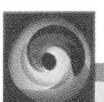

Table 30-1
Developmental Changes Affecting Self-Concept

Developmental Period	Changes Affecting Self-Concept	Implications for Nursing	Potential Causes of Disturbances in Self-Concept
Infancy	• No self-concept at birth • Beginning differentiation of self and nonself	• Teach parents the critical importance of providing consistent and affectionate parenting • Assess if the parents have reasonable expectations of the infant: sleeping, eating, other awake behaviors	• Unmet basic human needs • Lack of adequate body and sensory stimulation • Parents' lack of acceptance of the infant's appearance or behavior
Childhood	• An intact body is important to the young child, who fears bodily mutilation • During middle childhood, a sense of being trusted and loved, of being competent and trustworthy develops • Differences between self and others are strong	• If invasive procedures are indicated, explain simply to the child what is being done and offer the child support • Assess the parents' ability to provide the type of developmental environment in which the child's self-concepts can evolve positively	• Dysfunctional family • Too much or too little structure • Sensory perceptual impairments
Adolescence	• Development of secondary sex characteristics; rapid body changes • Emphasis on sexual identity • Parental influences on self-concept are often rejected; peers become more important; movement is toward development of own identity	• Assess adolescent's self-knowledge and understanding of body changes • Counsel adolescent regarding mature and healthy use of independence he or she craves • Provide anticipatory guidelines regarding hazards to life, health, human functioning	• Inability to accept body • Inability to resolve competing pulls to be both a child and an adult • Unhealthy peer pressure
Adulthood	• Society places emphasis on intactness of body, fitness, energy, sexuality, style, sophistication, beauty • Important to meet role expectations well	• Assess how realistic the adult's expectations are and the incentive they provide for growth and development • Assist patient to deal constructively with negative influences in self-image • Preretirement counseling	• Inability to fulfill conflicting role expectations • Failure to accept role responsibility (eg, parenting responsibilities) • Unreasonable expectations • Irreversible body change related to trauma, illness • Unsatisfying job • Failure to develop new goals to give meaning and purpose to life
Later years	• Declining physical and possibly mental abilities	• Assess how the older person is adjusting to effects of aging • Counsel regarding meaningful use of time • Explore resources	• Loss of significant work (retirement); feelings of uselessness • Death of spouse, significant others • Diminished physical attractiveness, strength, overall health • Multiple stressors • Fear of dependency

tient's responses in relation to observations made about the patient and what is known about the patient from other sources. (See the accompanying box, Applying Learning to Practice: Promoting Health.) When the nursing assessment reveals a clustering of these behaviors, it is important to discuss this finding with the patient. This is especially true when there is a discrepancy between the patient's words and behavior. "You've told me that you feel in control of your situation right now and are committed to the treatment plan, but I notice you've broken three therapy

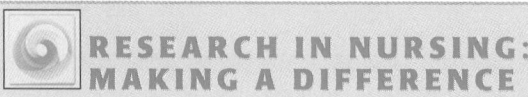

RESEARCH IN NURSING: MAKING A DIFFERENCE

Promoting Enhanced Self-Concept Through Social Support

Social support has been demonstrated to have a positive influence on the experience of dealing with illness. Elements of social support include provision for attachment and intimacy, being an integral part of a group, opportunity for nurturant behavior, reassurance of worth, and availability of informational, emotional, and material help. Whereas some individuals have excellent natural support networks, others have few supports to facilitate coping in times of illness.

Related Research
Cudney, S. A., & Weinert, S. C. (2000). Computer-based support groups: Nursing in cyberspace. *Computers in Nursing, 18*(1), 35–43.
The focus of this study is the Nurse Monitor role in a project whose overall goal is to use telecommunica-

tion technology to provide information and support to rural middle-aged women living with chronic illness who are unable to participate in a more traditional face-to-face support group. A supportive community was created by means of the use of telecommunication technology that can reach geographically isolated individuals. The study explores the effects of participation in these support groups on the women's psychosocial health.

Relevance for Practice
Nurses can now "be there" for people who are underserved or live in areas isolated from medical centers and traditional health services by means of outreach support programs linked electronically by personal computers.

appointments this month, and you did mention that you are drinking more heavily. . . ."

Personal Identity

When assessing self-concept, the information needed first is the patient's description of self. **Personal identity** describes an individual's conscious sense of who he or she is. "How would you describe yourself to others?" The nurse pays special attention to the labels used by the patient and the order in which they appear. A simple exercise consists of asking patients to "Make a list of ten labels that you believe identifies yourself (for example, student, Italian American, opera fan, premed major). Put the most important label first and then list the others in order of decreasing importance. (What if the order were reversed?) To

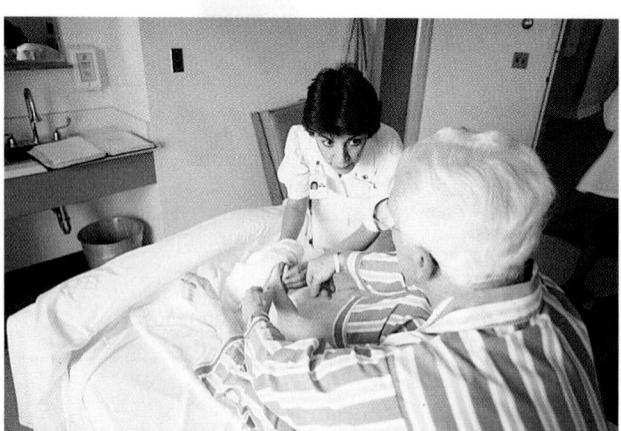

Figure 30-2
An illness or alteration in function may present a dilemma for the patient and affect his or her self-concept.

what extent do you think your way of organizing information about yourself affects your behavior?"

It is important to discover whether individuals are comfortable with their perceived identity. Developmental changes, trauma, and cultural and gender dissonance may all place a patient at risk for personal identity disturbances.

Patient Strengths

Many patients focus naturally on their deficiencies; asking pointed questions about personal strengths can help a patient identify positive factors:

> "What are some of your personal strengths . . . qualities you are proud of . . . things you do well?"
> "What special talents or abilities do you have?"
> "What has helped you cope in the past when things were tough?"

Body Image

When a **body image** disturbance is suspected, the nurse carefully interviews and observes the patient to identify the nature of the threat to the person's body image (functional significance of the part involved, importance of physical appearance, and visibility of the part involved): the meaning the patient attaches to the threat; the adequacy of the patient's coping abilities; response of family members and significant others; and help available to the patient and his or her family.

The patient's response to the deformity or limitation is assessed, including changes in independence–dependence patterns and in socialization and communication.

Response to Deformity or Limitation

Adaptive responses: Exhibits signs of grief and mourning (shock, disbelief, denial, anger, guilt, acceptance)

APPLYING LEARNING TO PRACTICE

The Nurse as Role Model

Before nurses can successfully identify and resolve self-concept disturbances in patients, they must be comfortable with themselves and possess an adequate self-concept. Important goals for nurses include the following:

- Identify basic unmet human needs, exploring positive means to meet these needs.
- Schedule time every day to meet personal needs.
- Assess the effect of feedback from significant others on self-esteem.
- Describe personal strengths accurately.
- Develop a realistic plan to achieve goals for personal growth and development.

Specific strategies for enhancing self-concept in relation to one's professional practice follow:

Dispel the myth that it is necessary to know all there is to know about nursing to be a good nurse. At no one point in time does any nurse ever have it all together. Acceptance of the need to learn new theories or new procedures frees you from having to practice defensively (ie, pretend to be on top of every new development) and is a great stimulus for professional growth and development.

Realistically evaluate strengths and weaknesses. Build a periodic review into your practice and be fair in your self-evaluation. "I think I'm giving better care than ever before and I know my patients are appreciative, but I'm sensing a lot of tension between myself and a couple of the other nurses. . . ."

Accentuate the positive. Many of us have a knack for forgetting the 99 things we did well and focusing on our one error. Errors need to be taken seriously and evaluated but not to the exclusion of overlooking positive accomplishments.

Develop a conscious plan for changing weaknesses into strengths. Professional growth and development depend on strong motivation to become better at what you do. "Realizing that I never know what to say when a patient receives bad news, I can try to avoid these patients or consciously plan to develop better interpersonal skills." Nurses are tremendous resources for each other. Tapping into each other's strengths is a great way to build self-esteem mutually. "You always seem to know the right thing to say or do with patients. Do you mind if I observe for a while and then 'try on' some of your behaviors?"

Work to develop team self-esteem. A basic interpersonal principle that seems to work well in practice is to offer to others what you want yourself. Because our sense of self is strongly influenced by the feedback we receive from others, positive reinforcement of our strengths and sincere offers to help correct deficiencies are needed by everyone.

Actively demonstrate your commitment to nursing and concern about nursing's public image. To feel good about yourself, you need to be able to experience pride in your profession. Active participation in professional organizations can offer many personal rewards—not the least of which is enthusiasm and pride in being a nurse. Monitoring the media's portrayal of nursing and providing appropriate feedback contributes to individual and corporate nursing self-esteem.

Maladaptive responses: Continues to deny and to avoid dealing with the deformity or limitation, engages in self-destructive behavior, talks about feelings of worthlessness or insecurity, equates deformity or limitation with whole person, shows a change in ability to estimate relationship of body to environment

Independence–Dependence Patterns

Adaptive responses: Assumes responsibility for care (makes decisions); develops new self-care behaviors; uses available resources; interacts in a mutually supportive way with family

Maladaptive responses: Assigns responsibility for his or her care to others; becomes increasingly dependent or stubbornly refuses necessary help

Socialization and Communication

Adaptive responses: Maintains usual social patterns; communicates needs and accepts offers of help; serves as support for others

Maladaptive responses: Isolates himself or herself; exhibits superficial self-confidence; is unable to express needs (becomes hostile, ashamed, frustrated, depressed)

Self-Esteem

When a patient has shared perceptions of self, the nurse questions if the patient likes himself or herself, if the patient is pleased with his or her expectations, and the progress the patient is making to realize these expectations.

"Tell me what you like about yourself."
"What would you change about yourself if you could?"

Using a graphic description of self-esteem as the discrepancy between the "real self" (what we think we really are) and the "ideal self" (what we think we would like to be or think we should be), the nurse can obtain a quick

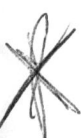

FOCUSED ASSESSMENT GUIDE

Self-Concept

Factors to Assess	High-Risk Factors	Questions and Approaches
Personal identity	• Developmental changes • Trauma • Gender dissonance • Cultural dissonance	How would you describe yourself to others? • Personal characteristics and traits • Strengths
Body image	• Loss of body part or function • Disfigurement • Developmental changes	Describe your body to me. What do you like most/least about your body? Is there anything about your body that you would like to change?
Self-esteem	• Unhealthy interpersonal relationships • Failure to achieve developmental milestones • Failure to achieve life goals • Failure to live up to personal moral code • Sense of powerlessness	Tell me something about your sense of satisfaction with yourself. Who would you like to be? Who or what has influenced your self-expectations? Are these expectations realistic? • *Significance:* What is your response when you feel unloved or unappreciated by those who are important to you? • *Competence:* How do you feel about your ability to do the things in life that are important to you? • *Virtue:* To what degree are you satisfied with the way you are able to live up to your moral standards? • *Power:* To what extent do you feel able to control what happens to you in life? How does this make you feel?
Role performance	• Loss of valued role • Ambiguous role expectations • Conflicting role expectations • Inability to meet role expectations	How do you feel about your ability to do all the things your roles demand of you? Are these roles satisfying for you?

indication of a patient's self-esteem by having the patient plot two points on a line—real self and ideal self (Fig. 30-3). The greater the discrepancy, the lower the self-esteem; the smaller the discrepancy, the higher the self-esteem.

A person's ideal self may differ dramatically from the current sense of self and positively or negatively influence behavior and personal development. If indicated, the nurse questions the patient about self-expectations:

"You've told me something about who you are, how you view yourself now. Tell me who you would like to be in the future."

"What life goals are important to you?"

"Where do you see yourself 5 years from now? In 10 years?"

"Are these expectations realistic?"

"Are your expectations stemming from who you would like to be or from who you think you should be?"

"Who or what has influenced your self-expectations?"

The nurse is assessing whether the patient possesses life goals that are positively motivating personal development. Unrealistic expectations need to be identified, and their source needs to be explored with the patient. For example:

"You seem to feel that it is necessary to be all things to all people—no matter what this costs you. How might this belief have developed? Is it helpful to you?"

"What I'm hearing is that your performance must always be perfect, that although you allow others to make mistakes, you cannot allow yourself this luxury. . . . Tell me more about this."

"Then, unless you graduate at the top of your class, you will not be satisfied? Why is this so important? Is this type of achievement realistic with your abilities? What will this success both benefit and cost you?"

"You state you have no goals for the future . . . when you wake up each morning what gets you out of bed? What keeps you moving?"

APPLYING LEARNING TO PRACTICE

Promoting Health

Self-Concept

Use the assessment checklist to determine how well you are meeting your need for positive self-concept. Then develop a prescription for self-care by choosing appropriate behaviors from the list of suggestions.

ASSESSMENT CHECKLIST

almost always | sometimes | almost never

☐ ☐ ☐   1. I have established appropriate expectations and goals for myself.

☐ ☐ ☐   2. I have effective and satisfying relationships with others.

☐ ☐ ☐   3. I cope effectively with change and loss.

☐ ☐ ☐   4. I accept and feel good about myself.

SELF-CARE BEHAVIORS

1. Accept normal variations in physical appearance and capabilities.
2. Use problem-solving and decision-making strategies to define expectations and set goals.
3. Set priorities and accept that no one person can be all things to all people.
4. Forget past mistakes; carrying around "excess baggage" is unhealthy.
5. Emphasize strengths and abilities in self.
6. Take an active part in group activities in school, work, church, or the community.
7. Volunteer time, talents, or services.
8. Avoid excessive alcohol and drugs.
9. Live life one day at a time.

If this exercise indicates the need for a more detailed assessment, the nurse next explores the concepts of significance, competence, virtue, and power.

Significance
"Are there people in your life with whom you share a close relationship?"

"Many people have 'people' problems. Are your relationships causing you any problems right now?"

"To what extent do you feel loved and approved of by the key people in your life?"

"Does it bother you when you feel unloved or when others fail to appreciate you?"

"In what ways do you let family members and friends know that you like them or are proud of their accomplishments?"

Competence
"What are the things you need to do to feel important?"

"Is anything interfering with your ability to execute these tasks?" ("How does this make you feel?")

"How important to you is it to feel that others value your work?"

Virtue
"Tell me something about the moral–ethical principles that govern your life."

"How must you live to describe yourself as a 'good' person?"

"How do you feel about your ability to live this way?"

"Describe any difficulties you experience in living up to your moral principles that you would like to discuss."

"In what ways can the nurses help you to live better according to your moral standards?"

Power
"How important is it to you to 'be in control' of your life (health)?"

"To what extent did you feel 'in control' of your life (health) before this illness (trauma, crisis, and so forth)?"

"To what extent do you feel 'in control' of your life (health) currently?"

"What is it that makes you feel not in control?"

"How might you change this? How can nurses help you to develop and gain more control?"

High self-esteem

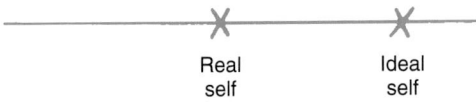

Real self   Ideal self

Low self-esteem

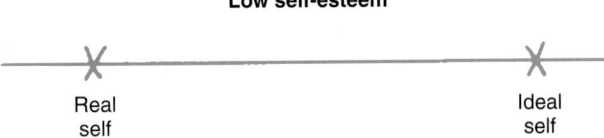

Real self   Ideal self

Figure 30-3
The patient who perceives his or her real self as relatively close to the ideal self has high self-esteem. The patient who perceives his or her real self as far from the ideal self has low self-esteem.

Role Performance

We all play many roles. Our ability to execute successfully societal expectations regarding role-specific behaviors, or our **role performance,** is easily compromised by illness and injury. If a nurse suspects this might be contributing to a self-concept disturbance, the following questions are indicated:

"What major roles describe you—son, daughter, spouse, parent, employer or employee, student, club member, and so on?"

"How important is it to you to be good in each of these roles?"

"Tell me how successful you think you are in each of these roles."

"What roles or expectations would you change if you could?"

"If you feel 'incompetent' or less than successful in some of these roles, why? What is preventing you from being more successful? What can you do about this? How might I help you?"

DIAGNOSING

Disturbances in Self-Concept as the Problem

Specific disturbances in self-concept that can be treated by independent nursing interventions receive one of four nursing diagnostic labels:

Body Image Disturbance: The state in which an individual experiences or is at risk for experiencing a disruption in the way one perceives one's body image

Self-Esteem Disturbance (Chronic Low Self-Esteem or Situational Low Self-Esteem): The state in which an individual experiences or is at risk for experiencing negative self-evaluation about self or capabilities

Altered Role Performance: The state in which an individual experiences or is at risk for experiencing a disruption in the way he or she perceives his or her role performance

Personal Identity Disturbance: The state in which an individual experiences or is at risk for experiencing an inability to distinguish between self and nonself (Carpenito, 1995)

Common etiologies and defining characteristics for these diagnoses are found in the accompanying box.

Disturbance in Self-Concept as the Etiology

Because disturbances in self-concept have the potential to affect so many other areas of human functioning, they may serve as etiologies for numerous problem statements. Examples of these follow:

Impaired Adjustment related to change in health status (increasing dependency, need for ongoing medical evaluation and treatment, and so forth)

Anxiety related to irreversible change in body image (eg, amputation, mastectomy, burn); delayed

development of secondary sex characteristics (body image); discrepancy between real and ideal self (self-esteem); perceived incompetence in important roles; loss of key roles (child or spouse dies, separation, retirement, graduation)

Ineffective Individual Coping related to inability to identify personal strengths, low self-esteem, "I know I can't manage this"; role conflict

Anticipatory or Dysfunctional Grieving related to change in body image, loss of key roles

Altered Health Maintenance related to low self-esteem—"Why bother?"

Hopelessness related to low self-esteem, overwhelming role demands, belief that nothing will change (destiny is controlled externally)

Knowledge Deficit: How to help children develop High Self-Esteem related to lack of experience with parenting

Noncompliance (specify) related to low self-esteem

Altered Parenting related to disturbance in role performance (rejection of parent role)

Posttrauma Response related to disturbance in personal identity

Self-Care Deficit related to learned helplessness, low self-esteem—"I can't"

Sensory/Perceptual Alterations related to disturbance in personal identity (ability to distinguish between self and nonself)

Altered Sexuality Patterns related to changed body image, disturbance in self-concept

Impaired Social Interaction or Social Isolation related to low self-esteem, disturbance in personal identity

Altered Thought Processes related to disturbance in personal identity

High Risk for Self-Directed Violence related to disturbance in self-concept, overwhelmed by failure to live according to moral-ethical standards

Important Distinctions

When assessment data point to an alteration in self-concept, the nurse's first task is to determine whether the altered self-concept is the problem, the cause of the problem (etiology), or merely a sign that a problem exists (defining characteristics). Self-concept data seem to fit well in all three categories. It is important that an accurate determination be made because this directs the goals developed for the patient and related nursing interventions. For example, the following three different diagnoses might be written for a 25-year-old woman who is recently divorced:

1. Self-Esteem Disturbance related to perceived failure in role of wife (recent divorce) as manifested by neglect of personal appearance and inability to accept positive reinforcement

Assessment data point to a disturbance in self-esteem as the priority problem. Nursing energies will be directed to helping the patient evaluate herself positively despite the stress of the divorce.

Nursing Diagnoses for Common Problems

Disturbances in Self-Concept

Problem	*Related Factors*	*Sample Defining Characteristics*
Body Image Disturbance	Irreversible changes in body image—amputation, mastectomy, hysterectomy, colostomy, scars, burns, disfiguring skin disorder	"Look at me. Nothing can ever be the same again. I feel less whole. When I look in the mirror, all I see is my (stump, missing breast, scar). I know when others look at me they feel repulsed or at the very least pity me."
	Effects of treatment (eg, braces, casts)	Thirteen-year-old female adolescent with scoliosis wearing a Milwaukee brace (covers pelvic area and has rods in the front and back that extend up to the chin): "I feel dumb in this thing . . . it's bad enough that my back is crooked but this makes me look like a freak. Besides, it's hot. Must I wear it to school?"
	Difficulty accepting development of secondary sex characteristics or delayed development of same	Fifteen-year-old male adolescent, sophomore in high school, height 5'1″, weight 88 lb; "When am I going to grow up and start looking like the other guys in my class?" No pubic hair; penis, testes, and scrotum are the same size and proportion as in childhood.
	Extreme thinness or obesity	Twenty-year-old woman, height 5'7″; weight 200 lb: "I hate my body . . . I've been fat all my life and I'm always on a diet. Why can't I be like everyone else?"
Self-Esteem Disturbance	Feeling unloved or unapproved of by significant others	Twelve-year-old son of parents in the process of getting a divorce: "No matter what I do to make my dad like me he acts like I don't exist. When he's home he fights with mom, but mostly he's away. I wouldn't even care if he yelled at me so long as he noticed me. I wonder why he doesn't like me?"
	Feelings of incompetence	Forty-two-year-old car salesperson, with company for 18 years: "What's wrong with me? I do my job, I'm also never absent, I have a good sales record, but I keep getting passed over for promotions. I think I'm too old to move to a different company, but I don't want to just sell cars for someone else for the rest of my life!"
	Failure to live according to personal moral ethical code	Thirty-three-year-old single female computer programmer: "I should have known I'd get pregnant—I deserve it. I knew I was wrong to go to bed with this guy. Basically I've tried to live the way I think I should all my life up until now. What if something's wrong with the baby because of my sin?"
	Powerlessness	Sixty-seven-year-old alert widow with degenerative joint disease: "It may be hard for me to move around now, but darn it—there's nothing wrong with my mind. The kids think they are helping me by making all my decisions, but they aren't. I'm not a doddering old lady in a nursing home."
Altered Role Performance	Rejection of role	Twenty-two-year-old mother 2 days after birth of her second son (first son is 15 months old): "I don't know who my husband got to watch our son. I never wanted to be a mother anyway. My husband and I have never had any time for ourselves—and things aren't going to get any better."

(continued)

Nursing Diagnoses for Common Problems *(Continued)*

Problem	*Related Factors*	*Sample Defining Characteristics*
Altered Role Performance	Role conflict Role fatigue Multiple life stressors	Twenty-one-year-old, full-time junior nursing student who failed a major exam; is married and the mother of an 18-month-old daughter; works every other weekend in a hospital as an electrocardiogram technician: "I'm trying so hard to get my grades up, but I don't know what else I can do. My husband seems to be losing patience with me more and more and I sometimes feel awful about neglecting my daughter. I'd stop working but we need the money. I want nursing so bad but I'm getting awfully tired."
	Changing personal resources (physical health, mental abilities, motivation)	Fifty-year-old college chemistry teacher begins exhibiting signs of early Alzheimer's disease; forgets where she is and what she is doing; began rambling in class and saying things that made no sense—much to the class's amusement. Later cried and called herself "stupid."
Personal Identity Disturbance	Unresolved crisis	Eighty-eight-year-old man who lost his wife 6 months ago; wife took care of all his needs; sits alone in the house all day: "We always did everything together. I wish I had died first. What shall I do?"
	Declining physical, mental, or sensory abilities	Same 88-year-old man 3 months after admission to long-term care institution, medical diagnosis "rule out depression/dementia"; has become increasingly withdrawn, never initiates conversation; responses to questions are sometimes inappropriate: "What do you mean, what's my name? Who cares? I want to go home to my wife."
	Rejection of membership in minority group	Fifteen-year-old Cambodian girl recently emigrated to the United States with family; in constant conflict with parents as she rejects her family's culture in hopes of fitting in with peer group: "Sometimes I feel like I no longer know who I am or how I should act. I feel lonely inside and afraid."

2. Altered Health Maintenance related to decreased self-esteem as manifested by failure to follow through on referrals (support group, stress-management class, and so forth); "Why bother? Nothing ever works for me anyway."

   Here, low self-esteem is contributing to the patient's problem of failing to follow through with health-seeking behaviors. Nursing energies will be best directed to improving the patient's use of health resources; one of the means used will be to help her to value herself enough to choose healthy behaviors.

3. Ineffective Individual Coping related to inability to accept recent divorce as manifested by low self-esteem statements: "I never should have gotten married—my mother said I'd be a rotten wife." "I know I can't make it on my own." "Why did he do this to me?"

   Here, low self-esteem statements are the cues that led to the identification of the problem statement. One of the criteria used to evaluate nursing intervention to increase the patient's coping skills will be a reduction in or elimination of low self-esteem statements.

PLANNING: EXPECTED OUTCOMES

Whenever nurses care for patients, nursing interventions need to be supportive of the following patient goals/outcomes. The patient will achieve the following:

- Describe self realistically, identifying both strengths and deficiencies
- Verbalize realistic expectations for self based on who he or she would like to be
- Verbalize that self is liked, or at least "OK"
- Communicate his or her feelings and needs in a way that is comfortable and effective in meeting needs
- Nurture relationships in which needs for love and worth are mutually met (significance)
- Assume role-related responsibilities with confidence (competence)

- Express satisfaction with ability to live according to one's moral-ethical standards (virtue)
- Demonstrate confidence in ability to accomplish what is desired (power)

Sample outcomes for patients with specific disturbances in self-concept follow:

- Describe the relation between self-concept and behavior
- Identify faulty thinking that reinforces a negative self-concept (distortions and denials, faulty categorizing, inappropriate standards)
- Integrate positive self-knowledge into self-concept
- Report feeling better about himself or herself

IMPLEMENTING

Nursing interventions to assist patients to develop and maintain a positive self-concept may vary tremendously from one patient to another. Nurses must be comfortable with their own self-image before they can address image problems in patients. Specific nursing strategies addressed in this section include helping patients identify and use personal strengths, helping high-risk patients maintain a sense of self, changing the self-concept, developing a positive body image, and working with parents and educators to develop self-esteem in children and adolescents. These and other nursing interventions are summarized in the accompanying NIC box.

Helping Patients Identify and Use Personal Strengths

When confronted with a major stressor, many people forget that they have histories of successful coping and numerous personal strengths. Patients at high risk for giving up are those with low self-esteem or multiple stressors perceived as being overwhelming.

Using the Nursing Interventions Classification (NIC)

Selected Self-Awareness Enhancement Activities

- Encourage patient to recognize and discuss thoughts and feelings
- Assist patient to realize that everyone is unique
- Assist patient to realize the impact of illness on self-concept
- Assist patient to change view of self as victim by defining own rights, as appropriate
- Assist patient to be aware of negative self-statements
- Assist patient to identify guilty feelings
- Explore with patient the need to control
- Assist patient to identify positive attributes of self

From McClosky, J., & Bulechek, G. (2000). *Nursing interventions classification (NIC)* (3rd ed.) (p. 574). St. Louis: C. V. Mosby. A full listing of nursing activities for each nursing intervention can be found in this book.

Although attributing strength to a patient sounds like something nurses would do naturally, nurses frequently fall into the trap of doing for patients (i.e., solving their problems, rather than helping them to identify and tap their personal power and strengths). Moreover, patients continually instruct nurses about how they should be perceived, and some patients successfully communicate a manipulative helplessness that encourages the nurse's taking charge. An appropriate nursing response in this case is, "I wonder why you want me to speak with your physician about treatment alternatives. I am sure you would feel much better hearing this information firsthand. If you'd like, I will stay here while you talk with the physician."

Patients experiencing powerlessness may need help to recognize their strengths (Fig. 30-4). Examples of personal strengths include a healthy functioning body, cognitive abilities, emotional strengths, communication strengths, other interpersonal skills; a sense of meaning and purpose in life; a belief system; a social support network; meaningful work, hobbies, and other interests; education; life experience; and a past history of effective coping. A good sense of humor, belief in a loving God, a healthy nutritional state, the ability to make decisions, and a sense of self-worth are all personal strengths that may better equip a person to respond to life's challenges.

Specific strategies nurses can use to help patients identify and use personal strengths include the following:

- Encouraging patients to identify their strengths
- Replacing self-negation with positive thinking (see the accompanying box)
- Noticing and reinforcing patient strengths
- Encouraging patients to will for themselves the strengths they desire and to try them on

Helping High-Risk Patients Maintain a Sense of Self

People who are acutely ill are often separated not only from their strengths but also from any real sense of self. One patient, a college president who was recovering from serious

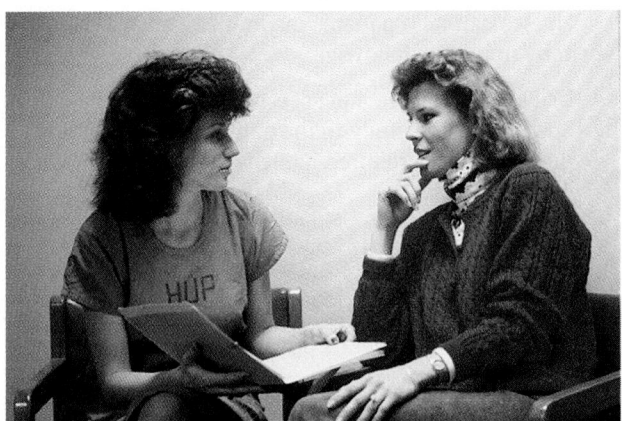

Figure 30-4
The nurse helps the patient recognize his or her self-worth and strengths that he or she possesses. (Photo by Gates Rhodes, Courtesy of School of Nursing, University of Pennsylvania.)

Exploring and Developing the Positive

Example: Twenty-year-old mother who perceives herself as "a failure in everything I try"; states husband feels childrearing is the woman's responsibility and she is terrified.

Immediate goal: Develop confidence in parenting skills, see herself as a good mother

- Explore and reinforce the patient's personal qualities and strengths that will help her to reach her goal.

  "You look like a natural mother when you hold your baby; some women are afraid at the beginning to even hold their infants."

  "That's good that you are talking with your baby. Babies quickly sense how a parent feels about them."

- Teach the patient how to substitute positive self-talk for negative self-talk.

  Negative self-talk (mother during feeding): "She's awfully fussy tonight, I mustn't be doing this right. . . . It was probably dumb luck that she took to breast so well this morning. . . ."

  New positive self-talk: ". . . but she fed so well this morning and the nurse said her weight is good. I wonder what else might be making her fussy . . . maybe she's wet. . . ."

complications after surgery for ovarian cancer, shared the following:

> When I first got sick it didn't matter how people treated me because I knew who I was. As I've grown sicker and weaker, I become whomever people make me. If a nurse walks in here and moves me like meat, I become a slab of meat. My sense of self seems more and more dependent on how people respond to me.

Nurses can help patients maintain a sense of self and worth by doing the following:

- Using looks, touch, and speech to communicate worth
- Speaking respectfully to the patient and addressing the patient by preferred name whenever entering the patient's room
- Offering the patient a simple explanation before initiating any procedure
- Moving the patient's body respectfully if the patient is unable to do this
- Respecting the patient's privacy and sensibilities

This type of caring does not require additional nursing time or energy. It does require from the nurse continual reaffirmation that nursing is a person-centered profession and that nothing is more important at any moment of a nurse's workday than the person being served.

Changing a Negative Self-Concept

The time is ripe for change when a patient realizes that a negative self-concept is hindering personal development. A nurse working in a setting that allows long-term nurse–patient relationships may intervene to assist the patient in modifying self-concept. At the outset, it must be remembered that the self-concept is firmly entrenched and that by nature it resists change. Helpful nursing interventions include the following:

- After the patient has identified faulty thinking patterns (negative self-talk) that reinforce the negative self-concept, teach the patient to "red flag" this behavior as soon as he or she is aware of it happening. The goal is to replace the negative self-talk with talk that will develop a more positive self-image.
- Help the patient explore the positive dimensions of himself or herself that he or she wishes to develop, and incorporate this new knowledge into the self-concept.

Developing a Positive Body Image

Interventions for body image disturbances vary according to the nature of the disturbance. Interventions may include any combination of the following:

- Establish a trusting relationship with the patient. Allow the patient to share his or her feelings openly. Sitting quietly by the patient for a few minutes with a few words such as, "How are things?" or "Gee, it must be hard to lie there after all you've been through. . ." communicates to the patient your willingness and readiness to share his or her experience.
- Support the patient through the various stages of loss, grief, and mourning (shock, disbelief, denial, anger, guilt, acceptance), remembering that there is no one right way to proceed through these stages. Rather, patients may move fluidly in and out of various stages, sometimes returning to earlier stages. Some patients may need to learn that it is okay to cry, to be angry, to feel depressed.
- Use play therapy with children so that they can describe their feelings and work through their grief using the nonthreatening medium of dolls or animals.
- Role-model for the patient a healthy acceptance of the patient's body. Be careful that facial expressions, words, or body positioning do not communicate to the patient disgust, fear, or rejection.
- While communicating support to the patient who is slow to develop and use appropriate self-care behaviors, firmly insist that the patient participate in his or her care to the extent that the patient is able. Whenever possible, provide the patient with honest answers to his or her questions or put the patient in touch with the appropriate person to give the answers.
- Strengthen the decision-making ability of the patient by honestly exploring alternatives; help the patient to imagine living with the consequences of different courses of action.
- Reinforce the patient's personal strengths and help the patient and family to identify all possible resources.
- Assess the response of the patient's significant others and intervene if they negatively influence the patient.

Developing Self-Esteem in Children, Adolescents, and Older Adults

Nurses who work in practice settings where they have access to groups of parents, adult caregivers, or teachers can offer specific guidelines for creating developmental environments that build high self-esteem. The accompanying box offers five strategies for building self-esteem in children. Because some parents and educators may not have experienced these aids to personal growth themselves, it is beneficial for the nurse to role-model these behaviors when interacting with children.

Important learning tasks for children include understanding and accepting oneself, feelings, and others; independence; goals and purposeful behavior; mastery, competence, and resourcefulness; emotional maturity; and choices and consequences.

The many losses associated with aging (eg, diminished strength and physical health, interpersonal losses, retirement, and shrinking income) make older adults especially

---

Building Self-Esteem in Children

Strategy One: Looking at the Positive and the Negative

Instruct parents to write an honest description of their child for a stranger. Next have the parents underline the child's positive and negative qualities.

To reinforce the positive qualities, (1) notice examples of ability in many different circumstances and point this out to the child; (2) find occasion to frequently and honestly praise the child; and (3) give the child an opportunity to show ability frequently.

To address the negative qualities constructively, ask: (1) What need is being expressed by this behavior? (2) Can I see a positive quality being expressed by this behavior? and (3) How can I help my child express this quality and meet her needs in a more positive way?

Reexamine the list of negative qualities and ignore those that are a matter of taste, preference, or personal style.

Strategy Two: Listening

The following guidelines can help parents to use listening to communicate to a child, "You are important. What you say matters to me. You matter to me."

1. Make sure that you are ready to listen.
2. Give your child your full attention.
3. Minimize distractions.
4. Be an active listener.
5. Invite your child to talk.

Listen for the point of a child's story ("What is she trying to tell me? Why is this important to him?"). Don't feel that you have to fix things. Listen for and respond to the feelings.

Strategy Three: Using the Language of Self-Esteem

Feedback that enhances self-esteem has three components: (1) a description of the behavior (describe the behavior without judging it); (2) your reaction to the behavior (language that shares something about your self); and (3) acknowledgement of the child's feelings. For example, "Thanks for playing with your brother tonight [description]. I was wondering how I was going to pay attention to our guests if he got fussy and was really grateful when I noticed that you kept him occupied and happy [reaction]. I know that there were other things you might have enjoyed doing more [acknowledgment]."

To give correction using the language of self-esteem, (1) describe the problematic behavior, (2) state a reason for the behavior change, (3) acknowledge the child's feelings, and (4) offer a clear statement of what is expected.

Attacking communications: "Don't let me ever hear you talk that way to your mother again."

Language of self-esteem: "I overheard you telling your mom that she should 'Get a life and get off your case.' [description]. When you talk like that it just makes people angry or sad, which isn't very helpful [reason for behavior change]. You probably feel like you are being picked on, and we may have some expectations that are different from those of your friends' parents. I hope you know that this is because we love you and want the best for you [acknowledgment]. In the future try to talk to others with the same respect you'd like others to show you [statement of expectation]."

Avoid using the following destructive language styles, which tear down self-esteem: overgeneralizations ("You *never* come home on time!"), the silent treatment, and vague or violent threats.

Strategy Four: Helping Children Meet Expectations

To help children meet expectations, (1) be sure that your expectations are reasonable and appropriate for your child's age; (2) plan ahead; (3) be clear about your expectations; (4) focus on the positive; (5) provide choices when possible; and (6) provide rewards.

Strategy Five: Promoting a Feeling of Success

To help children have the courage to try new types of experiences, which results from successfully meeting challenges, (1) let a child know what to expect; (2) let your child practice the necessary skills; (3) be patient; and (4) make it safe to fail.

(Material adapted from McKay, M., & Fanning, P. (1992). *Self-esteem* [2nd ed.]. Oakland, CA: New Harbinger Publications.)

vulnerable to disturbances in self-concept, particularly chronic low self-esteem. Society's generally negative view of aging compounds the problem. Nurses interacting with older adults need to understand that simple measures, such as addressing older patients respectfully, communicating that you take their concerns seriously, noticing and affirming their personal strengths, and interacting with them as individuals as opposed to members of a homogeneous group, can greatly enhance the older person's self-esteem. The accompanying box describes nursing interventions to promote self-esteem in older adults.

EVALUATING

Nurses who are sensitive to the relation between self-concept and general well-being consistently evaluate the effect the nursing plan of care has on the patient's self-concept. For example, while educating a patient with hypertension for whom lifestyle counseling was recommended, the nurse may detect that the patient is feeling extremely guilty about his or her smoking, dietary habits, and lack of exercise. "Why should I even try to change any of these things now? I made myself sick, so I may as well live with the punishment." If the plan of care is to be effective, the nurse must first help this patient value himself or herself sufficiently to want to make the necessary changes.

When the plan of care includes specific interventions to assist patients with disturbances in body image, self-esteem, role performance, and personal identity, the nurse listens carefully to the patient's self-report and observes patient behaviors to see if the disturbances are being resolved. Basically, the patient should be able to meet the following outcomes:

- Is comfortable with body image and able to use it effectively to meet human needs
- Is able to describe self positively
- Is able to meet realistic role expectations without undue anxiety and fatigue
- Is capable of interacting appropriately with environment while recognizing self to be a separate and distinct entity

See the accompanying Patient Care Study and Nursing Plan of Care.

Focus on the Older Adult

Nursing Strategies to Promote Self-Esteem in Older Adults

Personal Identity

- When an older person's sense of self is threatened, assist him or her to find meaning in the experience, to regain mastery to the extent that this is possible, and to evaluate realistically the adequacy of his or her coping strategy.
- Teach older people to identify and develop a game plan for confronting anxiety-producing situations.
- Help to identify and secure intervention for treatable depressions.
- Remedy treatable causes of self-identity disturbances, such as pain, abusive living arrangements, and substance abuse.

Body Image

- Notice and affirm positive physiologic characteristics of older adults.
- Teach preventive self-care measures that reduce discomforting signs of aging (eg, exercise, which maintains muscle mass and joint flexibility; proper nutrition; and basic hygiene and skin care measures).
- Explore new activities (including hobbies) that are within the changing physical capabilities of the older person.

Self-Esteem

- Assist older adults to identify and use personal strengths.

- Communicate that you value older people simply for who they are (unconditional affirmation)—know and use the name they prefer, ask them questions about their life, interests, or values.
- When appropriate, use the expertise of older people and ask their advice; let them know you value their life experience.
- Engage older people in activities in which they can be successful.
- Allow older people to make tough decisions and to confront challenging situations when appropriate; teach protective family members the value of older adults confronting situations that invite their continued growth.
- Empower older people to meet their own needs: provide necessary knowledge, teach new behaviors, instill the belief that they "can manage."

Role Performance

- Explore with older people the many roles they have fulfilled throughout their lifetime; invite reminiscences.
- Facilitate grieving over valued roles that are no longer able to be performed.
- Remedy, whenever possible, factors that prevent older people from engaging in valued roles.
- Explore new roles.

APPLYING LEARNING TO PRACTICE

Patient Care Study

Melissa Motsky is a 31-year-old married woman, mother of three children (aged 12, 10, and 8 years) and junior-level nursing student. She works every other weekend as a nurse's aide. She has just received a letter from the nursing division head informing her that she is in academic jeopardy and will fail out of the program unless her grades improve. She presents this to her adviser.

After talking with Ms. Motsky, who calls herself a failure and who cries as she describes her situation at home, her faculty adviser suspects a serious self-esteem problem and helps her to list factors contributing to her current sense of failure and low self-esteem. The following list is generated:

Significance

- – Receives little understanding, affection, approval from husband. "I stay with him because of the kids. I started back to school because I had to get out of the house and want to make something of myself. He doesn't understand this."
- + Children are very supportive but get impatient when I have to study and can't spend time with them."
- – Feels a failure in all the roles that are important to her—wife, mother, and, now, student. "I jeopardized everything to go back to school—if I fail, it's all over

for me. There just isn't enough time or energy to do anything well."
- + "They do love me at work, though, which makes me feel like nursing is what I should be doing."

Virtue

- – "I've always believed that hard work pays off and that if you were faithful to your duty you'd be rewarded by the 'good life'—I'm beginning to doubt that. Maybe I'm a fool for trying so hard."
- + "I do still try to live according to my beliefs and feel okay about this. I treat others as I'd like to be treated."

Power

- – "I always believed I could do anything I put my heart and soul into. But I can't seem to change my marriage, and if I fail out of school, that will be the end of all my dreams."

Key indicators of low self-esteem that also surfaced in the interview included overeating (10-lb weight gain during the past year); difficulty sleeping; fatigue; new sensitivity to criticism; and expressions of feeling unloved, alone, and no longer able to manage. Personal strengths included history of "can do" mentality, high motivation to succeed, and past history of success as mother and nurse's aide.

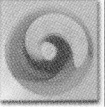

NURSING PLAN OF CARE
for Mrs. Motsky

Nursing Diagnosis	Situational Low Self-Esteem related to decreased sense of significance, competence, virtue, and power as manifested by expressions of being a failure, powerlessness, fatigue, tears, weight gain, low academic performance (test grades 68, 74)
Expected Outcome	By this time next month, 11/2/02, the client will demonstrate increased self-esteem by: • Expressing positive statements about herself

Nursing Interventions	Rationale	Evaluative Statement
Assist patient to rediscover and "own" personal strengths: identify personal qualities and strengths that have pleased her in the past and explore why this has changed; recommend that she make at least one positive statement about herself each morning and evening.	Patients can lose touch with their strengths, especially when multiple stressors seem to create impossible demands.	11/3/02 Goal partially met. Patient's statements are of the "This is good, *but* . . ." variety. "I think I'm doing better in school but I don't know if it will continue." *Recommendation:* Continue to identify and reinforce personal strengths. *C. Taylor, RN*
Consistently interact with the patient as if she had the power to weather the crisis successfully (ie, "will" strength to her). Role-model positive self-concept behaviors.	Once the patient senses that an authority believes in her power and expects her to use it, she may internalize this knowledge and act on it.	

(continued)

Expected Outcome   By this time next month, 11/2/02, the patient will demonstrate increased self-esteem by:

- Reporting ability to receive negative feedback without falling apart

Nursing Interventions	Rationale	Evaluative Statement
Explore with patient to what degree she allows the opinions of others to influence her self-concept.	Significance—sense of being loved and approved of by significant others—is a critical component of self-esteem.	11/3/02 Goal partially met. Patient reports being able to handle everything except putdowns from her husband.
Teach how the self-concept filters life experiences; thus, if I feel that I am a failure, I may interpret the words and behaviors of others as confirming this, even though that was not their intention.	Principle of self-consistency: once I am down, I may reinforce this by distorting what I feel, hear, and experience.	*Recommendation:* Explore origin of power she has given to her husband to influence her sense of self and what she wants to do about this.
Explore with the patient ways she can enhance her self-concept independently of others (eg, take time each day for herself). Encourage patient to draw on personal strengths.	This facilitates internal locus of control versus external. Spending time on self communicates that self is valuable.	*C. Taylor, RN*
Teach the patient how to analyze feedback constructively and respond appropriately; *cancel negative thinking.* For example, patient receives care plan back with many corrections and the notation, "sloppy work."	It is important to break the cycle of negative thinking, which reinforces negative self-concept.	
Maladaptive response: "She hates me. See, this proves I'll never be a good nurse. I wasted my time even doing this."		
Adaptive response: "I spent as much time as I had on this . . . now let me see what I did wrong. Maybe I should make an appointment with my instructor so she can show me how to improve."		

Expected Outcome   By this time next month, 11/2/02, the patient will demonstrate increased self-esteem by

- Getting a passing grade on her next quarterly examination

Nursing Interventions	Rationale	Evaluative Statement
Explore study skills with patient; recommend study group.	Poor study skills may also be contributing to her low academic performance. A study group will meet both her social and academic needs.	11/3/02 Goal met. Grade: 82 *C. Taylor, RN*

(continued)

Nursing Interventions	Rationale	Evaluative Statement
Discuss importance of how she *perceives* present situation. If present failures are equated with *defeat,* she may be unable to mobilize her resources to succeed; if present failures represent *challenge,* it may call forth her best efforts and result in success.	The meaning given to present stressor can dramatically affect the patient's response to it and condition her for success or failure.	
Discuss importance of breaking cycle of failure leading to another failure.	If this short-term goal is met, it will set the stage for future successes and contribute to the patient's positive self-concept.	

Expected Outcome	By this time next month, 11/2/02, the patient will demonstrate increased self-esteem by:
	• Verbalizing that the way she is living her life is okay

Nursing Interventions	Rationale	Evaluative Statement
Assist patient to examiner her moral–ethical standards; explore sources of these standards and whether the patient feels comfortable with them.	Moral–ethical standards may be uncritically internalized and place the patient in conflict.	11/3/02 Goal met. Patient stated: "I guess I'm living the best way I know how right now. If things are meant to be different someone is going to have to show me how."
Identify unrealistic standards; patient may need "permission" to be human.	Unrealistic standards (perfectionism, conventionality) may constantly undermine the patient's self-esteem.	*Recommendations:* Reinforce self-acceptance.
Refer if appropriate for counseling.	Support groups on campus (counseling centers, ministries) may be able to meet patient's needs.	*C. Taylor, RN*

Expected Outcome	By this time next month, 11/2/02, the patient will demonstrate increased self-esteem by:
	• Reporting two recent instances when personal power was effective in accomplishing desired goals

Nursing Interventions	Rationale	Evaluative Statement
Identify and affirm patient's use of personal power to accomplish goals.	A negative self-concept may deny or distort personal successes; outside intervention may be necessary to bring these to consciousness.	11/3/02 Goal met . . . with difficulty. Needed considerable prompting to identify successful use of her personal power. Was ready to attribute passing grade to luck rather than her own efforts.
		Recommendations: Have patient make daily record of her use of personal power and results.
		C. Taylor, RN

(continued)

NURSING PLAN OF CARE (Continued)
for Mrs. Motsky

Sample Documentation

10/2/02   Nursing

Melissa Motsky presented today after receiving academic jeopardy letter. She is strongly motivated to complete nursing program successfully and seems to have the ability to do this. Current multiple life stressors—lack of support from husband; need to mother three children (12, 10, 8); part-time nurse's aide job (necessary for financial reasons); and current academic jeopardy (test grades 68, 74) are all contributing to her low self-esteem and overwhelming sense of being a failure. We together developed a care plan that it is hoped will help her to do better academically as well as begin to feel better about herself. See attached. She will return 11/2/02 at 10 AM for follow-up.

C. Taylor, RN

SOAP Format
10/2/02, 12:30 pm, nursing

Academic jeopardy—Melissa Motsky
S: "I jeopardized everything to go back to school—if I fail, it's all over for me." Reports lack of support from husband; grief that she does not have enough time for children; failure of personal work ethic ("hard work pays off"); and sense of powerlessness.
O: Nursing II quarterly exam grades: 68, 74; weight gain of 10 lb during past year; facial and body expressions of fatigue, profuse tears
A: Disturbance in Self-Esteem related to decreased sense of significance, competence, virtue, and power
P: See attached plan of care.

C. Taylor, RN

Learning Outcomes

After completing this chapter, the learner should be able to accomplish the following:

1. Define key terms used in the chapter.
body image	role performance
global self	self-actualization
ideal self	self-concept
personal identity	self-esteem
2. Identify three dimensions of self-concept: self-knowledge, self-expectation, and self-evaluation (self-esteem).
3. Describe major steps in the development of self-concept.
4. Differentiate positive and negative self-concept and high and low self-esteem.
5. Identify six variables that influence self-concept.
6. Use appropriate interview questions and observations to assess a patient's self-concept.
7. Develop nursing diagnoses to identify disturbances in self-concept (body image, self-esteem, role performance, personal identity).
8. Describe nursing strategies that are effective in resolving self-concept problems.
9. Plan, implement, and evaluate nursing care related to select nursing diagnoses for disturbances in self-concept.

Critical Thinking Exercises

1. The personal strengths an individual recognizes, develops, and uses are powerful but subjective determinants of self-concept. Identify the strengths that have been major determinants of your self-concept (eg, power, intelligence, physical attractiveness, goodness, humor, "can-do" attitude) and explore how this is helping you to succeed in nursing. Discuss with another student ways in which nurses can assist patients to recognize, develop, and use personal strengths to cope better with the stress of injury and illness.
2. Role play with another student your responses to the following patients, and then reverse roles. Reflect on the effects different types of nursing presence and response have on a patient's self-concept. Discuss the nursing responses that would be most helpful to patients at risk for self-concept disturbances.

- A male patient who was recently passed over for a promotion states, "I can't believe I've got to deal with this ulcer . . it's just one more thing holding me back from succeeding in this business.
- An anorexic teenager tells you that she can't possibly eat the dinner you brought her, and states, "I can't do my usual workout in here, and look how fat I'm getting."

- A woman, after mastectomy, refuses to look at the incision site and notes, "If I can't bring myself to look at this, how can I ever expect my husband to want me again?"
- A resident in a nursing home says, "Don't trouble yourself about me. I'm sure you have lots of people to take care of who are more deserving of your time and attention."

Study Questions

1. Robert, aged 19 years, has Down syndrome and is mildly mentally retarded with an intelligence quotient of 82. He told his nurse, "I'm a good helper. You see I can carry these trays because I am so strong. But I'm not very smart so I have just learned to help with the things I know how to do." Robert most likely has
   a. a negative self-concept and low self-esteem
   b. a negative self-concept and high self-esteem
   c. a positive self-concept and fairly high self-esteem
   d. a positive self-concept and low self-esteem

2. Jerry was having academic difficulty in all his college courses, and during a counseling session, he was asked to make a list of 20 words that describe him. After 15 minutes, Jerry listed the following: 19 years old, male, named Jerry; and he declared he couldn't think of anything else. Jerry has demonstrated
   a. lack of self-esteem
   b. deficient self-knowledge
   c. unrealistic self-expectation
   d. inability to evaluate himself

3. Jerry, who is in counseling because he is having academic difficulty, was able to list only three facts, traits, or qualities to describe himself. His counselor then asked him to list facts, traits, or qualities that he would like to be descriptive of himself or that he thinks he should have. Jerry quickly listed 25, all of which were characteristic of a successful man. When asked if he knew anyone like this, he replied, "My father." This discrepancy between Jerry's description of himself as he is and as he would like to be indicates
   a. positive self-concept
   b. Jerry's modesty (lack of conceit)
   c. body image disturbance
   d. low self-esteem

4. David and his wife have decided that she will get a job so that David can go to pharmacy school as he has wanted to do for some time. Their three teenagers, who were involved in the decision, are also getting jobs to buy their own clothes. David plans to work 12 to 16 hours weekly. He states, "I was always an A student, but I may have to settle for Bs now because I don't want to neglect my family and I need to work a few hours so that my wife won't have to work overtime." David's self-expectations are
   a. realistic and positively motivating his development
   b. unrealistic and negatively motivating his development

   c. unrealistic but positively motivating his development
   d. realistic but negatively motivating his development

5. Which of the following statements made by a parent of a child you are seeing in clinic needs to be followed up with teaching about how to foster healthy development of the self in children?
   a. "I love my child so much I 'hug him to death' every day."
   b. "I think children need challenges, don't you?"
   c. "My husband and I both grew up in very restrictive families. We want our children to be free to do whatever they want."
   d. "My husband and I have different ideas about discipline, but we're talking this out because we know it's important for Johnny that we be consistent."

6. Which intervention would you take first to assist a woman who states that she feels incompetent as a mother of a teenage daughter?
   a. recommend that she discipline her daughter more strictly and consistently
   b. make a list of things her husband can do to help her improve
   c. assist the mother to identify both what she believes is preventing her success and what she can do to improve
   d. explore with the mother what the daughter can do to improve her behavior

7. Which of the following patients is least likely to develop problems related to self-concept?
   a. 55-year-old female television news reporter undergoing a hysterectomy (removal of uterus)
   b. young clergyperson whose vocal cords are paralyzed after a motorbike accident
   c. 32-year-old accountant who survives a massive heart attack
   d. 23-year-old model who has just learned that she has breast cancer

For questions 8 to 11, read the patient data below and use the following letters to indicate the diagnosis the data suggest (each response may be used only once):
a. Personal Identity Disturbance
b. Body Image Disturbance
c. Self-Esteem Disturbance
d. Altered Role Performance

8. Juanita Sanchez has only been in the United States 3 months and has recently suffered the loss of her husband and job. She states that nothing feels familiar, "I don't know who I am supposed to be here," and she misses home (Nicaragua) terribly.

9. Jim Boa, a sophomore in high school, has missed a great amount of school this year because of leukemia. He said he feels like he is falling behind in everything and misses "hanging out at the mall" with his friends most of all.

10. "Why did I have to be born into a family of big bottoms and short fat legs! No one will ever ask me out for a date . . . oh why can't I have long thin legs like everyone else in my class? What a frump I am."

11. Marissa Yule, a 33-year-old businessperson, is now in counseling attempting to deal with a long-repressed history of sexual abuse by her father. "I guess I should feel satisfied with what I've achieved in life, but I'm never content and nothing I achieve makes me feel good about myself. . . . I hate my father for making me feel like I'm no good. This is an awful way to live."

12. Nancy, 36 years of age, who was divorced 5 years earlier, entered the emergency department with severe burns and cuts on her face after an auto accident in a car driven by her fiancé of 3 months. Three weeks later, her fiancé has not yet contacted her. Nancy states that he is so busy and she is too tired to visit anyway. Nancy frequently lies with her eyes closed and head turned away. These data suggest that
    a. there is no disturbance in self-concept
    b. this patient has ego strength and high self-esteem but may have a disturbance of body image
    c. the area of self-esteem has very low priority at this time and should be ignored until much later
    d. it is probable that there are disturbances in self-esteem and body image

13. Which of the nursing interventions below is least likely to assist a severely ill patient with cancer to maintain a positive sense of self?
    a. making it a point to address the patient by name each time you enter the room
    b. fatiguing the patient as little as possible by performing all procedures in silence
    c. continuing to respect the patient's privacy and sensibilities
    d. offering the patient a simple explanation before moving her in any way

14. Doris, 16 years of age, has a nursing diagnosis of Body Image Disturbance related to severe acne. In planning nursing care, an appropriate goal for this nursing diagnosis is, "The patient will
    a. make above B grades in all tests at school"
    b. demonstrate by diet control and skin care increased interest in control of acne"
    c. report that she feels more self-confidence in her music and art, which she enjoys"
    d. express that she is very smart in school"

15. A 4½-year-old boy required stitches for a laceration on the eyebrow. After the doctor held him, visited with him, and explained what was going to be done and that his eye would get better and look just like it did before, the boy placed his hands under his hips as instructed and quietly permitted the procedure. He then expressed pride in himself. Evaluation of the effect of this healthcare experience is best expressed in which of the following?
    a. The doctor did an excellent job.
    b. The child's self-esteem was enhanced and fear of bodily mutilation decreased, and the parents were given an excellent role model.
    c. The child was made the center of attention and the situation exaggerated, thus encouraging the child to become self-centered.
    d. These interventions consumed too much physician time to be evaluated positively.

Answers With Rationale

1. The correct response is *c*. The data point to Robert's having a positive self-concept ("I'm a good helper") and fairly high self-esteem (realizes his strengths and limitations). The statement "But I'm not very smart" is accurate and is not an indication of a negative self-concept.

2. The correct response is *b*. Jerry's inability to list more than three items about himself indicates deficient self-knowledge. There are not enough data provided to determine whether he lacks self-esteem, has unrealistic self-expectations, or is unable to evaluate himself.

3. The correct response is *d*. Low self-esteem is characterized by great discrepancy between the ideal and real selves. There are no data in this item to suggest that Jerry has either a positive self-concept or a body image disturbance. The data do indicate something more serious than modesty.

4. The correct response is *a*. David's self-expectations are realistic, given his multiple commitments, and seem to be positively motivating his development.

5. The correct response is *c*. Each option with the exception of *c* correctly addresses some aspect of fostering healthy development in children. Because children need effective structure and development, giving them total freedom to do as they please may actually hinder their development.

6. The correct response is *c*. The first intervention priority with a mother who feels incompetent to parent a teenage daughter is to assist the mother to identify what is preventing her from being an effective parent and then to explore solutions aimed at improving her

parenting skills. The other interventions may prove helpful, but they do not directly address the mother's problem with her feelings of incompetence.

7. The correct response is *a*. Based simply on the facts given, the 55-year-old news reporter would be least likely to experience a body image or role performance disturbance because she is beyond her childbearing years and the hysterectomy should not impair her ability to report the news. The young clergyperson's inability to preach, the 32-year-old's massive myocardial infarction, and the model's breast resection have much greater potential to result in self-concept problems.

8. The correct response is *a*. An unfamiliar culture, coupled with traumatic life events and loss of husband and job, has resulted in this patient's total loss of her sense of self: "I don't know who I am supposed to be here." Her very sense of identity is at stake, not merely her body image, self-esteem, or role performance.

9. The correct response is *d*. Important roles for Jim are being a student and a friend. His illness is preventing him from doing either of these well. This self-concept disturbance is basically one that concerns role performance.

10. The correct response is *b*. Clearly, this patient's concern is with his or her body image.

11. The correct response is *c*. Marissa's self-concept disturbance is mainly one of devaluing herself and thinking that she is no good. This is a self-esteem disturbance.

12. The correct response is *d*. The traumatic nature of Nancy's injuries, her fiancé's failure to contact her, and Nancy's response, that is, her withdrawal, all point to potential problems with both body image and self-esteem. It is not true that self-esteem needs are of low priority.

13. The correct response is *b*. Each option, with the exception of *b*, should assist the patient to maintain a positive sense of self. Working in silence with the patient may be preferable to idle chatter, but the ideal is to address the patient by name, give simple explanations of procedures, and communicate that he or she is a person of worth by simple words of caring.

14. The correct response is *b*. All of these patient goals may be appropriate for Doris, but the only goal that directly addresses her body image disturbance is *b*.

15. The correct response is *b*. The physician enhanced the child's self-esteem by teaching him how to participate effectively, decreased his fear of bodily mutilation by telling him that his eyebrow would heal and look normal, and gave the parents an excellent role model.

Bibliography

Atwater, W. E. (1996). *Adolescence* (4th ed.). Upper Saddle River, NJ: Prentice-Hall.

Bello, L. K., & McIntire, S. N. (1995). Body image disturbances in young adults with cancer. *Cancer Nursing, 18*(2), 138–143.

Bensink, G. W., Godbey, K. L., Marshall, M. J., & Yarandi, H. N. (1992). Institutionalized elderly: Relaxation, locus of control, self-esteem. *Journal of Gerontological Nursing, 18*(4), 30–36.

Carpenito, L. J. (1995). *Nursing diagnosis: Application to clinical practice* (6th ed.). Philadelphia: J. B. Lippincott.

Coleman, J. C., Morris, C. G., & Glaros, A. G. (1990). *Contemporary psychology and effective behavior* (7th ed.). Glenview, IL: Scott, Foresman.

Coopersmith, S. (1967). *The antecedents of self-esteem.* San Francisco: Freeman.

Davidhizar, R. (1991). Ten strategies for increasing your self-confidence. *Imprint, 38*(3), 105–108.

LeMone, P. (1991). Analysis of a human phenomenon: Self-concept. *Nursing Diagnosis, 2*(3), 126–130.

Maslow, A. (1954). *Motivation and personality.* New York: Harper & Row.

McCloskey, J., & Bulechek, G. (2000). Nursing interventions classification (NIC) (3rd ed.). St. Louis: C.V. Mosby.

McKay, M., & Fanning, P. (1992). *Self-esteem* (2nd ed.). Oakland, CA: New Harbinger Publications.

Otto, H. (1965). The human potentialities of nurses and patients. *Nursing Outlook, 13*(8), 32–35.

Stein, K. F. (1995). Schema model of the self-concept. *Image— The Journal of Nursing Scholarship, 27*(3), 187–193.

Taylor, C. (1982). The need for self-esteem. In H. Yura & M. B. Walsh (Eds.). *Human needs 2 and the nursing process.* Norwalk, CT: Appleton-Century-Crofts.

Chapter 31
Stress and Adaptation

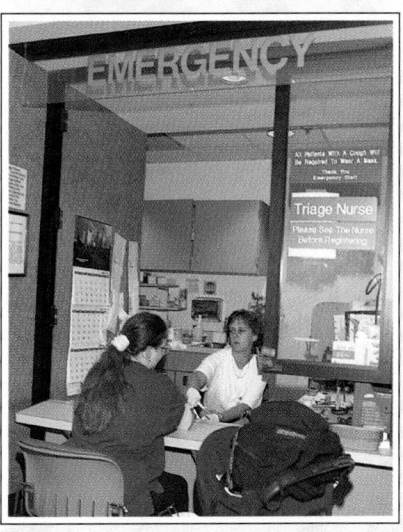

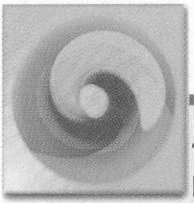

Thinking Critically About
Nursing's Blended Skills

Before reading this chapter, think about the types of blended skills you will need to respond to stress-related problems.

- A young pregnant woman is brought into the emergency room screaming "Save my baby! Save my baby!" She was in a motor vehicle accident and appears to have multiple injuries.

- Teachers invite you to speak to parents at a local elementary school. There have been two kidnappings of school-aged children in the neighborhood, and no one is feeling safe. Area parents are terrified and demanding assistance. You will be on a panel with local police and the school counselor. You are requested to offer practical suggestions for managing stress.

- A first-year college student comes to the student health center and reports experiencing flare-ups of her bowel disease related to the stresses of beginning college.

- Things have gotten a lot more hectic at work recently since two nurses who left were not replaced, and everyone's caseloads are heavier. You find yourself always eating on the run and have resumed smoking. You wake up tired in the morning and spend the day getting more tired.

What cognitive, technical, interpersonal, and ethical/legal skills do you think you will need to respond to the challenges described above?

tress is a part of life. Everyone feels stress at one time or another. Books and magazines are full of articles about stress, discussing everything from the negative stressful effects of performing one's job to the positive stress of holidays. Television advertisements for over-the-counter remedies promise fast relief from stress headaches and upset stomachs. Stress is blamed for excessive weight gain, drinking, and smoking as well as for divorce and child abuse. Feeling "stressed out" is common, and taking "stress breaks" to do physical exercise is recommended in many work settings. With stress such a part of everyday life, it is easy to see that any additional problem—such as a health problem—can increase the effects of stress on the person experiencing the problem.

Not only is stress a part of everyday experience, but a person's responses to stress are also necessary to life. Stress can have both positive and negative effects. Stress is produced by a change in the environment that is perceived as a challenge, a threat, or a danger. Stress affects the whole person in all the human dimensions (physical, emotional, intellectual, social, and spiritual). The perception of stress and the responses to it are highly individualized, not only from person to person but also from one time to another in the same person. Because stress is individual and holistic, there is no commonly accepted definition or measurement. Most simply, **stress** is a condition in which the human system responds to changes in its normal balanced state.

A **stressor** is anything that a person perceives as challenging, threatening, or demanding. Stressors may be either internal (such as an illness, a hormonal change, or fear) or external (such as loud noise or cold temperature). As with stress, the perception and effects of the stressor are highly

individual. Stressors themselves are neither positive nor negative, but they can have positive or negative effects as the person responds to change.

When a person is in a threatening situation, immediate responses occur. Those responses, which are often involuntary, are called *coping responses.* The change that takes place as a result of the response to a stressor is **adaptation**. Adaptation is, to some degree, an ongoing process as a person strives to maintain balance in his or her internal and external environments (Fig. 31-1). Adaptation also occurs in families and groups. Adaptation results in the following:

- Optimal functioning in all dimensions
- Normal growth and development
- Normal reactions to physical and emotional stress
- Ability to tolerate changing situations

Stress, stressors, and adaptation are all unique to each individual. The process of adapting to stress is constant and dynamic and is essential to the person's physical, emotional, and social well-being. Stress and adaptation are major components in health and illness. Nurses need to understand the concepts and dimensions of stress when providing nursing care to patients in all settings. Nurses themselves are subject to stress from the demands of their career, and they need to know healthy ways of responding. This chapter discusses stress from a holistic perspective, including both physical and psychological stress. Elements discussed include homeostasis, stress and adaptation, and nursing actions to promote stress reduction. The concluding case study illustrates how the nurse promotes coping and adaptation by the patient through knowledge of the causes of and patient's responses to stress and specific nursing interventions.

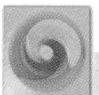

COGNITIVE SKILLS

- Basic knowledge about the relationship between stressors, stress, and adaptation
- Ability to integrate knowledge about healthy lifestyles, support systems, stress management techniques, and crisis intervention into nursing care
- Ability to recognize the warning signs when stressors are exceeding coping mechanisms—in self and others
- Knowledge of stress management resources within the community

TECHNICAL SKILLS

- Ability to use correctly the equipment necessary to diagnose and treat problems related to inadequate coping

INTERPERSONAL SKILLS

- Strong people skills; ability to communicate and interact effectively with patients and their caregivers; ability to establish trusting relationships—even in times of crisis
- Ability to "connect" with a public audience, to project competence and confidence, to motivate appropriate self-care and prevention skills

ETHICAL/LEGAL SKILLS

- Commitment to safety and quality; strong sense of responsibility, accountability
- Familiarity with agency policy and role responsibilities related to stress management

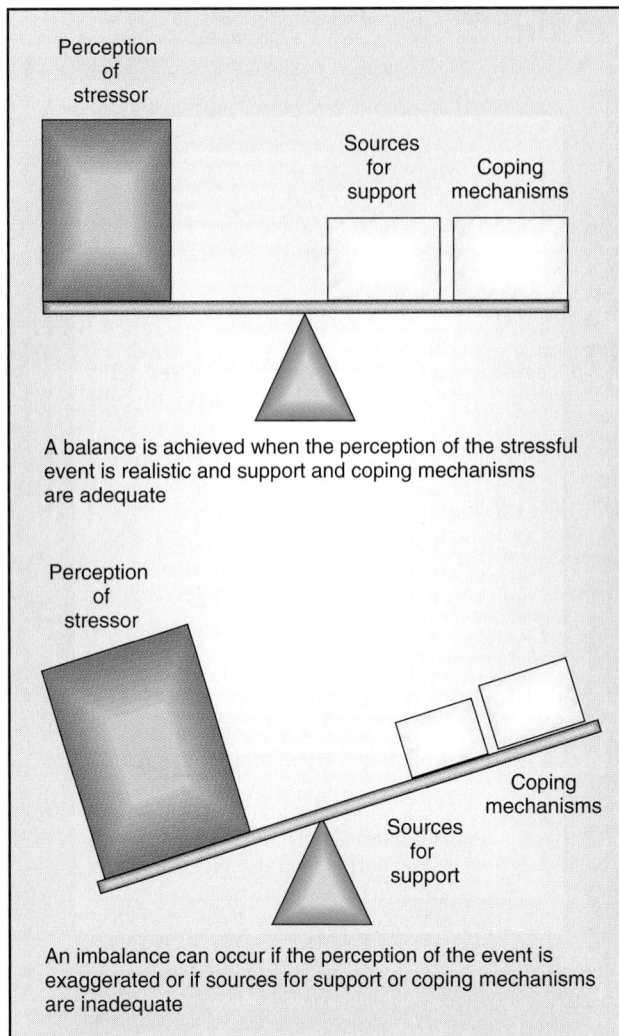

A balance is achieved when the perception of the stressful event is realistic and support and coping mechanisms are adequate

An imbalance can occur if the perception of the event is exaggerated or if sources for support or coping mechanisms are inadequate

Figure 31-1
A realistic perception of a stressful event, sources for emotional support, and appropriate coping mechanisms are components of a system of balances during stress.

⊚ Physiology of Stress and Adaptation

Our bodies are always interacting with a constantly changing environment. The environment includes the external environment, which surrounds our bodies, and the internal environment, which includes the mechanisms that regulate body functions and the fluids that surround body cells. To maintain health, the body's internal environment must remain in a balanced state. Various physiologic mechanisms within the body respond to internal changes to maintain relative constancy in the internal environment, called **homeostasis**.

Homeostasis

The specific concept of homeostasis was introduced by W. B. Cannon in 1939, although throughout history people have believed that health is the result of a balanced state.

Some of the most important people in medical history, including Hippocrates (the father of medicine) and Claude Bernard (the father of physiology), believed in and wrote about this balanced state. Originally the focus was on life processes that occur within the body, such as heart rate, blood pressure, and water balance. The concept of homeostasis has been expanded, however, to include both the internal and the external environment, both physiologic *and* psychological balance.

Physiologic Homeostasis
Long before you entered nursing, you knew that sweating when you were hot and shivering when you were cold occur to help maintain a stable body temperature. These are examples of homeostatic mechanisms that regulate the body's internal environment.

Homeostatic mechanisms are primarily controlled by the autonomic nervous system and the endocrine system. Involved to a lesser degree are the respiratory, cardiovascular, gastrointestinal, and renal systems. These mechanisms are self-regulating, occur without conscious thought, and usually function to correct abnormal conditions. On a simple level, they are like a thermostat regulating a furnace. When the temperature in a house falls below the preset temperature on the thermostat, the thermostat turns on the furnace, which heats the house to the desired temperature and then shuts off.

The regulatory mechanisms of the body are constantly reacting to changes to maintain homeostasis and health. The homeostatic mechanisms of the body systems are summarized in Table 31-1. They are important in understanding the consequences of both short-term and long-term stress, which can threaten physiologic homeostasis and result in illness (see the accompanying box for examples of illnesses associated with stress).

Psychological Homeostasis
To maintain mental well-being, humans also must maintain psychological homeostasis. As discussed in Chapter 2, each person needs to feel loved and a sense of belonging, to feel safe and secure, and to have self-esteem. When these needs are not met or a threat to need fulfillment occurs, homeostatic measures in the form of coping or defense mechanisms help return the person to emotional balance. Psychological homeostasis is discussed further later in this chapter.

Adaptive Responses to Stress

Everyone frequently encounters physical, psychological, and social changes in their internal and external environments. A person's perception of these changes may be conscious or unconscious. If the person has the necessary resources, adaptation takes place, and balance is maintained. If the resources cannot reestablish balance, a state of stress results. The person's responses and the degree of stress depend in part on the nature, intensity, timing, number, and duration of stressors. Adaptation to stress is also individualized by a person's age, developmental level, past

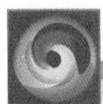

Table 31-1
Homeostatic Regulators of the Body

System	Action	Effect
Autonomic Nervous		
Parasympathetic—Functions under normal conditions and at rest (Cranial and sacral nerves)	• Regulates heart rate • Stimulates secretion of digestive juices and digestive tract smooth muscle • Stimulates insulin secretion	• Slows rate • Improves digestion, increases peristalsis • Increases uptake of glucose by cells
Sympathetic—Functions under stress conditions to bring about the fight-or-flight response	• Stimulates heart rate and force • Dilates skeletal muscle blood vessels • Dilates blood vessels to the brain • Stimulates release of glycogen stores	• Increases rate, strengthens contractions, increases cardiac output • Increases muscle strength • Increases mental alertness • Increases blood glucose levels
Endocrine		

Pituitary	• Secretes hormones:
	    Adrenocorticotropic hormone (ACTH)
	    Thyroid-stimulating hormone (TSH)
		• Stimulates the adrenal cortex
		• Stimulates the thyroid

Adrenals	• Medulla produces epinephrine and norepinephrine • Cortex secretes mineralocorticoids, glucocorticoids, and androgens	• Prepares the person for emergencies; supports the sympathetic system • Mineralocorticoid aldosterone regulates fluid and electrolytes • Glucocorticoids raise glucose levels (for energy) and increase resistance to physical stress
Thyroid	• Secretes thyroid hormone and calcitonin	• Regulates metabolic rate and growth
Other		
Cardiovascular	• Serves as transport system and pump	• Provides oxygen and nutrients and removes carbon dioxide and wastes from cells
Renal	• Filters, excretes, and reabsorbs metabolic products and water	• Maintains fluid, electrolyte, and acid–base balance
Respiratory	• Intake and output of oxygen and carbon dioxide	• Necessary for metabolism; helps maintain acid–base balance
Gastrointestinal	• Takes in food and fluids • Eliminates waste products	• Energy sources; maintains fluids and electrolytes

experiences, support systems, and coping mechanisms. Adaptive responses to health include the mind–body interaction, the local adaptation syndrome, the general adaptation syndrome, and coping/defense mechanisms.

Mind–Body Interaction
Consider the following examples of mind–body interaction.

• Tomorrow you are scheduled to take a final examination, and you must make a passing score to pass the course and remain in the nursing program. After being awake most of the night, you are unable to swallow any food for breakfast, have a rapid heartbeat, are filled with feelings of apprehension, and have diarrhea.

• Since his wife was killed in a car accident, Tom Green has been the sole support of his 4-year-old son, who is developmentally delayed and hyperactive. Tom has been coming to the neighborhood health clinic with increasing frequency the past 5 months, complaining of weight loss, headaches, and stomach pain.

These two examples illustrate the relationship between psychological stressors and the physiologic stress response. In the first example, as you begin the test and discover that you know most of the answers, your symptoms rapidly disappear. Tom's stress, however, is always present and long-term, increasing his risk for developing an illness.

Examples of Physical Illnesses Associated With Stress

Autoimmune disorders
  Graves' disease (hyperthyroidism)
  Rheumatoid arthritis
  Ulcerative colitis
  Psoriasis
  Myasthenia gravis

Cardiovascular disorders
  Hypertension
  Coronary artery disease

Respiratory disorders
  Asthma

Gastrointestinal disorders
  Esophageal reflux
  Constipation
  Diarrhea
  Ulcerative colitis

Why does this happen? Although the exact cause is not well understood, it is thought that humans react to threats of danger as if they were physiologic threats. A person perceives the threat on an emotional level, and the body prepares itself to either resist the danger or run away from it (the **fight-or-flight response**). Each person reacts in her or his own way. With prolonged stress, some may develop chronic diarrhea, whereas others may develop headaches. Such illnesses are real and are called **psychosomatic disorders** because the physiologic alterations are thought to be at least partially caused by psychological influences. The accompanying box lists physiologic indicators of stress.

Another component of mind–body interaction is the impact of life changes on a person. Researchers have found

Physiologic Indicators of Stress

Backache

Constipation or diarrhea

Dilated pupils

Dry mouth

Headache

Increased urination

Increased pulse, blood pressure, and respirations

Loss of appetite

Nausea

Sleep disturbances

Stiff neck

Sweaty palms

that the number of changes a person has in his or her life (both positive and negative) is correlated with illness. A life change is defined as an event in a person's life that requires energy for adaptation. When energy is expended to adapt to the event, the person's resistance to illness is lowered. For example, although a holiday celebration with family and friends is considered a positive event in one's life, stressful factors include the time necessary to prepare for the party, worrying about how everyone will get along, and trying to decide how much money to spend.

Physiologic Responses to Stress

As we have seen, there are both physical and emotional components in a person's response—or adaptation—to stress. The physiologic responses occur in what are called the local adaptation syndrome and the general adaptation syndrome.

Local Adaptation Syndrome

The **local adaptation syndrome** (LAS) is a localized response of the body to stress. It involves only a specific body part (tissue, organ) instead of the whole body. The stress precipitating the LAS may be traumatic or pathologic. LAS is a short-term adaptive response, primarily homeostatic. Although the body has many localized stress responses, the two most common responses that influence nursing care are the reflex pain response and the inflammatory response.

The **reflex pain response** is a response of the central nervous system to pain. It is rapid and automatic, serving as a protective mechanism to prevent injury. The reflex depends on an intact, functioning neurologic reflex arc and involves both sensory and motor neurons. For example, if you step into a bathtub of dangerously hot water, your skin senses the heat and immediately sends a message to the spinal cord. A message is then sent to a motor nerve, which activates the muscles in your leg to pull back your foot. All of this happens before you consciously realize that the water is too hot to be safe.

The **inflammatory response** is a local response to injury or infection. It serves to localize and prevent the spread of infection and promote wound healing. When you cut your finger, for example, you often develop the symptoms of the inflammatory response: pain, swelling, heat, redness, and changes in function. There are three phases in the inflammatory response:

1. In the first phase, bleeding is initially controlled by vasoconstriction (narrowing) of the blood vessels at the injury site. After the bleeding has been controlled, histamines are released and capillary permeability increases, allowing increased blood flow and white blood cells to the area. The blood flow then returns to normal, but the white blood cells remain to help resist infection.
2. During the second stage, exudate (made up of fluid, cells, and inflammatory byproducts) is released from the wound. The amount of exudate depends on the size, location, and severity of the wound.

3. During the third and final stage, damaged cells are repaired by either regeneration (replacement with identical cells) or formation of scar tissue. Some body tissues (skin, bone) are easily reproduced and regain their former function; others (nervous system, intestines) do not regenerate but form nonfunctional scar tissue.

General Adaptation Syndrome

The **general adaptation syndrome** (GAS) is a biochemical model of stress developed by Hans Selye (1976). The GAS describes the body's general response to stress, a concept essential in all areas of nursing care. There are three stages in the GAS (Fig. 31-2):

1. In the first stage, the *alarm reaction,* a person perceives a specific stressor, and various defense mechanisms are activated. The perception of threat may be conscious or unconscious. The autonomic nervous system initiates the fight-or-flight response, and hormone levels rise to prepare the body to react. This phase of the alarm reaction, called the *shock phase,* is characterized by an increase in energy levels, oxygen intake, cardiac output, blood pressure, and mental alertness. (If you recall the last time you almost had a car accident, you can easily identify these body reactions!) During the second phase of the alarm reaction, *countershock,* there is a reversal of body changes.
2. The second stage of the GAS is *resistance.* Having perceived the threat and mobilized its resources, the body now attempts to adapt to the stressor. Vital signs, hormone levels, and energy production return to normal. If the stress can be managed or confined to a small area (LAS), the body regains homeostasis. If the damage to the body is too great (eg, with severe injury and bleeding or a major illness such as cancer or a heart attack), the adaptive mechanisms fail, and the third phase of the GAS begins.
3. The third stage, *exhaustion,* results when the adaptive mechanisms are exhausted. Without defense against the stressor, the body may either rest and mobilize its defenses to return to normal or reach total exhaustion and die.

Although the alarm stage is short-term (minutes to hours), the length of the resistance and exhaustion stages varies greatly, depending on such variables as the severity and duration of the stressor, the previous health of the person, and the immediacy and effectiveness of healthcare interventions.

The GAS is a physiologic response to stress, but it is important to remember that the response results from either physical or emotional stressors. The stages occur with either physical or psychological damage to the person. Obvious examples are seen in patients with severe injury or an illness, but GAS is also a factor in mental illness, social isolation, and loss (or lack) of human relations.

Psychological Responses to Stress

Humans respond to threat—and stress—psychologically as well as physically. Various emotional responses may occur,

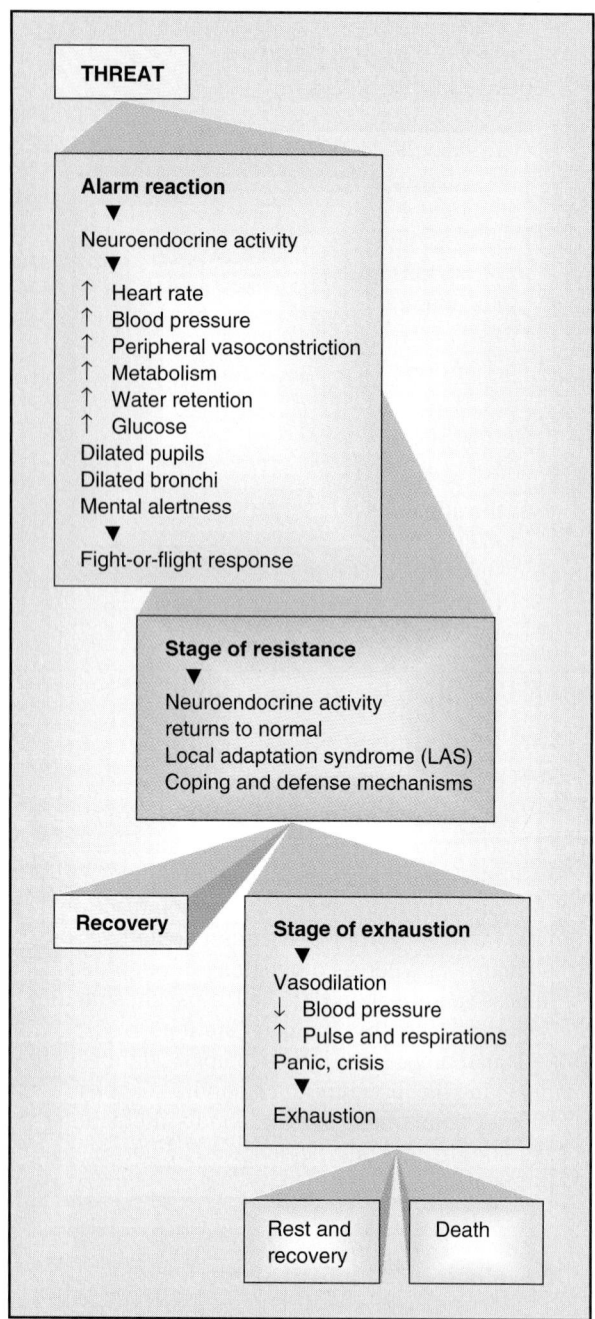

Figure 31-2
The general adaptation syndrome (general response to stress).

including depression and anger. The most common human response is **anxiety.** Anxiety is experienced at some time by all people and can involve one's body, self-perceptions, and social relationships. Anxiety is "a vague, uneasy feeling of discomfort or dread accompanied by an autonomic response; the source is often nonspecific or unknown to the individual; a feeling of apprehension caused by the anticipation of danger. It is an altering signal that warns of impending danger and enables the individual to take measures to deal with threat" (North American Nursing Diagnosis Association, 1999, p. 134). In contrast, fear (a feeling of dread) is a cognitive response to a known threat. Anxiety is the emotional response to that threat. Anxiety is often present before new experiences, such as starting college or beginning a new job, which may be perceived as a threat to one's identity and self-esteem.

The four levels of anxiety each have different effects:

Mild anxiety: Present in day-to-day living; increases alertness and perceptual fields (eg, vision and hearing) and motivates learning and growth. Although mild anxiety may interfere with sleep, it also facilitates problem solving. Mild anxiety is often manifested by restlessness and increased questioning.

Moderate anxiety: Narrows the person's perceptual fields so that the focus is on immediate concerns, with inattention to other communications and details. Moderate anxiety is manifested by a quivering voice, tremors, increased muscle tension, a complaint of "butterflies in the stomach," and slight increases in respirations and pulse.

Severe anxiety: Creates a very narrow focus on specific detail; causes all behavior to be geared toward getting relief. The person has impaired learning ability and is easily distracted. Severe anxiety is manifested by difficulty verbally communicating, increased motor activity, a fearful facial expression, headache, nausea, dizziness, tachycardia, and hyperventilation.

Panic: Causes the person to lose control and experience dread and terror. The resulting disorganized state is characterized by increased physical activity, distorted perception of events, and loss of rational thought. The person is unable to learn, concentrates only on the present situation, and often experiences feelings of impending doom. This level of anxiety can lead to exhaustion and death. Panic is manifested by difficulty verbally communicating, agitation, trembling, poor motor control, sensory changes, sweating, tachycardia, hyperventilation, dyspnea, palpitations, choking sensation, and sensations of chest pain or pressure.

At a mild level, anxiety can have a positive effect. For example, mild anxiety about an upcoming examination can motivate a student to do the required reading and review. Anxiety beyond that level is generally negative and has unpleasant effects. In an attempt to neutralize, deny, or counteract the anxiety, the person develops individual patterns of coping.

Coping Mechanisms

Mild anxiety is often managed without conscious thought by **coping mechanisms,** which are behaviors used to decrease stress and anxiety. Typical behaviors include the following:

- Crying, laughing, sleeping, cursing
- Physical activity, exercise
- Smoking, drinking
- Lack of eye contact, withdrawal
- Limiting relationships to those with similar values and interests

Moderate, severe, and panic levels of anxiety are greater threats and involve more complex coping mechanisms as the person strives to reduce the stress and anxiety. Many coping behaviors are learned, based on past experiences and sociocultural influences and expectations. Coping mechanisms used at higher levels of anxiety are categorized as task-oriented reactions or defense mechanisms.

Task-oriented reactions involve consciously thinking about the stress situation and then acting to solve problems, resolve conflicts, or satisfy needs. These reactions are as follows:

Attack behavior: Occurs when a person attempts to overcome obstacles to satisfy a need; may be constructive, with assertive problem solving, or destructive, with feelings and actions of aggressive anger and hostility

Withdrawal behavior: Involves physical withdrawal from the threat, or emotional reactions such as admitting defeat, becoming apathetic, or feeling guilty and isolated

Compromise behavior: Usually constructive; involves the substitution of goals or negotiation to fulfill one's needs partially

Defense Mechanisms

Other unconscious reactions, called **defense mechanisms,** often occur. These mechanisms protect one's self-esteem and are useful in mild to moderate anxiety. When extreme, they distort reality and create problems with relationships. At that point, the mechanisms become maladaptive instead of adaptive.

Common defense mechanisms are summarized here. You will learn more about them in your study of mental health nursing.

Compensation occurs when a person attempts to overcome a perceived weakness by emphasizing a more desirable trait or overachieving in a more comfortable area. For example, a student who has difficulty with academic subjects may excel at sports.

Denial occurs when a person refuses to acknowledge the presence of a condition that is disturbing. An ill person is in denial when refusing to accept a diagnosis or prognosis.

Displacement occurs when a person transfers (or displaces) an emotional reaction from one object or person to another object or person. For example, an employee who is angry with a coworker displaces anger by kicking a chair.

Introjection occurs when a person incorporates qualities or values of another person into his or her own ego structure. This is an important mechanism in the formation of the conscience during early childhood. An older sibling may, for instance, tell his preschool sister not to talk to strangers, expressing his parents' values to his smaller sister.

Projection occurs when a person's thoughts or impulses are attributed to another person, allowing intolerable feelings or motivation to be attributed to someone else. For example, a person who denies any sexual feelings for a coworker accuses her of sexual harassment.

Rationalization occurs when a person tries to give questionable behavior a logical or socially acceptable explanation. It amounts to behavior justification. For example, a patient may rationalize for forgetting an appointment with a healthcare practitioner by saying, "If patients didn't have to wait for 3 months to get an appointment, they would not forget them!"

Reaction formation occurs when a person develops conscious attitudes and behavior patterns that are opposite to what one really would like to do or feel. For example, a married woman is attracted to her husband's best friend but is constantly rude to him.

Regression occurs when a person returns to an earlier method of behaving. Children often demonstrate regressive behavior, such as soiling diapers and demanding a bottle, when they are ill.

Repression occurs when a person involuntarily excludes an anxiety-producing event from conscious awareness. This is the primary ego defense mechanism. As an extreme example, a father may not remember shaking his crying baby.

Sublimation occurs when a person substitutes a socially acceptable goal for one whose normal channel of expression is blocked. An individual who is aggressive toward others may, for example, become a star football player.

Undoing is an act or communication that is used to negate a previous act or communication. A parent who is verbally abusive to his or her child and then brings home presents the next day is undoing.

Effects of Stress

Stress affects all of the human dimensions. It strongly influences how one attains basic human needs; it is a factor in health and illness; and it becomes a component in family reactions to illness. Both long-term or prolonged stress and crisis situations may seriously affect a person's physical and emotional health.

Interactions With Basic Human Needs

Basic human needs, described in Chapter 2, are common to all people. Stress, too, is common to all people. Both need attainment and the adaptation to stress require energy, respond to internal and external environments, and motivate behaviors. As a person strives to meet basic human needs at each level, stress can be either a stimulus or a barrier.

How a person meets basic human needs and responds to stress is unique to the individual; both are modified by sociocultural backgrounds, priorities, and past experiences. In all people, the failure to meet needs results in an imbalance in homeostatic mechanisms and, eventually, illness. Stress affects a person and his or her attainment of basic human needs in different ways, as illustrated in the accompanying box.

Stress in Health and Illness

The health–illness continuum (described in Chap. 4) is also affected by stress. Health and homeostatic balance are at one extreme of the continuum; exhaustion and death are at the other extreme.

Stress in a healthy person may promote health and prevent illness. For example, the fear of developing lung cancer may motivate a person to stop smoking, or anxiety about baby care may prompt prospective parents to attend prenatal classes and read child care books. Stressors in health also facilitate normal growth and development, provide the stimulus for learning constructive adaptive behaviors, stimulate problem-solving abilities, encourage social relationships, and help develop spiritual strength.

The effects of stress on a sick or injured person are, in contrast, usually negative. Stress can cause illness; illness causes stress. The presence of an illness or a disability demands new coping skills at a time when homeostasis is challenged. The accompanying Research in Nursing box describes a study of the stressful life events, social support, and health status of rural older adults. Addi-

---

Effects of Stress on Basic Human Needs

Physiologic

Change in appetite, activity, or sleep

Change in elimination patterns

Increased pulse, respirations, blood pressure

Safety/Security

Feels threatened or nervous

Uses ineffective coping mechanisms

Is inattentive

Love/Belonging

Is withdrawn and isolated

Blames others for own faults

Demonstrates aggressive behaviors

Becomes overly dependent on others

Self-Esteem

Becomes a workaholic

Exhibits attention-seeking behaviors

Self-Actualization

Refuses to accept reality

Centers on own problems

Demonstrates lack of control

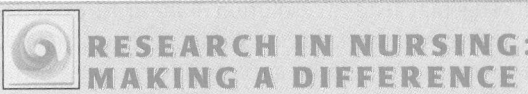

RESEARCH IN NURSING: MAKING A DIFFERENCE

Stress, Social Support, and Health in Rural Older Adults

About one third of adults older than 65 years of age live in rural areas, and these experience more physical disabilities and chronic illnesses than do urban older adults. Stress is a significant factor in the development of illness, but stress can be buffered by social support. Not much is known about the physical and mental health needs of rural older adults, nor about how comprehensive care can be planned and implemented to enhance the quality of life for this population.

Related Research

Johnson, J. E. (1998). Stress, social support and health in frontier elders. *Journal of Gerontological Nursing*, 24(5), 29–35.

This study was conducted to examine the stressful life events, social support, and perceived health status of older adults living in rural isolated areas of the Western United States. Data were collected about these factors from 82 participants. The most frequently reported stressful events were a lack of transportation, changes in eyesight, changes in hearing, loss of friends, loss of

family, loss of pet, loneliness, dependence on others, and loss of driver's license. Many of the participants had no one to depend on for assistance, and 68% rated their health as poor or very poor.

Relevance to Nursing Practice

This is an example of nursing research about groups of people who are little studied but who have many needs that can be met through nursing care. It is important for nurses to assess older adults carefully for levels of stress and support. Referrals to appropriate sources of help, such as a local minister, should be considered in the plan of care. Nurses should also explore ways to increase or strengthen rural older adults' social support systems, including maintaining telephone contact with family and friends, using available church transportation services, having pets, and using e-mail on the computer. Such interventions not only improve older adults' quality of life but also may enable them to continue living at home.

tionally, people who enter healthcare settings are subjected to situational stressors.

Adaptation to acute and chronic illness involves two sets of adaptive tasks: *general tasks* (as in the case of any situational stress) that involve maintaining self-esteem and personal relationships and preparing for an uncertain future, and *illness-related tasks*, which include the following (Moos, 1985):

- Losing independence and control
- Handling pain and incapacitation
- Facilitating body function recovery
- Dealing with the hospital environment
- Developing relationships with caregivers
- Controlling symptoms
- Carrying out medical treatment
- Confronting economic and family problems

Every situation is different, and each person perceives and reacts to stressors in an individual manner. There is no one best way to cope with a given situation. Nursing considerations include the person's major concern, specific illness, sociocultural background, and available resources. For example, an older woman may be anxious about the cost of treatment for her hip fracture, whereas her roommate, with the same injury, is seriously concerned about the care of her cats while she is in the hospital. As another example, Mary and Jane have both entered the hospital with the medical diagnosis of breast cancer. Mary is worried about possible disfigurement and death, but she be-

lieves that with the help of surgery and chemotherapy, she can overcome the cancer. Jane, on the other hand, comes from a community that has strong fundamental religious beliefs. She believes that the cancer is a punishment from God and refuses treatment, even though she fears death.

Family Responses to the Stress of Illness

The stress that affects an ill person also affects the person's family members or significant others. When the family is viewed as a system, the behavior of the individual is seen to be influenced by the family, and any alterations in the individual's behavior in turn affect the family. The family thus is an integral part in the assessment, planning, nursing interventions, and evaluation of actions to promote adaptation to stress.

The family of a person with an acute or chronic illness is subjected to various stressors, including the following:

- Changes in family structure and roles
- Isolation from the loved person
- Loss of control over normal routines
- Anger and feelings of helplessness and guilt
- Lack of information about care
- Concern for future economic stability

The family, both as individuals and as a unit, uses many of the same coping and defense mechanisms previously described. Family members may be overly protective, deny the seriousness of the illness, or blame healthcare providers for the patient's condition or behaviors. On the other hand, the family can provide the social support necessary to help the patient manage and adapt to stress. Emotional support from family members allows open expression of feelings and helps meet love and belonging needs. The inclusion of family members in problem solving, teaching and learning activities, and physical care helps both the patient and the family to maintain their self-esteem and feeling of worth.

Prolonged Stress

Prolonged or long-term stress is a serious threat to physical and emotional health. As the duration, intensity, or number of stressors increases, a person's ability to adapt is lessened. The failure of adaptive mechanisms is also influenced by a person's state of health and past experiences with stress.

Long-term stress affects physical status, increasing the risk for disease or injury. Recovery and return to normal function are also compromised by prolonged stress. High levels of stress are associated with cardiovascular disease, gastrointestinal disorders, and cancer. It is believed that these diseases are the result of various factors, including the effects of the fight-or-flight response, eating patterns, lifestyle, and coping mechanisms. A person who reacts to stress by overeating, smoking, becoming chemically dependent, or becoming hyperactive puts additional strain on the body. Homeostasis cannot be maintained, and illness results.

Reactions to home care of a family member for long periods also cause prolonged stress. Called **caregiver burden**, this stress response includes chronic fatigue, sleep problems, and increased incidence of stress-related illnesses, such as high blood pressure and heart disease.

Prolonged stress can seriously threaten mental health. As coping or defense mechanisms become ineffective, a person may try less effective coping patterns or maladaptive defense mechanisms. As anxiety increases despite these measures, the person may experience difficulties on the job, with personal relationships, and with self-esteem. These problems in turn act as additional stressors, and mental illness may result.

Crisis

A **crisis** is a disturbance caused by a precipitating event, such as a perceived loss, a threat of loss, or a challenge, that is perceived as a threat to self (Stuart & Sundeen, 1999). The person's usual methods of coping becoming ineffective, resulting in increasingly greater levels of anxiety. This failure produces high levels of anxiety, disorganized behavior, and an inability to function adequately.

After the precipitating event, the person's anxiety increases, and phases of the crisis emerge. First, the anxiety activates the person's usual methods of coping. If these are not effective, the person experiences more anxiety because the coping mechanisms are not working. As the crisis continues, the person tries new methods of coping or redefines

the threat. This may lead to resolution of the crisis or, if not effective, may result in severe or panic levels of anxiety. The crisis is more likely to be successfully resolved if the person realistically views the event, if effective coping mechanisms are present, and if situational support systems are available.

Crises may be maturational, situational, or adventitious. Maturational crises occur during developmental events that require role change, such as when a teenager moves into adulthood. Situational crises occur when a life event disrupts a person's psychological equilibrium, such as loss of a job or death of a loved family member. Adventitious crises are accidental and unexpected events, resulting in multiple losses and major environmental changes, such as fires, earthquakes, and floods that involve not only individuals but also entire communities. These types of crises are further described in the following section.

Factors Affecting Stress and Adaptation

Stress and adaptation are affected by the sources of stress, the types of stressors experienced, and personal factors.

Sources of Stress

Although there are an almost infinite number of sources of stress, they can be categorized into two broad areas. Both create major demands for adaptive responses. These sources are developmental stress and situational stress.

Developmental stress, or a **developmental crisis**, occurs as a person progresses through the normal stages of growth and development from birth to old age (these are described in Chaps. 9 and 10). Within each stage, certain tasks must be achieved to resolve the crisis and reduce the stress. Examples of developmental stress include the following:

- The infant learns to trust others.
- The toddler learns to control elimination.
- The school-aged child socializes with peers.
- The adolescent strives for independence.
- The middle adult accepts physical signs of aging.

Situational stress is different from developmental stress. It does not occur in predictable patterns as one progresses through life. Rather, situational stress can occur at any time, although the person's ability to adapt may be strongly influenced by his or her developmental level. Examples of situational stress (or crises), which may be either positive or negative, include the following:

- Illness or accidents
- Marriage or divorce
- Loss (belongings, relationships, family member)
- New job
- Role change

To further illustrate the positive or negative aspects of situational stress, consider pregnancy as an example. A young married couple may be overjoyed at the prospect of becoming parents, whereas an unmarried adolescent may be panic stricken when she discovers she is pregnant. The situations and the developmental levels of the young couple and the adolescent will have a major impact on the adaptations they will make. A person's physical and psychosocial capacities to cope with the situation depend not only on the stage of maturation but also on the support systems available.

Types of Stressors

Physiologic stressors have both a specific effect and a general effect. The specific effect is an alteration of normal body structure and function. The general effect is the stress response. Primary physiologic stressors include chemical agents (drugs, poisons), physical agents (heat, cold, trauma), infectious agents (viruses, bacteria), nutritional imbalances, hypoxia, and genetic or immune disorders.

There are an almost infinite variety of *psychosocial stressors,* which become so much a part of our daily lives that we often overlook them. To illustrate the many types of psychosocial stressors, consider the following categories, summarized from work by Antonovsky (1979):

- Accidents and their survivors, which cause stress for the victim, the person who caused the accident, and the families of both
- Stressful experiences of family members and friends
- Horrors of history, such as Nazi concentration camps, famine in Africa, and the effects of the atomic bomb on Hiroshima
- Fear of aggression or mutilation from others, such as muggings, rape, murder, and terrorist attacks
- Events of history that are brought into our homes through television, such as wars, earthquakes, and violence in schools
- Developmental and life crises
- Rapid changes in our world and the way we live, including changes in economic and political structures and technology

Psychosocial stressors include both real and perceived threats. The person's responses are continuous and include the individual coping mechanisms for responding to anxiety, guilt, fear, frustration, and loss. The mechanisms serve to maintain psychological homeostasis.

Personal Factors

A person's adaptation to stress—whether positive or negative—is influenced by a number of personal factors. One's physiologic reserve and genetic inheritance are important to maintaining homeostasis and adapting to stressors. The ability to adapt is decreased in the very young, the very old, and those with altered physical or mental health, who do not have the necessary physiologic reserve to cope with physical changes, such as dehydration or fluid excess. Adequate nutrition and sleep are necessary to enzyme function, immune responses, wound healing, and energy production and restoration. Malnutrition, dietary excess, and sleep deprivation all impair one's ability to

adapt to stress. Social factors and life events are also implicated in adaptation to stress, with people who have strong support systems and relationships better able to adapt to stress and remain healthy (Porth, 1998).

The Nursing Process

ASSESSING STRESS

Stress and anxiety are problems that nurses encounter in patients at all ages and in all settings. Stress is assessed through a health assessment, including a nursing history and physical assessment. Risk factors for or indicators of stress may be identified through standardized tests or open-ended questions to elicit information. The patient's willingness to share information is affected by the level of stress experienced as well as the coping or defense mechanisms in use.

Nursing History

The nursing history assists the nurse in identifying stressors and how the person perceives and copes with stress. Manifestations of anxiety, as well as questions and leading statements to identify stress and anxiety, are listed in the accompanying Focused Assessment Guide: Assessing Anxiety.

Physical Assessment

There are no specific guidelines for the physical assessment of stress. Physical indicators of stress, in addition to those listed in the Focused Assessment Guide, may include cardiac dysrhythmias, chest pain, headache, hyperventilation, diarrhea, tense muscles, and skin lesions such as eczema. These manifestations are the result of the mind–body interaction described earlier.

DIAGNOSING

When assessment data provide cues to a problem with stress that can be treated by nursing interventions, it is labeled with the nursing diagnosis *Anxiety.* Common etiologies for anxiety include conflicts about values and goals in life, threat to self-concept, threat of death, threat of or change in health status, threat to or change in environment or role, situational/maturational crisis, or unmet needs. Examples of other nursing diagnoses that are significant in patients or families having problems with stress are as follows:

Ineffective Individual Coping related to inability to maintain marriage
Defensive Coping related to loss of job and economic security
Altered Thought Processes related to panic state
Ineffective Denial related to continued smoking behavior

FOCUSED ASSESSMENT GUIDE

Assessing Anxiety

Assess the patient for:

- Subjective data: heart palpations; difficulty breathing; nausea; sleeping or eating problems; verbalizing sadness, apprehension, anger, mistrust, helplessness, hopelessness, changes in sexual function
- Objective data: dry mouth, increased perspiration, tremors, tachycardia, hypertension, crying, dilated pupils, restlessness, poor eye contact, quivering voice, slouched posture, pacing, rapid speech, lack of facial expression

Ask questions or make leading statements to elicit information; for example:

- You have been very quiet today . . . has anything happened since our last visit?
- It must be very frightening to learn that you have cancer.
- I notice that you seem upset . . . would you like to talk about it?
- What is causing you a problem at this time?
- How does your body feel when you are nervous?
- What has caused you to feel stressed in the past?
- What do you do to feel better when you feel anxious or stressed?

Decisional Conflict related to placement of parent in nursing home

Ineffective Family Coping: Disabling related to lack of knowledge about home care of child on ventilator

Stress may affect many other areas of human functioning. In the following nursing diagnoses, stress and anxiety are involved in the etiologies of other problems.

Altered Nutrition: Less Than Body Requirements related to inadequate caloric intake while striving to excel in gymnastics

Caregiver Role Strain related to long-term stress of care for parent with Alzheimer's disease

Social Isolation related to feelings of worthlessness and apprehension following failure in school

Spiritual Distress related to inability to accept diagnosis of terminal illness

Hopelessness related to presence of disabling physical injuries

Sleep Pattern Disturbance related to anxiety about terminally ill spouse

Examples of nursing diagnoses for common problems are outlined in the accompanying box.

PLANNING: EXPECTED OUTCOMES

The nurse plans and implements care to decrease anxiety and facilitate adaptation in the patient with anxiety. The expected outcomes of the plan must be mutually determined with the patient or family members. The expected outcomes of the plan of care may include that the patient will achieve the following:

- Decrease the level of anxiety by verbalizing feelings and using support systems
- Develop effective coping skills through problem-solving skills and anxiety-reducing techniques

- Describe a reduction in anxiety and an increase in comfort

IMPLEMENTING

Nurses may use a variety of interventions to help patients decrease stress and to facilitate coping. If the patient's anxiety seems too great or the nurse is uncomfortable with the interventions, a referral should be made. A referral may be made, for example, to a professional counselor, to individuals who have experienced the same type of surgery or health problem, or to the patient's rabbi, minister, or priest.

The following nursing interventions are discussed in this section: teaching healthy activities of daily living, encouraging use of support systems, and practicing stress management techniques. Methods should be carefully selected, based on the person's physical and emotional characteristics, family and social structure, and previously successful coping mechanisms. The accompanying box, Guidelines for Nursing Care, lists nursing interventions to reduce anxiety for patients as they enter a healthcare setting.

Teaching Healthy Activities of Daily Living

A person's normal lifestyle greatly influences his or her perceptions of and reactions to stressors. For example, a person who is overweight, sedentary, and chronically tired is at increased risk for developing an illness as a result of stress. These factors are also stressors and further increase the risk. Exercise, rest, and good nutrition are important components of stress reduction.

Exercise

Regular exercise helps to maintain physical and emotional health. The benefits of exercise include an improved musculoskeletal system, more effective cardiovascular func-

Nursing Diagnoses for Common Problems

Stress

Problem	*Related Factors*	*Sample Defining Characteristics*
Anxiety	Diagnosis of illness requiring surgery and fear of disfigurement	Newly diagnosed with breast cancer; pulse and respirations are increased above baseline; restless and unable to sleep; facial expression tense; states, "I can't get any rest because I'm so afraid of having surgery and losing my breast."
Impaired Adjustment	Refusal to follow prescribed treatment	Middle-aged man who had a serious myocardial infarction (heart attack) refuses to join a cardiac rehabilitation program and continues to smoke and eat high-fat foods.
Ineffective Individual Coping	Recent divorce and lack of support systems	"I just can't seem to handle things anymore. I know I smoke and drink too much, but I'm just so tired of being alone."
Ineffective Family Coping: Compromised	Spinal cord injury with loss of lower extremity function (paraplegia)	Mother of 19-year-old young man who has paraplegia from a diving accident refuses to let him provide self-care. She states, "I know he will be able to walk soon and he needs me to take care of him now."
Ineffective Family Coping: Disabling	Developmental delay Childhood autism	10-month-old infant with severe mental retardation has obvious malnutrition and signs of neglect.
Family Coping: Potential for Growth	Joins a support group for lung cancer that includes a stop smoking program	Wife of husband with lung cancer attends support group and takes pride in her support of his success in stopping smoking.
Ineffective Denial	Changes in size, shape, and color of a mole	Older adult man has large black lesion on forehead, states "Oh, I've had that for a long time—it's just a pimple."
Defensive Coping	Obesity	"I don't care if I'm fat. It's not my fault that I can't lose weight. I just don't have time to exercise, and I can't stand vegetables." Is 20% above standard weight for height.

tion, weight control, and relaxation. Exercise improves one's general sense of well-being, relieves tension, and enables one to cope better with day-to-day stressors. General health guidelines recommend that an exercise program consist of 30 to 45 minutes of activity three or four times a week. People who are overweight, chronically ill, or older than 35 years of age should have a thorough physical examination before beginning such a program. The type of exercise can be individualized to what one enjoys most—for example, walking, jogging, bicycling, swimming, or participating in sports such as golf or tennis.

Rest and Sleep

Rest and sleep help the body to maintain homeostasis and restore energy levels. Adequate rest can provide "insulation" against stress, but stress may interfere with one's ability to sleep. Although each person has individual needs, 7 to 8 hours sleep a day is recommended. Relaxation techniques can be helpful in health and illness to facilitate rest and sleep. Hospitalized patients may require additional nursing interventions to relieve pain and promote comfort to get needed rest.

Nutrition

Nutrition plays an active role in maintaining the body's homeostatic mechanisms and in increasing resistance to stress. Obesity and malnutrition are major stressors and greatly increase the risk for illness. People of all ages are encouraged to maintain a normal body weight and to follow these guidelines established by the U.S. Senate Committee on Nutrition and Human Needs:

- Reduce intake of salt, refined sugar, animal fat, and cholesterol.
- Eat more fruit, vegetables, and whole grains.
- Eat less red meat and more fish and poultry. Nutrition is discussed further in Chapter 41.

Encouraging Use of Support Systems

Support systems provide emotional support that helps a person identify and verbalize feelings associated with stress. Other valuable contributions include providing information and services, maintaining positive self-concept, and establishing an avenue for new relationships and social roles. Additionally, families and support groups provide an accepting environment, allowing the person to explore problem-solving methods and try out new coping skills. There are support groups for almost every situation. Examples include the following:

Alcoholics Anonymous
Overeaters Anonymous

Guidelines for Nursing Care

Reducing Anxiety in the Patient Entering the Healthcare Setting

Nursing Intervention	*Rationale*
• Assess physical status, sensory status, and cognitive status	• Altered responses to illness or injury, such as pain, nausea and vomiting, and dyspnea may increase anxiety and decrease the ability to be attentive and retain information. Impairments in function, such as vision, hearing, cognitive, or memory deficits, interfere with communications.
• Assess cultural/ethnic background, including beliefs about healthcare, dietary restrictions, and language spoken.	• Entering the healthcare system of a different culture is stressful; if a different language is used, communications and teaching are difficult.
• Assess past experiences with the healthcare system, including medical-surgical treatment for illness or injury.	• Expectations and perceptions of healthcare are influenced both positively and negatively by past experiences.
• Assess concerns and stressors.	• All people entering the healthcare system have an emotional response; additional stressors may increase anxiety.
• Assess amount and type of support systems available.	• Support from family and friends and belief in a higher being can provide strength in handling new or unfamiliar stressors; a lack of support can increase stress and decrease coping.
• Provide information about the environment: a. All healthcare providers should introduce themselves by name and title. b. Explain policies and routines. c. If the hospital is the setting, provide verbal and written guidelines for use of equipment, telephone, television, meals, and visiting hours.	• Providing information decreases the unknown and thus lessens anxiety.
• Provide and discuss the patient's rights specific to care in the agency or institution.	• Knowing one's rights within an unfamiliar setting enhances a sense of control and helps decrease anxiety.
• Mutually determine expected outcomes of the plan of care.	• Coping is enhanced when the patient participates in decision making; loss of control contributes to a feeling of powerlessness and increases anxiety.
• Provide information about all diagnostic procedures, surgical procedures, activity, and diet.	• Knowing the how, what, where, and why of what will be done allows a sense of control and decreases anxiety.
• Use verbal and nonverbal communication skills to convey genuine interest, concern for the patient's well-being, and empathic understanding.	• Effective communications facilitate verbalization of concerns, allowing interventions to decrease anxiety and provide comfort.

(Adapted from Carpenito, L. (1999). *Nursing care plans and documentation: Nursing diagnoses and collaborative problems* (3rd ed.). Philadelphia: Lippincott Williams & Wilkins.)

Weight Watchers
Parents Without Partners
Reach to Recovery (cancer)
Ostomy clubs
Child abuse support groups
Sudden infant death support groups
Stroke clubs
Assertiveness training groups

Encouraging Use of Stress Management Techniques

Stress creates emotional distress that often has outward symptoms. One person may have tension headaches; another becomes irritable; another clenches his or her fists. Many people take legal or illegal drugs, drink or smoke to excess, or eat compulsively. These behaviors can be modified and adaptive mechanisms strengthened through specific techniques aimed at managing stress. Only a few techniques are included here, but the literature describes many stress reduction methods, including exercise, prayer, art therapy, music therapy, massage, and therapeutic touch. Students are encouraged to learn different methods they can use for themselves and in varied clinical situations.

Relaxation

Relaxation techniques are useful in many situations—childbirth, pain, anxiety, sleeplessness, illness, anger—and other uses are being discovered. Relaxation promotes a body reaction opposite to that of the fight-or-flight response, decreasing respiratory, pulse, and metabolic rates; blood pressure; and energy use.

Relaxation can be taught to individuals or groups. It is especially helpful because it allows a person to control feelings and behaviors. Various techniques are used, but most involve rhythmic breathing, reduced muscle tension, and an altered state of consciousness (Stuart & Sundeen, 1998). Relaxation is discussed as a comfort measure in Chapter 40. Two relaxation activities, to be practiced three or four times at each session, are deep breathing and progressive muscle relaxation.

Deep Breathing

1. Sit comfortably and place your hands on your stomach. Inhale slowly and deeply, letting your abdomen expand as much as possible. Hold your breath for a few seconds.
2. Exhale slowly through your mouth, blowing through puckered lips. When your abdomen feels empty, begin again with the a deep inhalation.

Progressive Muscle Relaxation

1. Tighten your hand into a fist and notice how it feels. Hold the tension for a few seconds.
2. Loosen your grip, relax the muscles in your hand, and let the tension slip away.
3. Continue to tighten-hold-relax each muscle group: hands, arms, shoulders, face, chest, back, abdomen, legs, feet.

Meditation

Meditation has four components: quiet surroundings, a passive attitude, a comfortable position, and a word or mental image on which to focus. A person practicing meditation sits comfortably with closed eyes, relaxes each of the major muscle groups, and repeats the selected word silently with each exhalation. Alternatively, the person may focus on a pleasant scene and mentally place himself or herself in it while breathing slowly in and out. This exercise should be performed for 20 to 30 minutes twice a day.

Anticipatory Guidance

Anticipatory guidance focuses on psychologically preparing a person for an unfamiliar or painful event. Nurses use this technique to teach patients about procedures and the surgical experience. When patients know what to expect, their anxiety is reduced and their coping mechanisms are more effective. For example, before changing a dressing, teaching would include all the information about the pain involved—onset, severity, cause, and methods of relief. With this knowledge, the patient feels less threatened and tolerates the procedure more easily. A related process is anticipatory socialization, in which people prepare themselves for roles to which they aspire but do not yet occupy. This process may be used, for example, to prepare expectant parents for the role of parenting, thereby enhancing the potential of the child to experience normal growth and development.

Guided Imagery

In guided imagery, a person creates a mental image, concentrates on the image, and becomes less responsive to stimuli (including pain). The nurse sits by the patient and reads a description of a scene or an experience that the patient has described as happy, pleasant, or peaceful. The patient is then "guided" through the image. For example, using a soothing, soft voice, the nurse might start as follows: "You are floating in your swimming pool. The water is cool and comfortable. Birds are singing in the trees. The roses are perfuming the air." As the patient becomes more and more focused on the scene, the nurse need only verbally "paint the picture" at intervals.

Biofeedback

Biofeedback is a method of gaining mental control of the autonomic nervous system and thus regulating body responses, such as blood pressure, heart rate, and headaches. A measurement device (eg, skin temperature sensors) is used, and the patient tries to control the readings through relaxation and conscious thought. The feedback of the change in readings in a long-term process teaches the person to control physiologic functions that normally are considered involuntary responses. The process is still being researched.

Providing Crisis Intervention

As defined earlier, a crisis is a situation that cannot be resolved by usual coping mechanisms. As a result, a person is unable to function normally and requires interventions to regain equilibrium. **Crisis intervention** is a five-step, problem-solving technique designed to promote a more adaptive outcome, including improved abilities to cope with future crises. The steps are as follows:

1. *Identify the problem.* This may be more difficult than it appears; the cause of the crisis is often difficult for the person to identify accurately. Until it is clear, a solution is impossible.
2. *List alternatives.* All possible solutions to the problem need to be listed. An appropriate solution to a problem is much more likely if a substantial number of options are considered.
3. *Choose from among alternatives.* Each option needs to be carefully considered, using a "what would happen if I . . ." approach. The alternative chosen will be highly individualized, based on the person's priorities and values.

4. *Implement the plan.* The alternative chosen is put into action. The nurse may need to provide support and encouragement so that action is taken.
5. *Evaluate the outcome.* In this final step, the effectiveness of the plan needs to be carefully considered. If it did not work as well as expected, another alternative should be chosen. If it did work, it has the positive benefit of improving self-confidence and future problem solving.

The major factor in helping patients adapt to high levels of stress is to identify and plan individually for situations causing the stress. The following suggestions are useful:

- Help the person recognize his or her own stress level and specific responses to stress.
- Encourage a philosophy of accepting what cannot be changed and changing what cannot be accepted.
- Encourage the person to accept help from others—and to give support to others when needed.
- Encourage active but deliberate involvement in problem solving and decision making.
- Be an active listener, increasing the therapeutic relationship and communication.
- Provide health teaching about developmental crises and threatening events.

Stress in the Nursing Profession

Nursing involves activities and interpersonal relationships that are often stressful (Fig. 31-3). Activities identified as highly stressful include the following:

- Having to assume responsibilities for which one is not prepared
- Working with unqualified personnel
- Working in an environment in which supervisors and administrators are not supportive
- Caring for a patient during a cardiac arrest or for a patient who is dying
- Experiencing conflict with peers

The stress is even greater for two groups of nurses: new graduates, who must adjust to an environment different from what they experienced as students; and nurses who work in settings such as intensive care and emergency care. In the present healthcare reform climate, nurses are also stressed by healthcare institutions downsizing and increasing nurses' patient care assignments. They worry not only about the future of their positions but also about the safety of their patients. The anxiety is further complicated by the expectations of nurses: Even though they may have strong negative feelings and reactions, their role does not include behaviors and verbal expressions that are less than positive and supportive.

Student nurses also experience stress and may have difficulty adapting to the requirements and responsibilities of caring for others. Factors causing stress in student nurses include the following:

- Fear of failing the classroom or clinical laboratory components of each course

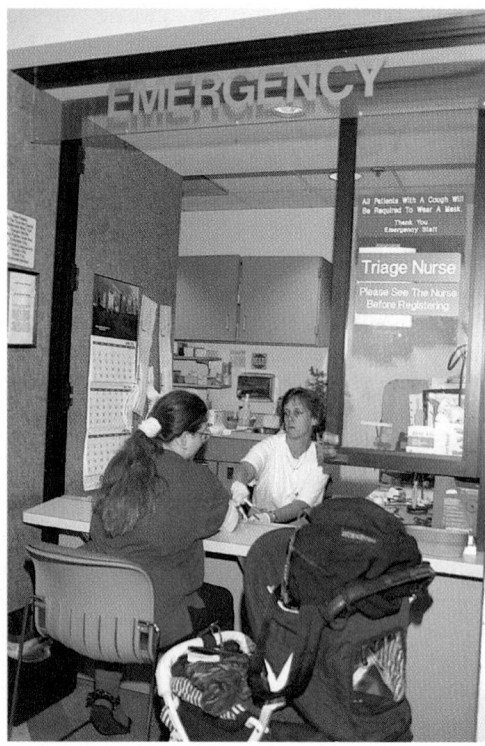

Figure 31-3
Some nursing specialties can be more stressful than others. To prevent burnout and alleviate personal stress, a nurse may need to work in another area of nursing temporarily or permanently. (Photo © Kathy Sloane.)

- Fear of failing the licensure examination after graduation
- Meeting the demands of the nursing program
- Fear of injuring patients
- Balancing work and study
- Meeting financial and family responsibilities

Most nurses and student nurses thoroughly enjoy their education and work and cope with physical and emotional demands effectively. Some, however, are overwhelmed over time and develop symptoms of anxiety and stress. The complex of behaviors is called burnout. **Burnout** can be compared with the exhaustion stage of anxiety and is characterized by a wide range of behaviors. Some try to become "supernurses," expecting perfection in themselves and others. Some withdraw and do only minimal work; still others resort to drugs or alcohol. Many nurses who are unable to handle the stress leave the profession.

What can graduate and student nurses do to help reduce stress and prevent burnout? The first step in preventing a stress level high enough to cause burnout is to identify and accept the stress. The same stress reduction techniques that are used for patients have positive benefits for nurses. The accompanying box provides suggestions for the nurse as a role model in alleviating stress. Other suggested activities to reduce stress are as follows:

- Get involved in constructive change, particularly if organizational activities cause you stress.

APPLYING LEARNING TO PRACTICE

The Nurse as Role Model

Nurses who design care for patients to reduce stress must also examine themselves as a factor in the success of that plan of care. Patients view nurses as role models in achieving healthy lifestyles. Nurses dealing with stresses from professional and personal aspects of their lives sometimes make inappropriate responses. The nurse who wishes to encourage adaptation to stress must demonstrate behaviors that support a healthy lifestyle. With that goal in mind, the nurse will do the following:

- Follow the recommendations of the food pyramid for proper nutrition

- Participate in regular exercise.
- Get adequate sleep and rest.
- Evaluate own use of drugs, nicotine, alcohol, and food as coping methods.
- Practice relaxation techniques regularly.
- Set aside time for activities that are fun.
- Focus on his or her own strengths and abilities.
- Learn to say "no" without feeling guilty or offering an excuse.

- Be supportive of other nurses, other healthcare personnel, and other student nurses; take time to give a compliment for something done well.
- Take time for relaxation—use break time to practice a relaxation technique that works, and go off the unit for lunch.
- Eat regularly, following recommended guidelines for nutrition.
- Carry out a regular exercise program—walk, jog, play tennis, play golf, play handball, join an aerobic dance class.
- Give yourself some time each day to unwind, relax, and do what you want—soak in a bubble bath, listen to music, read a novel.
- Learn something new—how to knit, make cane chairs, speak a foreign language, cook gourmet food.

- Develop assertiveness skills—learn to say no to additional tasks (you don't have to have an excuse—just say, "no, I can't do that"). Accept the fact that no one person is perfect or indispensable.
- Develop and maintain support systems and relationships at work and at home.

Nurses must accept that they have the same needs and are as individual as their patients. The nurse can assess his or her own stress levels and adaptation using the checklist in the accompanying box. By recognizing the early signs of stress and taking steps to reduce it, nurses can continue to be effective and productive as well as satisfied in the profession. (See the accompanying box, Developing Critical Thinking Skills.)

PROMOTING HEALTH

Stress and Adaptation

Use the assessment checklist to determine how well you are adapting to stress. Then develop a prescription for self-care by choosing appropriate behaviors from the list of suggestions.

Assessment Checklist

almost always / sometimes / almost never

☐ ☐ ☐ 1. I have realistic perceptions of new situations, self, and others.

☐ ☐ ☐ 2. I understand my own personal physical and emotional responses to stress.

☐ ☐ ☐ 3. I anticipate and prepare for change.

☐ ☐ ☐ 4. I have the ability to satisfactorily solve problems and make decisions.

Self-Care Behaviors

1. Accept as positive indicators of growth the changes that come with different parts and stages of life.

2. Maintain an open mind about change—change what you can, and accept what you cannot change.

3. Avoid self-defeating behaviors to cope with stress, such as smoking, alcohol, and drugs.

4. Practice methods of stress management that work best for you: relaxation techniques, exercise, hobbies.

5. Set realistic goals.

6. Develop problem-solving strategies for use in stressful situations.

7. Accept help from others.

8. Take life one day at a time.

Developing Critical Thinking Skills

Situation

You are a senior nursing student in your community health course. You have been assigned to visit and provide ongoing assessments for Charles Obedide, a 28-year-old man who was involved in a serious motorcycle accident a year ago and is paralyzed from the waist down. Charles initially participated fully in his rehabilitation and has been living independently in an apartment that is wheelchair accessible. However, a month ago, Charles was ill for 2 weeks, lost his job, and broke up with his girlfriend. When you made your last home visit, Charles was restless, had an increased pulse, and did little talking. At this visit, Charles is wearing dirty clothes and has a strong body odor, and there are several empty beer cans on the table in the kitchen. Charles begins to cry, saying, "I am so upset—I can't sleep or eat—I need help." What would you do?

1. **Identify Goal of Thinking**

   Identify the level of anxiety experienced by Charles and begin interventions to help Charles decrease his level of anxiety.

2. **Assess Adequacy of Knowledge**

   Pertinent circumstances: Charles has had numerous losses in the past year, including loss of body function and changes in body image. He has recently lost his job, a major source of economic support and self-concept. He lost his girlfriend, a major source of support. Previously, Charles was clean and well-groomed. There was no previous evidence of drinking. His parents live nearby and are supporting and loving.

   Prerequisite knowledge: Before you decide what to do in this situation, you need to assess the level of anxiety experienced by Charles. You need to know the typical behaviors of each level and be able to recognize that Charles has severe anxiety. You must recognize that Charles needs interventions to regain equilibrium.

   Room for error: Charles requires and has asked for help. You are unsure of your abilities to help

him to deal effectively with his anxiety. You realize that his frustration with the situation could make him angry. You also know that depression and the potential for self-violence are risks unless something is done to reduce his anxiety.

Time constraints: Although you are not certain about how serious his problem is, you understand that Charles needs help in reducing his anxiety soon. There is time for you to ask for guidance from your instructor.

3. **Address Potential Problems**

   There are several potential barriers to critical thinking in this situation. You realize Charles needs help in reducing his level of stress, which in turn causes you anxiety. You are also somewhat frightened about his appearance and behavior. You do not believe your own abilities are developed well enough to help Charles adequately, but at the same time, you do know he needs help.

4. **Consult Helpful Resources**

   Your best source of information is Charles himself. You ask him what you can do to help him. He replies, "Just get someone here to help me." You ask his permission to call his mother, and he agrees. His mother says she will be there in 5 minutes. You call your instructor, and she tells you to call the home health agency for further instructions.

5. **Critique Judgment/Decision**

   When his mother arrives, she says she had no idea he was so distressed. She talks to the home health agency staff, who report that they have called Charles's physician and will continue to follow up on needed care and referrals for professional counseling. You believe you made the right decisions: you identified that Charles needed help, you contacted his mother to provide support, you contacted your instructor, and you contacted the home health agency. You also remained calm during the situation, despite your own anxiety.

EVALUATING

The evaluation of the plan of care is based on the mutually established expected outcomes. It is important to observe both verbal and nonverbal cues when evaluating the usefulness of the plan. In general, the plan is considered to be successful if the patient and family achieve the following:

- Verbalize causes and effects of stress and anxiety

- Identify and use sources of support
- Use problem-solving to find solutions to stressors
- Practice healthy lifestyle habits and anxiety-reducing techniques
- Verbalize a decrease in anxiety and an increase in comfort

See the accompanying Applying Learning to Practice and Nursing Care of Plan boxes.

APPLYING LEARNING TO PRACTICE

Patient Care Study

Mei Fu is a 24-year-old graduate student. She is married and has two small children; her husband is also a graduate student. Although she lived in China until 3 years ago, she speaks English well. After several months of headaches and diarrhea, Mrs. Fu made an appointment at the student health clinic.

Assessment Findings

The nurse practitioner at the clinic conducted a health history and physical assessment of Mrs. Fu and noted the following data:

- Patient is a thin woman who appears her stated age. She is currently in school and expects herself to make the highest grades. She also cares for her two children and her husband. Although her husband encourages her to go to school, he believes it is the wife's responsibility to provide all child and house

care. She has had no previous serious illnesses or surgery.
- Patient reports having frequent headaches, rating the pain as a 3 on a scale of 0 (no pain) to 10 (worst possible pain). She also reports having 4 to 6 bowel movements each day, sometimes with abdominal cramping. The diarrhea does not seem to be related to any type of foods eaten. Both the headaches and the diarrhea have been present for the past 2 months. During the interview, the patient appeared restless and talked rapidly. Questions often had to be repeated.
- Physical assessment reveals slight tachycardia, a fine hand tremor, and visible perspiration. Large muscle groups are tense and fists clenched. No tenderness is noted on abdominal palpation. Pupils are equal in size and react to light and accommodation. Nasal mucosa is normal.

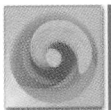

NURSING PLAN OF CARE
for Mrs. Fu

Nursing Diagnosis Anxiety related to stress of achievement in school and care of family as manifested by rapid speech, tachycardia, tremor, tense muscles, headache, and diarrhea.

Expected Outcome By her return appointment in 2 weeks, 10/20/01, Mrs. Fu will:
- Identify sources of and responses to stress

Nursing Interventions	Rationale	Evaluative Statement
Ask Mrs. Fu to keep a diary of hours spent in school-related activities and family care, number and times of headaches, and circumstances that occurred before diarrhea.	Identifying sources of stress and the physical responses to stress is the first step in planning coping strategies to reduce stress.	10/20/01 Goal met. Mrs. Fu kept a diary as requested. She identified that she does not have any time for herself. Her headaches are worse during the week. She often has diarrhea when papers are due or when her husband and children are demanding of her time.

S. Aird, RN, FNP

(continued)

NURSING PLAN OF CARE (Continued)
for Mrs. Fu

Expected Outcome

By her return appointment, 10/20/01, Mrs. Fu will:
- Identify sources of personal strength and support

Nursing Interventions	Rationale	Evaluative Statement
Ask Mrs. Fu to make a list of the people who are important to her and provide her comfort. Ask her to discuss how these people can help her cope with her situation. Ask Mrs. Fu to describe her strengths as a woman, a mother, a wife, and a student.	Identifying support people and areas of personal strength provides the patient with the means to manage stress and enhances self-concept.	10/20/01 Goal met. Mrs. Fu stated that her family is her greatest source of support, but they are in China and she misses them very much. She does have a very good friend who is also a good listener. She identified her strengths as being a person who cares for others and a good student. She said she is also a good artist, but has not had time for art for months. *S. Aird, RN, FNP*

Expected Outcome

By her return appointment, 10/20/01, Mrs. Fu will:
- Describe lifestyle changes that include eating a well-balanced diet with three meals a day, walking for 20 to 30 minutes four times a week, and sleeping restfully 7 hours a night

---

Nursing Interventions	Rationale	Evaluative Statement
Discuss with Mrs. Fu the food pyramid and the importance of eating foods from each group. Also discuss why she should eat three meals a day.	Adequate nutrition helps maintain the homeostatic mechanisms of the body and increases resistance to stress.	10/20/01 Goal met. Mrs. Fu was given a copy of the food pyramid, and food preparations were discussed. Although the Fu's have a healthy diet, Mrs. Fu often was too busy to eat more than a few bites. She said that she is making a big effort to eat three times a day.
Discuss with Mrs. Fu the benefits of regular exercise in reducing stress.	Exercise improves well-being, relieves tension, and facilitates coping with daily stressors.	She is walking to school and enjoys the time by herself. She arranged this time by asking her husband to take the children to school.
Discuss with Mrs. Fu the importance of sleep in reducing stress.	Adequate rest and sleep restore energy and facilitate coping with stressors.	She is sleeping better, and averages 7 hours most nights. *S. Aird, RN, FNP*

(continued)

NURSING PLAN OF CARE (Continued)
for Mrs. Fu

Expected Outcome

By her return appointment, 10/20/01, Mrs. Fu will:
* Practice relaxation for 20 minutes each day

Nursing Interventions	Rationale	Evaluative Statement
Teach and have Mrs. Fu practice progressive muscle relaxation. Suggest that she buy a tape to facilitate the technique (tapes for relaxation are widely available). Recommend that she plan a time when she can be alone and use 20 minutes to complete the technique.	Relaxation promotes a response opposite to the stress response; decreases heart rate, respiratory rate, blood pressure, and metabolic processes.	10/20/01 Goal met. Mrs. Fu said that at first she had difficulty in finding time to be alone, but she feels so much better after she relaxes that she insists on the time. She did buy a tape and says it helps her very much. *S. Aird, RN, FNP*

Expected Outcome

By her return appointment, 10/20/01, Mrs. Fu will:
* Report a decrease in headaches and diarrhea and an increase in her ability to provide self-care to manage stress

Nursing Interventions	Rationale	Evaluative Statement
Assess frequency and severity of headaches and bowel movements. Assess patient's self-report of coping with stressors.	Decreasing stress in daily life often is effective in decreasing physical responses. Self-care of stress is critical in effective management.	10/20/01 Goal met. Mrs. Fu reports she has noticed fewer headaches in the past week, and the diarrhea is almost gone. Mrs. Fu verbalized the importance of continuing to practice a healthy lifestyle and relaxation. She said she has spent time with her friend and has gotten out her sketch pad. She stated that she believes she can manage her life much better now. *S. Aird, RN, FNP*

Sample Documentation

10/06/01, 10 AM, nursing

Initial visit to student health center by Mrs. Fu to discuss physical problems of headache and diarrhea. History and physical assessment findings indicated large number of personal stressors, manifested by physical signs and symptoms. Assessment data supported nursing diagnosis: Anxiety related to stress of achievement in school and care of family. Discussion centered on identifying sources of stress, physical responses to stress, sources of support, and personal strength. Teaching strategies included diet, exercise, sleep, and progressive muscle relaxation. Patient's progress will be monitored at next visit on 10/20/01.

S. Aird, RN, FNP

Learning Outcomes

After completing this chapter, the learner should be able to accomplish the following:

1. Define the key terms used in the chapter.

   adaptation
   anxiety
   burnout
   caregiver burden
   coping mechanisms
   crisis
   crisis intervention
   defense mechanisms
   developmental crisis
   fight-or-flight response
   general adaptation syndrome
   homeostasis
   inflammatory response
   local adaptation syndrome
   psychosomatic disorders
   reflex pain response
   situational stress
   stress
   stressor

2. Describe the mechanisms involved in maintaining physiologic homeostasis.

3. Explain the interdependent nature of stressors, stress, and adaptation.

4. Compare and contrast developmental and situational stress, incorporating the concepts of physiologic and psychosocial stressors.

5. Describe the physical and emotional responses to stress, including mind–body interaction, local adaptation syndrome, general adaptation syndrome, and coping and defense mechanisms.

6. Discuss the effects of short-term and long-term stress on basic human needs, health and illness, and the family.

7. Integrate knowledge of healthy lifestyle, support systems, stress management techniques, and crisis intervention into hospital-based and community-based care.

8. Recognize and effectively cope with stress unique to the nursing profession.

Critical Thinking Exercises

1. Identify the nursing activities and relationships that cause you the most stress. What are your personal warning signs that a situation is becoming stressful? What do you do to decrease your level of stress? Who is most important in helping you do this?

2. List nursing interventions you would use to reduce stress in the following situations:

   - A newly married young woman who found a lump in her breast is having a breast biopsy
   - The parents of a 2-year-old who are sitting in the surgical waiting room as their child undergoes brain surgery
   - The daughter (and caretaker) of a woman with severe Alzheimer's disease

Study Questions

1. Stress is a condition in which the human system
   a. becomes increasingly disorganized
   b. responds to changes in its normal balanced state
   c. responds to negative changes in its internal environment
   d. is less likely to respond appropriately to stimuli
2. Which of the following is an external stressor?
   a. high environmental temperature
   b. changes in hormone levels
   c. fear of the dark
   d. having an infection of the intestine
3. The body maintains the internal environment at a constant state through
   a. internalization
   b. adaptation
   c. cellular integrity
   d. homeostasis
4. Which of the following is developmental stress?
   a. an infant learns to turn over
   b. a school-aged child learns how to add and subtract
   c. an adolescent gets a job
   d. a young adult has a variety of friends

5. The reflex pain response and the inflammatory response are examples of
   a. localized responses of the body to stress
   b. negative responses of the body to stress
   c. generalized responses of the body to stress
   d. ways in which the body controls stress
6. What response is expected during the shock phase of the general adaptation syndrome?
   a. decreasing pulse
   b. increasing sleepiness
   c. increasing energy levels
   d. slow respirations
7. A vague feeling of discomfort or dread with an unknown source is:
   a. fear
   b. concern
   c. panic
   d. anxiety
8. Toward the end of the semester, as final examinations near, you find yourself sleeping more than usual. This behavior is probably your form of a
   a. coping mechanism
   b. defense mechanism

c. offense mechanism
d. adapting mechanism

9. Your patient has just been diagnosed with cancer but responds as though this is an impossibility. Which of the defense mechanisms is being demonstrated here?
   a. projection
   b. denial
   c. displacement
   d. repression

10. Home care of patients by family members for long periods of time can cause long-term stress and increased risk for illness. The name for this stress response is
    a. home care chronicity
    b. patient burnout
    c. residual stress
    d. caregiver burden

11. All but one of the following responses are typical of relaxation techniques. Which is *not* typical?
    a. rhythmic breathing
    b. an increased pulse rate
    c. reduced muscle tension
    d. an altered state of consciousness

12. Which type of stress reduction activity would probably be most useful for patients before an unfamiliar or painful event?

a. progressive muscle relaxation
b. meditation
c. anticipatory guidance
d. biofeedback

13. What is the first step in crisis intervention through problem solving?
    a. identify the problem
    b. list alternatives
    c. implement a plan
    d. evaluate the outcome

14. Biofeedback is a method of gaining mental control of what part of the body?
    a. the skin
    b. the senses
    c. the autonomic nervous system
    d. the central nervous system

15. What type of setting is considered most stressful for nurses?
    a. cancer treatment centers
    b. nursing homes
    c. operating room
    d. intensive care units

Answers With Rationale

1. The correct answer is *b*. Individuals perceive and respond to stress in highly individualized ways. Stress evokes both positive and negative responses to changes in the internal and external environment.

2. The correct answer is *a*. Answers *b, c,* and *d* are all internal stressors.

3. The correct answer is *d*. To maintain health, the internal environment must remain in balance; this balance is maintained through various physiologic mechanisms as they respond to internal changes.

4. The correct answer is *c*. Although the other choices are milestones in a developmental age, the adolescent who gets a job is seeking independence, a major task for that level of growth and development.

5. The correct answer is *a*. The local adaptation syndrome is a localized response of the body to stress. These responses are homeostatic and short-term; the most common are the reflex pain response and the inflammatory response.

6. The correct answer is *c*. The body perceives a threat and prepares to respond by increasing the activity of the autonomic nervous and endocrine systems. The initial or shock phase is characterized by increased energy levels, oxygen intake, cardiac output, blood pressure, and mental alertness.

7. The correct answer is *d*. Panic is an experience of terror. A concern is a worry. Fear has a known cause. Only anxiety is a psychological response to an unknown threat.

8. The correct answer is *a*. Mild anxiety is often handled without conscious thought through the use of coping mechanisms, which are behaviors used to decrease stress and anxiety. Sleeping is a coping mechanism.

9. The correct answer is *b*. Denial occurs when a person refuses to acknowledge the presence of a condition that is disturbing.

10. The correct answer is *d*. Reactions to home care of family members for long periods of time, called caregiver burden, include chronic fatigue, sleep disorders, and increased incidence of stress-related illnesses, such as hypertension and heart disease.

11. The correct answer is *b*. No matter what the technique, relaxation involves rhythmic breathing, reduced muscle tension, and an altered state of consciousness.

12. The correct answer is *c*. Anticipatory guidance focuses on psychological preparation of the patient for an unfamiliar or painful event. When patients know what to expect, their anxiety is reduced and their coping mechanisms are more effective.

13. The correct answer is *a*. Although identifying the problem may be difficult, a solution to a crisis situation is impossible until the problem is identified.

14. The correct answer is *c*. Biofeedback is a method of gaining control of the autonomic nervous system and regulating body responses to stress such as increased blood pressure, increased heart rate, and headaches.

15. The correct answer is *d*. Patients in intensive care units have complex needs and are at greater risk for death; their care is often stressful.

Bibliography

Antonovsky, A. (1979). *Health, stress and coping.* San Francisco: Jossey-Bass.

Bennett, J. (1998). Fear of contagion: A response to stress? *Advances in Nursing Science, 21*(1), 76–87.

Benson, S. (1997). Editorial message. Coping with stress. *Images, 16*(1), 3.

Bernier, D. (1998). A study of coping: Successful recovery from severe burnout and other reactions to severe work-related stress. *Work & Stress, 12*(1), 50–65.

Carpenito, L. J. (1997). *Nursing diagnosis: Application to clinical practice* (7th ed.). Philadelphia: Lippincott-Raven.

Carpenito, L. J. (1999). *Nursing care plans and documentation: Nursing diagnoses and collaborative problems* (3rd ed.). Philadelphia: Lippincott Williams & Wilkins.

Dean, R. (1998). Occupational stress in hospice care: Causes and coping strategies. *American Journal of Hospice & Palliative Care, 15*(3), 151–154.

Fontaine, K. L., & Fletcher, J. S. (1999). *Mental health nursing* (4th ed.). Menlo Park, CA: Addison-Wesley.

Frasca-Beaulier, K. (1999). Interior design for ambulatory care facilities: How to reduce stress and anxiety in patients and families. *Journal of Ambulatory Care Management, 22*(1), 67–73.

Griffin, T., Wishba, C., & Kavanaugh, K. (1998). Nursing interventions to reduce stress in parents of hospitalized preterm infants. *Journal of Pediatric Nursing: Nursing Care of Children & Families, 13*(5), 290–295.

Griffiths, K. (1998). Stress and coping. *Assignment, 4*(1), 7–12.

Johnson, J. (1998). Stress, social support, and health in frontier elders. *Journal of Gerontological Nursing, 24*(5), 29–35.

Jones, D. (1998). When stress affects a child's colon. *Office Nurse, 11*(4), 22–24.

Lunney, M., & Myszak, C. (1997). Stress overload: A new diagnosis. In M. Rantz & P. LeMone (Eds.). *Classification of nursing diagnoses: Proceedings of the Twelfth Conference of the North American Nursing Diagnosis Association* (pp. 190–191). Glendale, CA: CINAHL Information Systems.

Marcus, I. (1997). Women & diabetes: Strategies for handling stress. *Diabetes Self Management, 14*(2), 40–42, 44–45.

McMahon, B. (1998). Calm down . . . stress is inevitable. *Nursing Standard, 13*(1), 18.

Moos, R. (1985). *Coping with physical illness* (2nd ed.). New York: Plenum.

North American Nursing Diagnosis Association. (1999). *Nursing diagnoses: Definitions & classification 1999–2000.* Philadelphia: Author.

Orme-Johnson, D., & Walton, K. (1998). All approaches to preventing or reversing effects of stress are not the same. *American Journal of Health Promotion, 12*(5), 297–299.

Porth, C. M. (1998). *Pathophysiology: Concepts of altered health states* (5th ed.). Philadelphia: Lippincott Williams & Wilkins.

Selye, H. (1976). *The stress of life.* New York: McGraw-Hill.

Strickland, D. (1998). Balancing life's choices—all dressed up and too many places to go. *AORN Journal, 68*(4), 634–636, 639–641.

Stevenson, J. (1998). Stress. High tension warnings. *Men's Health, 13*(7), 94.

Stuart, G., & Sundeen, S. (1999). *Principles & practice of psychiatric nursing* (5th ed.). St. Louis: C. V. Mosby.

Stuart, G., & Sundeen, S. (1998). *Nurse-client interaction: Implementing the nursing process* (6th ed.). St. Louis: C. V. Mosby.

Thomas, R. (1998). Technology, status, and stress. *Case Manager, 9*(5), 48–49.

Chapter 32
Loss, Grief, and Dying

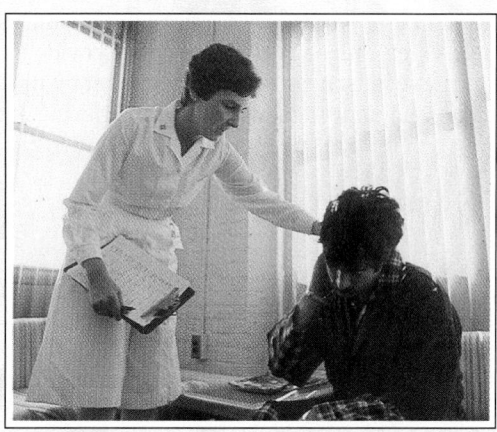

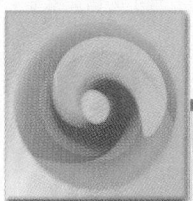

**Thinking Critically About
Nursing's Blended Skills**

Before reading this chapter, think about the types of blended skills you will need to respond to these problems.

- A college student tells the nurse in the student health center that she feels like she's been sad forever. Ever since her dad died of cancer when she was 8 years old, she and her mom had been "best friends." Last semester, her mother died instantly in a car crash. Ever since her mom's death she has had difficulty sleeping, eating, and studying. "Nothing seems to mean anything anymore. All I see is gray."

- Yvonne's labor started 7 weeks early, and she just delivered an infant who was immediately transported to a neonatal intensive care unit. Yvonne is 20 years old, single, and desperately wanting to be a mother. She had a normal pregnancy up to this point and was expecting a healthy baby girl. She was told that her baby has less than a 50% chance of surviving the next 24 hours.

- Manuel and his wife had just moved to a retirement community and were looking forward to traveling. Both were golf enthusiasts. Two months after they had settled in, Manuel's wife suffered a major stroke and is now unconscious in the hospital. Manuel sits at her bedside, holding her hand, crying. Manuel is being asked to make decisions about continuing aggressive life-sustaining treatment for his wife who suffered permanent neurologic damage. He has questioned whether or not his wife would be a potential organ donor.

- You inform Mr. Miller's doctor that Mr. Miller is asking to write an advance directive and wants a do-not-resuscitate order. The doctor tells you it's too early to talk about things like this, that such conversations tend to "depress patients."

- You find Mrs. Zhang, a nursing home resident with a do-not-resuscitate order, dead in her bed when you try to awaken her in the morning.

What cognitive, technical, interpersonal, and ethical/legal skills do you think you will need to respond to the challenges described above?

t any stage of one's life there is the potential for loss, grief, and death. This is especially true for the person experiencing altered health and for his or her family. A wide variety of losses may occur, including loss of a body part or function; loss of one's ability to care for oneself; loss of one's role as head of a family; and death, which may be the most difficult loss of all. Death may be as difficult for healthcare professionals as it is for surviving family members. The goals of nursing focus on health maintenance and health restoration, with an emphasis on facilitating maximum potential in wellness. Another function of the nurse, however, is to facilitate coping with disability and death. The nurse is often the key person in providing support and care when loss or death occurs. To provide effective care, the nurse must have accepted his or her own feelings about death and understand the stages of grieving and dying.

Loss and Grieving

Loss

Loss occurs when a valued person, object, or situation is changed or made inaccessible so that its value is diminished or removed. There are several types of loss, all of which everyone may experience at some time. **Actual loss** can be recognized by others as well as by the person sustaining the loss; loss of a limb, of a spouse, of a valued object such as money, and of a job are all examples of actual loss. **Perceived loss** is felt by the person but is intangible to others; loss of youth, of financial independence, and of a valued environment are examples of perceived loss. Directly related to actual and perceived loss are physical and psychological loss. A person who loses an arm in an automobile accident

suffers from both the **physical loss** of the arm and the **psychological loss** that may be caused by an altered self-image and the inability to return to his or her occupation. These losses are simultaneously physical, psychological, and actual. A person who is scarred but does not lose a limb may suffer a perceived and psychological loss of self-image.

Another type of loss is **anticipatory loss,** in which a person displays loss and grief behaviors for a loss that has yet to take place. Anticipatory loss is often seen in families of terminally ill patients and serves to lessen the impact of the actual loss of a family member.

Loss can have a tremendous impact on a person's development; conversely, age affects a person's reaction to loss (see Factors That Affect Grief and Death, later in this chapter). Although most adults can accept death on an intellectual level, they may have trouble dealing with it on an emotional level. The loss of a friend, a pet, or a job may help a person anticipate and cope with the loss of a spouse or other loved one.

Grieving

Grief is the emotional reaction to loss. It occurs with loss caused by separation as well as with loss caused by death. Many people who divorce experience grief; loss of a body part, a job, a house, or a pet may cause grief. **Bereavement** is the state of grieving during which a person goes through grief reaction. **Mourning** is the period of acceptance of loss and grief during which the person learns to deal with the loss.

Bereavement, which is experienced by both the patient and the family, may have profound health consequences that require additional care. Bereaved people often neglect

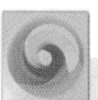

COGNITIVE SKILLS

- Basic knowledge about loss and grieving and the factors that affect loss, grief, and dying
- Knowledge about quality end-of-life outcomes and the competencies necessary for nurses to provide high-quality care to patients and families during the transition at the end of life
- Ability to use the nursing process to care for patients with problems related to loss, grief, and dying

TECHNICAL SKILLS

- Ability to use correctly the equipment and protocols necessary to diagnose and treat problems related to inadequate loss, grief, and dying
- Ability to perform postmortem care

INTERPERSONAL SKILLS

- Strong people skills; ability to communicate and interact effectively with patients and their caregivers; ability to establish trusting relationships—even in times of great crisis related to loss
- Ability to affirm dignity and worth in times of stress and grieving; ability to communicate caring
- Ability to facilitate decision making; ability to confront colleagues

ETHICAL/LEGAL SKILLS

- Commitment to safety and quality; strong sense of responsibility, accountability; strong advocacy skills
- Familiarity with federal and state legislation related to end-of-life care and organ donation and with agency policy and role responsibilities related to end-of-life care and organ donation

their health to an extreme, whereas mourning is characterized by a return to more normal living habits.

Grief Reactions

Grief is the emotional pain caused by a loss. Reactions to grief and dying are similar. The stages of these reactions overlap and vary among individuals. One person may skip a reaction stage, whereas another may repeat an earlier stage. Each person is different, and patients and family members may be at different reaction stages.

Engel (1964) was among the first to define stages of grief. Engel's six stages are (1) shock and disbelief, (2) developing awareness, (3) restitution, (4) resolving the loss, (5) idealization, and (6) outcome. Shock and disbelief are usually defined as refusal to accept the fact of loss, followed by a stunned or numb response: "No, not me." Developing awareness is characterized by physical and emotional responses such as anger, feeling empty, and crying: "Why me?" Restitution involves the rituals surrounding loss, and with death, includes religious, cultural, or social expressions of mourning, such as funeral services. Resolving the loss is dealing with the void left by the loss, and idealization is the exaggeration of the good qualities of the person or object lost, followed by acceptance of the loss and a lessened need to focus on it. Outcome is the final resolution of the grief process, including dealing with loss as a common life occurrence.

Kübler-Ross (1969), considered a pioneer in the study of grief and death reactions, defined five stages of reaction similar to those of Engel (see accompanying box). Other theorists describe similar stages. More important than the actual stages of any given grief reaction is the idea that grief is a process and that it varies from person to person.

Normal Versus Dysfunctional Grief

Both normal and dysfunctional grief may be delayed, and normal grief may be either abbreviated or anticipatory. Abbreviated grief is of short duration but is genuine; anticipatory grief occurs before the actual loss, as in the extended terminal illness of a family member. **Dysfunctional grief** is abnormal or distorted; it may be either unresolved or inhibited. In unresolved grief, a person may have trouble expressing feelings of loss or may deny them; unresolved grief also describes a state of bereavement that extends over a lengthy period. In inhibited grief, a person suppresses feelings of grief and may instead manifest somatic symptoms.

Assessment priorities, expected outcomes, and interventions for patients and families experiencing anticipatory grieving are illustrated in the accompanying box.

Dying and Death

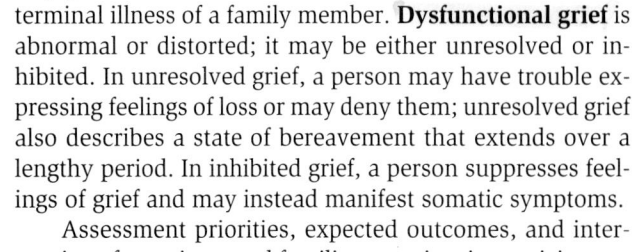

Dying may occur suddenly as a result of an accident, injury, or pathologic crisis, such as a heart attack; or it may occur after a prolonged experience of debilitating disease, such as cancer, acquired immunodeficiency syndrome (AIDS), or multiple sclerosis. Whereas some welcome death and even hasten death, choosing the time and manner of their dying, others fear death and will try anything to delay it. Given the choice, some choose to die at home surrounded by loved ones. Others die alone or in intensive care units surrounded by healthcare professionals and technologic equipment (see the accompanying Research in Nursing box). A patient's wishes should, if possible, be followed. Rights of dying people are listed in the accompanying box.

Signs of Impending Death

The clinical signs of impending or approaching death include inability to swallow; pitting edema; decreased gastrointestinal and urinary tract activity; bowel and bladder incontinence; loss of motion, sensation, and reflexes; elevated temperature, but cold or clammy skin; cyanosis; lowered blood pressure; noisy or irregular respiration; and Cheyne-Stokes respirations. The patient may or may not lose consciousness. It is often helpful to prepare family members and significant others for the transformations that signal impending death. Nuland's popular books entitled *How We Die* (1994) and *The Wisdom of the Body* (1997) are useful resources.

Definitions of Death

Death was defined in 1981 by the President's Commission for the Study of Ethical Problems in Medicine and Biomedical and Behavioral Research as follows:

> Death is present when an individual has sustained either (1) irreversible cessation of circulatory and respiratory functions, or (2) irreversible cessation of all functions of the entire brain, including the brain stem.

A Harvard University committee stated that the following characteristics must be present for at least 24 hours before death can be declared:

- Lack of receptivity and responsiveness
- Lack of movement or breathing

Grief and Death Reactions

Engel's Six Stages of Grief Reactions

1. Shock and disbelief
2. Developing awareness
3. Restitution
4. Resolving the loss
5. Idealization
6. Outcome

Five Stages of Kübler-Ross' Grief and Death Reactions

1. Denial and isolation
2. Anger why me?
3. Bargaining
4. Depression
5. Acceptance

Grieving

Grieving may be defined as the state in which an individual or family experiences a natural human response involving psychosocial and physiologic reactions to an actual or perceived loss (person, object, function, status, relationship). NANDA nursing diagnoses include the following:

Anticipatory Grieving: Intellectual and emotional responses and behaviors by which individuals work through the process of modifying self-concept based on the perception of potential loss (NANDA, 1994)

Dysfunctional Grieving: Extended, unsuccessful use of intellectual and emotional responses by which individuals attempt to work through the process of modifying self-concept based upon the perception of loss (NANDA, 1994)

Because nurses encounter patients dealing with anticipatory grieving more frequently than patients dysfunctionally grieving, assessment priorities, expected outcomes, and interventions will be given for anticipatory grieving.

Assessment Priorities

- Determine the exact nature of the anticipated or potential loss.
- Explore factors that are contributing to the importance or significance of the anticipated loss.
- Assess concerns, fears, feelings, and hopes related to the anticipated loss.
- Assess adequacy of knowledge and coping mechanisms.
- Recognize personal strengths and available resources, including present support system.

Expected Outcomes

The patient will:

- Express grief openly and progress through stages of grief with appropriate grief work
- Share concerns with significant others and seek needed help
- Make decisions about the future that advance best interests
- Demonstrate eventual resolution of grief by self-report, appearance, and resumption of usual activities of daily living

Interventions

Interventions for anticipatory grieving are determined by the type of loss (eg, body part; death of self, a significant other, or child), the extent of the loss to the individual and family, and what other support the individual or family has. Examples of interventions are the following:

- Use interpersonal skills to demonstrate empathy for patient's situation and commitment to patient's well-being.
- Encourage the patient to share concerns, feelings, fears, and hopes openly.
- Respond to inquiries honestly, compassionately, and in a manner that does not deprive the patients of realistic hope.
- Promote grief work through each stage of grieving (see box below). Support the patient and "nudge" the patient to begin the next stage of grieving as appropriate.
- Make appropriate referrals (see earlier listing of bereavement resources).
- Alert the patient who is moving through the grief work slowly of the signs of dysfunctional grieving and instruct about how to obtain help should this happen; referral for counseling may be indicated.

Stages of Grief and Related Grief Work

Denial

- Initially support and then strive to increase the development of awareness (when individual indicates readiness for awareness)

Isolation

- Listen and spend designated time consistently with person and family
- Offer the person and family opportunity to explore their emotions
- Reflect on past losses and acknowledge loss behavior (past and present)

Depression

- Begin with simple problem solving and move toward acceptance

- Enhance self-worth through positive reinforcement
- Identify the level of depression and indications of suicidal behavior or ideas
- Be consistent and establish times daily to speak with the person and family

Anger

- Allow for crying to release this energy
- Listen to and communicate concern
- Encourage concerned support from significant others as well as professional support

Guilt

- Listen and communicate concern
- Allow for crying
- Promote more direct expression of feelings
- Explore methods to resolve grief

(continued)

Grieving *(Continued)*

Fear	*Rejection*
• Help the person and family recognize the feeling • Explain that this will help cope with life • Explore the person's and family's attitudes about loss, death, etc.	• Allow for verbal expression of this feeling state to diminish the emotional strain • Recognize that expression of anger may create a rejection of self to significant others

(From Carpenito, L. J. [1995]. *Nursing diagnosis: Application to clinical practice* [6th ed.]. Philadelphia: J. B. Lippincott, pp. 421–422. Used with permission.)

• Lack of reflexes
• Flat encephalogram

In the United States, there are currently three definitions of death in the literature: the traditional heart–lung definition, the whole-brain definition, and the higher-brain definition.

Heart–lung death: the irreversible cessation of spontaneous respiration and circulation; the accepted criterion for death until the 1960s, emerged as a definition of death from the historical idea that the flow of body fluids was essential for life

Whole-brain death: the irreversible cessation of all functions of the entire brain, including the brain stem; this definition emerged in the 1960s from the belief that neocortical functioning is the key to the definition of a human being. Most protocols require two separate clinical examinations, including induction of painful stimuli, pupillary responses to

light, oculovestibular testing, and apnea testing. To enhance accuracy, standard practice is not to perform brain death testing while a patient is hypothermic, hypotensive, or under the influence of neuromuscular blocking agents or barbiturates.

Higher-brain death: the irreversible loss of all 'higher' brain functions, of cognitive function; this definition was suggested in the 1970s and emerged from the belief that the brain is more important than the spinal cord and that the critical functions are the individual's personality, conscious life, uniqueness, and capacity for remembering, judging, reasoning, acting, enjoying, worrying (Ott, 1995)

Responses to Dying and Death

Although each person reacts to the knowledge of impending death or to loss in his or her own way, there are similarities in the psychosocial responses to the situation.

RESEARCH IN NURSING: MAKING A DIFFERENCE

Promoting Quality End-of-Life Care

National studies continue to report poor patient and family satisfaction with end-of-life care in all settings.

Related Research
Kirchoff, K. T., Spuhler, V., Walker, L., Hutton, A., Cole, V., & Clemmer, T. (2000). Intensive care nurses' experiences with end-of-life care. *American Journal of Critical Care, 9*(1), 36–42.
The purpose of this project was to address end-of-life care by intensive care unit (ICU) nurses through focus groups with nurses and to listen to the stories of the people who are major witnesses and providers of that care. The research questions addressed in the study were: (1) What do ICU nurses consider "good" end-of-life care? (2) How do nurses describe their experiences of shifting from curative nursing interventions to end-of-life care? (3) What are ICU nurses' perceptions of

care dilemmas and barriers to providing quality end-of-life care? "Good" end-of-life care in the ICU was described as ensuring that the patient is as pain free as possible and that the patient's comfort and dignity are maintained. Involvement of the patient's family is crucial. A clear, accurate prognosis and continuity of care are important. Switching from curative care to comfort care is awkward.

Relevance to Nursing Practice
These researchers noted that disagreement among patients' family members or among caregivers, uncertainty about prognosis, and communication problems further complicate end-of-life care in ICUs. Changes in the physical environment, education about end-of-life care, staff support, and better communication would improve care of dying patients and their families.

The Dying Person's Bill of Rights

I have the right to be treated as a living human being until I die.

I have the right to maintain a sense of hopefulness, however changing its focus may be.

I have the right to be cared for by those who can maintain a sense of hopefulness, however changing this might be.

I have the right to express my feelings and emotions about my approaching death in my own way.

I have the right to participate in decisions concerning my care.

I have the right to expect continuing medical and nursing attention even though "cure" goals must be changed to "comfort" goals.

I have the right not to die alone.

I have the right to be free from pain.

I have the right to have my questions answered honestly.

I have the right not to be deceived.

I have the right to have help from and for my family in accepting my death.

I have the right to die in peace and dignity.

I have a right to retain my individuality and not be judged for my decisions, which may be contrary to beliefs of others.

I have the right to discuss and enlarge my religious and/or spiritual experiences, whatever these may mean to others.

I have the right to expect that the sanctity of the human body will be respected after death.

I have the right to be cared for by caring, sensitive, knowledgeable people who will attempt to understand my needs and will be able to gain some satisfaction in helping me face my death.

(Created at the workshop *The Terminally Ill Patient and the Helping Person,* in Lansing, Michigan, sponsored by the Southwestern Michigan Inservice Education Council and conducted by Amelia J. Barbus, Associate Professor of Nursing, Wayne State University, Detroit.)

Kübler-Ross has studied the emotional responses to death and dying in depth, and her findings have been used extensively by the nursing and other helping professions.

The stages of dying, much like the stages of grief, may overlap, and the duration of any stage may range from as little as a few hours to as long as a period of months. The process varies from person to person. Some people may be in one stage for such a short time that it seems as if they skipped that stage. Sometimes, a person returns to a previous stage.

According to Kübler-Ross, the stages of dying are (1) denial and isolation, (2) anger, (3) bargaining, (4) depression, and (5) acceptance.

Denial and isolation: In the denial and isolation stage, the patient denies that he or she will die, may repress what is discussed, and may isolate self from reality. The patient may think, "They made a mistake in the diagnosis. Maybe they mixed my records with someone else's."

Anger: The patient expresses rage and hostility in the anger stage and adopts a "why me?" attitude. "Why me? I quit smoking and I watched what I ate. Why did this happen to me?"

Bargaining: The patient tries to barter for more time. "If I can just make it to my son's graduation I will be satisfied. Just let me live until then." Many patients put their personal affairs in order, make wills, and fulfill last wishes, such as trips, visiting relatives, and so forth. It is important to meet these wishes, if possible, because bargaining helps patients move into later stages of dying.

Depression: In the depression stage, the patient goes through a period of grief before death. The grief is characterized by crying and not speaking much. "I waited all these years to see my daughter get married. And now I may not be here to see her walk down the aisle. I can't bear the thought of not being there for the wedding—and of not seeing my grandchildren."

Acceptance: When the stage of acceptance is reached, the patient feels tranquil. She or he has accepted death and is prepared to die. The patient may think, "I've tied up all the loose ends—made the will, made arrangements for my daughter to live with her grandparents. Now I can go in peace knowing everyone will be fine."

Terminal Illness

In the case of a **terminal illness,** an illness in which death is expected within a limited space of time, the physician is usually responsible for deciding what and how much the patient should be told. The nurse, clergyperson, and other healthcare professionals may be involved with this decision and in discussing the patient's condition with him or her. Most patients want to know their diagnosis and prognosis as soon as possible, so that they can both come to grips with it and take care of business and personal affairs. Even more important is a description of how the disease is likely to play out and what this will mean for the patient. All who are involved with the patient's care should know exactly what the patient and the family have been told;

members of the patient's healthcare team need to communicate among themselves. Cultural influences may dictate how much information is desired and which family members are to be informed.

Impact on Patient

Many patients realize without being told that they are suffering from a terminal illness; this realization is often picked up from nonverbal communication by their families and by healthcare professionals. Patients must be allowed to go through the stages of the grieving process and to make decisions about their care, and they must be supported in their decision making. Competent patients have the right to consent to and refuse any and all indicated medical treatment—even that which is life-sustaining—and should be made aware of this right. In the past, patients and family members complained about receiving care they did not want and of not being allowed to die. In today's climate of cost-conscious decision making, some patients and family members are complaining that they are being denied costly life-sustaining treatment because of inadequate personal funds or insurance or because they are deemed a poor "investment" of scarce resources.

Impact on Family

The family and significant others of terminally ill patients should be encouraged to participate in planning the patient's care. Healthcare personnel should be available to discuss the patient's condition with family members and should offer support and care as the family begins the grieving process. The family may want to make arrangements with the patient for funeral or memorial services, depending on which stage of grief both the patient and the family members are in.

Palliative Care

Palliative care means taking care of the whole person—body, mind, spirit—heart and soul. It looks at dying as something natural and personal. The goal of palliative care is to give patients with life-threatening illnesses the best quality of life they can have. Palliative care is sometimes called hospice care. See the accompanying box, which illustrates the five principles of palliative care.

Ethical and Legal Dimensions

Multiple treatment options and sophisticated life-support technologies may make it difficult to draw the line between promoting life and needlessly prolonging the dying process. In these cases, healthcare decision making is complicated for patients and healthcare professionals alike. The increasing popularity of the "managed death" concept and calls to legalize physician-assisted suicide and physician-administered lethal injections ("aid in dying") pose new ethical challenges. As patients and families struggle with end-of-life treatment decisions, they are increasingly looking to nurses for information, advice, and support. See the accompanying boxes, which highlight nursing care priorities and related Internet resources for patients and families experiencing conflict about decision making.

Five Principles of Palliative Care

1. Palliative care respects the goals, likes, and choices of the dying person and his or her loved ones . . . helping them to understand the illness and what can be expected from it, and to figure out what is most important during this time.
2. Palliative care looks after the medical, emotional, social, and spiritual needs of the dying person . . . with a focus on making sure he or she is comfortable, not left alone, and able to look back on his or her life and find peace.
3. Palliative care supports the needs of family members . . . helping them with the responsibilities of caregiving and even supporting them as they grieve.
4. Palliative care helps to gain access to needed healthcare providers and appropriate care settings . . . involving various kinds of trained providers in different settings, tailored to the needs of the patient and his or her family.
5. Palliative care builds ways to provide excellent care at the end of life . . . through education of care providers, appropriate health policies, and adequate funding from insurers and the government.

Used with permission. The Robert Wood Johnson Foundation, Last Acts Palliative Care Task Force, "Five Principles of Palliative Care," 1999. Special supplement to *Advances*, 2, 3

Patients have a legally and morally protected right to consent to and refuse any and all indicated medical therapies. Legal foundations for the patient's freedom to choose include the common law right of self-determination and the constitutionally supported right of privacy. The ethical and legal implications of nursing are discussed in general in Chapters 6 and 7. Select counseling and advocacy responsibilities are described in Chapters 22 and 23. A discussion of nursing's ethical and legal responsibilities in end-of-life care follows.

Advance Directives

Decisions about healthcare are becoming increasingly complex. Patients, family members, and healthcare professionals alike are voicing frustration as they grapple with complex decisions about prolonging life. Some of the most difficult cases involve patients who are no longer able (competent) to indicate their treatment preferences. Two kinds of written **advance directives** can minimize difficulties by allowing individuals to state in advance what their choices would be for healthcare should certain circumstances develop. Living wills provide specific instructions about the kinds of healthcare that should be provided or foregone in particular situations. A durable power of attorney for healthcare appoints an agent the person trusts to make decisions in the event of

Decisional Conflict

Patients and the surrogate decision makers for incompetent patients frequently feel overwhelmed when they need to make life-and-death decisions about end-of-life care. The NANDA diagnosis for this response follows:

Decisional Conflict: The state of uncertainty about course of action to be taken when choice among competing actions involves risk, loss, or challenge to personal life values (NANDA, 1994)

Assessment Priorities

The objective of assessment is to identify individuals and families who are at high risk for decisional conflict and to provide the support they need to make appropriate end-of-life care decisions that advance the patient's interests before problems develop. Potential problems when this need is overlooked include postponement of decision making, which interferes with the patient receiving optimal care; vacillation in decision making, which disturbs continuity of care for the patient; and escalation of conflict concerning decision making, which may result in a standoff between participating parties—the patient, individual family members, and healthcare professionals.

- Detect difficulties with making decisions: fear; insufficient or erroneous information; inadequate support; conflict between religious convictions, personal moral beliefs, and choice one wants to make; reluctance to assume responsibility for making life-and-death decision.
- Identify what is causing the decision making to be hard for the patient or family and what type of information or support could reverse this.
- Identify potential conflicts between what the patient wants and what his or her family or caregivers believe should be done.
- Observe the patient or his or her surrogate decision makers for physical signs of distress that reflect feeling overwhelmed by the decision that needs to be made: signs of fatigue and general exhaustion; signs of agitation and distress; signs of growing anger and alienation.
- Read the chart carefully to identify decisions that are pending and note the lack of movement toward a decision or toward resolution of existing conflict.

Expected Outcomes

The morally and legally valid decision-maker will achieve the following:

- Describe care options (including the option of nontreatment), listing the advantages and disadvantages of each

- Seek clarification of options, if necessary, and whatever support is needed
- Express fears, concerns, and hopes
- Make an informed and voluntary choice
- Make end-of-life decisions that reflect the patient's values and goals, advancing his or her interests
- Make end-of-life decisions that are consistent with the aims of medicine and nursing

Interventions

Nursing measures revolve around identifying and supporting the morally and legally valid decision maker. The following should be considered:

- Competent patients—those who can (1) understand the information needed to make the decision, (2) reason in accord with a relatively consistent set of values, and (3) communicate a preference— have the right to consent to and to refuse any and all indicated medical treatment.
- Surrogates of previously competent patients are to be guided by what is known about the patient's values and preferences. These surrogates may be designated in an advance directive, or there may be state or province law designating a hierarchy of surrogates, such as spouse, parent, adult child, sibling; the morally valid surrogate is the one who best knows the patient and the patient's preferences.
- Surrogates deciding for a never-competent patient (child or profoundly retarded adult) must be guided by a determination of what is in the patient's best interests by referring to more objective and socially shared values.

The nurse clarifies the goal of treatment (cure, stabilization of functioning, preparation for a comfortable and dignified death) and makes sure that treatment decisions are consistent with this goal. Nursing intervention may be helpful in making sure that everyone is clear about the goal of care and changes in the goal of care as the patient's condition changes. Because some physicians are reluctant to accept preparation for a comfortable, dignified death as an appropriate goal of medicine, some patients have received unwanted care that needlessly prolonged their dying. Conversely, decisions are being made today for financial and other reasons that deprive patients of wanted end-of-life care.

The nurse serves as an advocate for the patient and the family unless what the patient or family wants violates the profession of nursing and nursing's code of ethics or one's own conscience. Interventions include the following:

(continued)

Decisional Conflict *(Continued)*

- Providing whatever information and support the patient or family needs to make an informed and voluntary decision
- Referring the patient or family to sources that can clarify problematic aspects of the decision, such as religious authority, ethicist, legal counsel
- Identifying and addressing coercive influences on decision making, being sensitive to cultural norms; for example, whereas a controlling husband may be violating his wife's freedom to make autonomous choices in one culture, in another, it is customary for the husband (or male elder in the family) to make choices for a woman.

Documentation of end-of-life care preferences of competent, or previously competent, patients is important. This includes a written record of communication, a living will, durable power of attorney for healthcare, and a medical advance directive. These preferences must be communicated to those who are ordering care.

- Mediating sources of conflict
- Referring patient or family to ethics consult team or ethics committee if conflict cannot be resolved

Internet Resources for End-of-Life Care

- *Aging With Dignity:* A not-for-profit organization founded to affirm and safeguard human dignity and to promote better care of the dying. Makes available the "Five Wishes" living will.
  http://www.agingwithdignity.org
- *Choice in Dying:* A national, not-for-profit organization devoted to right-to-die issues and end-of-life decision making. The site features a wide range of educational materials as well as state-specific advance directives that can be downloaded from the site at no charge.
  http://www.choices.org
- *End of Life Physician Education Resource Center* (EPERC): A central repository for educational materials and information about end-of-life (EOL) issues.
  http://www.eperc.mcw.edu
- *Last Acts:* A call-to-action campaign to improve care at the end of life. Its goals are to bring death-related issues out in the open and help individuals and organizations pursue better ways to care for the dying.
  http://www.lastacts.org
- *Supportive Care of the Dying: A Coalition for Compassionate Care:* Thirteen Catholic healthcare organizations and the Catholic Health Association have joined together to promote culture change that will bring supportive care, compassionate relief of suffering, and pain and symptom management to persons with life-threatening illness and their caregivers. The overall goal of the coalition is to develop and test innovative projects and to provide support to member organizations as they initiate systemic change in the care of persons affected by life-threatening illness.
  http://www.careofdying.org

the appointing person's subsequent incapacity. A combination directive is illustrated in Figure 32-1.

Many means have been suggested to ensure that adult patients have an opportunity to learn about and use advance directives to indicate their wishes about life-prolonging treatment and to appoint surrogate decision makers should they lose decision-making capacity. Nurses have an important role to play in facilitating this dialogue. In the United States, the Patient Self-Determination Act of 1990 requires all hospitals to inform their patients about advance directives. Because the status of advance directives varies from state to state, it is important for nurses to be familiar with federal and state law concerning these directives. Nurses can also be instrumental in developing institutional policies that ensure that patients on admission are encouraged to talk with family, significant others, and healthcare professionals about their treatment preferences.

Assisted Suicide and Direct Voluntary Euthanasia

Euthanasia may be simply defined as good dying. Until recently, most societies maintained that the distinction between killing and allowing to die was morally relevant. This meant that withholding or withdrawing medically ineffective or disproportionately burdensome therapies was morally and legally justified even when this hastened or directly caused a patient's death. On the other hand, killing a patient by administering a lethal injection or carbon monoxide—even when performed with compassionate intent at the request of a patient—was deemed both immoral and illegal. Some are questioning the validity of this distinction today, and there are efforts to legalize **assisted suicide** and **active euthanasia** in numerous countries. In the United States, physician-assisted suicide is legal in Oregon.

It is important for nurses to understand the arguments for and against assisted suicide and direct voluntary euthanasia. These are briefly listed in the accompanying box.

In 1994, the American Nurses Association issued position statements claiming that assisting in suicide and participating in active euthanasia are in violation of the Code

(text continues on page 736)

D.C., Maryland and Virginia

ADVANCE DIRECTIVE

My Durable Power of Attorney for Health Care, Living Will and Other Wishes

I, _____ , write this document as a directive regarding my medical care.

Put the initials of your name by the choices you want.

PART 1. MY DURABLE POWER OF ATTORNEY FOR HEALTH CARE.

_____ I appoint this person to make decisions about my medical care if there ever comes a time when I
cannot make those decisions myself:

NAME _____ PHONE HOME _____ WORK _____

ADDRESS _____

_____

If the person above cannot or will not make decisions for me, I appoint this person:

NAME _____ PHONE HOME _____ WORK _____

ADDRESS _____

_____

_____ I have not appointed anyone to make health care decisions for me in this or any other document.

***I want the person I have appointed, my doctors, my family, and others to be guided by the decisions I
have made below:***

PART 2. MY LIVING WILL.

These are my wishes for my future medical care if there ever comes a time when I can't make these decisions
for myself.

A. **These are my wishes if I have a *terminal condition*:**
   Life-Sustaining Treatments

   _____ I do not want life-sustaining treatments (including CPR) started. If life-sustaining treatments are
   started, I want them stopped.
   _____ I want life-sustaining treatments that my doctors think are best for me.

   _____ Other wishes: _____

   Artificial Nutrition and Hydration

   _____ I do not want artificial nutrition and hydration started if it would be the main treatment keeping me
   alive. If artificial nutrition and hydration
   is started, I want it stopped.
   _____ I want artificial nutrition and hydration even if it is the main treatment keeping me alive.

   _____ Other wishes: _____

   Comfort Care

   _____ I want to be kept as comfortable and free of pain as possible, even if such care prolongs my dying
   or shortens my life.

   _____ Other wishes: _____

B. **These are my wishes if I am ever in a *persistent vegetative state*:**

   Life-Sustaining Treatments

   _____ I do not want life-sustaining treatments (including CPR) started. If life-sustaining treatments are
   started, I want them stopped.
   _____ I want life-sustaining treatments that my doctors think are best for me.

   _____ Other wishes: _____

Figure 32-1

Example of an advance directive. (Used with permission of District of Columbia Hospital Association, Washington, DC.)

Artificial Nutrition and Hydration

_____ I do not want artificial nutrition and hydration started if it would be the main treatment keeping me alive.
If artificial nutrition and hydration is started, I want it stopped.
_____ I want artificial nutrition and hydration even if it is the main treatment keeping me alive.

_____ Other wishes: _____

Comfort Care

_____ I want to be kept as comfortable as possible, even if such care prolongs my dying or shortens my life

_____ Other wishes: _____

C. **Other Direction**

You have the right to be involved in all decisions about your medical care, even those parts not dealing with terminal conditions or persistent vegetative states. If you have wishes not covered in other parts of this document, please indicate them here.

_____

_____

PART 3. OTHER WISHES.

A. **Organ Donation**
_____ I do not wish to donate any of my organs or tissues.
_____ I want to donate all of my organs and tissues.
_____ I only want to donate these organs and tissues: _____

_____ Other wishes: _____

Autopsy
_____ I do not want an autopsy.
_____ I agree to an autopsy if my doctors wish it.

_____ Other wishes: _____

If you wish to say more about any of the above choices, or if you have any other statements to make about your medical care, you may do so on a separate sheet of paper. If you do so, put here the number of pages you are adding: _____

PART 4. SIGNATURES.

You and two witnesses must sign this document for it to be legal.

A. **Your Signature**

By my signature below I show that I understand the purpose and the effect of this document.

SIGNATURE _____ DATE _____

ADDRESS _____

B. **Your Witnesses' Signatures**
I believe the person who has signed this advance directive to be of sound mind, that he/she signed or acknowledged this advance directive in my presence, and that he/she appears not to be acting under pressure, duress, fraud or undue influence. I am not related to the person making this advance directive by blood, marriage or adoption, nor, to the best of my knowledge, am I named in his/her will. I am not the person appointed in this advance directive. I am not a health care provider or an employee of health care provider who is now, or has been in the past, responsible for the care of the person making this advance directive.

Witness #1

SIGNATURE _____ DATE _____

ADDRESS _____

Witness #2

SIGNATURE _____ DATE _____

ADDRESS _____

Figure 32-1 (Continued)

Assisted Suicide and Direct Voluntary Euthanasia: Arguments For and Against

Arguments in Favor of Assisted Suicide and Direct Voluntary Euthanasia

1. It is a beneficent and compassionate act.
2. It respects autonomy by preserving the patient's control of the manner, method, and timing of death.
3. It takes the matter outside the reach of "medical power" and scrupulosity.
4. It prevents the injustice that allows some patients to choose death by refusal of life-support measures, while denying others the right to do so by active euthanasia.
5. In a pluralistic society, euthanasia must be accepted, whatever its intrinsic morality, because states have no moral justification for intruding into such private decisions.

Proponents of involuntary euthanasia argue that, in addition, it is irrational to afford rights of personhood to anencephalics or patients in a permanent vegetative state and unjust to deny them the right to die to which they are entitled. They argue that beneficence to patient, family, and healthcare professionals, as well as conservation of society's resources, make involuntary euthanasia a positive moral duty of physicians.

Arguments Against Assisted Suicide and Direct Voluntary Euthanasia

1. It undermines the value of, and respect for, all human life.
2. Guidelines cannot avoid "sliding down the slippery slope" to involuntary euthanasia and selective devaluation of the lives of the most vulnerable among us.
3. Euthanasia should be unnecessary because the major reasons for requesting it—intolerable pain and fear of overtreatment—can now be handled by better palliative care, analgesia, and advance directives.
4. A focus on euthanasia will deviate attention from other valuable palliative techniques.
5. If euthanasia is legal, it is predicted patients will feel a subtle pressure to conform so as to relieve the economic and emotional burdens they impose on family and friends.
6. Euthanasia is socially destructive: it undermines trust in physicians and healthcare professionals, desensitizes society to killing, and imperils the grounds already gained in legitimizing passive euthanasia.
7. Many Americans hold the religious belief that human life is the gift of the Creator and that humans are its stewards but not its absolute masters.

(Adapted from Pellegrino, E. D. [1991]. Ethics. *Journal of the American Medical Association, 265*[23], 3118–3119.)

---

for Nurses, the ethical traditions and goals of the profession, and its covenant with society. Nurses can expect to be confronted by patients who seek their assistance in ending their life. Unless nurses think through this issue carefully, they will be unprepared to respond to the request, "Nurse, please help me die."

Do-Not-Resuscitate or No-Code Orders

To prevent the improper use of cardiopulmonary resuscitation, which is designed to prevent unexpected death, some physicians will write do-not-resuscitate (DNR), or no-code, on the chart of a patient if the patient or surrogate has expressed a wish that there be no attempts to resuscitate the patient in the event of cardiopulmonary resuscitation. Many physicians are reluctant to write these orders, especially when this issue is a source of conflict between the patient and family or between individual family members. In these cases, a physician who believes the patient will not benefit from resuscitative measures may verbally indicate to the nurse that only a slow-code (or "show-code") should be called; that is, in the case of cardiopulmonary or respiratory arrest, calling a code and resuscitating the patient are to be delayed until these measures will be ineffectual. Slow-codes are never good practice, and many

healthcare institutions now have policies forbidding their use. It is likely that a nurse could be charged negligent in the event of a slow-code and resultant patient death.

The standard of care still obligates healthcare professionals to attempt resuscitation if a patient stops breathing or his or her heart stops (cardiopulmonary arrest) and there is no order to the contrary. For this reason, it is important for nurses to clarify a patient's code status if the probable benefits of resuscitation are negligible or if the nurse has reason to believe a patient would not want to be resuscitated. Many states now allow patients living at home to craft special orders that allow emergency technicians (EMTs) called to the home in the event of cardiopulmonary arrest to respect the patient's wishes not to be resuscitated.

Comfort Measures Only and Other Special Orders

A **do-not-resuscitate order** means simply that—that no attempts are to be made to resuscitate a patient who stops breathing or whose heart stops beating. When a discussion is taking place about resuscitation, it is appropriate to question aggressive treatment in general, for example, the use of dialysis, ventilatory support, artificial nutrition and hydration, blood transfusions, antibiotics and other medications, and surgery. Whereas some patients may want aggressive treatment and such treatment is medically beneficial, other patients may be at a point in their illness at which they choose to terminate all life-sustaining measures. There is no moral obligation to initiate or continue the use of life-sustaining treatment that is minimally effective or disproportionately burdensome. Law may place constraints on those who may decide to withhold or withdraw life-sustaining treatment for incompetent patients. Nurses should be familiar with pertinent federal and state law and the policies in their institution or agency concerning the withholding or withdrawing of life-sustaining treatment. Nurses should also be familiar with the forms used to indicate patient preferences about end-of-life care. A **comfort-measures-only order** is written to indicate that the goal of treatment is a comfortable, dignified death and that further life-sustaining measures are no longer indicated. A **do-not-hospitalize order** is being used by patients in nursing homes and other residential settings who have elected not to be hospitalized for further aggressive treatment.

Terminal Weaning

Terminal weaning is the gradual withdrawal of mechanical ventilation from a patient with a terminal illness or an irreversible condition with poor prognosis. In some cases, competent patients decide that they wish their ventilatory support ended; more often, the surrogate decision makers for an incompetent patient determine that continued ventilatory support is futile. Although it may be expected that a patient will not be able to survive the weaning, death is never a certain outcome, and it is not unusual for a patient to initiate spontaneous respirations once ventilatory support is withdrawn and live for several hours to several days. Competent patients and family members should be prepared for all possibilities. Nursing's role in the event of a terminal weaning is to participate in the decision-making process by offering helpful information about the benefits and burdens of continued ventilation and a description of what to expect if terminal weaning is initiated. Supporting the patient's family and managing sedation and analgesia are critical nursing responsibilities; unfortunately, many agencies and institutions do not have policies. If involved in terminal weaning, consult the literature (Campbell, 1994; Rushton & Terry, 1995).

Death Certificate

United States law requires that a death certificate be prepared for each person who dies. The law specifies what information needs to be supplied. Death certificates are sent to local health departments, which compile many statistics from the information. The mortician assumes responsibility for handling and filing the death certificate with proper authorities. A physician's signature is required on the certificate, as well as that of the pathologist, the coroner, and others in special cases. The nurse's responsibility is to ensure that a death certificate has been signed by the physician.

Organ Donation

Patients who express a wish to donate functional organs, such as heart, corneas, liver, lungs, and kidneys, can fill out an organ donor consent card (Fig. 32-2). The family

Signed by the donor and the following two witnesses in the presence of each other:

Signature of Donor ______ Date of Birth of Donor ______

Date Signed ______ City and State ______

Witness ______ Witness ______

This is a legal document under the Uniform Anatomical Gift Act or similar laws in all 50 states. For further information call

Delaware Valley TRANSPLANT PROGRAM

800 KIDNEY-1
2401 Walnut St., Suite 404
Philadelphia, PA 19103

UNIFORM DONOR CARD

Print or type name of donor ______

In the hope that I may help others, I hereby make this anatomical gift, if medically acceptable, to take effect upon my death. The words and marks below indicate my desires.

I give: a)______any needed organs or parts
b)______only the following organs or parts

Specify the organ(s) or part(s) ______

for the purpose of transplantation, therapy, medical research or education;
c)______my body for anatomical study if needed

Limitations or special wishes, if any ______

Figure 32-2
Example of an organ donor card.

of a deceased patient also may decide to donate the patient's functional organs. The nurse should be able to review options and provide consent forms to interested patients and their families. Until recently, most organs were retrieved from totally brain-dead patients. New protocols for retrieving organs from non–heart-beating cadavers are raising multiple practice concerns. Comprehensive attention to optimal patient and family care at the time of withdrawal of life-sustaining therapy needs to remain nursing's priority. The scarcity of organs has resulted in legislation mandating hospitals and other healthcare agencies to notify transplantation programs of potential donors.

Autopsy

An autopsy is an examination of the organs and tissues of a human body after death. Consent for autopsy is a legal requirement. The closest surviving family member or members usually have the authority to determine whether an autopsy is performed. Some religious groups prohibit autopsies except for legal purposes.

It is commonly the physician's responsibility to obtain permission for an autopsy. Sometimes, the patient may grant this permission before death. The nurse can assist by explaining the reasons for an autopsy. Many relatives find comfort when they are told that the knowledge gained from an autopsy may contribute to advances in medical science as well as establish the exact cause of death.

If death is caused by accident, suicide, homicide, or illegal therapeutic practice, the coroner must be notified, according to law. The coroner may decide that an autopsy is advisable and can order that one be performed, even though the patient's family has refused consent. In some cases, a death that occurs within 24 hours of admission to the hospital must be reported to the coroner.

Factors That Affect Grief and Dying

Many factors, including age, family relationships, socioeconomic position, and cultural and religious influences, affect a person's reaction to and expression of grief, and like the stages of grief reaction, they vary from person to person.

Developmental Considerations

Children do not understand death on the same level as adults do, but their sense of loss is just as great. Both terminally ill children and their siblings are likely to talk and ask questions about death in an attempt to understand it. Terminally ill children of all ages require parental love and support as well as social interaction with other children. Death of a parent or another significant person can retard a child's development or may cause the child to regress developmentally. Children need to go through the same grief reactions as adults to accept such a loss and maintain emotional well-being.

The loss of a parent by a middle-aged adult helps to prepare the adult for the loss of a spouse or significant other and to accept his or her own eventual death. Older people may lose a spouse or friends and relatives their own age. As this happens, they reminisce about life, put their lives and the purpose of living in perspective, and prepare themselves for their own inevitable death.

Family

Roles within families are important factors that affect reactions to and expressions of grief. For example, the eldest sibling may feel a need to "be strong" and therefore may not grieve openly; a person who loses a spouse may display the same type of behavior to "protect the children."

The death of a child is usually a devastating experience for her or his family. The family needs time to accept the reality of the situation, opportunities to talk and to be listened to, and the experience of expressing themselves behaviorally in a nonjudgmental environment. The family of a terminally ill child may express feelings of guilt by wondering if they were responsible for the impending death. A sibling may suppress a guilt feeling for having wished the ill child (or a parent) dead.

Socioeconomic Factors

A bereaved family may suffer more acutely if there is no health or life insurance or pension after the death of the family provider. Such families face not only the loss of a loved one but also an economic loss that may further disrupt family life. Older people especially may be placed in a difficult position because the death of a spouse may result in a source of retirement income for the surviving spouse being either diminished or cut off. This reduction in income may lead to loss of home, community, and support systems.

Cultural Influences

Both the physical and emotional manifestations of grief may be culturally influenced. Clinical symptoms of grief include repeated somatic distress, tightness in the chest, choking or shortness of breath, sighing, empty feeling in the abdomen, loss of muscle power, and intense subjective distress. Other symptoms include vomiting, dizziness, fainting, fatigue, weight loss, headaches, and chest pains.

Culture also influences a person's expression of grief. In many families in the Western culture, grief is a private matter that is shared only with the family. As such, many people internalize their feelings of grief and may not express their feelings of loss to others. On the other hand, cultural background may necessitate that the patient's and family's public display be emotional and distressed, with loud weeping and moaning.

Although sex roles have become more unified in the past few decades, male and female reactions to death may differ. The widow who has a job may not be as emotionally distraught as the woman who has needed her husband for support. Likewise, the widower who has not taken care of the children or the house may view the future more bleakly than the man who has cooked meals and changed diapers. Some ethnic traditions may be ingrained in certain people, and the woman may be expected to be weak and need support, whereas the man may be expected to be emotionally supportive. This varies from culture to culture and from person to person.

Religious Influences

Faith and religious practices play an important role in the expression of grief and provide comfort and solace to the person experiencing loss. Many people who have put spiritual matters in the background of their lives have found death to be an impetus for a return to earlier practices of religion. At the same time, others may blame God for the death of their loved one and turn away from God (see Chap. 35.)

Cause of Death

Death may result from various causes, and the grief response often depends on the cause. Many deaths are sudden and involve shock as well as normal grieving in the survivors. Death from disease generates several types of response, including belief that the death is a punishment (eg, when AIDS was first diagnosed in homosexuals and drug users), terror and panic (eg, when people are reminded of the devastation caused by plagues of earlier centuries), and guilt (eg, when family and friends believe that they could have prevented the death). Accidental death is often associated with feelings of bad luck. The guilt response can be enormous, especially when children die as the result of an accident. Death while defending a country usually is viewed by most of society as honorable and necessary. Violent deaths occur daily, especially in the larger cities of North America. Suicide accounts for a great number of violent deaths; in fact, among teenagers, it has become a major concern. It is also believed that many accidental deaths are actually suicides.

The Nurse as Role Model

Holistic care of the terminally ill patient and family almost always involves some personal emotional investment. It is unrealistic and unfair to expect nurses to handle circumstances surrounding death without feelings. The best policy seems to be taking the time to explore one's own feelings and express them (see the accompanying Applying Learning to Practice: Promoting Health box). The nurse who neglects to deal with personal feelings about life, dying, and death is in a questionable position to analyze and consider the needs of patients facing death. Therefore, a nurse's own feelings play a major role in determining how he or she cares for a patient with a terminal illness. The following are some personal questions the nurse should use to help clarify feelings about finiteness of self:

- If I could control the events that result in my own death, where would I want to be? What cause of death would I choose? Whom would I want to have present during my terminal illness?

- What fears do I have about death?
- How would I answer these same questions for a patient for whom I have been caring?
- How could I improve the quality of care for a terminally ill patient for whom I am caring?
- If I were a member of the patient's family, what things would I want a nurse to do for me?

The nurse who cares for a patient for an extended period will undergo a grief reaction when the patient dies. Grief after the death of a patient is natural, and the nurse should allow himself or herself to go through the grieving process rather than shut off the grief. The nurse should also address personal health needs.

Nurses caring for patients experiencing loss, grief, dying, and death will be effective role models if they can achieve the following goals:

- Identify personal losses that are influencing current state of well-being and identify and utilize effective coping strategies
- Communicate openly with patients about their losses and invite a discussion of the adequacy of their coping mechanisms
- Respond genuinely to the concerns and feelings of dying patients and their families; do not be afraid to cry with patients and to allow feelings to show
- Value time spent with patients and family members in which supportive presence is the primary intervention

---

APPLYING LEARNING TO PRACTICE

Promoting Health

If a past or current loss is influencing your everyday functioning, use the assessment checklist to see how well you are responding to the losses in your life. Then develop a prescription for self-care by choosing appropriate behaviors from the list of suggestions.

ASSESSMENT CHECKLIST

almost always / sometimes / almost never

1. I can name the personal losses that are presently influencing my state of well-being.

2. I have a plan for coping with these losses that is in place and helping me to cope.

3. I understand the importance of grieving, and I actually set time aside for this self-care measure.

4. I am comfortable with my feelings and am able to give them expression.

5. There is someone who knows and accepts me well enough to allow me to share openly and honestly.

SELF-CARE BEHAVIORS

1. Make a list of the losses that are interfering with your present state of well-being. These may include the loss of health; valued role, image/reputation, relationship; material object; job; person.

2. Determine whether or not you are addressing these losses in a conscious fashion, and identify coping strategies that may be of help.

3. Try implementing a "tried and true" or new coping strategy.

4. Talk about one of these losses with a friend, religious leader, or counselor/therapist. Assess your comfort level in sharing your feelings openly. Ask the person you are sharing with how they think you are responding.

5. Be honest about any maladaptive coping strategies you may be using to cope, such as addictions, apathy ("Who cares?"), withdrawal and passivity, depression, acting out. Get any help you need to replace these maladaptive coping measures.

The Nursing Process

The nursing process is a helpful tool when caring for patients who are grieving or dying and their families and significant others. The accompanying display presents the competencies necessary for nurses to provide high-quality care to patients and families during the transition at the end of life.

ASSESSING

Focused assessment for those experiencing loss, grief, and dying is directed toward determining the adequacy of the patient's and family's knowledge, perceptions, coping strategies (see Chap. 31), and resources. Pertinent interview questions are in the accompanying Focused Assessment Guide. Physical assessment of both the dying patient and of concerned family, friends, and family caregivers is essential to diagnosing some problems.

DIAGNOSING

The data the nurse collects about how a patient or the patient's caregivers are responding to loss, actual or anticipated, or impending death, may lead to several different nursing diagnoses.

Response to Loss as the Problem

Nursing diagnoses that specifically address human responses to loss and impending death in the problem statement include the following: Impaired Adjustment, Caregiver Role Strain, Decisional Conflict, Ineffective Denial, Ineffective Coping, Anticipatory or Dysfunctional Grieving, Hopelessness, Ineffective Management of Therapeutic Regimen, and Powerlessness. Sample defining characteristics for these diagnoses appear later in the box in the Implementing section.

Response to Loss as the Etiology

Difficulty responding to loss or impending death may also affect other areas of human functioning and result in different diagnoses. Examples of nursing diagnoses for which the experience of loss is the etiology follow:

Anxiety related to inability to predict how the last stage of illness will play itself out

Altered Comfort related to complications of chemotherapy for end-stage breast cancer

Altered Family Processes related to stress of caring for dying mother

Fatigue related to constant demands of caring for dying family member

Fear related to perceived loss of control and increasing need to be dependent in final stages of illness

---

Competencies Necessary for Nurses to Provide High-Quality Care to Patients and Families During the Transition at the End of Life

1. Recognize dynamic changes in population demographics, healthcare economics and service delivery that necessitate improved professional preparation for end-of-life care.
2. Promotes the provision of comfort care to the dying as an active, desirable, and important skill and an integral component of nursing care.
3. Communicate effectively and compassionately with the patient, family and healthcare team members about end-of-life issues.
4. Recognize one's own attitudes, feelings, values, and expectations about death and the individual, cultural, and spiritual diversity existing in these beliefs and customs.
5. Demonstrate respect for the patient's views and wishes during end-of-life care.
6. Collaborate with interdisciplinary team members while implementing the nursing role in end-of-life care.
7. Use scientifically based standardized tools to assess symptoms (eg, pain, dyspnea [breathlessness], constipation, anxiety, fatigue, nausea/vomiting, and altered cognition) experienced by patients at the end of life.
8. Use data from symptom assessment to plan and intervene in symptom management using state-of-the-art traditional and complementary approaches.
9. Evaluate the impact of traditional, complementary, and technological therapies on patient-centered outcomes.
10. Assess and treat multiple dimensions, including physical, psychological, social, and spiritual needs, to improve quality at the end of life.
11. Assist the patient, family, colleagues, and self to cope with suffering, grief, loss, and bereavement in end-of-life care.
12. Apply legal and ethical principles in the analysis of complex issues in end-of-life care, recognizing the influence of personal values, professional codes, and patient preferences.
13. Identify barriers and facilitators to patients' and caregivers' effective use of resources.
14. Demonstrate skill at implementing a plan for improved end-of-life care within a dynamic and complex healthcare delivery system.
15. Apply knowledge gained from palliative care research to end-of-life education and care.

(Used with permission. American Association of Colleges of Nursing [1999]. Competencies necessary for nurses to provide high-quality care to patients and families during transition at the end of life.)

FOCUSED ASSESSMENT GUIDE

The Experience of Loss, Grief, Dying, and Death

Assessment Priorities

Patient and family's understanding of medical condition and prognosis

Patient and family's attitude toward death and dying

Patient's preferences concerning death: desire to be at home or in a hospital or hospice setting; decisions concerning aggressiveness of treatment, resuscitation, advanced life support, organ donation, etc.

For the incompetent patient: existence of advance directive *[It is critical that the authorized decision maker be known to all members of the healthcare team]*

Religious beliefs

Cultural influences

Stage of grief and death reaction (denial and isolation, anger, bargaining, depression, acceptance)

Adequacy of coping behaviors

Adequacy of resources

Physiologic needs of the patient: personal hygiene, pain control, nutritional and fluid needs, movement, elimination and respiratory care needs

Psychological needs of the patient and family: fear of the unknown, pain, separation, leaving loved ones, dependence; loss of dignity; unfinished business; powerlessness

Spiritual needs of the patient and family: need for meaning and purpose, for love and relatedness, for forgiveness, for hope.

Factors to Assess	Questions and Approaches
Adequacy of knowledge base	What have you been told about your condition? What do you know about this condition? Please describe what you have been told about your treatment options. Is there anything you don't understand about what your doctor is recommending? What else would you like to know about your present condition and treatment options? Do you know how to contact your doctor and to get the information you need/desire? *Objective is to identify whether or not the knowledge the patient and family possess will allow them to make informed decisions that will serve their best interests.*
Realism of expectations/perceptions	Have you had any previous experiences with this condition or with the death of someone you love? What are your expectations in this case? How do you see the next few weeks (days) playing out? What are your fears, hopes, concerns, worries? What good do you think might be happening in the midst of all this? *Objective is to discover whether the patient and family have unrealistic expectations or misperceptions about the diagnosis, prognosis, and care options that will interfere with their decision making and coping.*
Adequacy of coping strategies	Dealing with our own dying is a once-in-a-lifetime experience, and sometimes we begin the process feeling totally unprepared. Tell me something about how you think you are coping with all this. How well do you think those around you are coping? How can I help you develop or tap the resources that will help you to cope better? *Objective is to identify whether the patient and the patient's family are using effective coping strategies. If you detect problems, try to identify coping strategies they have used effectively in the past. Also identify and address destructive habits that have not served them well in the past such as addictions, destructive relationships, passivity, acting out. Creatively problem-solve about new strategies they might try.*
Adequacy of resources	What is helping you to get through this? Do you think the resources available to you are adequate? If the sky was the limit, what help would you wish for? What is interfering with your getting the help you need? What are some of the community resources that might be of help to you? Are you using these?

(continued)

Factors to Assess	Questions and Approaches
	Objective is to assess the adequacy of the human, financial, spiritual, and psychological resources available to the patient. Questions should be directed to determining what, if anything, is interfering with the patient using whatever resources are available to facilitate coping.
Physical response	A physical assessment of the patient and the patient's family and caregivers should be performed to detect problems with coping that result in fatigue, decreased energy, decreased self-care (deficient grooming, unplanned weight loss), and other maladaptive responses.

Knowledge Deficit related to lack of experience of ever having to care for dying family member at home

Noncompliance related to denial of gravity of illness and impending death

Self-Esteem Disturbance related to inability to accept need for assistance as disease progresses

Spiritual Distress related to inability to reconcile diagnosis and pain with belief in a loving God

Self-Care Deficit related to waning strength as terminal illness progresses

PLANNING: EXPECTED OUTCOMES

Nursing care should be directed toward the achievement of the following goals or outcomes for grieving and dying patients and their families. The patient or family will achieve the following:

* Demonstrate freedom to express feelings, needs, fears, and concerns
* Identify and use effective coping strategies
* Accept need for help as appropriate and use available resources
* Make healthcare decisions reflecting personal values and goals; ultimately feel peaceful about role in decision making
* Declare preferences regarding treatment options
* Report sufficient relief of pain to interact meaningfully with family and to attend to everyday concerns
* Experience a dignified and comfortable death
* Family or significant others: resolve grief after a suitable period of mourning and resume meaningful roles and daily activities

The patient and the family should take an active role in planning for care. Such planning takes the patient's preferences into consideration, facilitates the acceptance of death by the patient and the family, and provides interventions to meet holistic needs.

IMPLEMENTING

The nurse's aims in caring for dying patients and their families include facilitating coping of the dying person and family and promoting health and preventing illness of the family. The accompanying boxes feature nursing diagnoses for common problems related to death and dying as well as specific NIC dying care activities.

Developing a Trusting Nurse–Patient Relationship

Communication is a lifelong need up to the moment of death and should be maintained at all times with the patient and family. To develop meaningful communications, the nurse must develop a trusting relationship with the patient. This relationship is explored throughout this text. The nurse needs to develop listening skills and the ability to recognize both verbal and nonverbal cues given by the patient and family. These skills are discussed in Chapter 21.

The nurse should be willing to discuss the patient's fears and doubts openly and to serve as a nonjudgmental listener. A caring nurse feels at ease in crying with the grieving person and sharing experiences with fears, loneliness, and death. This allows the griever the freedom to express his or her deepest concerns. Nonverbal communication is equally important. A smile, a touching hand or stroke, and eye-to-eye contact are all meaningful. The warmth behind the gesture and the honest concern of the nurse are what count.

The sense of hearing is believed to be the last sense to leave the body; many patients retain a sense of hearing almost to the moment of death. It is kind and thoughtful of the nurse to speak to the comatose patient and to encourage family members to do likewise. The nurse should explain to the patient the nursing care being given and the noises in the unit.

Explaining the Patient's Condition and Treatment

All involved healthcare personnel should know exactly what the patient and family have been told. Telling them different things puts the nurse and other team members at cross-purposes and sets up distrust in the family. Because patients and families often direct questions about the patient's prognosis to the nurse, it is up to the nurse to take the initiative in determining a means to be consistent in terminology, prognosis, and description of progress.

Nursing Diagnoses for Common Problems

Loss and Impending Death

Problem	*Related Factors*	*Sample Defining Characteristics*
Impaired Adjustment	Newly diagnosed terminal illness	"This can't be happening to me. . . . I know I'm going to die. . . . Why should I try and fight this? Mother fought this same diagnosis and died, why should I hope to be any different?"
Caregiver Role Strain	Hospital discharged dying patient because of inadequate insurance	Spouse has dark circles under eyes, reports unable to sleep through night, decreased appetite, and general lack of energy. "I want to do everything I can for Tony, but I feel so overwhelmed. . . . I don't think anyone prepared me for everything I now find myself needing to do for him. . . . I'm always afraid that I'll hurt him or do something wrong." "I don't want to complain, but I miss being able to go out with my friends. Last week I didn't even get to church because Tony wasn't feeling well Sunday morning and asked me not to leave. . . . Sometimes I think I'll just go crazy."
Decisional Conflict	Repeat hospitalizations for aspiration pneumonia and new inability to swallow	Family has requested ethics consult because they are split about pending decisions for initiation of artificial nutrition and hydration and advisability of future hospitalizations and continued aggressive treatment; patient has Alzheimer's disease and has been in a nursing home for last 5 years.
Ineffective Coping	Inability to accept death of 42-year-old son who died of a heart attack 2 years ago; failure of coping mechanisms that worked in the past	70-year-old widow who lived alone with son until his death 2 years ago has become a recluse and eats just enough to keep herself alive, seems to exist on gin, cigarettes, and chocolate. "Mothers aren't supposed to outlive their children . . . why didn't God take me first? I just want to die and be with Bernie. . . ."
Ineffective Denial	Inability to believe that she has AIDS and that husband was bisexual	Patient who is just "getting her life back in order" (left abusive husband 1 year ago and is newly happily remarried) learns that she has AIDS. "This can't be happening to me . . . after all I've been through . . . I hear what you are saying but I don't believe you . . . there must be some mistake. . . ." Breaks next appointment and refuses to respond to repeated urgings to seek treatment.
Anticipatory Grieving	Knowledge that fetus is anencephalic	"I don't know how this can be happening to us. . . . We've tried to do everything right. . . . We've waited for this baby for so long. . . . It's hard to believe that our baby won't be normal and that if what the doctors say is true she will only live for a few hours or days at most. . . ."
Dysfunctional Grieving	Inability to accept death of anencephalic infant; no grief resolution	Two years after birth of anencephalic infant who died 3 days after delivery, couple has failed to come to peace with child's death; divorce impending; wife has lost 15 pounds, and her husband complains that she "really let herself go, she quit her job, mopes around the house all day, and isn't interested in anything anymore."
Hopelessness	Inability to accept son's diagnosis of leukemia and favorable prognosis linked to knowledge of death of neighbor's son who had similar diagnosis	"Don't be leading us on. . . . We know what leukemia means, we have neighbors who lost a son to leukemia. . . . It's not true that you can treat this. . . ." Parents refuse to believe favorable prognosis; after hearing diagnosis, they become apathetic and withdrawn. "Marge and Joe tried to do everything to save their son and failed, why should we even try? Nothing else in our lives has worked out."

(continued)

Nursing Diagnoses for Common Problems *(Continued)*

Loss and Impending Death

Problem	*Related Factors*	*Sample Defining Characteristics*
Ineffective Management of Therapeutic Regimen (also, Powerlessness)	Suddenness of injury and inability to prepare sufficiently to provide needed in-home care	"One minute our life was perfect and then, WHAM, all of a sudden everything went wrong. If only my husband hadn't gone out that night and if only he could get his leg back. I should be doing more to help him but I just want to sit and cry. This isn't what I bargained for when we got married. I don't think I can spend the rest of my life with a cripple." Home health nurse notes that neither the patient nor his wife is following through with recommended exercises, and he has broken several appointments at the rehabilitation center. Both the patient and his wife seem to have given up and express no interest in therapeutic regimen.

The patient's condition and treatment should be explained to both the patient and the family. Patience is required during explanations. They may be so grieved by the diagnosis that they do not hear all the information that is shared with them. The nurse can question them to learn how much they have retained. Then, the information they missed can be repeated. Care options, as well as the expected outcomes of each option, should be fully explained.

Teaching Self-Care and Promoting Self-Esteem

The patient should be encouraged to retain independence and decision making as long as possible. Personal hygiene practices and self-feeding should also be managed by the patient as long as possible. After the patient is confined to bed, the creative nurse and family caregivers should attempt to find self-care activities the patient can perform. When physical abilities fail, determining when to take medication, for example, may be all the control the patient can retain.

Having familiar objects in view can help make the patient feel more comfortable and secure. Whether the patient is at home or in a healthcare agency, it is desirable to have the environment reflect personal preferences. This gives the patient some degree of control when health and other activities of daily living have slipped out of the patient's reach, and supports self-esteem.

In the transition from independence to interdependence and ultimately to dependence, the patient may experience depression and express frustration and grief about "being a burden." It is crucial for professional and nonprofessional caregivers to respond to the dying patient as a person of worth whose life has meaning and value. Chapter 14 discusses practical ways nurses can use looks, touch, words, and actions to communicate respect and caring.

Teaching Family Members to Assist in Care

Preparing family members to assist in nursing care competently and confidently yields benefits to both the patient and family members. The patient is comforted by having loved ones near; family members are comforted by knowing that they helped comfort the patient. Family members providing nursing care to the patient must be supervised by the nurse.

Family members may not want to provide care themselves but may want to know what to expect and how they can psychologically aid the patient. The nurse can help by explaining the patient's condition, what treatment the patient is undergoing, and what result the family can expect from the treatment. Knowing the facts may help family members to cope better with impending loss.

Meeting the Needs of Dying Patients

Physiologic Needs

Physiologic care of the patient involves meeting physical needs such as personal hygiene, pain control, nutritional and fluid needs, movement, elimination, and respiratory

---

Using the Nursing Interventions Classification (NIC)

Selected Dying Care Activities

- Monitor patient for anxiety
- Monitor mood changes
- Communicate willingness to discuss death
- Encourage patient and family to share feelings about death
- Support patient and family through stages of grief
- Monitor pain
- Monitor deterioration of physical and/or mental capabilities
- Facilitate obtaining spiritual support for patient and family
- Include the family in care decisions and activities, as desired

From McClosky, J., & Bulechek, G. (2000). *Nursing interventions classification* (NIC) (3rd ed.) (p. 262). St. Louis: C. V. Mosby. A full listing of nursing activities for each nursing intervention can be found in this book.

care. Personal hygiene includes cleanliness of the skin, hair, mouth, nose, and eyes. Frequent baths and linen changes may be necessary. The mouth and nose should be kept free of mucus, and secretions should be wiped from the eyes. The physician will determine the medication and dosage needed for pain control, but the patient's wishes should be considered. (See Chap. 40 for a further discussion of pain control.) Some patients prefer and are able to control their own medication. Many dying patients suffer from malnutrition and dehydration, and nutritional and fluid needs must be addressed. The patient may require nutritional support but should be encouraged to take sips of water if still able to swallow. The dying patient may also elect to forego artificial nutrition and hydration because the burdens of feeding and hydrating artificially may outweigh the benefits. See the classic article by Zerwekh (1983) for a discussion of these benefits and burdens. Periodic movement should also be allowed; regular changes of position help prevent pressure ulcers. Problems with elimination include the development of incontinence, constipation, and urinary retention. Absorbent pads or a nearby bedpan may be used for incontinent patients; laxatives or enemas may be used for relieving constipation; and catheterization may be required for urinary retention. Bed linens should be changed often. Respiratory care can be provided by repositioning the conscious patient in semi-Fowler's position; the unconscious patient should be positioned in a semiprone position that allows drainage of saliva and mucus. Oxygen therapy may be necessary for some patients.

Psychological Needs

When people speak of their fears of death, responses typically include fear of the unknown, pain, separation, leaving loved ones, loss of dignity, loss of control, and unfinished business. Kübler-Ross believes that there is still another, more overwhelming and more significant fear that often is repressed and unconscious: that of the catastrophic, destructive force that has befallen a person and that the person cannot change. Kübler-Ross points out that terminally ill people communicate this fear of a destructive force but do so largely through symbolic language. A person may use nonverbal language, such as a facial expression, a particular kind of hand clasp, or, in the case of children, drawings and manner of play with toys. Verbal communication may also be used symbolically. Two nurses have provided an excellent study of the special awareness, needs, and communications of the dying (Callanan & Kelley, 1992).

A fear of isolation, of having to face death alone, is a primary concern of the dying patient. The nurse supports the patient by indicating his or her presence, giving full attention, and showing that he or she cares. The presence of family members in the room should be encouraged. Reminiscences should be shared.

Sexual Needs

Dying patients and their sexual partners may feel uncomfortable discussing their sexual needs. Frequently, partners may wish to be physically intimate with the dying person but are afraid of "hurting" him or her and also afraid that an open expression of sexuality is somehow "inappropriate" when someone is dying. Nurses who are sensitive can help by en-

couraging discussion and by suggesting ways to be physically intimate that will meet the needs of both partners. A loving foot massage or tender, cradling body embrace may be exactly what a dying person needs in his or her last moments.

Spiritual Needs

Many terminally ill patients find great comfort in the support they receive from their religious faith. The nurse should aid in obtaining the services of clergy as each situation indicates.

Although not all patients follow specific spiritual or religious beliefs, most require some form of spiritual care. Most patients need to feel that their lives have meaning; many feel a need for hope in the face of death. The nurse should not impose his or her beliefs on the patient but should let the patient know that his or her beliefs are important. The nurse should arrange for visits from a spiritual adviser if desired. Spiritual needs are discussed more fully in Chapter 35.

Meeting Family Needs

The nurse can provide care for the family facing loss by listening to the family's concerns. Family members need to verbalize their worries and fears, and nurses and other healthcare personnel can provide support by being nonjudgmental listeners. Likewise, nursing care of the grieving family involves communication and listening. Application of communication skills discussed in Chapter 21 and earlier in this section aids the nurse in being a nonjudgmental listener; feedback to the family can be provided by summarizing or paraphrasing, without questioning the validity of the family's emotions. All family members, including children, should be part of the grieving process.

In some instances, the nurse spends more time with the relatives than with the patient, such as when the patient becomes comatose. Family members may need to be reminded to get rest and to eat. Too many visitors may tire the patient; when explanations are offered, most relatives readily understand this. When they want to remain at the hospital, they should be directed to a quiet place where they may relax.

The reality of death can be made less painful by preparing the family ahead of time. When the process has been explained to the family, they are better prepared to understand the needs of and to support the dying person.

The steps of the grieving process should be explained to all family members ahead of time, so that they will recognize the specific stages as they experience them and understand that the process is normal. They will be able to recognize that other members of the family are going through the same stages, perhaps at different times. This preparation allows for better understanding and communication within the family.

Death creates a change in family roles. As one person (the dying person) leaves a role, adjustments must be made within the family to compensate. Each member plays a part in that compensation. The nurse can help with these adjustments.

Responding to Requests for Suicide Assistance

Attempts to legalize assisted suicide and the media's portrayal of suicide as a defining heroic act are resulting in more and more nurses being confronted with requests for suicide assistance. Each nurse should carefully weigh the arguments for and against assisted suicide presented earlier in this chapter and know where he or she stands regarding the morality and legality of this intervention. What we believe influences what we do and do not say to patients and the way we say it. It also influences what we include in our range of therapeutic options.

Regardless of one's beliefs about the legality of assisted suicide, nurses must join other healthcare professionals in addressing the human responses that underlie requests for suicide assistance. Nursing is well positioned to offer leadership in meeting the following human needs:

> Fear of losing control
> Fear of not being "allowed" to die or of being encouraged to die prematurely
> Fear of intractable pain and overwhelming suffering
> Fear of becoming increasingly dependent
> Fear of loss of human dignity
> Fear of an endless succession of meaningless days
> Fear of dying alone
> Economic fears

Providing Postmortem Care

When a patient dies, the nurse's responsibilities include caring for the patient's body, caring for the family, and discharging specific legal responsibilities. The latter involve ensuring that a death certificate is issued and signed, labeling the body, and reviewing organ donation arrangements, if any.

Care of the Body
After the patient has been pronounced dead, the nurse is responsible for preparing the body for discharge. The body is placed in normal anatomic position to avoid pooling of blood, soiled dressings are replaced, and tubes are removed. In most cases, it is unnecessary to wash the body; the mortician normally attends to this. Some religions strictly forbid washing of the body, whereas in others, it must be performed by a special person. In cultures in which the family's washing of the deceased's body is considered the last service a family can give a loved one, the family should be given the necessary supplies and left alone in the room with the body. If an autopsy is to be performed, any tubes that were in place should not be removed. In such cases, the nurse should follow the hospital's policy.

The nurse is legally responsible for placing identification tags on both the shroud or garment the body is clothed in and the ankle to ensure that the body can be identified even if it is separated from its shroud. The nurse should also place an identification tag on the patient's dentures or other prostheses to ensure that these are received by the mortician. The patient's body may have to be placed in the hospital's morgue refrigerator if mortuary arrangements were not made before the patient's death. The importance of proper and complete identification cannot be overemphasized.

If the patient died of a communicable disease, the body may require special handling to prevent the spread of that disease. Requirements for such handling are usually specified by local law and are contingent on the disease-causing organism, mode of transmission, and other characteristics.

Care of the Family
After a patient has died, the nurse provides support and care to the patient's family. See the accompanying box: Through the Eyes of a Student. In most cases, this involves listening to the family's expressions of grief, loss, and helplessness. Because comforting words are often difficult to find, the nurse should offer solace and support by being an attentive listener. Family members may need to see the patient's body to accept the death fully; in such cases, the nurse should arrange for family members to view the body before it is discharged to the mortician.

Sudden death creates unique problems for the family. In the case of sudden injury or illness, the physical needs of the patient are paramount to the healthcare team. This means that family members are not provided as much emotional support or information as they would be if the patient's illness were prolonged, nor are they permitted to exercise as many options regarding the patient's care. The family that loses a member unexpectedly has not had an opportunity to begin the grieving process or to share in grieving with the deceased person. Family members should be allowed to express grief and should be given emotional support. Most often, the family is in the emergency department waiting room when death is confirmed. They are stunned, bewildered, and numb. They should not be rushed from the waiting room, but rather provided a private place to begin their grieving. The nurse should acknowledge their shock and listen to their grief. The family needs guidance in making plans and help in making decisions.

It is proper for the nurse who was caregiver or who took care of the patient for a prolonged period to attend the funeral. It also is appropriate for the nurse to make a follow-up call to the patient's family after the funeral or memorial service to offer both concern and care for the family's well-being. Follow-up visits are important to give support to the family. If the nurse assesses that the family is not coping well (dysfunctional grief), appropriate referral should be made.

Care of Other Patients
Because it is not unusual for nurses in institutional settings to provide care to more than one patient at a time, after the death of one patient, the nurse must continue to provide care to the other patients. Other patients are often aware of a death and may need to be consoled; this is particularly true of a patient who has shared a room with the deceased patient. Other patients may have grief reactions and should be supported through the grief process by the nurse. Death of a patient may cause depression in other patients and may make them more aware of their own future deaths.

EVALUATING

The plan of nursing care for dying patients is effective if patients meet the outcome of a comfortable, dignified death and family members resolve their grief after a suitable time of mourning and resume meaningful life roles and activities. See the accompanying Applying Learning to Practice and Nursing Plan of Care boxes.

(*text continues on page 750*)

Through the Eyes of a Student

We had had several day-shift clinical rotations, but this was our first evening clinical experience. We were unsure as to what the evening would be like. We knew the evening would provide us with a new outlook on nursing, but we were not prepared for what unfolded.

I had been taking care of a patient when another nursing student asked if I would check in on her patient while she had her dinner break. This patient was known to each of the students because we all had the pleasure of caring for him. I was told he was lying in bed watching television and that he had changed his code status to "DNR" (do not resuscitate) just that day. When I went to check on him, I found him lying in bed but not watching television. His eyes were closed as if he were sleeping peacefully. I spoke his name several times without a response. At the same time, I was also checking for a radial pulse. When I couldn't find his pulse, I swiftly walked to find the instructor. Together we went back to him and assessed his condition. There were no radial or carotid pulses. His chest was not rising and the instructor listened to his heart with a stethoscope. There wasn't a heartbeat. I stood there feeling helpless and low-spirited. This was a man to whom we had all grown close. His family came to see him and to say a few final words. Tears were shed not only by his family but by those of us who had cared for him.

Our first evening clinical was an extremely emotional night. We were all quiet as we walked down the hallway to go home. The student who was caring for him that night was stopped by his daughter and two young granddaughters. One granddaughter was wearing his hat and the other was carrying his belt. This man's daughter was broken-hearted by his death, yet needed to know that he wasn't alone when he died. The student told her that I had been the one with him. The daughter seemed relieved to know that he was not by himself when he died.

As I look back on that evening, I'm sad that this man is no longer with us. I did not know him for very long, but he touched me in a way that helped me understand the true meaning of nursing: not only to care for the sick, disabled, or enfeebled, but also to be human and offer support for grieving families.

—Joyce A. Shearman, Delaware County Community College, Media, Pennsylvania

APPLYING LEARNING TO PRACTICE

Patient Care Study

The Espositas have been married for 19 years and have two children, Jorge, who is 16, and Marita, who is 13. It has been 2 years since Mrs. Esposita was diagnosed with ovarian cancer, and this period has been difficult for the entire family. She has had several hospitalizations because of bowel obstructions and returned home more debilitated each time. At present, she is extremely cachexic and in the end stage of her illness. She initially tried aggressive treatment, and several chemotherapy regimens failed. During her last hospitalization 2 months ago, a decision was made not to continue aggressive therapy, and Mrs. Esposita insisted on returning home to die.

The nurse who has been visiting Mrs. Esposita at home asked for assistance from her colleagues in devising a plan of care for Mr. Esposita. Until now, Mrs. Esposita wanted nothing to do with the local hospice because of a reported "bad experience" a neighbor had. Her insurance will not provide for all the home nursing care she needs, and her husband and children have been trying to meet her needs for nursing as well as run the house and meet their own needs. A demanding woman, Mrs. Esposita never seems satisfied with anything anyone does, and the family is looking utterly frustrated, angry, and fatigued. Jorge is coping by "opting out"; he frequently spends the night with friends and doesn't even call home to report on his whereabouts. Marita's grades have fallen, and she has dropped out of cheerleading and other school activities so that she can take care of her mother. Mr. Esposita, who has been silent until now, recently confided that he doesn't know how much longer he can go on this way, and seemed horrified to hear himself say, "I just wish she would die already and get this all over with!" He is very concerned about the changes in his children and feels powerless to change what is happening. For her part, Mrs. Esposita seems oblivious to her family's needs and, even in her weakened state, multiplies pleas for assistance. She seems to be afraid of dying and never wants to be left alone.

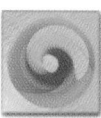

NURSING PLAN OF CARE
for Mrs. Esposita and Her Family

Nursing Diagnosis

Caregiver Role Strain related to multiple losses and burdens associated with caregiving responsibilities as manifested by self-report, breakdown in family relationships, fatigue, and anger.

Expected Outcome

- Mr. Esposita will talk openly about his feelings and share his frustrations about his present situation

Nursing Interventions	Rationale	Evaluative Statement
Plan visits for when there is time for private conversation with Mr. Esposita; initiate conversations by telling him that it is not unusual for family caregivers to feel fatigued, powerless, frustrated, angry, and emotionally distant. Encourage him to talk about what he is feeling: "You seemed surprised at yourself when you said that you wished your wife would 'just die.' This isn't an unusual wish for someone in your situation. . . . Tell me more about what you are feeling now. . . ."	This will normalize what Mr. Esposita is experiencing and communicate that someone cares about him and about what he is experiencing. Simply giving voice to what he is feeling and sharing this with a healthcare professional may help him to accept and address what he takes to be negative and possibly shameful feelings.	10/15/02 Goal partially met. Mr. Esposita states that he feels better now that he is sharing some of what he's been holding in for such a long time, but he still believes that if he was really a good husband he wouldn't feel this way. Also states that it is hard for him to find words to express everything that he is feeling. *Revision:* Continue to encourage Mr. Esposita to talk about what he is experiencing and provide a private opportunity for this to happen. *E. McLoughlin, RN*

Expected Outcome

- By 10/17/02 Mr. Esposita will develop a realistic caregiving plan that matches his ability to care with his wife's need for care and that identifies other resources for his wife's unmet needs.

Nursing Interventions	Rationale	Evaluative Statement
Assist Mr. Esposita to identify what his wife's actual needs for care are; how much of this care it is reasonable to expect the family to provide; and other potential caregiving sources.	Mr. Esposita may need "permission" to *not* meet his wife's unrealistic needs. The nurse's authority may be useful in helping him to believe that he can be a good and faithful husband and still fail to meet her expectations. Identifying other caregiving resources will ensure that Mrs. Esposita's needs will be met.	10/17/02 Goal not met. To date, Mr. Esposita has been unable to identify any additional caregivers for Mrs. Esposita and continues to feel the need to assume all responsibility for her care when he is home. *Revision:* Bring list of community resources to Mr. Esposita, including church group, and plan with him to contact these sources. Reinforce that it is OK to ask for help. *E. McLoughlin, RN*
Explain to Mrs. Esposita that her family may not be able to meet all her needs for care but that every effort will be made to ensure these needs are met by other caregivers.	Even if the nurse's sympathies are with the family, it is critical to communicate to the patient that you are committed to her and intent on doing all in your power to ensure that her needs are met. If the patient's needs are met, it will improve her relationships with her family.	

(continued)

NURSING PLAN OF CARE (Continued)
for Mrs. Esposita and Her Family

Nursing Interventions	Rationale	Evaluative Statement
Assist Mr. Esposita to identify and use new resources: identify at least one new support person who can sit with Mrs. Esposita and relieve the family of some of this burden; explore the family's reluctance to use hospice and evaluate other community resources. Use appropriate referrals.	The family may be feeling unnecessarily overwhelmed because they have failed to explore the availability of other resources. A gentle push may be needed to make this happen. If a "sitter" can be obtained for several hours in the evening, this would give Mr. Esposita time after work to do something with his children or for himself.	

Expected Outcome
- By 10/20/02 Mr. Esposita will report feeling more in control and less depressed and angry

Nursing Interventions	Rationale	Evaluative Statement
Lead Mr. Esposita in a discussion that aims to identify everything that is making him feel powerless; then list those factors over which he has no control and those he can influence or change.

Provide opportunities for Mr. Esposita to control decision making over those aspects of his life and his wife's care for which he can exert control. Affirm constructive decision making and ask him how it feels to be "back in control" of at least some aspects of his life. Discuss with Mr. Esposita those factors he can change, and assist him in making decisions. | This will break the cycle of his thinking that there is nothing at present over which he can exert control. Simply making the list is a first step toward taking action.

This is an example of "guided discovery"; you are allowing Mr. Esposita to experience himself as once again in charge and to allow this experience to define his self-image. Reinforcement of his success affirms his self-image of one who is in charge. Types of support that can be given to caregivers include emotional (concern, trust), appraisal (affirms self-worth), informational (useful advice), and instrumental assistance or tangible goods. | 10/20/02   Goal met. Mr. Esposita reports that even though most of his situation remains unchanged, he no longer feels powerless and is less depressed and angry. He expressed gratitude for this intervention and says it has given him new energy.

E. McLoughlin, RN |

Sample Documentation

10/17/02, 12 PM, Nursing

Met with Mr. Esposita this morning and talked about the plan to identify other caregivers who might be able to "sit" with his wife on some evenings in order to give him time to do things for his children and himself. He reported no progress in identifying anyone but also stated that he hadn't really made any efforts to locate someone: "Who would want to help us? Besides, I wouldn't want to inflict my wife and her moods on anyone right now." I explained that there are many individuals and groups who provide exactly this type of assistance and that his wife's moods were not uncommon for someone in her situation. We then made a list of possible caregiver resources, including some family members who had earlier expressed an interest in helping out, the parish nurse service from his church, and finally the local hospice. If the first two sources do not work out, will explore family reluctance to use hospice resources more carefully because this may be their best hope. Will evaluate progress made on 10/21/02.

E. McLoughlin, RN

Learning Outcomes

After completing this chapter, the learner should be able to accomplish the following:

1. Define key terms used in the chapter.

active euthanasia	dysfunctional grief
actual loss	grief
advance directive	loss
anticipatory loss	mourning
assisted suicide	palliative care
bereavement	perceived loss
comfort-measures-only order	physical loss
	psychological loss
death	terminal illness
do-not-hospitalize order	terminal weaning
do-not-resuscitate order	

2. Differentiate the types of loss.
3. Describe the grief process and the stages of grief.
4. Describe Kübler-Ross's stages of dying.
5. Compare and contrast three definitions of death.
6. Identify ethical and legal issues concerning end-of-life care.
7. Identify six factors that affect loss, grief, and dying.
8. Describe physiologic, psychological, and spiritual care of a dying patient and family.
9. Use the nursing process to plan and implement care for dying patients and their families.
10. Articulate and defend a personal response to a patient's plea, "Please help me die."
11. List the clinical signs of approaching death.
12. Outline nursing responsibilities after death.
13. Discuss the role of the nurse in caring for a patient's family.

Critical Thinking Exercises

1. Recall personal losses (family member, friend, job, opportunity) and recollect what you were experiencing at the time. Try to remember what your expectations were from those you looked to for support, and how your ability to cope was influenced by whether those expectations were met. Remembering that no two people respond to loss in exactly the same way, develop a list of nursing measures to help patients dealing with loss. Compare your list with other students and incorporate their ideas.

2. Compare and contrast the care a patient dying of cancer would receive in a critical care unit and at home with hospice care. Identify the advantages and disadvantages of each. Use your analysis to help you describe these options to prospective patients. Role play a situation with a peer in which you counsel a woman with cancer who is told that cure is no longer an option and that she has less than 6 months to live.

Study Questions

1. A woman who is firmly committed to natural childbirth and who has attended each natural childbirth class in preparation for her experience of labor and delivery undergoes a cesarean delivery when her fetus displays signs of distress. Inconsolable, she cries and calls herself a failure as a mother. Her loss may best be described as
   a. actual
   b. perceived
   c. psychological
   d. combination of above
2. The period of acceptance of loss and grief during which the person learns to deal with experienced loss is best termed
   a. anticipatory grieving
   b. bereavement
   c. mourning
   d. stages of death and dying
3. When you interview an 82-year-old resident in a nursing home, she tells you that she has never gotten over the death of her son who died 20 years ago. She reports that her life fell apart after that and she never again felt like herself or was able to enjoy life. This type of grief is best described as
   a. abbreviated
   b. anticipatory
   c. dysfunctional
   d. inhibited
4. A patient with AIDS whom you have been visiting at home tells you, "I'm no longer afraid of dying. I think I've made my peace with everyone and I'm actually ready to move on." This reflects his progress to which stage of death and dying?
   a. acceptance
   b. anger
   c. bargaining
   d. denial
5. When you next visit this dying patient with AIDS, he breaks down and cries and tells you that it is unfair that he should have to die now when he's finally made peace with his family and wants to live. You are shocked by this change in his mood. Your best reply would be
   a. "You can't be feeling this way. You have to proceed through the stages of dying in an orderly progression, and you've just moved backward."
   b. "It does seem unfair . . . tell me more about how you are feeling. . . ."

c. "You'll be all right . . . who knows how much time any of us has to enjoy relationships with those we love. You are lucky to have had the opportunity to make your peace."

d. "Tell me about your pain. Did it keep you awake last night?"

6. Which definition of death is gaining in popularity as more people believe that critical human functions are personality, conscious life, and the capacity for remembering, judging, reasoning, acting, enjoying, and worrying?

a. heart–lung death

b. higher-brain death

c. personhood death

d. whole-brain death

7. If your patient tells you that he has no one he trusts to make healthcare decisions for him in the event that he becomes incapacitated, you should help him to prepare

a. combination advance medical directive

b. durable power of attorney for healthcare

c. living will

d.

8. Which of the following nurse responses would be endorsed by the American Nurses Association?

a. A nurse promises a dying patient that he will do everything possible to keep her comfortable but that he cannot administer an injection or overdose to cause her death.

b. A nurse tells a dying patient who is on a ventilator that under no condition can he be removed from the ventilator because this is active euthanasia and it is expressly forbidden by the Code for Nurses.

c. After exhausting every intervention in her bag of tricks to keep a dying patient comfortable the nurse says, "I think you are now at a point where I'm prepared to do what you've been asking me. Let's talk about when and how you want to die."

d. In response to a patient who asks for assistance in committing suicide a nurse replies, "I'm personally opposed to assisted suicide but I'll find you a colleague who can help you."

9. You are caring for a comatose patient whose primary diagnosis is breast cancer but who has suffered multiple complications and who is now in the end stages of her illness. She has been in the medical intensive care unit for 3 weeks. Her husband tells you that he and his wife often talked about the end of her life and that she was very clear about not wanting aggressive treatment that would merely prolong her dying. You both agree that this seems to be all that therapy is now doing for her. Which of the following orders would you recommend the husband speak to her physician about

a. comfort-measures-only

b. do-not-hospitalize

c. do-not-resuscitate

d. slow-code-only

10. If you are involved in the terminal weaning of a patient, you will want to do all of the following except

a. participate in the decision-making process by offering the family information about the advantages and disadvantages of continued ventilatory support

b. explain to the family what will happen at each phase of the weaning and offer support

c. check the orders for sedation and analgesia and make sure that the anticipated death is comfortable and dignified

d. tell the family that death will occur almost immediately after the patient is removed from the ventilator

11. All of the following diagnoses may apply to a young couple who gave birth to a premature infant with serious respiratory problems who has been in the neonatal intensive care unit for the last 3 months. The couple has a 22-month-old son at home. Which diagnosis best fits the following set of assessment data: report of chronic fatigue and decreased energy, guilt about neglecting son at home, shortness of temper with one another, apprehension about continued ability to go on this way?

a. anticipatory grieving

b. ineffective coping

c. caregiver role strain

d. powerlessness

12. Which of the nursing actions described below would you correct if you saw a nursing assistant doing this?

a. talking to a comatose patient

b. sitting on the bed of a dying patient holding her hand and crying

c. agreeing with the daughter of a dying resident with Alzheimer's disease that the burdens associated with artificially feeding her father may outweigh the benefits

d. telling a dying patient to sit back and relax and that she will wash him because it's easier that way

13. Which of the following nursing actions violates the standards of caring for the body after a patient has been pronounced dead?

a. keeping the patient in a comfortable sitting position until the family has arrived and said their good-byes

b. placing identification tags on both the shroud and the ankle

c. removing soiled dressings and tubes

d. preparing to transfer the body to the morgue

14. The family of a patient who has just died requests to be alone with the body and asks for supplies to wash the body. You know that the mortician usually washes the body. Your best response is

a. inform the family that there is no need for them to wash the body since the mortician does this

b. explain that hospital policy forbids their being alone with the deceased patient and that hospital supplies are only to be used by hospital personnel

c. give the supplies but watch the family so that nothing unusual happens

d. provide the requested supplies and ask if this request is linked to their religious or cultural customs and if there is anything else you can do to be of assistance

15. A 70-year-old woman who has had a number of strokes refuses further life-sustaining interventions, including artificial nutrition and hydration. She is competent, understands the consequences of her actions, is not depressed, and persists in refusing treatment. Her doctor is adamant that she cannot be allowed to die this way and her daughter agrees. An ethics consult has been placed. Who is the appropriate decision maker?

a. patient

b. daughter

c. doctor

d. ethics consult team

Answers With Rationale

1. The correct answer is *d*. Each of the above are only partially correct because there are elements of the loss of the type of delivery she values, which are actual, perceived, and psychological.

2. The correct answer is *c*. Mourning is defined as the period of acceptance of loss and grief during which the person learns to deal with experienced loss. The text offers other definitions for anticipatory grieving, bereavement, and the stages of death and dying.

3. The correct answer is *c*. Abbreviated grief and anticipatory grief are both types of normal grief, and given the length of time this resident's grief has lasted and its effects on her life, it is not normal. Because she is able to give expression to her grief, inhibited grief is not the correct answer. By a process of elimination, the correct answer is dysfunctional grief.

4. The correct answer is *a*. The patient's statement does not reflect anger, bargaining, or denial; hence, by a process of elimination, acceptance is the correct choice.

5. The correct answer is *b;* you want to validate that you have heard what the patient is saying and invite him to share more of his feelings, concerns, and fears. You do not want to offer false reassurance *(c)*, nor use diversion *(d):* both of these strategies would communicate your lack of interest in what he is really feeling. It is simply not true that people have to move through these stages in an orderly fashion *(a)*.

6. The correct answer is *b* because the functions described are controlled by the cortex, or higher brain. There is no such thing as personhood death.

7. The correct answer is *c*. The living will is a document whose precise purpose is to allow individuals to record specific instructions about the type of healthcare they would like to receive in particular end-of-life situations. Both the combination directive and the durable power of attorney involve appointing someone to make decisions—something this patient is reluctant to do.

8. The correct answer is *a*. The American Nurses Association states that nurse-assisted suicide and participation in active euthanasia violates the Code for Nurses and the ethical traditions of the profession. This makes *c* and *d* incorrect because it does not matter if a nurse's personal morality allows him or her to accept assisted suicide. Removing ventilatory support is not necessarily active euthanasia and is not expressly forbidden by the Code for Nurses.

9. The correct response is *a*, comfort-measures-only order, because she would want all aggressive treatment to be stopped at this point and all care to be directed to a comfortable, dignified death. Because she is already in the hospital, there is no need for *b* at this point, and a do-not-resuscitate order is not sufficiently comprehensive. One should never recommend performing a slow-code-only order because it violates good practice.

10. The correct answer is *d; a, b,* and *c* are all nursing interventions that should be carried out by the nurse involved in terminal weaning. Because there are no guarantees how any patient will respond once removed from a ventilator, and because it is possible for the patient to breathe on his or her own and live for hours, days, and, rarely, even weeks, the family should definitely not be told that death will occur immediately.

11. The correct answer is *c;* although it is true that each of the diagnoses listed might apply to the couple described, the defining characteristics for the NANDA diagnosis Caregiver Role Strain fit the set of assessment data provided.

12. The correct answer is *d*. The answers *a* and *b* are acceptable and desirable nursing interventions, and if the nursing assistant is experienced, he or she may very well be in a position to do *c*. Because it is good to encourage dying patients to be as active as possible for as long as possible, it is generally not good practice to perform basic self-care measures the patient can perform simply because it is "easier" to do it this way.

13. The correct answer is *a*. The other answers are all indicated nursing interventions and consistent with standards of care. Because the body should be placed in normal anatomic position to avoid pooling of blood, leaving the body in a sitting position is contraindicated.

14. The correct answer is *d*. The answer *a* ignores the needs of the family and reflects an ignorance of or insensitivity to cultural and religious practices; *b* is simply not true; and *c* presumes that the family is up

to no good purpose and, unless you have reason to suspect something out of the ordinary, is simply uncalled for.

15. The correct answer is *a*. Because this patient is competent, she has the right to refuse therapy that she finds to be disproportionately burdensome, even if this hastens her death. Neither her daughter nor her doctor has the authority to assume her decision-making responsibilities unless she asks them to do this. The ethics consult team is not a decision-making body; it can make recommendations but has no authority to order anything.

Bibliography

American Association of Colleges of Nursing. (1999). Competencies necessary for nurses to provide high-quality care to patients and families during the transition at the end of life.

American Geriatrics Society Ethics Committee. (1995). The care of dying patients: a position statement from the American Geriatrics Society. *Journal of the American Geriatrics Society, 43*, 577–578.

American Geriatrics Society Public Policy Committee. (1991). Voluntary active euthanasia. [Position statement]. *Journal of the American Geriatrics Society, 39*(8), 826.

American Nurses Association. (1991). *Position statement on promotion of comfort and relief of pain in dying patients.* Washington, DC: Author.

American Nurses Association. (1995). *Position statement on assisted suicide.* Washington, DC: Author.

Badger, J. M. (1994). Reaching out to the suicidal patient. *American Journal of Nursing, 94*(3), 24–31.

Beauchamp, T. L., & Veatch, R. M. (1996). *Ethical issues in death and dying* (2nd ed.). Upper Saddle River, NJ: Prentice Hall.

Bramwell, L., MacKenzie, J., Laschinger, H., & Cameron, N. (1995). Need for overnight respite for primary caregivers of hospice patients. *Cancer Nursing, 8*(5), 337–343.

Brown, P. S., & Sefansky, S. (1995). Enhancing bereavement care in the pediatric ICU. *Critical Care Nurse, 15*(5), 59–64.

Callanan, M., & Kelley, P. (1992). *Final gifts.* New York: Poseidon Press.

Campbell, C. S. (1992). Religious ethics and active euthanasia in a pluralistic society. *Kennedy Institute of Ethics Journal, 2*(3), 253–277.

Campbell, M. L. (1994). Terminal weaning. *Nursing, 24*(9), 34–39.

Carpenito, L. J. (1995). *Nursing diagnosis: Application to clinical practice* (6th ed.). Philadelphia: J. B. Lippincott.

Catholic Health Association. (1993 March). Care of the dying: A Catholic perspective. [Special Section]. *Health Progress,* 34–38.

Dyer, I. D. (1993). Breaking the news: Informing visitors that a patient died. *Intensive Critical Care Nurse, 9*(1), 2–10.

Edwards, B. S. (1994). When the family can't let go. *American Journal of Nursing, 94*(1), 52–56.

Ehrle, R. N., Shafer, T. J., & Nelson, K. R. (1999). Determination and referral of potential organ donors and consent for organ donation: Best practices—a blueprint for success. *Critical Care Nurse, 19*(2), 21–33.

Engel, G. L. (1964). Grief and grieving. *American Journal of Nursing, 64*(9), 93–98.

Furukawa, M. M. (1996). Meeting the needs of the dying patient's family. *Critical Care Nurse, 16*(1), 51–62.

The Hastings Center. (1987). *Guidelines on the termination of life-sustaining treatment and the care of the dying.* Bloomington, IN: Indiana University Press.

Holmquist, M., Chabalewski, F., Blount, T., Edwards, V. M., & Pietroski, R. (1999). A critical pathway: Guiding care for organ donors. *Critical Care Nurse, 19*(2), 84–98.

Irish, D. P., Lundquist, K. F., & Nelsen, V. J. (Eds.). (1993). *Ethnic variations in dying, death, and grief.* Washington, DC: Taylor & Francis.

Kass, L. R. (1993 January/February). Is there a right to die? *Hastings Center Report,* 34–43.

Kirchoff, K. T., Spuhler, V., Walker, L., Hutton, A., Cole, V., & Clemmer, T. (2000). Intensive care nurses' experiences with end-of-life care. *American Journal of Critical Care, 9*(1), 36–42.

Kübler-Ross, E. (1969). *On death and dying.* New York: Macmillan.

Lauterbach, S. S. (Ed.). (1995). The experience of loss. *Holistic Nursing Practice, 9*(3).

Martocchio, B. C. (1985). Grief and bereavement: Healing through hurt. *Nursing Clinics of North America, 20*(2), 327–341.

McCue, J. D. (1995). The naturalness of dying. *Journal of the American Medical Association, 273*(13), 1039–1043.

Murphy, P. A., & Price, D. M. (1995). "ACT": Taking a positive approach to end-of-life care. *American Journal of Nursing, 95*(3), 42–43.

North American Nursing Diagnosis Association. (1994). *NANDA nursing diagnoses: Definitions and classifications 1995–1996.* Philadelphia: Author.

Nuland, S. B. (1994). *How we die.* New York: Alfred A. Knopf.

Nuland, S. B. (1997). *The wisdom of the body.* New York: Alfred A. Knopf.

Ott, B. B. (1995). Defining and redefining death. *American Journal of Critical Care, 4*(6), 476–480.

Ott, B. (1999). Advance directives: The emerging body of research. *American Journal of Critical Care, 8*(1), 514–519.

Pellegrino, E. D. (1991). Ethics. *Journal of the American Medical Association, 265*(23), 3118–3119.

Pellegrino, E. D. (2000). Decisions to withdraw life-sustaining treatment. *Journal of the American Medical Association, 283*(8), 1065–1067.

President's Commission for the Study of Ethical Problems in Medicine and Biomedical and Behavioral Research. (1981). *Defining death.* [Pub. No. 81-600150]. Washington, DC: U.S. Government Printing Office.

Quill, T. E. (1993). Doctor, I want to die. Will you help me? *Journal of the American Medical Association, 270*(7), 870–876.

Rasmussen, B. H., Norberg, A., & Sandman, P. O. (1995). Stories about becoming a hospice nurse. *Cancer Nursing, 18*(5), 344–354.

Rushton, C., & Terry, P. B. (1995). Neuromuscular blockade and ventilator withdrawal: Ethical controversies. *American Journal of Critical Care, 4*(2), 112–115.

Saver, C. L. (1994). Decoding the ACLS algorithms. *American Journal of Nursing, 94*(1), 27–36.

Schwarz, J. K. (1999). Assisted dying and nursing practice. *Image—The Journal of Nursing Scholarship, 31*(4), 367–373.

Sullivan, J., Seem, D. L., & Chabalewski, F. (1999). Determining brain death. *Critical Care Nurse, 19*(2), 37–46.

Taylor, C. (1995). Medical futility and nursing. *Image—The Journal of Nursing Scholarship, 27*(4), 301–306.

Vergara, M., & Lynn-McHale, D. J. (1995). Ethical issues. Withdrawing life support: Who decides? *American Journal of Nursing, 95*(11), 47–49.

Zerwekh, J. V. (1983). "The dehydration question?" *Nursing, 13*(1), 47–51.

Zerwekh, J. (1994). The truth-tellers: How hospice nurses help patients confront death. *American Journal of Nursing, 94*(2), 31–34.

Chapter 33
Sensory Stimulation

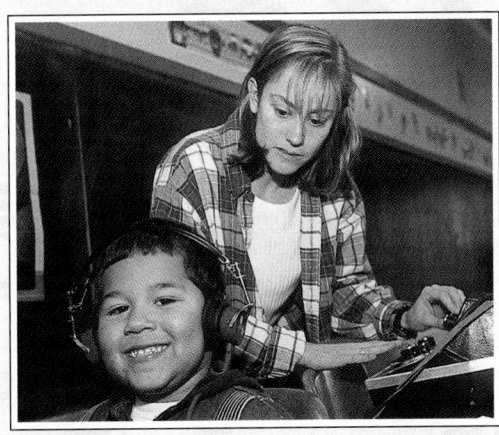

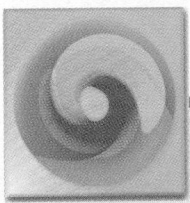

Thinking Critically About
Nursing's Blended Skills

Before reading this chapter, think about the types of blended skills you will need to respond to sensory problems.

- The Kleins are adopting a 14-month-old infant from China. They are warned that she is likely to arrive with developmental delays related to the nonstimulating environment in the orphanage.

- Mr. Pirolla, aged 77 years, has macular degenerative disease and is experiencing progressive loss of vision. Recently, his wife has noticed that he is also having difficulty hearing. They present in the geriatric assessment clinic because of her concerns that he no longer wants to leave the house, and both their social lives are suffering.

- Nancy Tider begs you to "get the doctor to do something" about her dad (aged 92 years) who continues to drive even though his vision is severely impaired. "I keep waiting for the call telling me he's killed himself or someone else!"

- Ori Soltes, aged 54 years, is in the intensive care unit after a motor vehicle crash that resulted in internal injuries as well as fractures. On the fifth day after the crash, he began to exhibit transient episodes of acute confusion. His wife is scared.

What cognitive, technical, interpersonal, and ethical/legal skills do you think you will need to respond to the challenges described above?

A person's senses are vital to survival, growth and development, and the experience of bodily pleasure. For example, awareness of the intensities and sources of sound, ways to control noise, and the assessment of patients' perceptions of and responses to sound can provide nurses with a basis for therapeutic manipulation of the environment.

Many of the patients nurses encounter have impaired sensory functioning, which places them at high risk for injury and altered growth and development and decreases their well-being. Moreover, the stress of illness or trauma and the need for diagnosis and treatment may quickly result in sensory deprivation or overload, with serious disturbances in visual, perceptual, cognitive, or emotional functioning.

Study of this chapter provides knowledge of the process of sensation, the role of the arousal mechanism, sensory alterations, and factors affecting sensory stimulation. Practical suggestions are given for performing an assessment of sensory functioning. Examples are given of nursing diagnoses identifying specific sensory/perceptual alterations, as are many diagnoses describing the effects of altered sensory functioning on other areas of human functioning. Patient goals for preventing and managing sensory alterations are described. Specialized nursing interventions for vision- or hearing-impaired, confused, and unconscious patients are presented.

The Sensory Experience

Components and Conditions

The two components of any sensory experience are reception and perception. Sensory **reception** is the process of receiving data about the internal or external environment through the senses. The senses by which individuals maintain contact with the external environment are vision (**visual**), hearing (**auditory**), smell (**olfactory**), taste (**gustatory**), and touch (**tactile**). The kinesthetic and visceral senses arise internally from muscles and hollow organs, respectively, and are the basic orienting systems. (**Kinesthesia** refers to awareness of positioning of body parts and body movement; **visceral** pertains to inner organs.) **Stereognosis** is the sense that perceives the solidity of objects and their size, shape, and texture. Sensory **perception** is the conscious process of selecting, organizing, and interpreting data from the senses into meaningful information. Perception is influenced by the intensity, size, change, or representation of stimuli as well as by past experiences, knowledge, and attitudes.

For a person to receive data necessary to experience the world, four conditions must be met:

- A **stimulus**—an agent, act, or other influence capable of initiating a response by the nervous system—must be present.

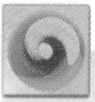

COGNITIVE SKILLS

- Knowledge of factors contributing to sensory alterations and of nursing interventions to prevent sensory alterations (in the intensive care unit), stimulate the senses (of the adopted infant and Mr. Pirolla), and assist patients with sensory difficulties
- Knowledge of how to meet the safety needs of individuals with impaired perception (Nancy's dad and Mr. Pirolla)

TECHNICAL SKILLS

- Ability to use the nursing process to identify and treat problems related to sensory alterations

INTERPERSONAL SKILLS

- Strong people skills; ability to empathize with and to communicate and interact effectively with patients and their caregivers, which will be particularly challenging when establishing

relationships with the Pirollas, Nancy's dad, and Mr. and Mrs. Soltes

- Ability to establish trusting relationships—even in times of crisis
- Teaching and counseling skills to prepare the Klein's to assume new parenting skills with confidence
- Ability to coordinate the efforts of the healthcare team and community resources to meet the needs of these patients and their family caregivers

ETHICAL/LEGAL SKILLS

- Knowledge of professional responsibilities and ability and willingness to meet these responsibilities in a legally defensible manner (familiarity with agency policy and role responsibilities related to managing sensory alterations)
- Human caring, compassion, and strong sense of accountability for delivering quality care

- A receptor or sense organ must receive the stimulus and convert it to a nerve impulse.
- The nerve impulse must be conducted along a nervous pathway from the receptor or sense organ to the brain.
- A particular area in the brain must receive and translate the impulse into a sensation.

Arousal Mechanism

To receive stimuli and respond appropriately, the brain must be alert or aroused. The **reticular activating system** (RAS), a poorly defined network that extends from the hypothalamus to the medulla, mediates arousal. The optimal arousal state of the RAS is a general drive state called **sensoristasis.** Nerve impulses from all the sensory tracts reach the RAS, which then selectively allows certain impulses to reach the cerebral cortex and be perceived. The mesencephalic portion of the RAS appears to be the center of the system, and stimulation of this area produces the most pronounced and long-lasting effects on the cerebral cortex (Fig. 33-1). With its many ascending and descending connections to other areas of the brain, the RAS serves to monitor and regulate incoming sensory stimuli and thereby maintain, enhance, or inhibit cortical **arousal.** States of awareness are described in the accompanying box.

A stimulus must be variable or irregular to evoke a response. The body quickly adapts to constant stimuli; thus,

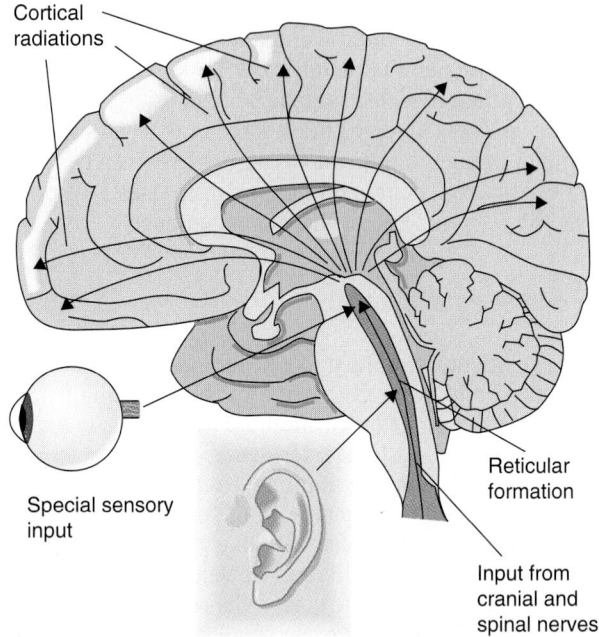

Figure 33-1

Nerve impulses from all the sensory tracts reach the reticular activating system (RAS), which then selectively allows certain impulses to reach the cerebral cortex and to be perceived.

States of Awareness

Conscious States

Delirium	Disorientation, restlessness, confusion, hallucinations, agitation, alternating with other conscious states
Dementia	Difficulties with spatial orientation, memory, language, changes in personality
Confusion	Reduced awareness, easily distracted, easily startled by sensory stimuli, alternates between drowsiness and excitability; resembles minor form of delirium state
Normal consciousness	Aware of self and external environment, well-oriented, responsive
Somnolence	Extreme drowsiness, but will respond normally to stimuli
Chronic vegetative state	Conscious but unresponsive, no evidence of cortical function

Unconscious States

Asleep	Can be aroused by normal stimuli (light touch, sound, etc.)
Stupor	Can be aroused by extreme and/or repeated stimuli
Coma	Cannot be aroused and does not respond to stimuli (coma states can be further subdivided according to the effect on reflex responses to stimuli) (see Glasgow Coma Scale, Chapter 25)

the repeated stimulus of a continuing noise, such as city traffic, or a noxious odor eventually goes unnoticed. This phenomenon is termed *adaptation.* Impulses that are not acted on when received may be used at a later date. The memory process involves the storage of that material. For example, thought and memory are used when a new sensory experience occurs and the organism uses a response based on previous knowledge and experience.

Sensory Alterations

When a patient is admitted to a health agency, he or she is confronted with stimuli that are different in quality and quantity to the accustomed stimuli. For example, a patient confined to bed rest may receive many fewer stimuli, whereas one undergoing multiple diagnostic tests may receive a greater than normal level of sensory input. These and other typical experiences are likely to result in the patient's having sensory alterations. Behavioral changes in hospitalized patients have been reduced because more attention is being paid to the use of color and sound and increased privacy and social interaction. Factors contributing to severe sensory alteration (intensive care unit psychosis) include sensory overload, sensory deprivation, sleep deprivation, and cultural care deprivation. Table 33-1 provides an overview of sensory deprivation and sensory overload with related nursing interventions. The accompanying Research in Nursing box addresses the experiences of patients in intensive care units.

Sensory Deprivation

Sensory deprivation results when a person experiences decreased sensory input or input that is monotonous, unpatterned, or meaningless. With decreased sensory input, the RAS is no longer able to project a normal level of activation to the brain, and the individual may hallucinate simply to maintain an optimal level of arousal. Factors placing a patient at high risk for sensory deprivation include the following:

- An environment with decreased or monotonous stimuli (institutionalized patients, patients confined to a small living area at home, patients on bed rest or in isolation, and so on)
- Impaired ability to receive environmental stimuli (patients with sensory alterations: impaired vision or hearing; patients with bandages or casts that interfere with vision, hearing, or tactile stimulation; patients with affective disorders who "close out" the environment, and so on)
- Inability to process environmental stimuli (patients with spinal cord injuries or brain damage, patients who are confused or disoriented, patients taking prescribed or recreational drugs that affect the central nervous system)

Effects of sensory deprivation include perceptual, cognitive, and emotional disturbances.

Perceptual responses: inaccurate perception of sights, sounds, tastes, smells, and body position, coordi-

nation, and equilibrium; mild to gross distortions ranging from daydreams to hallucinations

Cognitive responses: inability to control the direction of thought content; decreased attention span and ability to concentrate; difficulty with memory, problem solving, and task performance

Emotional responses: inappropriate emotional responses, including apathy, anxiety, fear, anger, belligerence, panic, or depression; rapid mood changes (see Table 33-1 for additional information)

Sensory Overload

Sensory overload is the condition that results when a person experiences so much sensory stimuli that the brain is unable to respond meaningfully to or ignore the stimuli. The person feels out of control and may exhibit all of the manifestations observed in sensory deprivation. The amount and quality of stimuli necessary to produce overload may differ greatly from one individual to another and are influenced by factors such as age, culture, personality, and lifestyle.

In some patients, especially those coming from a quiet environment with unvarying stimuli, the experience of being hospitalized quickly results in sensory overload. In such patients, the brain is assaulted by the constant presence of strangers who not only demand to be spoken to but also touch and poke at the body; by the strange sights, odors, sounds, and feels of the unfamiliar environment; by the constant presence of pain or discomfort from dressings, intravenous lines, drainage tubes, or endotracheal tubes; and by the ever-present worries about the meaning and course of the illness. Nursing assistance is directed to reducing distressing stimuli and helping the patient to gain control over the environment (see Table 33-1).

Cultural Care Deprivation

Sensory deprivation, sensory overload, and sleep deprivation are all related to or affected by an individual's cultural practices, values, and beliefs. Kloosterman (1991) suggests that the concept missing in current practices concerning severe sensory alteration is "culturally congruent care." **Cultural care deprivation** is described as "a lack of culturally assistive, supportive, or facilitative acts" (p. 121). The nurse who is sensitive to the patient's culture attempts to determine what constitutes acceptable levels of stimuli from the patient's viewpoint. For example, in certain cultures, touching is viewed as a natural and welcome custom, whereas other cultures may view it as insulting or offensive. Kloosterman noted that different cultures have rules on how, where, and for what purpose the human body may be touched. Similarly, patients may find comfort in cultural and religious symbols of care and healing that are absent in a hospital environment.

Sensory Deficits

Impaired or absent functioning in one or more senses is termed *sensory deficit.* Examples of sensory deficits include impaired sight and hearing, altered taste, numbness

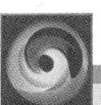

Table 33-1
Overview of Sensory Deprivation and Sensory Overload

Sensory Deprivation   Insufficient quantity or quality of stimuli; may result from decreased sensory input or monotonous, unpatterned, and unmeaningful input

Defining Characteristics	Contributing Factors	Patients at Risk
Physical behaviors: drowsiness, excessive yawning *Escape behaviors:* eating, exercising, sleeping, running away to escape the deprived environment *Changes in perception:* unusual body sensations; preoccupation with somatic complaints (dry mouth, palpitations, difficulty breathing, nausea); change in body image; illusions and hallucinations *Changes in cognitive behavior:* decreased attention span, inability to concentrate, decreased problem solving and task performance *Changes in affective behavior:* crying, increased irritability and annoyance over small matters, confusion, panic, depression	*Decreased environmental stimuli:* institutionalized environment; separation from significant others and usual sources of stimuli; treatments that decrease access to stimuli, such as bed rest or isolation *Impaired ability to receive environmental stimuli:* impaired vision, hearing, taste, smell, touch resulting from treatments such as bandages or body casts that interfere with reception of stimuli, or as a result of depression and other affective disorders *Inability to process environmental stimuli:* spinal cord injuries, brain damage, confusion, dementia, medications that depress the central nervous system	Institutionalized patients, especially those in long-term care settings Patients with communicable disease (eg, AIDS) Patients confined to bed Patients with sensory alterations (eg, impaired vision or hearing, or patients with eye patches or body casts) Patients who are depressed Patients from a different culture Patients with a disturbance of the nervous system

Nursing Interventions

Maintain sufficient level of arousal by increasing sensory stimuli from all sensory modalities:
- Instruct the patient in self-stimulation methods: counting, singing, reading, reciting poetry.
- Structure meaningful tangible stimuli into patient's external environment; include a variety of people, ideas, sensations, a pet may provide excellent stimulation.
  - *Visual stimulation*
      Colorful sheets, pajamas, robes
      Colorful uniform tops for the nurse
      Face-to-face human contact
      Clocks, calendars, wrist watches
      Pictures, flowers, greeting card
  - *Auditory stimulation*
      Call person by name
      Conversation that communicates caring as well as orients patient
      Reading to the patient
      Television, radio
  - *Gustatory and olfactory stimulation*
      Attention to oral hygiene and properly fitting dentures
      Food of different textures, colors, temperatures served attractively
      Smelling food before eating it and recalling pleasurable aromas from the past
      Seasoning foods or having favorite foods brought from home
  - *Tactile stimulation*
      Backrubs   Foot soaks
      Turning and repositioning   Hugs
      Passive range-of-motion exercises   Touching of arms or shoulders
      Hair brushing, combing, washing
  - *Cognitive input*
      Orient patient to environment
      Encourage patient participation in self-care
      Discuss current events or patient's occupation, hobbies, or interests
      Reinforce reality without arguing with a patient who is hallucinating. "No, I don't see a man standing there but the linen hamper may be confusing you."

(continued)

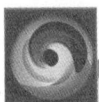

Table 33-1 (Continued)

- *Emotional input*
  Encourage patient to share fears, concerns, and perceptions; reassure patient that illusions and misperceptions do occur with sensory deprivation
- Incorporate culturally assistive, supportive, facilitative acts into nursing care.
- *Caution:* Because it can be difficult to distinguish the behavioral manifestations of sensory deprivation from sensory overload, introduce more stimulation cautiously. If the added stimulation only increases the patient's maladaptive behaviors, consider reducing sensory input because the patient may be experiencing sensory overload.

Sensory Overload Excessive stimuli over which an individual feels little control; brain is unable meaningfully to respond to or ignore stimuli

Defining Characteristics	Contributing Factors	Patients at Risk
Similar to those observed in sensory deprivation

Elderly patients and patients who have suffered a stroke are more likely to experience a confusion or agitation. Young patients are more likely to seek the comfort of their parents' embrace to block out sensory overload. | *Increased internal stimuli:* pain, pressure and discomfort of intrusive tubes (eg, intravenous lines [IVs], catheters; endotracheal tubes, nasogastric tubes), worry about state of health or need to make treatment decisions

Increased external stimuli: unfamiliar healthcare environment, such as lights, noises, sounds, odors, movement, and constant presence of strangers, many of whom touch the body; intrusive procedures such as diagnostic tests and treatments; scratchy linens

Inability perceptually to disregard or selectively ignore some stimuli: nervous system disturbances, medications such as caffeine that stimulate the central nervous system arousal mechanism | Acutely or chronically ill patients

Patients in pain

Patient with intrusive monitoring or treatment equipment

Hospitalized patients, especially those in critical care settings

Patients with disturbances of the nervous system |

Nursing Interventions

- Provide a consistent, predictable pattern of stimulation to help the patient develop a sense of control over the environment.
- Offer simple explanations before procedures, tests, and examinations.
- Establish a schedule with the patient for routine care such as eating, bathing, turning, positioning, coughing, and exercising.
- Speak calmly with the patient and move slowly; communicate confidence.
- Explore with the patient what stimuli are most distressing and develop a plan to reduce or eliminate these (eg, incoming phone calls, visitors); ear plugs or pain medication may be indicated.
- Be careful not to cause sensory deprivation
- Identify and, wherever possible, eliminate culturally inappropriate stimuli.

(Adapted from Lee, K. A. [1991]. Sensory overload, sensory deprivation, and sleep deprivation. In M. L. Patrick, S. I. Woods, R. F. Craven, J. S. Rokosky, & P. M. Bruno [Eds.], *Medical-surgical nursing* [2nd ed.]. Philadelphia: J. B. Lippincott.)

and paralysis that results in altered tactile perception, and impaired kinesthetic sense. These deficits may be reversible or permanent, may occur gradually or all at once, and may be present at birth or evolve later. It is important for nurses to be aware of a patient's sensory deficits and to determine whether the patient is able to compensate for the deficit. Illness and hospitalization may threaten a patient's usual adaptive patterns and require new self-care abilities. Patients with evolving deficits will

require assistance in coping and in learning to compensate skillfully.

Factors Affecting Sensory Stimulation

There appears to be considerable variation in the amount of stimuli different individuals consider optimal. Factors influencing the amount and quality of stimuli needed to

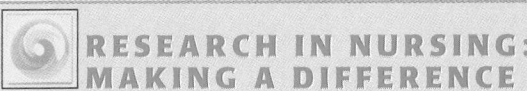

RESEARCH IN NURSING: MAKING A DIFFERENCE

Promoting Improved Intensive Care Experiences

Critical care staff may have difficulty comprehending how patients experience a stay in an intensive care unit. Barriers to the usual means of achieving shared understanding, such as patients' inability to speak because of intubation or fluctuating levels of consciousness, led these authors to search the literature for systematic research into patients' perceptions of critical care.

Related Research
Stein-Parbury, J., & McKinley, S. (2000). Patients' experiences of being in an intensive care unit: A select literature review. *American Journal of Critical Care, 9*(1), 20–27.
The authors reviewed a total of 26 research studies on patients' experiences of being in an intensive care

unit. Patients recalled not only experiences that were negative but also ones that were neutral or positive. Positive experiences included a sense of safety and security promoted especially by the nurses. Negative experiences included impaired cognitive functioning and discomforts, such as problems with sleeping, pain, and anxiety. The review indicates steps that critical care staff can take to develop better ways to understand patients' experiences.

Relevance to Nursing Practice
This is an excellent example of using research findings to improve practice: to improve the quality of patients' experiences and to reduce anxiety and offset potential adverse effects of being a patient in an intensive care unit.

---

maintain cortical arousal include developmental considerations, culture, personality and lifestyle, stress, and illness and medication.

Developmental Considerations

Different types of sensory stimulation are needed for growth as sensory receptors and organs and the nervous system mature. Although the newborn is capable of rudimentary perceptual discriminations at birth, many neural pathways are immature and must be stimulated to develop, become refined, and function adequately. Appropriate stimulation includes soothing; holding; rocking and changes of position (tactile and kinesthetic sensations); singing and being talked to (auditory sensations); and changing patterns of light and shade, such as through the use of mobiles and bright objects (visual sensations). Developmentally appropriate play develops the child's muscles and coordination, provides an outlet for surplus physical energy, develops communication skills, furnishes sources of learning, acts as a stimulant to creativity, develops social skills, teaches sex roles, provides an outlet for the release of emotional energy, and develops self-insights.

Sensory functioning tends to decline progressively throughout adulthood as the result of aging or chronic illness. The adult may experience the need to compensate for the loss of one type of stimulation by increasing other sources of sensory stimuli. See the accompanying box, Focus on the Older Adult.

Culture

An individual's culture may dictate the amount of sensory stimulation considered normal. For example, the amount of touching a child experiences in a Puerto Rican family

may be different from that experienced by a child in a German family. Similarly, male and female roles may be culturally defined; for example, although the male is expected to respond to the challenge of out-of-the-home sensory stimuli, the female who attempts to do so may be scorned if her place is considered to be in the home. Ethnic norms, religious norms, income group norms, and the norms of subgroups within a culture all influence the amount of sensory stimulation sought by an individual and perceived as meaningful.

Personality and Lifestyle

Apart from a person's culture, different personality types demand different levels of stimulation. One person may thrive on a steady stream of fast-paced changes and excitement, whereas another may feel best when daily routines are rigidly structured and life sends no challenges necessitating changes. Lifestyle choices can dramatically influence the quantity and quality of stimuli received by an individual. The nurse who elects to work in the emergency room of a large city hospital is exposed to vastly different stimuli than the nurse making home visits in a rural setting.

Stress

Increased sensory stimulation may be sought during periods of low stress simply to maintain cortical arousal. During high-stress periods, multiple stressors may already be overloading the sensory system, and decreased sensory stimulation is desired. The stress of physical illness, pain, hospitalization, testing, surgery, and treatment may provide more stimulation than an individual can process and respond to without assistance.

Focus on the Older Adult

The senses of vision, hearing, and touch (and to a lesser degree, taste and smell) all decline with age. Moreover, many of the chronic illnesses experienced by elderly people impair sensory functioning. Common sensory problems include vision problems, such as cataracts; **presbyopia** (condition of aging in which decreased elasticity of the lens hinders accommodation to close vision); glaucoma and macular degeneration; hearing problems, such as **presbycusis** (age-related hearing loss in which there is decreased ability to distinguish higher frequencies); diminution of touch with diabetes and cerebrovascular disease; and altered body sense or awareness associated with restricted mobility and arthritis, cardiovascular and respiratory diseases, and neurologic disorders involving some degree of paralysis.

Selected Nursing Interventions

- Make every effort to correct patient's sensory impairments (eg, medical evaluation and treatment of sensory deficits; correct use and care of eyeglasses, contact lenses, hearing aids, ambulation aids).
- Ensure that the patient has adequate periods of rest and that daytime activities prevent boredom and cat-napping. Discourage the use of sedatives. Assess the effect on the central nervous system of any other medications the patient is taking.

- Implement the plan to increase sensory stimulation (see Stimulating the Senses box). Homebound or institutionalized older people may benefit greatly from visits by children. Pet therapy is an excellent source of stimulation. Simple activities like rolling a colorful, large, soft ball among four people seated at a table can effectively stimulate multiple senses (vision, hearing, touch, kinesthetic) for confused patients. Exercise classes for elderly patients also provide excellent stimulation.
- Make a concerted effort to increase the patient's mobility and encourage changes in the environment. Use family and community resources to get the homebound patient out of the house. Implement a plan to assist institutionalized patients to visit other parts of the institution, to get outside, and to participate in scheduled social events. Volunteers may be extremely helpful once committed to a plan of action.
- When interacting with the older patient, communicate that the patient is important and valued and make your expectations known.
- Avoid endorsing confusion. Gently reorient the patient to reality whenever delusional statements are made.
- Keep the environment safe for the patient.

Illness and Medication

Illness can affect the reception of sensory stimuli and their transmission and perception. Medications that alert or depress the central nervous system may interfere with the perception of sensory stimuli. Certain medications may also contribute to impaired sensory functioning by decreasing reception (eg, captopril, an antihypertensive agent, can cause taste alteration.

The Nursing Process

Before reading this section, review the box, Applying Learning to Practice: The Nurse as Role Model.

ASSESSING

When assessing a patient for sensory disturbances, the nurse interviews the patient and examines him or her for sensory

APPLYING LEARNING TO PRACTICE

The Nurse as Role Model

Sensitivity to the important role sensory functioning plays in a person's well-being guides the nurse to promote personal well-being. Awareness of one's own sensory functioning and the stimulation in one's own life is a stepping stone to providing proper stimulation to patients. The nurse works to achieve the following goals:

- Evaluate the quantity and quality of sensory stimuli present in both the home and at work

- Identify stimuli important to self-development as a person (mental, physical, and spiritual health) and as a professional nurse
- Manipulate the environment to decrease distressing stimuli and increase positive stimuli
- When practicing nursing, be conscious of the need to promote optimal sensory functioning in patients

deficits and manifestations of sensory deprivation or overload. Examination of the patient's environment is included in the assessment to determine whether it is providing adequate sensory stimulation for healthy development.

Assessing the Sensory Experience

The assessment may be structured using the components of the sensory experience—stimulation, reception, and transmission–perception–reaction. These components are outlined in the accompanying Focused Assessment Guide. Because patients may adapt to sensory impairments, it may be helpful to include someone the patient knows well (eg, spouse or parent) in the assessment to see if that person has noticed behavioral characteristics in the patient that suggest a sensory disturbance (eg, "I've noticed he turns the television volume much louder than ever before").

Stimulation

Assess whether there have been any recent changes in sensory stimulation, for example, reduction of stimulation from one or more sensory modalities ("Since my husband died, no one touches me anymore. It sounds crazy, but I'm hungry to be touched!") or new or unusual stimulation ("Ever since my granddaughter moved in with me, my house is always noisy. I can't stand the constant noise and her smoking."). Assess whether the type of stimulation present is developmentally appropriate. High-risk patients for problems related to stimulation include children in nonstimulating environments, older people, terminally ill patients, patients on bed rest, patients in isolation, and patients requiring intensive nursing in a critical care setting.

Reception

Assess for anything that may interfere with sensory reception, and describe any corrective devices the patient uses for sensory impairments (eyeglasses, contact lenses, hearing aids). The reception section of the Focused Assessment Guide highlights assessment strategies for each sense. Patients at high risk for reception problems include people with visual, auditory, or other sensory impairments.

Transmission–Perception–Reaction

High-risk patients for transmission–perception–reaction problems include confused patients and patients with nervous system impairments. Everyday interactions afford the nurse multiple opportunities to assess patients' abilities to transmit, perceive, and react to stimuli.

Defining Characteristics of Sensory Deprivation and Overload

Complete the assessment of the patient's sensory functioning by assessing for specific indicators of sensory deprivation or overload (see Table 33-1), including boredom, inactivity, slowness of thought, daydreaming, increased sleeping, thought disorganization, anxiety, panic, illusions, and hallucinations. It is important to know the patient's usual state to be able to identify changes stemming from sensory deprivation or overload.

Physical Assessment

Physical examination skills related to the senses are discussed in Chapter 25. Ear and eye tests, whether performed by a physician or nurse, should be considered when planning care. Problems with the neurologic system indicate the necessity of further assessment of the sensory experience.

DIAGNOSING

Sensory/Perceptual Alterations as the Problem

When assessment data point to sensory disturbances that can be treated independently by nursing interventions, nursing diagnoses are developed and labeled. The North American Nursing Diagnosis Association (1999) recognizes the following diagnostic labels for sensory/perceptual problems:

- *Sensory/perceptual alterations:* A state in which the individual or group experiences or is at risk for a change in the amount, pattern, or interpretation of incoming stimuli. These alterations may be further specified as visual, auditory, gustatory, olfactory, tactile, or kinesthetic. Sensory deprivation, sensory overload, and uncompensated sensory loss may also be used to further specify the sensory/perceptual alteration and in some cases may be the etiology.
- *Acute confusion:* The abrupt onset of a cluster of global, transient changes and disturbances in attention, cognition, psychomotor activity level of consciousness, or sleep–wake cycle
- *Chronic confusion:* An irreversible, long-standing, or progressive deterioration of intellect and personality characterized by decreased ability to interpret environmental stimuli or decreased capacity for intellectual thought processes and manifested by disturbances of memory, orientation, and behavior.
- *Impaired memory:* The state in which an individual experiences the inability to remember or recall bits of information or behavior skills. Impaired memory may be attributed to pathophysiologic or situational causes that are either temporary or permanent.

Common etiologies for sensory/perceptual alterations include the following:

- Altered environmental stimuli: excessive or insufficient
- Altered sensory reception, transmission, or integration
- Chemical alterations: endogenous (eg, electrolytes) or exogenous (eg, drugs)
- Psychological stress

Sample nursing diagnoses in which the sensory/perceptual alteration is the problem are listed in the accompanying box.

FOCUSED ASSESSMENT GUIDE

Sensory Stimulation

Factors to Assess	Questions and Approaches
Stimulation	"Does your current environment overly, insufficiently, or appropriately stimulate you?"
	"Are you bored? Why?"
	"Are you able to read? Watch television? Knit? Why not?"
	"Are there other people in your home during the day? Do you spend much time together? How do you spend the time?"
	"Who visits you while you are in the hospital?"
	Note reduction in the patterns or meaningfulness of stimulation in each sensory modality; changes in stimulation other than decreases (eg, new or unusual stimulation); or developmental appropriateness of stimulation.
Reception	"Does anything interfere with the functioning of your senses?"
	"Describe any corrective devices you use for sensory impairments."
Assess for visual disturbances.	"Please read my name tag (or this page of print)."
	Note if the patient can correctly identify objects directly in front of the eyes as well as those requiring peripheral vision.
	Note eye rubbing; squinting; movements indicating faulty vision (bumping into furniture, overreaching or underreaching for objects); changes in the appearance of the eye (cataracts, swelling); and complaints of eye pain, spots, halos, or other visual disturbances.
Assess for auditory disturbances.	"Repeat the words that I will speak softly close to each ear."
	Note if the patient is able to hear equally well from both ears, distinguish voices, locate the direction of a sound, if the patient needs to face the person speaking and relies on lip reading, if the patient's responses to questions include blank looks, many nods, smiling, or inappropriate responses indicating faulty hearing.
	Note complaints of ringing or buzzing in ears.
Assess for gustatory (taste) disturbances.	"Close your eyes, stick out your tongue, and tell me if what I place on your tongue is sweet, sour, bitter, or salty."
	"Have you been experiencing any strange tastes (bitter, metallic) or aftertastes lately?"
	Note if the patient is able to differentiate sweet, sour, bitter, or salty tastes or reports unusual, persistent taste sensations.
	Note deficient oral hygiene, ill-fitting dentures, braces, or anything else that might contribute to gustatory disturbances.
Assess for olfactory (smell) disturbances.	"Close your eyes and tell me what you smell."
	"Have you smelled odors lately that others cannot smell, or have you been especially sensitive to odors?" Note if the patient can correctly identify common odors (coffee, vanilla) or has noticed increased sensitivity to odors.
Assess for tactile (touch) disturbances.	"Close your eyes and tell me when you feel something (brush skin with cotton ball), if what you feel is dull or sharp (use both ends of safety pin), hot or cold (use items from food tray). Now, keep your eyes closed and tell me what I am placing in your hand (coin, cotton ball, paper clip)."
	Note if the patient can correctly sense touch and distinguish sharp and dull, hot and cold, and different shapes.
	Note if the patient reports decreased sensation in any part of the body; numbness, pins and needles, tingling; or abnormal sensitivity to pain or touch.

(continued)

FOCUSED ASSESSMENT GUIDE (Continued)

Sensory Stimulation

Factors to Assess	Questions and Approaches
Assess for kinesthetic and visceral disturbances.	Note if the patient withdraws from being touched.
	"Have you noticed any changes in the way you perceive your body?"
	"Do you feel any unusual pressure or pain inside your body?"
	Note if the patient seems unsure of his or her body parts or body position and if he or she experiences new internal sensations (fullness, pressure, pain).
Transmission–perception–reaction	"Are you aware of any problems with your nervous system?"
	"Have you found it difficult to communicate verbally?"
	Note consciousness, orientation, appropriateness of responses, ability to perform usual self-care activities, ability to follow simple commands, decision-making abilities, pathology affecting central nervous system, or prescribed or recreational drug use that affects the central nervous system.
Behavioral manifestations of sensory deprivation or overload	
Perceptual responses	Mild to gross sensory distortions (illusions, hallucinations)
Cognitive responses	Thought disorganization, slowness of thought, decreased attention/concentration, difficulty with problem solving and task performance
Emotional responses	Rapid mood changes, anxiety, panic

Sensory/Perceptual Alterations as the Etiology

Because sensory/perceptual alterations affect many other areas of human functioning, they serve as etiologies for multiple problem statements. Examples of these follow:

- Activity Intolerance related to impaired balance and coordination (kinesthetic alteration)
- Anxiety related to paranoia stemming from hearing impairment, sensory deprivation (specify setting), sensory overload
- Impaired Verbal Communication related to difficulty receiving, transmitting, and perceiving sensory stimuli
- Ineffective Individual Coping related to sensory overload (multiple stressors)
- Diversional Activity Deficit related to impaired vision or hearing
- Altered Growth and Development related to nonstimulating home environment
- High Risk for Injury related to decreased or impaired sensation (specify visual, auditory, tactile, kinesthetic)
- Knowledge Deficit: Means to Compensate for Sensory Impairment (blindness, deafness, and so forth) related to lack of previous experience with this problem, unavailability of resources
- Knowledge Deficit: Providing a Developmentally Stimulating Environment related to lack of experience with children's growth and development
- Impaired Physical Mobility related to impaired balance and coordination (kinesthetic alteration)
- Altered Parenting: Failure to Provide Stimuli for Growth related to lack of knowledge, decreased motivation to provide for child's growth and development
- Powerlessness related to inability to interact meaningfully with environment
- Self-Care Deficit: (specify) related to visual impairment, auditory impairment, tactile impairment
- Body Image Disturbance related to kinesthetic impairment (distorted sense of body parts), sensory deprivation
- Self-Esteem Disturbance related to sensory/perceptual alterations (specify visual, auditory, and so forth)
- Altered Role Performance related to sensory/perceptual alteration (blindness, deafness, and so forth)
- Personal Identity Disturbance related to sensory deprivation or overload
- Sexual Dysfunction related to decreased sensation
- Impaired Skin Integrity related to absent tactile sensation (injury)
- Sleep Pattern Disturbance related to sensory deprivation or overload
- Impaired Social Interaction related to inability to receive and process interactional stimuli
- Social Isolation related to visual or auditory impairment
- Altered Thought Processes (specify: illusions, hallucinations, decreased attention or concentration, and so forth) related to sensory deprivation or overload

PLANNING: EXPECTED OUTCOMES

In whatever setting nurses encounter and care for patients, optimal sensory stimulation is a priority, and nursing care

FOCUSED ASSESSMENT GUIDE

Sensory/Perceptual Alterations

Problem	Related Factors	Sample Defining Characteristics
Sensory/Perceptual Alteration: Sensory Deficit or Excess		
Visual	Eye patches after surgery	"I never realized before how sight-dependent I am. I don't know what time of day it is now unless I have the radio on or smell food coming in."
		"It's frightening not to know who is in my room and what they are doing."
		Patient observed sitting in room with blank facial expression; frequently comments on how bored he or she is and how slowly time is passing; hesitant to move about room without assistance although he or she has been oriented repeatedly
Auditory	Effects of aging	"You're right. I don't always hear what people are saying anymore so I try not to get involved in conversations. If people insist on talking, I just nod and hope I'm giving the right response."
		Able to hear moderately spoken word close to right ear; cannot hear same from left ear; often startled when someone approaches from left side
		Sits close to television and radio; loud volume, no history of hearing testing
Gustatory or olfactory	Chemotherapy	"I always seem to have a bitter taste in my mouth now and can't stomach certain foods at all that I used to enjoy, like beef, tomatoes, coffee. . . . I also can't take sweets, and I used to be a real sweets junkie."
		"Sometimes the very smell of certain foods or even the thought of eating nauseates me."
		Patient has been receiving vincristine (cancer chemotherapeutic agent) for past 3 months; some nausea and vomiting; history of poor oral hygiene
Tactile	Psychological stress	"I don't know why I feel this way, but I'm hypersensitive to touch. If anyone even brushes against me I feel burning pain. Even the weight of my clothes against my skin bothers me. I'm trying to move my body as little as possible and keep it protected—but that's obviously impossible when even a breeze assaults me."
		Patient observed holding the body stiffly looking like he or she does not know what to do with the arms and legs; dressed only in a loose-fitting outfit; reports that he or she sits at home all day afraid to go out
Kinesthetic	Clinitron bed therapy	"I've been in this bed for 2 weeks now and I've lost all sense of my body . . . it's a curious weightless feeling that I have . . . sort of like floating in Jell-O. I'm no longer sure where my body begins and ends, and when I try to lift an arm or leg I feel like I'm in slow motion. I hope I'll be able to walk when I get out of here."

(continued)

FOCUSED ASSESSMENT GUIDE (Continued)

Sensory/Perceptual Alterations

Problem	Related Factors	Sample Defining Characteristics
Sensory/Perceptual Alteration: Sensory Deprivation	Isolation	"One of the worst things that has happened to me since I found out I had AIDS is that everyone is afraid of me—and no one touches me. I'm so lonely. I've always needed a lot of people around."
		"Here in the hospital I think I'm going crazy. I can't leave this room. Everyone who comes in looks the same dressed in those yellow gowns. Lately I've seen some bizarre things that I know can't be real. I look at the clock and it turns into a swirling sun with a sad face that keeps coming closer and closer to me and I'm terrified I'll burn up if it gets too close. That's crazy, isn't it? I'm really losing it now."
		Disturbed sleep for past 2 weeks; during the day yawns excessively and cat-naps; limited attention span; states he or she is unable to concentrate on anything.
Sensory/Perceptual Alteration: Sensory Overload	Trauma of rape and aftercare	"When is everyone going to stop touching me? First he wouldn't stop. Now everyone here is poking at me, looking at me, asking me hundreds of questions. . . . Why did I have to report this and come to the hospital? Oh please leave me alone. Get out of here everyone."

is supportive of the following patient goals/outcomes. The patient will achieve the following:

- Live in a developmentally stimulating and safe environment
- Exhibit a level of arousal that enables the brain to receive and meaningfully organize patterns of stimulation
- Demonstrate intact functioning of the senses: vision, hearing, taste, smell, touch, kinesthetic and visceral awareness
- Maintain orientation to time, place, and person
- Respond appropriately (verbally and nonverbally) to sensory stimuli while executing self-care activities

Patients with impaired sensory functioning require individualized goals similar to the following. The patient will achieve the following:

- Report feeling safe and in control of the environment
- Describe different types of meaningful stimuli present in the environment
- Demonstrate (describe) appropriate self-care behaviors for visual impairment, hearing impairment, or other sensory impairment
- Verbalize acceptance of the sensory deficit

IMPLEMENTING

The nurse can assist patients to improve sensory functioning by teaching patients and significant others means to stimulate the senses, teaching patients with intact and impaired senses appropriate self-care behaviors, and interacting therapeutically with impaired patients. Safety is always a special concern for patients with sensory alterations. Nurses are responsible for ensuring that the patient's environment is as free of danger as possible and for assisting the patient to develop new self-care behaviors to compensate for sensory impairments. Safety considerations are discussed in Chapter 26. In this section, the nursing interventions described are preventing sensory alteration, stimulating the senses, meeting the needs of vision- and hearing-impaired people, communicating with a confused person, and communicating with an unconscious person. Communication guidelines for patients with sensory deficits are also highlighted in Chapter 21.

Preventing Sensory Alteration and Stimulating the Senses

The most effective means by which sensory alteration can be managed is prevention. The key to prevention is, with the patient's help, to create a functional and meaningful environment while keeping limitations in mind. The creation of such an environment requires careful observation, analysis, and creative planning.

Numerous nursing measures can be considered in planning care. Appropriate measures for implementing depend on the circumstances. Well-being is promoted by offering care that provides rest and comfort (see Chaps. 39

and 40). Patient discomfort should be controlled whenever possible. The nurse should be aware of the need for sensory aids and prostheses, such as eyeglasses, contact lenses, hearing aids, dentures, canes, and artificial limbs, and these should be made available as needed. Social activities, as shown in Figure 33-2, help to stimulate the senses and mind. Family members may participate in or encourage these activities. Physical activity and exercise, which help maintain normal sensory perceptions and decrease the likelihood of sensory alteration, should be encouraged (exercises are discussed in Chap. 38).

As many senses as possible should be stimulated. Varied sights, sounds, smells, body positions, and textures can be helpful in providing a variety of sensations. For example, music therapy was found to have beneficial effects for mechanically ventilated patients on selected psychophysiologic variables (heart rate, respiratory rate, and mood state). It was found that listening to music ameliorated the stress response and promoted nonpharmacologically induced relaxation for the study subjects. Critical care nurses can be confident in implementing this nonpharmacologic, independent intervention to promote relaxation without worry of untoward side effects, which are sometimes caused by pharmacologic sedation (Chlan, 1995). Cultural factors are taken into consideration when stimulating senses and when offering nursing care. This is especially important when caring for patients from cultures different from the nurse's own culture.

Teaching About Sensory Experiences

Teaching is a significant nursing responsibility. The nurse can help prepare patients for sensory experiences. An informed patient is better able to handle fears, frustration, and confusion; therefore, procedures are explained before being instituted. Explanations also help prevent the patient from feeling that his or her space and body are being invaded.

Individuals experiencing perceptual and thought distortions should have the opportunity to acknowledge that fact. To discuss such experiences and be reassured that these experiences are normal and usually temporary generally eases anxiety.

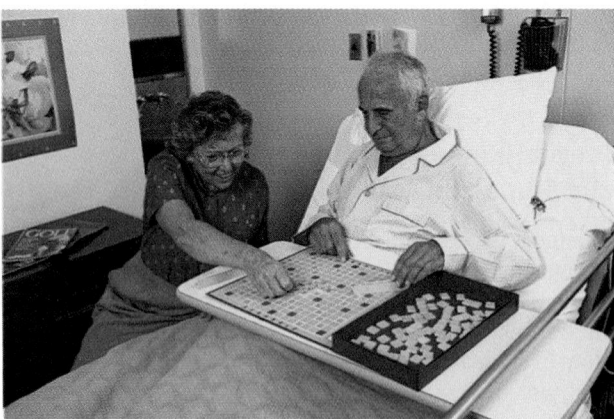

Figure 33-2
The nurse helps the patient find methods for stimulating his or her senses. Family members may participate in sensory activities.

Patients and family members can be guided in sensory self-stimulation, and parents can be aided in stimulation of newborns, infants, and children. The accompanying box, Stimulating the Senses, gives helpful suggestions for teaching patients about sensory stimulation and includes suggestions that the nurse can use in a variety of situations.

Meeting the Needs of Visually Impaired Patients

It is necessary for the nurse to check with the physician to discover if a visual problem is temporary, permanent, partial, or complete and the degree to which the problem is likely to affect the patient's everyday functioning. The nurse cannot develop a realistic teaching plan or plan of care without this information.

The nurse's first priority is to teach patients self-care behaviors to maintain vision and prevent blindness. Lindberg and Kruszewski (1983) offered the following suggestions:

- Avoid rubbing eyes.
- Avoid eyestrain.
- Avoid damage from ultraviolet rays.
- Protect eyes from foreign bodies.
- Keep eyeglasses clean, protected, adjusted.
- Avoid nonprescription eyedrops and seek attention for symptoms.
- Avoid cleaning eyes or contact lenses with soiled articles.
- Use caution with aerosol sprays.
- Use caution with ammonia, lye, and so on.
- Visit your physician frequently if you are prone to eye problems.
- Know the danger signals that indicate serious eye problems: persistent eye redness; pain or discomfort, especially after injury; visual disturbances; crossing eyes; growth on or near the eyes; discharge or increased tearing; and pupil irregularities.

The following guidelines are recommended for communicating with patients who are visually impaired:

- Acknowledge your presence in the patient's room. Identify yourself by name.
- Speak in a normal tone of voice. Remember that the blind person is unable to pick up most nonverbal cues during communication.
- Explain the reason for touching the person before doing so.
- Keep the call light or bell within easy reach of the person and place the bed in the lowest position.
- Orient the person to sounds in the environment.
- Orient the person to the arrangement of the room and its furnishings. Clear pathways for the person and do not rearrange furnishings. Clarify this fact with housekeeping personnel also.
- Assist with ambulation by walking slightly ahead of the person, allowing the person to grasp your arm.
- Stay in the person's field of vision if he or she has partial or reduced peripheral vision.
- Provide diversions using other senses.
- Indicate to the person when the conversation has ended and when you are leaving the room.

Stimulating the Senses

	Teaching Patients	*Nursing Interventions*
Vision	Surround yourself with different colors and with an environment that changes (walk through a mall, sit by a window where you see people come and go). Develop a sensitivity to changes in nature (weather patterns, dawn-to-night cycle, changing seasons, changes in a plant or animal). Use visual devices to keep oriented (watches, calendars, newspaper, television). Use crossword puzzles and games to stimulate mental activities. Create favorite scenes in your mind, paying attention to tiny details.	Wear visually stimulating and comforting colors. Keep meaningful visual stimuli such as photos, greeting cards, toys, or flowers near patient. Position patients with impaired mobility where they can see out a window or watch local traffic on the unit.
Hearing	Decrease or eliminate distressing auditory stimuli (change bedroom, talk with family members about noise of stereos and other such equipment, use earplugs, use headphones to listen to soft music). Develop sensitivity to different sounds (music, chirping birds, night sounds, different voices). Use the telephone to maintain contact with family and friends. Use television, radio, cassettes to keep current and to stimulate mental activities. Recall favorite sounds of the past with the situations in which they were heard.	Speak in a warm and pleasant tone and communicate caring to the patient. Use your voice to orient patient to environment and current situation (eg, procedure, treatment). Avoid speaking about the patient to others within the patient's hearing. Remember that patients overhearing snatches of conversation outside their room often presume it is about *them!* Decrease extraneous noise (intercom, movement of carts, loud conversations of staff); use carpets and sound-absorbing material whenever possible.
Taste	Experiment with foods of different tastes (seasonings), colors, temperature, and textures; realize that as taste buds age, things will no longer taste the same. Practice thorough oral hygiene and have regular dental examinations. Recall foods that tasted especially good in the past and the events surrounding these tastes (eg, grandparent baking cookies or homemade bread).	Consult with the dietitian about preparing meals with varied taste sensations; serve meals attractively. Perform routine oral hygiene for patients who are unable to do this for themselves.
Smell	Consciously savor smells that are pleasant; decrease or eliminate noxious odors. Recall pleasant aromas or smells from the past and the events surrounding them (eg, smell of the ocean as the vacation house was neared, smell of fresh pine in the house at Christmas, the body scent of a loved person or animal).	Keep the patient's room well ventilated, using opportunities when the patient is out of the room to air it out. Remove dressings, drainage, and any equipment with odors from the patient's room as quickly as possible. Encourage patients to focus on pleasant or familiar smells, such as coffee, newspaper, or flowers. Avoid wearing heavy perfumes.

(*continued*)

Stimulating the Senses *(Continued)*

	Teaching Patients	*Nursing Interventions*
Touch	Consciously surround yourself with different textures and let yourself feel and enjoy them (scratchy afghan; a puppy's moist, wet tongue; soft petal of a flower; smooth silk scarf; mug of hot chocolate). Allow these textures to evoke memories of past tactile experiences (grandchild's hug may bring back memories of hugs from own children, scrap of fabric may recall a prom dress or wedding gown or baby blanket). Recognize need to be touched and tell someone, "I need a hug today!" Receive tactile stimulation from a pet.	Include different textures in the patient's environment (silky pillow sham from home, soft sheepskin, wooly blanket). Respect the patient's need and desire to be touched or not touched (touch the patient's forearm or shoulder, hug the patient). Use physical care (bath time, foot soaks, hair care, back massages, turning and positioning, passive range of motion) to provide tactile stimulation. Limit intrusive procedures and times when the patient needs to be uncomfortably manipulated.
General Nursing Strategies in the Hospital or Other Residential Care Setting		Encourage the patient to participate in activities that require exploration of the environment (exercise, feeling, tasting, touching, moving, listening). Use conversation to explore areas of interest to the patient. Encourage the patient to share feelings. Familiarize the environment by encouraging the patient to wear own clothes and keep personal items nearby. Suggest the use of self-stimulation techniques—humming, singing, whistling, reciting, memory review, and problem solving.

Meeting the Needs of Hearing Impaired Patients

Temporary hearing losses are most often conductive in nature, that is, they are due to a problem with the external or middle ear (wax buildup, foreign-body obstruction, infection). Sensorineural hearing losses are caused by inner ear or central nervous system problems and may not be totally correctable. Health teaching to prevent hearing problems includes the following recommendations from Lindberg and Kruszewski (1983, pp. 307, 312):

- Avoid excessive noise.
- Avoid inserting sharp objects into ears.
- Avoid excessive cleaning of ears.
- Avoid practices that can cause infection; treat infection early.
- Know the symptoms of hearing loss: asking frequently that statements be repeated, inability to hear at a distance, need to see the person who is talking, leaning forward or turning an ear toward the speaker, answering inappropriately, talking too loudly, inability to carry on a phone conversation, strained facial expression.

The following are recommended guidelines for communicating with people with hearing deficits:

- Orient the person to your presence before initiating conversation. This may be done by moving so you can be seen or by gently touching the person.
- Decrease background noises (television, radio) if possible before you speak.
- Make sure that hearing aids (if applicable) are working optimally.
- Position yourself so that the light is on your face and the person can see your lips and expressions.
- Talk directly to the person while facing him or her or angle the chair so that your voice reaches the ear that hears best. If the person is able to lip-read, use simple sentences and speak in a quiet, natural manner and pace. Be aware of nonverbal communication.
- Do not chew gum, cover your mouth, or turn away when talking with the person.
- Demonstrate or pantomime ideas you wish to express, as appropriate.
- Use sign language or finger spelling, as appropriate.
- Write any ideas that you cannot convey to the person in another manner.

Aids for hearing impaired individuals include: TDD (telecommunication devices), infrared systems, computers, voice amplifiers, amplified telephones, low-frequency door bells and telephone ringers, closed-caption TV decoders, flashing alarm clocks, and flashing smoke detectors.

Communicating With a Confused Patient

The patient who lacks the mental ability to process environmental stimuli may be aware of this inability and find it frustrating. This patient needs the nurse's support to make adjustments to this limitation. Other patients may be oblivious of the deficiency. In both instances, the nurse must protect the safety of the patient while providing optimal sensory stimulation. Nursing interventions include the following:

- Using frequent face-to-face contact to communicate the social process (use touch when appropriate, walk arm in arm, hug, give a back rub)
- Speaking calmly, simply, and directly to the patient and allowing sufficient time for the patient to think before responding
- Orienting and reorienting the patient to the environment and filling the patient's personal space with as many personal objects as possible
- Using conversation, watches, clocks, calendar, newspaper, television, radio, and other such devices to orient the patient to time, place, and person
- Clearly communicating that the patient is expected to perform all self-care activities of which the patient is capable
- Keeping the emphasis on patient strengths rather than on deficiencies and verbally reinforcing strengths
- Offering the patient simple explanations for care, new activities, and so on
- Varying environmental stimuli gradually while keeping the environment structured enough that the patient feels comfortable and at home
- Using objects from the patient's past (baseball, picture of a train, photograph) to spark reminiscences and discussions
- Reinforcing reality if the patient is delusional

Specific intervention suggestions for caring for confused older adults were given the box, Stimulating the Senses. A list of selected cognitive stimulation activities may be found in Chapter 21.

Communicating With an Unconscious Patient

The following are recommended guidelines for communicating with an unconscious patient:

- Be careful of what is said in the person's presence. Hearing is believed to be the last sense lost in the unconscious person, and therefore the person is often likely to hear what is being said, even though there does not appear to be a response.
- Assume the person can hear you. Talk with the person in a normal tone of voice about things you would ordinarily discuss.
- Speak to the person before touching. Remember that touch can be an effective means of communicating with the unconscious person.
- Keep environmental noises at as low a level as possible. This helps the person focus on the communication.

EVALUATING

While implementing a plan of nursing care designed to decrease excessive sensory stimuli or increase meaningful stimuli, the nurse evaluates the effectiveness of the plan by observing for a decrease in the behavioral manifestations of sensory deprivation or overload. It may be concluded that the plan of care is working if a patient who had begun to withdraw and spend most of the day lying in bed with a blank facial expression appears more alert and begins to initiate conversations and to take an interest in personal care. The nurse also evaluates the patient's ability to interact appropriately with the environment while practicing necessary self-care behaviors. The patient's achievement of desired outcomes is evaluated at established times.

The nurse also evaluates the patient's need for nursing versus his or her ability to manage the plan of care independently. Ideally, the patient and family learn to manipulate the environment to promote optimal sensory stimulation for growth and development. Patients with specific sensory impairments are evaluated for their knowledge of the impairment, acceptance and management of the treatment regimen, and ability to perform necessary self-care activities. See the accompanying Applying Learning to Practice: Patient Care Study and Nursing Plan of Care boxes.

(*text continues on page 774*)

APPLYING LEARNING TO PRACTICE

Patient Care Study

Two days ago, Mrs. Philomela Palikias delivered by cesarean birth a 32-week-old, small-for-gestational-age infant girl weighing 3 lb, 8 oz. Because of her size and respiratory distress, the infant was placed in the neonatal intensive care unit (NICU). Postpartal assessments indicate that Ms. Palikias's physical progress is satisfactory. However, the nurses are concerned about her mental status. Ms. Palikias arrived in the United States 3 months ago with her husband. Both speak only Greek and neither has family in the United States.

Recorded in the patient's progress notes the evening of her second postpartal day is the following nursing assessment:

12/4/02, 9 PM, nursing
Patient refused to get out of bed again this evening—demonstrates no interest in seeing baby; to date has not ambulated to NICU. Refusing to learn and participate in self-care activities—expressing breast milk or performing perineal care. Nurses throughout the day reported sudden mood changes—apathy, frustration, panic, and hostility. Unable to find someone who speaks Greek to serve as translator. Husband does not speak English but appears concerned about his wife.

N. Gable, RN

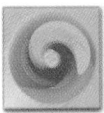

NURSING PLAN OF CARE
for Mrs. Palikias

Nursing Diagnosis	Sensory/Perceptual Alteration: Mixed Sensory Deprivation and Overload related to unfamiliar hospital environment (different culture) and stress of cesarean birth and infant's prematurity as manifested by patient not demonstrating interest in baby or self-care activities; limited ability to concentrate on new tasks (pericare, expressing breast milk); sudden mood changes—apathy, frustration, panic, hostility
Expected Outcome	Before discharge, the patient will: • Demonstrate increased comfort in the hospital environment (decreased or absent mood swings—apathy, frustration, panic, hostility)

Nursing Interventions	Rationale	Evaluative Statement
Secure assistance of an interpreter and work with the interpreter to do the following:		12/6/02 Goal met. Patient is quiet but no longer apathetic, fearful, or hostile. Moving about in hospital with more confidence.
• Orient the patient to her surroundings (explaining reasons for equipment, procedures, treatment)	Sensory deprivation results from *meaningless,* unpatterned stimuli; once the patient understands her environment, she can respond to it appropriately.	*N. Gable, RN*
• Reassure the patient that what she is experiencing is normal given her recent stresses (moving to new country, cesarean birth of first child, infant's prematurity)	Patients experiencing strange perceptual, cognitive, and affective responses to sensory deprivation and overload often fear they are going crazy and hesitate to share their feelings.	
• Determine the patient's needs	The patient herself is best able to voice her needs.	
Have the interpreter teach the nurse several Greek words and make recommendations about how the patient can personalize her environment, such as having her husband provide her with usual food, music, and other familiar items.	Contributing to sensory deprivation is the absence of familiar sounds (native languages, sights, tastes, or scents). Having access to familiar food and the like may reduce sensory deprivation.	
See if the interpreter can explain usual customs regarding childbirth and aftercare in Greece.	Including culturally familiar childbirth and aftercare customs in the plan of care enhances patient well-being and cooperation in the plan of care.	
Limit the number of nurses and other persons interacting with the patient; attempt to have the same nurse caring for her each shift.	A trusting nurse–patient relationship can develop.	
Schedule care to allow for uninterrupted periods of sleep and rest.	Sleep deprivation contributes to other sensory alterations.	

(continued)

NURSING PLAN OF CARE (Continued)
for Mrs. Palikias

Expected Outcome	Before discharge, the patient will:
	• Resume independent self-care activities

Nursing Interventions	Rationale	Evaluative Statement
Use services of interpreter to teach patient importance of ambulating and becoming independent again in self-care measures.	Regaining independence enhances patient's sense of well-being.	12/6/02 Goal partially met. Patient is ambulating, but she resists pericare and is fearful when expressing breast milk.
Have interpreter write simple directions for follow-up care, times when baby may be visited after patient is discharged, and so on. Share these instructions with the patient's husband.	Cognitive responses to sensory deprivation and overload include decreased attention span and concentration and problem-solving ability. Written instructions and husband's knowledge reinforce the patient's learning.	*Recommendation:* Continue teaching with assistance of interpreter. *N. Gable, RN*
See if husband has bilingual friends or work acquaintances who might be willing to help the patient when she gets home until she has established a comfortable routine of care for the baby and is knowledgeable about community resources.	Careful discharge planning is necessary to ensure that the patient can manage new parenting responsibilities in an unfamiliar country.	

Expected Outcome	Before discharge, the patient will:
	• Demonstrate interest in her baby by visiting the neonatal intensive care unit, holding the baby, expressing her milk, and other such activities.

Nursing Interventions	Rationale	Evaluative Statement
Learn and respect cultural norms for new mothering behaviors.	Nursing care that is not culturally sensitive is deficient.	12/6/02 Goal met. Patient is now visiting baby in the unit on her own. *N. Gable, RN*
Assist the patient to ambulate to unit to see the baby; if interpreter is available, have the person explain equipment surrounding the baby and answer the patient's questions about the baby.	The patient may be refusing to visit the unit to protect herself from barrage of frightening stimuli (sensory overload); the goal is for her to become familiar with the unit so she is able to focus on bonding with her daughter.	

Sample Documentation	***Traditional Note Format***
	12/5/02, 10 AM, nursing
	First session with interpreter and patient at 9 AM. Patient's face brightened as soon as she heard someone speak to her in Greek. Basically, patient shared she did not care too much about what was happening to her but she was terrified about the baby and afraid of what everyone was doing to the baby. Directed interpreter to orient patient to her environment, daily routine, and NICU. Patient appeared anxious when she first saw baby but looked content when able to hold her. Schedule teaching session for tomorrow AM when interpreter will come for 1 hour. Patient currently resting comfortably. *N. Gable, RN*

(*continued*)

NURSING PLAN OF CARE (Continued)
for Mrs. Palikias

Sample Documentation

SOAP Format

12/5/02, 9 PM, nursing

Sensory/Perceptual Alterations: Mixed Sensory Deprivation and Overload related to unfamiliar hospital environment stress of cesarean birth and infant's prematurity

S: —

O: Cried after husband left this evening; refused postpartal check; turned away from nurses

A: Still feels overwhelmed by newness of all that is happening to her and tries to shut out what she cannot handle

P: Continue to intervene with help of interpreter; focus on helping patient develop more control over her situation; proceed at slow pace; referral to social services for follow-up care.

N. Gable, RN

Learning Outcomes

After completing this chapter, the learner should be able to accomplish the following:

1. Define key terms used in the chapter.

arousal	sensoristasis
auditory	sensory deprivation
cultural care deprivation	sensory overload
gustatory	sensory/perceptual
kinesthesia	alterations
olfactory	stereognosis
perception	stimulus
presbycusis	tactile
presbyopia	visceral
reception	visual
reticular activating system	

2. Describe the four conditions that must be met in each sensory experience.

3. Explain the role of the reticular activating system in sensory experience.

4. Identify etiologies and perceptual, cognitive, and emotional responses to sensory deprivation and sensory overload.

5. Perform a comprehensive assessment of sensory functioning using appropriate interview questions and physical assessment skills.

6. Develop nursing diagnoses that correctly identify sensory/perceptual alterations that may be treated by independent nursing intervention.

7. Describe specific nursing interventions to prevent sensory alterations, to stimulate the senses, and to assist patients with sensory difficulties.

8. Develop, implement, and evaluate a plan of nursing care to help patients meet individualized sensory/perceptual outcomes.

Critical Thinking Exercises

1. Describe the practical measures you would take to stimulate the senses of the following sensory-impaired patients. Think carefully about the special sensory needs that accompany different conditions.
   - A deaf child
   - A confused older adult
   - An adult male who has just lost his sight
   - A premature infant whose skin is extremely fragile

2. Visit a critical care unit with other students and list all the factors that contribute to sensory overload or deprivation. Try to identify how the critical care culture evolved in ways that are actually harmful to patients. Discuss which of these factors are unavoidable and which could be modified to better meet patient needs. Identify individualized nursing strategies to minimize sensory overload and deprivation.

Study Questions

1. The major components of any sensory experience are
   a. the kinesthetic and visceral senses
   b. reception and perception
   c. the intensity, size, change, or representation of stimuli
   d. vision, hearing, smell, taste, and touch

2. Four conditions necessary for a person to receive data and experience the world are
   a. a stimulus, a receptor, an intact nerve pathway, and a functioning brain
   b. the visual, auditory, olfactory–gustatory, and tactile senses
   c. the basic orienting systems arising from muscles, joints, hollow organs, and movement
   d. the reticular activating system, variable stimuli, memory, and motivation

3. By monitoring and regulating incoming sensory stimuli, this system maintains, enhances, or inhibits cortical arousal:
   a. general adaptation system
   b. kinesthetic/visceral system
   c. reticular activating system
   d. sensory/perceptual system

4. You notice that Mr. Wong, who has cataracts, is sitting closer to the television than usual. The etiology of his sensory problem is
   a. altered environmental stimuli
   b. altered sensory reception
   c. altered nerve impulse conduction
   d. altered impulse translation

5. Should you learn that Mr. Wong, who is 85 years old, also has presbycusis, you would want to
   a. obtain large-print written material
   b. speak distinctly using lower frequencies
   c. decrease tactile stimulation
   d. initiate a safety program to prevent falls

6. Peter Almone is in the last stages of AIDS, which is now affecting his brain as well other major organ systems. He confides to you that he feels terribly alone because most of his friends are afraid to visit. The etiology of his sensory alterations is most likely related to
   a. stimulation
   b. reception
   c. transmission–perception–reaction
   d. all of the above

7. Which of the following factors is least likely to place a patient at high risk for sensory deprivation?
   a. an environment with decreased or monotonous stimuli
   b. impaired ability to receive environmental stimuli
   c. impaired ability to process environmental stimuli
   d. impaired ability to respond to environmental stimuli

8. Which of the following patients is at greatest risk for sensory deprivation?
   a. an elderly man confined to bed at home after a stroke
   b. an adolescent in an oncology unit working on homework supplied by friends
   c. a woman in labor
   d. a toddler in a play room awaiting same-day surgery

9. A patient in an intensive care burn unit for 1 week is in pain much of the time and has his face and both arms heavily bandaged. His wife visits every evening for 15 minutes at 6, 7, and 8 PM. A heart monitor beeps for a patient on one side, and another patient moans frequently. These data suggest that the patient probably
   a. has sufficient sensory stimulation
   b. has deficient sensory stimulation
   c. has excessive sensory stimulation
   d. has both sensory deprivation and overload

10. Richard's spinal cord was severed, and he is paralyzed from the waist down. In making an assessment of this patient, it is most important to assess which component of the sensory experience?
    a. transmission of tactile stimuli
    b. adequate stimulation in the environment
    c. reception of visual and auditory stimuli
    d. general orientation and ability to follow commands

11. An 11-year-old 6th grader whose grades have dropped has difficulty completing her work on time, frequently rubs her eyes, and squints. Her visual acuity on a Snellen's eye chart was 160/20. Based on these data, the most appropriate nursing diagnosis is
    a. Knowledge Deficit related to visual impairment
    b. Altered Role Performance (Student) related to visual impairment
    c. Body Image Disturbance related to visual impairment
    d. Altered Growth and Development related to visual impairment

12. Of the four items listed below, the best nursing intervention to prevent sensory alterations for a man with a severe hearing deficit who reads lips well is to
    a. turn the radio or television volume up very loud and close the door to his room
    b. prevent embarrassment and emotional discomfort as much as possible
    c. provide daily opportunity for him to participate in a social hour with six or eight people
    d. encourage daily participation in exercise and physical activity

13. In a boarding home where most patients have slight to moderate visual or hearing impairment and some

are periodically confused, the nurse's first priority in caring for sensory concerns is to
a. maintain safety and prevent sensory deterioration
b. insist that every patient participate in as many self-care activities as possible
c. emphasize and reinforce individual patient strengths
d. encourage reminiscence and life review in groups

14. The nursing diagnosis for 8-month-old Sally was Sensory/Perceptual Alterations: Sensory Deprivation related to inadequate parenting. Since that time, both parents have attended parenting classes. However, both parents work while Sally stays with her 86-year-old grandmother who is visually impaired. The parents provide appropriate stimulation in the evening. At an evaluation conference at age 11 months, Sally lay on the floor sucking her thumb and rocking her body. Her facial expression was dull, and she vocalized only in a low monotone ("uh-h-h"). Your best evaluation concerning Sally's sensory deprivation is that

a. her parents lack motivation to provide necessary stimulation
b. her grandmother is unable to improve Sally's care
c. Sally's sensory deprivation is still severe
d. this is normal behavior for a child of Sally's age

15. Which of the following nursing interventions should not have been implemented for an elderly woman in a nursing home who walked out the door unobserved and was was hit by a car? The nursing diagnosis was Sensory/Perceptual Alterations: Chronic Sensory Deprivation related to the effects of aging.
a. Ignore when the patient is confused or go along to prevent embarrassment.
b. Encourage self-care and independent decisions.
c. Take walks around the grounds and to the garden daily.
d. Provide daily contact with children, community people, and pets.

Answers With Rationale

1. The correct response is *b*. Reception and perception are the major components of any sensory experience. All other choices are merely part of the sensory experience.

2. The correct response is *a*. A stimulus, a receptor, an intact nerve pathway, and a functioning brain are the four conditions necessary for a person to receive data and experience the world.

3. The correct response is *c*. The reticular activating system maintains, enhances, or inhibits cortical arousal by monitoring and regulating incoming sensory stimuli.

4. The correct response is *b*. Cataracts are interfering with the patient's ability to receive visual stimuli—altered sensory reception. The nature of incoming stimuli, the conduction of nerve impulses, and the translation of incoming impulses in the brain are not a problem here.

5. The correct response is *b*. Presbycusis is a normal loss of hearing as a result of the aging process. Speaking distinctly in lower frequencies is indicated. The other choices refer to interventions for other sensory problems.

6. The correct response is *d*. This patient is receiving decreased environmental stimuli (eg, from his friends); is more than likely experiencing problems with reception because of major organ involvement; and his impaired brain function will impair impulse transmission–perception–reaction.

7. The correct response is *d*. The other options all pertain to components of the sensory experience that, if impaired, may place a patient at high risk for sensory deprivation. An impaired ability to respond to environmental stimuli places a patient at risk for problems other than sensory deprivation.

8. The correct response is *a*. The patient confined to bed rest at home is at risk for greatly reduced environmental stimuli. The other patients are all in environments where environmental stimuli are at least adequate.

9. The correct response is *d*. This patient's bandages may result in deficient sensory stimulation (sensory deprivation), and the monitors and other sounds in the intensive care burn unit may cause a sensory overload. All other options are incomplete responses.

10. The correct response is *a*. Below-the-waist paralysis makes the transmission of tactile stimuli a problem. Although the other options may be assessed, they are indirectly related to his paralysis.

11. The correct response is *b*. An important role for an 11-year-old is that of student. Her impaired vision is clearly disturbing her role performance as a student, as evidenced by her lower grades. Although the other options may also represent accurate diagnoses for this patient, they do not flow from the data that were presented.

12. The correct answer is *c*. Providing daily opportunities for this patient to participate in a social hour builds on his strength of being able to lip-read and provides sufficient sensory stimulation to prevent sensory deprivation resulting from his hearing loss.

13. The correct answer is *a*. Safety is a basic physiologic need that must be met before higher-level needs, such as love and belonging, self-esteem, and self-actualization, can be met.

14. The correct response is *c*. Although the data show that the parents have been motivated to improve their parenting skills, it is clear from the data presented that Sally's sensory deprivation is still severe. The data suggest that the grandmother is not improv-

ing Sally's care, but there is nothing to suggest that she is unable to do so if shown how.

15. The correct response is *a*. Even if well motivated, ignoring a patient's confusion to prevent embarrass-

ment may be dangerous, as it was in this case in which the appropriate safety precautions were never implemented. The other options are all appropriate for this patient.

Bibliography

Broussard, A. B. (1990). Incorporating infant stimulation concepts into prenatal classes. *Journal of Obstetric, Gynecologic, and Neonatal Nursing, 19*(5), 381–387.

Chlan, L. L. (1995). Psychophysiologic responses of mechanically ventilated patients to music: A pilot study. *American Journal of Critical Care, 4*(3), 233–238.

Fine, J. I., & Rouse-Bane, S. (1995). Using validation techniques to improve communication with cognitively impaired older adults. *Journal of Gerontological Nursing, 21*(6), 39–45.

Glynn, N. J. (1992). The music therapy assessment tool in Alzheimer's patients. *Journal of Gerontological Nursing, 18*(1), 3–9.

Hall, G. R., & Wakefield, B. (1996). Confusion in the elderly. *Nursing 96, 26*(7), 32–37.

Hancock, C. K., Munjas, B., Berty, K., & Jones, J. (1994). Altered thought processes and sensory perceptual alterations: A critique. *Nursing Diagnoses, 5*(1), 26–30.

Harrison, L. L., & Woods, S. (1991). Early parental touch and preterm infants. *Journal of Obstetric, Gynecologic, and Neonatal Nursing, 20*(4), 299–306.

Janken, J. K. (1990). Auditory sensory/perceptual alteration: Suggested revision of defining characteristics. *Nursing Diagnosis, 1*(4), 147–154.

Kloosterman, N. D. (1991). Cultural care: The missing link in severe sensory alteration. *Nursing Science Quarterly, 4*(3), 119–122.

Larsen, P. D., Hazen, S. E., & Hoot Martin, J. L. (1997). Assessment and management of sensory loss in elderly patients. *AORN Journal, 65*(2), 432–437.

Lindberg, J. B., & Kruszewski A. Z. (1983). Special senses and the environment. In J. Lindberg, M. Hunter, & A. Kruszewski (Eds.). *Introduction to person-centered nursing* (pp. 297–315). Philadelphia: J. B. Lippincott.

Lindblade, D. D., & McDonald, M. (1995). Removing communication barriers for the hearing-impaired elderly. *MEDSURG Nursing, 4*(5), 379–385.

Martini, F. H., & Timmons, M. J. (1995). *Human anatomy.* Englewood Cliffs, NJ: Prentice-Hall.

McConnell, E. A. (1996). Caring for a patient who has a vision impairment. *Nursing 96, 26*(5), 28.

Moore, J. R., & Gilbert, D. A. (1995). Elderly residents: Perceptions of nurses' comforting touch. *Journal of Gerontological Nursing, 21*(1), 6–13.

North American Nursing Diagnosis Association. (1999). *NANDA nursing diagnoses: Definitions and classifications 1999–2000.* Philadelphia: Author

Oehler, J. M. (1991). Beyond technology: Meeting developmental needs of infants in NICUs. *Maternal–Child Nursing, 16*(3), 148–151.

Palumbo, M. V. (1990). Hearing access 2000: Increasing awareness of hearing impaired. *Journal of Gerontological Nursing, 16*(9), 26–31, 37–38.

Pope, D. S. (1995). Music, noise, and the human voice in the nurse–patient environment. *Image—The Journal of Nursing Scholarship, 27*(4), 291–296.

Poroch, D. (1995). The effect of preparatory patient education on the anxiety and satisfaction of cancer patients receiving radiation therapy. *Cancer Nursing, 18*(3), 206–214.

Seyfrit, M. (1995). Going blind. *American Journal of Hospice and Palliative Care, 12*(3), 31–40.

Snyder, M., Egan, E. C., & Burns, K. R. (1995). Interventions for decreasing agitation behaviors in persons with dementia. *Journal of Gerontological Nursing, 21*(7), 34–40.

Standley, J. M., & Moore, R. S. (1995). Therapeutic effects of music and mother's voice on premature infants. *Pediatric Nursing, 21*(6), 509–512.

Suedfeld, P. (1985). Stressful levels of environmental stimulation. *Issues in Mental Health Nursing, 7*(1/4), 83–104.

Wang, J. F. (1995). Caregiver–child interaction in Japan, Taiwan, and the United States. *Journal of Obstetric, Gynecologic, and Neonatal Nursing, 24*(4), 353–361.

Zahr, L. K., & Balian, S. (1995). Responses of premature infants to routine nursing interventions and noise in the NICU. *Nursing Research, 44*(3), 179–185.

Chapter 34
Sexuality

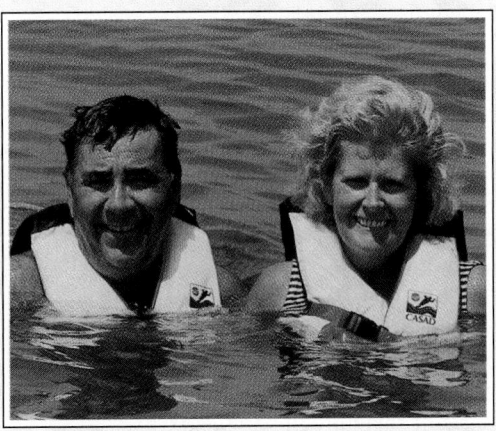

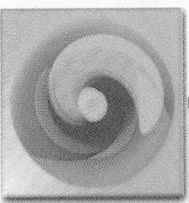

Thinking Critically About
Nursing's Blended Skills

Before reading this chapter, think about the types of blended skills you will need to meet the sexual needs of patients.

- You are invited to speak to a college audience on the topic of "date rape."

- A self-help group for parents of teenagers with Down syndrome invites you to come to one of their meetings to discuss how they can best promote the "sexual health" of their children.

- Idelle, the 40-year-old wife of a patient who has just had a heart attack, confides to you: "Well I guess this dooms me to celibacy! We weren't doing much before the infarct, and I guess now we won't be doing anything at all." Upon questioning, she reveals that her sexual drive is in "high gear" and she feels "deprived." "Fantasy only takes you so far."

- A surgeon of the opposite gender makes sexually inappropriate remarks to you at work and tells you that he/she would love to get you alone for awhile. You feel increasingly uncomfortable when assigned to work with this surgeon.

What cognitive, technical, interpersonal, and ethical/legal skills do you think you will need to respond to the challenges described above?

Sexuality is a concern in professional nursing care because sexuality permeates an individual's life, both in illness and in health. Sexuality is the degree to which a person exhibits and experiences maleness or femaleness physically, emotionally, and mentally. Sexuality is defined not only by a person's genitalia but also by attitudes and feelings. It can also be defined as learned behaviors in how a person reacts to his or her own sexuality and by how one behaves in relationships with others. Culture profoundly influences learned behaviors about sexuality. Sexuality is an integral part of a person's identity and is present in one's demeanor through actions, communications, and physical appearances.

This chapter discusses sexual health, reproductive anatomy and physiology, the sexual response cycle, and factors that affect sexuality. Obtaining a sexual history as part of a comprehensive patient history is presented, as well as interview questions that specifically address a patient with a sexual dysfunction. Nursing priorities with regard to assessment of the reproductive system are presented. Analysis of assessment data is discussed, with examples of corresponding nursing diagnoses. The patient care study and nursing plan of care provide the nurse with examples of how the information presented in the chapter can be used in a clinical setting to nurture and promote aspects of sexuality in patients.

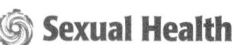 Sexual Health

The World Health Organization defines **sexual health** as "the integration of the somatic, emotional, intellectual and social aspects of sexual being, in ways that are positively enriching and that enhance personality, communication, and love (1975, p.6). Because our sexuality is so basic to our sense of self, successful nurses need to value sexuality as a critical element of health and well-being in general and be skilled in using conversation to identify and meet problems related to sexual self-concept, body image, and sexual identity.

Sexual identity encompasses a person's self-identity, biologic sex, gender identity, gender-role behavior or orientation, and sexual orientation or preference. **Biologic sex** is the term used to denote chromosomal sexual development: male (XY) or female (XX), external and internal genitalia, secondary sex characteristics, and hormonal states. **Gender identity** is the inner sense a person has of being male or female, which may be the same as or different from biologic gender. **Gender role behavior** is the behavior a person conveys about being male or female, which, again, may or may not be the same as biologic gender or gender identity (Pillitteri, 1995).

People experience sexual gratification in many ways, and what is considered "normal" differs from one individ-

COGNITIVE SKILLS

- Strong knowledge base of human sexuality, including anatomy and physiology, growth and development, sexual myths, and current issues of sexuality
- Ability to integrate knowledge about sexual health into nursing care
- Ability to identify patients with problems related to sexuality and to develop and implement appropriate plans to address these problems
- Strong assessment skills of interviewing a patient with concerns of sexuality
- Teaching skills to provide patients with necessary information and skills

TECHNICAL SKILLS

- Ability to use correctly the products and equipment necessary to meet the sexual needs of patients

INTERPERSONAL SKILLS

- Interpersonal communication skills to build rapport with college students, parents of children with Down syndrome, Idelle and her husband, and your surgeon colleague
- Nonjudgmental attitude to avoid bias, which would impede trusting nurse–patient and nurse–colleague relationships
- Counseling skills to diffuse patient anxiety over sexual growth and development
- Sense of own sexuality and comfort with sexual issues

ETHICAL/LEGAL SKILLS

- Commitment to safety and quality; strong sense of responsibility, accountability
- Familiarity with agency policy and role responsibilities related to meeting the sexual needs of patients
- Knowledge of how to respond to sexual harassment in the workplace

ual to another and among cultures. **Sexual orientation** refers to the preferred gender of the partner of an individual. The origins of sexual orientation are unknown, but there are studies claiming a genetic basis. Certainly, some sexual preferences are culturally determined and may be dictated by opportunity.

- A **heterosexual** is one who experiences sexual fulfillment with a person of the opposite gender.
- A **homosexual** is one who experiences sexual fulfillment with a person of the same gender. Homosexual males often use the term "gay"; homosexual females use the term "lesbian." Heterosexuality and homosexuality can be placed at opposite ends of a continuum with many variations in between.
- A **bisexual** is a person who finds pleasure with both opposite-sex and same-sex partners. Homosexual or heterosexual people may have bisexual relationships at times.
- A **transsexual** is a person of a certain biologic gender with the feelings of the opposite sex. The person feels trapped within the body of the wrong sex. The reason, or etiology, behind this is unknown, although many factors are believed to be involved. For many transsexuals, the solution is to change their bodies to match their inner feelings through surgery and hormone therapy.
- A **transvestite** is an individual who desires to take on the role or wear the clothes of the opposite sex. Most transvestites are heterosexual, and many keep their lifestyle hidden.

Physiology

Female

The female genitalia are represented by both internal and external structures. The appearance of the external genitalia (illustrated in Fig. 25-46 in Chap. 25) varies slightly among individuals.

External Genitalia

The mons pubis is actually a pad of fatty tissue that lies over the part of the bony pelvis called the symphysis pubis. In the physically mature female, the mons pubis is covered with coarse pubic hair. It contains many nerve endings that make the mons pubis sensitive to touch and pressure. The labia majora consist of two rounded folds of fatty tissue. The outer lips separate downward from the mons pubis and meet again below the vaginal introitus. The labia majora contain a multitude of sebaceous and sweat glands. They respond to touch during sexual activity. The labia minora are the smaller lips located within the labia majora. They are thin and sensitive structures and are pale pink in color. When stimulated by touch, the labia minora may turn a darker pink or even red owing to the presence of many blood vessels. The labia minora have no hair and are smooth in texture.

The clitoris is found above the urinary meatus at the joining of the labia minora, called the clitoral hood. The cli-

toris is a small, button-like structure similar to the male penis in its reaction to stimuli. The clitoris contains erectile tissue, blood vessels, and nerves. It is extremely sensitive. The opening of the vagina lies between the urinary meatus and the anus. It may contain a structure called the hymen, which is a thick membrane with no apparent function. At one time, the hymen was thought to represent virginity (not having experienced sexual intercourse); however, this is erroneous. Remnants, or "tags," of the hymen may be noted at the vaginal introitus in both sexually active and inactive women.

Internal Genitalia

The internal genitalia—the ovaries, fallopian tubes, uterus, and vagina—are located deep within the pelvis of the female. The female body normally contains two ovaries, one on each side of the body. The ovaries closely resemble an almond in size and shape. At the time of a female child's birth, each ovary contains some 200,000 to 400,000 follicles. This number steadily decreases until puberty, when 100,000 to 200,000 follicles remain, and the number continues to decline over the reproductive years. The process of ovulation is discussed later in this chapter. The ovaries also secrete the hormones estrogen and progesterone.

The fallopian tubes are slender structures that extend from either side of the uterus and end in a fringed fashion near each ovary. Their function is to transport a mature ovum (female reproductive cell) from an ovary to the uterus. Fertilization of the ovum by a sperm usually occurs in the tube. The fertilized ovum then travels the rest of the way to the uterus, where it implants. An unfertilized ovum travels the same path but does not implant. It is eventually expelled from the body during the menses. Because the lumen of each tube is so narrow, it can easily be damaged by the effects of infection and surgery.

The uterus is a pear-shaped organ about 3 inches long located between the urinary bladder and the rectum. Its primary purpose is to house and nurture a pregnancy (the condition of carrying a developing embryo in the uterus). The uterus comprises three layers: the outermost layer, the perimetrium, consists of elastic tissue; the middle layer, the myometrium, is muscular; and the innermost layer, the endometrium, comprises tissue that thickens and sloughs off with the menses. The cervix is the structure at the lower portion of the uterus that connects the uterus and the vagina. The cervix is usually closed. However, during the birth process, it dilates and thins out extensively to permit the birth of a baby. The cervix is a smooth, pink-colored structure that possesses few nerve endings. When touched, the sensation resembles that of touching the end of one's nose.

The vagina is a tubular, hollow organ that lies between the urinary urethra and the rectum. Its size and shape are individual among women. The walls of the vagina are composed of rugae, or ribbed tissue. The vagina serves three purposes: it is (1) a receptacle for the penis during sexual intercourse, (2) a birth canal for the passage of a baby, and (3) an exit for menstrual flow from the uterus. During sexual activity, the walls of the vagina secrete, or "sweat," a thin watery material, sometimes in copious amounts. This lubrication is necessary for the comfortable placement and movement of the penis in the vagina.

Breasts

Although the breasts are not considered part of the internal or external genitalia, they are an important aspect of the female's physical sexuality. The breasts consist of fatty and glandular tissues and the nipples. Their size and shape vary widely among women. The nipples are pale to deep pink in color. Caressing of the breasts can be pleasurable during sexual activity, and many women can be brought to orgasm by this action alone.

Menstrual Cycle

Menstruation is a cycle during which the body prepares for the presence of a fertilized ovum. Each cycle is about 28 days long but may vary from as short as 21 days to as long as 40 days. The first menstrual period, called **menarche,** is experienced at about 12 years of age; again, the age of menarche is individual and may occur anywhere between 8 years and 17 years of age. **Menopause,** the cessation of a woman's menstrual activity, occurs between the ages of 45 and 55 years. The woman may experience irregular menses over time before menstruation ends.

The menstrual cycle is controlled by a series of reactions that rely on feedback from the ovaries to the pituitary gland. Actually, two cycles occur simultaneously: one in the ovaries and one in the uterus (Fig. 34-1).

In the ovaries, in a typical 28-day cycle, the phase from day 4 to 14 is called the follicular phase. During this phase, a number of follicles mature, but only one produces a mature ovum. At the same time, in the uterus, the endometrium is becoming thick and velvety in preparation for receiving a fertilized egg. This phase in the uterus is called the proliferation phase. Ovulation generally occurs on day 14. The mature ovum ruptures from the follicle and the surface of the ovary and is swept into the fallopian tube. If sperm are present, the ovum is fertilized at this time. Some women can detect ovulation by the presence of a sharp, cramping pain over the ovulating ovary; this pain is called mittelschmerz, or middle pain, because it occurs in the middle of the cycle. From day 15 to day 28, the phase in the ovaries is called the luteal phase. The leftover empty follicle fills up with a yellow pigment and is then called the corpus luteum, or yellow body. The purpose of the corpus luteum is to produce hormones that encourage a fertilized egg to grow. If fertilization does not occur, the corpus luteum begins to disintegrate. During the luteal phase in the ovaries, the uterus also undergoes changes. This phase is called the secretory phase. The endometrial lining becomes thick. However, in the absence of a fertilized egg, the corpus luteum dies and the endometrial lining disintegrates. At day 28, the menses, or the menstrual flow, begins as a result of the uterus shedding the useless portion of its endometrium.

The menses lasts for 3 to 7 days, the average length of flow being 5 days. The menstrual discharge is a bloody fluid that also contains endometrial debris, mucus, and enzymes. It is odorless until exposed to the air, when a light,

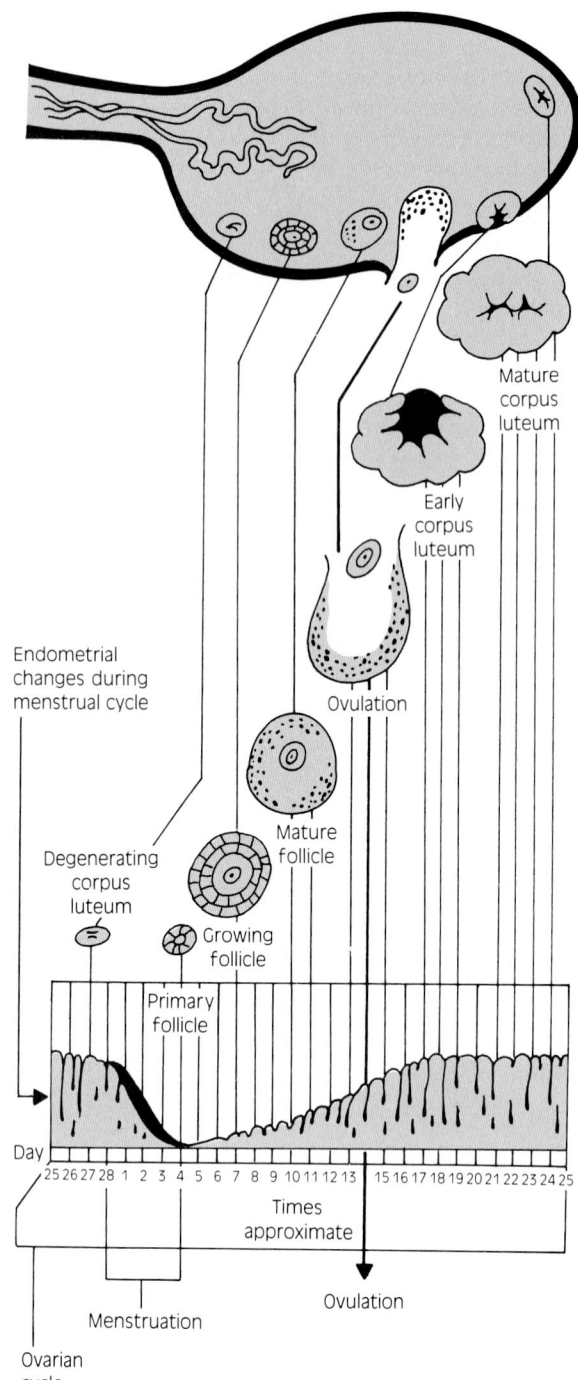

Figure 34-1

Schematic representation of one ovarian cycle and the corresponding changes in the endometrium.

fleshy, pungent odor may be noticed by the woman. Deodorized pads and tampons do little to minimize odor and can cause a chemical irritation to the vulva and vagina. Good hygiene and regular bathing are much more effective during the menses to prevent odor. Normal blood loss averages between 30 and 80 mL. Pads and tampons should be changed frequently to prevent odor and irritation from wetness. Women using tampons should be advised to read and follow the manufacturer's suggestions to reduce the risk for toxic shock syndrome. Usually, the flow is the heaviest and is bright red in color on the first day or two of the menses, gradually tapering off in amount to light brown staining. Many women experience some degree of discomfort either premenstrually or at the time of the menses.

There is no scientific rationale supporting abstinence from sexual activity during the menses. Many women enjoy sex during the menses owing to the increase in vascularity in the pelvic region, which heightens enjoyment. Men may also enjoy the warm wetness the menstrual flow provides to the vagina. If the flow is heavy, a diaphragm can be used to hold back the flow until sexual activity ceases, or a towel can be placed under the woman's buttocks to protect bedding. Women who experience abdominal cramping during the menses, or dysmenorrhea, find that sexual activity and orgasm relieve their discomfort.

Premenstrual (Tension) Syndrome

Menstrual cycle–related distress, commonly called **premenstrual (tension) syndrome** (PMS), reportedly occurs in 50% to 90% of the female population. PMS is characterized by the appearance of one or more of the following several days before the onset of menstruation: irritability, emotional tension, anxiety, mood changes, headache, breast tenderness, and water retention. Although it is often used to explain unusual behavior (and has been used as a legal defense), its etiology is still uncertain (both physiologic and psychogenic theories have been postulated), as are its effects on women's roles and relationships. Most of the current PMS literature perpetuates a twofold myth: (1) biology and physiology are destiny (many females do and should experience premenstrual distress), and (2) female biology and physiology result in psychiatric disorder, destruction, and violence (Winter, Ashton, & Moore, 1991). Nurses have a great role to play in researching PMS and ensuring that women and the public correctly understand its effects.

Male

Unlike female genitalia, the male genitalia (illustrated in Fig. 26-47 in Chap. 25) are found primarily outside the body. The testes, which are about the size of walnuts, feel smooth and are freely movable within the scrotum. The scrotum is the loose, baglike structure that houses the testes. Normally, two testes are present. The testes produce sperm and the hormones necessary for the maintenance of male sex characteristics. The primary hormone secreted by the testes is testosterone, which is responsible for a man's deep voice, beard growth, and body hair.

The scrotum hangs between a man's upper thighs. The area around the base of the penis and the scrotum is covered with pubic hair. The looseness of the scrotum is intentional to provide expansion and contraction. When exposed to cool temperatures, the scrotum contracts and draws the testes closer to the body for warmth. In warm temperatures, the scrotum become loose and allows the testes to hang farther away from the heat of the body. The testes are sensitive organs and can suffer discomfort, sometimes extreme, if handled roughly or jostled. It is important that a man wear a properly fitted athletic support, or jockstrap, when engaged in strenuous physical activity. However, the continuous use of a support can cause the temperature within the scrotum to rise and the delicate sperm to die because of constant exposure to high temperatures. Snug-fitting garments such as tight jeans can have the same effect on a man's fertility. The scrotum can be a source of sexual pleasure when lightly stroked, fondled, or caressed during sexual activity.

Tubules from the testes drain into the epididymis, which in turn drains into the vas deferens and ejaculatory ducts. These ducts then drain directly into the urethra. It is believed that the vas deferens acts as a reservoir for sperm between ejaculations.

The seminal vesicles, prostate gland, and Cowper's glands produce a liquid called seminal plasma. The seminal plasma and the sperm collectively make up the semen. The plasma aids in the transport of sperm and also provides energizing nutrients for the sperm. It contains a form of sugar (fructose), mucus, salts, water, base buffers, and coagulators to aid the sperm in their journey. Semen is a thick, creamy white fluid with the consistency of mucus or egg whites. The normal amount of semen per ejaculate is 2 to 6 mL. A fertile man dispels 120 to 160 million sperm per ejaculate. Cowper's glands produce small droplets of fluid during sexual activity that neutralize the acidity of the male urethra and aid in the transport of sperm. This fluid may contain sperm. Therefore, contraceptive measures, if used, must be taken before this fluid can be introduced into the woman's vagina.

The penis is a tubular structure located above the scrotum. It functions to eliminate urine from the bladder, to ejaculate semen and impregnate a woman, and as a sex organ for sexual pleasure. It consists of the shaft and the glans (head of the penis). In the uncircumcised male, the glans is covered by loose skin (foreskin) that can be retracted. In the circumcised male, the foreskin has been surgically removed, and the glans is exposed. Penis size and shape vary among individuals. Normally, the penis is soft and flaccid and $2\frac{1}{2}$ to 4 inches long. The dimensions of the penis in no way dictate the man's ability to perform effectively during sexual activity. When an erection occurs, the blood vessels in the shaft of the penis become congested, and the penis becomes hard and erect. The size of the penis during an erection may increase to $5\frac{1}{2}$ to 7 inches in total length. The penis, particularly the glans, is extremely sensitive to stimulation. Stroking and handling of the shaft of the penis are also pleasurable during sexual activity. Stimulation to prompt the penis to an erection is varied. A full bladder on awakening in the morning can cause an erection. Fantasy, memories of a past sexual encounter, and accidental brushing by an attractive stranger can all lead to an erection. An erection in the male does not always signify desire for sexual activity. Exposure of the male patient by the nurse during a bed bath may cause an erection. An erection is a normal physiologic response and not something the man can voluntarily control. The erection ceases if no further stimulation is added.

Ejaculation is the expulsion of semen by the rhythmic contractions of the penis. The penis engages in short, jerky movements that produce a spurt of semen with each motion. The period of ejaculation is short, and the penis becomes flaccid after ejaculation. Many males, particularly adolescent boys, may experience a phenomenon known as nocturnal emission, or "wet dream." These ejaculatory episodes occur during sleep without physical stimulation. They are perfectly normal and do not represent any sort of deviation.

Male breasts contain little real breast tissue, but they still may be stimulated during sexual activity. Although the area of sensitivity is usually limited to the nipple and areola, its stimulation can be as pleasurable an experience for the male as it is for a female.

⑤ Sexual Response Cycle

The physiologic responses to sexual activity of female and male are more similar than different (Fig. 34-2). Also, body response is essentially the same regardless of the source of

stimulation; that is, fantasy, masturbation, and sexual intercourse between two individuals can all bring about the same body reactions. The sexual response cycle is not limited to the genital organs but is a total-body response that causes many physiologic changes throughout the body. The cycle has four phases: (1) excitement, (2) plateau, (3) orgasm, and (4) resolution; there is a smooth progression from one phase to the next. Although only physiologic response is discussed here, the emotional and mental involvement of sexual response contributes a great deal to the pleasure and satisfaction of sexual activity.

The human body contains many **erogenous zones**, areas that, when stimulated, cause sexual arousal and desire. The genitals are an obvious source of sexual pleasure for both men and women, but other areas of the body are also considered erogenous zones. The skin of the body is the largest erogenous zone. Other areas include the ears, lips, thighs, and breasts. Some people can reach orgasm simply by stimulation of erogenous zones other than the genitals. The most important body organ for sexual arousal and stimulation is the brain. It allows individuals freedom to enjoy a sexual experience but also may prevent satisfaction by inhibitions, doubts, and guilt.

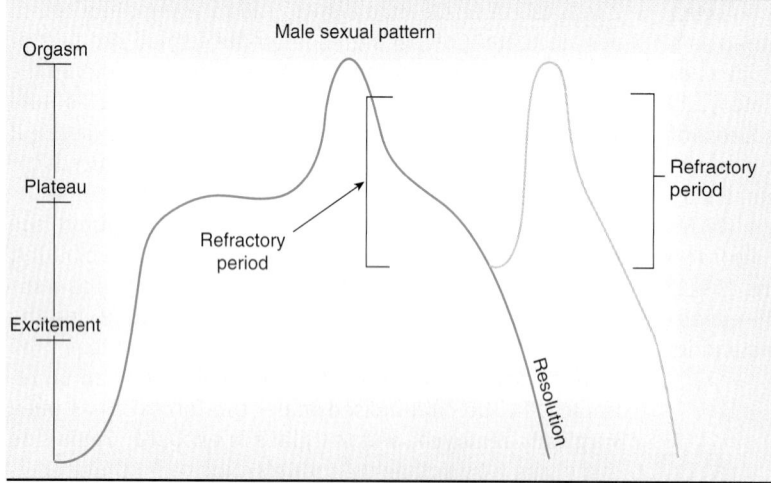

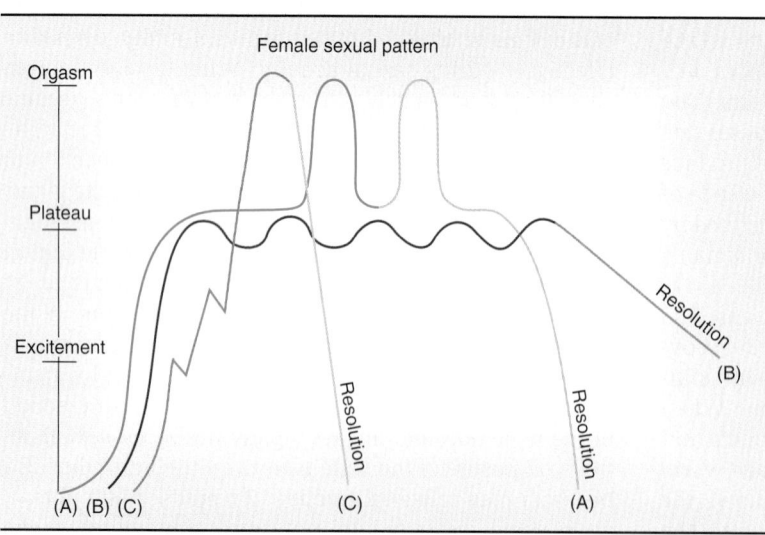

Figure 34-2

Male and female sexual response patterns. There are three female patterns shown. (**A**) Steady progression to plateau stage is followed by intense orgasm; subsequent orgasms may occur; resolution is slower. (**B**) Slower progression to plateau stage is followed by minor surges toward orgasm, causing prolonged pleasurable feelings without definitive orgasm; resolution is slowest. (**C**) Rapid progression to plateau stage with some peaks and dips; one intense orgasm follows with rapid resolution. This most closely resembles the male pattern. (Reeder, S. J., & Martin, L. L. L. [1992]. *Maternity nursing* [17th ed.]. Philadelphia: J. B. Lippincott.)

Excitement

The *excitement phase* is initiated by erotic stimulation and arousal. Some of the physiologic changes common in both men and women include increase in heart rate and blood pressure and the appearance of a pink flush to the skin. This sex flush, which is more evident in women than in men, spreads over the face, neck, back, and upper torso of the body. Congestion of the genitals with increased blood flow begins in the excitement phase and causes even more arousal. The length of the excitement phase varies greatly among individuals and even from one experience to another. Women usually enjoy a more prolonged period of stimulation than do men.

During the excitement phase, the breasts of the woman swell and the nipples become erect and hard to the touch. Lubrication of the vagina seeps to the outside of the body along the vulvar creases and makes stimulation of the genitals more pleasurable by decreasing friction. The upper two thirds or so of the vagina enlarge and expand. The clitoris enlarges and emerges slightly from the clitoral hood. The labia also enlarge and separate and turn a deep rosy red in color with arousal.

The first obvious sign of arousal in the man is an erection of the penis caused by increased pelvic congestion of blood. The scrotum noticeably elevates, thickens, and enlarges. The skin of the penis and scrotum turns a deep reddish purple in response to congestion and arousal. Male nipples may also harden and become erect.

Plateau

The intensity of the *plateau phase* is greater than that of excitement but not enough to begin orgasm. Desire and arousal continue to build and intensify. The length of time of this phase varies from a few minutes to 15 to 20 minutes. In the female, the clitoris retracts and disappears under the clitoral hood. It is thought that the clitoris performs in this mysterious way as the body's protection against overstimulation. In the male, secretions from Cowper's glands may appear at the glans of the penis during the plateau phase.

Orgasm

The term **orgasm** defines the climax and sexual explosion of the tension built over the preceding phases. Orgasm lasts a matter of seconds, but it is an extremely intense reaction. Characteristic of the orgasm phase are the involuntary spasmodic contractions of the genital organs. The number of contractions felt by the individual depends on the intensity of the orgasm.

The *orgasm phase* in the female begins with a heightened feeling of physical pleasure followed by overwhelming release and involuntary contractions of the genitals. Loss of muscular control can also be seen in spastic contractions and twitching of the arms and legs. The number of contractions can be as few as 4 or as many as 20. Areas of the body that contract spasmodically are the uterus, anal sphincter, rectum, and urethral sphincter. It is believed that women achieve orgasm in a variety of ways. Although some women can achieve orgasm by penile thrusting in the vagina alone, most women need clitoral stimulation to reach orgasm.

Involuntary spasmodic contractions of the genitals occur in the male during orgasm. These occur in the penis, epididymis, vas deferens, and rectum. The male orgasm is most often accompanied by ejaculation of semen from the urinary meatus of the penis. It is not necessary for ejaculation and orgasm to occur simultaneously; rather, it is a coincidence that the two events usually happen at the same time.

Resolution

The *resolution phase* is characterized by a return to normal body functioning present before the excitement phase. Feelings of relaxation, fatigue, and fulfillment are common. Some people may also have a need to be held, fondled, and caressed. Physical demonstrations of affection may initiate the sexual response cycle once again. The woman is physiologically capable of immediate response to sexual stimulation. Because of this, many women can achieve multiple orgasms. The man experiences a period during which he is incapable of sexual response, called the refractory period. The length of the refractory period is individual; it may be a few minutes or even days before the man's body responds readily to continued sexual stimulation.

Sexual Expression

The methods by which people gain satisfaction through sexual stimulation are varied. Touch, smell, sight, sounds, feelings, thoughts, and fantasy can all contribute to sexual fulfillment in any form of expression chosen by individuals. Feelings of love for another person are closely associated with desire.

Forms of sexual stimulation include kissing, hugging, stroking, squeezing, breast stimulation, manual stimulation of the genitals, oral–genital stimulation, and anal stimulation. Sexual stimulation may be physical or psychological. Erotic stimulation through the use of films, magazines, and photographs is common. *Fetishism*, usually practiced by a male, is sexual arousal with the aid of an inanimate object not generally associated with sexual activity. Items such as shoes, leather, rubber, and women's undergarments may be used.

Masturbation

Masturbation is a technique of sexual expression in which an individual practices self-stimulation. Many myths and misinformation surround the issue of masturbation. Masturbation is a means of learning what is preferred by a person during stimulation and what feels good. Men masturbate by holding and stroking the shaft of the penis. Women find manual stimulation of the clitoris enjoyable, although variations of technique are numerous. People masturbate regardless of sex, age, or marital status. People may not masturbate because of a sense of guilt or wrongness associated with self-stimulation. Masturbation is not "dirty" and will not lead to blindness, nor will it cause insanity.

Sexual Intercourse

Heterosexual genital intercourse is the most common image that comes to mind when sexuality is mentioned. The act of intercourse (coitus or copulation) usually begins by stimulation of the senses in some way, followed by a period of activity known as foreplay. Petting is part of foreplay and can be simple stroking of the breasts, arms, back, and neck without genital involvement or may lead to mutual masturbation and orgasm.

The act of placing the penis in the vagina, penile–vaginal intercourse, can be accomplished by various positions. The most common position in Western cultures is the missionary position, which places the woman horizontally under the man. (This position was named *missionary* by the Polynesians because it was the preferred position used for intercourse by religious missionaries.) Other positions may be more stimulating and comfortable. Clitoral stimulation is difficult to achieve in the missionary position. Lying side by side, female on top, and rear entry are some examples of coital positions that make clitoral stimulation more successful. Some people are sexually inhibited and may need permission to engage in alternative sexual positions.

When the penis is pushed into the vagina, the man begins rhythmic thrusting movements of his hips to stroke the penis back and forth along the vaginal walls. The woman may match her partner's hip movements with movements of her own body. These movements continue until orgasm is attained by one person or both. Simultaneous orgasms, or both people attaining orgasm at the same moment, are difficult to achieve. Preoccupation with attaining simultaneous orgasms may disrupt the ultimate intimacy and satisfaction possible during the coital experience. The period after coitus is just as significant as the events leading up to it. Caressing, hugging, and kissing actually deepen the intimacy shared by the couple and should be nurtured and not rushed.

Anal intercourse, the act of inserting the penis into the anus and rectum of a partner, is the other form of intercourse. Commonly practiced by gay men, it is also used by heterosexual couples. Once the penis (or any object) is placed in the rectum, it should not be introduced into the vagina without thorough cleansing because many organisms present in the rectum can cause subsequent vaginal infections. Care should be exercised to avoid injury to the delicate rectal mucosa, and lubrication is essential for comfort. Condoms are now recommended for both types of intercourse to prevent sexually transmitted diseases.

Oral–Genital Stimulation

Stimulation by using the mouth and tongue on the genitals may be used during foreplay or as a method to reach orgasm. *Cunnilingus* is stimulation of the female genitals by licking and sucking the clitoris and surrounding structures. *Fellatio* is stimulation of the male genitals by licking and sucking the penis and surrounding structures. These techniques may be used singularly or simultaneously (*soixante-neuf*).

Celibacy

Celibacy is abstinence from genital sexual activity. Celibacy may be practiced for many reasons. Dissatisfaction with the harmful consequences of the "sexual revolution" of the 1960s is leading an increasing number of adolescents and adults to choose celibate lifestyles. Many members of religious orders and institutes live celibate lives to commit themselves to nonexclusive love relationships and to nonphysical types of generativity.

Alternative Forms of Sexual Expression

Voyeurism is the achievement of sexual arousal by looking at the body of another. Some voyeurs develop complex means to spy on others that involve a violation of the observed's privacy rights.

Sadism refers to the practice of gaining sexual pleasure while inflicting abuse on another person. *Masochism* refers to gaining sexual pleasure from the humiliation of being abused. When practiced together, the act is called *sadomasochism*. It may involve being tied up, biting, hitting, spanking, whipping, pinching, and other activities.

Pedophilia is a term used to describe the practice of adults gaining sexual fulfillment by sexual acts with children.

Factors Affecting Sexuality

Many factors influence and affect a person's sexuality and thus differentiate personal feelings regarding sexuality. That is, the brain, rather than the genitals, plays the most significant role in how people perceive themselves as sexual beings.

Developmental Considerations

The process of human development affects the psychosocial, emotional, and biologic aspects of life, and these in turn affect an individual's sexuality. Sexuality is the only distinguishing trait present at conception. From birth onward, gender, or sex, influences behavior throughout life. See Table 34-1 for a summary of sexuality throughout the life span and nursing implications for each stage.

Culture

The manner in which sexuality is perceived by a society in turn influences the individual. Every culture has its own norms regarding sexual identity and behavior. To some degree, culture dictates the duration of sexual intercourse, methods of sexual stimulation, and sexual positions. In some cultures, women may be expected merely to tolerate

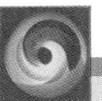

Table 34-1
Developmental Aspects of Sexuality Through the Life Span

Stage	Characteristics	Nursing Implications and Teaching Guidelines
Infancy: Birth to 18 mo	<ul><li>Needs affection and tactile stimulation</li><li>Boys have penile erections, and girls have orgasmic potential</li><li>Gradually can differentiate self from others</li><li>Obtain pleasure from touching genitals</li><li>Dressed according to gender</li><li>Toys are gender related</li></ul>	<ul><li>Avoid early weaning to prevent oral deprivation.</li><li>Encourage parents to provide ample physical touch, deprivation of which may cause physical and mental underdevelopment.</li><li>Self-manipulation of genitals is normal behavior; avoid denoting this as "bad."</li><li>Avoid confusion of sex by consistent use of male or female role reinforcement.</li></ul>
Toddler: Age 1–3 yr	<ul><li>Establishes control over bowels and bladder</li><li>Both sexes enjoy fondling genitals</li><li>Able to identify own gender</li><li>Develops vocabulary related to anatomy</li></ul>	<ul><li>Allow toddler to designate his or her readiness to toilet-training. Strict measures may lead to compulsive behaviors later.</li><li>Punishment of genital fondling may lead to guilt and shame regarding sexual behavior later in life.</li><li>Use proper terms for body parts.</li></ul>
Preschooler: Age 4–6 yr	<ul><li>By age 6, sexuality has been internalized and preference for sexual partners determined</li><li>Methods of play and dress are in accordance with gender</li><li>Enjoys exploring body parts of self and playmates</li><li>Engages in masturbation</li></ul>	<ul><li>Parents may cause anxiety in the child by intolerance of inconsistency of sex-role behavior.</li><li>Negative overreaction by parents of child's masturbating behavior can lead to a belief that the genitals and sex are bad and dirty.</li></ul>
School-age: Age 6–10 yr	<ul><li>There is attachment to the parent of the opposite sex</li><li>Tendency toward having same-sex friends</li><li>Curiosity about sex and sharing of fears</li><li>Increasing self-awareness</li></ul>	<ul><li>Same-sex preference for relationships is not related to heterosexual or homosexual tendencies.</li><li>Give child the information desired in a clear, factual form. May look to peers for information that may be incorrect.</li></ul>
Preadolescence: Age 10–13 yr	<ul><li>Puberty begins for most boys and girls with development of secondary sex characteristics</li><li>Menarche takes place</li><li>May test behavioral limits</li></ul>	<ul><li>Information is necessary regarding body changes to alleviate fears. This information should be given to the young person before pubertal changes begin.</li><li>Parents need to find a satisfactory middle ground for role setting. Rules that are either too rigid or too lenient can interfere with the development of self-confidence and internal value system.</li><li>Treat body image changes with a positive attitude to prevent poor self-image.</li></ul>
Adolescence: Age 13–19 yr	<ul><li>Begins to develop opposite-sex relationships</li><li>Sexual fantasies are common</li><li>Masturbation is common</li><li>May begin to partake in sexual activity ranging from light to heavy petting to full genital intercourse</li><li>Girls concerned with reputations and self-image</li><li>Boys preoccupied with competitiveness of sexual activity</li><li>Incidence of adolescent pregnancies is increasing</li></ul>	<ul><li>Parents share their beliefs and moral value systems with their children.</li><li>Teenagers may share their feelings with parents. Not taking them seriously may lead to lack of trust and communication gap.</li><li>Teens need information regarding contraceptive measures and the potential for contracting sexually transmitted diseases.</li></ul>

(continued)

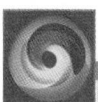

Table 34-1 (Continued)

Stage	Characteristics	Nursing Implications and Teaching Guidelines
Young adulthood: Age 20–35 yr	• Premarital sex is common • Although many young adults choose cohabitation instead of marriage, most marry and begin families before age 30 yr • Knowledge regarding sexual response and activity increases pleasure of relationship • May experiment with various sexual expressions • Develops own value system and respects values of other people • Many couples share financial responsibilities as well as household tasks	• Encourage communication between partners regarding sexual needs and differences. • Teach use of abstinence and contraceptive measures to prevent unwanted pregnancies. • Counsel against promiscuous behavior to guard against sexually transmitted diseases and loss of trust of partner • Daily communication is necessary to vent stresses and work out difficulties.
Adulthood: Age 35–55 yr	• Bodily changes as a result of menopause • Couples focus on quality rather than quantity of sexual experiences • Divorce is common • Grown children begin their own lives and sexual experiences • Sexual satisfaction may actually increase because of loss of fear of pregnancy	• Both men and women need positive reinforcement of what is good about themselves and their relationships. • Teach parents that *empty nest syndrome* (feelings of loss caused by children leaving) is common. Accentuate positive aspects of this situation. • Encourage couple to use this period as one of renewal for themselves.
Late adulthood and elderly: Age 55 yr and older	• Orgasms may become shorter and less intense in both men and women • Vaginal secretions decrease, and period of resolution in men lengthens • May feel need to conform to stereotypes regarding the aging process and cease sexual activity • Fear of loss of sexual abilities	• Sexual activity need not be hindered by age. • Teach couples that adaptation to bodily changes is possible with use of comfortable positions for intercourse and increased time for stimulation. • Teach alternatives to coitus, such as caressing, hugging, and stroking, when coitus is impossible because of illness or disability. • Couples who have been consistently sexually active throughout their lives may continue their intimate relationship for as long as they desire.

sex, whereas in others, the woman's participation is encouraged.

Religion

Some view organized religion as having a generally negative effect on the expression of sexuality. Many forms of sexual expression other than male–female coitus are considered unnatural by some religions. Also, over time, the concept of virginity came to be synonymous with purity, and sex became synonymous with sin. Double standards and rigid regulations have inflicted a considerable amount of guilt and anxiety on many individuals. A number of sex-

ual dysfunctions can be related to the individual's anguish over the negative connotation of sex as dictated by some religious groups. Most major religions are reexamining their teachings on sexuality in response to challenges posed by their members. Many have recognized the importance of solid sex education within the realm of the church.

Ethics

Healthy sexuality depends on freedom from guilt and anxiety. What one person believes is wrong may be perfectly natural and correct to another. Some individuals, however, may feel that certain forms of sexual expression are bizarre and the people who participate in them are perverted. If the sexual expression is performed by consenting adults, is not harmful to them, and is practiced in privacy, it is not considered a deviant behavior. Individuals should personally decide with which aspects of sexual expression they are comfortable. Frequently, all an individual needs to alleviate guilt and consequently enhance sexual satisfaction is permission from a healthcare professional to engage in a different form of expression.

Lifestyle

Modern lifestyles greatly affect sexuality and its expression. Both men and women are exposed to stress, and many are under considerable strain to perform and function in the workplace as well as at home. Stressors may be external, such as job and financial demands, or internal, such as a competitive nature. These varied responsibilities place a time restraint on communication between a couple as well as on the energy level and motivation for sexual satisfaction. Although some couples view sexual activity as a release from the stressors of everyday life, most place sex far from the top of the list of things to do. It is crucial to a relationship's survival that a couple set aside priority time—if not for lovemaking, then for intimate, quiet contact.

Health State

A healthy body, mind, and emotions are necessary for sexual wellness. Any trauma or stress that interferes with an individual's ability to perform daily functions certainly also affects the expression of sexuality. Illness is no exception.

Chronic Pain

Many chronic illnesses are accompanied by constant pain, and an individual with persistent pain may not desire any sexual contact. However, the desire for human warmth and contact does not cease because of pain. Altered or modified positions for coitus are sometimes necessary; these are discussed in more detail later in this section.

Diabetes Mellitus

Diabetes mellitus is a hormonal disease in which the body is deficient in the amount of insulin secreted by the pancreas. Although almost all hormonal disorders affect sexuality in some way, diabetes is the most prevalent and well known. *Erectile dysfunction*, or **impotence**, is a great concern among diabetic men. Treatment to date depends largely on the degree of erectile ability lost. Some men may be candidates for a penile prosthesis, which was developed in 1973. The prosthesis is surgically implanted below the base of the penis, and inflation of the device produces an erection when sexual activity is desired. Pharmacologic management (eg, sildenafil citrate [Viagra]) may also be indicated.

It is not uncommon for diabetic women to experience loss of capacity for orgasm (*orgasmic dysfunction*). Difficulty experiencing arousal and loss of vaginal lubrication

have also been reported. Frequent *Monilia* species infections of the vagina are also common and cause discomfort during coitus.

Cardiovascular Disease

Cardiovascular disease is prevalent in North America. It is known that the sexual response cycle can greatly increase the demands of the heart and other structures. A person with a cardiovascular disease may experience much anxiety over the effect the illness will have on sexuality and sexual functioning.

Hypertension

The most significant difficulty a hypertensive person faces regarding sexuality is that the medication used to control the disease frequently causes a change in sexual functioning. These sexual dysfunctions may be relieved by modifying the dose of the medication or switching to a different medication.

Myocardial Infarction (Heart Attack)

The primary goal after a myocardial infarction (MI) is to allow the heart ample time to heal. Activities of daily living, including sexual activity, should be resumed gradually, and stressors such as overexertion, alcohol consumption, and emotional upheavals should be avoided. In an uncomplicated MI, sexual activity may begin at about the third week of recovery, beginning with masturbation to partial erection in the male. Generally, this activity is gradually increased until 3 months after the MI, when sexual intercourse may be resumed. A comfortable position that places the least stress on the affected partner should be assumed.

Diseases of the Joints and Mobility

Joint diseases and disorders affect young and old people. Pain, fatigue, stiffness, and loss of range of motion can accompany any of the dozens of known diseases of the joints. The disease itself does not affect sexual functioning, although the manifestation of it can cause discomfort and anxiety.

Surgery and Body Image

Surgery is performed to remove diseased tissue and repair body organs, usually requiring an incision with resulting scars. The most devastating kinds of surgery are those used to remove cancerous tissue and surrounding structures. The patient is almost always distressed about a diagnosis of cancer and possible death. After surgery, people need to cope and adjust to major alterations to their bodies. Changes in body image also affect a person's self-perception as a sexual being.

Mastectomy is a surgical procedure to remove a breast and its surrounding tissue. After such surgery, a woman's return to sexual functioning depends on many factors, such as support of her partner, the value placed on the breast by the man or woman, and fear of discomfort during sexual activity.

An *ostomy* is a surgical opening placed on the outside of the body to allow for the passage of secretions and elimination into a closed drainage bag. The grief over the loss of the natural means to eliminate waste, such as urine or feces, accompanies learning to live with an obvious artificial device. Many people are anxious as to how this apparatus will affect their sexual lives and how accepting sexual partners will be of it.

Spinal Cord Injuries

Thousands of people are victims of spinal cord injuries each year as a result of various types of accidents. This type of injury almost always results in some degree of permanent disability. Such people face multiple adaptations in normal living styles, including those related to mobility, bowel and bladder control, sexual functioning, and role expectations. The extent of remaining sexual response after a spinal cord injury depends primarily on the level and extent of the injury. Ejaculation and orgasm are most likely to remain with low spinal injuries. Women are more likely to experience orgasm than men but complain more about the lack of physical sensations during the excitement phase than do men. Many people find that other erogenous zones become more easily stimulated after the injury.

Mental Illness

Various psychological and physical disorders can cause mental illness. The mind plays a powerful role in sexuality, and any disruption of its functioning will no doubt cause a disturbance in some way to sexual functioning. Even a disorder such as mild depression can affect desire and sexual functioning. Sometimes, it is difficult for the partner of a patient who has developed a mental illness to continue the sexual relationship. People afflicted with Alzheimer's disease can lose the memory of any contact with a partner or spouse. At times, patients with mental illness act out in a sexual manner, such as touching themselves or discarding their clothing at inappropriate times and places.

Sexually Transmitted Diseases

The term *sexually transmitted disease* (STD) is used to describe diseases that are almost always transmitted through direct sexual contact. Table 34-2 lists the more common types of STDs and their signs and symptoms. The number of cases and varieties of STDs has increased over the years, and many are at epidemic proportions. STDs are hard to control because the partner or partners also need treatment; this is usually difficult if the partner is promiscuous or a one-time contact. It is believed that to have sexual contact with one person is also to have sexual contact with everyone else that person has had contact with in the past. The only clear way to avoid exposure to an STD is for a virginal person to have sexual contact with another virgin. Some STDs can be treated easily and effectively, whereas others have long-standing implications. For instance, women may suffer severe consequences from an STD by developing pelvic inflammatory disease (PID); the resulting adhesions cause much damage to delicate reproductive structures and may lead to infertility. Furthermore, other STDs, such as ac-

quired immunodeficiency syndrome (AIDS), are deadly because there is no cure.

Medications

Some medications have side effects that may affect sexual functioning. Illegal drugs are used by some people because of their reputed ability to heighten the sexual experience; these drugs can have serious and even deadly side effects of their own. Table 34-3 lists some of the categories of medications and their possible effects on sexual functioning.

The Nurse as Role Model

A nurse's attitudes, biases, and prejudice regarding sexuality are readily transmitted to patients through his or her actions, manner of speech, avoidance of certain circumstances, and types of discussion (see the accompanying box, Developing Critical Thinking Skills on p. 794). The level of knowledge a nurse has about sexual issues can inhibit or promote discussion of sexual health. The nurse who does not have a sound knowledge base of reproductive anatomy and physiology, sexual response, sexual expression, and other issues surrounding sexuality will be unable to assess, teach, or counsel effectively the patient with sexual concerns. The nurse must also feel comfortable with himself or herself as a sexual being (see the accompanying box, Applying Learning to Practice: Promoting Health on p. 795).

Nursing goals to enhance interactions with patients and to promote individual sexual health are as follows. The nurse will be able to achieve the following:

- Feel comfortable as a sexual being
- Develop self-awareness regarding sexual topics
- Develop communication skills that promote discussion of sexual concerns with patients
- Identify patients with problems related to sexuality and intervene competently and comfortably to meet these needs
- Practice responsible sexual expression

Sexual Harassment

Nurses in different types of healthcare settings have experienced work-related sexual harassment. **Sexual harassment** may be defined as "any unwelcome verbal or physical advance or sexually explicit statement—such as leers, pats, grabs, jokes, requests for dates, and even rape—that interferes with your ability to do your job by making you feel humiliated, intimidated or uncomfortable" (Horsley, 1990, p. 69). It is important for nurses to recognize that harassment can often be effectively stopped when confronted early. Horsley gives the following specific measures to stop harassment:

Confrontation: Look the harasser in the eye and tell him or her you do not like this behavior and want it to stop.

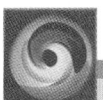

Table 34-2
Sexually Transmitted Diseases

Disease	Characteristics
Acquired immunodeficiency syndrome (AIDS)	• Human immunodeficiency virus (HIV) • Positive ELISA and Western Blot tests • Incidence high in IV drug users and homosexual and bisexual men; increased heterosexual transmission • Fatigue, diarrhea, weight loss, enlarged lymph nodes, fever, anorexia, and night sweats
Cervical intraepithelial neoplasia (CIN) Cervical cancer	• Abnormal Pap smears • Women with multiple sex partners, women who began sexual activity before age 18, and women whose partners have multiple female partners • Asymptomatic • Possible vaginal bleeding or spotting
Chlamydia trachomatis Nongonococcal urethritis (NGU) *Chlamydia*	• The most prevalent STD to date • Intracellular bacteria • Vaginal discharge, burning on urination, urinary frequency, dysuria, and urethral soreness • Many women do not have symptoms.
Cytomegalovirus (CMV)	• A virus in the same family as herpes and Epstein-Barr • May be asymptomatic or may be confused with another disease such as pneumonia, mononucleosis, or hepatitis • Not exclusively sexually transmitted.
Nonspecific vaginitis *Gardnerella vaginalis*	• Mixed anaerobic bacteria • Foul-smelling, thin, grayish white vaginal discharge • Male partners do not have symptoms.
Neisseria gonorrhoeae "The clap" or "the drip" Gonorrhea	• Gram-negative bacteria • Both men and women may not have symptoms. • Symptoms in men: purulent penile discharge, dysuria, frequency of urination • Symptoms in women: dysuria, abnormal menses, vaginal discharge, pelvic inflammatory disease • Symptoms of pharyngitis if oral sex practiced • May be accompanied by chlamydial infection • Detected by gonorrhea culture of cervix or penile discharge from men • Newborns exposed at birth are at risk for blindness and pneumonia. • Untreated gonorrhea can result in infertility, skin rash with lesions, and acute arthritis.
Herpes simples virus type 1 and 2 "Cold sores" Herpes	• A DNA virus • Lesions develop mostly in oral and genital areas. • Appear as single or multiple painful vesicles, which rupture and form ulcer-like lesions; these form scabs as they heal. • First infections last about 10 to 14 days, whereas subsequent infections are shorter in duration. • Recurrences are usually preceded by prodromal symptoms of tingling and fullness.
Human papilloma virus (HPV) Condylomata acuminata Genital warts Venereal warts	• A DNA virus • Pale, soft, papillary lesions found around the internal and external genitalia and perianal and rectal areas of the body; vary in size • Profuse watery vaginal discharge, dyspareunia, intense pruritus, and vulvar irritation • Women with HPV are at risk for cervical cancer. • Male partner may or may not have lesions.

(continued)

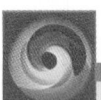

Table 34-2 (Continued)

Disease	Characteristics

Treponema pallidum
Syphilis
	• A spirochete detected through serologic blood test (VDRL, RPR, STS)
	• Three stages to disease if left untreated
	  Primary: Single painless genital lesion 10 days to 3 months after exposure
	  Secondary: Generalized skin rash, enlarged lymph nodes, fever that may appear 2 to 4 weeks after appearance of primary lesion; may last for several years
	  Latent: Usually no clinical symptoms present for as long as 20 years; may continue to involve and damage neurologic and cardiovascular organs; dementia, confusion, paralysis, and paresis may occur

Trichomoniasis "Trich" *Trichomonas vaginalis*	• Protozoan with flagella • Identified on wet-mount microscopic examination of vaginal discharge • May be identified on Pap smear • Usually asymptomatic in male patients • Foul-smelling vaginal discharge, thin, foamy, and green in color, causes itching of vulva and vagina, burning on urination and dyspareunia; "strawberry" cervix may be seen on speculum examination

(Data from Baldwin, K., & Goodwin, K. [1985]. The Papanicolaou smear. *Journal of Nurse–Midwifery 30*[6]: 327–331; Bourcier, K., & Seidler, A. [1987]. *Chlamydia* and condylomata acuminata; An update for the nurse practitioner. *Journal of Obstetric, Gynecologic, and Neonatal Nursing 16*[1], 17–21; Fromer, M. [1983]. *Ethical issues in sexuality and reproduction.* St. Louis: C. V. Mosby; Hatcher, R., et al. [1986]. *Contraceptive technology.* New York: Irvington.)

Documentation: Document specific instances of harassment (words and acts, your response, date, time, place, and the names of any witnesses). Put the details of these incidents in a letter and send it to the harasser, indicating that you do not like this behavior and want it to stop. Send the letter by way of registered mail.

Written complaint: If the behavior does not stop, submit a written complaint to administration (use appropriate channels).

Government complaint: If all else fails, file a complaint with the Equal Employment Opportunity Commission.

The Nursing Process

ASSESSING

Sexual History

The comprehensive health history should include information regarding a patient's reproductive and sexual health, depending on the circumstances in which the patient is receiving care. As a rule, three general categories of patients should have a sexual history recorded by the nurse:

• Any inpatient or outpatient patient who is receiving care for pregnancy, STD, infertility, or contraception
• Any patient who is experiencing sexual dysfunction
• Any patient whose illness will affect sexual functioning and behavior in any way

Information is best obtained from the patient by beginning with nonthreatening questions and progressing to more sensitive concerns (see the accompanying Focused Assessment Guide). Patients usually have no difficulty answering questions regarding their bodies and general reproductive issues such as, "When did your menstrual periods first begin?"

Nurses should explain to patients that this information may be helpful in assisting them in the plan of care and in identifying any sexual problems or concerns. It is an excellent opportunity for the nurse to teach by helping the patient confront fears. Watts (1979) suggested four general levels of sexual history:

Level 1: Sexual history as part of a comprehensive health history—obtained by a nurse
Level 2: Sexual history—obtained by a nurse with education and training in sexuality
Level 3: Sexual problem history—obtained by a sex therapist
Level 4: Psychiatric/psychosocial history—obtained by a psychiatric nurse clinician

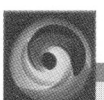

Table 34-3
Medications and Their Effects on Sexual Functioning

Drug	Effect on Sexual Functioning
Amyl nitrite	Peripheral vasodilator used in the past for treating angina; has become popular as sex enhancer among male homosexuals in particular; when inhaled at time of orgasm, the resulting vasodilation is felt to cause an intensified orgasmic release. Loss of erection, hypotension, and faintness may occur.
Anticonvulsants	Dilantin (phenytoin) has sedative effects, which may decrease desire and reduce sexual response.
Antidepressants Tricyclic compounds Monoamine oxidase inhibitors Lithium carbonate	Similar to antihypertensive drugs. Male impotence is significant. Male impotence and ejaculatory dysfunction in 25% to 30% of men. Decreases serum testosterone in men. Some antidepressants have been found to cause prolonged painful erections known as *priapism;* one such drug is trazodone.
Antihistamines	May have sedative effect that decreases desire; may also cause decreased vaginal lubrication.
Antihypertensives Methyldopa Clonidine Reserpine	 May decrease desire in both male and female patients. Erectile failure in 24% of men; no adverse effect on female patients. Decreased desire in women; erectile and ejaculation dysfunctions in men.
Antipsychotics	Causes decreased desire in 10% to 20% of patients; may also cause erection and ejaculatory dysfunctions. Small amount of the antipsychotic drug may be found in the semen. The partner may experience resulting genital rash. Wear condoms while on therapy.
Antispasmodics	These drugs relax smooth muscle; male impotence may occur.
Barbiturates	In low initial doses, sexual pleasure may be increased due to loss of inhibitions. However, long-term use commonly causes decreased desire and orgasmic dysfunction. Male impotence is not uncommon.
Cocaine	Reported to increase quality of sexual experience. Chronic use, however, results in sexual dysfunction and loss of desire in both men and women.
Ethyl alcohol	In moderate amounts, decreases inhibitions and consequently improves sexual functioning. Continued consumption decreases sexual functioning. Chronic alcoholics are impotent and often sterile. Testicular damage and permanent dysfunction are common. Female alcoholics experience decreased desire and orgasmic dysfunction.
Marijuana	Release of inhibitions may cause feeling of increased sexual functioning. Marijuana users have increased incidence of decreased desire and male impotence.
Narcotics	Serious impairment of sexual functioning with increased dependence. Erectile and ejaculatory dysfunctions common in men. Testosterone levels and amount of semen decreased. High incidence of decreased desire occurs in both men and women.

(Data from Fuentes, R. [1983]. Sexual side effects. What to tell your patients, what not to say. *RN, 46*[2], 34–41; Woods, N. F. [1984]. *Human sexuality in health and illness.* St. Louis, MO: C. V. Mosby.)

Each level acquires more specific information from the patient regarding sexual health and also requires the interviewer to have more sophisticated preparation and skills. The professional nurse usually performs a sexual history on level 1.

The nurse sets the tone or atmosphere for the interview. The nurse's attitudes will greatly affect the patient's response to the sexual history, and patients will be more cooperative if they sense the nurse's security and ease during the interview. Privacy is essential for the sexual history; doors should be closed and no interruptions allowed. The nurse sits close to the patient and speaks in a quiet, relaxed, objective tone of voice. Eye contact and open body posture are used. The patient needs to know what will happen to this information and who will have access to it. The nurse needs to explain to the patient that no one will have access to this information unless it is significant to the patient's care. Reproductive health information should be obtained from the patient first, followed by the patient's sexual health history. The best approach is to begin with general open-ended questions and progress to more specific ones. The nurse should use the language used by the patient. If

Developing Critical Thinking Skills

Situation

A 33-year-old Caucasian male with AIDS who is living alone at home asks you, the visiting nurse, about the nurse who was substituting for you during your vacation. "I don't like to complain, but he was overly friendly—if you get what I mean. . . . I wasn't comfortable with the way he was touching me and I'd rather not have help with my bath than have him back here." You have to decide how to respond.

1. **Identify Goal of Thinking**

   Clarify what the patient is saying and make a judgment about the behavior behind his concern so that you can respond appropriately.

2. **Assess Adequacy of Knowledge**

   Pertinent circumstances: You have been visiting the patient for the last 2 months following his discharge from a local hospital because of AIDS-related complications. Apart from his clinical picture, you know very little about the patient, who has always seemed private and reserved during your visits. You "feel sorry" that the patient is as sick as he is at this point in his life, and your instinct is to trust him. You really don't know the colleague who was substituting for you because he is a "new hire."

   Prerequisite knowledge: Before you can make a judgment about the patient's concern, you need to know more about what actually happened between him and your colleague. You do not know your colleague well because he is a "new hire" and has only been working in the agency for 3 months. You have heard reports that he is gay. You know that the patient is single but do not know his sexual orientation. You will need to talk with your colleague to get his description of his encounter with the patient. You will also need to know more about what touch means to both the patient and your colleague because culture and individual preference can profoundly influence the meaning different individuals give to touch.

   Room for error: Life and death do not hinge on how you respond to this patient. However, the well-being of the patient and your colleague's reputation are at stake, so the matter is grave.

   Time constraints: You must make some immediate response to the patient. Because you do not have sufficient information to judge what happened, you should not feel pressured to make a definitive response. The patient's well-being will not be jeopardized if you postpone a complete response until you have investigated the complaint.

3. **Address Potential Problems**

   The most serious obstacles to critical thinking in this situation would be false assumptions you (and the patient) might have about homosexuality in general and male homosexual nurses in particular, and the failure to reason carefully about the situation. Your tendency to "go to bat" for patients and to believe whatever a patient tells you "no matter what" may result in your unfairly and prematurely judging a colleague.

4. **Consult Helpful Resources**

   Your colleague is the first resource you should consult because you need to hear his side of the event before you can think critically about what happened. When you do meet with him, he thanks you for bringing up the subject because he was similarly disturbed by his encounter with this patient. "I guess I'm a touchy-feely kind of guy and generally find that patients respond well to human touch. In the past, patients have told me how much it means to them to have someone massage their back, stroke a forearm, or greet them with a hug. Touch is certainly a big part of the 'therapeutic package' I give each of my patients. I did sense rather quickly, though, that Jim didn't like to be touched and modified my approach. My sense, from a few comments he made, is that he's probably homophobic [afraid of homosexuals]."

   After listening to your colleague, you decide you need to learn more about touch, touch as a therapeutic intervention, and homophobia. You can consult the literature or local experts.

5. **Critique Judgment/Decision**

   Wanting to explore the situation more fully, you responded to the patient initially by saying, "I am sorry that you felt uncomfortable by my colleague's care. I want to talk with him about his sense of what happened and will then discuss this with you when I return on Wednesday." After talking with your colleague you are reasonably assured that he was not intending, inappropriately, to communicate anything of a sexual nature to the patient. On your return visit to the patient you inform him about your research and judgment and say, "Touch can mean different things to different people. My sense is that Dave simply wanted to communicate that he cares. If he is going about this in the wrong way, he wants to know what he should be doing differently. We certainly don't want this to be a problem for you or any other patient. Would you like to talk more about this or to file a report?"

(continued)

🌀 🌀 🌀 **Developing Critical Thinking Skills (Continued)**

You initially think you have three options: (1) to agree at the outset that your colleague has behaved in a sexually inappropriate and unprofessional manner, (2) to investigate the incident and conclude that your colleague was in the wrong, or (3) to investigate the incident and conclude that your colleague was in the right. You chose the third and are relieved when the patient seems to accept your explanation. Two months later,

when you receive a similar complaint from another male patient, you are troubled. You realize now that there was a fourth option, and that this is the one you should have taken. Convinced by your colleague's sincerity and good intent, you might nonetheless have informed Dave that you need to communicate this patient concern to your supervisor so that if future incidence are reported there will be a record of repeat complaints.

not, patients may be reluctant to tell the caregiver that they do not understand certain terms for fear of appearing ignorant or foolish. For example, the patient may choose the term "come" to mean climax or orgasm.

It is useful to begin questions with "many people like" or "many people feel." This gives patients security in knowing they are not alone in how they feel and are encouraged to talk about their problems or concerns. An example of this type of questioning is the following: "Many people feel that it's helpful to discuss your concerns about sex with your partner. What do you think about this?"

One helpful means to obtain information about sexual problems follows:

Description of the problem: "How would you describe the problem?"
Onset and cause of the problem: "What do you think caused the problem or what was happening when you first noticed it?"

Past attempts at resolution: "What have you tried in the past to correct the problem?"
Goals of the patient: "What do you wish to accomplish?"

A narrative form of recording a sexual history is generally used because it allows the interviewer to document the data in many of the patient's own words. If a patient is seeking help for a sexual problem, a more specific format will be used in recording information obtained by a skilled therapist (see the accompanying box, Focus on the Older Adult).

Sexual Dysfunction

Sexual dysfunction is a problem that prevents an individual or couple from engaging in or enjoying satisfactory sexual intercourse and orgasm. Dysfunctions may occur as a result of physiologic malfunctions, conflicts with cultural

---

APPLYING LEARNING TO PRACTICE

Promoting Health

Sexuality

Use the assessment checklist to determine how well you are meeting your sexuality needs. Then develop a prescription for self-care by choosing appropriate behaviors from the list of suggestions.

ASSESSMENT CHECKLIST

almost always | sometimes | almost never

☐ ☐ ☐ 1. I feel good about my sexual identity.

☐ ☐ ☐ 2. I have satisfying relationships with others.

☐ ☐ ☐ 3. I accept sexual needs as a normal part of life.

☐ ☐ ☐ 4. I am comfortable with physical actions that indicate love and belonging (such as touching and hugging).

SELF-CARE BEHAVIORS

1. Avoid stereotyping typical gender roles.

2. Learn the biologic aspects of sexual functioning.

3. Ask questions about sexual needs and sexual activity when necessary.

4. Enjoy close relationships with others who love you.

5. Give a hug to someone you love.

6. Accept touch from others as a sign of caring and affection.

7. Practice safer sex (eg, use contraceptives or condoms, and choose partner carefully).

8. Recognize how age, illness, or disability influences sexual needs and expression.

FOCUSED ASSESSMENT GUIDE

Sexuality

Factors to Assess	Questions and Approaches
Reproductive history	Ask women their date of menarche, date of last menstrual period, duration and length of flow in days, number of pregnancies, living children, miscarriages, abortions, method of birth control. Ask men the number of children they have fathered and method of birth control used. Ask both men and women of childbearing age if they have any concerns about their fertility and determine whether there is any interest in the new reproductive technologies and genetic testing options.
History of sexually transmitted diseases	"Do you or a sexual partner have a history of sexually transmitted diseases? Many people today have questions about sexually transmitted diseases that they are reluctant to express. Do you have any questions? Have you noticed any signs that might indicate a problem?"
History of sexual dysfunction	"Have you ever experienced a problem such as erectile dysfunction, failure to achieve orgasm, or pain during intercourse?"
Sexual self-care behaviors	"Do you perform the breast-self exam [testicular-self exam] on a monthly basis? When was your last gynecologic [urologic] examination (Pap smear, mammogram)? Is there a family history of breast disease, ovarian cancer, testicular cancer, colon cancer? With all the attention on safer sex today and responsible parenting, many people have questions about their sexual self-care behaviors. Do you have any such concerns?" [It is important for nurses to ascertain whether patients possess the knowledge, attitudes, and skills necessary to promote their own sexual health and that of others.]
Sexual self-concept	
Sexual identity	"How do you feel about yourself as a man or woman? Is anything changing the way you feel about yourself?"
Sexual body image	"Many people have concerns about their sexual body image. Are you comfortable with your physical maleness or femaleness? Have you experienced any physical changes (eg, baldness, weight loss or gain, impotence, menopause, mastectomy, hysterectomy, sterilization) that are troubling to you?"
Sexual self-esteem	"We all have certain expectations of ourselves. Are you comfortable with the way you are currently expressing yourself sexually and meeting your sexual needs?"
Sexual role performance	"Has anything interfered with your ability to be a spouse, sexual partner, parent (any other valued sex-related roles)?"
Sexual functioning	"It's not unusual for people with health concerns [name specific medical problem, if appropriate] to have questions related to sexuality and sexual functioning. Do you have any questions or concerns that I can help you with? Has anything [if appropriate, substitute the name of a specific disease, surgery, or medication] changed your ability to function sexually?" [Asking patients if they have questions about resuming their usual sexual activity is an appropriate part of discharge planning for many patients.]

norms, interpersonal problems, or any combination of these. Anxieties and fears concerning the sexual act are almost always present. Patients with severe sexual dysfunctions require intensive professional therapy from a qualified sex therapist. A few of the major dysfunctions are briefly discussed here and in Table 34-4.

Male Sexual Dysfunctions

Erectile failure, also called impotence, is the inability of a man to attain or maintain an erection to such an extent that he cannot have satisfactory intercourse. Common causes of impotence (which may be physiologic or psychological) include various illnesses, treatments for these illnesses, and personal anxieties. The medication *Viagra* has revolutionized treatment for erectile dysfunction.

Premature ejaculation is the condition when a man consistently reaches ejaculation or orgasm before or soon after entering the vagina. The result is that his partner usually does not have time to reach sexual satisfaction. Causes of the problem are rarely physical in nature.

Focus on the Older Adult

*Talking With Elderly People
About Sexuality*

The many losses associated with aging leave older people with special needs for love and affection. Unfortunately, many healthcare professionals simply assume that older people have no health concerns related to sexuality. Factors that can inhibit sexual activity in older adults include the following:

- Societal expectations that sexual activity somehow belongs to the young and beautiful
- Rigid moral principles
- Decreased self-esteem
- Physical factors: age-related body changes, the effects of fatigue, illness, medications
- The attitudes of healthcare professionals who ignore or demean expressions of sexual needs by older people
- Institutional factors, such as policies preventing sexual activity between competent, consenting older adults

Nurses who are sensitive to these factors can initiate a discussion about sexuality with older patients by asking the following questions. If questioning results in the older person's discomfort, do not press for information not needed for medical reasons.

"Many older people talk about feeling lonely. Are there people with whom you feel close who meet your needs for love and affection?"

"Are you sexually active currently?" [or] "Are you comfortable with your current level of sexual activity?"

"Is there anything interfering with your ability to be as sexually active as you would like? Physical limitations? Attitudes, beliefs, values? No partner?" [In a long-term care setting, institutional factors may inhibit sexual activity.]

"In what physical ways do you express and receive affection?" [kissing, hugging, handholding, coitus, oral or manual genital stimulation]

"Do you have concerns about sexually transmitted diseases?"

"Is there any information you would like from me that would help you to better meet your needs for love and affection?" "Are there any questions or concerns you have that we haven't addressed?"

Retarded ejaculation, also called ejaculatory incompetence, refers to a man's inability to ejaculate into the vagina or delayed intravaginal ejaculation. The causes of this problem are similar to those of impotence. When it occurs after having experienced normal ejaculations, the cause is most probably due to interpersonal problems.

Female Sexual Dysfunctions

Inhibited sexual desire consists of an inhibition in sexual arousal so that congestion and vaginal lubrication are absent or minimal. Causative factors may be anxiety, negative emotions, fear, interpersonal problems, or physical factors.

Orgasmic dysfunction is defined as the inability of a woman to reach orgasm. The causes are similar to those of inhibited sexual desire.

Dyspareunia is painful intercourse. Although it is most often described by women, some men may also suffer from this disorder. The cause is usually physical in nature, although psychological problems such as fear and anxiety can cause pain in some women.

Vaginismus is a rare condition in which the vaginal opening closes tightly and prevents penile penetration. Vaginismus is due to involuntary spastic contractions of muscles at and around the vaginal opening and the levator ani muscles. The cause of vaginismus may be physical, psychological, or both.

Vulvodynia, a chronic vulvar discomfort or pain characterized by burning, stinging, irritation, or rawness of the female genitalia that interferes with sexual activity, is particularly problematic because little is known about its cause or treatment.

Physical Assessment

Physical examination of the reproductive or genitourinary system for either male or female patients is necessary under the following circumstances:

- As part of a routine physical examination
- Annual women's healthcare, including Pap smear
- Suspicion of an STD
- Suspicion of pregnancy
- Work-up for infertility
- Unusual lump, discharge, or unusual appearance of the genital organs noticed by the patient
- Request for birth control
- Change in urinary function

The examiner may routinely perform a complete physical examination along with assessment of the reproductive system if the patient has not had contact with the healthcare system within 1 year or if assessment findings of a complete examination would be useful in diagnosing an ailment or complaint of the patient. See Chapter 25 for a detailed description of how to examine the female and male genitalia.

The nurse should initially ask whether the patient has experienced this type of examination in the past if this information is not evident by the patient's records. Depending on the patient's knowledge base, the nurse

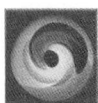

Table 34-4
Sexual Dysfunction and Nursing Assessment

Sexual Dysfunction	Assessment Priorities
Male	
Erectile failure (impotence)	• History of diabetes, spinal cord trauma, cardiovascular disease, surgical procedure, alcoholism • Use of certain medications such as antihypertensives, antidepressants, or illicit drugs • Determine degree of mental depression that may be present • Obtain specific information regarding the degree of impotence, length of time of disorder, continuing life factors
Premature ejaculation	• Assess what patient defines as his dysfunction and ability to control ejaculation • Assess any causative relationship factors, such as anxiety, guilt, lack of time, new partner, and so on
Retarded ejaculation	• History of neurologic disorders, Parkinson's disease, or use of certain medications • Same assessment priorities as for premature ejaculation
Female	
Inhibited sexual desire	• Use of oral contraceptives or other hormonal therapy, use of alcohol or certain medications • History of sexual abuse, rape or incest, depression, or other sexual dysfunctions • Assess any other contributing or relationship factors.
Orgasmic dysfunction	• Assess knowledge level regarding sexual response cycle and anatomy • Assess communication pattern between patient and her partner • Assess usual sexual pattern and behavior between patient and her partner • Assess any other contributing factors
Dyspareunia	• History of diabetes, hormonal imbalance, vaginal infection, endometriosis, urethritis, cervicitis, or rectal lesions • Use of antihistamines, alcohol, tranquilizers, or illicit drugs • Assess patient's ability for vaginal lubrication during sexual act • Assess patient's use of coital positions • Assess use of cosmetic or chemical irritants to genitals, such as deodorant tampons, contraceptive creams, or jellies or condoms • Physical assessment of internal and external genitalia • Assess any other contributing factors
Vaginismus	• Assess knowledge regarding anatomy and sexual response • Assess pattern of sexual activity: how often, level of arousal, orgasm • Assess presence of other sexual dysfunctions • History of sexual abuse, trauma, or rape • Assess patient's feelings regarding her partner • Assess any other causative factors, such as fear of pregnancy, anxiety, guilt • Physical assessment of internal and external genitalia

should explain the progressive steps of the examination and what the patient may feel during the examination. This will give the patient some feeling of control and security during the examination. The nurse's responsibilities during an examination of the reproductive system are as follows:

• To provide information to the patient regarding the examination
• To teach the patient
• To provide support for the patient during the examination
• To assist the examiner, if appropriate, with any procedures or laboratory studies

DIAGNOSING

Nursing diagnoses written to address problems of sexuality belong to one of two categories:

Altered Sexuality Patterns: The state in which an individual experiences or is at risk for a change in sexual health. Sexual health is the integration of somatic, emotional, intellectual, and social aspects of sexual being in ways that are enriching and that enhance personality, communication, and love.

Sexual Dysfunction: The state in which an individual experiences or is at risk for change in sexual function that is viewed as unrewarding or inadequate.

A related diagnosis is Rape-Trauma Syndrome.

Sexual Dysfunction as the Problem

Before a nursing diagnosis can be made regarding a sexual problem, the assessment data collected by the nurse must be carefully reviewed to determine whether the situation can be corrected by independent nursing interventions. Although many problems of sexuality experienced by a patient in a healthcare situation are amenable to nursing action, some require the expertise of other specialties. For example, an impotent diabetic patient who would benefit from a penile implant needs medical consultation. A patient with a serious sexual dysfunction or one who practices a destructive sexual expression needs intensive therapy by a clinical psychologist, sex therapist, or counselor. Appropriate referrals by the nurse should follow the identification of such problems.

Sexual dysfunction may be specified as erectile failure (impotence); premature ejaculation; retarded ejaculation; inhibited sexual desire; orgasmic dysfunction; vaginismus; or dyspareunia. Common etiologies for sexual dysfunction include effects of medication (specify); effects of alcohol consumption; effects of disease process (specify); history of abuse (specify rape, incest); feelings of depression; guilt; anxiety; fear of rejection; miscommunication with partner; fear of pain; effects of birth control method (specify); lack of knowledge; or effects of surgical procedure (specify).

The nursing diagnosis Altered Sexuality Patterns can be further specified by loss of desire (to abstinence); increased desire (to promiscuity); or change in sexual expression. Common etiologies for Altered Sexuality Patterns include stress (lifestyle, job, family, finances, marital conflict); isolation from partner; effects of pregnancy (specify); feelings of depression; loss of privacy; loss of communication with partner; relationship change (new partner); effects of disease process (sexual position, frequency, mode of expression); change in body image; change in self-concept; or loss of partner. A representative sample of some nursing diagnoses concerning sexuality is given in the accompanying display.

Sexual Dysfunction as the Etiology

Changes in sexuality can affect other areas of human functioning. In the following nursing diagnoses, problems of sexuality are the etiology of another problem:

Impaired Adjustment related to loss of sexual partner, loss of sexual body part

Anxiety related to fear of pregnancy, loss of sexual functioning or desire, effects of disease process on sexual functioning

Pain related to sexual position, penile penetration, effects of genital surgery, lack of vaginal lubrication

Ineffective Individual Coping related to effects of body image on sexual expression, change in sexual partner

Fear related to pain during sexual intercourse, history of sexual abuse

Anticipatory Grieving related to loss of sexual functioning, effects of surgical excision of genital body part

Altered Growth and Development related to sexual exploitation or abuse, sexual guilt, effects of hormonal imbalance, lack of information about sexuality

Knowledge Deficit (specify: Contraceptive Methods, Spread of STDs, Sexual Response, Genital Anatomy, Modes of Sexual Expression, Self-Examination, Effects of Disease or Medications) related to misinformation, sexual myths, lack of interest in learning, cognitive limitation

Body Image Disturbance (specify: Surgical Excision of Genital Body Part, Loss of or Gain in Body Weight) related to fear of rejection

Impaired Social Interaction related to effects of marital separation or divorce

Social Isolation related to fear of contraction of STD, fear of sexual encounter

PLANNING: EXPECTED OUTCOMES

Nurses should value sexuality as an important aspect of who the patient is and how the patient is identified as a unique human. Specific patient goals/outcomes to promote sexual health follow. The patient will achieve the following:

- Define individual sexuality
- Establish open patterns of communication with significant others
- Develop self-awareness and body awareness
- Describe responsible sexual health self-care practices, identifying appropriate resources
- Practice responsible sexual expression (eg, by 5/1/02, the patient will use rubber condoms with all sexual encounters)

Specific patient goals/outcomes will depend on the nature of the patient's problem or concern. Expected outcomes should be patient oriented, that is, something the patient desires to do or has the ability to accomplish. For example, it is not enough to advise a method of birth control; rather, the nurse needs to know which method the patient is motivated and able to use.

IMPLEMENTING

Establishing a Trusting Nurse–Patient Relationship

It is impossible to address or help a patient's sexuality if trust has not been developed between the nurse and the patient (see the accompanying box, Through the Eyes of a Student). The nurse needs to project an objective, nonthreatening, and nonjudgmental attitude and an aura of confidentiality. Anticipating patient concerns and needs through awareness of his or her behavior and verbal and nonverbal cues also helps the patient trust the nurse later on with information

Nursing Diagnoses for Common Problems

Sexuality

Problem	*Related Factors*	*Sample Defining Characteristics*
Sexual Dysfunction: Erectile Failure	Use of antihypertensive medication	• 45-year-old man with 3-year history of hypertension • Maintained normotensive on reserpine, 0.25 mg daily • "I have had trouble keeping an erection. My wife and I haven't made love in months. We don't talk about it anymore. I guess that part of my life is over." • Patient appears resigned and saddened.
Sexual Dysfunction: Dyspareunia	Effects of menopausal process	• 54-year-old woman whose last menses was 1 year ago • "Whenever my husband and I make love, my vagina burns and stings." • States decrease in vaginal lubrication during past several months
Altered Sexuality Patterns: Change in Sexual Expression	Loss of privacy due to hospitalization	• 23-year-old man hospitalized for past 6 weeks with injuries resulting from car crash; has been in traction for fractured right femur • "I can't take this place anymore! Everyone barges in here whenever they want to—nobody cares about my feelings—a guy can't even act like a guy around here. I wish I could be alone with my wife for a while with no interruptions."
Altered Sexuality Patterns: Loss of Desire	Change in body image due to body-altering surgery	• Surgery for bowel cancer with construction of permanent colostomy 1 month ago • "I know the colostomy was necessary to save my life, but it is so disgusting. I'll never be able to have a relationship with my husband again. It's a real turn-off to me—just imagine what he'll think—how can I expect him to want to make love to a freak?"
Alteration in Comfort: Pain	Abduction of hips in sexual positioning	• 60-year-old woman with history of osteoarthritis for 6 years • "The act of intercourse hurts my hips so bad that I'm in pain the whole next day. I don't want to stop having intercourse with my husband, but I'm going to have to if this pain gets worse." • Patient states that the missionary position is the only position used during sex with her husband throughout their 40-year-marriage.

of an intimate nature. It is important to establish respect for the individual and empathy before sexual topics are discussed. An empathic nurse considers all of an individual's circumstances and life experiences and views them from a therapeutic, not a pitying, approach. Only when the nurse is accepted as a trusted, caring person will the patient relay details of his or her private life, including concerns of a sexual nature.

Teaching About Sexuality and Sexual Health

Most nursing interventions pertaining to a patient's sexuality encompass teaching to promote sexual health. Major goals of patient teaching are a change in knowledge, a change in patient attitude, or a change in behaviors. In some situations, patients need assistance in defining or redefining their sexuality and its importance to their lives.

Through the Eyes of a Student

I knew it was going to happen sooner or later. Male nurses are not unheard of in this day and age, but some people just aren't yet ready for us. Especially Ethel, a 68-year-old black woman with a deep religious conviction. I concluded this because she called on Jesus for help when I told her that I was her student nurse for the day, and that I would be giving her a bath.

"You're my nurse?" she said. "Help me, Jesus. . . . No, no, you just go on and help somebody else, honey. I've already had my bath," she insisted.

Accordingly, I told her she was mistaken and that I understood her anxiety. Then I proceeded to exaggerate the truth by saying that I had done this before, when really I had given baths before, but not to members of the opposite sex. She thought *she* was having anxiety!

Next I asked my instructor, Lynn, for help. She quickly assessed the situation and tried to comfort Ethel by vouching for my professional character and abilities, but still no go. Then I tried appealing to her logic.

"This is a hospital where male doctors examine you all the time. Why is this any different?" I asked. "Because you are *not* a doctor" was her logical reply.

I felt inadequate. I could not give this woman the care she needed because of my gender. Luckily, in the next bed, Michele was about to give her patient a bath. She offered to give Ethel her bath if I would help her with her patients.

Consequently, Ethel got her bath, and I learned that a nurse has to be flexible as well as willing to ask for and accept help when the patient's quality of care is at stake. This is something I hope to remember throughout my nursing career.

—DANIEL E. ZIROLLI,
DELAWARE COUNTY COMMUNITY COLLEGE,
MEDIA, PENNSYLVANIA

Offering information, dispelling fears, and providing positive reinforcement are some ways nurses can assist patients to increase their knowledge about their bodies and sexual functioning. Patients may need assistance in modifying behaviors or learning new skills to increase the quality of sexual health and functioning.

Correcting Sexual Myths and Promoting Body Awareness

Many people believe things about sex that they have heard from family or friends or as part of their culture that are simply not true or not based on scientific data. The nurse may refute sexual myths (Table 34-5) and teach factual information during the assessment or while providing care.

Patients may need assistance in becoming familiar with what they believe and feel about their sexual selves. The nurse can be helpful in a situation in which a patient has difficulty accepting or developing his or her sexuality by promoting self-confidence and a good self-concept in the patient. When patients feel comfortable about themselves and their sensual feelings, they can begin to focus on how they feel about their sexual functioning and specific sexual expressions.

Getting to know one's physical body is important to healthy sexual development. Every man and woman, sexually active or not, needs to be aware of the appearance of his or her individual genitalia. Some people, because of their background, feel ashamed and repulsed by their bodies; others feel that touching the body is dirty and may feel guilt and anxiety in stimulating themselves. Patients need assistance in improving body awareness if any of these issues are present. Patients become accustomed to looking at their bodies by looking at nonthreatening anatomy first and then proceeding to the genitals. This can be done in the shower or with the use of a mirror. Knowing what looks normal can be of great importance in reporting the development of an unusual appearance later on. After patients have developed some degree of comfort in looking at their bodies, they can progress to experiencing touch. Again, patients should progress from nonthreatening parts of the body until the genitals can be touched without stress.

A good exercise for women in developing body awareness is the use of Kegel exercises. These exercises promote good vaginal tone by localizing and strengthening the pubococcygeal muscle. A woman can locate this muscle by stopping a stream of urine midway through urination. Contracting this muscle can be repeated at any time of the day in any circumstance because its performance is undetectable. Women who practice Kegel exercises have found that sexual satisfaction is greatly improved.

Teaching Self-Examination

It is important for both men and women to learn to examine themselves through inspection and palpation of sexual body parts. Many conditions, some life-threatening, can be detected when self-examination is performed. Early detection of cancer is crucial to its control and cure. The presence of some STDs may also be detected by self-examination.

Breast Self-Examination

The importance of breast self-examination (BSE) lies in its routine monthly performance, which helps the person to become familiar with what is normal. BSE should be performed after each menses or once a month for a postmenopausal woman. Any contact with a female patient in

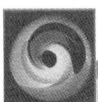

Table 34-5
Sexual Myths and Facts to Refute Them

Sexual Dysfunction	Assessment Priorities
Each person is born with a certain amount of sexual drive, which if overdrawn in youth leaves little reserve for later years.	Actually, the correlation between sexual activity and length of time it persists throughout life is just the opposite. The more consistently sexually active a person is, the longer the activity continues into the later years of life.
The need for expressing one's sexuality becomes less important in the latter half of one's life.	Physiologically, sexual desire and ability do not decrease markedly after middle age. The expression of one's sexuality, as an integral part of development, follows the overall pattern of health and physical performance.
Sexual abstinence is necessary in training for sports.	Physiologically, the achievement of orgasm is rarely more demanding than most activities encountered in daily life. The desire for sleep that often follows is most commonly due to factors other than physical exhaustion from sexual activities. There is no scientific evidence that sex "weakens" a person.
Excessive sexual activity can lead to mental illness.	The biologic significance of human sexuality has no greater effect on total development than any other necessary biologic function. There is no scientific basis for believing that one will develop a mental or physical illness with excessive or no sexual activity.
Wet dreams are indicators of sexual disorders.	Erotic dreams that culminate in orgasms are normal common physiologic phenomena in at least 85% of men. They can occur at any age after puberty. Some women also report in clinical studies that their sexual dreams culminate in orgasm. In women, this phenomenon is believed to increase with advancing age.
Because of the anatomic nature of the sex organs, women are passive and men are aggressive.	Physiologic studies disprove this myth by showing the woman to be far from passive. Maximum gratification requires each partner to be both passive and aggressive in participating mutually and cooperatively.
It is unnatural for a woman to have as strong a desire for sex as a man—women should not enjoy sex as much as men.	These myths have been reinforced by a society that has traditionally taught women that they are to suppress sexual desires to gain love, security, and society's respect, based on the assumption that it is the basic nature of women to be submissive, dependent, and subordinate. Physiologic studies indicate that, in some respects, the woman's sex drive is not only as strong but may be even stronger than that of the man.
Women who have multiple orgasms or who readily come to climax are nymphomaniacs or promiscuous.	Physiologic studies at this time suggest that we do not know women's sexual potential; these studies indicate that there is a wide range of intensity and duration of orgasmic experience, and the potential for multiple or frequent orgasms within a brief period is not at all uncommon. Therefore, women normally may have greater orgasmic capacity than men with regard to duration and frequency of orgasm.
There is a difference between vaginal orgasm and clitoral orgasm.	Physiologic misunderstanding has produced the myth of separate clitoral and vaginal orgasms rather than their interrelations. Female orgasm is normally initiated by clitoral stimulation, but because it is a total-body response, there are marked variations in intensity and timing. There is no reason to believe that the female response to the sex act is due to a vaginal rather than a clitoral orgasm.
A mature sexual relationship requires the man and woman to achieve simultaneous orgasm.	Although simultaneous orgasm may be desirable, it is unrealistic. Often, it is possible only under the most ideal circumstances and is not a determinant of sexual achievement or of satisfaction (except to someone who accepts this as dogma).
It is dangerous to have intercourse during menstruation.	Because the source of the menstrual flow is from the uterus rather than the vagina, there is no basis for concern about tissue damage to the vagina. Actually, the desire for sex increases during the menses as a result of increased pelvic vasocongestion. There is no physiologic basis for abstinence during the menses.
The larger penis has greater possibilities for producing orgasm in the woman.	Physiologically, there is practically no relation between the size of a man's penis and his ability to satisfy a woman sexually. Furthermore, there is little correlation between penile size and body size and their relation to sexual potency.
The face-to-face coital position is the proper, moral, and healthy one.	Recent knowledge of human sexual practices dispels this myth with the recognition that there is no normal or single most acceptable sexual position. Whatever position offers the most pleasure and is acceptable to both partners is correct for them. Any variation is normal, healthy, and proper if it satisfies both partners.
The ability to achieve orgasm is an indicator of a person's sexual responsiveness.	Achievement of a satisfactory sexual response is the result of numerous physical, psychological, and cultural influences. Too often, the physical fact of orgasm (or lack of orgasm) is taken to be symbolic of sexual responsiveness and seen out of context of the entire relationship between man and woman.

the healthcare delivery system should include assessment of her knowledge and practice of BSE. See the accompanying Research in Nursing box.

The steps in performing BSE are shown in Figure 34-3 and are as follows:

1. Stand before a mirror with hands on hips to inspect the breasts. Look for the presence of indentations, dimpling, or odd position of a nipple. Any discharge from a nipple is abnormal unless the woman is nursing. Changes in size or shape of breasts should be reported.

2. Lie on the bed with a small pillow under the shoulder on the side of the breast to be examined and the arm over the head. Using the opposite hand, palpate the breast starting at the outer edge of the breast, using small circular motions of the flat portions of the fingers. Work inward in a clockwise manner toward the nipple. The nipple should be gently squeezed to detect the presence of any discharge. This procedure should be repeated for the opposite breast. Any unusual lump or tenderness should be reported to a healthcare professional.

Testicular Self-Examination

Male patients need to be taught to perform monthly assessment of the testicles. Although testicular cancer is not widespread, it can be easily detected, and its prognosis is good if found early. A good time to examine the testes is during a shower, when the scrotum becomes warm and loose. Men should also be taught the importance of examining their breasts.

The steps in testicular self-examination (TSE), shown in Figure 34-4, are as follows:

1. The thumb and the fingers of each hand are used to palpate each testicle simultaneously. The patient should systematically palpate the testes for the presence of lumps or differences in texture. The testes should feel smooth.

2. The epididymis is palpated above each testicle. The epididymis feels soft and not as smooth as a testicle.

3. The spermatic cord, or vas deferens, extends upward from the scrotum toward the base of the penis and should be palpated for firmness and smoothness in texture.

Considering Contraception

Patients choose **contraception** for many reasons and may contact healthcare providers for information on birth control or contraceptive methods. Some people use contraception for the orderly spacing of pregnancies in a family. Others use a contraceptive method to prevent pregnancy from occurring until a family is desired. Some people choose a permanent method to prevent pregnancy from ever occurring. Factors that affect choice of a contraceptive method include age, marital status, desire for future pregnancy, religious beliefs, level of education, cost, and ease of use. Other considerations are the woman's knowledge about available methods, her perceptions of the various methods, and, in many cases, her previous experience with contraception.

The safest and most effective method available to prevent a pregnancy is sexual abstinence. For many people, however, this is not an acceptable method. All contraceptive methods have distinct advantages and disadvantages. It is the responsibility of the nurse to understand and explain thoroughly the available methods so that the patient can choose one that will best meet his or her unique situation

---

RESEARCH IN NURSING: MAKING A DIFFERENCE

Promoting Breast Health Education and Screening

Millions of people today are using the Internet to gather information to manage their health. Potentially, these individuals are a rich source of research data. Nurses knowledgeable about the advantages and disadvantages of collecting research data using the Internet will have an innovative way to reach both a national and international population of women while containing research costs.

Related Research

Thomas, B., Stamler, L. L., Lafreniere, K., & Dumala, R. (2000). The Internet: An effective tool for nursing research with women. *Computers in Nursing, 18*(1), 13–18.
This study outlines the methodology of using the Internet to survey an international population of

women about their perceptions of breast health education and screening. A large population of women from North America and elsewhere was reached through the establishment of a website with linkages to other sites frequented by women. Anonymity was guaranteed, and simple instructions were provided at the site. Investigators found the Internet to be an appropriate medium for health-related research that also garnered national and international media interest.

Relevance for Practice

The increased use of electronic networking and collaborative problem solving through various national and international linkages may be the hallmark of healthcare professionals in the 21st century.

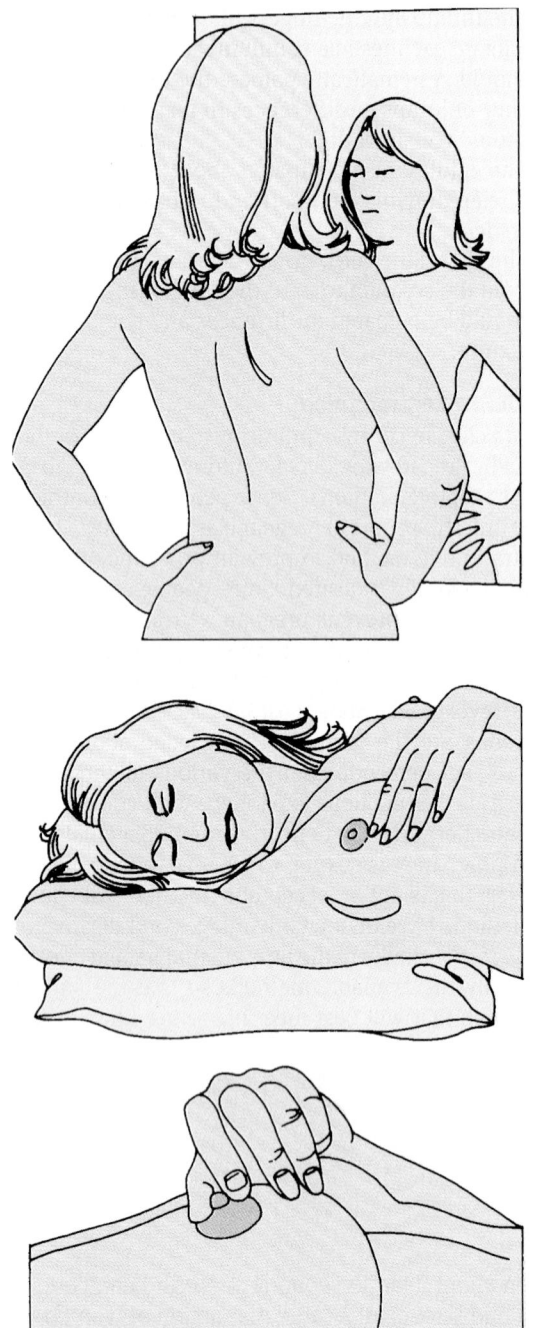

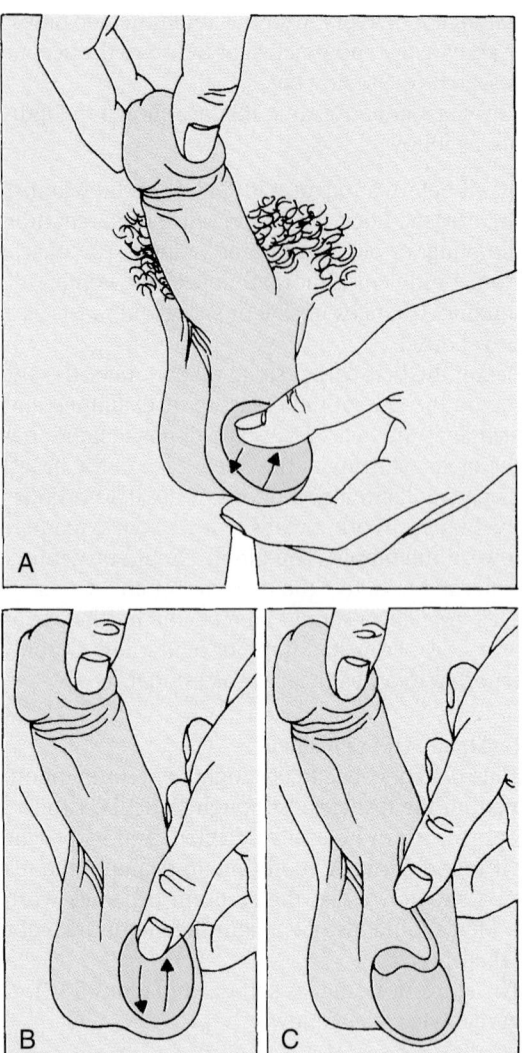

Figure 34-3
Breast self-examination is to be performed once a month. It is begun with inspection using a mirror. Attention is given to contours of the breast and to the skin. Pressing down on the hips serves to tense pectoralis major muscles to inspect for any retraction of the skin. Palpatory examination is performed in a supine position with the side to be examined elevated on a pillow or blanket. Self-examination is completed with a squeeze of the nipple to detect abnormal discharge.

Figure 34-4
Testicular self-examination is to be performed once a month. A convenient time is after a warm bath or shower when the scrotum is relaxed. Both hands are used to palpate the testis; the normal testicle is smooth and uniform is consistency. (**A**) With the index and middle finger under the testis and the thumb on top, roll the testis gently in a horizontal plane between the thumb and fingers, feeling for any evidence of a small lump or abnormality. (**B**) Follow the same procedure for palpation in the vertical plane. (**C**) Locate the epididymis (cordlike structure on the top and back of the testicle that stores and transports sperm). Repeat the examination for the other testis; it is normal to find one testis larger than the other. Any evidence of a small, pea-sized lump should be checked by a physician. It may be due to an infection or a tumor growth.

and needs (see the accompanying box, Knowledge Deficit: Contraceptive Methods).

Natural Family Planning

Natural family planning methods are available to everyone, but using them effectively requires motivation and understanding of male and female reproductive anatomy and physiology. There are four basic natural family planning methods: *calendar* (rhythm method), *basal body temperature* (BBT), *ovulation* (Billing's method), and *symptothermal.*

The rhythm, or calendar, method is based on a woman's monthly menstrual cycle in determining safe and unsafe days. It is an inappropriate method for a woman with irregular cycles. The unsafe days are regarded as periods for sexual abstinence because they are optimal for conception.

Knowledge Deficit: Contraceptive Methods

Assessment Priorities

- Determine past use of contraceptive methods.
- Assess effectiveness and satisfaction with past methods.
- Assess the patient's current knowledge of contraceptive methods.
- Assess frequency of the patient's sexual activity.
- Identify any methods that are unacceptable to the patient.
- Assess motivation of the patient to use certain methods.
- Assess the patient's level of comfort with manipulation of genital body parts.
- Obtain complete patient history and perform a physical examination if indicated.

Expected Outcomes

The patient will achieve the following:

- Choose a contraceptive method that the patient is motivated to use.
- List the adverse effects or danger signs associated with the contraceptive method.
- List the steps needed to use the contraceptive method effectively.
- Use the contraceptive with every act of sexual intercourse.
- Choose a back-up method.
- Report back to the healthcare setting for follow-up as directed.

Nursing Interventions

- Describe in terms at the patient's level of understanding each contraceptive method for which the patient needs information (give objective information in matter-of-fact manner to avoid bias by nurse).
- Describe the effectiveness of each method and side effects or possible complications.
- Instruct the patient in the use of a chosen method, giving step-by-step instructions.
- Advise the patient of the importance of having a back-up method on hand.
- Instruct the patient in the use of the back-up method.
- Have the patient obtain a physical examination if indicated by the chosen contraceptive method (eg, the pill).
- Instruct the patient to report back in a specified period for follow-up of use of method if indicated (follow-up visits to a healthcare facility are important, particularly if a patient elects to use the pill).

The BBT method is based on the body's response to hormones and ovulation. The woman takes and records her temperature on awakening every morning. A sudden drop in temperature indicates ovulation. This method restricts sexual activity to the second half of the menstrual cycle after ovulation has occurred. The Billing's method is based on the changes in the cervical mucus throughout the menstrual cycle. As ovulation occurs, the mucus changes considerably in consistency, becoming sticky, clear, and slippery like an egg white. This method requires the woman to be aware of and have the ability to assess her cervical mucus. The symptothermal method combines a number of signs of ovulation, including the rise in BBT, changes in cervical mucus, and variations of the cervix. Both the ovulation and symptothermal methods can be effective in avoiding pregnancy if mutual understanding, support, and motivation exist between the woman and her partner (Fehring, 1991).

Coitus interruptus, one of the oldest and most widely used contraceptive methods, is the withdrawal of the penis from the vagina before ejaculation. Its drawbacks include the possibility of the presence of sperm in Cowper's gland secretions before ejaculation and the stress it places on the man's sexual experience.

Barrier Methods

Barrier methods include the condom, diaphragm, cervical cap, and vaginal sponge used in combination with a spermicidal agent. The *diaphragm* has been used in various forms since ancient times. It is currently marketed as a large, dome-shaped device made of latex rubber that mechanically prevents semen from coming into contact with the cervix. It is also used to hold a quantity of spermicidal jelly in place against the cervix. The diaphragm is placed in the vagina before sexual activity. It fits between the pelvic notch at the front of the vagina to behind the cervix at the back. It should not be detected by either the woman or her partner when correctly situated in the vagina. A diaphragm must be individually fitted at a pelvic examination. The woman needs to be familiar with her body and able to handle her genitals for diaphragm placement and removal. The diaphragm must be worn during each episode of sexual activity and consistently used with a spermicidal agent.

The traditional *condom*, or "rubber," is used by men, although it is appropriate for a woman to have them available for her partner's use. The condom is rolled over the erect penis and collects the semen after ejaculation occurs. If the condom does not have a nipple receptacle end, leave a small space at the end of the condom to collect sperm (this prevents breakage). Condoms are available over the counter and have had a surge of popularity with the recent increase in incidence of AIDS and other STDs among single people. A new female condom, known as the *vaginal pouch*, may offer women greater protection from STDs than male condoms and equal protection from unwanted pregnancy.

The *cervical cap* is not universally available. Its mechanism of action is similar to that of the diaphragm. The cervical cap is a thimble-shaped rubber device that is placed over the cervix and may be left there for up to 3 days at a time. Not all women can wear a cervical cap because of individual anatomic differences. There is some evidence to suggest that the cervical cap can cause cervical inflammation and increase the risk for pelvic infection.

Spermicides are used with barrier methods but can also be used alone. Spermicides come in creams, jellies, foams, and suppositories. Although readily available, spermicides are not as effective alone as when combined with another method, such as a diaphragm or a condom.

The *vaginal sponge* is a barrier method that contains a spermicide. It has been available over the counter for several years. The sponge not only acts as a barrier between the semen and the cervix but also serves as a reservoir to hold semen. The vaginal sponge carries some risk of toxic shock syndrome (TSS) and is contraindicated for use in women who have a past history of TSS. It is important for women who use the vaginal sponge to follow package directions carefully and to remove the sponge within 24 hours. The vaginal sponge is about as effective as the diaphragm.

Intrauterine Device

The *intrauterine device* (IUD) is an object that is placed by a physician or nurse practitioner within the uterus to prevent implantation of fertilized ovum. The precise mechanism by which it works is unknown. Although it has a high effectiveness rate and requires little care or motivation on the part of the patient, the IUD has many serious side effects and resulting complications. It is an excellent method for women who have completed their families but are not ready or willing to take the final step toward sterilization. Owing to the litigation resulting from complications caused by the IUD, it has been taken off the market by most IUD-producing pharmaceutical companies. Although the IUD may reappear in the future, all women who currently have an IUD in place should seek assistance from a healthcare provider to have it removed. Women wearing a Progestasert IUD should check for the presence of the string in the vagina after every menses and should have the IUD replaced every year.

Hormonal Methods

Hormonal methods are based on the feedback mechanism of hormones of the menstrual cycle. Synthetic estrogens and progestin chemical compounds are used in the form of a pill, shot, or implant to prevent ovulation.

The *oral contraceptive* ("the pill") is the most common contraceptive method and the most popular method for women in their twenties. Most of the harmful side effects and dangers associated with taking the pill are related to the estrogen component. However, most pills currently available contain a small dose of 35 mg of estrogen. The pill has many beneficial noncontraceptive effects. It has been shown to protect women against the development of breast, ovarian, and endometrial cancer. Taken consistently and as prescribed, the pill is almost 100% effective in guarding against pregnancy. However, the cost may be prohibitive to some women. The woman must also be motivated to take a pill every day at the same time. A health history and physical examination by a healthcare provider are necessary to obtain a prescription for oral contraceptives. Some women should not take the pill in the presence of certain physiologic disorders or diseases. Smoking increases the risks associated with oral contraceptives.

Vaccines

As this text goes to print, there is news that a contraceptive vaccine is being developed that would make the woman's egg immune to sperm and confer immunity for about 3 years with an 85% effectiveness rate.

Sterilization

Although male and female sterilization methods can be surgically reversed, the results are not always satisfactory, and these methods should therefore be regarded as permanent and irreversible. Sexual desire and ability are unaffected by sterilization.

Sterilization in the woman is accomplished by surgically severing the fallopian tubes. This procedure is known as a *tubal ligation* and prevents travel of the ovum down the tube. Tubal ligation is usually performed on an outpatient basis. Some physicians can also perform the tubal ligation under local anesthesia. Postoperative care and recovery time are required after a tubal ligation.

Sterilization in the man is accomplished by surgically severing the vas deferens, which prevents sperm from entering the semen. The *vasectomy* is usually performed in a physician's office under local anesthesia. It is important that the man know that he and his partner must use an alternative form of contraception until he has produced two semen analyses with zero sperm. It usually takes about 4 to 6 weeks for all stored sperm to be eliminated from the ductal system of the male.

Coerced Contraception

Implantable long-lasting contraceptives that gradually release progestin for up to 5 years, such as Norplant, are currently available. Because effectiveness does not depend on patient compliance and use can be monitored easily by checking for the implants in the woman's arm, Norplant immediately initiated controversy in the press, legislative arena, and courts for fear it might be used for coerced contraception. Some suggested the use of financial incentives for welfare recipients who agreed to use Norplant; others recommended its use as part of a sentence or plea agreement for offenses such as child abuse, child endangerment, and murder. At issue is whether an individual's right to privacy outweighs the state's interest in limiting unwanted pregnancies.

Future Trends

Almost 40 million women in the United States are at risk for unintended pregnancy. More than half of the 6.3 million pregnancies that occur annually in the United States are unintended. Of this number, nearly half occur in women who currently use some means of birth control. In view of the fact that unintended pregnancies are as likely to end in abortion as in birth, there is a clear need to focus on unintended pregnancy prevention. Future trends in contraception are likely to be shaped in part by increased awareness of STDs and continuation of the AIDS pandemic. For at-risk women, the emphasis will be on a highly effective primary means of contraception used in conjunction with a barrier method, such as the condom, to prevent STDs.

Facilitating Coping With Special Sexual Needs

The nurse can do much for patients to facilitate their coping with sexual concerns generated by diseases and their treatments. Anticipatory guidance and information should be offered to the patient. The importance of open communication with the partner should be stressed. The nurse should include the partner in teaching. Discussion about possible sexual positions is useful and can aid in eliminating pain during coitus. The patient can use drawings in selecting possible sexual positions. The patient will also find that intercourse may be more comfortable if pain medication is taken before beginning any sexual activity.

When teaching patients about medications, it is important to include known possible sexual alterations to prevent future anxiety and also depression. Patients should alert their physicians if these side effects are experienced. Often, a drug dosage can be modified or the drug changed if sexual functioning is affected; otherwise, patients may opt to discontinue the medication on their own rather than sacrifice optimal sexual functioning, if this is an important aspect of life.

Nurses also need to be aware of the special concerns and issues surrounding the care of a homosexual patient. Homosexuals have the same right to healthcare, information, and confidentiality as do heterosexuals.

Teaching Responsible Sexual Expression

Patients need to know how best to gain satisfactory sexual experiences and yet behave responsibly in their activities. Responsible sexuality encompasses these major areas: the form of sexual expression, the prevention of unwanted pregnancy, the prevention of spread of STDs, and sex education.

The form of sexual expression used by patients should not inflict unwanted harm on themselves or others. When the sexual expression encroaches on the rights of others, it is neither healthy nor desirable. Sexual acts that violate another's rights are usually considered to be acts of aggression or hostility rather than stemming from sexual need or desire. Acts of rape in particular are motivated by the need to dominate and humiliate the victim.

The prevention of an unwanted pregnancy must be a conscious decision. Anyone considering the possibility of a sexual encounter who is unprepared for pregnancy should refrain from intercourse or obtain a contraceptive method either from a healthcare provider or from the pharmacy; it is too late to think about contraception during sexual intercourse. To practice responsible sexuality, the contraceptive method must be used consistently and according to instructions.

The incidence of the various STDs is widespread. The only absolute method to avoid an STD is to remain a virgin until marriage, to marry a person who is a virgin, and thereafter never to have sex with anyone else. When this is impractical, other practices that can decrease a person's exposure to STDs are the following:

- The patient should limit the number of sexual partners. The risk for an STD rises with the addition of each new partner.
- If a partner has symptoms of an STD, the patient should abstain from any sexual activity.
- If the patient is in doubt about possible exposure, or she should report to a healthcare facility for examination.
- If the patient does contract an STD, all partners should be notified and advised to seek treatment.
- The use of condoms is advocated for protection against STDs as well as against pregnancy. The patient should keep a box of condoms on hand if monogamy is not practiced within the relationship.

Sex education is critical to healthy sexual development and safe sexual behaviors. See the accompanying box on teaching safe sex activities. Information received from peers and friends is almost always inadequate and erroneous. Parents should be taught to answer children's questions immediately and accurately.

Advocating Sexuality Needs of Patients

A hospital experience or institutionalization puts a strain on a person's individuality and sexual self. Illness may diminish feelings of sexual desire. Therefore, it can be a sign of a patient's improving health if sexual interaction is desired with the partner. This necessitates anticipatory guidance on the part of the nurse because many patients

Using the Nursing Interventions Classification (NIC)

Selected Teaching: Safe Sex Activities

- Discuss patient's attitudes about various birth control methods
- Instruct patient on the use of effective birth control methods, as appropriate.
- Incorporate religious beliefs into discussion of birth control, as appropriate.
- Discuss abstention as a means of birth control, as appropriate.
- Encourage patient to be selective when choosing sexual partners, as appropriate.
- Stress the importance of knowing the partner's sexual history, as appropriate.
- Instruct patient on low-risk sexual practices, such as those that avoid bodily penetration or the exchange of bodily fluids, as appropriate.
- Instruct patient on the importance of good hygiene, lubrication, and voiding after intercourse, to decrease susceptibility to infections.
- Plan sex education classes for groups of patients as appropriate.

(From McCloskey, J., & Bulechek, G. [2000]. *Nursing interventions classification [NIC]* [3rd ed]. [p. 654]. St. Louis: C. V. Mosby. A full listing of nursing activities for each nursing intervention can be found in this book.)

may hesitate to make such a request for fear of being ridiculed. Often, a patient merely desires the privacy to hold and caress the partner. The intimacy of this act often fulfills feelings of longing to be needed and loved.

There are many ways nurses can advocate for a patient's sexual needs. Some may seem obvious and commonplace, whereas others may necessitate nurses' coming to terms with their own sexuality (see the accompanying box, Advocating Patients' Sexual Needs).

Counseling the Patient Regarding Sexuality

Not all patients with sexual concerns need intensive therapy. Some patients benefit greatly from the presence of another to listen to verbally expressed concerns. Voicing their concerns allows patients the opportunity to put information into perspective and gain a clearer focus on what the problem really is and how to solve it. Nurses counseling patients need to refrain from offering their own advice because what is right for one person may be wrong for another. Also, offering false reassurances, such as "It will be all right," is unproductive. Rather, the nurse needs to adopt an objective, empathic, and receptive attitude to facilitate an open communication between nurse and patient.

Annon (cited in Hatcher et al., 1990) developed a model, termed PLISSIT, for counseling to be used by therapists and nontherapists for patients with sexual problems. The four stages to this model, each increasing in intensity

Advocating Patients' Sexual Needs

- All patients should be accepted as sexual beings with the right to be treated with dignity and with sensitivity to their feelings.
- All patients have the right to some degree of privacy.
    Anticipate the patient's desire for privacy by the simple act of drawing a curtain or closing a door.
    Patients should be given the option of wearing their own sleepwear to promote sexual identity.
- Potentially shaming situations for the patient should be anticipated.
    Give information regarding what the procedure is and why it needs to be done, and acknowledge that the patient's embarrassment is normal and understandable.
- Healthcare providers should not simply take for granted that patients do not mind intrusive or embarrassing procedures performed on their bodies and private parts.
- Patients have a right to question the physician regarding sexual needs or future sexual functioning.
    Anticipate these questions for the patient.

    Ask patients if they have any concerns regarding sexuality that can be answered by the nurse. Nurses can interface with the physician to obtain information required by the patient.
- The atmosphere in healthcare settings needs to allow for sexual expression between patients and their partners.
- Confidentiality is a right of every patient.
    Do not promise confidentiality if that promise cannot be kept.
    Allow no one access to the patient's personal records who is not directly involved in the patient's care.
    Allow no information regarding patients to escape into idle conversation.
- All patients should be referred to formally as Mr., Mrs., Miss, Ms., according to the patient's preference.
- Visitors, including a visiting spouse, should be referred to as people with genders, rather than as "the visitor."
- Patients should be allowed to keep some personal possessions, if it is practical to do so.

Model for Counseling Patients With Sexual Problems (PLISSIT)

P—*Permission giving:* The nurse may make a suggestion that the patient can use. Permission giving is not the same as advice. Permission giving implies giving the patient freedom to choose to do something that the authority figure (such as a nurse) deems to be a positive alternative. It may be something the patient wanted to do all along. For example,

Patient: "Aren't some sexual positions perverted?" *Nurse:* "Many people enjoy using different positions for sex. Some positions are more pleasurable to some couples than others. You and your partner have the right to use any position for sex that you desire."

LI—*Limited information:* Specific factual information is required by the patient. It often involves some aspect of anatomy and physiology or the specifics of certain sexual expressions.

SS—*Specific suggestions:* Patients need very specific instructions regarding a useful technique. Many patients have a sexual dysfunction for which they are seeking intervention and correction.

IT—*Intensive therapy:* Used primarily by therapists, it involves issues such as marriage, self-concept, and sexual desire, to name a few. If the first three levels of counseling presented were unsuccessful, intensive therapy is indicated.

with the seriousness of the patient's problem, are listed in the accompanying box.

EVALUATING

To evaluate the plan of care for the patient's sexuality needs, the nurse needs to use information from the patient for most patient goals/outcomes. It is unrealistic and inappropriate for the nurse to evaluate the patient by observing the patient's expression of his or her sexuality. However, the nurse can evaluate how the patient is progressing toward sexuality-oriented goals by appearance, level of self-confidence, and manner. For example, a patient who has expressed feelings of anxiety in the past over a sexual concern should be observably more confident and free of anxiety if patient goals are being met. The nurse also needs to question the patient about progress toward goals. Some goals need to be "stepping stones" because not all problems are easily resolved with one-time intervention and direction.

One line of questioning when evaluating a patient's progress is as follows: "In what ways have you been able to achieve [orgasm, increased desire, comfortable intercourse, erection]?" "What methods seemed most effective?" "Which were not?" "What do you think should be the next step?" The nurse should determine from this interaction with the patient whether something more needs to be accomplished. It is not enough to assume that because a set of goals has been met, the patient is satisfied with the results. See the accompanying Applying Learning to Practice: Patient Care Study and Nursing Plan of Care boxes.

APPLYING LEARNING TO PRACTICE

Patient Care Study

Pete is a 13-year-old adolescent boy attending the area health clinic. He is nervous as he explains to the nurse his need for healthcare. He has noticed "sticky white stuff" around his penis and bedclothes on arising some mornings and fears he may be ill. Pete has also expressed concern about his lack of knowledge regarding sexuality. He has heard a lot of stories from his friends but does not feel he can talk to his parents because the subject has never been broached at home. Also, although Pete is a virgin, he is beginning to feel pressured by his friends, who boast of many sexual experiences.

After spending time in conversation with Pete, the nurse gathered the following data:

- Pete is experiencing nocturnal emissions and has little scientific knowledge about their source.
- Pete is anxious because of the stories regarding sex he has heard from his friends.

- There is no communication or dialogue at home with parents about issues of sexuality.
- Pete is having feelings of insecurity and anxiety about his present virginal status, which he feels he should change.
- Peer pressure from friends is also a concern.

Plan of Nursing Care

The nurse will work together with Pete to develop a plan of care to correct misinformation and relieve his anxiety. Planning will be directed toward correcting myths and supplying Pete with accurate information. Because Pete has a negligible knowledge base on sexuality, the plan of care will allow for ongoing sessions to augment the initial information. The nurse should outline this plan with Pete to be certain it is acceptable to him.

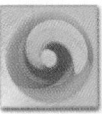

NURSING PLAN OF CARE
for Pete

Nursing Diagnosis	Knowledge Deficit: Adolescent Sexuality Concerns related to misinformation and absent family-based sex education as manifested by self-report
Expected Outcome	By the end of the teaching session, the patient will: • Describe the nature of nocturnal emissions

Nursing Interventions	Rationale	Evaluative Statement
Assess patient's present knowledge base on nocturnal emission and the source of his information.	It is necessary to discover what the patient does know and to build on that knowledge.	8/1/02 Goal met. Patient able to describe the source of nocturnal emissions. *R. Gordon, RN*
Use terms that the patient has used and language at the level of the patient's understanding.	This facilitates comprehension.	
Teach the patient about nocturnal emissions: • Nocturnal emissions, or "wet dreams," are normal in men of all ages, and they are particularly common in the teenage years. They are not the result of disease. • They occur during sleep as the result of erotic dreams. The "white sticky stuff" is the result of ejaculation of semen from the penis. • This is an involuntary action over which the male has no control.	Knowledge decreases anxiety.	

Expected Outcome	By the end of the teaching session, the patient will: • Differentiate sexual myths from sound knowledge

Nursing Interventions	Rationale	Evaluative Statement
Assess what patient has heard from peers regarding sexual information:	The nurse can then specifically address the myths to which the patient has been exposed.	8/1/02 Goal met. Patient was able to differentiate between truth in sexual issues and what is myth. *R. Gordon, RN*
Myth 1: "A large penis is better for sex than a small one." *Truth:* No relation exists between the size of a penis and the man's ability to perform sexually. When a penis becomes erect, it reaches sufficient size to engage in sexual intercourse.	This enables the patient to develop a positive sexual body image based on fact.	

(continued)

NURSING PLAN OF CARE (Continued)
for Pete

Nursing Interventions	Rationale	Evaluative Statement
Myth 2: "Jerking off causes blindness. It is a dirty habit." *Truth:* Masturbation or self-stimulation is a natural and healthy outlet for sexual urges. Men and women of all ages masturbate. Masturbation can also teach the person what feels good and what does not. Every person has the right to masturbate if he or she wishes to do so.	The patient is given permission to engage in a sexual activity of a masturbatory nature.	
Myth 3: "It looks bad for a guy to be a virgin—everybody's doing it." *Truth:* No one, whether male or female, should feel pressured into sexual activity at any age. Engaging in sexual activity carries with it a great deal of responsibility and concerns of pregnancy and spread of sexually transmitted diseases (STDs). No one needs to know of another person's status if the person chooses not to discuss it.	The patient is given permission to abstain from sexual activity and not to feel pressured by friends. Almost 39% of teens have had sex by age 16 years.	

Expected Outcome   By the end of the teaching session, the patient will:
- List the positive aspects of abstinence in a sexual relationship

Nursing Interventions	Rationale	Evaluative Statement
Assess the patient, including previous discussion of sexual myths and knowledge.	Giving the patient all the information necessary allows him to make an informed decision.	8/1/02 Goal partially met. Patient able to list verbally all positive aspects of abstinence but is still undecided.
Instruct the patient on the positive aspects of abstinence, including the following: • Engagement in any sexual activity should be a personal decision and not the result of pressure from friends. • Abstinence will guarantee protection from pregnancy and from most sexually transmitted diseases.	Many young people think they are immune to the consequences of their actions. Therefore, it is important to stress that pregnancy and STDs are very probable results of sexual intercourse.	*Revision:* Reinforce to patient that this is a personal decision that he can make for himself with a good knowledge base. Also, he does not have to make a firm decision for or against abstinence immediately. He should take time to think about this information. *R. Gordon, RN*

(continued)

NURSING PLAN OF CARE (Continued)
for Pete

Nursing Interventions	Rationale	Evaluative Statement
• People can show affection for each other without sexual involvement.	It is difficult to understand and undertake all the implications of a sexual relationship during the teenage years. The patient learns that a successful sexual relationship requires intimacy, love, and sharing; it should not be merely an outlet for sexual feelings.	
• Every person has the right to say no.	The patient has permission to refuse an activity in which he is not sure he wishes to engage.	

Expected Outcome By the end of the teaching session, the patient will:
• Describe the correct use of rubber condoms

Nursing Interventions	Rationale	Evaluative Statement
Assess what the patient knows about rubber condoms and their use.	Since patient is undecided about whether to initiate a sexual relationship in the future, it is prudent to give him information to protect against pregnancy and STDs.	8/1/02 Goal met. Patient successfully listed the steps in using a condom. *R. Gordon, RN*
Inform the patient that rubber condoms are available over the counter in drug stores. Prices vary according to type and style.	Patient should know where to purchase condoms and the variety available.	
Teach patient the steps in using rubber condoms:	Patient should know how to use condoms safely.	
• Roll condom onto the penis as soon as it becomes erect.	Protects against sperm from secretions from Cowper's glands	
• If condom does not have a nipple receptacle end, leave a small space at end of condom to collect semen.	Provides a pocket to collect semen and prevents breakage	
• Immediately after ejaculation, remove penis and condom from vagina by holding onto base of condom.	Prevents spillage of semen into the vagina	
• Discard condom.	Condoms are not meant to be reused. A new condom is used for each act of intercourse.	
Advise the patient to use a condom with every act of intercourse. Spermicides used with condom increase effectiveness.	To be as effective as possible, the condom should be used with every act of intercourse. The rubber condom used with spermicide is effective against pregnancy and the spread of STDs. The woman's use of a spermicide foam in the vagina increases effectiveness.	

(continued)

NURSING PLAN OF CARE (Continued)
for Pete

Expected Outcome	By the end of the teaching session, the patient will:
	• Express a decrease in anxiety

Nursing Interventions	Rationale	Evaluative Statement
Assess patient's anxiety level by verbal and nonverbal behavior.	Patient was anxious when he came into clinic. It is important to evaluate level of anxiety before he leaves. If he is still anxious, reassessment should occur because plan of care may have been unsuccessful.	8/1/02 Goal met. Patient expressed relief that he is normal. Would like to bring a friend to next session.

Future teaching sessions to include these topics identified by patient:

- STDs, particularly AIDS
- Pregnancy—occurrence and prevention
- Sexual expression
- Further discussion of sexual myths

R. Gordon, RN

Sample Documentation

8/1/02, 11 AM, nursing

Nursing consultation with 13-year-old patient regarding anxiety about cause and source of nocturnal emissions. Patient also expressed concern about sexual myths he has heard from friends. Stated that much peer pressure exists to become sexually active. Patient admits to possessing little knowledge regarding sexual issues. Feels he cannot discuss sexuality with parents because it is not a topic that has been brought up in the past at home. Will conduct initial teaching session with patient to provide information and decrease anxiety about priority concerns. Patient is willing to return to clinic for at least three more teaching sessions to expand knowledge base of sexuality.

R. Gordon, RN

Learning Outcomes

After completing this chapter, the learner should be able to accomplish the following:

1. Define key terms used in the chapter.

biologic sex	menopause
bisexuality	menstruation
contraception	orgasm
erogenous zones	premenstrual (tension)
gender identity	syndrome
gender role behavior	sexual dysfunction
heterosexuality	sexual harassment
homosexuality	sexual health
impotence	sexual orientation
masturbation	sexuality
menarche	transsexual
	transvestite

2. Describe male and female reproductive anatomy and physiology.

3. Describe the sexual response cycle, differentiating male and female responses.
4. Identify factors that affect an individual's sexuality.
5. Perform a sexual assessment using suggested interview questions and appropriate physical assessment skills.
6. Describe types of sexual dysfunctions and assessment priorities for each.
7. Develop nursing diagnoses identifying a problem with sexuality that may be remedied by independent nursing actions.
8. Describe five areas in which the nurse can provide the patient with education to promote knowledge of sexuality.
9. Plan, implement, and evaluate nursing care related to selected nursing diagnoses involving problems of sexuality.

Critical Thinking Exercises

1. Role play with another student the interview you would use to obtain a sexual history from the following individuals. Think about how you modified the interview in each situation and why. Identify what made you feel uncomfortable as either the nurse or the patient. Discuss how you can best address this discomfort.

   • Mother voices concern that her 9-year-old son is frequently playing with his penis.
   • Adult man appears distressed when he notes that he has suddenly become impotent with his partner of many years.
   • A high school girl shares with you that her mother tells her something is wrong with her because she is only attracted to women.
   • A new resident in a nursing home complains that he misses his privacy and has nowhere to make love.

2. Describe how you would respond to a newly diagnosed HIV-positive woman with multiple partners who tells you that it is none of your business how she acquired the virus or what she plans to do now that she has it. Think carefully about what is at stake in terms of your response.

Study Questions

1. The female counterpart to a male penis is the
   a. clitoris
   b. vagina
   c. hymen
   d. labia majora

2. Fertilization of the ovum by the sperm usually occurs in the
   a. uterus
   b. fallopian tube
   c. ovary
   d. vagina

3. The primary hormone secreted by the testes is
   a. estrogen
   b. progesterone
   c. semen
   d. testosterone

4. The sexual response cycle is
   a. limited to the genitalia
   b. a total-body response
   c. limited to the erogenous zone
   d. divided into two phases: excitement and resolution

5. Male orgasm always consists of
   a. ejaculation of semen
   b. 15 to 20 contractions
   c. involuntary spasmodic contractions of the genitals
   d. 4 to 10 contractions

6. A 16-year-old girl confides to the school nurse, "Something must be wrong with me. I'm the only one in my class who doesn't have her period yet." The nurse's best initial response is to
   a. recommend a thorough medical examination to rule out medical disease
   b. explain that menarche can be experienced as early as 8 years and as late as 17 years of age
   c. question her about life stresses that might be retarding the start of her period
   d. question her about the age at which her mother, maternal grandmother, and aunts experienced menarche

7. You are asked, "Is it okay to enjoy intercourse during menses?" Your answer is best based on the knowledge that
   a. there is no scientific rationale to support abstinence from sexual activity during menses
   b. intercourse during menses is more likely to damage sensitive tissues in the vagina
   c. women should not have intercourse during the time of the month when they are "unclean"
   d. women have been oppressed for too long and need to regain control of their bodies

8. When exposure of a male patient during the bed bath results in an erection, the best nursing response is to
   a. explain that this is a natural physiologic response and offer to leave the room if the patient wishes
   b. leave the room quickly to allow the patient to regain control
   c. state firmly that this behavior makes you uncomfortable and that you expect it to stop
   d. ask that patient if he is experiencing anxiety about his ability to be sexually active after his illness

9. When a young mother confides to you that she is concerned about her toddler who frequently fondles his genitals, you should
   a. explain that it is not too early to begin teaching the youngster what is "bad" or unacceptable behavior
   b. stress the importance of the parent's "setting limits" by using negative reinforcement
   c. explain that it is perfectly natural for toddlers to enjoy fondling their genitals
   d. stress that this may signal a medical or psychiatric problem that requires evaluation

10. A 77-year-old patient asks you if you think it's wrong for her to masturbate. Your best response is
    a. "I thought you were too old for that!"
    b. "Do you really do that?"
    c. "How do you feel about it?"
    d. "Why don't you ask your physician?"

11. The statement below that reveals a correct knowledge of sexuality is
    a. "My small penis makes it hard for me to satisfy a woman sexually."
    b. "Because sex 'weakens a person,' the coach insists we abstain before big games."
    c. "Something must be wrong with me. I know women aren't supposed to enjoy sex as much as men."
    d. "I think all the attention being paid to achieving simultaneous orgasms is misplaced."

12. Which of the following statements indicates a need for contraceptive teaching?
    a. "Because breastfeeding isn't a foolproof contraceptive, we plan to use a condom as soon as we are sexually active again."
    b. "My partner always withdraws before ejaculation, so we are not worried about pregnancy."
    c. "My husband and I are highly motivated to make natural family planning work so that we can have our children when we are ready."
    d. "I understand that I should always use a spermicidal agent with my diaphragm."

13. When teaching young patients about sexually transmitted diseases, it is important to communicate that

    a. abstinence is an unrealistic, old-fashioned idea
    b. having sexual contact with one person is to have contact with everyone else with whom that person has had sexual contact
    c. adolescents are less likely to contract a sexually transmitted disease because they are generally healthier than adults
    d. with prompt medical treatment, all sexually transmitted diseases can be cured without long-standing complications

14. In 1974, the American Psychiatric Association removed which of the following from the category of mental illness?
    a. transsexuality
    b. bisexuality
    c. homosexuality
    d. heterosexuality

15. During the admission history, Mrs. Victor tells you that she experiences extreme pain during intercourse. An appropriate nursing diagnosis would be
    a. Fear related to pain during sexual intercourse
    b. Body Image Disturbance related to painful intercourse
    c. Ineffective Individual Coping related to pain
    d. Pain related to dyspareunia

Answers With Rationale

1. The correct response is *a*. The clitoris is the female counterpart to the male penis because they are similar in their reaction to stimuli. The vagina, hymen, and labia majora are not similarly responsive to stimuli.

2. The correct response is *b*. Fertilization of the ovum by the sperm usually occurs in the fallopian tube, not in the uterus, ovary, or vagina.

3. The correct response is *d*. The primary hormone secreted by the testes is testosterone, not estrogen or progesterone (female sex hormones). Semen, seminal plasma, and sperm are not hormones.

4. The correct response is *b*. The sexual response cycle is clearly a total-body response and is not limited to the genitalia nor to the erogenous zones. There are more than two phases in the sexual response cycle.

5. The correct response is *c*. By definition, the male orgasm always consists of involuntary spasmodic contractions of the genitals. The other options are all possible but unnecessary.

6. The correct response is *b*. The nurse's first priority is to inform the patient that, at 16 years of age, she is still within the normal age span for experiencing menarche (8 to 17 years). Once this is done, a more detailed history may be taken.

7. The correct response is *a*. If a patient asks about enjoying intercourse during the menses, it is important to base your response on fact (there is no scientific rationale to support abstinence from sexual activity during menses) rather than on a religious, cultural, or personal belief. Option *b* is simply false.

8. The correct response is *a*. Explaining to the patient that this is a natural physiologic response and giving him time to regain control will decrease any embarrassment he is experiencing. Option *b* (leaving the room without comment) might be interpreted as signifying disapproval. Option *c* clearly communicates disapproval, and option *d* is premature.

9. The correct response is *c*. The appropriate response to this mother's concern is the factual information that this is developmentally appropriate behavior. Options *a* and *b* communicate incorrectly that this is abnormal behavior that ought to be curbed. Option *d* is false.

10. The correct response is *c*. Option *a* is based on the myth that elderly people do not have any sexual needs. Option *b* implies disapproval. Option *d* refers to the physician a question the nurse should be able to answer. Asking the patient how she feels (option *c*) opens the door for a frank discussion of the patient's concerns and will surface any false information or negative beliefs the patient holds.

11. The correct response is *d*. Placing too much attention on achieving simultaneous orgasm can detract from the overall sexual experience. The other options are all common sexual myths.

12. The correct response is *b*. Withdrawing before ejaculation is no guarantee that no sperm have been released because, during sexual activity, Cowper's glands produce small droplets of fluid that may contain sperm. The other options are all statements that

reveal a correct understanding of contraceptive measures.

13. The correct response is *b*. Having sexual contact with one person is to have contact with everyone else that person has had contact with is the only factually correct response. Option *a* may be held by some nurses but is a personal belief that many would challenge. Options *c* and *d* are false.

14. The correct response is *c*. Homosexuality was removed from the category of mental illness in 1974 by the American Psychiatric Association.

15. The correct response is *d*. The data point to a nursing diagnosis of Pain related to dyspareunia (painful intercourse). The patient has not mentioned fear, and no data point to a disturbance in body image or to ineffective coping.

Bibliography

Alteneder, R. R. (1997). Addressing couples' sexuality concerns during the childbearing period: Use of PLISSIT model. *Journal of Obstetric, Gynecologic, and Neonatal Nursing, 26*(6), 651–658.

Brady, M. (1998). Female genital mutilation. *Nursing 98, 28*(9), 50–51.

Carter, J., & Verhoef, M. J. (1995). Efficacy of self-help and alternative treatments of premenstrual syndrome. *Women's Health Issues, 4*(3), 130–137.

Cholewinski, J. T., & Burge, J. M. (1990). Sexual harassment of nursing students. *Image—The Journal of Nursing Scholarship, 22*(2), 106–110.

Cole, F. L., & Slocumb, E. M. (1995). Factors influencing safer sexual behaviors in heterosexual late adolescent and young adult collegiate males. *Image—The Journal of Nursing Scholarship, 27*(3), 217–223.

Doyle, D., Bisson, D., Janes, N., Lynch, H., & Martin, C. (1999). Human sexuality in long-term care. *Canadian Nurse, 95*(1), 26–29.

Fehring, R. J. (1991). New technology in natural family planning. *Journal of Obstetric, Gynecologic, and Neonatal Nursing, 20*(3), 199–205.

Fuentes, R. J., Rosenberg, J. M., & Marks, R. G. (1983). Sexual side effects: What to tell your patients, what not to say. *Registered Nurse, 46*(2), 34–41.

Harbin, R. E. (1995). Female adolescent contraception. *Pediatric Nursing, 21*(3), 221–226.

Hatcher, R., Guest, S., Stewart, F., Stewart, G. K., Trussell, J., Cerel, S., & Kates, W. (1990). *Contraceptive technology* (15th ed.). New York: Irvington.

Hofland, S. L., & Powers, L. (1996). Sexual dysfunction in the menopausal woman: Hormonal causes and management issues. *Geriatric Nursing, 17*(4), 161–165.

Horsley, J. E. (1990). Don't tolerate sexual harassment at work. *RN, 53*(1), 69, 72, 75.

Kaye, J., Donald, C. G., & Merker, S. (1994). Sexual harassment of critical care nurses: A costly workplace issue. *American Journal of Critical Care, 3*(6), 409–415.

McGrory, A. (1995). Education for the menarche. *Pediatric Nursing, 21*(5), 439–443.

MacLaren, A. (1995). Primary care for women: Comprehensive sexual health assessment. *Journal of Nurse-Midwifery, 40*(2), 104–119.

Pillitteri, A. (1995). *Maternal and child health nursing* (2nd ed.). Philadelphia: J. B. Lippincott.

Smith, L. L., Taylor, B. B., Keys, A. T., & Gornto, B. A. (1997). Nurse-patient boundaries. Crossing the line: How to recognize signs of professional misconduct and intervene effectively. *American Journal of Nursing, 97*(12), 26–31.

Staff. (1993). American Academy of Pediatrics Committee on Adolescence: Homosexuality and adolescence. *Pediatrics, 92*, 631–633.

Stockard, S. (1991). Caring for the sexually aggressive patient: You don't have to blush and bear it. *Nursing, 21*(11), 72–73.

Thomas, B., Stamler, L. L., Lafreniere, K., & Dumala, R. (2000). The Internet: An effective tool for nursing research with women. *Computers in Nursing, 18*(1), 13–18.

Varnhagen, C. K. (1991). Sexually transmitted diseases and condoms: High school students' knowledge, attitudes, and behaviors. *Canadian Journal of Public Health, 82*(2), 129–132.

Warner, P. H., Rowe, T. (1999). Shedding light on the sexual history. *American Journal of Nursing 99*(6), 34–41.

Williams, A. B. (1992). The epidemiology, clinical manifestations and health maintenance needs of women infected with HIV. *Nurse Practitioner, 17*(5), 27–44.

Winter, E. J. S., Ashton, D. J., & Moore, D. L. (1991). Dispelling myths: A study of PMS and relationship satisfaction. *Nurse Practitioner, 16*(5), 34–45.

Woods, N. F. (1984). Human sexuality in health and illness. St. Louis: C. V. Mosby.

World Health Organization. (1975). *Education and treatment in human sexuality: The training of health professionals.* Geneva: Author.

Chapter 35
Spirituality

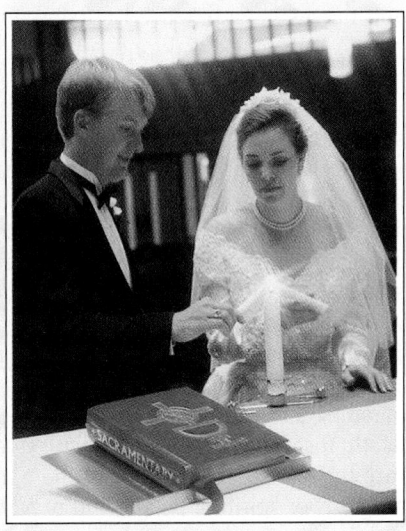

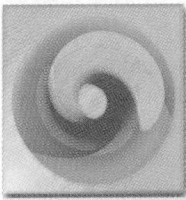

**Thinking Critically About
Nursing's Blended Skills**

Before reading this chapter, think about the types of blended skills you will need to promote spiritual health and well-being in your professional practice.

- Five-year-old Anna asks you where her mommy is now. Anna's mother died of breast cancer.

- The O'Malleys ask you what kind of God allows young people to drink and drive and kill other young people. Their daughter was killed in a fatal motor vehicle accident on her prom night. The student driver of the car that killed her was intoxicated. He is now critically ill, and his family is similarly in shock and grieving.

- The Kisons have been trying to get pregnant for 5 years without success. They are desperate to have a child and consult an infertility specialist. Mrs. Kison reports that their families are very religious and their church does not approve of in vitro fertilization. "If we conceived this way and anything ever happened to our child, I would know that God is punishing us for breaking his law."

- Mrs. Zeuner tells you that she hasn't been able to get out to church since her husband was discharged from the hospital. Her husband has advanced Alzheimer's disease and requires constant supervision. "I really miss the support I received from our congregation. It was the one thing in the past that kept me going."

What cognitive, interpersonal, and ethical/legal skills do you think you will need to respond to the challenges described above?

The "spirit" dimension of the person was recognized in ancient cultures. "The dual roles of priest and physician were generally held by one individual, and thus the functions and dictates of religion (pertaining to the spirit) and medicine (pertaining to the body) were closely interwoven" (O'Brien, 1982, p. 85). Over the years, however, medicine and religion evolved separately. Not until the holistic health movement took root was the person once again viewed as an integrated whole of body, mind, and spirit. Healthcare practitioners began again to probe the relationships among physical, psychological, and spiritual health.

Nursing has always had a strongly holistic tradition, and nurses have practiced nursing with sensitivity to the physical, psychosocial, and spiritual needs of people (see the accompanying box, Six Basic Spiritual Needs of Americans). According to Shelly and Fish (1988), there are three **spiritual needs** underlying all religious traditions and common to all people: (1) need for meaning and purpose, (2) need for love and relatedness, and (3) need for forgiveness. Although nurses may differ in their beliefs about how involved they should become in meeting patients' spiritual needs, it is impossible to nurse individuals well while ignoring the spiritual dimensions of health. Nurses can assist patients to meet spiritual needs by offering a compassionate presence; assisting in the struggle to find meaning and purpose in the face of suffering, illness, and death; fostering relationships (with God/humans) that nurture the spirit; and facilitating the patient's expression of religious or spiritual beliefs and practices.

Study of this chapter provides the student with a knowledge base of spirituality, spiritual health, and spiritual care. Practical suggestions for performing a spiritual assessment are given, along with specific interview questions. Sample nursing diagnoses are developed for common problems of **spiritual distress** (spiritual pain, alienation, anxiety, guilt, anger, loss, and despair). Related patient and nursing goals and specific nursing strategies for promoting spiritual health are described. The concluding patient care study illustrates how the nurse's knowledge of spirituality may be combined with skilled nursing interventions and caring to resolve spiritual distress successfully.

Spirituality and Faith

Although the terms spirituality, religion, and faith are used interchangeably by some, there are distinctions. **Spirituality** is anything that pertains to a person's relationship with a nonmaterial life force or higher power. Whereas one person describes spirituality in terms of coming to know, love, and serve God, another speaks of transcending the limits of body and experiencing a universal energy. Spirituality is not something that runs parallel to the rest of human life. Rather it is, in the words of theologian Karl Rahner:

> . . . simply the ultimate depth of everything spiritual creatures do when they realize themselves—when they laugh or cry, accept responsibility, love, live and die, stand up for truth, break out of preoccupation with themselves to help the neighbor, hope against hope, cheerfully refuse to be embittered by the stupidity of daily life, keep silent, not so that evil festers in their hearts, but so that it dies there—when, in a word, they live as they would like to live in opposition to selfishness and to the despair that always assails us (1971, p. 229).

Spirituality may include **religion**, which refers to an organized system of beliefs about a higher power. Religions are often characterized by set forms of worship, spiritual practices, and codes of conduct. Thus, a person may be deeply spiritual yet not profess a religion. The fact that people do not belong to an organized religion should not be interpreted by the nurse to mean that they have no spiritual needs. **Faith** generally refers to a confident belief in something for which there is no proof or material evidence. It can involve a person, idea, or thing, and it is usually followed by action related to the ideals or values of that belief.

COGNITIVE SKILLS

- Basic knowledge about the influence of religion and spirituality on everyday living, health, and illness
- Understanding of the factors that influence spiritual development and spiritual health
- Knowledge of how to use the nursing process to meet spiritual needs and to prevent and resolve spiritual problems

INTERPERSONAL SKILLS

- Strong people skills; ability to communicate and interact effectively with patients and their

caregivers; ability to establish trusting relationships—even in times of crisis
- Ability to be a healing presence to others searching for meaning and purpose, love and belonging, forgiveness in their own lives

ETHICAL/LEGAL SKILLS

- Commitment to safety and quality; strong sense of responsibility, accountability
- Familiarity with agency policy and role responsibilities related to meeting spiritual needs

Six Basic Spiritual Needs of Americans

George Gallup, who is chair of the George H. Gallup International Institute, recently identified six basic spiritual needs of contemporary Americans. His conclusions are based on a variety of religious research and were presented in a speech given at a meeting of the Theological Students Fellowship, Princeton Theological Seminary, on December 10, 1990.

The need to believe that life is meaningful and has a purpose. During a time when sociologists observe an obsession with self in America, 70% of Americans nevertheless believe it is important that life is meaningful and has a purpose. Yet as many as two thirds of people interviewed believe that "most churches and synagogues today are not effective in helping people find meaning in life." Here is a basic need apparently being only partially met. The fact is, significant numbers of people find churches irrelevant, unfulfilling, and boring.

The need for a sense of community and deeper relationships. "Radical individualism" continues to have a hold on the religious lives of Americans. Most Americans, for example, believe that one can be a good Christian or Jew if one does not attend church or synagogue. One of the poignant consequences of this separateness is loneliness. As we have discovered from surveys, as many as 3 people in 10 say they have been lonely "for a long period of time" in their lives, with half of these people saying this experience has affected their thoughts "a great deal."

The need to be appreciated and respected. This is certainly a basic and fundamental need, yet as many as one third of the American people have a low sense of self-worth or self-esteem, as a direct consequence of not being loved or appreciated. Low self-esteem brings with it a host of social problems, including alcohol and drug abuse, child and spouse abuse, lawlessness, and crime. Significantly, surveys suggest that the closer people feel to God, the better they feel about themselves. They are also more satisfied with their lives than are others, are more altruistic, enjoy better health, and have a happier outlook. Furthermore, it has been found that experiencing the closeness of God is a key factor in the ability of people to forgive themselves and others.

The need to be listened to—to be heard. Americans overwhelmingly think the future of the church will be shaped to a greater extent by the laity than by the clergy. In specific terms, this means that the laity should play a greater role in the church, freeing up clergy to perform what the laity expects of them: to listen to people's religious needs and to provide spiritual counseling and inspiration. When the "unchurched" in one survey were asked what would most likely draw them back in the community of active worshippers, the lead reason given was "if I could find a pastor or rabbi with whom I could share my religious needs and doubts."

The need to feel that one is growing in faith. People like to feel that they are maturing spiritually; we go through passages in our faith lives, just as we do in our secular lives. It would appear that, basically, people aspire to lead good lives. Significant numbers of people have given thought to living a worthwhile life, to their relationship to God, to the basic meaning and value of their lives, and to developing their faith. People need help in understanding the significance of these experiences and in building on them.

The need for practical help in developing a mature faith. There is an urgent need to work toward closing the gap between belief and practice—to turn professed faith into lived-out faith.

(Used with permission.)

An **atheist** is a person who denies the existence of a God; an **agnostic** is one who holds that nothing can be known about the existence of a God. The agnostic and the atheist are guided by philosophies of living that do not include a religious faith. They deserve respect for what they choose to believe, just as do those who accept a particular religious creed.

Spirituality and Everyday Living

Spiritual beliefs and practices are associated with all aspects of a person's life, including health and illness. Aspects of a person's life commonly influenced by spirituality and religion include relationships with others, daily living habits, required and prohibited behaviors, and the general frame of reference for thinking about oneself and the world.

Religious influences may be life affirming or life denying. Life-affirming influences enhance life, give meaning and purpose to existence, strengthen one's feelings of self-worth, encourage self-actualization, and are health giving and life sustaining. Life-denying influences restrict or enclose life patterns, limit experiences and associations, place burdens of guilt on individuals, encourage feelings of unworthiness, and are generally health denying and life inhibiting.

Spirituality, Health, and Illness

Spiritual beliefs are of special importance to nurses because of the many ways they can influence a patient's level of health and self-care behaviors.

Guide to Daily Living Habits

Certain practices generally associated with healthcare may have religious significance for a patient. For example, many religions prescribe dietary requirements and restrictions. Acceptable birth-control practices are determined by some religious faiths, as are some types of medical treatments.

Source of Support

It is common for many people to seek support from their religious faith during times of stress. This support is often vital to the acceptance of an illness, especially if the illness brings with it a prolonged period of convalescence or indicates a questionable outcome. Prayer, devotional reading, and other religious practices often do for the person spiritually what protective exercises do for the body physically (Fig. 35-1). The accompanying box describes how one religion, Buddhism, sees the divine grounding for all human experience, including suffering.

Source of Strength and Healing

The values derived from religious faith cannot be enumerated or evaluated easily. However, the effects attributable to faith are constantly in evidence to healthcare workers. People have been known to endure extreme physical distress because of strong faith. Patients' families have taken on almost unbelievable rehabilitative tasks because they had faith in the eventual positive results of their effort.

Source of Conflict

There are times when religious beliefs conflict with prevalent healthcare practices. For example, the doctrine of the Jehovah's Witnesses prohibits blood transfusions. In the Islamic religion, humans are regarded as largely helpless in controlling their environment, and illness is accepted as their fate rather than something against which action might be taken. Some Navajo Indians use a lengthy religious ceremony to cure certain diseases, such as tuberculosis. For some people, illness is viewed as punishment for sin and is therefore inevitable.

Such beliefs may require the healthcare worker to modify a treatment plan to accommodate the person's religion. In some instances, acknowledgment of the patient's

---

The Center Point That Grounds Us . . .

. . . I could scarcely make out the large sitting Buddha near the entrance of the house. But what caught my attention was the metal circle with spokes resembling a wheel, hanging over the figure of the Buddha. . . . I asked our host about the wheel. I was told it represented our eternal journey in this life and continuing into the next. Buddha's teachings say that life is suffering. We cannot avoid suffering as we move around the rim of the wheel, which represents perpetual change and the transitory nature of life. But the wheel also symbolizes wholeness or completion because the wheel revolves around the center axis that does not move. That center point represents the presence of the divine. If we remain aware of this center point, we are strengthened for whatever lies ahead.

. . . It is this center point that grounds us in the midst of the many changes in our lives. It is at the center point where we experience the energy and power that turns the wheel. It is at this center point that we connect with the Everywhere Spirit. When we rest in the center point, we find that we have come home again to the place from which we started. But because of the journey, it is as if we had arrived home for the first time. In our journey around the circles of life, we become new persons over and over again.

(From Susan Gregg-Schroeder, *The Journal of Fellowship in Prayer*, April 1999.)

---

religious convictions and efforts by health practitioners to accommodate the patient's beliefs can result in quality healthcare without violating the person's religious practices. In other situations, an objective explanation of alternative treatments and the predicted consequences of each may help the patient determine acceptable therapy. Whatever the person's decision about healthcare, the nurse should remember that each person is unique and has a right to pursue his or her own convictions, even though they may differ from those of the healthcare provider.

Major Religions

Nurses care for people from many different religious traditions. Although it is impossible for nurses to be knowledgeable about all religions, nurses are better able to meet the spiritual needs of patients when they understand the patient's religious beliefs and practices. These can directly influence the patient's response to illness and suffering, self-care practices such as diet and hygiene, birth and death rituals, gender roles, spiritual practices, and moral codes. A brief illustration of the beliefs and health practices of major religious traditions in the United States is displayed in Table 35-1. Nurses who are unfamiliar with a patient's religion can gain valuable knowledge by reading (see Carson's *(text continues on page 823)*

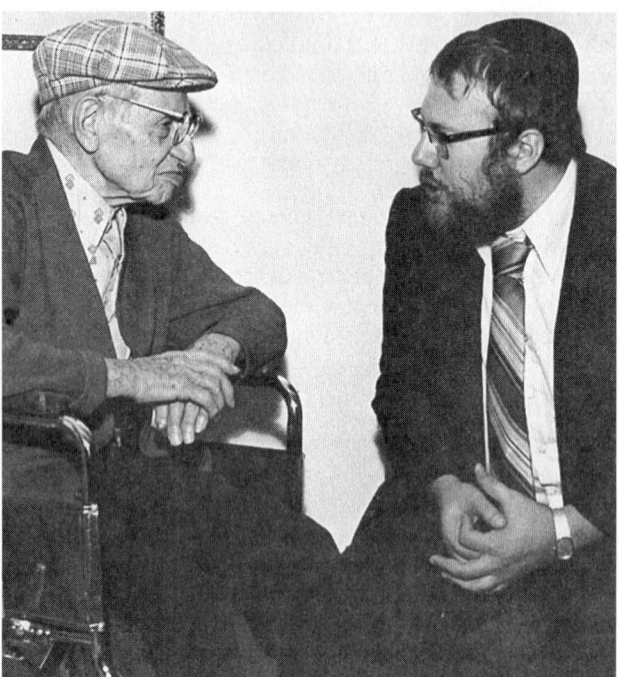

Figure 35-1
The rabbi's visit is important for this resident of a geriatric center.

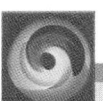

Table 35-1
Beliefs and Healthcare Practices of Major Religious Traditions in the United States

Religion	Beliefs	Select Healthcare Practices
Adventist	Believe in the individual's choice and God's sovereignty. The body is believed to be the temple of the Holy Spirit.	• The taking of all narcotics and stimulants is prohibited because the body is the temple of the Holy Spirit and should be protected. Many groups prohibit meat. • Many regard Saturday as the Sabbath. • Approach to healthcare is holistic.
American Muslim Mission	Accept the Koran as their sacred scripture (see Islam); most stress the importance of cooperation among blacks in business and education to build self-esteem.	• Members are encouraged to obtain healthcare provided by members of the black community. • Major tenets involve prayer rituals, dietary restrictions (prohibitions against pork and alcohol), hygiene (extreme cleanliness), lifestyle modifications, and marital faithfulness.
Baha'i International Community	Believe in a basic harmony between religion and science	• Seek out competent medical care and pray for health. • Obligatory prayers, holy days, and the 19-day fast • Permanent sterilization is prohibited, and abortion is discouraged.
Buddhism	Buddha or "the Great Physician" taught the Four Noble Truths to indicate the range of "suffering," its "origin," its "cessation," and the "way" that leads to its cessation. The real cause of human suffering is ignorant craving. The Noble Eightfold Path, which consists of right views, aspirations, speech, conduct, mode of livelihood, effort, mindfulness, and concentration, leads to the cessation of suffering.	• Buddhist hospitals for sick humans and sick animals antedated anything similar found in the West. • Buddhists do not outwardly proclaim healing through faith. However, spiritual peace and liberation from anxiety attained through the awakening to Buddha's wisdom may be an important factor in expediting healing and the recovery process. • Accepts modern science. The doctrine of avoidance of extremes is applied to the use of drugs, blood, vaccines. • Buddhism does not condone taking lives of any form. • Check with the patient about any special diet restrictions and the observance of holy days.
Christian Scientist	They deny the existence of health crises; sickness and sin are errors of the human mind and can be overcome by altering thoughts, not by using drugs or medicines.	• They will use orthopedic services to set a bone but decline drugs and, in general, other medical or surgical procedures. • They do not allow hypnotism or any form of psychotherapy, which alters the "Divine Mind." • A Christian Science Practitioner may be called to administer spiritual support. • Alcohol and tobacco are not used.
Church of Jesus Christ of Latter Day Saints (Mormons)	Devout adherents believe in divine healing through the "laying on of hands," though many do not prohibit medical therapy. The Church maintains an extensive and well-funded welfare system, including financial support for the sick.	• Disapprove of alcohol, tobacco, and caffeinated beverages. • A special undergarment worn by some members should be removed only in an emergency.

(continued)

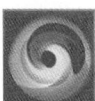

Table 35-1 (Continued)

Religion	Beliefs	Healthcare Practices
Confucianism	Inherent in Confucianism is the appreciation of life and the desire to keep the body from untimely or unnecessary death.	• Appreciate life and desire to keep the body from untimely or unnecessary death. • Historically emphasized public health solutions to impending health problems.
Daosim (Taoism)	Health is a manifestation of the harmony of the universe, obtained through the proper balancing of internal and external forces. Implicit throughout the Daoist tradition is the tendency to understand salvation in the biomedical sense of health and qualitative improvement and prolongation of human life. The universal principle of the Tao is the mysterious biologic and spiritual life rhythm or order of nature.	• There is a "medicinal" concern for maintaining and prolonging human health and life (*sheng*). Knowing and living a natural life—following the Tao—is the secret of both health and sagehood. • Long tradition of seeking pragmatic medical techniques, along with its religious techniques of meditation and ritual for establishing a harmony of body and spirit, humanity, and nature (holistic approach)
Hinduism	Doctrine of Transmigration. Moral factors, linked with the all-embracing doctrine of "karma," were believed to be significant in promoting health or causing disease.	• Hindu medicine shows a surprising openness to new ideas, at least in respect to practical treatment. • Many Hindu dietary restrictions conform to individual sect doctrine. • The nurse administering medications should avoid touching patient's lips. • Certain prescribed rites are followed after death; disposal of the body is by cremation.
Jehovah's Witnesses	They oppose the "false teachings" of other sects; opposition often extends to modern science, including medicine.	• Blood transfusions violate God's laws and therefore are not allowed. Alternative treatments include use of nonblood plasma expanders, surgical techniques to decrease blood loss, and autotransfusions through use of a heart–lung machine. • The courts have not supported the right of Jehovah Witness parents to refuse life-saving treatment for their children. • Use of alcohol and tobacco are discouraged.
Judaism	Formation closely bound with a divine revelation and with commitment to obedience to God's will. The Hebrew Bible is the authority, guide, and inspiration of the many forms of religion of the Jews (currently Reform, Conservative, and Orthodox).	• For observant Jews: special needs in the areas of diet, birth rituals, male and female contact, and death. • Treatment and procedures should not be scheduled on the Sabbath.
Islam	Allah, one God, who is only one, all seeing, all hearing, all speaking, all knowing, all willing, all powerful Must be able to practice the Five Pillars of Islam May have a fatalistic view of health	• Obligatory prayers, holy days, and fasting (Ramadan), and almsgiving • Koranic law and customs that influence birth, diet (eating pork and drinking alcohol are forbidden), care of women, death and prayer rituals • Women are not allowed to make independent decisions, and husbands need to be present when consent is sought.

(continued)

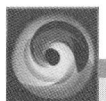

Table 35-1 (Continued)

Religion	Beliefs	Healthcare Practices
Native American Religions	Difficult to generalize; notion of cosmic harmony, emphasis on directly experiencing powers and visions and a common view of the cycle of life and death. Death is not the end but the beginning of new life (reincarnation or transcendent hereafter).	• Rituals mark important life changes: birth, puberty, initiation rites, death • Medicine men and women have specialized spirits from whom they receive the mission to cure • Common therapeutic measures: sucking, blowing, and drawing out with a feather fan
Protestantism	Worship of the one God revealed to the world through Jesus Christ. Love of neighbor is a central tenet. Other beliefs include sin, redemption, salvation, and a final accounting with God. Care of sick encouraged. God the author and giver of life is also the healer. Most accept modern medical science.	• Religious practices vary according to denomination, may include prayer, faith healing, "laying on of hands," and anointing. • Sacraments: baptism, communion, confirmation
Roman Catholicism	Worship of the one God revealed to the world through Jesus Christ. Love of neighbor is a central tenet. Other beliefs include sin, redemption, salvation, and a final accounting with God. Care of sick encouraged. God the author and giver of life is also the healer. Human life is a gift of God. Many take an antiabortion stance; most accept modern medical science.	• Importance of private devotions and Mass attendance on Sunday • Seven sacraments (importance of baptism, eucharist, penance, and the anointing of the sick) • Dietary habits • Sexual ethical norms • Only natural means of birth control; abortion, euthanasia, and sterilization are forbidden
Unification Church	God is the living, eternal person who represents universal love and care. God created the world and humans to reflect his nature. The goal of the Unification Church is to unite Christians everywhere as one family under God.	• Most members are still healthy young adults. There is little information available on their interactions with the healthcare team.
Unitarian Universal Association of Churches and Fellowships	Encourage creativity, reason, and living an ethical life. No member is required to adhere to a given creed or set of religious beliefs. The inherent worth and dignity of every person is affirmed.	• Free to accept what they take to be best for their health.

[1989] *Spiritual Dimensions of Nursing Practice*) and through discussion with the patient and the patient's family and spiritual adviser. Never presume to know what a patient's religious beliefs are upon learning that a patient is, for example, Jewish or Muslim because many religious groups and individuals work out their own set of beliefs and practices.

Religion and Law, Ethics, and Medicine

Christian Scientists, Jehovah's Witnesses, and members of faith-healing groups are among those challenging the intricate web of rights and responsibilities among individual, society, church, and state. These religious bodies are asking for protection, under the veil of religious freedom, of their right to exercise individual decisions in accordance with scriptural interpretations, even though those decisions may result in the individual's own death or that of a family member, including a child. The most troubling cases are those in which treatable problems, such as bacterial meningitis, diabetes, and bowel obstruction, resulted in the death of minors whose parents chose religious means of healing over traditional medicine. The American Pediatrics Academy is urging that all child abuse, neglect, and medical neglect statutes be applied without potential or actual exemption for religious beliefs.

Perhaps even more troubling for nurses are situations in which family members insist on care deemed medically futile (ie, the likelihood of medical benefit is virtually nonexistent) because they believe that God is going to work a miracle. In these cases, simple nursing measures, such as turning or bathing patients, become occasions of pain and torment to both the patient and nurse. Nurses are forced to administer care that they take to be cruel and abusive to conscious patients whose agonized dying is being needlessly prolonged. Unfortunately, there are no clear guidelines for drawing the line between promoting life and prolonging the dying process. Although nurses always have the moral right to withdraw from administering care that violates their personal moral code, this does not resolve the problem for the patient. More dialogue is needed on the interaction between religion and law, ethics, and medicine. Ideally, the religious freedom of patients and their families is respected, as is the moral autonomy of caregivers and the integrity of the healing professions.

Factors Affecting Spirituality

Among the many factors that can influence a person's spirituality, the most important are developmental considerations, family, ethnic background, formal religion, and life events.

Developmental Considerations

Because spirituality has to do with the nonmaterial realm of being, a child must have some capacity for abstract thought before beginning to understand the spiritual self. This is not to say that spirituality is meaningless for children.

David Heller (1985) interviewed 40 children aged 4 to 12 years who were affiliated with one of four major religions—Judaism, Roman Catholicism, Protestantism, or Hinduism—and discovered that the children had definite perceptions of God. Central themes in all the children's descriptions included the following:

* Notion of a God who works through human intimacy and the interconnectedness of lives
* Belief that God is involved in self-change and growth and transformations that make the world fresh, alive, and meaningful
* Attributing to God tremendous and expansive power and then showing considerable anxiety in the face of this power
* Image of light

As the child matures, life experiences usually influence and mature spiritual beliefs. With advancing years, the tendency to think about life after death prompts some individuals to reexamine and reaffirm their spiritual beliefs. Chapter 8 describes the stages of faith development.

Family

A child's parents play a key role in the development of the child's spirituality. What is important is not so much what parents teach a child about God and religion but rather what the child learns about God, life, and self from parents' behavior.

Ethnic Background

Religious traditions differ among ethnic groups. There are clear distinctions between Eastern and Western spiritual traditions as well as among those of individual ethnic groups, such as Native Americans. A person's culture and formal religion have much to do with whether the basic approach to religion is doing something, being someone, or continually striving for harmony (see the accompanying box, Cultural Care).

Formal Religion

Each of the major religions discussed earlier in this chapter has several characteristics in common:

* Basis of authority or source of power
* A portion of scripture or sacred word
* An ethical code that defines right and wrong
* A psychology and identity, so that its adherents fit into a group and the world is defined by the religion
* Aspirations or expectations
* Some ideas about what follows death

Life Events

Both positive and negative life experiences can influence spirituality and, in turn, are influenced by the meaning a person's spiritual beliefs attribute to them. For example, if two women who believe in a loving God both lose a child in a car accident, one may bitterly deny God's existence, whereas the other may spend more time in prayer asking God to help her. Similarly, a chain of successful life experiences (marriage, promotion) may cause one person to assume success and experience no need for God, whereas for another, it occasions deep gratitude and rejoicing.

The Nursing Process

Before reading further, use the accompanying Applying Learning to Practice exercises to see how well you are meeting your own spirituality needs; also see the accompanying Research in Nursing box.

Cultural Care

After a year of legal struggles that took the case all the way to the U.S. Supreme Court, the parents of a Vietnamese refugee defeated an attempt by social workers to force their son to have corrective surgery on his two clubfeet. The surgery would have shattered the Hmong family's religious beliefs. They believe their son Kou was born with clubfeet so that a warrior ancestor whose own feet were wounded in battle could be released from a sort of spiritual entrapment. They do not regard Kou's clubfeet as a deformity but as a sign of good luck, and they think their son is special because of it.

(From Kurtzman, L. [1990, December 22]. Surgery for boy, 7, blocked. *Philadelphia Inquirer*, p. 3A.)

APPLYING LEARNING TO PRACTICE

The Nurse as Role Model

Three spiritual needs are common to all people—the need for meaning and purpose, the need for love and relatedness, and the need for forgiveness (Shelly & Fish, 1988). These needs are common to nurses, whether they observe an established religion, believe in a spiritual essence, or recognize a field of power. As the nurse develops plans to be a spiritual role model to patients, the nurse develops goals for self. The nurse will accomplish the following:

- Hold spiritual beliefs that meet his or her need for meaning and purpose, love and relatedness, and forgiveness
- Derive from these beliefs strength for everyday living, especially when confronting pain, suffering, and death in his or her professional practice

- Set aside regular periods to nurture his or her spiritual self
- Demonstrate in his or her interactions with others peace, inner strength, warmth, joy, caring, and creativity
- Respect the spiritual beliefs and practices of others even when they are different from the nurse's own
- Increase his or her knowledge of how the spiritual beliefs of patients influence their lifestyles, responses to illness, healthcare choices, and treatment options
- Demonstrate sensitivity to the spiritual needs of patients
- Develop successful nursing strategies to assist patients in spiritual distress

ASSESSING

Nursing History

Because a person's spirituality and religious beliefs have the potential to influence every aspect of being, an assessment of the patient's spirituality should be included in each comprehensive nursing history. Helpful assessment guides are offered by Stoll (1979), O'Brien (1982), and Shelly & Fish (1988). Data are gathered about the patient's spiritual beliefs and practices, the effect of these beliefs on everyday living, spiritual distress, and spiritual needs. Sample questions are listed in the accompanying Focused Assessment Guide.

The following questions are from O'Brien's Spiritual Assessment Guide (1982, p. 102):

Spiritual pain: Do you ever feel hurt or pain associated with the spiritual or religious beliefs that you hold? Do you feel pain related to uncertainty or nonbelief?
Spiritual alienation: Do you frequently feel far away from God? Does it seem that he is remote and far removed from your everyday life?
Spiritual anxiety: Are you afraid that God might not take care of your needs? That he might not be there when you need him?
Spiritual guilt: Have you ever done things that God would be angry at you for? Are you feeling badly

APPLYING LEARNING TO PRACTICE

Promoting Health

Spirituality

Use the assessment checklist to determine how well you are meeting spirituality needs. Then develop a prescription for self-care by choosing appropriate behaviors from the list of suggestions.

ASSESSMENT CHECKLIST

almost always / sometimes / almost never

1. I am comfortable with my spiritual beliefs and values.
2. My beliefs meet my needs for love, belonging, forgiveness, meaning, and purpose.
3. I respect the belief systems of others.
4. I derive sufficient strength from my religious beliefs to meet each day's challenges.

SELF-CARE BEHAVIORS

1. Explore personal values and beliefs of self and others.
2. Explore practices that are spiritually supportive.
3. Respect the belief systems of others.
4. Practice loving relationships with self and others.
5. Seek spiritual assistance to help cope with stress, crisis, or loss.

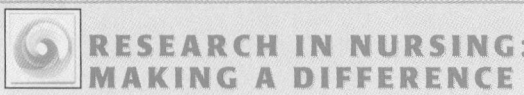

RESEARCH IN NURSING: MAKING A DIFFERENCE

Promoting Spiritual Health

Although not all nurses may or must feel comfortable in providing spiritual care, the assessment of a patient's spiritual needs is a professional responsibility.

Related Research
O'Brien, M. E. (1999). *Spirituality in nursing* (pp. 80–81, 88–115). Boston: Jones and Bartlett.
O'Brien examined the concept of spirituality as related to nursing practice in a qualitative exploratory descriptive study of 66 nurse administrators, educators, researchers, and practitioners. A focused interview guide of 12 items related to spirituality and the practice of nursing was developed. Ultimately, an overall construct describing the association between spirituality and nurse–patient relationship emerged from analysis of the data and was labeled "The Nurse: The anonymous minister." This construct, which identifies the nurse's frequently unrecognized role in spiritual ministry, consists of three dominant themes: A Sacred Calling, Nonverbalized Theology, and Nursing Liturgy.

Relevance to Nursing Practice
Contemporary holistic healthcare mandates attention to the problems and concern of the spirit as well as to those of the body and mind.

---

about things that you have done or failed to do in your life?

Spiritual anger: Are you angry at God for allowing you to be ill? Do you ever feel like blaming God for your illness? Do you think God is unfair to you?

Spiritual loss: Do you ever feel that you have lost God's love? That you have broken or weakened your relationship with God? Has God turned his back on you?

Spiritual despair: Do you ever feel that there is no hope of having God's love? Of pleasing him? That God does not love you anymore?

FOCUSED ASSESSMENT GUIDE

Spirituality

Factors to Assess	Questions and Approaches
Spiritual beliefs	"Are there particular spiritual or religious beliefs that are important to you? Have these beliefs changed recently? Is your illness challenging these beliefs? Do your religious beliefs in any way dictate a course of action that puts you in conflict with what your physicians are recommending?"
Spiritual practices	"Describe your usual spiritual practices and anything interfering with your ability to perform them. Can I help in any way to secure the aids necessary for these practices (prayer shawl, Bible, crystals, beads, icon)?"
Relation between spiritual beliefs and everyday living	"Describe ways your spiritual beliefs affect everyday living (daily schedule, diet, hygiene, sense of self and the world, relationships). Do you find this influence to be healthy (life affirming) or destructive (life denying)?"
Spiritual deficit or distress	"Are your spiritual beliefs currently causing you any distress?"
Spiritual needs	"In what ways can I and the other nurses help you to meet your spiritual needs?" "Would you like me to contact your spiritual adviser or the hospital's pastoral care minister?"
Need for meaning and purpose	"In what ways do your religious beliefs help or hinder you to understand your current situation and face it with peace and courage?"
Need for love and relatedness	"In what ways do your religious beliefs help or hinder you to meet your need to love and be loved?"
Need for forgiveness	"In what ways do your religious beliefs help or hinder you to feel at peace?"
Significant behavioral observations	Be alert to sudden changes in spiritual practices, mood changes, sudden interest in spiritual matters, and sleep disturbances—all of which may point to unresolved spiritual needs.

If the patient shares a spiritual problem, remember to use interview questions to determine the specific nature of the problem, its probable causes, related signs and symptoms, when it first began and how often it occurs, how it affects everyday living, the severity of the problem and whether it can be treated independently by nursing or needs to be referred, and how well the patient is coping with the problem.

Nursing Observation

Because many patients may find it difficult to talk about their spiritual beliefs and problems, the nurse also observes the patient's behavior for signs of spiritual distress. A family member or close friend may share significant observations.

> "He's been awfully moody since his heart attack . . . I can't believe the change in him."
>
> "I've never seen my father so depressed. He's never in his life been away from the synagogue at Passover. I don't know how to help him."

Significant behavioral observations include sudden changes in spiritual practices (rejection, neglect, fanatical devotion); mood changes (frequent crying, depression, apathy, anger); sudden interest in spiritual matters (reading religious books or watching religious programs on television, visits to clergy); and disturbed sleep. A nurse who observes these behaviors should follow up with appropriate interview questions. Often, problems with spiritual distress do not surface until well after a patient's admission history and examination. Effective questions include the following:

> "You've been lying there so quietly . . . what are you thinking about?"
>
> "After all you've been through, you must have done a good bit of soul searching. . . . Experiences like these are enough to shake anyone's faith—how is yours holding up?"

DIAGNOSING

The nurse uses each phase of the nursing process when identifying and treating spiritual problems categorized as nursing diagnoses. The North American Nursing Diagnosis Association (NANDA, 1994) diagnoses are as follows:

> *Spiritual Distress*: Disruption in the life principle that pervades a person's entire being and that integrates and transcends one's biologic and psychosocial nature.
>
> *Potential for Enhanced Spiritual Well-Being*: The process of an individual's developing/unfolding of mystery through harmonious interconnectedness that springs from inner strengths.

Spiritual distress may be further specified as spiritual pain, alienation, anxiety, guilt, anger, loss, or despair (O'Brien, 1982). Common etiologies for spiritual distress include inability to reconcile current life situation (eg, illness, death of loved person, divorce) with spiritual beliefs ("God is all powerful, all loving, all wise, and he cares about me") or separation from the religious community or supports. Sample nursing diagnoses of spiritual distress are presented in the accompanying box.

Spiritual distress may affect other areas of human functioning. In the following nursing diagnoses, spiritual distress is the etiology of another problem.

> Impaired Adjustment to Illness related to inability to reconcile illness with spiritual beliefs
>
> Ineffective Individual Coping related to loss of religion as primary support (feels abandoned by God)
>
> Fear related to feeling unprepared for death and afterlife experience
>
> Dysfunctional Grieving: Despair related to belief that religion is meaningless
>
> Hopelessness related to belief that no one cares—including God
>
> Powerlessness related to feeling victimized by a tyrannical and arbitrary God
>
> Self-Esteem Disturbance related to failure to live according to dictates of religion
>
> Sexual Dysfunction related to values conflict
>
> Sleep Pattern Disturbance related to spiritual distress
>
> Risk for Self-Directed Violence related to feeling that life is meaningless

PLANNING: EXPECTED OUTCOMES

Nurses who are sensitive to the role spiritual beliefs play in influencing both a person's thoughts about self and the world and interactions with the world value spiritual health. Their interactions with any patient who values spirituality are supportive of the following patient goals/outcomes. The patient will achieve the following:

- Identify spiritual beliefs that meet needs for meaning and purpose, love and relatedness, and forgiveness
- Derive from these beliefs strength, hope, and comfort when facing the challenge of illness, injury, or other life crisis
- Develop spiritual practices that nurture communion with inner self, with God, and with the world
- Express satisfaction with the compatibility of spiritual beliefs and everyday living

Goals and expected outcomes for patients in spiritual distress need to be individualized and may include some of the following. The patient will achieve the following:

- Explore the origin of spiritual beliefs and practices
- Identify factors in life that challenge spiritual beliefs
- Explore alternatives given these challenges: deny, modify, or reaffirm beliefs; develop new beliefs
- Identify spiritual supports (eg, spiritual reading, faith, community)
- Report or demonstrate a decrease in spiritual distress after successful intervention

IMPLEMENTING

A variety of interventions are available to the nurse who wishes to help patients meet spiritual needs. Like other nursing skills, these interventions need to be practiced before the nurse is able to use them confidently, competently, and at the

Nursing Diagnoses for Common Problems

Spiritual Distress*

Problem	*Related Factors*	*Sample Defining Characteristics*
Spiritual pain	Inability to accept death of son	A 46-year-old woman, agnostic, only son died 6 months ago (lung cancer)
		"I've often wondered throughout my life if there is a God—thought maybe if I had tried harder I'd have recognized him. Now I don't care if God exists or not because if he allows this I don't want to know him."
		"My son was my whole life; there's nothing left for me to live for."
		Lost 10 lb in 6 months since son died; leaves home only when necessary to purchase food, go to bank, and engage in other routine activities.
Spiritual alienation	Separated from "faith community"	A 72-year-old Orthodox Jewish man, recently admitted to Protestant nursing home following 3-week hospitalization for stroke
		"I guess Yahweh has written me off; first the stroke that killed half my body and then I'm abandoned here where I can't even observe the Sabbath."
		"I want to go home."
Spiritual anxiety	Challenged belief and value system	A 37-year-old previously healthy male executive recovering from massive myocardial infarction
		"My parents were strict Methodists, but when I left home for college I stopped going to church . . . never gave it much thought . . . there was always something else to do. I started going again but it never meant much."
		"I haven't exactly done anything awful but I've also not been a saint and I find myself wondering if there is a God, what does he think of me."
		"Funny, I guess I thought I'd live forever. I sure never thought about dying and what happens after that."
		Often observed lying quietly in bed awake; asked to see minister.
Spiritual guilt	Failure to live according to religious rules	A 23-year-old, single, Baptist woman being treated for premenstrual syndrome
		"I was raised in a strict Baptist home but had to leave . . . I needed more room to be me. I like life here at the university but there's a restlessness in me I can't describe. I've dated several men, one or two I really liked, but I always do something to mess up the relationship. It would kill my mother if she knew I lived with Gary for 3 months."
		"What it really comes down to is my own sense of betraying myself, my family, and my religion. Who am I anyway?"
Spiritual anger	Inability to accept illness	A 38-year-old homosexual man recently diagnosed with AIDS
		"My parents are fundamentalists . . . all I ever heard at home was how much Jesus loves me . . . all the while my mom was beating the daylights out of me. . . . Does he love me? Does he love me so much that he had my parents throw me out when I finally told them I was gay? Does he love me so much that I got AIDS and now no one comes near me?"
		Facial features are tight; body held rigidly; speech is sharp, appears angry with God, the world, himself.

(continued)

Nursing Diagnoses for Common Problems *(Continued)*

Spiritual Distress*

Problem	*Related Factors*	*Sample Defining Characteristics*
Spiritual loss	Terminal illness; anticipatory grieving; inability to find comfort in religion	A 40-year-old mother of three sons who was diagnosed with ovarian cancer 18 months ago; currently in advanced stage of disease
		"I've tried hard to do it all right . . . I read my Bible, prayed every day, went to church each Sunday, loved my husband and kids . . . why is this all happening to me? Why must I lose it all? Where is God now that I need him? Some mornings I wish I could shoot myself and end it all—instead another day drags on. Who can help me?"
		Cries frequently, no longer interested in everyday activities of family, no interest in praying, told family not to have pastor call anymore. "No one can help now."
Spiritual despair	Feeling that no one (not even God) cares	A 92-year-old frail widow who lives alone in a two-room apartment; crippled with arthritis; has two married sons she has not seen for years.
		Says to community nurse who visits every week, "No one should have to live like this. If it weren't for the neighbor who comes on Saturday with a few groceries and you I'd be dead. I guess that would be for the best. It's been a long time since I felt like my living or dying would matter to anyone. Because I'm 92 now I guess even God doesn't want me. Couldn't you do something to put me out of my misery?"

* NANDA-approved nursing diagnosis label.

right moment. In this section, the following nursing interventions are presented: offering supportive presence, facilitating the patient's practice of religion, nurturing spirituality, praying with a patient, counseling the patient spiritually, contacting a spiritual counselor, and resolving conflicts between treatment and spiritual beliefs. See the accompanying box for a list of selected spiritual support activities.

Offering Supportive Presence

A nurse's gift of supportive presence must underlie all other types of intervention to meet spiritual needs. Supportive presence communicates value and respect (Fig. 35-2). Chapter 21 presents basic communication skills helpful in establishing this type of presence.

The patient who senses that the nurse is sincerely concerned and committed to helping meet human needs is better able to participate in the plan of care. Patients who experience respect and affirmation from other humans find it easier to hold spiritual beliefs that meet their needs for meaning and purpose, love and relatedness, and forgiveness.

Facilitating the Practice of Religion

The following are means the nurse can use to help the patient continue normal spiritual practices in the unfamiliar environment of the hospital or care center:

Using the Nursing Interventions Classification (NIC)

Selected Spiritual Support Activities

- Be open to patient's expressions of loneliness and powerlessness
- Encourage chapel service attendance, if desired
- Encourage use of spiritual resources, if desired
- Refer to spiritual advisor of patient's choice
- Use values clarification techniques to help patient clarify beliefs and values, as appropriate
- Be available to listen to patient's feelings
- Express empathy with patient's feelings
- Assure patient that nurse will be available to support patient in times of suffering
- Be open to patient's feelings about illness and death

(From McClosky, J., & Bulechek, G. [2000]. *Nursing interventions classification [NIC]* [3rd ed.] [p. 607]. St. Louis: C. V. Mosby. A full listing of nursing activities for each nursing intervention can be found in this book.)

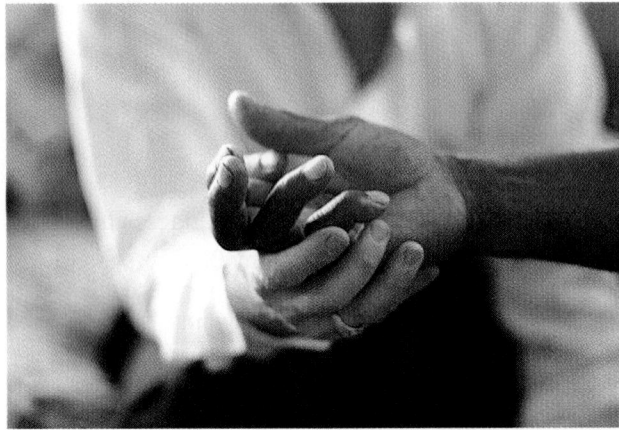

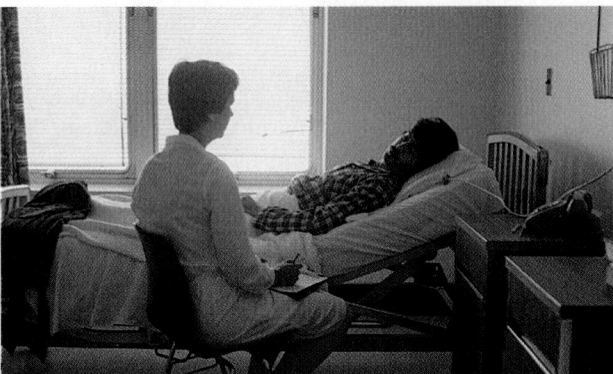

Figure 35-2
The nurse offers supportive presence by holding the patient's hand to show that he or she is sincerely concerned or simply by being present to communicate value and respect.

- Familiarize the patient with religious services and materials available within the institution.
- Respect the patient's need for privacy or quiet during periods of prayer.
- Assist the patient to obtain devotional objects and protect them from loss or damage.
- Arrange for the patient wishing to receive the sacraments to do so.
- Attempt to meet the patient's religious dietary restrictions.
- Arrange for the patient's minister, priest, or rabbi to visit if the patient so wishes.

If the patient has a conflict between spiritual beliefs and the proposed medical therapy, the nurse can assist the patient in discussing this with the physician.

The ill patient in the home may not be able to attend services or meetings to which the patient is accustomed. The nurse can aid the patient in finding ways to express his or her spiritual needs. Other sections in the remainder of this chapter can be used in the home, hospital, or care center in helping patients meet their spiritual needs. Recent research findings support the importance and value of caregivers' spirituality, yet as a resource, it is often overlooked (Kaye & Robinson, 1994). Nurses should consider using interventions that enhance a caregiver's ability to

take part in church activities to satisfy their spiritual needs and to work with church groups to secure helpful services. Using clergy, prayer, forgiveness, and spiritual reading materials as resources for caregivers may also be helpful.

Nurturing Spirituality

Some patients experiencing a need to get in touch with their spiritual self and to nurture their spiritual development may look to the nurse for direction. The person who lives life enmeshed in the action and noises of society may feel strangely uncomfortable when illness forces self-introspection. The nurse can be helpful in recommending means to develop a relationship with one's inner world and manifest spiritual energy in one's outer world (Hill & Smith, 1990). The accompanying box lists ways to develop one's inner world and to manifest this energy to the outside world.

Promoting Meaning and Purpose

- Explore with the patient what has given the patient's life meaning and purpose up to the present, sources of meaning for other people, and possible meanings for the patient's current experience of illness, pain, suffering, or impending death.
- Refer the patient to a spiritual adviser if the patient wishes this.
- Explore with the patient spiritual practices from which strength and hope might be derived (eg, prayer or reading scripture or other spiritual books).
- Recommend that the patient read spiritual biographies or Harold Kuschner's (1983) book *When Bad*

Using the Nursing Interventions Classification (NIC)

Ways to Develop a Relationship With One's Inner World

- Prayer
- Reflection or "quiet listening to one's essence"
- Communion with nature through walks in the park, woods, beach
- Enjoyment of music, drama, art, dance
- Inner dialogues with oneself or with a higher being
- Dream analysis

Ways to Manifest Spiritual Energy in One's Outer World

- Loving relationships with others
- Service to others in need
- Forgiveness of others
- Empathy, compassion, and hope
- Laughter, joyous expressions
- Participation in church services and activities and social gatherings

(From Hill, L., & Smith, N. [1990]. *Self-care nursing* [2nd ed.]. New York: Appleton & Lange.)

Things Happen to Good People (available in paperback in most bookstores).

- Refer the patient to the appropriate support groups (eg, self-help groups for people with stroke, cancer, and so on).

Promoting Love and Relatedness

- Treat the patient at all times with respect, empathy, and genuine caring.
- Encourage the patient to talk about relationships with others and to identify the origin of negative beliefs about people.
- Encourage conversation about God as the patient knows and experiences God (if God is part of the patient's spiritual beliefs). If appropriate, introduce or reinforce the belief that God is a loving and personal God who is concerned about the patient.
- Whenever possible, encourage and facilitate visits from the patient's family, friends, and spiritual adviser.

Promoting Forgiveness

- Offer a supportive presence to the patient that demonstrates your acceptance of the patient.
- Explore with the patient the importance of learning to accept oneself and others, including both strengths and limitations.
- Explore negative images of God and others that make it difficult for the patient to seek forgiveness and to believe that the patient is forgiven.
- Explore the patient's self-expectations and assist the patient to determine how realistic these are.
- Allow the patient to verbalize shame, guilt, and anger and counsel about the importance of expressing negative emotions in healthy ways. Refer the patient to a spiritual adviser, if appropriate.
- Offer the patient examples of how feelings of unforgiving toward others can end up hurting only the one who cannot forgive.

Praying *With* Patients

Patients accustomed to regular periods of prayer but who feel too ill to pray as they would like or who enjoy praying with others may ask the nurse to pray with them or hope that the nurse will suggest this. Because there are many forms of prayer—quiet reflection, silent communion with God or higher power, reading or recitation of formal prayers, silent or loud calling on God or conversation with God, or reading religious materials—the nurse can take the lead from the patient by asking, "How would you like us to pray?" The religious background of the patient is considered along with the type of prayers that have been meaningful in the past. It is also helpful to ask the patient if there is a particular prayer request.

The nurse unaccustomed to praying aloud or in public may find it helpful to have a Bible passage or formal prayer readily available. The prayer may also be a simple expression aloud of the patient's needs and hopes. A sample follows:

> Lord God, our Creator and Healer, I entrust Mrs. Smith and her family to your loving care . . . bring peace to her mind and health and strength to her body. . . . Be with

her [as her treatment begins today, as she goes for surgery, and so on]. . . . We remember all your blessings to us in the past and thank you. . . . We are confident of your help now as we claim your promises.

Prayer should not block communication with the patient. Praying before a patient feels ready to pray may communicate to the patient a lack of interest in the patient's feelings. Because prayer often evokes deep feelings, the nurse should be prepared to spend time with the patient after sharing prayer to respond to these feelings.

Praying *for* Patients

With research beginning to suggest links between prayer and physical, mental, and spiritual health (Fish, 1995), arguments are being made that healthcare professionals have an obligation to pray *for* as well as *with* their patients. At the present time, no one is claiming that healthcare professionals are negligent if they fail to pray for patients. This, may, however, be an effective intervention strategy. At the very least, nurses ought to be mediators of the spiritual resources patients and their families need.

Counseling Patients Spiritually

The patient who feels that the nurse is sensitive to spiritual needs and comfortable in his or her own spirituality may choose to share spiritual concerns with the nurse rather than with a religious counselor. The nurse who feels able to counsel the patient may assist the patient to accomplish the following:

- Articulate spiritual beliefs
- Explore the origin of the patient's spiritual beliefs and practices
- Identify life factors that challenge the patient's spiritual beliefs (cause spiritual distress)
- Explore alternatives given these challenges: modify lifestyle; deny, modify, or reaffirm beliefs; develop new beliefs
- Develop spiritual beliefs that meet needs for meaning and purpose, care and relatedness, forgiveness

To be an effective spiritual counselor, the nurse must be open to different spiritual beliefs and forms of spiritual expression and supportive of the patient's efforts to nurture spiritual growth.

Contacting a Spiritual Counselor

Not every nurse feels comfortable in the role of spiritual counselor. The nurse may suggest that the patient talk to a spiritual counselor. When a patient expresses a desire to speak to his or her spiritual counselor, the nurse helps make the appropriate referral. The nurse may offer to contact the patient's own spiritual adviser. Other options are to contact the healthcare facility's pastoral ministry department or use a referral list of clergy in the local community. If a representative of the patient's own religion is unable to visit within the hospital at a particular time, the nurse may suggest a visit from a clergyperson from another faith. Such a suggestion may be welcomed by the patient, depending on the situation and the immediacy of the need.

The nurse in a care center can assist the spiritual counselor by making the counselor feel welcome, answering questions about the patient, directing the counselor to the patient, and ensuring that the patient is ready to receive the counselor. Preparations of the patient's room for the visit may vary, but the following are generally recommended practices:

- The room should be orderly and free of unnecessary equipment and items.
- There should be a seat for the religious counselor at the bedside or near the patient so that both can be comfortable during the visit.
- The top of the bedside table should be free of items and covered with a clean, white cover if a sacrament is to be administered.
- The bed curtains should be drawn to provide privacy if the patient is in a unit with other patients and is unable to be moved to a more private setting.

Some patients and spiritual advisers may value the nurse's participation in prayers, rituals, or the administration of sacraments. When a nursing diagnosis of spiritual distress is made, the nurse and the religious counselor can often collaborate on the plan of care and reinforce each other's efforts to assist the patient to meet goals/outcomes.

Resolving Conflicts Between Spiritual Beliefs and Treatments

Both the patient and members of the patient's family may experience conflict between a particular spiritual belief or religious law and a proposed medical treatment or health option. The patient may want the nurse's assistance when conferring with the spiritual adviser about a particular procedure. The nurse's role is to assist the patient in obtaining the information needed to make an informed decision and to support the patient's decision making. Because what the nurse says and the way it is said may powerfully influence the patient's decision, it is important for the nurse to maintain objectivity. Conflicts that resist resolution may be referred to an ethics committee or consult team. See Chapter 6.

EVALUATING

The nurse working with a patient and family to achieve specified goals/outcomes to meet spiritual needs can use each patient interaction to evaluate the plan of care. Necessary to the evaluation are sensitivity to what the patient is saying and not saying and observation of the patient when alone as well as when interacting with the family and nurses.

In general, the nurse evaluates the patient's ability to accomplish the following:

- Identify some spiritual belief that gives meaning and purpose to everyday life
- Move toward a healthy acceptance of the current situation: illness, pain, suffering, impending death
- Develop mutually caring relationships
- Reconcile any interpersonal differences causing the patient anguish
- Verbalize satisfaction with relationship with God (if this is important)
- Express peaceful acceptance of limitations and failings
- Express ability to forgive others and to live in the present
- Demonstrate an "interior state of peace and joy; freedom from abnormal anxiety, guilt, or a feeling of sinfulness; and a sense of security and direction in the pursuit of one's life goals and activities" (O'Brien, 1982, p. 98)

The nurse helps the patient to determine whether spiritual beliefs are generally life affirming or life denying and whether there is harmony between these beliefs and the patient's everyday life experiences. See the accompanying Applying Learning to Practice: Patient Care Study and Nursing Plan of Care boxes.

APPLYING LEARNING TO PRACTICE

Patient Care Study

Mr. Gargan is a 38-year-old divorced man on a step-down unit after treatment for a myocardial infarction. He owns a small car dealership. His religion is listed as Protestant. Frequently unable to sleep at night, Mr. Gargan often talks with the night nurse and once asked, "Did you ever give much thought to whether or not there is a God?" Sensing much concern behind this question, the nurse asks specific questions to determine whether the patient has spiritual needs that are not being met.

Patient Care Study

12/26/02, 2 AM
Patient again unable to sleep and initiated discussion about God. States was raised in a Lutheran home where everyone went to church on Sunday and tried to live according to God's commandments. Upon leaving home, he stopped going to church (was never a value for his wife) and simply has not given much thought to religion—too busy running his business. Until now has not experienced any need for God. "But when I think how close I was to dying and that I've no idea what to expect after death—I'm actually scared. Do others feel this way?" Wants to explore religious beliefs—feels lack in his life. Said he would like to talk with hospital minister—will arrange for tomorrow.

E. Nolan, RN

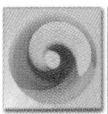

NURSING PLAN OF CARE
for Mr. Gargan

Nursing Diagnosis	Spiritual Distress: Anxiety related to concerns about relationship with God as manifested by self report
Expected Outcome	Before discharge, the patient will: • Identify his religious beliefs

Nursing Interventions	Rationale	Evaluative Statement
Assist the patient to (1) identify the spiritual beliefs he had as a child and the origin of these beliefs; (2) evaluate these beliefs in terms of his life experiences; and (3) reaffirm, modify, or reject these beliefs or develop new spiritual beliefs.	Life experiences may challenge religious beliefs that were uncritically held as a child.	12/30/02 Goal partially met. Patient states he has a much clearer concept of God and no longer fears that God will reject him for ignoring him for so long . . . but believes he also has a lot to learn. *E. Nolan, RN*
Assist the patient to assess whether his newly articulated spiritual beliefs are life affirming or life denying and the degree to which they meet his needs for meaning and purpose, love and relatedness, and forgiveness.	Because spiritual beliefs can exert positive (life-affirming) and negative (life-denying) influences on a person's life, individuals should have some criteria to use when evaluating their beliefs.	
Refer the patient to the hospital minister for assistance with the above.	Patient may value speaking with a minister.	

Expected Outcome	Before discharge, the patient will: • Reconcile his life up until the present with God

Nursing Interventions	Rationale	Evaluative Statement
Reassure the patient that many persons get involved in day-to-day living to the extent that they forget about God and that in some religions persons believe that God uses illness and other stressors to invite people to rethink their spiritual beliefs. In these traditions, God is often pictured with open arms waiting to welcome a child home.	Images of a stern and unyielding God ready to strike down transgressors may contribute to a patient's spiritual distress.	12/30/02 Goal met. "This minister has really helped. I wish I had talked to him a long time ago. I've carried so much guilt about my divorce and some other things—thought God would never forgive me. I feel so much more at peace now." *E. Nolan, RN*
Refer the patient to a spiritual advisor for help in experiencing forgiveness if he mentions guilt feelings.	Guilt often inhibits persons from seeking and experiencing the forgiveness they desire.	
Communicate to the patient the importance of people accepting themselves—with all their strengths and weaknesses.	Many persons have unrealistic self-expectations.	

(continued)

NURSING PLAN OF CARE (Continued)
for Mr. Gargan

Expected Outcome	Before discharge, the patient will:
	• Verbalize that his spiritual beliefs have become a source of strength and peace rather than anxiety

Nursing Interventions	Rationale	Evaluative Statement
Encourage the patient to compare the role of spiritual beliefs in his life before, during, and after hospitalization.	This highlights the positive and negative roles spiritual beliefs can play. It may motivate the patient to continue searching if he values his present experience.	12/30/02 Goal met. "It's good to be able to feel more peaceful about whatever the future brings. I'm anxious to get out of here because there's a lot I want to do with God's help."
		E. Nolan, RN

Expected Outcome	Before discharge, the patient will:
	• Increase night sleep to at least 6 undisturbed hours

Nursing Interventions	Rationale	Evaluative Statement
Nurse on the 11 to 7 shift checks on patient at beginning of shift to make sure he is comfortable and ready for sleep.	Nursing supervision of the patient at bedtime rules out other factors that may interfere with sleep.	12/30/02 Goal met. Patient slept last night from midnight to 6 AM. Will continue to monitor.
		E. Nolan, RN
Use power of suggestion to enhance sleep. "I'm sure when I check back you'll be sound asleep."	Suggestion has been shown to enhance the therapeutic effect of other interventions.	
If sleep remains disturbed, try relaxation exercises or guided imagery (see Chap. 31).	As spiritual anxiety decreases, sleep should improve. If sleep does not improve, other contributing factors and interventions will need to be explored.	

Sample Documentation	12/27/02 3 PM, Nursing
	B. Hanks, Protestant minister, here to see patient at 1 PM. Afterward, patient said he felt "a whole lot better." Reported minister had assured him that many people in the hospital with a serious illness go through exactly what he is experiencing now—and this thought seemed to decrease much of his anxiety. Minister had reinforced nurse's suggestion that he explore his religious beliefs and he has already jotted down some thoughts. "I knew you fixed bodies in hospitals but didn't know you fix souls, too." Patient looking forward to minister's visit tomorrow.
	E. Nolan, RN

Learning Outcomes

After completing this chapter, the learner should be able to accomplish the following:

1. Define key terms used in the chapter:

    agnostic   spiritual beliefs
    atheist   spiritual distress
    faith   spirituality
    religion   spiritual needs

2. Identify three spiritual needs believed to be common to all people.

3. Describe the influences of spirituality on everyday living, health, and illness.

4. Differentiate life-affirming influences of religious beliefs from life-denying influences.
5. Distinguish the spiritual beliefs and practices of the major religions practiced in the United States.
6. Identify five factors that influence spirituality.
7. Perform a nursing assessment of spiritual health, using appropriate interview questions and observation skills.
8. Develop nursing diagnoses that correctly identify spiritual problems.
9. Describe nursing strategies to promote spiritual health and state their rationale.
10. Plan, implement, and evaluate nursing care related to select nursing diagnoses involving spiritual problems.

Critical Thinking Exercises

1. Assess your spiritual well-being, that is, to what extent are you currently able to meet your needs for love and belonging, meaning and purpose, and forgiveness? If confronted with a life-threatening or chronic illness, would you be able to draw on religion or spirituality as a source of strength? Are there any special skills you believe you need to develop to better meet the spiritual needs of your patients? Compare your responses to those of your classmates and explore reasons for the differences you encounter.
2. Poll your classmates and see if they agree strongly, agree, disagree, or disagree strongly with the following statements. Discuss reasons for the differences in your answers and how this is likely to affect your professional practice.

- Prayer has the power to heal physical, mental, and spiritual illness.
- Nurses who do not pray for their patients are deficient professional caregivers.
- Nurses who do not offer to pray with their patients are deficient professional caregivers.

3. How would you respond to a patient who tells you that he isn't very religious but is now wondering if there is a God, and if so, where he stands in relation to God now that his life is in jeopardy? Think about how your personal experience of religion/spirituality colors you response and determine whether your personal experience of religion/spirituality has prepared you well to respond to these queries.

Study Questions

1. Which of the following statements most correctly differentiates between an agnostic and an atheist?
   a. The terms are used interchangeably, both believing there is no God.
   b. An agnostic denies that humans can know anything about God's existence, whereas an atheist denies God's existence.
   c. They both deny the need for a philosophy of living to guide their life.
   d. No aspect of an atheist's life is influenced by spirituality, whereas an agnostic has spiritual values.
2. A nurse who was raised a strict Roman Catholic stated she couldn't assist patients with their spiritual distress because she recognizes only a field power in each individual. She said, "My parents and I hardly talk because I've deserted my faith. Sometimes I feel real isolated from them and also God—if there is a God." Analysis of these data reveals which unmet spiritual need?
   a. need for meaning and purpose
   b. need for forgiveness
   c. need for love and relatedness
   d. need for strength for everyday living
3. Which statement is true concerning the influence of spirituality and religion on the various aspects of a person's life?
   a. All aspects of life may be influenced by spirituality.
   b. Activities of daily living (eating, bathing, sleeping, dressing) are rarely influenced by religion.

   c. Work and recreation are not influenced by religion.
   d. Whereas physical illness is seldom influenced by religion, mental illness frequently is.
4. A patient whose last name was Goldstein was served on a paper plate a kosher meal ordered from a restaurant because the hospital made no provision for kosher food or dishes. Mr. Goldstein became angry and accused the nurse of insulting him. "I want to eat what everyone else does—and give me decent dishes." Analysis of these data reveals that
   a. the nurse should have ordered kosher dishes also
   b. the staff must have behaved condescendingly or critically
   c. Mr. Goldstein is a problem patient and difficult to satisfy
   d. Mr. Goldstein was stereotyped and not consulted about his dietary preferences
5. You are least likely to encounter resistance to emergency life-saving surgery for a patient from which of the following families?
   a. Christian Scientist family
   b. Faith Assembly Healer family
   c. Jehovah's Witness family
   d. Orthodox Jewish family
6. When the family desires baptism for an infant, it is imperative that the nurse provide for baptism to be done because

    a. baptism frequently postpones or prevents death or suffering

    b. it is legally required that nurses provide for this care when the family makes this request

    c. it is a nursing function to assure the salvation of the baby

    d. lack of baptism when desired may increase the family's sorrow and suffering

7. Because the capacity for abstract thought develops as a child grows older, spirituality is understood differently by children of different ages. Which of the following statements is false?

    a. Spirituality and perception of God is meaningless for the 4- to 5-year-old.

    b. Even young children, 4 to 5 years of age, have definite perceptions of God and forms of worship.

    c. Children's perceptions of their "spiritual self" mature as they mature.

    d. Children, 5 to 11 years of age, may show anxiety concerning the power they believe God has.

8. The most important source of learning about his or her own spirituality for a child is

    a. his or her church or religious organization

    b. what parents say about God and religion

    c. how parents behave in relationship to one another and their children, to others, and to God

    d. the spiritual adviser for the family

9. Even though a detailed nursing history in which spirituality is assessed is taken on admission, problems with spiritual distress may not surface until days after admission. The probable explanation is that

    a. patients usually want to conceal information about spiritual needs

    b. patients are not concerned about spiritual needs until after their spiritual adviser visits

    c. family members and close friends often initiate spiritual concerns

    d. illness increases spiritual concerns, which may be difficult for patients to express in words

10. When a patient needs spiritual counseling, the nurse who is comfortable with his or her own spirituality should

    a. always call the patient's own spiritual adviser

    b. consult with the patient about the spiritual adviser with whom he or she wishes to counsel

    c. attempt to counsel the patient and, if unsuccessful, make a referral

    d. advise the patient and spiritual adviser concerning health options and the correct decision

11. When assessment data point to a spiritual problem that can be treated by independent nursing intervention, it receives the NANDA-approved diagnostic label

    a. Spiritual Alienation

    b. Spiritual Despair

    c. Spiritual Distress

    d. Spiritual Pain

12. A patient states she feels so isolated from her family and church and even God "in this huge medical center so far from home." An appropriate goal for the patient to relieve her spiritual distress is as follows. The patient will

    a. express satisfaction with the compatibility of her spiritual beliefs and everyday living

    b. identify spiritual beliefs that meet her need for meaning and purpose

    c. express peaceful acceptance of limitations and failings

    d. identify spiritual supports available to her in this medical center

13. A man who is a declared agnostic is extremely depressed after losing his home, his wife, and his children in a fire. His nursing diagnosis is Spiritual Distress: Spiritual Pain related to inability to find meaning and purpose in his current condition. The most important nursing intervention to plan is to

    a. ask the patient which spiritual adviser he would like you to call

    b. recommend that the patient read spiritual biographies or religious books

    c. explore with the patient what, in addition to his family, has given his life meaning and purpose in the past

    d. introduce the belief that God is a loving and personal God

14. After having an abortion, the patient told the visiting nurse, "I shouldn't have had that abortion because I'm Catholic, but what else could I do? I'm afraid I'll never get close to my mother or back in the Church again." She then talked with her priest about this feeling of guilt. Which evaluation statement shows a solution to the problem?

    a. Patient states, "I wish I had talked with the priest sooner. I now know God has forgiven me and even my mother understands."

    b. Patient has slept from 10 PM to 6 AM for three consecutive nights without medication.

    c. Patient has developed mutually caring relationships with two women and one man.

    d. Patient has identified several spiritual beliefs that give purpose to her life.

15. Mr. Brown's teenage daughter had been involved in shoplifting. He expressed much anger toward her and stated he could not face her, let alone discuss this with her. "I just will not tolerate a thief." Which of the following nursing interventions would you take to assist Mr. Brown with his deficit in forgiveness?

    a. Assure him that many parents feel the same way.

    b. Reassure him that many teenagers go through this kind of rebellion and that it will pass.

    c. Assist the patient to identify how unforgiving feelings toward others only hurt the one who cannot forgive.

    d. Ask him if he is sure he has spent sufficient time with his daughter.

Answers With Rationale

1. The correct response is *b.* It is factually correct that an agnostic denies that humans can know anything about God's existence, whereas an atheist denies God's existence. The other options are factually incorrect.

2. The correct response is *c.* The data point to an unmet spiritual need to experience love and belonging given her estrangement from her family and God after her leaving the church. The other options may represent other needs this patient has, but the data provided do not support them.

3. The correct response is *a.* It is true that spirituality can influence all aspects of a person's life, including activities of daily living, work and recreation, and all types of illnesses. The other options are incomplete or false.

4. The correct response is *d.* The nurse jumped to the premature and false conclusion with this patient on the basis of his name alone that he would want a kosher diet.

5. The correct response is *d.* There is no teaching in the Hebrew scriptures that prohibits emergency life-saving surgery. On the contrary, most Orthodox Jews would be highly motivated to have the surgery because of the high value attached to preserving life. All of the other groups mentioned might have religious grounds for refusing surgery.

6. The correct response is *d.* Failure to ensure that an infant baptism is performed when parents desire it may greatly increase the family's sorrow and suffering, and this is an appropriate nursing concern. Whether baptism postpones or prevents death and suffering (option *a*) is a religious belief that is insufficient to bind all nurses. There is no legal requirement regarding baptism; option *b* is false. Although some nurses may believe part of their role is to assure the salvation (option *c*) of the baby, this function would understandably be rejected by many.

7. The correct response is *a.* It is false that spirituality and perception of God is meaningless for the 4- to 5-year-old. All the other options are factually correct.

8. The correct response is *c.* Children learn most about their own spirituality from how their parents behave in relationship to one another, their children, others, and God. Less important sources of learning are each of the other options.

9. The correct response is *d.* It is factually correct that illness surfaces and may increase spiritual concerns, which many patients find difficult to express. The other options do not correspond to actual experience.

10. The correct response is *b.* Even when a nurse feels comfortable discussing spiritual concerns, he or she should always check first with patients to determine the spiritual adviser with whom they wish to counsel. Calling the patient's own spiritual adviser (option *a*) may be premature if it is a matter the nurse can handle. Options *c* and *d* deny patients the right to speak privately with their spiritual adviser from the outset, if this is what they prefer.

11. The correct response is *c.* The only NANDA-approved nursing diagnosis among the options is Spiritual Distress. The other options may be further specifications of the broader diagnosis Spiritual Distress.

12. The correct response is *d.* Each of the four options represents appropriate spiritual goals. Identifying spiritual supports available to her in the medical center demonstrates a decreased sense of isolation.

13. The correct response is *c.* The nursing intervention of exploring with the patient what, in addition to his family, has given his life meaning and purpose in the past is more likely to correct the etiology of his problem, Spiritual Pain, than any of the other nursing interventions listed.

14. The correct response is *a.* Because this patient's nursing diagnosis is Spiritual Distress: Guilt, an evaluative statement that demonstrates a diminishment of guilt is necessary. Only option *a* directly deals with guilt.

15. The correct response is *c* because this is the only nursing intervention that directly addresses the patient's unmet spiritual need concerning forgiveness. Options *a* and *b* may make him feel better initially, but neither option addresses his need to forgive. Option *d* is likely to make him feel guilty.

Bibliography

Andrews, M. M., & Hanson, P. A. (1995). Religion, culture, and nursing. In M. M. Andrews & J. S. Boyle (Eds.), *Transcultural concepts in nursing care.* Philadelphia: J. B. Lippincott.

Burnhard, P. (1987). Spiritual distress and the nursing response: Theoretical considerations and counseling skills. *Journal of Advanced Nursing, 12*(3), 377–382.

Callahan, D., & Campbell, C. S. (Eds.). (1990). Theology, religious traditions, and bioethics: A special supplement. *Hastings Center Report, 20*(6), 18–19.

Carson, V. B. (1989). *Spiritual dimensions of nursing practice.* Philadelphia: W. B. Saunders.

Charnes, L. S. (1992). Meeting patients' spiritual needs: The Jewish perspective. *Holistic Nursing Practice, 6*(3), 64–72.

Clark, C., & Heidenreich, T. (1995). Spiritual care for the critically ill. *American Journal of Critical Care, 4*(1), 77–81.

Coles, R. (1990). *The spiritual life of children.* Boston: Houghton Mifflin.

Cutcliffe, J. R. (1995). How do nurses inspire and instill hope in terminally ill HIV patients? *Journal of Advanced Nursing, 22,* 888–895.

Dossey, B. (Ed.). (1989). Spirituality and healing. *Holistic Nursing Practice, 3*(3) [entire issue].

Dossey, B. M., & Dossey, L. (1998). Attending to holistic care. *American Journal of Nursing, 98*(8), 35–38.

Fish, S. (1995). Can research prove that God answers prayer? *Journal of Christian Nursing, 12*(1), 24–27, 46.

Fitchett, G. (1993). *Assessing spiritual needs: A guide for caregivers.* Minneapolis: Augsburg.

Fowler, J. W. (1981). *Stages of faith: The psychology of human development and the quest for meaning.* San Francisco: Harper-Collins.

Gaskins, S., & Forte, L. (1995). The meaning of hope: Implications for nursing practice and research. *Journal of Gerontological Nursing, 21*(3), 17–24.

Goddard, N. C. (1995). "Spirituality as integrative energy": A philosophical analysis as requisite precursor to holistic nursing practice. *Journal of Advanced Nursing, 22*(4), 808–815.

Gregg-Schroeder, S. (April 1999). A transforming experience: Circles of Life. *Journal of Fellowship in Prayer,* 23–25.

Hauerwas, S. (1990). *Naming the silences: God, medicine, and the problem of suffering.* Grand Rapids: Erdmans.

Heller, D. (1985). The children's God. *Psychology Today, 19*(12), 22–27.

Hill, L., & Smith, N. (1990). *Self-care nursing* (2nd ed.). New York: Appleton & Lange.

Hungelmann, J., et al. (1989). Development of the JAREL spiritual well-being scale. In NANDA (Eds.), *Classification of nursing diagnosis: Proceedings of the eighth conference* (pp. 393–398). Philadelphia: J. B. Lippincott.

Kaye, J., & Robinson, K. M. (1994). Spirituality among caregivers. *Image—The Journal of Nursing Scholarship, 26*(3), 218–221.

Kuschner, H. S. (1983). *When bad things happen to good people.* New York: Avon.

Macrae, J. (1995). Nightingale's spiritual philosophy and its significance for modern nursing. *Image—The Journal of Nursing Scholarship, 27*(1), 8–10.

Manson, C. H. (1995). Prayer as a nursing intervention. *Journal of Christian Nursing, 12*(1), 4–8.

McHolm, F. A. (1992). A nursing diagnosis validation study: Defining characteristics of spiritual distress. In R. M.

Carroll-Johnson (Ed.), *Classification of nursing diagnosis: Proceedings of the ninth conference* (pp. 112–119). Philadelphia: J. B. Lippincott.

Miles, A. (199). When faith is used to justify helping victims of family violence. *American Journal of Nursing, 99*(5), 32–35.

Miller, M. A. (1995). Culture, spirituality and women's health. *Journal of Obstetric, Gynecologic, and Neonatal Nursing, 24*(3), 257–263.

Murray, R. B., & Zentner, J. P. (1989). *Nursing assessment and health promotion strategies throughout the lifespan* (4th ed.). New York: Appleton-Lange.

North American Nursing Diagnosis Association. (1994). *NANDA nursing diagnoses: Definitions and classifications* 1995–1996. Philadelphia: Author.

O'Brien, M. E. (1982). The need for spiritual integrity. In H. Yura & M. Walsh (Eds.), *Human needs 2 and the nursing process* (pp. 81–115). Norwalk, CT: Appleton-Century-Crofts.

O'Brien, M. E. (1999). *Spirituality in nursing.* Boston: Jones and Bartlett.

O'Neill, D. P., & Kenny, E. K. (1998). Spirituality and chronic illness. *Image—The Journal of Nursing Scholarship, 30*(3), 275–280.

Parrinder, G. (Ed.). (1983). *World religions.* New York: Facts on File Publications.

Rahner, K. (1971). How to receive a sacrament and mean it. *Theology Digest, 19,* 229.

Shaffer, J. L. (Ed.). (1989). Spirituality and healing. *Holistic Nursing Practice, 3*(3) [entire issue].

Shelly, J., & Fish, S., (1988). *Spiritual care: The nurse's role* (3rd ed.). Downer's Grove, IL: InterVarsity Press.

Starck, P. L., & McGovern, J. P. (Eds.). (1992). *The hidden dimension of illness: Human suffering.* New York: National League for Nursing Press.

Stoll, R. I. (1979). Guidelines for spiritual assessment. *American Journal of Nursing, 79*(9), 1574–1577.

Sumner, C. H. (1998). Recognizing and responding. *American Journal of Nursing, 98*(1), 26–31.

Widerquist, J., & Davidhizar, R. (1994). The ministry of nursing. *Journal of Advanced Nursing, 19*(4), 647–652.

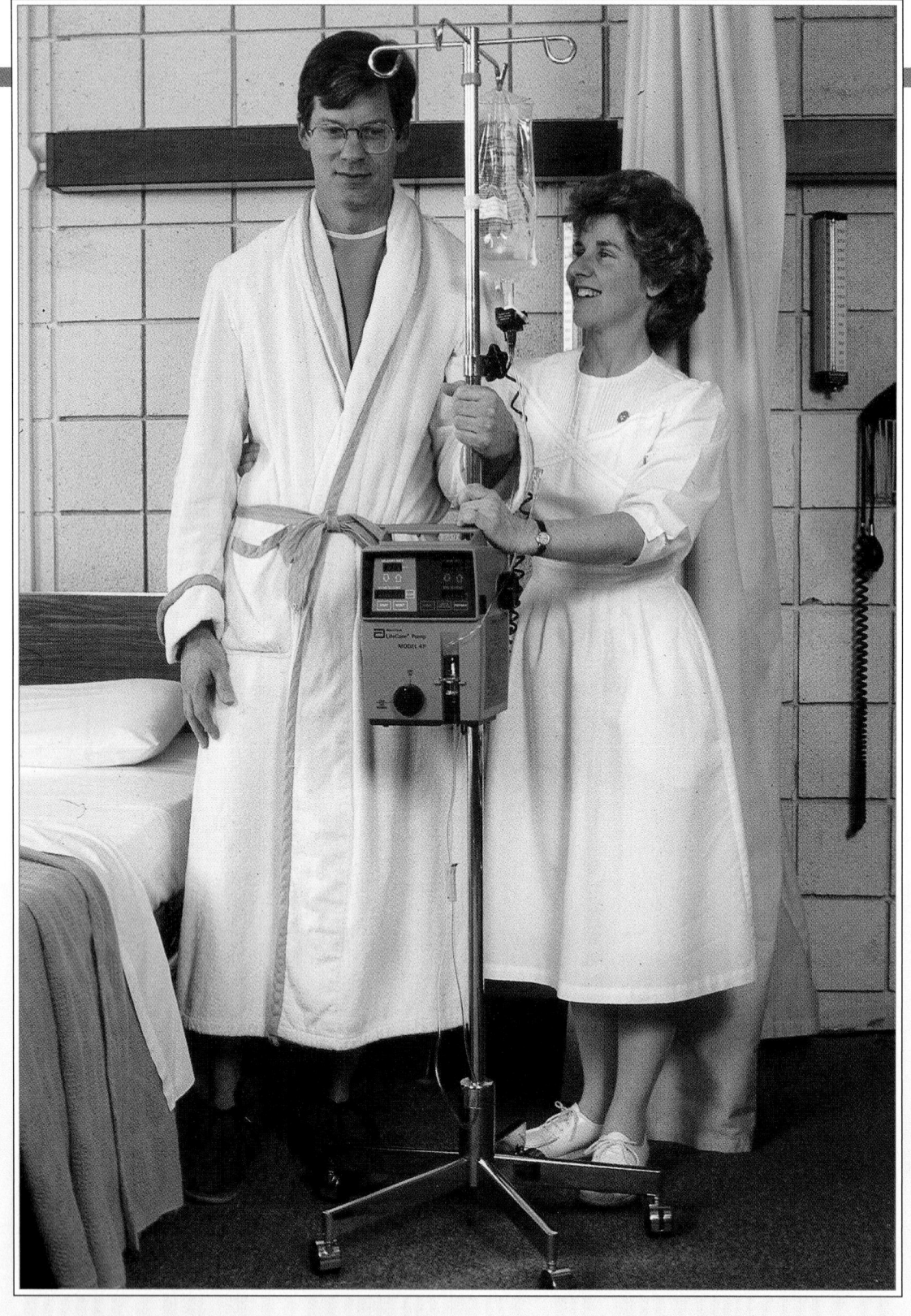

UNIT VIII

Promoting Healthy Physiologic Responses

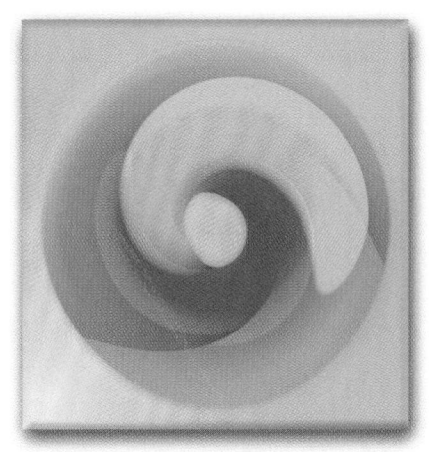

". . . what nursing has to do is to put the patient in the best condition for nature to act upon him."

Florence Nightingale (1820–1910)
a philosopher, theorist, statistician, humanitarian, and inspirational leader who founded modern nursing through a systematic method of training well-qualified nurses; also initiated important reforms in military sanitation and hospital construction that greatly improved patient survival

The art and science of caring are blended when nurses implement actions to meet basic human needs and to promote healthy physiologic responses. The chapters in Unit VIII focus on information and guidelines essential to nursing practice in a wide variety of clinical settings and involving both healthy and ill patients of all ages. Included are nursing interventions to promote safety and comfort and to meet basic physiologic needs—hygiene, activity and rest, nutrition, elimination, oxygenation, and fluid–electrolyte balance.

Each basic physiologic need is discussed, first, with a review of concepts pertinent to the specific area of human function and response, and then with an examination of factors that affect need satisfaction. The steps of the nursing process are used to provide guidelines and information necessary for making accurate assessments; establishing goals; and planning, implementing, and evaluating specific nursing interventions to meet needs and promote wellness.

The chapters in Unit VIII enable the beginning nurse caregiver to integrate the knowledge and skills necessary to promote healthy physiologic responses in patients in any practice setting. Nursing process skills are further refined to ensure that care is holistic, comprehensive, and individualized.

Chapter 36
Hygiene

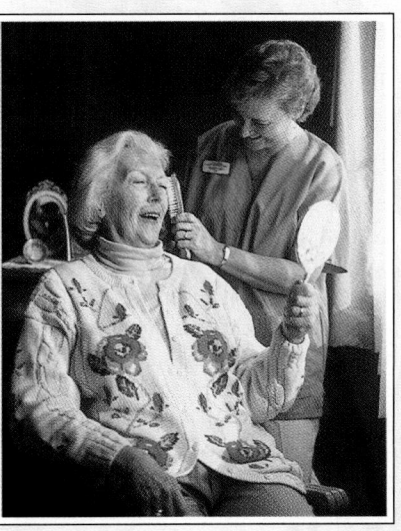

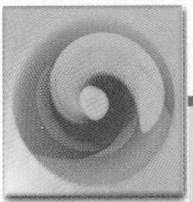

**Thinking Critically About
Nursing's Blended Skills**

Before reading this chapter, think about the types of blended skills you will need to assist patients effectively with hygiene measures.

- Jean and Bob are the proud new parents of twins. Neither patient has siblings, and both report no experience in childcare. They seem afraid to hold their babies—let alone bathe them!

- Another nurse asks you why you still bother to give patients back massages. "No one does that anymore. I tell patients they can pay for a massage therapist if they want to be massaged."

- Mrs. Della Pia had a new stroke, which left the right side of her body paralyzed. She is being discharged from the hospital and will now live with her daughter, who will be her primary caretaker. Her daughter is eager to learn everything she can about how she can best help her mom. Among her questions is, "What's the best way to keep her clean?"

- John Doe is a homeless man who was found unconscious on the street and brought to the emergency room. It appears that he has not bathed for days. No one wants to touch him.

What cognitive, technical, interpersonal, and ethical/legal skills do you think you will need to respond to the challenges described above?

easeres for personal cleanliness and grooming that promote physical and psychological well-being are called *personal hygiene*. Personal hygiene practices vary widely among people. The time of day one bathes and how often a person shampoos his or her hair or changes the bed linens and sleeping garments are relatively unimportant. What is important is that personal care be carried out conveniently and frequently enough to promote personal hygiene.

Well people are ordinarily responsible for their own hygiene. In some cases, the nurse may assist a well person through teaching to develop personal hygiene habits the person may lack.

Illness, hospitalization, and institutionalization generally require modifications in hygiene practices. In these situations, the nurse helps the patient to continue sound hygienic practices and can teach the patient and family members, when necessary, regarding hygiene. Nurses assisting patients with basic hygiene should respect individual patient preferences and give only the care that patients cannot or should not provide for themselves.

This chapter discusses multiple factors that affect personal hygiene and nursing measures that promote personal hygiene. A practical guide for assessing the adequacy of personal hygiene behaviors is presented. Because the data the nurse collects when assisting with hygiene may lead to identifying multiple nursing diagnoses and collaborative problems, samples of these are provided. Patient goals are presented, as are specific nursing strategies used when performing care of the skin; mouth; eyes, ears, and nose; feet; and perineal and vaginal areas.

The concluding patient care study on feminine hygiene illustrates how the nurse uses knowledge of personal hygiene practices and the integumentary system along with specific nursing interventions to resolve nursing diagnoses successfully and to promote the patient's general sense of well-being.

Physiology of the Skin and Its Appendages

Integument refers to the skin. The *integumentary system* is made up of the skin, the subcutaneous layer directly under the skin, and the appendages of the skin, that is, the hair, glands in the skin, and the nails. The skin is one of the body's vital organs and is essential for maintaining life.

The skin has two layers. The superficial portion, the **epidermis**, is composed of layers of stratified epithelial cells. These cells are fused to form a protective, waterproof layer of keratin material. Epithelial cells have no blood vessels of their own and depend on underlying tissues for nourishment and waste removal. When well nourished, epithelium regenerates relatively easily and quickly.

The second layer of skin, the **dermis**, consists of smooth, muscular tissue; nerves; hair follicles; certain glands and their ducts; arteries, veins, and capillaries; and fibrous, elastic tissue. Each hair consists of the shaft, which projects through the dermis beyond the surface of the skin, and the hair follicle, which lies in the dermis. The dermis rests on a subcutaneous fatty tissue layer that anchors the skin layers and serves as a heat insulator for the body. This

COGNITIVE SKILLS

- Basic knowledge about hygiene, hygiene measures, massage, and the products and equipment that facilitate care
- Knowledge about common problems of the skin and mucous membranes and how to treat them
- Ability to identify patients with self-care deficits related to hygiene and to develop and implement appropriate plans to address these deficits

TECHNICAL SKILLS

- Ability to use the products and equipment correctly that are necessary to meet the hygiene needs of patients

INTERPERSONAL SKILLS

- Strong people skills; ability to communicate and interact effectively with patients and their caretakers while assisting with hygiene measures

- Ability to use the time spent assisting patients with hygiene measures to communicate that you care about the patients and are committed to their health and well-being
- Ability to encourage patients and their caretakers, as appropriate, and colleagues in learning new self-care measures related to hygiene.

ETHICAL/LEGAL SKILLS

- Commitment to safety and quality; strong sense of responsibility and accountability
- Ability to delegate the provision of basic hygiene measures to unlicensed assistive personnel and to supervise this care according to agency protocol
- Ability to document problems with hygiene and nursing's response according to agency policy

fatty tissue layer contains blood and lymph vessels, nerves, and fat cells. The two main layers of skin and the subcutaneous layer compose the integumentary system.

The skin covers the entire body and is continuous with mucous membranes at normal body orifices. A cross-section of normal skin is illustrated in Figure 36-1. Glands in the skin include the sebaceous glands, the sweat glands, and the ceruminal glands. The **sebaceous glands** secrete an oily substance called *sebum*, which lubricates the skin and hair and keeps the skin and scalp pliant. The sweat glands secrete perspiration. The **cerumen** (ear wax) in the external ear canals, consisting of a heavy oil and brown pigment, is secreted by *ceruminal glands*.

Functions of Skin and Mucous Membranes

The skin serves six major functions, described in Table 36-1. Mucous membranes line body cavities that open to the outside of the body and can also be found in the digestive tract, the respiratory passages, and the urinary and reproductive tracts. Epithelium covers the mucous membrane surfaces and contains cells that secrete mucus. Connective tissue lies beneath the epithelium. Mucous membranes have receptors that offer the body protection; for example, an irritating substance in the upper respiratory tract causes a person to sneeze, and food caught in the larynx or trachea causes a person to cough. Sneezing and coughing are protective

mechanisms that help rid the body of foreign materials. Mucous membranes are insensitive to temperature, except in the mouth and rectum, but are sensitive to pressure. Mucous membranes also function to absorb substances from their surface; for example, digested food is absorbed through the mucous membrane in the small intestine.

Principles of Skin Care

Knowledge of the functions of the skin and mucous membranes and of factors affecting them includes an understanding of certain basic principles that become important in the care of the skin and mucous membranes:

- *Unbroken and healthy skin and mucous membranes serve as the first lines of defense against harmful agents.*
- *Resistance to injury of the skin and mucous membranes varies among people.* Factors influencing resistance include the person's age, the amount of underlying tissues, and illness conditions.
- *Adequately nourished and hydrated body cells are resistant to injury.* The better nourished the cell, the better its ability to resist injury and disease.
- *Adequate circulation is necessary to maintain cell life.* The cells are inadequately nourished and wastes are poorly removed when circulation is impaired for any reason.

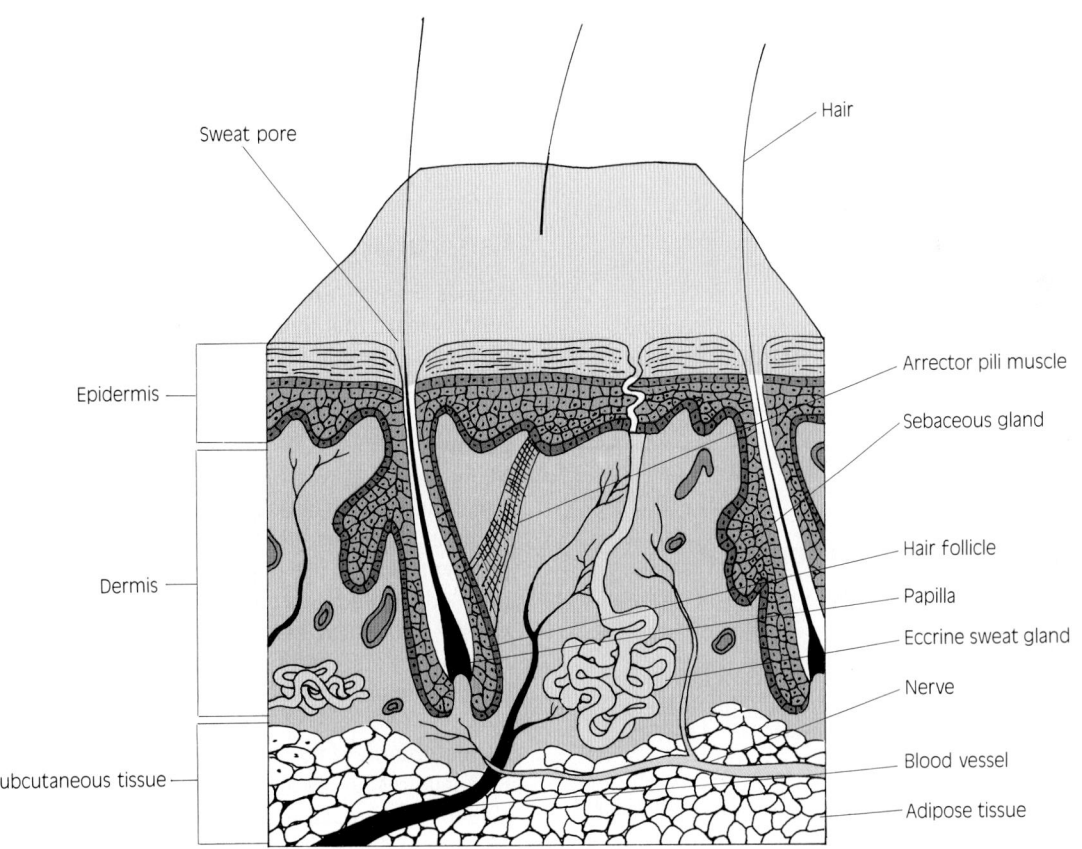

Figure 36-1
A cross-section of normal skin.

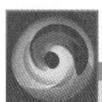

Table 36-1
Functions of the Skin

Function	Mechanisms
The skin protects the body	Invasion of the body by bacteria is prevented by intact skin. Injury to underlying tissues and organs is decreased by intact skin.
The skin helps regulate body temperature	The production of perspiration and its loss by evaporation help cool the body.
	Much heat is lost from the body by radiation and by conduction when the blood supply to the skin is increased by vasodilation.
	Lack of perspiration and vasoconstriction help the body retain heat.
	The phenomenon of producing gooseflesh, which is caused by contraction of pilomotor muscles in the skin, helps conserve body heat because the hair standing on end forms a layer of air on the body for insulation.
The skin is a sense organ	There are receptors for pain, touch, pressure, and temperature in the skin that help the body receive stimuli from the environment.
The skin is an excretory organ	Water, salts, and nitrogenous wastes are lost from the skin, although in much smaller quantities than are lost from the kidneys.
The skin helps maintain water and electrolyte balance	The escape of excess water and electrolytes from the body is prevented by the skin.
The skin produces and absorbs vitamin D	A precursor for vitamin D is present in the skin, which, in conjunction with ultraviolet rays from the sun, produces vitamin D.

Factors Affecting Skin Condition and Personal Hygiene

Skin Condition

A person's developmental stage and health affect skin condition in various ways.

Developmental Considerations

- An infant's skin and mucous membranes are easily injured and subject to infection. Careful handling of infants is required to prevent injury and infection of the skin and mucous membranes.

- A child's skin becomes increasingly resistant to injury and infection. However, the skin requires special care because of the toilet and play habits of children.
- An adolescent's skin ordinarily has enlarged sebaceous glands and increased glandular secretions, caused by hormonal changes in the body. These characteristics predispose adolescents to acne (discussed later in this chapter).
- Secretions from the skin glands are at their maximum during adolescence and continue until about 50 years of age.
- Changes that occur in the skin with aging are discussed in the accompanying box, Focus on the Older Adult. These changes are irreversible. Brown spots, called *liver spots*, often appear. They may begin appearing as early as 35 years of age and tend to become more numerous and larger with aging. These spots result from exposure to the wind and sun and are unrelated to the liver.

Health State

- Very thin and very obese people tend to be more susceptible to skin irritation and injury.
- Fluid loss through fever, vomiting, or diarrhea reduces the fluid volume of the body and is called *dehydration*. Dehydration makes the skin appear loose and flabby.
- Excessive perspiration, often associated with being ill, predisposes the skin to breakdown, especially in skin folds.
- *Jaundice*, a condition caused by excessive bile pigments in the skin, results in a yellowish skin color. The skin is often itchy and dry in patients with jaundice.
- Diseases of the skin often cause lesions that require special care in personal hygiene and therapeutic regimens.

Personal Hygiene

Nurses caring for patients from diverse backgrounds quickly learn that hygiene practices vary widely among individuals. The following factors may influence personal hygiene behaviors.

Culture

Many people in North America place a high value on personal cleanliness and feel unclean unless they shower or bathe at least once daily. Many consider bathing incomplete without the use of products to reduce or mask normal body odors. People from many other cultures often find a weekly bath sufficient and may feel no need to mask normal body odors. Culture may also influence whether bathing is a private or communal activity (Freeman, 1997).

Socioeconomic Class

Financial resources often define the hygiene options available to individuals. A person renting a room in a boarding house may have limited or no access to a tub or shower and may have limited finances for the purchase of soap, shampoo, shaving cream, and deodorant. Homeless peo-

Focus on the Older Adult

Older skin is different from younger skin. The visible changes may vary considerably based on intrinsic (natural aging) factors and extrinsic (environmental factors).

Skin Alterations Due to Aging	Implications for the Older Adult
Subcutaneous and dermal tissue become thin.	Skin is thinner, is more easily injured, has less capacity to insulate, and wrinkles.
Activity of sebaceous and sweat glands decreases.	Perspiration is decreased, skin becomes dryer, and pruritus (itching) may occur.
Cell renewal is shorter.	Healing time is delayed.
Melanocytes (cells that make the pigment that colors hair and skin) decline in number.	Hair becomes gray-white and skin may be unevenly pigmented.
Vascularity decreases to the skin.	Skin temperature is cooler, and pallor may be apparent.
Nail growth rate diminishes.	Nails become soft and tear easily.
Collagen fiber is less organized.	Skin loses elasticity.

ple, who often carry all their belongings in a car or shopping cart, may welcome the warm running water and soap available in roadside or public restrooms. Other people may refrain from using public restrooms because they are perceived as being dirty.

Spiritual Practices

Religion may dictate ceremonial washings and purifications, sometimes as a prelude to prayer or eating. For example, in the orthodox Jewish tradition, ritual baths are required for women after childbirth and menstruation. In some religions, contact with a deceased person or a deceased animal may make a person "unclean."

Developmental Level and Knowledge Level

Children learn different hygiene practices while growing up. Family practices may dictate morning or evening baths, the frequency of shampooing, feelings about nudity, frequency of clothing changes, and so on. Adolescents may experience a need to change hygiene measures from those of childhood, such as beginning to take more frequent hot showers. Older people often experience a need to decrease bathing frequency and the use of deodorant soaps to avoid excessively drying the skin.

Health State

Disease or injury may adversely affect a person's ability to perform hygiene measures or motivation to follow usual hygiene habits. Weakness, dizziness, and fear of falling may prevent an individual from entering a tub or shower or from bending to wash the lower extremities. Illness may also create a demand for new or modified hygiene measures.

Personal Preferences

People have different personal preferences with regard to hygiene practices. Showers versus tub baths, bar soap ver-

sus liquid soap, and washing to wake oneself or to relax before sleep are examples of personal preferences. One's self-concept and sexuality are also personal influences on hygiene.

Basic Skin Care and Personal Hygiene

The Nursing Process

Before attempting to teach patients healthy hygiene practices, nurses should evaluate their own practices. See the accompanying box, Applying Learning to Practice.

ASSESSING

Nursing History

Bathing practices and cleansing habits and rituals vary widely. A clear threat to health must exist before a nurse decides that an individual's hygiene practices are inadequate. The nurse assessing the adequacy of a patient's hygiene practices evaluates whether the patient has the knowledge, attitude, skills, and resources to care for the skin and mucous membranes. See the Focused Assessment Guide in the accompanying box.

The patient should be questioned about any past or current problems, (eg. rashes, lumps, itching, dryness, lesions). When skin problems are present, the patient should be asked the following:

How long have you had this problem?
Does it itch or bother you?
How does it bother you?
Have you found any care helpful in relieving these
    symptoms?

APPLYING LEARNING TO PRACTICE

The Nurse as Role Model: Personal Hygiene

Nurses consistently serve as role models for patients in regard to personal hygiene. If unable to meet the following goals, you may wish to take the time now to examine your own hygiene practices.

- The nurse's physical appearance and body scents give evidence of adequate hygiene practices:
  - Hair is clean and neatly styled.
  - Skin is clean.
  - Mouth evidences satisfactory oral hygiene.
  - Nails are neatly manicured.
  - Body is free of unpleasant odors.

- The nurse's diet and exercise habits contribute to clean and intact skin.
- The nurse brushes teeth after each meal, flosses daily, and goes to the dentist for a checkup at least annually.
- The nurse's care of patients demonstrates an appreciation for the relationship between hygiene and overall well-being.
- The nurse consistently uses appropriate aseptic safeguards (ie, handwashing, use of gloves) to prevent the transmission of microorganisms.

Sample entries in documentation of a nursing history follow:

> *Hygiene:* "Showers twice daily, once in the morning and after working out in the evening. Skin tends to be very dry, and moisturizing creams are used daily. Aveeno Oilated baths p.r.n. Allergic to deodorant soaps."
>
> *Integument:* "History of athlete's foot since high school days with outbreaks every 2 to 3 months. Knowledgeable about appropriate foot care. Uses Tinactin cream (topical fungicidal agent) and Mexsana medicated powder (topical protectant)."

Physical Assessment

The inspection and palpation skills used to assess the integumentary system are described in detail in Chapter 25. Nurses assisting patients with basic hygiene measures have an excellent opportunity to examine the patients' skin carefully. Many individuals are unaware of skin lesions, such as precancerous moles, which, if untreated, could prove fatal. Early detection and treatment of skin problems are important nursing functions.

In examining the skin, the nurse pays careful attention to cleanliness, color, texture, temperature, turgor, moisture, sensation, vascularity, and the presence of lesions. If a lesion is detected, the nurse documents the type, color, size, distribution and grouping, location, and consistency. Terminology helpful in describing these findings is presented in Chapter 25. General guidelines for assessing the skin are as follows:

- Proceed systematically in head-to-toe fashion.
- Use a good source of light, preferably daylight.
- Compare bilateral parts for symmetry.
- Use standard terminology to report and record findings.
- Allow data obtained in the nursing history to direct the skin assessment.

- Identify any variables known to cause skin problems, such as deficient self-care abilities; immobility; malnutrition; decreased hydration; decreased sensation; vascular problems (altered tissue perfusion or venous return); or presence of irritants (body secretions or excretions on the skin, other chemicals, mechanical devices).

Because lifestyle factors, changes in health state, illness, and certain diagnostic and therapeutic measures may adversely affect the skin, the nurse needs to identify high-risk populations and perform the appropriate skin assessment. Knowing *when* to perform the skin assessment and incorporating this into the patient's plan of care is as important as knowing *how* to do this well. Table 36-2 identifies sample factors that place an individual at risk for skin alterations.

Sample entries under integumentary system in documentation of the nursing examination follow:

> "Skin is pink, warm, dry, and elastic; no petechiae, lesions, or excoriation; multiple moles of small size and regular border and surface."
>
> "Red, macular rash generalized over trunk and thighs; semiconfluent lesions measure 1 to 2 mm; abrupt onset."

DIAGNOSING

A careful assessment of the skin and mucous membranes may lead to the identification of numerous patient problems that can be classified as nursing diagnoses. Problems concerning deficient hygiene are categorized as self-care deficits. Self-Care Deficit diagnoses address four specific activities necessary to meet daily needs: feeding, bathing and hygiene, dressing and grooming, and toileting. It is important to identify the cause of these problems correctly. If hygiene is deficient because of insufficient knowledge, health education may quickly remedy the problem. If, however, the individual gives low priority to hygiene or lacks the physical ability

FOCUSED ASSESSMENT GUIDE

Hygiene Practices

Factors to Assess	Questions and Approaches
Daily and weekly bathing habits	Tell me about your daily and weekly bathing habits.
	Are there special bathing or hygiene products you routinely use or can't use?
	How can nurses best help you to meet your hygiene needs?
Factors interfering with hygiene practices (sensory, cognitive, endurance, mobility, or motivation)	What recently or in the past has interfered with your hygiene practices?
	Does anything interfere with your ability to be as clean as you would like?
History of skin or mucous membrane problems (nature, onset of problem and frequency, causes, severity, symptoms, interventions attempted, and results)	Describe any skin problems with rashes, lumps, itching, dryness, lesions, ecchymosis, or masses.
	What have you used to relieve these symptoms?
Special hygiene practices	
• Mouth	How do you clean your teeth and gums?
	How often do you have a dental examination?
	Do you have any dental appliances?
	Are there any tender areas or lesions in your mouth?
• Eyes, ears, and nose	Do you wear glasses or contact lenses to improve your vision?
	Do you wear a hearing aid?
	Have you experienced any discharge or bleeding from or swelling of your eyes, ears, or nose?
• Hair	Have you noticed any unusual dryness of the scalp or changes in hair texture and amount?
• Feet and nails	Is the appearance of the nails normal?
	How do you normally care for and clean your nails?
	Is the skin intact on the feet?
	Have you noticed any swelling of one or both feet?
	Do you wear any special shoes?
• Perineum	Have you noticed any unusual discharge, swelling, itching, or inflammation?
	Are you able to complete your own perineal care?
	Do you follow any special hygiene practices during menstruation?
	What type of feminine hygiene products (eg, pads, tampons, douches) do you use?

to perform hygiene measures, these problems must be addressed before health education can be effective.

Sample nursing diagnoses related to hygiene and skin problems follow:

- Bathing/Hygiene Self-Care Deficit related to sensory, cognitive, endurance, mobility, or motivation deficits
- Pain related to skin or mucous membrane alterations
- Ineffective Individual Coping related to chronic skin problems
- Altered Health Maintenance (eg, dental caries, periodontal disease, halitosis) related to deficient oral hygiene practices
- Knowledge Deficit related to new therapeutic regimen to manage skin or mucous membrane alteration

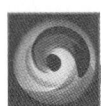

Table 36-2
Factors Placing an Individual at Risk for Skin Alterations

Factor	Nursing Implications
Lifestyle Variables	
Homosexual male, with a history of multiple sexual partners; drug users; hemophiliacs; bisexual male; partners of the above	• These patients are at high risk for acquired immunodeficiency syndrome (AIDS). • Assessment needs to include careful examination of the skin for purple blotches that may be indicative of Kaposi's sarcoma.
Occupation that gives a fair, thin-skinned individual prolonged exposure to the sun	• Places individual at high risk for developing skin cancer, which has an excellent prognosis if detected and treated in its early stages but which may be fatal if treatment is delayed. • Assessment needs to include careful examination for a sore that does not heal or a change in size or color of a wart or mole.
Changes in Health State	
Dehydration or malnutrition	• If fluid, protein, and vitamin C intake is deficient, skin loses elasticity and becomes prone to breakdown. • Nursing care is directed toward preventing skin breakdown: frequent changes of patient's position with skin assessment at each change, special mattresses and protection of bony prominences, use of lotions, attention to fluid and nutritional status.
Reduced sensation (paralysis, local nerve damage, circulatory insufficiency)	• Patient's inability to sense temperature extremes, pressure, friction, and other such factors can easily result in injury. • Nursing care incorporates special attention to safety.
Illness	
Diabetes mellitus	• Numerous factors combine to cause skin problems in diabetic patients: cuts and sores that do not heal, lesions on the lower extremities that ulcerate and become necrotic, recurrent bacterial and fungal infections. • The diabetic patient must be taught special hygiene measures to prevent trauma to the skin and learn to assess the skin carefully to detect any alteration.
Diagnostic Measures	
Gastrointestinal (GI) series	• The GI cleansing preparations administered to patients having GI studies done may result in diarrhea, which irritates the sensitive skin in the peri-anal area—especially if the patient had bouts of diarrhea before the studies; anticipating the problem, noting redness and inflammation, and beginning warm baths and ointments are welcome nursing measures that patients may be too embarrassed to seek.
Therapeutic Measures	
Bed rest	• Bed rest predisposes patients to skin breakdown; the harsh detergents used on hospital laundry compound this problem. • Pressure points need to be examined frequently and protected.
Casts	• Casts easily irritate the skin; careful assessment, covering the rough edges of the cast, and skin care are indicated.
Aquathermia unit	• Wet heat has therapeutic benefit but, if applied to the skin for too long, may macerate the skin; follow protocol in length of application, examine skin carefully between treatments, and allow to dry.
Medications	• Medications may cause allergic skin reactions, such as rashes. • When evaluating the patient's response to a new drug, examine the skin for redness and itching.

- Impaired Physical Mobility related to painful foot condition (calluses, corns, plantar warts)
- Altered Oral Mucous Membrane related to inadequate oral hygiene, stomatitis, malnutrition, or dehydration
- Risk for Infection related to broken skin or traumatized tissue
- Body Image Disturbance related to visible integumentary problems, body odors
- Altered Sexuality Patterns related to fear of transmitting or acquiring sexually transmitted disease, painful genital lesions
- Impaired Skin Integrity related to altered circulation, nutrition and fluid deficit or excess, impaired mobility, irritants (chemical, thermal, mechanical, radiation)
- Risk for Impaired Skin Integrity related to immobility, use of physical restraints, use of an aquathermia device, dehydration, bladder and/or bowel incontinence
- Impaired Social Interaction related to negative body image (eg, acne, alopecia)
- Impaired Swallowing related to reddened, irritated oropharyngeal cavity
- Impaired Tissue Integrity (eg, cornea, mucous membrane, integumentary, or subcutaneous) related to altered circulation, nutrition or fluid deficit or excess, impaired mobility, irritants (chemical, thermal, mechanical, radiation)

In certain situations, a wellness nursing diagnosis may be appropriate as the patient progresses toward an increased level of health awareness and wellness. An example of a wellness diagnosis is as follows:

Potential for Enhanced Oral Hygiene Practices

Additional diagnoses related to specific body parts are discussed later in this chapter.

Data collected during the nursing assessment may also lead to the identification of a collaborative problem. A nurse caring for a patient receiving intravenous chemotherapy should carefully check the infusion site every shift, knowing that phlebitis commonly occurs with certain chemotherapeutic agents. Careful preparation and administration of the drug according to the manufacturer's instructions, adherence to nursing protocols for the maintenance of intravenous infusions, and ongoing nursing assessment may decrease the likelihood of phlebitis. If redness, warmth, tenderness, or swelling is noted with any intravenous infusion, immediate collaborative intervention is indicated.

Similarly, a nurse may notice a 1.5-cm mole with an irregular border on a patient's back during a bath. Prompt reporting of this finding to the physician may lead to the detection and early, successful treatment of the medical diagnosis of malignant melanoma.

PLANNING: EXPECTED OUTCOMES

The plan of nursing care identifies nursing measures to assist the patient to develop or maintain hygiene practices that contribute to a sense of well-being. Appropriate expected outcomes include the following. The patient will achieve the following:

- Verbalize feeling comfortable and clean
- Participate fully in necessary hygiene measures according to cognitive, sensory, mobility, and endurance abilities
- Maintain intact skin and mucous membranes
- Demonstrate correct skin care measures (when indicated)
- Demonstrate signs of healing in existing lesions

Expected outcomes related to specific body parts are presented later in this chapter.

IMPLEMENTING

When performing general personal hygiene skills, nurses respect patients' personal preferences in hygiene measures, allow and encourage as much self-care as patients can perform, meet patients' needs for privacy, and promote physiologic and psychological wellness. The following sections discuss general hygiene measures, including providing scheduled care, helping with bathing, massaging, bedmaking, and providing environmental care. Hygiene related to specific body areas is discussed later in this chapter.

Providing Scheduled Hygienic Care

When patients require nursing assistance with personal hygiene, it is important to schedule this care at regular intervals. In most hospitals and long-term care settings, the following types of hygienic care are provided. These are individualized according to the patient's personal and cultural preferences.

Early Morning Care
Shortly after awakening, the patient is assisted with toileting if necessary and then provided with comfort measures to refresh the patient and prepare him or her for breakfast (or diagnostic tests). Nursing measures include washing the face and hands and providing mouth care. If needed, supplies necessary for morning care can be ordered at this time.

Morning Care (AM Care)
After breakfast, the nurse completes morning care. Depending on the patient's self-care abilities, the nurse offers assistance with toileting, oral care, bathing, back massage, special skin care measures (eg, pressure ulcer), hair care (includes shaving if indicated), cosmetics, dressing, and positioning for comfort. Cosmetics, if desired, can enhance morale in an ill patient. Agency policies are followed for refreshing or changing bed linens, and the patient's bedside area is tidied. When morning care is completed, the patient should feel refreshed and be in a comfortable and safe environment.

Morning care is often characterized as self-care, partial care, or complete care. *Self-care* patients are capable of managing their personal hygiene independently once oriented to the bathroom. These patients should still be offered a back massage and receive quality nursing time directed to assessing their day-to-day needs. *Partial care* patients most often receive morning hygiene care at the bedside or seated near the sink in the bathroom and usually require assistance with body areas that are difficult to reach. *Complete care* patients require nursing assistance with all aspects of personal hygiene. A complete bed bath is done, or the patient is taken to the shower or tub.

Afternoon Care (PM Care)

Because hospitalized patients frequently receive visitors in the afternoon or evening or use this time to rest when not scheduled for tests or therapies, the nurse should ensure the patient's comfort after lunch and offer assistance to nonambulatory patients with toileting, handwashing, and oral care. Straightening bed linens and helping patients with mobility problems to reposition themselves comfortably are other welcome nursing measures.

Hour of Sleep Care (hs Care)

Shortly before the patient retires, the nurse again offers assistance with toileting, washing of face and hands, and oral care. Because many patients find that a back massage helps them to relax and fall asleep, this should be offered routinely. Soiled bed linens or clothing should be changed and the patient positioned comfortably. The call light and any other objects the patient desires (eg, urinal, radio, water glass) should be within easy reach.

As Needed Care (prn Care)

In addition to scheduled care, the nurse offers individual hygiene measures as needed. Some patients require oral care every 2 hours. Patients who are *diaphoretic* (sweating profusely) may need their clothing and bed linens changed several times a shift. At other times, a nurse may decide to forego hygienic measures because the patient's need for undisturbed rest may be a higher priority.

Helping With Bathing

Bathing serves a variety of purposes, including the following:

- It cleanses the skin.
- It acts as a skin conditioner.
- It helps relax a restless person.
- It promotes circulation by stimulating the skin's peripheral nerve endings and underlying tissues.
- It serves as a musculoskeletal exercise through activity involved with bathing and thus improves joint mobility and muscle tonus.
- It stimulates the rate and depth of respirations.
- It promotes comfort through muscle relaxation and skin stimulation.
- It provides the person with sensory input.
- It helps improve self-image.
- It gives the nurse an excellent opportunity to strengthen the nurse–patient relationship, to observe the patient's physiologic and emotional status closely, to teach the patient as indicated, and to

demonstrate that the nurse cares for the patient and is interested in the patient's general welfare.

The simple act of bathing a patient is a vital and caring intervention. In recent years, this basic personal care measure has often been assigned to an unlicensed staff member rather than the professional nurse. It has become a task to be accomplished rather than an opportunity for therapeutic individualized intervention. Although hygiene measures are increasingly being performed by unlicensed assistive personnel, the nurse is responsible for ensuring that hygiene measures were satisfactorily performed. Refer to Chapter 18 for a discussion of the nurse's accountability when care is delegated. Nurses whose primary focus is the patient, however, can use their expertise and sensitivity to meet bathing needs and deliver quality patient care (Hektor & Touhy, 1997). See the accompanying box, Through the Eyes of a Student.

Shower and Tub Baths

A shower or tub bath is the preferred method of bathing for hospitalized people who are ambulatory. Even though most patients can for the most part do this on their own, the nurse still has the following responsibilities:

- Check to see that the bathroom is available, clean, and safe. Showers and tubs should have mats or nonskid strips to prevent patients from slipping and falling.
- Ensure that necessary articles, such as soap, a washcloth, a towel, and a gown, are available for the patient.
- Provide for a place for a weak or physically disabled patient to sit in a shower. Most health agencies have a stool or chair that can be used in a shower, and handheld shower heads may facilitate the process. Some nurses have reported that a commode chair with the pan removed serves effectively as a shower chair, and it offers the patient more support than a stool or chair.
- Assist patients to the shower or bathroom, as indicated. Patients who are beginning ambulation often need assistance to help prevent falling and fainting.
- Check to see that the water temperature is safe and comfortable, 43° to 46°C (110° to 115°F). The lower temperature is recommended for children and elderly patients.
- Help the patient get in and out of a bathtub, as indicated. Have the patient grasp hand rails at the side of the tub, or place a chair at the side of the tub. The patient sits on the chair and eases to the edge of the tub. After putting both feet into the tub, it is then relatively easy for the patient to reach the opposite side and ease down into the tub. The patient may kneel first in the tub and then sit in it; this process can be reversed to leave the tub in the same manner. Use a hydraulic lift, when available, to lower and lift a helpless, heavy patient in and out of a tub.
- Ensure privacy for patients who can safely shower or bathe independently. See to it that a call device is handy so that the patient can obtain help if necessary.

Through the Eyes of a Student

I entered the room with a feeling of dread. How could I possibly bathe the sick, elderly, helpless woman lying in this hospital bed? I had never bathed anyone older than age 2 years, other than myself, of course. How would I be able to move her limp, seemingly lifeless old body? What would an 85-year-old body look like? I could not imagine. I've read all the manuals that describe this procedure, I know what to do, so why am I so nervous? I must be worried that I will hurt her in some way. Maybe she has not been cared for properly before and her hygiene is poor. Well, I might as well get this over with because I'll be doing it the rest of my life. I've got to learn sometime.

I've mustered up enough courage to enter my patient's room. Michelle, her primary nurse, offers to help me because the patient is so difficult to move. Boy, am I relieved! Right before Michelle and I are about to begin, my patient, Mrs. Ash, asks for her teeth. I assume this must mean her dentures and reassure her that I have not seen them but will be happy to look for them as soon as we have completed her bath. Michelle and I each take a side and begin to bathe her. It's truly amazing how those range-of-motion exercises come to mind so easily. I had thought they were long forgotten with the rest of the past semester. Wouldn't my instructors love to hear me now! Suddenly Mrs. Ash yells, "I need the bed pan!" "Oh no!" I thought, as I rushed to the bathroom with soapy gloved hands trying frantically to locate her bed pan before there could be an accident. Michelle, who remained calm during my frenzy, simply stated, "Don't worry, she has an indwelling catheter. She says that every time I bathe her." I knew she had a catheter, how did I forget? Somewhat humbled, I returned to the procedure. I really wanted to put some lotion on her skin because it was so dry. When we were ready to do her back, we prepared to lift her. I pulled her toward me, and Michelle was to continue the bath. We were not prepared for what we saw underneath. Firmly cushioned in Mrs. Ash's lower left buttock were none other than her dentures! On removing them, Michelle and I had to smile at the periodontal grin implanted on Mrs. Ash's bottom. Michelle then asked her how her teeth had gotten to the location where we found them. All she seemed to know was that she needed those teeth back in her mouth STAT! She snatched the dentures from Michelle's hand and attempted to insert them. Michelle and I in unison blurted out, "*No, Mrs. Ash, please wait until we clean your teeth before you put them back in your mouth!*" Mrs. Ash, somewhat confused, begrudgingly handed over her teeth to be cleaned. Michelle had the honors while I finished the last touches of good hygiene for Mrs. Ash.

What a difference cleanliness can make, not only for the patient but also for me, the student nurse. I felt better knowing that Mrs. Ash was clean and that this procedure was behind me. And to think that I was apprehensive! This was definitely an interesting learning experience.

—Marilyn Johnson,
Holy Family College, Philadelphia

- Keep the bathroom door unlocked. Health personnel should be able to enter with ease if the patient needs help. A sign hung on the door ensures privacy. Never leave children alone in the bathroom.
- Help wash and dry areas of the body that the patient cannot reach, such as the back.

Figure 36-2 illustrates several features that add to the safety of a patient who takes a shower or tub bath.

Bed Baths

Some patients must remain in bed as a part of their therapeutic regimen but are still able to bathe themselves. The nurse helps these patients take a bath in bed in several ways:

- Provide the patient with articles for bathing. Provide a basin of water that is a comfortable and safe temperature. Place these items conveniently for the patient on a bedside stand or overbed table.
- Provide privacy for the patient. See to it that the call device is within reach.
- Remove the top linens from the patient's bed and replace them with a bath blanket.

- Place cosmetics in a convenient place for the patient's use. Provide a mirror, a good light, and hot water for patients who wish to shave with a razor.
- Assist patients who cannot bathe themselves completely. For example, some patients are able to wash only the upper parts of the body. The remainder of the bath is then completed by nursing personnel.

Bathing procedures for patients who require total nursing assistance vary among health agencies. The one described in Procedure 36-1 is offered as a guide. It assumes that the patient can be raised or lowered in bed and that, although the patient may have limited movement, it is possible for the nurse to manage the patient alone.

The Bag Bath

Some healthcare agencies recommend use of the "bag bath" as an alternative to the traditional bed bath. This self-contained bathing system consists of a plastic bag containing 8 to 10 premoistened washcloths. The bag bath is warmed

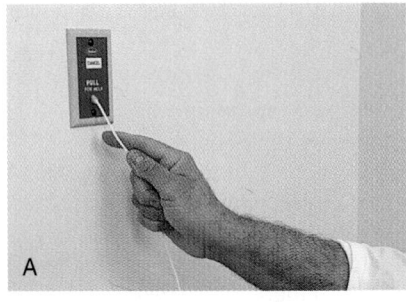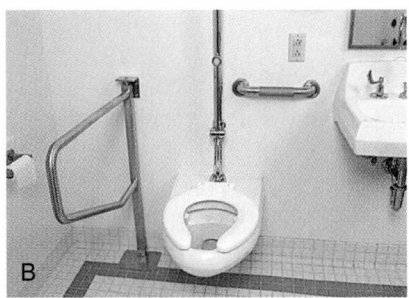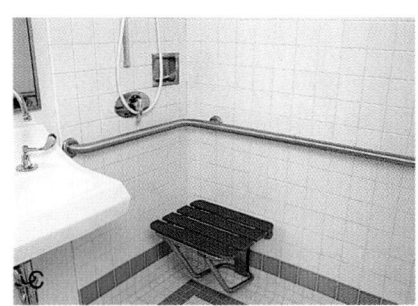

Figure 36-2
Examples of features that add to the safety of a patient in bed: (**A**) a call bell equipped with a pull cord, (**B**) hand rails for use with the commode, and (**C**) a shower equipped with a safety seat. (Photos © B. Proud.)

for a short time (about a minute and a half) in a microwave; experimenting may be needed to find the appropriate time for warming the washcloths to a safe temperature. Each part of the patient's body is cleansed with a fresh cloth. The skin is allowed to air dry (for about 30 seconds) so that the emollient ingredient of the cleaner remains on the skin. Feedback about this procedure has been overwhelmingly positive. Staff value the time savings when compared with a traditional bed bath and find it effective and easy to perform. Most patients have commented favorably on the bag bath. Patients with mild to moderate skin impairments demonstrated an improved skin condition from consistent use of the bag bath. Figure 36-3 shows a nurse preparing to give a bag bath to a patient.

Assisting With Antiembolism Stockings

Antiembolism stockings are often used for patients with limited activity to help prevent phlebitis and thrombi formation (described in Chap. 38). Manufactured by several companies, they are made of elastic material and are available in either knee-high or thigh-high length. Antiembolism stockings help force blood in superficial veins of the legs to deeper veins, prevent stagnation of blood in the veins of the legs, and promote venous return to the heart. A physician's order is required for their use.

Antiembolism stockings should always be removed during morning care, the legs inspected, and the stockings reapplied before the patient is out of bed, as shown in Procedure 36-2. General nursing guidelines for assisting with antiembolism stockings follow:

- Measure the patient's leg to determine the proper size stocking. The manufacturer whose stockings are being used gives directions for measuring. Some stockings fit either leg; others are designated right or left. An improperly fitting stocking is uncomfortable, ineffective, and may even harm the patient.
- Be prepared to apply the stockings in the morning before the patient is out of bed and while the patient is supine. If the patient is sitting or has been up and about, have the patient lie down with legs and feet well elevated for at least 15 minutes before applying the stockings. After the leg vessels are congested with blood, the effectiveness of the stockings is defeated.

- Do not massage the legs. If a clot is present, it may break away from the vessel wall and circulate in the bloodstream.
- Check the legs regularly for redness, blistering, swelling, and pain. Some people recommend checking the legs at least once every 8 hours; others recommend twice a day. The stockings should be removed completely once a day to bathe the legs and feet.
- Launder the stockings as necessary but at least every 3 days. Soiled stockings irritate the skin. The stockings should be dried on a flat surface to prevent them from stretching.

Several manufacturers produce men's and women's hose that apply pressure to the legs from the foot to midthigh or higher. Some apply mild pressure; others apply pressure equivalent to that of an elastic bandage. Stockings are available in a variety of colors so that in ambulatory patients other stockings are not needed to cover them. Many people who are on their feet or remain in one position a great deal, such as homemakers, nurses, salespeople, and business people, find them useful. The stockings should be fitted correctly to the person's measurements. Also, they should be applied immediately on awakening, before getting out of bed and before the legs are in a dependent position.

Applying Intermittent Pneumatic Compression Stockings

Intermittent pneumatic compression stockings may be used in conjunction with antiembolism stockings. They require a physician's order and are often prescribed for high-risk surgical patients, individuals with chronic venous disease, and patients at risk for deep-vein disorders. They consist of a knee-length or thigh-high cuff that is connected to hoses and a pump apparatus. Sequential compression stockings promote venous return by simulating the normal muscle-pumping action in the legs. These stockings are described further in Chapter 29.

Massaging the Back

A backrub generally follows the patient's bath. This acts as a general body conditioner. It can be used to relieve muscle tension and promote relaxation. Giving a backrub pro-

(*text continues on page 860*)

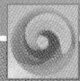

PROCEDURE 36-1
Giving a Bed Bath

Equipment

Wash basin
Soap and dish
Washcloths
Bath blanket
Gown or pajamas

Bed linen
Towels (2)
Disposable gloves—for anal and
    perineal care (optional for
    remainder of bath)

Personal hygiene supplies—
    deodorant, lotion, and others
Bedpan or urinal
Laundry bag or cart

Action	Rationale
1. Discuss procedure with the patient and assess the patient's ability to assist in the bathing process as well as personal hygiene preferences. Review the patient's chart for any limitations in physical activity.	This discussion promotes reassurance and provides knowledge about the procedure. Dialogue also encourages patient participation and allows for individualized nursing care.
2. Bring necessary equipment to the bedside stand or overbed table. Remove sequential compression devices and antiembolism stockings from lower extremities according to agency protocol.	Bringing everything to the bedside conserves time and energy. Arranging items nearby is convenient, saves time, and helps prevent unnecessary stretching and twisting of muscles on the part of the nurse. Most manufacturers and agencies recommend removal of these devices during the bath to allow for assessment.
3. Close the curtains around the bed and close the door to the room if possible.	This ensures the patient's privacy and lessens the possibility of loss of body heat during the bath.
4. Offer the patient the bedpan or urinal.	Voiding or defecating before the bath lessens the likelihood that the bath will be interrupted because warm bath water may stimulate the urge to void.
5. Wash your hands.	Handwashing deters the spread of microorganisms.
6. Raise the patient's bed to the high position.	Having the bed in a high position prevents strain on the nurse's back.
7. Lower the side rail nearer to you and assist the patient to the side of the bed where you will work. Have the patient lie on his or her back.	Having the patient positioned near the nurse and lowering the side rail help prevent unnecessary stretching and twisting of muscles on the part of the nurse.
8. Loosen top covers and remove all except the top sheet. Place bath blanket over the patient and then remove the top sheet while the patient holds the bath blanket in place. If linen is to be reused, fold it over a chair. Place soiled linen in the laundry bag.	The patient is not exposed unnecessarily, and warmth is maintained. If a bath blanket is unavailable, the top sheet may be used in place of the bath blanket.
9. Assist the patient with oral hygiene, as necessary, and as described in Procedure 36-5.	This helps maintain teeth and gums in good condition, alleviates unpleasant odor and taste, and may improve appetite. Some patients may prefer oral care after the bath is completed.
10. Remove the patient's gown and keep the bath blanket in place. If patient has an intravenous line and is not wearing a gown with snap sleeves, remove the gown from the other arm first. Lower the intravenous container and pass the gown over the tubing and the container. Rehang the container and check the drip rate.	This provides uncluttered access during the bath and maintains warmth of the patient. Intravenous fluids must be maintained at the prescribed rate.

(continued)

PROCEDURE 36-1

Giving a Bed Bath (Continued)

11. Raise the side rail. Fill the basin with a sufficient amount of comfortably warm water (between 43° and 46°C [110° to 115°F]).Change as necessary throughout the bath. Lower the side rail closer to you when you return to the bedside to begin the bath.

Warm water is comfortable and relaxing for the patient. It also stimulates circulation and provides for more effective cleansing. Side rails maintain patient safety.

12. Fold the washcloth like a mitt on your hand so that there are no loose ends, as illustrated.

Having loose ends of cloth drag across the patient's skin is uncomfortable. Loose ends cool quickly and feel cold to the patient.

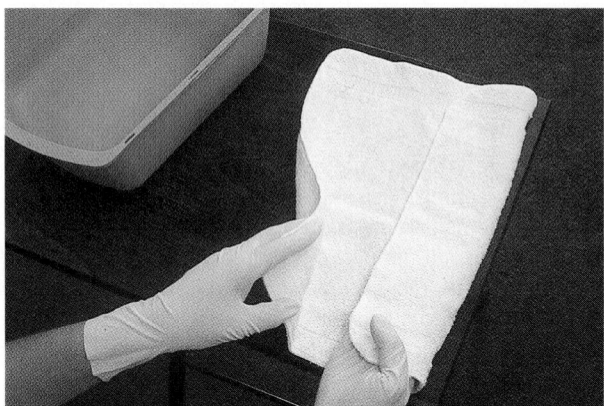

Action 12: Folding washcloth in thirds around hand to make a bath mitt.

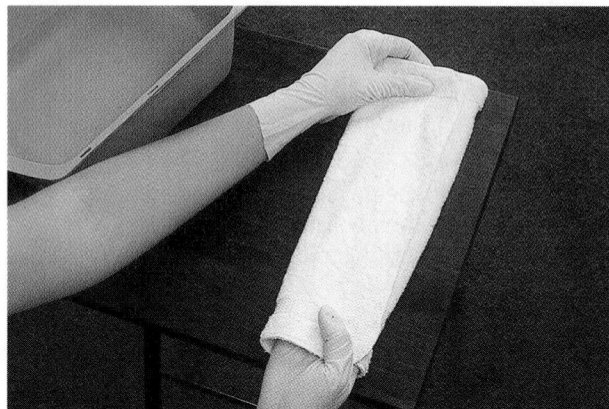

Action 12: Straightening washcloth before folding into mitt.

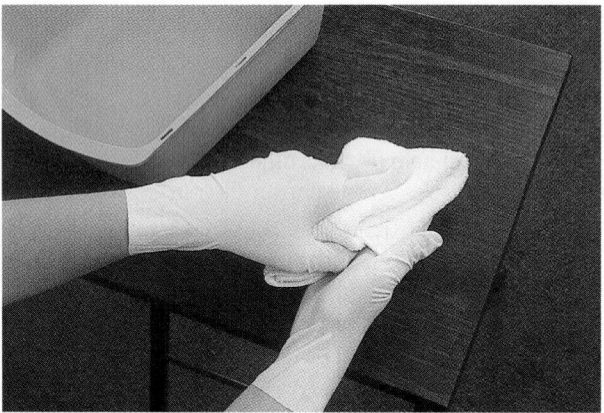

Action 12: Folding ends over and tucking ends under folded washcloth over palm.

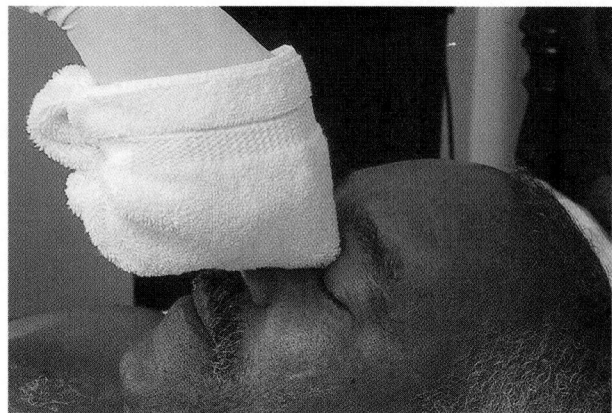

Action 14: Washing from the inner corner of the eye outward.

13. Lay a towel across the patient's chest and on top of the bath blanket.

This prevents chilling and keeps the bath blanket dry.

14. With no soap on the washcloth, wipe one eye from the inner part of the eye, near the nose, to the outer part. Rinse or turn the cloth before washing the other eye.

Rinsing or turning the washcloth prevents spreading organisms from one eye to the other. Soap is irritating to the eyes. Moving from the inner to the outer aspect of the eye prevents carrying debris toward the nasolacrimal duct.

(continued)

PROCEDURE 36-1

Giving a Bed Bath (Continued)

15. Bathe the patient's face, neck, and ears, avoiding soap on the face if the patient prefers.

Soap can be drying and may be avoided as a matter of personal preference.

16. Expose the far arm of the patient and place the towel lengthwise under it. Using firm strokes, wash the arm and axilla, rinse, and dry.

The towel helps to keep the bed dry. Washing the far side first eliminates contaminating a clean area once it is washed. Gentle friction stimulates circulation and muscles and helps remove dirt, oil, and organisms. Long, firm strokes are relaxing and more comfortable than short, uneven strokes.

17. Place a folded towel on the bed next to the patient's hand and put the basin on it. Soak the patient's hand in the basin. Wash, rinse, and dry the hand.

Placing the hands in the basin of water is an additional comfort measure for the patient. It facilitates a thorough washing of the hands and between the fingers and aids removal of debris from under the nails.

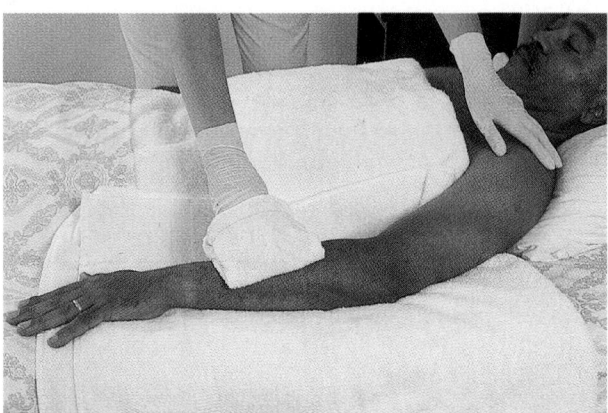

Action 16: Exposing the far arm and washing.

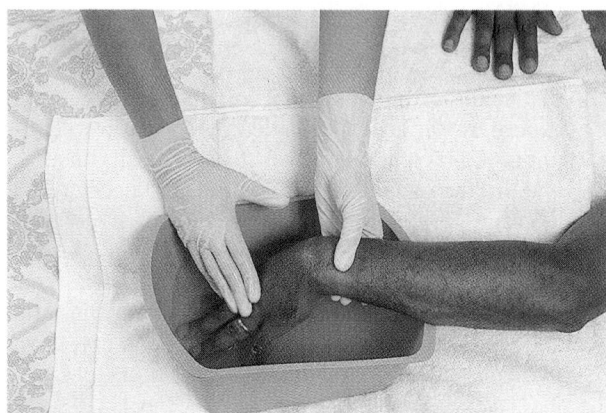

Action 17: Soaking hand in basin.

18. Repeat actions 16 and 17 for the arm nearer to you. (An option for the shorter nurse or one prone to back strain might be to bathe one side of the patient and move to the other side of the bed to complete the bath.)

19. Spread a towel across the patient's chest. Lower the bath blanket to the patient's umbilical area. Wash, rinse, and dry the patient's chest. Keep the patient's chest covered with the towel between the wash and rinse. Pay special attention to skin folds under the breasts of patients.

Exposing, washing, rinsing, and drying one part of the body at a time avoids unnecessary exposure and chilling. Skin-fold areas may be sources of odor and skin breakdown if not cleansed and dried properly.

20. Lower the bath blanket to the patient's perineal area. Place a towel over the patient's chest.

Keeping the bath blanket and towel in place avoids exposure and chilling.

21. Wash, rinse, and dry the patient's abdomen. Carefully inspect and cleanse the umbilical area and any abdominal folds or creases.

Skin-fold areas may be sources of odor and skin breakdown if not cleansed and dried properly.

(continued)

PROCEDURE 36-1

Giving a Bed Bath (Continued)

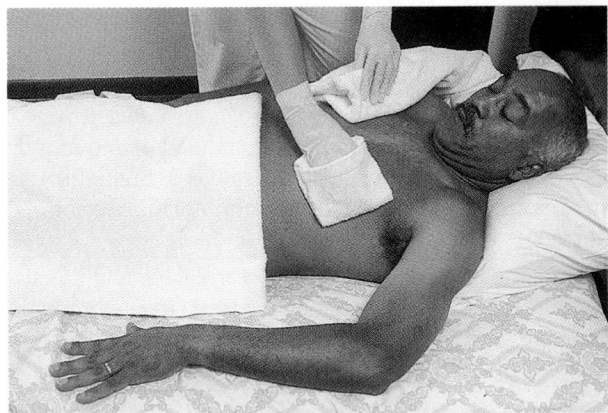

Action 19: Washing the chest area, including the axillae.

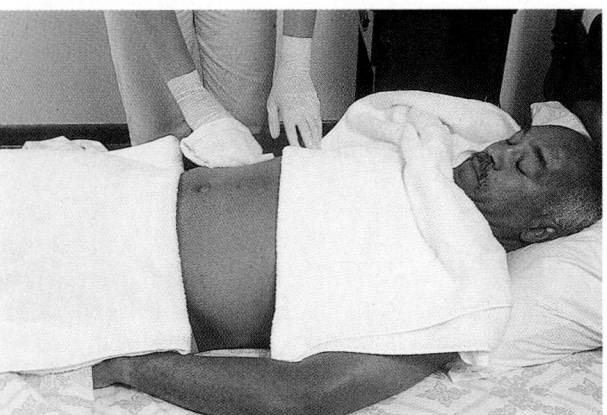

Action 21: Washing the abdomen, with perineal and chest areas covered.

22. Return the bath blanket to its original position and expose the far leg of the patient. Place the towel under the far leg. Using firm strokes, wash, rinse, and dry the patient's leg from ankle to knee and knee to groin.

23. Fold a towel near the patient's foot area and place the basin on it. Place the patient's foot in the basin while supporting the patient's ankle and heel in your hand and the leg on your arm. Wash, rinse, and dry, paying particular attention to the area between the toes.

24. Repeat actions 22 and 23 for the other leg and foot.

25. Make sure the patient is covered with the bath blanket. Change water at this point or earlier if necessary. Assist the patient onto his or her side.

The towel protects linens and prevents the patient from feeling uncomfortable from a damp or wet bed. Washing from ankle to groin with firm strokes promotes venous return.

Supporting the patient's foot and leg helps reduce strain and discomfort for the patient. Placing the feet in a basin of water is comfortable and relaxing and allows for a thorough cleaning of the feet and the areas between the toes and under the nails.

The bath blanket maintains warmth and privacy. Clean, warm water prevents chilling and maintains the patient's comfort.

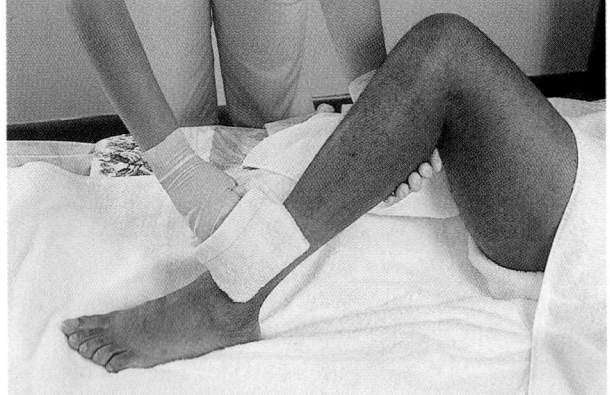

Action 22: Washing and drying far leg, keeping other leg covered.

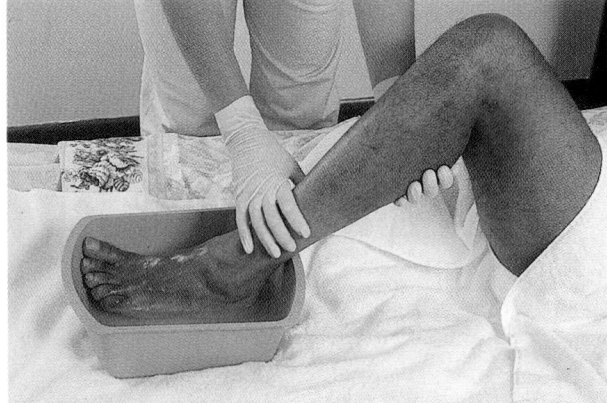

Action 23: Soaking the foot in basin.

26. Assist the patient to a prone or side-lying position. Position the bath blanket and towel to expose only the back and buttocks.

Positioning of the towel and bath blanket protects the patient's privacy and provides warmth.

(continued)

Giving a Bed Bath (Continued)

27. Wash, rinse, and dry the patient's back and buttocks area. Pay particular attention to cleansing between gluteal folds and observe for any indication of redness or skin breakdown in the sacral area.

Fecal material near the anus may be a source of micro-organisms. Prolonged pressure on the sacral area or other bony prominences may compromise circulation and lead to development of decubitus ulcer.

28. If not contraindicated, give the patient a backrub, as described in Procedure 40-1. Back massage may be given also after perineal care.

A backrub improves circulation to the tissues and is an aid to relaxation. A backrub may be contraindicated in patients with cardiovascular disease or musculoskeletal injuries.

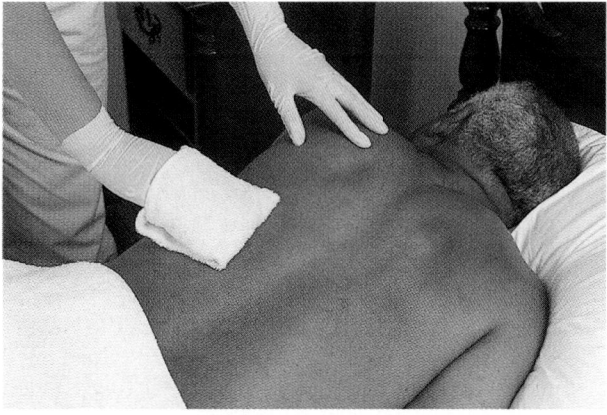

Action 27: Washing the upper back.

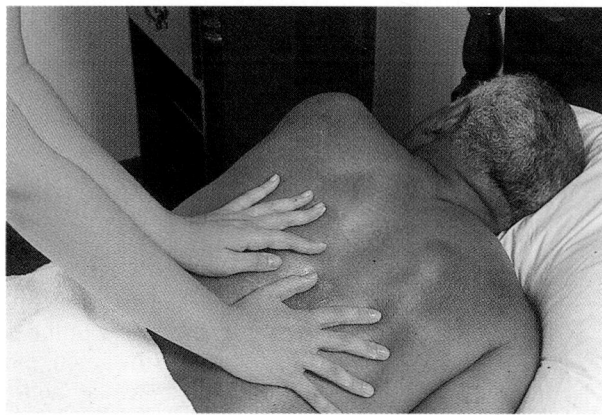

Action 28: Giving a backrub, after washing lower back.

29. Refill basin with clean water. Discard washcloth and towel.

The washcloth, towel, and water are contaminated after washing the patient's gluteal area. Changing to clean supplies decreases the spread of organisms from the anal area to the genitals.

30. Clean the patient's perineal area or set up the patient so that he or she can complete perineal self-care (see Fig. 36-9).

Providing perineal self-care may decrease embarrassment for the patient. Effective perineal care reduces odor and decreases the chance of infection through contamination.

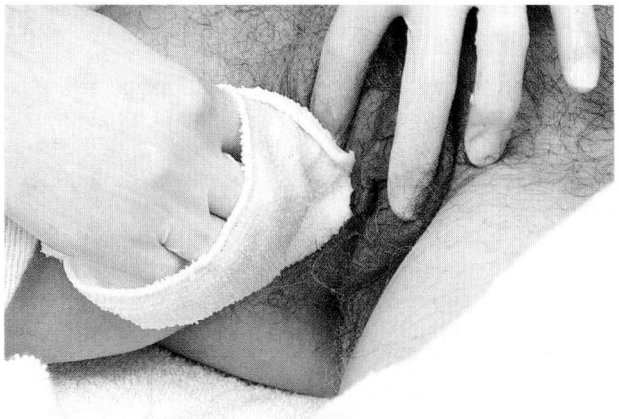

Action 30: Cleansing the perineal area.

(*continued*)

PROCEDURE 36-1

Giving a Bed Bath (Continued)

31. Help the patient put on a clean gown and attend to personal hygiene needs.

This provides for the patient's warmth and comfort.

32. Protect the pillow with a towel, and groom the patient's hair, as described in the text.

33. Change bed linens, as described in Procedures 36-3 and 36-4.

34. Record any significant observations and communication on the patient's chart.

A careful record is important for planning and individualizing the patient's care.

Age Considerations

When bathing an infant or young child, have supplies within easy reach and support or hold the child securely at all times to ensure safety. Never leave the child alone.

Check temperature of water, particularly before bathing an older patient because sensitivity to temperature may be impaired.

An older patient who is not incontinent may not require a full bed bath with soap and water every day. If dry skin is a problem, water and skin lotion or bath oil may be used on alternate days.

Special Considerations

Removal of gown if patient has an intravenous line necessitates taking the gown off, uninvolved arm first, and then threading the intravenous tubing and bottle or bag through the arm of the gown after the affected arm has been removed from the gown. To replace the gown, place the clean gown on the unaffected arm first and thread intravenous tubing and bottle or bag from inside the arm of the gown on the involved side. *Never* disconnect intravenous tubing to change a gown because this causes a break in a sterile system and introduces the potential for infection.

Lying flat in bed during the bed bath may be contraindicated for certain patients. Position may have to be modified to accommodate their needs.

Home Care Considerations

Evaluate the safety of the bathing area in the home. Tub mats, adhesive strips, grab bars, and shower stools are helpful accessories to prevent falls.

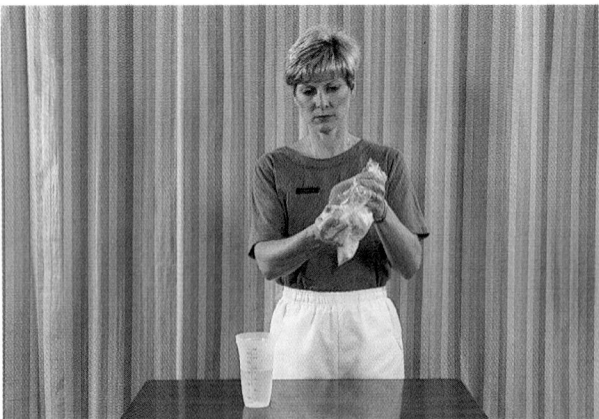

Figure 36-3
After warming the "bag bath" in the microwave, the nurse further mixes the solution with the disposable cloths to distribute warmth evenly.

vides an opportunity for the nurse to observe the skin for signs of breakdown. It improves circulation and provides a means of communication with the patient through the use of touch.

Because some patients may consider the backrub a luxury and be reluctant to accept it, the nurse should communicate its importance and value to the patient. An effective backrub should take 4 to 6 minutes to complete. A lotion for massaging the back is usually used. For the comfort of the patient, the lotion should be warmed before it is applied to the back. The nurse should be aware of the patient's medical diagnosis when considering giving a backrub. A backrub is contraindicated, for example, when the patient has had back surgery or has fractured ribs. Position the patient on the abdomen or, if this is contraindicated, on the side for a backrub. Recommended techniques for administering a backrub are outlined in

PROCEDURE 36-2

Applying Antiembolism Stockings

Equipment

Elastic stockings (in correct size)
For knee-high stockings:
  • Measure from heel to popliteal space

  • Measure circumference of calf at widest point
Measuring tape
Talcum powder (optional)

For thigh-high stockings:
  • Measure from heel to gluteal fold
  • Measure circumference of calf and thigh at widest point

Action	Rationale
1. Explain the rationale for use of elastic stockings to the patient.	Explanation encourages the patient's cooperation.
2. Wash your hands.	Handwashing deters the spread of microorganisms.
3. Assist the patient to the supine position. If the patient has been sitting or walking, it is necessary to have him or her lie down with the legs and feet well elevated for at least 15 minutes before applying the stockings.	Dependent position of legs encourages blood to pool in the veins.
4. Provide privacy. Expose legs one at a time, and powder lightly unless patient has dry skin. If the skin is dry, a lotion may be used. Powders and lotions are not recommended by some manufacturers.	Powder and lotion reduce friction and make application of stockings easier.
5. Place hand inside stocking and grasp heel area securely. Turn stocking inside out to the heel area.	Inside-out technique provides for easier application and less compromising of circulation to the extremity from bunched elastic material.

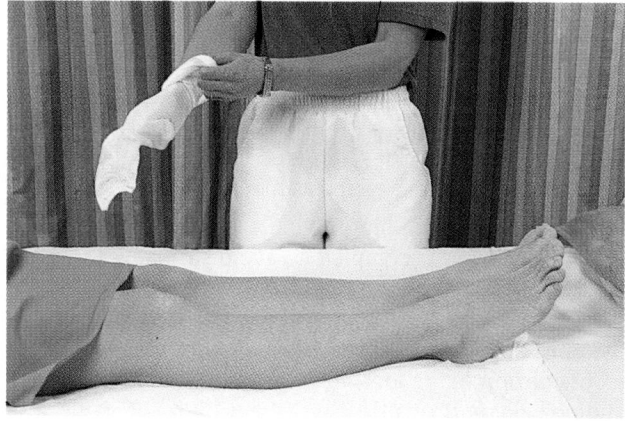

Action 5a: Inserting hand into stocking to grasp heel area.

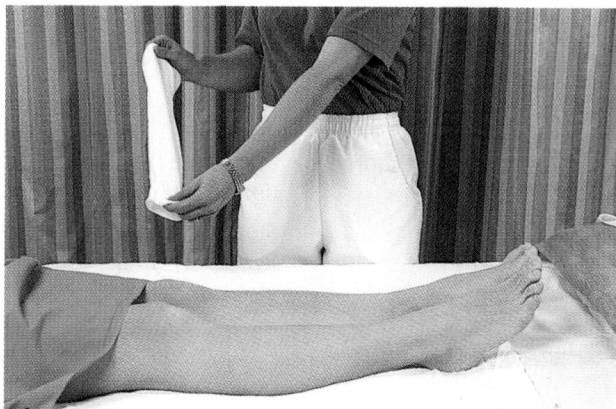

Action 5b: Turning stocking inside out to the heel pocket area.

6. Ease the foot of the stocking over the patient's foot and heel. Check that patient's heel is centered in heel pocket of stocking.	Wrinkles and improper fit interfere with circulation.
7. Using your fingers and thumbs, carefully grasp the edge of the stocking and pull it up smoothly over the ankle and calf until entire stocking is turned right side out. Pull forward slightly on toe section. Repeat for the other leg. Caution the patient not to roll stockings partially down.	Easing the stocking carefully into position ensures proper fit of the stocking to the contour of the leg. Rolling stockings may have a constricting effect on veins. Loosening the toe section provides for comfort in that area.

(continued)

PROCEDURE 36-2

Applying Antiembolism Stockings (Continued)

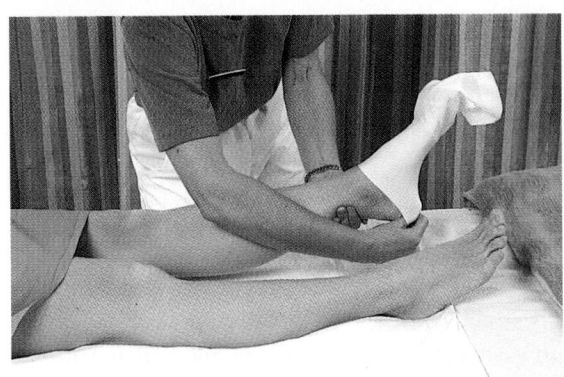

Action 6: Stretching stocking open and easing the foot of the stocking over the patient's foot.

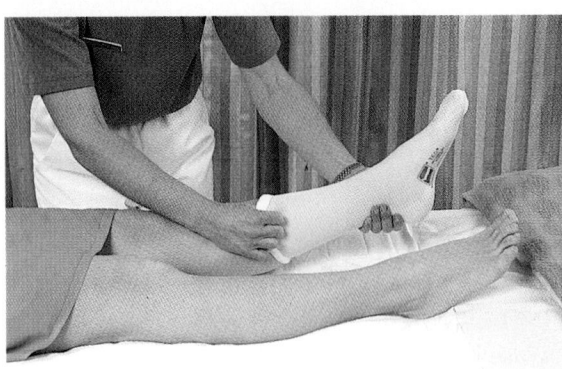

Action 7: Grasping top of stocking to pull up over calf.

8. Wash your hands.

9. To remove stocking, grasp the top of the stocking with your thumb and fingers and smoothly pull the stocking off inside out to heel. Support the patient's foot and ease stocking over it.

10. Remove stockings once every shift for 20 to 30 minutes. Wash and air dry as necessary (according to manufacturer's directions).

11. Record the application of elastic stockings as well as assessment of the patient's circulatory status and skin condition.

Handwashing deters the spread of infection.

This preserves elasticity and contour of the stocking.

This allows observation of the patient's circulatory status and condition of the skin on the lower extremity.

This provides accurate documentation of the procedure.

Home Care Considerations

Make sure that the patient has an extra pair of stockings ordered during the hospitalization before discharge (for payment and convenience purposes).

Stockings may be laundered with other "white" clothing. Avoid excessive bleach. Remove from dryer as soon as "low heat" cycle is complete to avoid shrinkage. May also be air dried.

Special Considerations

At times, despite the use of elastic stockings, a patient may develop thrombophlebitis. A positive Homans' sign (pain on dorsiflexion of the foot) may be an indication of a deep thrombosis or development of a blood clot in the calf.

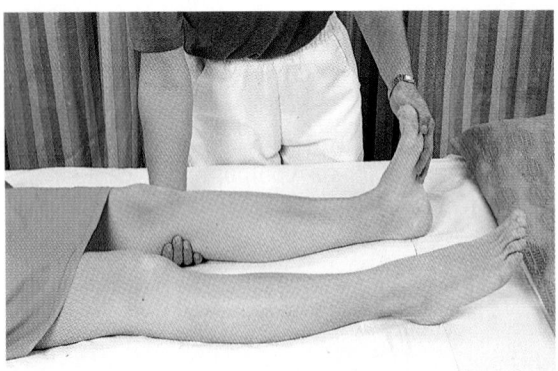

Special consideration: Checking Homan's sign.

Chapter 40 in Procedure 40-1. See also the accompanying Research in Nursing box.

Bedmaking

It is usual procedure to change bed linens after the bath, but some agencies change linens only when soiled. The bed is made for the ambulatory patient in the manner described in Procedure 36-3. If the patient is bedridden, the occupied bed is made according to Procedure 36-4.

There are minor variations in the procedure for making an occupied bed. However, these small differences have no real effect on the patient's comfort. In some instances, it is necessary for nurses to devise unique ways to change the linens on a patient's bed because of the nature of the patient's condition, orthopedic appliances on the bed, or treatments that may be in progress. See the accompanying box, Through the Eyes of a Student.

Providing Environmental Care

Bedside Unit

Because the environment contributes positively or negatively to the patient's sense of well-being, the nurse ensures that the *bedside unit*, the furnishings and equipment in the space surrounding the patient's bed, is clean, safe, and pleasant. Basic furniture includes the bed, overbed table, bedside stand, and chairs. Standard equipment in the healthcare environment includes the call light, oxygen, suction, and electrical outlets; light fixtures; bath basin; emesis basin; bedpan or urinal; water pitcher and glass; and bed linens. A nursing responsibility is ensuring that necessary equipment and items are in their proper place and functioning properly.

Because patients' personal items are generally stored in the bedside stand, the nurse should request permission from alert patients before opening the stand to obtain the bath basin, lotion, or other items. When assisting with hygiene, respecting the patient's right to privacy and ownership of personal goods decreases the patient's sense of powerlessness.

Before leaving the bedside unit, it is good nursing practice to say to the patient, "Is there anything else I can do to make you more comfortable?" Checking with the patient can correct for any oversight and communicates genuine caring. Limits may need to be set for manipulative patients regarding what comfort and hygiene measures the nurse is able to perform.

Elements of a safe bedside unit include the following:

- Patient call light functioning and always within reach
- Bed positioned properly and at the appropriate height
- Side rails safely used when indicated
- Principles of medical asepsis followed
- Electrical equipment safely grounded
- Uncluttered walk space

Elements of providing a comfortable bedside unit include attention to ventilation, odors, room temperature, lighting, and noise.

Ventilation and Odors

Because of pathogens and unpleasant odors associated with body secretions and excretions (ie, urine, stool, vomitus, draining wounds, or body odors), good ventilation in patient rooms is imperative. Odors may be decreased by promptly emptying bedpans, urinals, and emesis basins and by being careful not to dispose of soiled dressings or anything with a strong odor in the waste receptacle in the patient's room. Deodorizers may need to be used.

(*text continues on page 868*)

RESEARCH IN NURSING: MAKING A DIFFERENCE

Using Massage to Reduce Agitation

Traditionally, back massage completes the bed bath and promotes relaxation. The therapeutic effects of massage also make it beneficial in a variety of situations. Researchers questioned whether the episodes of agitated behavior that are common in patients with Alzheimer's disease might respond positively to massage techniques.

Related Research
Rowe, M., & Alfred, D. (1999). The effectiveness of slow-stroke massage in diffusing agitated behaviors in individuals with Alzheimer's disease. *Journal of Gerontological Nursing, 25*(6), 22–34.

This study measured the effectiveness of slow-stroke massage administered by caregivers to reduce agitated behavior in a patient with Alzheimer's disease in a home setting. Family caregivers were instructed in the techniques of slow-stroke massage, which they administered during a 10-day treatment period for a maximum time of 7.5 minutes each massage session. The massage was scheduled before patient activities that predictably resulted in agitation. The massage session diffused the more physical expressions of aggression (pacing, wandering, and resisting) but was less effective against verbal displays of agitation. Poorly managed agitated behavior has a negative effect on the ability of family caregivers to continue to care for their family member at home.

This simple technique has the potential to calm agitated patients and possibly allow them to remain in a familiar environment for a longer period of time. Sometimes, the simplest nursing action can prove to be an effective, caring intervention.

PROCEDURE 36-3

Making an Unoccupied Bed

Equipment

Two large sheets (or one large sheet and one fitted sheet)
Drawsheet (optional)
Blankets

Bedspread
Pillowcases
Linen hamper or bag
Bedside chair

Protective Pad (optional)
Disposable gloves (use if linens are soiled)

Action	Rationale
1. Wash your hands.	Handwashing deters the spread of microorganisms.
2. Assemble equipment and arrange on a bedside chair in the order in which items will be used.	Organization facilitates performance of task.
3. Adjust the patient's bed to the high position, and drop the bed side rails.	Having the bed in the high position and the side rails down reduces strain on the nurse while working.
4. Check bed linens for the patient's personal items and disconnect call bell or any tubes from bed linens.	It is costly and inconvenient when personal belongings are lost.
5. Loosen all linen as you move around the bed from the head of the bed on the far side to the head of the bed on the near side.	Loosening the linen helps prevent tugging and tearing on linen. Loosening the linen and moving around the bed systematically reduce strain caused by reaching across the bed.
6. Fold reusable linens, such as sheets, blankets, or spread, in place on the bed in fourths and hang them over a clean chair.	Folding saves time and energy when reusable linen is replaced on the bed. Folding linens while they are on the bed reduces strain on the nurse's arms. Some agencies change linens only when soiled.
7. Snugly roll all of the soiled linen inside of the bottom sheet and place directly into the laundry hamper. Do not place them on the floor or on furniture. Do not hold soiled linens against your uniform.	Rolling soiled linens snugly and placing them directly into the hamper helps prevent the spread of organisms. The floor is heavily contaminated; soiled linen will further contaminate furniture. Soiled linen contaminates the nurse's uniform, and this may spread organisms to another patient.

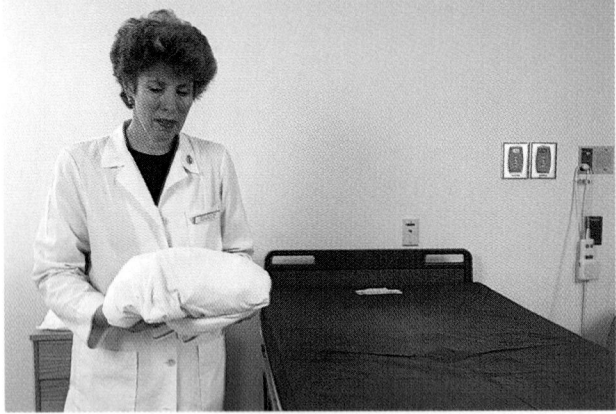

Action 7: Bundling soiled linens in bottom sheet and holding away from body.

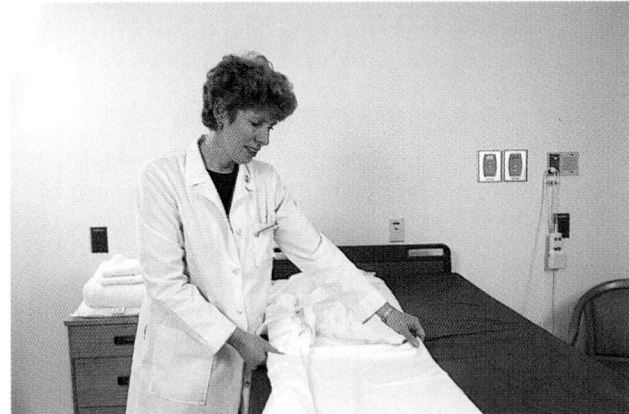

Action 9: Placing clean linens to begin bed making.

8. If possible, shift mattress up to the head of the bed.

This allows more foot room for the patient and moves the mattress against the head of the bed.

(continued)

PROCEDURE 36-3

Making an Unoccupied Bed (Continued)

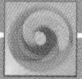

9. Place the bottom sheet with its center fold in the center of the bed and high enough to have a sufficient amount of the sheet to tuck under the head of the mattress.

Opening linens on the bed reduces strain on the nurse's arms and diminishes the spread of organisms.

10. Place the drawsheet with its center fold in the center of the bed and positioned so it will be located under the patient's midsection. If a protective pad is used, place it over the drawsheet in the proper area. Not all agencies use drawsheets routinely. The nurse may decide to use one.

When a patient soils the bed, drawsheets can be changed without the bottom and top linens on the bed. Having all bottom linens in place before tucking them under the mattress avoids unnecessary moving about the bed. A drawsheet is also an aid when moving the patient in bed.

11. Tuck the bottom sheet securely under the head of the mattress on one side of the bed, making a corner according to agency policy. A mitered corner is shown in the illustrations. Using a fitted bottom sheet eliminates the need to miter corners. Tuck the remaining bottom sheet and drawsheet securely under the mattress. (At this point, before moving to the other side of the bed, top linens may be placed on the bed, unfolded, and secured, allowing the entire side of the bed to be completed at one time as shown in the illustrations.)

Making the bed on one side and then completing the bed on the other side saves time. Having bottom linens free of wrinkles reduces discomfort to the bedridden patient.

12. Move to the other side of the bed to secure bottom linens. Secure bottom sheet under the head of the mattress and miter the corner. Pull remainder of sheet tightly and tuck under mattress. Do the same for the drawsheet.

This rids bottom linens of any wrinkles that can cause discomfort for the patient.

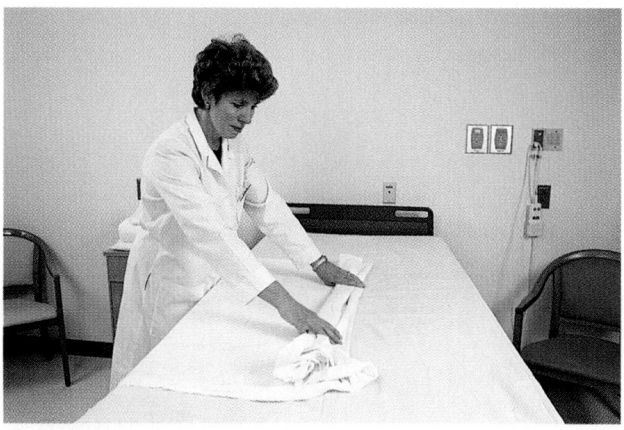

Action 10: Placing the drawsheet on the bed.

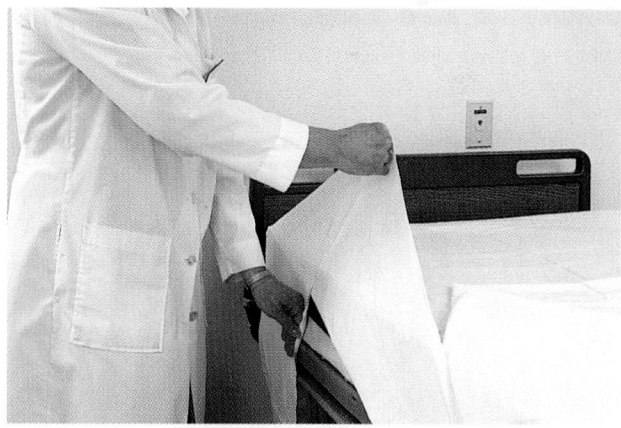

Action 11a: Beginning to make mitered corner by creating a triangular fold.

(continued)

Making an Unoccupied Bed (Continued)

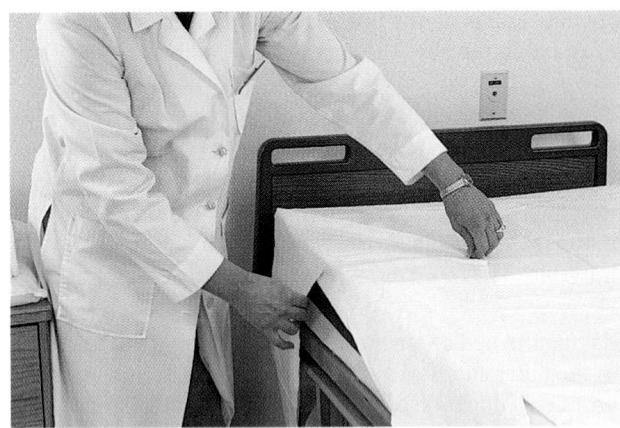

Action 11b: Laying triangular fold on top of bed.

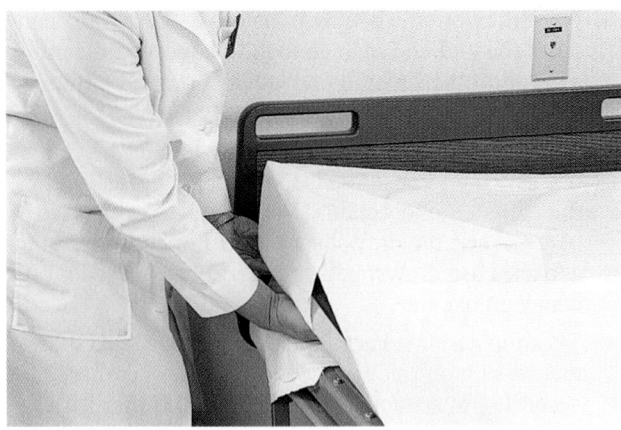

Action 11c: Tucking end of sheet under mattress.

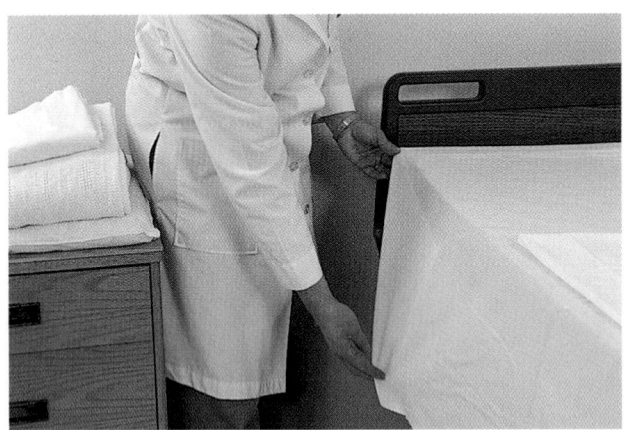

Action 11d: Folding triangular linen fold down over side of mattress.

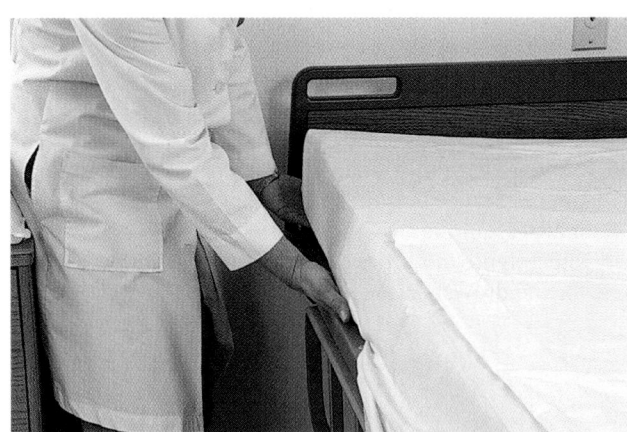

Action 11e: Tucking end of triangular linen fold under mattress to complete mitered corner.

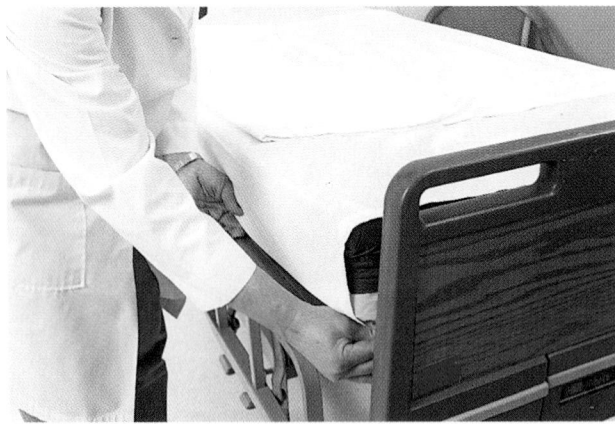

Action 11f: Tucking sheet snugly under foot of mattress.

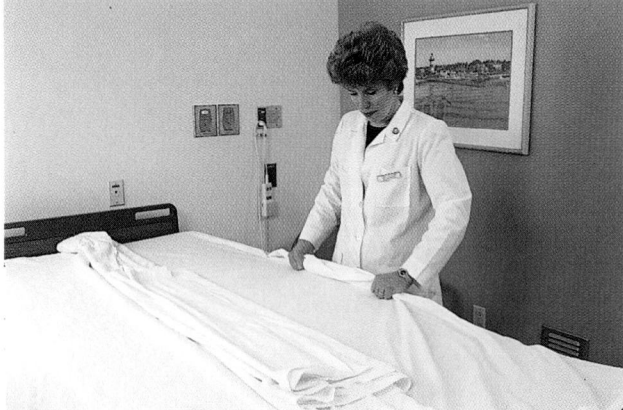

Action 12: Pulling bottom sheet tightly on opposite side of bed.

(continued)

13. Place the top sheet on the bed with its center fold in the center of the bed and with the top of the sheet placed so that the hem is even with the head of the mattress. Unfold the top sheet in place, as illustrated. Follow same procedure with top blanket or spread, placing the upper edge about 6 inches below the top of the sheet.

Opening linens by shaking them spreads organisms into the air. Holding linens overhead to open them causes strain on the nurse's arms.

14. Tuck the top sheet and blanket under the foot of the bed on the near side. Miter the corners.

This saves time and energy and keeps the top linen in place.

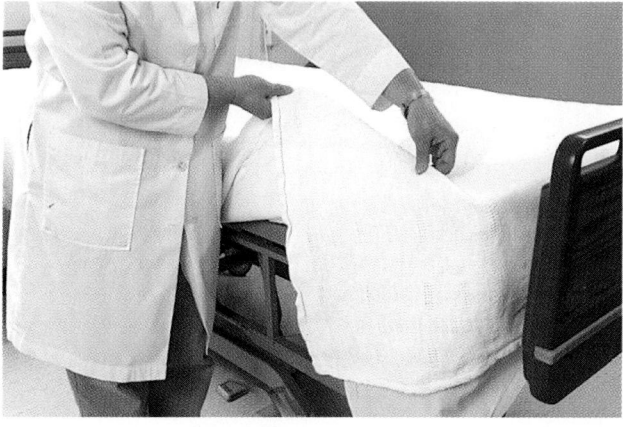

Action 14: Mitering the corner of the top sheet and spread.

15. Fold the upper 6 inches of the top sheet down over the spread and make a cuff.

This makes it easier for the patient to get into bed and pull the covers up.

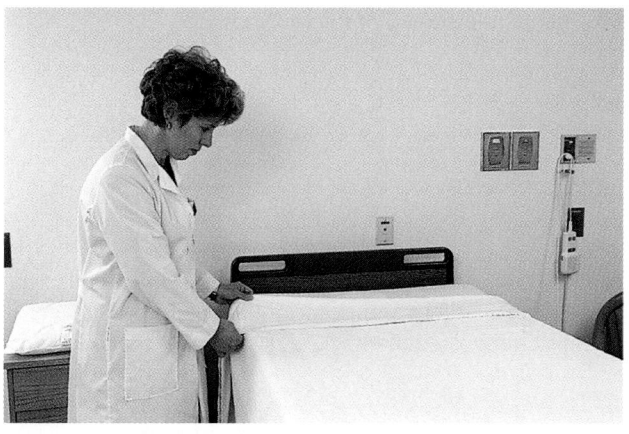

Action 15: Cuffing top linens.

16. Move to the other side of the bed and follow the same procedure for securing top sheets under the foot of the bed and making a cuff.

Working on one side of the bed at a time saves energy and is more efficient.

(continued)

PROCEDURE 36-3

Making an Unoccupied Bed (Continued)

17. Place the pillows on the bed. Open each pillowcase in the same manner as opening other linens. Gather the pillowcase over one hand toward the closed end. Grasp the pillow with the hand inside the pillowcase. Keeping a firm hold on the top of the pillow, pull the cover onto the pillow.

Opening linens by shaking them causes organisms to be carried around on air currents. Covering the pillow while it rests on the bed reduces strain on the nurse's arms and back.

18. Place the pillow at the head of the bed with the open end facing toward the window.

This provides for a neater appearance.

19. Fan-fold or pie-fold the top linens.

Having linens opened makes it more convenient for the patient to get into bed.

20. Secure the signal device on the bed according to agency policy.

Having the signal device handy for the patient makes it possible for the patient to call for assistance as necessary.

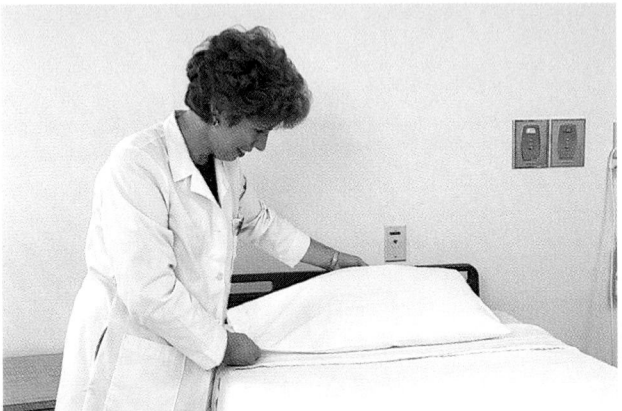

Action 18: Placing pillow on bed.

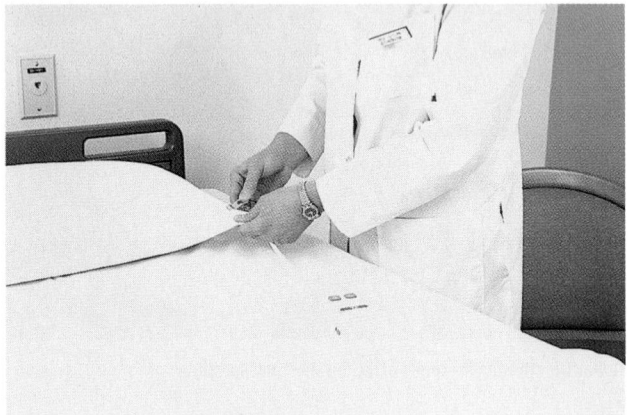

Action 20: Securing the signal device to the bed.

21. Adjust the bed to the low position.

Having the bed in the low position makes it easier and safer for the patient to get into bed.

22. Dispose of soiled linen according to agency policy. Wash your hands.

This deters the spread of microorganisms.

Room Temperature

Whenever possible, patient preferences (which may vary widely) should determine the room temperature. In general, the room temperature should be between 20° and 23°C (68° and 74°F).

Lighting and Noise

Because many patients find it difficult to sleep in a healthcare facility and may need to be disturbed frequently for assessment or treatment purposes, nurses should be careful to reduce harsh lighting and noises whenever possible. However, adequate lighting must be provided for all nursing procedures. Whenever possible, conversations should not be carried on immediately outside the patient's

room. Many patients find this stressful both because the noise disturbs them and because they believe whatever is being said involves them.

Beds

Because many people who are ill spend a large portion of the day—if not the entire day—in bed, the bed is an important part of the patient's environment. Nursing responsibilities include ensuring a safe and comfortable bed.

Bed Safety

The typical hospital bed has a motorized metal frame in three sections, which allows the height of the bed to be
(text continues on page 872)

PROCEDURE 36-4
Making an Occupied Bed

Equipment

Two large sheets (or one large sheet
    and one fitted sheet)
Drawsheet or lift pad
Disposable gloves (use if linens are
    soiled)

Blanket (optional)
Bedspread
Pillowcases
Linen hamper or bag (optional)
Bedside chair

Protective pad (optional)
Bath blanket (optional)

Action	Rationale
1. Explain the procedure to the patient. Check the patient's chart for limitations on the patient's physical activity.	This facilitates patient cooperation and determines level of activity.
2. Wash your hands.	Handwashing deters the spread of microorganisms.
3. Assemble equipment and arrange on the bedside chair in the order the items will be used.	Organization facilitates performance of task.
4. Close door or curtain.	This provides for privacy.
5. Adjust the patient's bed to the high position. Lower the side rail nearest you, leaving the opposite side rail up. Place the bed in the flat position unless contraindicated.	Having the bed in the high position reduces strain on the nurse while working. Having the mattress flat facilitates making a wrinkle-free bed.
6. Check bed linens for patient's personal items and disconnect the call bell or any tubes from bed linens.	It is costly and inconvenient when personal items are lost. Disconnecting tubes from linens prevents discomfort and accidental dislodging of the tubes.
7. Place a bath blanket, if available, over the patient. Have the patient hold onto the bath blanket while you reach under it and remove top linens. Leave the top sheet in place if a bath blanket is not used. Fold linen that is to be reused over the back of a chair. Discard soiled linen in a laundry bag or hamper.	This provides warmth and privacy.

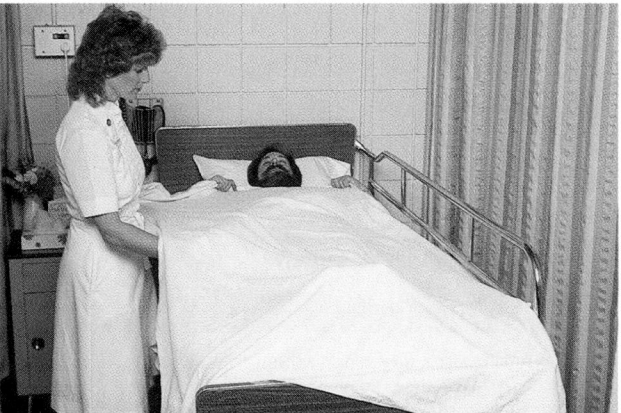

Action 7: Removing top linens from under bath blanket.

8. If possible and another person is available to assist, grasp mattress securely and shift it up to the head of the bed.	This allows more foot room for the patient and positions the mattress against the head of the bed.

(continued)

9. Assist the patient to turn toward the opposite side of the bed and reposition the pillow under the patient's head.

This allows the bed to be made on the vacant side.

10. Loosen all bottom linens from the head and sides of the bed.

This facilitates removal of linens.

11. Fan-fold soiled linens as close to the patient as possible.

This facilitates removal of linens when the patient turns to the other side.

12. Use clean linen and make near side of bed following actions 9, 10, and 11 of Procedure 36-3. Fan-fold the clean linen as close to the patient as possible.

This positions clean linen to make the side of the bed.

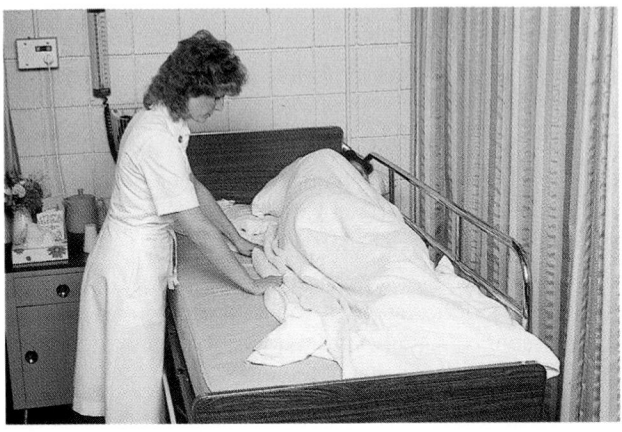

Action 11: Moving soiled linen as close to patient as possible.

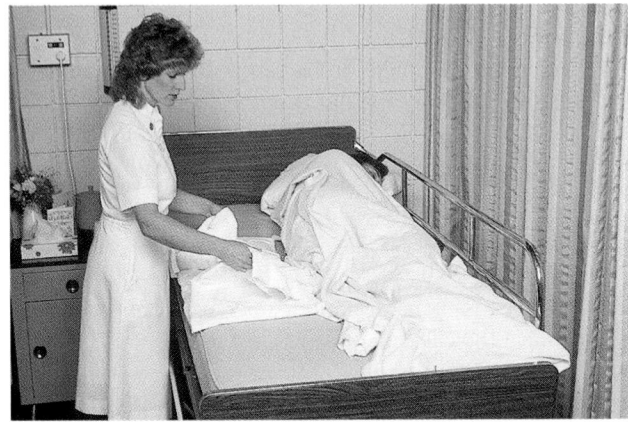

Action 12: Opening and folding clean linens.

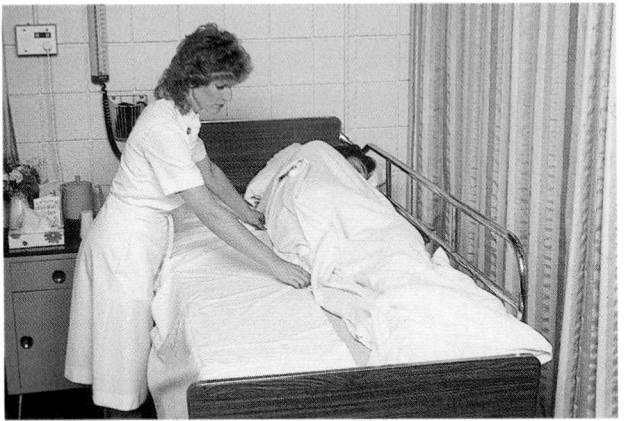

Action 12: Aligning clean bottom sheet on half of bed.

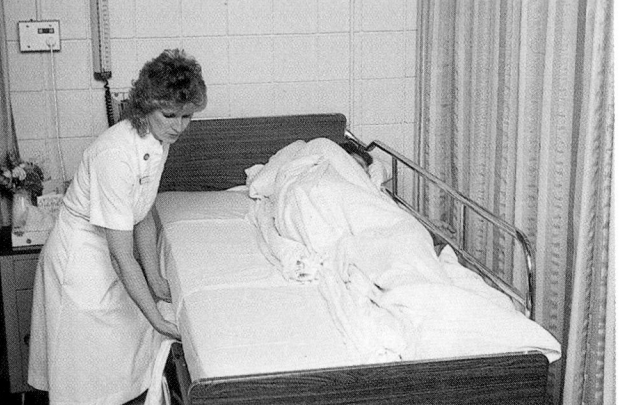

Action 12: Tucking bottom sheet and drawsheet tightly.

13. Raise the side rail. Assist the patient to roll over the folded linen in the middle of the bed toward you. Reposition the pillow and bath blanket or top sheet. Move to the other side of the bed and lower the side rail.

This ensures patient safety. The movement allows the bed to be made on the other side. The bath blanket provides warmth and privacy.

(continued)

PROCEDURE 36-4

Making an Occupied Bed (Continued)

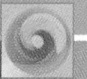

14. Loosen and remove all bottom linen. Place these in a linen bag or hamper. Hold soiled linen away from your uniform.

Proper disposal of soiled linen prevents spread of microorganisms.

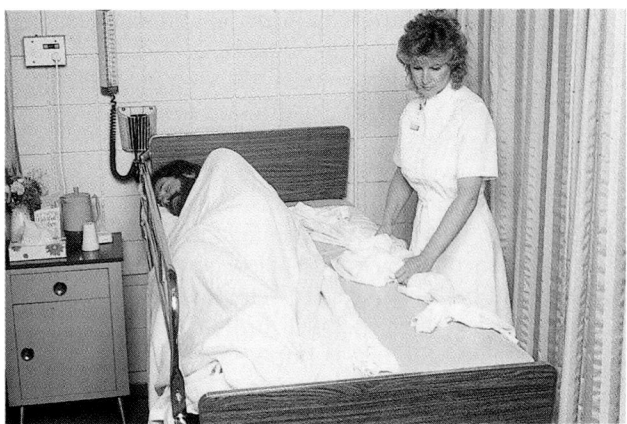

Action 14: Removing soiled bottom linens from other side of bed.

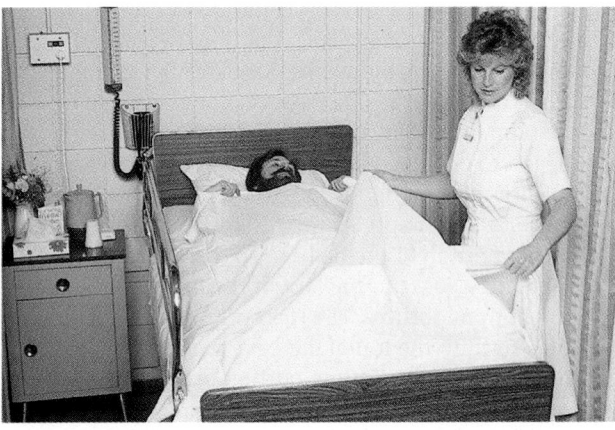

Action 17: Removing the bath blanket from under the top linens.

15. Ease the clean linen from under the patient. Pull taut and secure the bottom sheet under the head of the mattress. Miter corners. Pull the side of the sheet taut and tuck under the side of the mattress. Repeat this with the drawsheet.

This removes wrinkles and creases in the linens, which are uncomfortable to lie on.

16. Assist the patient to return to the center of the bed. Remove the pillow and change the pillowcase before replacing, with open end facing toward the window.

This provides for a neater appearance.

17. Apply top linen so that it is centered and top hems are even with the head of the mattress. Have the patient hold onto the top linen so the bath blanket can be removed.

This allows bottom hems to be tucked securely under the mattress and provides for privacy.

18. Secure top linens under the foot of the mattress and miter corners. Loosen top linens over the patient's feet by grasping them in the area of the feet and pulling gently toward the foot of the bed.

This provides for a neat appearance. Loosening linens over the patient's feet gives more room for movement.

19. Raise the side rail. Lower bed height and adjust the head of the bed to a comfortable position. Reattach call bell and drainage tubes.

This provides for the patient's safety.

20. Dispose of soiled linens according to agency policy. Wash your hands.

This prevents spread of microorganisms.

Home Care Considerations   Use of a synthetic sheepskin, a soft bath blanket, or flannelette blanket as a bottom sheet may solve the problem of "coldness" for elderly patients with vascular problems or arthritis.

Through the Eyes of a Student

One of my first patients was a man in his late 60s who had suffered a stroke. I was assigned to care for him, and his care included a bed bath and complete linen change—with him *in the bed.* I was determined to complete this task totally on my own, without asking anyone for help. This was my first mistake.

The patient yelled obscenities at me and had very rough mannerisms. I kept thinking to myself, "I must treat him with gentle care and not show any fear." Inside I was shaking furiously.

I managed to complete his bath and then began to change the sheets. I helped the patient to turn to one side, tucking the dirty linens close to him. I applied the fitted sheets to the upper portion of the bed . . . so far, so good. Immediately going to the foot of the bed, I applied the bottom portion. The top portion popped off—I ran to the top of the bed, reapplied the top portion—the bottom portion popped off—I reapplied it. . . . I must have spent 15 minutes running back and forth trying to get both ends to stay on. By this time sweat was pouring off my face.

When I finally cried "Uncle," I discovered that certain fitted sheets just didn't fit all the mattresses. The usual routine in this case is to walk to the linen closet and get another fitted sheet. That probably takes about 15 seconds!

—Linda A. Keough, Delaware County Community College, Media Pennsylvania

raised or lowered and the head and foot to be adjusted. Nurses need to know how to operate the bed and explain it to the patient. Bed positions are described in Chapter 38. Hospital beds can also be ordered for use in the home. Because certain positions may actually be harmful to some patients, the patient and family should be instructed about advisable bed positions and the use of the bed controls. Hospital beds are generally 66 cm (26 inches) from the floor. This is higher than most beds at home and enables the nurse or caregiver to reach the patient without undue musculoskeletal strain.

Whenever the patient's condition indicates the need for upper or lower side rails, these should be used to provide assistance with moving in bed and to prevent dangerous falls by an unconscious patient (refer to Chap. 26 for additional discussion about the use of side rails). The wheels or casters on the hospital bed should be locked whenever the bed is stationary to prevent the bed from slipping away from a patient moving from the bed to an upright position or being transferred to a stretcher. The headboard of most hospital beds is removable to allow close patient contact in an emergency situation. Before leaving the patient's bedside, ensure the following:

- The bed is in its lowest position.
- The bed position is safe for the patient.
- The bed controls are functioning (bed is electrically safe).
- Side rails (upper and lower) are raised if indicated.
- The wheels or casters are locked.

Bed Comfort

The hospital mattress is firm and generally covered with a water-repellent material that can be easily wiped down with a bactericidal solution between patients. A variety of therapeutic beds and mattresses are available to reduce or relieve the effects of pressure on the skin (Fig. 36-4; these are discussed in more detail in Chap. 38).

Agency policies usually dictate the availability and use of bed linens. Bed linens include mattress covers, sheets, drawsheets, incontinence pads, pillow cases, blankets, bedspreads, and bath blankets. Towels, washcloths, and patient gowns are often included in linen packs. In some settings, making the bed is not a nurse's responsibility. However, ensuring patient comfort is always a priority in nursing, and this often involves creating a comfortable bed environment. Before leaving a patient, the nurse should ensure the following:

- Linens are clean and wrinkle free.
- The patient feels comfortably warm.
- Pressure points of patients with a nursing diagnosis of Risk for Impaired Skin Integrity are protected from rough sheets, hem edges, and water-repellent materials.

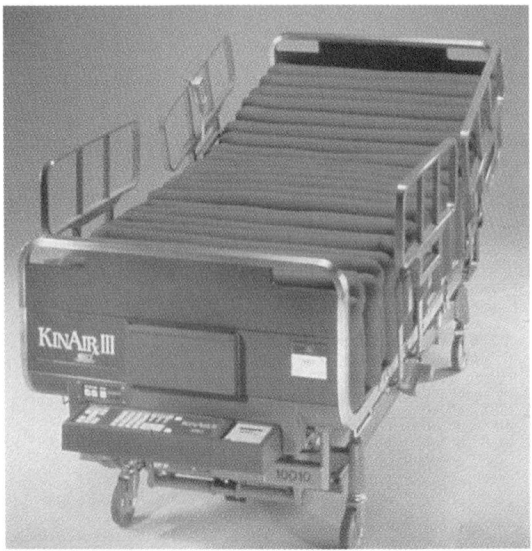

Figure 36-4
This special bed is an air-flotation, low-air-loss support surface that provides pressure relief. In this KinAir III there is a microprocessor computer control panel that controls air flow and temperature precisely. A built-in digital scale and heater are included. The bed also has a quick-release level for CPR. (Photo courtesy of KCI Therapeutic Services, San Antonio, TX.)

Teaching Patients About Skin Care

Occasionally, patients ask for specific information; otherwise, the nurse can share information with the patient during assessment and care procedures. The following section concerns skin care and skin problems.

Soaps and Detergents

A wide variety of soaps and detergents are available. Expensive cleansing agents, however, have not been found better than less expensive ones. For most people, the best way to cleanse the skin is with soap or detergent and water. Soaps are often made from vegetable and animal fats, whereas most detergents are made from petroleum derivatives. People who are sensitive to soap often find they can use detergents without difficulty.

Deodorants and Antiperspirants

Perspiration is essentially odorless, although it contains some waste products, such as uric acid and ammonia. The odor of perspiration occurs when bacteria, normally present on everyone's skin, act on the skin's normal secretions.

Keeping the body and clothing clean is the best way to prevent body odors. Deodorants and antiperspirants may be used *after* the skin is clean. Deodorants mask odor and antiperspirants are intended to reduce the amount of perspiration. They act as astringents and tend to close the exits of the sweat glands. Antiperspirants and deodorants should be used with care and according to directions to prevent irritation of the skin. They are contraindicated in some situations, such as before mammography and during the postoperative period for a mastectomy patient.

Cosmetics

Cosmetics frequently enhance the appearance of clean and healthy skin, although certain cultural and religious groups may discourage their use. Cosmetics used judiciously help disguise blemishes, improve skin coloring, and make wrinkles appear less obvious.

Periodically, cosmetics containing harmful ingredients, have appeared on the market. The nurse should be alert to such agents and help consumers avoid their use. The U.S. Department of Health and Human Services, Food and Drug Administration (FDA), enforces federal laws on the purity of foods, drugs, and cosmetics and on the advertising claims of their manufacturers. The FDA is a good source of information.

Cosmetics often become contaminated with bacteria and fungi. It is best to discard cosmetics after they are about 4 months old, especially those applied near the eyes. Makeup applicators and puffs should be kept immaculately clean. Cosmetics should not be shared.

Common Skin Problems

Assessment frequently reveals dry skin, acne, and skin rashes. Table 36-3 summarizes recommended treatments for these skin problems.

Pressure ulcers are areas of cellular **necrosis** caused by the lack of blood circulation to the involved area. At best, they are extremely painful and debilitating to patients; at worst, they may be life-threatening. Preventing pressure ulcers whenever possible and identifying and treating them at the earliest stage possible are critical nursing responsibilities. This topic is explored in detail in Chapter 37.

EVALUATING

Daily contacts with the patient while performing hygiene measures enable the nurse to evaluate frequently whether the patient is meeting hygiene goals. Evaluative criteria include the following:

- Level of patient's participation in hygiene program
- Elimination of, reduction in, or compensation for factors interfering with the patient's independent execution of hygiene measures (eg, weakness, decreased motivation, lack of knowledge)
- Achievement of expected outcomes related to specific skin problems by giving attention to the healing of skin lesions, by eliminating or reducing causative factors, and by the patient managing the prescribed treatment program independently

Oral Care

The mouth is the first part of the alimentary canal and an important part of the respiratory system. The ducts of the salivary glands open into the vestibule of the mouth. The teeth and the tongue are accessory organs in the mouth and play an important role in beginning digestion by breaking up food particles and mixing them with saliva. Saliva is also important as a mechanical cleaner of the mouth.

General good health is as essential as cleanliness for maintaining a healthy mouth and teeth. For example, the relationship between good teeth and a diet sufficient in calcium and phosphorus, along with vitamin D, which is necessary for the body to use these minerals, is well established.

There are several benefits to maintaining good oral hygiene and dental care. There is aesthetic value in having a clean and healthy mouth. Having one's own teeth contributes to an intact body image. The beginning of the digestive process and gustatory pleasure are enhanced when the mouth and teeth are in good condition.

The Nursing Process

ASSESSING

Nursing History

Identify the patient's normal oral hygiene practices and the variables influencing these practices. Note the history of any oral problems and related treatments.

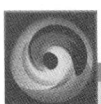

Table 36-3
Skin Care Problems

Skin Problem	Definition	Treatment
Dry Skin	Is characteristically flaky and is easily susceptible to injury and irritation	• Bathe less frequently. • Rinse off soaps and detergents well. • Use a superfatted soap (eg, Dove) for cleansing. • Avoid wearing wool garments because they tend to irritate the skin. • Use a humidifier to add moisture to the air. • Increase fluid intake when the skin is dry. • Use an emollient to soften, soothe, and protect dry skin after it is cleansed. • Use creams to clean skin that is dry or allergic to soap.
Acne	A condition that is particularly bothersome during adolescence. Hormones cause enlargement of the sebaceous glands and an increase in glandular secretions. Blackheads and pustules appear when secretions become blocked in the sebaceous ducts. Inflammation with infection can also occur.	• Infected areas should not be squeezed or picked because this can spread the infection and cause scarring. • Wash skin and shampoo hair with soap or detergent and hot water to remove oil and debris. • Avoid oily cosmetics, cleansing creams, and emollients. • Use cosmetics sparingly to avoid further blockage of the sebaceous ducts. • Eliminate foods that aggravate the condition. • Physician may recommend combination therapies that control manifestations of acne but result in *erythema* (redness) and skin peeling. Sun exposure may also be dangerous and should be avoided.
Skin rashes	Eruptions or inflammations of the skin that may be found anywhere on the body. May be precipitated by skin contact with an allergen, overexposure to sun, systemic causes (eg, reaction to a medication). May be described as flat or raised, pruritic or non-pruritic, localized or systemic, or dry or wet.	• Wash area thoroughly with mild cleansing agent and rinse well. • Use a moisturizing lotion on a dry rash to prevent itching and promote healing. • Use a drying agent on a wet rash. • Tepid baths may relieve inflammation and itching. • Antiseptic sprays or lotions may be useful in lessening itching, promoting healing, and preventing skin breakdown. • Over-the-counter products such as Caladryl lotion and hydrocortisone cream may prove useful. • Avoid exposure to causative agent if it is known. • See physician if symptoms do not respond to treatment.

Identify any variables known to cause oral problems, such as deficient self-care abilities, poor nutrition or excessive intake of refined sugars, family history of periodontal disease, or ingestion of chemotherapeutic agents that produce oral lesions. Patients at high risk for oral problems include those who are seriously ill, comatose, dehydrated, confused, depressed, or paralyzed. Patients who are mouth breathers, who can have no oral intake of nutrition or fluids, who have nasogastric tubes or oral airways in place, and who have had oral surgery are also at increased risk.

Physical Assessment

Examine the lips for color, moisture, lumps, ulcers, lesions, and edema. Examine the buccal mucosa for color, moisture, lesions, nodules, and bleeding. Examine the color of the gums and surface of the gums for lesions, bleeding, edema, and exudate. Examine for loose, missing, or carious (decayed) teeth. Note the presence of dentures or other orthodontic devices. Examine the tongue for color, symmetry, movement, texture, and lesions. Examine the hard and soft palates for intactness, color, patches, lesions, and petechiae.

Examine the oropharynx for movement of the uvula and condition of tonsils, if present. Note unusual mouth odors. Assess adequacy of mastication and swallowing. Chapter 25 further describes nursing assessment of the oral cavity.

When inspecting the oral cavity, the nurse frequently observes oral problems that at best are benign and only mildly annoying to patients but that may also be life-threatening. It is imperative to identify the problem and its cause and to initiate the appropriate treatment. This may require consultation with a dentist or physician.

Dental Caries

The decay of teeth with the formation of cavities is called **caries**. Caries result from the failure to remove **plaque**, an invisible, destructive, bacterial film that builds up on everyone's teeth and eventually leads to the destruction of tooth enamel. A successful plaque-fighting program includes elimination of sweet snacks between meals, such as soft drinks, candy, gum, jams, and jellies; thorough cleansing; and regular dental checkups. The use of antiplaque fluoride toothpastes, mouth rinses, and flossing helps prevent dental caries.

Periodontal Disease

The major cause of tooth loss in adults older than 35 years of age is gum disease. **Gingivitis** is an inflammation of the *gingiva*, the tissue that surrounds the teeth.

Pyorrhea, or *periodontal disease*, is a marked inflammation of the gums and also involves the alveolar tissues. Symptoms include bleeding gums; swollen, red, painful gum tissues; receding gum lines with the formation of pockets between the teeth and gums; pus that appears when gums are pressed; and loose teeth. If unchecked, plaque builds up and, along with dead bacteria, forms hard deposits called **tartar** at the gum lines. The tartar attacks the fibers that fasten teeth to the gums and eventually attacks bone tissue also. The teeth then loosen and fall out. A strong mouth odor (**halitosis**) or persistent bad taste in the mouth may be the first indication of periodontal disease. Regular dental treatment by a dentist is imperative.

Other Oral Problems

Other oral problems that the nurse may observe when inspecting the oral cavity include the following:

* *Stomatitis* is an inflammation of the oral mucosa with numerous causes, such as bacteria, virus, mechanical trauma, irritants, nutritional deficiencies, and systemic infection. Symptoms may include heat, pain, increased flow of saliva, and halitosis.
* *Glossitis* is an inflammation of the tongue that can be caused by vitamin B_{12}, folic acid, and iron deficiencies.
* *Cheilosis* is an ulceration of the lips (reddened fissures at the angles of the mouth) most often caused by vitamin B complex deficiencies (especially riboflavin).
* *Dry oral mucosa* may simply be related to dehydration or may be caused by mouth breathing, an alteration in salivary functioning, or certain medications (eg, anticholinergic drugs).

* *Oral malignancies* appear as lumps or ulcers; it is crucial that these be distinguished from benign mouth problems because early detection may be the difference between cure and radical dissecting surgery or death. Teach patients if they notice white or red patches, persistent sores, swelling, bleeding, numbness, or pain in the mouth to see their dentist immediately.

DIAGNOSING

Make a judgment about the adequacy of the patient's oral hygiene practices, identifying any factors contributing to deficiencies. An example is as follows:

Self-Care Deficit: Oral Hygiene related to low value attached to regular brushing, flossing, and dental examinations

Identify actual or potential oral problems that nurses can treat, noting contributing factors. Identify unhealthy patient responses to oral problems. Examples include the following:

* Pain related to chemotherapy-induced oral ulceration
* Risk for Infection related to breaks in oral mucosa and inadequate secondary defenses
* Altered Nutrition: Less Than Body Requirements related to painful oral lesions (ill-fitting dentures, gingivitis)
* Altered Oral Mucous Membrane related to dehydration (ineffective oral hygiene, medication)
* Impaired Swallowing related to neuromuscular impairment
* Body Image Disturbance related to loss of teeth, halitosis, or dental caries

PLANNING: EXPECTED OUTCOMES

Identify nursing measures to help the patient develop or maintain oral hygiene practices to promote oral health and general well-being and resolve identified nursing diagnoses. Plan for the following patient outcomes. The patient will achieve the following:

* Have lips, oral mucosa, gums, and tongue that are intact, moist, and free of inflammation and lesions
* Have clean teeth (or dentures)
* Demonstrate the ability to masticate and swallow food
* Demonstrate signs of healing of oral lesions
* Demonstrate correct oral hygiene measures—brushing and flossing
* Verbalize importance of fluoride use and regular dental examinations

Pertinent nursing measures to include in the plan of care are the following:

* Teach proper brushing and flossing techniques; instruct patients about fluoride use and the importance of regular dental examinations.
* Teach correct denture care or provide this when necessary.

- Perform mouth care for the unconscious patient (clean the mouth with swabs dipped in dilute mouth rinse or in normal saline solution; suction as necessary to prevent aspiration; apply a petroleum jelly to the lips).
- Perform mouth care for patients with oral lesions (cleanse to prevent infection and numbing if indicated to encourage eating).

In the plan of care, identify any supplies needed to carry out the specified oral care and the timing and frequency of oral hygiene measures.

IMPLEMENTING

While carrying out the plan of care, the nurse uses each nurse–patient interaction for ongoing assessment of the patient's oral cavity and evaluation of the adequacy of the plan of care. Techniques for administering and teaching oral care are described in this section. Sample documentation of oral hygiene care follows:

> 10/20/01 Patient generally breathes with mouth open. Sores present on palate, teeth, gums, and oral mucosa. Toothettes dipped in normal saline used for cleansing every 4 hours. Lubricating jelly to lips.
>
> D. Sadowski, RN

Administering Oral Hygiene

The mouth must be cared for even during illness. However, there are times when care must be modified to meet the specific needs of a patient. If the patient is able to assist with mouth care while bedridden, the nurse provides necessary materials (Procedure 36-5). If the patient is helpless, the nurse needs to make certain that the patient's mouth receives care as often as necessary to keep it clean and moist, as often as every 1 or 2 hours if necessary. This is especially true for patients who are unable or are not permitted fluids by mouth. Procedure 36-6 gives techniques for administering oral hygiene to dependent patients. Normal saline solution is recommended when giving oral care to dependent patients. The nurse should wear disposable gloves. Moisten the mouth with water, if allowed, and lubricate the lips sufficiently frequently to keep the membranes well moistened.

The procedure for cleaning the mouth thoroughly is more important than the agent used. This supports the personal experience of many people that no mouthwash, breath freshener, ointment, or paste replaces a thorough mechanical cleaning of the oral cavity.

Denture Care

Having dentures out of the mouth for long periods allows the gum line to change, thus affecting their fit. If the patient has been instructed to remove dentures while sleeping, a disposable denture cup is convenient and easy to use. Dentures should not be wrapped in toilet tissue or disposable wipes because these are likely to be thrown away. It is recommended that dentures be stored in water to prevent drying and warping of plastic materials.

Patients with dentures are more likely to keep them in the mouth when dentures are kept clean. If the patient cannot care for them, the nurse is responsible for ensuring that dentures are clean. Care should be exercised when handling a patient's dentures. They represent a considerable financial investment, and damage or loss is expensive. When cleaning dentures, don gloves and hold them over a basin of water or a sink lined with a washcloth or soft towel (Fig. 36-5) so that if they slip from your grasp, they will not fall onto a hard surface and break. Cool or lukewarm water should be used to cleanse them. Hot water may warp the plastic material from which most dentures are made. The use of a brush and a nonabrasive powder or paste is also recommended. Dentures may be soaked in commercial preparations to help remove stains and hardened particles. The dentures are rinsed well after cleaning. The patient should be given the opportunity to rinse his or her mouth before the dentures are replaced.

Teaching Oral Hygiene

Toothbrushing and Flossing

A toothbrush should be small enough to reach all teeth. The bristles should be sufficiently firm to clean but not so firm that they are likely to injure tooth enamel and gum tissue. Brushes should be cleaned and dried between uses. Most damage is done by bacteria directly after eating. Therefore, it is ideal to brush the teeth immediately after eating or drinking. The tongue should also be cleaned with the brush.

Automatic toothbrushes, electric or battery operated, have been found to be simple to use and as good as hand brushes for removing debris and plaque. Waterspray units are available to assist with oral hygiene. However, if an undue amount of water pressure is used, particles of debris may be forced into tissue pockets, and damage may occur to gum tissue. Therefore, it is recommended that their use be discussed with a dentist.

The toothbrush cannot effectively reach areas between the teeth where food lodges; hence, flossing once a day is recommended. The practice not only removes what the brush cannot but also helps to break up colonies of bacteria. The accompanying box, Guidelines for Nursing Care: Flossing, illustrates a flossing technique.

Toothpastes and powders aid the brushing process and usually have a pleasant taste that encourages brushing, especially by children. Most dentifrices are safe to use, but those containing harsh abrasives may scratch the enamel of the teeth and therefore are not recommended. Salt or sodium bicarbonate are far less expensive than proprietary products on the market and just as effective for short-term use, but they lack fluoride and should not be used exclusively. Dentifrices containing stannous fluoride and antiplaque rinses have proved effective in helping to decrease dental caries and hence are recommended by many dentists.

Mouthwashes

An offensive breath odor or halitosis is often systemic in nature. For example, the odor of onions and garlic on the breath comes from the lungs, where the oils are being removed from the bloodstream and eliminated with respiration. A mouthwash cannot remove halitosis when odors are being eliminated by respiration.

PROCEDURE 36-5

Assisting the Patient With Oral Care

Equipment

Toothbrush	Towel	Denture cup
Toothpaste	Mouthwash (optional)	Denture cleaner
Emesis basin	Dental floss (optional)	4 × 4 gauze
Glass with cool water	Denture-cleansing equipment	Washcloth or paper towel
Disposable gloves	(if necessary)	Petroleum jelly (optional)

Action	**Rationale**
1. Explain the procedure to the patient.	Explanation facilitates cooperation.
2. Wash your hands. Don disposable gloves if assisting with oral care.	Handwashing deters the spread of microorganisms. Gloves protect the nurse from exposure to blood and blood-borne infections.
3. Assemble equipment on an overbed table within the patient's reach.	Organization facilitates performance of task.
4. Provide privacy for the patient.	Patient may be embarrassed if cleansing involves removal of dentures.
5. Lower side rail and assist patient to sitting position if permitted, or turn the patient onto the side. Place the towel across the patient's chest. Raise the bed to a comfortable working position.	The sitting or side-lying position prevents aspiration of fluids into the lungs. The towel protects the patient from dampness.
6. Encourage the patient to brush own teeth or assist if necessary:	
a. Moisten the toothbrush and apply toothpaste to bristles.	Water softens the bristles.
b. Place brush at a 45-degree angle to gum line and brush from gum line to crown of each tooth. Brush outer and inner surfaces. Brush back and forth across biting surface of each tooth.	This facilitates removal of plaque and tartar. The 45-degree angle of brushing permits cleansing of all surface areas of the tooth.

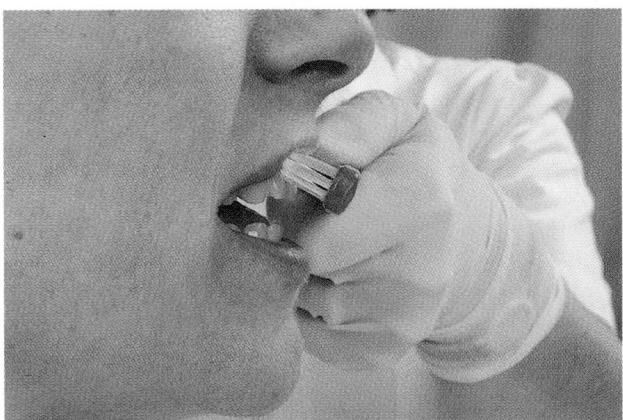

Action 6b: Placing brush at 45-degree angle to the gum line.

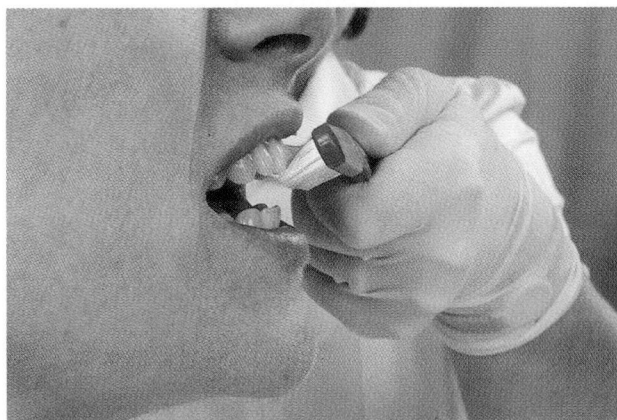

Action 6b: Brushing from the gum line to the crown of each tooth.

(continued)

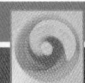

PROCEDURE 36-5

Assisting the Patient With Oral Care (Continued)

c. Brush tongue gently with toothbrush.

d. Have the patient rinse vigorously with water and spit into emesis basin. Repeat until clear. Suction may be used as an alternative for removal of fluid and secretions from mouth.

e. Assist the patient to floss teeth if necessary.

f. Offer mouthwash if the patient prefers.

7. Assist the patient with removal and cleansing of dentures if necessary:
   a. Apply gentle pressure with 4 × 4 gauze to grasp upper denture plate and remove. Place it immediately in the denture cup. Lift the lower denture using slight rocking motion, remove, and place in the denture cup.
   b. If the patient prefers, add denture cleanser to the cup with water and follow directions on preparation or brush all areas thoroughly with toothbrush and paste. Place paper towels or washcloth in sink while brushing.
   c. Rinse thoroughly with water and return dentures to the patient.
   d. Offer mouthwash so patient can rinse his or her mouth before replacing dentures.
   e. Apply petroleum jelly to lips if needed.

8. Remove equipment and assist the patient to a position of comfort. Record any unusual bleeding or inflammation. Raise side rail and lower the bed.

9. Remove disposable gloves from inside out and discard appropriately wash your hands.

This removes coating on the tongue. Gentle motion does not stimulate gag reflex.
The vigorous swishing motion helps to remove debris. Suction is appropriate if swallowing reflex is impaired or absent.

Flossing aids in removal of plaque and promotes healthy gum tissue.
Mouthwash leaves a pleasant taste in the mouth.

Rocking motion breaks suction between the denture and gum. Using 4 × 4 gauze prevents slippage and discourages spread of microorganisms.

Dentures collect food and microorganisms and require daily cleansing. Paper towels or washcloth in the sink protects against breakage.

Water aids in removal of debris and acts as a cleansing agent.
Mouthwash leaves a pleasant taste in the mouth and removes food particles, thus permitting proper fit.
Petroleum jelly prevents cracking and drying of lips.

This promotes oral hygiene and provides for oral assessment. Elevated side rails and lowered bed position maintain safety for bedridden patients.

This protects the nurse from contact with any microorganism. Handwashing deters spread of microorganisms.

If the cause of halitosis is poor oral hygiene, cleaning reduces the odor. Commercial mouthwashes may be helpful. If concentrated mouthwashes are used frequently for debilitated patients, however, they may injure oral tissue.

EVALUATING

At designated intervals, evaluate whether the patient has met the goals established during planning and revise the care plan if indicated. An example follows:

10/26/01 Goal partially met. Patient's oral mucosa is intact, but thick, dry secretions continue to build on oral mucosa and gums despite every-4-hour care.
Revision: Increase frequency of oral hygiene to every 2 hours. Instruct family.

N. Glynn, RN

 ## Care of the Eyes, Ears, and Nose

The Nursing Process

ASSESSING

Nursing History

Identify any special eye, ear, or nose care the patient performs. Include the use and care of visual aids or prostheses (glasses, contact lenses, artificial eye) and hearing aids. Note any history of eye, ear, and nose problems and related treatments.

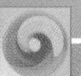

PROCEDURE 36-6

Providing Oral Care for the Dependent Patient

Equipment

Toothbrush
Toothpaste
Emesis basin
Disposable gloves
Cup with cool water
Towel
Mouthwash
Normal saline solution

Denture-cleansing equipment
  (if necessary)
Denture cup
Washcloth or paper towel
Sponge toothette or tongue blades
  padded with 4 × 4 gauze
  sponges

Irrigating syringe with rubber tip
  (optional)
Petroleum jelly
Suction catheter with suction
  apparatus (optional)

Action	Rationale
1. Explain the procedure to the patient.	Explanation facilitates cooperation.
2. Wash your hands and don disposable gloves.	Handwashing and disposable gloves deter the spread of microorganisms.
3. Assemble equipment on overbed table within reach.	Organization facilitates performance of task.
4. Provide privacy for the patient. Adjust the height of the bed to a comfortable position. Lower one side rail and position the patient on the side with the head of the bed lowered. Place the towel across the patient's chest and emesis basin in position under the chin.	The side-lying position with head lowered prevents aspiration of fluid into lungs. Towel and emesis basin protects patient from dampness.
5. Open the patient's mouth and gently insert a padded tongue blade between the back molars if necessary.	Padded tongue blade keeps mouth open for easier cleaning and prevents the patient from biting the nurse's fingers.

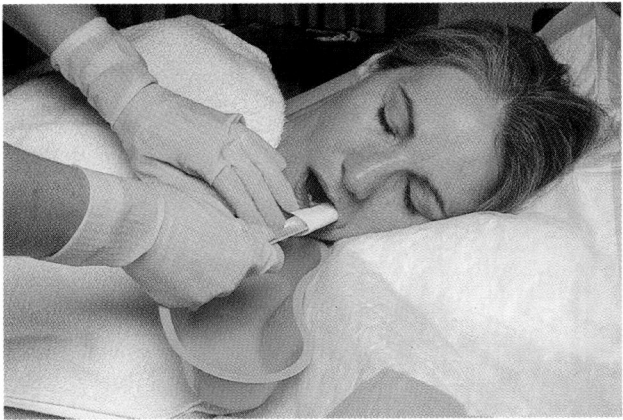

Action 5: Gently inserting padded tongue blade between back molars.

6. If teeth are present, brush carefully with toothbrush and paste. Remove dentures if present and clean before replacing (see action 7 of Procedure 36-5). Use toothette or gauze-padded tongue blade moistened with normal saline or dilute mouthwash solution to gently cleanse gums, mucous membranes, and tongue.	Toothbrush or padded tongue blade provides friction necessary to clean areas where plaque and tartar accumulate. Hydrogen peroxide is considered an irritant and no longer recommended. The mechanical action of cleansing is more important than the solution.

(continued)

PROCEDURE 36-6

Providing Oral Care for the Dependent Patient (Continued)

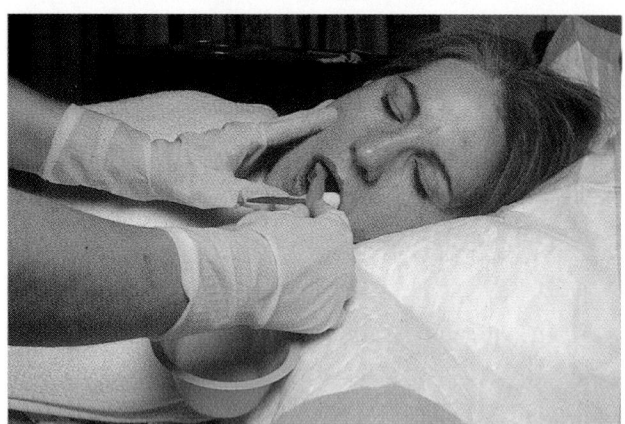

Action 6: Carefully brushing patient's teeth.

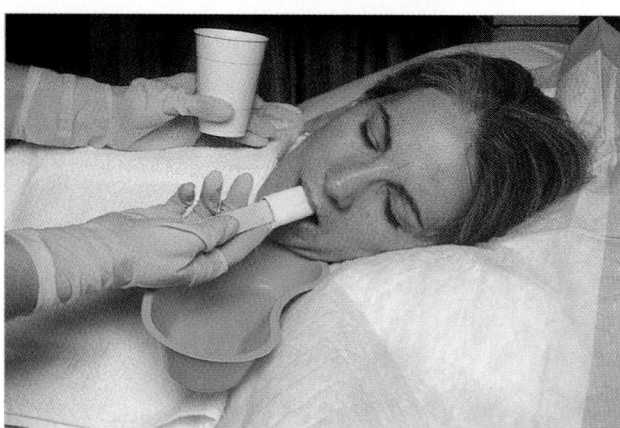

Action 6: Using moistened padded tongue blade to cleanse gums, mucous membranes, and tongue.

7. Use gauze-padded tongue blade dipped in mouthwash solution to rinse the oral cavity. If desired, insert the rubber tip of the irrigating syringe into the patient's mouth and rinse gently with a small amount of water. Position the patient's head to allow for return of water or use suction apparatus to remove the water from oral cavity.

Rinsing helps to cleanse debris from the mouth. Solution that is forcefully irrigated may cause aspiration.

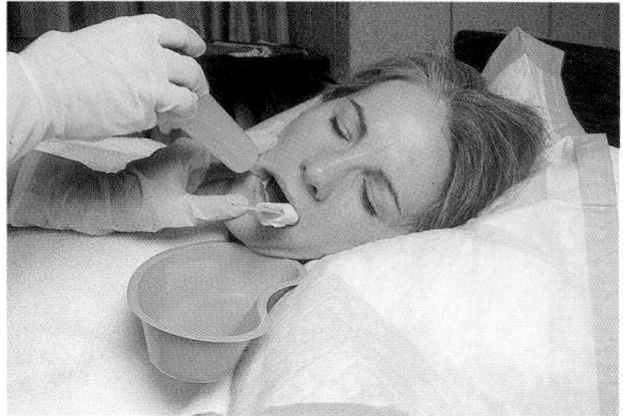

Action 7: Using irrigating syringe and a small amount of water to rinse mouth.

8. Apply petroleum jelly to the patient's lips.

This prevents drying and cracking of lips.

9. Remove equipment and return the patient to a position of comfort. Raise the side rail and lower the bed. Record any unusual bleeding or inflammation.

This promotes oral hygiene and provides for oral assessment. Raised side rail and lowered bed maintain patient safety.

10. Wash your hands.

Handwashing deters spread of microorganisms.

Special Considerations

A patient receiving chemotherapy medication may have bleeding gums and extremely sensitive mucous membranes. Use a soft sponge toothette for cleaning or substitute a salt water rinse (½ teaspoon salt in 1 cup of warm water) for brushing of teeth.

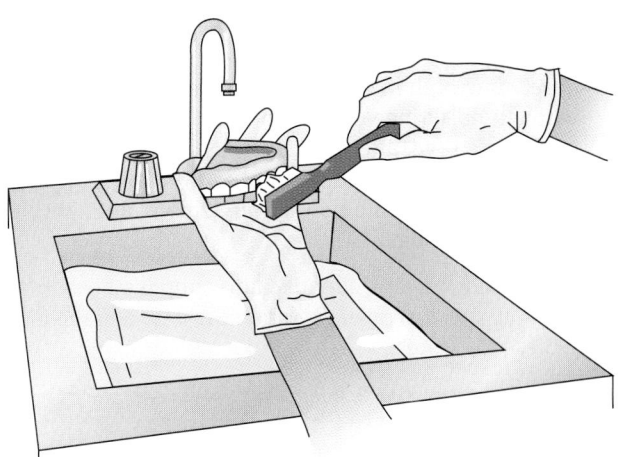

Figure 36-5
Proper method of cleaning dentures.

Physical Assessment

During the eye examination, note the position, alignment, and general appearance of the eye. Check that eyelashes are equally distributed and curl outward. Note the presence of lesions, nodules, redness, swelling, crusting, flaking, excessive tearing, or discharge of eyelids. Check the color of the conjunctivae, presence of blink reflex, and visual acuity (ability to read newsprint).

In the ear examination, note the position, alignment, and general appearance of the ear. Pay particular attention to a buildup of wax in the canal, dryness, crusting, or the presence of any discharge or foreign body. Check hearing acuity. About one third of older adults have at least one ear obstructed by a wax buildup, and this frequently causes hearing loss that can be reversed (Stone, 1999).

During examination of the nose, note its position and general appearance, patency of the nostrils, and presence of tenderness, dryness, edema, bleeding, discharge, or secretions. Refer to Chapter 25 for additional information related to nursing assessment of the eyes, ears, and nose.

DIAGNOSING

Make a judgment about the adequacy of the patient's self-care practices related to eye, ear, and nose care, identifying any factors that contribute to deficiencies. The following are some examples of nursing diagnoses related to eye, ear, and nose care:

> Self-Care Deficit: Artificial Eye Care related to Knowledge Deficit

Identify actual or potential eye, ear, and nose problems that nurses can treat, noting contributing factors. Identify

---

Guidelines for Nursing Care

Flossing

- Wear gloves when flossing a patient's teeth.
- Keep about 1 to 1½ inches of floss held taut between the fingers.
- Do not force the floss between the teeth; insert it gently by moving it back and forth where teeth touch each other.
- Move the floss up and down while using both fingers, first on the side of one tooth and then on the side of the other tooth, until the surfaces are squeaky clean.

- Go to the gum tissue with the floss but not into the gum because this may result in discomfort, soreness, or bleeding.
- Advance the floss from one hand to the other to bring up a fresh section of floss when it has become frayed or soiled.
- Rinse the mouth well with water after flossing to remove food particles and plaque that have been loosened. Also, rinse after eating when flossing or brushing is impossible.

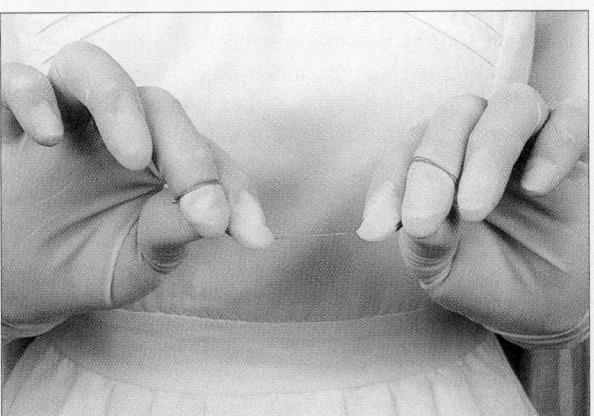

Securing floss around the fingers.

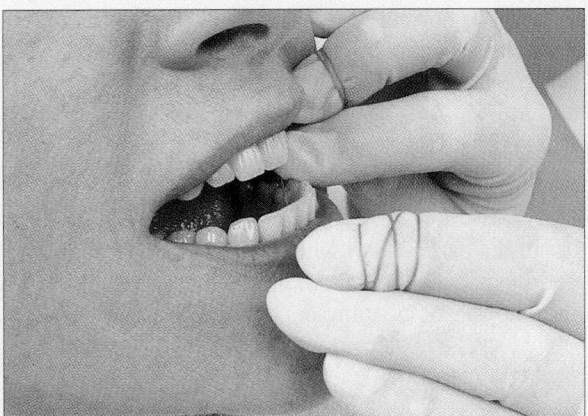

Inserting floss between the teeth.

unhealthy patient responses to eye, ear, and nose problems, such as the following:

- Sensory/Perceptual Alterations (Visual, Auditory, or Olfactory) related to psychologic stress
- Altered Health Maintenance related to perceptual impairment (visual or auditory)
- Impaired Social Interaction related to visual or auditory impairment
- Fear related to sudden loss of vision or hearing
- Anticipatory Grieving related to increasing visual or auditory impairment
- Risk for Injury related to visual impairment

PLANNING: EXPECTED OUTCOMES

Identify nursing measures that will help the patient develop or maintain care measures that contribute to healthy eye, ear, and nose functioning and to the patient's general sense of well-being. Plan for the following patient outcomes. The patient will achieve the following:

- Demonstrate healthy functioning of eyes, ears, and nose
- Have eyes, ears, and nose that appear clean
- Show signs of healing (if realistic, specify these signs) of sensory impairment (visual, auditory, olfactory), or seek aids appropriate to impairment
- Demonstrate correct eye, ear, and nose care measures, including the proper use and care of visual or auditory aids

Pertinent nursing measures to include in the plan of care are as follows:

Eye

- Clean the eye from the *inner canthus* (angle of the eye closest to the nose where the upper and lower lids meet) to the *outer canthus* (lateral angle of the eye where the upper and lower lids meet) using a wet, warm washcloth, cotton ball, or compress to soften crusted secretions. Carefully avoid cross-contamination.
- When the blink (corneal) reflex is decreased or absent (eg, in a comatose patient), use artificial tear solution or normal saline at least every 4 hours to keep the eyes moist and protected from drying; a protective shield may be necessary to keep the lids closed.
- Offer correct eyeglass, contact lens, or artificial eye teaching and care.

Ear

- Clean the external ear with a washcloth-covered finger, instructing the patient never to insert an object into the ear for cleaning purposes. Use of cotton-tipped swabs is discouraged because they may impact cerumen.
- Assist with the softening and removal of excessive wax deposits.
- Offer hearing aid teaching and care.

Nose

- Clean the nose by instructing the patient to blow the nose while both nares are patent (nasal suctioning with a bulb syringe may be indicated) unless contraindicated (eg, after brain surgery or head trauma).
- Remove crusted secretions around the nose and protect this tissue with a non–water-soluble ointment (eg, petroleum jelly).

In the plan of care, identify any supplies needed to carry out the specified eye, ear, and nose care and the timing of these measures.

IMPLEMENTING

Carry out plan of care, remembering to use each nurse–patient interaction for ongoing assessment of the patient's eyes, ears, and nose and for evaluation of the adequacy of the plan of care. The following sections describe select nursing measures related to eye, ear, and nose care. Sample documentation of eye care follows:

> 10/20/01 Patient states, "I can't believe they expect me to take care of this eye. I don't want to touch it." Has not participated in artificial eye care to date. Patient encouraged to verbalize concerns about artificial eye and assist with care.
>
> S. Cohen, RN

Cleaning the Eyes

Normally, the eyes are clear and kept clean with lacrimal secretions. During illness, the eyes may produce more secretions than normal and appear glasslike. The following techniques are recommended when secretions adhere to the eyelashes and become dry and crusty or when discharge is present:

- Wear gloves during the cleaning procedure.
- Use water or normal saline and cotton balls or a clean washcloth or compress to clean the eyes. Boric acid solution, once popular for cleaning the eyes, is no longer recommended because of its toxicity when absorbed through mucous membranes. The eyes are never cleaned with soap because of its irritating effects on eye tissues.
- Position the patient on the same side as the eye to be cleaned so that solution and debris do not run across the bridge of the nose and contaminate the other eye.
- Dampen a cotton ball with the solution of choice and wipe once while moving the cotton ball from the inner canthus to the outer canthus of the eye. This technique minimizes forcing debris into the area drained by the nasolacrimal duct. Discard the used cotton ball.
- Continue this technique, using one cotton ball for each stroke, until the eye is clean.
- Turn the patient to the opposite side and clean the other eye in the same manner.
- Wipe the lashes dry with a paper tissue or a clean washcloth, exposing a clean area of the tissue or cloth with each stroke.

Caring for the Unconscious Patient's Eyes

Patients with diminished or absent blink (corneal) reflexes and patients whose eyelids remain open require frequent eye care (at least every 4 hours). If the eye is not kept moist, corneal ulceration may result from excessive drying of the eye. Nursing measures include using saline or artificial tears to lubricate the eye and a protective eye shield to keep the eye closed.

Providing Care of Eyeglasses

Eyeglasses are essential for many people and represent a considerable financial investment. The nurse should take precautions to prevent their breakage or loss. Patients needing glasses should be encouraged to wear them to avoid eye strain.

Plastic lenses are popular because they are considerably lighter in weight than glass lenses while correcting vision just as well as glass. One disadvantage of plastic is that the material scratches easily.

Eyeglasses should be cleaned over a terry towel, so that if they slip, they will not become scratched or broken. Glasses are cleaned with warm water and soap or using a special cleansing preparation. Hot water may warp plastic lenses and frames. The glasses should be rinsed well when cleansed with soap and water. They should be dried with a clean, soft cloth, such as a cotton handkerchief or cotton napkin. Paper products are made of wood pulp and are likely to scratch the lenses. Eyeglasses should not be cleaned with a dry paper tissue or cloth.

Providing Care of Contact Lenses

A contact lens is a small disc worn directly on the eyeball. It stays in place by surface tension of the eye's tears. Contact lenses are either hard or soft. The older hard lenses are not gas permeable, whereas newer ones are gas permeable and more comfortable because they allow oxygen to pass directly through the lens to the cornea. Soft lenses are of a plastic material that absorbs water to become soft and pliable. They are brittle when dehydrated and absorb water when placed in solution, usually normal saline, or when in contact with tears. Soft lenses may be used for daily wear or extended wear. Disposable soft lenses are also available.

People wearing contact lenses need to take special precautions to keep them free of microorganisms that may lead to eye infections and to use them in a manner that does not injure or scratch the surface of the eye. Hands must always be washed before touching eye surfaces and lenses. Lens wearers need to be cautious about eye irritation in the presence of noxious vapors or smoke. The lenses should not contact cosmetics, soaps, or hair sprays because eye irritation may result. It is recommended that any adverse reaction to their use be reported to the prescribing physician immediately.

The cornea, which consists of dense connective tissue, does not have its own blood supply. It is nourished primarily by oxygen from the atmosphere and from tears. When wearing contact lenses, the cornea requires more than its normal supply of oxygen because its metabolic rate increases. To allow the cornea to receive a maximal supply of oxygen, hard lenses should be removed before sleeping and should not be worn more than 12 to 16 hours. Extended-wear soft lenses can be left in place for 1 to 30 days, depending on the manufacturer. It is recommended that extended-wear lenses be cleansed at least once weekly. The time that disposable soft lenses should be worn also varies according to the type and the manufacturer. A new type of disposable lens is replaced daily, while other options include lenses that can be worn day and night for 7 days or those worn during waking hours only for 14 days. Excessive tearing, pain, and redness signal the need to remove lenses.

There may be times when the nurse may be required to remove lenses if a patient cannot do so. To leave them in place for long periods could result in permanent eye damage. This may occur, for example, when the nurse is attending an unconscious patient.

Before removing hard or gas-permeable lenses, the nurse should use gentle pressure to center the lens on the cornea. A small suction device can also be used in an emergency situation to remove gas-permeable or hard lenses. Figure 36-6 demonstrates removal of hard and soft lenses. Once removed, the lenses should be identified as being for the right or left eye because the two lenses are not necessarily identical. The nurse should not try to remove lenses, however, if an eye injury is present, because of the danger of additional injury.

Providing Care of an Artificial Eye

Most patients who wear an artificial eye prefer to take care of it themselves, and they should be encouraged to do so when possible. The necessary equipment includes a small basin, soap and water for washing, and solution for rinsing the prosthesis. Normal saline or tap water can be used for rinsing. Most people have their own method for cleaning the eye socket and the area around it. The nurse should ask the patient how he or she does this and make it possible for the patient to continue with the usual practice. The patient should be lying down so that the eye does not accidentally fall to the floor. The socket is ordinarily flushed with normal saline before the eye is replaced.

Providing Ear Care

Other than cleaning the outer ears, little is needed for routine hygiene of the ear. After the ears are washed, they should be dried carefully with a soft towel so that water and cerumen (wax) are removed by capillary action. Forcing the towel into the ear for drying or using a cotton-tipped applicator may aid in the formation of wax plugs. Using bobby pins, hairpins, paper clips, or fingernails to remove wax from the ear is extremely dangerous because these may injure or puncture the eardrum (refer to

Removing hard contact lenses

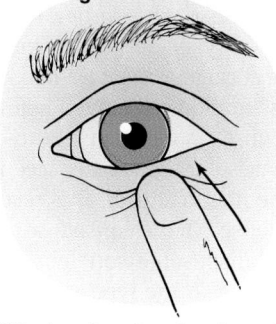

If the lens is not centered over the cornea, apply gentle pressure on the lower eyelid to center the lens.

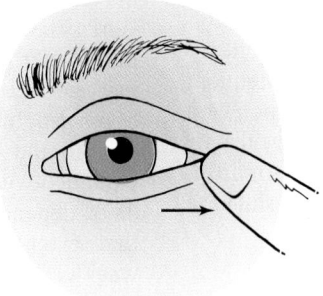

Gently pull the outer corner of the eye toward the ear.

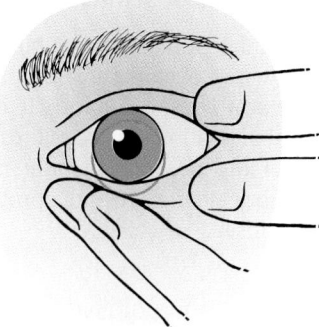

Position the other hand below the lens to receive it and ask the patient to blink.

Or

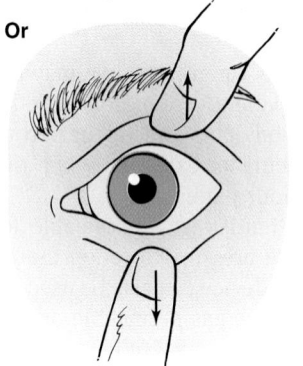

Gently spread the eyelids beyond the top and bottom edges of the lens.

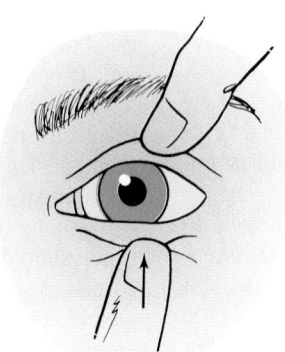

Gently press the lower eyelid up against the bottom of the lens.

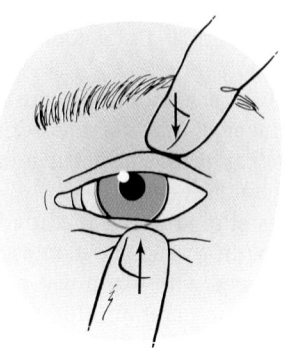

After the lens is tipped slightly, move the eyelids toward one another to cause the lens to slide out between the eyelids.

Removing soft contact lenses

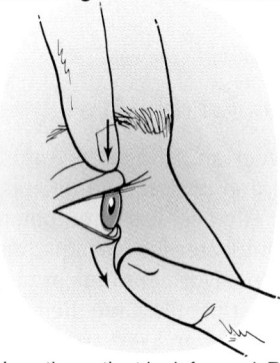

Have the patient look forward. Retract the lower lid with one hand. Using the pad of the index finger of the other hand, move the lens down to the sclera.

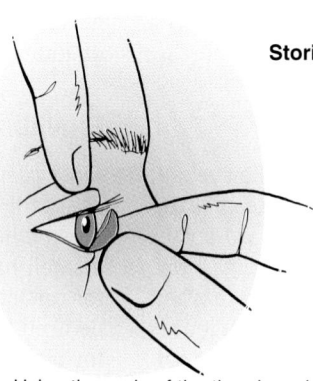

Using the pads of the thumb and index finger, grasp the lens with a gentle pinching motion and remove.

Storing lenses

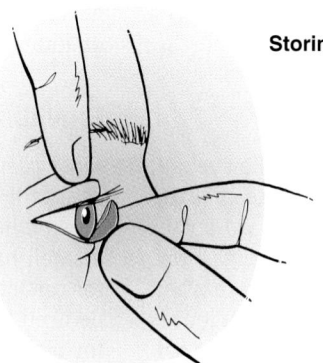

Because lenses may be different for each eye, storage cases are marked L and R, designating left and right lenses. It is important to place the first lens in its designated cup in the storage case before removing the second lens to avoid mixing them up.

Figure 36-6
Removing contact lenses.

the accompanying box for selected standardized nursing interventions for care of the ear).

Hearing Aids

If the patient uses a hearing aid, batteries should be checked routinely and the ear pieces or ear mold cleaned daily with mild soap and water. A whistling sound that is audible when the hearing aid is held in the hand with the power on and the volume high indicates that the battery is functioning properly. Refer to Chapter 21 for strategies nurses can use to facilitate communication with a hearing-impaired patient. If hearing loss is mild and the patient is not using a hearing aid, the following suggestions may help to improve hearing and should be included in any health teaching:

- Avoid noisy places for conversation.
- Choose well-lighted places where it is easier to look at the speaker's face, lips, and hands for cues to the conversation.

Using the Nursing Interventions Classification (NIC)

Ear Care

- Monitor for drainage from ears, as appropriate.
- Avoid placing sharp objects in the ear.
- Determine if cerumen in the ear canal is causing pain or hearing loss.
- Instill mineral oil in the ear to soften impacted cerumen before irrigation.
- Irrigate the ear canal with a Water-Pik (or similar device) on a low setting, using warm water (80° to 90°F), as appropriate.
- Demonstrate proper technique for ear irrigation to caregiver, as appropriate.

From McClosky, J., & Bulechek, G. (2000). *Nursing interventions classification (NIC)* (3rd ed). (p. 265). St. Louis: C. V. Mosby. (This text provides a full listing of nursing activities for each nursing intervention.)

- Cup your hand behind your ear.
- Ask people to face you when they are speaking to you.
- Ask people to repeat what they said, if it was not clear to you, and to speak slowly.
- Consider buying amplitude devices so that you can hear your television and radio without turning up the sound (Eliopoulos, 1997).

Figure 36-7 illustrates several types of hearing aids.

Providing Nose Care

The best way to clean the nose is to blow it gently. Both nostrils should be open while doing this. Closing one nostril adds to the danger of forcing debris into the eustachian tubes. Irrigations are usually contraindicated because of the possible danger of forcing material into the sinuses.

If the external nares are crusted, applying mineral or cottonseed oil helps to soften and remove the crusts. Disposable paper tissues are recommended for nasal secretions. A cotton applicator may be used to clean the nares, but with great care to avoid injury. The applicator should never be introduced into the nares.

EVALUATING

At designated intervals, evaluate whether the patient has achieved the outcomes established during planning. Revise the plan of care if indicated. An example follows:

> 10/24/01 Goal met. Patient demonstrated correct care (cleaning) of artificial eye for the past two mornings. States, "I guess I should be happy to be alive and still able to see."
>
> N. Glynn, RN

Hair Care

Hair is an accessory structure of the skin. Good general health is essential for attractive hair and skin, and cleanliness is a positive influence. Illness affects the hair, especially when endocrine abnormalities, increased body temperature, poor nutrition, or anxiety and worry are present. Changes in

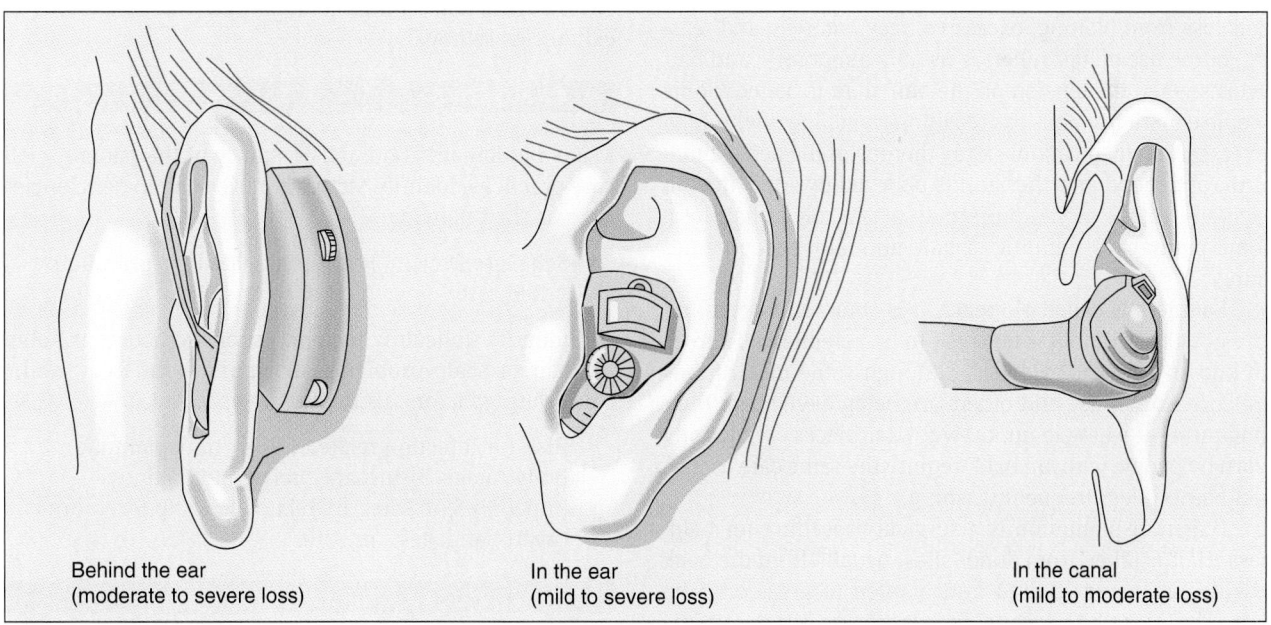

Behind the ear
(moderate to severe loss)

In the ear
(mild to severe loss)

In the canal
(mild to moderate loss)

Figure 36-7
Several types of hearing aids.

the color or condition of the hair shaft are related to changes in hormonal activity or to changes in the blood supply to hair follicles.

The Nursing Process

Nursing History

Identify the patient's usual hair and scalp care practices, including styling preferences. Note any history of hair or scalp problems; possible causes of changes in the distribution, texture, or amount of hair; and related treatments.

Identify any factors known to cause hair or scalp problems or that require special care-deficient self-care abilities, immobility, malnutrition, and treatments known to result in hair loss (eg, certain chemotherapeutic agents).

Physical Assessment

Assess the condition of the hair (texture, cleanliness, oiliness) and scalp (scaling, lesions, inflammation, infection).

Dandruff

Dandruff is a condition characterized by itching and flaking of the scalp that may be further complicated by the embarrassment it causes. Persistent, severe cases usually require medical attention. Daily brushing and shampooing with a medicated shampoo may be all that is needed to keep the scalp free of dandruff.

Hair Loss

Hair growth and hair loss are ongoing, daily processes. Hair loss from plaiting, excessive back combing and teasing, or the use of hair rollers is usually temporary, and hair returns when the tension on the hair shaft is halted. Some people experience hair loss resulting from illness with high fever, certain medications, x-ray therapy of the head, childbirth, or general anesthesia. It is believed by some that an excessive intake of vitamin A may play a role in hair loss. Some permanent thinning of hair normally accompanies aging.

Baldness is called **alopecia**. It is common in men but rare in women, and it is believed to be hereditary. There is no known cure for baldness, although some medications are currently in use and others are being developed; their long-term efficacy is unknown. Hairpieces, frequently worn by people who are bald, require the same care as normal hair but less frequent washing.

Hair transplantation is a surgical procedure for baldness. Hair is taken from donor sites, usually from the back or sides of the scalp, and transplanted to areas with no hair. The procedure is long and expensive but reportedly has decided benefits for people who find baldness psychologically unpleasant. Complications include serious scalp infections.

Pediculosis

Infestation with lice is called **pediculosis**. There are three common types of lice: *Pediculus humanus capitis*, which infests hair and scalp; *P. humanus corporis*, which infests the body; and *Phthirus pubis*, which infests the shorter hairs on the body, usually the pubic hair and the axillary hair. Lice lay eggs, called nits, on the hair shafts. *Nits* are white or light gray and look like dandruff, but they cannot be brushed or shaken off the hair. Frequent scratching and scratch marks on the body and the scalp suggest the presence of pediculosis. Although anyone may become infested with lice, the continued presence of pediculosis is usually a result of uncleanliness. Pediculosis can be spread directly by contact with infested areas or indirectly through clothing, bed linen, brushes, and combs. Teaching patients, especially children, not to share personal items is a good way to prevent transmission. The linens and personal care items of a patient with pediculosis require separate and careful handling to prevent spread from person to person.

Several commercial preparations, called *pediculicides,* are available for the treatment of pediculosis, some of which destroy the nits as well as the lice. Several treatments are usually necessary before all the nits are destroyed. The procedures and the medications used for the treatment of pediculosis vary among health agencies. The infested hair may be shaved, especially when pubic hair and axillary hair are infested. Partners must be notified in all cases of pubic infestation.

Ticks

Ticks are important because they can transmit serious diseases such as Lyme disease, Rocky Mountain spotted fever, and tularemia. Ticks should never be forcibly pulled out of the skin because the sucking apparatus may remain in the skin and cause an infection. Because oil suffocates the tick, covering the tick with mineral oil or a lubricating jelly facilitates its removal.

Make a judgment about the adequacy of the patient's self-care practices. Identify factors contributing to deficiencies, such as the following:

Self-Care Deficit: Hair Care related to continuous bed rest

Identify unhealthy patient responses, actual or potential hair or scalp problems, that nurses can treat, noting contributing factors. Examples are as follows:

- Risk for Infection related to hair transplantation
- Body Image Disturbance related to baldness
- Impaired Skin Integrity related to scalp laceration (head bandages), pruritus

Identify nursing measures that will assist the patient to develop or maintain needed hair and scalp care practices or that otherwise resolve nursing diagnoses. Specify any special products needed for hair care. Plan for the following expected outcomes. The patient will achieve the following:

- Have clean hair
- Demonstrate decreased or absent scalp lesions (or infestation)
- Verbalize satisfaction with appearance
- Participate in hair and scalp care as able

IMPLEMENTING

Carry out the plan of care, remembering to use scheduled hygienic care interactions for ongoing assessment of the patient's hair and scalp and for evaluating the adequacy of the plan of care. The following sections give suggestions for grooming hair, shampooing hair, caring for beards and mustaches, and assisting with unwanted hair removal.

Grooming the Hair

There are many cultural overtones associated with hair; moreover, styles also change within a culture from decade to decade. The nurse shows consideration when she grooms the patient's hair in the style preferred by the patient. Daily brushing of the hair helps to keep it clean and distributes oil along the shaft of each hair. Brushing also stimulates the circulation of blood in the scalp. Hair that becomes entangled is difficult to comb. Combing of tiny sections of hair at a time may be necessary if a patient's hair has not been combed for even 1 day. The best way to protect long hair from matting and tangling is to ask the patient for permission to braid it. Patients usually consent to the procedure if it provides them with more comfort. Parting the hair in the middle on the back of the head and making two braids, one on either side, prevents the discomfort of lying on one heavy braid on the back of the head.

Occasionally, a patient's hair is almost hopelessly matted, and cutting the hair may be necessary. Before a patient's hair is cut, it is usual procedure to have the patient sign a written consent. It is also recommended that the nurse discuss the necessity for cutting the hair with an immediate member of the patient's family.

The care of a person with kinky hair usually requires special attention. The hair is normally dry and curly and becomes easily matted and tangled. The comb used for arranging the hair should have widely spaced teeth and is worked through the hair from the neckline upward toward the forehead.

Some individuals may choose to have their hair straightened. Even after this process, it may be difficult to untangle hair of a person who is confined to bed. Some African Americans style their hair in small braids. The braids are not undone for shampooing and may need to have a lubricant or oil applied daily to prevent hair strands from breaking.

Shampooing the Hair

The hair is exposed to the same dirt and oil as the skin. It should be washed as often as necessary to keep it clean. The comb and the brush should be washed each time the hair is washed and as frequently as necessary between

shampoos. Many health agencies have beauticians and barbers to assist with the care of the patient's hair, including shampooing. However, this convenience does not relieve the nurse of responsibility.

Before shampooing the hair, it is recommended that the nurse, or the patient if able, brush and comb the hair well to stimulate the scalp and undo tangled hair. The patient may then shampoo the hair while showering, if able. In some hospitals, a physician's order is required for shampooing a patient's hair.

The following techniques are recommended for shampooing the hair of a person on bed rest whether at home or in the hospital:

- Prepare several pitchers of water of a suitably warm temperature for a thorough washing and rinsing, shampoo, one or two towels for drying, and a receptacle to receive wash and rinse water.
- Place a protective pad and a plastic hair washing tray if one is available (Fig. 36-8) under the head.
- Place the patient in a position over the pad so that there is constant drainage of water directed into the receptacle.
- Wet the hair, apply shampoo, and massage the scalp well while washing the hair.
- Rinse the hair and reapply shampoo for a second washing, if indicated.
- Rinse the hair thoroughly after washing it with soap and water.
- Apply conditioner if requested.
- Dry the hair as quickly as possible to prevent the patient from becoming chilled and arrange the hair according to the patient's preference.

Dry Shampoo

Dry shampoos cannot replace the cleaning benefits of regular shampoos , but they are helpful in removing at least some of the dirt, oils, and odors from the hair of patients too ill or

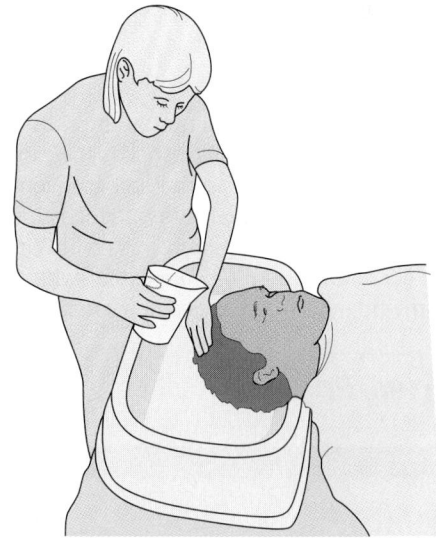

Figure 36-8
A nurse uses a protective pad and plastic tray when shampooing a patient's hair.

incapacitated to have a wet shampoo. Dry shampoos or powders are not recommended for people with kinky hair because of their normally dry hair and scalp. The dry shampoo or powder is applied and then combed or brushed from the hair. The teeth of the comb can then be pulled through gauze, which helps remove and capture the powder.

Caring for Beards and Mustaches

Most patients with beards or mustaches are able to groom them independently. Dependent patients require nursing assistance to keep the beard and mustache clean, especially after eating. For no reason should a nurse trim or shave off a patient's beard or mustache without the patient's consent.

Shaving

An electric shaver is usually recommended when the patient is receiving anticoagulant therapy or has a bleeding disorder. Blade razors tend to give a closer shave than electric razors, but many patients find electric razors convenient and practical. They are especially convenient for ill and bedridden patients. The technique for shaving patients who are unable to shave themselves is described in the Guidelines for Nursing Care box.

EVALUATING

At designated intervals, evaluate whether the patient has achieved the outcomes established during planning and revise the plan of care if indicated. An example follows:

> 10/27/01 Goal partially met. Patient reports that she is uncomfortable wearing a wig but feels better since its purchase.
> *Revision:* Because patient still has many questions about effects of chemotherapy, continue teaching and use opportunities to build self-esteem.
>
> V. Henderson, RN

⑨ Nail and Foot Care

The nails are an accessory structure of the skin composed of epithelial tissue. The body of the nail is the exposed portion; the root lies in the skin in the nail groove where the nail grows and is nourished. Healthy nailbeds have a pink color and are convex and evenly curved. With certain pathologic conditions, and to some extent with aging, the nails become ridged and areas become concave.

The Nursing Process

ASSESSING

Nursing History

Identify the patient's normal nail and foot care practices, the type of footwear worn, and any history of nail or foot problems and their related treatments. Foot problems, par-

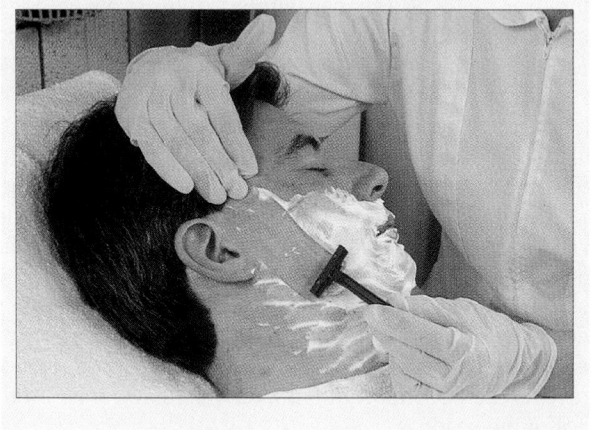

Guidelines for Nursing Care
Shaving

- Wear gloves because contact with blood is possible if any skin nicks occur.
- Apply shaving cream or a warm soap lather to the skin to soften the facial hair and prevent pulling.
- Pull the skin of the face so that it is taut.
- Use short, firm strokes in the direction of hair growth. Patients can often give suggestions on how they shave.
- Wash the patient's face of residual lather and dry.
- Apply aftershave lotion if patient requests it. Aftershave preparations tend to make the patient feel refreshed and have a cosmetic rather than a therapeutic effect.

ticularly common in people with diabetes mellitus and peripheral vascular disease, often require hospitalization (Halpin-Landry & Goldsmith, 1999). A proactive educational approach can prevent many of the serious complications (eg, ulcers, lower extremity amputations) associated with foot problems.

Identify any variables known to cause nail and foot problems, such as deficient self-care abilities, vascular disease, arthritis, diabetes mellitus, history of biting nails or trimming them improperly, frequent or prolonged exposure to chemicals or water, trauma, ill-fitting shoes, or obesity.

Physical Assessment

Examine nails for intactness and cleanliness; note capillary refill and the contour of the nailbed; observe the nail base for redness, swelling, bleeding, discharge, and tenderness. Examine the feet for cleanliness and intactness of skin, and note the presence of any swelling, inflammation, lesions, tenderness, or orthopedic problems. Examine carefully the skin between the toes. Refer to Chapter 25 for additional information on techniques for assessing the nails and feet.

Make a judgment about the adequacy of the patient's self-care practices related to nail and foot care, identifying any factors that contribute to deficiencies. An example is as follows:

> Self-Care Deficit: Diabetic Foot Care related to knowledge deficit and weakened physical state

Identify actual or potential nail or foot problems that nurses can treat, noting contributing factors. Identify unhealthy patient responses to these problems, for example:

- Pain related to corns (calluses, plantar warts, ingrown nails) in foot
- Impaired Physical Mobility related to painful foot condition (specify)
- Risk for Infection related to traumatized nail base or deficient nail or foot care
- Impaired Skin Integrity related to altered circulation to feet

Identify nursing measures that will assist the patient to develop or maintain healthy nail and foot care practices. Plan for the following expected outcomes. The patient will achieve the following:

- Have intact, clean, and manicured nails
- Have intact, clean, and lesion-free foot skin
- Have reduced or absent nail and foot problems (specify: calluses, corns, plantar warts, ingrown nails, athlete's foot)
- Demonstrate correct nail and foot care measures
- Verbalize nails and feet contribute to general sense of comfort and well-being

Pertinent nursing measures to include in the plan of care are as follows:

- Soaking nails and feet and assisting with cleaning of nails and trimming nails (if not contraindicated)
- Massaging the feet to promote relaxation and comfort
- Teaching correct nail and foot care

In the plan of care, identify any supplies needed to carry out the specified nail and foot care and the timing of these measures.

Carry out the plan of care, remembering to use bath times to assess continually the status of the patient's nails and feet and to evaluate the adequacy of the plan of care. Techniques for providing fingernail and foot care are described in the following sections. Sample documentation of foot care follows:

> 10/20/01 Patient states, "I guess I cut that nail too short—it's been hurting for 2 months now." Great toe on right foot is swollen, red, and painful. Skin at base of nail is white. Limps when walking. After bath, patient soaked right foot and dried it carefully.
>
> A. Jones, RN

Providing Care of Fingernails

The following are recommended techniques for the care of fingernails:

- File the nails to form an oval at the ends. Do not trim so far down on the sides that injury to the skin and cuticle occurs.
- Remove hangnails, which are broken pieces of cuticle, by cutting them off. Take special care to avoid injury to tissue with the cuticle scissors.
- *Gently* push cuticles back off the nail after they are soft and pliable after a soaking in warm water.
- Push back cuticles with a blunt instrument or a terry cloth.
- Apply an emollient to the cuticle to help prevent hangnails.
- Clean under the nails with a blunt instrument or the large end of a toothpick, being careful to prevent injuring the area where the nail is attached to the underlying tissue.

Splitting and peeling of the nails are usually caused by dryness. It is helpful to avoid contact with soap and water as much as possible, use a good hand cream frequently, and avoid the use of nail polish and polish remover, both of which have a tendency to dry the nails.

Providing Foot Care

Proper foot care is important at any age. It becomes even more so with aging and when such conditions as circulatory disturbances or diabetes mellitus are present. Refer to the accompanying Guidelines for Nursing Care for techniques related to foot care.

At designated intervals, evaluate whether the patient has achieved the expected outcomes established during planning and revise the plan of care if indicated. An example follows:

> 10/24/01 Expected outcome met. Patient correctly verbalized rationale for diabetic foot care program and expressed interest in attending the diabetic classes.
>
> A. Diaz, RN

Perineal and Vaginal Care

The perineal area is dark, warm, and often moist, which favors bacterial growth. The patient who cannot clean the perineal area needs the nurse's assistance for this important part of personal hygiene. Neglecting cleaning the perineal area of the patient who is unable to provide self-care often results in physical and psychological discomfort for the patient, a breakdown in the skin, and offensive odors.

Guidelines for Nursing Care

Foot Care

- Bathe the feet thoroughly in a mild soap and tepid water solution. Avoid soaking the feet. Be sure to clean the interdigital area.
- Rinse the feet to remove soap residue that can dry and irritate the skin.
- Dry feet thoroughly, including the area between the toes.
- Apply a water-soluble lotion to feet if they are dry. Include the area between the toes.
- Use an antifungal foot powder if necessary to prevent fungal infections, such as athlete's foot.
- For diabetic patients, file the nails; avoid using scissors or nail clippers, which may slip and injure tissues. Nondiabetic patients should avoid digging into or cutting the toenails at the lateral corners when trimming the nails.
- Do not cut off corns or calluses. Commercial removers should be avoided because they may contain ingredients that can lead to development of infection and ulcers. Consult a *podiatrist*, a physician who treats foot disorders, when corns or calluses are present.
- Explain the dangers of going barefoot. Skin on the feet may be injured, or athlete's foot may be acquired in public showers.
- Wear appropriate footwear. Break in new shoes gradually. Improperly fitting shoes can lead to corns, calluses, bunions, and blisters. The soles should be flexible and nonslippery and the heel heights should be safe and offer appropriate support. Shoes with rough ridges, wrinkles, or tears in the linings should be discarded or repaired.
- Wear cotton socks that provide warmth and absorb perspiration.
- Avoid wearing knee-high stockings, and do not sit with the knees crossed because this can obstruct the circulation to the lower extremities and feet.
- Prop the feet up above the level of the hips a few minutes several times a day if the feet swell.
- Avoid using heating pads and hot-water bottles because of the danger of blistering and burning the feet.
- Report any signs of foot problems to your physician. This is especially important for patients with diabetes.

The Nursing Process

ASSESSING

Nursing History

Note any history of perineal or vaginal problems and related treatments. Identify any variables known to cause perineal or vaginal problems or to create a need for special care: urinary or fecal incontinence; indwelling Foley catheters; childbirth; rectal or genital surgery; and diseases such as urinary tract infection, diabetes mellitus, and certain sexually transmitted diseases (STDs) such as herpes.

Physical Assessment

Examine the male genitalia for lesions, swelling, inflammation, excoriation, tenderness, and discharge (amount, color, odor, and source); examine the female genitalia (pubic area, labia, clitoris, urinary meatus, and perineum) for color, size, lesions, masses, swelling, inflammation, excoriation, tenderness, and discharge (amount, color, odor, and source). Examine the anal area for cracks, nodules, distended veins, masses, or polyps; note strong perineal odors. Refer to Chapter 25 for additional perineal assessment information.

DIAGNOSING

Make a judgment about the adequacy of the patient's perineal (vaginal) self-care practices, identifying any factors that contribute to deficiencies. An example is as follows:

> Self-Care Deficit: Perineal Care related to cognitive impairment

Next, identify actual or potential perineal and vaginal problems that nurses can treat, noting contributing factors, and identify unhealthy patient responses to these problems. Examples of these are as follows:

- Pain related to excoriated perineal area
- Risk for Infection related to patient's deficient perineal hygiene
- Knowledge Deficit: Advisability of using deodorized feminine hygiene products related to inexperience and a desire to "be clean"
- Disturbance in Body Image related to genital lesions
- Altered Sexuality Patterns related to painful genital lesions
- Risk for Impaired Skin Integrity related to urinary and fecal incontinence

PLANNING: EXPECTED OUTCOMES

Identify nursing measures that will assist the patient to develop or maintain healthy perineal (vaginal) care practices that will contribute to the patient's general sense of well-being. Plan for the following patient outcomes. The patient will achieve the following:

- Demonstrate clean perineal area with skin intact
- Demonstrate signs of healing of perineal lesions or excoriations (discharge is decreased or absent)
- Demonstrate correct perineal and vaginal hygiene measures

The following are pertinent nursing measures to include in the plan of care:

- Cleaning the male genitalia (penis, scrotum, perineum, and rectal area) or the female genitalia (pubic area, labia, clitoris, urinary meatus, perineum, and rectal area)
- Instructing the patient on perineal hygiene practices

IMPLEMENTING

Carry out the plan of care, remembering to use bath time, when appropriate, for ongoing assessment of the patient's perineum and for evaluation of the adequacy of the plan of care. Procedures for perineal and vaginal care are described in the following sections. Sample documentation of teaching care of genitalia follows:

10/20/01 Child presented with large amount of smegma under the foreskin and painful urination. Mother and child were instructed in the need and correct technique for cleansing the uncircumcised penis. Child correctly returned the demonstration.

L. Woo, RN

Providing Perineal Care

It is not always possible for male nurses to attend to male patients and female nurses to attend to female patients. When the perineal cleaning is carried out in a matter-of-fact and dignified manner, patients generally do not find care by a person of the opposite gender to be offensive or embarrassing.

Some nurses use a sitz tub to clean the patient's perineal and anal areas. The portable type is especially handy when it is cumbersome to move a patient to a stationary sitz tub. The procedure may be carried out while the patient remains in bed. The following techniques are recommended to administer perineal care to patients (Fig. 36-9):

- Assemble supplies and provide for privacy.
- Explain the procedure to the patient and don disposable gloves.
- Wash and rinse the groin area (both male and female patients).
- Always proceed from the least contaminated area to the most contaminated area. For a female patient, spread the labia and move the washcloth from the pubic area toward the anal area to prevent carrying organisms from the anal area back over the genital area. Use a clean portion of the washcloth for each stroke. For a male patient, move the washcloth in a spiral motion from the tip of the penis down its length toward the pubic area.
- In an uncircumcised male patient, retract the foreskin (prepuce) while washing the penis. Rinse well with plain water.
- Rinse the washed areas well with plain water.
- Pull the uncircumcised male patient's foreskin back into place over the glans penis to prevent constriction of the penis, which may result in edema and tissue injury.
- Wash and rinse the male patient's scrotum. Handle the scrotum, which houses the testicles, with care because the area is sensitive.
- Dry the cleaned areas and apply an emollient as indicated. Powder the area only if the patient requests it. For the female patient, powder may become a medium for the growth of bacteria.

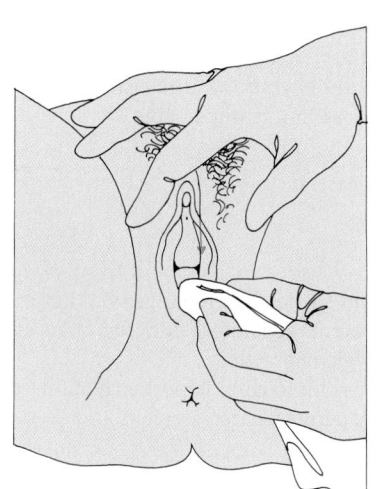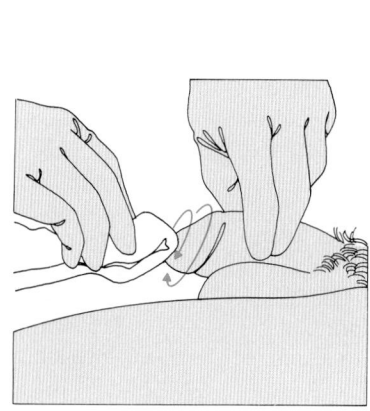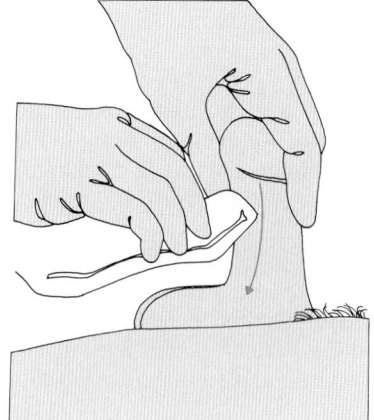

Figure 36-9
Performing normal perineal care.

- Turn the patient on his or her side and continue with cleansing the anal area. Continue in the direction of least contaminated to most contaminated area. In the female, cleanse from the vagina toward the anus. In both female and male patients, change the washcloth with each stroke until the area is clean. Rinse and dry the area.
- If the patient has an indwelling catheter and the agency recommends daily care for the catheter, it is usually done after perineal care. Agency policy may recommend use of an antiseptic cleaning agent (eg, povidone-iodine) or plain soap and water on a clean washcloth. Put on clean gloves before cleaning the catheter. Cleanse 6 to 8 inches of the catheter, moving from the meatus downward. Be careful not to pull or tug on the catheter during the cleaning motion. Inspect the meatus for drainage and note the characteristics of the urine. A physician's order is required if antibiotic ointment is applied to the meatus after cleansing. Additional information involving care of an indwelling catheter is discussed in Chapter 42. The accompanying box, Guidelines for Nursing Care, presents general adaptations for hygiene care in the home environment.

Providing Vaginal Care

In normal, healthy women, regular daily internal douching is believed unnecessary and unwise. The practice tends to remove normal bacterial flora from the vagina, and if the solution is high in acid content, it may irritate or injure normal cells. Although douching may occasionally be ordered to treat a vaginal infection, it is not recommended as a routine hygiene measure. Vaginal mucous secretions are odor free until they combine with air and body perspiration. Using plain soap and water is the most effective means to control odor.

Deodorants to control odor around the vaginal orifice are unnecessary and should not be placed on sanitary napkins or tampons. Although these deodorants do not contain aluminum salts, which are irritating to the mucous membrane, they are intended for external use only. Some have been reported as possibly harmful when sprayed into the vagina. Repeated use is not generally recommended because of reported irritation and rashes, nor should they be used on broken skin areas. No therapeutic benefit from their use has been proved to date. These special deodorants cannot replace cleanliness of the area. (See the accompanying box, Applying Learning to Practice.) Medical attention is recommended when discharge or irritation and itching around the vaginal orifice persist.

EVALUATING

At designated intervals, evaluate whether the patient has achieved the expected outcomes established during planning, and revise the plan of care if indicated. An example follows:

> 11/20/01 Outcome partially met. Child returned to clinic with clean perineal area and relief of painful urination.

Guidelines for Nursing Care

Hygiene Needs: General Adaptations for the Home Environment

- Use plastic trash bags or a plastic shower curtain liner to protect the mattress when bathing or shampooing a patient in bed. Disposable washcloths may also be an option to consider. A large plastic container or baby bathtub can effectively serve as a shampoo basin.
- Teach patient and caregiver how to administer oral care and care for dentures. A recent weight loss due to illness can result in dentures that no longer fit properly. Inform the patient that a dentist can reline the dentures for better fit or measure the patient for a new set.
- Review care and cleaning procedures for contact lenses with patient and caregiver. Check that lens case is clearly marked so that each lens is placed in its suitable case (right or left).
- Remind patients or caregivers at home to ask the telephone company about special equipment that can help a hearing-impaired person hear the phone ringing and carry on a phone conversation more easily.
- If linens are soiled with blood or body fluids, instruct family members to wear gloves when handling them. They should be rinsed first in cold water, and then washed separately from other household wash, using hot water, laundry detergent, and bleach.
- Teach family member or caregiver how to perform comfort measures, such as a backrub.
- Instruct caregivers or patients at home with an indwelling catheter to wash the urinary meatus and perineal area twice daily with soap and water. The anal area should also be cleansed after each bowel movement. Careful handwashing is imperative.

Mother reports child spends half the time with her and half with father (parents separated) and that father is uncommitted to hygiene practices.

Revision: Stress again to child importance of retracting foreskin during perineal care.

C. Moser, RN

See the accompanying Applying Learning to Practice and Nursing Plan of Care.

APPLYING LEARNING TO PRACTICE

Many women have concerns about feminine hygiene. Personal healthcare practices are influenced by past experiences, cultural knowledge, and societal expectations. It is important for women to feel comfortable with their bodies and to be knowledgeable about self-care practices that promote health and well-being and prevent infection and disease. Use the following assessment checklist to determine how well you are meeting your own need for feminine hygiene, if appropriate. Then develop a prescription for self-care by choosing appropriate behaviors from the list of suggestions.

ASSESSMENT CHECKLIST

almost always / sometimes / almost never

☐ ☐ ☐ 1. I feel comfortable with my body and accept its uniqueness.

☐ ☐ ☐ 2. I am knowledgeable about feminine hygiene practices and products.

☐ ☐ ☐ 3. I value preventive measures that promote health and reduce the likelihood of infection.

☐ ☐ ☐ 4. I understand that changes in vaginal discharge, pain, and bleeding may indicate pathology or disease or may be normal.

☐ ☐ ☐ 5. I am not uncomfortable seeking professional help when symptoms occur.

SELF-CARE BEHAVIORS

1. Wash the perineal area at least once daily. Towels and washcloths should be clean and never shared.

2. Always wipe from front to back after voiding and defecation to avoid introducing bacteria into the vagina or urethra.

3. Avoid sprays, soaps, powders, deodorants, tampons, and pads that are perfumed or irritating in any way.

4. Avoid clothing that is too tight and wear underpants and pantyhose that have a cotton crotch.

5. Avoid douching because it can strip the vagina of its normal flora and introduce bacteria.

6. Change tampons regularly. Use good handwashing technique before and after insertion.

7. Seek professional assistance to distinguish normal symptoms from pathology.

8. Schedule a yearly gynecologic examination with a healthcare professional you trust.

APPLYING LEARNING TO PRACTICE

Patient Care Study

Glenda Davis is a nurse practitioner who works in a campus health clinic at a state university. Frequently women ask her questions about feminine hygiene. Realizing that each woman who presents with a question probably represents many other women with similar unvoiced questions, she decides to develop an insert entitled *Self Care: Feminine Hygiene* for the campus newspaper. The information she plans to include and the population she will address in her checklist are based on the following assessment data:

- Heterogeneous female population is of various ages, cultures, religions, sexual orientation, and family and lifestyle backgrounds.

- Knowledge about feminine hygiene varies widely from almost no knowledge to students who are well read or members of women's health professions.

- Students who present with questions are mostly concerned about the risk of acquiring an STD or the dangers of certain products (eg, tampons and toxic shock syndrome) or have questions related to intercourse and contraception.

- Numerous students report to the clinic with vaginal infections and urinary tract infections.

- Interest is high; ability to comprehend written materials is high.

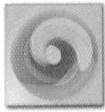

NURSING PLAN OF CARE
for Female University Students

Nursing Diagnosis

Self-Care Deficit: Feminine Hygiene related to knowledge deficit as manifested by female students presenting to the campus clinic with questions about feminine hygiene; high incidence of vaginal and urinary tract infections; negative attitudes about feminine body frequently expressed.

Expected Outcome

Students will:
- Express positive body image, valuing their uniqueness

Nursing Interventions	Rationale	Evaluative Statement
With each student who presents at the clinic for help with a gynecologic concern or problem, take the time to assess her knowledge of the female body and her acceptance of her body and comfort with it.	The women's health movement has encouraged women to feel ownership of their bodies, to appreciate their uniqueness as women, and to increase their awareness of their physical bodies and the feelings associated with them. Many women still feel that the genital area and cyclic phenomena such as the menstrual cycle and the female sexual response cycle are "dirty," and symptoms in this area may evoke fear, guilt, anxiety, and shame.	*Six-month evaluation:* 6/30/01 Goal partially met: students are beginning to discuss gynecologic concerns more freely, yet great hesitance persists. *Revision:* Continue to help women to know, understand, and accept their bodies and to talk about their bodies. Make this a priority of the nursing staff at the clinic. *G. Davis, RN*
Counsel appropriately.	It is important for nurses to provide women with information about their bodies.	

Expected Outcome

Students will:
- Correctly describe feminine hygiene self-care behaviors they are willing to incorporate into their daily lifestyles

Nursing Interventions	Rationale	Evaluative Statement
Assess with each patient her knowledge of feminine hygiene practices (correct any misconceptions) and motivation to use them consistently.	Many women have never been instructed about feminine hygiene, and harmful practices may be "picked up" from the media and other sources (eg, the use of frequent douching and deodorants to eliminate normal body odors).	6/30/01 Goal met. Following publication of the *Self-Care: Feminine Hygiene* feature and one-on-one counseling using this printed handout, patients are knowledgeable about preventive hygiene measures. *G. Davis, RN*
Address specific concerns related to menstruation, intercourse, other maturational events.	Maturational events, such as menstruation, becoming sexually active, and pregnancy, may result in a need for new or modified hygiene practices.	
Teach the importance of using preventive hygiene measures to reduce the likelihood of acquiring a urinary tract or vaginal infection. Distribute the *Self-Care: Feminine Hygiene* handout and discuss this with the patient.	It is better to prevent a genitourinary infection than to treat it.	

(continued)

NURSING PLAN OF CARE (Continued)
for Female University Students

Expected Outcome

Campus health clinic records will:
- Demonstrate a reduction in both new and recurrent genitourinary infections

Nursing Interventions	Rationale	Evaluative Statement
Educate women regarding preventive hygiene measures (refer to the *Self-Care* handout).	It is better to prevent a genitourinary infection than to treat it.	6/30/01 Goal met. Six months after publication and use of the *Self-Care: Feminine Hygiene* handout, the incidence of genitourinary infections is reduced 10%. Will continue to keep education in this regard a priority.
Educate women to distinguish normal from abnormal findings (vaginal discharge, pain, bleeding, problems with urination) and to seek help when appropriate. Nursing measures include teaching preventive measures, instructing in recognition of symptoms, and assisting with self-care activities to prevent and treat infections, including the securing of assistance when indicated.	Early treatment of genitourinary infections reduces the likelihood of residual problems.	*G. Davis, RN*
Document new and recurrent genitourinary infections; identify predisposing factors.	Documentation facilitates ongoing management of a recurring problem.	

Sample Documentation

6/15/01   Nursing

Student visited clinic and expressed need for information about feminine hygiene practices in general as well as those specific hygiene measures for use after intercourse. Also related concern about contracting an STD from partners. Reported that she became sexually active this year and has sexual intercourse once or twice weekly. Stated that "many of my friends use douches" and questioned whether any particular douche products are recommended. We discussed the *Self-Care: Feminine Hygiene* handout and reviewed various healthcare practices. Clarified for student her misconception regarding the advisability of douching. Also counseled her about her right to talk with a sexual partner about STDs and previous contacts with infected individuals. Advised that she refrain from contact or use a condom when she has intercourse. Student reported feeling more "in charge" of body and better able to care for it. Discussed all topics on plan of care and encouraged her to revisit clinic in 6 months for further clarification and evaluation.

G. Davis, RN

Learning Outcomes

After studying this chapter, the learner should be able to accomplish the following:

1. Define the key terms used in the chapter.

alopecia	necrosis
caries	pediculosis (lice)
cerumen	plaque
dermis	podiatrist
epidermis	pyorrhea
gingivitis	sebaceous glands
halitosis	tartar
integument	

2. List five functions of the skin, three factors influencing the skin's condition, and four basic principles that guide practices of skin care.

3. Identify factors affecting skin condition and personal hygiene.
4. Assess the integumentary system and the adequacy of hygiene self-care behaviors using appropriate interview and physical assessment skills.
5. Develop nursing diagnoses related to deficient hygiene measures.
6. Describe the priorities of scheduled hygienic care, early morning care, morning care, afternoon care, and evening care.
7. Identify at least four reasons for including the back massage in daily nursing care.
8. Demonstrate techniques used when assisting patients with hygiene measures, including those used when administering various types of baths and those used in cleaning each part of the body.
9. Describe agents commonly used on the skin and scalp and precautions to observe in their use.
10. Plan, implement, and evaluate nursing care for common problems of the skin and mucous membranes.

Critical Thinking Exercises

1. Practice the art of back massage with a willing partner until you feel comfortable and confident including this nursing measure in your routine care. Discuss with other students the therapeutic benefits of massage, and identify nursing situations for which it may be the primary therapy.
2. Interview people of different ages and cultural backgrounds about their essential hygiene practices. Ask specific questions about the type of nursing assistance they would require if hospitalized and unable to meet their hygiene needs independently. Are there special products or equipment they would need? To what extent are nurses obliged to respect the hygiene preference of different patients?

Study Questions

1. An older patient's skin requires special care because
   a. subcutaneous fat increases
   b. sebaceous glands secrete more oil
   c. the skin becomes increasingly dry
   d. the skin thickens
2. An appropriate nursing intervention for a patient wearing antiembolic stockings is to
   a. measure legs before applying stockings to assure proper fit
   b. apply stockings while the patient is sitting in a chair
   c. massage the legs when the stockings are removed
   d. leave stockings in place for 1-week intervals
3. During a bath, the nurse observes that a patient has dry skin. The nurse's best action is to
   a. bathe the patient more frequently
   b. use an emollient on the dry skin
   c. massage the skin with alcohol
   d. discourage fluid intake
4. An adolescent patient discusses her acne condition with the nurse. The nurse recommends that the patient
   a. wash the skin frequently using soap
   b. use cosmetics liberally to cover blackheads
   c. use emollients on the area
   d. squeeze blackheads as they appear
5. A marked inflammation of the gums involving the alveolar tissue is referred to as
   a. glossitis
   b. caries
   c. cheilosis
   d. pyorrhea
6. A priority nursing action when administering oral care to a dependent patient is to
   a. assist the patient to the dorsal recumbent position
   b. wear disposable gloves
   c. use a firm toothbrush to cleanse teeth and gums
   d. irrigate forcefully with hydrogen peroxide
7. Mr. James has an eye infection with a moderate amount of discharge. To clean his eyes, the nurse should
   a. use hydrogen peroxide
   b. wipe from the outer canthus to the inner canthus
   c. position him on the same side as the eye to be cleansed
   d. use only one cotton ball per eye
8. The nurse's responsibility when giving foot care to an older patient includes
   a. using scissors to correct an ingrown toenail situation
   b. trimming toenails as short as possible
   c. using an alcohol rub if the feet are dry
   d. bathing the feet at least daily
9. Providing perineal care to a patient requires that the nurse
   a. use a clean portion of the washcloth for each stroke
   b. proceed from most contaminated to least contaminated area
   c. use sterile gloves
   d. leave the foreskin undisturbed in an uncircumcised male
10. A nurse is caring for an 80-year-old patient who requires total assistance with his personal and oral hygiene. He is thin, has few visitors, and prefers to remain in bed in a semisitting position. The priority nursing diagnosis is

a. Risk for Impaired Skin Integrity related to immobility

b. Bathing/Hygiene Self Care Deficit related to decreased strength and endurance

c. Social Isolation related to lack of visitors

d. Activity Intolerance related to generalized weakness

11. An older patient with an unsteady gait requests a tub bath. The nurse is aware that

a. Alpha-Keri oil should be added to the water to prevent dry skin

b. the patient should lock the door to guarantee privacy

c. the patient will require assistance in and out of the tub to prevent falling

d. the water temperature should be very warm because the patient chills easily

12. During morning care, the patient asks the nurse to shave him with a disposable razor. Before shaving him, the nurse should

a. have him sign a permission form

b. check to see if the patient is taking anticoagulants

c. indicate that only a family member may shave a patient

d. position him flat in bed

13. To remove gas-permeable contact lenses from an unresponsive patient, the nurse

a. gently irrigates the eye with an irrigating solution from the inner canthus outward

b. grasps the lens with a gentle pinching motion

c. dons sterile gloves before attempting the procedure

d. ensures that the lens is centered on the cornea before gently manipulating the lids to release the lens

14. To remove a patient's gown when she has an intravenous line, the nurse

a. temporarily disconnects the intravenous tubing at a point close to the patient and threads it through the gown

b. cuts the gown with scissors

c. threads the bag and tubing through the gown sleeve, keeping the line intact

d. temporarily disconnects the tubing from the intravenous container and threads it through the gown

15. When making an occupied bed, it is important for the nurse to

a. keep the bed in the low position

b. use a bath blanket or top sheet for warmth and privacy

c. constantly keep side rails raised on both sides

d. move back and forth from one side to the other when adjusting the linens

Answers With Rationale

1. The correct response is *c*. With age, the skin becomes increasingly dry, subcutaneous fat decreases, sebaceous glands secrete less oil, and the skin becomes thinner.

2. The correct response is *a*. The legs should always be measured according to manufacturer's directions before ordering antiembolism stockings. Stockings may be uncomfortable if applied while the patient is sitting because leg veins are apt to be congested. Massage is dangerous because it may cause a clot to break away and circulate in the bloodstream. Stockings should always be removed once daily.

3. The correct response is *b*. An emollient soothes dry skin, whereas frequent bathing increases dryness, as does alcohol. Discouraging fluid intake leads to dehydration and, subsequently, dry skin.

4. The correct response is *a*. Washing the skin frequently with soap removes oil and debris, whereas liberal use of cosmetics and emollients can clog the pores. Squeezing blackheads is always discouraged because it may lead to infection.

5. The correct response is *d*. Pyorrhea is a marked inflammation of the gums, whereas caries refers to the presence of tooth decay. Cheilosis is ulceration of the lips, and glossitis is an inflammation of the tongue.

6. The correct response is *b*. Disposable gloves provide a barrier to protect the nurse and patient. The dorsal recumbent position is unsafe because the patient may easily aspirate any secretions or fluids. A soft tooth-brush is recommended to avoid causing irritation and bleeding, and forceful irrigation is never safe. Water would be the choice for any gentle irrigation.

7. The correct response is *c*. Positioning on the same side as the involved eye discourages any contamination of the other eye. Water or normal saline should be used for cleansing the eye of any discharge, and one cotton ball should be used for each stroke. Always cleanse from the inner canthus to the outer canthus to avoid forcing debris into the nasolacrimal duct.

8. The correct response is *d*. An older patient should have foot care once daily. Correcting an ingrown toenail situation should be done by a podiatrist, and trimming the toenails may require a physician's order. Additionally, cutting the toenails as short as possible exposes tender areas to friction and may lead to the skin being cut during trimming. Alcohol is drying and should not be used when dry skin is usually already a problem.

9. The correct response is *a*. Using a clean portion of the washcloth for each stroke prevents contamination of other areas. Cleansing should always proceed from the least contaminated to the most contaminated area. Clean gloves, not sterile gloves, are used to provide perineal care, and the foreskin in an uncircumcised male should be pulled back to allow cleansing underneath and then gently returned to its former position.

10. The correct response is *a*. Although Bathing/Hygiene Self Care Deficit, Social Isolation, and Activity Intolerance may be appropriate nursing diagnoses for this patient, the priority at this time is Risk for Impaired Skin Integrity. A break in his skin, such as that from a pressure ulcer, may lead to infection. At his age, this could be life-threatening.

11. The correct response is *c*. Safe nursing practice requires that you assist a patient with an unsteady gait in and out of the tub. Alpha-Keri oil is dangerous for this patient because it makes the tub slippery. Although privacy is important, if the patient locks the door, the nurse cannot help if there is an emergency. The water temperature should be comfortably warm at 43° to 46°C. Older patients have an increased susceptibility to burns.

12. The correct response is *b*. A patient who is taking anticoagulants should be shaved with an electric razor rather than a blade razor. Shaving a patient does not require permission and can be completed by either the caregiver or a family member. A shave is best completed with the patient in a Fowler's or semi-Fowler's position to prevent soap and water from running behind the patient's head.

13. The correct response is *d*. To remove hard contact lenses, the upper and lower eyelids are gently maneuvered to help loosen the lens and slide it out of the eye. The lens must be situated on the cornea, not the sclera, before removal. An attempt to grasp a hard lens might result in a scratch on the cornea. Clean gloves are optional if drainage is present.

14. The correct response is *c*. Threading the bag and tubing through the gown sleeve keeps the system intact. Opening an intravenous line causes a break in a sterile system and introduces the potential for infection. Cutting a gown off is not an alternative except in an emergency.

15. The correct response is *b*. Using the bath blanket or top sheet keeps the patient warm and provides privacy. Keeping the bed in the low position and working over raised side rails may strain the nurse's back. Continually moving back and forth to tuck and arrange linen is time-consuming and disorganized.

Bibliography

Bennett, J. (1999). Activities of daily living: Old-fashioned or still useful? *Journal of Gerontological Nursing, 25*(5), 22–29.

Blawat, D., & Banks, P. (1997). Comforting touch: Using topical-skin preparations. *Nursing, 27*(5), 46–48.

Cavendish, R. (1998). Clinical snapshot: Adult hearing loss. *American Journal of Nursing, 98*(8), 50–51.

Cavendish, R. (1999). Clinical snapshot: Periodontal disease. *American Journal of Nursing, 99*(3), 36–37.

Eliopoulos, C. (1997). *Gerontological Nursing* (4th ed.). Philadelphia: Lippincott-Raven.

Freeman, E. (1997). International perspectives on bathing. *Journal of Gerontological Nursing, 23*(5), 40–44.

Halpin-Landry, J., & Goldsmith, S. (1999). Feet first: Diabetes Care. *American Journal of Nursing, 99*(2), 26–33.

Hektor, L., & Touhy, T. (1997). The history of the bath: From art to task. *Journal of Gerontological Nursing, 23*(5), 7–15.

Hess, C. (1999). Caring for a diabetic ulcer. *Nursing, 29*(5), 70–71.

Hoeffer, B., Rader, J., McKenzie, D., Lavelle, M., & Stewart, B. (1997). Reducing aggressive behavior during bathing cognitively impaired nursing home residents. *Journal of Gerontological Nursing, 23*(5), 16–23.

Kovach, C., & Meyer-Arnold, E. (1997). Preventing agitated behaviors during bath time. *Geriatric Nursing, 18*(3), 112–114.

Kraker, K., & Vajdik, C. (1997). Designing the environment to make bathing pleasant in nursing homes. *Journal of Gerontological Nursing, 23*(5), 50–51.

McCloskey, J., & Bulechek, J. (1996). *Nursing Interventions Classification (NIC)* (2nd ed.). St. Louis: C. V. Mosby.

McConnell, E. (1998). Communicating with a hearing-impaired Patient. *Nursing, 28*(1), 32.

North American Nursing Diagnosis Association. (1999). *NANDA nursing diagnoses: Definitions & classification, 1999–2000.* Philadelphia: Author.

Pyle, M., Massie, M., & Nelson, S. (1998). A pilot study on improving oral care in long-term care settings. *Journal of Gerontological Nursing, 24*(10), 35–38.

Skewes, S. (1997). Bathing: It's a tough job! *Journal of Gerontological Nursing, 23*(5), 45–49.

Stone, C. (1999). Preventing cerumen impaction in nursing facility residents. *Journal of Gerontological Nursing, 25*(5), 43–45.

Whitmyer, C., Terezhalmy, G., Miller, D., & Hujer, M. (1998). Clinical evaluation of the efficacy and safety of an ultrasonic toothbrush system in an elderly patient population. *Geriatric Nursing, 19*(1), 29–33.

Chapter 37
Skin Integrity and Wound Care

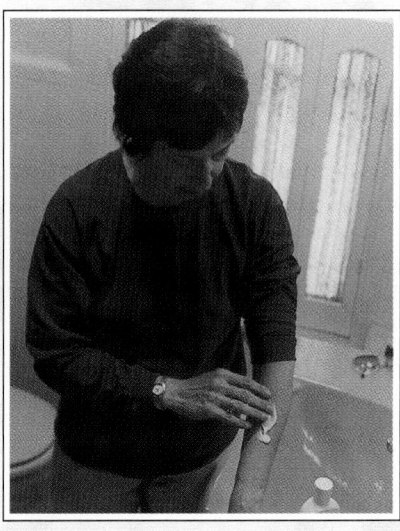

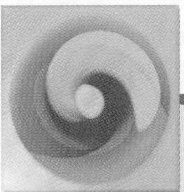

Thinking Critically About
Nursing's Blended Skills

Before reading this chapter, think about the types of blended skills you will need to diagnose and treat patients with alterations in skin integrity.

- A 5-week-old infant, small for gestational age and born at only 28 weeks' gestation, is in the neonatal intensive care unit on a respirator with chest tubes in place and intravenous lines. Maintaining skin integrity is a constant challenge.

- A 17-year-old boy is admitted to a rehabilitation hospital after a diving accident that left him quadriplegic. Skin over several of his pressure points is observed to be red.

- Called to visit a bed-bound elderly woman being cared for by a nephew in her own home, you discover a large pressure ulcer over the sacrum. The ulcer is about 3 inches across and at least 1 inch deep. There is purulent drainage. The nephew says he does the best he can, but it is obvious that the woman is undernourished and that her gown and sheets are soiled.

- Nurses groan when they realize Mr. Lee is returning to their unit. Only 5 feet and 4 inches tall, he weighs more than 300 pounds. Unfortunately, he acquired an infection in his bone that has not responded to treatment. During his last admission, he developed several areas of skin breakdown.

What cognitive, technical, interpersonal, and ethical/legal skills do you think you will need to respond to the challenges described above?

A **wound** is a disruption in the normal integrity of the skin. (The structures, function, and physiology of the skin are described in Chap. 36). The nurse cares for wounds as one aspect of the nursing care given to patients with wounds. In other words, it is the *patient* to whom care is given. With the nursing process, an individualized plan of care is developed to assess the patient, to identify and prevent complications, to implement and evaluate skills essential to wound care, and to provide physical and emotional support to facilitate healing, adaptation, and self-care. Wound care may be required in any healthcare setting, and increasingly complex wounds are being cared for at home. Nurses need to know how to assess and implement care for patients and their wounds with knowledge and skill.

Because the skin is the body's first line of defense, an intact skin surface has added significance. Altered skin integrity is potentially dangerous and can be life-threatening. It is especially serious among older adults, patients who are immobile, those with chronic health problems, and those in critical care settings. This chapter discusses both acute surgical wounds and pressure ulcers. Surgical wounds are those that result from surgical incisions and include those wounds that are unintentional but have been cleaned and sutured.

Wound Classification

An *intentional wound* is the result of planned therapy or treatment that requires invasive measures. Intentional wounds include those that result from surgery, intravenous therapy, and lumbar puncture. The wound edges are clean, and bleeding is usually controlled. Because the wound was made under sterile conditions with sterile supplies and skin preparation, the risk for infection is decreased, and healing is facilitated.

Unintentional wounds occur from unexpected trauma, such as from accidents, forcible injury (such as stabbing, gun shots), and burns. Because the wounds occur in an unsterile environment, contamination is likely. Wound edges are usually jagged, multiple trauma is common, and bleeding is uncontrolled. These factors create a high risk for infection and a longer healing time.

An *open wound* occurs from intentional or unintentional trauma. The skin surface is broken, providing a portal of entry for microorganisms. Open wounds may be accompanied by bleeding, tissue damage, and increased risk for infection. A *closed wound* results from a blow, force, or strain caused by trauma such as a fall, an assault, or a motor vehicle accident. The skin surface is not broken, but soft tissue is damaged, and internal injury and hemorrhage may occur.

Wounds may also be clean or contaminated, and superficial or deep. Many wounds are described with multiple characteristics; for example, an intentional wound to remove the appendix is usually a clean, open wound. In comparison, after an automobile accident, a person may have an unintentional, open laceration considered to be contaminated.

Wound Healing

The healthy body has the ability to protect and restore itself. Increasing the blood supply to the damaged area, walling off and removing cellular and foreign debris, and initiating cellular development are all aspects of the body's healing process. The healing process occurs normally,

COGNITIVE SKILLS

- Basic knowledge of the anatomy and physiology related to skin integrity and wound healing
- Knowledge of how to prevent, diagnose, and treat pressure ulcers and other skin alterations
- Familiarity with effective skin, pressure ulcer, and wound care products and equipment

TECHNICAL SKILLS

- Ability to use correctly the products, protocols, and equipment necessary to prevent and treat pressure ulcers and other skin alterations

INTERPERSONAL SKILLS

- Ability to establish trusting professional relationships that enlist patients and their caretakers in a plan to prevent or treat pressure ulcers and other skin alterations
- Ability to work collaboratively with the interdisciplinary team to prevent and treat skin alterations

ETHICAL/LEGAL SKILLS

- Commitment to safety and quality; strong sense of responsibility and accountability for skin and wound care
- The ability to document skin care according to agency policy

without assistance, although interventions can help to support the process. For example, keeping the injured area free of debris by proper cleaning helps to promote tissue healing, as does positioning the wounded area to promote circulation to that part.

Wound healing involves the following principles:

- The body's ability to handle altered skin integrity depends on the extent of the damage and the person's general state of health. The capacity to deal adequately with a wound is limited when a healthy person sustains a massive injury, when the patient has a chronic illness or a depressed immune system, or when the patient is very young or very old.
- The body's response to a wound is more effective if proper nutrition has been maintained. Undernourished patients are at greater risk for developing a wound infection because they have difficulty mounting their cell-mediated defense system associated with T-lymphocyte activity, and some leukocytic functions are diminished in the presence of protein deficiency. Although the role of fatty acids in wound healing is not well understood, certain quantities of glucose are necessary to meet the energy requirements for wound healing. Various vitamins, minerals, and trace elements are also needed for efficient wound healing. Vitamin A is necessary for collagen synthesis and epithelialization. Vitamin B complex serves as a cofactor of enzyme reactions needed for wound healing. Vitamin C is needed for collagen synthesis, capillary formation, and resistance to infection. Vitamin K is needed for the synthesis of prothrombin. Zinc, copper, and iron assist in collagen synthesis. Manganese serves as an enzyme activator.
- The body responds systematically to trauma in any of its parts. For example, a surgical incision can cause a variety of systematic reactions, including increased body temperature, increased heart and respiratory rates, anorexia or nausea and vomiting, musculoskeletal tension throughout the body, and hormonal changes.
- An adequate blood supply is essential for the body's normal response to any injury. The blood brings increased numbers of leukocytes, erythrocytes, and platelets to the site of injury. Antibodies also are carried by the plasma. Increased circulation to the injured part removes toxins and debris and provides needed nutrients and oxygen. Areas of the body with a good blood supply, such as the head and the neck, heal faster than areas in which the blood supply is not as great, such as the distal part of an extremity.
- Intact skin and mucous membranes are the first line of defense against microorganisms. A break in the integrity of the skin or mucous membranes increases the risk for infection. Surgical asepsis is used in caring for a wound to minimize the possibility of pathogens entering the site. Careful handwashing before caring for a wound is probably the single most effective method for preventing wound infections.

- Normal healing is promoted when the wound is free of foreign material. Excessive exudate, dead or damaged tissue cells, pathogenic organisms, or embedded fragments of bone, metal, glass, or other substances may all be foreign materials. In some situations, the body walls off a collection of pus or another foreign body, and healing occurs around it. This localized collection of pus is called an *abscess*.

Phases of Wound Healing

Wound healing is a process of tissue repair involving tissue response to injury. All wounds follow the same phases in healing, although differences occur in the length of time required for each phase and in the extent of granulation tissue formed. The phases of wound healing are inflammation, fibroplasia, and maturation. Each phase is controlled and regulated by substances called *growth factors*. These hormone-like substances interact with specific surface cell receptors to control the wound healing process (Steed, 1997).

Inflammatory Phase

The inflammatory phase begins with the incision for surgery and lasts through the third or fourth postoperative day. The two major physiologic activities are hemostasis and phagocytosis. The inflammatory response is immediate and prepares the tissues for healing.

An injury to the skin initiates the local adaptation syndrome (described in Chap. 31). First, there is an immediate and brief constriction of blood vessels, allowing clotting of blood to seal the wound. This is followed by vasodilation, allowing increased blood flow to the area, which permits white blood cells (leukocytes) to invade the area of injury and engulf bacteria and debris. About 24 hours after injury, large phagocytic cells (macrophages) enter the area and secrete an angiogenesis factor that stimulates the formation of epithelial buds at the end of injured vessels so that reanastomosis can occur. During the inflammatory phase, the patient has a generalized body response, including a mildly elevated temperature, leukocytosis, and generalized malaise.

Fibroplasia (Proliferation) Phase

The fibroplasia phase begins on about day 3 or 4 and can last up to day 21. Fibroblasts rapidly synthesize collagens and ground substance. These two substances form the scaffold for the final repair of the wound. A thin layer of epithelial cells formed across the wound during the inflammatory phase; now, capillaries grow across the wound. This revascularization brings oxygen and nutrients required for continued healing. Fibroblasts also migrate from the bloodstream into the wound, depositing fibrin that stretches through the clot. A thin layer of epithelial cells forms across the wound, and blood flow across the wound is reinstituted. The new tissue, called **granulation tissue**, is highly vascular and reddish and bleeds easily.

building up of tissue

The systemic symptoms now typically disappear. During this phase, adequate nutrition and oxygenation, as well as prevention of strain on the suture line, are important patient care considerations.

Maturation (Remodeling) Phase

The final stage of healing begins about 3 weeks after the injury and can continue for as long as 1 to 2 years. Collagen that was haphazardly deposited in the wound is remodeled, making the healed wound stronger and more like adjacent tissue. New collagen continues to be deposited, which compresses the blood vessels in the healing wound, so that the scar eventually becomes a flat, thin, white line. The **scar** is avascular collagen tissue that does not sweat, grow hair, or tan in sunlight.

Wound Healing Processes

Wounds heal by one of three processes—primary, secondary, or tertiary healing (sometimes also called primary, secondary, or tertiary intention) (Fig. 37-1). Most surgical incisions and small sutured lacerations heal by *primary healing*. The wound is a clean, straight line with little loss of tissue. All wound edges are well approximated with su-

tures. These wounds normally heal rapidly with minimal scarring. *Secondary healing* takes place in large wounds that have considerable tissue loss, so that the edges cannot be approximated. Healing occurs by formation of granulation tissue. Because the wounds are more open, there is a greater chance of infection, healing time is longer, and scars are larger. *Tertiary healing* occurs when the interval between the wound's occurrence and its suturing is extended. This delay allows access for pathogens, so that there is an increased risk for infection. There is also a greater inflammatory reaction and more granulation tissue compared with healing by primary or secondary intention; hence, scars are larger and less likely to shrink to a flat line.

Factors Affecting Wound Healing

Wound healing is affected by a variety of factors. These factors include age, circulation to and oxygenation of tissues, condition of the wound, and overall patient health.

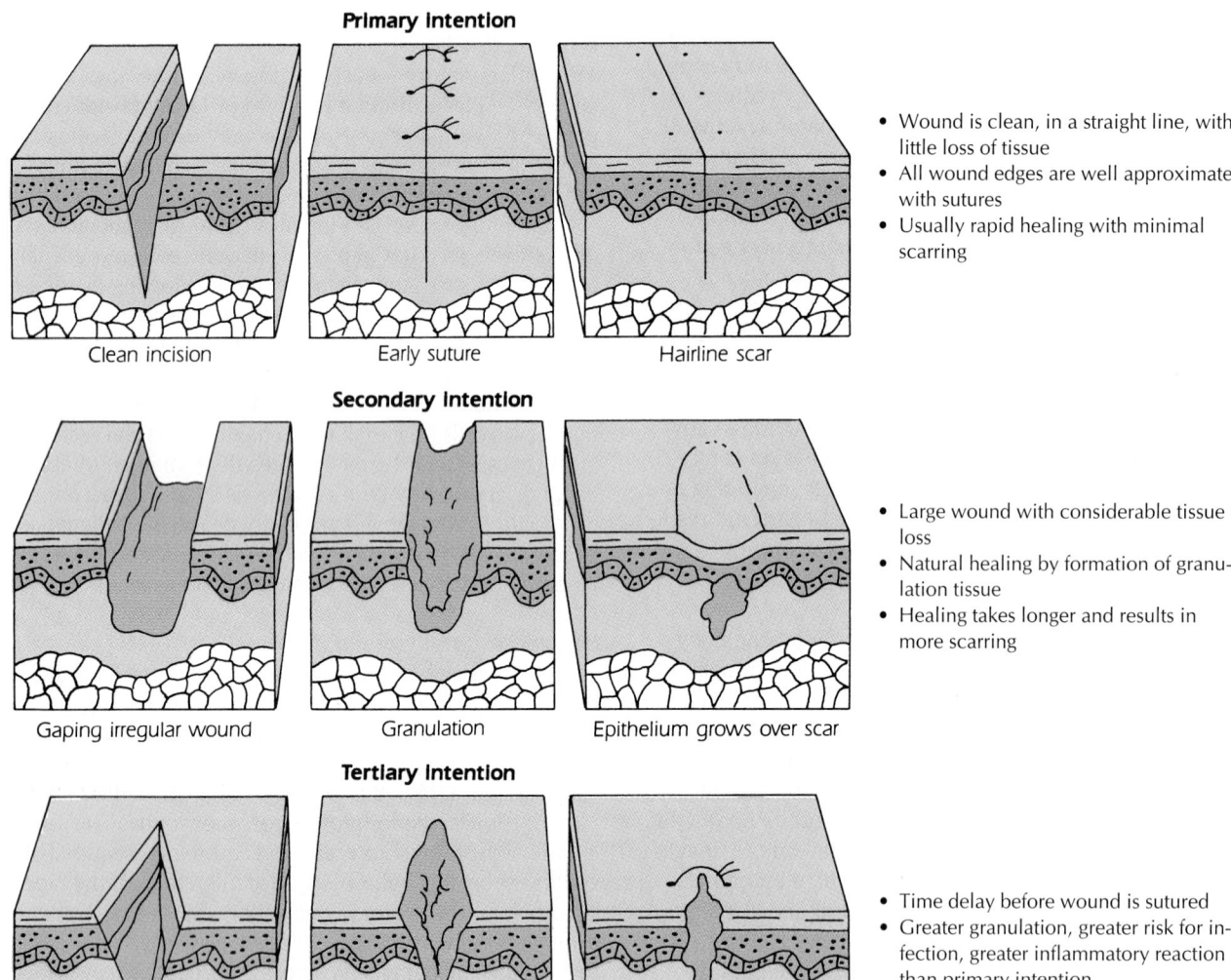

Primary Intention

Clean incision   Early suture   Hairline scar

- Wound is clean, in a straight line, with little loss of tissue
- All wound edges are well approximated with sutures
- Usually rapid healing with minimal scarring

Secondary Intention

Gaping irregular wound   Granulation   Epithelium grows over scar

- Large wound with considerable tissue loss
- Natural healing by formation of granulation tissue
- Healing takes longer and results in more scarring

Tertiary Intention

Wound   Increased granulation   Late suturing with wide scar

- Time delay before wound is sutured
- Greater granulation, greater risk for infection, greater inflammatory reaction than primary intention
- Late suturing and more scarring

Figure 37-1
Processes of wound healing.

Age

Children and healthy adults heal more rapidly than older adults, in whom physiologic changes caused by aging result in diminished fibroblastic activity and circulation. Older adults are more likely to have one or more chronic illnesses, with pathologic changes that impede the healing process (see the accompanying box, Focus on the Older Adult).

Circulation and Oxygenation

A number of physical conditions can affect wound healing. The presence of large amounts of subcutaneous and tissue fat (which has fewer blood vessels) in obese people may slow wound healing because fatty tissue is more difficult to suture, is more prone to infection, and takes longer to heal. Circulation may be impaired in older adults and in people with peripheral vascular disorders, cardiovascular disorders, hypertension, or diabetes mellitus. Oxygenation of tissues is decreased in people with anemia or chronic respiratory disorders and in those who smoke.

Wound Condition

The specific condition of the wound affects how quickly and effectively it heals. For example, large, contaminated, infected wounds or wounds that retain foreign bodies heal slowly. Some wounds may fail to heal.

Overall Patient Health

Patients who have inadequate nutrition, are taking steroid drugs, or require postoperative radiation therapy are at high risk for delayed healing and wound complications. The presence of a chronic physical illness (such as cardiovascular disease or diabetes mellitus) can negatively affect wound healing.

Wound Complications

Wound complications include infection, hemorrhage, dehiscence, and evisceration. These complications increase the risk for generalized illness and death, lengthen the patient's need for healthcare interventions, and add to healthcare costs.

Infection

Bacteria can invade a wound at the time of trauma, during surgery, or at any time after the initial wound. A contaminated wound is more likely to become infected, as is a surgical wound in a procedure that involves the intestines, in which the risk for contamination with fecal material is high. Symptoms of wound infection usually become apparent within 2 to 7 days after the injury or surgery, often after the patient is at home. Symptoms of infection include purulent drainage; increased drainage, pain, redness, and swelling in and around the wound; increased body temperature; and increased white blood cell count. Nursing care of infected wounds is discussed later.

Hemorrhage

Hemorrhage may occur from a slipped suture, a dislodged clot from stress at the suture line or operative site, infection, or the erosion of a blood vessel by a foreign body (such as a drain). The dressing (and the wound under the dressing if possible) should be checked frequently during the first 48 hours after surgery and no less than every 8 hours thereafter. If excessive bleeding does occur, additional sterile pressure dressings or packing may be necessary, fluid replacement is probably necessary, and surgical intervention may be required.

Dehiscence and Evisceration

Dehiscence and evisceration (Fig. 37-2) are the most serious postoperative wound complications. **Dehiscence** is the partial or total disruption of wound layers. **Evisceration** is the protrusion of viscera through the incisional area. Patients at greater risk for these complications include those who are obese or malnourished, have infected wounds, or have excessive coughing, vomiting, or straining. An increase in the flow of serosanguineous fluid from the wound between postoperative days 4 and 5 is a clue to impending dehiscence. The patient may say that "something has suddenly given way." If dehiscence or evisceration occurs, the wound area should be covered with sterile towels soaked in 0.9% sodium chloride solution, and the physician should be notified immediately. Both these situations are emergencies that require prompt preparation for surgical repair.

Focus on the Older Adult

Factors That Affect Wound Healing in Older Adults

Changes in Skin

- Skin loses turgor and is more fragile
- There is increased risk for further injury from cleaning agents and tape.

Nutrition

- Decreased secretion of enzymes and absorption of nutrients and minerals may have potential risk for altered nutrition, which would delay wound healing.

Potential for Infection

- Age reduces antibody production and functioning of the endocrine system, both of which increase susceptibility to infection.
- The incidence of chronic illnesses that compromise circulation and oxygenation of tissues (such as diabetes mellitus and cardiovascular problems) further decreases resistance to infection.

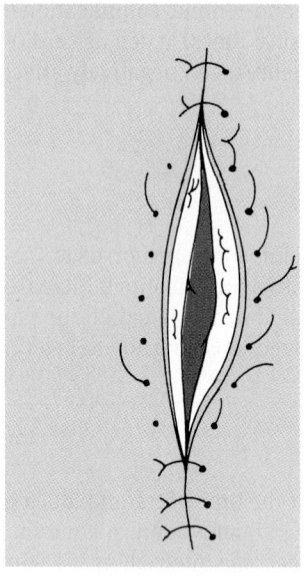 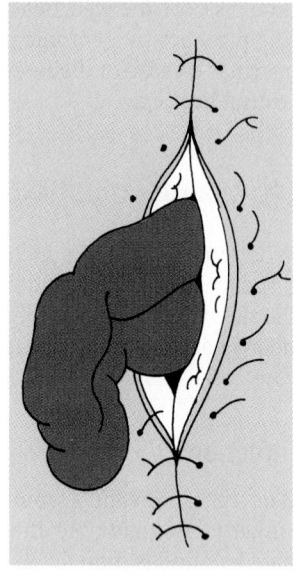

Dehiscence   Evisceration

Figure 37-2
Wound complications.

Psychological Effects of Wounds

Because the skin is a sensory organ and plays a major role in the way we communicate with others and feel about ourselves, wounds require adaptation in the emotional as well as the physical dimension. Although stress and adaptation vary greatly among individuals, actual and potential emotional stressors are common in all patients with wounds. These stressors include pain, anxiety, fear, and alterations in body image.

Pain

Pain is part of almost any trauma, from a small cut on the finger to a large abdominal incision made during bowel surgery. Although pain can be considered a physical complication, it has a large psychological component as well. Pain from wounds is often increased by activities such as ambulating, coughing, moving in bed, and dressing changes. The actual pain may be worsened by the patient's anticipatory apprehension of such activities. Nursing interventions to reduce pain through skill and explanations can greatly reduce emotional stress.

Anxiety and Fear

Anxiety and fear are common responses to a wound. Patients are apprehensive about the possibility of the wound opening, how much privacy will be lost as the wound is cared for, and how they and others will react to the appearance and smell of the wound. As nurses care for patients with wounds, it is important to be accepting and empathic, to encourage expression of feelings, to answer questions accurately and honestly, and to avoid excessive exposure of body parts when giving wound care.

Alterations in Body Image

Everyone's body image is of a whole entity. When the skin and tissues are traumatized, that image is changed, and the person must adapt and reformulate the concept of self. Wounds and scars that are visible to others, especially on the face, can leave the patient with feelings of being conspicuous and ugly and of less worth. Large scars, such as from removal of a breast or from a colostomy opening, can seriously affect the person's sexuality, social relationships, and self-concept. Referral to support groups or counselors may be necessary to facilitate coping and acceptance of changes in body structure or function.

The Nursing Process

ASSESSING THE WOUND

Wounds are assessed by inspection (sight and smell) and palpation for appearance, drainage, and pain. Included in the assessment are sutures, any drains or tubes, and manifestations of complications.

Appearance

Assess for the approximation of wound edges, color of the wound and surrounding area, drains or tubes, sutures, and signs of dehiscence or evisceration. The wound edges should be clean and well approximated, with a crust along the wound edges. The wound's edges are initially reddened and slightly swollen, but by the end of about a week, the skin should be closer to normal in appearance and the wound edges should be healed together. Skin surrounding the wound may at first be bruised, but this too returns to normal as blood is reabsorbed. If an infection is present, the wound is swollen, has increased redness, and feels hot. If dehiscence is impending or present, the wound edges are separated.

Wound Drainage

During the first two phases of wound healing, the inflammatory response results in **exudate** from the wound. The exudate is composed of fluid and cells that escape from blood vessels and are deposited in or on tissue surfaces. This exudate is called *wound drainage* and is described as *serous*, *sanguineous*, or, if infected, *purulent*:

Serous—composed primarily of the clear, serous portion of the blood and from serous membranes. Serous drainage is clear and watery.
Sanguineous—consists of large numbers of red blood cells and looks like blood. Bright red sanguineous drainage is indicative of fresh bleeding, whereas darker drainage indicates older bleeding.

Purulent—made up of white blood cells, liquefied dead tissue debris, and both dead and live bacteria. Purulent drainage is thick, often has a musty or foul odor, and varies in color (such as dark yellow or green), depending on the causative organism.

Drainage may be a mixture of these three types. Surgical wounds most commonly have a mixture of serum and red blood cells, called *serosanguineous* drainage.

Assess the amount, color, odor, and consistency of wound drainage. The amount and color depend on the wound location and size, with larger wounds having more drainage. Drainage can be assessed on the wound, on the dressings, in drainage bottles or reservoirs, or, depending on the location of the wound and the amount of drainage, under the patient.

Pain

If the patient has increased or constant pain from the wound, further assessments should be made. Pain, especially when accompanied by an increased or purulent flow

of drainage, may indicate delayed healing or the presence of an infection. Incisional pain is usually most severe for the first 2 to 3 days and then progressively diminishes.

Sutures and Staples

Skin sutures, which may be black silk, synthetic material, metal staples, fine wire, or metal skin clips, are used to hold tissue and skin together. Retention sutures are used to provide extra support for obese patients and for wounds with increased risk for dehiscence (Fig. 37-3).

Sutures are removed when enough tensile strength has developed to hold the wound edges together during healing. This stage varies from patient to patient, depending on age, nutritional status, and wound location. Silk sutures should be removed within 6 to 8 days to prevent suture marks, even though collagen formation and remodeling takes at least 21 days altogether. That means the scar may still stretch and widen after the silk sutures have been removed. Special subcutaneous techniques have now been developed to minimize this problem. Small wound closure strips of adhesive (Steri-Strips) may be applied directly to

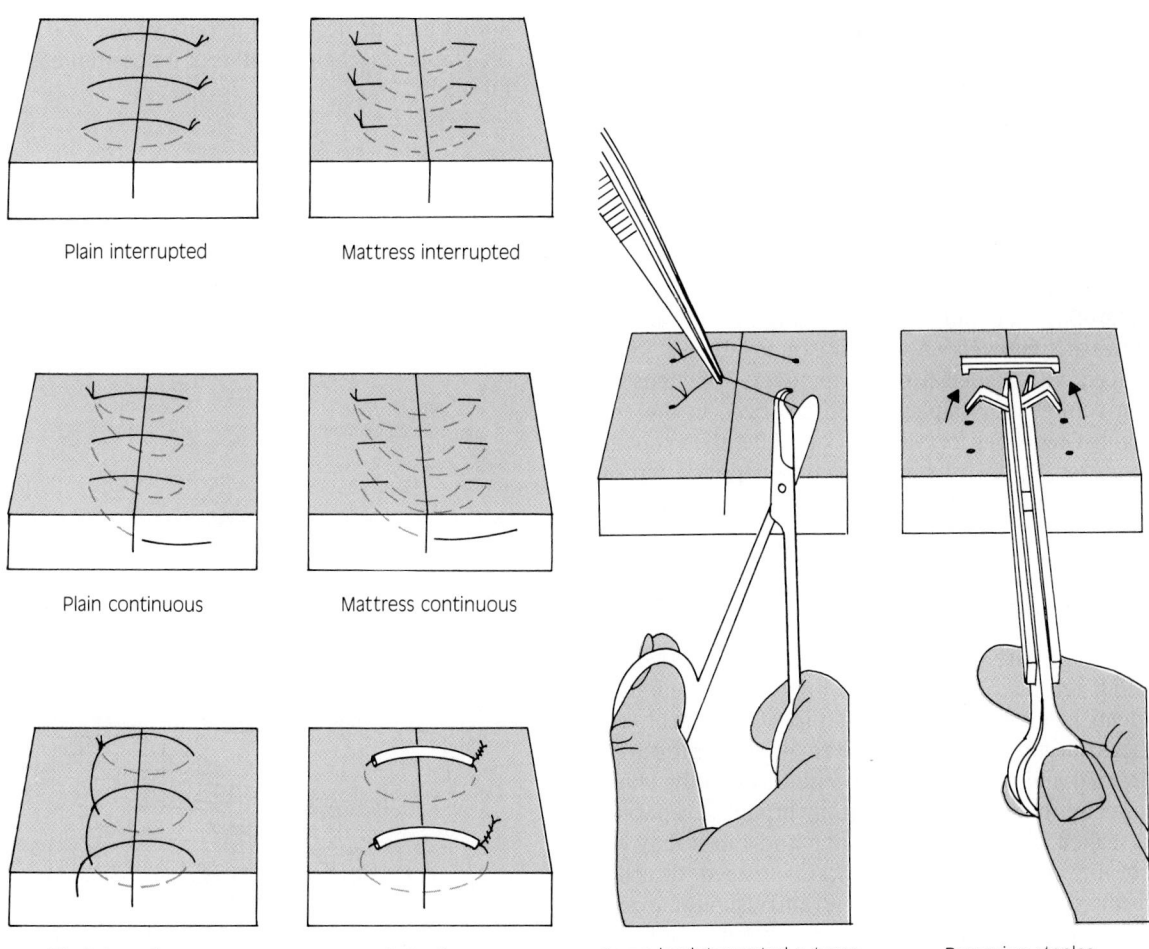

Types of sutures

Plain interrupted   Mattress interrupted

Plain continuous   Mattress continuous

Blanket continuous   Retention

Removing interrupted sutures   Removing staples

Figure 37-3
Types of sutures and techniques for removal.

Guidelines for Nursing Care

Removing Staples and Sutures

The removal of staples or sutures may be done by the physician or by the nurse with a physician's order. Agency protocol should be followed, but general guidelines are as follows:

- Use sterile techniques, following recommended CDC guidelines for care of wounds.
- Wash hands before and after the procedure.
- Explain the procedure to the patient. Describe the sensation that will be experienced as a pulling or slightly uncomfortable experience.
- Use proper technique to remove and dispose of old dressings.
- Clean the incision from the center of the wound outward, using hospital policy and procedure for type of agent.
- Remove every other suture or staple to be sure wound edges are healed; if they are, remove remaining sutures or staples as ordered.
- Remove or reapply dressing, depending on physician preference and agency policy.
- Some physicians order Steri-Strip application to the healed wound after removal of staples or sutures to give additional support to the wound as it continues to heal. Follow agency protocol and physician preference for placement of these tapes.

Specifics for Suture Removal

1. Use a sterile suture removal kit.
2. Using the sterile forceps, grasp the knot of the first suture and gently lift the knot.
3. Using the sterile scissors, cut one side of the suture below the knot close to the skin.
4. Grasp the knot with the forceps and pull the cut suture through the skin (be sure to pull through the healed wound only the portion of the suture that has been inside the tissue).

Specifics for Staple Removal

1. As directed on the package, gently position the sterile staple remover under the staple to be removed.
2. Firmly close the staple remover to straighten the staple ends (do not lift upward while disengaging staple ends).
3. Carefully lift upward with the closed staple remover to remove the staple from the incision line. It may be necessary to remove one end of the staple and then the other if it does not easily lift out.

the wound to help hold it together. Unless otherwise directed, Steri-Strips are not removed during wound care.

Sutures are removed with a suture removal set; staples are removed with a special staple remover. The steps in removing sutures and staples are summarized in the accompanying Guidelines for Nursing Care. After the removal of skin sutures, Steri-Strips are sometimes applied across the healing wound to give additional support as it continues to heal.

Drains and Tubes

Drains and tubes are inserted into or near a wound when it is anticipated that a collection of fluid in a closed area would delay healing. After a surgical procedure, the physician places one end of the tube or drain in or near the area to be drained and passes the other end through the skin, either directly through the incision or through a separate opening called a *stab wound*. Drains and tubes may or may not be sutured in place; drains placed directly through the wound (eg, a Penrose drain) usually have a large safety pin in the part outside the wound to prevent them from slipping back into the incised area and are not sutured (Fig. 37-4). Tubes that are connected to suction or that have a built-in reservoir to maintain constant low suc-

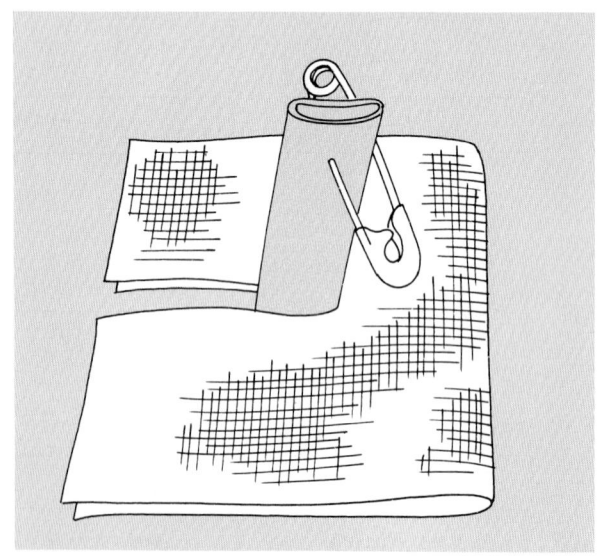

Figure 37-4
Penrose drain.

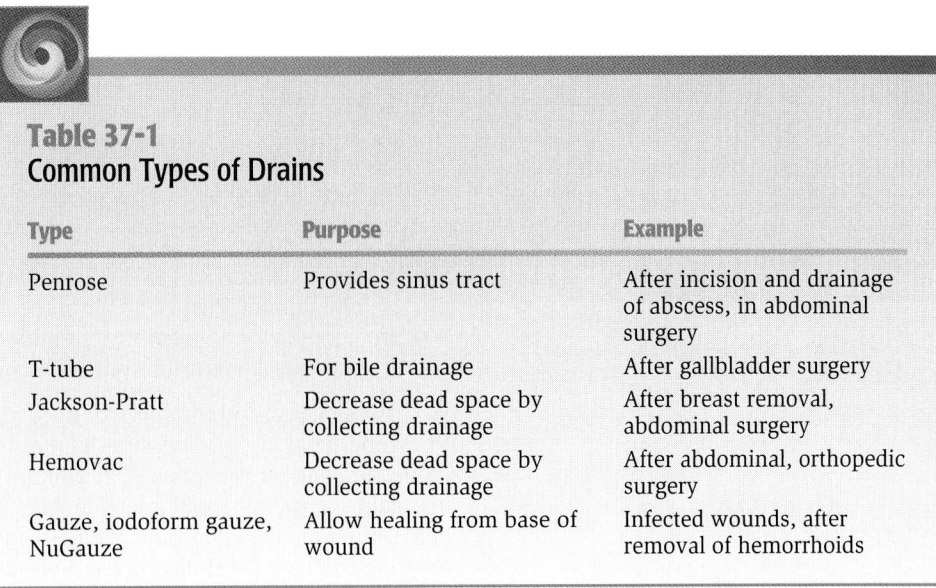

Table 37-1
Common Types of Drains

Type	Purpose	Example
Penrose	Provides sinus tract	After incision and drainage of abscess, in abdominal surgery
T-tube	For bile drainage	After gallbladder surgery
Jackson-Pratt	Decrease dead space by collecting drainage	After breast removal, abdominal surgery
Hemovac	Decrease dead space by collecting drainage	After abdominal, orthopedic surgery
Gauze, iodoform gauze, NuGauze	Allow healing from base of wound	Infected wounds, after removal of hemorrhoids

tion are usually sutured to the skin (eg, a Jackson-Pratt drainage tube or a Hemovac). It is important to know which type of drain or tube was inserted during surgery, so that accurate assessment can be made. The patency and placement of tubes or drains are included in wound assessment. Table 37-1 describes the purpose and common use of selected drains and tubes.

Related Assessments

In addition to assessments of the wound, the nurse evaluates the patient's general condition and laboratory test results. *Infection* may cause generalized malaise, increased pain, anorexia, and an elevated body temperature and pulse rate. Laboratory data indicating an infection are an elevated white blood cell count and, if a wound culture has been done, a causative organism. *Hemorrhage* is further identified by restlessness, thirst, anxiety, a drop in systolic blood pressure, increased pulse and respiratory rates, decreased urinary output, and decreased hemoglobin and hematocrit.

DIAGNOSING IN WOUND CARE

The patient with a wound is at risk for or has several alterations in health that are supported by assessment. One of the most appropriate North American Nursing Diagnosis Association (NANDA) nursing diagnoses is Altered Skin Integrity, defined as a state in which an individual has altered epidermis or dermis. Other NANDA nursing diagnoses related to wound care follow:

- Risk for Infection related to obesity and contamination during automobile accident causing thoracic wound
- Pain related to presence of large midline abdominal incision
- Ineffective Airway Clearance related to high abdominal incision and refusal to cough and deep breathe after surgery

- Delayed Surgical Recovery related to wound complications of evisceration and infection
- Anxiety related to possible loss of employment as a result of inability to work after emergency surgery
- Body Image Disturbance related to presence of wound extending from hairline to chin on left side of face

PLANNING: EXPECTED OUTCOMES FOR WOUND CARE

The plan of care is directed toward facilitating the patient's return to health by providing interventions that facilitate wound healing, reduce the risk for complications, and promote psychosocial adaptation. In planning for appropriate expected outcomes, the patient will achieve the following:

- Remain free of symptoms of infection
- Verbalize that pain management regimen relieves pain to an acceptable level
- Follow recommended schedule and techniques for coughing and deep breathing
- Use recommended relaxation methods to reduce anxiety levels
- Be discharged to home within established parameters
- Demonstrate appropriate wound care measures before discharge
- Verbalize understanding of symptoms to report and necessary follow-up care

IMPLEMENTING WOUND CARE

In caring for the patient with a wound, the nurse carries out interventions to promote wound healing, prevent further injury or alteration in skin integrity, prevent infection, promote physical and emotional comfort, and facilitate coping. The interventions are focused on the nursing diagnosis Impaired Skin Integrity, defined as a state in which an individual has altered epidermis or dermis (NANDA,

1999). The accompanying box, Incision Site Care, provides guidelines for wound care interventions.

Using Dressings

The goal of wound care is to promote tissue repair and regeneration so that skin integrity is restored. The two methods of caring for wounds are the closed method, in which a **dressing** is used as a protective cover over the wound, and the open method, in which no dressing is used.

Most dressings, especially those used for surgical wounds, consist of three layers. The dressing applied directly over the wound, called the *contact layer,* allows drainage to pass into the middle layer. This layer should be able to be removed without causing further tissue damage. The middle layer dressing absorbs the drainage, and the outer layer keeps the two inner layers in place. There are many different types of dressings, but all have essentially the same purposes:

- Provide physical, psychological, and aesthetic comfort
- Remove necrotic tissue
- Prevent, eliminate, or control infection
- Absorb drainage
- Maintain a moist wound environment
- Protect the wound from further injury
- Protect the skin surrounding the wound

Dressings can rub or stick to the wound, causing further superficial injury. Dressings can also create a warm, damp, and dark environment—all conducive to the growth of organisms and potential infection. Most wounds are covered with a dressing, and nurses are responsible for most dressing changes. The following sections deal with the supplies needed for dressing changes, guidelines for prevention of infection, and procedures for changing selected types of dressings.

Dressing Supplies

The items needed for a dressing change may be gathered individually or may be packaged in a sterile dressing tray, depending on the healthcare setting. Some hospital units have special dressing carts to keep all dressing supplies in one area. Wound care in the home may depend on the supplies provided by the patient or family.

The supplies needed vary with the type, location, and amount of wound drainage; the nursing plan of care should include specifics about each patient's dressing procedure and supplies. Materials and supplies include cleaning agents, materials to cover the wound (the dressing), and materials used to secure the dressing and support the wound.

Cleaning Agents

Although various antiseptic cleaning agents could be used to clean a wound, sterile 0.9% sodium chloride solution is usually the agent of choice. Some authorities question the use of any agent other than 0.9% sodium chloride solution because of the caustic effect of other agents on skin, tissues, and granulation tissue.

Types of Dressings

The number and types of dressings used depend on the location and size of the wound as well as the amount and type of drainage. The incision line is often covered with sterile petrolatum gauze or a special gauze called Telfa. Telfa's shiny outer surface is applied to the wound and allows drainage to pass through and be absorbed by the center absorbent layer. Both these protective dressings prevent outer dressings from adhering to the wound and causing further injury when removed.

Gauze dressings are commonly used to cover wounds. These dressings come in various sizes (2 × 2 inches, 4 × 4 inches, and 4 × 8 inches) and are commercially pack-

---

Using the Nursing Interventions Classification (NIC)

Incision Site Care

Definition

Cleansing, monitoring, and promoting healing in a wound that is closed with sutures, clips, or staples.

Activities

- Explain the procedure to the patient, using sensory preparation.
- Inspect the incision site for redness, swelling, or signs of dehiscence or evisceration.
- Note characteristics of any drainage.
- Monitor the healing process in the incision site.
- Cleanse the area around the incision with an appropriate cleansing solution.
- Swab from the clean area toward the less clean area.
- Monitor incision for signs and symptoms of infection.
- Use sterile, cotton-tipped applicators for efficient cleansing of tight-fitting wire sutures, deep and narrow wounds, or wounds with pockets.
- Cleanse the area around any drain site or drainage tube last.
- Apply closure strips, as appropriate.
- Apply antiseptic ointment, as ordered.
- Remove sutures, staples, or clips, as indicated.
- Change the dressing at appropriate intervals.
- Apply an appropriate dressing to protect the incision.
- Facilitate the patient's viewing of the incision.
- Instruct the patient on how to care for the incision during bathing or showering.
- Teach the patient how to minimize stress on the incision line.
- Teach the patient and/or family how to care for the incision, including recognizing signs and symptoms of infection.

From McClosky, J., & Bulechek, G. (2000). *Nursing interventions classification* (3rd ed.). (p. 396). St. Louis: C. V. Mosby.

aged as single units or in packs. Special gauze dressings (eg, Sof-Wick) are precut halfway to fit around drains or tubes. Larger dressings (8 × 10 bandages, abdominal pads [ABDs], Surgi-Pads) are placed over the smaller gauze dressings and absorb drainage and protect the wound from contamination or injury.

Transparent dressings (eg, Op-Site) are applied directly over a small wound or tube; these dressings are occlusive, decreasing the possibility of contamination while allowing visualization of the wound. This type of dressing is often used over intravenous sites, subclavian catheter insertion sites, and healing wounds.

Tape

There are many kinds of tape, ranging in width from 2 to 4 inches (1-inch wide tape is the most commonly used). Table 37-2 summarizes the types and purposes of different tapes.

Cleaning a Wound and Applying a Clean Dressing

The nurse prepares the patient for the dressing change before starting the procedure by explaining what will be done. Proper screening is needed to provide privacy. The patient is helped into a position that is comfortable and also convenient for changing the dressing. The area is exposed while maintaining proper draping.

It is important to use appropriate aseptic techniques when changing the dressing, especially to wash hands thoroughly before and after changing dressings and to follow standard precautions. Among the most common causes of nosocomial infections is carelessness in practicing asepsis when changing dressings.

The wound is cleaned and the dressing changed as described in Procedure 37-1. The nurse has an excellent opportunity for teaching while changing the dressing, which is especially important when the patient will be changing dressings at home. The patient should be encouraged to help as much as possible, beginning with such assistance as preparing adhesive strips.

A patient may be disturbed by the sight of the wound. The nurse should listen carefully to what the patient is saying and observe nonverbal communication as well. In some instances, the patient may not want to look at the wound, particularly with a wound that involves a change in normal body functions or appearance, such as a wound resulting from the removal of a breast, the amputation of an extremity, or the placement of a tube in a draining wound. With patience and emotional support, patients usually become accustomed to the wound in time.

There is no standard frequency for how often dressings should be changed. It depends on the amount of drainage, the physician's preference, and the nature of the wound. It is customary for the physician to perform the first dressing change, usually within 24 to 48 hours after surgery. Thereafter, nurses change the dressings as needed or daily. The frequency of dressing changes should be noted on the patient's care plan.

Applying Bandages and Binders

Bandages and binders are used to secure dressings, apply pressure, and support the wound. **Bandages** are strips of cloth, gauze (eg, roller gauze, Kerlix, Kling), or elasticized material (eg, Ace bandages) used to wrap a body part. They come packaged in rolls and vary in width from 1 to 6 inches. **Binders** are designed for a specific body part and include slings, abdominal binders, chest binders, and T-binders. They may be made of cloth (flannel, muslin) or of an elasticized material that fastens together with Velcro.

Following are guidelines for applying bandages and binders:

- Prolonged heat and moisture on the skin may cause skin breakdown. The area to be covered should be

(*text continues on page 912*)

Table 37-2
Types of Tape

Type	Purpose
Adhesive (can cause occlusion, allergy, skin maceration, shearing)	Used for strength, support, and economy • To secure dressings and splints • To strap joints to prevent athletic injuries • To immobilize or stabilize body parts • To provide pressure • To approximate wound edges
Paper, plastic, acetate	Increased comfort, decreased allergic and skin problems • To close small wounds • To secure dressings
Microfoam	Used for compression or pressure dressings

PROCEDURE 37-1

Cleaning a Wound and Applying a Sterile Dressing

Equipment

Sterile gloves
Gauze dressings or squares
Sterile dressing set or suture set
    (contains scissors and forceps)
Cleaning solution
Clean disposable gloves
Sterile basin (optional)

Sterile drape (optional)
Plastic bag for soiled dressings
Waterproof pad
Bath blanket
Tape or ties
Surgi-pads or ABDs

Additional dressing supplies as
    needed or ordered (antiseptic
    ointments, extra dressings)
Acetone or adhesive remover
    (optional)
Sterile normal saline (optional)

Action	Rationale
1. Explain the procedure to patient.	An explanation encourages patient cooperation and reduces apprehension.
2. Gather equipment.	Provides for organized approach to task
3. Wash your hands.	Handwashing deters spread of microorganisms.
4. Check physician's order for dressing change. Note whether drain is present.	Clarifies type of dressing
5. Close door or curtain. Use bath blanket as needed when exposing area to be redressed. Position waterproof pad under patient if desired.	Provides for privacy and warmth
6. Assist patient to comfortable position that provides easy access to wound area.	Provides for comfort
7. Place opened, cuffed plastic bag near working area.	Soiled dressings may be placed in disposal bag without contaminating outside surfaces of bag.
8. Loosen tape on dressing. Use adhesive remover if necessary. If tape is soiled, don gloves.	It is easier to loosen tape before putting on gloves.
9. Don clean disposable gloves, and remove soiled dressings carefully in a clean to less clean direction. Do not reach over wound. Check position of drains before removing dressing. If dressing is adhering to skin surface, it may be moistened by pouring a small amount of sterile saline onto it. Keep soiled side of dressing away from patient's view.	Protects the nurse from handling contaminated dressings. Cautious removal of dressing is more comfortable for patient and ensures that drain is not removed if one is present. Sterile saline provides for easier removal of dressing.
10. Assess amount, type, and odor of drainage.	Wound healing process or presence of infection should be documented.
11. Discard dressings in plastic disposal bag. Pull off glove inside out and drop it in bag.	Prevents spread of microorganisms by contaminated dressings
12. Using aseptic technique, open sterile dressings and supplies on work area.	Supplies are within easy reach, and sterility is maintained.
13. Open sterile cleaning solution, and pour over gauze sponges in plastic container or over sponges placed in sterile basin.	Sterility of dressings and solution is maintained.
14. Don sterile gloves.	Maintains surgical asepsis.

(continued)

Cleaning a Wound and Applying a Sterile Dressing (Continued)

15. Clean wound or surgical incision. Use sterile forceps if desired.

    a. Clean from top to bottom or from center outward.   Clean from least to most contaminated area.
Previously cleaned area is not recontaminated.

    b. Use one gauze square for each wipe, discarding each square by dropping into plastic bag. Do not touch bag with forceps.

    c. Clean around drain, if present, moving from center outward in a circular motion. Use one gauze square for each circular motion.   Move from least to most contaminated area.

    d. Dry wound using gauze sponge and same motion.   Moisture provides medium for growth of microorganisms.

    e. Apply antiseptic ointment if ordered.   Growth of microorganisms may be retarded and healing process improved.

16. Apply a layer of dry, sterile dressings over wound. Use sterile forceps if desired.   Primary dressing serves as a wick for drainage.

17. Use sterile scissors to cut sterile 4 × 4 gauze square to place under and around drain if one is present or use precut sterile gauze.   Drainage is absorbed, and surrounding skin area is protected.

18. Apply second gauze layer to wound site.   Provides for increased absorption of drainage

19. Place Surgi-pad or ABD dressing over wound as outermost layer.   Wound is protected from microorganisms in environment.

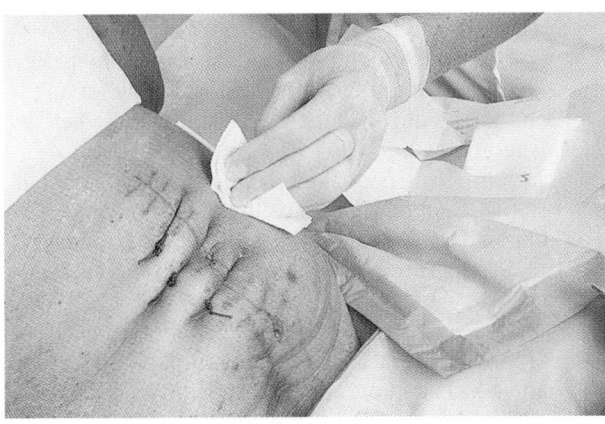

Action 15: Cleaning a surgical incision.

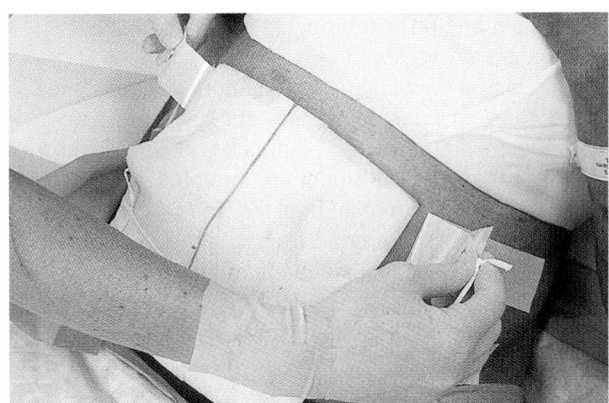

Action 19: Applying Montgomery straps over outer layer of dressing.

20. Remove gloves from inside out, and discard them in plastic waste bag. Apply tape or tie existing tapes to secure dressings.   Tape is easier to apply after gloves have been removed.

21. Wash hands. Remove all equipment, and make patient comfortable.   Prevents spread of microorganisms

22. Check dressing and wound site every shift. Record dressing change and appearance of wound, and describe any drainage in chart.   Provides accurate documentation of procedure

(continued)

PROCEDURE 37-1

Cleaning a Wound and Applying a Sterile Dressing (Continued)

Age Considerations   To keep a dressing intact or to prevent contamination of wound and supplies on an infant or young child, it may be necessary to restrain the child's hand. An old stocking or piece of stockinette may be used to encircle child's hand and then may be secured to the bed or crib with a tie or safety pin. Care must be taken not to compromise circulation to that extremity.

Home Care Considerations   Reinforce need for thorough handwashing before and after dressing change.

Have plastic bag available for safe disposal of soiled dressings and equipment.

Boil any nondisposable equipment (eg, forceps) for 10 minutes to ensure sterility after washing carefully in warm soapy water.

Inform patient about availability of disposable wound care supplies.

Special Considerations   Patient must be instructed that any break or interruption in the suture line may require immediate intervention and that the surgeon should be notified immediately. Instruct patient and family about significant changes that need to be reported to the nurse or physician.

Encourage splinting of wound during activity (coughing, sneezing, sudden movement, or change in position).

---

cleaned and dried thoroughly before applying a bandage or binder.

- Bandaging the body part in the normal functioning position prevents deformities and discomfort.
- The bandage or binder is applied with sufficient pressure to provide the amount of immobilization or support desired, to remain in place, and to secure a dressing when present. Pressure should not be so great, however, that circulation in the body part involved is impeded.
- The tension of all bandage turns should be equal, and unnecessary and uneven overlapping of turns should be avoided.
- After application, circulation and comfort are assessed at regular intervals.

Applying Roller Bandages

A roller bandage is a continuous strip of material wound on itself to form a cylinder or roll (Fig. 37-5). Plain gauze, elastic webbing, and stretchable roller bandages are made in various widths and lengths. To begin, the free end is held in place with one hand while the other hand passes the roll around the body part. After the bandage is anchored, the roll is passed or rolled around the body part, taking care to exert equal tension in all turns. It is easier to keep tension equal by unwinding the bandage gradually and only as it is required. There should be even overlapping of one half to two thirds the width of each bandage, except for the circular turn. The basic turns for roller bandages are as follows:

Circular turn. The bandage is wrapped around the body part with complete overlapping of the previous bandage turn. This is used primarily for anchoring a bandage where it is begun and where it is terminated.

Spiral turn. The bandage ascends in a spiral manner so that each turn overlaps the preceding one by one half or two thirds the width of the bandage. The spiral turn is useful for the wrist, the fingers, and the trunk.

Figure-of-eight turn. The figure-of-eight turn consists of making oblique overlapping turns that ascend and descend alternately. It is effective for use around joints, such as the knee, the elbow, the ankle, and the wrist.

Recurrent-stump bandage. After a few circular turns to anchor the bandage, the initial end of the bandage is placed in the center of the body part being bandaged, well back from the tip to be covered. The bandage is passed back and forth over the tip, first on the one side and then on the other side of the center piece of bandage. Figure 37-5 shows how to apply a recurrent bandage to a stump, using the figure-of-eight turn to finish the bandage. Recurrent bandages are used for fingers, for the head, and for the stump of an amputated limb.

When removing a roller bandage, it is best to cut the bandage with a bandage scissors to prevent excessive manipulation of the part. Cut on the side opposite the injury or the wound, from one end to the other, so that the bandage

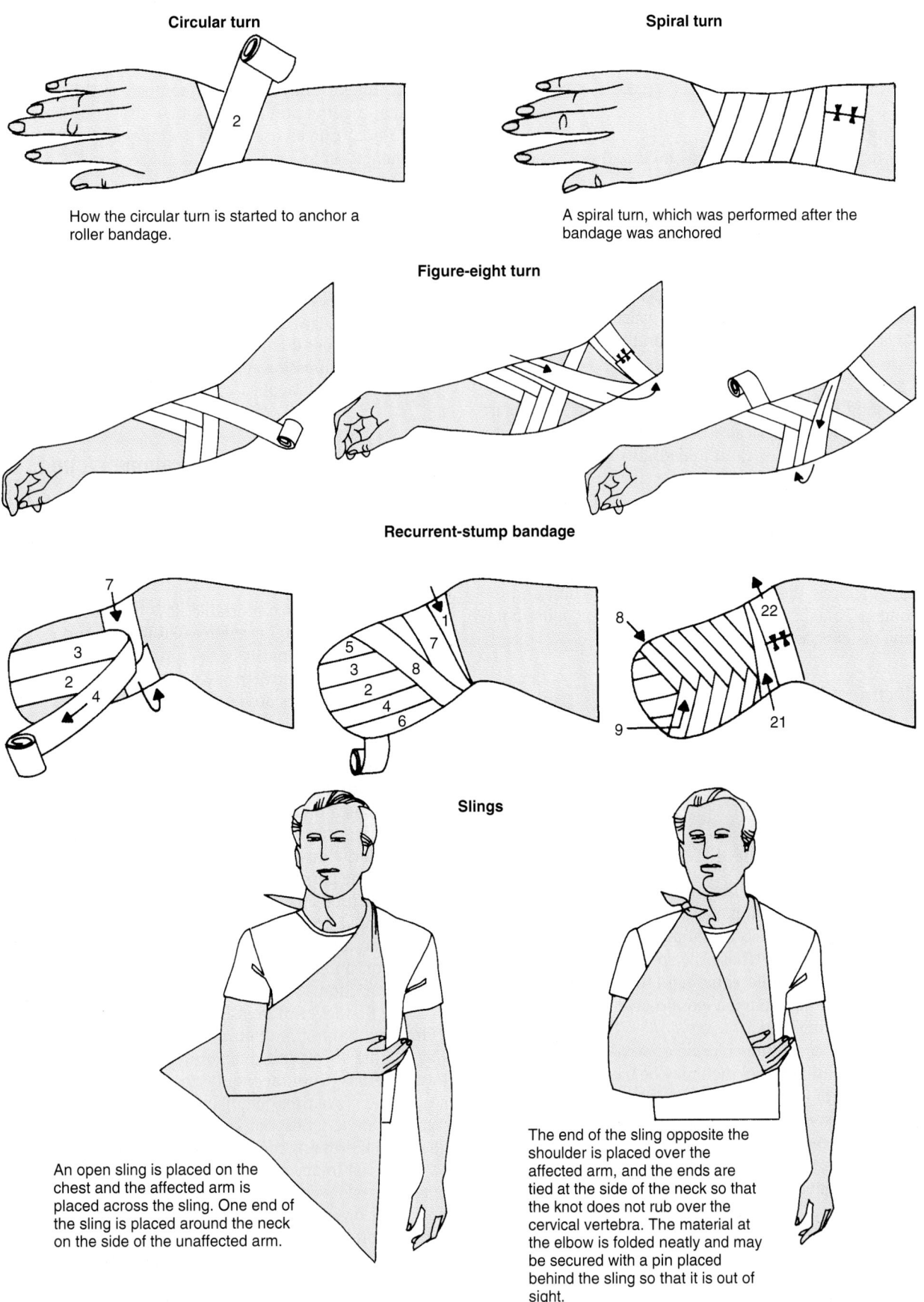

Circular turn

How the circular turn is started to anchor a roller bandage.

Spiral turn

A spiral turn, which was performed after the bandage was anchored

Figure-eight turn

Recurrent-stump bandage

Slings

An open sling is placed on the chest and the affected arm is placed across the sling. One end of the sling is placed around the neck on the side of the unaffected arm.

The end of the sling opposite the shoulder is placed over the affected arm, and the ends are tied at the side of the neck so that the knot does not rub over the cervical vertebra. The material at the elbow is folded neatly and may be secured with a pin placed behind the sling so that it is out of sight.

Figure 37-5

Techniques for applying various bandages.

can be folded open for its entire length. If the bandage is to be reused, it may be unwound by keeping the loose end together and passing it as a ball from one hand to the other while unwinding it.

Applying Binders

Of the many different kinds of binders, those used most commonly are described here.

T-Binders

T-binders are used to secure dressings on the rectum and perineum and in the groin. The single T-binder is used for female patients, and the double T-binder is used for male patients. The belt is passed around the waist and secured, and the tails are passed between the legs and fastened to the belt.

Sling

A sling is used to support an arm. Most healthcare agencies use commercial strap slings or sleeve slings. In the home, a large piece of cloth folded into a triangle can be used as a sling.

Straight Binders

A straight binder is a straight piece of material, usually about 15 to 20 cm (6 to 8 inches) wide and long enough to more than circle the torso. It is used for the chest and the abdomen. Straight binders may be pinned or, more commonly, fastened with Velcro.

Collecting a Wound Culture

If assessment of the wound indicates a possible infection, a specimen of the drainage is obtained and sent to the laboratory for culture and sensitivity, as outlined in Procedure 37-2.

Irrigating and Packing a Wound

An irrigation is a directed flow of solution over tissues. The purposes of an irrigation include cleaning the area of pathogens and other debris and applying local heat or an antiseptic to the area. Nonsterile solutions are used if the wound is closed. Sterile equipment and solutions are required for irrigating an open wound, even in the presence of an existing infection.

Sterile 0.9% sodium chloride or sterile water, an antiseptic, or an antibiotic solution may be used, depending on the condition of the wound and the prescription. A sterile, large-volume syringe is used. Packing is sometimes placed in wounds after irrigation to allow granulation tissue and healing by secondary intention to take place. The techniques for irrigating a wound and inserting packing are described in Procedure 37-3.

Documenting Wound Care

The nurse documents assessments and interventions each time wound care is given. If drainage is present, the kind and amount are described. If the patient has a complicated dressing, details for caring for the wound should be described in the care plan. Many patients have preferences for when dressings are changed and how the dressings are best arranged. They may become distressed if one nurse uses one method and another nurse uses a different one, even if both nurses use proper technique. An example of documentation follows:

> 1/12/93, 1 PM, nursing
>
> Sterile dressing change of midline abdominal incision. Old dressing moderately saturated with serosanguineous drainage. Four-inch midline abdominal incision cleaned with sterile 0.9% saline. Wound edges well approximated; skin sutures intact. Crust along suture line, edges of incision slightly edematous and dark pink. Penrose drain present in lower one fourth of incision. New dressing applied, using Telfa, four 4×4 pads, and two ABDs applied with nonallergenic tape.
>
> A. Bowman, RN

Changing a Dressing for a Draining Wound

The basic care of a draining wound is similar to that of a wound with little or no drainage. The following techniques are important in caring for a draining wound.

Promoting Comfort

If wound care is uncomfortable, it is best to administer a prescribed analgesic or sedative 30 to 45 minutes before changing the dressing. It is also preferable to change the dressing midway between meals so that the patient's appetite and mealtimes are not disturbed.

Maintaining Skin Integrity

A protective ointment or paste may be applied to cleaned skin surrounding the draining wound. The ointment or paste acts as a protective barrier to prevent skin irritation and excoriation from wound drainage. Protecting the skin is particularly important if the drainage period may be prolonged or the person's skin is especially susceptible to irritation. The protective ointment or paste should be removed at least daily, and the skin should be cleaned thoroughly. It is best to remove the protective material with a minimal amount of rubbing to prevent epithelial cells from being injured by friction.

The first layer of dressing material applied directly to a draining wound is often nonabsorbent but hydrophilic (ie, capable of carrying moisture). This type of material allows drainage from the wound to move into overlying absorbent layers of dressing, helping prevent maceration and reinfection. It tends not to stick to the wound, making changing a dressing more comfortable for the patient.

Material to absorb and collect drainage is then placed over the first layer of nonabsorbent material. This material wicks out drainage by capillary action, or *capillarity*. Absorbent cotton has far greater capillarity than untreated cotton. Therefore, cotton-lined gauze sponges soak up more liquid than unlined sponges. Loosely packed gauze, the threads of which act as numerous wicks, enhances capillarity and directs drainage upward and away from the wound. Fluffed and loosely packed dressings are more absorbent

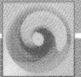

PROCEDURE 37-2
Collecting a Wound Culture

Equipment

Sterile Culturette tube with enclosed
    swab (or culture tube with
    individual swabs)

Sterile gloves
Clean disposable gloves
Plastic bag for soiled dressing

Label for Culturette tube
Laboratory requisition with rubber
    band or plastic bag

Action	Rationale
1. Explain the procedure to patient.	An explanation encourages patient cooperation and reduces apprehension.
2. Gather equipment.	Provides for organized approach to task
3. Wash your hands.	Handwashing deters spread of microorganisms.
4. Don clean disposable gloves. Remove dressing and assess wound and drainage (see Procedure 37-1, actions 5 to 11).	Protects nurse from handling contaminated dressings
5. Using aseptic technique, don sterile gloves and clean wound (see Procedure 37-1, action 15). Remove sterile gloves.	Previous drainage and skin flora are removed.
6. Twist cap to loosen swab in Culturette tube, or open separate swab and remove cap from culture tube, keeping inside uncontaminated.	Supplies are within easy reach, and sterility is maintained.
7. Don clean glove or new sterile glove, if necessary.	Use of Culturette does not require immediate contact with skin or wound. If contact with wound is necessary to collect specimen, wear sterile glove on that hand.
8. Carefully insert swab into drainage and roll gently. Use another swab if collecting specimen from another site.	Cotton tip absorbs wound drainage. This prevents cross-contamination of wound.
9. Place swab in Culturette tube, being careful not to touch outside of container. Twist cap to secure.	Outside of container is protected from contamination with microorganisms.
10. If using Culturette tube, crush ampule of medium at bottom of tube.	Swab with drainage can be surrounded by culture medium.

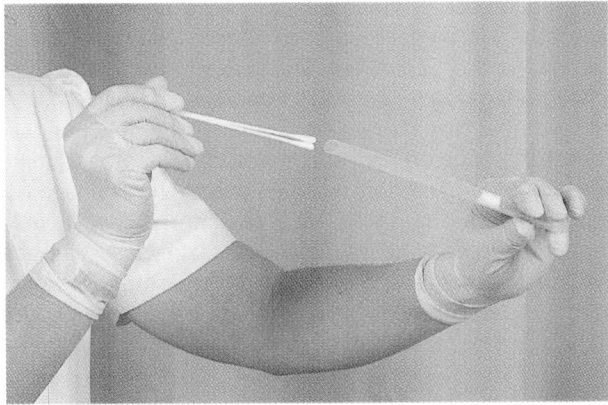

Action 9: Placing swab in a Culturette tube.

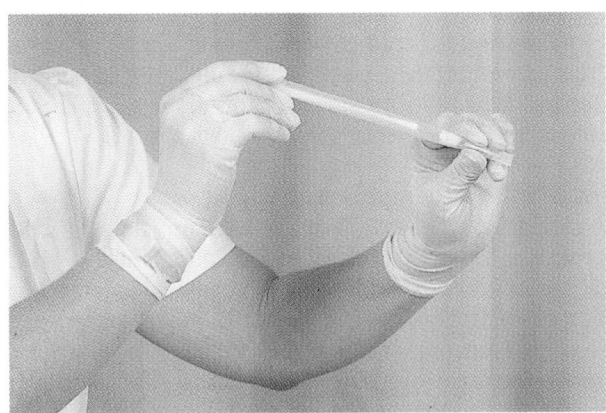

Action 10: Crushing ampule of medium at bottom of tube. (PHOTOS © B. PROUD.)

(continued)

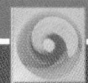

11. Remove gloves from inside out, and discard them in plastic waste bag.

Prevents spread of microorganisms

12. Wash your hands.

Handwashing deters the spread of microorganisms.

13. Apply clean dressing to wound (see Procedure 37-1, actions 16 to 20).

Drainage from wound is absorbed.

14. Wash your hands. Remove all equipment and make patient comfortable.

Handwashing deters the spread of microorganisms.

15. Label specimen container appropriately (patient's name, date, time, nature of specimen). Attach laboratory requisition to tube with rubber band or place tube in plastic bag with requisition attached. Send to laboratory within 20 minutes.

Ensures proper identification of specimen. Overgrowth of other organisms can interfere with test results if specimen remains at room temperature for extended period.

16. Record collection of specimen, appearance of wound, and description of drainage in chart.

Provides accurate documentation of procedure

than tightly packed dressings. The number of gauze sponges used in the dressing depends on the amount of drainage. The top of the dressing may be further protected by surgical or abdominal pads, which are thick, absorbent pads that help to absorb profuse drainage.

Because a draining wound requires more frequent changes of dressing than a wound without drainage, Montgomery straps are recommended to secure the dressing (Fig. 37-6). These straps do not require changing with each dressing, as tape strips do. Montgomery straps can be made or are available commercially. If made of tape, the adhesive end of the strap is placed on the skin well away from the wound. The end of the strap near the wound remains free because the adhesive side is turned back on itself. Gauze or woven strips passed through eyelets or openings are tied over the dressing. When the dressing is changed, the strips are untied and turned back to allow for wound care.

Preventing Infection and Promoting Healing

In caring for wounds, the nurse uses principles of both medical and surgical asepsis. Precautions should be taken to prevent infection of the wound by following Centers for Disease Control and Prevention (CDC) guidelines.

Contamination occurs through a moist medium. Microorganisms can move from the external surface through the dressing to the wound if a dressing remains in place until it is saturated. Microorganisms can also move from the wound to the outer surface of a saturated dressing. For these reasons, dressings should not be allowed to become saturated. They should either be replaced with fresh dressings or be reinforced with additional dressings before drainage causes saturation.

A rubber tubular drain (Penrose), a sump tube, or a catheter may be placed in a wound to promote exudate drainage. Care must be used so that these devices are not dislodged when dressings are changed. If a Penrose drain is ordered to be shortened each day, grasp the end of the drain with sterile forceps, pull it out a short distance while using a twisting motion, and cut off the end of the drain with sterile scissors. A sterile safety pin (or Klip) is often placed at the end of the drain so that it cannot slip down into the wound.

Closed drainage systems are used more often than incisional drains like the Penrose drain. Some studies show that the infection rate is cut nearly in half when drains are placed only when necessary and through a separate stab wound rather than in the incision itself. Closed drainage systems consist of a drain connected to an electric suction machine or a portable closed drainage suction system (Fig. 37-7).

Portable closed drainage systems have directions for their use printed on the container itself. The nurse should not touch the open port when emptying the drainage because reflux of drainage from a contaminated port could contaminate the wound. The closed drainage system prevents potential microorganisms from entering the wound from saturated dressings. Closed drainage systems also allow accurate measurement of drainage.

Changing Dressings in Special Situations

Infected Wounds

The CDC recommends special techniques for the care of extensive wounds with purulent drainage. In particular, wounds infected with *Staphylococcus aureus*, beta-hemolytic

(*text continues on page 919*)

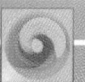

PROCEDURE 37-3

Irrigating a Sterile Wound

Equipment

Sterile irrigation set (basin, container for irrigant, irrigating syringe)
Prescribed irrigating solution (warmed to body temperature or 34°–37°C [93.2°–98.6°F])
Sterile soft catheter (optional)
Plastic bag for soiled dressings

Sterile gloves
Clean disposable gloves
Sterile dressing set or suture set (contains scissors and forceps)
Waterproof pad
Sterile gauze and surgipads or ABDs (for dressing change)

Packing gauze (as specified by physician)
Gown (optional)
Goggles (optional)
Bath blanket
Tape

Action	Rationale
1. Explain procedure to patient. Check physician's order for irrigation.	Explanation facilitates patient cooperation. Clarifies procedure and type of supplies required.
2. Gather equipment.	Provides for organized approach to task
3. Wash your hands.	Handwashing deters spread of microorganisms.
4. Close door or curtain. Use bath blanket as needed when exposing wound site.	Provides for privacy and warmth
5. Position patient so that irrigating solution will flow from upper end of wound toward lower end. Place waterproof pad under patient.	Gravity directs flow of liquid from least contaminated to most contaminated area. Waterproof pad protects patient and bed linens.
6. Warm sterile irrigating solution to body temperature.	Warmed solution is more comfortable for patient and promotes vasodilation.
7. Place opened, cuffed plastic bag near working area. Don gown and goggles if recommended.	Soiled dressings and packing may be placed in disposal bag without contaminating outside surfaces of bag. Gown protects uniform from contamination if splashing should occur. Goggles protect mucous membranes of eyes from contact with irrigant fluid.
8. Loosen tape on dressing, and put on clean gloves to remove soiled dressings.	Nurse is protected from handling contaminated dressings.
9. Assess amount, type, and odor of drainage. Observe condition of wound.	Provides information about wound healing process or presence of infection.
10. Discard dressings in plastic disposal bag. Remove gloves inside out and drop in bag.	Spread of microorganisms by way of contaminated dressings is prevented.
11. Using aseptic technique, open sterile dressings and supplies on work area.	Supplies are within easy reach and sterility is maintained.
12. Pour armed sterile irrigating solution into sterile container. Amount may vary from 200 to 500 mL depending on size of wound.	Facilitates wound irrigation.

(continued)

PROCEDURE 37-3

Irrigating a Sterile Wound (Continued)

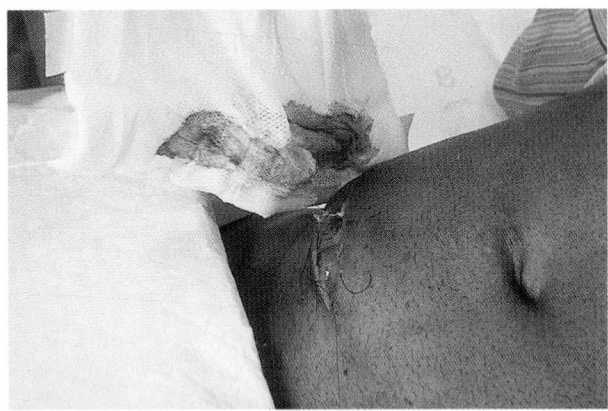

Action 9: Assessing wound drainage.

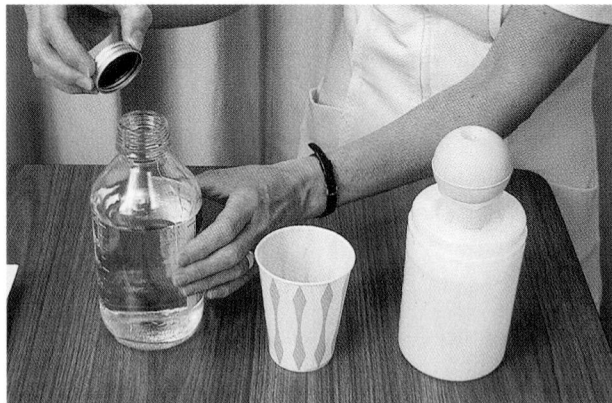

Action 12: Preparing sterile irrigating solution.

13. Put on sterile gloves.

14. Position the sterile basin below the wound to collect irrigation fluid with nondominant hand.

15. Use dominant hand to fill syringe with irrigant. Gently direct a stream of solution into wound, keeping tip of syringe 1 inch (2.5 cm) above upper tip of wound. If using a catheter tip on syringe, insert it gently into wound to point of resistance.

Maintains surgical asepsis

Irrigation is facilitated and patient and bed linens are protected from contaminated fluid.

Debris and contaminated solution flow from least contaminated to most contaminated area. Catheter allows introduction of irrigant into wound with small opening or one that is deep.

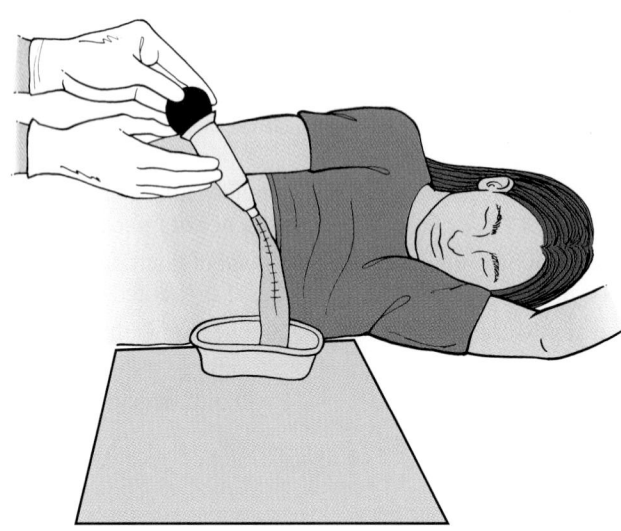

16. Continue irrigation until solution returns clear. Try to maintain a steady flow of solution.

17. Dry area around wound with a sterile gauze sponge.

18. Apply layers of sterile dressing.

Irrigation removes exudate and debris.

Moisture provides medium for growth of microorganisms.

Drainage is absorbed and surrounding skin area is protected.

(continued)

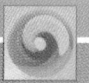

PROCEDURE 37-3

Irrigating a Sterile Wound (Continued)

19. Remove gloves, and discard them in plastic waste bag. Apply tape to secure dressings.

Tape is easier to apply after gloves have been removed.

20. Wash hands. Remove all equipment, and make patient comfortable.

Prevents spread of microorganisms

21. Check dressing and wound site every shift. Record dressing change, appearance of wound, and describe any drainage in chart.

Provides for accurate documentation of procedure

Special Considerations

If insertion of packing is ordered:
- Use sterile forceps to insert sterile packing into wound gently.
- Be careful not to pack wound excessively because this may impede blood flow and delay healing.
- Cut packing with sterile scissors if necessary.
- Allow a small strip of packing to protrude from small and deep wounds to facilitate removal.

---

streptococcus, and *Clostridium perfringens* (gas gangrene) require these special techniques. When the causative organism is unknown, the CDC advises the use of these techniques for all infected and extensive wounds with purulent drainage:

- Wash hands before wound care.
- Wear a gown while caring for the patient's wound. This gown need not be sterile unless there is danger of carrying organisms on a clean gown to an already debilitated patient.
- Wear a mask while caring for the wound.

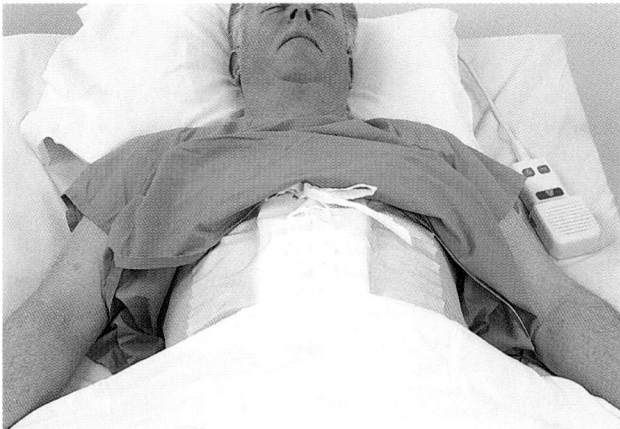

Figure 37-6
Montgomery straps make it possible to care for a wound without removing adhesive strips with each dressing change. (Photo © B. Proud.)

- Be prepared with two pairs of sterile gloves, and change gloves between the removal of the old dressing and the application of the new dressing.
- Wash hands thoroughly between glove changes. An antimicrobial soap is recommended by many healthcare agencies.
- Use a no-touch technique when handling soiled dressings. Lift soiled dressings with a clamp or forceps. This prevents contamination of the hands.
- Place soiled dressings in a moisture-proof bag, which is then closed securely, double-bagged, and incinerated without being opened.
- Wash the hands again thoroughly after completing wound care. If organisms accumulate on the hands because proper technique was broken, the organisms not only are likely to be carried to others but eventually may also become resident flora on the nurse's hands.

Open Wounds

Recommendations for the treatment of open wounds facilitate healing. Research supports the harmful effects of treatments such as the use of full-strength povidone-iodine (Betadine) and of wet-to-dry dressings. Each wound is individually evaluated, and one (or more) of a variety of choices for dressing is made.

A moist (rather than wet) packing for open wounds is recommended. Cellular migration needed for tissue repair and healing is enhanced by a moist surface. Packing material is soaked in a solution (0.9% sodium chloride solution is the solution of choice) and then wrung out so that it is only slightly moist. Packing is applied loosely and only to the edges of the wound, and it is then covered

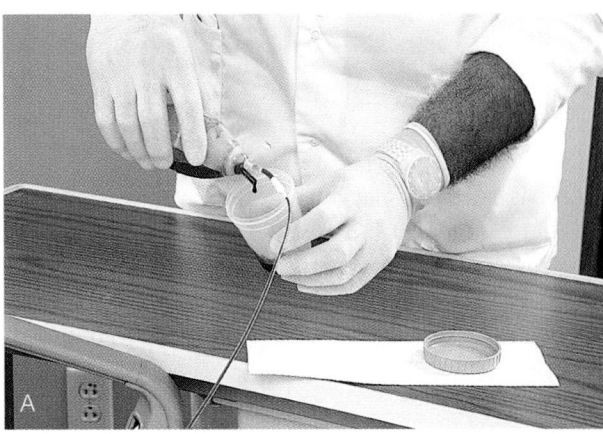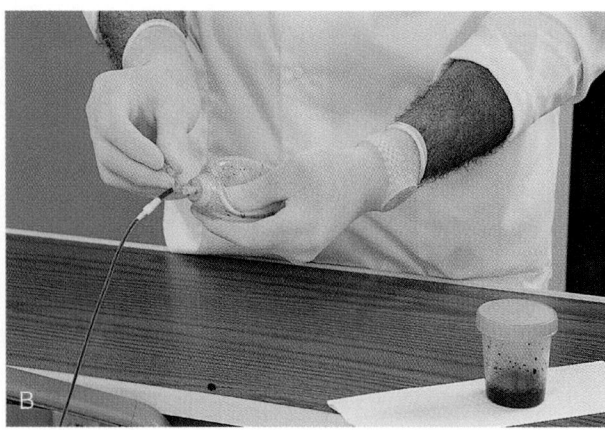

Figure 37-7
The Jackson-Pratt drain is a closed drainage system. The nurse empties the drain (**A**) and reapplies suction by compressing the drain reservoir before connecting it to the drain tubing (**B**). (Photo © B. Proud.)

with a secondary dressing to absorb drainage. If the packing dries, it should be soaked with 0.9% sodium chloride solution before removal.

The RYB color classification (Stotts, 1990) can be used in implementing care for open wounds. The classification based on the following:

R = red = protect
Y = yellow = cleanse
B = black = débride

The classification, with related interventions, is based on the assessment of the color of the wound, as follows:

- Red wounds are in the proliferative stage of healing and are the color of normal granulation tissue. Wounds in this stage need *protection* by nursing interventions that include gentle cleansing, use of moist dressings, application of a transparent or hydrocolloid dressing, and changing of the dressing only when necessary.
- Yellow wounds are characterized by oozing from the tissue covering the wound, often accompanied by purulent drainage. To *cleanse* these wounds, nursing interventions include irrigating the wound; using wet-to-moist dressings; using nonadherent, hydrogel, or other absorptive dressings; and consultation with the physician for the use of a topical antimicrobial medication to decrease the growth of bacteria.
- Black wounds are covered with thick eschar (necrotic tissue), which is usually black but may also be brown, gray, or tan in color. The eschar must be *débrided* (removed) before the wound can heal. These wounds are most often cared for by advanced practice nurses who are educated in the care of more complex wounds. The eschar may be removed by sharp débridement (using a scalpel or scissors to cut away the dead tissue), mechanical débridement (scrubbing the wound or applying a wet-to-moist dressing), chemical débridement (using collagenase enzyme agents), or autolytic débride-

ment (using dressing that contains wound moisture to help the body produce enzymes to break down the eschar). After débridement, the wound is treated as a yellow wound, and as healing progresses, a red wound.

Many wounds have red, yellow, and black components and are categorized as mixed wounds. When all colors are present, the wound is treated first for the most serious color (black), followed by yellow, and finally red.

Chronic Wounds

Many types of special moisture-retentive dressings are used to facilitate healing, especially in chronic wounds, as described in the following sections.

Transparent Films

These semipermeable dressings (eg, Acu-derm, Bioclusive, Op-Site, Tegaderm) allow an exchange of oxygen between the wound and the environment, protect against contamination, and maintain a moist wound environment. They are used for wounds with minimal drainage and may remain in place from 24 to 72 hours.

Absorptive Fillers

Included as absorptive dressings are karaya powder, dextranomer beads, and copolymer starches (eg, Bard absorption dressing, Chronicure, DuoDerm, HydraGran, Debrisan). These dressings, which absorb drainage and maintain a moist surface by forming a gelatinous mass, are most often used for deep wounds with heavy drainage. They conform to the shape of the wound and can remain in place for up to 24 hours. They must be irrigated from the wound when changed.

Alginates

These masses of fibers (eg, Curasorb, Kaltostat, Sorbsan) form a moisture-retentive gel on contact with exudate. They are used for wounds with moderate to heavy exudate and require a secondary dressing to hold them in place.

Hydrocolloids

Hydrocolloid dressings (eg, DuoDerm, Tegasorb, Restore, Comfeel) are wafer-shaped dressings that come in many shapes and thicknesses. They absorb drainage, maintain a moist wound surface, and decrease the risk for infection. They are used for shallow wounds with minimal drainage and may remain in place for 3 to 7 days (Fig. 37-8). Polyurethane dressings are nonadhesive hydrocolloid dressings that must be taped down to prevent wound contamination because they do not adhere to the wound surface. They may be used in conjunction with packing for deep, open wounds.

Hydrogels

Hydrogel dressings (eg, Aquasorb, Biolex, ClearSite, Nugel, Vigilon) are oxygen permeable and nonadhesive and maintain moisture. They may consist of powders, pastes, or beads and may remain in place for 8 to 48 hours. They are used for wounds with minimal exudate.

Synthetic Barrier Dressings

Synthetic barrier dressings are pastes that dry to form transparent, semipermeable dressings. Pores in the dried paste allow drainage to move from the wound to an absorbent dressing.

Newer biologic-biosynthetic products include Apligraf, Inerspan, and Regranex (Beaumont & Anderson-Dam, 1998). Apligraf is living skin derived from donor tissue that is used for chronic leg ulcers, acting as a skin graft to facilitate wound closure. Inerspan is a platelet-derived growth factor used for leg ulcers, burns, abrasions, skin tears, and chronic wounds. Regranex is a growth factor that stimulates the formation of new granulation tissue. It is used for leg ulcers.

Vacuum-Assisted Closure Therapy

Vacuum-assisted closure (VAC) therapy is the application of negative pressure to pull the cells closer together. This allows the epithelial cells to multiply rapidly and form

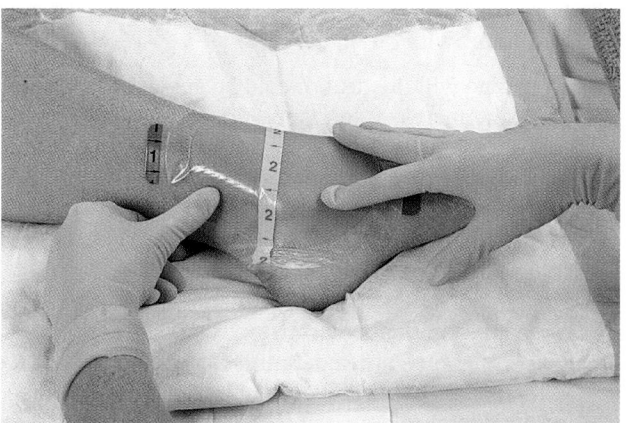

Figure 37-8
For proper wear, the hydrocolloid dressing must be sized generously, allowing at least a 1-inch margin of healthy skin around the wound. (Photo © B. Proud.)

granulation tissue so that healing can begin. It also increases cell proliferation, stimulates blood flow to wounds, and stimulates the growth of new blood vessels. This painless procedure is used on chronic open wounds, surgical incisions with dehiscence, and stage III and IV pressure ulcers.

Teaching for Home Care of a Wound

With increased ambulatory surgery and earlier discharge of patients from inpatient settings to home care, teaching patients and their families about wound care is important. Although a nurse may be needed to change dressings and provide wound care in complex situations, family members often do the procedure. To provide the continuity of care that is necessary to prevent infection and promote healing, the nurse must include teaching about wound care as part of discharge planning and in interactions with home care patients and families.

Each of the following components should be included in the teaching plan; the patient or family member who will be changing the dressing should demonstrate proper techniques in wound care and dressing change.

- Dressing materials can be purchased from pharmacies, drug stores, discount stores, and medical supply stores. The cost and ease of use should be considered.
- Signs and symptoms of infection (increased body temperature; malaise; reddened wound edges; drainage that is thick, green, odorous, or increased in amount; increased pain) should be reported immediately to the healthcare provider.
- Eating well-balanced meals and drinking fluids are important to wound healing. The diet should be high in proteins, zinc, iron, and vitamins.
- Modifying activities of daily living and exercise patterns may be necessary until healing is completed.
- Disposable gloves should be worn when changing the dressing, and hands should be washed before donning and after removing the gloves.
- The old dressing should be placed in a plastic bag or wrapped in several layers of newspaper before disposal in a trash container.

EVALUATING WOUND CARE

The plan of care for the patient with a wound is evaluated based on the expected outcomes. Evaluation is ongoing throughout the care of the patient, with the plan being effective if no complications have occurred during wound healing, the wound is progressing through the healing stages, and the patient or family has the knowledge and skills necessary for wound care at home.

Applying Heat and Cold as Nursing Interventions

Heat and cold are applied to a part or all of a patient's body to bring about a local or systemic change in body temperature for various therapeutic purposes. Physiologic responses to heat and cold are modified by the method and duration of application, the degree of heat and cold applied, the patient's age and physical condition, and the amount of body surface covered by the application. Nurses use heat and cold as nursing interventions in both hospital and community-based settings.

Heat and cold cause local and systemic effects. Body temperature is regulated by cells in the hypothalamus in response to signals from thermal (heat and cold) receptors located close to the skin's surface. Stimulation of these receptors sends sensory messages to the anterior hypothalamus to initiate mechanisms to dissipate heat (through vasoconstriction and shivering). Pain receptors, also located near the skin's surface, are also affected by heat and cold.

The nurse's aims in applying heat and cold are (1) to promote wound heating, (2) to facilitate comfort, (3) to use knowledge and skill in carrying out the application, and (4) to follow safety measures.

Effects of Applying Heat

Heat dilates peripheral blood vessels, a mechanism that helps to dissipate heat from the body to the environment. Vasodilation also increases local blood flow. In turn, the supply of oxygen and nutrients to the area is increased, and venous congestion is decreased. Reduced viscosity of blood and increased capillary permeability improve the delivery of leukocytes and nutrients while also facilitating the removal of wastes and prolonging clotting time. These actions, combined with increased tissue metabolism, accelerate the inflammatory response to promote healing. Heat reduces muscle tension to promote relaxation and helps to relieve muscle spasms and joint stiffness. Heat also helps relieve pain by stimulating specific nerve fibers, closing the gate that allows transmission of pain stimuli to centers in the brain. Because of these local physiologic effects, heat in various forms is used to treat infections, surgical wounds, inflamed tissue, arthritis, joint and muscle pain, dysmenorrhea, and chronic pain.

The systemic effects of extensive, prolonged heat are increased cardiac output, sweating, increased pulse rate, and decreased blood pressure. This response occurs as application of heat to a large body area increases the blood flow to that area while decreasing it to another part of the body (in effect, causing hypovolemic shock).

Effects of Applying Cold

Cold constricts peripheral blood vessels, reducing blood flow to tissue and decreasing the local release of pain-producing substances such as histamine, serotonin, and bradykinin. This action in turn reduces the formation of edema and inflammation. Decreased metabolic needs and capillary permeability, combined with increased coagulation of blood at the wound site, facilitate the control of bleeding and reduce edema formation. Cold also reduces muscle spasm, alters tissue sensitivity (producing numbness), and promotes comfort by slowing the transmission of pain stimuli. Cold, for these effects, is used after direct trauma, for dental pain, for muscle spasms, after sprains,

and to treat some chronic pain syndromes. Extensive cold produces systemic effects of increased blood pressure, shivering, and goose bumps. Although shivering is a normal body response to cold, prolonged cold may cause tissue injury.

Physiologic Considerations

The rebound phenomenon is important to the therapeutic value of heat and cold and to the safety of patients receiving such therapy. Heat produces maximum vasodilation in 20 to 30 minutes; if heat is continued beyond that time, tissue congestion and vasoconstriction occur (for unknown reasons). With cold, maximum vasoconstriction occurs when the skin reaches 15°C (60°F), then vasodilation begins.

The ability of the body to adapt to heat and cold is an important consideration in providing or teaching patients to apply heat or cold. Heat and cold skin receptors are initially strongly stimulated by sudden changes in temperature. For the first few seconds after being stimulated, the response decreases rapidly; it then decreases more slowly for the next 30 minutes, as the receptors adapt to the temperature. A hot application, even if the temperature remains constant, does not feel as warm after adaptation has taken place. Patients must be informed that increasing the temperature or lengthening the time of application can seriously damage tissues.

Applying Heat and Cold

The Nursing Process

ASSESSING FOR HEAT AND COLD APPLICATIONS

Before initiating applications of heat or cold, the nurse assesses the patient's physical and mental status, the condition of the body area to be treated with heat or cold, and the condition of the equipment to be used. Those factors that influence the tolerance of heat and cold need to be carefully considered and are the bases for the following considerations with rationale:

- How long will the heat or cold be applied? Prolonged exposure increases tolerance, and rebound effects are undesirable.
- What body part is involved? Some body areas are more sensitive to thermal changes.
- Is the skin intact? Open tissue or abraded skin is more sensitive to thermal changes.
- How large is the area? Applications of heat or cold to large areas of the body cause systemic responses and lower tolerance of temperature change.
- What is the patient's age? Infants, children, and older adults do not tolerate temperature changes as well as adults.
- What is the patient's physical condition? Patients with certain alterations in health have reduced response to or tolerance of thermal changes.

Assessing Physical and Mental Status

Assessing the patient's physical status includes a health history and physical examination. A history of cardiovascular or peripheral vascular impairment, sensory impairment, and alterations in mental status (such as confusion or decreased level of consciousness) indicates caution when using heat or cold because of the danger of tissue damage. Heat should not be applied to an open wound immediately after the trauma; during hemorrhage; over noninflammatory edema; to an acutely inflamed area, a localized malignant tumor, the testes, or the abdomen of a pregnant woman; or over metallic implants. Cold should not be used for open wounds or for patients with impaired peripheral circulation or allergy to cold.

Assessments include response to stimuli (sharp and dull), color and appearance of body tissues, circulation (pulses, blanching sign, temperature, and color), level of consciousness, and orientation.

Assessing the Area of Application

Baseline assessments are used to ensure safety and to evaluate outcomes of therapy. The risk for damage to tissues is increased if the area is traumatized or has altered integrity (assess for open lesions, blisters, wounds, edema, bleeding, or drainage) or altered circulation (assess color, temperature, pulses, and sensation). As with any assessment, bilateral body parts are compared for changes. Tissue that has decreased or absent pulses, is pale or cyanotic, and feels cold has decreased circulation. This increases the risk for injury from heat and cold.

Ongoing assessments of the application area are made to ensure patient safety and comfort. Undesired responses to heat include localized redness, blistering, and pain (symptoms of burning) as well as systemic responses of hypotension and changes in consciousness. Localized responses to prolonged cold include pallor, cyanosis, numbness, and pain.

Assessing the Condition of Equipment

The nurse is responsible for checking the equipment used and for maintaining patient safety. Included is the condition of cords, plugs, and heating or cooling elements; the presence of fluid leaks; and the distribution and constancy of temperature.

DIAGNOSING FOR HEAT AND COLD APPLICATIONS

The patient's response to the heat or cold indicates possible nursing diagnoses. Collaborative problems include potential complications—hypothermia (specify body part), hyperthermia (specify body part), impaired circulation, tissue injury, and neurovascular deficits.

The following are examples of nursing diagnoses that might be indicated:

- Risk for Altered Peripheral Tissue Perfusion related to use of ice packs to reduce edema after fractured left tibia and known decreased peripheral circulation
- Anxiety related to lack of knowledge about treatment of infected wound on right upper arm with hot soaks
- Risk for Infection related to daily débridement of lacerations of left hand followed by hot soaks
- Risk for Injury related to decreased thermal perception and the application of a heat lamp to legs every 4 hours
- Pain related to thrombophlebitis of left lower leg requiring use of aquathermia heating pad.

PLANNING: EXPECTED OUTCOMES OF APPLYING HEAT AND COLD

Heat and cold are used for a wide variety of therapeutic purposes that are an essential part of planning individualized care and form the basis for patient outcomes. When applications of heat or cold are part of a plan of care, the following outcomes are appropriate (specific outcomes should be chosen based on the purpose of the application). The patient will achieve the following:

- Verbalize increased comfort, as evidenced by decreased muscle spasms, increased ability to rest, decreased local inflammation, and decreased edema
- Have evidence of wound healing
- Verbalize and demonstrate safe hot or cold application

IMPLEMENTING HEAT AND COLD APPLICATIONS

Heat and cold are applied by both moist and dry applications, using many forms and methods. The prescription for the heat application should include the type of application, the body area to be treated, and the frequency and length of time for the applications.

Patient Teaching

As with any other procedure, the nurse explains the purpose and steps of the application and the sensations that will be experienced. In the hospital, provide a timer or clock and have the call light in reach. In the home, teach the patient or family member to check the equipment each time to ensure that it is in good working order; to avoid lying or leaning on the equipment; to cover the heating device with a protective cloth; to apply heat only for the prescribed time period; and to report any changes in sensation or discomfort to the healthcare provider.

Applying Heat

Heat is applied by both dry and moist methods. Hot water bottles, electric heating pads, aquathermia pads, or chemical heat packs provide local heat by conduction (see Procedure 37-4). Dry heat by radiation is provided by heat lamps or heat cradles. Moist heat by conduction is provided by hot compresses or packs, sitz baths, or soaks.

PROCEDURE 37-4

Applying an External Heating Device

Equipment

Hot water bag
Cover for bag
Water at the appropriate temperature:
  46.1° to 51.6°C (115° to 125°F)
    for older children and
    adults

40.5° to 43.3°C (105° to 110°F)
  for infants, young children,
  elderly people, diabetic
  patients, unconscious
  patients
Bath thermometer

Aquathermia pad
Electrically controlled unit
Distilled water
Cover for pad
Gauze bandage or tape
  (to secure pad)

Action	Rationale
1. Explain the procedure to the patient.	Facilitates cooperation and provides reassurance for patient
2. Assess condition of skin where heat is to be applied.	Impaired circulation may affect sensitivity to heat. Elderly people and very young children have the least tolerance to applications of heat.
3. Assemble necessary equipment, and close door or curtain if privacy is desired.	Organization facilitates performance of task.
4. Wash your hands.	Handwashing deters the spread of microorganisms.

Hot Water Bag

Action	Rationale
5. Check temperature of water with bath thermometer or test on inner wrist. Rinse bag with water, empty, and then fill.	This provides for application of heat within the acceptable range for individual. Rinsing bag with warm water warms the rubber.
6. Fill hot water bag one-half to two-thirds full.	Hot water bottle molds more easily to area and puts less pressure on site.
7. Expel remaining air from bag in one of two ways: Place the bag on a flat surface, permit the water to come to the opening, and then close the bag; or, hold the bag up, twist the unfilled portion to remove the air, and then close the bag. Fasten top securely. Check for leaks.	Air reduces pliability of bag. Securing the top prevents leakage of water and discomfort for patient.
8. Cover bag with towel or other protector, and apply hot water bottle to prescribed area.	Protects skin from direct contact with rubber. Heat travels by conduction from one object to another.
9. Assess condition of skin and patient's response to heat at frequent intervals. Do not exceed prescribed length of time for application of heat. Remove hot water bag if excessive swelling, redness, or pain occurs, and report to physician.	Maximum therapeutic effects from application of heat occur within 20 to 30 minutes. Extended use of heat (beyond 45 minutes) results in tissue congestion and vasoconstriction. This *rebound phenomenon* results in increased risk to patient of burns from application of heat.
10. After removal, record patient's response and dispose of equipment appropriately.	Provides for accurate documentation of procedure
11. Wash your hands.	Handwashing deters the spread of microorganisms.

Aquathermia Pad

Action	Rationale
12. Check that distilled water is at appropriate level. Use key to adjust temperature at 40.6°C (105°F) if it has not already been preset. Plug in unit, and warm pad before use.	Water temperature is regulated by key. Presetting the temperature eliminates risk of patient adjusting the temperature.

(continued)

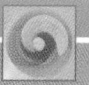

PROCEDURE 37-4

Applying an External Heating Device (Continued)

13. Cover pad with pillowcase or other protector, and apply to prescribed area. Do not allow patient to lie on pad if applying to back. Patient should assume prone position and place aquathermia pad on back.

Protects skin from direct contact with rubber or source of heat. Pressure reduces dissipation of heat.

14. Secure with gauze bandage or tape. Never use safety pins to hold pad in place.

Hold pad in position on patient. Pins may puncture and damage the pad.

15. Same as actions 9 to 11.

Same as actions 9 to 11.

Dry Heat

Hot Water Bags or Bottles

Hot water bags have disadvantages: they may leak, their weight often makes them uncomfortable, and there is a danger of burns from improper use. They are, however, relatively easy and inexpensive to use (see Procedure 37-4).

Electric Heating Pads

The electric heating pad can be used to apply dry heat locally. It is easy to apply, relatively safe to use, and provides constant and even heat. Improper use can, however, result in injury. The following are recommended techniques for using an electric heating pad:

- Avoid pins to secure a heating pad. There is a danger of electric shock if a pin touches a wire.
- Place a covering over the pad, preferably one that is moisture proof. Prevent wet and moist conditions around the pad. Short-circuiting the heating element may cause an electric shock to occur. The heat pad should not be covered too heavily. Heat may accumulate and burn the patient when it cannot dissipate normally from the pad.
- Place a heating pad anteriorly or laterally to, not under, the body part. If the heating pad is between the patient and the mattress, there may be inadequate heat dissipation. This could cause the patient or bed linens to be burned.
- Use a heating pad with a selector switch that cannot be turned up beyond a safe temperature. After heat has been applied and a certain amount of adaptation of heat receptors takes place, the patient often increases the heat when the switch is not permanently preset because the pad does not seem sufficiently warm. Many people have been burned by turning up the heat in an electric pad because they thought that the pad was too cool.
- Assess the skin at regular intervals for the effects of excessive exposure to heat.
- Be sure to check agency protocol for use of heating pads; a release form may need to be signed.

Aquathermia Pads

Aquathermia (Aqua-K) pads are commonly used in healthcare agencies for various health problems, including back pain, muscle spasms, thrombophlebitis, and mild inflammation. These devices are safer than a heating pad but still must be checked carefully. Guidelines for using aquathermia pads are as follows (see also Procedure 37-4):

- The temperature setting is usually set and locked before application.
- If the distilled water in the reservoir runs low, more is added at the top of the control unit. Tap water is not used. Fill two thirds of the control unit. Tighten the cap and then loosen it one-quarter turn to allow heat expansion.
- Place the unit above the patient so that gravity will help make the water flow.
- Plug in the unit and let it warm for 2 minutes, making sure that the temperature does not exceed 40.6°C (105°F).
- An application should last only 20 to 30 minutes.
- Assess the patient's skin frequently.

Heat Lamps

Heat lamps provide dry heat to increase circulation to a small area, such as a pressure ulcer. They are available with either infrared or regular 40- to 60-watt bulbs. The lamps (often gooseneck type) are placed 46 to 76 cm (18 to 30 inches) from the area to be treated and applied for 15 to 20 minutes. Precautions for use are as follows:

- Clean and dry the area before the treatment to prevent burning.
- Do not cover the lamp or place it under bedclothes.
- Assess skin exposed to heat every 5 minutes.

Heat Cradles

A heat cradle is a metal half-circle frame that encloses the body part to be treated with heat. A series of 25-watt bulbs, 16 to 18 inches (41 to 46 cm) from the patient, provides heat over a larger area. The cradle may be covered with a sheet. Treatments usually last for 15 minutes.

Precautions should be taken to prevent burning, as for a heat lamp.

Hot Packs

Commercial hot packs provide a specified amount of dry heat for a specific period. Instructions on the package describe how to activate the pack, either by striking it on a firm surface or by squeezing or kneading it.

Moist Heat

Warm Moist Compresses

Sterile warm moist compresses are used on wounds to promote circulation and wound healing (especially if infected) and to reduce edema. To maintain heat—because moist heat evaporates and cools rapidly—the compresses must be changed frequently and covered with a heating agent (hot water bottle, heating pad, Aqua-K pad) or plastic wrap. Procedure 37-5 describes the application of warm sterile compresses to an open wound.

Sitz Baths

As a mean of applying tepid or hot water to the pelvic or rectal area, patients are placed in a tub filled with sufficient water to reach the umbilicus. These baths are called sitz baths. Special tubs and chairs or basins that fit onto the toilet seat are available. They are designed so that the patient's buttocks fit into a rather deep seat that is filled with water of the desired temperature; the legs and feet remain out of the water. The basins are disposable and economical for home or healthcare agency use. A regular bathtub is not as satisfactory for a sitz bath because the heat causes generalized vasodilation, altering the effect desired.

The following are recommended techniques for administering a sitz bath:

- Test the water on a sitz bath with a thermometer before the patient enters the tub. If the purpose of the sitz bath is to apply heat, water at a temperature of 34° to 37°C (109° to 115°F) for 15 minutes produces relaxation of the parts involved after a short initial period of contraction. Warm water should not be used if considerable congestion is already present.
- If the purpose of the sitz bath is to produce relaxation or to help to promote healing in a wound by cleaning it of discharge and debris, water at a temperature of 34° to 37°C (93° to 99°F) is used. Check agency protocols for the correct temperature.
- Assist the patient into the tub and position him or her properly. The patient should be able to sit in the basin or tub with his or her feet flat on the floor. There should be no pressure on the sacrum or thighs.
- Wrap a blanket around the shoulders to protect the patient from feeling chilly and from exposure.
- Observe the patient closely for signs of weakness and fatigue. Discontinue the bath if he or she exhibits faintness, pallor, a rapid pulse rate, or nausea.
- Test the water in the tub several times, and keep it at the desired temperature. Additional hot water may be added by pouring it slowly from a pitcher or by

opening the hot water faucet a little bit. The water should be agitated by stirring it as hot water is added to prevent burning the patient.
- Do not leave the patient alone unless it is safe to do so.
- Help the patient out of the tub when the bath is completed. A sitz bath should take 15 to 30 minutes. Help the patient dry, and cover him or her adequately.

Warm Soaks

The immersion of a body area into warm water or a medicated solution is called a *soak*. The purposes of soaks vary: to increase blood supply to a locally infected area; to aid in cleaning large, sloughing wounds, such as burns; to improve circulation; and to apply medication to a locally infected area. A soak has the added advantage of making manipulation of a painful area much easier because the body part is buoyed up by the weight of water it displaces. General guidelines for administering a warm soak include the following:

- If a soak is prescribed for a large wound, such as might cover an entire arm or lower leg or even an area of the torso, a compromise with sterile technique is usually made. The container into which the body area is placed is sterilized before use if possible; if not, the container should be cleaned scrupulously. Tap water may be used for soaks because it is accepted as being free from pathogens.
- Unless the temperature of the soak is prescribed otherwise, a range of 40.5° to 43°C (105° to 109°F) is considered physiologically effective and comfortable for the patient.
- The container holding the fluid should be positioned so that the part to be immersed is comfortable and the patient is in good body alignment.
- During the treatment, which usually takes 15 to 20 minutes per soak, the temperature should be kept as constant as possible. This may be done by discarding some of the fluid every 5 minutes and replacing it or by adding solutions at a higher temperature while agitating the water. The patient must remove the extremity from the soak while replacing or adding fluids.

Applying Cold

Dry Cold

Ice Bags

Ice bags have essentially the same disadvantages as hot water bags, but they are also a relatively easy and inexpensive way to apply cold to an area. The following are recommendations for the use of an ice bag:

- Fill the bag with small pieces of ice to about two-thirds full. This makes the bag light in weight. Ice chips, rather than cubes, make it easier to mold the bag to a body part.
- Remove air from the ice bag in the same manner as removing air from a hot water bag.

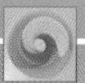

PROCEDURE 37-5

Applying Warm Sterile Compresses to an Open Wound

Equipment

Prescribed solution (warmed to about 40° to 43°C [105° to 110°F])
Sterile container for solution
Sterile gauze dressings or compresses

Sterile gloves
Clean disposable gloves
Waterproof pad
Dry bath towel
Bath blanket

Tape or ties
Aquathermia or external heating device (optional)
Sterile bath thermometer (if available, to check temperature of solution)

Action	Rationale
1. Assess patient for any circulatory impairment to area where compress is to be applied (numbness, tingling, impairment in temperature sensation, or cyanosis).	Circulatory impairment may interfere with patient's ability to perceive heat and place him or her at risk of injury from the application of heat.
2. Check physician's order for warm compresses. Explain procedure to patient.	An explanation encourages patient cooperation and reduces apprehension.
3. Gather equipment.	Provides for organized approach to task
4. Wash your hands.	Handwashing deters spread of microorganisms.
5. Close door or curtain. Use bath blanket as needed when exposing area for application of warm compresses. Position waterproof pad under patient.	Provides for privacy and warmth
6. Assist patient to comfortable position that provides easy access to area.	Allows comfort and ease of application of compresses
7. Place opened, cuffed plastic bag near working area.	Soiled dressings may be placed in disposal bag without contaminating outside surfaces of bag.
8. Prepare aquathermia pad or external heating device (optional).	External heating device allows compress to retain heat for longer interval.
9. Using sterile technique, open dressings, and warmed solution. Pour solution into sterile container, and carefully drop gauze for compresses into sterile solution.	Sterile technique is used for warm moist compresses to an open wound.
10. Don clean disposable glove, and remove any dressing carefully. Discard dressing in disposable plastic bag. Pull off soiled glove inside out, and drop it in bag.	Prevents spread of microorganisms by contaminated dressings
11. Assess wound healing or presence of infection.	Document condition of wound before application of compress.
12. Don sterile gloves.	Gloves maintain surgical asepsis.
13. Retrieve sterile compress from warmed solution, and squeeze moisture from it. Apply carefully, and gently mold around wound. Be alert for patient's response to heat.	Excess moisture may contaminate surrounding area and is uncomfortable for patient. Molding compress to skin promotes retention of warmth around wound site.
14. Cover the gauze compresses with dry bath towel, and secure in place if necessary.	Towel provides additional insulation.
15. Apply aquathermia pad or external heating device over towel (optional).	Controls temperature and extends therapeutic effect of compress.
16. Monitor condition of skin and patient's response to warm compress at frequent intervals.	Impaired circulation may affect sensitivity to heat.

(continued)

PROCEDURE 37-5

Applying Warm Sterile Compresses to an Open Wound (Continued)

17. After 30 minutes (or time ordered by physician), remove warm compress. Carefully observe condition of skin around wound and patient's response to application of heat.

Maximum therapeutic effects of heat occur within 20 to 30 minutes. Extended use of heat (beyond 45 minutes) results in tissue congestion and vasoconstriction. This *rebound phenomenon* results in increased risk to patient of burns from application of heat.

18. Apply sterile dressing to wound (see Procedure 37-1).

Dressing protects wound from microorganisms in environment.

19. Dispose of equipment appropriately. Wash hands.

Deters spread of microorganisms

20. Record patient's response and condition of wound and surrounding skin area.

Provides for accurate documentation of procedure

- After securing the cap, test the ice bag for leaks and wipe off excess moisture.
- Place a cover on the ice bag to provide comfort and to absorb moisture that may accumulate on the outside of the bag.
- Apply an ice bag for 30 minutes and then remove it for about an hour before reapplying it. This technique prevents the effects of prolonged exposure to cold.
- In an emergency in the home setting, a sack of frozen vegetables (such as peas) makes a good substitute for an ice bag.

Cold Packs

Commercially prepared ice packs are available in many healthcare agencies and may be purchased commercially. These bags are sealed containers filled with a nontoxic substance. The bags are frozen in the freezer of a refrigerator. An advantage of these bags is that the frozen solution remains pliable and can be easily molded to fit a body part. They are covered with a ribbed cotton sleeve so that the bag can be slipped onto an extremity, or the bag can simply be placed on a body part, such as the head. Some of the bags cannot be reused.

Cooling Blankets

Body temperature may be lowered by placing the patient on a special hypothermia blanket or pad. This apparatus has coils through which refrigerated solution is circulated. (It operates much like an Aqua-K heating unit, except that the liquid is cooled instead of heated.) This method of reducing high body temperature may be used in place of a sponge bath.

Moist Cold

Cold Compresses

Moist, cold local applications are called *cold compresses*. They might be used for an injured eye, a headache,

a tooth extraction, and sometimes for hemorrhoids. The texture and thickness of the material used depend on the area to which it is to be applied. For example, eye compresses could be prepared from surgical gauze compresses, which have a small amount of cotton filling. A washcloth makes an excellent compress for the head or the face.

The material used for the application is immersed in a clean basin that contains pieces of ice and a small amount of water. The compress should be wrung thoroughly before it is applied to avoid dripping, which is uncomfortable for the patient and may also wet the bed or clothing. The compresses should be changed frequently. The application should be continued for 20 minutes and repeated every 2 to 3 hours. Ice bags or commercial devices for keeping the compresses cold decrease the frequency with which the compresses must be changed.

Alcohol or Cold Sponge Bath

Alcohol or cold sponge baths are used to reduce body temperature. Plain water may be used, but alcohol added to water makes the temperature more easy to tolerate for most patients and removes heat from skin surfaces rapidly. Cold water often produces a strong initial reactionary effect, which elevates the temperature even further. This is observed when the patient shivers and has gooseflesh.

The following techniques are recommended for administering an alcohol or cold-water sponge bath:

- Prepare a water and alcohol solution at about 29.5° to 32°C (85° to 89.6°F). If plain water is used, prepare it at a temperature of about 29.5°C (85°F), but add ice chips to bring the temperature down while bathing the patient until the water temperature reaches about 18°C (64.4°F).
- Protect the patient's bed with moisture-proof material.
- Prepare several ice bags. One ice bag is placed on the patient's head to promote comfort; others are placed

in the groin and axillary areas, where blood vessels are close to the skin surface. The ice bags help to cool the patient further.

- Cover the patient properly to prevent shivering as various parts of the body are exposed for bathing.
- Sponge the face, neck, arms, and legs for 3 to 5 minutes and back for 10 minutes. The anterior chest and abdomen are usually not sponged. Cover, but do not dry, each part as it is sponged. Evaporation of moisture on the skin helps to reduce body temperature.
- Move from one part of the body to another, and continue the bathing for 25 to 30 minutes. If the bath is short in duration, the body does not adjust to the coolness; it then reacts to conserve heat, and the patient's temperature may go even higher.
- Check the patient's color and pulse rate during the bath. If the patient becomes pale or cyanotic or if the pulse rate increases or becomes irregular, discontinue the bath.
- Pat rather than rub to dry the patient after the bath is completed. The friction of rubbing may raise body temperature.
- Check the patient's body temperature about 30 minutes after the bath to evaluate its effectiveness.

EVALUATING HEAT AND COLD APPLICATIONS

The expected outcomes of the applications of heat and cold as part of a plan of care are used to evaluate the effectiveness of the planned interventions. Although the specific outcomes depend on the purpose of the application, nursing care is considered effective if the patient is able to:

- Verbalize increased comfort
- Verbalize increased ability to rest and sleep
- Demonstrate evidence of wound healing
- Demonstrate a decrease in symptoms of inflammation and edema
- Verbalize and demonstrate safe hot and cold applications

Pressure Ulcers

A **pressure ulcer** is defined by the Agency for Health Care Policy and Research (AHCPR) as any lesion caused by unrelieved pressure that results in damage to underlying tissue (U.S. Department of Health and Human Services [USDHHS], 1994). The terms *pressure ulcer, decubitus ulcer,* and *bedsore* are synonymous. The term *decubitus* derives from a Latin word meaning lying down, although lying down does not in itself cause a decubitus ulcer, and a patient need not be bedridden to develop one. Therefore, most people prefer the term *pressure ulcer* because pressure is the most prominent underlying cause.

Pressure ulcers are one of the most common skin disruptions and are costly in terms of healthcare expenditures. The incidence in hospitalized patients is about 3.5% to 29% and in long-term care facilities, about 23%. Statistics

are not available for home care patients, but they too are at risk for pressure ulcers. When pressure ulcers occur, aggressive intervention and treatment can spare the patient unnecessary pain and discomfort, prevent further tissue deterioration, hasten wound healing, and save millions of healthcare dollars.

Pathology of Pressure Ulcer Development

Pathologic changes at a pressure ulcer site result from blood vessel collapse caused by pressure, usually from body weight. **Necrosis**, or death of cells, eventually occurs, leading to the characteristic ulcer. Two mechanisms contribute to pressure ulcer development: (1) external pressure that compresses blood vessels, and (2) friction and shearing forces that tear and injure blood vessels.

External Pressure

Pressure ulcers usually occur over bony prominences where body weight is distributed over a small area without much subcutaneous tissue to cushion damage to the skin. Common sites for pressure ulcers are illustrated in Figure 37-9. Of the susceptible areas, most pressure ulcers occur over the sacrum and coccyx, followed by the trochanter and the calcaneus (heel). One may form in as short a time as 1 to 2 hours if the person has not moved for an extended period of time.

The major predisposing factor for a pressure ulcer is pressure over an area, which results in occluded blood capillaries and poor circulation to tissues. This lack of sufficient circulation causes necrosis and ulcer formation. The skin can tolerate considerable pressure without cell death but for short periods only. Duration is more important than the amount of pressure in the formation of a pressure ulcer. Most pressure ulcers develop within 2 weeks of admission to a healthcare facility.

Friction and Shearing Forces

Friction occurs when two surfaces rub against each other. The injury resembles an abrasion and can also damage superficial blood vessels directly under the skin. A patient who lies on wrinkled sheets is likely to sustain tissue damage as a result of friction. The skin over the elbows and heels often suffers injury when patients lift and help move themselves up in bed with the use of their arms and feet. Friction burns can also occur on the back when patients are pulled or slid over sheets when moved up in bed or transferred onto a stretcher.

A **shearing force** results when one layer of tissue slides over another layer. Shearing forces are often responsible for deep pressure ulcers. The small blood vessels and capillaries in the area are stretched and may even tear, resulting in a decrease in circulation to the tissue cells under the skin. Figure 37-10 illustrates how shearing forces occur. Patients who are pulled rather than lifted when moved up in bed or from bed to chair or stretcher are at risk for injury from shearing forces. A patient who is partially sitting up in bed is susceptible when skin sticks to the sheet and underlying tissues move downward with the

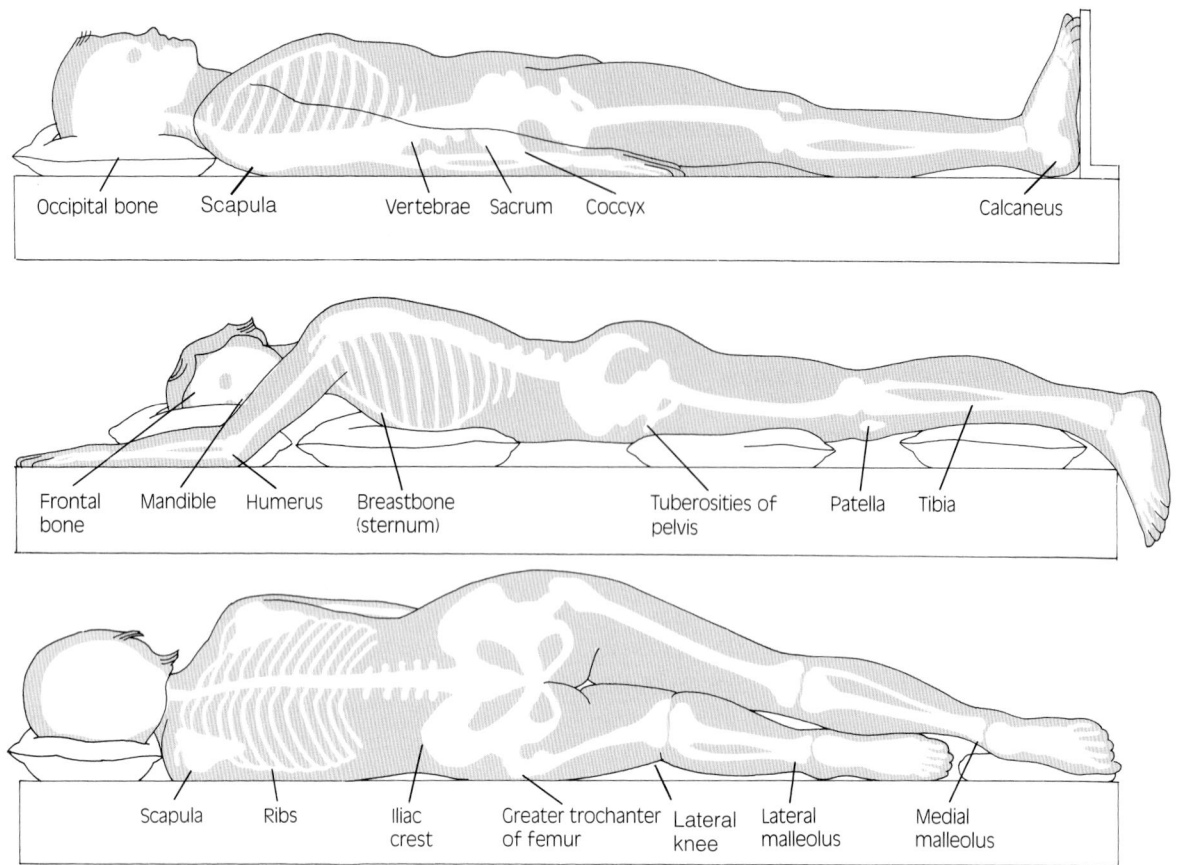

Figure 37-9
Common sites for development of pressure ulcers.

body toward the foot of the bed. This may also occur in a patient who sits in a chair but slides down.

Factors Affecting Pressure Ulcer Development

Usually, a combination of causes, in addition to pressure, friction, and shearing, contribute to ulcer development. These include mobility and immobility, nutrition and hydration, skin moisture, mental status, and age.

Mobility and Immobility

Someone who sits or lies most of the time is at risk for a pressure ulcer because immobility causes prolonged pressure on body areas. Ambulatory people do not develop this injury because no part of the body suffers from prolonged pressure. When asleep, well people tend to move about in bed freely. Unconscious and paralyzed patients are subject to pressure ulcers if allowed to remain in any one position. So too are emotionally depressed people who do not ordinarily move much. Additional factors that cause immobility and may result in this serious problem are lengthy surgery and the use of tranquilizers or sedatives.

Nutrition and Hydration

Malnutrition predisposes a person to pressure ulcer formation because poorly nourished cells are easily damaged. For example, vitamin C deficiency causes capillaries

to become fragile, with resultant poor circulation to the area. Protein deficiency leading to a negative nitrogen balance, electrolyte imbalances, and insufficient caloric intake also predisposes the skin to injury. The condition of the teeth or fit of dentures may also exacerbate the problem of inadequate dietary intake. Dehydration as well as edema can interfere with circulation and subsequent cell nourishment.

Moisture on the Skin

Prolonged moisture on the skin reduces the skin's resistance to trauma. Warmth increases the cells' demands for oxygen. Therefore, moisture and warmth eventually lead to cell destruction, especially when pressure is present. When skin is damp, less friction is required to blister and abrade skin. It is believed that the moisture associated with urinary incontinence increases the risk for skin damage more than is accounted for by the chemical irritation from the ammonia in the urine. If personal hygiene is poor, the skin contains many organisms that thrive in the warm, moist environment; this increases the risk for a pressure ulcer that will become infected.

Mental Status

The more alert an individual is, the more likely he or she is to protect skin integrity by relieving pressure periodically and maintaining adequate skin hygiene. Apathy, confu-

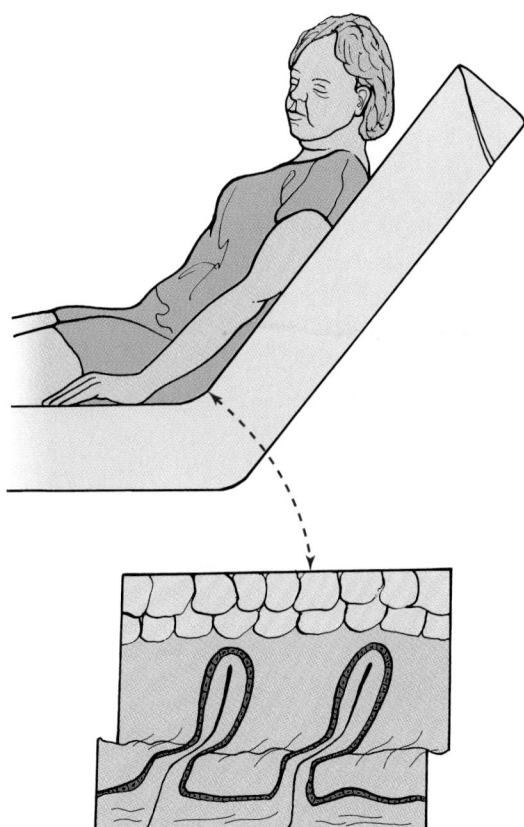

Figure 37-10
Shearing force can occur when a patient is moved carelessly or slides down in bed. Friction causes resistance on the surface layers of the skin, while underlying tissue moves in the direction of the body movement. Capillaries in underlying tissue are stretched and torn in pressure areas by opposing forces of movements.

sion, or a comatose state can diminish these self-care abilities and increase the likelihood of skin breakdown.

Age

Older people are at a greater risk for pressure ulcers because the aging skin is more susceptible to injury. The box, Focus on the Older Adult, outlines the risk factors that predispose older adults to pressure ulcers. Chronic and debilitating diseases, more common in this age group, may adversely affect skin nourishment. Destruction of tissues that leads to pressure ulcers becomes relatively easy when illness causes an elevated temperature and normal function of body cells is altered in any way.

Pressure Ulcer Staging

Appropriate intervention depends on early recognition of the stage of development of the pressure ulcer. To improve the quality of care and save healthcare dollars, the USDHHS (1994) addressed the treatment of pressure ulcers. Differentiation of the four stages and a visual representation of differences among the stages are presented in Table 37-3.

The first sign that a pressure ulcer may be developing is blanching (becoming pale and white) of the skin over the

area under pressure. Insufficient blood circulation makes the skin appear paler than areas where circulation is adequate. This local anemia resulting from poor circulation is called **ischemia.**

When pressure is relieved, ischemia is rapidly followed by *hyperemia.* The area appears red and feels warm. **Reactive hyperemia** is the occurrence of a blanchable reddening of the skin when pressure is removed. The body literally floods the area with blood to nourish and remove wastes from the cells. Reactive hyperemia is *not* a stage I pressure ulcer. With reactive hyperemia, after a patient who has been lying supine for 2 hours is repositioned onto the side, any reddened area should fade within 1 to $1\frac{1}{2}$ hours. In patients with darkly pigmented skin, hyperemia may best be detected by touch. The skin feels warm, or some change in color is detected. A stage II pressure ulcer is superficial and may present as a blister or abrasion. Damage to the subcutaneous tissue indicates a stage III lesion, and the extensive destruction associated with full-thickness skin loss is categorized as a stage IV pressure ulcer. This staging process has several limitations. If eschar is present, it may be difficult to stage a pressure ulcer. **Eschar** is a thick, leathery scab or dry crust that is necrotic and must be removed before staging can accurately be determined. Patients with casts, orthopedic devices, or support stockings require routine assessment of areas where inadequate circulation may be a contributing factor to development of a pressure ulcer.

The Nursing Process

ASSESSING THE RISK FOR OR ACTUAL PRESSURE ULCERS

Most pressure ulcers in adults can be prevented. It is a nursing priority to perform a comprehensive assessment in all settings and identify patients at risk, predisposing factors, or actual pressure ulcers.

All assessment data need to be reassessed regularly to ensure that patients receive healthcare interventions that prolong and enhance the quality of their life.

Nursing History

The nursing history includes questions about the appearance of the skin and patient activities that may contribute to altered skin integrity. It is often a combination of risk factors that places the patient at greatest risk for a pressure ulcer.

The nurse questions the patient and family caregiver about recent changes in the appearance or condition of the skin and any skin care regimens. It is important to assess activity status, nutritional state, changes in elimination patterns, and presence of pain associated with altered skin integrity. Nurses have long recognized that patients with a pressure ulcer experience pain. It is important to assess whether dressing changes, position in bed or in a chair, or movement elicit any subjective or objective expressions of pain. Even if pain is never verbalized or expressed, the nurse

Table 37-3
Comparison of Stages of Pressure Ulcers

Stage I

Nonblanchable erythema of intact skin: the heralding lesion of skin ulceration. Note: Reactive hyperemia can be present for ½ to ¾ as long as the pressure occluded blood flow to the area. This should not be confused with a stage I pressure ulcer.

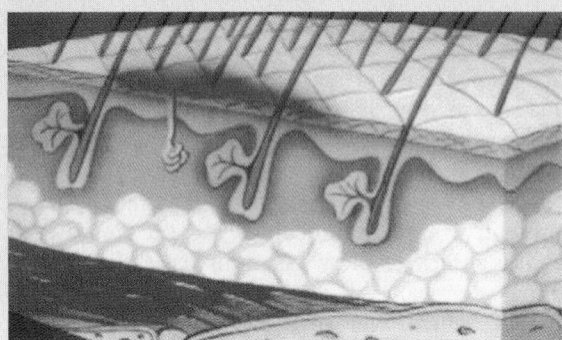

Pressure-relieving measures:
- Frequent turning
- Pressure-relieving devices
- Positioning

Stage III

Full-thickness skin loss involving damage or necrosis of subcutaneous tissue that may extend down to, but not through, underlying fascia. The ulcer presents clinically as a deep crater with or without undermining of adjacent tissue.

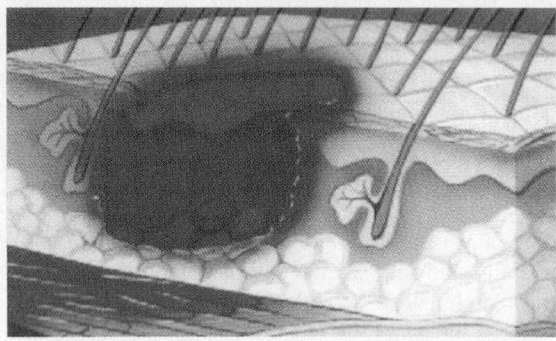

Requires débridement, which can be accomplished by one of the following:
- Wet-to-dry dressings
- Surgical intervention
- Proteolytic enzymes

Stage II

Partial-thickness skin loss involving epidermis and/or dermis. The ulcer is superficial and presents clinically as an abrasion, blister, or shallow crater.

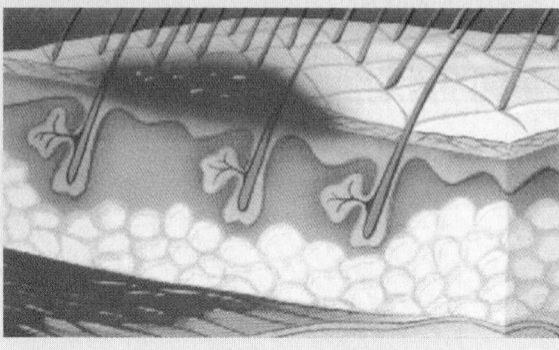

Maintenance of a moist healing environment:
- Saline or
- Occlusive dressing that promotes natural healing but prevents formation of a scar

Stage IV

Full-thickness skin loss with extensive destruction, tissue necrosis, or damage to muscle, bone, or supporting structures (eg, tendon or joint capsule). Sinus tracts may also be associated with stage IV ulcers.

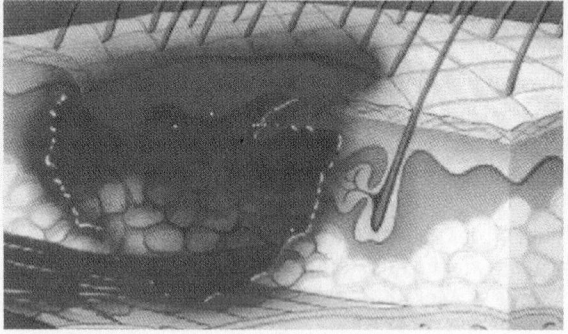

Wounds are treated in the following manner:
- Covered with nonadherent dressing
- Changed every 8–12 hours
- May require skin grafts

From U.S. Department of Health and Human Services. Agency for Health Care Policy and Research. (1992). *Pressure ulcers in adults: Prediction and prevention.* Rockville, MD: DHHS, and Porth, C. (1994). *Pathophysiology: Concepts of altered health states.* Philadelphia: JB Lippincott.

should assume that pain is a definite possibility and focus on comfort needs. Severe pain may actually slow the healing process by interfering with the immune system response (O'Hanlon-Nichols, 1995). Specific nursing assessments to validate the pain experience are included in Chapter 40.

Patients with pressure ulcers are often cared for in the home. It is imperative that the nurse assess the educational needs of the patient and family and their ability to understand, participate in, and adhere to a treatment regimen. Assessment should include the following areas:

- Mental status, learning ability, and communication skills
- Social support systems
- Goals, values, and lifestyle
- Culture and ethnicity
- Stressors
- Personal strengths and resources

The accompanying Focused Assessment Guide provides additional suggestions for gathering a nursing history.

Physical Assessment

Physical assessment of the skin is included as part of the initial database collection (skin assessment is described in Chap. 25). All at-risk patients should have a systematic skin inspection, including bony prominences, at least once a day. Weekly inspections are recommended by the AHCPR to monitor the progress and evaluate the effectiveness of treatment of a documented ulcer, whatever the setting. Documentation of these assessments ensures continuity of care and becomes the foundation for the skin care plan. All caregivers in the home or healthcare agency need to be aware of assessment criteria.

According to the AHCPR Clinical Practice Guideline (USDHHS, 1994), skin assessment for a pressure ulcer specifically includes inspection of the following:

- Location of any lesion or ulcer
- Estimation of the stage
- Dimensions of the ulcer: length, width, depth
- Presence of any abnormal pathways in the wound:
  Sinus tract—a cavity or channel underneath the wound that has the potential for infection
  Tunneling—a passageway or opening that may be visible at skin level, but with most of the tunnel under the surface of the skin
  Undermining—areas of tissue destruction underneath intact skin along wound margins
  Visible *necrotic tissue* (tissue that has died); necrotic tissue that is in the process of separating from viable portions of the body is referred to as *slough*.
- Presence of an exudate
- Presence or absence of granulation tissue
- Visible evidence of **epithelialization**

Figure 37-11 illustrates the various types of tissue a nurse may observe during assessment of a wound, and the accompanying box describes pressure ulcer measurement.

Assessing Mobility

Assessing a patient's mobility status includes evaluating the patient's ability to move, turn, and reposition the body. A patient who is confined to bed or a chair or has limited range of motion is at greater risk for pressure ulcer. This assessment of activity status is done upon admission to the healthcare facility or during the initial home care interview. The nurse also observes any assistive devices that the patient uses to maintain a level of mobility and activity. Additional suggestions for gathering information about mobility are described in Chapter 38.

Assessing Nutritional Status

The importance of sound nutrition in the prevention and treatment of a pressure ulcer is well established. Older adults, in particular, need adequate nutrition for optimal health and wound healing. Nutritional assessment is described in Chapter 41. The AHCPR guidelines (USDHHS, 1994) suggest the following laboratory criteria as assessment data indicating that a patient is nutritionally at risk:

- Albumin level < 3.5 mg/dL (normal, 3.5–5 mg/dL)
- Total lymphocyte count < 1800/mm³ (normal, 1000–4000/mm³)
- Body weight decrease of more than 15%

Assessing Moisture and Incontinence

Many studies have documented that moisture makes the skin more susceptible to injury. Whether the moisture is from perspiration, wound drainage, urine, or stool, the skin is compromised. Moisture can create an environment in which microorganisms can multiply and the skin is more likely to blister, suffer abrasions, and become *macerated* (softening or disintegration of the skin in response to moisture). Chapter 42 has additional assessment information related to incontinence.

Assessment Forms

An aggressive approach to prevent a pressure ulcer or manage the care of a patient who already has impaired skin integrity begins with a risk assessment form, which must be simple to use, reliable, and cost-effective. The Norton scale and the Braden scale are two assessment forms often used (see the accompanying box). Neither tool is ideal, but both can efficiently and systematically identify patients at high risk for a pressure ulcer.

Agencies use different approaches after a patient at risk has been identified. Many healthcare facilities use a special pressure ulcer assessment form. (The sample is included in the AHCPR guideline.) Signs placed outside the room or attached to medical records indicate the need for ongoing assessment and special attention to skin integrity.

DIAGNOSING FOR PRESSURE ULCERS

Impaired Skin Integrity is a common NANDA nursing diagnosis for patients with a pressure ulcer. The stage of the pressure ulcer, however, should be a factor in determining the nursing diagnosis. Stage I and II pressure ulcers have

FOCUSED ASSESSMENT GUIDE

Skin Integrity

Factors to Assess	Questions and Approaches
• Overall appearance of skin	Are there any areas of your skin that are discolored?
	Is there any difference in skin temperature anywhere on your body?
	How does your skin feel in relation to moisture? Dry? Clammy? Oily?
	Is this a change from normal?
	Are there any areas on your body where your skin seems paper-thin?
	Have you noticed any swelling in your feet? Around your ankles? In your fingers?
	Tell me about your bathing routine.
	Are there any skin products that you routinely use? Are there any that you are unable to tolerate? What happens?
• Recent changes in skin condition	Have you noticed any sores anywhere on your body?
	Do you ever notice redness over a bony area when you stay in one position for a while?
	Does the reddened area disappear after a short time?
	Is the skin broken?
	Do you have any drainage from this area?
	Has the sore changed in size?
• Contributing factors	
• Activity/Mobility	Do you need assistance to walk and move?
	Are you confined to a chair? Bed?
	Can you change your position whenever you want?
	Specifically, what kind of help do you need?
• Nutrition	Have you gained weight recently? Lost weight recently?
	Do you eat well-balanced meals?
	Do you drink adequate amounts of fluid every day?
	Do you take any vitamins? Food supplements?
	Has the doctor ever told you that you were anemic?
	Do you prepare your own meals?
	Do you need help to eat?
	Do you wear dentures? Do they fit?
	Do you have any difficulty swallowing?
• Pain	If you have a sore anywhere, is it painful?
	Does anything help relieve the pain?
	Are you currently taking any medication for pain?
• Elimination	Have you noticed any changes in your usual bowel and bladder patterns? Any problems with incontinence?
	Have you ever used any briefs or pads to help with an incontinence problem?

superficial skin damage; for them, Impaired Skin Integrity is the appropriate choice. Stage III and IV pressure ulcers include full-thickness skin loss and damage to underlying tissue; therefore, the diagnosis Impaired Tissue Integrity is more appropriate.

Nursing diagnoses pertaining to the presence of pressure ulcers include the following:

- Risk for Impaired Skin Integrity
- Risk for Impaired Tissue Integrity

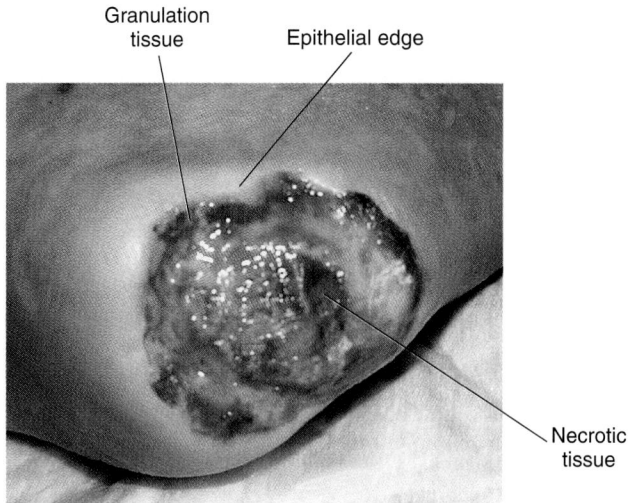

Figure 37-11
A chronic wound with various types of wound surface tissue.

- Risk for Infection
- Impaired Bed Mobility
- Altered Tissue Perfusion
- Pain
- Altered Nutrition: Less than body requirements

Measurement of a Pressure Ulcer

In addition to assessing location, stage, drainage, and types of tissue present in the wound, it is imperative that nurses accurately and consistently measure a pressure ulcer. Effective treatment is dependent on precise assessments. The nurse should document the following:

Size of the Wound

- Draw the shape and describe it.
- Measure the length, width, and diameter (if circular).

Depth of the Wound

- Moisten a sterile swab with saline and insert it gently into the wound at a 90-degree angle with the tip down.
- Mark the point on the swab that is even with the surrounding skin surface.
- Remove the swab and measure the depth with a ruler.

Presence of Undermining, Tunneling, or Sinus Tract

- Insert a saline-moistened sterile swab under the wound edge.
- Apply gentle pressure and assess for any abnormal pathways.
- *Never use force when probing with the swab.*
- Measure the location and depth of penetration.

PLANNING: EXPECTED OUTCOMES FOR PREVENTING OR CARING FOR PRESSURE ULCERS

Whenever nurses care for patients who have or are at risk for impaired skin integrity, nursing measures support the following patient outcomes. The patient will achieve the following:

- Participate in the prescribed treatment regimen to promote wound healing
- Demonstrate progressive healing of the pressure ulcer
- Demonstrate increase in body weight and muscle size
- Remain free of infection at the site of the pressure ulcer
- Develop no new areas of skin breakdown
- Demonstrate self-care measures necessary to prevent development of a pressure ulcer (if able)

An additional expected outcome may be appropriate for family members who function as the primary caregivers for a person at risk for a pressure ulcer:

- Family members will demonstrate care measures necessary to prevent development of a pressure ulcer.

IMPLEMENTING TO PREVENT OR CARE FOR PRESSURE ULCERS

Preventing Pressure Ulcers

Many pressure ulcers can be prevented, but some high-risk individuals may develop pressure ulcers that continue to worsen despite aggressive nursing intervention. The AHCPR (USDHHS, 1992) recommends a series of interventions to prevent injury to the skin and promote optimal health. These protocols, displayed in the accompanying Guidelines for Nursing Care, also provide the basis for an educational program that promotes ongoing implementation of preventive measures by caregivers in the home.

Protecting the Skin From External Mechanical Forces

To protect patients at risk from the adverse effects of pressure, implement an every-2-hour turning schedule in the healthcare setting. Encourage home care patients and caregivers to change body position at least every 2 hours when seated in a chair or bedridden (a written schedule or kitchen timer may be helpful) Some clinicians believe that older patients have less tissue tolerance and should be repositioned more frequently if redness on bony prominences is noted (Maklebust, 1995). The oblique position is an alternative to the side-lying position and results in significantly less pressure on the trochanter area.

Positioning devices such as pillows or foam wedges can prove helpful to keep body weight off bony prominences. For example, a standard pillow placed under the calves effectively raises the heels off the bed and alleviates pressure. Ring cushions, or "donuts," were previously thought to protect reddened areas from additional pressure; however, *donut-type devices cause increased venous pressure and should never be used.* The effects of

Examples of Pressure Ulcer Risk Assessment Tools

Braden Scale

Assess the patient for each category, assign a score, and total the score. A score of 16 or less is considered high risk for pressure ulcer development.

Sensory Perception	Moisture	Activity	Mobility	Nutrition	Friction and Shear
No impairment—4	Rarely moist—4	Walks frequently—4	No limitations—4	Excellent—4	No apparent problem—3
Slightly limited—3	Occasionally moist—3	Walks occasionally—3	Slightly limited—3	Adequate—3	Potential problem—2
Very limited—2	Moist—2	Chairfast—2	Very limited—2	Probably inadequate—2	Problem—1
Completely limited—1	Constantly moist—1	Bedfast—1	Immobile—1	Very poor—1	
Total: _____	Total: _____	Total: _____	Total: _____	Total: _____	Total: _____

Grand total: _____

Norton Scale

A score of 14 or less indicates risk for pressure ulcers; a score under 12 indicates high risk.

Physical Condition	Mental Condition	Activity	Mobility	Continence
Good—4	Alert—4	Walks—4	Full—4	Good—4
Fair—3	Apathetic—3	Walks with help—3	Slightly limited—3	Occasional incontinence—3
Poor—2	Confused—2	Sits in chair—2	Very limited—2	Frequent incontinence—2
Very poor—1	Stuporous—1	Remains in bed—1	Immobile—1	Urine & fecal incontinence—1
Total: _____	Total: _____	Total: _____	Total: _____	Total: _____

Grand total: _____

shearing force can be minimized by limiting the amount of time the head of the bed is elevated (when possible). Positioning devices and techniques maintain posture and distribute weight evenly for patients in a chair. Using a trapeze or bed linen to assist transfer and position changes prevents friction on the skin. Pressure-relieving support surfaces, such as a foam overlay, static flotation mattress, alternating air mattress, low-air-loss bed, and air-fluidized bed, are available, but there is disagreement about which are most appropriate for a patient at risk. The type of support surface used must be individualized to the patient's needs. Because none of these devices totally relieves pressure, position changes at regular intervals must still be done.

Teaching Patients and Families About Prevention

Teaching patients and caregivers how to prevent pressure ulcers requires a comprehensive, organized educational effort. Initially, the healthcare provider presents basic information that explains the terminology, identifies risk factors, explains where and how pressure ulcers develop, and describes various prevention strategies and options. Illustrated instructions written at the level of the learner are a valuable resource. The AHCPR's booklet *Patient Guide for Preventing Pressure Ulcers* outlines specific care measures related to each risk factor and emphasizes the importance of personal involvement in care and treatment decisions; it is available for distribution to consumers. The previously mentioned protocols listed in the Guidelines for Nursing Care box also serve as a model for development of a teaching plan that incorporates basic principles and targets individuals at risk. As new information becomes available, education for prevention of pressure ulcers should be updated.

Pressure Ulcer Care

Despite prevention tactics, pressure ulcers may develop in certain high-risk patients. Aggressive treatment measures by the nurse or caregiver are the key to effective manage-

Guidelines for Nursing Care

Preventing Pressure Ulcers

Action	Rationale
Assess the skin of patients at risk on a daily basis. Pay particular attention to bony prominences.	Careful documentation of skin inspection is essential for formulating and evaluating an individualized plan of care.
Cleanse the skin routinely and whenever any soiling occurs. Use a mild cleansing agent, minimal friction, and avoid hot water.	Frequent cleansing limits exposure to environmental contaminants and the chemical irritants found in body waste products. Water that is just slightly warm causes less trauma to fragile skin and a mild cleansing product is less drying to the skin.
Maintain higher humidity in the environment and use skin moisturizers for dry skin.	Many older patients prefer overheated settings that promote dry skin. Humidification is effective in controlling dry skin. Moisturizers control the manifestations of dry skin and help to keep the skin intact.
Avoid massage over bony prominences.	Massage, in general, promotes relaxation, but massage over bony prominences may worsen soft tissue damage already present.
Protect the skin from moisture associated with episodes of incontinence or exposure to wound drainage.	Research indicates that the moisture associated with incontinence is responsible for skin breakdown. Underpads and briefs that absorb moisture and present a quick-drying surface to the skin can be used to keep the skin drier.
Minimize skin injury from friction and shearing forces by using proper positioning, turning, and transferring techniques. Use lubricants, protective films, dressings, and padding to diminish the effects of friction on the skin.	Proper positioning, turning techniques, lubricants, and protective dressings decrease friction between the skin and bed linens or contact surface, reducing the chance of injury.
Investigate reasons for inadequate dietary intake of protein and calories. Administer nutritional supplements or more aggressive nutritional intervention as needed.	Research has indicated that adequate dietary intake is a factor in preventing the development of a pressure ulcer and facilitating wound healing.
Continue efforts to improve mobility and activity. If this is unrealistic, attempt to maintain current level of activity, mobility, and range of motion.	An individualized activity regimen is essential to promote intact skin and prevent the hazards of inactivity and immobility.
Document measures used to prevent pressure ulcers and the results of these interventions.	Documentation of interventions and outcomes ensures continuity of care and facilitates collaboration with other caregivers.

ment. Patients, family members and other caregivers, and healthcare providers collaborate to decide appropriate treatment goals. The 1994 AHCPR guideline on *Treatment of Pressure Ulcers* specifically outlines measures for treating a pressure ulcer that reflect current knowledge and research (USDHHS, 1994).

Cleaning the Pressure Ulcer

A pressure ulcer that is clean and free of infection should demonstrate some degree of healing within 2 to 4 weeks. Experts agree on the following protocol for wound cleansing:

- Clean the wound with each dressing change.
- Use careful, gentle motion when using cleaning materials (eg, gauze) to minimize trauma.
- Avoid using harmful cleaners or antiseptic agents (eg, povidone-iodine, hydrogen peroxide) because they damage cells needed for healing.
- Use 0.9% sodium chloride to irrigate and clean most pressure ulcers.
- Use an irrigating device that produces enough pressure to clean the wound adequately without damaging tissue (see accompanying box).

Effective Irrigation Pressure

- For irrigation to clean a wound effectively and safely, the pressure or force of the irrigation must measure between 4 and 15 pounds per square inch (psi).
- Irrigation pressure below 4 psi is ineffective (eg, using a bulb syringe).
- Irrigation pressure above 15 psi may cause trauma and force bacteria into the wound.
- The following types of equipment deliver from 4 to 15 psi, which is adequate to clean a wound:

    Piston irrigating syringe with catheter tip (60 mL)

    Syringe (35 mL) with a 19-gauge needle or angiocath

    Water Pic set at the lowest setting (#1)

From U.S. Department of Health and Human Services, Agency for Health Care Policy and Research. (1994). *Treatment of Pressure Ulcers.* Rockville, MD: DHHS.

- Report when thick exudate or necrotic tissue is present in the wound. (Whirlpool treatments may be ordered until the ulcer is considered clean, or surgical excision of necrotic tissue may be necessary.)

Dressing the Pressure Ulcer

According to the AHCPR (USDHHS, 1994), the cardinal rule when dressing a pressure ulcer is to *keep the ulcer tissue moist and the surrounding skin dry.* Recommendations for wound dressing include the following:

- Use dressings that continuously keep the wound moist. Wet-to-dry dressings should be used only for **débridement** (cleaning away of devitalized tissue and foreign matter from a wound, accomplished by various methods).
- Keep the intact, healthy skin surrounding the ulcer dry because it is susceptible to breakdown. Place the moist dressing only on the wound surface. Use a skin sealant or moisture-barrier ointment on the surrounding skin and the least amount of tape that is necessary.
- Select a dressing that absorbs exudate, if present, but still maintains a moist environment for healing.
- When choosing a dressing, consider the amount of nursing time required for using the various types of dressings that maintain a moist wound environment.
- Pack wound cavities loosely with dressing material. Overpacking the wound may increase pressure and interfere with tissue healing.

- Tape the edges of a dressing that is near the anus (frame the dressing like a picture) to keep it intact, and monitor it on a frequent basis.

Controlling Infection

CDC guidelines or body substance isolation (BSI) precautions and good handwashing technique must be followed to prevent infection (see Chap. 27 for barrier techniques and handwashing recommendations). AHCPR guidelines (USDHHS, 1994) state that clean gloves and clean dressings may be used to treat pressure ulcers as long as the agency infection control procedures are followed. Sterile instruments must be used for débridement purposes. An alternate method for dressing change that combines sterile and nonsterile technique, referred to as the *no-touch technique,* consists of the following steps:

1. Use two pairs of nonsterile gloves, sterile 4 × 4 pads, and sterile 0.9% sodium chloride.
2. Discard first set of gloves after soiled dressing is removed. Wash hands.
3. Open sterile supplies using sterile technique.
4. Put on clean gloves and pour sterile 0.9% sodium chloride directly on the wound using an emesis basin to collect drainage.
5. Pick up sterile gauze and bunch ends backward toward your hand, keeping the front center of the gauze untouched.
6. Clean the wound moving from the center outward using a fresh gauze pad for each motion.
7. Dry the surrounding skin also.
8. Redress the wound by picking up gauze sponges by the corner and placing the untouched side over the pressure ulcer.
9. Cover with a transparent dressing; secure edges with tape; and write date, time, and initials on the dressing.

Teaching for Home Care

The patient and caregivers must be involved in the plan of care and should understand causative factors for the pressure ulcer. Teach good handwashing techniques and the signs of infection. Provide the patient and caregivers simple, easy-to-read instructions. Encourage frequent consultation with the primary healthcare provider about the progress of wound healing and products used. Assess the patient's nutritional status and suggest consultation with a dietitian for dietary deficiencies.

If dressing changes or wound care are painful, teach patients and caregivers to take a pain medication 30 to 60 minutes before the procedure. Emphasize the importance of handwashing before and after the dressing change. When removing a soiled dressing at home, a small plastic sandwich bag can be used to cover the hand. The dressing is lifted off with the covered hand and the plastic bag turned inside out over the hand and soiled dressing before careful disposal.

Providing Care in Other Treatment Options

When other treatments have failed, surgery may be considered as an option. Direct closure of the wound, skin grafting, or various skin flap procedures are surgical procedures that may be used based on the patient's condition and the severity of the ulcer. After surgery, the nurse must vigilantly protect the surgical site from pressure and contamination.

Several other treatment modalities are being investigated. They include electrical stimulation, hyperbaric oxygen, laser irradiation, ultrasound, and miscellaneous topical agents and systemic drugs.

EVALUATING PRESSURE ULCER CARE

When evaluating the effectiveness of a plan of care designed to prevent the development of pressure ulcers or treat those already present, the nurse uses each nurse–patient interaction to check whether the patient has met the individualized expected outcomes in the plan of care. Nursing care is considered effective if the patient, family member, or caregiver expresses satisfaction with preven-

tion and treatment measures and is able to accomplish the following:

- Participate effectively in preventive and treatment regimens
- Prevent development of any additional areas of skin breakdown
- Demonstrate progressive healing of pressure ulcer
- Improve overall physical condition (including nutritional state and mobility status)
- Remain free of infection at any pressure ulcer site
- Communicate need for additional support (environmental, physical, psychosocial)
- Respond effectively to the teaching strategies and plan

Color photographs are an excellent method of evaluating progression of wound healing, allowing comparison of the pressure ulcer at the initial assessment with the recovery stages. Evaluation is a continuous process that involves ongoing assessment and revised plans and implementations.

(*text continues on page 942*)

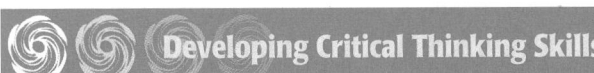

Developing Critical Thinking Skills

Situation

During both clinical days in one week you (a female student) have been assigned to care for a middle-aged woman who has had a breast removed because of cancer. The patient, Mrs. Nola, is an attractive woman who is usually cheerful and eager to get better and return home. However, on both days she turned her head away and would not look at the incision when her dressing was changed. She tells you that she "just can't stand to look at herself." Her husband has left the room during the dressing changes after telling you that "it makes me sick to see what happened to my wife." Mrs. Nola is to be discharged to her home the next day and needs to learn how to provide self-care for her wound. What do you do?

1. **Identify Goal of Thinking**

   Determine the most effective way of ensuring wound care and at the same time assisting Mrs. Nola in accepting her altered self-image.

2. **Assess Adequacy of Knowledge**

   Pertinent circumstances: The diagnosis of cancer was made only one day before the surgical removal of the breast. The patient is to be discharged to her home the next day. The wound from her mastectomy has not completely healed and will require dressing changes for another 3 or

4 days. Mrs. Nola has had a disfiguring surgery and is coping with not only a change in body image but also the diagnosis of cancer. She has never before been seriously ill nor had surgery. She has a strong, loving relationship with her husband, but he is unable to deal with the physical disfigurement at this time.

Prerequisite knowledge: Before you decide what to do in this situation, you need to know at what level Mrs. Nola is in coping with the diagnosis of cancer. If she is still in denial about the disease, it is likely that she is also denying the surgical procedure and the changes in her body. You will need to review responses to the diagnosis of cancer as well as the stages of grief and loss. You will have to learn what her sources of support are and how she can best access and use them. You will need to assess how best to help her achieve wound care in the face of her continued refusal even to look at the wound.

Room for error: If she is forced to look at the wound or made to feel inadequate because of her inability to do so, she will feel threatened and most likely will become angry in response to the perceived threat.

Time constraints: Some decision about wound care must be made before her discharge the next day.

Developing Critical Thinking Skills (Continued)

3. Address Potential Problems

There are several potential obstacles to critical thinking in this situation. As a student, you want to exhibit safe, knowledgeable care, and the importance of teaching for home care has been an emphasis in this course. As a woman, you have a sense of what the loss of a breast must mean. Having had a family member die of cancer, you find yourself wanting to do everything for Mrs. Nola. As a novice in nursing, you find it difficult to handle these emotional components of patient care and find yourself wanting to scold both the patient and her husband for being so silly about something as simple as a dressing.

4. Consult Helpful Resources

You must first understand the loss and grief Mrs. Nola is experiencing, and you must then relate that to her response to self-care of the wound. Your best source of information about her coping methods and sources of personal strength is Mrs. Nola herself. You also discuss the most effective way of providing wound care at home with your instructor and the case manager for Mrs. Nola.

5. Critique Judgment/Decision

After talking to Mrs. Nola, your instructor, and the case manager, you mutually agree that Mrs. Nola cannot be hurried into acceptance of her medical diagnosis or her body changes. The case manager consults with Mrs. Nola's physician, who writes an order for a home health nurse to visit for the next 4 days and complete the dressing change. After talking with Mrs. Nola, you identify that she is still very much in denial. You discuss with her the possibility of having a visitor from "Reach to Recovery," a support group for women with breast cancer who have had a mastectomy. Mrs. Nola tells you that she thinks she would like to talk to someone with the same problem, and you call a referral for her. When you tell Mrs. Nola that a home health nurse will be visiting her for the first few days at home to change her dressing, tears come into her eyes. She says "I am so scared, I just don't know what to do." You realize that insisting that Mrs. Nola do her own dressing would have been extremely stressful for her, and that you would have considered the wound as more important than the patient. When you share the situation in postconference, your clinical group supports your decision.

APPLYING LEARNING TO PRACTICE

PATIENT CARE STUDY

Mary Biesicker, who is 84 years of age, has been cared for at home by her daughter since being hospitalized last year for a stroke or cerebrovascular accident. During the past several months, Mary has been confined to her bed, has had minimal appetite, and has occasionally been confused and disoriented. During the past week, she has had several episodes of bowel and bladder incontinence. Her daughter also reports that Mary has developed a "blister on her lower back at the end of her backbone." She is scheduled for an assessment visit by the nurse from a local home care agency because her daughter is finding it increasingly difficult to care for her mother alone.

The nurse's initial assessment of Mary, relative to skin integrity, revealed the following:

Skin status: Presence of a nickel-sized open area on the sacrum (stage II pressure ulcer), 2 cm in diameter and 1 cm in depth. No abnormal pathways noted. Reddened area (0.5 cm) surrounding lesion. No drainage noted. Reddened area (2.5 cm) also noted on right elbow. Skin dry over all body surfaces.

Nutritional status: Daughter states "usual weight is 115–120 lb, and she has definitely lost some weight." Poor skin turgor.

Elimination status: Wearing "adult diaper," diaper damp with urine and small amount of light brown liquid stool

Activity status: Lying quietly in bed, moans when area around lesion is palpated.

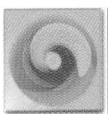

NURSING PLAN OF CARE
for Mary Biesicker

Nursing Diagnosis

Impaired Skin Integrity related to mechanical factors, inactivity, altered nutritional intake, and incontinence *as manifested by* stage II pressure ulcer on sacral area and reddened area on right elbow

Expected Outcome

6/6/02—at daily observation (or weekly in the home setting), the patient will:
- Experience reduction of pressure on bony prominences (absence of any additional reddened areas)

Nursing Interventions	Rationale	Evaluative Statement
Assess skin for development of any pressure areas (use agency tool).	Pressure results in poor circulation that causes skin breakdown.	*Six-month evaluation:* 6/13/02 Goal met. Patient has been turned from side to side every 2 hours. Reddened area on right elbow measures 1.25 cm in diameter. No new reddened areas observed.
Avoid sitting or lying on a pressure ulcer.	This facilitates pressure relief in the area and allows blood to reenter capillaries and provide oxygen to the area.	
Reposition from side to side at least every 2 hours.	The duration of pressure is more devastating to skin than the amount of pressure.	*Recommendation:* Arrange for delivery of hospital bed with overbed trapeze setup. Secure a home health aide for limited period of time to assist with repositioning during the night and allow daughter time to rest.
Use pillows to maintain side-lying or oblique position in bed and support right ankle off bed surface.	Pillows relieve pressure on lesion and areas at risk and promote improved circulation to those areas.	
Place foam overlay mattress on bed.	Static device provides support and relieves pressure on skin surface.	*M. Lieb, RN*

Expected Outcome

6/6/02—at weekly observation, the patient will:
- Demonstrate a reduction in the size of the stage II pressure ulcer on sacrum

Nursing Interventions	Rationale	Evaluative Statement
Assess condition of pressure ulcer at time of dressing change (refer to previous assessments).	Signs of infection and deterioration can be recognized and treatment plan revised.	6/13/02 Goal met. Pressure ulcer has decreased slightly in size—1.7 cm in diameter, depth remains the same. No apparent infection noted. Will continue with present treatment regimen.
Irrigate wound with normal saline using a 60-mL piston syringe with a catheter tip.	Normal saline cleanses the wound without harming tissues.	
Dry skin thoroughly surrounding the ulcer.	Moisture makes intact skin more susceptible to injury.	*M. Lieb, RN*
Apply moisture-retentive dressing (Tegasorb).	Moisture-retentive dressings create a healing environment by allowing epithelial cells to bridge the wound gap and close it.	
Use clean technique for the dressing change.	In the home, the risk is minimal for cross-contamination of micro-organisms.	

(continued)

NURSING PLAN OF CARE (Continued)
for Mary Biesicker

Expected Outcome

6/6/02—at weekly visit, the patient/caregiver will:
- Demonstrate skills required to promote skin integrity and care for a pressure ulcer

Nursing Interventions	Rationale	Evaluative Statement
Assess caregiver's (daughter) motivation and ability to manage treatment regimen.	Motivation influences readiness to learn and contributes to positive learning outcomes.	6/13/02 Goal partially met. Daughter able to recognize appearance of pressure areas on skin. Stated she would like to review treatment routine again. Daughter performed assessment and dressing change satisfactorily with nurse in attendance. Clarified and reviewed written instructions again. Daughter states, "I feel much more confident now."
Instruct daughter about causes, skin assessment techniques, and individualized treatment regimen. Provide written instructions and illustrations when possible.	A clear concise teaching guide provides consistent education and is available for reinforcement.	
Provide information about community resources available for assistance with care of mother.	Resources provide opportunity for support and problem solving.	
		M. Lieb, RN

Sample Documentation

6/20/02 Home care visit (nursing)

Mrs. Biesicker was revisited in her home for continued assessment and treatment of pressure ulcer. Nursing diagnosis: Impaired Skin Integrity related to pressure, inactivity, inadequate nutritional intake, and incontinence. According to daughter, patient was turned and repositioned every 2 hours. Foam mattress and pillow supports used for support and pressure reduction. Dressing on pressure ulcer changed. Wound cleansed with normal saline, intact skin surrounding wound, and Tegasorb dressing applied. Granulation tissue noted in wound bed, no evidence of drainage or reddened area around wound. Ulcer has decreased to 1½ cm in size. Reddened area not apparent on right elbow. Reviewed written instructions with daughter for 6/23/02 to discuss healthcare options. Will continue current plan of care and visits every other day.

M. Lieb, RN

Learning Outcomes

After completing this chapter, the learner should be able to accomplish the following:

1. Define key terms used in this chapter.

bandage	friction
binder	granulation tissue
débridement	ischemia
dehiscence	necrosis
dressing	pressure ulcer
epithelialization	reactive hyperemia
eschar	scar
evisceration	shearing force
exudate	wound

2. Discuss the processes involved in wound healing.
3. Describe factors that affect wound healing.
4. Accurately assess and document the condition of wounds.
5. Implement dressing changes for different kinds of wounds.
6. Apply heat and cold effectively and safely.
7. Provide information to patients and caregivers for self-care of wounds at home.
8. Identify patients at risk for a pressure ulcer.
9. Describe the four stages of pressure ulcers.
10. Provide nursing interventions to prevent or minimize pressure ulcers in adults.
11. Follow guidelines for cleaning and dressing a pressure ulcer.

Critical Thinking Questions

1. How would you individualize your teaching about needed supplies, wound care, and resources for the following patients:
    - A homeless man admitted to the hospital for gangrene of the big toe. The toe has been amputated.
    - A teenage gang member treated in the emergency department for a superficial (but long) knife wound.
    - An infant who has had abdominal surgery and is now having diarrhea.
    - A frail, 80-year-old man who needs daily dressing changes on a draining wound, who lives with his blind wife.

2. Describe the nursing interventions you would include in a plan of care to prevent pressure ulcers in the following patients:
    - A middle-age woman, 70 pounds over normal body weight, who has a fractured femur and is recovering at home (she lives alone).
    - A 90-year-old man with cognitive impairment who is bedfast.
    - A 17-year-old girl who is paralyzed from the waist down after a diving accident and is wheelchair dependent.

Study Questions

1. After a surgical incision, a patient often has an elevated body temperature and generalized malaise. These manifestations most often occur during which phase of wound healing?
    a. inflammatory
    b. primary
    c. fibroplasia
    d. maturation

2. Which of the following terms should be used to document wound drainage that is thick, odorous, and green?
    a. serous
    b. sanguineous
    c. serosanguineous
    d. purulent

3. Your patient who has a large abdominal wound suddenly calls out for help because she feels as though something is falling out of her incision. When you inspect the incision, you find the wound to be gaping open with tissue bulging outward. You immediately report this as:
    a. an overproduction of granulation tissue
    b. wound dehiscence with evisceration
    c. a normal response to a large wound
    d. an unknown complication

4. Sara Liu, 16 years of age, was in an automobile accident and received a wound across her nose and cheek. After surgery to repair the wound, Sara says, "I am so ugly now." Based on this statement, what nursing diagnosis would be appropriate?
    a. Pain
    b. Altered Skin Integrity
    c. Altered Body Image
    d. Altered Thought Processes

5. Which action is believed to be of most use in preventing wound infections?
    a. using sterile dressing supplies
    b. suggesting dietary supplements
    c. applying antibiotic ointment
    d. careful handwashing

6. During a dressing change, the nurse observes what appears to be reddish pink tissue in the wound. This is most likely
    a. a sign of infection
    b. eschar
    c. exudate
    d. granulation tissue

7. Which of the following therapeutic interventions uses moist heat?
    a. a sitz bath
    b. an aquathermia pad
    c. a heat lamp
    d. a commercial hot pack

8. The most common site for a pressure ulcer to develop is the
    a. occipital area
    b. sacrum
    c. sternum
    d. humerus

9. The key factor contributing to the cause of a pressure ulcer is
    a. moisture
    b. incontinence
    c. pressure
    d. malnutrition

10. Which hospitalized patient is most at risk for a pressure ulcer?
    a. a 70-year-old patient with a fractured hip
    b. a 45-year-old woman recovering from gallbladder surgery
    c. a 16-year-old male paraplegic who suffered a spinal cord injury
    d. a 50-year-old patient who suffered a mild stroke

11. After an initial assessment, the nurse documents the presence of a reddened area that has blistered. According to recognized staging systems, this ulcer is classified as
    a. stage I
    b. stage II
    c. stage III
    d. stage IV

12. An older invalid patient sits and slumps in her chair most of the day. She is most likely to develop a pressure ulcer because of
    a. malnutrition
    b. shearing forces
    c. edema
    d. a chronic disease
13. The nurse assesses a stage III pressure ulcer. The nurse has observed
    a. redness that persists when pressure is relieved
    b. an open lesion with subcutaneous tissue exposed
    c. a necrotic area extending through the fascia to bone
    d. a reddened area with an abrasion

14. A priority nursing action to prevent a patient from developing a pressure ulcer is
    a. use waterproof material on the bed
    b. massage any reddened area frequently
    c. use an air-inflated ring to relieve pressure on areas
    d. use a mild soap when cleansing the skin
15. Usual treatment for a stage II pressure ulcer is
    a. a moisture-retentive dressing
    b. surgical débridement
    c. exposure to a heat lamp four times daily
    d. whirlpool treatment twice daily

Answers With Rationale

1. The correct answer is *a*. Systemic manifestations occur as a result of the inflammatory response to the altered skin and tissue integrity. Primary is not a phase of wound healing. Systemic manifestations do not usually continue into the fibroplasia and maturation phases of wound healing.
2. The correct answer is *d*. Purulent drainage is the result of an infection and is thick, odorous, and colored. Serous draining is clear and watery. Sanguineous drainage contains blood. Serosanguineous drainage is a combination of serous and sanguineous, commonly found in wound drainage.
3. The correct answer is *b*. The wound complications of dehiscence and evisceration are manifested by a wound that opens up and has viscera protruding. These are serious complications, requiring immediate care.
4. The correct answer is *c*. Wounds cause emotional as well as physical stress. Based on Sara's statement, the correct nursing diagnosis is Altered Body Image.
5. The correct answer is *d*. Although all of the answers may help in preventing wound infections, careful handwashing (medical asepsis) is the most important.
6. The correct answer is *d*. Granulation tissue is new tissue composed of many small blood vessels, is pinkish red in color, and fills an open wound when it starts to heal. Eschar is thick, dry, necrotic tissue. An infection in a wound is usually accompanied by other signs of inflammation. A wound exudate is a fluid that accumulates in the wound.
7. The correct answer is *a*. All the other responses are examples of dry heat.
8. The correct response is *b*. All sites involve bony prominences, but the sacrum is the most common area where pressure ulcers develop.
9. The correct response is *c*. Pressure interferes with circulation to the cell, resulting in cell death. Moisture, incontinence, and malnutrition predispose a patient

to altered skin integrity, making the skin more susceptible to injury.
10. The correct response is *a*. An older patient with a fractured hip already has age-related skin changes that, coupled with some degree of immobility, make that person a likely candidate. The two middle-aged patients should not suffer any extended period of inactivity. Even though a spinal cord injury may cause immobility, a 16-year-old is usually well developed muscularly and in good health and is probably able to use his arms to aid in movement.
11. The correct answer is *b*. A stage II pressure ulcer is superficial and presents clinically as an abrasion, ulcer, or shallow crater.
12. The correct answer is *b*. Sitting slumped in a chair for an extended period can easily result in shearing force, causing a pressure ulcer. Malnutrition, edema, and the presence of chronic disease may certainly be risk factors for the development of a pressure ulcer, but the most likely cause in this situation is shearing force.
13. The correct answer is *b*. A stage III pressure ulcer is an open lesion that exposes subcutaneous tissue. Redness that persists is stage I, a reddened area that has an abrasion is stage II, and stage IV would involve a necrotic area extending through the fascia to the bone.
14. The correct answer is *d*. A mild soap is less irritating. The skin should be rinsed and dried thoroughly. Waterproof materials may cause the patient to perspire; massage is not recommended for areas that are already traumatized; and air-inflated rings place additional pressure and compromise circulation to the area where they are used.
15. The correct response is *a*. A moisture-retentive dressing provides a moist environment for wound healing. A heat lamp or irrigation with povidone-iodine (Betadine) is no longer recommended, and surgical débridement is used for stage III and IV pressure ulcers.

Bibliography

Beaumont, E., & Anderson-Dam, M. (1998). Technology scoreboard. Wound care science at the crossroads. *American Journal of Nursing, 98*(12), 16–21.

Bergman-Evans, B., Cuddigan, J., & Bergstrom, N. (1994). Clinical practice guidelines: Prediction and prevention of pressure ulcers. *Journal of Gerontological Nursing, 20*(9), 19–26.

Bergstrom, N., Braden, B., Laguzza, A., & Holman, V. (1987). The Braden scale for predicting pressure sore risk. *Nursing Research, 36*(4), 205–210.

Carpenito, L. (1997). *Nursing diagnosis: Application to clinical practice* (7th ed.). Philadelphia: Lippincott-Raven.

Ebner, C. (1996). Cold therapy and its effect on procedural pain in children. *Issues in Comprehensive Pediatric Nursing, 19,* 197–208.

Gray, M. (1998). A report card on wound care research: Support surface issues and beyond. *Journal of WOCN, 25*(6), 269–270.

Herlihy, D., & Schroeder, B. (1998). Principles of wound care. *Home Health Focus, 5*(6), 41, 43.

Hess, C. (1998). Wound care. Treating a stage 3 pressure ulcer. *Nursing, 28*(2), 20.

Kiernan, M. (1998). Post-operative wound care. *Community Nurse, 4*(8), 48–49.

Krasner, D., & Kane, D. (Eds.) (1997). *Chronic wound care: A clinical source book for healthcare professionals* (2nd ed.). Wayne, PA: Health Management Publications.

Krasner, D., & Kennedy, K. (1994). Using the no-touch technique to change a dressing. *Nursing, 24*(9), 50–52.

Lait, M., & Smith, L. (1998). Wound management: A literature review. *Journal of Clinical Nursing, 7*(1), 11–17.

Lehman, C. (1998). Preventing pressure ulcers with something old and SUMPINU. *Nursing, 28*(6), 32-14, 32-16.

Maklebust, J. (1997). Pressure ulcers: Decreasing the risk for older adults. *Geriatric Nursing, 18*(6), 250–254.

Maklebust, J. (1995). Pressure ulcer: What works. *RN, 58*(9), 46–50.

McCloskey, J.C., & Bulechek, G.M. (2000). *Iowa Intervention Project: Nursing Interventions Classification (NIC)* (3rd ed.). St. Louis: C. V. Mosby.

McConnell, E. (1992). Clinical do's and don'ts: How to apply an ice bag, ice collar, or ice glove. *Nursing92, 22*(7), 18.

McConnell, E. (1997). Clinical do's and don'ts: Using dry heat to promote healing. *Nursing97, 27*(5), 22.

McDowell, J., McFarland, E., & Nalli, B. (1994). Use of cryotherapy for orthopedic patients. *Orthopedic Nursing, 13*(5), 21–24.

Myrer, J., Measom, G., Durrant, E., & Fellingham, G. (1997). Cold- and hot-pack contrast therapy: Subcutaneous and intramuscular temperature changes. *Journal of Athletic Training, 32*(3), 238–241.

Nanneman, D. (1991). Thermal modalities: Heat and cold. A review of physiologic effects with clinical applications. *American Association of Occupational Health Nursing, 39*(2), 22.

North American Nursing Diagnosis Association. (1999). *NANDA nursing diagnoses: Definitions and classification 1999–2000.* Philadelphia: Author.

Norton, D., McLaren, R., & Exton-Smith, A. (1975). An investigation of geriatric nursing problems in hospital. London: Churchill Livingstone. (Original work published in 1962.)

O'Hanlon-Nichols, T. (1995). Commonly asked questions about wound healing. *American Journal of Nursing, 95*(4), 22–24.

Pieper, B., Sugrue, M., Weiland, M., Sprague, K., & Heitman, C. (1998). Risk factors, prevention methods, and wound care for patients with pressure ulcers. *Clinical Nurse Specialist, 12*(1), 7–14.

Rice, R. (1997). Trends in skin care and pressure management in the home. *Geriatric Nursing, 18*(6), 282–284.

Rolstad, B. (1998). At a glance: Wound dressings and their functions. *Nursing, 28*(11), 32-12.

Smith-Temple, J., & Johnson, J. (1998). Pressure ulcer management. *American Journal of Nursing, 98*(2), 16D–16G.

Spencer, R. T., Nichols, L. W., Lipkin, G. B, Sabo, H. M., & Bergan, F. W. (1993). *Clinical pharmacology and nursing management* (4th ed.). Philadelphia: J. B. Lippincott.

Steed, D. (1997). The role of growth factors in wound healing. *Surgical Clinics of North America, 77*(3), 575–586.

Stotts, N. (1990). Seeing red, yellow, and black: The three-color concept of wound care. *Nursing, 20*(2), 59–61.

Sussman, C., & Bates-Jensen, B. (1998). *Wound care: A collaborative practice manual for physical therapists and nurses.* Gaithersburg, MD: Aspen.

Thomas, S. (1998). The importance of secondary dressings in wound care. *Journal of Wound Care, 7*(4), 189–192.

Turner, S. (1998). Home care 101: Infection control in wound care. *Home Care Nurse News, 5*(8), 1, 3.

U.S. Department of Health and Human Services, Agency for Health Care Policy and Research (1992). *Pressure ulcers in adults: Prediction and prevention.* Rockville, MD: Author.

U.S. Department of Health and Human Services, Agency for Health Care Policy and Research. (1994). *Treatment of pressure ulcers.* Rockville, MD: Author.

Chapter 38
Activity

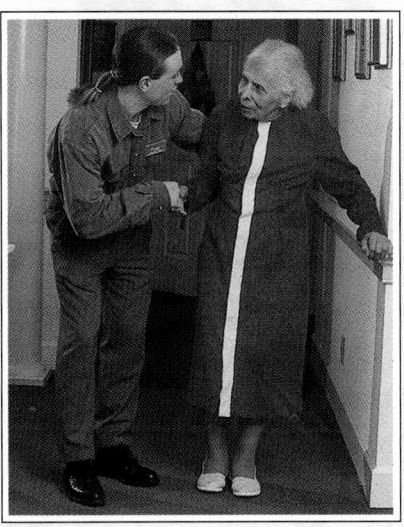

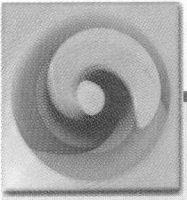

Thinking Critically About
Nursing's Blended Skills

Before reading this chapter, think about the types of blended skills you will need to care for patients with fitness goals or problems related to positioning, activity, or mobility.

- You have been invited to speak to a breast cancer survivor group that meets monthly about fitness programs.

- When you visit an elderly couple in their home, the wife complains about her joints aching all the time because of the physical wear and tear on her joints related to caring for her husband since his stroke. When you observe her helping her husband with position changes, you immediately see problems.

- A child in the pediatric unit suffered closed head trauma after a skiing accident. Unconscious at present, she may or may not regain consciousness. You want to keep her body in correct alignment and maintain normal range of joint motion.

- You work in a rehabilitation hospital and help patients transfer all day long. Recently, a nurse on your unit seriously injured her back. You've experienced some back pain yourself and realize you've been taking your good health for granted.

What cognitive, technical, interpersonal, and ethical/legal skills do you think you will need to respond to the challenges described above?

Most healthy individuals take the ability to move for granted. People simply expect our amazingly complex musculoskeletal and nervous systems to work together smoothly and on command to enable us to stand upright, to walk, and to reach for and grasp what we want. People usually give little thought to caring for the systems that promote and coordinate healthy movement until disuse, trauma, or illness cripples some aspect of movement. Although some people value exercise and fitness, many people live overwhelmingly inactive lifestyles that limit their ability to experience and enjoy life to its fullest and that openly invite degenerative and chronic diseases such as hypertension, ischemic heart disease, or diabetes.

The ability to move is closely related to the fulfillment of other basic human needs. Although breathing continues during rest, movement facilitates pulmonary functioning and increases peripheral blood flow. Because regular exercise contributes to the healthy functioning of each body system and, conversely, immobility negatively affects each body system, nurses actively promote exercise to promote wellness, prevent illness, and restore health. It is generally accepted that more serious health consequences are related to a sedentary lifestyle than there are risks related to exercise.

This chapter describes the physiology of movement, the principles of body mechanics, and factors affecting body alignment and mobility. A comprehensive section on exercise differentiates types of exercise, explores the role of exercise in disease prevention and health promotion, notes risks related to exercise, and assists in the design of individualized exercise programs. The effects of immobility on body systems are discussed along with related nursing interventions. A practical guide for assessing body alignment and mobility states is included with pertinent interview questions and physical assessment techniques. Analysis of patient mobility data may lead to the nursing diagnoses of Impaired Physical Mobility or Activity Intolerance or to diagnoses identifying effects of mobility problems on other areas of human functioning. Examples of nursing diagnoses are included. Expected outcomes are identified, and specific nursing strategies are presented. The concluding patient care study illustrates how the nurse uses knowledge of body mechanics and mobility along with specific nursing interventions to promote fitness and to resolve mobility problems.

Physiology of Movement

Purposeful, coordinated movement of the body requires the integrated functioning of the musculoskeletal and nervous systems. The following sections review the physiology of movement.

Skeletal System

The framework of bones and cartilage that protects our organs and allows us to move is called the *skeletal system*. Functions of this system include the following:

- It supports the soft tissues of the body (maintains body form and posture).
- It protects the delicate structures of the body (brain, lung, heart, spinal cord).
- It furnishes surfaces for the attachments of muscles, tendons, and ligaments, which in turn pull on the individual bones and produce movement.
- It has storage areas for mineral salts and fat.
- It produces blood cells (hematopoiesis).

COGNITIVE SKILLS

- Basic knowledge of the physiology of movement, the principles of body mechanics and factors affecting body alignment and mobility, and complications related to immobility
- Knowledge of how to design and implement a plan of care to prevent complications related to immobility and to treat mobility problems
- Ability to work with individuals to devise fitness goals and related programs

TECHNICAL SKILLS

- Ability to use correctly the protocols, products, and equipment necessary to promote body alignment and prevent or treat complications related to immobility

INTERPERSONAL SKILLS

- Strong people skills; ability to encourage individuals to value fitness and to participate actively in fitness measures
- Ability to work collaboratively with team members to achieve fitness and mobility goals

ETHICAL/LEGAL SKILLS

- Commitment to safety and quality; strong sense of responsibility, accountability
- Strong commitment to patient advocacy
- Familiarity with nursing responsibilities to prevent and treat complications related to immobility as specified by agency policy
- Ability to document nursing care related to problems of mobility or activity intolerance according to agency policy

The 206 bones in the human body are classified by their shape. *Long bones*, which are found in the upper and lower extremities (eg, humerus and femur), contribute to height and length. *Short bones*, located in the wrist and ankle, contribute to movement. *Flat bones* are relatively thin (eg, ribs and several of the skull bones) and contribute to shape (structural contour). *Irregular bones* are all those bones not included in the preceding classifications (eg, bones of the spinal column and jaw).

Because bones are too rigid to bend without damage, all movements that change the positions of the bony parts of the body occur at joints. The terms *articulation* and *joint* refer to the area where a bone come into close contact with another bone. Joints are classified according to the amount of movement they permit. Of concern are the freely movable joints, called *diarthroses* or *synovial joints*, in which there is a space between the articulating bones. Movements possible at diarthric joints include abduction, adduction, flexion, extension, and rotation. Special movements of the forearm,

ankle, and clavicle include supination, pronation, inversion, and eversion. These movements are defined in Table 38-1 and illustrated in Procedure 38-2 later in the chapter. Types of freely movable joints include the following:

Ball-and-socket joint: The rounded head of one bone fits into a cuplike cavity in the other; flexion–extension, abduction–adduction, and rotation can occur (eg, shoulder and hip joints).

Condyloid joint: The oval head of one bone fits into a shallow cavity of another bone; flexion–extension and abduction–adduction can occur (eg, wrist joint).

Gliding joint: Articular surfaces are flat; flexion–extension and abduction–adduction can occur (eg, carpal bones of wrist and tarsal bones of feet).

Hinge joint: A spool-like surface of one bone fits into a concave surface of another bone; only flexion–extension can occur (eg, elbow, knee, and ankle joints).

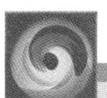

Table 38-1
Terms Commonly Used to Describe Body Positions and Movements

Term	Definition and Example
Abduction	Lateral movement of a body part away from the midline of the body. *Example:* A person's arm is abducted when it is moved away from the body.
Adduction	Lateral movement of a body part toward the midline of the body. *Example:* A person's arm is adducted when it is moved from an outstretched position to a position alongside the body.
Circumduction	Movement of the distal part of the limb to trace a complete circle while the proximal end of the bone remains fixed. *Example:* The leg is outstretched and moved in a circle.
Flexion	The state of being bent. *Example:* A person's cervical spine is flexed when the head is bent forward chin to chest.
Extension	The state of being in a straight line. *Example:* A person's cervical spine is extended when the head is held straight on the spinal column.
Hyperextension	The state of exaggerated extension. It often results in an angle greater than 180 degrees. *Example:* A person's cervical spine is hyperextended when looking overhead, toward the ceiling.
Dorsiflexion	Backward bending of the hand or foot. *Example:* A person's foot is in dorsiflexion when the toes are brought up as though to point them at the knee.
Plantar flexion	Flexion of the foot. *Example:* A person's foot is in plantar flexion in the footdrop position.
Rotation	Turning on an axis; the turning of a body part on the axis provided by its joint. *Example:* A thumb is rotated when it is moved to make a circle.
Internal rotation	A body part turning on its axis toward the midline of the body. *Example:* A leg is rotated internally when it turns inward at the hip and the toes point toward the midline of the body.
External rotation	A body part turning on its axis away from the midline of the body. *Example:* A leg is rotated externally when it turns outward at the hip and the toes point away from the midline of the body.
Special Movements	
Pronation	The assumption of the prone position. *Examples:* A person is in the prone position when lying on the abdomen; a person's palm is prone when the forearm is turned so that the palm faces downward.
Supination	The assumption of the supine position. *Examples:* A person is in the supine position when lying on the back; a person's palm is supine when the forearm is turned so that the palm faces upward.
Inversion	Movement of the sole of the foot inward (occurs at the ankle)
Eversion	Movement of the sole of the foot outward (occurs at the ankle)

Pivot joint: A ringlike structure that turns on a pivot; movement is limited to rotation, for example, turning a doorknob (eg, joints between the atlas and axis and between the proximal ends of the radius and the ulna).

Saddle joint: Bone surfaces are convex on one side and concave on the other; movements are side to side and back and forth (eg, joint between the trapezium and metacarpal of the thumb).

The strength and flexibility of the skeletal system also depend on ligaments, tendons, and cartilage. *Ligaments* are tough fibrous bands that bind joints together and connect bones and cartilage. *Tendons* are strong, flexible, inelastic fibrous bands that attach muscle to bone. *Cartilage* is nonvascular connective tissue found in the joints as well as in the nose, ear, thorax, trachea, and larynx.

Muscular System

Bones and joints provide form to the body and serve as the levers and fulcrums that make body movement possible. It is the contraction and relaxation of skeletal muscles, however, that actually produces movement as the muscles pull on bones. The excitability, contractility, extensibility, and elasticity of muscles enable them to perform three important functions for the body through contraction:

* Motion
* Maintenance of posture (skeletal muscle contractions hold the body in stationary positions)
* Heat production (skeletal muscle contractions produce heat and help maintain body temperature)

The three types of muscles are (1) skeletal, (2) cardiac, and (3) smooth or visceral muscles. The skeletal muscle system includes the skeletal muscle tissue and connective tissue that comprise individual muscle organs, such as the biceps. Movement results from a skeletal muscle contracting and exerting force on a tendon, which in turn pulls on a bone. Muscles have two differing points of attachment: (1) the attachment of a muscle to the more stationary bone is called the *point of origin,* and (2) the attachment to the more movable bone is the *point of insertion.* Between these two points is the fleshy "belly" of the muscle. Figure 38-1 illustrates the relationship of skeletal muscles to bones and the use of bones as levers and of joints as fulcrums to produce body movement.

Nervous System

The skeletal and muscular systems cannot produce purposeful movement without a functioning nervous system. Nerve impulses stimulate muscles to contract. More specifically:

* The afferent nervous system conveys information from receptors in the periphery of the body to the central nervous system (eg, light pressure on nose).
* Nerve cells called *neurons* conduct impulses from one part of the body to another.

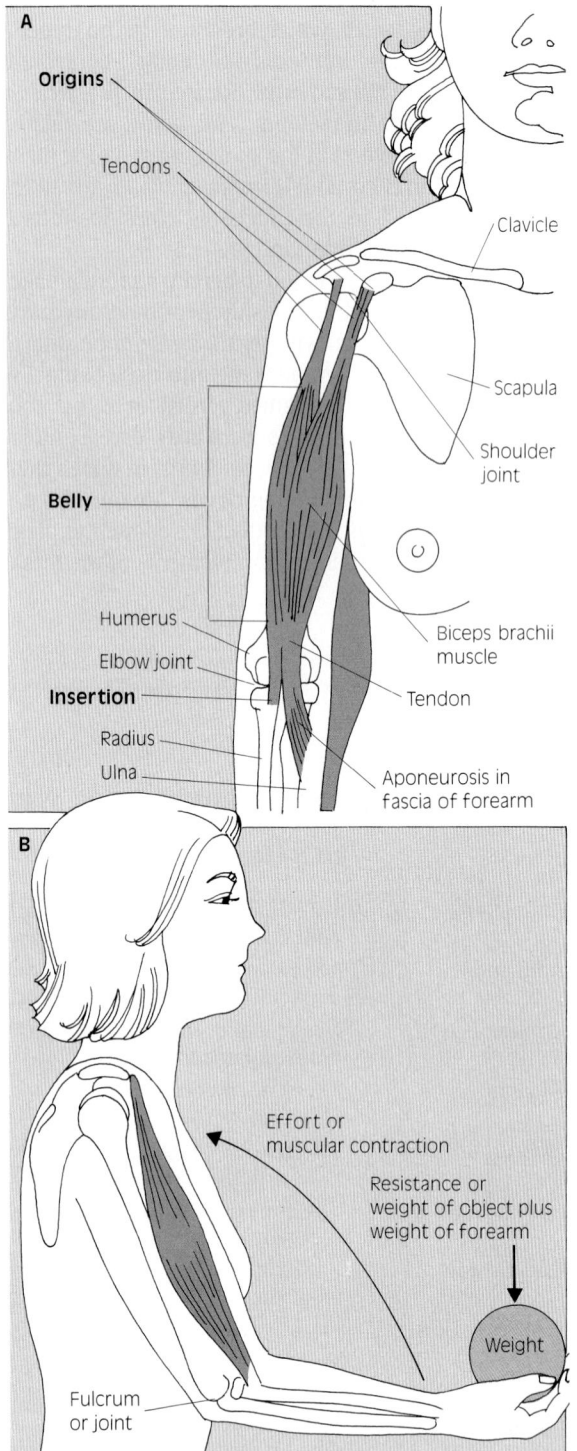

Figure 38-1
Relationship of skeletal muscles to bones. (*Top*) Skeletal muscles produce movements by pulling on bones. (*Bottom*) Bones serve as levers, and joints act as fulcrums for the levers. The lever and fulcrum principle is illustrated by the movement of the forearm lifting a weight.

* This information is processed by the central nervous system (CNS), leading to a response (eg, "There is a fly on my nose. I want to brush it off.").
* The efferent system conveys the response from the CNS to skeletal muscles by way of the somatic ner-

vous system (eg, muscles in the arm, wrist, and hand contract, and the fingers brush the fly from the face).

Body Mechanics

Body mechanics is the efficient use of the body as a machine and as a means of locomotion. Body mechanics is directly related to the effective functioning of the body. The principles of body mechanics should be correctly used in every activity and even during rest periods.

Because correct use of body mechanics is another phase of illness prevention and health promotion, the nurse has a major responsibility to teach good body mechanics both directly and indirectly by example (see the accompanying box, The Nurse as Role Model: Activity). To be able to evaluate the patient's musculoskeletal needs, the nurse must understand and use correct body mechanics. Every activity in which the nurse engages requires understanding and using these principles, from as simple an activity as moving a chair to lifting a patient out of bed.

Orthopedics means the correction or prevention of disorders of body structures used in locomotion. Nurses have long recognized that basic orthopedic principles apply in all areas of nursing, not just to patients with bone fractures or other pathologic skeletal changes. For example, a person who has a sedentary occupation and engages in little physical activity may have poorly developed muscles. A patient who is on complete bed rest is in danger of losing muscle tonus. **Tonus** is the term used to describe the state of slight contraction—the usual state of skeletal muscles. If bed rest is prolonged, there is danger of developing contractures if the patient does not have exercise and joint motion and if good posture is not maintained. The functioning of various internal body processes is also influenced by position and movement or by their absence.

Concepts of Body Mechanics

Concepts most helpful to the understanding of body mechanics are body alignment, balance, and coordinated movement.

Body Alignment or Posture

Good posture, or good body alignment, is that alignment of body parts that permits optimal musculoskeletal balance and operation and promotes healthy physiologic functioning. A person in correct alignment is experiencing no undue strain on the joints, muscles, tendons, or ligaments while balance is maintained. The criteria for correct alignment in the standing, sitting, and reclining positions are described in the assessment section later in this chapter.

Balance

A body in correct alignment is balanced. An object is balanced when its center of gravity is close to its **base of support,** the line of gravity goes through the base of support, and the object has a wide base of support. The **center of gravity** of an object is the point at which its mass is centered. In humans, the center of gravity when standing is located in the center of the pelvis about midway between the umbilicus and the symphysis pubis. The **line of gravity** is a vertical line that passes through the center of gravity. The base of support is the foundation that provides for an object's stability. The wider the base of support and the lower the center of gravity, the greater the stability of the object. Figure 38-2 illustrates body balance.

Nurses can increase body balance when working by spreading their feet farther apart (broadening the base of support) and by flexing their hips and knees (lowering the center of gravity). These two simple maneuvers are important principles in body mechanics by which nurses can decrease musculoskeletal strain. This type of injury can occur when there is excessive stretching or overexertion of a muscle or muscle–tendon unit. Musculoskeletal strain most commonly affects the lower back and cervical spine region. Trauma to the musculoskeletal system is discussed later in the chapter.

Coordinated Body Movement

Because nurses providing direct patient care must frequently use their body to assist in positioning, turning, and lifting both patients and equipment, it is important to do

---

APPLYING LEARNING TO PRACTICE

The Nurse as Role Model: Activity

Nurses who wish to role-model healthy mobility behaviors to patients demonstrate a commitment to using the principles of body mechanics in both their leisure and work activities and to exercising regularly to promote fitness. Because nurses who work closely with patients providing physical care are at high risk for developing musculoskeletal problems if they do not use their bodies properly, they also have a personal reason for being attentive to the use of good body mechanics. Similarly, the work of nursing places heavy demands on a nurse's psychic and physical energy; the nurse who is physically fit is better able to respond to these challenges. Nurses who are effective role models easily meet the following goals:

- Consistently use sound principles of body mechanics in both leisure and work activities
- Incorporate regular periods of physical exercise into lifestyle (minimum of three 30- to 45-minute exercise sessions weekly)
- Demonstrate a preference for an active versus a sedentary lifestyle (eg, use stairs in preference to elevators, walk rather than drive short distances, balance active leisure alternatives with sedentary options)
- Appear physically fit to patients and colleagues (appropriate weight for height; adequate muscle mass, tone, and strength; perform work activities without becoming short of breath or excessively fatigued)

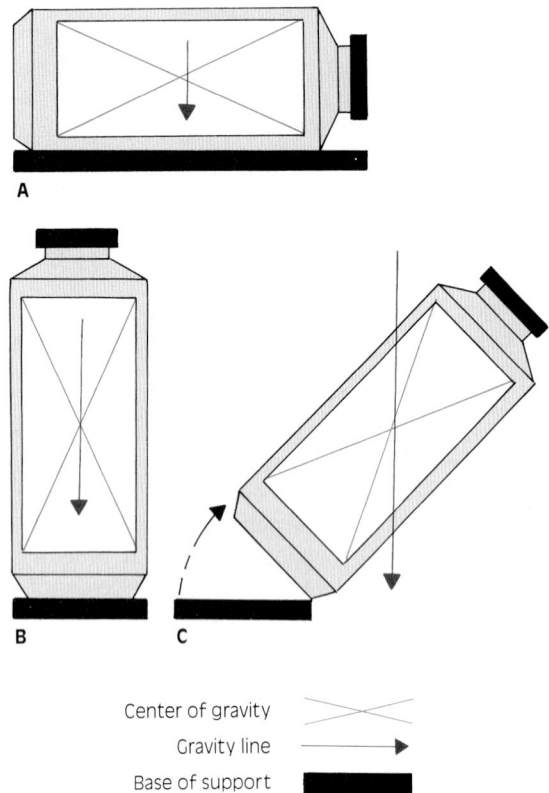

Center of gravity

Gravity line

Base of support

Figure 38-2

The effect of the base of support and gravity on balance is shown. (**A**) The line of gravity passes through the wide base of support. This object is the most stable of the three. (**B**) The line of gravity also passes through the base support, although the base is narrower. This object is less stable than the one above it. (**C**) The line of gravity does not pass through the base of support. This object is unstable.

this knowledgeably to avoid musculoskeletal strain and injury. This work is facilitated when nurses use major muscle groups rather than weaker ones and take advantage of the body's natural levers and fulcrums. For example, rather than attempt to push a patient to the opposite side of the bed, the nurse flexes the knees, positions the forearms above and below the patient's buttocks (preferably under a pull sheet), and rocks backward, sliding the patient toward self. This one coordinated movement illustrates the following principles:

- The nurse is using major muscle groups—flexors, extensors, and abductors of the thighs; flexors and extensors of the knees; flexors and extensors of the upper and lower arms—rather than weaker ones.
- Use of the arm bones as levers and the elbows as fulcrums facilitates lifting a weight against resistance (force of gravity)—the lever and fulcrum principle (see Fig. 38-1).
- Using a pull sheet and smooth, dry, firm bed foundation decreases the effects of friction, which increases the amount of effort required to move an object. Rough, wet, or soiled surfaces can contribute to friction's effect.

- By positioning the arms under the patient's center of gravity (hips) and sliding the body back toward himself or herself, the nurse is working close to the object to be moved and decreasing the effort involved.

Postural Reflexes

Integrated functioning of the musculoskeletal and nervous systems is essential for body alignment and balance. Postural tonus, the sustained contraction of select skeletal muscles that keeps the human body in an upright position against the force of gravity, depends on the functioning of several postural reflexes:

Labyrinthine sense: This sense of position and movement is provided by the sensory organs in the inner ear, which are stimulated by body movement (changes in head position) and transmit these impulses to the cerebellum.

Proprioceptor or kinesthetic sense: This informs the brain of the location of a limb or body part as a result of joint movements stimulating special nerve endings in muscles, tendons, and fascia.

Visual or optic reflexes: Visual impressions contribute to posture by alerting the person to spatial relationships with the environment (nearness of ceilings, walls, furniture, condition of floor, and so on).

Extensor or stretch reflexes: When extensor muscles are stretched beyond a certain point (eg, when knees buckle under), their stimulation causes a reflex contraction that aids a person to reestablish erect posture (eg, straighten the knee).

Application of Body Mechanics

The body mechanics guidelines listed below are important for nurses and others engaged in physical activity both at home and at work. It is not uncommon to hear nurses who are retiring or leaving the profession cite back injuries as an influencing factor. In 1997, 43% of practicing RNs sustained a work-related back injury that required time off from work or restrictions in activity (Sheehan, 1999). The following are techniques to prevent back stress that should be included routinely in injury prevention programs:

- *Develop a habit of erect posture* (correct alignment) and, whenever necessary, begin activities by broadening the base of support and lowering the center of gravity.
- *Use the longest and the strongest muscles of the arms and the legs to help provide the power needed in strenuous activities.* The muscles of the back are less strong and more easily injured when used improperly.
- *Use the internal girdle and a long midriff to stabilize the pelvis and to protect the abdominal viscera* when stooping, reaching, lifting, or pulling. The internal girdle is made by contracting the gluteal muscles in the buttocks downward and the abdominal muscles upward. It is helped further by making a long midriff. This is done by stretching the muscles in the waist. Figure 38-3 illustrates the internal girdle.

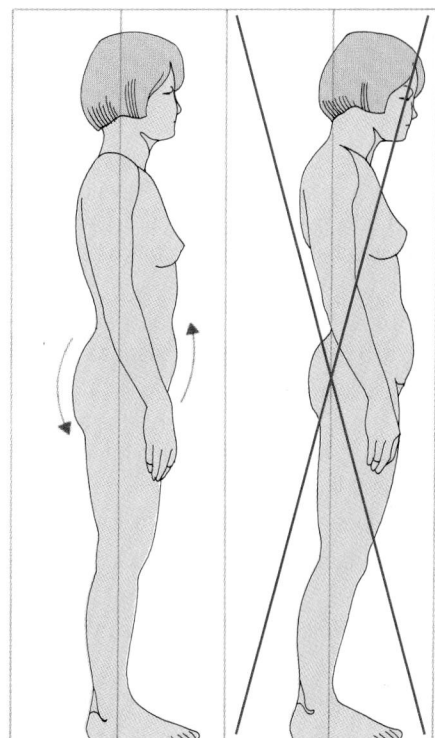

Figure 38-3
(*Left*) Internal girdle "on." Abdominal muscles contracted, giving a feeling of upward pull, and gluteal muscles contracted, giving a downward pull. (*Right*) Slouch position, showing abdominal muscles relaxed and body out of good alignment.

- *Slide, roll, push, or pull an object rather than lift it* to reduce the energy needed to lift the weight against the pull of gravity.
- *Use the weight of the body to push an object* by falling or rocking forward and to pull an object by falling or rocking backward.
- *Spread the feet apart to provide a wider base of support* when increased stability of the body is necessary.
- *Flex the knees, put on the internal girdle, and come down close to an object that is to be lifted.*

Nurses who consciously develop good habits can demonstrate to others proper ways of using the musculoskeletal system (refer to the accompanying box, Applying Learning to Practice: Promoting Health). In the home, nurses can model proper body mechanics when they assist patients to dress, help them move, or perform care. Caregivers in the home need reminders that preventing back problems is more effective than treating them after they occur.

- *Work as closely as possible to an object that is to be lifted or moved.* This brings the body's center of gravity close to that of the object being moved, thereby permitting most of the burden to be borne by the leg and arm muscles rather than the back. Figure 38-4 illustrates a proper and an improper way to pick up an object.
- *Use the weight of the body as a force for pulling or pushing,* by rocking on the feet or leaning forward or backward. This reduces the amount of strain placed on the arms and the back.

Factors Affecting Body Alignment and Mobility

Numerous factors, including growth and development, physical health, mental health, lifestyle variables, attitude and values, fatigue and stress, and external factors such as weather, influence an individual's posture, movement, and daily activity level.

Developmental Considerations

A person's age and degree of neuromuscular development markedly influence body proportions, posture, body mass, movements, and reflexes. To promote neuromuscular development in patients of all ages and to facilitate each patient's use of the body to perform self-care actions, nurses need to be familiar with developmental variations in body proportions and neuromuscular development. These variations are presented in Table 38-2 with related nursing assessment priorities and nursing interventions.

Figure 38-4
(*Left*) A good position for lifting is illustrated. This person is using the long and strong muscles of the arms and legs and holding the object so that the line of gravity falls within the base of support. (*Right*) This is an incorrect position for lifting because pull is exerted on the back muscles and leaning causes the line of gravity to fall outside the base.

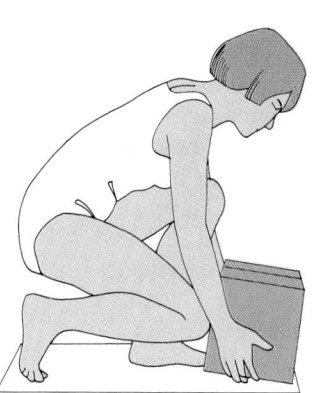
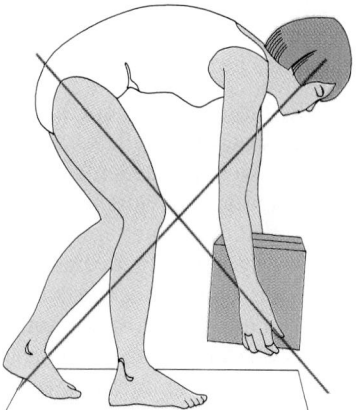

APPLYING LEARNING TO PRACTICE

Promoting Health

Exercise

Use the following assessment checklist to determine how well you are meeting your need for exercise. Then develop a prescription for self-care by choosing appropriate behaviors from the list of suggestions.

Assessment Checklist

almost always sometimes almost never

☐ ☐ ☐ 1. My lifestyle demonstrates that I place a high value on exercise as a component of wellness (eg, I use stairs instead of elevators).

☐ ☐ ☐ 2. I exercise for 30 to 45 minutes three or four times per week.

☐ ☐ ☐ 3. I have sufficient energy for each day's tasks.

☐ ☐ ☐ 4. I maintain my target weight.

Self-Care Behaviors

1. Decide to make the most of everyday opportunities for exercise: use stairs instead of elevators, walk instead of ride, park the car farther from your destination than usual and walk the distance briskly, and so forth.

2. Choose exercise activities you enjoy and plan three or four 30- to 45-minute exercise sessions weekly.

3. Obtain medical clearance for exercise if you fall in a high-risk group. Learn and observe the appropriate exercise safeguards (eg, wear running shoes with the proper support).

4. Alternate types of exercise to avoid boredom.

5. Use part of your lunchtime for brisk walking or other exercise.

6. Invite a friend to exercise with you so you have the added support of a buddy.

7. Join a spa, health club, or exercise group.

8. Build up exercise sessions gradually to avoid overexertion and injury to muscles.

9. Evaluate your lifestyle to see what prevents you from exercising regularly and address these factors (low value attached to health or exercise, low motivation, lack of time, lack of rest, or faulty nutrition).

Physical Health

Problems in the musculoskeletal or nervous systems can have a negative influence on body alignment and movement. Similarly, illness or trauma involving other body systems may interfere with movement because of either the underlying pathology or the treatment regimen. Nurses need to become sensitive to how both acute and chronic health problems affect a patient's general appearance (posture, body proportions, and movements) and ability to move purposefully to perform the activities of daily living. When assessing a patient's response to a mobility deficit, the nurse accomplishes the following:

- Reinforces behaviors that promote healthy functioning (eg, congratulates a patient who manages transfers well despite left-sided weakness or paralysis)
- Corrects behaviors that compound the mobility deficit over time (eg, a patient with arthritis who severely restricts movement because of joint stiffness and tenderness learns successful adaptive strategies that can be shared with other patients and families; or energy conservation measures are used by patients with emphysema who have greatly decreased activity tolerance)

Musculoskeletal Problems

Congenital or Acquired Postural Abnormalities

A newborn with congenital hip dysplasia or a clubfoot, a teenager with scoliosis (lateral curvature of the spine), and an older person with kyphosis (increased convexity in the curvature of the thoracic spine) are all experiencing postural abnormalities that affect their appearance and mobility. Nursing responsibilities may include the following:

- Early detection and referral of these problems
- Exploration and selection of patient education, counseling, and support as treatment options
- Careful attention to positioning, transfers, and exercise
- Education of the patient and family regarding safe self-care activities

Problems With Bone Formation or Muscle Development

Problems with bone formation may include any of the following:

- *Congenital problems,* such as achondroplasia, in which premature bone ossification leads to dwarfism, or osteogenesis imperfecta, which is characterized by excessively brittle bones and multiple fractures both at birth and later in life

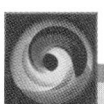

Table 38-2
Activity Variations Based on Developmental Level: Assessment Priorities and Nursing Interventions

Developmental Level	Assessment Priorities	Nursing Interventions
Infant		
• Periods of activity and alertness alternate with quiet periods and sleep • At 3 months: may raise chest and head when prone • By 5 months: head control usually achieved	**3 to 6 mo** • Ability to sit • Head control **6 to 9 mo** • Sits steadily • Rolls over • Creeps on all fours • Pulls to a standing position • Has improved hand–eye coordination **9 to 12 mo** • Progresses toward unassisted walking • Is able to pick up small objects	• Encourage parents to examine their baby (eg, count fingers and toes) • Respond to concerns that parents have about minor variations in newborn's appearance or behavior • Emphasize that individual variation in activity patterns and neuro-muscular development should be expected
Toddler		
• Gross and fine motor development continue rapidly • By 15 months: most can walk unassisted • At 18 months: most can run • At 2 years: can jump • At 3 years: most can stack blocks, string large beads, work simple puzzles, and dress themselves	• Assess progress in walking, running, and jumping • Assess small muscle coordination (eg, ability to dress themselves, wash hands, brush teeth) • Distinguish slow developers who fall within normal range from those with developmental lags	• Help parents to learn and accept their child's uniqueness. • Teach parents the importance of providing a safe environment. • Enthusiastically reinforce and praise toddler's mastery of new skills. • Set limits so that toddler does not overextend himself or herself in drive for mastery of skills.
Child		
• Muscles, bones, and nervous system develop, allowing greater gross and fine motor control **Common Activities** • By age 4: negotiate stairs, walk backward, and hop on one foot • By age 5: skip, jump rope, and jump off heights of several steps • Able to manipulate writing materials • Has acquired all basic mechanisms for physical locomotion	• Use developmental charts to assess gross and fine motor development	• Teach parents that attitudes about the body and exercise are developed during this period. • Counsel as appropriate.
Adolescent		
• Size increases: growth spurt • Secondary sex characteristics appear • If physically fit: can be a time of boundless energy and great athletic performance • If inactive: may begin a lifelong pattern of unhealthy behavior	• Determine activity level and type of regular exercise • Evaluate safety of recreational choices • Screen for scoliosis (lateral curva-ture of the spine). • Examine muscle mass, tone, and strength and joint mobility.	• Lifestyle counseling regarding the importance of exercise and fitness is critical. • Encourage to exercise regularly if necessary. • Caution about gauging physical limits and not "pushing too hard."

(continued)

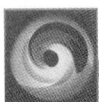

Table 38-2 (Continued)

Developmental Level	Assessment Priorities	Nursing Interventions
Adult • Stands and sits erect and is capable of balanced and coordinated, purposeful movement • During pregnancy: center of gravity shifts because of developing fetus • Activity levels vary greatly	• Assess balance between activity and rest in person's lifestyle. • Note any lifestyle factors or illnesses that interfere with mobility or ability to carry out activities of daily living.	• Fitness counseling is important. • Clarify misconceptions about exercise. • Design and monitor safe exercise programs. • Those with mobility alterations may require special care.
Older Adult • Increased convexity in the thoracic spine (kyphosis) from disk shrinkage and decreased height • Flexed posture • Loss of muscle tone • Subcutaneous fat loss • Arthritic joint changes may be present	• Assess general ease of movement and gait. • Assess alignment. • Check joints and their function. • Assess muscle mass, tone, and strength.	**Teach and Counsel About:** • Importance of regular exercise • Need to maintain proper weight • Need for high protein, calcium, and vitamin D–enriched diet • Pacing activities • Using assistive devices safely when needed • Safety-proof homes to reduce falls

- *Diet-related problems*, for example, vitamin D deficiency, which results in deformities of the growing skeleton (rickets)
- *Disease-related problems*, such as in Paget's disease, in which excessive bone destruction and abnormal regeneration result in skeletal pain, deformities, and pathologic fractures
- *Age-related problems*, such as osteoporosis, in which bone destruction exceeds bone formation and in which the resultant thin, porous bones fracture easily

The muscular dystrophies are a group of genetically transmitted disorders that have in common progressive degeneration and weakness of skeletal muscles. They vary in terms of the muscle groups involved and their clinical course. Myasthenia gravis is a weakness of the skeletal muscles caused by an abnormality at the neuromuscular junction that prevents muscle fibers from contracting.

Nursing responsibilities for patients with problems of bone formation and muscle development and functioning include the following:

- Careful collaboration with the physician and healthcare team to determine the motor capacities of the individual
- Patient and family education aimed at developing optional mobility

The nurse must be knowledgeable about the underlying disease process and be able to position, lift, transfer, and exercise the patient safely, with attention to patient comfort.

Problems Affecting Joint Mobility

Inflammation, degeneration, and trauma can all interfere with joint mobility. The term *arthritis* describes more than 20 diseases, all characterized by inflammation in one or more joints and possibly pain and stiffness in adjacent body parts. *Degenerative joint disease*, also termed *osteoarthritis*, is a noninflammatory, progressive disorder of movable joints, particularly weight-bearing joints, characterized by the deterioration of articular cartilage and pain with motion. Spurs form, which restrict joint movement. Trauma to a joint may result in either a *sprain*, in which the wrenching or twisting of a joint results in a partial tear or rupture to its attachments, or a *dislocation*, the displacement of a bone from a joint with tearing of ligaments, tendons, and capsules. Any condition restricting joint mobility has potentially crippling effects.

Nurses caring for patients with joint problems work collaboratively with physicians and physical therapists to maintain joint mobility. Patient education is directed to the patient's mastery of an exercise and care program, which fosters tissue repair and maximal independence in activities of daily living.

Problems Affecting the Central Nervous System

A problem in any of the principal parts of the brain or spinal cord involved with skeletal muscle control can affect mobility:

The *cerebral motor cortex* assumes the major role of controlling precise, discrete movements. A cerebrovascular accident (stroke) or head trauma may damage the motor cortex and produce temporary or permanent voluntary motor impairment.

Basal ganglia integrate semivoluntary movements such as walking, swimming, and laughing. In Parkinson's disease, there is progressive degeneration of the basal ganglia of the cerebrum. Unnecessary skeletal movements result in tremors and muscle rigidity, which interfere with voluntary movement.

The *cerebellum* assists the motor cortex and basal ganglia by making body movements smooth and coordinated. In multiple sclerosis, the myelin sheaths of neurons in the CNS deteriorate to hardened scars or plaques.

Plaque formation in the cerebellum may produce lack of coordination of one hand.

The *pyramidal pathways* convey voluntary motor impulses from the brain through the spinal cord by way of two major pathways: (1) the pyramidal pathway and (2) the extrapyramidal pathway. With trauma to the spinal cord, transection of these motor pathways results in complete bilateral loss of voluntary movement below the level of the trauma.

The overwhelming complaint of patients with injury to the CNS is that no one talks with them (or with their families) about how the disease may progress and affect their functioning. Nurses caring for these patients need to be knowledgeable about the pathology and clinical course of these diseases in order to give appropriate patient education and counseling.

Trauma to the Musculoskeletal System

Injury to the musculoskeletal system can result in fractures and soft tissue injuries. A *fracture* is a break in the continuity of a bone or cartilage. It may result from a traumatic injury or some underlying disease process. Healing requires realignment of the bone fragment, immobilization, and restoration of the bone's function. Soft tissue injuries include sprains, strains, and dislocations. (Dislocations and sprains are discussed above under Problems Affecting Joint Mobility.) A *strain*, the least serious of these injuries, is a stretching of a muscle. Nurses need to be knowledgeable in first-aid measures for musculoskeletal trauma as well as in acute and rehabilitative care.

Problems Involving Other Body Systems

The pathology of numerous other acute and chronic illnesses may also affect mobility. Chronic obstructive lung disease and conditions such as ascites may alter posture. Any illnesses that interfere with oxygenation at the cellular level decrease the amount of oxygen available to the muscles for work and thus decrease activity tolerance. These illnesses include anemia, angina, cardiac dysrhythmias, congestive heart failure, and chronic obstructive pulmonary disease. Diseases characterized by negative nitrogen balance (eg, anorexia nervosa and certain cancers) result in muscle wasting and decreased physical energy for movement and work. Symptoms accompanying many illnesses, such as fatigue, muscle aches, and pain, may also immobilize patients. Bed rest is an important component of treatment for many diseases or trauma states, such as myocardial infarction, surgery, and fractures. Although rest is essential for the healing process, immobility may cause its own problems (Table 38-3). Nurses need to be vigilant in determining the effects of any injury or illness on mobility and in providing care to facilitate optimal mobility.

Mental Health

Just as an individual's physical health influences body appearance and movement, so also does the person's mental health. Bodily processes tend to slow down in depression, and there is a lack of visible energy and enthusiasm. The depressed person often sits with head bowed and shoulders slumped and may lack the energy to eat or even to use the toilet. Even facial movement may be decreased to the point at which the individual's face registers no emotion (termed a *flat affect*). On the other hand, nondepressed individuals are more likely to have erect posture and animated facial features.

Lifestyle Variables

Whether an individual has an active or sedentary lifestyle is influenced by many factors. Among the most important are the individual's occupation, leisure activity preferences, and cultural influences. Because most professional occupations as well as many blue-collar jobs are sedentary, individuals wishing to exercise regularly need to plan leisure activities that give the body a workout. Cultural influences may encourage or discourage exercise. For example, it is popular for both male and female professionals to engage in aerobic exercise. In the not-so-distant past, it was considered unladylike for women to be involved in most sports activities. Nurses, particularly those involved in community health activities, need to consider appropriate forms of exercise and geographic location before making recommendations to patients from diverse cultures. Commonly prescribed exercises, such as jogging, tennis, or even walking, may be viewed as white, middle-class choices and prove unsafe in a high-crime area. An exercise prescription for a Native American, for example, might suggest exploring nearby mountain areas, hunting, or even participation in Native American dances as more acceptable methods to increase activity level. Other lifestyle variables that influence mobility include the person's diet and smoking history.

Attitude and Values

In some families, such as those who hike, swim, or play ball together, children learn early to value regular exercise. As these children mature, they often continue to value exercise and find new ways to incorporate regular exercise into their daily routine. Similarly, children may be raised in sedentary families where watching sports is the closest anyone comes to exercise. This attitude may also be internalized for a lifetime. Many individual values also influence the exercise options people make. Older people who integrate a planned exercise regimen into their daily routine benefit physiologically and report improved self-esteem (see the accompanying Research in Nursing box).

Individuals who place a high value on physical attractiveness may be highly committed to regular exercise

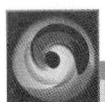

Table 38-3
Comparison of Effects of Exercise and Immobility on Body Systems

Effects of Exercise	Effects of Immobility
Cardiovascular System	**Cardiovascular System**
↑Efficiency of heart	↑Cardiac workload
↓Resting heart rate and blood pressure	↑Risk for orthostatic hypotension
↑Blood flow and oxygenation of all body parts	↑Risk for venous thrombosis
Respiratory System	**Respiratory System**
↑Depth of respiration	↓Depth of respiration
↑Respiratory rate	↓Rate of respiration
↑Gas exchange at alveolar level	Pooling of secretions
↑Rate of carbon dioxide excretion	Impaired gas exchange
Gastrointestinal System	**Gastrointestinal System**
↑Appetite	Disturbance in appetite
↑Intestinal tone	Altered protein metabolism
Urinary System	Altered digestion and utilization of nutrients
↑Blood flow to kidneys	**Urinary System**
↑Efficiency in maintaining fluid and acid–base balance	↑Urinary stasis
↑Efficiency in excreting body wastes	↑Risk for renal calculi
Musculoskeletal System	↓Bladder muscle tone
↑Muscle efficiency	**Musculoskeletal System**
↑Coordination	↓Muscle size, tone, and strength
↑Efficiency of nerve impulse transmission	↓Joint mobility, flexibility
Metabolic System	Bone demineralization
↑Efficiency of metabolic system	↓Endurance, stability
↑Efficiency of body temperature regulation	↑Risk for contracture formation
Integument	**Metabolic System**
Improved tone, color, turgor, resulting from improved circulation	↑Risk for electrolyte imbalance
Psychological Well-Being	Altered exchange of nutrients and gases
Energy, vitality, general well-being	**Integument**
Improved sleep	↑Risk for skin breakdown and formation of decubitus ulcers
Improved appearance	
Improved self-concept	**Psychological Well-Being**
Positive health behaviors	↑Sense of powerlessness
	↓Self-concept
	↓Social interaction
	↓Sensory stimulation
	Altered sleep–wake pattern
	↑Risk for depression

because it helps produce the body they want. Another individual may exercise because of the desire for physical strength, relating strength with power. Someone more disposed to intellectual pursuits may perceive body development as simply wasting time that could be better used to develop the mind.

Fatigue and Stress

Chronic stress may deplete body energy to the point that fatigue makes even the thought of exercise overwhelming. Ironically, regular exercise is energizing and can better equip a person to deal with daily stresses. At the same time,

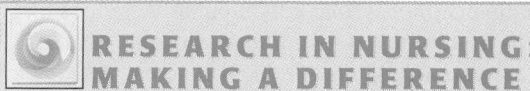

RESEARCH IN NURSING: MAKING A DIFFERENCE

Supporting Positive Self-Care Practices in Older Adults

The positive effects of exercise have often been documented. An active lifestyle is particularly important for older adults as they strive to stay healthy and remain independent. In an effort to promote these positive outcomes, nurses attempt to identify the specific self-care activities that support wellness in this population.

Related Research
Clark, C. (1998). Wellness self-care by healthy older adults. *Image–The Journal of Nursing Scholarship, 30*(4), 351–355.
In this descriptive study, a small sample (*N* = 28) of older adults ranging in age from 57 to 83 years, who were active members of their communities, responded to a questionnaire about self-care behaviors. In addition to their age, participants were asked to report

specific health promotion activities and the relationship between their self-care procedures and their functional ability or attitudes. Areas surveyed included activity, nutrition, rest and sleep, stress management, safety, supportive relationships, energy and independence, quality of life, and zest for living. An active lifestyle was viewed by all respondents as the key to managing stress and enhancing well-being. This pattern of behavior has implications for nurses, who can make significant contributions to the well-being of this growing population group. Nurses will be challenged to provide the health education necessary to encourage older individuals to achieve maximal benefits from exercise. Changing lifestyle behavior to include participation in regular physical exercise is also beneficial in improving an older adult's ability to function independently.

---

excessive exercise may stress the body and lead to injury as well as to fatigue.

External Factors

Many external factors can influence mobility. Among these, weather probably exerts the greatest influence. A brisk, clear day is invigorating and invites increased activity. High humidity and high temperatures, on the other hand, discourage extra movement. Sufficient financial resources for exercise memberships and equipment, safe outdoor parks and sports areas, the availability of malls for early-morning walkers, support people, and occupational or insurance rewards for exercise can all encourage regular exercise. Discouraging factors include insufficient funds, air pollution, unsafe neighborhoods, lack of free time, and lack of support and reinforcement.

Exercise

Active exertion of muscles involving the contraction and relaxation of muscle groups is termed **exercise**. Each of the many different types of exercise can produce different physiologic and psychological benefits.

Types of Exercise

Muscle Contraction
Exercise may be categorized according to the type of muscle contraction involved as being isotonic, isometric, or isokinetic (Fig. 38-5).

Isotonic exercise involves muscle shortening and active movement. Examples include carrying out activities of daily living, independently performing range-of-motion exercises, and swimming, walking, jogging, and bicycling. Potential benefits include increased muscle mass, tone, and strength; improved joint mobility; increased cardiac and respiratory function; increased circulation; and increased osteoblastic or bone-building activity. When the nurse or family member performs passive range-of-motion exercises for a patient, the patient's muscles do not exert effort, and potential benefits are reduced to improved joint mobility and increased circulation.

Isometric exercise involves muscle contraction without shortening (ie, there is no movement or a minimum shortening of muscle fibers). Examples include contractions of the quadriceps and gluteal muscles. Potential benefits are increased muscle mass, tone, and strength; increased circulation to the exercised body part; and increased osteoblastic activity. Nurses encourage both isotonic and isometric exercises for hospitalized patients with limited mobility.

Isokinetic exercise involves muscle contractions with resistance, varying at a constant rate produced by a device with a capacity for variable resistance. Examples include rehabilitative exercises for knee and elbow injuries. Using the isokinetic device, the person takes the muscles and joint through a complete range of motion without stopping, meeting resistance at every point.

Body Movement
Exercise activities may also be categorized according to the type of body movement involved and the health

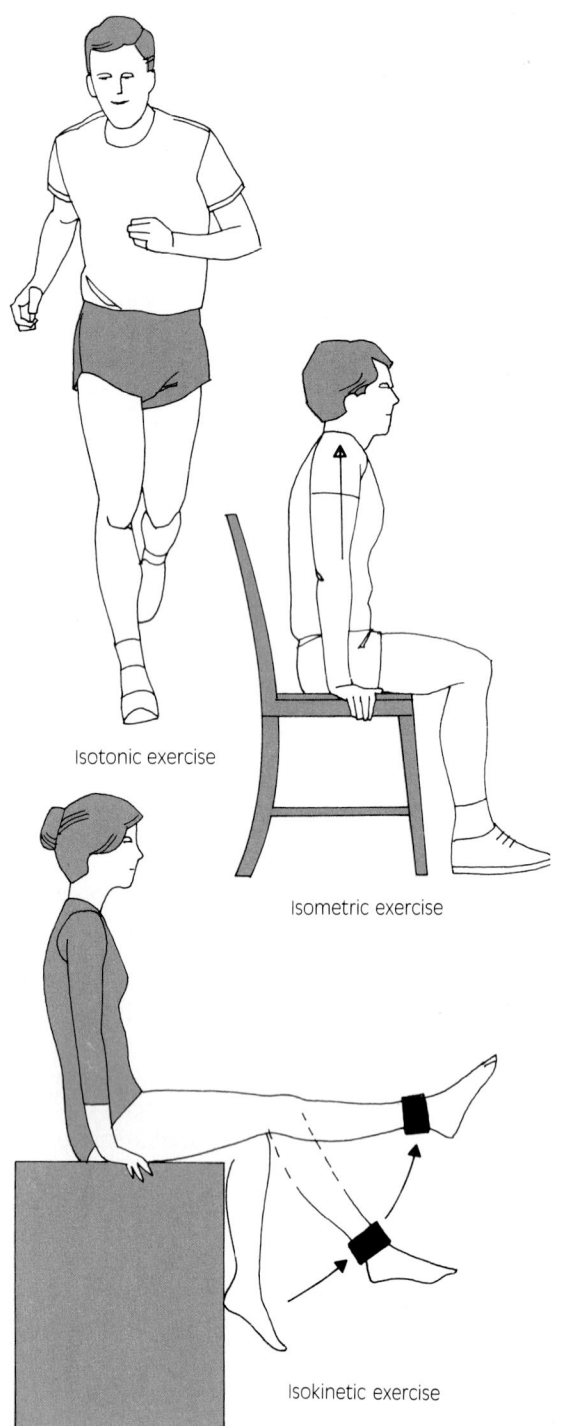

Figure 38-5
Three types of exercise. *Isotonic* involves muscle shortening and active movement. *Isometric* involves muscle contraction without shortening. *Isokinetic* involves muscle contraction with resistance.

benefits they produce. Types of exercise include the following:

> *Aerobic exercise:* sustained (often rhythmic) muscle movements that increase blood flow, heart rate, and metabolic demand for oxygen over time, pro-

moting cardiovascular conditioning. Activities that may be aerobic are swimming, walking, jogging, cross-country skiing, aerobic dance, bicycling, jumping rope, and racquetball. (Aerobic exercise may be further distinguished as having high or low impact. The number of injuries, such as shin splints, related to high-impact aerobic workouts led to the development of low-impact workouts that place less stress on the musculoskeletal system.)

> *Stretching exercises:* movements that allow muscles and joints to be stretched gently through their full range of motion, increasing flexibility. Specific warm-up and cool-down exercises, hatha yoga, and some forms of dance are examples. Benefits include increased range of joint movements, improved circulation and posture, and relaxation.

> *Strength and endurance exercises:* a variety of muscle-building programs. Weight training, calisthenics, and specific isometric exercises can build both strength and endurance, increasing the power of the musculoskeletal system and generally improving the whole body. They may or may not have aerobic benefit.

> *Movement and activities of daily living:* housecleaning, running after playful toddlers, climbing stairs instead of riding in elevators, and so on. These all have an effect on health. Increased fitness does not require a gym (Kenney, 1997).

Effects of Exercise and Immobility on Major Body Systems

The human body was designed for motion, and regular exercise is necessary for its healthy functioning. Individuals who choose inactive lifestyles or who are forced into inactivity by illness or injury place themselves at high risk for serious health problems. The effects of both regular exercise and immobility on major body systems are explored in the following sections and outlined in Table 38-3. Just as individuals differ in the benefits they receive from exercise, complications resulting from immobility differ in their occurrence and severity according to the patient's age and overall health state.

Cardiovascular System
Effects of Exercise

To meet the demand for oxygen created by the rhythmic contraction and relaxation of skeletal muscle groups, the supply of oxygenated blood to skeletal muscle needs to be increased. The cardiovascular system meets this challenge by increasing the heart rate, increasing the contractile strength of the myocardium, and increasing stroke volume (volume of blood ejected), thus increasing cardiac output. Arterial (systolic) blood pressure is increased, and blood is shunted from the nonexercising tissues to the heart and muscles. Exercise also improves venous return because the contracting muscles compress superficial veins and push blood back to the heart against gravity. Over time, with cardiovascular conditioning, regular exercise produces the following benefits:

- Increased efficiency of the heart
- Decreased heart rate and blood pressure
- Increased blood flow to all body parts
- Increased circulating fibrinolysin (substance that breaks up small clots)

Effects of Immobility

The primary and serious effects of immobility on the cardiovascular system include increased cardiac workload, orthostatic hypotension, and venous thrombosis. Immobility results in an increased workload for the heart. It has been demonstrated that the heart works more when the person is immobile because the skeletal muscles that normally compress valves in the leg veins and help to pump the blood back to the right side of the heart do not adequately contract. There is less resistance offered by the blood vessels and blood pools in the veins, thus increasing the venous blood pressure and changing the distribution of blood in the immobile person. As a result, the heart rate, cardiac output, and stroke volume increase.

Immobility predisposes the patient to thrombi formation because of venous stasis, especially in the legs, where normal muscular activity helps move blood toward the central circulatory system. Thrombus formation is also caused by an increased rate in the coagulation of blood, one reason being that during periods of immobility, calcium leaves bones and enters the blood, where it has an influence on blood coagulation.

An immobile person is more susceptible to developing orthostatic hypotension. The person tends to feel weak and faint when this condition occurs. See Chapter 24 for additional discussion of orthostatic hypotension.

Respiratory System
Effects of Exercise

The respiratory and cardiovascular systems work together to make increased oxygen available to the muscles. During exercise, the depth of respiration, respiratory rate, gas exchange at the alveolar level, and rate of carbon dioxide excretion are increased. Over time, regular exercise leads to improved pulmonary functioning.

Effects of Immobility

The effects of immobility on the respiratory system are related to decreased ventilatory effort and increased respiratory secretions. Immobility causes a decrease in the depth and rate of respirations, in part because of a reduced need for oxygen by body cells. When areas of lung tissues are not used over time, atelectasis may occur. *Atelectasis* is an incomplete expansion or collapse of lung tissue. Immobility results in a poor exchange of carbon dioxide and oxygen, upsets their balance in the body, and results eventually in an acid–base imbalance.

When a person is immobile, the movement of secretions in the respiratory tract is decreased, resulting in the pooling of secretions and in respiratory tract congestion. These conditions predispose the person to respiratory tract infections. *Hypostatic pneumonia* is a type of pneumonia that results from inactivity and immobility. The situation worsens when the person is dehydrated or using pharmaceutical agents that increase the tenacity of secretions, depress the coughing mechanism, and depress respirations.

Decreased movement in the thoracic cage during respirations also occurs with immobility. This decrease may be due to loss of tonus in muscles involved with respirations, pressure on the chest wall because of the patient's position in bed, and depression of the respiratory apparatus by various pharmaceutical agents.

Musculoskeletal System
Effects of Exercise

The rhythmic contraction and relaxation of muscle groups during exercise result in increased muscle mass, tone, and strength and increased joint mobility. The more a person exercises, the more strength he or she has to exercise or work in the future. Regular exercise produces the following benefits:

- Increased muscle efficiency (strength) and flexibility
- Increased coordination
- Increased efficiency of nerve impulse transmission

Regular exercise is also believed to slow the effects of aging (ie, it helps prevent osteoporosis associated with aging).

Effects of Immobility

Effects of immobility on the musculoskeletal system are rapidly seen in patients confined to bed. People attempting to walk after several days of bed rest are often surprised to find how weak their legs have become. Immobility (musculoskeletal disuse) leads to decreased muscle size **(atrophy)**, tone, and strength; decreased joint mobility and flexibility; bone demineralization; and limited endurance, resulting in problems with activities of daily living.

Immobility is often the cause of **contractures**, which are permanent contraction states of muscle (muscle shortening), and **ankylosis,** which is a consolidation and immobilization of a joint. Contractures result from atrophy of muscles with resulting incompetence and from a decrease in the muscle's strength, coordination, and endurance. A joint can be permanently fixed when ankylosed.

The process of bone demineralization **(osteoporosis)** is also increased in immobile patients. Normally, the stress and strain of weight-bearing activity stimulate bone formation and balance this natural destruction of bone. With immobility, however, bone formation slows while breakdown increases, with a net loss of bone calcium, phosphorus, and matrix. This condition, *disuse osteoporosis*, is characterized by bones that may be either spongy or brittle. Bone demineralization may result in pathologic fractures related to the bone's brittleness; bone deformities related to the bone's sponginess; arthropathy (joint disease) related to calcium depletion in the joints; and renal calculi (stones) related to the excessive excretion of calcium through the kidneys and urinary tract.

Metabolic System
Effects of Exercise

The metabolic rate increases during exercise so that sufficient glucose and fatty acids can be converted to provide the energy needed for increased muscle function. During strenuous exercise, the metabolic rate can increase to up to 20 times normal. Increased body heat and waste products are also produced. With regular exercise the body develops the following:

- Increased efficiency of metabolic system
- Increased efficiency of body temperature regulation

Effects of Immobility

Because the resting body requires less energy, the cellular demand for oxygen is decreased, leading to a decreased metabolic rate. In many immobilized patients, however, factors such as fever, trauma, chronic illness, or poor nutrition can actually increase the body's metabolic demands and increase *catabolism* (the breakdown of the body's protein stores to provide energy to meet the body's energy requirements). If unchecked, this process results in muscle wasting. When more protein is being broken down than manufactured, the body excretes more nitrogen than it takes in, and *negative nitrogen balance* occurs. Anorexia, or decreased appetite, often accompanies and compounds this problem. Negative nitrogen balance and poor nutrition thus worsen the muscle atrophy and weakness already resulting from immobility. Numerous fluid and electrolyte imbalances, alterations in the exchange of nutrients and gases at the cellular level, and gastrointestinal problems can all result from metabolic disturbances.

Gastrointestinal System
Effects of Exercise

During exercise, blood is shunted away from the stomach and intestines to the exercising muscles. With regular exercise, the following occur:

- Appetite is increased.
- Intestinal tone is increased, which improves digestion and elimination.

Effects of Immobility

Immobility leads to disturbances in appetite, decreased food intake, altered protein metabolism, and poor digestion and utilization of food. If individuals increase food intake while decreasing energy expenditure, weight gain will result.

Normal muscular activity in the gastrointestinal tract also slows down in an immobile person, which often results in constipation, poor defecation reflexes, and an inability to expel feces and gas adequately.

Urinary System
Effects of Exercise

Regular exercise increases blood circulation, including improved blood flow to the kidneys. This allows the kidneys to maintain the body's fluid balance and acid–base balance more efficiently and to excrete body wastes.

Effects of Immobility

In a nonerect patient, the kidneys and ureters are level, and urine stays longer in the renal pelvis before being expressed against gravity into the ureters and bladder. Urinary stasis favors the growth of bacteria that, when present in sufficient quantities, may cause urinary tract infections. Poor perineal hygiene, incontinence, decreased fluid intake, or an indwelling Foley catheter can increase the risk for urinary tract infection in an immobile patient.

Immobility also predisposes the patient to renal calculi, or kidney stones, which are a consequence of high levels of urinary calcium; urinary retention and incontinence resulting from decreased bladder muscle tone; the formation of alkaline urine, which facilitates growth of urinary bacteria; and decreased urinary volume.

Skin
Effects of Exercise

Increased circulation resulting from regular exercise nourishes the skin and promotes its general health.

Effects of Immobility

In older or debilitated immobile patients, the impaired circulation that accompanies immobility may result in serious skin breakdown. Prolonged pressure over bony prominences produces areas of breakdown, or pressure ulcers, which can progress from stage 1, redness, to stage 4, destruction of subcutaneous tissue and muscle. Pressure ulcers are described in detail in Chapter 37.

Psychosocial Outlook
Effects of Exercise

Some of the most important benefits of regular exercise are psychological:

- Increased energy, vitality, and general well-being
- Improved sleep
- Improved appearance (body image)
- Improved self-concept
- Increased positive health behaviors

Effects of Immobility

When a person can no longer move the body purposefully and needs to depend on someone else for assistance with simple self-care activities, the person's sense of self is often threatened. Skeletal deformities can influence body image; an inability to meet role expectations can decrease self-concept; and a prolonged period of lying dependent in bed can lead to feelings of worthlessness and diminished self-esteem.

Immobility can produce exaggerated emotional responses to the stresses of everyday living. People who become apathetic, possibly because of decreased sensory stimulation, often exhibit altered thought processes. Lack of mobility can also diminish an individual's opportunities to interact socially and deprive that person of normal support systems. Coping difficulties are common for both immobilized patients and their families. Furthermore, the amount of time immobilized patients spend resting often disrupts their usual sleep–wake patterns and may interfere with both the quantity and quality of their sleep.

Role of Exercise in Preventing Illness and Promoting Wellness

Promoting exercise and emphasizing wellness behaviors are challenging opportunities for nurses. Nurses are committed to assisting and supporting patients to make lifestyle changes that improve the patients' health and well-being. As researchers focus on the potential of regular exercise activities to slow the aging process, nurses intervene to prevent the deleterious effects associated with decreased physical activity.

Although there is no evidence that exercise prevents the occurrence of chronic disease, clinical improvement has been noted when older patients participate in regular exercise activities. See the accompanying box, Focus on the Older Adult, for a summary of the benefits of exercise and specific precautions related to exercise for this age group.

Risks Related to Exercise

Among the reasons many people offer for not exercising is fear of experiencing personal harm. Nurses need to respond to these fears with realistic knowledge of the risks associated with exercise and specific prevention strategies.

Avoiding Exercise
The greatest risk associated with exercise is viewing it as too much of a chore and avoiding it.

Precipitating a Cardiac Event
Although the risk of exercise precipitating a major cardiac event in a healthy individual is minimal, the risk is much higher for individuals with known or documentable cardiovascular disease. Thus, a preexercise medical examination, medical supervision during exercise, and an individually designed exercise plan are recommended for sedentary people older than 35 years of age and for any person with a past or current cardiovascular condition.

Orthopedic Discomfort and Disability
The most common injuries associated with exercise are orthopedic problems caused by irritation of bones, tendons,

---

Focus on the Older Adult
Exercise and Activity

Regular exercise is beneficial for all age groups. Older adults, particularly, demonstrate positive results from a program of regular physical activity that is appropriate for their age and health status.

Benefits that can result from regular physical activity include the following:

- Cardiovascular improvements
  Decreased blood pressure
  Decreased heart rate
  Improved circulation
  Decreased cholesterol level
  Decreased body weight
- Respiratory improvements
  Increased vital capacity
  Increased endurance
- Musculoskeletal improvements
  Increased muscle strength
  Improved stability of gait
  Improved range of motion
  Increased flexibility
  Decreased back and joint pain
  Improved posture
- Psychosocial and cognitive improvements
  Improved ability to manage stress
  Improved memory
  Increased self-esteem
  Increased opportunities for socialization

- Other improvements
  Improved sleep
  Improved bowel function
  Improved energy level

Special precautions for older adults before and during exercise include the following:

- Before exercise
  Obtain physician's approval and directions for exercise program.
  Wait until 2 hours after eating before exercising.
  Perform warm-up exercises before beginning activity.
  Wear proper footwear and appropriate clothing.
  Provide for sufficient hydration.
  Avoid extreme temperatures if exercising outdoors.
- During exercise
  Avoid sudden position changes
  Maintain heart rate at lower end of target zone specified by physician.
  Check pulse at regular intervals while exercising.
  Avoid exercise if weak or ill.
  Stop exercising if chest pain or difficulty breathing occurs and consult with physician before resuming activity.

ligaments, and sometimes muscles. This irritation may result from added weight-bearing stress or from collision with the ground, an object, or another person. Patients should be taught when injured to follow the guideline of the acronym RICE: *rest, ice, compression,* and *elevation.* While the injured area is rested, ice should be applied to minimize pain and edema. Application of an ace bandage for compression and elevation of the injured area help to reduce edema. A physician should be contacted immediately to diagnose the extent of the injury. Exercise should not be continued until the injury is healed.

Other Health Problems

Other types of health problems may be associated with different types of exercise, depending to a large extent on external factors (temperature on a given day, humidity, pollution index, safety of the neighborhood) as well as internal factors (age, history of previous injury, overuse, obesity, health history). Examples of other health problems related to exercise include heat exhaustion or heat stroke, exercise-induced asthma, and chest pain related to overexertion.

The Nursing Process

ASSESSING

The comprehensive nursing assessment uses both interview and physical assessment skills to elicit data about the patient's mobility status. When alterations in a patient's physical or mental health state result in impaired mobility, additional specific assessment skills are needed.

Nursing History

During the nursing history, the nurse interviews patients regarding their daily activity level, endurance, exercise and fitness goals, mobility problems, physical or mental health alterations that affect mobility, and external factors affecting mobility. It is important to question patients about their fitness goals. This interviewing strategy communicates to patients that you expect them to be exercising and is itself a powerful teaching tool.

The accompanying Focused Assessment Guide illustrates elements common to a mobility status history. When a problem exists, the nurse assesses the nature of the problem, its onset and frequency, known causes, its severity and symptoms, its effects on everyday functioning, and the interventions attempted by the patient and the results.

Physical Assessment

Physical assessment of mobility status includes an assessment of general ease of movement and gait; alignment, joint structure, and function; muscle mass, tone, and strength; and endurance. Table 38-4 provides normal findings and significant alterations. The nurse performing this assessment directs attention to both structure and function. The

patient's ability to stand, walk, sit up, and grasp are important because these enable the patient to wash, dress, and feed himself or herself and perform other basic activities of daily living. Refer to Table 38-5 for assessment priorities related to specific problems associated with immobility.

General Ease of Movement and Gait

The nurse begins the examination of an ambulatory patient the moment the patient walks into the room. Voluntarily controlled, fluid, and coordinated body movements are keys to the integrated functioning of the skeletal, skeletal muscle, and nervous systems. Common involuntary movements that may be observed include *tremors* (continuous quivering of whole muscles or major portions of a muscle) and *tics* (irregularly occurring spasmodic movements such as winking, grimacing, or shoulder shrugging) (Porth, 1998).

The nurse also notes whether the patient's body movements are quick and sure or slow and deliberate. These observations communicate both a sense of the person's emotional status and self-care abilities.

The gait of the ambulatory patient is also noted. The patient's movements while walking should be coordinated and the posture well balanced. The arms should swing freely in a rhythm alternating with the legs. Figure 38-6 illustrates stance and swing, the two phases of the normal gait. The heel of the right foot strikes the ground (stance), while the toe of the left foot pushes off and leaves the ground, moving the leg from behind to in front of the body (swing). While one leg is in the stance phase, the other is in the swing phase. Gait abnormalities are important because they may place the individual at risk for injury and also because they may indicate intoxication or a neuromuscular disorder

If a patient uses a wheelchair, brace, cane, walker, or crutches to assist with ambulation, this should be noted. The nurse also determines whether this aid is meeting the patient's needs and is being used safely.

Alignment

Correct body alignment permits optimal musculoskeletal balance and operation and promotes good physiologic functioning. Deviations in body alignment may result from chronic poor posture, trauma, muscle damage, or nerve dysfunction. Fatigue and a person's mental and emotional status may also influence alignment. Alignment may be observed when a patient is standing, sitting, or lying (Fig. 38-7). The nurse notes whether the patient is able to maintain correct alignment independently.

Correct body alignment when standing is as follows:

- The head is held erect.
- The face is in the forward position, in the same direction as the feet.
- The chest is held upward and forward.
- The spinal column is upright, and the curves of the spine are within normal limits.
- The abdominal muscles are held upward and the buttocks downward.

FOCUSED ASSESSMENT GUIDE

Mobility and Exercise

Factors to Assess	Questions and Approaches
Daily activity level	Describe the activities you normally carry out during a routine day. What type of physical exercise is a part of your daily lifestyle? • Activities of daily living • Type, frequency, duration of physical exercise • Past history of activity and exercise; recent changes
Endurance	Describe how much and what type of activity makes you tired. • History of dizziness, dyspnea, frequent pauses in activity to rest, or marked increase in respiratory rate after moderate activity
Exercise/fitness goals	What exercise or fitness goals are you currently working on? • Attitudes about exercise and physical fitness • Knowledge of the benefits of exercise • Motivation to exercise • Current exercise and fitness goals
Mobility problems	Do you experience any problems with movement or with more vigorous activity or exercise? If yes, please describe these problems. • Nature of the problem • Onset of disturbance and frequency • Known causes • Severity • Symptoms • Effect of problem on everyday functioning • Interventions attempted and results
Physical or mental health alterations	Are there any physical or mental health problems that may be affecting your mobility? Tell me about them. • Decrease of strength or endurance (eg, myocardial infarction, congestive heart failure, cardiomyopathy, chronic obstructive pulmonary disease, cancer, gastrointestinal disorders) • Neuromuscular impairment (multiple sclerosis, Parkinson's disease, spinal injuries) • Musculoskeletal impairment (arthritis, fractures, muscular dystrophy) • Perceptual or cognitive impairment (cerebrovascular accident, brain tumor or trauma, vision disorders) • Pain or discomfort (burns, rheumatoid arthritis, chronic pain syndrome, postoperative pain) • Depression or severe anxiety (neurosis, schizophrenia)
External factors affecting mobility	Is there anything else you can think of that limits your ability to get around? • Environmental factors (stairs, lack of railings or other assistive devices, unsafe neighborhood) • Financial resources

• The knees are extended—not bent or hyperextended in the knee-locked position.
• The feet are at right angles to the lower legs.
• The line of gravity goes through the center of the knees and in front of the ankle joints.
• The base of support is on the soles of the feet, and weight is distributed through the soles and heels.

Correct body alignment when sitting is similar to correct alignment when standing except that the hips are flexed, the knees are flexed and not crossed, and the base of support is on the buttocks and upper thighs. The popliteal area should be free of the edge of the chair to prevent circulatory stasis and possible nerve injury.

Joint Structure and Function

The nurse uses inspection and palpation skills to examine joints, their range of motion, and the surrounding tissue. **Range of motion** is the complete extent of movement of

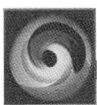

Table 38-4
Overview of the Physical Assessment of Mobility Status

Component	Normal Finding	Significant Alterations
General ease of movement	Body movements are: • Voluntarily controlled (purposeful) • Fluid • Coordinated	Involuntary movements: • Tremors • Tics • Chorea • Athetosis • Dystonia • Fasciculations • Myoclonus • Oral–facial dyskinesias
Gait and posture	Head erect, vertebrae are straight Knees and feet point forward Arms at side with elbows flexed Arms swing freely in alternation with leg swings While one leg is in the stance phase, the other is in the swing phase	Abnormalities of gait and posture: • Spastic hemiparesis • Scissors gait • Steppage gait • Sensory ataxia • Cerebellar ataxia • Parkinsonian gait • Gait of old age • Use of assistive devices for ambulation
Alignment	Independent maintenance of correct alignment: • In the standing and sitting position, a straight line can be drawn from the ear through the shoulder and hip • In bed, the head, shoulders, and hips are aligned	Abnormal spinal curvatures Inability to maintain correct alignment independently
Joint structure and function	Absence of joint deformities Full range of motion	Limitation in the normal range of motion Increased joint mobility Swelling or tenderness in or around the joint Heat or redness Crepitation Deformities Muscle atrophy, nodules, skin changes Asymmetry of involvement
Muscle mass, tone, and strength	Adequate muscle mass, tone, and strength to accomplish movement and work	Atrophy, hypertrophy Hypotonicity (flaccidity), spasticity Paresis or paralysis
Endurance	Ability to turn in bed, maintain correct alignment when sitting and standing, ambulate, and perform self-care activities	Physiologic or psychological inability to tolerate an increase in activity: • Significantly increased pulse, respiration, blood pressure after rest • Shortness of breath, dyspnea • Weakness • Pallor • Confusion • Vertigo

which a joint is normally capable. Procedure 38-2 later in this chapter illustrates the range of motion of selected joints. When assessing joint mobility, Weber and Kelley (1998) and O'Hanlon-Nichols (1998) have recommended nurses note the following:

• Size, shape, color, and symmetry of joints. Note any masses, deformities, or muscle atrophy.

• Range of motion of each joint.
• Any limitation in the normal range of motion or any unusual increase in the mobility of a joint (instability). Range of motion varies among individuals and decreases with aging.
• Muscle strength when performing range-of-motion exercises against resistance.

(*text continues on page 969*)

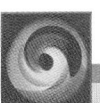

Table 38-5
Selected Nursing Diagnoses, Assessment Priorities, Expected Outcomes, and Nursing Interventions

Problems Related to Immobility	Etiologies	Assessment Priorities	Expected Outcomes	Nursing Interventions
Cardiovascular				
Activity Intolerance: Increased Cardiac Workload	Supine position contributes to greater volume of circulating blood, which must be pumped by the heart; decreased vascular resistance	Assess apical and peripheral pulses. Note increased heart rate, weakened peripheral pulses. Note presence of edema.	Patient will maintain baseline vital signs. Patient will show signs of adequate venous return (absence of dependent edema, thrombi, emboli)	Encourage patient to sit in Fowler's position. Avoid activities that increase intrathoracic pressure (eg, Valsalva maneuver)
Altered Tissue Perfusion: Thrombus Formation	Venous stasis due to lack of muscle contraction in the legs. Increased blood coagulation because calcium moves from bones into circulation. External pressure on the veins (eg, from knee gatch on bed)	Assess for complaints of pain, especially calf pain, and signs of inflammation. Compare one extremity to the other. Measure calf or thigh circumference daily (mark place to measure).		Encourage active exercise of legs three to four times daily. Elevate legs periodically. Avoid prolonged knee and hip flexion. Apply TEDS if ordered. Never rub or massage the legs—especially if patient complains of pain.
Risk for Injury: Orthostatic Hypotension	Skeletal muscle weakness and decreased vessel tone. Hypovolemia	Assess for complaints of dizziness or fainting. Compare BP before position change with BP after position change.	Patient will change from a lying to a sitting or standing position safely, without injury.	Have patient sleep sitting up or in an elevated position (if not contraindicated). Change position gradually. Encourage leg exercises. Avoid Valsalva maneuver.
Respiratory				

Ineffective Breathing Pattern	Limited chest expansion
	    Prolonged sitting or lying
	    Muscle disuse or atrophy
	    Loss of muscle coordination
	    Medications that decrease respiratory effort
		Assess rate, rhythm, quality of respirations. Assess symmetry of chest wall movements.	Patient will maintain baseline respiratory rate and depth. Patient coughs and deep breathes every 1 to 2 hours.	Change position every 2 hours. Encourage deep breathing and coughing every 1–2 hours. Remove abdominal binders every 2 hours to allow for deep breathing.

Ineffective Airway Clearance	Altered function of mucous membranes and cilia. Decreased position changes. Ineffective coughing due to weakness, pain. Dehydration	Assess breath sounds over the entire lung region. Note any adventitious breath sounds. Assess sputum (C&S may be ordered). Percuss chest.	Patient's lungs will be clear to auscultation. Patient will remain free of signs of respiratory infection.	See nursing interventions for Ineffective Breathing Pattern. Keep patient well hydrated. Initiate chest physiotherapy. Suction as needed.

(continued)

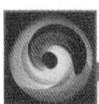

Table 38-5 (Continued)

Problems Related to Immobility	Etiologies	Assessment Priorities	Expected Outcomes	Nursing Interventions
Impaired Gas Exchange (O_2/CO_2 ratio)	Decreased respiratory movement Pooling of secretions	Note any changes in behavior or mental status. Compare clinical picture with changes in ABGs, pulse oximetry, PFTs.	Patient will maintain an adequate O_2/CO_2 exchange.	See nursing interventions for Ineffective Breathing Pattern and Ineffective Airway Clearance.
Musculoskeletal				
Risk for Activity Intolerance (Self-Care Deficits) Impaired Physical Mobility	Decreased muscle mass, tone, and strength (atrophy) Contractures Stiffness and pain in the joints Limited range of motion Decreased endurance	Assess for weakness, fatigue, muscle, or joint pain or tenderness. Assess for decreased muscle mass, decreased muscle tone and strength. Note contractures of ankyloses.	Patient will maintain adequate muscle strength and joint mobility to perform basic self-care activities.	Incorporate ROM exercises and isometric setting exercises into daily routine (at least three to four times daily).
Risk for Injury: Pathologic Fractures	Excessive bone demineralization (disuse osteoporosis)	Bone demineralization is not detectable through physical assessment. Relate clinical picture to blood chemistries (note elevated serum calcium and phosphorus levels).	Patient will remain free of contractures, ankyloses, pathologic fractures.	Increase patient's activity tolerance gradually. Progress to independence in all self-care activities.
Metabolic				
Altered Nutrition: Less Than Body Requirements Altered Nutrition: More Than Body Requirements Fluid Volume Excess: Dependent Edema	Negative nitrogen balance Anorexia Imbalance between calories ingested and burned off Fluid shifts because of negative nitrogen balance	Assess diet history. Monitor intake and output. Compare clinical picture to laboratory studies that evaluate fluid and electrolyte status. Evaluate muscle atrophy. Assess skin turgor and wound healing.	Patient will maintain appropriate weight for height. Patient's fluid output will approximately equal output. Patient's electrolyte values and serum protein will fall within normal range. Patient's skin will demonstrate adequate turgor.	Provide patient with high-protein, high-calorie diet. Explore parenteral and enteral alternatives if patient is unable to eat. Serve small, frequent feedings in pleasant environment. Monitor intake and output.
Gastrointestinal				
Constipation	Decreased gastric motility and muscle tone Decreased fluid intake	Assess frequency and consistency of bowel movements. Examine for bowel sounds, abdominal tone, and anal sphincter tone.	Patient will have a formed, semisolid stool every 1 to 3 days. Patient will be free of signs of fecal impaction.	Respect usual elimination schedule. Offer assistance with bedpan or commode and provide privacy. Increase fluid intake and roughage.

(continued)

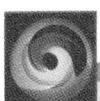

Table 38-5 (Continued)

Problems Related to Immobility	Etiologies	Assessment Priorities	Expected Outcomes	Nursing Interventions
Urinary				
Altered Urinary Elimination Urine Retention Risk for Infection: Urinary Tract	Renal calculi Urinary stasis	Assess voiding patterns—time and amount. Question about urgency, dysuria, pain. Monitor fluid output. Examine for bladder distention. Examine urine for cloudiness or odor (C&S if indicated)	Patient will maintain usual voiding pattern. Patient will be free of renal calculi. Patient will be free of signs of urinary tract infection.	Keep patient well hydrated. Maintain usual voiding pattern. If needed, provide assistance with bedpan or urinal—respect patient's privacy.
Skin				
Impaired Skin Integrity (pressure ulcer)	Decreased local blood circulation to the tissues Prolonged pressure on the skin	Examine skin, especially pressure points, for beginning stages of breakdown with each position change (at least every 2 hours). Assess for factors that place patient at high risk for breakdown (eg, malnutrition and incontinence).	Patient's skin will show no signs of breakdown.	Reposition patient in correct alignment at least every 1–2 hours. Protect pressure points (eg, heel and elbow protectors). Decrease effects of shearing force. Keep skin clean and dry. Keep bed linens dry and free of wrinkles.
Psychological and Social				
Self-Esteem Disturbance Powerlessness Impaired Social Interaction Altered Thought Processes Knowledge Deficit Ineffective Individual Coping Ineffective Family Coping Sleep Pattern Disturbance	Inability to move voluntarily Dependency on others Inability to fulfill role expectations Pain experience Skeletal deformities Exaggerated emotional and behavioral responses Decreased ability to learn and retain information. Increased need for sleep and napping.	Assess patient for changes in behavior, emotional status, and mental abilities. Assess adequacy of the patient's and family's coping. Assess sleep–wake patterns. Explore with patient and family possible reasons for these changes.	Patient will identify personal strengths. Patient will verbalize positive body image. Patient will describe successful coping strategies. Patient will demonstrate ability to problem solve.	Explore immobility effects on mental status and behavior. Explore means to meet needs for socialization. Increase stimuli to maintain orientation. Encourage patient to be as independent as possible. Challenge patient intellectually. Explore impact of patient's illness on family and counsel appropriately.

BP, blood pressure; TEDS, thromboembolis disease stockings; C&S, culture and sputum; ABGs, arterial blood gas levels; PFTs, pulmonary function tests; ROM, range of motion.

- Any swelling, heat, tenderness, pain, nodules, or crepitation (palpable or audible crunching or grating sensation produced by motion of the joint).
- Compare findings in one joint with those of the opposite joint.

Muscle Mass, Tone, and Strength

Adequate skeletal muscle mass, tone, and strength are prerequisites to body movement and work performance. Mass refers to muscle size. *Atrophy* describes muscle mass that is decreased through disuse or neurologic impairment.

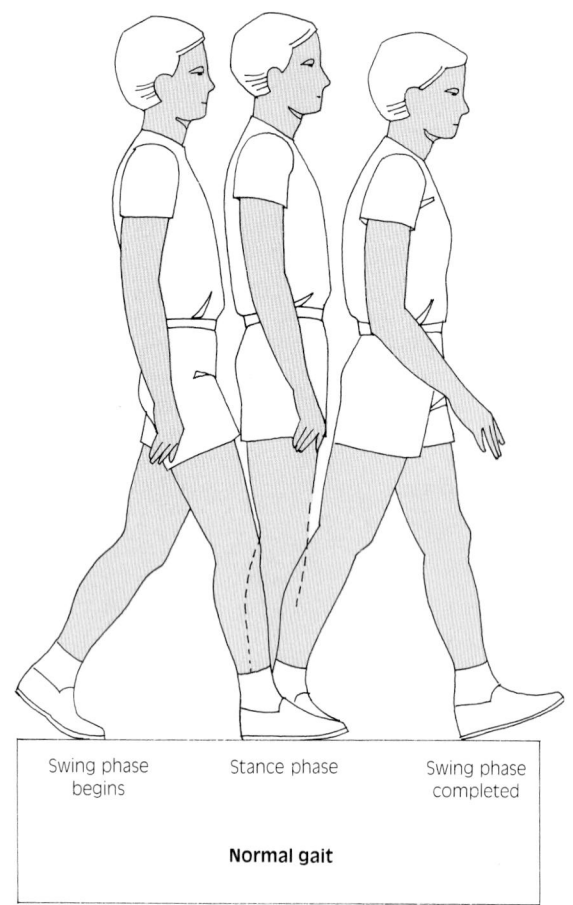

Swing phase begins   Stance phase   Swing phase completed

Normal gait

Figure 38-6
The stance and swing phases of normal gait.

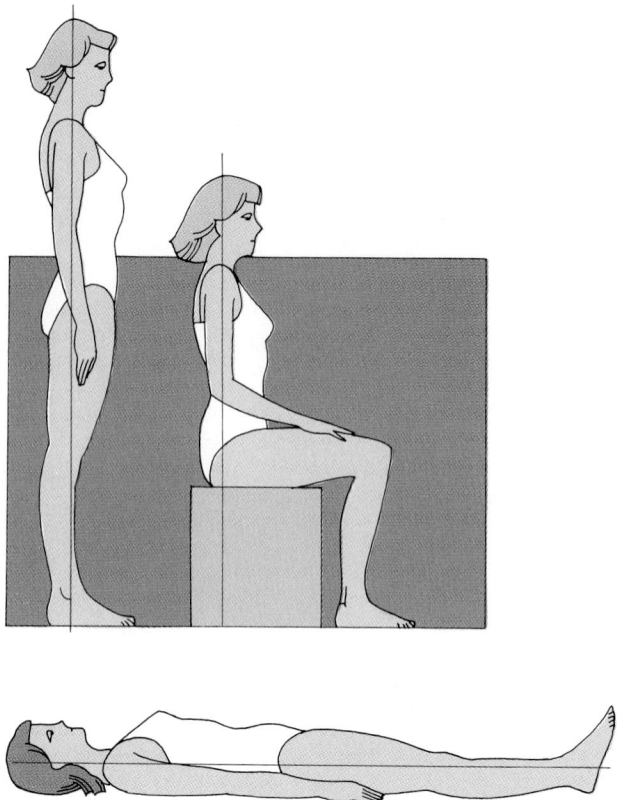

Figure 38-7
Adequate posture. In the sitting and standing positions, a straight line can be drawn from the ear through the shoulder and hip. In bed, the head, shoulders, and hips are aligned.

Hypertrophy refers to increased muscle mass resulting from exercise or training. The examiner assesses muscle mass throughout the body and may also compare one muscle group to another using tape measurements. Patients experiencing muscle wasting as a result of a chronic disease process such as cancer may report visible changes in muscle mass.

The slight residual tension that remains in a resting normal muscle with an intact nerve supply is termed *muscle tone*. Muscle tone may be assessed by flexing and extending the elbow or knee and noting the degree of resistance to these movements. Decreased tone, hypotonicity, or **flaccidity** results from disuse or neurologic impairments. **Spasticity**, increased tone that interferes with movement, is also caused by neurologic impairments.

Muscle *strength* varies greatly from one individual to another and within the same individual and is affected by muscle use. Muscle strength is tested by asking the patient to move actively against resistance. For example, the patient may be instructed to push the examiner's palms apart or to push the foot against the examiner's palm. When comparing muscle groups, remember that a person's dominant side tends to be stronger.

Impaired muscle strength or weakness is termed *paresis*. The absence of strength secondary to nervous impairment is *paralysis. Hemiparesis* refers to weakness of one half of the body, and *hemiplegia* is paralysis of one half of the body. *Paraplegia* is paralysis of the legs, and *quadriplegia* is paralysis of the arms and legs.

Nursing's concern is that the patient's muscle strength is adequate for the performance of tasks the patient deems necessary. For example, a patient whose primary means of ambulation is a wheelchair requires upper body strength.

Endurance

When assessing *endurance*, the nurse evaluates the patient's ability to turn in bed, maintain correct alignment when sitting or standing, ambulate, and perform self-care activities. When a physical or psychological factor is believed to be affecting endurance, the nurse accomplishes the following:

- Takes the vital signs while the patient is at rest
- Instructs the patient to perform the activity (eg, ambulation)
- Observes the patient's response during and after the activity
- Takes the vital signs immediately after the activity
- Reassesses the vital signs after the patient has rested for 3 minutes

Significant findings indicating that a person's exercise tolerance has been reached include noticeably increased pulse, respirations, and blood pressure; shortness of breath; dyspnea; weakness; pallor; confusion; and vertigo.

DIAGNOSING

The nurse must recognize cues that indicate both potential and actual problems when analyzing data about a patient's mobility status. Because the problems associated with immobility can seriously undermine the patient's well-being and often require complex and costly treatment, nursing energies are directed to preventing these problems whenever possible. The plan of care for the patient with an alteration in mobility should include nursing diagnoses that identify the complications of immobility for which the patient is at greatest risk.

Nursing diagnoses specifically addressing problems of mobility include Activity Intolerance and Impaired Physical Mobility. Examples of pertinent etiologies and defining characteristics are listed in the accompanying box.

Examples of nursing diagnoses that describe the effect of immobility on body systems are included in Table 38-5. Selected assessment priorities, expected outcomes, and nursing interventions are also included. Additional nursing diagnoses related to a patient's mobility alterations on other areas of human functioning follow. This list is by no means exhaustive—multiple etiologies are possible for many of these problem statements.

Pain related to inability to change body position independently

Pain: Joint related to limited range of motion and muscle atrophy

Impaired Walking related to development of footdrop

Impaired Transfer Ability related to generalized weakness

Altered Health Maintenance related to lack of mobility to procure needed services—no support people

Impaired Home Maintenance Management related to immobility

Noncompliance With Exercise Prescription related to decreased endurance, decreased motivation

Self-Care Deficit: Bathing/Hygiene, Feeding, Dressing/Grooming, Toileting related to physical weakness (decreased muscle mass and strength), altered mobility (upper or lower extremities)

Sexual Dysfunction related to neuromuscular impairment

Collaborative problems related to the effect of immobility on body systems include the following:

Potential complication: thromboemboli/deep-vein thrombosis

Potential complication: hypoxemia secondary to pneumonia

For patients who are incorporating some form of exercise in their daily routine, the following wellness diagnoses may be appropriate:

Potential for Enhanced Activity Level

Potential for Enhanced Compliance With Exercise Regimen

Nursing Diagnoses for Common Problems

Mobility

Problem	Related Factors	Sample Defining Characteristics
Activity Intolerance	Any condition that interferes with the transport of oxygenated blood to tissue (eg, cardiac problems such as congestive heart failure and arrhythmias; respiratory problems, especially chronic obstructive pulmonary disease; circulatory problems; diabetes mellitus) Any condition that causes fatigue (depression, pain, sleep disturbances, prolonged bed rest, sedentary lifestyle)	Decreased ability to perform basic self-care activities: turning in bed, changing position, ambulating, washing, dressing, eating, and so on Altered response to activity: • Dyspnea, shortness of breath, excessive increase in respiratory rate • Weak pulse, excessive increase in pulse rate, change in rhythm • Blood pressure that fails to increase with activity or that decreases • Weakness, pallor, confusion, vertigo
Impaired Physical Mobility	• Neuromuscular impairment (arthritis, stroke, Parkinson's disease) • Musculoskeletal impairment • Decreased strength and endurance • Pain or discomfort • Depression	• Physical inability to move purposefully or a reluctance to move • Limited range of motion • Decreased muscle mass, tone, or strength • Therapy-related restrictions on movement (eg, an order for bed rest, traction, cast, or splints)

If the patient is not experiencing any mobility problems, expected patient outcomes are directed toward the promotion of physical fitness. For example, the patient will achieve the following:

• Follow a program of regular physical exercise that improves cardiovascular function, endurance, flexibility, and strength

To achieve this long-term expected outcome, numerous short-term expected outcomes may be needed. An example follows.

By the next visit, 2/20/01, the patient will:

• Identify four personal benefits of regular exercise
• Describe an exercise program (activities, frequency, duration) the patient is willing to follow
• Identify his or her own target heart range
• Obtain medical clearance for the exercise program if at high risk for complications
• List support systems that will reinforce exercise efforts

Patients at high risk for specific mobility problems require different expected outcomes. The patient will achieve the following:

• Demonstrate correct body alignment whenever observed (alignment)
• Adhere to an every-2-hour positioning schedule (alignment)
• Demonstrate full range of joint motion (joint mobility)
• Demonstrate adequate muscle mass, tone, and strength to perform functional activities of daily living (muscle mass, tone, and strength)

Specific expected outcomes for patients at risk for complications related to immobility may be found in Table 38-5. Goals for more specific problems (eg, for the patient learning to walk with crutches or needing to master transfer techniques with only upper body mobility) need to be individualized.

Nursing strategies designed to promote correct body alignment, mobility, and fitness are described in the following sections. Techniques for positioning patients; performing range-of-motion exercises; moving, lifting, and ambulating patients; and designing exercise programs are included.

Positioning Patients

Positioning that maintains correct body alignment and facilitates physiologic functioning contributes to the patient's psychological and physical well-being. The force of gravity pulls parts of the body out of alignment unless adequate support is provided. Various positions are therefore protective in nature only when the patient is positioned properly.

Common Devices to Promote Correct Alignment

Many devices can help maintain good body alignment and muscle tonus while the patient is in bed and alleviate discomfort or pressure on various parts of the body.

Pillows

Pillows are used primarily to provide support or to elevate a part. Pillows of different sizes are useful for different body parts. Those intended for the head are usually full-sized or large-sized pillows. Small pillows are ideal for support or elevation of the extremities, shoulders, or incisional wounds. Specially designed heavy pillows are useful to elevate the upper part of the body when an adjustable bed is unavailable, such as at home.

Mattresses

For a mattress to be comfortable and supportive, it must be firm but have sufficient "give" to permit good body alignment. A patient who must remain in a bed with a nonsupportive mattress might well complain of backache and other discomforts.

A well-made and well-supported foam-rubber mattress retains a uniform firmness. This mattress is made of natural or synthetic rubber or a combination of both. A large volume of air is incorporated. The foam-rubber mattress conforms to the contours of the body and provides support at all points. Its greatest advantage is that it does not form slopes and valleys as inner-spring mattresses are likely to do. Moreover, foam-rubber mattresses do not create as much pressure against bony prominences, such as the ankles, the elbows, the scapulae, and the coccyx. Special mattresses, pads, and types of beds used to help prevent pressure ulcers are discussed in Chapter 37.

Adjustable Bed

The head of an adjustable bed can be elevated to the desired degree. This positioning is discussed later in the chapter. The foot of an adjustable bed can also be elevated as desired. Some adjustable beds allow the bed to be "broken," or gatched, so that the mattress is flexed at the level of the knees. This position is rarely recommended or is used only for brief periods because it can cause pressure on the popliteal space behind the knee, resulting in impaired circulation to the lower extremity and an increased risk for clot formation.

The adjustable bed can also be changed so that the distance of the bed to the floor can be altered. The patient can get in and out of bed easier when the bed is in the lowest position. The higher positions are used by healthcare workers so that they do not strain their backs while giving bed care. General guidelines for safe use of beds are discussed in Chapter 36.

Bed Side Rails

One of nurses' greatest safety concerns is to prevent patients from falling out of bed. The use of side rails requires explanation to patients and their families and must follow the protocol of the healthcare agency. They help to remind patients that they are not in their usual environment, should they awaken during the night and wish to get out of bed. Side rails also make it possible for a patient to roll from one side to the other or to sit up without calling for assistance. This in itself is a good activity: it helps the patient retain or regain muscle efficiency.

Bed side rails may not deter some patients from getting out of bed. Many a patient has crawled over the foot of the bed. It is recommended that side rails extend only for three fourths of the length of the mattress. Then, if side rails are in use and patients do attempt to get out of bed, they do not have to climb over the side rail or the foot of the bed and further increase the danger of falling. For patients who sleep restlessly or have frequent involuntary movements of the extremities and may be in danger of harming themselves against the side rails, protective padding may be ordered. Safe use of side rails is discussed in Chapter 26.

Trapeze Bar

A *trapeze bar* (Fig. 38-8) is a hand grip suspended from a frame near the head of the bed. The patient can grasp the bar with one or both hands and then raise the trunk from the bed. The trapeze makes moving and turning considerably easier for many patients and facilitates transfers into and out of bed. It can also be used to perform exercises that strengthen some muscles of the upper extremities (eg, biceps).

Additional Equipment

The greatest danger to the feet occurs when they are unsupported in the dorsiflexion position. The toes drop downward, and the feet are in plantar flexion. Because of the pull of gravity, this position of the feet occurs naturally when the body is at rest. If maintained for extended periods, plantar flexion can cause an alteration in the length of muscles, and the patient may develop a complication called **footdrop**. In this position, the foot is unable to maintain itself in the perpendicular position, heel–toe gait is impossible, and the patient experiences extreme difficulty in walking. The use of a foot support, such as a foot boot, helps avoid this complication. Figure 38-9 demonstrates a foot in plantar flexion versus the dorsiflexion position maintained by wearing a high-top canvas sneaker.

If top bedding must be kept off the patient's lower extremities, a device called a cradle is used. A *cradle* is usu-

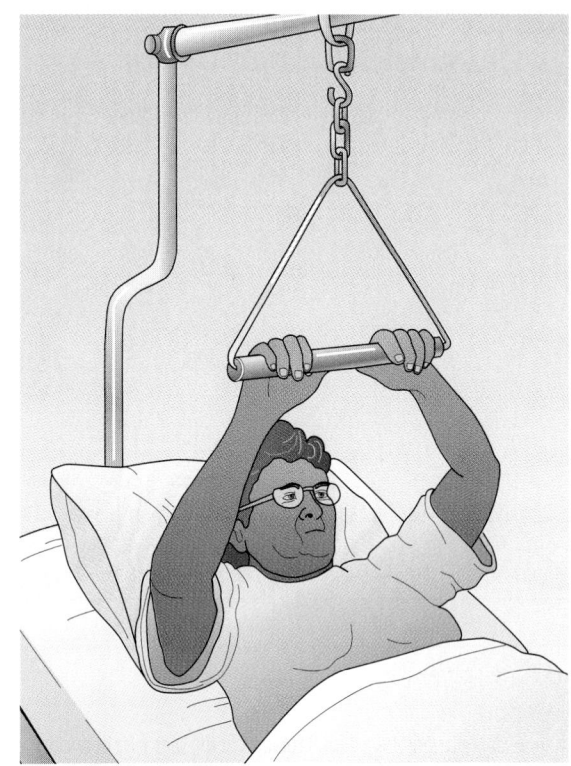

Figure 38-8
A trapeze device makes it possible for the patient to lift part of the body from the bed, thus facilitating turning and moving up in bed.

ally a metal frame that supports the bed linens away from the patient while providing privacy and warmth. There are any number of sizes and shapes of cradles. If used, the cradle should be fastened securely to the bed so that it does not slide or fall on the patient.

Sandbags can be used to immobilize an extremity and support body alignment. They have greater value when available in various sizes. When properly filled, they are not hard or firmly packed. They should be pliable enough to be shaped to body contours to give support. They should be placed so that they do not create pressure on a bony prominence.

Trochanter rolls are used to support the hips and legs so that the femurs do not rotate outward. Figure 38-10

Figure 38-9
(*Left*) Plantar flexion occurs when the foot is not supported. (*Right*) When high-top sneakers support the feet, the dorsiflexion position is maintained.

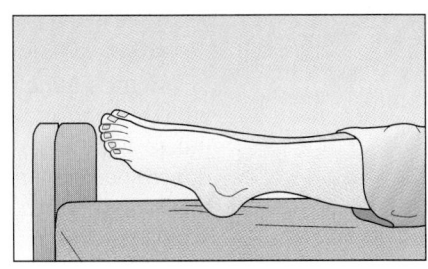

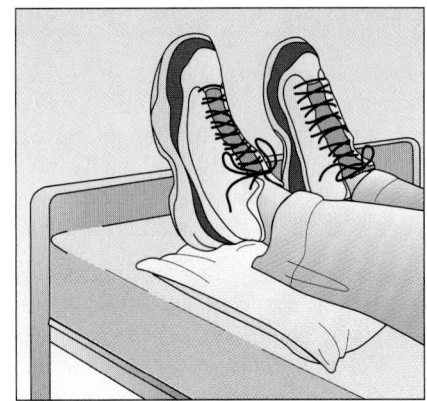

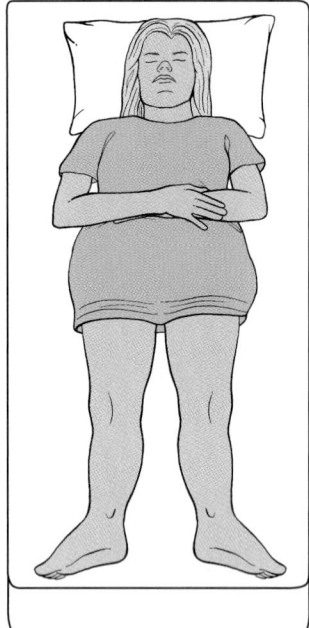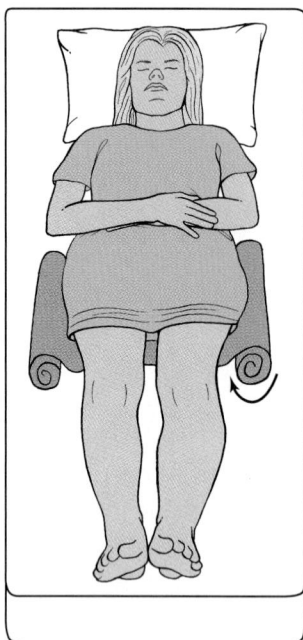

Figure 38-10
Trochanter rolls prevent the external rotation of the hips of a bedridden patient. The patient is placed on a folded sheet so that the top edge is at the hips and the lower edge is about one third of the way down the thighs. Towels or a bath blanket is rolled under each side until the roll is snugly against the patient's hips and thighs. The support cannot unroll, and the weight of the patient keeps it secure.

illustrates and describes how to use trochanter rolls. Properly placed pillows can also be used to help prevent the thighs from turning outward, but they tend to slip out of place and require frequent adjustment to be effective.

If a patient is paralyzed or unconscious, hand–wrist splints or hand rolls may be necessary to provide a means for keeping the thumb in the correct position, that is, slightly adducted and in apposition to the fingers. A hand roll can be created by folding a washcloth, rolling it, and securing it in place with tape. Once placed against the palm of the hand, it can effectively keep the hand in a functional position (Fig. 38-11). A commercial plastic or aluminum splint may be used to hold the thumb in place regardless of the hand position. Patients who are not moving their fingers should be encouraged to do finger exercises, with special attention to having the thumb touch the tip of each finger.

Protective Positioning

Patients accustomed to an active lifestyle who generally use only a bed for sleep are often unaware of the importance of correct body alignment and regular position changes when on prescribed bed rest. Whenever possible, nurses should teach both the patient and family the following:

- Correct positioning techniques
- The need to change positions frequently, at least every 2 hours
- The importance of using the time allotted to position changes to exercise the extremities and to assess and

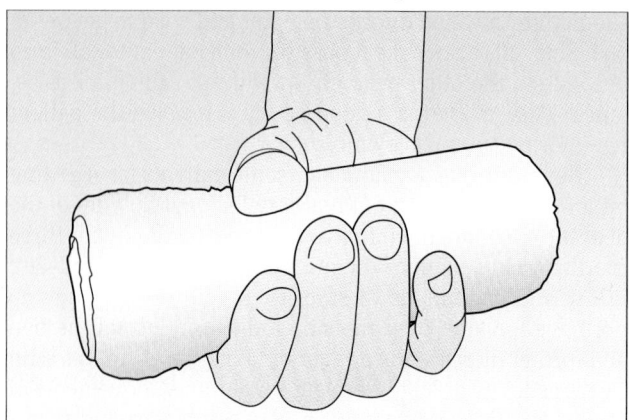

Figure 38-11
A hand roll holds the hand in functional position.

massage pressure areas (reddened areas should not be massaged.)

When the patient is unable to change position independently, a turn schedule should be posted at the bedside so that nurses assist with and document the rotation of positions. Table 38-6 describes nursing measures to prevent complications associated with common bed positions.

Fowler's Position

The semisitting position is called *Fowler's position* and calls for the head of the bed to be elevated 45 to 60 degrees. This position is often used to promote cardiac and respiratory functioning because abdominal organs drop in this position and thereby provide maximal space in the thoracic cavity. This is also the position of choice for eating, conversation, vision, and urinary and intestinal elimination.

Variations of Fowler's position include high Fowler's and low Fowler's or semi-Fowler's position. In the high Fowler's position, the head of the bed is elevated 90 degrees. When a bedside table with a pillow on top of it is placed in front of the patient in high Fowler's position, the patient can lean forward and rest the arms on the pillow, assuming a posture that allows for maximal lung expansion. In low Fowler's or semi-Fowler's position, the head of the bed is elevated only 30 degrees. In Fowler's position, the buttocks bear the main weight of the body. Other skin areas that require assessment and massage include the heels, the sacrum, and the scapulae. The correct positioning and nursing actions to prevent complications associated with Fowler's position are presented in Table 38-6.

Supine or Dorsal Recumbent Position

In the *supine position*, the patient lies flat on the back with the head and shoulders slightly elevated with a pillow unless contraindicated. The pillow under the head and upper shoulders may not be allowed after a spinal anesthetic or surgery on the spinal vertebrae. Table 38-6 describes nursing actions to prevent complications associated with this position and illustrates correct alignment in the supine position.

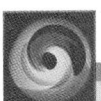

Table 38-6
Common Bed Positions and Protective Nursing Actions

Position	Complication to Be Prevented	Suggested Preventive Actions
Fowler's Position	Flexion contracture of the neck	Allow the head to rest against the mattress or be supported by a small pillow only.
	Exaggerated curvature of the spine	Use a firm support for the back; position the patient so that the angle of elevation starts at the hips.
	Dislocation of the shoulder	Support the forearms on pillows to elevate them sufficiently so that no pull is exerted on the shoulders.
	Flexion contracture of the wrist	Support the hand on pillows so that it is in natural alignment with the forearm.
	Edema of the hand	Support the hand so that it is slightly elevated in relation to the elbow.
	Flexion contractures of the fingers and abduction of the thumbs	Provide hand–wrist splints if necessary.
	Impaired lower extremity circulation and knee contracture, pressure on heels	Elevate the knees for only brief periods; place one or two pillows under the lower legs from below the knees to the ankles; avoid pressure on the popliteal vessels; avoid using the knee gatch.
	External rotation of the hips	Use trochanter roll.
	Footdrop	Support the feet in dorsal flexion. Use footboard; high-top sneakers can also be used.
Protective Supine Position	Exaggerated curvature of the spine and flexion of the hips	Provide a firm supportive mattress; use a bed board if necessary.
	Flexion contracture of the neck	Place pillows under the upper shoulders, the neck, and the head so that the head and the neck are held in the correct position.
	Internal rotation of the shoulders and extension of the elbows (hunch shoulders)	Place pillows or arm supports under the forearms so that the upper arms are alongside the body and the forearms are pronated slightly.
	Flexion of the lumbar curvature	Place rolled towel or small pillow under lumbar curvature if needed.
	Extension of the fingers and abduction of the thumbs (clawhand deformities)	Use hand–wrist splints if appropriate.
	External rotation of the femurs	Place sandbags or a trochanter roll alongside the hips and the upper half of the thighs.
	Hyperextension of the knees	Place a pillow under the lower legs from below the knees to the ankles.
	Footdrop	Use a footboard or make an improvised firm foot support to hold the feet in dorsal flexion; high-top sneakers may also be recommended.

(continued)

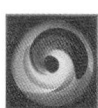

Table 38-6 (Continued)

Position	Complication to Be Prevented	Suggested Preventive Actions
Protective Side-Lying or Lateral Position 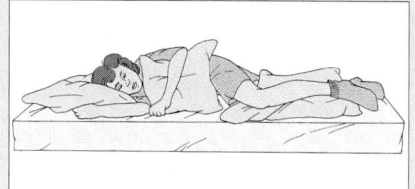	Lateral flexion of the neck	Place a pillow under the head and the neck.
	Inward rotation of the arm and interference with respiration	Place a pillow under the upper arm; lower arm should be flexed and positioned comfortably.
	Extension of the finger and abduction of the thumbs	Provide hand–wrist splint if necessary.
	Internal rotation and adduction of the femur	Use one or two pillows as needed to support the leg from the groin to the foot.
	Twisting of the spine	Ensure that the two shoulders are aligned with the two hips.
Protective Sims' Position 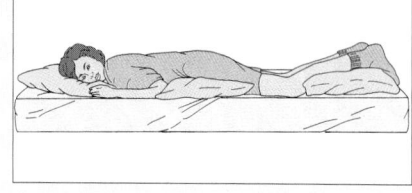	Lateral flexion of the neck	Place a small pillow under the head unless the drainage of oral secretions is desired.
	Damage to nerves and blood vessels in the axillae of the lower arm	Carefully position lower arm behind and away from the patient's back.
	Internal shoulder rotation and adduction	Abduct the upper shoulder slightly so that shoulder and elbow are flexed; place a pillow between the chest and upper arm.
	Internal rotation and adduction of the hip; lumbar lordosis	Place a pillow under the upper flexed leg from the groin to the foot.
	Twisting of the spine	Ensure that the two shoulders are aligned with the two hips.
	Footdrop	Support the lower foot in dorsal flexion with a sandbag.
Protective Prone Position 	Flexion on the cervical spine	Place a small pillow under the head.
	Hyperextension of the spine; impaired respirations	Place some suitable support under the patient between the end of the rib cage and the upper abdomen if this facilitates breathing and if there is space there.
	Footdrop	Move the patient down in bed so that the feet are over the mattress, or support the lower legs on a pillow just high enough to keep the toes from touching the bed.

Side-Lying or Lateral Position

In the *side-lying position*, the patient lies on the side and the main weight of the body is borne by the lateral aspect of the lower scapula and the lateral aspect of the lower ilium. Because many people routinely fall asleep in the side-lying position, this is a comfortable alternate to the supine position for the patient on bed rest. Although it relieves pressure on the scapulae, sacrum, and heels and allows the legs and feet to be comfortably flexed, support pillows are needed for correct positioning. Table 38-6 describes and illustrates the protective side-lying position.

The *oblique position* is recommended as an alternative to the side-lying position because it places significantly less pressure on the trochanter region. The patient turns toward the side with the hip on the top leg flexed at a 30-degree angle and the knee flexed at 35 degrees. The calf of the upper leg is positioned slightly behind the body's midline. Pillows support the patient's back and calf of the top leg (Fig. 38-12).

A variation of the lateral position is Sims' position. In this position, the patient again lies on the side, but the lower arm is behind the patient and the upper arm is flexed at both the shoulder and the elbow. Because in this position the main body weight is borne by the anterior aspects of the humerus, clavicle, and ilium, the major pressure points differ from those in the lateral and other bed-lying positions (see Table 38-6).

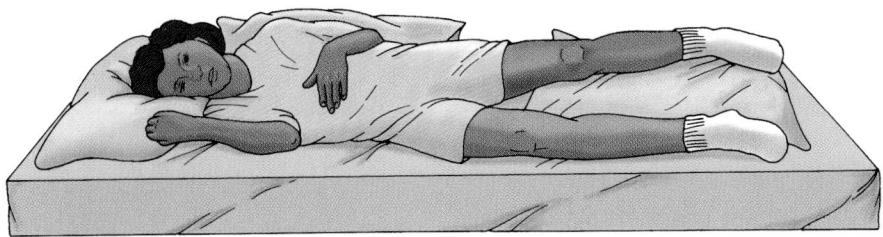

Figure 38-12
Modified lateral position (oblique position) is an alternative to the side-lying position and results in significantly less pressure on the trochanter area.

Prone Position

In the *prone position*, the person lies on the abdomen with the head turned to the side. The body is straightened out in the prone position because the shoulders, head, and neck are in an erect position, the arms are easily placed in correct alignment with the shoulder girdle, the hips are extended, and the knees can be prevented from flexing or hyperextending. When patients on bed rest use this position periodically, it helps to prevent flexion contractures of the hips and knees. However, the pull of gravity on the trunk when the patient lies prone produces a marked lordosis or forward curvature of the lumbar spine. The position is thus contraindicated for people with spinal problems. The pull of gravity on the feet may result in plantar flexion unless the legs and feet are positioned carefully. Table 38-6 illustrates correct alignment in the prone position and describes nursing activities to prevent complications. Placing a patient in the prone position requires that the nurse and an assistant move the person as far as is safely possible onto his or her side, facing the direction that the person will be turned, and near the edge of the level bed. While maintaining the patient securely in that position, pillows can be situated alongside the trunk and upper and lower extremities. Once the patient is gently turned face down, the pillows can be readjusted for comfort and support.

Turning the Patient in Bed

Frequently, a patient cannot turn in bed without assistance. Nurses need to use their knowledge of correct body mechanics and correct alignment to turn the patient from the back onto the side, from the back onto the abdomen, and from the abdomen onto the back. The technique for turning a patient in bed is described and illustrated in Procedure 38-1. Mastering this turning technique helps nurses adhere to an every-2-hour turn schedule for an immobile patient.

Assisting With Range-of-Motion Exercises

Range of motion is the complete extent of movement of which a joint is normally capable. Engaging in routine tasks, such as bathing, eating, dressing, and writing, helps use muscle groups that keep many joints in effective range of motion. When all or some of normal activities of daily living are impossible, attention should be given to the joints not being used at all or to those that are limited in their use.

Unless contraindicated, active, active-assistive, or passive range-of-motion exercises should be encouraged regularly and included in the patient's plan of care. In **active exercise**, the patient independently moves joints through their full range of motion (isotonic exercise). In *active-assistive exercise*, the nurse may provide minimal support, whereas in **passive exercise**, the patient is unable to move independently, and the nurse moves each joint through its range of motion. Both active and passive exercises improve joint mobility and increase circulation to the affected part, but only active exercise increases muscle mass, tone, and strength and improves cardiac and respiratory functioning. Thus, exercises should be as active as the patient's physical condition permits. It is also helpful to teach isometric exercises to patients to increase muscle mass, tone, and strength.

Directives should be included in the nursing plan of care for range-of-motion exercises. The nursing orders should explain what, how, and when, so that all who care for the patient observe the same routine. In some institutions, nurses work closely with physiotherapists in designing and implementing exercise programs. The following are basic guidelines for the nurse when helping to put the patient's joints through range of motion:

- Teach the patient what exercise is being undertaken, why, and how it will be done. A show-and-tell technique is often helpful.
- Avoid overexertion and using exercises to the point that the patient develops fatigue. The exercises are not to exhaust or tax the patient. Certain exercises may need to be delayed until the patient's condition allows.
- Avoid neck hyperextension and attempts to achieve full range of motion in all joints with older patients. These movements may prove painful. Encourage adequate range of motion in those joints necessary to perform activities of daily living.
- Start gradually and work slowly. All movements should be smooth and rhythmic. Irregular and jerky movements are uncomfortable for patients.
- Move each joint until there is resistance but not pain. Uncomfortable reactions should be reported and exercises halted until further instructions are obtained.
- While exercising joints, use a variety of support measures to prevent muscle strain or injury to the patient (Fig. 38-13):
  - *Cupping*—placing a cupped hand under the joint to support it (eg, under the elbow)
  - *Cradling*—supporting the joint with one hand while cradling the distal portion of the extremity with the remaining arm (eg, the calf or forearm might be cradled while the knee or elbow is supported)
  - *Supporting* the joint by holding the adjacent distal and proximal muscular areas (indicated when a

PROCEDURE 38-1

Turning a Patient in Bed

Action	Rationale
1. Explain the procedure to the patient.	This facilitates the cooperation of the patient.
2. Wash your hands.	Handwashing deters the spread of microorganisms.
3. Raise the bed to your waist level. Adjust to flat position or as low as the patient can tolerate. Lower side rail nearest you and raise the opposite side.	This position facilitates the turning maneuver and minimizes strain on the nurse yet keeps the patient safe.
4. Position the patient closer to the far side of the bed in the supine position.	The patient will be in the center of the bed after turning is accomplished.
5. Place the patient's arms across the chest and cross the patient's far leg over the near one.	This facilitates the turning motion and protects the patient's arms during the turn.
6. Stand opposite the patient's center with your feet spread and one foot ahead of the other. Tighten your gluteal and abdominal muscles and flex your knees.	This positions the turner opposite the center of the body mass. It places the nurse in a stable position with good body alignment and prepared to use large muscle masses to turn the patient.

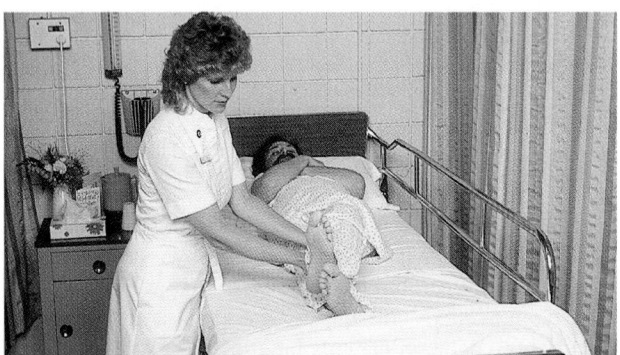

Action 5: Positioning patient's arms and legs.

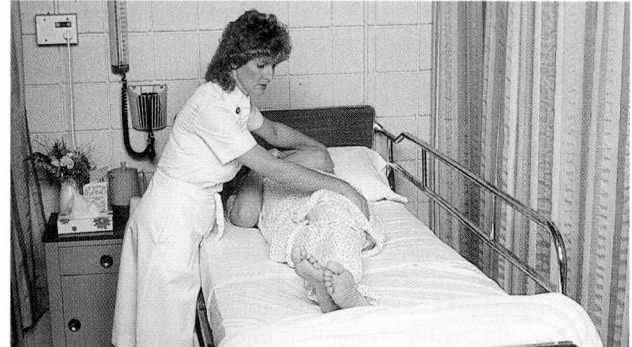

Action 6: Preparing to turn patient.

Action	Rationale
7. Position your hands on the patient's far shoulder and hip and roll the patient toward you.	This maneuver supports the patient's body and makes use of the nurse's weight to assist with turning.
8. Make the patient comfortable and position in proper alignment.	This ensures that the patient will be able to maintain desired position.

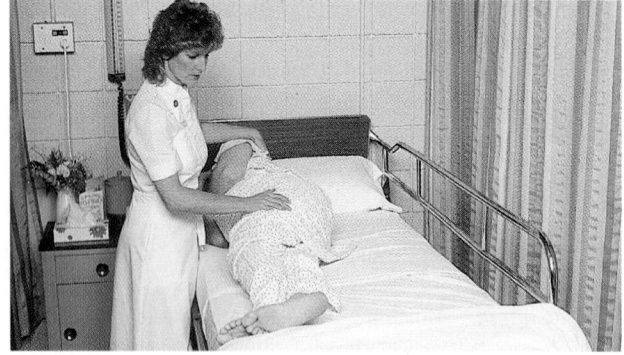

Action 7: Turning patient.

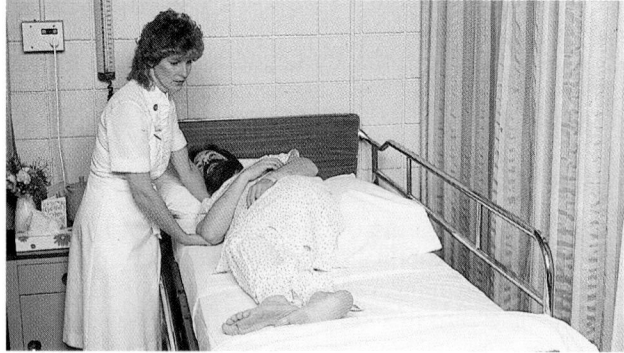

Action 8: Making patient comfortable.

Action	Rationale
9. Readjust the bed height and position and raise side rail if appropriate.	This ensures the patient's safety.
10. Wash your hands.	Handwashing deters the spread of microorganisms.

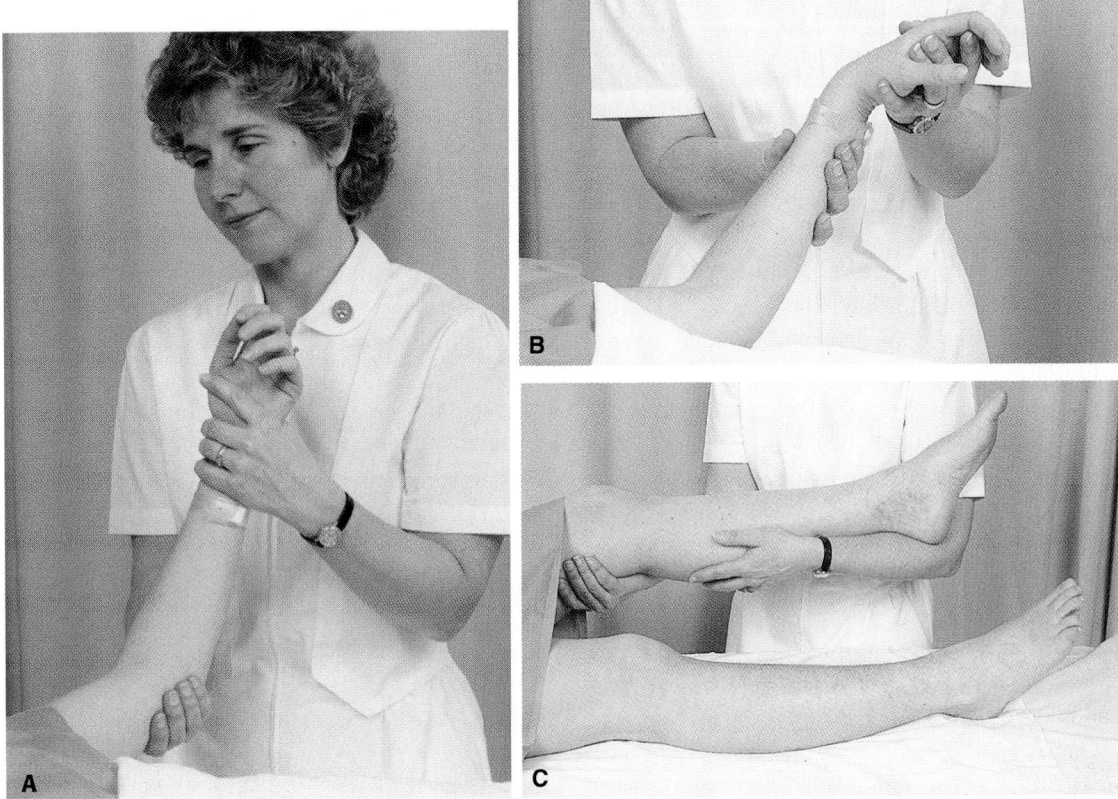

Figure 38-13
Support measures used to prevent muscle strain or injury to the patient during range-of-motion exercises (**A**) using a cupped hand to support a joint; (**B**) cradling the distal portion of an extremity; and (**C**) supporting the joint by holding the distal and proximal areas adjacent to the joint.

joint is painful); grasping muscle groups or major tendons is likely to cause injury to the tissues.

- Return the joint to a neutral position, that is, its normal position of alignment, when finishing each exercise.
- Keep friction at a minimum when moving extremities to avoid injuring the skin.
- Use range-of-motion exercises twice a day, and do the exercises regularly to build up muscle and joint capabilities. Each exercise is carried out two to five times. Many of the exercises can be carried out when the patient is being bathed and become part of that procedure. Routine tasks, such as eating, dressing, self-bathing, and writing, also help to put certain joints through range of motion and should be encouraged.
- Expect the patient's respiratory and heart rate to increase during exercising, which is good. These rates should return to usual resting levels within 3 minutes. If they do not, the exercises are probably too strenuous for the patient.
- Use passive exercises as necessary, but encourage active exercises of the same kind when the patient is able to do so independently. Exercises should continue at home after a period of hospitalization, as necessary.

The goal of range-of-motion exercises is to keep the patient in the best possible physical state when bed rest is necessary. When range-of-motion exercises are not considered as routine measures, the patient's physician should be consulted. Procedure 38-2 illustrates the normal movements incorporated in passive range-of-motion exercises.

Moving and Lifting the Patient

Frequently, it is necessary to move a helpless patient. The patient must be kept in good alignment and protected from injury while being moved. Nurses should follow these recommended guidelines when moving and lifting patients:

- Know the patient's medical diagnosis, capabilities, and any movement not allowed. Place braces or any device the patient wears before helping from bed.
- Plan carefully what you will do before moving or lifting a patient. Assess the mobility of attached equipment. You may injure the patient or yourself if you have not planned well. If necessary, enlist the support of another nurse. This reduces the strain on everyone involved.
- Explain to the patient what you plan to do. Then, use what abilities the patient has to assist you. This technique often decreases the effort required and the possibility of injury to you.
- If the patient is in pain, administer the prescribed analgesic sufficiently in advance of the transfer to allow the patient to participate in the move comfortably.

(*text continues on page 984*)

PROCEDURE 38-2

Assisting With Passive Range-of-Motion (ROM) Exercises

Action	Rationale
1. Explain the procedure to the patient.	This facilitates the patient's cooperation.
2. Wash your hands.	Handwashing deters the spread of microorganisms.
3. Raise the bed to your waist level. Adjust to flat position or as low as patient can tolerate.	This position minimizes strain on the nurse.
4. Begin ROM exercises at the patient's head and move down one side of the body at a time.	Systematic progression ensures that all body parts are exercised.
5. Perform each exercise two to five times, moving each joint in a smooth and rhythmic manner.	Repeated movement of muscles and joints improves flexibility and increases circulation to the body part.
6. Protect joint during ROM exercises (see Fig. 38-13).	This prevents muscle strain or injury to the joint.
7. Progress through ROM exercises for each joint.	

Head

- *Flexion*—move chin down to rest on chest.
- *Extension*—return head to normal upright position.
- *Lateral flexion*—tilt head as far as possible toward each shoulder.

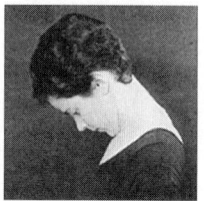
Flexion

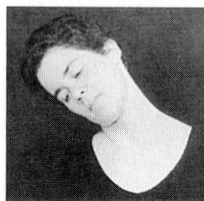
Lateral flexion

Neck

- *Rotation*—move the head from side to side bringing chin toward shoulder.

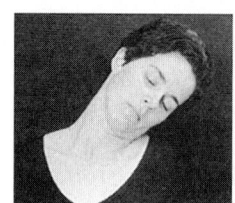
Lateral flexion

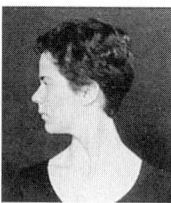
Rotation

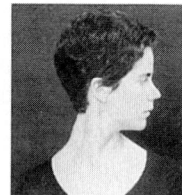
Rotation

Shoulder

- *Flexion*—start with arm at side and lift arm forward to above head.
- *Extension*—return arm to starting position at side of body.

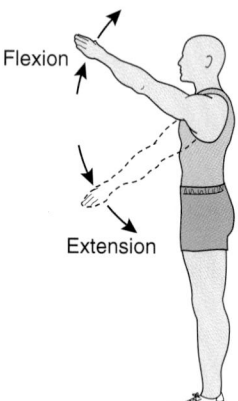
Flexion
Extension

(continued)

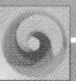

PROCEDURE 38-2

Assisting With Passive Range-of-Motion (ROM) Exercises (Continued)

- *Abduction*—start with arm at side and move laterally to upright position above head.
- *Adduction*—lower arm to original position and move across body as far as possible.
- *Internal and external rotation*—raise arm at side until upper arm is on line with shoulder. Bend elbow at a 90-degree angle and move forearm upward and downward.

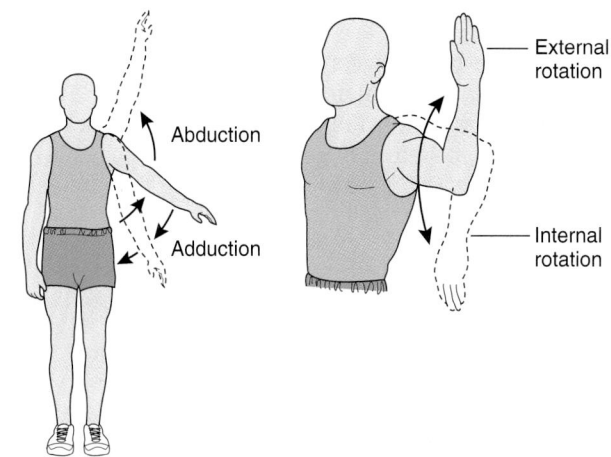

Elbow

- *Flexion*—bend elbow and move lower arm and hand upward toward shoulder.
- *Extension*—return lower arm and hand to original position while straightening elbow.

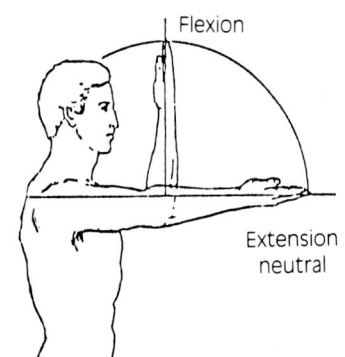

Forearm

- *Supination*—rotate lower arm and hand so palm is up.
- *Pronation*—rotate lower arm and hand so palm is down.

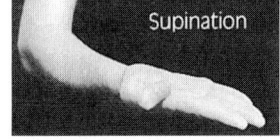

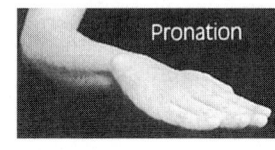

Wrist

- *Flexion*—move hand downward toward inner aspect of forearm.
- *Extension*—return hand to neutral position even with forearm.
- *Hyperextension*—move dorsal (upper) portion of hand backward as far as possible.

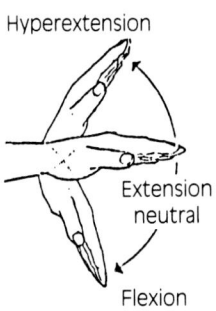

(continued)

PROCEDURE 38-2

Assisting With Passive Range-of-Motion (ROM) Exercises (Continued)

Fingers

- *Flexion*—bend fingers in to make a fist.
- *Extension*—straighten fingers out.
- *Abduction*—spread fingers apart.
- *Adduction*—return fingers until they are together.
- *Opposition of thumb to fingers*—touch thumb to each finger on hand.

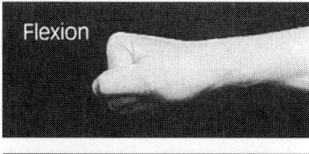

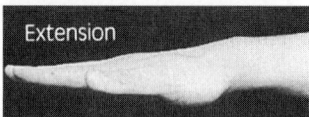

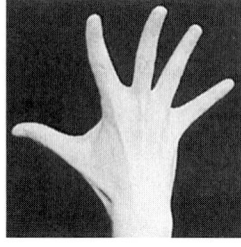

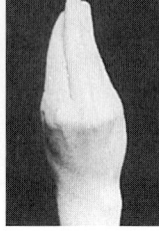

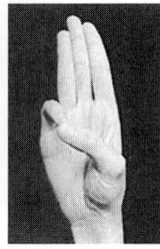

Abduction   Adduction   Apposition of thumb to finger

Hip

- *Flexion*—with leg extended, lift upward.
- *Extension*—return leg to original position next to other leg.
- *Abduction*—lift leg laterally away from body.
- *Adduction*—return leg toward other leg and lift beyond it if possible.
- *Internal rotation*—turn foot and leg toward other leg.
- *External rotation*—move foot and leg outward away from other leg.

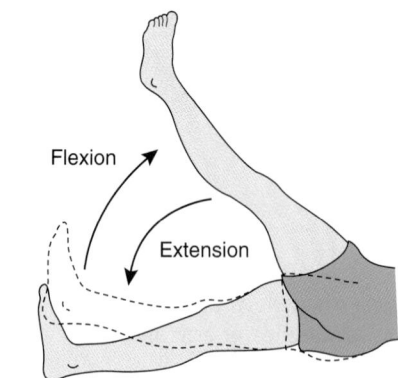

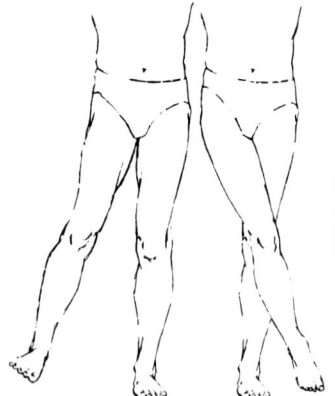

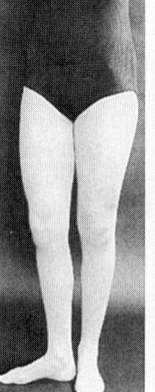

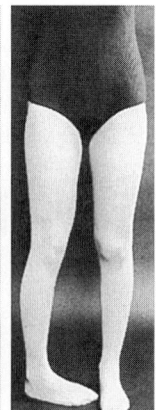

Abduction   Adduction   External rotation   Internal rotation

(continued)

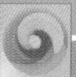

Assisting With Passive Range-of-Motion (ROM) Exercises (Continued)

Knee

- *Flexion*—bend leg, bringing heel toward back of leg.
- *Extension*—return leg to straight position.

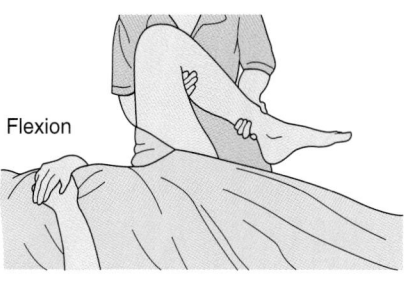

Flexion

Flexion

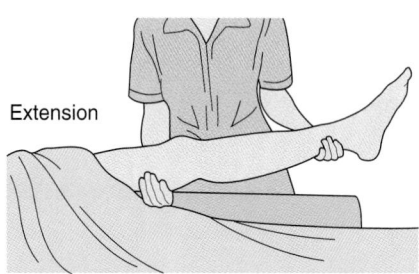

Extension

Flexion

Ankle

- *Dorsiflexion*—move foot up and back until toes are upright.
- *Plantar flexion*—move foot with toes pointing downward.
- *Inversion*—turn sole of foot toward the middle.
- *Eversion*—turn sole of foot outward.

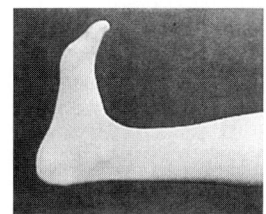

Dorsiflexion

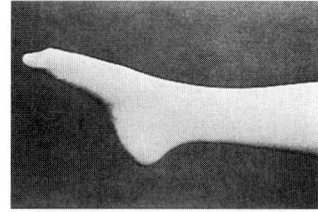

Plantar flexion

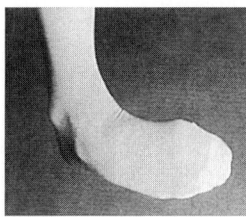

Inversion

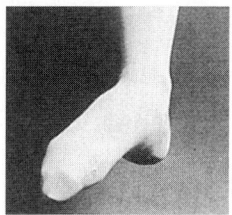

Eversion

Toes

- *Flexion*—curl toes downward.
- *Extension*—straighten toes out.
- *Abduction*—spread toes apart
- *Adduction*—bring toes together.

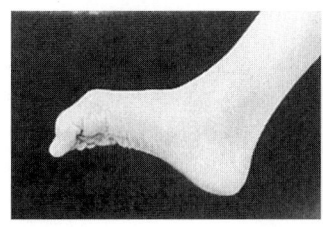

Flexion

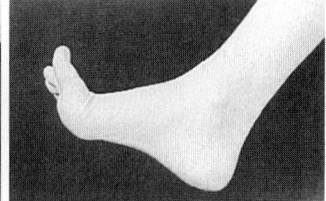

Extension

(continued)

PROCEDURE 38-2

Assisting With Passive Range-of-Motion (ROM) Exercises (Continued)

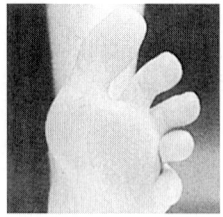 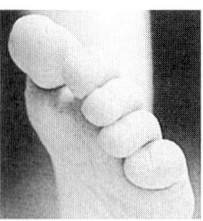

Abduction   Adduction

8. Return patient to comfortable position.	This promotes rest and sleep.
9. Readjust the bed height and position and raise side rail if it is appropriate.	This ensures the patient's safety.
10. Wash your hands.	Handwashing deters the spread of microorganisms.

- Remove any obstacles that may make moving and lifting inconvenient.
- Elevate the bed as necessary so that you are working at a height that is comfortable and safe for you.
- Lock the wheels of the bed, wheelchair, or stretcher so that they do not slide while you are moving the patient.
- Observe the principles of body mechanics while you work to prevent injuring yourself.
- Be sure the patient is in good body alignment while being moved and lifted to protect the patient from strain and muscle injury.
- Support the patient's body well. Avoid grabbing and holding an extremity by its muscles.
- Avoid friction on the patient's skin during moving. Friction can be reduced by sprinkling powder or cornstarch on bed linens and on the patient's skin.
- Move your body and the patient in a smooth, rhythmic motion. Jerky movements tend to put extra strain on muscles and joints and are uncomfortable for the patient.
- Use mechanical devices such as a Hoyer lift or turning board when available for moving patients. Be sure that you understand how the device operates and that the patient is properly secured and informed of what will occur. Patients who do not understand or are afraid may be unable to cooperate and may suffer injury as a result.
- Be realistic about how much you can safely do without injury. Two small people cannot lift or move an obese patient without risking muscle strain and injury.

Nurses who retire from or leave nursing often cite back injuries as an influencing factor. Nurses may incur back in-juries as a result of poor body mechanics or become injured when a patient falls. Back injuries are the most frequent cause of nurses' workers compensation claims (Ellis & Hartley, 1998; Skewes, 1997). Many other nurses do not file incident reports but say they have had episodes of occupation-related back problems and accept back pain as a routine consequence of the job—which it need not be. Transferring patients from a wheelchair to the bed, toilet, or scale chair and any transfers related to bathing are listed as the most physically stressing tasks (Skewes, 1997). Other variables that can lead to back injuries for healthcare workers include:

- Uncoordinated lifts
- Height–weight differential among the lifters
- Lifting when fatigued
- Lifting after recent recovery from a back injury
- Lack of training in proper body mechanics

Techniques to prevent back stress should be included routinely in injury prevention programs. Additional emphasis in the nursing curriculum on principles of body mechanics and patient-lifting techniques may also help improve the nursing environment.

Moving the Patient Up in Bed

Children and light-weight adults are relatively easy to slide toward the head of the bed without the assistance of a second person. The nurse places one arm under the patient's neck and grasps the patient's far shoulder with the hand. The other arm is placed under the patient's thighs. With knees and hips flexed, the nurse moves the patient closer to the nurse's side of the bed. On a count of three, the nurse moves the patient toward the head of the bed while the patient assists the movement either by pushing with the feet or by using an overbed trapeze. A technique used to move a patient up in bed when the patient is able to assist and two nurses are available is described and illustrated in Procedure 38-3.

Moving the Patient From Bed to Stretcher

Considerable care must be taken when moving a patient from a bed to a stretcher, or vice versa, to prevent injury to the patient. If the patient is unconscious or helpless, additional nurses are needed to support the extremities and the head. These skills are described in Procedure 38-4. For patients who are obese, use of a transfer board or roller board facilitates the move from stretcher to bed and helps ensure that the patient's body is properly aligned during the transfer (see Special Considerations in Procedure 38-4). When returning the patient to the bed from the stretcher, the same techniques are used. The carriers should first move the patient from the stretcher onto the edge of the bed. Then one member of the team supports the patient on the edge of the bed to ensure the patient does not fall off while the other two team members go around to the opposite side of the bed and place their arms underneath the patient. After the two people on the opposite side of the bed have a good grip on the patient, the third person joins them and assists in sliding the patient to the center of the bed.

Sometimes, patients must be lifted and carried. This can be done by means of a three-carrier lift. If done properly, the patient will feel secure, and those lifting will not suffer strain. The three-carrier lift is described and illustrated in Procedure 38-4 under Special Considerations. The three-carrier lift is used in various other situations, such as lifting a patient who has fallen to the floor and is unable to get up independently or lifting a patient out of a chair into the bed.

For patients who present special problems because of their excessive weight or a cast, it may be necessary to have an additional person to support the heaviest or most cumbersome part of the patient. The people distribute their arms while carrying so that the heaviest part is well supported.

Moving the Patient From Bed to Chair

Safety and comfort are key concerns when the nurse assists the patient out of bed. Preliminary assessment of vital signs provides baseline data, and subsequent recordings determine the effect of this activity on the patient. The position of the nurse as he or she prepares to move the patient and placement of the chair are critical elements in the transfer. The patient's apparel should be sufficient to prevent embarrassment and provide warmth yet not impede movement. The technique for assisting a patient to transfer from bed to chair is described in Procedure 38-5.

It is possible for only one person to get a helpless patient from a bed to a chair, although it is safer and simpler with two people. The one-person technique is valuable for nurses to know for the home care of invalids and for emergency use. More than one person should be available if the bed and chair seat are not the same height. The technique for two nurses transferring a patient is described in Procedure 38-6.

Logrolling a Patient

When a patient has a spinal injury or is recovering from neck, back, or spinal surgery, it is necessary to keep the body in straight alignment when turning the patient. Two or three nurses can accomplish this safely by logrolling a patient (Fig. 38-14). Following are guidelines for using this technique:

* Use a drawsheet if possible to facilitate smooth movement.
* Have the patient cross his or her arms on the chest.
* Place a pillow between the knees.
* Two nurses should stand on one side of the bed opposite the direction the patient will be turned. The third helper stands on the other side.
* Fanfold or roll the drawsheet tightly against the patient and carefully slide him or her to the side of the bed toward the two nurses.
* One helper should then move to the other side of the bed.
* Holding the rolled drawsheet taut to support the body, turn the patient as a unit toward the two nurses. Everyone moves on a predetermined signal.
* Use pillows to support the patient on his or her side in straight alignment.
* Raise the side rails, lower the bed, and place the call signal within the patient's reach.

Using a Hydraulic Lift

A hydraulic device, such as the Hoyer lift, can safely transfer an immobile or obese patient from bed to chair. One person may operate the device, but two are preferable. The manufacturer's instructions should be carefully reviewed before attempting the procedure. Generally, the patient is positioned supine in the center of the sling. Chains or straps from the hydraulic mechanism are attached to the sling; the patient is raised to a sitting position, lifted clear of the bed, and slowly lowered into the chair (Fig. 38-15). Many caregivers do not readily use a hydraulic lift because the lift was not readily available or they view the procedure as too time-consuming.

Helping Patients Ambulate

Fortunately for most patients, prolonged periods of bed rest are no longer considered necessary during most illnesses. Activity, even as mild as a stroll around the room, down the hall, from the bedroom to the living room, or out into the yard, is a protective measure for the body.

Physical Conditioning

Patients who are not confined to bed for long periods, who sleep well, and who experience possibly short periods of rest during the day may not require special considerations for increased physical activity in preparation for ambulation. However, others have to be prepared for the day when ambulation is resumed. Certain exercises that strengthen the overall efficiency of the musculoskeletal system can be done in bed.

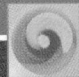

PROCEDURE 38-3

Assisting a Patient Up in Bed (Two Nurses)

Action	Rationale
1. Explain the procedure to the patient.	This facilitates cooperation of the patient.
2. Wash your hands.	Handwashing deters the spread of microorganisms.
3. Raise the bed to a comfortable position for you. Adjust the bed to flat position if the patient can tolerate it. With two nurses on opposite sides of the bed, lower the side rails.	This position facilitates moving the patient and minimizes strain on the nurse.
4. Remove the pillow and place it at the head of the bed.	This reduces friction and protects the patient's head from striking the top of the bed.
5. Place drawsheet on bed under the patient's midsection.	Drawsheet supports the patient's weight and reduces friction during the lift.
6. If able to assist, have the patient flex the knees and place feet flat on the bed.	The patient is prepared to push upward by using a major muscle group.
7. Fold the patient's arms across the chest and instruct patient to flex the neck with chin on the chest.	This provides assistance, reduces friction, and prevents hyperextension of the neck.

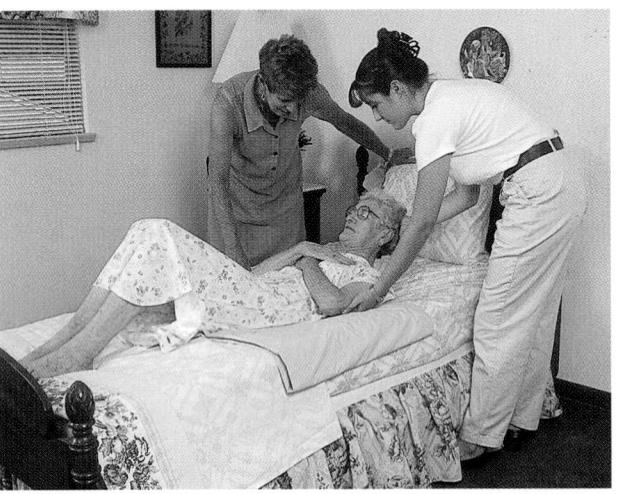

Action	Rationale
8. Stand opposite the patient's center with your feet spread and turned toward the head of the bed. Position one foot slightly forward.	This positions the mover opposite the center of the body mass. It places both nurses in a stable position with good alignment.
9. Fold or bunch drawsheet close to the patient before grasping it securely and preparing to move patient.	This brings the patient's center of gravity closer to each nurse and provides for a secure hold.

(continued)

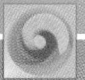

PROCEDURE 38-3

Assisting a Patient Up in Bed (Two Nurses) (Continued)

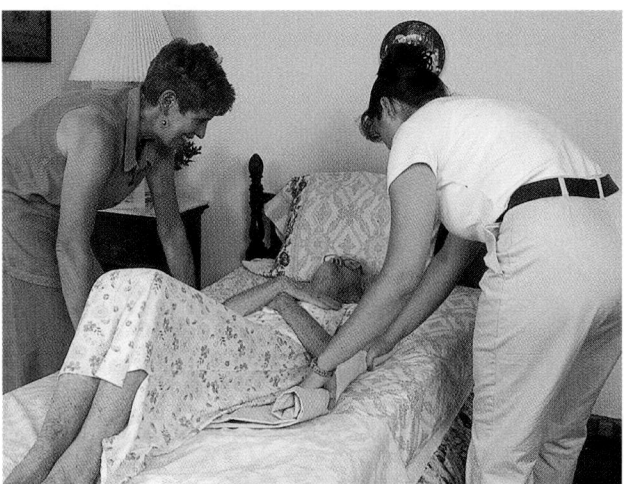

Action

10. Shift your weight back and forth from back leg to front leg, and on count of three, move the patient upward in bed. If possible, the patient can assist the move upward by pushing with the legs. Repeat if necessary.

11. Assist the patient to a comfortable position. Reposition the pillow. Raise the side rail and adjust the bed position if necessary.

12. Wash your hands.

Rationale

The rocking motion uses the nurse's weight to counteract the patient's weight as the nurses move the patient up in bed. If the patient assists, less effort is required by the nurses.

This ensures the patient's safety.

Handwashing deters the spread of microorganisms.

Special Considerations   Two nurses may also move a patient up in bed by interlocking their arms under the patient's shoulders and thighs and lifting as described above.

Quadriceps Drills (Sets)

Quadriceps drills are an isometric exercise—an exercise in which muscle tension occurs without a significant change in the length of the muscle. One of the most important muscle groups used in walking is the quadriceps femoris. This muscle group helps extend the leg and flexes the thigh. To help reduce weakness and make first attempts at walking easier, bedridden patients should be encouraged to contract this muscle group frequently. Following are techniques for quadriceps drills:

- Have the patient contract or tighten the muscles on the front of the thighs. The patient has the feeling of pushing the knees downward into the mattress and pulling the feet upward.
- Have the patient hold the position just described while counting slowly to four, and then relax the muscles for an equal count. Emphasize that relaxation is important to prevent muscle fatigue.

- Caution the patient not to hold his or her breath during these exercises to avoid straining the heart.
- Teach the patient to do quadriceps drills two or three times each hour, four to six times a day.
- Instruct the patient to stop the exercise short of muscle fatigue.

The muscles in the buttocks can be exercised in the same way by pinching the buttocks together and then relaxing them. This is called *gluteal setting.* Tightening and holding the abdominal muscles for 6 seconds and then relaxing them also strengths this muscle group to facilitate walking.

Pushups

The muscle strength of the arms and shoulders may also need improvement before the patient is ready to be out of bed. Exercises should improve the strength needed to
(*text continues on page 992*)

Transferring a Patient From Bed to Stretcher

Action	Rationale
1. Explain the procedure to the patient.	This facilitates the cooperation of the patient.
2. Wash your hands.	Handwashing deters the spread of microorganisms.
3. Move the bed and equipment in the room to make room for the stretcher. Make sure that assistants are available. Close the door or curtain.	This facilitates transfer movement and provides for privacy.
4. Raise the bed to the same height as the stretcher and adjust the head of the bed to the flat position if the patient can tolerate it. Lower side rails.	Pushing and pulling require less effort than lifting, This position facilitates moving the patient.
5. Place a drawsheet under the patient if one is not already there. Use the drawsheet to move the patient to the side of the bed where the stretcher will be placed.	This facilitates movement of the patient to the stretcher.
6. Position stretcher next to the bed and parallel to it. Lock wheels on the stretcher and bed. Remove the pillow from the bed and place it on the stretcher.	Positioning of the stretcher and locking the wheels facilitate safe transfer of patient.
7. To move the patient: a. The first nurse should kneel on far side of the bed away from the stretcher. Position the knee at the upper torso closer to the patient than the other knee. Grasp the drawsheet securely.	The nurse uses a major muscle group to assist in movement. The nurse's flexed hips help avoid back injury.
b. The second nurse should reach across the stretcher and grasp the drawsheet at the head and chest areas of the patient.	This promotes safe transfer by supporting the patient's head and upper body.
c. The third nurse should reach across the stretcher and grasp the drawsheet at the patient's waist and thigh area. Ask the patient to fold arms across the chest.	This supports the lower part of the patient's body for safe transfer.
d. At a signal given by the first nurse, the second and third nurses pull while the first nurse lifts the patient from the bed to the stretcher.	Working in unison distributes the work of moving the patient and facilitates the transfer.

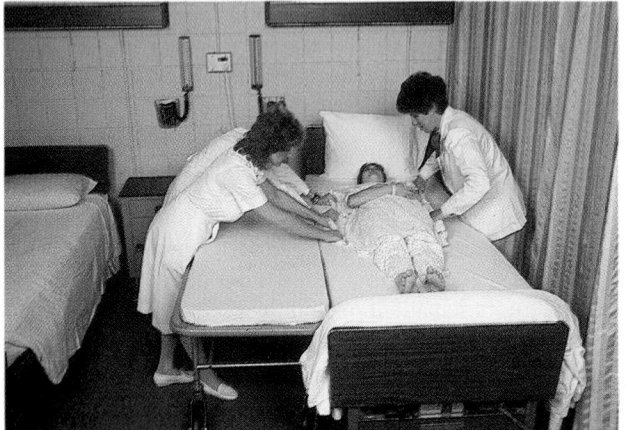

Action 5: Using drawsheet to move patient to side of bed.

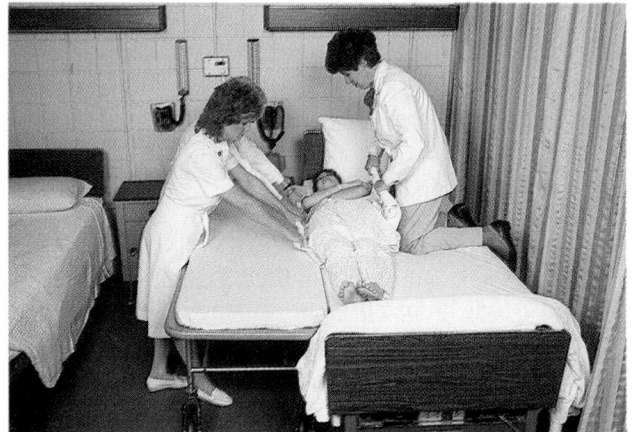

Action 7: Moving patient to stretcher.

Action	Rationale
8. Secure the patient on the stretcher until side rails are raised. Assist the patient to a comfortable position with the covering in place. Leave the drawsheet in place for transfer back to bed.	This ensures patient safety and comfort.
9. Wash your hands.	Handwashing deters the spread of microorganisms.

(continued)

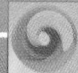

Transferring a Patient From Bed to Stretcher (Continued)

Special Considerations

- A long polyethylene board with handgrips on the edges may be used to assist with the transfer:
  - Turn the patient on his or her side with the back toward the stretcher.
  - Position the transfer board lengthwise and midway between the bed and stretcher.
  - Return the patient to his or her back with a bottom sheet or drawsheet between the patient and the board.
  - Using the sheet, slide the patient across the transfer board and onto the stretcher.
  - Reposition the patient on the stretcher, remove the board, and secure with safety belts and side rails.

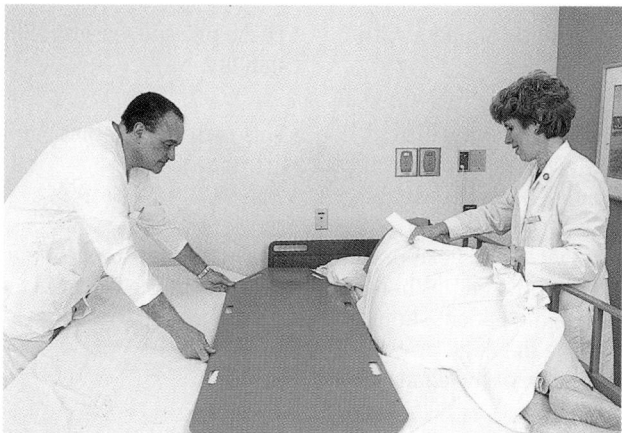

Special Considerations: Using a transfer board to facilitate moving the client from bed to stretcher.

- A three-carrier lift may also be done to move a patient from bed to stretcher:
  - Each person must support one section of the patient's body—head, shoulders, and chest; hips; and thighs and legs.
  - Slide your arms under the patient as far as possible and on signal, simultaneously roll the patient toward your chests.
  - On signal, stand up and steady the patient against your chests.
  - Step back together, pivot around to the stretcher, and, on signal, lower the patient onto the stretcher.

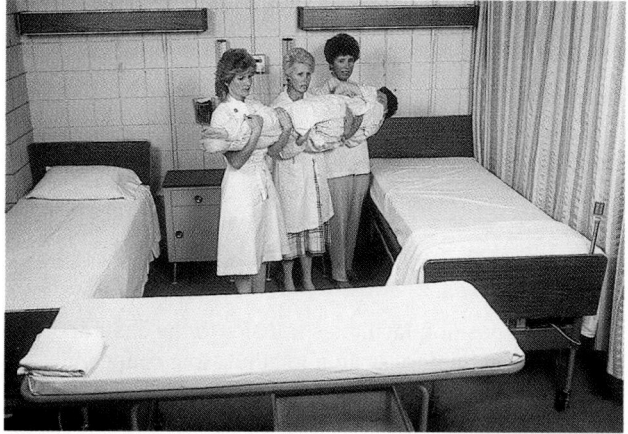

Special Considerations: Pivoting to stretcher.

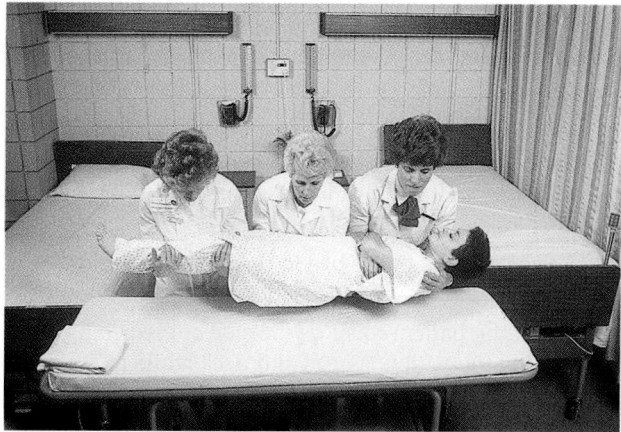

Special Considerations: Lowering patient to stretcher.

PROCEDURE 38-5

Assisting a Patient to Transfer From Bed to Chair

Action	Rationale
1. Explain the procedure to the patient. Offer bedpan.	This facilitates cooperation of the patient. Empty bladder will increase patient comfort.
2. Wash your hands.	Handwashing deters the spread of microorganisms.
3. Assess the patient's ability to assist with transfer. Move equipment as necessary to make room for the chair. Close the door or curtain.	This ensures patient safety and facilitates the transfer. Closing the door or curtain provides for privacy.
4. Place the bed in the low position.	This facilitates transfer to chair.
5. Assist the patient to put on a robe and slippers with nonskid soles.	These provide warmth. Slippers provide protection and stability.
6. Position the chair at the bedside:	
a. *For a patient with unimpaired mobility:* Bring chair close to the bedside facing the foot of the bed and, if possible, brace the back of the chair against a bedside table.	This increases stability and ensures patient safety during the transfer.
b. *For a patient with impaired mobility:* Position the chair facing the head or foot of the bed. When sitting on the side of the bed, the patient should be able to steady self by using the hand on the unaffected side to grasp the arm of the chair.	This uses the strong side to provide balance and improve stability during the transfer.

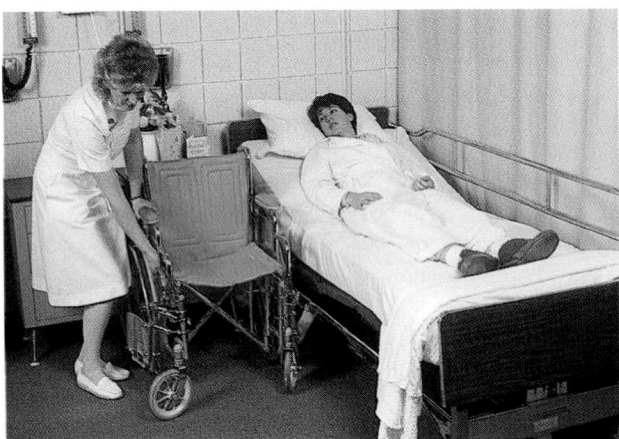

Action 6: Placing chair at bedside.

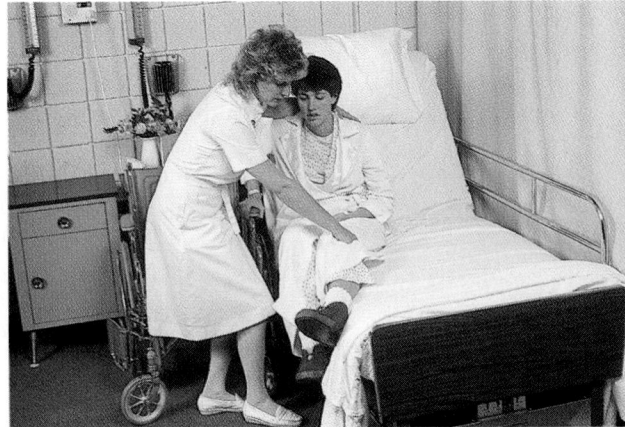

Action 9: Supporting patient while moving legs off bed.

Action	Rationale
7. Lock the wheels on the chair and bed if appropriate. Raise the foot pedals on the wheelchair to the up position.	This ensures patient safety.
8. Raise the head of the bed to the highest position.	Moving from the sitting to the standing position requires less energy.
9. Assist the patient to sit on the side of the bed by supporting the patient's head and neck while moving the patient's legs off the bed to dangle. Steady the patient in that position for a few minutes.	The sitting position facilitates transfer to the chair and allows the circulatory system to adjust to a change in position.

(continued)

PROCEDURE 38-5

Assisting a Patient to Transfer From Bed to Chair (Continued)

10. Assist the patient to the standing position:
    a. *For a patient with unimpaired mobility:* Face the patient and brace your feet and knees against the patient. Place your hands around the patient's waist while the patient holds onto you between the shoulders and the waist. Use your legs to help you raise the patient to the standing position.

    b. *For a patient with impaired mobility:* Face the patient and brace your feet and knees against the patient, especially against the affected extremity. Place your hands around the patient's waist. The patient may place the unaffected arm around your shoulder or use the unaffected arm to reach for the arm of the chair and to push up while raising to the standing position.

11. Pivot the patient (on the unaffected limb if applicable) into position in front of the chair with legs positioned against the chair.

This provides for stability and for use of major muscle groups to facilitate movement. Allowing the patient to grasp the nurse around the neck could injure the nurse if the patient should fall.

This provides for stability and makes use of the unaffected extremities to facilitate movement.

This provides security and proper position before sitting.

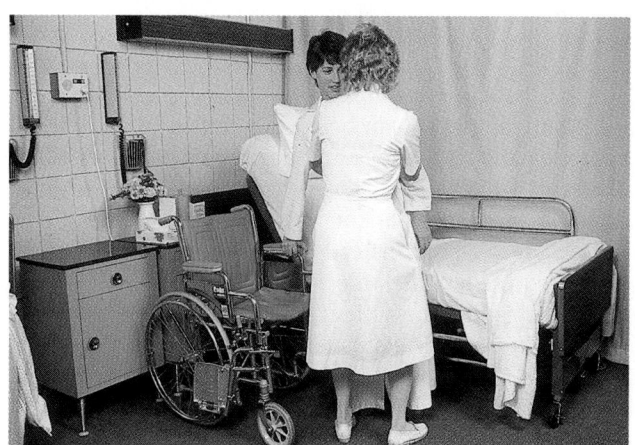

Action 10b: Assisting patient to stand.

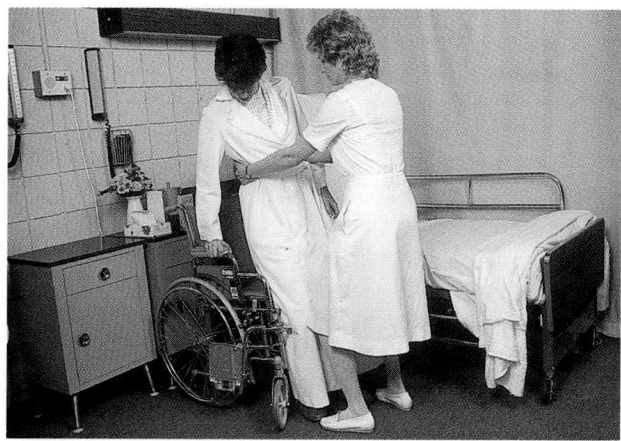

Action 12: Bracing patient's knees while lowering patient to chair.

12. The patient may use one arm (the unaffected limb if applicable) to place on the arm of the chair and steady self while slowly lowering to the sitting position. Continue to brace the patient's knees with your knees and flex your own hips and knees when seating the patient.

13. Adjust the patient's position using pillows where necessary. Cover the patient and use restraint if necessary. Position the call bell so it is available for use.

14. Wash your hands.

15. Document the patient's tolerance of the procedure and length of time in the chair.

The patient uses own arm for support and stability. The nurse flexes the knees and hips to use a major muscle group to aid in movement and reduce strain on the back.

This maintains proper body alignment and provides for comfort and safety.

Handwashing deters the spread of microorganisms.

This provides accurate documentation and ensures continuity of care.

(continued)

PROCEDURE 38-5

Assisting a Patient to Transfer From Bed to Chair (Continued)

Special Considerations

- A walking or transfer belt may be used to assist the transfer. With the belt secure around the patient's waist, the nurse can grasp the belt on both sides (or use handles if they are available) and assist the patient to stand and move to the chair.
- A sliding board may also be used to ease the patient who cannot stand into a chair.

---

hold onto or get into a chair and to move about better. They are part of the preparation for patients who must learn to walk on crutches.

A trapeze attached to the bed of a patient who has limited use of the lower part of the body helps the patient to move about in bed and strengthens muscles in the upper part of the body. However, this does not strengthen the triceps, which is the muscle group necessary for crutch walking or for moving from a bed to a chair. More suitable exercises are *pushups,* which are done as follows:

- While sitting up in bed without support, the patient can do pushup exercises to strengthen the triceps. Instruct the patient to lift the hips off the bed by pushing down with the hands on the mattress. If the mattress is too soft, a block of books can be placed on the bed under the patient's hands.
- Pushups may also be done with the patient lying in bed on the abdomen. Instruct the patient to place the hands near the outstretched body at about shoulder level, with palms down on the mattress and elbows bent sharply. Then have the patient straighten the elbows to lift the head and shoulders off the bed.
- Pushups may also be done when the patient sits in an armchair or wheelchair. The patient places the hands on the arms of the chair and then raises the body out of the seat.

Pushups should at first be done three or four times a day, with the number increased as upper body strength is increased.

Dangling

Dangling refers to the position in which the person sits on the edge of the bed with legs and feet over the side of the bed. This exercise helps prepare patients for being out of bed. It is carried out as follows:

- Place the patient in the sitting position in bed for a few minutes. This will accustom the patient to this position and help prevent feelings of faintness.
- Place the bed in the low position or have a footstool handy on which the patient can rest the feet while dangling.
- Move the patient toward the side of the bed near you so that you do not stretch and strain while turning the patient.

- Pivot the patient a quarter of a turn by supporting the shoulders and legs. Swing the patient's legs over the side of the bed. The patient may place his or her hands on your shoulders.
- Rest the patient's feet on the floor or on a footstool. This gives a sense of security, and the patient is less likely to slide from the bed.
- Have the patient pick up and put down the feet alternately in a marching motion. This promotes circulation in the legs.
- Remain with the patient and be ready to put the patient in a lying position if he or she feels faint, to prevent falling out of bed.

Daily Activities for Purposeful Exercise

Many activities can be carried out in ways that encourage patients to move and thereby gain the benefit of exercise. For example, the bedside stand can be positioned so that the patient must use shoulder and arm muscles to reach it, instead of placing it so that little effort is required to take things from it. The signal cord can be placed so that the patient must move either the arm or shoulder to reach it. Patients can be encouraged to sit up and reach for the overbed table, to pull it close, and then to push it back in place. Patients can be encouraged to try to wash their back independently. Patients can put on socks while still in bed. There are innumerable ways in which patients can be helped to exercise, and when they understand the purpose, they often adopt other exercises for themselves.

In a hospital setting, activities of daily living may be one of the few independent activities that a patient can perform. It is vital that the nurse allows the patient to do as much as he or she can accomplish independently while offering encouragement and praise. "Learned dependency," which often occurs with the geriatric population, can lead to a decrease in self-esteem and depression. Nurses should collaborate with the occupational therapist when necessary to determine types of adaptive equipment that would help the patient achieve maximal functional independence. The accompanying box provides examples of available adaptive equipment. Providing the necessary adaptive tools, coupled with encouraging independence, will create the optimal outcome.

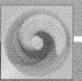

PROCEDURE 38-6

Transferring a Dependent Patient From Bed to Chair (Two Nurses)

Action	Rationale
1. Explain the procedure to the patient.	This facilitates cooperation of the patient.
2. Wash your hands.	Handwashing deters the spread of microorganisms.
3. Move equipment as necessary to make room for the chair. Close the door or curtain. Assist the patient to put on a robe and slippers.	This ensures patient safety and facilitates transfer. It provides for privacy and warmth.
4. Move the patient to the near side of the bed and cross the patient's arms across the chest if possible. Lock the wheels of the bed.	This requires less effort to move the patient. Locked wheels will prevent the bed from moving if the patient leans against it.
5. Position the chair next to the bed near the upper end and with the back of the chair parallel to the head of the bed. (If wheelchair, remove the armrest closer to the bed if possible.) Lock the wheels if appropriate.	Positioning the chair next to the bed facilitates easier movement into the chair.
6. Adjust the bed to a comfortable level for nurses or at the level of the armrest if one is present on the chair.	This facilitates transfer with minimal muscle strain on the nurses.

7. Prepare to lift the patient from the bed to the chair:
  a. The first nurse should stand behind the chair. Slip the arms under the patient's axillae and grasp the patient's wrists securely.
  b. The second nurse should face the wheelchair and support the patient's knees by placing the arms under them.
  c. On a predetermined signal, both nurses flex their hips and knees and simultaneously lift the patient gently to the chair.
	Two people lifting the patient distributes weight and decreases the effort needed for transfer.

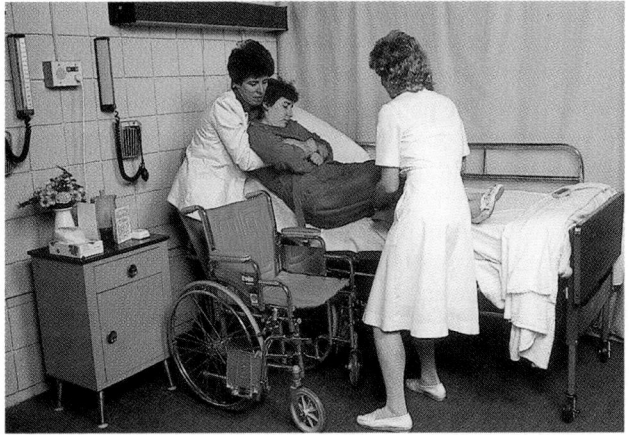

Action 7a & b: First nurse slips arms under patient's axillae and grasps wrists; second nurse support patient's knees.

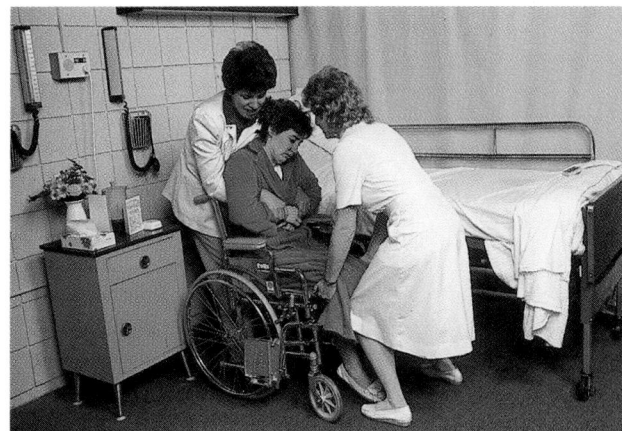

Action 7c: Lowering patient into chair.

Action	Rationale
8. Adjust the patient's position using pillows where necessary. Cover the patient and use restraint if necessary. Position the call bell so it is available for use.	This maintains proper body alignment and provides for comfort and safety.
9. Wash your hands.	Handwashing deters the spread of microorganisms.
10. Document the patient's tolerance of the procedure and length of time in the chair.	This provides accurate documentation and ensures continuity of care.

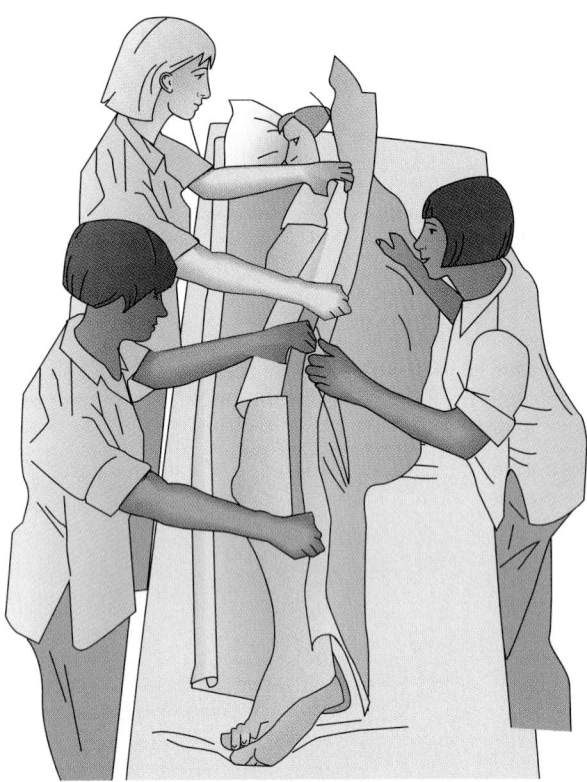

Figure 38-14
Logrolling by two or three nurses aids in turning a patient with a spinal injury. One nurse stands on the side, holding the draw-sheet taut. The patient is moved toward the other two nurses on a predetermined signal.

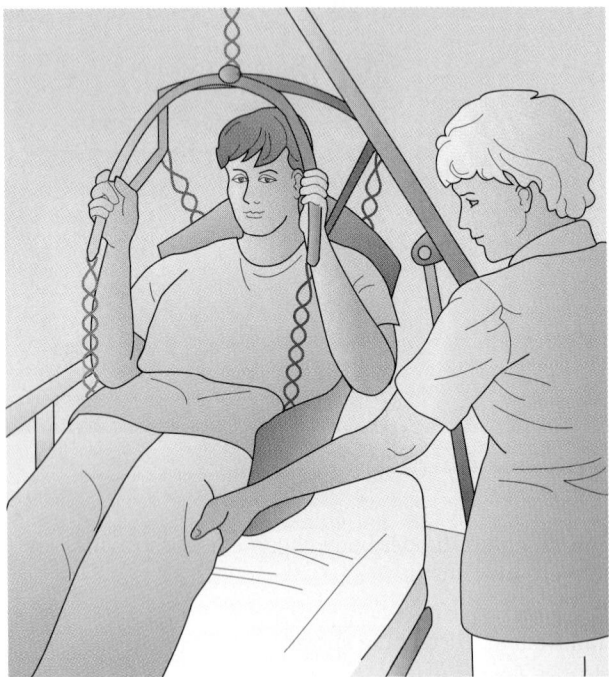

Figure 38-15
A hydraulic lift is used to transfer an immobile or obese patient. The patient is raised to a sitting position suspended just above the bed; then the patient is transferred, and the sling with the patient is lowered onto the seat.

> ### Adaptive Equipment to Assist With Activities of Daily Living
>
> - Long-handled bath sponges
> - Reachers
> - Long-handled shoe horns and sock aids
> - Elastic shoe laces
> - Utensils that are enlarged, specially angulated, or have special grips
> - Velcro devices
> - Feeding devices such as plates or bowls with suction-cup bottoms
> - Splints and positioning equipment
> - Environmental adaptations

Assisting the Patient to Walk

Many patients who have been confined to bed for an extended period find that they must almost learn to walk all over again. Often, nurses play a major role in the patient's recovery and mental outlook, hope, and faith, especially when the patient must adhere to a rigid and often difficult schedule of reeducating muscle groups. A patient who is able to raise the leg only 2.5 cm (1 inch) from the bed possesses sufficient power to begin walking.

Because muscle reeducation is a major task, the patient needs the assistance of experts in physical medicine. However, nurses can assist patients out of bed and help them walk when a physical therapist is not present. Nurses should also plan to walk with a patient who is walking for the first few times after a period of bed rest.

Before getting the patient out of bed, the nurse does the following:

- Assesses the patient's ability to walk and need for assistance (one nurse, two nurses, walker, cane, walking belt, or crutches)
- Explains to the patient exactly what is to be done: transfer technique from bed to erect position, projected distance to be ambulated, assistance available and the correct manner of using it; instructs the patient to alert the nurse immediately if feeling dizzy or weak
- Ensures that the patient has a clear path for ambulation

The nurse then slowly assists the patient to an erect position for ambulation, pausing after the patient is seated at the edge of the bed and again after the patient first stands to ensure that the patient feels steady. The nurse reminds the patient to take deep breaths to promote good aeration of the lungs while walking. Patients who are fearful of walking often tend to look at their feet and may need to be reminded to stand erect and to hold their head high to achieve the full benefits of walking. Because patients who are walking for the first time after prolonged bed rest often feel faint or weak, a short distance should be planned. As this distance is increased, it is helpful to have chairs readily available should the patient need to rest. Should a patient faint or begin to fall while walking, the nurse stands with feet apart to create a wide base of support and rocks the pelvis out on the side facing the patient. With arms under the patient's axillae and encircling the patient, the nurse slides the patient down the nurse's own body to the floor, carefully protecting the patient's head (Fig. 38-16). If the patient is wearing a walking belt, the nurse can use the belt to ease the patient backward against her own body and gently ease the patient to the floor while protecting the patient's head. When two nurses are assisting a patient who starts to fall or faint, they both should use one hand to support the patient under the axillae and grasp the patient's hand or wrist with their other hands. After they have steadied the patient, they can slowly lower him or her to a chair or the floor (see Fig. 38-16). These maneuvers should be practiced before they are needed in an emergency situation.

One-Nurse Assist

Patients who require minimal nursing assistance may ambulate well with the nurse walking alongside. The nurse best supports the patient by standing at the patient's side and placing both hands at the patient's waist. By supporting the patient at the waist, the nurse helps the patient maintain an erect posture and is prevented from pulling the patient unintentionally to one side. Use of a walking belt snugly secured around the patient's waist also provides this type of support. The nurse grasps the belt securely in the back and walks behind and slightly to the side of the patient (Fig. 38-17).

Frequently, it is necessary to assist the patient to ambulate with intravenous (IV) therapy equipment. The nurse should secure a portable IV pole that moves easily. The patient ambulates with the assistance of the nurse and the portable IV pole. The nurse needs to secure all the equipment before ambulating and to be alert for any tension or sudden action that might dislodge or interfere with the infusion (Fig. 38-18A). The nurse should also consider reviewing this technique with family members who are assisting with ambulation and are unfamiliar with how to steady the patient, maneuver equipment, and navigate through crowded or narrow areas.

When a patient has weakness or paralysis on one side, the nurse usually stands on the weaker or affected side and stabilizes the patient by putting one arm around the patient's waist. Support for the patient's weak arm can be accomplished by placing the nurse's other arm around the inner aspect of the patient's upper arm in the axilla area or using the nurse's hand to support the patient's forearm and hand (see Fig. 38-18B). Supporting the patient's weak arm in the axillary area allows the nurse to support the patient's weight more easily and ease him or her to the floor should the patient feel faint. A transfer belt should always be used with patients who are unstable. A two-nurse assist is the safer method when the nurse is uncertain of the patient's ability to ambulate.

Two-Nurse Assist

There are two methods of ambulation that two nurses can safely use to support a patient. In the first, the nurses stand at the patient's sides with their near hands grasping the inferior aspect of the patient's near upper arm and their far hands holding the patient's lower arm or hand. The second position provides more support to the patient but requires the three people involved to be of similar height. The nurses again position themselves at the patient's sides, slipping their near arms under the patient's arms and around the patient's back, grasping one another's wrists. The patient stretches the arms around the nurses' shoulders and the nurses grasp the patient's hands with their far hands. In both positions, the nurses and the patient step in unison (see Fig. 38-17).

Figure 38-16
(**A**) One nurse guiding a patient to the floor. (**B**) Two nurses lowering a patient to the floor.

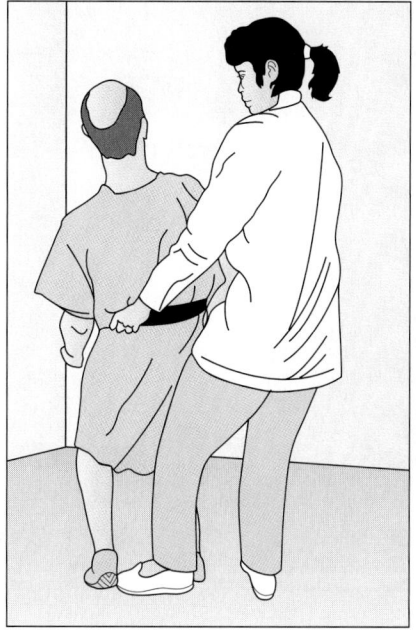

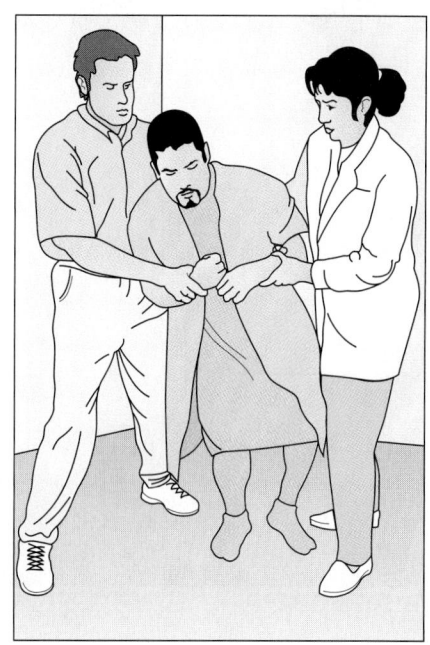

A

B

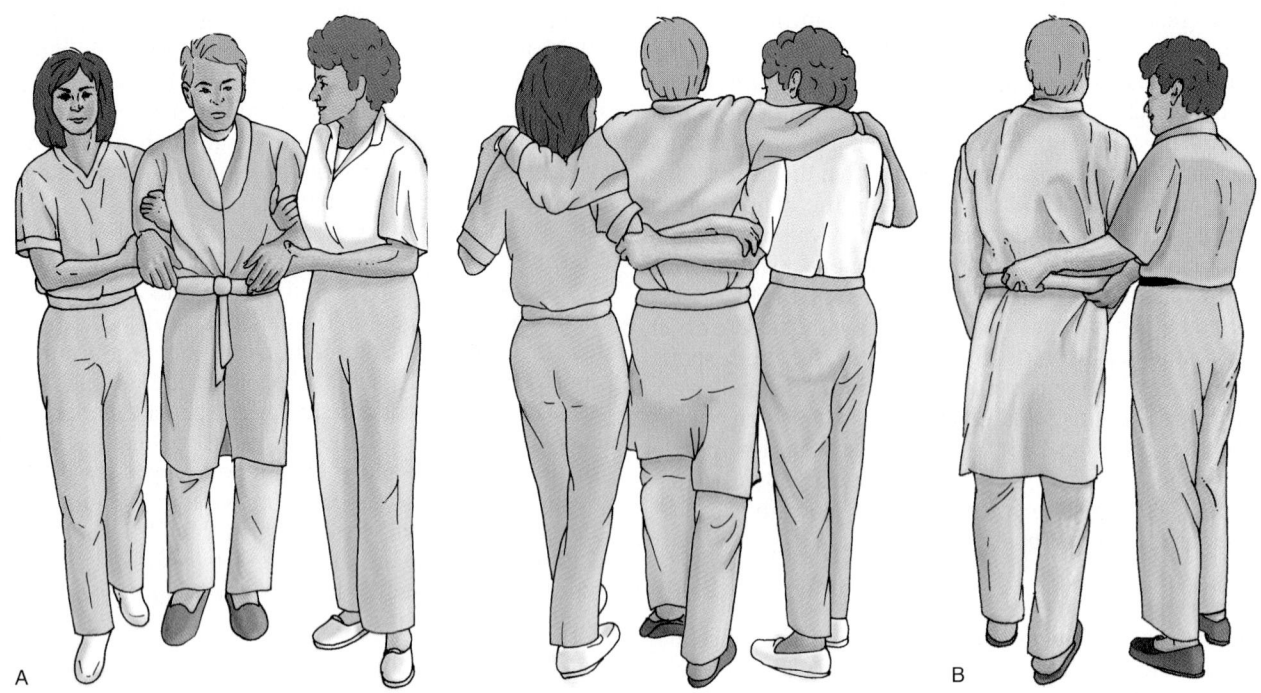

Figure 38-17
(**A**) Assisting a patient to ambulate. Two techniques for two nurses to safely assist a patient to ambulate. (**B**) The nurse using a walking belt to support a patient while walking.

Using Mechanical Aids for Walking

Various devices can assist a patient with walking. The most common are walkers, canes, braces, and crutches. Most often, a patient is fitted for a device and instructed in its use in the department of physical medicine or phys-

ical therapy. In this instance, nursing's concern is chiefly to reinforce the teaching the patient has received and to ensure that the patient continues to use the device properly to assist in safe ambulation. In some healthcare settings, however, nurses may be responsible for fitting

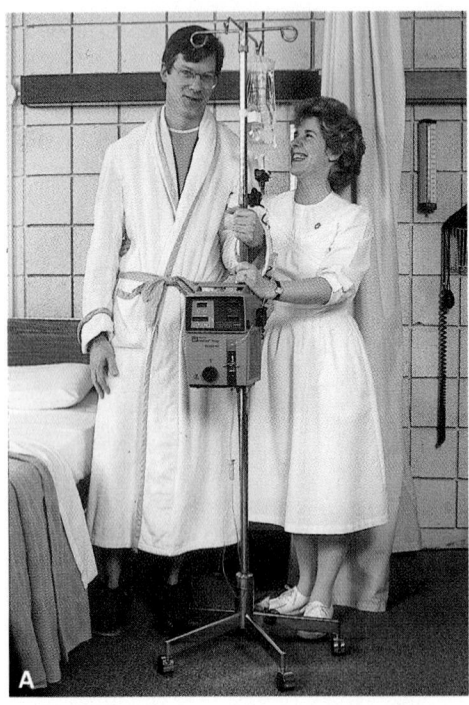

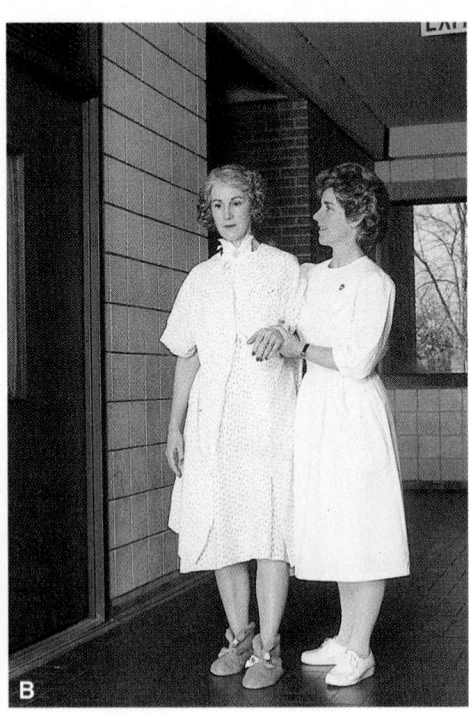

Figure 38-18
(**A**) Ambulating a patient who needs additional support. The nurse assists the patient to ambulate with a portable IV pole. (**B**) The nurse assists the patient with weakness or paralysis on one side to ambulate by supporting the patient on the affected side. (Photographs © B. Proud.)

patients with the device. Whenever a nurse assesses a patient who has been using a walker, cane, brace, or crutches over time, it is important to determine whether the device is still needed, whether it continues to meet the patient's needs, and whether the patient continues to use it properly.

Some elderly patients consider the use of a mobility aid a visible symbol of weakness or an indication of decline in capabilities and loss of independence. Many patients refuse to use them and keep them out of sight. If the mobility aid is intended for short-term use (eg, after hip replacement surgery), the response is usually more positive. Nurses need to be sensitive to a patient's perspective regarding these devices and focus on the meaning the aid has for the patient rather than simply emphasizing how to use it. It is imperative to allow patients some control over their mobility decisions while still ensuring a safe environment (Rush & Ouellet, 1997).

General guidelines for helping patients who need the assistance of a walker, cane, brace, or crutches are as follows:

- Whenever possible, instruct the patient and family members in the correct use of the device before it is needed (eg, before surgery). If family members are knowledgeable, they can reinforce the teaching as needed.
- When ready to begin ambulation with the new device, make sure the patient is wearing rubber-soled, well-fitting shoes and that there is a clear path for ambulation (clean, flat, dry, and well lit). If the patient is at high risk for falls, use a walking belt for added support.
- Before moving, make sure the patient is steady on the feet when standing; instruct the patient to stand erect, looking straight ahead. The nurse should walk behind and slightly to one side of the patient (in cases of hemiparesis or hemiparalysis, walk on the patient's affected side). Should the patient lose balance, be prepared to grasp the patient's shoulder and the transfer belt to steady the patient.

Walker

A *walker* is a light-weight metal frame (usually aluminum) with four legs (Fig. 38-19A). The walker provides a sense of security and support. There are several types of walkers, specified according to the arm strength and balance of the patient.

When the patient stands between the back legs of the walker, the walker should extend from the floor to the patient's hip joint; the patient's elbows should be flexed about 30 degrees. The walker's rubber tips should be intact to prevent slipping. Generally, the patient lifts the walker ahead of himself or herself and steps into it. Instructions for a patient using a walker should include the following:

- Wear nonskid shoes or slippers.

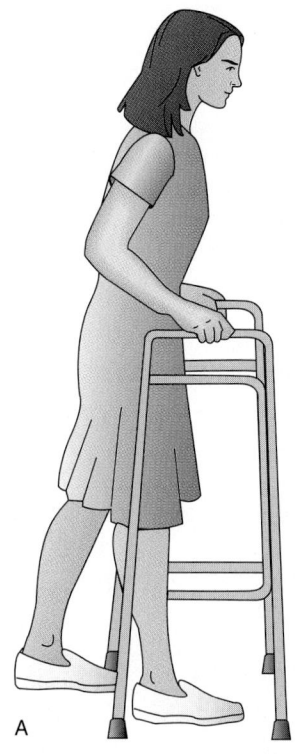
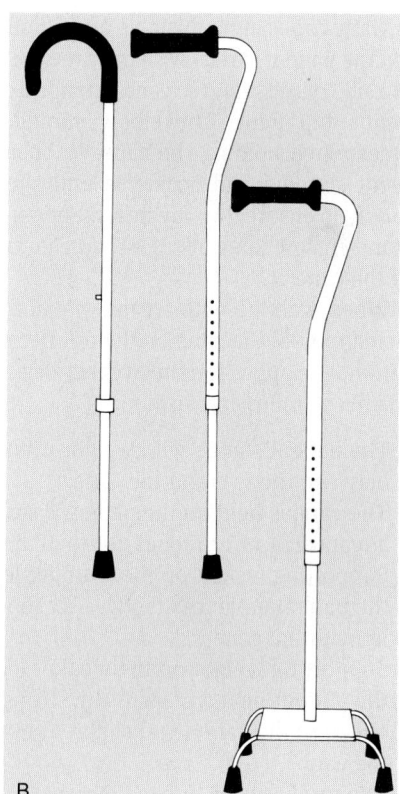

Figure 38-19
(**A**) Mechanical aids to walking. A walker is a lightweight metal frame with a broad, four-point base of support. The walker should be adjusted to the height of the patient's hip joint so that the patient's elbows are flexed about 30 degrees. (**B**) Three types of canes. Single-ended canes with half-circle handles are recommended for patients requiring minimal support. Single-ended canes with straight handles are recommended for patients with hand weakness. Three- or four-prong canes are recommended for patients with poor balance.

A

B

- When rising from a seated position, use the chair arms for support. Once standing, place one hand at a time on the walker and move forward into it.
- If one leg is impaired, move that leg and the walker forward together for 6 to 8 inches. Move the unaffected leg forward once body weight is securely supported by the walker and the impaired leg. Older patients frequently develop dangerous walking patterns with a walker and may require close observation.
- Never use a walker on stairs (Stewart & Murray, 1998).

Canes

Canes come in three variations (see Fig. 38-19B):

- Single-ended canes with half-circle handles are recommended for patients requiring minimal support and those who will be using stairs frequently.
- Single-ended canes with straight handles are recommended for patients with hand weakness because the handgrip is easier to hold; they are not recommended for patients with poor balance.
- Canes with three or four prongs or legs to provide a wide base of support (tripod or quad cane) are recommended for patients with poor balance. Instruct the patient to use a cane with as small a base as possible and eventually to progress to a single-ended cane if possible. The smaller the base, the less the patient relies on the cane for support.

Many canes are adjustable and should be fitted so that when the patient stands with the cane's tip 4 inches (10 cm) to the side of the foot, the cane extends from the floor to the patient's hip joint. The elbow should be flexed thirty degrees when holding the cane. Rubber tips on the cane prevent slipping and accidents and should be inspected regularly to ensure they are intact. Patients should be taught to stand erect when walking with a cane and not to lean out over the cane.

When walking with a cane, patients are generally instructed to hold the cane on the unaffected side to provide additional support for the weaker leg. Ambulation proceeds in the following fashion:

1. The patient stands with weight evenly distributed between the feet and the cane.
2. The cane is held on the patient's stronger side and is advanced 4 to 12 inches (10 to 30 cm).
3. Supporting weight on the stronger leg and the cane, the patient advances the weaker foot forward, parallel with the cane.
4. Supporting weight on the weaker leg and the cane, the patient next advances the stronger leg forward ahead of the cane (heel slightly beyond the tip of the cane).
5. The weaker leg is moved forward until even with the stronger leg, and the cane is once again advanced as in step 2.

When less support is required from the cane, the patient can advance the cane and weaker leg forward while the stronger leg supports the patient's weight. Patients should be taught to position their canes within easy reach when they sit down so that they can rise easily.

Braces

Braces that support weakened leg muscles are available in many variations. Nursing responsibilities include learning with the patient when the brace is to be worn and the correct technique for applying the brace; monitoring the patient's correct use of the brace; and observing for any untoward problems the brace might cause (eg, skin irritation). Muscle changes such as those occurring with growth and development or brought about by illness (atrophy) may result in the brace needing to be refitted to maintain its effectiveness.

Crutches

Sometimes, it is necessary for patients to use crutches for a time to avoid using one leg or to help strengthen one or both legs. This procedure is taught best by a physical therapist; however, nurses are often called on to measure patients for crutches and to teach them to use them. Even if a patient is being taught to crutch walk by a physical therapist, the nurse needs to understand the patient's progress and the gait being taught. The nurse must often guide the patient at home or in the hospital after the initial teaching is completed. The two types of crutches most commonly used are the underarm or axillary crutches and the forearm support crutches (Fig. 38-20).

Measuring for Axillary Crutches. The following techniques can be used to measure the patient for axillary crutches:

- Have the patient lie flat in bed on the back wearing the shoes to be used when walking.
- Measure the distance from the anterior fold of the axilla straight down to the heel, and then add 2.5 cm (1 inch).
- With the patient standing, position the crutch pad three finger-widths below the axilla with the bottom tip of the crutch placed diagonally out to a point 10 to 15 cm (4 to 6 inches) to the side of the heel.
- To obtain an approximate crutch length, use the patient's height and subtract 16 inches (40 cm).
- After the crutches have been adjusted to the proper length, have the patient stand to adjust the handgrips. Secure the handgrips while the patient grasps them in the hands with elbows slightly bent and wrists bent backward.
- Teach the patient that the support of body weight should come primarily on the hands and arms while using the crutches, not in the axillary areas, where pressure may damage nerves and cut off circulation. Also, the crutches should not be forced into the axillae each time the body moves forward.

It is important that axillary crutches are properly fitted and used correctly to prevent damage to nerves and

the crutches placed in the patient's hands. Next, standing slightly away from the wall, the patient should sway on the crutches from side to side. This accustoms the hands and the arms to weight bearing.

Next, the patient should be asked to lean against the wall and pick one crutch up about 15 cm (6 inches) from the floor and then place it down. This should be repeated with the other crutch, and the whole exercise should be done six to eight times. Then, still leaning against the wall, the patient should pick up both crutches from the floor and place them down. This too should be repeated several times.

These exercises make it possible to judge the patient's ability to hold and manage the crutches without the risk of moving. If judged capable, the patient proceeds to the practice of a gait. If possible, it is recommended that the patient begin with the four-point gait. Patients using axillary crutches need to be carefully screened for cardiovascular problems and advised to ambulate slowly to reduce cardiovascular stress.

Crutch Gaits. Before moving into one of the gaits, the patient assumes the *tripod position*, or basic crutch stance (Fig. 38-21). Placing the crutches 15 cm (6 inches) in front of the feet and 15 cm to the side of each foot creates a triangle that provides a wide base of support. The nurse instructs the patient to maintain erect posture with the head held straight and eyes facing forward.

There are five crutch gaits: four-point, three-point, two-point, swing-to, and swing-through. These gaits are described here and their patterns outlined in Figure 38-22.

In *four-point gait*, weight bearing is permitted on both legs. The pattern is shown in Figure 38-22, beginning at the bottom of the figure. In *two-point gait*, weight bearing is also permitted on both feet. The pattern is a speed-up of the four-point gait. In *three-point gait*, weight bearing is permitted on only one foot; the other foot cannot support, but acts as a balance. The *swing-to gait* requires that both crutches move ahead together and the body weight is lifted by the arms and

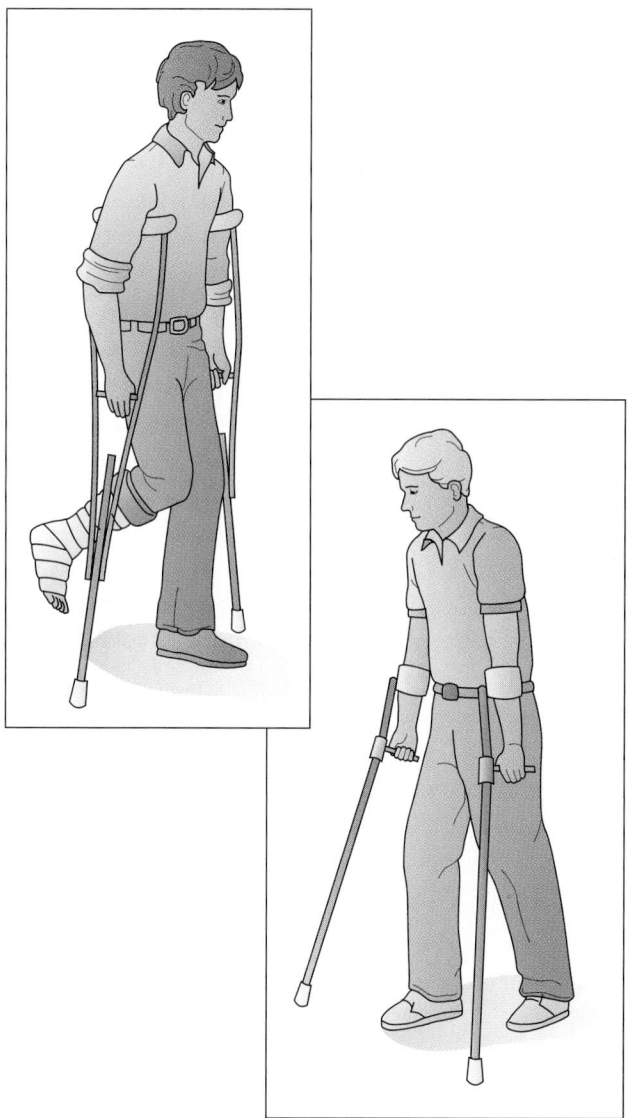

Figure 38-20
Axillary and forearm support crutches.

circulation in the axillae from being cut off and to provide well-balanced support. Forearm support crutches have no axillary support. A supportive frame extends beyond the handgrip for the lower arm to help guide the crutch. These crutches are more likely to be used by patients who have permanent limitations and will always need crutch assistance for ambulation.

Exercises to Prepare for Crutch Walking. Before trying to use the crutches, several exercises will help the patient become more confident and skillful. The patient begins by strengthening the arm and the shoulder muscles. The pushup exercise described earlier is most helpful. The muscles of the hand must also be strengthened. Squeezing a rubber ball 50 times a day by flexing and extending the fingers helps to do this.

The patient should be assisted into a chair that is close to the wall and then helped to stand against the wall, with

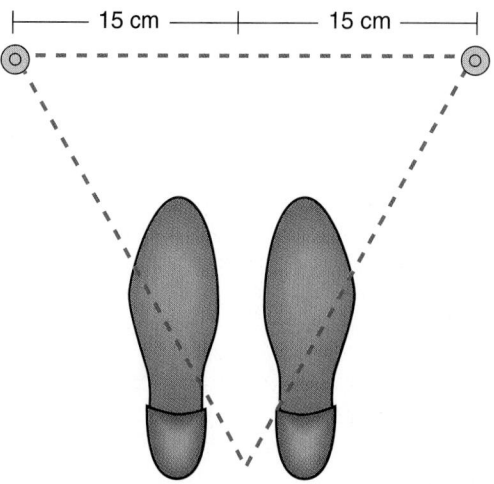

Figure 38-21
The tripod position is the initial crutch stance from which the person advances.

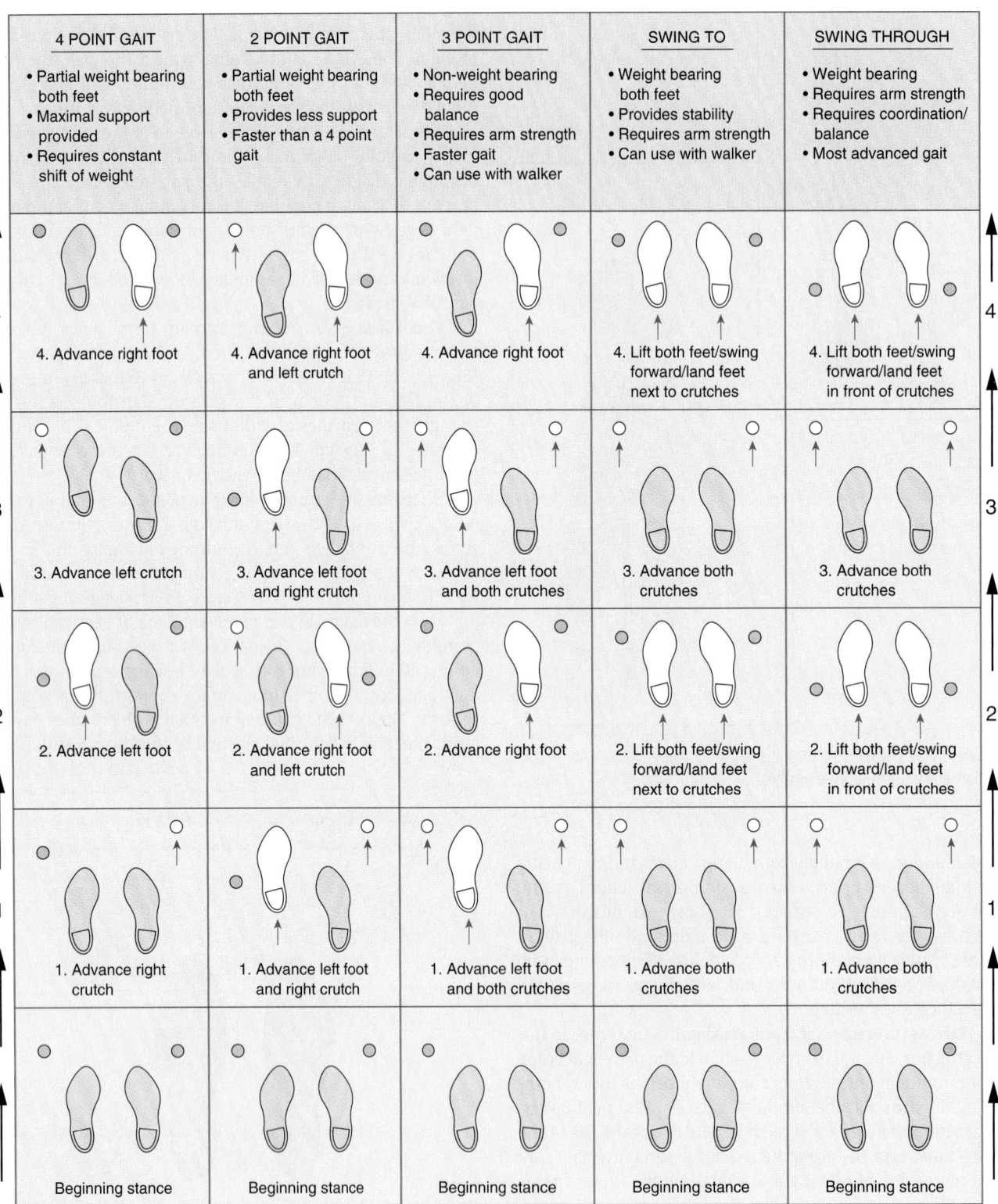

Figure 38-22
Crutch gaits. *Shaded* areas are weight-bearing. *Arrow* indicates advance foot or crutch.

swung *to* the crutches. In *swing-through gait* the body weight is swung *through* and beyond the crutches. The swing gaits require strength and coordination and are frequently used by patients with hip and leg paralysis. A disadvantage of these two gaits is that they do not simulate normal walking. Extended use leads to atrophy of the muscles in the lower extremity that are not being used.

Instructions for crutch walking should also include practice and demonstration of the safe technique for moving up and down stairs. One technique involves advancing the unaffected leg first up the stairs and past the crutches. The patient's body weight is then transferred to the unaffected leg and the crutches are then positioned on either side of the unaffected leg. When coming down the stairs, move the affected leg and crutches first followed by the unaffected one (Fig. 38-23). An easy way to teach the patient to remember this technique is the statement, "The good leg goes up, the bad leg goes down."

When a railing is available, the patient can use another technique to climb and descend stairs. This technique involves using one hand to grasp the railing firmly while the other hand grasps both crutches held together at the handgrips and under the axilla and uses them for support. While holding securely onto the rail, move the uninjured leg up one step, straighten it, and move the injured leg and the crutches onto the same step. When moving down the stairs, one hand should always be on the railing while the other hand again steadies both crutches under the arm using the handgrips. The crutches and the injured leg should move together down one step, followed by the uninjured leg.

Designing Exercise Programs

The benefits of exercise for each of the major body systems are so important that designing individualized exercise programs for patients is an important nursing responsibility. Such a program should incorporate activities of daily living and planned exercise sessions. Depending on the patient's physical condition, exercise is designed to promote optimal fitness.

The individual's commitment to a program of regular exercise depends on the following:

- Knowledge of the benefits of exercise and problems related to immobility
- Appreciation of the fact that in society, sedentary lifestyles are common and most people must consciously choose to exercise
- Belief that each person is responsible for his or her own health and that exercise is essential to one's well-being

Nurses can foster a commitment to regular exercise by teaching and counseling patients about exercise. To do this, nurses need knowledge of the types and benefits of exercise as well as of the risks associated with exercise.

Nurses working with a patient to develop an individualized exercise prescription use the following process:

- Explore the patient's fitness goals, interests, skills, exercise opportunities, and exercise capacity.
- Assist the patient in obtaining medical clearance for exercise.

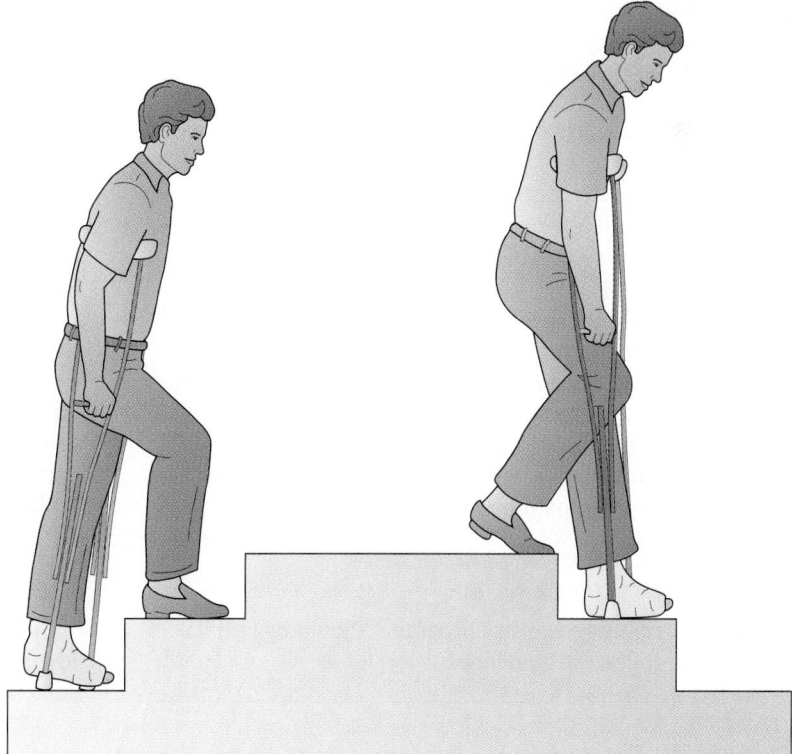

Figure 38-23
Stairs can be dangerous for the person navigating them; therefore, the proper method must be learned. Illustrated here is one of the methods, using both crutches: The good leg goes up; the bad leg comes down.

- Explore feasible exercise activities with the patient, considering the health benefits sought, the time involved, cost, any need for special equipment, precautions, and risks.
- Develop an exercise program that specifies warm-up and cool-down activities (walking, stretching) and three or four major exercise activities from which the patient can choose. Specify the frequency, duration, and intensity of the exercise activity. The recommended frequency for most types of exercise is at least three times a week (but may work up to five or six times a week). For recommended duration and intensity, a person should be able to speak normally without getting out of breath or should maintain a *target heart rate* (60% to 90% of maximal heart rate [220 minus age]).
- Encourage the patient to complement the exercise program with everyday activities that require exercise.
- Try to identify with the patient any potential threats to the exercise program's successful implementation. Plan support strategies.
- Use ongoing evaluation to determine whether the exercise prescription is meeting the patient's needs and whether the patient is adhering to the prescription.

The accompanying box identifies characteristics of a successful exercise program and prevention strategies to avoid the risks associated with exercise.

Advanced age has traditionally been associated with a decline in muscle strength and reticence to exercise. Maintaining balance during exercise is frequently a concern of patients and caregivers. The accompanying box lists NIC standardized nursing interventions that help the patient maintain a sense of balance. Research has demonstrated that an exercise program consisting of low-intensity aerobic activities improves flexibility, benefits the cardiovascular system, and contributes to a sense of well-being (Jones & Jones, 1997). An ongoing program of exercise for older patients also promotes confidence, offers opportunities for socialization, and fosters continued independence while lessening the potential for falls and other factors that often lead to nursing home admission.

Teaching Exercise Benefits to Populations at Risk

Promoting health and wellness is an activity by which nurses can significantly contribute to the well-being of all populations. Assessment and intervention priorities that promote positive health behaviors for each developmental stage were outlined in Table 38-2 earlier in this chapter. As life expectancy continues to increase, nursing activities will increasingly focus on teaching that regular exercise is a positive factor contributing to longevity. In addition to improving the quality of life, exercise plays an important role in the prevention or slowing of osteoporosis. This crippling disease causes up to 1.3 million fractures each year, and regular weight-bearing exercise plays

---

Characteristics of a Successful Exercise Program

- The program is individually designed (considers the individual's fitness goals, interests, skills, exercise opportunities, and exercise capacity).
- The program specifies warm-up and cool-down activities and a variety of major exercise activities—variety is preferable to a single-exercise activity.
- The program specifies frequency, intensity, and duration of exercise.
- The program is convenient to perform, compatible with the individual's lifestyle, and fun!
- The individual in such a program should understand the program and feel confident that exercise will result in definite health benefits.

Prevention Strategies to Avoid Risks Associated With Exercise

People beginning exercise programs should be familiar with the following guidelines:

- Obtain a preexercise medical examination and medical supervision during exercise if older than age 35 years and sedentary or if there is any past or current cardiovascular condition.
- Begin a new exercise program slowly and allow your body's support structure time to accommodate to the new stress.
- Know your body and respect its limitations. Never force a joint beyond its natural range of motion.
- Respect fatigue. Whenever you feel tingling, pain, or burning in a muscle, stop and rest the muscle for 15 minutes before continuing to exercise.
- Follow the safety guidelines for specific exercises; for example, joggers are advised to run on soft surfaces as opposed to cement or asphalt, to wear well-constructed shoes with thick soles and arch supports, and to run in a safe environment with a low pollution index.

Using the Nursing Interventions Classification (NIC)

Exercise Therapy: Balance

- Determine patient's ability to participate in activities requiring balance
- Evaluate sensory functions (eg, vision, hearing, and proprioception)
- Dress patient in nonrestrictive clothing
- Provide safe environment for practice of exercises
- Encourage patient to maintain wide base of support, if needed
- Assist to stand (or sit) and rock body from side to side to stimulate balance mechanisms
- Assist patient to practice standing with eyes closed for short periods at regular intervals to stimulate proprioception
- Monitor patient's response to balance exercises

(From McCloskey, J., & Bulechek, G. [2000]. *Nursing interventions classification [NIC]* [3rd ed]. [p. 321]. St. Louis: C. V. Mosby. A full listing of nursing activities for each nursing intervention can be found in this book.)

an important role in preserving bone mass (Darovic, 1997). Nurses can help older patients use physical exercise to avert or alleviate the effects of this debilitating aging process.

EVALUATING

When evaluating the effectiveness of a plan of care designed to help patients enhance, maintain, or regain mobility and fitness goals, the nurse uses each nurse–patient interaction to evaluate the patient in the following respects:

- General ease of movement and gait
- Body alignment
- Joint structure and function
- Muscle mass, tone, and strength
- Endurance

An excellent time to assess these essential ingredients of well-being is when the patient is performing simple everyday tasks such as ambulating, undertaking hygiene measures, dressing, and eating. Because illness and enforced inactivity can affect these tasks negatively, ongoing evaluation is necessary if serious problems are to be avoided.

See the accompanying Applying Learning to Practice: Patient Care Study and Nursing Plan of Care boxes.

(*text continues on page 1009*)

APPLYING LEARNING TO PRACTICE

Patient Care Study

Quan Hong Nguyen is an alert, 57-year-old married man who was admitted to the hospital with a diagnosis of right cerebrovascular accident or brain attack secondary to thrombosis. He has a history of hypertension. This is his second hospital day, and the attending physicians have termed the stroke a *completed stroke;* that is, Mr. Nguyen's neurologic deficits have been unchanged for 2 days, and he is believed to be ready for more aggressive rehabilitative treatment. On hospital day 2, an assessment of Mr. Nguyen's mobility status and ability to participate in activities of daily living revealed the following data:

- *Mental status*—basically alert and able to follow simple commands; expresses his needs verbally when encouraged, but speech is slow; seems forgetful of usual routine for basic self-care activities
- *Neuromuscular status*—hemiplegia; severe motor and sensory deficits of the left side of the face and the left arm and leg

- *Muscle mass, tone, and strength*—well-developed muscles in all extremities; history of a lifetime of sports, most recently played tennis two to four times weekly; decreased muscle tone (hypotonicity, flaccidity) in left arm and leg motor function is absent in left arm and very weak in left leg; strong motor function on right extremities; incapable of weight-bearing on left side; incapable of independent turning, sitting, standing, transferring, or ambulation
- *Joint mobility*—decreased on left side; otherwise full range of motion; no contractures
- *Endurance*—fatigues quickly (eg, during complete bath)
- Some deficit in spatial-perceptual orientation (eg, ignores objects on his left side), but it is difficult to assess this completely yet

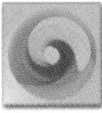

NURSING PLAN OF CARE
for Quan Hong Nguyen

Nursing Diagnosis	Impaired Physical Mobility (turning in bed, sitting, standing, transferring, and ambulating) related to left hemiplegia and weakness as manifested by: motor function absent in left arm and weak in left leg, decreased joint mobility in left extremities, fatigue
Expected Outcome	1/25/01 Whenever observed, the patient will: • Be in correct body alignment with (1) each joint on the left side higher than the joint proximal to it and (2) supportive devices in place (bed board, footboard, trochanter roll, hand–wrist splint, shoulder sling, pillows)

Nursing Interventions	Rationale	Evaluative Statement
At each position change (as dictated by every-2-hour turn schedule posted at the bedside), make sure that the patient is in correct alignment. Follow agency positioning guidelines for the supine, side-lying (lies on unaffected side), and prone positions.	Correct positioning prevents contractures, relieves pressures, and maintains alignment. • Positioning each joint higher than the preceding one prevents edema and its resulting fibrosis. • Placing the patient in the prone position for 30 minutes two or three times daily helps prevent knee and hip flexion contractures.	1/27/01 Goal being met. Every-2-hour positioning schedule being followed with patient in correct body alignment to prevent contractures. *S. Beecher, RN*
Use the following supportive devices: firm mattress, footboard, trochanter roll, shoulder sling when patient is in upright position, volar resting splint, and pillows.	Support devices aid in maintaining the patient in correct positioning. • Firm mattress provides skeletal support. • Footboard during flaccid period prevents footdrop, heel cord shortening, and plantar flexion. • Trochanter roll prevents external rotation of hip when patient is in dorsal position. • Shoulder sling during flaccid period prevents shoulder subluxation and shoulder–hand syndrome. • Volar resting splint supports the wrist and hand in a functional position. • A pillow in the axilla of the left side prevents adduction of the affected side.	
Teach both the patient and family the importance of correct positioning.	Teaching promotes self-care and lays the foundation for successful rehabilitation.	
Allow the family to participate in helping the patient to get comfortable in the different positions.	Involving the family in the patient's care facilitates the coping process.	

(continued)

NURSING PLAN OF CARE (Continued)

for Quan Hong Nguyen

Expected Outcome

By hospital day 7, 1/30/01, the patient will:
- Replace the passive range-of-motion exercises the nurse is now performing four times daily to all joints with (1) the patient's active exercise of the left arm and left leg and (2) the patient's active range-of-motion exercises for all other joints

---

Nursing Interventions	Rationale	Evaluative Statement
Assess the patient's knowledge of the importance of exercise and ability and motivation to exercise.	Unless the patient understands the reason for exercise and is physically, mentally, and attitudinally capable of exercise, he will not follow through.	1/30/01 Goal partially met. Patient has successfully demonstrated complete set of range-of-motion exercises (to both left and right sides); however, he tires during the exercises and stops unless verbally encouraged.
Teach the patient how to exercise his left arm and leg by using his unaffected (right) extremities.	Active exercise maintains joint mobility, prevents contracture development in the paralyzed extremity, prevents further deterioration of the neuromuscular system, helps to regain motor control, and increases circulation.	*Revision:* Monitor patient's exercise four times daily; continue to enlist family's support.
Demonstrate a complete set of range-of-motion exercises to the patient and family and have the patient return the demonstrations.	Involving the family helps ensure the success of the exercise program because it requires a big time and effort commitment.	*S. Beecher, RN*

Expected Outcome

By hospital day 7, 1/30/01, the patient will:
- Perform quadriceps, gluteal, and abdominal settings five times daily

---

Nursing Interventions	Rationale	Evaluative Statement
Teach the patient and family how to tighten the quadriceps, gluteal, and abdominal muscles and hold them for 6 seconds (slow count to 4) before relaxing. A 2-minute rest should be allowed between contractions and the patient cautioned not to hold his breath during these exercises because this places strain on the heart. The exercises should be stopped short of muscle fatigue.	These exercises will maintain muscle mass, tone, and strength (while the patient is on bed rest); and prevent atrophy. They also increase circulation to the exercised body parts.	1/30/01 Goal partially met. Patient has demonstrated exercises correctly; however, he needs to be reminded to perform them. Family is effective in this regard.
		Revision: Compliment family on excellent job they are doing and reinforce importance of exercise to maximize rehabilitative potential.
		S. Beecher, RN

Expected Outcome

By hospital day 7, 1/30/01, the patient will:
- Participate in the every-2-hour positioning schedule by assisting with turning to the degree he is able

---

Nursing Interventions	Rationale	Evaluative Statement
Teach the patient how he can help to reposition himself by grabbing onto the side rail with his right hand and also by placing his unaffected leg under the left one to move himself.	The more the patient can do independently, the more in control he will feel. These activities will pave the way to increasing independence in self-care activities.	1/27/01 Goal met. Patient consistently assists in repositioning. Seems pleased to be able to help the nurses in this way.
		S. Beecher, RN

(continued)

NURSING PLAN OF CARE (Continued)
for Quan Hong Nguyen

Expected Outcome	By hospital day 7, 1/30/01, the patient will:
	• Demonstrate a safe pivot transfer from bed to chair and chair to bed

Nursing Interventions	Rationale	Evaluative Statement
Assess the stage of recovery of muscle function.	Most patients will begin to show signs of spasticity with exaggerated reflexes within 48 hours—this denotes progress. If muscles are still flaccid after several weeks, prognosis for regaining function if poor.	1/30/01 Goal met. Patient can safely transfer from bed to chair and chair to bed but requires nursing assistance. *S. Beecher, RN*

Expected Outcome	By hospital day 7, 1/30/01, the patient will:
	• Demonstrate standing balance

Nursing Interventions	Rationale	Evaluative Statement
Assess activity tolerance by taking vital signs before attempting balance training and transfers.	Vital signs and the patient's physical condition should be assessed before a new activity, during the activity, and shortly afterward to assess activity tolerance.	1/30/01 Goal not met. Patient has not demonstrated standing balance; falls to left side without nursing support. *Revision:* Allow more time for goal achievement. *S. Beecher, RN*
Precede transfers with balance training. Assist the patient to a sitting position at the edge of the bed and observe for steadiness and the ability to maintain an erect posture.	The patient needs sitting and standing balance before progressing to harder tasks. Dizziness or syncope may signal vasomotor instability.	
Place the chair by the bed on the patient's unaffected side and assist the patient to dress. Initially, the nurse helps the patient to stand by placing his or her right knee against the patient's strong knee, grasping the patient around the waist with both arms, and pulling the patient forward while rocking back on the left leg (nurse's knees are slightly flexed).	This prevents the patient's knees from buckling and the pressure of the nurse's knee forces the patient to straighten the strong knee and bear weight on it. In this position, the patient's feet cannot slip forward. In this position, the nurse is using good principles of body mechanics.	
Once the patient is standing, assess standing balance and observe for signs of activity intolerance (pallor, shortness of breath, excessive increase in pulse rate, perspiration). Direct the patient to (1) grab the far arm of the chair with his strong arm, (2) turn on his strong foot, and (3) sit down. The nurse's right leg and the patient's strong leg are used as a pivot.	Using the unaffected extremity facilitates movement and provides stability.	

(continued)

Nursing Interventions	Rationale	Evaluative Statement
Pivot patient out of bed to chair three times a day (may pivot out of bed to bedside commode). Gradually increase time in chair based on patient's tolerance. Correctly align patient in chair using supportive devices as necessary.	Increasing exercise to the patient's tolerance level promotes improved muscle strength and maintenance of range of motion.	

Expected Outcome	On discharge to rehabilitation center, the patient will: • Be free of contractures

Nursing Interventions	Rationale	Evaluative Statement
Implement previously stated nursing actions.	These actions promote independence and return to activities of daily living.	1/30/01 Goal met. Patient has no contractures. *S. Beecher, RN*

Nursing Diagnosis:	Self-Care Deficit (all basic self-care activities) related to decreased alertness and left-sided motor and sensory deficits as manifested by: inability to use left arm (is right-handed), inability to ambulate, forgetfulness, fatigue.
Expected Outcome	By hospital day 7, 1/30/01, the patient will: • Demonstrate beginning ability to resume self-care activities despite motor and sensory deficits of left side; use right arm to (1) assist in morning hygiene; (2) feed himself (finger foods, beverages); and (3) exercise

Nursing Interventions	Rationale	Evaluative Statement
Continue to assess extent of patient's motor and sensory deficits and ability to perform self-care activities.	This facilitates recognition of any recovery of function and allows setting of appropriate goals.	1/29/01 Goal met. for the past 2 days, patient has washed his left arm, abdomen, and legs; combed his hair; fed himself; and performed range-of-motion exercises. *S. Beecher, RN*
Set realistic short-term goals for each sessions with patient and reward progress: "This morning we'll see how much of your bath you are able to manage yourself!" "It must feel good to be able to do this for yourself again."	Adding *realistic* new tasks for each day gives the patient a goal to work toward; a pattern of *noticed* success encourages continued efforts.	
Approach patient from his unaffected side, and place call light, bedside table, phone, and so on, on this side.	This helps the patient to compensate for alterations in sensory perception.	
Teach patient how to transfer all self-care activities to the unaffected side and how to use one-handed techniques and adaptive equipment.	There is never only one way to do anything.	

(continued)

NURSING PLAN OF CARE (Continued)
for Quan Hong Nguyen

Nursing Interventions	Rationale	Evaluative Statement
Encourage patient to brush his teeth, comb his hair, bathe and feed himself, and to assist in toileting. Explain to the family why it is critical to allow him to do these things himself, even if movements are tiring, clumsy, and initially frustrating.	This improves the patient's sense of control of his own activities of daily living and improves morale.	
Continually reevaluate the patient's need for gentle care versus firm, directive encouragement. Involve the family in this process.	Emotional lability is common after stroke. Patients fluctuate between heroic efforts toward independent self-care and whining demands to be totally cared for. The appropriate nursing response varies from moment to moment and runs the range of tender care to unrelenting firm direction. All nursing responses need to communicate the nurse's sincere care for the patient and commitment to developing his best potential.	

Expected Outcome	On discharge to rehabilitation center, the patient will:
	• Show signs of physical and mental readiness to acquire increasing independence in self-care

Nursing Interventions	Rationale	Evaluative Statement
Implement previously stated nursing actions.	These actions help the patient toward regaining control of his daily living and improve morale.	1/31/01 Goal met. Patient's muscle strength and joint mobility maintained during hospitalization. Patient is now participating in self-care activities and is eager to learn skills to become more independent. *S. Beecher, RN*

Sample Documentation	1/25/01 3 PM, Nursing
	Dr. Steel examined the patient at 1 PM and noted he is now in "completed stroke stage and ready for more aggressive rehabilitative treatment." This was explained to patient, his wife, and son. The patient smiled and seemed to understand that he is out of immediate danger. Initial instructions given to the patient on how he can assist with position changes and actively exercise his left arm and leg. Correctly demonstrated these maneuvers with verbal cuing. Motor function still absent in left arm and weak in left leg. Plan of care revised to incorporate new exercise goals. *Susan Beecher, RN*

Learning Outcomes

After completing this chapter, the learner should be able to accomplish the following:

1. Define the key terms used in this chapter.

active exercise	isokinetic exercise
ankylosis	isometric exercise
atrophy	isotonic exercise
base of support	line of gravity
body mechanics	osteoporosis
center of gravity	passive exercise
contractures	range of motion
exercise	spasticity
flaccidity	tonus
footdrop	

2. Describe the role of the skeletal, muscular, and nervous systems in the physiology of movement.

3. Identify seven variables that influence body alignment and mobility.
4. Differentiate isotonic, isometric, and isokinetic exercise.
5. Describe the effects of exercise and immobility on major body systems.
6. Assess body alignment, mobility, and activity tolerance, using appropriate interview questions and physical assessment skills.
7. Develop nursing diagnoses that correctly identify mobility problems amenable to nursing therapy.
8. Use proper body mechanics when positioning, moving, lifting, and ambulating patients.
9. Design exercise programs.
10. Plan, implement, and evaluate nursing care related to select nursing diagnoses involving mobility problems.

Critical Thinking Exercises

1. Pretend that you have a mobility impairment (ie, you have to use crutches or a walker, cane, or wheelchair), and attempt to perform your usual daily activities, ideally including visiting a public place such as a school or mall. How did you feel about the restriction of your movement? How can nurses best assist patients who are coping with these restrictions? How did the public respond to your impairment, and what effects might such responses have on individuals with mobility impairments? Are public spaces adequately adapted to meet the needs of those with mobility impairments? What measures are needed to address any deficiencies? Did you identify any safety needs?

2. Suppose a friend is confined to bed for several months after a motorcycle accident that resulted in severe orthopedic and internal injuries. What nursing measures would you recommend to avoid the hazards of immobility?

Study Questions

1. The strong, flexible, inelastic fibrous bands that attach muscle to bone are
   a. tendons
   b. ligaments
   c. cartilage
   d. joints
2. Nurses spread their feet apart when they prepare to help raise a patient from a chair. The most important reason for doing this is to
   a. use the body's weight to assist movement
   b. make a long midriff
   c. provide a wide base of support
   d. facilitate use of the stronger back muscles
3. A patient performs rehabilitative exercises with resistance after a knee injury. This type of exercise is referred to as
   a. isotonic
   b. isokinetic
   c. isometric
   d. aerobic
4. The expected result when more protein is broken down than is manufactured is
   a. fluid volume excess
   b. a contractor

   c. osteoporosis
   d. negative nitrogen balance
5. An immobile patient experiences multiple urinary tract infections. Urinary bacteria are more likely to grow when urine is
   a. alkaline
   b. dilute
   c. aromatic
   d. acidic
6. Mr. Brown is experiencing some difficulty breathing. The nurse most appropriately assists him into the
   a. dorsal recumbent position
   b. lateral position
   c. Fowler's position
   d. Sims' position
7. While doing range-of-motion exercises with a bedridden patient, the nurse is aware that
   a. neck hyperextension should be encouraged, particularly in older people
   b. exercises should be continued until the patient is fatigued
   c. exercises should be done frequently to lessen pain for the patient

d. each joint is exercised to the point of resistance but not pain

8. The nurse is assisting a patient with conditioning exercises to prepare for ambulation. The nurse correctly instructs the patient to
   a. do full-body pushups in bed six to eight times daily
   b. breathe in and out smoothly during quadriceps drills
   c. dangle on the side of the bed for 30 to 60 minutes
   d. allow the nurse to bathe the patient completely to prevent fatigue

9. In many situations, a patient has sufficient strength to walk if he or she can
   a. lie prone for 1 hour
   b. bathe himself or herself
   c. raise the foot off the bed 1 inch
   d. sit up in bed for 1 hour

10. Mrs. Eden tells the nurse she feels faint while walking in the corridor with the nurse. The nurse
    a. instructs the patient to quicken her pace so they can return to her room
    b. leaves her momentarily to find another nurse to help
    c. advises her to look down at her feet to help maintain her balance
    d. guides her to a chair in the corridor and eases her onto it to rest

11. When using a cane for maximal support, the nurse is aware that the patient should
    a. hold the cane on the weaker side
    b. distribute weight evenly between the feet and the cane
    c. keep the elbow that is holding the cane straight and stiff
    d. advance the weaker foot ahead of the cane

12. One technique the nurse can use when measuring a patient for axillary crutches is
    a. measure from axilla to heel while the patient is lying on his back in bed with his shoes on and add 1 inch
    b. have the patient stand with feet separated 12 inches and arms extended at shoulder height
    c. measure the distance from the shoulder to the heel and add 4 inches
    d. measure the distance from the anterior fold of the axilla diagonally to a point 12 inches from the heel

13. When using the swing-through crutch gait, the patient should
    a. bear weight on the unaffected foot
    b. bear weight on both feet
    c. simulate normal walking as closely as possible
    d. move the right crutch and left foot forward at the same time

14. When working with an older patient to develop an exercise program, the nurse would recommend
    a. a frequency of six times a week
    b. exercising to the point of breathlessness when trying to speak
    c. maintaining a target heart rate of 220 plus age
    d. medical clearance before beginning the program

15. A bedridden patient who is blind is admitted to a healthcare facility from his or her home with pressure ulcers on the sacral area. A priority nursing diagnosis is
    a. Risk for Altered Body Temperature related to stage 2 pressure ulcer
    b. Impaired Skin Integrity related to immobility
    c. Feeding Self-Care Deficit related to blindness
    d. Activity Intolerance related to prolonged bed rest

Answers With Rationale

1. The correct response is *a*. Tendons are the strong fibrous bands that attach muscle to bone. Ligaments bind joints together and connect bones and cartilage, whereas cartilage is nonvascular connective tissue found in the joints as well as in the nose, ear, thorax, trachea, and larynx.

2. The correct response is *c*. Spreading the feet apart broadens the base of support and lowers the center of gravity. The muscles of the back are not as strong as the long muscles of the arms and legs, and making a long midriff is accomplished by stretching the muscles in the waist. Rocking on the feet or leaning forward or backward uses the weight of the body as a moving force.

3. The correct response is *b*. Isokinetic exercise involves muscle contraction with resistance, whereas isotonic exercise involves muscle shortening and active movement. Isometric exercise involves muscle contraction without shortening, and aerobic exercise is sustained muscle movements that increase blood

flow, heart rate, and metabolic demand for oxygen over time, promoting cardiovascular conditioning.

4. The correct response is *d*. Negative nitrogen balance results when the body excretes more nitrogen than it takes in. Contractures are permanent contraction states of muscles, and osteoporosis involves bone demineralization. Fluid volume excess is indirectly related to protein manufacture or breakdown.

5. The correct response is *a*. Bacteria grow more easily in alkaline urine than acidic urine. Whether urine is dilute or aromatic is not a factor in bacteria growth.

6. The correct response is *c*. Fowler's position promotes maximal breathing space in the thoracic cavity and is the position of choice when someone is having difficulty breathing. Lying flat on the back or side or Sims' position would not facilitate respiration and would be difficult for the patient to maintain.

7. The correct response is *d*. Joints should never be exercised to the point of pain or fatigue. Joints should be exercised slowly, smoothly, and rhythmically.

Neck hyperextension should be avoided in older patients and may prove painful.

8. The correct response is *b*. The patient should never hold his or her breath during exercise drills because this places a strain on the heart. Pushups are usually done three or four times a day and involve only the upper body. Dangling for 30 to 60 minutes is unsafe. The nurse encourages the patient to be as independent as possible to prepare for return to normal ambulation and activities of daily living.

9. The correct response is *c*. Being able to raise the foot 1 inch off the bed frequently indicates sufficient strength for walking. Lying prone, bathing himself or herself, or sitting up in bed do not necessarily indicate the muscle coordination and strength necessary in the lower limbs for walking.

10. The correct response is *d*. Guiding the patient to a chair in the hall and easing her into it is the safest action. Asking her to walk faster and leaving her alone are definitely unsafe actions. If the patient looks down at her feet, she may become dizzy and unbalanced.

11. The correct response is *b*. The patient's weight should be evenly distributed between his or her feet and the cane. Holding the cane on the weaker side is difficult and unsafe. The elbow should be flexed at a 30-degree angle when holding the cane.

12. The correct response is *a*. Axillary crutches should be measured when the patient is lying flat in bed with his or her walking shoes on. The distance is measured from the anterior fold of the axilla straight down to the heel, and then adding 2.5 cm (1 inch). Or, measure the distance from the anterior fold of the axilla diagonally out to a point 10 to 15 cm (4 to 6 inches) away from the heel, allowing 3 finger-widths distance from the crutch top to the axilla.

13. The correct response is *a*. With the swing-through gait, weight-bearing is permitted only on one foot. A disadvantage of this gait is that is does not simulate normal walking. Both crutches are brought forward at the same time, and then both legs swing through and between the crutches, with weight-bearing returning to the unaffected leg.

14. The correct response is *d*. Patients older than 35 years should always get medical clearance before initiating an exercise program. Frequency is initially three times a week, and exercise should be maintained so that the patient is able to talk without becoming breathless. The target heart rate is calculated as 60% to 90% of the maximal heart rate (220 minus age).

15. The correct response is *b*. The priority nursing diagnosis for this patient at this moment is Impaired Skin Integrity related to immobility. An end result of the immobility is the development of a pressure ulcer. The other nursing diagnoses may be appropriate but are not the priority on admission to the healthcare facility.

Bibliography

Bennett, J. (1999). Activities of daily living: Old-fashioned or still useful? *Journal of Gerontological Nursing, 25*(5), 22–29.

Darovic, G. (1997). Caring for patients with osteoporosis. *Nursing, 27*(5), 50–51.

Eliopoulos, C. (1997). *Gerontological nursing* (4th ed.). Philadelphia: Lippincott Williams & Wilkins.

Ellis, J., & Hartley, C. (1998). *Nursing in today's world* (6th ed.). Philadelphia: Lippincott Williams & Wilkins.

Garcia, A., Broda, M., Frenn, M., Coviak, C., Pender, N., & Ronis, D. (1997). Gender differences: Exercise beliefs among youths. *Reflections, 23*(1), 21–23.

Jones, J., & Jones, K. (1997). Promoting physical activity in the senior years. *Journal of Gerontological Nursing, 23*(7), 40–48.

Kenney, W. (Ed.) (1997). *American College of Sports Medicine fitness book.* Champaign, IL: Human Kinetics.

Kriska, A., & Rexroad, A. (1999). The role of physical in minority populations. *Women's Health Issues, 8*(2), 98–103.

McCloskey, J., & Bulechek, J. (1996). *Nursing Interventions Classifications (NIC)* (2nd ed.). St. Louis: C. V. Mosby.

North American Nursing Diagnosis Association. (1999). *NANDA nursing diagnoses: Definitions & classification 1999–2000.* Philadelphia: Author.

O'Hanlon-Nichols, T. (1998). Basic assessment series: Adult musculoskeletal system. *American Journal of Nursing, 98*(6), 48–52.

Porth, C. (1998). *Pathophysiology: Concepts of altered health status* (5th ed.). Philadelphia: Lippincott Williams & Wilkins.

Rubenstein, L., & Nahas, R. (1998). Primary and secondary prevention strategies in the older adult. *Geriatric Nursing, 19*(1), 11–18.

Rush, K., & Ouellet, L. (1997). Mobility aids and the elderly client. *Journal of Gerontological Nursing, 23*(1), 7–15.

Sheehan, J. (1999). If you injure your back on the job. *RN, 62*(8), 63–65.

Shoemaker, M. (1998). Living with a leg immobilizer. *Nursing, 28*(8), 32hn9.

Skewes, S. (1997). Bathing: It's a tough job! *Journal of Gerontological Nursing, 23*(5), 45–49.

Stewart, K., & Murray, H. (1997). How to use crutches correctly. *Nursing, 27*(5), 32hn20–32hn22.

Stewart, K., & Murray, H. (1998). How to use a walker correctly. *Nursing, 28*(9), 32hn22–32hn23.

Weber, J., & Kelley, J. (1999). *Health assessment in nursing.* Philadelphia: Lippincott Williams & Wilkins.

Chapter 39
Rest and Sleep

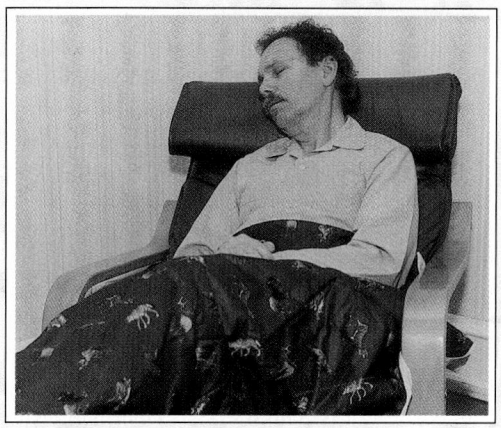

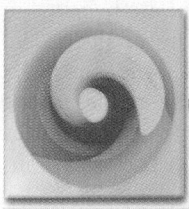

**Thinking Critically About
Nursing's Blended Skills**

Before reading this chapter, think about the types of skills you will need to care effectively for
patients with rest and sleep needs or problems.

- Mrs. Clark complains to the nurse that her 16-year-old son always seems to be tired. "When he
  was small, I could never get him to sleep. Now all he wants to do is sleep. It's all I can do to get
  him up for school each morning."

- A growing number of complaints from family members of patients in the intensive care unit has
  resulted in your being asked to head a task force to study whether the unit environment and
  work patterns are interfering with patients being able to get the rest they need.

- Administering a sleeping pill to one elderly resident in the nursing home you hear, "I don't know
  why they give me these pills. They don't do anything. I'm up half the night trying to fall asleep
  and then I'm no sooner asleep when I wake up and spend the rest of the early morning trying to
  fall back asleep. I wish you could find something to knock me out for at least a couple of hours."

- Jean is a cancer patient who is taking hourly oral pain medications around the clock. This is the
  only schedule that keeps her alert and her pain in check. She lives alone. A small beeper alerts
  her to take her medication and she wakens easily even when asleep. Recently she described
  herself as being "emotionally fragile" to her physician and was told, "No wonder. You haven't
  had more than an hour of undisturbed sleep for the last 2 months!" She asks your help.

*What cognitive, technical, interpersonal, and ethical/legal skills do you think you
will need to meet the needs of the patients described above?*

On the average, people spend one third of their lives asleep. Although the exact purpose of sleep is unclear, the functions of sleep are usually characterized as being protective and restorative. The advice that "everything will look better after a good night's sleep" is based on the belief that sleep accomplishes the following:

- Restores physical well-being
- Relieves stress and anxiety
- Restores the ability to cope and to concentrate on activities of daily living

In this chapter, rest connotes a condition in which the body is in a decreased state of activity with the consequent feeling of being refreshed. Many factors affect a person's ability to rest. Adults juggling the demands of their job and family responsibilities often find little opportunity for rest and relaxation during the course of a day. When rest is possible, the environment is not always conducive to physical and mental relaxation. Suggestions for preparing a restful environment and promoting relaxation are discussed later in the chapter.

Sleep is a state of rest accompanied by altered consciousness and relative inactivity. Sensitivity to external stimuli is diminished during sleep, but this can readily be reversed. Sleep is a complex rhythmic state involving a progression of repeated cycles, each representing different phases of body and brain activity.

Most people can fall asleep easily and remain asleep until the desired waking time. On the other hand, some individuals rarely fall asleep without a struggle, and even then their sleep is fragmented. Many people have sleep disturbances that go undetected for years, progressively undermining their energy and destroying their sense of self. Sleep loss that results in fatigue and decreased competence

may be a contributing factor in accidents. The National Highway Traffic Safety Administration in collaboration with the National Center on Sleep Disorder Research (NHTSA & NCSDR, 1999) estimated that 40,000 nonfatal injuries and 1,550 fatalities annually can be attributed to drowsy drivers. Also, the discomfort produced by physical and mental illness and the need for hospitalization and treatment may interfere dramatically with a patient's ability to sleep. Consequently, nurses need to be vigilant in detecting and treating sleep disturbances.

Study of this chapter provides the nurse with knowledge of the functions and physiology of sleep and factors affecting sleep. Practical suggestions for performing a comprehensive sleep assessment are included. Sample interview questions for a general sleep history are presented, along with information on sleep diaries and pertinent physical assessment data. The importance of analyzing these data is explained along with numerous examples of nursing diagnoses. Expected patient outcomes and specific nursing strategies for promoting rest and sleep are described. The concluding patient care study illustrates how the nurse's knowledge of rest and sleep, combined with skilled nursing interventions and caring, can successfully resolve sleep problems.

Physiology of Sleep

Two systems in the brain stem, the reticular activating system and the bulbar synchronizing region, are believed to work together to control the cyclic nature of sleep. The reticular formation is found in the brain stem. It extends upward through the medulla, the pons, the midbrain, and into the hypothalamus. It is composed of many nerve cells and fibers. The fibers have connections that relay im-

COGNITIVE SKILLS

- Knowledge of the functions and physiology of sleep and the variables that influence rest and sleep—including developmental variables
- Knowledge of how to use the nursing process to identify patients at risk for sleep disorders and to implement a plan of care to prevent or resolve sleep problems
- Knowledge of how to change a system (intensive care) to promote rest and sleep

TECHNICAL SKILLS

- Strong assessment skills to diagnose rest and sleep alterations
- Competence in particular skills may be needed (eg, how to monitor sleep apnea, sleep–wake cycles)

INTERPERSONAL SKILLS

- Strong people skills to establish trusting relationships with both the patients and their families
- A good working relationship with colleagues to implement changes in the intensive care unit environment if these prove to be necessary

ETHICAL/LEGAL SKILLS

- First and foremost, a strong sense of accountability for the health and well-being of these individuals; a commitment to getting them the help they need to achieve their rest and sleep goals—within the scope of your nursing responsibilities and available resources
- A willingness to hold colleagues accountable for safe and good-quality practice

pulses into the cerebral cortex and into the spinal cord. The reticular formation facilitates reflex and voluntary movements as well as cortical activities related to a state of alertness. During sleep, the reticular system experiences few stimuli from the cerebral cortex and the periphery of the body. Wakefulness occurs when the reticular system is activated with stimuli from the cerebral cortex and from periphery sensory organs and cells (Fig. 39-1). For example, an alarm clock awakens us from sleep to a state of consciousness when we realize that we must prepare ourselves for the day. Sensations such as pain, pressure, and noise produce wakefulness by means of peripheral organs and cells. Wakefulness is activated by the cerebral cortex and body sensations. During sleep, stimuli from the cortex are minimal.

The hypothalamus has control centers for several involuntary activities of the body, one of which concerns sleeping and waking. Injury to the hypothalamus may cause a person to sleep for abnormally long periods.

Various neurotransmitters are involved with the sleeping process. Norepinephrine and acetylcholine, followed by dopamine, serotonin, and histamine, are involved with excitation. Gamma-aminobutyric acid appears to be necessary for inhibition. However, research has yet to prove exactly how biochemical changes and hormones function in sleep.

Circadian Rhythms

Rhythmic biologic clocks are known to exist in plants, animals, and humans. Influenced by both internal and external factors, they regulate certain biologic and behavioral functions in humans. Some cycles are monthly, such as a woman's menstrual cycle. **Circadian rhythms** complete a full cycle every 24 hours. Fluctuations in a person's heart rate, blood pressure, body temperature, hormone secretions, metabolism, and performance and mood depend in part on circadian rhythms.

Sleep is one of the body's most complex biologic rhythms. *Circadian synchronization* exists when an individual's sleep–wake patterns follow the inner biologic clock. When physiologic and psychological rhythms are high or most active, the person is awake, and when these rhythms are low, the person is asleep. Although light and dark appear to be powerful regulators of the sleep–wake circadian rhythm, they do not exert primary control. The regulating mechanism is the person's individual biologic clock, which is subject to occupational demands, social pressures, and so forth. Nurses who work the night shift may routinely sleep from 2 to 8 PM, and peak physiologic activity may occur between 10 PM and 6 AM during work. Problems of desynchronization occur when sleep–wake patterns are frequently altered and the person attempts to sleep during high-activity rhythms or to work when the body is physiologically prepared to rest.

Stages of Sleep

Research reveals that there are two major stages of sleep: **non–rapid eye movement** (NREM) sleep and **rapid eye movement** (REM) sleep. These stages have been studied and analyzed with the help of the *electroencephalograph* (EEG), which receives and records electrical currents from the brain; the *electrooculogram* (EOG), which is a recording of eye movements; and the *electromyograph* (EMG), which records muscle tone (Fig. 39-2).

NREM Sleep

NREM sleep consists of four stages. Stages I and II, consuming about 5% to 50%, respectively, of a person's sleep, are light sleep, and the person can be aroused with relative ease. Stages III and IV, each composing about 10% of total sleep time, are deep-sleep states, termed **delta sleep** or *slow-wave sleep*. The arousal threshold (intensity of stimulus required to awaken) is usually greatest in stage IV NREM. Throughout the stages of NREM sleep, the parasympathetic branch of the autonomic nervous system dominates, and decreases in pulse, respiratory rate, blood pressure, metabolic rate, and body temperature are observed. Characteristics of the four stages of NREM sleep are summarized in Table 39-1.

REM Sleep

It is more difficult to arouse a person during REM sleep than during NREM sleep. In normal adults, the REM state consumes 20% to 25% of a person's nightly sleep. People who are awakened during the REM state almost always report that they have been dreaming. Many researchers state that everyone dreams; those people who say they do not simply are unable to recall their dreams.

During REM sleep, the pulse, respiratory rate, blood pressure, metabolic rate, and body temperature increase,

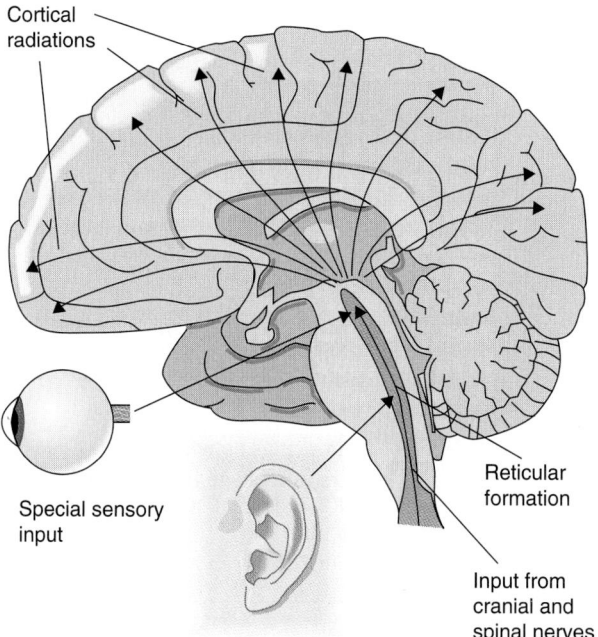

Figure 39-1
Nerve impulses from all the sensory tracts reach the reticular activating system (RAS), which then selectively allows certain impulses to reach the cerebral cortex and to be perceived.

Cortical radiations

Special sensory input

Reticular formation

Input from cranial and spinal nerves

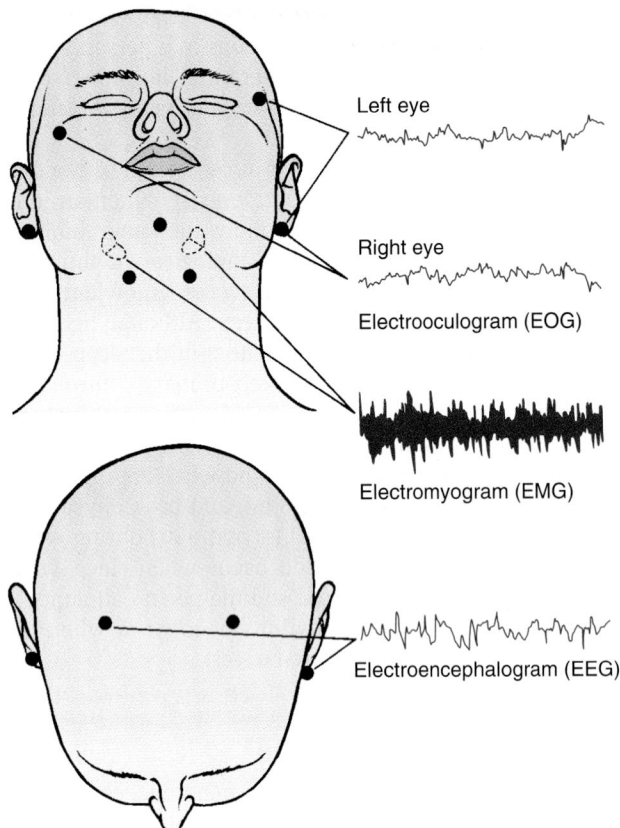

Figure 39-2
Sleep laboratory evaluation. Sleep is determined in the laboratory by measuring the electrical activity of the brain and muscles and the movement of the eyes, using techniques of electro-oculography, electromyography, and electroencephalography.

whereas general skeletal muscle tone and deep tendon reflexes are depressed. REM sleep is believed to be essential to mental and emotional equilibrium and to play a role in learning, memory, and adaptation.

A person who is deprived of REM sleep for several nights generally then spends more time in REM sleep on successive nights. This phenomenon is termed *REM rebound* and allows the total amount of REM sleep to remain fairly constant over time. Characteristics of REM sleep are included in Table 39-1.

Sleep Cycle

Normally during a **sleep cycle**, a person passes consecutively through the four stages of NREM sleep. This pattern is then reversed, and the person returns from stage IV to stage III to stage II. Instead of reentering stage I and awakening, the person enters into the REM stage of sleep, after which he or she reenters NREM sleep at stage II and returns to stages III and IV. If a person is awakened from sleep at any time, he or she returns to sleep again by starting at stage I of NREM sleep.

Most people go through four or five cycles of sleep each night. On the average, each cycle lasts about 90 to 100 minutes. The cycles tend to become longer as morning approaches. Ordinarily, more sleep occurs in the delta stage

Table 39-1
Characteristics of NREM and REM Sleep

NREM Sleep

Stage	Characteristics
I	The person is in a transitional stage between wakefulness and sleep
	The person is in a relaxed state but still somewhat aware of the surroundings.
	Involuntary muscle jerking may occur and waken the person.
	The stage normally lasts only minutes.
	The person can be aroused easily.
	This stage constitutes only about 5% of total sleep.
II	The person falls into a stage of sleep.
	The person can be aroused with relative ease.
	This stage constitutes 50% to 55% of sleep.
III	The depth of sleep increases, and arousal becomes increasingly difficult.
	This stage composes about 10% of sleep.
IV	The person reaches the greatest depth of sleep, which is called *delta sleep*.
	Arousal from sleep is difficult.
	Physiologic changes in the body include the following:
	Slow brain waves are recorded on an EEG.
	Pulse and respiratory rates decrease.
	Blood pressure decreases.
	Muscles are relaxed.
	Metabolism slows and the body temperature is low.
	This constitutes about 10% of sleep.

REM Sleep

Eyes dart back and forth quickly.
Small muscle twitching, such as on the face
Large muscle immobility, resembling paralysis
Respirations irregular; sometimes interspersed with apnea
Rapid or irregular pulse
Blood pressure increases or fluctuates
Increase in gastric secretions
Metabolism increases; body temperature increases
Encephalogram tracings active
REM sleep enters from stage II of NREM sleep and reenters NREM sleep at stage II: arousal from sleep difficult
Constitutes about 20% to 25% of sleep

in the first half of the night, especially if one is tired or has lost sleep.

Figure 39-3 illustrates the normal sleep pattern of young adults. Variations in the sleep cycle occur according to age, as Figure 39-4 illustrates.

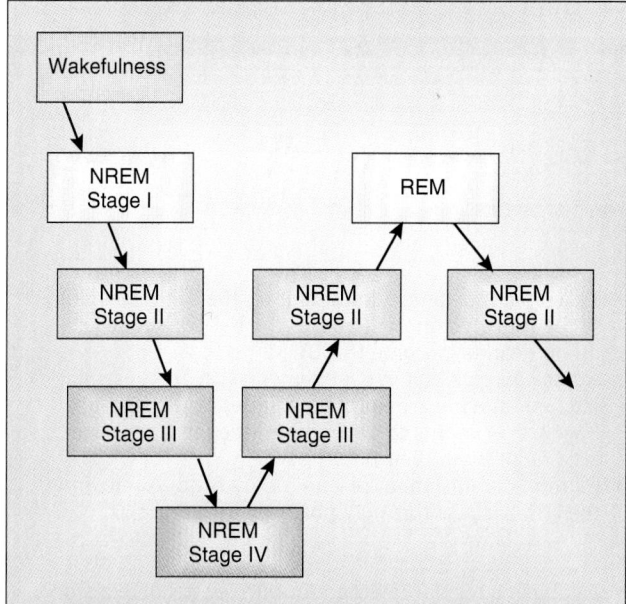

Figure 39-3
A single normal sleep cycle. In the normal nocturnal pattern, the shaded cycle is repeated four or five times. Periods of REM sleep generally increase in duration, and periods of deep sleep (stage IV) progressively decrease as morning approaches.

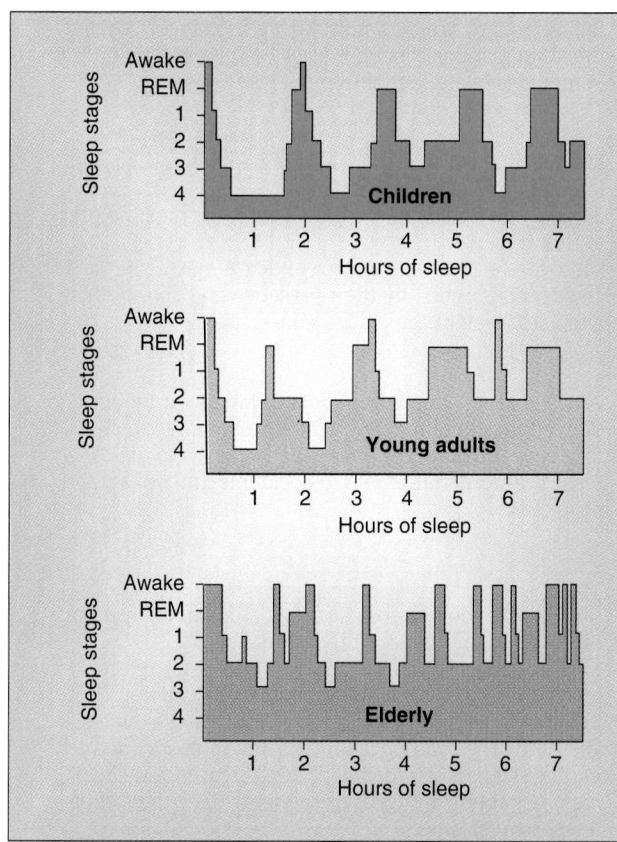

Figure 39-4
A comparison of developmental differences in NREM and REM cycles during nocturnal sleep for children, young adults, and older people.

Sleep Requirements and Patterns

For no known reason, 8 hours of sleep a night has been the accepted standard, despite obvious variances seen in the general population. There is no rigid formula for normal periodicity and duration of sleep. It is important, however, that each person follow a pattern of rest that maintains well-being.

Despite individual variations, some generalities can be stated. On the average, infants sleep from 14 to 20 hours each day. Growing children require from 10 to 14 hours of sleep. Adults average 7 to 9 hours. Those who are able to relax and rest easily, even while awake, often find that less sleep is needed, whereas others may find that more sleep is required to overcome fatigue. Fatigue can be considered a normal, protective body mechanism and nature's warning that sleep is necessary. Chronic fatigue, however, is abnormal and is often a symptom of illness.

Sleep patterns of older people vary. However, older people often need more time to fall asleep, wake earlier and more frequently during the night, and are less able to cope with changes in their usual sleep patterns than younger people. Many older individuals nap during the day, which often results in sleeping fewer hours at night.

Patterns of sleep periodicity appear to be learned. For example, most people learn to sleep at night and to be awake and work during the day. However, many night workers learn to sleep equally well during the day.

Factors Affecting Sleep

A variety of factors influence both the quality and quantity of sleep.

Developmental Considerations

Variations in sleep patterns are related to age. These are presented with related nursing interventions in Table 39-2.

Physical Activity

Activity and exercise increase fatigue and, in many instances, promote relaxation that is followed by sleep. It appears that physical activity increases both REM and NREM sleep.

Psychological Stress

Illness and various life situations that cause psychological stress tend to disturb sleep. Generally, psychological stress affects sleep in two ways: (1) the person experiencing stress may find it difficult to obtain the amount of sleep he or she needs, and (2) REM sleep decreases in amount, which tends to add to anxiety and stress.

Motivation

A desire to be wakeful and alert helps overcome sleepiness and sleep. For example, a tired person may be wakeful and alert when at a party or when attending an interesting play or concert. The opposite is also true: when there is minimal motivation to be awake, sleep generally follows. For example, a student who is bored and disinterested in a lecture or class may doze during the lecture.

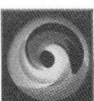

Table 39-2
Developmental Patterns of Sleep

Sleep Pattern	Nursing Implications
Infants	
• *Newborn:* sleeps an average of 16 hours/24 hours; averages about 4 hours at a time • Each infant's sleep pattern is unique. On the average, infants sleep 10–12 hours at night with possibly several naps during the day. • Usually by 8–16 weeks of age, an infant sleeps through the night. • REM sleep constitutes much of the sleep cycle of a young infant.	• Teach parents to position infant on the back. Sleeping in the prone position increases the risk for sudden infant death syndrome (SIDS). • Advise parents that eye movements, groaning, grimacing, and moving are normal activities at this age. • Encourage parents to have infant sleep in a separate area rather than their bed. • Caution parents about placing pillows, quilts, etc. in the crib because this may pose a suffocation risk.
Toddlers	
• Need for sleep declines as this stage progresses. May initially sleep 12 hours at night with two naps during the day and end this stage sleeping 8 hours a night and napping once during the day • May begin to resist naps and going to bed at night • May move from crib to youth bed or regular bed	• Establish a regular bedtime routine (eg, reading a story, singing a lullaby, saying prayers). • Advise parents of the value of a routine sleeping pattern with minimal variation. • Encourage attention to safety once child moves from crib to bed. If child attempts to wander out of room, a folding gate may be necessary across the door of their room.
Preschoolers	
• Children in this stage generally sleep 9–16 hours at night, with 12 hours being the average. • The REM sleep pattern is similar to that of an adult. • Daytime napping decreases during this period and most children by the age of 5 years no longer nap. • May continue to resist going to bed at night.	• Encourage parents to continue bedtime routines. • Advise parents that waking from nightmares or night terrors (awakening screaming about 20 minutes after falling asleep) are common during this stage. Waking the child and comforting him or her generally helps. Sometimes use of a nightlight is soothing.
School-Aged Children	
• Younger school-aged children may require 10–12 hours nightly, whereas older children in this stage may average 8 to 10 hours • Sleep needs usually increase when physical growth peaks.	• Discuss the fact that the stress of beginning school may interrupt normal sleep patterns. • Advise that a relaxed, bedtime routine is most helpful at this stage. • An awareness of the concept of death may occur at this stage, and parents, by their presence and support, can alleviate some of the child's concerns.
Adolescents	
• Sleep needs of teenagers vary widely. The growth spurt that normally occurs at this stage may necessitate the need for more sleep; however, the stresses of school, activities, and part-time employment may cause adolescents to have a restless sleep. • Many adolescents do not get enough sleep.	• Advise parents that complaints of fatigue or inability to do well in school may be related to not enough sleep. *Excessive daytime sleepiness (EDS)* may also make the teenager more vulnerable to accidents and behavioral problems.
Young Adults	
• The average amount of sleep required is 8 hours, but in fact, many young adults require less sleep. • Sleep is affected by many factors: physical health, type of occupation, exercise. Lifestyle demands may interfere with sleep patterns. • REM sleep averages about 20% of sleep.	• Developing good sleep habits has a positive effect on health, particularly as an individual ages. • If loss of sleep is a problem, the nurse can explore lifestyle demands and stress as possible causes. • Relaxation techniques and stress-reduction exercises should be tried rather than resorting to medication to induce sleep. Sleep medications decrease REM sleep, may be habit forming, and frequently lose their effectiveness over time.

(continued)

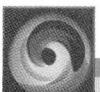

Table 39-2 (Continued)

Sleep Pattern	Nursing Implications
Middle-Aged Adults • Total sleep time decreases during these years with a decrease in stage IV sleep. • The percentage of time spent awake in bed begins to increase.	• Individuals become more aware of sleep disturbances during this period. • Encourage adults to investigate consistent sleep difficulties to exclude pathology or anxiety and depression as causes. • Encourage adults to avoid use of sleep-inducing medication on a regular basis.
Older Adults • An average of 5–7 hours of sleep is usually adequate for this age group. • Sleep is less sound, and stage IV sleep is absent or considerably decreased. Periods of REM sleep shorten. • Elderly people frequently have great difficulty falling asleep and have more complaints of problems sleeping. • Decline in physical health, psychological factors, effects of drug therapy (eg, nocturia), or environmental factors may be implicated as causes of inability to sleep.	• A comprehensive nursing assessment and individualized interventions may be effective in the long-term care of this age group. • Emphasize concern for a safe environment because it is not uncommon for older people to be temporarily confused and disoriented when they first awake. • Sedatives should be used with extreme caution because of declining physiologic function and concerns about polypharmacy. • Encourage people to discuss sleep concerns with their physicians.

Cultural Implications

Nurses should recognize that the individual's cultural beliefs and practices can influence rest and sleep. Although their developmental stages are similar, children's bedtime rituals, sleeping place, and pattern of sleep may vary according to culture. An older Asian patient may choose herbal tea rather than a sleeping medication to promote relaxation and sleep. A cultural orientation toward privacy and quiet makes sleep difficult in a busy special care unit where male and female patients sleep in close proximity. Nursing interventions that are sensitive to the patient's culture need to be included in the plan of care for preparing the patient for an evening's sleep.

Diet

It has long been believed that the dietary amino acid l-tryptophan acts to promote sleep. A small protein snack before bedtime used to be recommended frequently for patients with insomnia. As nutritionists have studied the effects of various foods on mood, however, new information has emerged. Protein may actually increase brain energy alertness and concentration, whereas carbohydrates appear to affect brain serotonin levels and promote feelings of calmness and relaxation. A small protein and carbohydrate snack may be effective.

Alcohol Intake

Alcoholic beverages, when used in moderation, appear to help induce sleep in some people. However, large quantities have been found to limit REM and delta sleep. This effect may partially explain the phenomenon of hangover after excessive alcohol consumption.

Caffeine-Containing Beverages

Caffeine is a central nervous system stimulant. For many people, beverages containing caffeine interfere with the ability to fall asleep. Examples of beverages containing caffeine include coffee, tea, and most cola drinks. Chocolate also contains caffeine.

Smoking

Nicotine has a stimulating effect, and smokers usually have a more difficult time falling asleep. They are more easily aroused once asleep and may describe themselves as light sleepers. Eliminating cigarette smoking after the evening meal appears to improve the smoker's ability to fall asleep, and people usually report improved sleep patterns after nicotine use is discontinued. Total withdrawal from smoking may be associated with temporary sleep disturbances. Patients who stop smoking often have more daytime sleepiness and report significantly more restlessness at night. Whether this is a short-term effect or is related to nicotine's effect on the central nervous system is uncertain.

Environmental Factors

Most people sleep best in their usual home environments. Sleeping in a strange or new environment tends to influence both REM and NREM sleep.

Lifestyle

Various lifestyle factors can affect a person's ability to sleep well. People working a shift other than the day shift must reorganize their priorities, or sleep difficulties may occur. Sleep disorders are the major problem associated with shift work, but shift work can also result in anxiety, personal conflicts, loneliness, gastrointestinal symptoms, and substance abuse. Developing a sleep pattern is especially difficult if the shift changes periodically. Sleep can be affected by watching some types of television shows, participation in stimulating outside activities, and one's level of activity or exercise. One's abilities to relax from work-related pressures and to put aside home stresses are also important factors in the ability to fall asleep (see the accompanying box, Applying Learning to Practice: The Nurse as Role Model: Rest and Sleep).

Exercise

Moderate exercise is a healthy way to promote sleep, but exercise that occurs within a 2-hour interval before normal bedtime can hinder sleep. The fatigue that results from normal work activities or exercise is believed to contribute to a restful sleep, whereas excessive exercise or exhaustion can negatively impact on the quality of sleep.

Illness

Illness is a physiologic and psychological stressor and therefore influences sleep. Certain illnesses are more closely related to sleep disturbances than others. Several examples follow.

Gastric secretions increase during REM sleep. Many people with peptic ulcers wake at night with pain. They find that eating a snack or using antacids to help neutralize stomach acidity often help to relieve discomfort and promote sleep.

The pain associated with diseases of the coronary arteries and the occurrence of myocardial infarctions is more likely with REM sleep. Epilepsy seizure attacks are most likely to occur during NREM sleep and appear to be de-

pressed by REM sleep. Liver failure and encephalitis tend to cause a reversal in day–night sleeping habits. Hypothyroidism tends to decrease the amount of NREM sleep, especially stages II and IV.

Chronotherapeutics is a growing field of study that involves the strategic use of time in medicine. Researchers have determined that certain treatments for disease are more effective when body rhythms are taken into account. The administration of a larger midafternoon dose of asthma medication may more effectively prevent attacks that commonly occur at night during sleep. Timing of antihypertensive medication may need adjustment to provide peak protection during early-morning hours, when heart attacks are more common. Cancer chemotherapy appears to be less toxic when administered at certain times of the day. Attention to biologic rhythms may influence drug tolerance and effectiveness of medication (Cowley, 1996).

Medications

Sleep quality is also influenced by certain drugs. Drugs that decrease REM sleep include barbiturates, amphetamines, and antidepressants. McKenry and Salerno (1998) list diuretics, antiparkinsonian drugs, some antidepressants and antihypertensives, steroids, decongestants, caffeine, and asthma medications as additional common causes of sleep interference. Chloral hydrate and zolpidem tartrate (Ambien) appear to influence the quality of sleep least and promote normal sleep.

Common Sleep Disorders

A nurse who interviews a patient to obtain a sleep history needs to understand common sleep disturbances to recognize significant data. The most recent classification of sleep disorders devised by the American Sleep Disorders Association includes four major categories of disturbances, as follow:

* Dyssomnias
* Parasomnias

APPLYING LEARNING TO PRACTICE

The Nurse as Role Model: Rest and Sleep

It is difficult for patients to work collaboratively with a nurse to achieve sleep and rest goals when the nurse's appearance and behavior demonstrate inadequate rest and sleep. Because professional, personal, and family demands can all outrank sleep on a nurse's list of priorities, nurses often find themselves showing up for work with inadequate rest and energy. Nurses who value their own well-being and who wish to be role models of healthy sleep self-care behaviors must develop lifestyles supportive of the following goals. The nurse will do the following:

* Routinely obtain the amount of sleep necessary to provide energy for the next day's work (specify number of hours)
* Incorporate three to four periods of regular exercise into each week
* Perform some relaxing activity 1 hour before retiring
* Evaluate the use of nicotine, caffeine, alcohol, and any pharmacologic sleep aids
* When possible, limit shift rotations and working two shifts back-to-back to prevent disrupting usual circadian rhythm

- Sleep disorders associated with medical or psychiatric disorders
- Other proposed disorders (Phipps, Sands, & Marek, 1999).

This classification system has been developed based on current and ongoing research, and all disorders have not yet been clearly defined. The more common sleep disorders are the dyssomnias and parasomnias. **Dyssomnias** are sleep disorders characterized by insomnia or excessive sleepiness. **Parasomnias** are patterns of waking behavior that appear during sleep. A brief description of these disturbances follows.

Insomnia

Insomnia is characterized by difficulty falling asleep, intermittent sleep, or early awakening from sleep. Usually, people complaining of insomnia have been observed to fall asleep more quickly and sleep more than they report they do. However, the condition can lead to such distress that further wakefulness results. It is the most common of all sleep disorders.

Individuals older than 60 years of age, women (especially after menopause), and persons with a history of depression are more likely to experience insomnia. This sleep disorder can also occur during periods of stress, in situations involving some change in the normal environment, jet lag, and in association with medication side effects. A person with insomnia often reports feeling tired, lethargic, and irritable during the day. Difficulty concentrating is also a common manifestation. *Hypersomnia* is a condition characterized by excessive sleep, particularly during the day. Although this may result from a medical condition, it frequently occurs as a coping mechanism when someone has no desire or energy to face a new day.

If the insomnia is transient or intermittent, treatment is usually unnecessary because episodes last for only a short period of time. Chronic insomnia lasts for longer than 3 to 4 weeks and may even continue throughout life. Depression is a common cause of chronic insomnia. Behavioral factors such as the misuse of alcohol or caffeine are also frequently implicated. Identifying and stopping these behaviors may reduce or eliminate the insomnia. Sedative hypnotics may be prescribed, but only short-term use is recommended at the lowest dose. Moderate-intensity exercise programs have proved effective for older adults (King & Oman et al., 1997). Nondrug therapies, such as sleep restriction, relaxation techniques, and sleep hygiene education, have provided significant improvement in people with chronic insomnia without causing major adverse effects (Winslow & Jacobsen, 1997). The accompanying research in nursing box focuses on a practical nursing intervention aimed at reducing sedative use in older adults.

Narcolepsy

Narcolepsy is a condition characterized by an uncontrollable desire to sleep. A person with narcolepsy can literally fall asleep standing up, while driving a car, in the middle

---

RESEARCH IN NURSING: MAKING A DIFFERENCE

Using Protocols That Enhance Sleep in Hospitalized Elderly Patients

Although sleep disturbances may occur at any age, it has been documented that older adults often experience difficulty achieving a restful sleep. Nurses recognize that insomnia is a common problem in older hospitalized patients and that sedative-hypnotic drugs (SHDs) are commonly prescribed to induce sleep for this population. The nurse plays a pivotal role in exploring alternative interventions that can successfully promote relaxation and sleep without concern about serious adverse effects from SHDs in this vulnerable population.

Related Research
McDowell, J., Mion, L., Lydon, T., & Inouye, S. (1998). A nonpharmacological sleep protocol for hospitalized older patients. *Journal of the American Geriatrics Society, 46*(6), 700–705.
In an effort to reduce the use of SHDs in acutely ill older adults, nurses tested the effectiveness of nonpharmacologic measures to induce sleep on 111 hospitalized adults who averaged 79 years of age.

Alternative measures consisted of a 5-minute slow-stroke back massage, a warm cup of herbal tea or milk, and the opportunity to listen to relaxation tapes using a head set or bedside cassette tape player. If these interventions proved ineffective after 1 hour, the nurse administered prescribed medications to induce sleep. Results of this study confirmed that this sleep protocol reduced use of SHDs by 23% in this group and had a beneficial effect on the quality of their sleep.

Relevance to Nursing Practice
By incorporating these simple sleep protocol measures into the nursing care plan, nurses can provide nonpharmacologic alternatives for older patients who are at increased risk for side effects from SHDs. Patient-focused care requires that nurses weigh the benefits of these nontoxic interventions against the daytime drowsiness and impairment in function that frequently accompany use of sleep-inducing medications.

of a conversation, or while swimming. Individuals with narcolepsy tend to fall asleep quickly, find it difficult to wake up, sleep fewer hours than others, and sleep restlessly. It is considered a neurologic disorder. The condition usually begins in susceptible people during adolescence or early adulthood and continues through life.

Sleepiness during the day is often the first symptom of narcolepsy and usually precedes by several years any difficulty with nighttime sleep. Common features of narcolepsy include the following:

* *Sleep attacks:* irresistible urge to sleep regardless of type of activity
* *Cataplexy:* sudden loss of motor tone that may cause the person to fall asleep
* *Hypnagogic hallucinations:* nightmares or vivid hallucinations
* *Sleep-onset REM periods:* during a sleep attack, the person moves directly into REM sleep
* *Sleep paralysis:* skeletal paralysis that occurs during the transition from wakefulness to stage I

Any combination of two symptoms helps to confirm the diagnosis. Undiagnosed, a narcoleptic person is potentially dangerous to self and others. A central nervous system stimulant (eg, methylphenidate [Ritalin]) that causes wakefulness is used to control narcolepsy. People using such drugs should take them faithfully because if they are discontinued, the uncontrollable desire to sleep returns.

Sleep Apnea

Sleep apnea refers to periods of no breathing between snoring intervals. The person may not breathe for periods of 10 to 20 seconds to as long as 2 minutes. During long periods of apnea, there is a drop in the oxygen level of the blood, the pulse usually becomes irregular, and the blood pressure often increases. Many people experience sleep apnea without symptoms. Although it occurs most commonly in middle-aged men who are obese and have short thick necks, women and people of other ages may also experience it. Obstructive sleep apnea (OSA) can result when the airway is occluded as a result of collapse of the hypopharynx (Fig. 39-5) or from other structural abnormalities, such as enlarged tonsils and adenoids, deviated nasal septum, and thyroid enlargement. Some investigators have theorized that sleep apnea may explain certain cases of death that occur during sleep. *Polysomnography* is the only certain method of diagnosing sleep apnea. This sleep study consists of an EEG recording of the stages of sleep and any episodes of apnea, continuous monitoring of arterial oxygen saturation, and an electrocardiogram (ECG) to detect any cardiac dysrhythmia.

People with obstructive sleep apnea may become irritable during the day, fall asleep during monotonous activities, have difficulty concentrating, and exhibit slower reaction times. They are also more likely to be involved in motor vehicle accidents. Alcohol, tobacco, and sleeping pills increase the breathing disruption that occurs in sleep apnea and should be avoided.

Treatment of moderate OSA may consist of removing the tonsils or using an oral appliance when sleeping. If this

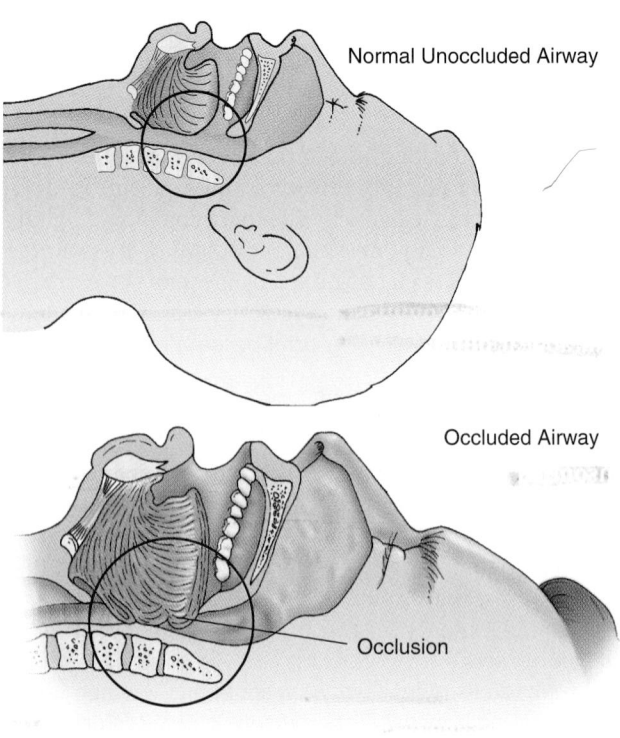

Figure 39-5
Obstructive sleep apnea occurs when the airway is occluded due to collapse of the hypopharynx. Normally the airway remains open during sleep (*see inset*).

is ineffective, continuous positive airway pressure (CPAP) may be recommended. CPAP is noninvasive and consists of a mask connected to an air pump that is worn during sleep. This device delivers positive air pressure that holds the airway open. Many patients discontinue use of CPAP because of a sensation of claustrophobia, discomfort exhaling against air inflow, or dryness and skin irritation. If conservative treatment methods fail, surgery that removes soft tissue at the back of the mouth may be an option. This surgery is not without risks, and people with OSA need continued support (Forth, 1998).

Restless Leg Syndrome

Although restless leg syndrome is a common sleep disorder that affects millions, many healthcare workers are unaware of its existence. People with **restless leg syndrome** are unable to lie still and report experiencing unpleasant creeping, crawling, or tingling sensations in the legs. Usually, these sensations are in the calf, but they may occur anywhere from the ankle to the thigh. Patients describe an irresistible urge to move the legs when these sensations occur. Massaging the legs, walking, doing knee bends, and moving the legs can sometimes bring relief. Research continues concerning additional treatment options, but the following may prove effective:

* Eliminate use of caffeine, tobacco, and alcohol.
* Take a mild analgesic at bedtime provided it is compatible with the current medical regimen.

● Use antiembolism stockings at the onset of symptoms (Boucher, 1997)

The Restless Legs Foundation is a support group available for the millions of people with this disorder who suffer from chronic sleep loss.

Sleep Deprivation

Sleep deprivation refers to a decrease in the amount, consistency, or quality of sleep. It may result from decreased REM sleep or NREM sleep. Total sleep deprivation is rarely seen other than in experimental settings. There are many causes, and the manifestations progress from irritability and impaired mental abilities to a total disintegration of personality. In general, the effects of sleep deprivation become increasingly apparent after 30 hours of continual wakefulness. Partial sleep deprivation may result in loss of concentration, inattention, and impaired information processing and pose serious safety risks. *Excessive daytime sleepiness,* a form of partial sleep deprivation, impairs performance at times when individuals need to be alert. The strange environment of the hospital, physical discomfort and pain, the effects of medications, and the need for 24-hour nursing care may also contribute to sleep deprivation in hospitalized patients.

It is unclear whether irreversible damage to body tissue results from prolonged or chronic sleep deprivation. However, sleep deprivation clearly produces changes in physical and mental functioning, supporting the belief that sleep is essential for well-being.

Parasomnias

Parasomnias are patterns of waking behavior that appear during sleep. Common examples include **somnambulism** (sleepwalking); sleeptalking; nocturnal erections; bruxism (grinding of teeth during sleep); and **enuresis** (bedwetting during sleep). They are more commonly seen in children. Although parasomnias are commonly outgrown before adulthood, concern for safety and prevention of injury is paramount.

The Nursing Process

ASSESSING

Sleep History

Interview questions help identify the patient's sleep–wakefulness patterns, the effect of these patterns on everyday functioning, the patient's use of sleep aids, and the presence of sleep disturbances and contributing factors. The sleep history may be brief (four questions) if the patient's sleep is adequate and poses no problems, or it may be more detailed. When the patient's response to any of the interview questions indicates a potential problem, open-ended questions may be used to gather more data (see the accompanying Focused Assessment Guide).

If the patient is being admitted to a care facility, it is important to assess his or her usual times for retiring and waking, bedtime rituals, and preferences regarding sleep

environment so that these can be incorporated into the plan of care, if possible. The nurse's sensitivity to small matters can make the difference between a patient's good night's sleep and no sleep. The checklist in Applying Learning to Practice: Promoting Health encourages the caregiver to evaluate personal behaviors related to sleep and rest.

When a sleep disturbance is noted, the history should include the following:

● The nature of the problem
● Its cause
● The related signs and symptoms
● When it first began and how often it occurs
● How it affects everyday living
● The severity of the problem and whether it can be treated independently by nurses or needs to be referred to another professional
● How the patient is coping with the problem and the success of any treatments attempted

The patient may request the assistance of a bed partner to aid in data collection and provide more accurate information regarding his or her sleep patterns. The patient's record may also contain pertinent information (eg, a history of illnesses that influence sleep).

Sample records of a sleep history in a comprehensive nursing assessment are as follows:

> Reports needs 8 to 9 hours of sleep to feel his best and usually gets this without problem. Generally retires at 11:30 PM and rises at 7:30 AM. No special sleep rituals.
> Mother reports toddler has erratic sleep patterns. May nap at any time in the afternoon or evening and sleep from 1 to 3 hours. Depending on nap, goes to bed anywhere from 7 to 11 PM and sleeps about 11 to 13 hours. Resists falling asleep and wants "water, story, snack, kisses, etc." Parents' lifestyle is constantly changing—little consistency for the child regarding sleep expectations.

Sleep Diary

A sleep diary or log provides more specific data on the patient's sleep–wakefulness patterns over a long period. The diary generally is kept for 14 days and includes the following:

1. A graph of the total number of hours of sleep per day. Depending on the nature of the problem, graphs may be made of the number of undisturbed hours of sleep, number of awakenings, and so forth.
2. A daily record of the following:
   ● Time patient decided to retire
   ● Time patient actually tries to fall asleep
   ● Approximate time patient falls asleep
   ● Time of any awakenings during the night and when sleep was resumed
   ● Time of awakening in the morning
   ● Presence of any stressors patient believes are affecting his or her sleep

FOCUSED ASSESSMENT GUIDE

Rest and Sleep

Factors to Assess	Questions and Approaches
Usual sleep–wakefulness pattern: Recent changes	
• Usual sleeping and waking times	How many hours of sleep do you usually get in a day?
	Do you wake up earlier in the morning than you would like and find it difficult to fall back asleep?
	Have there been any recent changes in your usual sleep–wake patterns? If yes, describe them and tell me if they are causing any problems for you.
	Do you usually go to bed and wake up about the same time each day?
• Number of hours of undisturbed sleep	How have you been sleeping?
	Do you have any difficulty falling asleep?
	Do you wake up frequently during the night?
	Do you dream at night?
	Are your dreams frightening?
• Quality of sleep	How much sleep do you think you need to feel rested?
• Number and duration of naps	Do you take naps throughout the day?
Effect of sleep pattern on everyday functioning	In what way does the sleep you get each day affect your everyday living?
	Has this sleep disturbance caused any change in your sex life?
• Energy level (ability to perform activities of daily living)	Do you feel rested and ready to start the day when you wake up?
	Are there times during the day or certain activities when you feel especially tired?
	What happens when you don't get enough sleep?
	Are you having difficulty concentrating?
Sleep aids	
• Means of relaxing before bedtime	What do you do to relax before you get ready for bed?
• Bedtime rituals	Describe what you usually do to help yourself fall asleep.
• Sleep environment	Tell me how you like your room (lights, noises, ventilation, position of door, temperature) and bed (mattress, pillows, blankets) when you are sleeping.
• Pharmacologic aids	Do you take any medications to help you sleep?
	Are you taking any medicine at all?
Sleep disturbances and contributing factors	
• Nature of the sleep disturbance	Tell me about your sleep problem.
• Onset of disturbance	How often does it occur?
• Causes (physical, psychosocial, medicine related)	Are you doing anything differently now that might be causing the problem?
• Severity	Do you wake up gasping for air?
• Symptoms	Do you snore?
	Do you recall changing your position frequently during the night?
• Interventions attempted and results	What have you been doing to deal with the problem?

APPLYING LEARNING TO PRACTICE

Promoting Health

Rest and Sleep

Use the assessment checklist to determine how well you are meeting needs for rest and sleep. Then develop a prescription for self-care by choosing appropriate behaviors from the list of suggestions.

Assessment Checklist

almost always | sometimes | almost never

☐ ☐ ☐ 1. I feel rested and refreshed when I get up in the morning.

☐ ☐ ☐ 2. I have energy to carry out normal activities of daily living.

☐ ☐ ☐ 3. I understand the normal changes in sleep and rest requirements and patterns that occur with aging.

☐ ☐ ☐ 4. I set aside time for quiet recreation and restful activities each day.

Self-Care Behaviors

1. Follow a regular routine for bedtime and morning awakening.
2. Accept individual differences in need for sleep.
3. Use relaxation exercises to relax before bedtime, especially if feeling stressed.
4. Avoid caffeine, smoking, and alcohol before bedtime.
5. Adjust bedcoverings, room temperature, and lighting to your preferences.
6. Eat a small carbohydrate snack before going to bed.
7. Be aware of the potential dangers of sleeping pills.
8. Use some part of each day for quiet, enjoyable activities, such as crafts, hobbies, reading, watching television, listening to music, visiting with friends.

- A record of any food, drink, or medication patient believes has positively or negatively influenced his or her sleep (include time of ingestion)
- Record of physical activities—type, duration, and time
- Record of mental activities—type, duration, and time
- Record of activities performed 2 to 3 hours before bedtime, bedtime rituals, changes in sleep environment
- Presence of any worries or anxieties patient believes are affecting his or her sleep

It is helpful if the patient has a bed partner who can assist with the diary. The patient needs to understand that the diary is simply a diagnostic tool. If keeping the diary causes too much stress for the patient and further interferes with his or her ability to sleep restfully, it should be discontinued. The sleep diary summarizes information regarding a person's sleep–wake pattern and may indicate activities and behaviors that affect the quality and quantity of sleep.

Physical Assessment

Physical findings in the physical assessment may either confirm that the patient is getting sufficient rest to provide energy for the day's activities or validate the existence of a sleep disturbance that is decreasing the quantity or quality of sleep. Key findings include diminished energy level (presence of physical weakness, fatigue, lethargy), facial characteristics (narrowing or glazing of eyes, swelling of eyelids, decreased animation), or behavioral characteristics (yawning, rubbing eyes, slow speech, slumped posture). Physical data suggestive of potential sleep problems (eg, obesity, enlarged neck, deviated nasal septum) may also be noted.

If the nurse or a bed partner is able to observe the patient sleeping, other sleep characteristics to assess include restlessness, sleep postures, and sleep activities such as snoring or leg jerking (nocturnal myoclonus).

Snoring

Snoring is caused by an obstruction to the air flow through the nose and mouth. Other than disturbing others in the same bedroom, snoring is not ordinarily a sleeping disorder. However, snoring accompanied by apnea can present a problem. When snoring changes from the characteristic sawing-wood sound to a more irregular silence followed by a snorting, this indicates obstructive apnea.

Nocturnal Myoclonus

Observed in 10% to 20% of chronic insomniacs, **nocturnal myoclonus** involves marked muscle contraction that results in the jerking of one or both legs during sleep. The jerking lasts about 28 seconds on the average, may arouse the sleeper, and contributes to insomnia.

DIAGNOSING

Sleep Pattern Disturbance as the Problem

When assessment data point to a sleep problem that is amenable to nursing therapy, it receives the label Sleep Pattern Disturbance and may then be further specified:

Insomnia: Difficulty Falling Asleep
Insomnia: Difficulty Remaining Asleep
Insomnia: Premature Awakening
Sleep Deprivation
Altered Sleep–Wake Patterns

Common etiologies for sleep pattern disturbances include the following:

- Physical discomfort or pain
- Emotional discomfort or pain caused by anxiety and stress
- Changes in bedtime rituals or sleep environment
- Disruption of circadian rhythm
- Exercise just before sleep
- Caffeine, nicotine, or alcohol after dinner
- Drug dependency and withdrawal
- Symptoms of physical illness

Sample nursing diagnoses in which the sleep disturbance is the primary problem are presented in the accompanying box.

Sleep Pattern Disturbance as the Etiology

Sleep pattern disturbances may affect many other areas of human functioning. In the nursing diagnoses that follow, the sleep pattern disturbance is the cause of another problem:

> Anxiety related to inability to fall asleep, inability to control behavior while asleep, sleep apnea—threat of death
>
> Activity Intolerance related to sleep deprivation
>
> Fatigue related to prolonged excessive role demands
>
> Ineffective Individual Coping related to insomnia: insufficient quantity and quality of sleep
>
> Fear related to narcoleptic patient's potential to harm self or others
>
> Impaired Gas Exchange related to sleep apnea (oxygen saturation of the blood)
>
> Risk for Injury related to somnambulism, narcolepsy, sleep apnea
>
> Knowledge Deficit (specify: eg, nonpharmacologic remedies for insomnia) related to misinformation, lack of interest in learning, cognitive limitation
>
> Self-Esteem Disturbance related to effects of sleep deprivation (eg, sleep apnea syndrome)
>
> Anxiety related to nocturnal enuresis
>
> Impaired Social Interaction related to excessive daytime sleeping, sleep deprivation
>
> Altered Thought Processes related to chronic insomnia, sleep deprivation

Important Distinctions

Because the *problem statement* of the nursing diagnosis identifies what is wrong with the patient and suggests the expected outcomes and the *etiology* of the problem directs nursing interventions, it is important for the nurse analyzing the assessment data to decide whether the sleep data indicate the problem, contribute to a different problem, or are signs or symptoms of the problem. Sleep data potentially fit in all three categories. For example, when altered sleep–wake patterns are assessed in a graduate nurse who is getting adjusted to a new full-time job, shift work, and increased independence, three different diagnoses might be written:

Sleep Pattern Disturbance: Altered Sleep–Wake Pattern (Insomnia) related to shift work and stress of new job as manifested by complaints of always feeling tired and not getting enough sleep. The altered sleep–wake pattern is the problem statement; priority nursing energies are directed to changing this pattern and to helping the patient achieve both the necessary quantity and quality of sleep.

Ineffective Individual Coping related to multiple stresses of new job and altered sleep–wake pattern (sleep deprivation) as manifested by statements such as, "I don't know how much longer I can do this," "I'm always tired, and all I want to do is sleep," "I'm so grouchy—people must hate me!" Here, the altered sleep–wake pattern is just one of the factors contributing to the patient's problem of ineffective coping; priority nursing energies are directed toward improving the patient's coping skills by teaching the patient how to increase the quantity and quality of sleep.

Ineffective Individual Coping related to multiple stressors and lack of distressing rituals as manifested by inability to fall asleep (altered sleep–wake pattern), excessive fatigue, and feelings that personality is changing. In this instance, the altered sleep–wake pattern is merely a symptom of the patient's actual problem—ineffective coping; it is expected that when the coping problem is resolved, the symptom will disappear.

None of the preceding diagnoses is more correct than the others. With each patient, the nurse must make a decision with each cluster of significant data and identify the key problem, contributing factors, and related signs and symptoms. The exact nature of the nursing diagnosis directs the nursing interventions.

PLANNING: EXPECTED OUTCOMES

Rest and sleep are essential components of well-being. Planning for patient care, especially in a healthcare facility, involves planning with the patient suitable measures to promote rest and sleep. Whenever nurses care for a patient, nursing measures support the following expected patient outcomes. The patient will achieve the following:

- Maintain a sleep–wake pattern that provides sufficient energy for the day's tasks
- Demonstrate self-care behaviors that provide a healthy balance between rest and activity
- Identify stress-relieving rituals that enable falling asleep more easily
- Demonstrate decreased signs of sleep deprivation
- Verbalize feeling less fatigued and more in control of life activities

IMPLEMENTING

Usually, sleep problems are not the primary reason for a patient's interaction with the healthcare system. Often, the

Nursing Diagnoses for Common Problems

Sleep

Problem	Related Factors	Sample Defining Characteristics
Sleep Pattern Disturbance: Difficulty Falling Asleep	Worries about family and lack of destressing rituals	• "At least four or five nights a week I lay in bed awake for 3 or 4 hours before I finally fall asleep. Sometimes it is 2 or 3 in the morning and I'm still awake worrying about the kids. I've tried getting up and reading or paying my bills, but even that doesn't make me sleepy." • Reports problem falling asleep for past 6 months; is widowed and very concerned about two teenage sons. Never sleeps until both sons are home. States she does nothing special to relax. Feels her worries are "her business"—no support person with whom she shares these.
Sleep Pattern Disturbance: Difficulty Remaining Asleep	Noise of hospital environment and need for periodic treatments	• Admitted to hospital 3/6/01; cholecystectomy 3/7/01 • "I don't think I've had one decent night's sleep since my surgery. I've been falling asleep about 9 PM and then someone wakes me up for my medicine. I just about get back to sleep and someone's putting the light on to poke at my dressing or to check this tube. I know I'm getting grouchy." • Orders include every-4-hour vital signs; nursing assessment of the incision, nasogastric tube, intravenous therapy; and medication for pain and for sleep.
Sleep Pattern Disturbance: Premature Awakening	Barbiturate dependency and lack of knowledge of nonpharmacologic aids for insomnia	• Patient has history of mild to moderate depression, related to loss of job and perceived role inadequacy, for the past 3 years; has been taking secobarbital (Seconal), a barbiturate hypnotic, 100 mg by mouth nightly for the past year and a half. • "I seem to be waking up earlier and earlier, can't fall back asleep, and I start each day feeling like I have a hangover." • "I'd like to get off these drugs, but I'm terrified that without them I won't sleep at all."
Sleep Pattern Disturbance: Excessive Daytime Sleeping	Effects of biologic aging (moderate increase in stage I and II sleep; slow-wave sleep, stages III and IV, decreases by 50% or more)	• Male patient aged 74, complains during his annual physical that he seems to be napping more during the day, yet when he tries to fall asleep at night he often cannot. • "I'm spending more time in bed, but I'm less rested. Worst of all is not knowing whether or not I'll be awake enough to drive my car or enjoy a good card game."
Sleep Pattern Disturbance: Altered Sleep–Wake Patterns	Frequent rotations of shift and overtime	• Graduate nurse, 24 years old, who has been working on a busy medical floor for 6 months; rotates 11–7 and 7–3 shifts; recently a problem with staffing has necessitated frequent rotations. Patient often volunteers (two or three times a week) for overtime. • "I don't know what is wrong with me. I'm so tired anymore and don't feel at all like myself. All I want to do when I'm off is to sleep—but often I can't fall asleep when I lay down. Please help!"

nurse's attitude communicated to the patient is key in the detection of a sleep problem. Patients who believe the nurse is generally concerned about their well-being are not reluctant to discuss their insomnia or their concern about a child who is a bedwetter. Fundamental to the success of any nursing measure to correct a sleep problem is the patient's belief that the nurse cares and will provide extra help to promote rest and sleep. The accompanying box lists a selection of standardized nursing interventions from the Nursing Interventions Classification (NIC) that aid in the promotion of sleep.

Preparing a Restful Environment

A comfortable bed helps promote rest and sleep. The bottom linen should be tight and clean. The upper linen, while secure, should allow freedom of movement and should not exert pressure, especially over the legs and feet. Good alignment of the body is conducive to relaxation. For patients who must assume unusual positions because of their illness, ingenuity and skill are necessary to minimize muscle strain and discomfort. For example, patients who must remain in the orthopneic position to aid breathing should be well supported in a manner that relieves muscle strain.

A quiet and darkened room with privacy is relaxing for nearly everyone. In a strange environment, unfamiliar noises, such as people walking by or entering and leaving the room and the sounds of elevator doors, bring complaints from most hospitalized patients. Although some of these sound sources are difficult for the nurse to control, every effort should be made to reduce disturbances and to promote relaxation and sleep.

The temperature of the room, the amount of ventilation, and the amount of bed covering are matters of individual choice. The patient's wishes should be met when at all possible. Many older patients are unable to sleep if they feel cold. Thermal blankets or comforters, insulated bed socks, cotton flannel sheets, leg warmers, long underwear, and a stockinette cap help patients stay warm and promote comfort and sleep. Refer to the accompanying box for additional suggestions for older adults.

Using the Nursing Interventions Classification (NIC)

Sleep Enhancement

- Approximate patient's regular sleep–wake cycle in planning care.
- Determine the effects of the patient's medications on sleep pattern.
- Adjust environment (eg, light, noise, temperature, mattress, and bed) to promote sleep.
- Encourage patient to establish a bedtime routine to facilitate transition from wakefulness to sleep.
- Facilitate maintenance of patient's usual bedtime routines, presleep cues/props, and familiar objects (eg, for children, a favorite blanket/toy, rocking, pacifier, or story; for adults, a book to read, etc.) as appropriate.
- Instruct patient to avoid bedtime foods and beverages that interfere with sleep.
- Instruct patient how to perform autogenic muscle relaxation or other nonpharmacologic forms of sleep inducement.
- Initiate/implement comfort measures of massage, positioning, and affective touch.
- Discuss with patient and family comfort measures, sleep-promoting techniques, and lifestyle changes that can contribute to optimal sleep.

McClosky, J., & Bulechek, G. (2000). *Nursing interventions classification (NIC)* (3rd ed.) (p. 602). St. Louis: C. V. Mosby. A full listing of nursing activities for each nursing intervention can be found in this book.

Focus on the Older Adult
Promoting Sleep

Nonpharmacologic measures to promote improved sleep in older patients include the following:

- Establish a daily schedule for waking and sleeping.
- Exercise daily, preferably not near bedtime.
- Avoid napping during the day.
- Avoid food, beverages, or OTC medications that contain caffeine in the evening.
- Consume alcohol only in small amounts and not before bedtime.
- Refrain from cigarette smoking in the evening.
- Eat a light meal for dinner.
- Eat a light carbohydrate snack at bedtime if hungry.
- Use relaxation methods at bedtime (eg, deep breathing, relaxation exercises, soothing music, massage, reading).
- Maintain comfortable temperature and reduced noise level in sleeping area.
- Keep to usual waking time every day even if previous night's bedtime was later than usual or sleep was restless.
- Get out of bed if unable to fall asleep within 30 minutes and go into another room. Engage in a nonstimulating activity, such as reading and return to bed when drowsy.
- Use bed only for sleeping or sexual activity.

Promoting Bedtime Rituals

Most people have bedtime rituals to help them relax and promote sleep. Reading, listening to the radio, watching television, talking to a family member, and praying are common before-sleep activities. Children may take a favorite doll, stuffed toy, or blanket to bed; listen to a bedtime story; kiss everyone good night; and say prayers before bed. Readiness for sleep follows a personal hygiene routine for many people, such as brushing teeth, washing hands and face, voiding, or taking a bath or shower. Snacks are important elements in the bedtime rituals of many children and adults. Although it is true that eating the wrong foods may produce a bad night's sleep, going to bed hungry may also interfere with sleep.

The nurse should be alert to the patient's bedtime rituals and make every effort to observe them as far as possible to promote relaxation and sleep. These rituals should appear in the patient's plan of care so that all health personnel can observe them.

Offering Appropriate Bedtime Snacks and Beverages

Because carbohydrates seem to help promote sleep, there currently appears to be justification for offering a snack or beverage high in carbohydrates before bedtime, such as toast, a small bagel, crackers, or a glass of fruit juice, if this is allowed in the patient's regimen. An alcoholic beverage helps to promote sleep for some people, but generally alcohol after dinner should be avoided because it may interrupt the normal sleep cycle and interfere with deep sleep. For most patients, beverages containing caffeine should be avoided for at least 4 to 5 hours before bedtime. It is a good idea for the patient to take fluids during the day and to avoid excessive fluid intake before bedtime to help prevent having to use the bathroom during the night.

Promoting Relaxation

One can relax without sleeping, but sleep rarely occurs until one is relaxed. Stress and anxiety interfere with a person's ability to relax, rest, and sleep. Effective means for dealing with worries include dealing with problems as they arise; conditioning oneself to consider stressful issues only at certain times; teaching oneself that worrying never solves problems and is counterproductive; and giving the worries over to another (eg, a trusted family member, friend, caregiver, or God). The distraction and relaxation techniques described in Chapters 31 and 40 may be beneficial for a patient whose worries are contributing to a sleep disturbance. Backrubs, warm baths, and face washing if the patient is bedridden are typical nursing measures to help patients relax. The technique for back massage is described in Procedure 40-1 in Chapter 40.

Promoting Comfort

One of the greatest deterrents to rest and sleep is pain, and pain commonly occurs in illness. Depending on the cause and severity of the discomfort or pain, appropriate nursing measures include remaining with a lonely and frightened child or adult, using the simple strategy of caring presence and touch, offering a back massage, obtaining an extra blanket, or administering an analgesic. These and other nursing techniques to promote comfort are described in Chapter 40. However, a nurse must be sensitive to the patient's discomfort in order to recognize and relieve it.

Respecting Normal Sleep–Wake Patterns

Every effort should be made to allow the patient to experience his or her normal period of sleep. In many instances, it is not necessary to insist that all patients retire and awaken at specific times. For example, is there a good reason to wake a patient at 7 AM if the patient ordinarily sleeps until 9 AM? It is also recommended that a patient's normal napping habits be followed when possible. REM sleep is more common during morning naps, whereas NREM sleep is more common during naps later in the day. With this knowledge, the nurse can help the patient plan napping periods that best fit individual needs and that interfere least with nighttime sleeping.

Scheduling Nursing Care to Avoid Unnecessary Disturbances

Common patient complaints are that they are awakened to take sleeping pills and are aroused in the early morning to prepare for breakfast long before it is served. These common complaints should be considered when planning care that will help most to promote rest and sleep.

Every effort should be made to time care during periods when the patient is normally awake. When this cannot be done, it is preferable to avoid awakening the patient during REM sleep, when the rapid eye movements can be observed. Because a patient's need for sleep is important, nursing priorities should be examined. For example, the nurse should consider whether checking a vital sign or carrying out a particular nursing measure is more important than the patient's sleep (see Developing Critical Thinking Skills).

Using Medications to Produce Sleep

Medications for sleep are often ordered for patients. Sedative-hypnotics induce sleep; antianxiety drugs reduce anxiety and tension. The sleep produced by sedative-hypnotics is an unnatural sleep, however. All these drugs disturb either REM or NREM sleep to some degree. Although most sedative-hypnotics provide several nights of excellent sleep, the medication often loses its effect after 1 or 2 weeks. At this point, many people increase the dosage of the medication or complement the drug with alcohol. The combination of a sedative-hypnotic and an over-the-counter antihistamine (eg, Benadryl) may intensify depression of the central nervous system, leading to additional safety concerns (Winslow & Jacobsen, 1997).

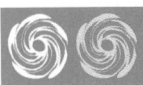 **Developing Critical Thinking Skills**

Situation

You have just arrived on the unit and checked your clinical assignment. You have two patients today and about 30 minutes before preconference. Your routine is to review their charts for pertinent information, go and introduce yourself to them, and take their morning vital signs before preconference. With 10 minutes to spare, you visit your second patient and find that he is sound asleep. Remembering that he had a fractured hip repaired 2 days ago and that the night nurse had stated in his note that the patient was restless and awake until 4:00 AM, you are reluctant to awaken him. On the other hand, at your midterm conference your instructor commented that you need to improve your organizational skills. If you don't have your vital signs recorded until after preconference, then breakfast arrives, doctors make rounds, and you're that much further behind in your morning care and documentation. When you look at the flow sheet at the foot of the bed, you note that the last set of vitals were taken at 12:00 midnight and were within normal limits. You're attempting to reconcile several things—the importance of these morning vital signs, the patient's need for sleep, and your need to accomplish your tasks on time and receive a good evaluation. What should you do?

1. **Identify Goal of Thinking**

   Determine whether it is more important to awaken your patient for morning vital signs or let him sleep at least until after your preconference.

2. **Assess Adequacy of Knowledge**

   Pertinent circumstances: Your patient had major surgery 2 days ago, did not have a restful night, but is sleeping peacefully now. You realize that his vital signs can be an important indicator of a complication. You also need to accomplish your tasks in a timely and organized manner.

   Prerequisite knowledge: To make your decision, you need knowledge about his postoperative condition, and assessment data that indicate he is recovering or developing a complication. You are aware that sleep is vital to promote tissue repair, physical recovery, and mental well-being. You also need to review the tasks that you need to accomplish this morning and decide how and if priorities could be shifted.

   Room for error/time constraints: Will a delay in taking vital signs cause injury to this patient? You are not planning to omit this task but just questioning whether to postpone it and allow the patient to have some additional sleep.

3. **Address Potential Problems**

   Waking your patient for vital signs may be disturbing for him and interfere with his need for rest. A decision to postpone morning vital signs might also cause several problems. If the patient has developed a complication such as an infection, his elevated temperature may go undetected for at least another hour. By the time you come out of preconference, the patient may be eating his breakfast, which further delays recording of vital signs. You perceive that you are already falling behind on your schedule and are really intent on completing your responsibilities on time today.

4. **Consult Helpful Resources**

   Before you make your decision, you should check the patient's flow sheet and note whether the previous set of vital signs were within normal limits. The primary nurse and your instructor may also help you sort through your priorities in this situation.

5. **Critique Judgment/Decision**

   You have two choices here. If you wake your patient up and take his vital signs, you are disturbing him when he is sleeping soundly, risking the fact that he may be angry with you but are on schedule for the day's activities. By postponing his vital signs at least until after postconference, you provide additional rest for the patient but know that you are already behind schedule and worry that your instructor will view you as disorganized. After reviewing your options and checking his chart again, you decide to allow him to sleep and plan to take them as soon as possible after your preconference. During preconference, when your instructor reviews your priorities for the day, she comments positively that you have individualized care based on your particular patient's needs at the moment. In your mind, you determine that the vital signs are your next priority and will take minimal time, and you should still be able to complete care and documentation in a competent manner and on time.

Because of its sedative effect, the antidepressant trazodone is often prescribed for elderly patients. The low incidence of cardiovascular and anticholinergic effects make this drug a safer alternative for elderly individuals with insomnia (Clark, Queener, & Karb, 1997). Vigorous nursing intervention is needed to prevent a patient from developing a pattern of drug dependency and alcohol abuse.

Nurses also need to be alert to the dangers of withdrawal symptoms that can accompany the abrupt cessation of barbiturate sedative-hypnotics. Progressive withdrawal symptoms include weakness, tremulousness, restlessness, insomnia, increased pulse and heart rates, anxiety, convulsions, psychosis, continued seizures, and death.

Medications used to induce sleep may produce daytime drowsiness and a morning hangover effect. Some people counteract this side effect by taking illicit drugs such as amphetamines, or "uppers." The antianxiety medications, once hoped to be the answer to the sleeping pill dilemma, are increasingly found to cause physical and psychological dependence.

Sleep medications are often ordered on a p.r.n. (as needed) basis. The nurse should administer these medications only when indicated and always with full knowledge of their limitations. Thorough patient teaching should accompany their use. Nurses should aid patients in developing other self-care strategies, including developing healthy sleep and lifestyle behaviors.

Teaching About Rest and Sleep

A well-informed person is better able to cope with distressing situations. Teaching patients and their families about the nature of rest and sleep and their importance to well-being is an important nursing function. Teaching should include aspects of normal variations in sleep patterns and common measures to promote relaxation and sleep. Also, the plan of care should be discussed with the patient for acceptability. If a sleep disorder becomes a problem and common nursing measures are inadequate, the nurse may need to recommend the services of health practitioners especially prepared to deal with them.

EVALUATING

The nurse evaluates the effectiveness of the plan of care to promote rest and sleep by checking whether the patient has met the individualized expected outcomes specified in the plan. Nursing care is considered effective if the patient is able to achieve the following:

- Verbalize feeling rested or having had a restful night's sleep
- Identify factors that interfere with or disrupt the normal sleep pattern
- Use techniques that effectively promote sleep and provide a restful environment
- Concentrate and function effectively during waking hours
- Eliminate behaviors related to sleep deprivation

See the accompanying boxes, Applying Learning to Practice and Nursing Plan of Care.

APPLYING LEARNING TO PRACTICE

PATIENT CARE STUDY

Mr. Bitner is an alert, widowed, 86-year-old African American man who was admitted to a nursing home 2 months ago. He is ambulatory and performs most of his self-care. His admitting medical diagnoses include diabetes mellitus and hypertension. He adds to this list "a touch of arthritis." His daughter complains to the charge nurse that her dad seems to be spending more and more time during the day napping and that he says he does not sleep well at night. A comprehensive sleep assessment of Mr. Bitner after his daughter's expression of concern reveals the following data.

Sleep–Wakefulness Pattern
- Patient goes to bed between 8 and 9 PM and gets out of bed between 7 and 8 AM because the staff are getting his roommate out of bed at this time. He states he never falls asleep before midnight because he always watched the late news at home. He usually wakes twice during the night to void and often cannot go back to sleep.
- During the day, patient is frequently observed dozing in his chair. If not discouraged, he returns to his room midmorning and afternoon for a 1-hour nap.

Effect of Sleep Pattern on Everyday Living
- Patient states: "I'm always tired. I don't seem to have much energy anymore."

- Patient has not socialized yet with other residents and, without strong encouragement, does not participate in group activities.
- From his point of view, life holds little reason for him to be awake. "I worked for the railroad for almost 50 years and I never overslept once."

Sleep Aids
- Patient denies ever using medication to fall asleep. States he often relaxed at home in the evening with a couple of beers.
- Patient likes a dim light on during the night so that he can find the bathroom easily and likes his bedroom door ajar.
- Patient sleeps with two blankets and is often still cold.

Sleep Disturbances and Contributing Factors
- Patient states: "Ever since my wife died, I'm just not getting enough sleep, and since I came here it's worse. I don't know why I don't fall asleep when I go to bed or why I wake up so much. It sure makes the nights long."
- Patient has no regular periods of exercise and drinks black coffee with every meal and one or two diet colas in the evening.

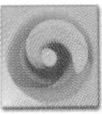

NURSING PLAN OF CARE
for Mr. Bitner

Nursing Diagnosis	Sleep Pattern Disturbance: Difficulty Falling Asleep and Remaining Asleep related to new sleep environment and schedule, evening caffeine intake, and insufficient meaningful daytime activity
Expected Outcome	By the next monthly assessment, 1/20/01, the patient will: • Retire after viewing the 11 PM news in the TV room with Mr. Sparter

Nursing Interventions	Rationale	Evaluative Statement
Assess advisability of reestablishing Mr. Bitner's usual retiring pattern of going to bed after the 11 PM news. Assess how patient spends the time from the evening meal to 11 PM—explore relaxing alternatives with him. Investigate possibility that he and Mr. Sparter might become social partners.	Strengthens the natural rhythm of his sleep–wake cycle. Elimination of evening naps will facilitate his falling asleep more easily.	1/18/01 Goal met. Patient does not go to bed until after the news and has been observed talking with Mr. Sparter. *Recommendation:* Continue to develop evening activities with him—he finds that the time after supper "drags." *M. LeBon, RN*

Expected Outcome	By the next monthly assessment, 1/20/01, the patient will: • Report that he falls asleep within 1 hour of getting into bed

Nursing Interventions	Rationale	Evaluative Statement
Continue to assess how long it takes patient to fall asleep after getting into bed. Explore with patient means to relax before falling asleep—deep breathing, imagery, prayer. Teach the importance of using the bed only as a place to sleep. Advise patient when he cannot sleep to get out of bed and to go to another room where he can perform some monotonous activity (watching television, listening to radio).	In elderly patients, stage I time is increased. Activities that calm and relax the person prepare the body for sleep. This maintains the bed as a powerful stimulus for sleep and helps to prevent "conditioned" insomnia ("Well, here I am in bed now and I know sleep won't come").	1/18/01 Goal partially met. Three or four nights a week, he falls asleep within 30 minutes of going to bed. States he really misses comfort of his wife. *Revision:* Investigate patient's sense of loss and need for touch. May be a good candidate for pet therapy program. *M. LeBon, RN*

Expected Outcome	By the next monthly assessment, 1/20/01, the patient will: • Decrease nighttime awakenings to one, after which he returns to a sound sleep

Nursing Interventions	Rationale	Evaluative Statement
Assess and manipulate factors that contribute to nighttime awakenings: • Need to void (time of day diuretic is taken, amounts of fluid intake in the evening) • Roommate's wakefulness, snoring, or need for care • Uncomfortableness in strange environment • Comfort (eg, temperature)	Individualizing the patient's bedtime environment and meeting comfort needs (warmth, soft light, and so forth) promote sleep onset and maintenance.	1/18/01 Goal partially met. Nighttime awakenings vary from none to three nightly. See previous revision. *M. LeBon, RN*

(continued)

NURSING PLAN OF CARE (Continued)
for Mr. Bitner

Nursing Interventions	Rationale	Evaluative Statement
Teach patient how, on awakening, to concentrate on breathing until he falls back to sleep.	This uses the power of positive thinking to facilitate return to sleep.	

Expected Outcome   By the next monthly assessment, 1/20/01, the patient will:
- Attend the center's exercise sessions Monday through Friday at 10 AM

Nursing Interventions	Rationale	Evaluative Statement
Assess whether patient understands the relation between daily exercise and his ability to sleep.	Regular exercise throughout the day is known to increase physical fatigue and to promote sleep. Exercise or stimulating activities immediately before retiring interfere with sleep's onset.	1/20/01 Goal met. Patient has become an enthusiastic participant in exercise sessions—attends daily.
Determine how his exercise needs can best be met (ie, through a group program or an individualized program of walking, or other program)	Exercise program must be individualized based on physical state and interests of patient.	*M. LeBon, RN*
Use positive verbal reinforcement to communicate to patient that someone cares that he is using positive means to remedy his sleep disturbance and increase his well-being.	Activity provides the opportunity for socialization and improvement of a self-image.	
Encourage patient's daughter to go for walks with him when she visits and to question him about his exercise program.	Communications and interaction with family members helps the elderly patient to maintain self-esteem and to feel valuable and loved.	

Expected Outcome   By the next monthly assessment, 1/20/01, the patient will:
- Substitute caffeine-free beverages for coffee and cola at supper and evening snack

Nursing Interventions	Rationale	Evaluative Statement
Assess patient's willingness to substitute caffeine-free beverages for coffee and cola.	Caffeine is a stimulant that can cause difficulty sleeping.	1/20/01 Goal met. Patient now drinks decaffeinated coffee with meals and milk in the evening. Dislikes caffeine-free sodas.
Consult with dietary department and his daughter about options. Experiment with options until his preferences are determined.	Caffeine-free versions of beverages are often available and can be used based on patient acceptance.	*M. LeBon, RN*
Gradually reduce his caffeine intake, especially from evening meal onward. Offer a carbohydrate evening snack.	Carbohydrate snack appears to promote sleep.	

(continued)

NURSING PLAN OF CARE (Continued)
for Mr. Bitner

Sample Documentation

12/20/01   Nursing

Family conference to discuss Mr. Bitner's sleep disturbance—initiated by daughter's concern. Present were Mr. Bitner and his daughter (A. Jelner), K. Behner (social worker), W. Quing (activity director), and M. LeBon (primary nurse). Primary nurse presented findings from comprehensive sleep assessment: Nursing diagnosis: Sleep Pattern Disturbance: Difficulty falling asleep and remaining asleep related to new sleep environment and schedule, evening caffeine intake, and insufficient meaningful daytime activity. Discussion centered on strategies to help Mr. Bitner develop interests in the center, including possibilities for increased physical exercise; decrease his evening caffeine intake (daughter to bring noncaffeine colas); and reestablish usual retiring and waking times. See plan of care. Patient's progress will be evaluated at next monthly assessment, 1/20/01.

M. LeBon, RN

Learning Outcomes

After completing this chapter, the learner should be able to accomplish the following:

1. Define the key terms used in this chapter.
circadian rhythm	rapid eye movement
delta sleep	sleep
dyssomnias	rest
enuresis	restless leg syndrome
insomnia	sleep
narcolepsy	sleep apnea
nocturnal myoclonus	sleep cycle
non–rapid eye movement	sleep deprivation
sleep	somnambulism
parasomnias	
2. Describe the functions and physiology of sleep.
3. Identify variables that influence rest and sleep.
4. Describe implications for nursing for age-related differences in the sleep cycle.
5. Perform a comprehensive sleep assessment using appropriate interview questions, a sleep diary when indicated, and physical assessment skills.
6. Describe common sleep disorders, noting key assessment criteria.
7. Develop nursing diagnoses that correctly identify sleep problems that may be treated through independent nursing interventions.
8. Describe nursing strategies to promote rest and sleep and identify their rationale.
9. Plan, implement, and evaluate nursing care related to select nursing diagnoses involving sleep problems.

Critical Thinking Exercises

1. Interview three adults of varying ages (young, middle, and elderly) about their sleep and rest patterns, using the focused assessment guide in this chapter. Explore the special problems experienced by each of the adults, the efficacy of self-help measures they are using to cope, and helpful nursing interventions.
2. Interview three practicing nurses who are recent graduates, using the focused assessment guide in the text. Ask them if they are getting adequate rest; what factors are compromising their rest (eg, working double or rotating shifts); how any lack of rest is affecting their practice; and what self-help measures are indicated. Discuss with your classmates the situation of practicing nurses with sleep alterations, the factors that place nurses at risk for sleep alterations, and what students can learn to lower their risk.

Study Questions

1. A patient's body temperature is 37.2°C (99°F) in the late afternoon. This is most likely
   a. a sign of an infection
   b. normal circadian rhythm
   c. hyperpyrexia
   d. due to a warm environment
2. Muscle tone is recorded by the
   a. electroencephalograph (EEG)

b. electrocardiogram (ECG)

c. electrooculogram (EOG)

d. electromyograph (EMG)

3. The nurse observes some involuntary muscle jerking in her sleeping patient. The patient is most likely in
   a. stage I NREM sleep
   b. stage II NREM sleep
   c. stage IV NREM sleep
   d. REM sleep

4. The nurse observes a slight increase in her patient's vital signs when she assesses them while the patient is sleeping during the night. According to his stage of sleep, the nurse expects that
   a. he is aware of his surroundings at this point
   b. he is in delta sleep at this time
   c. it would be most difficult to awaken him at this time
   d. this is most likely an NREM stage

5. How many cycles of sleep does a person typically go through each night?
   a. 2
   b. 4 or 5
   c. 10
   d. 20 to 25

6. While discussing factors that induce sleep with an older patient, the nurse teaches her that
   a. a cup of regular tea may induce sleep
   b. large quantities of alcohol promote a deep sleep
   c. the amount of REM sleep decreases with age
   d. physical activity decreases REM and NREM sleep

7. A patient falls asleep in the middle of a conversation. This disorder is called
   a. hypersomnia
   b. narcolepsy
   c. somnambulism
   d. sleep apnea

8. A sleep diary is a diagnostic tool that
   a. is generally kept for 1 week
   b. includes a record of daily physical activity
   c. includes a record of body temperature taken each evening
   d. reports only subjective information about sleep activities

9. To help Mr. Yang get to sleep, the nurse suggests that he
   a. follow his usual bedtime routine if possible

b. drink two or three glasses of water at bedtime

c. have a large snack at bedtime

d. take a sedative-hypnotic every night at bedtime

10. The most common complaint of patients visiting sleep disorder clinics is
    a. hypersomnia
    b. narcolepsy
    c. chronic insomnia
    d. enuresis

11. A prolonged pattern of REM deprivation may result in
    a. symptoms of psychosis
    b. increased episodes of dreaming
    c. decreased sensitivity to pain
    d. increased mental alertness

12. Active dreaming occurs during
    a. stage II NREM
    b. stage III NREM
    c. stage IV NREM
    d. REM sleep

13. Illness is a stressor and can influence sleep during various stages. An example is that
    a. asthma attacks appear to occur less frequently during stage IV NREM sleep
    b. a person with heart disease is more likely to have chest pain during NREM sleep
    c. an epileptic patient is more likely to have seizures during REM sleep
    d. an increase in gastric secretion in a person with an ulcer will most likely occur during NREM sleep

14. Caffeine is a known stimulant, and its intake should be
    a. avoided at least 30 minutes before bedtime
    b. combined with milk to counteract its effect
    c. avoided at least 4 to 5 hours before bedtime
    d. encouraged during waking hours to counteract effects of sleeplessness

15. Medications that induce sleep (sedative-hypnotics) may disturb REM or NREM sleep. The nurse should be aware that
    a. they should be taken with alcohol for increased effect
    b. these medications usually become ineffective after several weeks
    c. they can usually be given at intervals during the night
    d. they should be combined with daytime use of amphetamines to counteract any hangover effect

---

Answers With Rationale

1. The correct response is *b*. A slight increase in body temperature in the late afternoon is a normal circadian rhythm. This slight variation from normal does not necessarily mean an infection is present, nor is it hyperpyrexia (high fever). A warm environment might possibly cause an elevation in body temperature, but the most likely cause is normal circadian rhythm.

2. The correct response is *d*. An EMG measures muscle tone, whereas an EEG records electrical currents from the brain. An EOG is a recording of eye movements, and an ECG records cardiac activity.

3. The correct response is *a*. Involuntary muscle jerking occurs in stage I NREM sleep. In the other stages, the muscles proceed from a relaxed state to large muscle immobility.

4. The correct response is *c*. During REM sleep, it is difficult to arouse a person, and the vital signs increase. Delta sleep is NREM stage III and IV sleep.

5. The correct response is *b*. A person goes through probably four or five cycles of sleep each night, with each cycle lasting 90 to 100 minutes.

6. The correct response is *c*. Regular tea has caffeine and increases alertness, and large quantities of alcohol limit REM and delta sleep. Physical activity increases both REM and NREM sleep.

7. The correct response is *b*. Narcolepsy is an uncontrollable desire to sleep. Hypersomnia refers to excessive sleep, somnambulism is sleepwalking, and sleep apnea is a period where breathing ceases between snoring.

8. The correct response is *b*. A sleep diary includes activities during the day because they have an effect on sleep, is usually kept for at least 14 days, and is more helpful if objective comments from a bed partner are included. A record of body temperature is insignificant.

9. The correct response is *a*. Drinking two or three glasses of water at bedtime will probably awaken the patient during the night to void. A large snack may be uncomfortable right before bedtime, and taking a sedative-hypnotic every night disturbs REM and NREM sleep. The sedative also loses its effectiveness shortly.

10. The correct response is *c*. Chronic insomnia is the most common reason that people visit a sleep disorder clinic.

11. The correct response is *a*. Prolonged episodes of REM deprivation may cause symptoms of psychosis. REM deprivation results in an absence of episodes of dreaming and sensitivity to pain increases, and the person is less mentally alert.

12. The correct response is *d*. Active dreaming occurs during REM sleep.

13. The correct response is *a*. Chest pain occurs more frequently during REM sleep. Epileptic seizures occur more frequently during NREM sleep, and gastric secretions increase during REM sleep.

14. The correct response is *c*. Caffeine should be avoided at least 4 to 5 hours before bedtime. Milk does not counteract its effect, and caffeine use is never recommended, even during waking hours.

15. The correct response is *b*. Sedative-hypnotics should never be taken with alcohol because alcohol potentiates their effect. They are usually ordered only at bedtime and may have one repeat order if the patient cannot fall asleep. However, they are not given at intervals during the night. Amphetamine use is never recommended.

Bibliography

Beck-Little, R., & Weinrich, S. (1998). Assessment and management of sleep disorders in the elderly. *Journal of Gerontological Nursing, 24*(4), 21–29.

Boucher, M. (1997). Restless legs syndrome. *Home Healthcare Nurse, 15*(8), 551–556.

Clark, J., Queener, S., & Karb, V. (1997). *Pharmacologic basis of nursing practice* (5th ed.). St. Louis: C. V. Mosby.

Cowley, G. (1996, March 11). Timing is everything. *Newsweek*, 68.

Eisenhauer, L., Nichols, L., Spencer, R., & Bergan, F. (1998). *Clinical pharmacology & nursing management* (5th ed.). Philadelphia: Lippincott Williams & Wilkins.

Eliopoulos, C. (1997). *Gerontological nursing* (4th ed.). Philadelphia: Lippincott Williams & Wilkins.

Forth, R. (1998). Common questions about obstructive sleep apnea. *American Journal of Nursing, 98*(2), 60–64.

Johnson, J. (1996). Sleep problems and self-care in very old rural women: Nursing implications. *Geriatric Nursing, 17*(2), 72–74.

King, A., Oman, R., et al. (1997). Moderate-intensity exercise and self-rated quality sleep in older sleep: A randomized controlled trial. *Journal of the American Medical Association, 277*(1), 32.

McCloskey, J., & Bulechek, J. (1996). *Nursing interventions classification (NIC)* (2nd ed.). St. Louis: C. V. Mosby.

McKenry, L., & Salerno, E. (1998). *Pharmacology in Nursing* (20th ed.). St. Louis: C. V. Mosby.

NHTSA & NCSDR Program to Combat Drowsy Driving (1997). *Report to the House and Senate Appropriations Committees describing collaboration between National Highway Traffic Safety Administration and National Center on Sleep Disorders research.* National Heart, Lung, and Blood Institute.

North American Nursing Diagnosis Association. (1999). *NANDA nursing diagnoses: Definition & classifications, 1999–2000.* Philadelphia: Author.

Phipps, W., Sands, J., & Marek, J. (1999). *Medical-surgical nursing: Concepts & clinical practice* (6th ed.). St. Louis: C. V. Mosby.

Pillitteri, A. (1999). *Maternal & child health nursing* (3rd ed.). Philadelphia: Lippincott Williams & Wilkins.

Porth, C. (1998). *Pathophysiology: Concepts of altered health states* (5th ed.). Philadelphia: Lippincott Williams & Wilkins.

Schnelle, J., Alessi, C., Al-Samarrai, N., Fricker, R., & Ouslander, J. (1999). The nursing home at night: Effects of an intervention on noise, light, and sleep. *Journal of the American Geriatrics Society, 47*(4), 430–438.

Tabloski, P., Cooke, K., & Thoman, E. (1998). A procedure for withdrawal of sleep medication in elderly women who have been long-term users. *Journal of Gerontological Nursing, 24*(9), 20–28.

Thorpy, M. (1994). Classification of sleep disorders. In Kryger, M., Roth, T., & Dement, W. (Eds.). *Principles and practice of sleep medicine* (pp. 426–436). Philadelphia: W. B. Saunders.

Williams, P., et al. (1999). Fatigue in mothers of infants discharged to the home on apnea monitors. *Applied Nursing Research, 12*(2), 69–77.

Winslow, E., & Jacobsen, A. (1997). Nondrug therapies help patients with insomnia. *American Journal of Nursing, 97*(6), 23.

Wong, D. (1997). *Essentials of pediatric nursing* (5th ed.). St. Louis: C. V. Mosby.

Chapter 40
Comfort

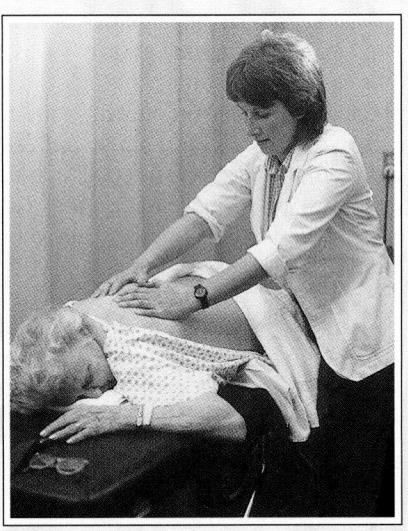

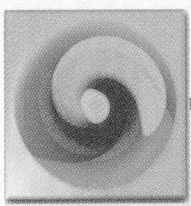

**Thinking Critically About
Nursing's Blended Skills**

Before reading this chapter, think about the types of skills you will need to meet the comfort needs of those entrusted to your care.

- For years, many routine invasive procedures in the neonatal intensive care unit were performed without anesthesia because no one really knew how much pain newborns experienced, and the newborns were not able to speak for themselves. Although analgesics are now routinely used, many clinicians continue to have unanswered questions about the comfort needs of newborns. You are meeting with a group of nurses and medical residents to research the topic and the adequacy of the care measures.

- A woman with chronic low back pain asks you what nonpharmacologic pain management modalities she can try.

- Billy is a 6-year-old patient with leukemia who has just had a bone marrow transplantation. He cries frequently and begs you to make him feel better. His parents are quick to tell you when they think he is in pain.

- Mr. Plachutta believes that he is experiencing terrible cancer pain because of sins in his past life. When you suggest trying different measures to alleviate his pain, he rejects your efforts and tells you he can "bear the pain."

- A physician colleague recommends increasing a patient's morphine to lethal doses saying, "No one should have to suffer like this."

What cognitive, technical, interpersonal, and ethical/legal skills do you think you will need to meet the needs of the patients described above?

person in pain often experiences it as an all-consuming reality and wants only one intervention—pain relief. If pain relief were as simple as rubbing a back or administering a prescribed analgesic, nursing's task would be easy. However, no two people experience pain exactly the same way. Differences in individual pain perception and response to pain, as well as the multiple and diverse causes of pain, require highly specialized abilities of the nurse seeking to promote comfort and relieve pain. The most essential of these are the nurse's belief that the patient's pain is real, willingness to become involved in the patient's pain experience, and competence in developing effective pain management regimens. Although pain is often an all-consuming priority for patients, it is frequently a low priority for nurses because it is intangible. Unfortunately, it is easier to ignore a patient's poorly communicated pain than it is to ignore a dressing that needs to be changed, a patient who requires assistance with ambulation, or a prescribed medication. Nurses who somehow manage to practice nursing while remaining insensitive to the comfort needs of their patients do a grave disservice to these patients and to the nursing profession itself.

Nurses are not alone in undervaluing the need for pain management. Although pain is a common reason for seeing a physician and taking medication, medical science is still ill equipped to deal with its widespread occurrence. For patients with cancer, the chronic pain that often accompanies this disease significantly affects the quality of life. Results of one study indicated that 7 of 10 patients with severe pain associated with metastatic cancer would consider suicide if they were unable to obtain adequate pain relief (Strevy, 1998). Scientists and clinicians have united in their efforts to ensure that management of pain, in its many facets, receives a high priority in our healthcare system. New advances in understanding and treating pain have focused on the real possibility of controlling most human pain. The Joint Commission on Accreditation of Healthcare Organizations (JCAHO) supports the patient's right to pain management and recently published revised standards for assessment and management of pain in hospitals, ambulatory care settings, and home care settings (Acello, 2000; Pasero, Gordon, & McCaffery, 1999). The JCAHO recommendations include teaching all patients to use a pain-rating scale and determining a pain-rating goal with each patient. Also, according to the JCAHO guidelines, if a facility does not have the resources to treat a patient's pain adequately, the patient must be referred to a facility that does (Acello, 2000).

This chapter discusses the pain experience and factors that influence it. A detailed guide to assessing pain is presented, along with numerous examples of nursing diagnoses and specific nursing strategies for promoting comfort and assisting patients to achieve pain management goals. The guidelines for management of acute pain and cancer pain developed by the Agency for Health Care Policy and Research (AHCPR) are presented as standards for effective pain management by nurses (AHCPR, 1992, 1994). The concluding patient care study illustrates how, with knowl-

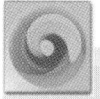

COGNITIVE SKILLS

- Knowledge about the pain experience and factors that influence pain experience (Mr. Plachutta's religious beliefs)
- Knowledge of effective pharmacologic and nonpharmacologic pain relief measures
- Knowledge of how to use the nursing process to identify patients at risk for pain and to implement a plan of care to prevent or resolve pain problems

TECHNICAL SKILLS

- Knowledge of how to use and document the equipment and protocols related to effective pain management protocols

INTERPERSONAL SKILLS

- Strong people skills to establish trusting relationships with each of the individuals described above, including the infants' parents
- Special interpersonal competence to relate to 6-year-old Billy, who most likely has limited

understanding of why he hurts, and to Mr. Plachutta, who may believe that he does not deserve compassionate care

- The ability to confront the physician who is contemplating euthanizing (lethal dose of morphine) your patient to prevent her suffering

ETHICAL/LEGAL SKILLS

- First and foremost, a strong sense of accountability for the health and well-being of these individuals; a commitment to getting them the help they need to achieve their comfort goals—within the scope of your nursing responsibilities and available resources
- A willingness to hold colleagues accountable for safe and good quality practice—especially in the nursery, where the infants cannot advocate for themselves
- A knowledge of the ethical and legal principles that guide decision making about pain management and appropriate treatment modalities

edge of and sensitivity to the patient's pain experience, nurses use specific nursing interventions to resolve pain problems successfully.

The Pain Experience

Pain is an elusive and complex phenomenon, and despite its universality, its exact nature remains a mystery. It is one of the human body's defense mechanisms that indicates the person is experiencing a problem. The definition of pain that is probably of greatest benefit to nurses and their patients is that offered by Margo McCaffery (1979): "Pain is whatever the experiencing person says it is, existing whenever he (or she) says it does" (p. 11). This definition rests on the belief that the only one who can be a real authority on whether, and how, an individual is experiencing pain is that individual.

Pain is present whenever a person says it is, even when no specific cause of the pain can be found. Health practitioners must rely on the patient's description of the pain because it is a subjective symptom that only the patient can identify and describe.

Categories of Pain

Pain may be classified according to source (nociceptive, neuropathic, and psychogenic), referral, or duration (acute and chronic).

Source of Pain

Pain that is usually acute and transmitted after normal processing of noxious stimuli is termed **nociceptive**. It may be categorized as cutaneous, deep somatic, or visceral in nature. **Cutaneous** (or superficial) **pain** usually involves the skin or subcutaneous tissue. A paper cut that produces sharp pain with a burning sensation is an example of cutaneous pain. Deep **somatic pain** is diffuse or scattered and originates in tendons, ligaments, bones, blood vessels, and nerves. Strong pressure on a bone or damage to tissue that occurs with a sprain causes deep somatic pain. **Visceral pain** is poorly localized and originates in body organs in the thorax, cranium, and abdomen. This pain occurs as organs stretch abnormally and become distended, ischemic, or inflamed. A reflex contraction or spasm of the abdominal wall, called *guarding*, may occur as a protective mechanism to prevent additional trauma to underlying structures.

Neuropathic pain results from an injury to or abnormal functioning of peripheral nerves or the central nervous system. The exact cause of neuropathic pain is unknown, and it can occur in many forms. Neuropathic pain can be of short duration or lingering and is often described as burning or stabbing (Rhiner & Kedziera, 1999). **Allodynia,** a characteristic feature of neuropathic pain, is pain that occurs after a normally weak or nonpainful stimuli, such as a light touch or a cold drink. Numerous pain syndromes have been identified that produce neuropathic pain. Several common examples are included in Table 40-1. All of

these pain syndromes are capable of causing severe pain. Because appropriate treatment of these syndromes is often delayed as a result of misdiagnosis, nursing can play an important role in their early detection.

Pain may originate from physical causes; that is, a physical cause for the pain can be identified. Pain may also have a psychogenic origin (**psychogenic pain**); that is, a physical cause for the pain cannot be identified. However, it has been observed that a pure origin is probably rare, and pain usually has both physical and psychogenic components. Furthermore, pain that results from a mental event can be just as intense as pain that results from a physical event.

Referred Pain

Referred pain is perceived in an area that is distant from its point of origin. Pain associated with a myocardial infarction, or heart attack, is frequently referred to the neck, shoulder, or arms (often the left arm). Referred pain is transmitted to a cutaneous (skin) site different from where it originated. This is possible because the pain can travel to other areas of the body innervated by the affected nerve root. Figure 40-1 illustrates cutaneous areas to which pain from various organs is usually referred.

Duration of Pain

Perhaps the most common distinction is between acute and chronic pain. **Acute pain** is generally rapid in onset, varies in intensity from mild to severe, and may last from a brief period up to any period less than 6 months. Acute pain is protective in nature; that is, it warns the individual of tissue damage or organic disease. After its underlying cause is resolved, acute pain disappears. Causes of acute pain include a pricked finger, sore throat, or surgery.

Chronic pain is pain that may be limited, intermittent, or persistent but that lasts for 6 months or longer and interferes with normal functioning. Commonly, people with chronic pain experience periods of **remission** (when the disease is present but the person does not experience symptoms) or **exacerbation** (the symptoms reappear). Pain associated with cancer or other progressive disorders is termed *chronic malignant pain*, and pain in people whose tissue injury is nonprogressive or healed is termed *chronic nonmalignant pain*. When pain is resistant to therapy and persists despite a variety of interventions, it is referred to as **intractable**. Patients have difficulty describing chronic pain because it may be poorly localized, and healthcare personnel have difficulty assessing it accurately because of the unique responses of individual patients to persistent pain. Most pain researchers agree that persistent or recurrent chronic pain is more common in people older than 60 years of age (Davis, 1997). According to Loeb (1999), about 45% to 80% of elderly patients residing in long-term care facilities have significant pain that negatively affects the quality of life. Unlike acute pain, chronic pain is often perceived as meaningless and may lead its host to withdrawal, depression, anger, frustration, and dependency. Management of patients with chronic pain can be adversely affected by the misconceptions and personal

Table 40-1
Common Pain Syndromes

Pain Syndrome	Description
Causalgia	Pain occurs in the area of a partially injured peripheral nerve (the most common lesions are of the brachial plexus or median or sciatic nerve). The pain is described as burning, severe, diffuse, and persistent and occurs most commonly on the palms of the hands, soles of the feet, and in the digits. Allodynia is a common feature.
Postherpetic neuralgia	Pain syndrome follows an acute central nervous system infection, such as herpes zoster (shingles). The herpes syndrome is characterized by a vesicular eruption and neuralgic pain, which is usually unilateral and encircles the body in bandlike clusters. The severity of the pain may be mild to severe. Intractable pain may persist for months to years.
Phantom limb pain	May occur in any person who has had a body part amputated either surgically or traumatically. Pain varies and may be a severe, burning, fiery sensation; crushing; cramping; a sense that the limb is edematous; or a sensation that the limb is being twisted and distorted. It may be triggered by the sensation of touching the stump, the occurrence of another illness, fatigue, atmospheric changes, and emotional stress.
Thalamic syndrome	Syndrome characterized by severe, spontaneous, and often continuous pain. The pain is often accompanied by a myriad of symptoms that may result from damage caused by a cerebrovascular accident or brain attack.
Trigeminal neuralgia	Paroxysms of lightening-like stabs of intense pain in the distribution of one or more divisions of the trigeminal nerve, the fifth cranial nerve. Pain is usually experienced in the mouth, gums, lips, nose, cheek, chin, and surface of the head and may be triggered by everyday activities like talking, eating, shaving, or brushing one's teeth.
Diabetic neuropathy	A common complication of long-term diabetes mellitus. Metabolic and vascular changes result in damage to peripheral and autonomic nerves. Sensory loss can result when peripheral nerves are involved and eventually leads to injury progressing to infection and gangrene. Symptoms include sensations of numbness, prickling, or tingling (paresthesias).

Adapted from Price, S., & Wilson, L. (1997). *Pathophysiology: Clinical concepts of disease processes.* St. Louis: C. V. Mosby.

biases of caregivers. Individuals with chronic pain may be viewed in general by healthcare personnel as hysterical personalities, malingerers, or hypochondriacs. On the other hand, nurses who have experienced chronic pain or struggled through the experience with a loved one have a special awareness of its debilitating, destructive nature. Nurses need an awareness of their own personal feelings toward pain and the factors that affect pain if they are to assess and manage their patient's pain creatively and effectively (refer to the accompanying box, Applying Learning to Practice: The Nurse as Role Model: Comfort).

The Pain Process

The mechanism or process of pain is believed to involve four stages: transduction, transmission, modulation, and perception of pain (Phipps, Sands, & Marek, 1999).

Transduction

The activation of pain receptors is referred to as *transduction*. It involves conversion of painful stimuli into electrical impulses that travel to the spinal cord at the dorsal horn. Additionally, when the threshold of perception for pain has been reached and when there is injured tissue, it

is believed that the injured tissue releases chemicals that excite or activate nerve endings. A damaged cell releases histamine, which excites nerve endings. Lactic acid accumulates in tissues injured by lack of blood supply and is believed to excite nerve endings and cause pain or to lower the threshold of nerve endings to other stimuli (eg, heat or pressure). Other substances are also released that stimulate nociceptors or pain receptors. These include bradykinin, prostaglandins, and substance P:

- *Bradykinin,* a powerful vasodilator that increases capillary permeability and constricts smooth muscle, plays an important role in the chemistry of pain at the site of an injury even before the pain message gets to the brain. It also triggers the release of histamine and, in combination with histamine, produces the redness, swelling, and pain typically observed when an inflammation is present.
- *Prostaglandins* are hormone-like substances that send additional pain stimuli to the central nervous system.
- *Substance P* is believed to act as a stimulant at pain receptor sites and may directly influence the inflammatory response in local tissues (Porth, 1998).

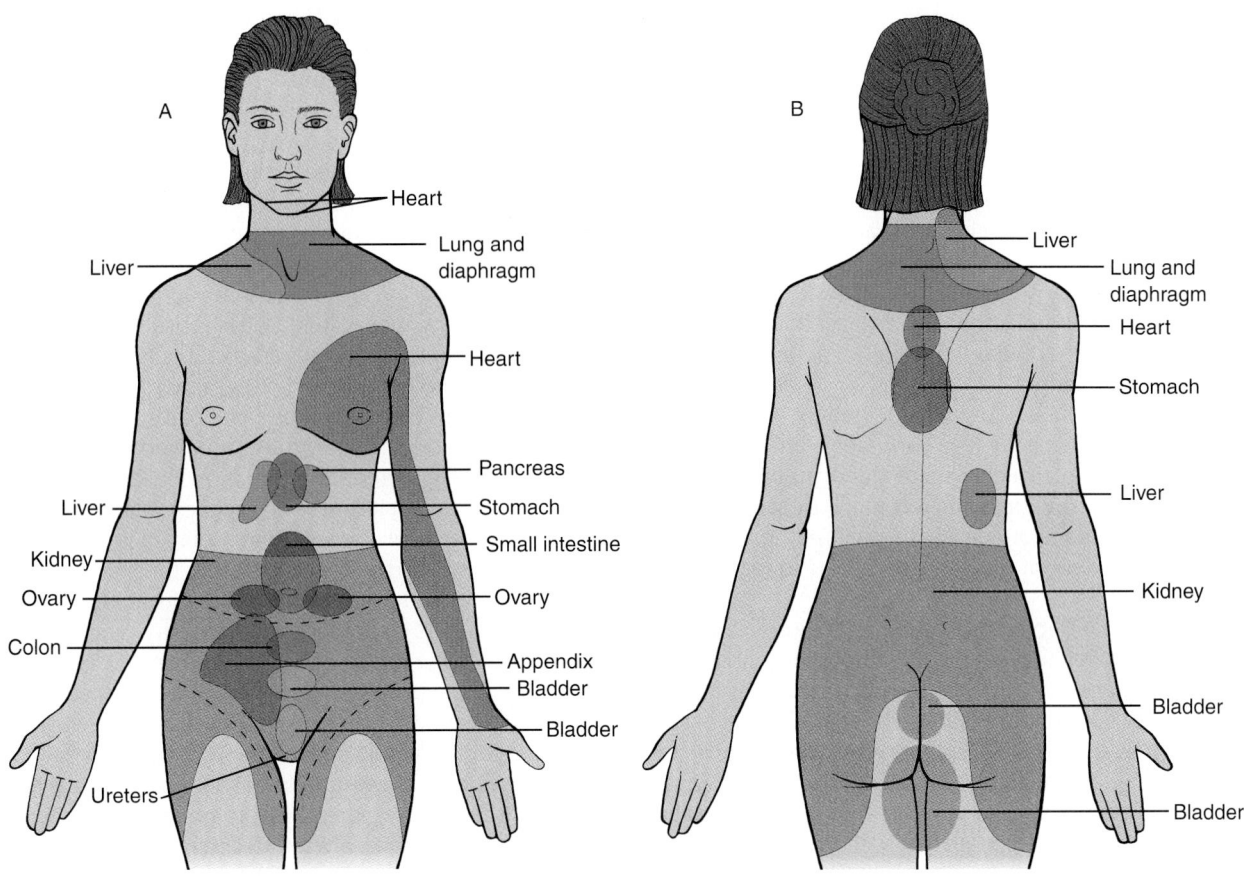

Figure 40-1
These drawings representing the anterior (**A**) and posterior (**B**) views of the body illustrate areas to which various
organs refer pain.

APPLYING LEARNING TO PRACTICE

The Nurse as Role Model: Comfort

The nurse who wishes to role-model healthy pain management behaviors to patients does the following:

- Balances work and leisure activities to promote optimal personal well-being (consistently communicates to self "I care about you!")
- Respects pain as the body's means of signaling that all is not well
- Treats what is producing pain as opposed to simply trying to eradicate pain
- Uses an effective coping model (pain view and view of self) when responding to personal pain
- Routinely incorporates comfort measures into nursing care
- Practices nursing sensitive to the pain needs of patients and is committed to pain relief

- Communicates to patients the belief that their pain experience is real and that help is available
- Assigns high nursing priority to assisting patients (and family members) to develop effective pain management strategies compatible with their belief systems
- Designs varied pain management programs that incorporate noninvasive and invasive interventions; works collaboratively with other health professionals
- Supports pain management programs with attention to the patient's overall nutrition, hydration, elimination, rest, activity, and stimulation
- Continuously updates knowledge of pain theories, assessment strategies, and treatment modalities

Prostaglandins, substance P, and serotonin (a hormone that can act to stimulate smooth muscles, inhibit gastric secretion, and produce vasoconstriction) are **neurotransmitters,** substances that either excite or inhibit target nerve cells.

Receptors in the skin and superficial organs, although incapable of responding selectively, may also be stimulated by mechanical, thermal, chemical, and electrical agents. Friction from bed linens and pressure from a cast are mechanical stimulants. Sunburn and cold water on a tooth with caries are thermal stimulants. An acid burn is the result of a chemical stimulant. The jolt of a static charge is an electrical stimulant.

Stretching of the hollow viscera, pulling on the omentum, and muscle spasms result in pain. Some investigators believe that at least some of the deep-lying organs have their own individual pain receptors, the uterus being an example. Some organs, such as the lungs, are insensitive to pain because of the absence of nociceptors or pain receptors.

It has been observed that pain may be present without injury and may not be present with injury. Therefore, tissue injury does not necessarily accompany pain in all instances. For example, tissue injury is present when the patient experiences pain because of a first- or second-degree burn. On the other hand, although physiologic changes do occur, tissue injury or destruction is not necessarily present when the patient has a headache caused by psychological tension. In addition, the intensity of pain may not be correlated to the seriousness of a particular condition giving rise to the pain. For example, a patient may not experience pain until the ravages of a malignancy are beyond control, whereas the severe pain that usually accompanies a bunion does not indicate a very serious pathology.

Transmission of Pain Stimuli

Pain sensations are conducted along pathways that have been rather clearly defined in certain areas but are still somewhat questionable in other areas. There are no specific pain organs or cells in the body. Rather, an interlacing network of undifferentiated free nerve endings receives painful stimuli. Free nerve ending pain receptors include the afferent (those fibers carrying impulses from the pain receptors toward the brain) fast-conducting A-delta-fibers and the slow-conducting C-fibers. The larger A-delta-fibers transmit acute, well-localized pain, whereas the smaller C-fibers convey diffuse, visceral pain that is often described as burning and aching. It is estimated that there are several million of these nerve endings in the body. They are numerous in the layers of the skin and in some internal tissues, such as the joint surfaces. In the deeper tissues of the body, the pain receptors are diffusely but unevenly spread.

A protective pain reflex is responsible for withdrawal of an endangered tissue from a damaging stimulus. Sensory impulses travel over A-fibers through the dorsal root ganglion to the dorsal horn of the spinal cord. At this point, the sensory nerve impulse synapses with a motor neuron, and the impulse is carried along efferent nerve pathways back to the site of the painful stimulus in a reflex arc. This results in an immediate muscle contraction that removes the injured part from the source of the pain.

Somatic sensation is carried to the dorsal gray horn cells of the spinal cord, then to the spinothalamic tract, and eventually to the cerebral cortex. Although the autonomic nervous system is an efferent system—that is, it carries impulses from the central nervous system—pain sensations from the viscera apparently course along the autonomic system. Through that system, these sensations from deeply-lying structures reach the spinal cord by way of the dorsal roots and then continue along the same pathways as sensations from the skin and superficial body structures. Pain impulses are also carried by the cranial nerve to the central nervous system. There is integration of the sensory impulses of pain along its entire central nervous system route, but the highest level of integration occurs in the cortex. Figure 40-2 illustrates the transmission of the pain sensation, the initiation of the protective reflex response, and conscious awareness of the location, intensity, and quality of the pain after the impulse reaches the cortex.

Stimulation of sensory receptors and intactness of their nerve supply are neither necessary nor sufficient conditions for pain. It would appear that a receptor for pain and a nerve route that eventually carries the impulse to the brain are necessary when pain is present, yet it is well known that this is not always necessary. The pain that is often referred to an amputated leg where receptors and nerves are clearly absent is a real experience for the patient. This type of pain is called **phantom pain** or phantom limb pain and is without demonstrated physiologic or pathologic substance. One theory suggests that sensory misrepresentations from the missing limb may still remain in the brain and cause the phantom pain.

Gate Control Theory of Pain

The **gate control theory** of pain describes the transmission of painful stimuli and recognizes a relation between pain and emotions. The theory states that certain nerve fibers, those of small diameter, conduct excitatory pain stimuli toward the brain, but nerve fibers of a large diameter appear to inhibit the transmission of pain impulses from the spinal cord to the brain. There is a gating mechanism that is believed by some to be located in substantia gelatinosa cells in the dorsal horn of the spinal cord. The exciting and inhibiting signals at the gate in the spinal cord determine the impulses that eventually reach the brain. Thus, only a limited amount of sensory information can be processed by the nervous system at any given moment. When too much information is sent through, certain cells in the spinal column interrupt the signal as if closing a gate. The brain can also influence the gating mechanism. Past experiences and learned behaviors, which are interpreted by the brain, have the effect of regulating or adjusting the eventual behavioral responses to pain. Thus, the gating mechanism appears to be influenced by the amount of activity in large and small afferent fibers in addition to nerve impulses that descend from the brain. This helps explain why similar painful stimuli are interpreted differently by different people. Although not everyone accepts the gate control theory, it appears to explain why mechanical and electrical interventions or heat and pressure may effectively relieve pain. Nursing measures, such as massage or a warm compress to a painful lower back area, stimulate large nerve fibers to close the gate, thus blocking pain impulses from that area. Figure 40-3 illustrates the gate control theory of pain.

Perception of Pain

The perception of pain involves the sensory process when a stimulus for pain is present. It includes the person's interpretation of the pain. The threshold of perception is the lowest intensity of a stimulus that causes the subject to recognize pain. This threshold is remarkably similar for everyone. Still, it is theorized by at least some authorities that the phenomenon of adaptation does occur; that is, the **pain threshold** can be changed within a certain range. This phenomenon has been studied, for example, when prisoners of war reported that the pain of repeated torture was not as acute as it would have been under different circumstances. Many factors might well have played a role, but at least some adaptation appears likely.

Adaptation may also be demonstrated when a person's hand is immersed in warm water. A sensation of pain eventually occurs as the water is heated. However, the person can tolerate a higher temperature as water is gradually heated to the pain level than if the hand had been plunged into hot water without any preparation.

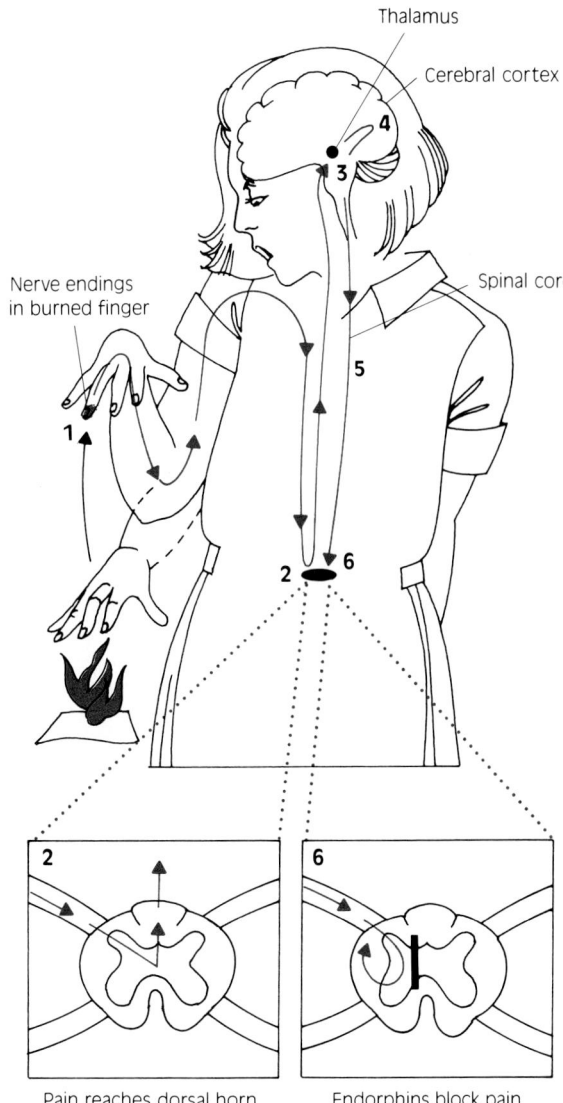

Figure 40-2

Pain sensation and relief. (1) Pain's path begins as a message is received by nerve endings in a burned finger. Potent chemicals (substance P, bradykinin, prostaglandins) are released, sensitizing the nerve endings, helping to transmit the pain message from the injured finger toward the brain, and setting the stage for healing (inflammatory response). (2) The pain signal from the burned finger travels as an electrochemical impulse along the length of the nerve to the dorsal horn on the spinal cord (a region that runs the length of the spine and receives signals from all over the body). (3) The message is relayed to the thalamus, a sensory center in the brain where sensations like heat, cold, pain, and touch first become conscious. (4) It then travels on to the cortex, where the intensity and location of pain are perceived. Little is known about factors that influence the individual's perception of pain at this point, the meaning attributed to the pain, and the voluntary responses elicited. (5) Pain relief begins as a signal from the brain descends by way of the spinal cord. (6) In the dorsal horn, chemicals like endorphin S are released to diminish the pain message from the injured finger. (Adapted from Unlocking pain's secrets. [1984, June 11]. *Time,* pp. 58–66.)

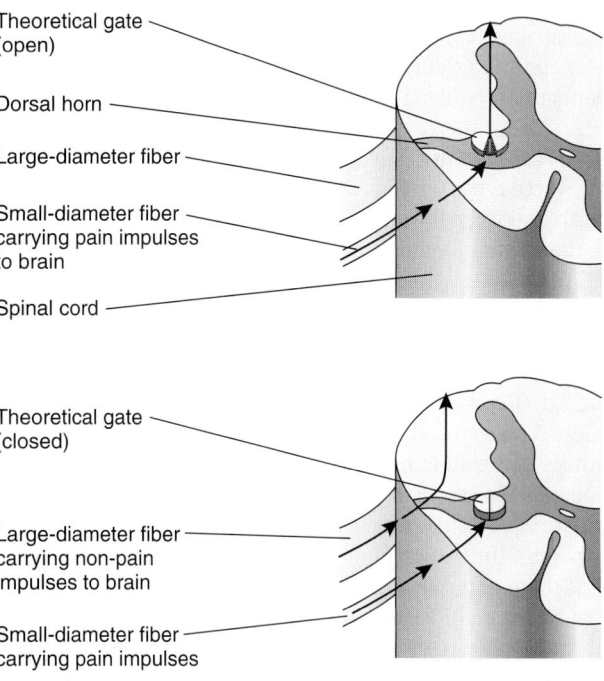

Figure 40-3

An illustration of the gate control theory of pain.

Modulation of Pain

The sensation of pain appears to be regulated or modified by substances called neuromodulators. **Neuromodulators** are endogenous opioid compounds, meaning they are naturally present, morphine-like chemical regulators in the spinal cord and brain. They appear to have analgesic activity and alter the perception of pain. It is believed that these endogenous opioid compounds produce their analgesic effects by binding to specific opioid receptor sites throughout the central nervous system and blocking release or production of pain-transmitting substances. Both pain and stress appear capable of activating the endogenous opiate system.

Endorphins and enkephalins are opioid neuromodulators. **Endorphins** are produced at neural synapses at various points in the central nervous system pathway. They are powerful pain-blocking chemicals that have prolonged analgesic effects and produce euphoria. It is suggested that endorphins may be released when certain measures are used to relieve pain, such as skin stimulation and relaxation techniques, and when certain pain-relieving drugs are used. Many questions remain about endorphins. **Enkephalins**, which are widespread throughout the brain and dorsal horn of the spinal cord, are considered less potent than endorphins. It is believed that enkephalins reduce pain sensation by inhibiting the release of substance P from the terminals of afferent neurons. **Dynorphin**, a recently discovered endorphin, has the most potent analgesic effect.

Pain is a highly personal experience. A person learns to know what causes unpleasantness and what to interpret as pain. Each person's interpretation is influenced by background, such as how he or she has experienced and dealt with pain in the past and what cultural factors have taught about pain. Through past experiences, each person also learns to differentiate among the various types of pain and to associate pain with certain descriptive words. Table 40-2 lists common definitions for additional terms used by patients to describe pain.

Responses to Pain

The three types of responses to pain are physiologic, behavioral, and affective. Examples of these responses are listed in the accompanying box, Common Responses to Pain.

The severity of pain and its duration affect responses to pain. Mild pain experienced briefly may produce little or no behavioral response, whereas intense pain experienced briefly usually results in reflex action to escape the cause. Pain that continues for a relatively short time, such as for a few days or a week, is often accepted by the patient without its being all consuming. The patient expects relief and believes the cause is self-limiting. However, anxiety is ordinarily present. On the other hand, chronic pain tends to consume the entire person. It demands total attention so that the patient has limited resources to take care of other matters of daily living. It is physically and emotionally exhausting and tends to result in depression and irritability. Chronic fatigue usually accompanies chronic pain.

Lack of an obvious response to pain does not mean the patient is without pain. Careful assessment is especially important to understand what the patient is experiencing.

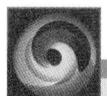

Table 40-2
Additional Terms Used by Patients to Describe Pain

Quality

Sharp	Pain that is sticking in nature and that is intense
Dull	Pain that is not as intense or acute as sharp pain, possibly more annoying than painful. It is usually more diffuse than sharp pain.
Diffuse	Pain that covers a large area. Usually, the patient is unable to point to a specific area without moving the hand over a large surface, such as the entire abdomen.
Shifting	Pain that moves from one area to another, such as from the lower abdomen to the area over the stomach.

Other terms used to describe the quality of pain include sore, stinging, pinching, cramping, gnawing, cutting, throbbing, shooting, viselike pressure.

Severity

Severe or excruciating Moderate Slight or mild	These terms depend on the patient's interpretation of pain. Behavioral and physiologic signs help assess the severity of pain. On a scale of 1 to 10, slight pain could be described as being between about 1 and 3; moderate pain, between about 4 and 7; and severe pain, between about 8 and 10.

Periodicity

Continuous	Pain that does not stop
Intermittent	Pain that stops and starts again
Brief or transient	Pain that passes quickly

Factors Affecting the Pain Experience

Many factors influence the comfort status of a person at any given moment. When an individual experiences pain, almost anything can influence how the painful stimulus is transmitted to the brain, how it is perceived, and the response that is made to it.

Culture

Because cultural norms dictate much of our daily behavior, attitudes, and values, it is natural that culture influences the individual's response to pain. It is important for nurses to un-

Common Responses to Pain

Behavioral (Voluntary) Responses

Moving away from painful stimuli

Grimacing, moaning, and crying

Restlessness

Protecting the painful area and refusing to move

Physiologic (Involuntary) Responses

*Typical Sympathetic Responses When Pain
Is Moderate and Superficial*

Increased blood pressure

Increased pulse and respiratory rates

Pupil dilation

Muscle tension and rigidity

Pallor (peripheral vasoconstriction)

Increased adrenalin output

Increased blood glucose

*Typical Parasympathetic Responses When Pain
Is Severe and Deep*

Nausea and vomiting

Fainting or unconsciousness

Decreased blood pressure

Decreased pulse rate

Prostration

Rapid and irregular breathing

Affective (Psychological) Responses

Exaggerated weeping and restlessness

Withdrawal

Stoicism

Anxiety

Depression

Fear

Anger

Anorexia

Fatigue

Hopelessness

Powerlessness

standing of cultural influences on pain tolerance, expressions of pain, and alternative practices used to manage pain.

Ethnic Variables

Much research has been done on cultural influences on pain. The classic study on behavioral responses to pain present in groups of people of similar ethnic origin was done by Zborowski (1969). He studied men in the 1950s and 1960s in four cultural groups—"Old American" (American-born, white, Protestant, and without identification with any foreign group), Jewish, Italian, and Irish. According to Zborowski, Old American and Irish men typically minimized and controlled their expression of pain, whereas Jewish and Italian men tended to be more vocal and outwardly emotional with their expressions of pain. The ethnic clusters today have become increasingly complex and multidimensional (Juarez, 1997). Healthcare providers increase their respect and sensitivity for diversity if they understand the effects of cultural concepts and ethnicity on the pain experience. Table 40-3 describes typical pain responses in selected ethnocultural groups. The nurse working with other ethnic groups can find pertinent studies in the literature. Additional information on cultural influences on pain is presented in Chapter 3.

Family, Gender, and Age Variables

Variables related to culture are family, gender, and age. An individual's response to pain or their symptoms may be affected or influenced by the response of family members. Also, spouses may reinforce pain behavior in their partners. Children growing up in different families may quickly learn to ignore pain, to exploit pain as a means to secure the attention and services of family members, or to value pain as a means the body uses to teach important truths. Family size and birth order do not appear to be significant in distinguishing chronic pain sufferers.

Similarly, children may learn that there are gender differences in pain expression; whereas it may be acceptable for a little girl to run home crying with a scraped knee, a little boy may be told that he should be brave and not cry. Adult men and women may hold onto gender expectations regarding pain communication and incorrectly interpret the presence or absence of pain expressions in others. Vallerand (1995) reviewed the literature on gender differences in pain in an effort to determine any effect on clinical practice. Research has indicated that women are more comfortable communicating the discomfort associated with pain, but this ability to verbalize their emotions may cause some to view the pain as psychologically based. Several studies report that pain in women needs to be addressed more aggressively because their pain management is consistently reported as inadequate.

In addition, different age groups have different beliefs and norms regarding pain sensation and response. At one time, the infant's inability to communicate pain led healthcare practitioners to the erroneous assumption that pain sensation was diminished or absent. More recently, it has been demonstrated that infants and small children are

derstand that there are ways other than their own of responding to pain. Nurses, as a subculture, value self-control and the ability to function under stress and may expect patients in pain to display a similarly calm, objective, uncomplaining approach to pain. It is particularly important to avoid stereotyping responses to pain because the nurse frequently encounters patients who are in pain or anticipating that it will develop. A form of pain expression that is frowned on in one culture may be desirable in another cultural group. The nurse studies cultural variations to develop an under-

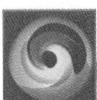

Table 40-3
Pain Expression in Selected Ethnocultural Groups

Ethnic Group	Response to Pain
African Americans	Often viewed as a sign of illness or disease Some believe that suffering and pain are inevitable. Spiritual and religious beliefs may contribute to high tolerance for pain. Some believe that praying and laying on of hands may aid in deliverance from pain and suffering.
Arab Americans	Often view pain as unpleasant and something that should be controlled Tend to express pain openly with family members but may act in a more restrained manner in the presence of health professionals Usually expect positive response from Western medical interventions to control pain
Chinese Americans	Expressions of pain are usually similar to those of Americans Often believe pain is related to the influence of imbalances in the yin and yang Usually cope with pain by using externally applied oils and massage as well as warmth, sleeping on the area of pain, relaxation, and aspirin
Greek Americans	*Ponos* (pain) is viewed by most as an evil that needs to be eradicated. Physical and emotional pain are usually shared with the family. Family is considered a resource for pain relief because they act as advocates and provide emotional support.
Mexican Americans	Most delay seeking medical help for pain and hope, instead, that it will go away; consider it a necessary part of life Seem to experience more pain than other ethnic groups but report it less frequently Often see a direct relationship between pain and suffering and immoral behavior
Navajo Indians	Do not usually openly express their pain or request pain medication Adequate pain control is often difficult because they may mask the actual intensity of their pain. May prefer herbal medicines and use them without the knowledge of the healthcare provider

Adapted from Purnell, L., & Paulanka, B. (1998). *Transcultural health care.* Philadelphia: F. A. Davis.

sensitive to and experience pain. Among older people, pain has often been viewed as a natural component of the aging process and may be ignored or undertreated by healthcare providers. On the other hand, conditions normally painful in young adults (eg, myocardial infarction) may present minimal pain complaints in older people. That an older person does not complain of pain may indicate that he or she fears the treatment for the pain or just refuses to give in to the pain (AHCPR, 1992). For many elderly people, pain has become accepted as a daily occurrence and is regarded as normal and untreatable (Davis, 1997). These variables, which influence pain sensation, perception, and response, make pain assessment a complex task for the nurse.

Religious Beliefs

Religious beliefs may powerfully influence the individual's experience of pain. In some religions, individuals view pain and suffering not as good in themselves but as a means of purification or of making up for individual and community sin. This meaning helps the individual to cope with pain and becomes a source of strength. Patients with this belief may refuse analgesics and other pain relief measures, feeling that

this lessens their offering. On the other hand, illness and pain may also be viewed as punishment from a vengeful God. Individuals may find their faith shaken and question the existence of a loving God. How can belief in a loving God be compatible with their present experience of pain? Anger, resentment, and depression may then compound the pain experience. Patients may find it helpful to confer with a spiritual adviser about their pain experience.

Environment and Support People

An individual's environment and the presence or absence of caring support people may also influence the experience of pain. Many people find that the strangeness of the healthcare environment, especially the lights, noise, and constant activity of a critical care unit, compounds the experience of pain. The sense of powerlessness that accompanies admission to an institution may decrease the individual's ability to cope with pain. Depersonalization or separation from a favorite pillow, pet, or source of music may further decrease the person's sense of comfort. For some, the presence of a loved family member or friend is essential to their sense of well-being. Others prefer to be alone when in pain and may become agitated in the presence of a family member.

Some patients may use their pain to acquire secondary gains, such as special attention and services from their families. Because this tendency, if unchecked, usually leads to resentment and anger in family members and their eventual avoidance of the patient, the nurse should intervene and attempt an honest discussion of this problem.

Anxiety and Other Stressors

Anxiety, which is almost always present when pain is anticipated or being experienced, tends to increase the perceived intensity of pain. The threat of the unknown is ordinarily more devastating and anxiety producing than a threat for which one has been prepared. Studies have indicated that patients who were taught preoperatively about what to expect postoperatively did not require as much medication for pain as those who had similar operative procedures but were not taught preoperatively.

Pain is ordinarily aggravated when anxiety, muscular tension, and fatigue are present. A vicious circle can easily develop when pain interferes with rest and relaxation, and tension and fatigue almost always aggravate the discomfort. The rested and relaxed person can often cope with great discomfort.

An individual who is greatly fatigued and who has no competing demands requiring attention may experience pain acutely. For example, many people have discovered that the pain of a footache or ingrown toenail that was only mildly annoying during the day's work becomes unbearable at night when there is nothing else to distract the mind from the pain.

Past Pain Experience

Whether an individual has experienced pain in the past and the qualities of that experience profoundly affect new pain experiences in the following ways:

- Some patients have never known severe pain and have no fear of pain, not realizing how intense the sensation can be.
- Some patients have experienced severe acute or chronic pain in the past but received immediate and adequate pain relief. These patients are generally unafraid of pain and initiate appropriate requests for assistance.
- Some patients have known severe pain in the past and were unable to secure relief. Even the suggestion of new pain can throw these patients into a frenzy of fear and feelings of despair and hopelessness.
- An individual whose past pain experience led to correction of unhealthy behavior and produced a greater sense of health and well-being may respect and value pain and consider the meaning and significance of a new pain carefully.
- In general, people who have experienced more pain than usual in their lifetimes tend to anticipate more pain and to exhibit increased sensitivity to pain.

- Some pain memories are virtually unerasable, and new contact with conditions similar to those that caused the earlier pain can provoke a violent response.

The Nursing Process

ASSESSING THE PAIN EXPERIENCE

Because the pain experience is unique to each individual, the nurse who wants to help the patient achieve pain control needs sophisticated pain assessment skills. It is necessary to assess all factors that affect the pain experience—psychological, emotional, and sociocultural as well as physiologic. Pain is complex and difficult to interpret and requires a reliable assessment tool. The accompanying Applying Learning to Practice: Promoting Health checklist allows the nurse to assess his or her personal responses to comfort needs.

Pain as the Fifth Vital Sign

In an effort to improve patients' quality of life and make pain management a priority, the American Pain Society is encouraging caregivers to include assessment for pain as the fifth vital sign (Pasero, 1997b). Routine measurement of vital signs accompanied by a pain assessment raises awareness of the existence of pain, places additional emphasis on optimizing pain relief, and moves patients more quickly toward comfort and recovery. The Department of Veterans Affairs has announced a new pain management initiative that commits additional funds to pain research and education at Veterans Administration facilities and includes routine assessment of pain as the fifth vital sign (Ventura, 1999).

Misconceptions

Many patient misconceptions interfere with the patient's ability to communicate pain:

- The doctor has ordered pain-relieving medication for me, which I will be given routinely.
- If I ask for something for my pain, I may become addicted to the medication.
- Sometimes it's better to put up with the pain than to deal with the side effects of the pain medication.
- I should somehow be able to control my pain. It is immature to talk about pain.
- It is better to wait until the pain gets really bad before asking for help. If I take the medication now for moderate pain, it won't relieve severe pain later on.
- I don't want to bother anyone—I know how busy they are.
- It's natural for me to have pain after surgery. After a few days, I should notice it lessening.

APPLYING LEARNING TO PRACTICE

Promoting Health

Comfort

Use the assessment checklist to determine how well you are meeting comfort needs. Then develop a prescription for self-care by choosing appropriate behaviors from the list of suggestions.

Assessment Checklist

almost always | sometimes | almost never

☐	☐	☐	1. I seek medical attention when pain persists.
☐	☐	☐	2. I am aware of my usual behavioral responses to pain.
☐	☐	☐	3. I use stress reduction techniques regularly.
☐	☐	☐	4. I am able to have a restful sleep at night.
☐	☐	☐	5. I have a positive outlook about my present situation.
☐	☐	☐	6. I am aware of how to use distraction strategies to deal with pain

Self-Care Behaviors

1. Obtain a medical evaluation when acute or chronic pain is present.
2. Control stress in the environment.
3. Avoid excessive fatigue.
4. Practice stress reduction or diversionary behaviors when pain is present.
5. Become aware of personal preconceived notions that affect your perception of pain in others.

Additional misconceptions and prejudices about pain and pain relief that hamper the nurse's assessment and treatment of the patient with pain have been summarized by McCaffery and Pasero (1999) and are presented in Table 40-4.

Components of Pain Assessment

Various forms used to help guide the assessment of pain have been described in the nursing literature. The primary purposes of using a guide to assess pain are to eliminate guesswork and biases when dealing with the patient's pain, to understand what the person is experiencing, to analyze findings that will help prepare an appropriate nursing response to the patient's pain, and to facilitate improved outcomes, such as fewer complications, shorter hospital stays, and improved quality of life.

Characteristics of pain generally assessed include the following:

- The patient's verbalization and description of the pain
- Duration of the pain
- The location of the pain
- The quantity and intensity of the pain
- The quality of the pain
- Chronology of the pain
- Aggravating factors
- Physiologic indicators of pain
- Behavioral responses
- The effect of the pain experience on activities and lifestyle

A comprehensive pain assessment must also include discussion of the patient's expectations for pain relief. The patient and healthcare team need to select a realistic goal or a number on the pain scale that is acceptable and satisfactory and facilitates recovery. This helps the patient recognize and report pain that is unacceptable and also allows caregivers to evaluate more readily the effectiveness of their pain management techniques. The accompanying Focused Assessment Guide suggests questions or approaches helpful in assessing the various pain factors.

Pain centers commonly ask patients to complete a self-questionnaire. The McGill-Melzack Pain Questionnaire is an example and requires that an individual check words that fit the description of the pain experience. Marks on a body figure also designate the location of the pain. Comparison of changes on subsequent questionnaires aid in determining an individual's improvement or regression. This comprehensive pain assessment is time-consuming and should be performed when the patient is more comfortable and better able to respond to questions. The AHCPR (1994) in its clinical practice guideline suggests use of an initial pain assessment tool (Fig. 40-4), which is brief and easily administered. For continual assessment of pain and evaluation of pain control measures, a pain scale allows the patient to rate effectively the pain he or she is experiencing on a continual basis. Figure 40-5 displays examples of several pain intensity rating scales. In descending order of importance, McCaffery (1997) ranks the basic methods of assessing an individual's pain:

- Patient's self-report
- Report of family member or other person close to the patient or caregiver who is familiar with the patient

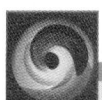

Table 40-4
Barriers to the Assessment and Treatment of Pain

Misconception	Correction
1. The best judge of the existence and severity of a patient's pain is the physician or nurse caring for the patient.	The patient is the authority about his or her pain. The patient's self-report is the most reliable indicator of the existence and intensity of pain.
2. Clinicians should use their personal opinions and beliefs about the truthfulness of the patient to determine the patient's true pain status.	Allowing each clinician to act on personal beliefs presents the potential for different pain assessments by different clinicians, leading to different interventions from each clinician. This results in inconsistent and often inadequate pain management. It is essential to establish the patient's self-report of pain as the standard for pain assessment.
3. The clinician must believe what the patient says about pain.	The clinician must accept and respect the patient's report of pain and proceed with appropriate assessment and treatment. The clinician is always entitled to his or her personal opinion, but this cannot be allowed to guide professional practice.
4. Comparable noxious stimuli produce comparable pain in different people. The pain threshold is uniform.	Findings from numerous studies have failed to support the notion of a uniform pain threshold. Comparable stimuli do not result in the same pain in different people. After similar injuries, one person may suffer moderate pain and the other severe pain.
5. Patients with a low pain tolerance should make a greater effort to cope with pain and should not receive as much analgesia as they desire.	A stoic response to pain is valued in this society and many others. Research shows that clinicians often do not like patients with a low pain tolerance. However, imposing these values on the patient and withholding analgesics is inappropriate.
6. There is no reason for patients to hurt when no physical cause for pain can be found.	Pain is a new science, and it would be foolish of us to think that we will be able to determine the cause of all the pains that patients report.
7. Patients should not receive analgesics until the cause of pain is diagnosed.	Pain is no longer the clinician's primary diagnostic tool. Symptomatic relief of pain should be provided while the investigation of cause proceeds. Early use of analgesics is now advocated for patients with acute abdominal pain.
8. Visible signs, either physiologic or behavioral, accompany pain and can be used to verify its existence and severity.	Even with severe pain, periods of physiologic and behavioral adaptation occur, leading to periods of minimal or no signs of pain. Lack of pain expression does not necessarily mean lack of pain.
9. Anxiety makes pain worse.	Anxiety is often associated with pain, but the cause-and-effect relationship has not been established. Pain often causes anxiety, but it is not clear that anxiety necessarily makes pain more intense.
10. Patients who are knowledgeable about opioid analgesics and who make regular efforts to obtain them are "drug seeking" (addicted).	Patients with pain should be knowledgeable about their medications, and regular use of opioids for pain relief is not addiction. When a patient is accused of "drug seeking," it may be helpful to ask, "What else could this behavior mean? Might this patient be in pain?"
11. When the patient reports pain relief after a placebo, this means that the patient is a malingerer or that the pain is psychogenic.	About one third of patients who have obvious physical stimuli for pain (eg, surgery) report pain relief after a placebo injection. Therefore, placebos cannot be used to diagnose malingering, psychogenic pain, or any psychological problem. Sometimes, placebos relieve pain, but why this happens remains unknown.
12. The pain rating scale preferred for use in daily clinical practice is the VAS.	For patients who are verbal and can count from 0 to 10, the NRS pain rating scale is preferred. It is easy to explain, measure, and record, and it provides numbers for setting pain-management goals.
13. Cognitively impaired elderly patients are unable to use pain rating scales.	When an appropriate pain rating scale (eg, 0–5) is used and the patient is given sufficient time to process information and respond, many cognitively impaired elderly patients can use a pain rating scale.

May be duplicated for use in clinical practice. From McCaffery, M., & Pasero, C. (1999). *Pain: Clinical manual* (p. 37). St. Louis: Mosby, Inc.

FOCUSED ASSESSMENT GUIDE

The Pain Experience

Factors to Assess	Questions and Approaches
Characteristics of the pain	
Location	"Where is your pain? Is it external or internal?" (Asking the patient with acute pain to point to the painful area with one finger may help to localize the pain. Patients with chronic pain may have difficulty trying to localize their pain, however.)
Duration	"How long have you been experiencing pain? How long does a pain episode last? How often does a pain episode occur?"
Quantity	Ask the patient to indicate the degree (amount) of pain currently experienced on the scale below:

```
0     1     2     3     4     5     6     7     8     9     10
No          Mild              Moderate        Severe          Pain as
pain                                                          bad as
                                                             it can
                                                             be
```

It is also helpful to ask how much pain the patient has (on the same scale) when the pain is at its least and at its worst:

Least _____ Worst _____

Quality	"What words would you use to describe your pain?" (Useful in research, this characteristic is least useful in day-to-day clinical practice.)
Chronology	"How does the pain develop and progress?" (If pattern can be identified, interventions early in a pain sequence will often be far more effective than those used after the pain is well established.) "Has the pain changed since it first began? If so, how?"
Aggravating factors	"What makes the pain occur or increase in intensity?"
Alleviating factors	"What makes the pain go away or lessen? What methods of relief have you tried in the past? How long were they used? How effective were they?" (Methods of relief currently in effect for hospitalized patients should be apparent from the chart. It is important to verify the use of current orders and their effectiveness with the patient. Outpatients may need to be asked to record a medication profile, a thorough and accurate account of all medications they are taking.)
Associated phenomena	"Are there any other factors that seem to relate consistently to your pain? Any other symptoms that occur just before, during, or after your pain?"
Physiologic responses	Signs of sympathetic stimulation commonly occur with acute pain.
Vital signs (blood pressure, pulse, respirations) Skin color Perspiration Pupil size Nausea	Signs of parasympathetic stimulation (decreased blood pressure and pulse, rapid and irregular respirations, pupil constriction, nausea and vomiting, and warm, dry skin) may be present, especially in prolonged, severe pain, visceral, or deep pain.
Muscle tension	Observe. Ask the patient whether he or she is aware of any tight, tense muscles.
Anxiety	Are signs of anxiety evident? (May include decreased attention span or ability to follow directions, frequent asking of questions, shifting of topics of conversation, avoidance of discussion of feelings, acting out, somatizing.)
Behavioral responses	
Posture, gross motor activities	Does patient rub or support a particular area? Make frequent position changes? Walk, pace, kneel, or assume a rolled-up position? Does patient rest a particular body part? Protect an area from stimulation? Lie quietly? (In acute pain, postural and gross motor activities are often altered; in chronic pain, the only signs of change may be postures characteristic of withdrawal.)

(continued)

FOCUSED ASSESSMENT GUIDE (Continued)

The Pain Experience

Factors to Assess	Questions and Approaches
Facial features	Does the patient have a pinched look? Are there facial grimaces? Knotted brow? Overall taut, anxious appearance? (A look of fatigue is more characteristic of chronic pain.)
Verbal expressions	Does the patient sigh, moan, scream, cry, repetitively use the same words?
Affective responses	
Anxiety	"Do you feel anxious? Are you afraid? If so, how bad are these feelings?"
Depression	"Do you feel depressed, down, or low? If so, how bad are these feelings? Are your feelings about yourself mostly good or bad? Do you have feelings of failure? Do you see yourself or your illness as a burden to those you care about?"
Interactions with others	How does the patient act when he or she is in pain in the presence of others? How does the patient respond to others when he or she is not in pain? How do significant others and caregivers respond to the patient when the patient is in pain? When the patient is not in pain?
Degree to which pain interferes with patient's life (use past performance as baseline)	"Does the pain interfere with sleep? If so, to what extent? Is fatigue a major factor in the pain experience? Is the conduct of intimate or peer relationships affected by the pain? Is work function affected? Participation in recreational–diversional activities?" (An activity diary is often helpful—sometimes crucial. One to several weeks of hourly activity recorded by the patient may be necessary. Levels of pain, intake of food, and sleep–rest periods are noted along with activities performed. Separate diaries for inpatient and outpatient episodes may be necessary because hospitalization markedly affects the nature and type of activities performed.)
Perception of pain and meaning to patient	"Are you worried about your illness? Do you see any connection between your pain and the nature or course of illness? If so, how do you see them as related? Do you find any meaning in your pain? If so, is this beneficial or detrimental to you? Are you struggling to find some meaning for your pain?"
Adaptive mechanisms used to cope with pain	"What do you usually do to relieve stress? How well do these things work? What techniques do you use at home to help cope with the pain? How well have they worked? Do you use these in the hospital? If not, why not?"
Goals	"What would you like to be doing right now, this week, this month, if the pain were better controlled? How much would the pain have to decrease (on the 0 to 10 scale) for you to begin to accomplish these goals?"

Adapted from Donovan, M.I., & Girton, S.E. (1984). *Cancer care nursing* (2nd ed.). Norwalk, CT: Appleton-Century-Crofts.

- Behaviors (restlessness, grimacing, crying, protecting the painful area)
- Physiologic measures (increased blood pressure and pulse)

Assessment in the Cognitively Impaired Patient

Assessment of pain in people who are cognitively impaired presents special challenges to nurses. It is generally recognized that cognitively impaired individuals are frequently undertreated because they may be unable to report pain verbally or describe the dimensions of their pain. Special efforts are needed to identify accurate means of assessing their pain. Parke (1998) concluded that gerontologic nurses used intuition, experience, and their long-term relationships with patients as a guide to validating pain cues and recognizing the presence of pain in a group of cognitively impaired older adults. Research by Feldt, Warne, and Ryden (1998) encouraged nurses to consider pain as a possible cause of aggressive behavior in cognitively impaired older adults. The combination of a history of pain, observations of a patient's pain by families and caregivers, and the presence of medical diagnoses associated with pain facilitated the development of a model for pain assessment in this population. To manage pain effectively, nurses must rely on their own careful assessments, their empathic qualities, and the expectation that a cognitively impaired patient will experience pain if a verbal patient usually reports this event as painful.

Assessment in a Child

In recent years, healthcare personnel have become much more concerned about addressing pain relief in infants and children (see the accompanying Research in Nursing box).

Date _____

Patient's name _____ Age _____ Room _____

Diagnosis _____ Physician _____

Nurse _____

1. LOCATION: Patient or nurse marks drawing.

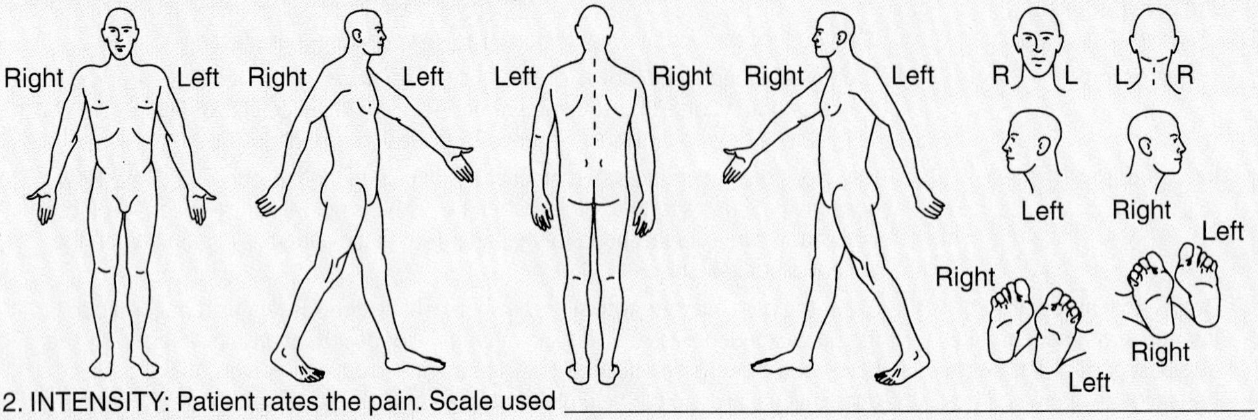

Right [figure] Left Right [figure] Left Left [figure] Right Right [figure] Left R [figure] L L [figure] R

Left Right

Right [figure] Left

Left

2. INTENSITY: Patient rates the pain. Scale used _____

Present: _____

Worst pain gets: _____

Best pain gets: _____

Acceptable level of pain: _____

3. QUALITY: (Use patient's own words, e.g., prick, ache, burn, throb, pull, sharp)

_____

4. ONSET, DURATION, VARIATION, RHYTHMS: _____

_____

5. MANNER OF EXPRESSING PAIN: _____

6. WHAT RELIEVES THE PAIN? _____

7. WHAT CAUSES OR INCREASES THE PAIN? _____

8. EFFECTS OF PAIN: (Note decreased function, decreased quality of life.)

    Accompanying symptoms (e.g., nausea) _____

    Sleep _____

    Appetite _____

    Physical activity _____

    Relationship with others (e.g., irritability) _____

    Emotions (e.g., anger, suicidal, crying) _____

    Concentration _____

    Other _____

9. OTHER COMMENTS: _____

_____

10. PLAN: _____

_____

May be duplicated for use in clinical practice. Adapted from McCaffery M, Pasero C: *Pain: Clinical manual*, p. 60. Copyright © 1999, Mosby, Inc.

Figure 40-4
Initial pain assessment tool.

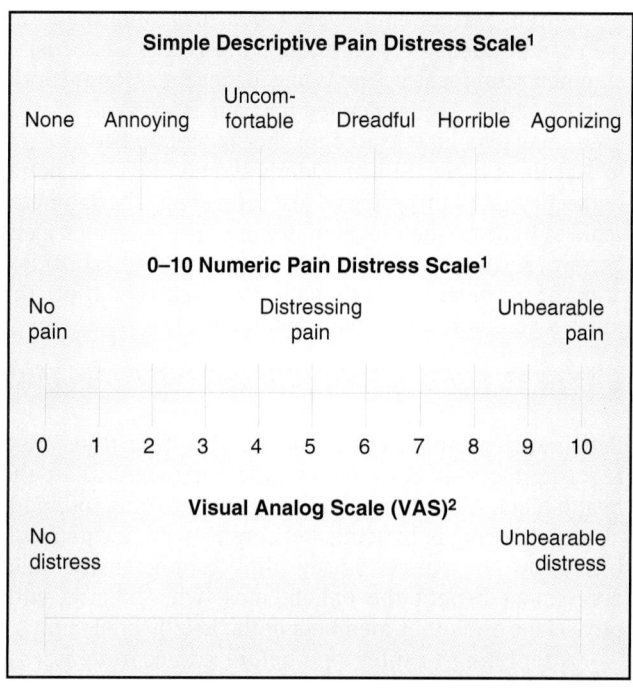

Simple Descriptive Pain Distress Scale[1]

None   Annoying   Uncom-   Dreadful   Horrible   Agonizing
                    fortable

0–10 Numeric Pain Distress Scale[1]

No   Distressing   Unbearable
pain   pain   pain

0   1   2   3   4   5   6   7   8   9   10

Visual Analog Scale (VAS)[2]

No   Unbearable
distress   distress

[1] If used as a graphic rating scale, a 10-cm baseline is recommended.
[2] A 10-cm baseline is recommended for VAS scales.

Figure 40-5
Pain distress scales. (From AHCPR, Acute Pain Management Guide Panel, 1992.)

It was formerly believed that young children lacked the neurologic development to sense pain the way adults do, and pain relief was not a priority when children were hospitalized. Young children frequently received no treatment for pain during entire hospital stays. Pain is frustrating for children because they are unable to understand the concept and cause of pain and may have difficulty describing it. Current methods of assessing and measuring children's pain frequently involve use of more than one technique for assessment. A pain history provides information about the language the child uses to indicate pain, how and to whom this pain is usually reported, and indications of previous pain experiences and coping strategies. Self-report is usually the most reliable account of pain, but the following observations may provide an indication of the presence and severity of pain in a child:

* Irritability and restlessness
* Crying, screaming, or other verbal expression of pain
* Grimacing, grinding of teeth, or clenching fists
* Touching of grabbing of painful body part
* Kicking, thrashing, or attempting to move away from a painful stimulus (Pillitteri, 1999)

Communication with parents, guardians, or other important family members is vital for accurate pediatric pain assessment and management. One commonly used pain assessment scale asks children to compare their pain to a

RESEARCH IN NURSING: MAKING A DIFFERENCE

Managing Pain in Children

Studies have consistently documented that pain relief in children is inadequate. Misconceptions unfortunately persist and can influence the nurse's decision to medicate a child for pain. Some of the misbeliefs that nurses have cited as reasons for undermedication of pain in children are that children do not feel pain as intensely as adults, children cannot remember pain, a quiet or active child is not in pain, children cannot tell where they hurt, and opiates frequently cause respiratory depression in children. As with adults, individual responses to pain are unique, and effective nursing measures must be varied and individualized.

Related Research
Jacob, E., & Puntillo, K. (1999). Pain in hospitalized children: Pediatric nurses' beliefs and practices. *Journal of Pediatric Nursing, 14*(6), 379–388.
This descriptive study investigated nurses' beliefs, perceptions, and documentation practices related to pain assessment and management of children's pain. The nurses who participated in this study were employed in a metropolitan pediatric healthcare facility. Most of the nurses surveyed agreed that pain assess-

ment is essential to relieve a child's pain effectively, but nursing documentation indicated that only one third to one half of children were actually being assessed for pain. There was disagreement among the nurses about whether they adequately prepared a child for a painful procedure. Most nurses, however, did feel that they could have a positive impact on how children cope with painful events. It was evident after this study that many of the misconceptions about pain in children appear to have been dispelled but that many nurses have not yet incorporated pediatric assessment tools into their practice.

Relevance to Nursing Practice
Until nurses routinely assess for pain in children and consider this assessment the "fifth vital sign," pain control for this group will be inadequate. Use of a standard pain assessment tool will facilitate communication and allow all nurses to address the presence of pain and modify their interventions if a child's pain is not adequately relieved. Consistent assessment and documentation appears to be the key to improved pain management strategies for children.

series of faces ranging from a broad smile to a tearful grimace. (Fig. 40-6 is an example of a pediatric pain assessment scale.) The Oucher pain scale, developed by Beyer and others (1992), combines a 0 to 100 scale that older children can use with six photographic images of children in pain for use with younger patients. Children may also be asked to record their pain experiences in a daily diary. Detecting and accurately assessing pediatric pain have resulted in new and innovative approaches toward pain control in children.

Assessment in the Older Patient

Because many older people have chronic disease, pain is a prevalent occurrence. Visual or hearing impairments may influence the assessment format. Multiple-drug regimens that are common in older people can also affect reliable reporting of pain. The AHCPR guidelines for management of acute and chronic pain (1992, 1994) summarize reasons that pain assessment is more complex in older people:

- There is a common belief that pain is an expected outcome of aging.
- Some caregivers mistakenly believe that older patients have a decreased sensitivity to pain and heightened pain tolerance.
- There is a fear among older patients that the admission of pain may limit independence.
- Pain is frequently considered an ominous sign—a forecast of serious illness or death.
- Terminology describing pain may vary significantly.
- The expression and interpretation of pain varies according to culture or ethnic group.
- Changing patterns or presentations of pain have been observed in older people.
- Boredom, loneliness, and depression may affect an older person's perception and report of pain.

Ferrell, Ferrell, and Rivera (1995) have indicated that pain can be adequately assessed in most older adults using common rating scales. The Wong/Baker Faces Rating Scale (see Fig. 40-6), recommended for pain assessment in children, may also be effective for this age group because a 0 to 5 scale is easier to use. Elderly women living at home with chronic pain preferred use of a Pain Thermometer scale to indicate their level of discomfort (Benesh, Szigeti, Ferraro, & Gullicks, 1997). Special attention and consideration of an older patient's pain can positively affect the nurse's ability to assess pain accurately.

DIAGNOSING

Pain is such a complex phenomenon that its analysis often requires the collaboration of different members of the health team. Although nursing has much to offer individuals experiencing both acute and chronic pain, the data collected by the nurse during the comprehensive pain assessment benefit the patient most when shared with physicians and other members of the healthcare team.

Attempting to intervene before an accurate assessment has been completed may mask the real cause of the patient's pain and lead to false assumptions and even further progression of symptoms and the disease process. The nurse who notes a pattern of headaches in a patient and relates this to the patient's description of recent stress (divorce, relocation, new job) may erroneously assume that the headaches are merely stress related and devise and implement a plan of relaxation exercises. A more careful analysis of patient data, however, may reveal that the headaches are of vascular origin and are migraine in nature and that medical intervention is indicated. The headaches may also be symptomatic of intracranial disease such as a brain tumor, in which case, delay in diagnosis could decrease the possibility of treatment and cure.

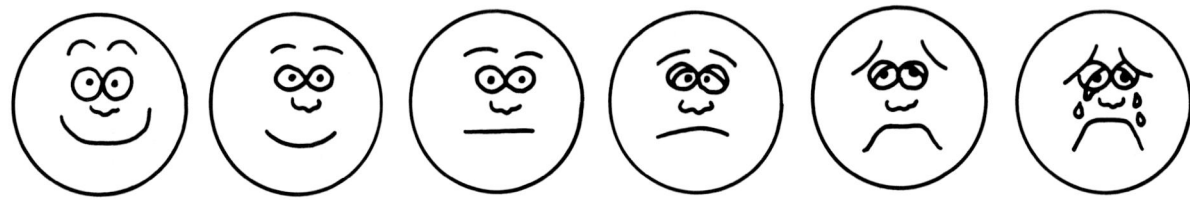

Figure 40-6
Wong/Baker Faces Rating Scale for use with children. (From Wong, D. Essentials of pediatric nursing [4th ed.]. St. Louis: C. V. Mosby.)
1. Explain to the child that each face is for a person who feels happy because he or she has no pain (hurt, or whatever word the child uses) or feels sad because he or she has some or a lot of pain.
2. Point to the appropriate face and state, "This face . . .":
   0—"is very happy because he [or she] doesn't hurt at all."
   1—"hurts just a little bit."
   2—"hurts a little more."
   3—"hurts even more."
   4—"hurts a whole lot."
   5—"hurts as much as you can imagine, although you don't have to be crying to feel this bad."
3. Ask the child to choose the face that best describes how he or she feels. Be specific about which pain (eg, "shot" or incision) and what time (eg, Now? Earlier before lunch?)

When a nursing diagnosis of acute or chronic pain is developed, the diagnostic statement and plan of care should identify the following:

- Type of pain
- Etiologic factors, to the extent that they are known and understood
- The patient's behavioral, physiologic, and affective responses
- Other factors affecting pain stimulus, transmission, perception, and response

Pain or Chronic Pain as the Problem

Many diagnoses can be developed for pain problems. The importance of the nurse identifying these problems and including them as priorities in the plan of care cannot be overstated. Examples of two-part nursing diagnoses follow. See the accompanying box for examples of defining characteristics of these diagnoses. In general, it is not recommended that the medical diagnosis be used as the etiology of the problem statement in the nursing diagnosis. However, when stating nursing problems of pain, it may be difficult to avoid this without sacrificing the specificity desired. Remember that the purpose of the etiology is to direct the nursing interventions.

Pain: Postoperative related to fear of taking prescribed analgesics

Pain related to fractured femur and multiple lacerations and unsuccessful attempts to determine effective analgesic

Pain related to prolonged labor (dystocia) and commitment to natural childbirth

Anxiety related to heightened pain anticipation from child's history of undergoing frequent painful procedures

Pain related to decreased blood supply to myocardium (angina)

Chronic Pain: Headache related to inadequate pain management secondary to belief that patient somehow "deserves" this pain

Chronic Pain related to inadequate pain management of metastatic cancer involving bone

Chronic Pain related to rheumatoid arthritis

Pain or Chronic Pain as the Etiology

Because the experience of pain affects so many other aspects of human functioning, pain may be the etiology of numerous other nursing diagnosis statements:

Ineffective Airway Clearance related to postoperative incisional pain

Anxiety related to pain anticipation and inadequate pain management in the past

Constipation related to chronic use of narcotic analgesics

Ineffective Family Coping: Disabling, related to father's inability to allow family to share his pain experience

Ineffective Individual Coping related to failure of chronic pain management strategies to date

Altered Health Maintenance related to loss of will to live secondary to prolonged chronic pain

Hopelessness related to belief that present pain means imminent death

Risk for Injury related to decreased pain sensation

Knowledge Deficit: Angina Pain Management related to belief that nothing will help the pain

Fatigue related to lack of relief from chronic pain

Fear related to possible significance of pain

Impaired Physical Mobility related to arthritic pain

Altered Nutrition: Less Than Body Requirements related to gastrointestinal distress

Self-Care Deficit: Dressing/Grooming related to painful movement of joints

Altered Sexuality Patterns related to painful intercourse

Sleep Pattern Disturbance: Inability to Fall Asleep related to pain's worsening at night

Risk for Spiritual Distress related to belief that God is unfairly causing this pain as some sort of undeserved punishment

Altered Thought Processes related to effects of chronic pain and overmedication

Risk for Self-Directed Violence related to loss of will to live with unrelieved chronic pain

PLANNING: EXPECTED OUTCOMES

After the diagnosis of a pain problem is made, it is critical for nurses to develop a plan of care that, when implemented, demonstrates nursing's commitment to assist the patient to develop effective pain management strategies.

Nursing measures are directed toward the achievement of the following patient goals for patients whose pain is acute in nature (ie, it is expected that with healing the pain will subside and eventually disappear). The patient will achieve the following:

- Describe a gradual reduction of pain using a scale ranging from 0 (no pain) to 10 (pain as bad as it can be)
- Demonstrate competent execution of successful pain management program (specify)

Chronic Pain

For patients whose pain is chronic in nature, an expected outcome may be contacting a hospice or a pain clinic. Hospice care (also mentioned in Chaps. 11 and 13) addresses the physical, spiritual, social, and economic needs of terminally ill patients and their families either in the home or a hospice center. Pain relief is a priority in this setting. Numerous outpatient centers are also available to support patients with chronic pain and improve their pain management through a variety of approaches. The physician, nurse, and other members of the healthcare team collaborate to develop the optimal pain treatment plan for each patient with chronic pain.

Nursing Diagnoses for Common Problems

Pain

Problem	Related Factors	Sample Defining Characteristics
Pain: Acute Postoperative	Fear of taking prescribed analgesics	• Recent cholecystectomy • Face is pale and drawn; vital signs elevated from baseline. • States, "I don't like to ask for anything for pain because I know people often get addicted."
Pain: Left Leg	Fractured femur and multiple lacerations; unsuccessful attempts to determine effective analgesic	• Recent motor vehicle accident • Grimaces whenever left leg is moved • Directs abusive language to anyone who touches left leg • Refused to have dressing changed on left leg • Reports analgesic "only takes the edge off" the pain
Pain	Prolonged labor (dystocia) and commitment to natural childbirth	• Admitted to labor unit 18 hours ago with moderate contractions 2 minutes apart • Strength of contractions weakening; progress of dilation and effacement slow; failure to progress • "I'll feel like a failure if I take anything for pain. I want to 'go natural.' I know I can do it. Besides, the drugs would only hurt my baby."
Pain: Heightened Anticipation	Child's history of undergoing frequent painful procedures	• Child diagnosed at age 3 years with acute nonlymphoid leukemia • History of bone marrow aspirations, spinal taps, platelet transfusions, chemotherapy, and other such procedures • Child "freezes" when unfamiliar healthcare worker enters room
Pain: Chest	Decreased blood supply to myocardium (angina) and fear	• "I never know when it will grab me next. I get this crushing pain in my chest and can't do anything. Usually one or two of those nitro tablets bring me relief. I'm always scared, though, that the pain won't go away."
Chronic Pain: Headaches	Inadequate pain management secondary to belief that somehow patient "deserves this pain"	• Reports history of migraine headaches for past 5 years • Never sought treatment • "My mother told me that we all get the pain in life that we deserve—goodness, I've been no saint."
Chronic Pain	Inadequate pain management of metastatic cancer involving bone	• "I can't help feeling, though, that no one is meant to live like this." • Diagnosed with cancer of bladder 2 years ago; presently metastatic spread to spine • Rates pain 10 on a scale of 1 (minimal) to 10 (greatest) • "I haven't been taking as much of this pain medicine as the doctor said I could because if I get used to it now nothing will work when the pain gets even worse later." • "When I told the nurse in the hospital about my pain she said I'd have to get used to it." • "I don't want to burden my wife and kids with my pain."
Chronic Pain	Rheumatoid arthritis and inappropriate activity during exacerbations	• Stiffness of joints. limitation of motion, heat, swelling, and tenderness • States pain is often intense after activity • "I can't accept not being able to do all I want to do for my husband and children."

After the plan of care is developed, the nurse implements the nursing strategies that are most likely to assist the patient to achieve pain relief goals whether at home or in a healthcare facility. Nursing interventions described in this chapter include establishing a trusting nurse–patient relationship; manipulating factors that affect the pain experience, initiating nonpharmacologic pain relief measures, managing pharmacologic interventions, reviewing additional pain control measures, considering ethical/legal responsibility to relieve pain, and teaching the patient about pain.

Establishing a Trusting Nurse–Patient Relationship

Most patients with pain feel better, suffer less, and experience less anxiety when they believe that a competent nurse cares about their experience of pain and is available for help and support. Without the confidence developed in a good nurse–patient relationship, nothing seems to work. With it, often amazing results have been obtained by using measures that ordinarily are only modestly effective. Measures that help strengthen the nurse–patient relationship and promote pain relief include discussing pain with the patient, allowing the patient to help choose a method of pain relief, and visiting and remaining with the patient in pain. These measures promote a collaborative relationship in which the patient's pain is treated with respect (see the accompanying box, Through the Eyes of the Patient).

Manipulating Factors Affecting the Pain Experience

Removing or Altering the Cause of Pain

Removing or altering the cause of the pain is ideal and sometimes possible. Ways of doing this include removing or loosening a tight binder, if permissible; seeing to it that a distended bladder is emptied; taking steps to relieve constipation and flatus; changing body positions and ensuring correct body alignment; and changing soiled linens and dressings that may be irritating the skin. A hungry or thirsty patient may need a snack or a drink to feel more comfortable.

Certain drugs are useful for removing or altering the intensity of painful stimuli. For example, drugs that decrease smooth muscle spasms in the gastrointestinal tract and those that decrease contractions of skeletal muscles reduce discomfort.

Altering Factors Affecting Pain Tolerance

As a result of the pain assessment and the trusting relationship he or she has established, the nurse is better able to identify those factors that are increasing the patient's pain experience and decreasing his or her pain tolerance. **Pain tolerance** is the point beyond which a person is no

Through the Eyes of the Patient

I've always thought of myself as a "take charge" kind of person. It's important for me in my business to be calm and always in control of my emotions. The "big C" changed everything for me. A recent hospitalization made me take time to think about what's happening to me.

Even in the hospital, I had a steady stream of visitors—some friends and some business associates. Even the mayor stopped by to see me! For all of them, I was my usual self—smiling, joking, and acting as if everything was normal. I made sure I took my pain medicine before they came. I kept all my fears about cancer and dying hidden behind my smiling face. I never broke down—not even in front of my wife! Men aren't supposed to cry, you know!

One nurse's simple gesture changed all that. One evening after all my visitors, my wife, and my son had left, she must have sensed something. She came over, stood next to me, put her arm around my shoulders and quietly said, "You know, Bob, it's alright to cry." It was like the dam opened up. I looked at her, my face cracked, and all of a sudden I couldn't stop sobbing. She must have known that I needed to talk about what was happening to me. I needed to say those words out loud to someone—"I'm afraid the pain will get too bad! I'm afraid of dying. I can't let my family see me this way!" She just let me cry, kept holding my hands, and just by being there and listening, helped me at that particular moment in ways that you will never know.

longer willing to endure pain. These factors should be alleviated whenever possible. For example, patients whose families have never acknowledged their pain and who have repeatedly been told that their pain is all in their head may experience a greater ability to deal with their pain when someone finally takes the pain seriously. Nursing measures include communication to the patient that responses to pain are acceptable as well as education of the patient's family.

Fatigue tends to increase pain, and promoting rest is then helpful. The patient in pain usually feels more comfortable when the environment is quiet and restful. Although sensory restrictions, such as eliminating unnecessary noise and bright lights, are usually indicated, it is rarely helpful to leave the patient alone in an environment with little sensory input. The patient is then more likely to focus on self and the discomfort.

Lack of knowledge, finding no meaning in the pain, being pessimistic about its relief, and fear may also interfere with the patient's ability to deal with pain. Common fears include a fear of losing control and embarrassing oneself by being unable to deal with the pain maturely and a fear of taking pain relief medication because this may be viewed as a sign of weakness or the medication may become addictive or lose its effectiveness later. Older patients, in particular, are frequently frustrated by similar concerns about pain management.

Initiating Nonpharmacologic Relief Measures

Although analgesics are usually the primary treatment of pain, there is a growing trend involving integration of complementary, nonpharmacologic measures with conventional medical treatment. AHCPR guidelines (1992, 1994) recommend use of these adjunct measures to complement drug regimens. These interventions are varied and can be practiced in all healthcare settings.

Distraction

Conscious attention often appears to be necessary to experience pain, whereas preoccupation with other things has been observed to distract the patient from pain. *Distraction* requires the patient to focus attention on something other than the pain. It is not entirely clear whether distraction raises the threshold of pain or increases pain tolerance. Many patients whose pain is relieved by distraction report being able to place pain in the periphery of awareness. This is compatible with the theory that if the reticular formation in the brainstem receives sufficient sensory input, it can ignore or block out select sensations such as pain. The Lamaze method of childbirth illustrates one common use of distraction.

Distraction alone may relieve mild pain but is best used before pain begins or soon thereafter. It has also proved effective when used with analgesics for treatment of a brief episode of severe pain (eg, pain that accompanies a diagnostic procedure). Distraction may also be used successfully with children.

Techniques that distract attention include the following:

- Visual distractions: counting objects, reading, or watching TV
- Auditory distractions: listening to music
- Tactile kinesthetic distractions: holding or stroking a loved person, pet, or toy; rocking; slow rhythmic breathing
- Project distractions: playing a challenging game, performing meaningful play or work

Humor

Humor can be an effective distraction, can help an individual cope with pain, and may even have a positive effect on the immune system. It has proved particularly effective before painful procedures, and many pain, cancer, and ambulatory care centers encourage patients to view humorous videos before a painful, tedious procedure (Pasero,

1998c). The accompanying box includes general guidelines for incorporating humor into patient care.

Music

Listening to music can relax, soothe, decrease pain, and provide distraction. By stimulating the release of en-

---

Using Humor to Help Patients Cope With Pain

Laughter is good medicine for our patients. Twenty years ago, Norman Cousins wrote his book, *Anatomy of an Illness as Perceived by the Patient: Reflections on Healing and Regeneration*. In this book, he recounted the value of humor and how 10 minutes of laughter gave him hours of pain-free sleep. Since then, there have been a number of studies on laughter in patient care situations. In one study, patients with chronic cancer pain rated laughter as the most effective self-initiated, nonpharmacologic measure they used to cope with pain. In another study, patients who listened to laughter-inducing tapes had higher pain thresholds, and this persisted for 10 minutes after the chuckling subsided. Some healthcare institutions have humor carts, humor baskets, and even humor rooms for patients. These may contain CDs, audiotapes, and videotapes of situation comedies; movies; stand-up comedy acts; and reading materials such as comic books and humorous magazines. Some carts even contain playful items, such as soap bubbles, wind-up toys, games, magic tricks, puppets, fingerpaints, and playdough—and this is not reserved for the pediatric ward. However, sources of humor should not be offensive (it is suggested that they have a "G" rating—for general audiences—and be age appropriate).

General guidelines for using humor with patients include using it only with those who are responsive to its use and wish to use it. Humor should not be used in patients with moderate to severe pain, nor should it be a replacement for pharmacologic analgesia. It is important, as it is in most nursing interventions, that the humor be patient specific. Thus, the nurse will need to determine what (or who, like Jack Benny or Lucille Ball or a Disney character) makes a patient laugh, how the patient has used humor or play in the past, and how it helped. Let the patient select the humorous materials, and when possible, incorporate strategies that include the patient's family and friends.

Nurses are often involved in procedures that are painful to their patients. Using humor is one nursing intervention that can be initiated after assessing the patient's interest and willingness and then evaluating its effectiveness.

Adapted from Rothrock, J. C. (1999). Laughter: The attitude worth catching. *First Hand, 14*(1), 5–6.

dorphins, music enhances one's sense of well-being and decreases the need for pain medication. Patients can select the music they prefer to be used for relaxation before, during, and after surgical experiences and to help focus on breathing techniques during labor. It has also proved effective to soothe agitated newborns and comatose patients (Strevy, 1999).

Imagery

Patients who use imagery, an example of mind–body interaction, to decrease pain sensation imagine something that involves one or all of the senses, concentrate on that image, and gradually become less aware of the pain. Imagery may be as simple as a child thinking of "happy things" (a beloved pet, lollipops, Christmas morning, grandmom's lap) or as involved as an adult recreating a favorite place and then experiencing the healing presence or touch of a loved person or the healing energies of nature in that setting. The imagery technique has also been used to create an image in which the cause of the pain is visualized and then overcome or counteracted by some more powerful image.

Imagery has been found to be more effective for patients with chronic pain than for patients with acute, severe pain. General techniques for successfully guiding a patient to use imagery include the following:

- Help the patient to identify the problem or goal.
- Suggest beginning the imagery with several minutes of focused breathing, relaxation, or meditation.
- Help the patient to develop images of the problem as well as personal internal resources (eg, coping strategies) and external healing therapies (eg, medications, treatments).
- Encourage images of the desired state of well-being at the end of the session.

If the patient becomes restless or upset, the imagery experience is terminated and attempted later when the patient seems better disposed. Guided imagery is also discussed in Chapter 31.

Relaxation

Relaxation techniques reduce skeletal muscle tension and lessen anxiety. By assisting the patient with relaxation techniques, the nurse acknowledges the patient's pain and expresses a willingness to help the patient relieve the distress caused by his or her pain. The positive effects of relaxation for the person with pain include the following:

- Improved quality of sleep
- Improved problem-solving ability
- Decreased fatigue
- Increased confidence and sense of self-control in coping with pain
- Lessening of the detrimental physiologic effects of continued or repeated stress from pain
- Distraction from pain
- Increased effectiveness of other pain relief measures

- Improved ability to tolerate pain
- Decreased distress or fear during anticipation of pain
- Reassurance that the nurse is aware of his or her problem and wants to help (McCaffery & Beebe, 1989)

Relaxation is most effective as a pain alleviator when combined with slow, deep, easy breathing from the abdomen or diaphragm while the eyelids are closed or with the individual focusing on a real or imagined fixed spot. Relaxation techniques are also discussed in Chapter 31.

Cutaneous Stimulation

The success of cutaneous stimulation (techniques that stimulate the skin's surface) in relieving pain is often explained on the basis of the gate control theory. The gate control theory of pain postulates that cutaneous nerve fibers are large-diameter fibers carrying impulses to the central nervous system. When the skin is stimulated, pain is believed to be controlled by closing the gating mechanism in the spinal cord. This decreases the number of pain impulses that reach the brain for perception. These techniques can be used in all healthcare settings to supplement a pain control regimen. Some forms of cutaneous stimulation include the following:

- Massage (with or without analgesic ointments or liniments containing menthol); see Procedure 40-1
- Application of heat or cold, or both intermittently (explained in detail in Chap. 37)
- Acupressure
- Transcutaneous electrical nerve stimulation (TENS)

Acupressure is a modern-day Western descendant of acupuncture. It involves the use of the fingertips to create gentle but firm pressure to usual acupuncture sites. This technique of holding and releasing various pressure points has a calming effect, most likely related to the body's release of endorphins and enkephalins. It is easy to learn, can be performed on oneself after demonstration and practice, and allows patients to participate in their own pain relief (Maxwell, 1997).

TENS is a noninvasive alternative technique that involves electrical stimulation of large-diameter fibers to inhibit transmission of painful impulses carried over small-diameter fibers. The TENS unit consists of a battery-powered portable unit, lead wires, and cutaneous electrode pads that are applied to the painful area (Fig. 40-7). It requires a physician's order. TENS therapy has reportedly been effective in reducing postoperative pain and improving mobility after surgery (AHCPR, 1992). Positive results have also been noted when it is used as an adjunct with physical therapy and for patients with low back pain. The TENS unit may be applied intermittently throughout the day or worn for extended periods of time, depending on the physician's order.

Cutaneous stimulation is limited in that unless the pain can be localized, it is most likely too diffuse to benefit from these techniques. In addition, most individuals cannot tolerate stimulation of the painful area; they may,

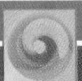

PROCEDURE 40-1

Giving a Back Massage

Equipment

Massage lubricant or lotion	Bath blanket
Powder	Towel

Action	Rationale
1. Explain the procedure and offer back massage to the patient.	Back massage can facilitate circulation and promote relaxation.
2. Wash your hands.	Handwashing deters the spread of microorganisms.
3. Close the curtain or door.	Privacy increases relaxation.
4. Assist the patient to the prone position or side-lying position with the back exposed from the shoulders to the sacral area. Use the bath blanket to drape the patient. Raise the bed to the high position and lower the side rail closest to you.	This position exposes an adequate area for massage with privacy and warmth maintained. Having the bed in the high position reduces back strain for the nurse.
5. Warm the lubricant or lotion in the palm of your hand or place the container in warm water.	Cold lotion causes chilling and uncomfortable sensation.
6. Using light gliding strokes (*effleurage*), apply lotion to patient's shoulders, back, and sacral area.	Effleurage relaxes the patient and lessens tension.
7. Place your hands beside each other at the base of the patient's spine and stroke upward to the shoulders and back downward to the buttocks in slow, continuous strokes. Continue for several minutes.	Continuous contact is soothing and stimulates circulation and muscle relaxation.
8. Massage the patient's shoulders, entire back, areas over iliac crests, and sacrum with circular stroking motion. Keep your hands in contact with the patient's skin. Continue for several minutes, applying additional lotion as necessary.	A firmer stroke with continuous contact promotes relaxation.
9. Knead the patient's skin by gently alternating grasping and compression motions (*pétrissage*).	Kneading increases blood circulation to areas.
10. Complete the massage with additional long stroking movements.	Long stroking motion is soothing and promotes relaxation.
11. During massage, observe the patient's skin for reddened or open areas. Pay particular attention to the skin over bony prominences.	Pressure may interfere with circulation and lead to development of decubitus ulcers. Backrub stimulates circulation to these areas.
12. Use the towel to pat the patient dry and to remove excess lotion. Apply powder if the patient requests it.	This provides additional comfort for the patient.
13. Wash your hands.	Handwashing deters the spread of microorganisms.
14. Assess the patient's response and record your observations on the patient's chart.	This provides accurate documentation of the procedure and condition of the patient's skin.

however, be helped by stimulation of the surrounding or contralateral area.

Acupuncture

Acupuncture is a technique that uses needles of various lengths to prick specific parts of the body to produce in-sensitivity to pain. The technique was developed in China and has been used for centuries in many Asian countries. It has gained acceptance in the Western world as an alternative intervention to help control discomfort from disorders such as headaches, menstrual cramps, postoperative dental pain, low back pain, and carpal tunnel syndrome.

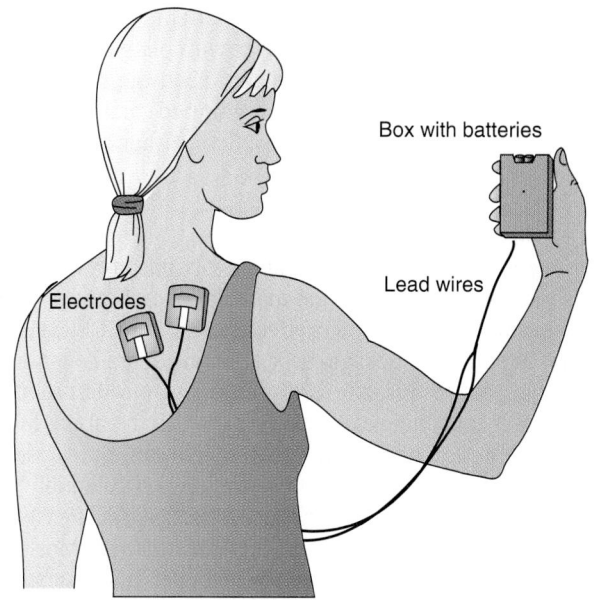

Figure 40-7
Three major components of a TENS unit with two electrodes placed on the upper back of the patient to relieve shoulder pain. This shows the size of the TENS unit in relation to an adult body, illustrating that it is small and portable. (From McCaffery, M., & Beebe, A. [1989]. Pain: Clinical manual for nursing practice. St. Louis: C. V. Mosby, p. 158.)

The relief of pain by acupuncture is generally explained on the basis of the gate control theory. Self-hypnosis may also account for some of acupuncture's success. Repeated treatments are often needed.

Percutaneous electrical nerve stimulation (PENS) is a new complementary therapy used particularly for the management of acute and chronic pain syndromes. This form of acupuncture combines the advantages of both electroacupuncture and TENS and consists of placement of needle probes into soft tissue to stimulate peripheral sensory nerves that relate to the area of injury or pain. The electrical stimulus that is delivered bypasses the skin barrier and goes directly to the involved nerve. The efficacy of PENS as a pain management technique is currently being investigated (White, Phillips, Proctor, & Craig, 1999).

Hypnosis

Hypnosis, a technique that produces a subconscious state accomplished by suggestions made by a hypnotist, has been used successfully in many instances to control pain. The person's state of consciousness is altered by suggestions so that pain is not perceived as it normally would be. According to many hypnotists, it also alters the physical signs of pain. Many people can be taught autohypnosis, that is, self-induced hypnosis, for the control of pain. It is generally believed that a successful response to hypnosis is related to the individual's openness to suggestion, belief that hypnosis will work, and emotional readiness.

Biofeedback

Biofeedback is a technique that uses a machine to monitor physiologic responses through electrode sensors on the patient's skin. The feedback signal or unit transforms the physiologic data into a visual display. Upon seeing pain-related responses, such as increased muscle tension or elevated blood pressure, the patient is taught to regulate this physiologic response and control pain by practicing techniques such as deep breathing exercises, progressive relaxation exercises, or visual imagery. Biofeedback decreases the individual's pain by reducing the anxiety associated with lack of control over bodily functions, distracts the person's attention from the pain to concentration on the person's inner state and the feedback signal, and reduces the cause of the pain. Eventually, the desired effect is for an individual to produce the expected effect without the use of the biofeedback machinery. Limitations of this method include the high degree of motivation needed and difficulty of maintaining control after the training program.

Therapeutic Touch

Therapeutic touch is an alternative therapy that involves using one's hands to direct an energy exchange consciously from the practitioner to the patient to facilitate healing or pain relief. It is viewed by many as a powerful adjunct to pain relief therapy. Patients who have received therapeutic touch report feeling relaxed and require less pain medication with longer periods of pain relief (Krieger, 1999). It is derived from the ancient practice of laying on of hands, but nurses skilled in therapeutic touch never actually touch their patients when administering this modality. Therapeutic touch was developed by nurses, does not require a physician's order, and can be used in any setting. Several recent studies have questioned the validity of this complementary therapy (Rosa et al., 1998; Glickman & Gracely, 1998), but nurses caring for patients with terminal diseases relate that therapeutic touch complements their efforts to alleviate suffering and promote comfort during the final stages of life.

Managing Pharmacologic Relief Measures

Whether pain is acute or chronic, measures exist to control most pain experiences. However, many misconceptions still exist about pain relief and, because of this, many people still receive inadequate pain treatment and suffer needlessly. The AHCPR guidelines focus on individualizing pain relief strategies and aggressively using pharmacologic measures. To make informed decisions and individualize care, nurses need updated information and ongoing education about drug therapy, the cornerstone of many pain treatment regimens. The AHCPR guidelines are a valuable resource for current knowledge and research on using drugs to control pain.

Analgesic Administration

An **analgesic** is a pharmaceutical agent that relieves pain. Analgesics function to reduce the person's perception of pain and to alter the person's responses to discomfort. There are three general classes of drugs used for pain relief:

- Nonopioid analgesics (acetaminophen and non-steroidal antiinflammatory drugs [NSAIDs])
- Opioids or narcotic analgesics (all controlled substances; eg, morphine, codeine, meperidine, methadone)
- Adjuvant drugs (anticonvulsants, antidepressants, and multipurpose drugs)

The nurse administering analgesics needs to combine a healthy respect for the drug being administered with thorough knowledge of its mechanism of action, side effects, and administration guidelines. This respect for the drug should result in analgesics being used wisely to produce their desired effect. Knowledge of common analgesics enables the nurse to tailor the patient's regimen and communicate professionally with physicians about a patient who is being undermedicated or who needs a different drug or route of administration. Nurses should not refrain from using analgesics or reduce their doses because of an unrealistic fear of their potency and side effects.

Repeated studies have demonstrated that pain is frequently undertreated. Physician, nurse, and patient variables all contribute to this outcome. Physicians often prescribe insufficient analgesic doses because of a tendency to overestimate the efficacy and duration of analgesics, underestimate the pain experience, and worry excessively about the possibility of respiratory problems and addiction. Nurses who ideally spend the most time with the patient and who are supposed experts in human responses (eg, the response to pain) often compound this problem by further reducing the insufficient analgesic dose or by not administering the medication at all. Nurse variables include the low priority nurses give to pain management; arbitrary pain assessments and erroneous judgments about a patient's pain and need for analgesia; and fear of being the person who administers the drug that causes respiratory depression or another serious side effect. The inability of many patients to discuss their pain and to request pain assistance perpetuates this problem.

Nonopioid Analgesics

Nonopioid analgesics are usually the drugs of choice for mild to moderate pain. The AHCPR guideline panels agree that the simplest dosage schedules and least invasive pain management modalities should be used first (AHCPR, 1992; 1994). Many times, these drugs alone can provide adequate pain relief; the NSAIDs also have an antiinflammatory effect (Peterson, 1997). Many of these medications are over-the-counter products; some are available by prescription only; and others are prepared in an injectable form. Some can cause gastric side effects, but these symptoms may be preventable if the drug is taken with food or antacids. Individual responses to the NSAIDs vary, but

these agents are contraindicated in patients with bleeding disorders (their action may interfere with platelet function) or probable infections (NSAIDs can mask the signs of an infection). The combination of nonopioid analgesics and opioids provides more analgesia than either drug taken alone.

Opioid Analgesics

According to the AHCPR panel, "opioids are the major class of analgesics used in the management of moderate to severe pain because of their effectiveness" (AHCPR, 1994, p. 49). In sufficient dosage, they are considered capable of relieving pain of virtually every nature. **Opioids** produce analgesia by attaching to opioid receptors in the brain. Morphine, the prototype opioid, is available in multiple dosage forms, has a fairly predictable action, and is relatively inexpensive. The most common side effects associated with opioid use are sedation, nausea, and constipation. Most adverse effects disappear with prolonged use, but if constipation persists, it usually responds to treatment with increased fluids and fiber and use of a mild laxative.

Respiratory depression is a commonly feared side effect of opioid use. In reality, it is an uncommon occurrence in long-term therapy because patients have usually developed a tolerance to the drug and its respiratory depressant effects. If respiratory depression is suspected, it is usually preceded by sedation. Nursing assessment using the numeric sedation scale that follows can determine those patients at risk for respiratory depression:

1 = awake and alert; no action necessary
2 = occasionally drowsy but easy to arouse; requires no action
3 = frequently drowsy and drifts off to sleep during conversation; decrease the opioid dose
4 = somnolent with minimal or no response to stimuli; discontinue the opioid and consider use of naloxone (McCaffery, 1997).

If respiratory depression is suspected and the opioid dose is withheld, the patient may be physically stimulated by shaking or using a loud sound, along with reminders every few minutes to breathe deeply. If this is ineffective, naloxone (Narcan), an opioid antagonist that reverses the respiratory-depressant effect of an opioid, can be used. Naloxone is administered intravenously very slowly. Within 1 to 2 minutes, the patient usually opens his or her eyes and is able to respond to the nurse. When the patient is alert again and the respiratory rate is greater than 9 breaths/min, the opioids may be resumed (McCaffery & Pasero, 1999).

Many myths and irrational fears persist concerning the use of opioid analgesics. Patients and caregivers cite fear of addiction as a reason for ineffective treatment of pain. Because of this, nurses are concerned about administering prescribed doses of opioids, physicians underprescribe pain medication, and patients refuse or take less than prescribed doses of the drugs. **Physical dependence** and tolerance are frequently confused with **addiction**. The accompanying box defines these terms. McCaffery and Ferrell (1999) report that fewer than 1% of patients with pain become addicted to opioids, yet many nurses surveyed seriously overestimated the likelihood of addiction when opioids are used for pain relief. Opioid tolerance and physical addiction are common with chronic opioid use, but this is not the same as the psychological dependence of addiction. The tolerance and physical dependence that can occur after 4 weeks of regular opioid use and result in a decrease in analgesic effect can be treated by increasing the dose until pain control is again apparent. AHCPR and the American Pain Society both recommend that opioid doses that are safe but ineffective can be increased by 25% to 50% to control pain that is unrelieved (McCaffery & Ferrell, 1999).

Adjuvant Drugs

Adjuvant drugs or analgesics are used to enhance the effect of opioids by providing additional pain relief. They may also reduce side effects from prescribed opioids or lessen anxiety about the pain experience. Commonly used adjuvant drugs include corticosteroids, anticonvulsants, and antidepressants.

General Principles for Administering Analgesics
Goals for Pain Relief

When using medications for pain relief, the nurse must first assess the patient's pain and understand the patient's goals for pain relief. In the home as well as in acute care settings, nurses provide quality nursing care when they empower patients to take charge of their pain relief measures. The following guidelines are recommended for effective, individualized pain management in any setting (McCaffery & Beebe, 1989; McCaffery, 1994):

- Review the pain scale of choice thoroughly.
- Discuss the benefits of using a pain scale.

Addiction, Physical Dependence, and Tolerance

Addiction or psychological dependence: pattern of compulsive drug use characterized by continued craving for an opioid and the need to use the opioid for effects other than pain relief

Physical dependence: physical phenomenon in which the body physiologically adapts to the presence of an opioid and suffers withdrawal symptoms if the opioid is suddenly withdrawn

Tolerance: a common physiologic result of chronic opioid use; it means that a larger dose of opioid is required to maintain the same level of analgesia

From AHCPR, Management of Cancer Pain Guideline Panel: Management of Cancer Pain. (1994). *Clinical practice guideline.* AHCPR Pub No 94-0592.Rockville, MD: Author.)

- Try various pain control measures.
- Use pain control measures before pain increases in severity.
- Ask the patient what has proved effective for pain relief in the past.
- Select and modify pain control measures based on the patient's response.
- Encourage the patient to try the pain treatment several times before labeling it ineffective.
- Be open-minded about alternative pain relief strategies.
- Be persistent.
- Be a safe practitioner.

Various organizations and groups have made recommendations for pain control in a variety of settings. These include the American Pain Society, the National Institutes of Health National Center for Nursing Research, and the American Nurses Association. The AHCPR is the major federal agency responsible for health services research and has issued guidelines for management of acute pain and cancer pain (see Fig. 40-10 later in this chapter) accompanied by pain control plans that facilitate participation of patients and their families as members of the healthcare team. These guidelines reflect the most current information on pain control. The revised JCAHO standards ensure that pain management is a quality assurance issue in healthcare agencies (Pasero, Gordon, & McCaffery, 1999).

In the home, oral morphine is still the drug of choice to control chronic pain and moderate to severe acute pain. This method is less expensive and easy to administer but requires that the patient can swallow and retain food and fluids. Accurate documentation is imperative to determine effectiveness of the current regimen or the need to change pain control measures if relief is not obtained. Effective patient and family teaching is the cornerstone of pain relief therapy in the home.

Ongoing Assessment

Just as the pain experience of each patient is unique, so too is the response of each patient to a prescribed analgesic. The nurse continually needs to evaluate whether the medication is producing the desired analgesic effect; identify changes in the patient's condition (correction or worsening of pathology, increased drug tolerance) that necessitate changes in the analgesic agent, dose, or route of administration; and identify the development of side effects of the analgesic that may warrant its discontinuance. As long as the patient's pain exists, ongoing assessment and documentation of pain control is imperative. The flow sheet in Figure 40-8 is an example of a pain control record used in a home setting. Fundamental to this assessment is the knowledge of the basic action, doses, routes of administration, side effects, and administration guidelines of the analgesic being administered.

Timing

Timing is an important consideration when administering analgesics. To time analgesics appropriately, the nurse

Pain Control Record

This is a record of how your pain medicines are working. Please keep this record until you and your nurse/doctor find the dose and frequency of medicine that provides satisfactory pain relief for you most of the time. After that, you only need to keep this record when you have problems related to your pain medicines.

Name: _____ *Martin* _____ Date: _*Friday*_

GOALS Satisfactory pain rating: _*5*_ Activities: _*Sleep through the night; walk around the house*_

My pain rating scale:

0	1	2	3	4	5	6	7	8	9	10

No pain — Moderate pain — Worst possible pain

Directions: Rate your pain before you take pain medicine and 1 to 2 hours later.

Time:	Pain rating:	Medicine I took:	Side effects (drowsy, upset stomach?)	Other:
12:15am	6	30 MSIR	No	
3	6	30		can't sleep
5:15	5	30		
8:30	6	30 + ibuprofen + MS Contin		staying in bed
10:30	4			MS IR 45 8 p.m. MS Contin 150 mg
11	6	45		
12	3			

If Pain is greater than __*5*__ , or if you have other problems with your pain medicine, call:

Nurse: Name/phone ____*C. Adams*____ *555-1234*____

Doctor: Name/phone ____*Jones*____ *555-4321*____

May be duplicated for use in clinical practice. From McCaffery M, Pasero C: *Pain: Clinical manual*, p. 88. Copyright © 1999, Mosby, Inc.
This patient has been receiving the following analgesics ATC every day: ibuprofen, 400 mg qid; amitriptyline, 100 mg HS; MS Contin, 100 mg q12h (8 AM and 8 PM). His supplemental (breakthrough, rescue) dose is morphine immedite release (MS IR), 30 mg PO q2h. He usually takes two supplemental doses a day. This has relieved his pain to a 3 or less, and he has been able to sleep through the night uninterrupted by pain and walk around his home. The record reveals that his pain ratings are now greater than 3 and that he is taking supplemental doses every 3 to 4 hours. Pain keeps him awake and he stays in bed. The patient talks with the nurse at 10:30 AM. The nurse contacts the physician and the decision is to increase his morphine doses by 50% to 45 mg MS IR q2h and to MS Contin 150 mg q12h. (This dose of MS Contin requires five 30-mg tablets. However, depending on the tablet strength the patient has on hand, the MS Contin dose may be slightly more or less than 150 mg.) When an opioid dose is safe but ineffective, a 50% increase will usually produce a moderate increase in pain relief. When the patient takes more than two supplemental doses during a 12-hour period, the controlled-release should be increased.

Figure 40-8
Patient control record—patient example.

needs to know the average duration of action for the drug and time administration so that the peak analgesic effect occurs when the pain is expected to be most intense. For example, an analgesic would be offered before ambulating a patient postoperatively.

A p.r.n. (as needed) drug regimen has not proved effective for people experiencing acute pain. In the early postoperative period, when pain is expected, this protocol may result in an intense pain experience for the patient. Later, however, in the postoperative course, a p.r.n. schedule may be acceptable to relieve occasional pain episodes. Continuous intravenous infusion of opioids has proved effective for the relief of acute postoperative pain. Patient-controlled analgesia (PCA) and epidural analgesia are discussed later in the chapter.

The p.r.n. protocol is totally inadequate for patients experiencing chronic pain. Regular administration of analgesics, or ATC administration (around the clock at regularly scheduled intervals), has been shown to offer superior pain management for chronic cancer pain. Long-acting controlled-release oral morphine or use of a fentanyl patch have proved effective for this type of pain. **Breakthrough pain** (a brief flare-up of moderate to severe pain that occurs even when the patient is taking ATC medication for persistent pain) is treated more effectively with supplemental doses of an opioid taken on a p.r.n. basis rather that an increase in the dose of ATC medication (Kedziera, 1998). It is best if the rescue medication is the same as that used for the ATC dose. The U.S. Food and Drug Administration has recently approved an immediate-release version of transdermal fentanyl that is called oral transmucosal fentanyl citrate (OTFC; Actiq). The raspberry-flavored preparation that is molded on a stick has a rapid onset of analgesic action and a short peak effect (Pasero & McCaffery, 1999).

Pain Treatment Regimens

Acute Pain Management

The AHCPR guideline (1992) on acute pain management places strong emphasis on the need for aggressive, individualized strategies that can minimize or eliminate acute pain and promote positive patient outcomes. Preventing pain is easier than treating it once it has occurred; pain control options should be discussed with patients before surgery, and the patient's responsibility regarding reporting pain should be addressed. Additional nursing interventions that can eliminate acute postoperative pain include maintaining a steady serum level of the analgesic (PCA or epidural analgesia can help here), treating adverse reactions quickly and aggressively, encouraging use of nondrug complementary therapies as adjuncts to the medical regimen, and expecting incident pain and dealing with it (Faries, 1998).

Undertreatment of pain that accompanies procedures, whether performed in a hospital, home, or outpatient clinic, is a common occurrence. If there is any doubt about the likelihood of pain resulting from a procedure, analgesia should be provided. It may be necessary in some instances, if the patient is unable to communicate verbally,

to provide a method for the patient to indicate that pain is occurring during a procedure. A simple raising of a finger or hand or squeeze of a squeak toy can alert the caregiver that analgesia is needed (Pasero, 1998b).

Cancer or Chronic Pain Management

Individuals with cancer sometimes suffer needlessly from pain. This pain, surprisingly, remains undertreated in both children and adults, and nurses need to act as advocates for pain relief for these patients. The AHCPR guideline on management of cancer pain (1994) aggressively supports treatment of the chronic pain associated with this disease using pharmacologic and nonpharmacologic approaches. Bral (1998) lists the four major principles that guide treatment for this chronic pain:

- Give medications orally, if possible.
- Administer medication ATC rather than on a p.r.n. basis.
- Adjust the dose to achieve maximum benefits with minimal side effects.
- Allow patients as much control as possible over their medication regimen.

In an effort to alleviate unnecessary pain and suffering, the World Health Organization (WHO) has devised a three-step analgesic ladder (Fig. 40-9) that recommends the appropriate progression of drugs and dosages that should be used to manage chronic pain effectively. Emphasis is on individualizing treatment and using the analgesic ladder to provide attentive, aggressive pain relief. The AHCPR flow

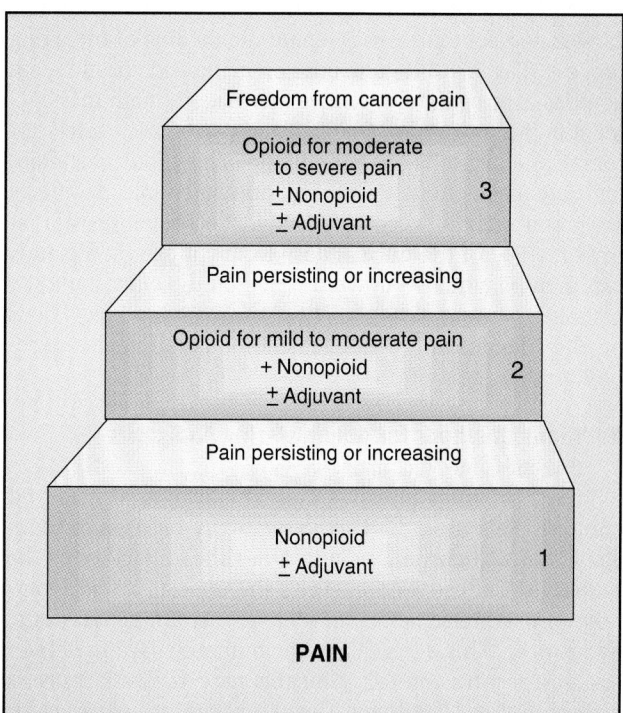

Figure 40-9

The WHO three-step analgesic ladder. (From World Health Organization. [1990]. Cancer pain relief and palliative care: Report of a WHO expert committee. WHO Tech Rep Series, No. 804. Geneva: WHO.)

chart (1994) for treatment of cancer pain (Fig. 40-10) incorporates these WHO recommendations.

Pain Treatment in Special Populations

Children

Effective pain management in children requires careful assessment; good communication between patient, family, and caregivers; and understanding of the actions and side effects of drugs used to relieve pain. The child is still the best source of information about the pain, and various assessment tools mentioned previously help to measure the intensity of the pain. In postoperative situations, children need analgesics ATC or by continuous infusion, and opioids are the drug of choice for moderate to severe pain. Pain management for cancer pain or chronic pain in children follows the prescription outlined in the WHO analgesic ladder. Withholding opioid drugs from children with cancer because of fear of addiction is unjustified because current knowledge does not indicate they are vulnerable to chemical dependence. Children also require pain management to minimize or alleviate the pain and distress associated with some procedures. Adequate education before the procedure and using drug and nondrug therapies to complement each other can take the pain and fear out of the experience. This is especially important for children with a chronic disease who must undergo multiple procedures as part of the treatment regimen (Faries, 1997).

Older Patients

Little research exists about pain management in older adults. Many healthcare providers, and older individuals as well, expect that pain is a natural outcome of the aging process. The AHCPR guidelines on acute and chronic pain emphasize a vigilant, attentive approach to pain management in this age group. Opioid drugs can be used safely for these patients as long as appropriate precautions are taken, pain is conscientiously assessed, and potential side effects are monitored. It is recommended that opioid doses start at 50% to 75% of the normal dose for a younger adult; they can then be adjusted upward based on the older patient's response (Pasero, 1998a). The accompanying box, Focus on the Older Adult, describes additional strategies pertinent to this age group.

Additional Methods for Administering Analgesics

Patient-Controlled Analgesia

PCA provides effective individualized analgesia and comfort. This drug delivery system may be used to manage acute and chronic pain in a healthcare facility or the home. PCA effectively relieves pain associated with operative procedures, labor and delivery, trauma situations, and cancer. This device is most commonly used to deliver analgesics intravenously, but the subcutaneous route is also an option. The most frequently prescribed drug for PCA administration is morphine. The PCA system consists of a portable infusion pump containing a reservoir or chamber for a syringe that is prefilled with the prescribed opioid. When the sensation of pain occurs, the patient pushes a button that activates the PCA device to deliver a small preset bolus dose of the analgesic. A lockout interval that is programmed into the PCA unit (usually, 5 to 10 minutes) prevents reactivation of the pump and administration of another dose during that period of time. The pump mechanism can also be programmed to deliver only a specified amount of analgesic within a given time interval (most commonly every hour or, occasionally, every 4 hours). These safeguards limit the possibility that a patient may overmedicate and provide time for the patient to evaluate the effect of the previous dose. Most pumps also have a locked safety system that prohibits any tampering with the device.

PCA has many advantages:

- Consistent analgesic blood level is maintained rather than the inconsistent analgesia obtained with periodic intramuscular injections, which results in sharp rises and falls of serum opioid levels.
- The analgesic is delivered intravenously so that absorption is faster and more predictable than with the intramuscular route.
- The patient is in charge of the pain management program.
- The patient tends to use less medication because it is self-administered before the pain becomes too severe.
- The patient is more satisfied and has improved pain relief.

An individual or child who is cognitively or physically unable to operate the PCA device may rely on a family member to act as pain manager. The nurse may also function in this role if a patient is incapable of managing PCA yet requires the consistent pain relief that this delivery system offers. A chemically dependent patient may qualify as a candidate for this pain relief strategy provided that expectations for its use are clearly stated. Careful documentation is required indicating specifically who is responsible and how the individual's pain is being managed.

Standardized nursing responsibilities are summarized in the accompanying Nursing Interventions Classification (NIC) box. Patients need instruction preoperatively if they are expected to use the PCA device postoperatively. Suitable candidates for this type of delivery system include individuals who are alert and capable of controlling the unit. Setting up the PCA system and ensuring that it is functioning properly are additional nursing activities. Figure 40-11 demonstrates a PCA device.

Epidural Analgesia

Epidural analgesia is being used more commonly to provide pain relief during the immediate postoperative phase (particularly after thoracic, abdominal, orthopedic, and vascular surgery) and for chronic pain situations. Epidural pain management is also being used more commonly with children with terminal cancer and with children undergoing hip, spinal, or lower extremity surgery

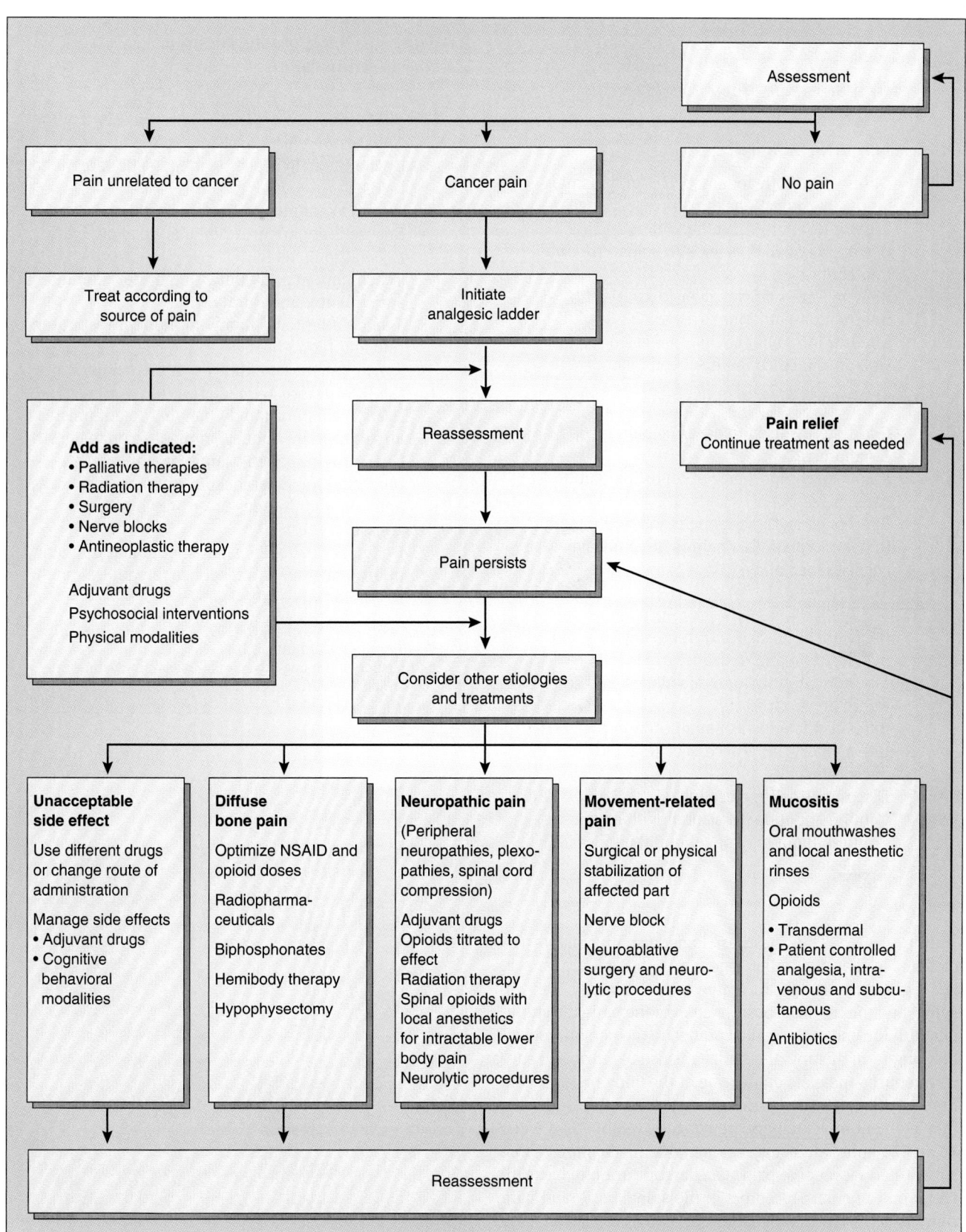

Figure 40-10
Flowchart: Continuing pain management in patients with cancer. (AHCPR: Management of Cancer Pain Guideline Panel, 1994.)

Focus on the Older Adult

Nursing Strategies for Pain Affecting Older Adults

Communication Difficulties

- Observe carefully for any behavioral manifestations or indications of pain (eg, change in activity level or grimacing with movement).
- Use open-ended questions to solicit information about pain.
- Rely on family or caregiver to assist with information-gathering process.
- Monitor for any behavior changes or confusion after medication has been taken.

Denial of Pain

- Clarify terms used to describe pain or discomfort.
- Emphasize importance of reporting pain to caregivers.
- Express concern about pain and willingness to help. Explain that pain is not a normal consequence of aging.

Altered Physiologic Response to Analgesics

- Be aware of dosage and frequency to avoid oversedation and toxicity.
- Monitor carefully for oversedation and respiratory depression.
- Explain side effects of analgesics to patient.
- Use memory aid if necessary to avoid overdosing.
- Discourage self-medication.
- Caution about use of alcohol with analgesics.
- Caution about driving when taking analgesics.

Using the Nursing Interventions Classification (NIC)

Patient-Controlled Analgesia (PCA) Assistance

- Collaborate with physicians, patient, and family members in selecting the type of narcotic to be used.
- Avoid use of meperidine (Demerol)
- Ensure that patient is not allergic to analgesic to be administered
- Teach patient and family to monitor pain intensity, quality, and duration
- Teach patient and family to monitor respiratory rate and blood pressure
- Teach patient and family members how to use the PCA device
- Assist patient or family member to administer an appropriate bolus loading dose of analgesic
- Consult with patient, family members, and physician to adjust lockout interval, basal rate, and demand dosage, according to patient responsiveness
- Document patient's pain, amount and frequency of drug dosing, and response to pain treatment in a pain flow sheet

McClosky, J., & Bulechek, G. (2000). *Nursing interventions classification (NIC)* (3rd ed.) (p. 496). St. Louis: C. V. Mosby. A full listing of nursing activities for each nursing intervention can be found in this book.

(Kubin, 1999). The anesthesiologist usually inserts the catheter in the midlumbar region into the epidural space. For temporary therapy, the catheter exits directly over the spine, and the tubing is positioned over the patient's shoulder with the end of the catheter taped to the person's chest. For long-term therapy, the catheter is usually tunneled subcutaneously and exits on the side of the body or on the abdomen (Fig. 40-12). Epidural catheters used for the management of acute pain are typically removed between 36 and 72 hours after surgery when oral medication can be substituted for relief of pain. The narcotic or opioid acts directly on the opiate receptors in the spinal cord, and pain relief is achieved with smaller doses and less severe side effects. The drug of choice is usually preservative-free morphine or fentanyl, and the medication can be administered as a single dose, by intermittent bolus injections, or by continuous infusion through a pump.

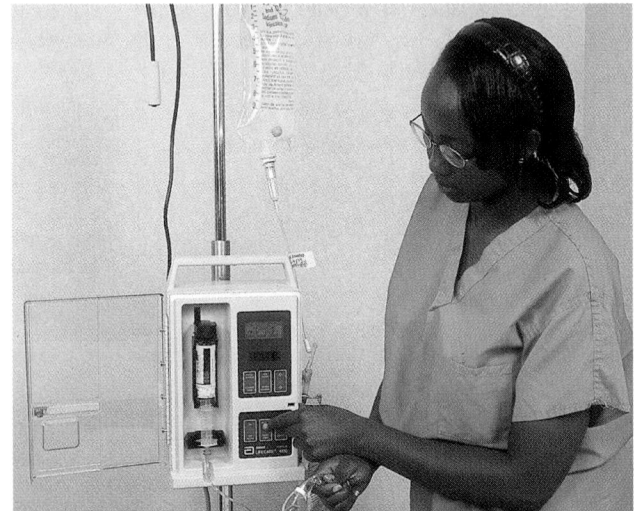

Figure 40-11

A patient-controlled analgesia unit allows the patient to regulate the intravenous infusion of small amounts of analgesic as needed. (Photo © B. Proud.)

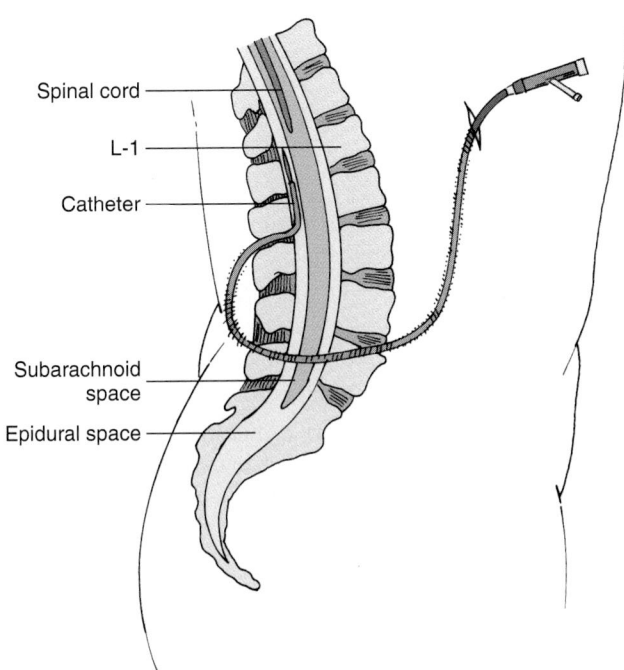

Figure 40-12
Placement of an epidural catheter for long-term use.

Nursing responsibilities vary among institutions but must include careful monitoring of the patient's response to therapy, with particular attention to the respiratory rate and pattern (refer to the accompanying Guidelines for Nursing Care for specific nursing interventions). Too much narcotic or a displaced catheter may allow the medication to have a depressant effect on the brainstem center, causing life-threatening respiratory depression. Other potential side effects include hypotension, pruritus, urinary retention, nausea and vomiting, and infection or contamination (Berkowitz, 1997).

Local Anesthesia

Anesthetic agents may be applied topically to the skin or mucous membranes or injected into the body to produce a temporary loss of sensation and motor and autonomic function in a localized area. The agents work by chemically blocking the nerve pathways involved in pain sensation and response and are sometimes called *nerve blocks*. Many people have experienced nerve blocks during dental work, when having a wound sutured, during delivery of a newborn, and for some minor surgical procedures. Nursing measures include noting any allergic responses the patient has had in the past to anesthetic agents, alerting the patient to the pain the initial injection of the anesthetic may cause if the physician does not numb the area first, offering emotional support to the patient during the procedure and observing for any untoward effects, and protecting the patient from injury until sensory and motor functions return. A topical anesthetic cream (such as EMLA, which contains lidocaine and

prilocaine) is usually an effective analgesic for children before painful procedures such as phlebotomy, spinal tap, or bone marrow aspiration (Pillitteri, 1999).

Teaching the Patient About Pain

A well-informed person can often cope better with the distress of pain and tends to experience less anxiety about pain. Teaching about pain should include family members so that they understand and may help the person in pain.

Following are examples of information to share with the patient and family to help them manage the pain experience:

- Review the purpose of a pain rating scale.
- Explain the specific pain rating scale that will be used.
- Discuss the concept of pain (functions, causes, types).
- Ask the patient to state two examples of pain that he or she has experienced.
- Have the patient practice using the pain rating scale on one of these examples.
- Help the patient set goals for comfort and optimal function or recovery (Pasero, 1997b).

Play may often be used effectively to discover a child's experience of pain and to teach the child how to cope with pain. Children are usually receptive to using dolls to act out pain experiences.

The Ethical/Legal Responsibility to Relieve Pain

Quality pain management results when patients have access to safe, effective pain relief measures. Healthcare providers, in addition to monitoring, delivering, and documenting administration of analgesics, also have responsibility to inform patients that effective pain relief is vital to their treatment. Patients also have the right to expect that their statements of pain will be heeded quickly. Institutions must assign and educate clinicians to address these issues in a timely, knowledgeable manner. The Rights of Patients With Pain displayed in the accompanying box recognizes the multidimensional aspects of the pain experience and an individual's right to have pain controlled as soon as possible.

The Placebo Controversy

The term **placebo** comes from the Latin word meaning "I shall please." It consists of an inactive substance often given to satisfy a person's demand for a drug. The person, unaware of the placebo's properties, may find it to be effective for the relief of pain because of the perception that it will provide comfort and because of belief in the person administering it. It is an injustice to judge a person experiencing relief from pain after the use of a placebo as a malingerer or as mentally ill. Various researchers have reported that a positive placebo effect may be related to a physiologic response (release of endorphins) or the pa-

Guidelines for Nursing Care

Caring for Patients Receiving Epidural Opioids

Nursing Action	Rationale
Verify the physician's order for analgesia, drug preparation, and rate of infusion with another RN.	Verification provides for safe administration of the correct dose at the correct rate.
Keep an ampule of 0.4 mg of naloxone (Narcan) and a syringe at the bedside.	Naloxone reverses the respiratory depressant effect of opioids.
Label tubing and pump apparatus "For Epidural Infusion Only."	Labeling prevents inadvertent administration of other intravenous medications through this setup.
Assess and record sedation level (using a sedation scale) and respiratory status q 1 h for the first 24 hours followed by q 4 h intervals (or according to agency policy). Notify MD for the following: sedation rating of 3, ↓ in depth and respiratory rate below 8 breaths/min.	Opioids can depress respiratory center in the medulla. Change in level of consciousness is usually the first sign of altered respiratory function.
Keep head of bed elevated 30 degrees unless this is contraindicated.	Elevation of the patient's head minimizes upward migration of opioid in the spinal cord, thus decreasing risk for respiratory depression.
Record level of pain and effectiveness of pain relief.	Referencing helps in determining need for subsequent "breakthrough" pain medication.
Monitor urinary output and assess for bladder distention.	Opioids can cause urinary retention.
Assess motor strength q 4 h.	Catheter may migrate into the intrathecal space and allow opioids to block transmission of nerve impulses completely through the spinal cord to the brain.
Monitor for side effects (pruritus, nausea, and vomiting).	Opioids may spread into the trigeminal nerve causing itching or result in nausea and vomiting due to slowed gastrointestinal function or stimulation of a chemoreceptor trigger zone in the brain. Medications are available to treat these side effects.
Assess for signs of infection at the insertion site.	Inflammation or local infection may develop at the catheter insertion site. Strict aseptic technique and sterile dressing and tubing changes according to agency policy can prevent this complication.
Do not administer any other narcotics or adjuvant drugs without approval of clinician responsible for epidural injection.	Additional medication may potentiate the action of the opioid, thus increasing the risk for respiratory depression.

tient's cultural expectations, attitudes, health beliefs, or anticipation of a positive response.

The use of placebos, however, raises serious ethical questions. Is lying to a patient justifiable? A nurse who administers a placebo must be willing to risk the possible consequence of the patient becoming aware of the duplicity and then refusing to trust the nurse or any other healthcare professional again. Patients who feel themselves to be in pain are vulnerable. If such a patient discovers a seeming plot to trick him or her into feeling better, it is unlikely that the patient will respect or appreciate the good intentions of the physicians and nurses involved. The long-term effects of this practice far outweigh any of its benefits. The consensus of the AHCPR Management of Cancer Pain Guideline Panel (1994) also clearly states that placebos should *not* be used in the management of cancer pain. Two nursing organizations, the Oncology Nursing Society and the American Nurses Association, oppose placebo use, and this practice may even violate state board of nursing policies (McCaffery, Ferrell, & Pasero, 1998). The nurse has firm legal and ethical grounds for refusing to administer a placebo.

The Rights of Patients With Pain

A Bill of Rights for People With Pain

1. I have the right to have my reports of pain accepted and acted on by healthcare professionals.
2. I have the right to have my pain controlled, no matter what its cause or how severe it may be.
3. I have the right to be treated with respect at all times. When I need medication for pain, I should not be treated like a drug abuser.

May be duplicated for use in clinical practice. From McCaffery, M., & Pasero, C. (1999). *Pain: Clinical manual* (p. 13.). Copyright © 1999, Mosby, Inc. St. Louis.

EVALUATING

As soon as a pain problem is identified and a treatment plan developed and implemented, evaluation becomes ongoing. Evaluation is directed toward the changing nature of the pain experience, the treatment modalities (pain management program), and the patient's and family's response to the plan of care, all of which overlap.

The Pain Experience

The pain the patient is experiencing may change in many ways, and the nurse must be careful not to make a judgment about this too quickly. For example, if the pain lessens in intensity or disappears, it may mean that the underlying cause of the pain is diminished or absent and that treatment should be stopped, or it may mean that the pain management program is effective and should be continued. When pain intensity increases, it may simply indicate the need for more aggressive therapy, or it may be a warning that the underlying pathology has changed or worsened and that new medical intervention is required. Often, a new problem amenable to treatment is masked by "old pain," and its detection may be delayed to the point that treatment is useless.

Treatment Modalities

The use of both noninvasive and invasive therapies must be continually evaluated to determine whether they are the best possible means the patient could use to obtain pain relief and whether they are effective with only minimal risk to the patient. Too often, a patient stays with the first analgesic prescribed without questioning whether it is the most effective drug for the particular pain, whether the dosage and timing guidelines are correct for the patient, and whether the analgesic is perhaps producing annoying or even harmful side effects that another drug would not produce. Similarly, one patient may take to progressive relaxation exercises and find them helpful, whereas another patient may obtain similar benefits from a daily walking program. Nursing time spent evaluating the effectiveness of each pain relief therapy is well spent and results in a pain management program that is truly individualized to the patient.

Patient and Family Response

Ultimately, the plan of care is unsuccessful unless the patient and family are satisfied with the results. A successful plan of care results in the achievement of specified patient goals that the patient values. Whenever possible, nursing care should terminate when the patient and family can independently direct the pain management program with the assistance of appropriate resources. See the Applying Learning to Practice and Nursing Plan of Care boxes.

APPLYING LEARNING TO PRACTICE

Patient Care Study

Carla Potter is a 26-year-old white woman. She is unmarried and has no children. She is employed at a large company as a computer programmer. During the past 7 months, she has been experiencing periodic fatigue, anxiety, irritability, depression, and mood swings. Her general health is excellent. The nurse practitioner at the gynecologist's office believes Ms. Potter may be suffering from premenstrual syndrome. The nurse practitioner who interviewed Ms. Potter noted the following data:

- Patient has generalized discomfort—fatigue, anxiety, irritability, depression, and mood swings—about 1 week before her menses; discomfort subsides after onset of menses.
- Discomforts are believed to be heightened by stress at work but do not depend on this. Patient denies any new or unusual stress in life but believes symptoms are affecting her job performance and relationships.
- Patient relates history of "bad cramps" ever since periods started. Patient lacks knowledge of appropriate dietary and stress management techniques.
- Patient relates she has occasionally taken some of her friend's "tranquilizers" to ease her through a bad day—but she prefers not to take medication.

Courtesy of Ruth E. Gordon, RNC, CRNP, DEd, Assistant Professor, Department of Nursing, Millersville University, Millersville, PA

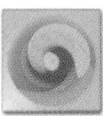

NURSING PLAN OF CARE
for Ms. Potter

Nursing Diagnosis   Ineffective Individual Coping related to discomforts of premenstrual symptoms as manifested by reports of fatigue, anxiety, irritability, depression, and mood swings

Expected Outcome   By the next monthly assessment, 10/30/01, patient will:
* Use relaxation techniques during periods of anxiety

Nursing Interventions	Rationale	Evaluative Statement
Assess patient's knowledge of relaxation techniques and motivation to use them.	Effective use of relaxation techniques requires a motivated patient.	10/30/01 Goal partially met, patient used relaxation techniques during two periods of anxiety. Was driving on expressway during another period of anxiety, which made relaxation difficult.
Instruct patient regarding the use of progressive relaxation exercises and controlled breathing during periods of anxiety. For example, "Find a quiet, comfortable place and sit down. Consciously contract and relax the muscles of the whole body starting at the head and neck and working down to the feet until completely relaxed. At the same time, take slow, rhythmic breaths. Continue until anxiety passes."	Relaxation and controlled breathing are used to decrease anxiety and increase coping mechanisms.	*R. Gordon, RNC*

Expected Outcome   By the next monthly assessment, 10/30/01, the patient will:
* Use a meal plan that includes three balanced meals per day and excludes caffeine, sugar, and sodium

Nursing Interventions	Rationale	Evaluative Statement
Assess patient's nutritional intake. Have patient identify current food preferences high in caffeine, sugar, and sodium and discuss substitutes. Teach patient rationale for decreasing intake of caffeine, sugar, and sodium.	Refined sugar and caffeine contribute to feelings of tension and irritability. Sodium contributes to water retention in the body.	10/30/01 Goal met. Patient used meal plan for three balanced meals per day and eliminated all sugar, caffeine, and sodium from diet.
Instruct patient in developing a meal plan that includes three balanced meals per day.	Balanced meals provide optimal nutrition.	*R. Gordon, RNC*

Expected Outcome   By the next monthly assessment, 10/30/01, the patient will:
* Incorporate exercise into routine

Nursing Interventions	Rationale	Evaluative Statement
Assess value patient attaches to physical fitness and regular periods of aerobic exercise; explore preferences.	Exercise can alleviate symptoms of depression, tension, anxiety, fatigue, and irritability. Exercise also serves as a distraction from discomforts.	10/30/01 Goal met. Patient includes daily brisk walk around her neighborhood in her routine.
Instruct patient in use of regular daily exercise; design exercise prescription.	The fitness produced by regular exercise contributes to self-esteem.	*R. Gordon, RNC*

(continued)

NURSING PLAN OF CARE (Continued)
for Ms. Potter

Expected Outcome	By the next monthly assessment, 10/30/01, the patient will:
	• Supplement her diet with 50 mg of vitamin B_6 daily

Nursing Interventions	Rationale	Evaluative Statement
Instruct patient on daily use of vitamin B_6.	Vitamin B_6 may be effective in relieving symptoms of irritability, fatigue, and depression.	10/30/01 Goal met. Patient supplements her diet daily with 50 mg of vitamin B_6.
		R. Gordon, RNC

Expected Outcome	By the next monthly assessment, 10/30/01, the patient will:
	• Continue use of daily record of premenstrual syndrome (PMS) symptoms

Nursing Interventions	Rationale	Evaluative Statement
Instruct patient to continue use of daily record of PMS symptoms throughout the menstrual cycle.	Record keeping allows evaluation of the effectiveness of care plan.	10/30/01 Goal met. Patient continued daily record, which illustrated drastic reduction in occurrence of PMS symptoms. Patient expressed delight in greater feeling of control she now has over how she feels. "I never realized that so many things affect my comfort level and health."
		R. Gordon, RNC

Sample Documentation	8/13/01 Nursing

Consultation with patient regarding apparent symptoms of PMS. She stated she experiences fatigue, anxiety, irritability, depression, and mood swings about 1 week before her menses. She states these symptoms interfere with her job performance and relationships. She also states that these symptoms seem to subside after onset of her menses. Patient admits to use of tranquilizers but prefers not to use medication. Advised patient to keep daily record of symptoms for one complete menstrual cycle. Patient indicated understanding of all instructions. She will return to office after completion of daily record for its analysis and to begin treatment, if indicated.

R. Gordon, RNC

Learning Outcomes

After completing this chapter, the learner should be able to accomplish the following:

1. Define the key terms used in the chapter.

acute pain	neuropathic pain
addiction	neurotransmitters
allodynia	nociceptive
analgesic	opioid
breakthrough pain	pain threshold
chronic pain	pain tolerance
cutaneous pain	phantom pain
dynorphin	physical dependence

endorphins	placebo
enkephalins	psychogenic pain
exacerbation	referred pain
gate control theory	remission
intractable	somatic pain
neuromodulators	visceral pain

2. Describe specific elements in the pain experience.
3. Compare and contrast acute and chronic pain.
4. Identify factors that may affect an individual's pain experience.
5. Obtain a complete pain assessment using appropriate interviewing and physical assessment skills.

6. Develop nursing diagnoses that correctly identify pain problems and demonstrate the relation between pain and other areas of human functioning.
7. Demonstrate the correct use of nonpharmacologic pain relief measures.
8. Administer analgesic agents safely to produce the desired level of analgesia without causing undesirable side effects.

9. Collaborate with the members of other health disciplines using different treatment modalities to promote pain relief.
10. Use teaching and counseling skills to empower patients to direct their own pain management programs.

Critical Thinking Exercises

1. Interview a nurse who specializes in pain management. Ask the nurse to describe the various physiologic and emotional responses to pain that she has observed in patients with acute and chronic pain. Question her about the different nursing interventions most likely to be effective for patients in general experiencing either acute or chronic pain. Inquire about specific pain management information and guidelines that she usually includes in discharge planning and teaching.
2. Consider what you personally believe about pain: what it is, what causes it, what is most likely to relieve it. Determine how pain is currently being managed within the tradition of Western medicine and what role nursing plays in keeping patients pain free. Visit nontraditional health centers where practitioners use a variety of noninvasive pain relief modalities, such as acupressure, relaxation techniques, imagery, and massage. In what ways, if any, has this new learning experience modified your beliefs about pain? Will it change your ability to design effective pain management regimens for your patients?

Study Questions

1. Abdominal pain that is difficult to localize is most likely categorized as
   a. causalgia
   b. visceral
   c. superficial
   d. psychogenic
2. Pain that is transmitted to a cutaneous site different from where it originates is termed
   a. transient pain
   b. superficial pain
   c. phantom pain
   d. referred pain
3. A patient who has fallen and injured his or her wrist carefully cradles it with the other hand. This response to pain is referred to as
   a. behavioral
   b. affective
   c. physiologic
   d. involuntary
4. To help relieve her pain, Ann concentrates on a favorite vacation setting. This is known as
   a. distraction
   b. relaxation
   c. recall
   d. imagery
5. Intractable pain is best described as being
   a. intermittent in nature
   b. resistant to treatment
   c. excruciating
   d. widespread

6. According to the gate control theory of pain, an effective nursing intervention for a patient with lower back pain is
   a. encouraging regular use of analgesics
   b. applying a K-pad to the area at prescribed intervals
   c. reviewing the pain experience with the patient
   d. ambulating the patient after medicating him or her
7. A physiologic response to moderate pain is
   a. increased blood pressure
   b. restlessness
   c. decreased pulse rate
   d. protection of the painful area
8. Mrs. Young is receiving ATC medication for treatment of terminal cancer. She has recently reported several episodes of breakthrough pain. What treatment is most effective to manage these sudden flare-ups of pain?
   a. Increasing the dose of her ATC medication.
   b. Restricting her physical activity.
   c. Nothing more can be done since her cancer is terminal.
   d. Supplementing with doses of a short-acting opioid.
9. When assessing pain in a child, the nurse needs to be aware that
   a. immature neurologic development results in reduced sensation of pain
   b. inadequate or inconsistent relief of pain is widespread

c. reliable assessment tools are currently unavailable

d. narcotic analgesic use should be avoided

10. Mr. Wright is recovering from abdominal surgery. When the nurse assists him to ambulate, she observes that he grimaces, moves stiffly, and becomes pale. She is aware that he has consistently refused his pain medication. A priority nursing diagnosis would be

   a. Acute Postoperative Pain related to fear of taking prescribed medications

   b. Impaired Physical Mobility related to surgical procedure

   c. Anxiety related to outcome of surgery

   d. Risk for Infection related to surgical incision

11. When planning strategies for pain control in older patients, the nurse should be aware that

   a. pain is a natural outcome of the aging process

   b. sensitivity to pain increases with age

   c. narcotic use should be avoided

   d. denial of pain may occur

12. Chronic pain is most effectively relieved when analgesics are administered

   a. on a p.r.n. (as needed) basis

   b. conservatively

   c. around the clock (ATC)

   d. intramuscularly

13. Using a placebo for pain control is

   a. a widespread practice

   b. consistently effective

   c. deceptive and unethical

   d. justified to determine whether the pain is real

14. The patient receiving epidural analgesia requires careful monitoring to prevent the occurrence of

   a. pruritus

   b. urinary retention

   c. nausea and vomiting

   d. respiratory depression

15. When assessing a patient receiving a continuous opioid infusion, the nurse immediately notifies the physician when the patient has

   a. a respiratory rate of 10 with respirations of normal depth

   b. a sedation level of 4

   c. mild confusion

   d. reported constipation

Answers With Rationale

1. The correct response is *b*. Visceral pain is poorly localized and can originate in body organs in the abdomen. Causalgia is pain that occurs in the area of injured peripheral nerves, whereas cutaneous pain is superficial and usually involves the skin or subcutaneous tissue. When a physical cause for the pain cannot be identified, it is known as psychogenic pain.

2. The correct response is *d*. Referred pain is perceived in an area distant from its point of origin, whereas transient pain is brief and passes quickly. Superficial pain originates in the skin or subcutaneous tissue. Phantom pain may occur in a person who has had a body part amputated, either surgically or traumatically.

3. The correct response is *a*. Protecting or guarding a painful area is a behavioral response. Affective responses are psychological ones, and examples of a physiologic or involuntary response would be increased blood pressure and dilation of the pupils.

4. The correct response is *d*. Imagery is a mind–body interaction that decreases pain sensation by focusing on pleasurable images. Distraction involves preoccupation with other things to relieve pain, and relaxation is a technique that reduces skeletal muscle tension and lessens anxiety. Recall is not a noninvasive relief measure.

5. The correct response is *b*. Intractable pain is severe pain that is resistant to relief measures. The other terms do not describe this resistance to treatment.

6. The correct response is *b*. Nursing measures such as applying warmth to the lower back stimulate the large nerve fibers to close the gate and block the pain. The other choices do not involve attempts to stimulate large nerve fibers that interfere with pain transmission as explained by the gate control theory.

7. The correct response is *a*. Increased blood pressure is a physiologic or involuntary response to moderate pain, whereas decreased pulse rate occurs when pain is severe and deep. Restlessness and protection of the painful area are behavioral responses.

8. The correct response is *d*. Breakthrough pain is best addressed by administering a short-acting opioid similar to her ATC medication. Increasing the dose of her ATC medication also increases her risk for developing adverse effects. All pain can be treated effectively, and limiting physical activity will not affect her breakthrough pain but may negatively effect her current lifestyle and self-esteem.

9. The correct response is *b*. Healthcare personnel are only now becoming aware of pain relief as a priority for children in pain. The evidence supports the fact that children do indeed feel pain, and reliable assessment tools are available specifically for use with children. Opioid analgesics may be safely used with children as long as they are carefully observed.

10. The correct response is *a*. Mr. Wright's immediate problem is his pain that is unrelieved because he refuses to take his pain medication for an unknown reason. The other nursing diagnoses are plausible but not a priority in this situation.

11. The correct response is *d*. Older people frequently deny pain because they view it as an ominous sign that may interfere with their independence. Pain sensitivity may

decrease with age, but even this assumption is unsafe, and it is not a natural outcome of the aging process. Opioid medications can be used if the older patient's response is carefully monitored and evaluated.

12. The correct response is *c*. The p.r.n. protocol is totally inadequate for patients experiencing chronic pain. ATN doses of analgesic are more effective, whereas conservative pain management for whatever reason may also prove ineffective. Intramuscular administration is not practical on a long-range basis for a patient with chronic pain.

13. The correct response is *c*. Using a placebo to control pain creates distrust in the nurse–patient relationship and is considered unethical behavior. It is not a widespread practice, is ineffective, and is never used to determine whether pain is real. Pain exists when the patient says it does.

14. The correct response is *d*. Too much of an opioid drug given by way of an epidural catheter or a displaced catheter may result in the occurrence of respiratory depression. Pruritus, urinary retention, and nausea and vomiting may occur but are not life-threatening.

15. The correct response is *b*. Sedation level is more indicative of respiratory depression because it usually precedes it. A sedation level of 4 calls for immediate action because the patient has minimal or no response to stimuli. A respiratory level of 10 with normal depth of breathing is usually not a cause for alarm. Mild confusion may be evident with the initial dose and then disappear; additional observation is necessary. Constipation should be reported to the physician, but is not the priority in this situation.

Bibliography

Acello, B. (2000). Meeting JCAHO standards for pain control. *Nursing, 30*(3), 52–54.

AHCPR, Acute Pain Management Guideline Panel (1992). *Clinical practice guideline, acute pain management: Operative or medical procedures and trauma.* AHCPR Pub. No. 920032. Rockville, MD: USDHHS.

AHCPR, Management of Cancer Pain Guideline Panel. (1994). *Clinical practice guideline, management of cancer pain.* AHCPR Pub. No. 940592. Rockville, MD: USDHHS.

American Pain Society Quality of Care Committee. (1995). Quality improvement guidelines for the treatment of acute pain and cancer pain. *Journal of the American Medical Association, 274*(23), 1874–1880.

Benesh, L., Szigeti, E., Ferraro, R., & Gullicks, J. (1997). Tools for assessing chronic pain in rural elderly women. *Home Healthcare Nurse, 15*(3), 207–211.

Berkowitz, C. (1997). Epidural pain control: Your job, too. *RN, 60*(8), 22–27.

Beyer, J., et al. (1992). The creation, validation, and continuing development of the Oucher: A measure of pain intensity in children. *Journal of Pediatric Nursing, 7*(5), 335.

Bral, E. (1998). Caring for adults with chronic cancer pain. *American Journal of Nursing, 98*(4), 27–32.

Davis, G. (1997). Chronic pain management of older adults in residential settings. *Journal of Gerontological Nursing, 23*(6), 16–22.

Derby, S. (1999). Opioid conversion guidelines for managing adult cancer pain. *American Journal of Nursing, 99*(10), 62–65.

Faries, J. (1997). Controlling pain: Assessing pediatric pain. *Nursing, 27*(8), 18.

Faries, J. (1998). Easing your patient's postoperative pain. *Nursing, 28*(6), 58–60.

Feldt, K., Warne, M., & Ryden, M. (1998). Examining pain in aggressive cognitively impaired older adults. *Journal of Gerontological Nursing, 24*(11), 14–22.

Ferrell, B., Ferrell, B., & Rivera, L. (1995). Pain in cognitively impaired nursing home patients. *Journal of Pain and Symptom Management, 8*(10), 591–598.

Glickman, R., & Gracely, E. (1998). Therapeutic touch: Investigation of a practitioner. *The Scientific Review of Alternative Medicine, 1*(2), 5.

Juarez, R. 1997. Culture and pain. In *Quality of life: A nursing challenge, 4*(4), 86–90. Bala Cywyd, PA: Meniscus Educational Institute.

Kedziera, P. (1998). The two faces of pain. *RN, 61*(2), 45–46.

Kettelman, K. (1999). Why give more morphine to a dying patient? *Nursing, 29*(11), 54–55.

Krieger, D. (1999). Therapeutic touch in hospice care. *American Journal of Nursing, 99*(4), 46.

Kubin, L. (1999). Managing pediatric epidural analgesia. *Nursing, 29*(2), 24-1–24-4.

Loeb, J. (1999). Pain management in long-term care. *American Journal of Nursing, 99*(2), 48–52.

Love, G. (2000). Electrifying news about iontophoresis. *Nursing, 30*(1), 48–49.

Maxwell, J. (1997). The gentle power of acupressure. *RN, 60*(4), 53–56.

McCaffery, M. (1979). *Nursing management of the patient with pain* (2nd ed.). Philadelphia: J. B. Lippincott.

McCaffery, M. (1994). Home health care update 94. Pain control: Keeping current. *Nursing, 24*(6), 51–52.

McCaffery, M. (1997). Pain management handbook. *Nursing, 27*(4), 42–45.

McCaffery, M., & Beebe, A. (1989). *Pain: Clinical manual for nursing practice.* St. Louis: C. V. Mosby.

McCaffery, M., Ferrell, B., & Pasero, C. (1998). When the physician prescribes a placebo. *American Journal of Nursing, 98*(1), 52–53.

McCaffery, M., & Ferrell, B. (1999). Opioids and pain management: What do nurses know? *Nursing, 29*(3), 48–52.

McCaffery, M., & Pasero, C. (1999). *Pain clinical manual* (2nd ed.). St. Louis: C. V. Mosby.

McClosky, J., & Bulechek, J. (1996). *Nursing interventions classification (NIC)* (2nd ed.). St. Louis: C. V. Mosby.

Melzak, R., & Wall, P. (1968). Gate control theory of pain. In A. Soulairac, J. Cahn & J. Carpentier (Eds). *Pain: Proceedings of the international association on pain.* Baltimore: Williams & Wilkins.

North American Nursing Diagnosis Association. (1999). *NANDA nursing diagnosis: Definitions & classification: 1999–2000.* Philadelphia: Author.

Parke, B. (1998). Realizing the presence of pain in cognitively impaired older adults. *Journal of Gerontological Nursing, 24*(6), 21–28.

Pasero, C. (1997a). Using local anesthetics to control procedural pain. *American Journal of Nursing, 97*(1), 17–18.

Pasero, C. (1997b). Pain ratings: The fifth vital sign. *American Journal of Nursing, 97*(2), 15–16.

Pasero, C. (1997c). Using the faces scale to assess pain. *American Journal of Nursing, 97*(7), 19–20.

Pasero, C. (1997d). Overcoming obstacles to pain assessment in elders. *American Journal of Nursing, 97*(9), 20.

Pasero, C. (1998a). How aging affects pain management. *American Journal of Nursing, 98*(6), 12–13.

Pasero, C. (1998b). Procedural pain management. *American Journal of Nursing, 98*(7), 18–20.

Pasero, C. (1998c). Is laughter the best medicine? *American Journal of Nursing, 98*(12), 12–14.

Pasero, C., Gordon, D., & McCaffery, M. (1999). JCAHO on assessing and managing pain. *American Journal of Nursing, 99*(7), 22.

Pasero, C., & McCaffery, M. (1999). Providing epidural analgesia. *Nursing,29*(8), 34–39.

Peloso, P. (2000). NSAIDs: A Faustian bargain. *American Journal of Nursing, 100*(6), 34–39.

Peterson, A. (1997). Analgesics. *RN, 60*(4), 51.

Phipps, W., Sands, J., & Marek, J. (1999). Medical-surgical nursing (6th ed.). St. Louis: C. V. Mosby.

Pillitteri, A. (1999). *Maternal & child nursing* (3rd ed.). Philadelphia: Lippincott Williams & Wilkins.

Porth, C. (1998). *Pathophysiology* (5th ed.). Philadelphia: Lippincott Williams & Wilkins.

Purnell, L., & Paulanka, B. (1998). Transcultural health care. Philadelphia: F. A. Davis.

Rhiner, M., & Kedziera, P. (1999). Managing breakthrough pain: A new approach. *American Journal of Nursing, 99* (Suppl 3), 3–13.

Rimmer, L. (1998). What every home healthcare nurse should know about complementary therapy. *Home Healthcare Nurse, 16*(11), 760–764.

Rosa, L. Rosa, E., et al. (1998). A close look at therapeutic touch. *JAMA, 279*(13), 1005.

Snelling, J. (1990). The role of the family in relation to chronic pain: Review of the literature. *Journal of Advanced Nursing, 15*(7), 771–776.

Strevy, S. (1998). Myths & facts about pain. *RN, 61*(2), 42–44.

Strevy, S. (1999). Listen to the music. *Nursing, 29*(4), 32-6-32-8.

Vallerand, A. (1995). Gender differences in pain. *Image—The Journal of Nursing Scholarship, 27*(3), 235–237.

Ventura, M. (1999). VA initiative focuses on pain management. *RN, 62*(5), 16.

White, P., Phillips, J., Proctor, T., & Craig, W. (1999). Percutaneous electrical nerve stimulation (PENS): A promising alternative-medicine approach to pain management. *American Pain Society Bulletin, 9*(2), 1–7.

Young, D. (1999). Acute pain management protocol. *Journal of Gerontological Nursing, 25*(6), 10–20.

Zborowski, M. (1969). *People in pain*. San Francisco: Jossey-Bass.

Chapter 41
Nutrition

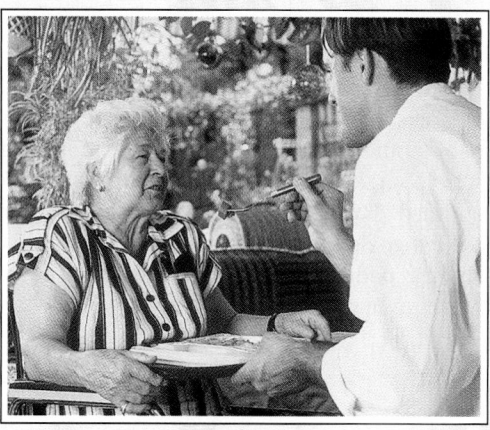

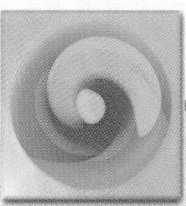

Thinking Critically About
Nursing's Blended Skills

Before reading this chapter, think about the types of skills you will need to meet the nutritional needs of the following people:

- Three-year-old Joey's mother tells you that she is at her "wits' end" trying to get him to eat a balanced diet. "My daughter ate whatever I placed in front of her. Joey will go a whole day eating only bananas or something else he likes. . . even when I threaten him!"

- At 5 feet 9 inches and 103 pounds, a 19-year-old college freshmen tells you that she feels and looks "fat" in spite of running 5 to 10 miles daily, lifting weights, and drastically reducing her nutritional intake.

- A 42-year-old male executive, newly diagnosed with high blood pressure and high cholesterol, confides that his health has been the last thing on his mind and that his health habits are less than admirable. "I usually eat on the run, often fast food, or big dinners with lots of alcohol. I can't remember the last time I worked out or did any exercise, unless running from my car to the train counts! I guess it's no wonder I've gained a few pounds over the years!"

- Another nurse tells you not to waste your time trying to feed Mrs. McLoughlin, a 92-year-old nursing home resident with dementia, because she clamps her mouth shut, spits out her food, or chokes each time anyone has tried. A review of her chart reveals a 20-pounds weight loss over the last 6 months.

What cognitive, technical, interpersonal, and ethical/legal skills do you think you will need to meet the needs of the patients described above?

Nutrition is a basic human need that changes throughout the life cycle and along the wellness–illness continuum. Food provides nutrition for both the body and the mind. Eating has evolved from being simply a necessity; it may be a source of pleasure, a pastime, a social event, a political statement, a religious symbol, a cultural emblem, or an integral component of medical treatment. As such, food, eating, and nutrition take on different meanings to different people, and changing a person's eating behaviors may be a difficult and slow process. Because nutrition is vital for life and health, and because poor nutrition can seriously decrease one's level of wellness, it is a vital component of nursing.

This chapter provides information about basic nutrition theory, focusing on the six classes of nutrients, energy balance, choosing an adequate diet, food patterns and habits, and factors that affect nutrition. Components of simple screening and in-depth nutritional assessments are outlined. Two sets of nursing diagnoses are provided, and patient goals for healthy nutrition are discussed. The concluding patient care study illustrates the significance of nutrition in nursing care.

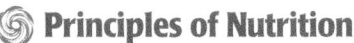 Principles of Nutrition

The science of **nutrition** encompasses the study of nutrients and how they are handled by the body as well as the impact of human behavior and environment on the process of nourishment. As such, this discipline involves physiology, psychology, and socioeconomics.

Nutrients are specific biochemical substances used by the body for growth, development, activity, reproduction, lactation, health maintenance, and recovery from illness or injury. Because the metabolic processes involved in these functions are complex, most nutrients work better together than they do alone. Also, nutrient needs change throughout the life cycle in response to changes in body size, activity, growth, development, and state of health.

Some nutrients are considered essential because they either are not synthesized in the body or are made in insufficient amounts; essential nutrients must be provided in the diet or through supplements. Essential nutrients that supply energy and build tissue (such as carbohydrates, fats, and protein) are referred to as *macronutrients*. *Micronutrients*, such as vitamins and minerals, are re-

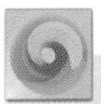

COGNITIVE SKILLS

- Basic knowledge about nutritional theory and the factors and variables that affect nutrition: How much does a 3-year-old need to eat to maintain nutritional balance? What is the best way to motivate 3-year-olds (or 42-year-olds!) to eat well?
- Knowledge about therapeutic nutrition (eg, anorexia: predisposing factors, clinical manifestations, effective treatment regimens, and treatment centers and resources; aging and dementia: ability to diagnose potential harms related to choking and to identify related interventions)

TECHNICAL SKILLS

- Strong nutritional assessment skills to diagnose nutritional alterations
- Competence in particular skills, such as how to perform intravenous therapy, the Heimlich maneuver, placement and maintenance of a feeding tube, and so forth

INTERPERSONAL SKILLS

- Strong people skills to establish trusting relationships with Joey, his mother, and the other patients

- Special interpersonal competence to help the college freshman and the executive to value making the life-style changes necessary to improve their nutritional status
- A good working relationship with colleagues to make sure that Mrs. McLoughlin's nutritional needs are met by all involved in her care

ETHICAL/LEGAL SKILLS

- First and foremost, a strong sense of accountability for the health and well-being of these individuals; a commitment to getting them the help they need to achieve their health goals—within the scope of your nursing responsibilities and available resources.
- A willingness to hold colleagues accountable for safe and good quality practice. If Mrs. McLoughlin's nutritional needs are not being met, this must be brought to everyone's attention, and a plan developed to redress this wrong.
- Knowledge of the ethical and legal principles that guide decision making about initiating or withholding artificial nutrition and hydration for someone like Mrs. McLoughlin.

quired in much smaller amounts to regulate and control body processes.

Nonessential nutrients do not have to be supplied through exogenous sources because they either are not required for body functioning or are synthesized in the body in adequate amounts. Some nutrients can be converted to others in the body. For instance, the body converts excess carbohydrates and protein into fat and stores them as triglycerides.

Of the six classes of nutrients, three supply energy (carbohydrates, protein, and lipids) and three are needed to regulate body processes (vitamins, minerals, and water).

Energy Balance

Energy in the diet is measured in the form of kilocalories, commonly abbreviated as **calories**, or cal. Only carbohydrates, protein, and fat provide energy; vitamins and minerals are needed for the metabolism of energy but do not provide calories. Total energy intake for a meal, a day, or longer can be calculated by using food composition tables: the values given for total calories for each food eaten can simply be added, or the grams of carbohydrate, protein, and fat for each food eaten can be added and multiplied by the appropriate calorie level (4, 4, and 9 cal, respectively).

Energy in the body is used to carry on any kind of activity, whether voluntary or involuntary. A person's total daily energy expenditure is the sum of all the calories used to perform physical activity, maintain basal metabolism, and digest, absorb, and metabolize food.

Basic Metabolic Requirements

Basal metabolism is the amount of energy required to carry on the involuntary activities of the body at rest, such as maintaining body temperature and muscle tone, producing and releasing secretions, propelling food through the gastrointestinal tract, inflating the lungs, and beating the heart. As the amount of energy used on physical activity declines, the proportion of calories used for basal metabolism increases; it accounts for more than half of most people's total energy requirements. Because of their larger muscle mass, males have a higher basal metabolic rate (BMR) than females. Other factors that increase BMR include growth, infections, fever, emotional tension, extreme environmental temperatures, and elevated levels of certain hormones, especially epinephrine and thyroid hormones. Aging, prolonged fasting, and sleep all decrease BMR. Most nutritionists agree that fasting or following a very-low-calorie diet (VLCD) defeats a weight loss plan because the body interprets this eating pattern as starvation and compensates by slowing down the resting metabolic rate, making it even more difficult to lose weight. BMR is about 1 cal/kg of body weight per hour for men and 0.9 cal/kg per hour for women.

Body Weight Standards

Ideal body weight (IBW) or healthy body weight is an estimate of optimal weight for optimal health. A general guideline, often called the *rule of thumb (ROT) method,* de-

termines ideal weight based on height. This formula is as follows:

For adult females:

100 lb (for height of 5 ft) + 5 lb for each additional inch over 5 ft

For adult males:

106 lb (for height of 5 ft) + 6 lb for each additional inch over 5 ft

(Add or deduct 10% from this figure based on body frame size.)

Using this method can result in unrealistically low figures for adults who are very short or very tall. (Height and weight tables commonly are used for infants and children.)

In the past, the 1983 Metropolitan Life Insurance Company height and weight table has consistently been the standard reference that nurses used for healthy body weight. The weight standards on the chart represent survey results of Americans who purchased life insurance and are adjusted according to height and frame size for the 25- to 59-year age bracket. Some difficulties with this measurement chart include the fact that minority populations are not represented, the calculated weights do not reflect body fat stores, and weights are calculated based on mortality statistics (Peckenpaugh & Poleman, 1999).

Although numerous tables and approaches have been devised for determining healthy body weight, many health experts now consider the body mass index (BMI) to be the most precise parameter. The BMI is a ratio of height to weight and more accurately reflects total body fat stores in the general population. The BMI does not differentiate according to sex, and is calculated in the following manner:

Using kilograms and meters:

$$\frac{\text{Weight in kilograms}}{\text{Height}^2 \text{ in meters}} \quad \begin{pmatrix} 2.2 \text{ lb} = 1 \text{ kg} \\ 39.37 \text{ inches} = 1 \text{ m} \end{pmatrix}$$

Using pounds and inches:

$$\frac{\text{Weight in pounds}}{\text{Height in inches}^2} \times 704.5$$

A quick method of determining BMI is displayed in Figure 41-1. According to these most recent guidelines published by the National Heart, Lung, and Blood Institute, a person with a BMI of 25 is considered overweight, whereas a BMI of 30 or greater indicates obesity. The first goal for individuals with a BMI of 25 to 29 should be to stop gaining weight, and if risk factors are present (eg, high blood pressure or high cholesterol), a weight loss of 10% is desirable. Many health practitioners use this more accurate weight calculation as an initial assessment of nutritional status.

Caloric Requirements

Just as healthy body weight or IBW can be determined in a variety of ways, so can a person's calorie requirements. One method appears in the accompanying box. After calorie requirements have been determined, adjustments can

Body Mass Index (BMI)														
	19	20	21	22	23	24	25	26	27	28	29	30	35	40
Weight (pounds)														
4'10"	91	96	100	105	110	115	119	124	129	134	138	143	167	191
4'11"	94	99	104	109	114	119	124	128	133	138	143	148	173	198
5'0"	97	102	107	112	118	123	128	133	138	143	148	153	179	204
5'1"	100	106	111	116	122	127	132	137	143	148	153	158	185	211
5'2"	104	109	115	120	126	131	136	142	147	153	158	164	191	218
5'3"	107	113	118	124	130	135	141	146	152	158	163	169	197	225
5'4"	110	116	122	128	134	140	145	151	157	163	169	174	204	232
5'5"	114	120	126	132	138	144	150	156	162	168	174	180	210	240
5'6"	118	124	130	136	142	148	155	161	167	173	179	186	216	247
5'7"	121	127	134	140	146	153	159	166	172	178	185	191	223	255
5'8"	125	131	138	144	151	158	164	171	177	184	190	197	230	262
5'9"	128	135	142	149	155	162	169	176	182	189	196	203	236	270
5'10"	132	139	146	153	160	167	174	181	188	195	202	207	243	278
5'11"	136	143	150	157	165	172	179	186	193	200	208	215	250	286
6'0"	140	147	154	162	169	177	184	191	199	206	213	221	258	294
6'1"	144	151	159	166	174	182	189	197	204	212	219	227	265	302
6'2"	148	155	163	171	179	186	194	202	210	218	225	233	272	311
6'3"	152	160	168	176	184	192	200	208	216	224	232	240	279	319
6'4"	156	164	172	180	189	197	205	213	221	230	238	246	287	328
	Normal						Overweight					Obese		

Height (left axis label)

Figure 41-1
Select your correct height, and move across the chart to your approximate weight. The appropriate body mass index is listed directly above this line. (From the National Heart, Lung, and Blood Institute, 1998.)

be made for weight gain or loss as needed. For instance, 1 lb (0.45 kg) of body fat equals about 3500 cal. Therefore, to gain or lose 1 lb (0.45 kg) in a week, daily calorie intake should be increased or decreased, respectively, by 500 cal (3500 cal divided by 7 days = 500 cal/d). Similarly, a weight gain or loss of 2 lb (0.9 kg) per week would require an adjustment of 1000 cal/d. Because it becomes increasingly difficult to plan an adequate diet as the calorie level drops, diets that result in more than a 2-lb (0.9-kg) weight loss per week are not recommended.

Energy Nutrients

Carbohydrates

Significance

Carbohydrates, commonly known as sugars and starches, are organic compounds composed of carbon, hydrogen, and oxygen. They serve as the structural framework of plants; the only animal source of carbohydrate in the diet is lactose, or "milk sugar."

The significance of carbohydrates cannot be overstated. Because they are relatively easy to produce and store, carbohydrates are the most abundant and least expensive source of calories in the diet worldwide. In fact, carbohydrate intake is correlated to income: as income increases, carbohydrate intake decreases and protein intake, a more expensive form of energy, increases. In countries where grains are the dietary staple, carbohydrates may contribute as much as 90% of total calories.

Classification and Metabolism

Depending on the number of molecules within the structure, carbohydrates are classified as either simple (monosaccharides and disaccharides) or complex (polysaccharides) sugars. Table 41-1 summarizes the sources, functions, and significance of dietary carbohydrates.

Carbohydrates are more easily and quickly digested than protein and fat. Ninety percent of carbohydrate intake is digested; the percentage decreases as fiber intake increases. All carbohydrates are converted to glucose so that they can be transported through the blood or used for energy. Glucose is an efficient fuel on which certain tissues, particularly the central nervous system, rely almost exclusively as an energy source. Glucose ingested in the diet is transported from the gastrointestinal tract, through the portal vein, to the liver. The liver stores glucose and regulates its entry into the blood. Hormones, especially insulin and glucagon, are responsible for keeping serum glucose levels fairly constant during both feasting and fasting.

Through a series of steps, cells oxidize (burn) glucose to provide energy, carbon dioxide, and water. Depending on a person's state of energy balance, the period between when carbohydrate is consumed and when it is used for energy may vary from minutes to months or longer. Unlike protein and fat, glucose is burned efficiently and completely and does not leave a toxic product for the kidneys to excrete.

When the supply of glucose exceeds what is needed for energy and to maintain serum levels, it is stored. If muscle or liver glycogen stores are deficient, glucose is con-

Method of Calculating Caloric Requirements

- Calculate the *resting energy equivalent* (REE), or the amount of calories necessary to maintain the body at rest. Because men usually have a greater muscle mass than women, their caloric requirements are slightly higher (1 cal/kg versus 0.9 cal/kg). A weight of 143 lb or 65 kg, is used for purposes of this calculation.

Male

65 kg × 1 cal/kg × 24 hr = 1560 cal/day

Female

65 kg × 0.9 cal/kg × 24 hr = 1404 cal/day

- Determine the calories needed for a specific activity level. The REE is multiplied by one of the following: light activity (REE × 0.55 to 0.65), moderate activity (REE × 0.65 to 0.7), heavy activity (REE × 0.75 to 1.0). Charts are available in most nutrition textbooks that define and give examples of each of the specific activity levels. For purposes of this calculation, 0.55 calories for light activity is used.

Male

1560 × 0.55 = 858 calories

Female

1404 × 0.55 = 772 calories

- Total the REE and calories needed based on activity level.

Male

1560 + 858 = 2418 calories

Female

1404 + 772 = 2176 calories

This is one method for calculating the energy requirements for a lightly active 143 pound man or woman.

(Adapted from Dudek, S. G. [1997]. *Nutrition handbook for nursing practice* [3rd ed.]. Philadelphia: Lippincott-Raven.)

verted to glycogen and stored (glycogenesis). Conversely, glycogen is broken down in time of need to supply a ready source of glucose (glycogenolysis). When glycogen stores are adequate, the body converts excess glucose to fat and stores it as triglycerides in adipose tissue.

Functions and Recommended Dietary Allowance

The primary function of carbohydrates is to supply energy. Except for undigestible fiber, all carbohydrates provide 4 cal/g, regardless of the source.

The **recommended dietary allowance (RDA)** of essential nutrients refers to recommendations for average daily amounts that healthy population groups should consume over time. Although an exact requirement for carbohydrates has not been established, at least 50 to 100 g is needed daily to prevent *ketosis* (an abnormal accumulation of ketone bodies that is frequently associated with acidosis). In terms of an optimal diet, most health experts recommend that carbohydrates provide 50% to 60% of the diet's total calories, mostly in the form of complex carbohydrates. Table 41-1 provides further information regarding the sources, functions, and significance of carbohydrates.

Protein

Significance

Protein is a vital component of every living cell. Within the human body, more than a thousand different proteins are made by combining various amounts and proportions of the 22 basic building blocks known as *amino acids*. Although amino acids, like carbohydrates, contain carbon, hydrogen, and oxygen, they differ in that amino acids also contain nitrogen. Nine amino acids are classified as essential because they cannot be synthesized in the body; the remaining amino acids are no less important, but because the body can make them if a supply of nitrogen is available, they are termed nonessential. Proteins are essential for the formation of all body structures, including genes, enzymes, muscle, bone matrix, and hemoglobin.

Classification and Metabolism

Dietary proteins may be labeled complete (high quality) or incomplete (low quality), based on their amino acid composition. *Complete proteins* contain sufficient amounts and proportions of all the essential amino acids to support growth, whereas *incomplete proteins* are deficient in one or more essential amino acids. Generally, animal proteins (eggs, dairy products, and meats) are complete, and plant proteins (grains, legumes, and vegetables) are incomplete. Because different sources of plant proteins lack different amino acids, a plant protein can be complemented and its quality made high by combining it with a different plant protein or by adding a small amount of an animal protein. Examples of complementary vegetable proteins include corn tortilla and refried beans and lentil rice soup. Complementary proteins that use a small amount of animal protein are cereal with milk, rice pudding, and a cheese sandwich.

Dietary protein is broken down into amino acid particles by pancreatic enzymes in the small intestine and are absorbed through the intestinal mucosa for transportation to the liver. In the liver, amino acids are recombined into new proteins or are released into the bloodstream for use in protein synthesis by tissues and cells. Excess amino acids are converted to fatty acids, ketone bodies, or glucose and are stored or used as metabolic fuel.

The body's protein tissues are in a constant state of flux: tissues are continuously being broken down (catabolism) and replaced (anabolism). *Nitrogen balance*, a comparison between catabolism and anabolism, can be measured by comparing nitrogen intake (protein intake) and nitrogen excretion (nitrogen lost in urine, urea, feces, hair, nails, and skin). When catabolism and anabolism are occurring at the same rate, as in healthy adults, the body is in a state of neutral nitrogen balance (ie, nitrogen intake equals nitrogen excretion). A positive nitrogen balance occurs when nitrogen intake is greater than excretion—for example, during periods of growth, pregnancy, lactation, and recovery from illness. A

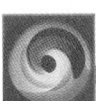

Table 41-1
Sources, Functions, and Significance of Carbohydrates, Protein, and Fat

Nutrient	Sources	Functions	Significance
Carbohydrates			
Simple sugars and starch	Fruits Vegetables Grains: rice, pasta, breads, cereals Dried peas and beans Milk (lactose) Sugars: white and brown sugar, honey, molasses, syrup	Provide energy Spare protein so it can be used for other functions Prevent ketosis from inefficient fat metabolism	Provide about 46% of the calories in the typical American diet; many believe carbohydrate intake should be increased to 50%–60% of total calories Low carbohydrate intake can cause ketosis; high simple sugar intake increases the risk for dental caries
Cellulose and other water-insoluble fibers	Whole wheat flour and wheat bran Vegetables: cabbage, peas, green beans, wax beans, broccoli, brussels sprouts, cucumber skins, peppers, carrots Apples	Absorb water to increase fecal bulk Decrease intestinal transit time	Is nondigestible; therefore, it is excreted Helps relieve constipation North Americans are urged to eat more of all types of fiber Excess intake can cause gas, distention, and diarrhea
Water-soluble fibers	Oat bran and oatmeal Dried peas and beans Vegetables Prunes, pears, apples, bananas, oranges	Slow gastric emptying Lower serum cholesterol level Delay glucose absorption	Help improve glucose tolerance in diabetics
Protein	Milk and milk products Meat, poultry, fish Eggs Dried peas and beans Nuts	Tissue growth and repair Component of body framework: bones, muscles, tendons, blood vessels, skin, hair, nails Component of body fluids: hormones, enzymes, plasma proteins, neurotransmitters, mucus Helps regulate fluid balance through oncotic pressure Helps regulate acid–base balance Detoxifies harmful substances Forms antibodies Transports fat and other substances through the blood Provides energy when carbohydrate intake is inadequate	Most North Americans consume twice the RDA (RNI) for protein Experts recommend that we eat less animal protein and more vegetable protein. Protein deficiency is characterized by edema, retarded growth and maturation, muscle wasting, changes in the hair and skin, permanent damage to physical and mental development (in children), diarrhea, malabsorption, numerous secondary nutrient deficiencies, fatty infiltration of the liver, increased risk for infections, and high mortality Except for elderly people, fad dieters, hospitalized patients, and people of low income, protein deficiency is rare in the United States and Canada

(*continued*)

Table 41-1 (Continued)

Nutrient	Sources	Functions	Significance
Fat	Butter, oils, margarine, lard, salt pork, salad dressings, mayonnaise, bacon Whole milk and whole milk products High-fat meats Nuts	Provides energy Provides structure Insulates the body Cushions internal organs Necessary for the absorption of fat-soluble vitamins	Fat supplies about 37% of total calories in the typical North American diet; experts suggest a reduction to 30% or less of total calories High-fat diets increase the risk for heart disease and obesity and are correlated with an increased risk for colon and breast cancers

(Dudek, S. G. [1997]. *Nutrition handbook for nursing practice* [3rd ed.]. Philadelphia: Lippincott-Raven.)

negative nitrogen balance, an undesirable state that occurs in situations such as starvation and the catabolism that immediately follows surgery, illness, trauma, and stress, indicates that more nitrogen is being excreted than consumed.

Functions and Recommended Dietary Allowance

The major function of protein is to maintain body tissues that break down from normal wear and tear and to support the growth of new tissue. Protein can be oxidized to provide 4 cal/g. Using protein for energy is more expensive both financially and physiologically than using carbohydrates; the nitrogen remaining after protein is metabolized burdens the kidneys and requires energy to be excreted. Like carbohydrates, protein consumed in excess of need can be converted to and stored as fat.

The RDA for protein for adults is 0.8 g/kg of desirable body weight, or about 44 g for the average woman and 56 g for the average man. Most health experts recommend that protein intake should contribute 10% to 20% of total caloric intake (Dudek, 1997). Table 41-1 summarizes the sources, functions, and significance of protein.

Hospitalized patients may be at risk for development of protein-calorie malnutrition (PCM) resulting from the stress of illness, surgery, or prolonged periods of time on simple intravenous solutions without oral intake. In developing countries, however, protein deficiency alone (kwashiorkor) or combined with calorie undernutrition (marasmus) is a leading cause of infant death. Signs and symptoms of protein deficiency include edema, retarded growth and maturation, mental apathy, muscle wasting, and changes in the hair and skin.

Fats

Significance

Fats in the diet, or **lipids**, are insoluble in water and, therefore, insoluble in blood. Like carbohydrates, they are composed of carbon, hydrogen, and oxygen. Ninety-five percent of the lipids in the diet are in the form of **triglycerides**, the predominant form of fat in food and the major storage form of fat in the body. Compound lipids (such as phospholipids, in which a lipid is combined with another substance) and derived lipids (such as cholesterol) constitute the remainder of the lipid intake.

Classification and Metabolism

Food fats contain mixtures of saturated and unsaturated fatty acids. The difference in degree of saturation depends on the amount of hydrogen in fat molecules. Saturated fats contain more hydrogen than unsaturated fats. Most animal fats are considered saturated and have a solid consistency at room temperature. Conversely, most vegetable fats are considered unsaturated, remain liquid at room temperature, and are referred to as oils. Saturated fats tend to raise serum cholesterol levels, whereas unsaturated fats lower serum cholesterol levels. When manufacturers partially hydrogenate liquid oils, they become more solid and more stable. This substance is referred to as *trans fat* (Liebman & Wootan, 1999). Trans fat raises serum cholesterol, and the U.S. Food and Drug Administration (FDA) may soon require that trans fat levels are included on all food labels.

Cholesterol is a fatlike substance found only in animal products. It is not essential that cholesterol be provided in the diet because the body synthesizes about twice as much cholesterol as most people in North America eat. Cholesterol is an important component of cell membranes and is especially abundant in brain and nerve cells. It also is used to synthesize bile acids and is a precursor of the steroid hormones and vitamin D. Although cholesterol serves many important functions in the body, high serum levels are clearly associated with an increased risk for atherosclerosis. To help lower serum cholesterol levels, researchers recommend limiting cholesterol intake, eating less total fat—especially saturated fat—eating more unsaturated fat, and increasing fiber intake, which increases fecal excretion of cholesterol.

Fat digestion occurs largely in the small intestine. Bile, secreted by the gallbladder, emulsifies fat to increase the surface area so that pancreatic lipase can break down fat more effectively. Through a complex series of events, most fats are absorbed into the lymphatic circulation with the help of a protein carrier and are transported to the liver. Of 100 g eaten, only about 3 g are excreted in the feces.

Functions and Recommended Dietary Allowance

Fats are the most concentrated source of energy in the diet, providing 9 cal for every gram. Fat increases the palatability of the diet (eg, to most people, filet mignon tastes better than flank steak) and has a high satiety value because it delays gastric emptying time. In the body, fat aids in the absorption of the fat-soluble vitamins and provides insulation, structure, and temperature control. Table 41-1 summarizes the sources, functions, and significance of fat.

Because fat can be synthesized in the body from carbohydrates and protein, an RDA for fat has not been established. Americans consume about 34% of their total caloric intake in the form of fat. Most experts agree that fat should not contribute more than 30% of the day's caloric intake, and saturated fat intake should be limited to less than 10% of total fat calories (Dudek, 1997).

Regulatory Nutrients

Vitamins, minerals, and water are regulatory nutrients because they are needed by the body for the metabolism of energy nutrients.

Vitamins

Vitamins are organic compounds needed by the body in small amounts. Most vitamins are active in the form of coenzymes, which, together with enzymes, facilitate thousands of chemical reactions in the body. Although vitamins do not provide energy (calories), they are needed for the metabolism of carbohydrates, protein, and fat. Because most vitamins are either not synthesized in the body or made in insufficient quantities, they are essential in the diet.

Vitamins are present in foods in only small amounts. Because vitamins may be destroyed by light, heat, and air and during preparation, fresh foods are higher in vitamins than processed foods. The exception is fortification, when vitamins that do not naturally occur in a food are added (eg, vitamin D–fortified milk).

In the United States, severe vitamin deficiencies are uncommon. Mild or subclinical deficiencies of vitamin A, vitamin C, folate, and vitamin B_6, however, may affect a significant proportion of the population, especially those who (1) are members of certain age groups or patient groups (infants, adolescents, pregnant and lactating women, and older people); (2) smoke, abuse alcohol, or use medications on a long-term basis; (3) are chronically ill, either physically or psychologically; or (4) are poor or finicky eaters, such as chronic dieters, strict vegetarians, and food faddists.

Vitamins are classified as either water soluble or fat soluble. *Water-soluble vitamins* include vitamin C and the B-complex vitamins. They are absorbed through the intestinal wall directly into the bloodstream. Although some tissues are able to hold limited amounts of water-soluble vitamins, they usually are not stored in the body. Deficiency symptoms are apt to develop quickly when intake is inadequate; therefore, a daily intake is recommended. Because water-soluble vitamins are not stored, amounts consumed in excess of need are excreted in the urine. Toxicities are not likely, although megadoses of certain water-soluble vitamins can be harmful.

Vitamins A, D, E, and K, the *fat-soluble vitamins*, are absorbed with fat into the lymphatic circulation; like fat, they must be attached to a protein to be transported through the blood. Secondary deficiencies of the fat-soluble vitamins can occur anytime fat digestion or absorption is altered, such as during malabsorption syndromes and pancreatic and biliary diseases. The body stores excesses of the fat-soluble vitamins mostly in the liver and adipose tissue. Because they are stored, a daily intake is not imperative, and deficiency symptoms may take weeks, months, or years to develop. Excessive intakes, particularly of vitamins A and D, are toxic.

Vitamins have been promoted as a "cure all" by many enthusiasts, and in fact, Americans spent about $5.7 billion in 1997 on vitamin supplements (Liebman, 1998). Many nutrition experts still believe that adequate amounts of most vitamins can be obtained from a healthy diet, but a growing body of scientific research indicates the benefits achieved with use of certain vitamin supplements. Although scrutiny and research continue about vitamin supplements and their long-term effects, most nutritionists agree that vitamins will never be a substitute for good nutrition and healthy lifestyle practices. Table 41-2 summarizes water- and fat-soluble vitamins.

Minerals

Minerals are inorganic elements found in all body fluids and tissues in the form of salts (eg, sodium chloride) or combined with organic compounds (eg, iron in hemoglobin). Some minerals function to provide structure within the body, whereas others help to regulate body processes. Because they are elements, minerals are not broken down or rearranged in the body but rather are contained in the ash that remains after digestion. Although excessive soaking and cooking in water can cause loss of minerals from food, minerals are commonly not destroyed by food processing. Calcium, phosphorus, and magnesium are considered *macrominerals* because they are needed by the body in amounts greater than 100 mg/day. Required intake of *microminerals*, or trace elements, is less than 100 mg/day. Iron, zinc, manganese, and iodine are examples of microminerals. Trace elements with an established RDA include iron, iodine, and zinc. Ranges of estimated safe and adequate daily intakes have been suggested for copper, manganese, fluorine, chromium, selenium, and molybde-

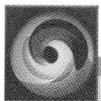

Table 41-2
Summary of Vitamins

Nutrient and Adult RDA*	Sources	Functions	Signs and Symptoms of Deficiency	Signs and Symptoms of Excess
Water-Soluble Vitamins				
Vitamin C (ascorbic acid) 60 mg (60–100 mg for smokers)	Citrus fruits, broccoli, green pepper, strawberries, greens	Collagen formation, antioxidant, enhances iron absorption	Scurvy, hemorrhaging, delayed wound healing	Kidney stones, scurvy on withdrawal, nausea, diarrhea
Vitamin B Complex				
Thiamin 1–1.4 mg	Pork, liver, whole and enriched grains, legumes	Coenzyme in key reactions that produce energy from glucose	Beriberi, mental confusion, fatigue	None known
Riboflavin 1.2–1.7 mg	Milk, organ meats, enriched grains, greens	Carbohydrate, protein, and fat metabolism	Ariboflavinosis—symptoms related to inflammation and poor wound healing	None known
Niacin 13–19 mg	Kidney, grains, lean meat, nuts	Carbohydrate, protein, and fat metabolism	Pellagra, dermatitis	Flushing and itching, nausea, vomiting
B_6 (pyridoxine) 1.6–2 mg	Yeast, banana, cantaloupe, broccoli, spinach	Coenzyme in protein, fat, carbohydrate metabolism	Anemia, CNS problems	Difficulty walking, numbness of feet and hands
Folate 180–200 µg	Green leafy vegetables, liver	RNA and DNA synthesis, formation and maturation of RBC	Macrocytic anemia: fatigue, weakness, pallor	None known
B_{12} (cobalamin) 2 µg	Only animal foods: organ meats, seafood	Coenzyme in protein metabolism and formation of heme portion of hemoglobin	Pernicious anemia (B_{12} deficiency related to impaired absorption due to lack of intrinsic factor)	None known
Pantothenic acid 4–7 mg	Liver, egg yolk, yeast	Carbohydrate, protein, and fat metabolism	None known	None known
Biotin 30–100 µg	Liver, egg yolk	Carbohydrate, protein, and fat metabolism	Deficiency produced by adding large amounts of raw egg white to a biotin-deficient diet	None known
Fat-Soluble Vitamins				
Vitamin A (retinol, retinal, retinoic acid) 800–1000 RE	Liver, carrots, egg yolk, fortified milk	Visual acuity in dim light, formation and maintenance of skin and mucous membranes	Night blindness, rough skin	Anorexia, loss of hair, dry skin, bone pain
Vitamin D (cholecalciferol, ergosterol) 5–10 µg	Sunlight, fortified milk, fish liver oils	Calcium and phosphorus metabolism, stimulates calcium absorption	Retarded bone growth, bone malformation	Excessive calcification of bones, renal calculi, nausea, headache
Vitamin E (tocopherol) 8–10 mg	Vegetable oils, wheat germ, whole grain products	Antioxidant, protects vitamin A, heme synthesis	Increased RBC hemolysis and macrocytic anemia in premature infants	Relatively nontoxic, although large doses can cause fatigue, diarrhea
Vitamin K 65–80 µg	Dark, green leafy vegetables; synthesized in intestines from gut bacteria	Synthesis of certain proteins necessary for blood clotting	Hemorrhagic disease of newborn, delayed blood clotting	Hemolytic anemia and liver damage with synthetic vitamin K

(Dudek, S. G. [1997]. *Nutrition handbook for nursing practice* [3rd ed.]. Philadelphia: Lippincott-Raven; and Williams, S. [1999]. *Essentials of nutrition and diet therapy* [7th ed.]. St. Louis: C. V. Mosby.)

num; no recommendations have been made for cobalt, nickel, vanadium, arsenic, and silicon. Macrominerals and microminerals are summarized in Table 41-3.

Water

As the major body constituent present in every body cell, water accounts for between 50% and 60% of the adult's total weight; infants have proportionately more water. About two thirds of the body's water is contained within the cells (intracellular fluid [ICF]); the remainder is called extracellular fluid (ECF), which includes all other body fluids, such as plasma and interstitial fluid. Total-body water and ECF decrease with age; ICF increases with an increase in body mass.

Water is more vital to life than food because it provides the fluid medium necessary for all chemical reactions, it participates in many reactions, and it is not stored in the body. Water acts as a solvent that dissolves many solutes, thereby aiding digestion, absorption, circulation, and excretion. Through evaporation from the skin, water helps to regulate body temperature. As a lubricant, water is needed for mucous secretions and between moving joints.

Sources of water in the diet include not only beverages but also solid foods, which contain from 10% to 98% water. Water is also produced through the metabolism of carbohydrates, protein, and fat. It leaves the body through urine, feces, expired air, and perspiration. Water intake (an average of 1500 to 3000 mL/day) usually equals water output. Water balance may be seriously affected when either intake (eg, in comatose states) or output (eg, in altered renal function, profuse perspiration, diarrhea, vomiting, fistulas, drainage tubes, hemorrhage, and severe burns) is altered.

How to Choose an Adequate Diet

An adequate diet provides a balanced intake of all essential nutrients in appropriate amounts; what constitutes an adequate diet is less obvious. Although a major problem in developing countries, malnutrition related to poor dietary intake is uncommon in the United States. Rather, nutritional concerns focus more on problems of overnutrition. Tools for planning or evaluating a diet for adequacy include the Food Guide Pyramid, the RDA, and dietary recommendations and guidelines issued from health and U.S. governmental agencies. The task of promoting health through proper nutrition has been made easier by labeling regulations that provide specific information about food contents and their comparison to recommended daily intakes.

Food Guide Pyramid

In response to the concerns of nutritionists and health officials, coupled with public interest in fitness and health, the U.S. Department of Agriculture developed the Food Guide Pyramid (Fig. 41-2). This graphic device places the grain and cereal group at the base of the pyramid, followed by the fruit and vegetable group, the meat and dairy groups, and a fat, oil, and sweets group at the peak. The intent of the pyramid is to emphasize the grain and cereal group as the basic food in the diet, with the less desirable groups playing a much smaller nutritional role. Each of these groups provides some nutrients, but all are required, in proper proportions, for a healthy diet.

The Food Guide Pyramid was designed to represent a total diet and to provide a firm foundation for health. It represents a focus on wellness and recognition of the role that food plays in prevention of such chronic disease threats as heart disease, high blood pressure, some types of cancer, diabetes, and obesity. The Food Guide Pyramid emphasizes the following (Peckenpaugh & Poleman, 1999):

Moderation: eat small amounts of those foods that are higher in fat and sugar
Variety: eat a number of different foods in each of the food groups
Balance: select foods that supply the required amounts of nutrients

Typical serving sizes are displayed in the box accompanying Figure 41-2.

Recommended Dietary Allowance

The RDA, prepared by the Committee on Dietary Allowances of the Food and Nutrition Board, represents average daily amounts of nutrients considered to be adequate to meet the known nutritional needs of practically all healthy people. Unlike a requirement, which is the amount of a nutrient needed to prevent a deficiency, an allowance has a safety factor built in to account for individual variations. Because the RDA is intended for populations and not individuals, some people may not be able to meet their individual requirements, despite consuming the RDA. Likewise, it is possible for some people to eat less than the RDA and still avoid deficiencies. Although the RDA is defined for age and sex and is revised about every 5 years as new information becomes available, it has not been established for all nutrients. Like the food pyramid approach, variety is recommended.

Dietary Recommendations

The dietary recommendations and guidelines proposed by numerous governmental and health agencies complement the food pyramid approach to diet planning and the RDA through their focus on avoiding nutritional excesses. Although these diet recommendations are not guaranteed to prevent diseases, many experts believe that most Americans can reduce their risk for chronic diet-related diseases, such as diabetes, certain types of cancer, and heart disease, by modifying the typical diet. The Public Health Service of the Department of Health and Human Services and the U.S. Department of Agriculture together update the *Dietary Guidelines for Americans* every 5 years. This document,

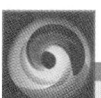

Table 41-3
Summary of Macrominerals and Microminerals

Nutrient and Adult RDA*	Sources	Functions	Signs and Symptoms of Deficiency	Signs and Symptoms of Excess
Macrominerals				
Calcium 800 mg (18–24 yr: 1200 mg)	Milk and dairy products, canned fish with bones, greens	Bone and tooth formation, blood clotting, nerve transmission, muscle contraction	Tetany, osteoporosis	Renal calculi in susceptible people
Phosphorus 800 mg (11–24 yr: 1200 mg)	Milk and milk products, soft drinks, processed foods	Bone and tooth formation, acid–base balance, energy metabolism	Hypophosphatemia: anorexia, muscle weakness	Hyperphosphatemia: symptoms of hypocalcemic tetany
Magnesium 280–350 mg	Green leafy vegetables, nuts, beans, grains	Bone and tooth formation, protein synthesis, carbohydrate metabolism	Hypomagnesemia: weakness, muscle pain, poor heart function	Hypermagnesemia: CNS depression, coma, hypotension
Sulfur (provided by adequate amounts of protein)	Meat, eggs, milk, dried peas and beans, nuts	Promotes certain enzyme reactions and detoxification reactions	None known	None known
Sodium 500 mg	Salt, processed foods	Major ion of extracellular fluid, fluid balance, acid–base balance	Hyponatremia: muscle cramps, cold and clammy skin	Edema, weight gain, high blood pressure if susceptible
Potassium 1600–2000 mg	Whole grains, fruits, leafy vegetables	Major ion of intracellular fluid, fluid balance, acid–base balance	Hypokalemia: muscle cramps and weakness, irregular heart beat	Hyperkalemia: irritability, anxiety, cardiac arrhythmia, heart block
Chlorine 750 mg (minimum requirement)	Salt	Component of HCl in stomach, fluid balance, acid–base balance	Hypochloremia: muscle spasms, alkalosis, depressed respirations	Hyperchloremia: acidosis
Microminerals				
Iron 10–15 mg	Liver, lean meats, enriched and whole-grain breads and cereals	Oxygen transport by way of hemoglobin, constituent of enzyme systems	Microcytic anemia, pallor, decreased work capacity, fatigue, weakness	Hemosiderosis; acute iron poisoning from accidental overdose leads to GI symptoms and possible shock
Iodine 150 mg	Iodized salt, seafood, food additives	Component of thyroid hormones	Goiter	Acne-like lesions
Zinc 12–15 mg	Oysters, liver, meats, dried peas and beans, nuts	Tissue growth, sexual maturation, immune response	Impaired growth, sexual maturation, immune system functioning	Anorexia, nausea, vomiting, diarrhea, muscle pain, lethargy
Copper 1.5–3 mg	Liver, shellfish, grains, dried peas and beans	Aids in iron metabolism and activity of some enzymes	Anemia, altered bone formation, hypercholesterolemia	Nervous system disturbances, vomiting
Manganese 2–5 mg	Whole grains, nuts, dried peas and beans, fruit	Part of enzymes needed for protein and energy metabolism	Poor reproductive performance, growth retardation	None known

(continued)

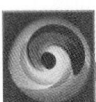

Table 41-3 (Continued)

Nutrient and Adult RDA*	Sources	Functions	Signs and Symptoms of Deficiency	Signs and Symptoms of Excess
Fluoride 1.5–4 mg (estimated safe, adequate intake)	Fluoridated water, fish, tea	Tooth formation and integrity, bone formation and integrity	Tooth decay; may increase risk for osteoporosis	Mottling and discoloration of tooth enamel
Chromium 50–200 µg	Whole grains, meats	Cofactor for insulin, proper glucose metabolism	Impaired glucose tolerance, insulin resistance	None known
Selenium 55–70 µg	Wheat (if grown in high-selenium soil), organ meats	Antioxidant	None known	Loss of hair, brittle fingernails, fatigue
Molybdenum 75–250 µg (estimated safe, adequate intake)	Liver, whole grains, dried peas and beans, organ meats	Oxidizes sulfur and products of sulfur metabolism	None known	Interferes with copper metabolism
Cobalt Unknown— apparently minute	Organ meats	Essential component of vitamin B_{12}	None known	None known

(Dudek, S. G. [1997]. *Nutrition handbook for nursing practice* [3rd ed.]. Philadelphia: Lippincott-Raven; and Williams, S. [1999]. *Essentials of nutrition and diet therapy* [7th ed.]. St. Louis: C. V. Mosby.)

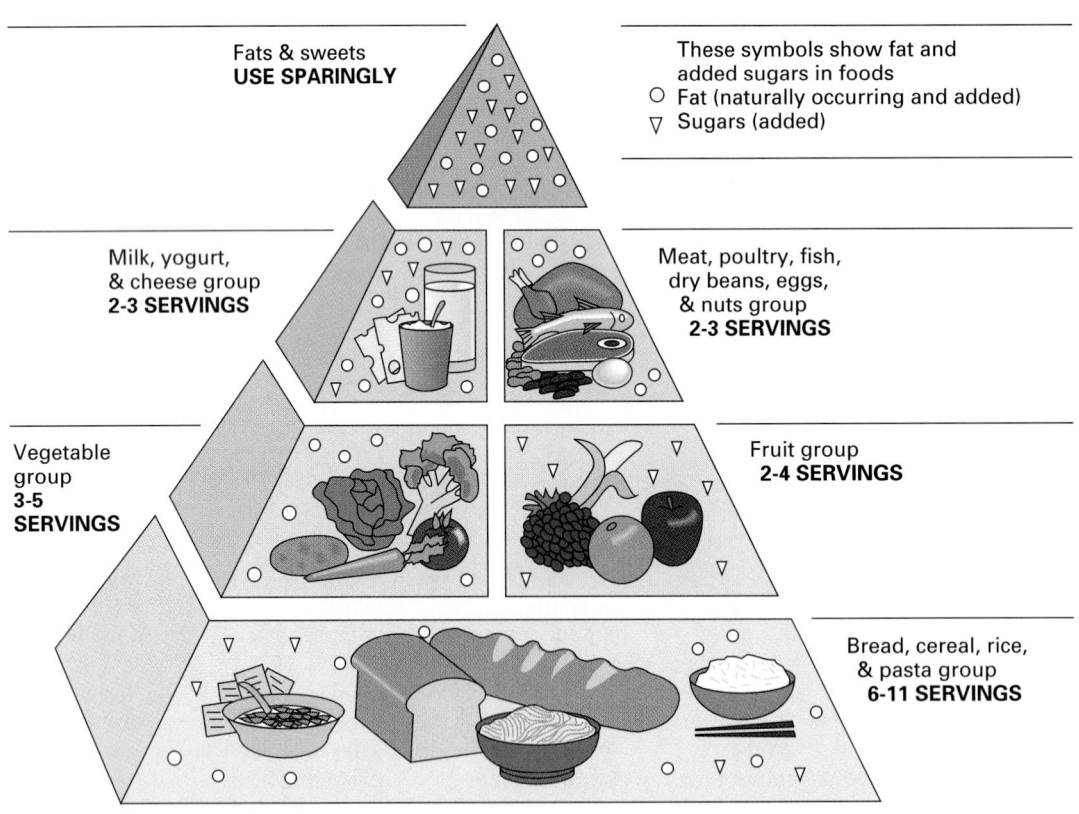

Figure 41-2
The Food Guide Pyramid. (Source: U.S. Department of Agriculture, April 1992.)

Food Guide Pyramid: Typical Serving Size

Bread, Cereal, Rice, & Pasta Group

1 slice of bread
½ cup of cooked rice, pasta, or cereal
1 ounce of ready-to-eat cereal
½ English muffin

Vegetable Group

½ cup of chopped raw or cooked vegetables
1 cup of leafy raw vegetables

Fruit Group

1 medium piece of fruit or melon wedge
¾ cup of juice
½ cup of canned fruit
¼ cup of dried fruit

Milk, Yogurt, & Cheese Group

1 cup of milk or yogurt
1½ ounces of natural cheese
2 ounces of processed cheese

Meat, Poultry, Fish, Dry Beans, Eggs, & Nut Group

2½ to 3 ounces of cooked lean meat, poultry, or fish
Count ½ cup of cooked beans, or 1 egg, or 2 tablespoons of peanut butter as 1 ounce of lean meat.

Fats & Sweets

Limit calories from these, especially if you need to lose weight.

(U.S. Department of Agriculture and the U.S. Department of Health and Human Services, 1992.)

---

entitled *Healthy People 2000,* includes seven broad nutritional challenges as part of overall strategies for health promotion. These guidelines were updated in 1995 (see accompanying box).

Food Labeling

Regulations that control food labels have always been controversial. In 1975, the FDA, a federal agency charged with protecting the U.S. food and drug supply, enacted legislation for a standardized label format that was considered a positive step toward educating the consumer about nutrition. Confusion and misinformation resulted as food manufacturers oversimplified or exaggerated health claims for their products. In 1990, Congress passed the Nutritional Labeling and Education Act, which required all foods, including fruits and vegetables, to be clearly labeled. Four broad categories are addressed in this legislation. They include nutrition labeling, serving sizes, descriptors, and health claims (Dudek, 1997). Consumers should be easily able to identify the amount of saturated fat and dietary fiber included in a product, in addition to viewing a listing of other nutritional information. Figure 41-3 illustrates a sample label with explanation of terms. All professional organizations agree that the food label is primarily a tool to educate the public about nutrition and a move toward ensuring that nutritional labeling is responsible and accurate. As mentioned previously, the FDA is currently considering a proposal that trans fat levels also be included on all food labels (Liebman & Wootan, 1999).

Factors Affecting Nutrition

Although nutritional adequacy is an important consideration in planning a diet, a person's food patterns and habits may have a greater impact on overall food intake. Food habits are a product of many evolving variables, such as physical factors (eg, geographic location, food technology, and income), physiologic factors (eg, health, hunger, and stage of development), and psychosocial factors (eg, culture, religion, tradition, education, politics, social status, food ideology, and learned aversions). Although not static, conservative traditional influences, like culture, geographic region, and religion, have a stabilizing effect on food habits.

Dietary Guidelines for Americans

- Eat a variety of foods.
- Balance the food you eat with physical activity; maintain or improve your weight.
- Choose a diet with plenty of grain products, vegetables, and fruits.
- Choose a diet low in fat, saturated fat, and cholesterol.
- Choose a diet moderate in sugars.
- Choose a diet moderate in salt and sodium.
- If you drink alcoholic beverages, do so in moderation.

(Report of the Dietary Guidelines Advisory Committee on the Dietary Guidelines for Americans. [1995]. U.S. Department of Agriculture and the U.S. Department of Health and Human Services.)

Total Fat

Aim low: Most people need to cut back on fat! Too much fat may contribute to heart disease and cancer. Try to limit your calories from fat. For a healthy heart, choose foods with a big difference between the total number of calories and the number of calories from fat.

Saturated Fat

A new kind of fat? No — saturated fat is part of the total fat in food. It is listed separately because it's the key player in raising blood cholesterol and your risk of heart disease. Eat less!

Cholesterol

Too much cholesterol — a second cousin to fat — can lead to heart disease. Challenge yourself to eat less than 300 mg each day.

Sodium

You call it "salt," the label calls it "sodium." Either way, it may add up to high blood pressure in some people. So, keep your sodium intake low — 2,400 to 3,000 mg or less each day.*

* The AHA recommends no more than 3,000 mg sodium per day for healthy adults.

Daily Value

Feel like you're drowning in numbers? Let the Daily Value be your guide. Daily Values are listed for people who eat 2,000 or 2,500 calories each day. If you eat more, your personal daily value may be higher than what's listed on the label. If you eat less, your personal daily value may be lower.

For fat, saturated fat, cholesterol and sodium, choose foods with a low % **Daily Value.** For total carbohydrate, dietary fiber, vitamins and minerals, your daily value goal is to reach 100% of each.

g = grams (About 28 g = 1 ounce)
mg = milligrams (1,000 mg = 1 g)

Nutrition Facts

Serving Size 1/2 cup (114g)
Servings Per Container 4

Amount Per Serving

		% Daily Value*
Calories 90	Calories from Fat 30	
Total Fat 3g		5%
Saturated Fat 0g		0%
Cholesterol 0mg		0%
Sodium 300mg		13%
Total Carbohydrate 13g		4%
Dietary Fiber 3g		12%
Sugars 3g		
Protein 3g		

Vitamin A 80%	•	Vitamin C	60%
Calcium 4%	•	Iron	4%

* Percent Daily Values are based on a 2,000 calorie diet. Your daily values may be higher or lower depending on your caloric needs:

		Calories	2,000	2,500
Total Fat	Less than		65g	80g
Sat Fat	Less than		20g	25g
Cholesterol	Less than		300mg	300mg
Sodium	Less than		2,400mg	2,400mg
Total Carbohydrate			300g	375g
Fiber			25g	30g

Calories per gram:
Fat 9 • Carbohydrate 4 • Protein 4

* More nutrients may be listed on some labels.

Serving Size

Is your serving the same size as the one on the label? If you eat double the serving size listed, you need to double the nutrient and caloric values. If you eat one-half the serving size shown here, cut the nutrient and caloric values in half.

Calories

Are you overweight? Cut back a little on calories! Look here to see how a serving of the food adds to your daily total. A 5'4", 138-lb. active woman needs about 2,200 calories each day. A 5'10", 174-lb. active man needs about 2,900. How about you?

Total Carbohydrate

When you cut down on fat, you can eat more carbohydrates. Carbohydrates are in foods like bread, potatoes, fruits and vegetables. Choose these often! They give you nutrients and energy.

Dietary Fiber

Grandmother called it "roughage," but her advice to eat more is still up-to-date! That goes for both soluble and insoluble kinds of dietary fiber. Fruits, vegetables, whole-grain foods, beans and peas are all good sources and can help reduce the risk of heart disease and cancer.

Protein

Most Americans get more protein than they need. Where there is animal protein, there is also fat and cholesterol. Eat small servings of lean meat, fish and poultry. Use skim or low-fat milk, yogurt, and cheese. Try vegetable proteins like beans, grains and cereals.

Vitamins & Minerals

Your goal here is 100% of each for the day. Don't count on one food to do it all. Let a combination of foods add up to a winning score.

Figure 41-3
Sample nutritional label with explanation of terms. (Source: American Heart Association.)

Physiologic Factors That Influence Nutrient Requirements

Developmental Considerations

Throughout the life cycle, nutrient needs change in relation to growth, development, activity, and age-related changes in metabolism and body composition. Periods of intense growth and development, such as during infancy, adolescence, pregnancy, and lactation, cause an increase in nutrient needs. Nutrient needs stabilize during adulthood, although older people may need more or less of some nutrients. Age influences not only nutrient requirements but also food intake. The consistency of food, eating patterns, and the significance of food change with physical and psychosocial development.

Infants

The period from birth to 1 year of age is the most rapid period of growth. Birth weight doubles in 4 to 6 months and triples by 1 year of age. Length increases 50% in the first year. Muscle control and the development of hand–eye coordination allow the infant to progress to sitting upright and self-feeding. The iron stores present at birth start to become depleted between 3 and 4 months of age. The immune system matures between 4 and 6 months of age.

Nutritional needs per unit of body weight are greater than at any other time in the life cycle. Breastfeeding is recommended as the major source of nutrition for the first 6 to 12 months of life. Supplements of vitamins may be prescribed. A variety of routine and special infant formulas are available if mothers choose not to breastfeed or if breastfeeding is contraindicated for some reason. Generally, solid foods are not introduced until 6 months of age, and by 1 year of age, the infant should be eating table food. Iron-fortified foods are recommended. Solid foods given too early may trigger allergic reactions.

Toddlers and Preschoolers

During this stage, the decrease in growth is dramatic. Mobility, autonomy, and coordination increase, as do muscle mass and bone density. Language skills improve, and the 3- to 5-year-old child also develops attitudes toward food.

Nutritionally, toddlers and preschoolers can feed themselves, verbalize food likes and dislikes, and occasionally use food to manipulate their parents. Appetite dramatically decreases and becomes erratic. Inappropriate use of food (ie, to punish, reward, bribe, or convey love) may lead to inappropriate food attitudes.

School-Aged Children

The 6- to 12-year-old child has an uneven, individualized, sometimes erratic growth pattern. Permanent teeth erupt as the digestive system matures. Socialization and independence increase. At this stage, the body accumulates reserves in preparation for the upcoming adolescent growth spurt.

Nutritional implications for the school-aged child focus on health promotion. Increasing energy requirements should be balanced with foods of high nutritional value. The appetite improves but may still be irregular. The parents' role as the primary regulator of food intake diminishes, and advertising has more of an impact on the child's food choices.

Adolescents

This is a period of rapid physical, emotional, social, and sexual maturation. It is also marked by intense psychosocial growth, family conflict, and social and peer pressure. The growth spurt begins at different ages among individuals. Girls begin menstruation and experience fat deposition, whereas males experience an increase in muscle mass, lean body tissue, and bones.

Nutrient needs, especially for calories, protein, calcium, and iron, increase to support growth. Weight consciousness becomes compulsive in 1 of 100 teenaged girls and results in *anorexia nervosa,* an eating disorder characterized by extreme weight loss, muscle wasting, arrested sexual development, refusal to eat, and bizarre eating habits. *Bulimia,* an eating disorder characterized by gorging followed by purging with self-induced vomiting, diuretics, and laxatives, also becomes more common in this age group. If a teenage pregnancy occurs, both mother and child are at increased nutritional risk. Nutritional needs may be harder to meet because fewer meals are eaten at home, and peer influence and busy schedules have an impact.

Adults

At this point in life, growth ceases. This age is also marked by a decline each decade in the basal metabolic rate (BMR). Adults may become more aware of the preventive role of exercise, or pressures of work and family may lead to a decline in physical activity and exercise.

Nutritional needs level off in adulthood, and fewer calories are required because of the decrease in BMR. If adjustments are not made, weight gain results.

Pregnant Women

During pregnancy, the fetus, maternal tissues, and placenta grow dramatically. Weight gain occurs, and gastrointestinal changes as a result of the pregnancy may result in nausea, vomiting, heartburn, or constipation. The quantity of milk produced depends on an adequate supply of nutrients.

Nutrient needs during pregnancy increase to support growth and maintain maternal homeostasis, particularly during the second and third trimesters. Key nutrient needs include protein, calories, iron, folic acid, calcium, and iodine. Caloric needs are higher for lactation than pregnancy, and the nutritional quality of breast milk is maintained at the expense of maternal nutrition if dietary intake is inadequate.

Older Adults

Because of the decreases in BMR and physical activity and loss of lean body mass, energy expenditure decreases. Loss of teeth and periodontal disease may make chewing more difficult. A decrease in peristalsis can result in constipation. Loss of taste between sweet and salty begins between 55 and 59 years of age, but discrimination between bitter and sour remains intact. The sensation of thirst also decreases. Degenerative diseases and the use of medications are more common with aging. It is not uncommon for social isolation, poor self-esteem, or loss of independence to affect nutritional intake negatively.

Because of the changes related to aging, the caloric needs of the body decrease. Foods that are difficult to chew may need to be eliminated, whereas an increase in fiber and fluid intake can relieve constipation. Elderly people are also prone to dehydration, and lack of interest in eating is common. Nutrient intake, digestion, absorption, metabolism, or excretion may be altered because of the physiologic changes common to this age.

The U.S. Department of Agriculture Human Nutrition Center on Aging at Tufts University recently developed a Modified Food Pyramid for adults 70 years of age and older who are relatively healthy and active (Russell, Rasmussen, & Lichtenstein, 1999). The base of the food pyramid is narrower to reflect the lower energy needs of this age group. Emphasis is on consuming nutrient-dense and high-fiber foods and water (Fig. 41-4). The flag atop the food pyramid

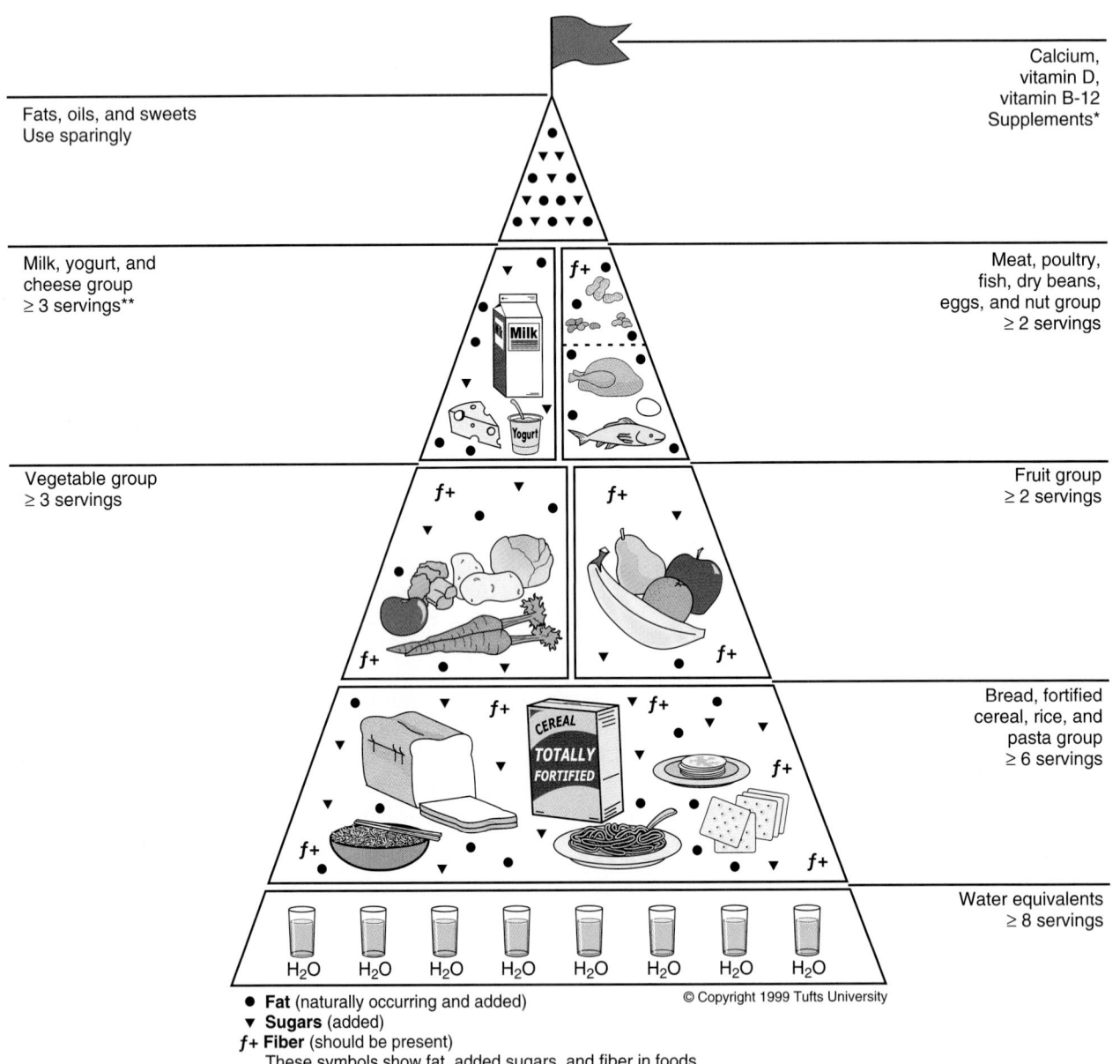

● **Fat** (naturally occurring and added)
▼ **Sugars** (added)
ƒ+ **Fiber** (should be present)
   These symbols show fat, added sugars, and fiber in foods
* Not all individuals need supplements; consult your healthcare provider
** ≥ Greater than or equal to

© Copyright 1999 Tufts University

Figure 41-4
Modified food pyramid for 70+ adults

serves as a reminder that calcium, vitamin D, and vitamin B_{12} supplements are frequently recommended for optimal nutrition in this population.

Sex

Men have somewhat different nutrient requirements from women related to differences in body composition and reproductive function. Their larger muscle mass translates into higher caloric and protein requirements (and therefore slightly higher needs for B vitamins that metabolize calories and protein) because muscle is more metabolically active than adipose tissue, of which women proportionately have more. Women of childbearing age have higher iron requirements related to menstruation.

State of Health

The alteration in nutrient requirements that results from illness and trauma varies with the intensity and duration of the stress. For instance, fevers increase the need for calories and water. Unlike fevers related to septicemia, however, fevers caused by a mild case of the flu require few dietary adjustments.

Trauma, like major surgery, burns, and crush injuries, is followed by hormonal changes that profoundly affect the body's use of nutrients. To preserve or replenish body nutrient stores and to promote healing and recovery, nutrient requirements increase dramatically in the adaptive phase after stress. In some cases of severe trauma, such as major burns, the rehabilitative phase of recovery, characterized by the gradual normalization of nutrient needs, may last for years.

Chronic disorders, like diabetes mellitus, renal disease, hypertension, heart disease, gastrointestinal disorders, and cancer, can alter nutrient requirements by influencing nutrient intake, digestion, absorption, metabolism, utilization, or excretion.

Alcohol Abuse

Alcohol can alter the body's use of nutrients, and thereby its nutrient requirements, by numerous mechanisms. The toxic effect of alcohol on the intestinal mucosa interferes with normal nutrient absorption: thus, requirements increase as the efficiency of absorption decreases. Need for B vitamins increases because they are used to metabolize alcohol. Alcohol can also influence nutrient metabolism by impairing nutrient storage, increasing nutrient catabolism, and increasing nutrient excretion. Alcohol abuse that results in liver damage has profound effects on the body's nutrient metabolism and requirements.

Medication

Many drugs have the potential to influence nutrient requirements. *Nutrient absorption* may be altered by drugs that (1) change the pH of the gastrointestinal tract, (2) increase gastrointestinal motility, (3) damage the intestinal mucosa, or (4) bind with nutrients, rendering them unavailable to the body. *Nutrient metabolism* can be altered by drugs that (1) act as nutrient antagonists, (2) alter the enzyme systems that metabolize nutrients, or (3) alter nutrient degradation. Some drugs alter the renal reabsorption of nutrients and therefore may increase or decrease *nutrient excretion*.

Megadoses of Nutrient Supplements

Because some nutrients compete against each other for absorption, an excess of one nutrient can lead to a deficiency (or increase the requirement) of another, especially if one is absorbed preferentially. For instance, a delicate balance exists between zinc and copper. People who take therapeutic levels of zinc run the risk of developing a copper deficiency—which is otherwise rare—unless they also increase their intake of copper.

Sociocultural and Psychological Factors

Religion

Nurses need to be aware of dietary restrictions associated with religions that might affect a patient's nutritional requirements. During the Lenten season, Roman Catholics, for example, fast on Ash Wednesday and Good Friday in addition to abstaining from meat on every Friday, and the nurse may recommend alternative food choices or meal patterns. Kosher dietary laws require special food preparation techniques and prohibit intake of pork and shellfish. The nurse must be conscious of the patient's religious affiliation and its impact on his or her nutritional regimen. Kosher diets and other special diets are available in hospitals, nursing homes, retirement homes, and programs such as Meals on Wheels.

Economics

The adequacy of a person's food budget affects dietary choices and patterns. The increasing cost of food, coupled with limited purchasing power, may result in a decrease in the nutritional quality of the diet. Many variables influence the types of foods purchased. Creative use of the food dollar means using unit pricing to determine cost per serving (eg, comparing the unit price of $.39 per serving with a similar product's $.42 per serving), selecting foods that contain adequate nutrients, and buying seasonal foods that are more economical and can be prepared easily at home. Avoiding convenience foods and meals purchased away from home saves food dollars.

Psychosocial Factors

Food plays multiple roles in the lives of most people. In addition to satisfying hunger and providing nutrition, food may signify a celebration, a social gathering, or a reward. Some people use various foods to indicate caring or to give comfort and reassurance during times of stress or unhappiness. Mealtime may evoke memories of family discussions, laughter, and enjoyable times. Some may remember conflicts associated with eating or avoid eating because it reminds them of their loneliness and isolation. Others, because of society's emphasis on being thin, may resort to fad or crash-reducing diets to resolve eating conflicts and lose weight rapidly. This initial weight reduction seldom is sustained for an extended period, and a cycle of yo-yo dieting frequently results. Drastic weight loss is followed by an eating binge that causes the dieter to regain all the lost weight and, possibly, some additional weight each time the sequence occurs. Nutritional deficiencies may occur and place the person at risk for other diseases. Losing weight and keeping it off require a change in eating habits as part of the overall commitment to health. Nurses can help by being aware of the multitudes of meanings that food has for people.

Two common eating disorders with psychological components are anorexia nervosa and bulimia. Although contrasts exist, there is also some overlap between these diseases. Both conditions are serious health and nutritional problems, and individuals with these disorders require professional help.

Cultural Factors

Nutritional diversity is common among cultural or ethnic groups. The variety and selections are unique to each group and represent their personal beliefs and customs. Culture influences what is eaten, how it is prepared, and what combinations of food are permitted. The variations in food choices within a culture also depend on income levels and availability of foods. Purnell & Paulanka (1998) mention the necessity of investigating a person's 24-hour food intake to identify and include culturally specific food choices in any therapeutic diet, thus improving compliance with the prescribed dietary modifications. Table 41-4 summarizes the food patterns of common ethnic groups.

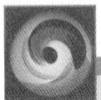

Table 41-4
Cultural Variations on Nutrition

Culture	Food Patterns	Additional Comments
Italian	• Bread and pasta are basic foods. • Use olive oil to prepare meats. • Cheese is main source of calcium.	• Milk is rarely consumed as a beverage. Red or white wine is consumed with dinner.
Chinese	• Use little milk or cheese. • Consume rice with most meals. • Use fresh foods that are stir-fried before serving. • Drink unsweetened green tea.	• Diet is high in fiber, low in fat, and may be deficient in protein. • Moderation is valued, and obesity is rare.
Japanese	• Rice may be eaten with every meal. • Seafood, especially raw fish, is the main protein source. • Main seasoning is soy sauce. • Tea is main beverage.	• Diet is low in fat but high in sodium. • Common methods of food preparation include broiling, steaming, boiling, and stir-frying.
Greek	• Cheese is a favorite food. • Yogurt is a popular source of calcium. • Lamb is the favorite meat.	• Consume relatively large quantities of sweets and snacks. • Consumption of meat is on the increase. • A meal is a family ritual.
Puerto Rican	• Steamed white rice is a staple. • Starchy vegetables (eg, breadfruit and viandas) and fruits such as plantains are popular. • Legumes are a good source of protein.	• Milk is rarely consumed as a beverage. • Food is frequently fried and cooked for a long period of time.
Mexican	• Consume many varieties of beans; little meat is used. • Drink little milk but consume large quantities of coffee. • Corn is the basic grain.	• Selection of hot and cold foods plays a role in body equilibrium. • Have a tendency to be lactose intolerant. • Diet is high in fiber and starch. • Lard is a basic cooking fat, and obesity is common.
African	• Favorite meats are pork and chicken. • Low intake of milk and dairy foods. • High intake of dark green, leafy vegetables.	• Diet tends to be high in fat and sodium. • Frying is a common method of preparation. • Obesity is common.

(Adapted from Dudek, S. G. [1997]. *Nutrition handbook for nursing practice* [3rd ed.]. Philadelphia: Lippincott-Raven; and Purnell, L., & Paulanka, B. [1998]. *Transcultural health care.* Philadelphia: F. A. Davis.)

Decreased Food Intake

Food intake may decrease for various reasons. **Anorexia**, or the lack of appetite, may be related to systemic and local diseases; numerous psychosocial causes, such as fear, anxiety, and depression; pain; and impaired ability to smell and taste—or it may occur secondary to drug therapy or medical treatments. Others who may have limited food intake include those who have difficulty chewing and swallowing, those who experience chronic gastrointestinal problems or undergo certain surgical procedures, and those on inadequate food budgets.

Increased Food Intake

Obesity presents a serious health problem physically, socially, and emotionally. **Obesity** is defined as body weight 20% or more above ideal weight or having a BMI of 30 or more. A positive caloric balance, resulting from an excess caloric intake or a decrease in energy expenditure, leads to the gradual accumulation of weight. This excess weight increases the risk for numerous medical problems; increases the risks associated with surgery; increases the risk for complications during pregnancy, labor, and delivery; and increases morbidity and mortality. Obese people are often discriminated against in social, educational, and employment settings. In a society that values thinness, obesity can cause one to feel desperate, frustrated, and rejected and to perceive oneself as being a failure. About half of Americans are considered obese (Gallagher, 1999). Numerous theories about the cause of obesity have been proposed. According to *genetic theories,* a low resting metabolic rate or an inherited family tendency contribute to obesity. *Physiologic factors* that have been implicated include an increased number of fat cells, a lowered body set-point, a decreased amount of brown fat that burns kilocalories, insulin resistance, and hormone imbalance. A food and family environment that encourages over-eating or a work environment where exercise is minimal are *environmental theories* that have been introduced. Additionally, many identify *psychological reasons* for obesity, including compulsiveness, using food to satisfy emotional needs, relying on food for compensation for lack of affection and companionship, and overeating as a release mechanism for boredom, anxiety, and feelings of inadequacy. Obesity is resistant to treatment, and weight loss is temporary at best unless behavior modification and exercise are incorporated into the dietary plan.

The Nursing Process

ASSESSING

Nutritional status has a significant impact on both health and disease. For well patients, good nutritional status can help to maintain health, promote normal growth and development, and protect against disease. During illness, good nutritional status can reduce the risk for complications and speed recovery time. Conversely, poor nutritional status can increase the risk for illness or death.

The nature of the nurse–patient relationship affords nurses the opportunity to incorporate nutritional assessment in the nursing process. Like other aspects of nursing care, nutritional assessment is a systematic approach used to identify the patient's actual or potential needs, formulate a plan to meet those needs, initiate the plan or assign others to implement it, and evaluate the effectiveness of the plan. As such, nutritional assessment is appropriate for all patients, although the level of assessment may range from simple screening to a comprehensive, in-depth assessment, depending on individual circumstances. Nurses can collect assessment data through history taking (dietary, medical, and socioeconomic data), physical assessments (anthropometric and clinical data), and laboratory data. An awareness of specific changes in older people that may reflect on the accuracy of the assessment process is necessary (see accompanying box).

Discussion continues among health experts about the most effective method to assess for the risk for nutritionally related complications. Some nutritionists state that a thorough physical assessment and nutritional history can more accurately determine the presence of malnutrition than a series of laboratory test results. Lyman & Marquardt (1997) reported on a nutrition screening tool that was developed to evaluate high-risk home care patients and has

---

Nutritional Assessment Considerations for Older Adults*

Biochemical Data

- Low serum albumin level (below 3.5 mg/dL) may be a reflection of the aging process rather than a nutritional risk factor. Albumin synthesis declines with age.
- Hemoglobin levels that are lower than normal may only reflect anemia observed in elderly people as part of the aging process.

Anthropometric Data

- Because of age-related changes in body composition, skin-fold measurements should be taken from several body sites.

Dietary Data

- Dietary recall may be inaccurate because of vision and memory problems.
- Question use of vitamin and mineral supplements.
- Gather information concerning medication regimen (prescribed and over-the-counter) to assess for food–drug interactions and adverse effects of medications.

* Specific clinical data for older adults may be found in the Focus on the Older Adult display.

proved to be reliable and valid. This approach incorporates a three-pronged assessment that raises patient awareness about nutrition; identifies risk factors and areas requiring nutritional counseling; and includes review of laboratory test results, medical regimens, and cognitive, functional, and emotional status. Nurses, by nature of their caring role and personal encounters, serve as nutritional role models and are ideally situated to identify nutritional needs and assess and monitor for nutritional risks (see the accompanying Applying Learning to Practice boxes).

Dietary Data

Dietary data may be collected from the patient or family and can be evaluated according to the food group approach, dietary guidelines, or the RDA, depending on the purpose of the assessment. Statistics indicate that as many as 50% of elderly people living independently may have nutritional deficiencies, and 20% of this group may in fact skip at least one meal a day (Dudek, 1997). After a screening tool identifies a patient at risk, such as in this group of older adults, it is imperative that a nutritional assessment be completed as a follow-up. When this is combined with other methods of assessing nutritional status, the nurse is better prepared to coordinate a focused strategy to combat malnutrition.

24-Hour Recall Method

The easiest way to collect dietary data is to obtain a 24-hour recall of all food and beverages the patient normally consumes during an average day. It includes the patient's usual portion sizes, meal and snack patterns, meal timing, and the place where food is eaten. Because this method relies on memory and accurate interpretation of portion sizes, the information may not be reliable.

Food Diaries

Food frequency questionnaires or food diaries may provide a better overall picture of nutrient intake because the patient records all food and beverages consumed in a specified period, usually 3 to 7 days.

Diet History

A more comprehensive approach to diet assessment is a full diet history. In addition to a 24-hour food recall and food frequency record, interview questions are geared to provide information on past and present food intake and habits. Sample questions are included in the accompanying Focused Assessment Guide.

The following findings are considered dietary risk factors for malnutrition (Cobb, 1997):

- Is severely underweight or overweight
- Has loss of 15% or more of body weight
- Has been NPO with simple intravenous therapy (eg, 5% dextrose and water) for longer than 5 days
- Has any condition that results in nutritional losses, such as diarrhea, vomiting, or burns
- Has any condition that results in increased metabolic needs, such as fever, burns, trauma, or wounds
- Is currently receiving medications that have catabolic effects, such as chemotherapy or neoplastic agents

Medical and Socioeconomic Data

Medical, social, and economic factors, as well as cultural and psychological influences, should be evaluated for their impact on nutritional requirements and food choices. A nutritional assessment should include information about the following (Dudek, 1997):

Medical Data

- Current illness as well as medical and surgical history
- Past and current drug history
- History of drug dependence or abuse
- Ability to chew and swallow, including condition of mouth, missing teeth, or dentures
- Appetite, food intolerance and allergies, and bowel habits

Social Data

- Age, gender, family history, lifestyle (eg, those at extremes in age are most at risk)
- Educational background
- Information about occupation, exercise and sleep pattern
- Religious affiliation, cultural and ethnic background
- Use of alcohol and tobacco

APPLYING LEARNING TO PRACTICE

The Nurse as Role Model: Nutrition

A nurse's credibility as a health practitioner may be severely questioned if he or she appears badly nourished or displays poor eating habits, weight problems, or other clinical signs of nutritional deficiencies. As a role model for health behaviors, the nurse should adopt the following goals:

- Attain and maintain ideal body weight.
- Use RDA guidelines for adequate nutrient intake.

- Maintain appropriate balance between food intake and exercise.
- Limit intake of alcohol, fats, sugar, salt, caffeine, and red meats.
- Eat foods high in fiber.

APPLYING LEARNING TO PRACTICE

Promoting Health

Nutrition

Use the assessment checklist to determine how well you are meeting your nutritional needs. Then develop a prescription for self-care by choosing appropriate behaviors from the list of suggestions.

ASSESSMENT CHECKLIST

almost always | sometimes | almost never

1. I know and use the recommended dietary guidelines and servings.
2. My weight is within 10% of the ideal for my height and body frame.
3. I maintain an appropriate balance between exercise and food intake.
4. I limit my fat, sugar, salt, and red meat intake.
5. I limit my caffeine intake.
6. I use alcoholic beverages in moderation.

SELF-CARE BEHAVIORS

1. Maintain desirable weight, eating a variety of foods in adequate amounts from each of the four food groups.
2. Eat slowly, take smaller portions, and avoid second helpings if trying to control overeating.
3. Eat a variety of foods low in calories and high in nutrients to lose weight.
4. Obtain medical clearance before starting a weight-loss program.
5. Avoid too many foods high in cholesterol (milk, egg yolk, organ meats, fats, oils); instead choose lean meat, fish, poultry, and beans.
6. Eat foods high in fiber: whole-grain breads and cereals, fruits, vegetables, dry beans.
7. Avoid excess use of salt and sugar.
8. Begin an exercise program, and maintain it.
9. Learn healthy eating habits; read labels, become familiar with healthy fast-food and restaurant menus, drink alcohol moderately (if at all).
10. Substitute healthy rewards for yourself that do not include high-calorie, low-nutrition snacks and beverages.

Economic Data
- Source of income
- Food budget

Anthropometric Data

Anthropometric measurements are used to determine body dimensions. In children, anthropometric measurements are used to assess growth rate; in adults, they can give indirect measurements of body protein and fat stores. For the data to be accurate and reliable, standardized equipment and procedures must be used, and the data must be compared with the appropriate reference standards for the patient's age and sex.

Height and weight, the most common anthropometric measurements, should be determined when the patient is admitted to the healthcare facility and periodically thereafter or assessed in a home care environment. A patient should be weighed on the same scale each time and at the same time of day, preferably before breakfast. Usual body weight should be compared with the BMI standard. Because actual weight may be inflated if the patient has edema, hydration status should be considered. Although self-reported weight may be recorded when actual weight is unobtainable, it is highly inaccurate and should be noted.

Additional anthropometric measurements include triceps skin-fold measurements, a measure of subcutaneous fat stores (Fig. 41-5); midarm circumference, a measure of skeletal muscle mass; and midarm muscle circumference, a measure of both skeletal muscle mass and fat stores. Reference standards have been determined for men and women for all three measures, as have figures representing 90%, 80%, 70%, and 60% of standard.

Clinical Data

Although signs and symptoms of malnutrition may be observed during a physical assessment (Table 41-5), they usually do not appear until malnutrition is advanced. In addition, further investigation is necessary to determine whether abnormal findings are actually caused by a nutritional deficiency, are possibly related to a nutritional deficiency, or are unrelated to nutritional status.

Biochemical Data

Laboratory tests, which measure blood and urine levels of nutrients or biochemical functions that depend on an adequate supply of nutrients, can objectively detect

---

FOCUSED ASSESSMENT GUIDE

Nutrition

Factors to Assess	Questions and Approaches
Usual dietary intake	Does your current intake differ from your usual intake?
	If so, is the reason a loss of appetite, changes in smell or taste, difficulty chewing and swallowing, hospitalization, a modified diet?
Food allergies or intolerances	Do you have any food allergies or intolerances?
Food preparation and storage	Who does the food shopping?
	Who prepares the meals?
	How is the food normally prepared? For instance, is food usually fried, baked, or broiled?
	Do you have adequate food storage space and preparation equipment?
Type of diet	Do you now or have you in the past followed a modified diet prescribed by a physician?
Dietary practices	Do you now or have you in the past used a fad diet, health foods, or self-prescribed supplements?
Eating disorder patterns	Do you view yourself as overweight?
	Do you weigh yourself frequently during one day?
	How is your appetite?
	Do you binge on large amounts of food in a short period?
	Have you ever caused yourself to vomit after eating a meal?
	Have you used laxatives, diuretics, or over-the-counter weight loss pills to lose weight?

---

nutritional problems in their early stages. Most routine biochemical tests measure protein status; measures of body vitamin, mineral, and trace element status are also available.

Hemoglobin, the oxygen-carrying protein of the red blood cells, and hematocrit, the volume of red blood cells packed by centrifugation in a given volume of blood, are measures of plasma protein also used to assess iron status. Protein status can also be determined by measuring serum albumin and transferrin levels and by a total lymphocyte count. The total lymphocyte count reflects immune status and is directly affected by impaired nutritional states. Albumin is an important laboratory value to assess over a period of time. The albumin level does not change with increasing age, but malnutrition and various disease states cause its level to decrease.

Twenty-four-hour urine tests used to measure protein metabolism are urine creatinine excretion and urine urea nitrogen. Urea, a breakdown product of amino acids, can be measured in the urine and blood. It reflects protein intake and the body's ability to detoxify and excrete this metabolic byproduct. Creatinine levels are directly proportional to the body's muscle mass, and a reduction in this value reflects severe malnutrition. These biochemical indicators with nutritional implications are summarized in the accompanying box.

DIAGNOSING

Assessment data may reveal actual or potential nutritional problems.

Altered Nutrition as the Problem

The following nursing diagnoses may be made when altered nutrition is the cause of the patient's disorder:

Altered Nutrition: Less Than Body Requirements related to NPO, inadequate tube feeding, prolonged use of a clear liquid diet, numerous food intolerance or allergies, excessive dieting, anorexia, chewing or swallowing difficulties, nausea, vomiting, chronic diarrhea, malabsorption, psychological eating disorders (anorexia nervosa, bulimia), alcoholism, metabolic and endocrine disorders, inappropriate use of supplements

Altered Nutrition: More Than Body Requirements related to overeating, inactivity, metabolic and endocrine disorders, inappropriate use of supplements

Altered Nutrition: Risk for More Than Body Requirements related to inappropriate eating, closely spaced pregnancies, metabolic and

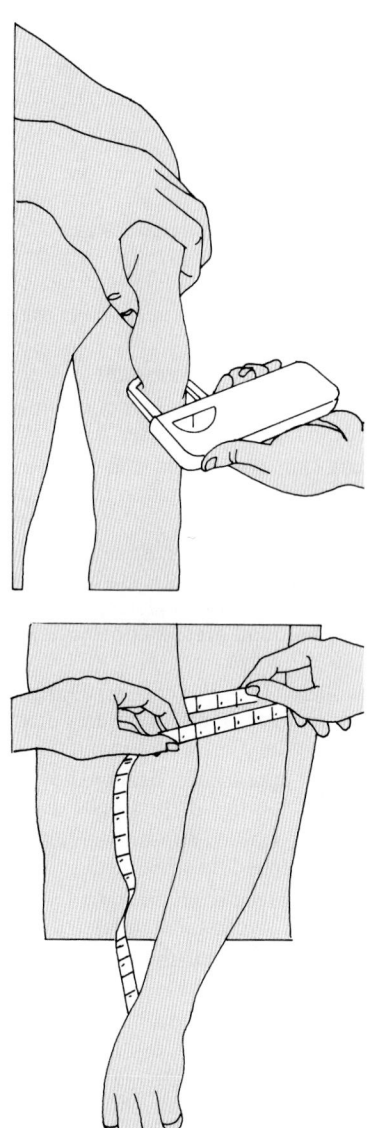

Figure 41-5
Two anthropometric measurements to assess nutritional status—triceps skin-fold measurement (*top*) and midarm muscle circumference (*bottom*).

endocrine disorders, inappropriate use of supplements

Samples of three of these diagnoses are given in the accompanying box.

Altered Nutrition as the Etiology

Nutritional problems may affect other areas of human functioning. In the following nursing diagnoses, the nutritional problem is the cause of another problem.

Activity Intolerance related to inadequate caloric intake, obesity, iron-deficiency anemia
Altered Dentition related to nutritional deficits
Altered Health Maintenance related to lack of knowledge about adequate nutrition

Anxiety related to obesity
Constipation related to inadequate fluid or fiber intake
Diarrhea related to overeating, excessive fiber intake, excessive sorbitol intake (sugar alcohol)
Fluid Volume Deficit related to inadequate fluid intake
Risk for Infection related to inadequate calorie intake, inadequate protein intake
Impaired Home Maintenance Management related to inability to purchase, store, or prepare food for family
Impaired Skin Integrity related to protein malnutrition, vitamin A deficiency
Knowledge Deficit related to new medical diet, nutrition misinformation, lack of interest in nutrition, intellectual deficit
Noncompliance to a particular diet order related to lack of motivation, misinformation
Self-Esteem Disturbance related to obesity
Sleep Pattern Disturbance related to excessive caffeine intake
Social Isolation related to obesity

Wellness Diagnosis

For patients who are incorporating sound nutritional practices in their daily routine, the following wellness diagnosis may be appropriate:

Potential for Enhanced Compliance with Low-Fat Diet Regimen

PLANNING: EXPECTED OUTCOMES

Expected outcomes are derived from the actual or potential nutritional problems diagnosed. General patient goals follow. The patient will achieve the following:

- Attain and maintain ideal body weight
- Eat a diet adequate but not excessive in all nutrients
- Eat a variety of food in each of three or more meals
- Follow the appropriate modified diet, when necessary, to restore health, avoid disease recurrences, and prevent or delay potential complications

IMPLEMENTING

Providing proper and adequate nourishment to the patient is a team effort implemented in a variety of settings. Diet orders are written by the physician, confirmed by the dietitian, and frequently explained to the patient by the nurse. The nurse may also be responsible for screening patients at home who are at nutritional risk, observing intake and appetite, evaluating the patient's tolerance, assisting the patient with eating, administering enteral and parenteral feedings, consulting with the dietitian and physician when dietary problems arise, addressing the potential for drug—nutrient reactions, obtaining more food or snacks for the patient when appropriate, monitoring food brought by visitors, and participating in nutrition education efforts.

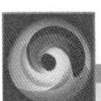

Table 41-5
Clinical Observations for Nutritional Assessment

Body Area	Signs of Good Nutritional Status	Signs of Poor Nutritional Status
General appearance	Alert, responsive	Listless, apathetic, and cachexic
General vitality	Endurance, energetic, sleeps well, vigorous	Easily fatigued, no energy, falls asleep easily, looks tired, apathetic
Weight	Normal for height, age, body build	Overweight or underweight
Hair	Shiny, lustrous, firm, not easily plucked, healthy scalp	Dull and dry, brittle, loss of color, easily plucked, thin and sparse
Face	Uniform skin color; healthy appearance, not swollen	Dark skin over cheeks and under eyes, flaky skin, facial edema (moon face), pale skin color
Eyes	Bright, clear, moist, no sores at corners of eyelids, membranes moist and healthy pink color, no prominent blood vessels	Pale eye membranes, dry eyes (xerophthalmia); Bitot's spots, increased vascularity, cornea soft (keratomalacia), small yellowish lumps around eyes (xanthelasma), dull or scarred cornea
Lips	Good pink color, smooth, moist, not chapped or swollen	Swollen and puffy (cheilosis), angular lesion at corners of mouth or fissures or scars (stomatitis)
Tongue	Deep red, surface papillae present	Smooth appearance, beefy red or magenta colored, swollen, hypertrophy or atrophy
Teeth	Straight, no crowding, no cavities, no pain, bright, no discoloration, well-shaped jaw	Cavities, mottled appearance (Fluorosis), malpositioned, missing teeth
Gums	Firm, good pink color, no swelling or bleeding	Spongy, bleed easily, marginal redness, recessed, swollen and inflamed
Glands	No enlargement of the thyroid, face not swollen	Enlargement of the thyroid (goiter), enlargement of the parotid (swollen cheeks)
Skin	Smooth, good color, slightly moist, no signs of rashes, swelling, or color irregularities	Rough, dry, flaky, swollen, pale, pigmented, lack of fat under the skin, fat deposits around the joints (xanthomas), bruises, petechiae
Nails	Firm, pink	Spoon shaped (koilonychia), brittle, pale, ridged
Skeleton	Good posture, no malformations	Poor posture, beading of the ribs, bowed legs or knock-knees, prominent scapulas, chest deformity at diaphragm
Muscles	Well developed, firm, good tone, some fat under the skin	Flaccid, poor tone, wasted, underdeveloped, difficulty walking
Extremities	No tenderness	Weak and tender, presence of edema
Abdomen	Flat	Swollen
Nervous system	Normal reflexes, psychological stability	Decrease in or loss of ankle and knee reflexes, psychomotor changes, mental confusion, depression, sensory loss, motor weakness, loss of sense of position, loss of vibration, burning and tingling of the hands and feet (paresthesia)
Cardiovascular system	Normal heart rate and rhythm, no murmurs, normal blood pressure for age	Cardiac enlargement, tachycardia, elevated blood pressure
GI system	No palpable organs or masses (liver edge may be palpable in children)	Hepatosplenomegaly

(Adapted from Dudek, S. G. [1997]. *Nutrition handbook for nursing practice* [3rd ed.]. Philadelphia: Lippincott-Raven.)

Biochemical Data With Nutritional Implications

- Hemoglobin (normal = 12–18 g/dL)
  decreased → anemia
- Hematocrit (normal = 40–50%)
  decreased → anemia
  increased → dehydration
- Serum albumin (normal = 3.3–5 g/dL)
  decreased → malnutrition (prolonged protein depletion), malabsorption
- Transferrin (normal = 240–480 mg/dL)
  decreased → anemia, protein deficiency
- Total lymphocyte count (normal = greater than 1800)

decreased → impaired nutritional intake, severe debilitating disease
- Blood urea nitrogen (normal = 17–18 mg/dL)
  increased → starvation, high protein intake, severe dehydration
  decreased → malnutrition, overhydration
- Creatinine (normal = 0.4–1.5 mg/dL)
  increased → dehydration
  decreased → reduction in total muscle mass, severe malnutrition

(Fischbach, F. [2000]. *A manual of laboratory and diagnostic tests* [6th ed.]. Philadelphia: Lippincott Williams & Wilkins.)

Teaching Nutritional Information

For the greatest chance of success, diet instructions should be individually tailored to the patient's lifestyle, intellectual ability, and level of motivation. Although strict guidelines and printed handouts may seem ideal, in practice, simplicity and compromise are often the keys to patient compliance. The accompanying box suggests standardized nursing interventions for nutritional counseling using the NIC terminology.

Nursing Diagnoses for Common Problems

Nutrition

Problem	*Related Factors*	*Sample Defining Characteristics*
Altered Nutrition: Less Than Body Requirements	Malabsorption	• "I seem to eat all day long and yet I keep losing weight." • Reports losing 15 lb within the past 3 weeks. Has 8 to 10 bowel movements daily of frothy, odorous stools that float. Fecal fat excretion test indicates steatorrhea. Patient appears fatigued and undernourished; muscle wasting is evident. Laboratory data reveal low serum albumin level (protein deficiency) and iron-deficiency anemia.
Altered Nutrition: More Than Body Requirements	Decreased thyroid function leading to a decrease in metabolism	• "I don't eat enough to keep a bird alive, but I just keep getting fatter and fatter. I don't know what else to do unless I stop eating altogether." • Patient reports a 10-lb weight gain within the past month despite following a 1200-calorie diet. Other symptoms noted include fatigue, amenorrhea, and dry skin. Laboratory data indicate low serum thyroxine (T_4) level, protein-bound iodine, and elevated serum thyroid-stimulating hormone and cholesterol levels. Radioactive iodine uptake was low.
Altered Nutrition: High Risk for More Than Body Requirements	Inappropriate use of supplements	• "I sent a sample of my hair away for a nutritional analysis, and the report came back saying that I should take supplements of zinc, iron, potassium, and magnesium." • For the past week, patient has been taking supplements of 500% of the RDA for zinc and magnesium. She takes twice as much iron as recommended, and large doses of potassium ad lib.

Using the Nursing Interventions Classification (NIC)

Nutritional Counseling

- Determine patient's food intake and eating habits.
- Establish realistic short-term and long-term goals for change in the nutritional status.
- Provide information, as necessary, about the health need for diet modification: weight loss, weight gain, sodium restriction, cholesterol reduction, fluid restriction, and so on.
- Help patient to consider factors of age, stage of growth and development, past eating experiences, injury, disease, culture, and finances in planning ways to meet nutritional requirements.
- Discuss patient's food likes and dislikes.
- Discuss food-buying habits and budget constraints.
- Discuss the meaning of food to the patient.
- Praise efforts to achieve goals.
- Provide referral or consultation with other members of the healthcare team, as appropriate.

(From McCloskey, J., & Bulechek, G. [2000]. *Nursing interventions classification [NIC]* [3rd ed.]. [p. 476]. St. Louis: C. V. Mosby. A full listing of nursing activities for each nursing intervention can be found in this book.)

Monitoring Nutritional Status

Nurses are aware that malnourished patients are more likely to have slower wound healing and develop complications. Prevention of malnutrition can have a positive effect on patient outcomes. In the hospital, shortened stays limit the time available for nutritional screening and intervention. Patients are often acutely ill and uninterested or unable to absorb and retain any nutritional instruction. It may also be difficult to include a family member or caregiver responsible for food preparation in scheduled teaching sessions. In many situations, the home healthcare nurse has the opportunity to have a significant impact on nutritional health. Instruction can be provided in a relaxed setting that allows insight into a patient's cultural orientation and family patterns and traditions. This environment also encourages modification and adjustments in the nurse's approach to nutritional instruction. The variety of community services and programs that are available to provide nutritional support to patients at home should be investigated. The accompanying box, Focus on the Older Adult, includes teaching content and strategies for the specific nutritional challenges facing the older adult.

Stimulating Appetite

Pain, illness, anxiety, and medications can contribute to anorexia and poor intake when in a healthcare facility or in the home. To the hospitalized patient, food and eating may take on much greater meaning. Loss of control over food choices, the way food is prepared, when and how food is served, and eating alone may do little to encourage normal eating. Every effort must be made to ensure that the proper food is not only served but also eaten. The additional time and attention nurses and caregivers spend when encouraging a person to eat may have a positive effect on dietary intake. The following measures may help to stimulate appetite in any setting:

- Serve small, frequent meals to avoid overwhelming the individual with large amounts of food.
- Solicit food preferences and encourage favorite foods from home or prepared when at home, if possible.
- Provide encouragement and a pleasant eating environment.
- Be sure that any prepared food looks attractive.
- Schedule procedures and medications at times when they are least likely to interfere with appetite.
- Control pain, nausea, or depression with medications.
- Offer alternatives for items that a person cannot or will not eat.
- Encourage or provide good oral hygiene.
- Remove clutter from the eating area.
- Keep eating area free from irritating odors.
- Arrange food tray so that an individual can easily reach food.
- Provide a comfortable position.

Assisting With Eating

The loss of independence that comes with the inability to self-feed can be a severe blow to a person's self-esteem. The following measures may help a person maintain dignity while being fed:

- Involve the person as much as possible. Solicit his or her preferences with regard to the order of items eaten and the eating pace.
- Engage the individual in pleasant conversation to ease tension.
- Place a napkin, not a bib, over the person's clothes for protection.
- Use straws or special eating utensils whenever possible.
- Ensure that if a person wears glasses, they are in place before mealtime.
- At the person's request, open containers, cut meat, or apply condiments to the prepared food.

Providing Nutrition in Special Situations

A variety of normal and modified diets are available in healthcare settings and may be prescribed for use at home. Normal or house diets are designed to maintain optimal nutritional status by providing adequate amounts of all nutrients. The diet's actual composition varies with the quantity and types of food selected; the average calorie content ranges from 1400 to 2500 cal.

Focus on the Older Adult

Nursing Strategies for Nutritional Problems Affecting Older Adults

Altered Ability to Chew Related to Loss of Teeth, Ill-Fitting Dentures, and Gingivitis

- Encourage and instruct patient to care for and retain own teeth and dentures.
- Encourage proper tooth-brushing and use of special toothpaste if gums and teeth are sensitive.
- Chop, shred, or puree foods that are difficult to chew.
- Select ground meat, fish, or poultry as protein sources more easily chewed.

Loss of Senses of Smell and Taste

- Serve food that is attractive and at proper temperature.
- Eat one food at a time rather than mixing foods.
- Serve foods with different textures and aromas.

Decreased Peristalsis in the Esophagus

- Avoid cold liquids.
- Avoid emotional upsets and stress-producing situations.
- Take anticholinergic drugs as ordered by physician.

Gastroesophageal Reflux

- Avoid overeating.
- Avoid juices, chocolate, and fat.
- Avoid alcohol and smoking.
- Elevate the head of the bed 30 to 40 degrees when sleeping.
- Lose weight if necessary.
- Avoid bending over.
- Take antacids or other medications as ordered by physician.

Decreased Gastric Secretions

- Chew food thoroughly.
- Eat meals on a regular schedule.
- Use antacids or other medications as prescribed by physician.
- Be alert for symptoms of deficiency of nutrients, particularly iron, calcium, fat, protein, and vitamin B_{12}.
- Ensure adequate intake of vitamin D for calcium absorption.

Slowed Intestinal Peristalsis

- Eat a high-fiber diet.
- Remain as active as possible.
- Increase fluid intake.
- Avoid laxative use.
- Eat meals at a regular time.
- Drink prune juice or eat prunes every morning.

Lowered Glucose Tolerance

- Eat more complex carbohydrates.
- Avoid sugar-rich foods.

Reduction in Appetite and Thirst Sensation

- Offer fluids at regular intervals and at preferred temperature.
- Be alert for symptoms of dehydration and electrolyte imbalance.
- Offer small meals at frequent intervals.

Nutritional Deficiencies Related to Alcohol Intake

- Encourage diet high in protein and carbohydrates.
- Offer small, frequent meals to maintain caloric intake.
- Restrict sodium and fluids if edema is present.
- Take multivitamin supplements as ordered by physician.

Loss of Appetite Associated With Depression and Loneliness

- Promote mealtime as a social event.
- Set an attractive table in a pleasant setting.
- Eat outdoors whenever possible.
- Invite guests as often as possible.
- Participate in special programs for senior citizens.

Physical Handicaps

- Open cartons and assist with setup of meal.
- Arrange for home-delivered meals.
- Conserve energy when preparing meals (sit on a stool, and so forth).
- Provide transportation and assistance to obtain food.

Low Income

- Buy specials when available at food store.
- Use generic brands.
- Use coupons.
- Cook larger quantities than necessary and freeze the leftovers for future use.
- Substitute eggs, skim milk powder, and beans for meat.

Malnutrition

- Eat essential foods first.
- Select nutrient-dense foods.
- Monitor for signs of nutritional deficiencies.
- Encourage eating by planning special events.

Drug–Nutrient Interactions

- Avoid unnecessary drugs.
- Be aware of drug actions and interactions.
- Check with pharmacist to determine if medication may or may not be taken with food.
- Assess for confusion and inability to manage medication regimen.

Liquid diets are used most often as transitional diets when eating resumes after acute illness, surgery, or parenteral nutrition. *Clear liquid diets* contain only foods that are clear liquids at room or body temperature—gelatin, fat-free broth, bouillon, ice pops, clear juices, carbonated beverages, regular and decaffeinated coffee, and tea. Because clear liquid diets are inadequate in calories, protein, and most nutrients, they should be progressed to more nutritious alternatives as soon as possible. *Full liquid diets* contain milk, plain frozen desserts, pasteurized eggs, cereal gruels, and milk and egg substitutes in addition to clear liquids. A full liquid diet contains liquids that can be poured at room temperature. High-calorie, high-protein supplements are recommended if the diet is used for more than 3 days.

Soft diets are usually regular diets that have been modified to eliminate foods that are hard to digest and to chew, including those that are high in fiber, high in fat, and highly seasoned. Soft diets are adequate in calories and nutrients and may be used on a long-term basis. Many nutritionists substitute low-fiber vegetables in place of purees.

Patients may be ordered *NPO* (nothing by mouth) for several reasons. Food is prohibited before surgery to prevent aspiration related to anesthesia, and after surgery until bowel sounds return. NPO may also be necessary for patients undergoing certain medical tests and for patients experiencing severe nausea and vomiting, an inability to chew or swallow, coma, various acute or chronic gastrointestinal abnormalities, and labor and delivery.

Well-nourished patients can easily withstand the stress of NPO for a short period, but being NPO for an extended period of time poses a nutritional challenge for many individuals. Patients with increased nutritional requirements and those who will be NPO for more than 2 days may require nutritional support from enteral or parenteral nutrition. The following measures may provide comfort to patients who are NPO:

- Encourage or provide good oral hygiene.
- Provide the patient with ice chips, sips of water, hard candies, or gum, as allowed.
- Urge the patient to avoid watching others eat. Suggest alternate activities at mealtimes.

Some patients may prefer a *vegetarian diet*. At least 12 million Americans follow some type of vegetarian food pattern (Peckenpaugh & Poleman, 1999). Meats are usually replaced with legumes, grains, and vegetables; if well planned, this type of diet can satisfy all nutritional requirements. People may choose to be vegetarians for a variety of reasons: religious preference, ethical belief that killing animals for food is unjust, fear of contamination with pesticides, or health concerns about the cholesterol and saturated fats found in meats. Vegetarian diets have a variety of formats and are more commonly followed by younger people. An individual who eats any animal product except red meat is at one end of the spectrum, with a Zen macrobiotic who consumes only brown rice and herb tea at the other end. Vitamin B_{12}, vitamin A, and iron are nutrients that may require supplementation in some vegetarian diets, but most vegetarian diets are not deficient in any nutrients. The nurse can support patients who follow a vegetarian diet by assisting them or their caregiver to select nutritious food items from the large variety of foods available within their dietary framework.

Providing Enteral Nutrition

Oral feeding is the preferred and most effective method of feeding patients. The next best method is the enteral route. **Enteral nutrition** involves passing a tube into the gastrointestinal tract to administer a formula containing adequate nutrients. This alternate feeding method may deliver total or supplemental nutrition over a short-term period or for longer intervals.

Providing Short-Term Nutritional Support

For short-term use (less than 6 weeks), a nasogastric or nasointestinal route is usually selected. A **nasogastric (NG) feeding tube** is inserted through the nose and into the stomach, whereas **nasointestinal (NI) tube** is passed through the nose and into the upper portion of the small intestine. Nasogastric feedings have the advantage of allowing the stomach to be used as a natural reservoir, regulating the amount of foods and liquids released into the small intestine. It is also thought that the presence of gastric acid in the stomach may decrease the risk for infection. The possibility of aspiration of tube feeding solution into the lungs is a disadvantage of this route. Patients with a dysfunctional gag reflex and those who are unable to have the head of the bed elevated during feedings are not candidates for nasogastric feeding. Occasionally, a smaller, softer, more pliable tube (eg, Dobbhoff tube) may be placed in the stomach or small intestine. The advantage of increased patient comfort with this tube is offset by difficulty checking tube placement. The nasal method of inserting a feeding tube, described in Procedure 41-1, requires skill and accuracy and is frequently done by the nurse.

A patient with a nasointestinal tube is at minimal risk for aspiration. When formula is delivered directly into the intestine, a type of *dumping syndrome* may develop because the pyloric valve in the stomach, which normally slows transit of food into the intestine, is bypassed. The volume of feeding distends the intestine and, combined with a hypoglycemic reaction, may result in symptoms of gas, bloating, crampy pain, weakness, and dizziness. Some medical conditions (delayed gastric emptying, gastric tumor) also necessitate the use of a nasointestinal tube.

Providing Long-Term Nutritional Support

When enteral feeding is required for a long-term period, an opening may be created into the stomach (gastrostomy) or into the jejunum (jejunostomy). The methods of accomplishing long-term feeding into the stomach include **percutaneous endoscopic gastrostomy (PEG)** or a surgically or laparoscopically placed gastrostomy tube. PEG tube insertion is popular because, unlike a gastrostomy tube, it usually does not require general anesthesia, can be safely inserted and removed at the bedside or in an outpatient setting, and is, therefore, more economical (O'Brien, Davis, & Erwin-Toth, 1999). Simply stated, positioning a PEG tube

PROCEDURE 41-1

Inserting a Nasogastric Tube

Equipment

Nasogastric tube of appropriate size
    (8 to 18 French)
Small basin filled with ice or warm
    water (optional)
Water-soluble lubricant
Tongue blade
Flashlight
Topical analgesic (optional)

Stethoscope
Normal saline solution (for irrigation
    only)
Asepto bulb syringe or Toomey
    syringe (20 to 50 mL)
Nonallergenic tape (1 inch wide)
Tissues
Glass of water with straw

Suction apparatus (if ordered)
Bath towel or disposable pad
Safety pin and rubber band
Clamp
Emesis basin
Disposable gloves
Tincture of benzoin

Action	Rationale
1. Check physician's order for insertion of nasogastric tube.	This clarifies procedure and type of equipment required.
2. Explain procedure to patient.	Explanation facilitates patient cooperation.
3. Gather equipment.	This provides for organized approach to task.
4. If nasogastric tube is rubber, place it in a basin with ice for 5 to 10 minutes or place a plastic tube in a basin of warm water.	Cold stiffens the rubber tube, making it easier to insert. Plastic tube may be placed in warm water to make it more flexible.
5. Assess patient's abdomen.	Assessment determines presence of bowel sounds and amount of abdominal distention.
6. Wash your hands. Don disposable gloves.	Handwashing deters the spread of microorganisms. Gloves protect from exposure to blood or body fluids.
7. Assist the patient to high Fowler's position, or 45 degrees, if unable to maintain upright position, and drape chest with bath towel or disposable pad. Have emesis basin and tissues handy.	Upright position is more natural for swallowing and protects against aspiration, if the patient should vomit. Passage of tube may stimulate gagging and tearing of eyes.
8. Check the nares for patency by asking the patient to occlude one nostril and breathe normally through the other. Select the nostril through which air passes more easily.	Tube passes more easily through the nostril with the largest opening.
9. Measure the distance to insert the tube by placing tip of tube at patient's nostril and extending to tip of earlobe and then to tip of xiphoid process. Mark tube with a piece of tape.	Measurement ensures that the tube will be long enough to enter the patient's stomach.

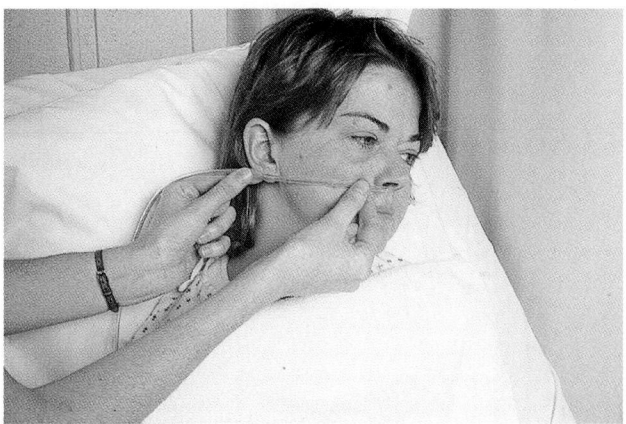

Action 9a: Measuring distance from nostril to tip of earlobe.

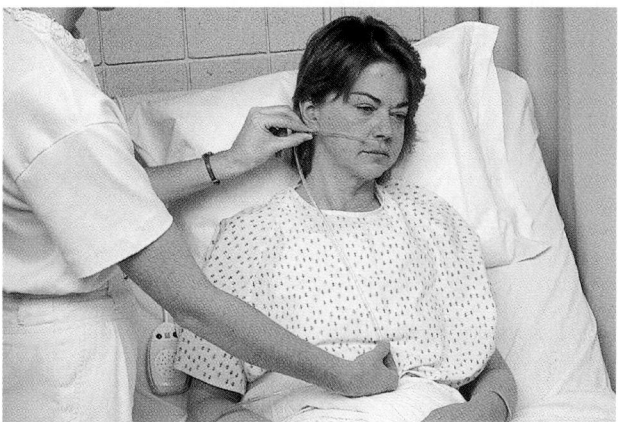

Action 9b: Measuring distance from earlobe to tip of xiphoid process.

(continued)

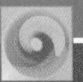

PROCEDURE 41-1

Inserting a Nasogastric Tube (Continued)

10. Lubricate the tip of the tube (at least 1–2 in) with a water-soluble lubricant. Apply topical analgesic to nostril and oropharynx or ask patient to hold ice chips in mouth for several minutes (according to physician's preference).

Lubrication reduces friction and facilitates passage of the tube into the stomach. Water-soluble lubricant will not cause pneumonia if tube accidentally enters the lungs. Topical analgesic or ice acts as a local anesthetic, reducing discomfort.

11. Ask the patient to lift the head, and insert the tube into the nostril while directing the tube downward and backward. The patient may gag when the tube reaches the pharynx.

Following the normal contour of the nasal passage while inserting the tube reduces irritation and the likelihood of mucosal injury. The gag reflex is readily stimulated by the tube.

12. Instruct the patient to keep head in upright or normal eating position. Encourage him or her to swallow even if no fluids are permitted. Advance the tube in a downward and backward direction when the patient swallows. Stop when the patient breathes. Provide tissues for tearing or watering of eyes. If gagging and coughing persist, check placement of tube with a tongue blade and flashlight. Keep advancing the tube until the tape marking is reached. Do not use force. Rotate the tube if it meets resistance.

Bringing the head forward helps close the trachea and open the esophagus. Swallowing helps advance the tube, causes the epiglottis to cover the opening of the trachea, and helps to eliminate gagging and coughing. Tears are a natural response as the tube passes into the nasopharynx. Excessive coughing and gagging may occur if the tube has curled in the back of throat. Forcing the tube may injure mucous membranes.

13. Discontinue the procedure and remove the tube if there are signs of distress, such as gasping, coughing, cyanosis, and the inability to speak or hum.

The tube is not in the esophagus if the patient shows signs of distress and is unable to speak or hum.

14. Determine that the tube is in the patient's stomach (these methods are appropriate for large-bore tubes but may be ineffective to check placement of small-bore, pliable tubes):
    a. Attach the syringe to the end of the tube and aspirate small amount of stomach contents.

The tube is in the stomach if its contents can be aspirated; pH of aspirate can then be tested to determine gastric placement.

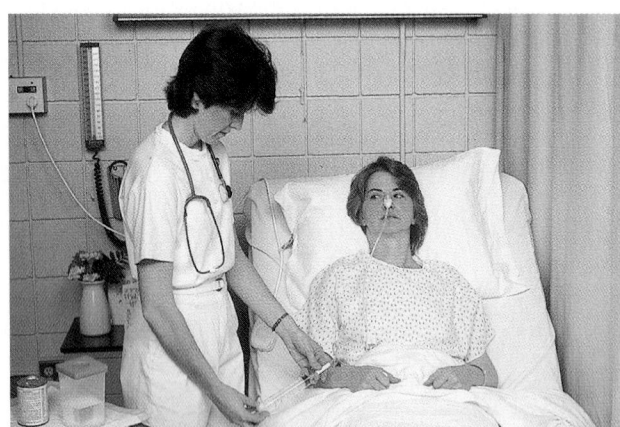

Action 14a: Aspirating gastric contents.

(continued)

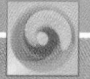

PROCEDURE 41-1

Inserting a Nasogastric Tube (Continued)

b. Measure the pH of aspirated fluid using pH paper or a meter.

The pH of gastric contents is acidic (4 or less), compared with an average pH of 7.0 or greater for respiratory fluid. Because pH of intestinal fluid also is slightly basic, this method will not effectively differentiate between intestinal fluid and pleural fluid.

c. Obtain radiograph of placement of tube (as ordered by physician).

Radiographic visualization is the most definitive measure to determine tube placement.

15. Apply tincture of benzoin to tip of nose and allow to dry. Secure the tube with tape to the patient's nose. Be careful not to pull the tube too tightly against the nose:

a. Cut a 4-inch piece of tape and split bottom 2 inches or use packaged nose tape for nasogastric tubes.

b. Place unsplit end over bridge of patient's nose.

c. Wrap split ends under the tubing and up and over onto the nose.

Tincture of benzoin facilitates attachment of tape. Constant pressure of the tube against the skin and mucous membranes causes tissue injury.

16. Attach tube to suction or clamp the tube and cap it according to the physician's orders.

Suction provides for decompression of stomach and drainage of gastric contents.

17. Secure tube to the patient's gown by using a rubber band or tape and a safety pin. If double-lumen tube is used, secure vent above stomach level. Attach at shoulder level.

This prevents tension and tugging on the tube. Securing the double-lumen tube above stomach level prevents seepage of gastric contents and keeps the lumen clear for venting air.

18. Assist with or provide patient with oral hygiene at regular intervals.

Oral hygiene keeps mouth clean and moist and promotes comfort.

19. Wash hands. Remove all equipment and make patient comfortable.

Handwashing deters the spread of microorganisms.

20. Record the insertion procedure, type and size of tube, and measure the tube from the tip of the nose to the end of the tube. Also document a description of gastric contents, and patient's response.

This facilitates documentation and provides for comprehensive care. Measurement of tube provides a baseline for future comparison.

Special Considerations

For insertion of a nasointestinal tube:

- Measure tube from tip of nose to ear lobe and from ear lobe to xiphoid process. Add 8 to 10 inches for intestinal placement. Mark tubing at desired point.
- Place patient on his or her right side. Nasointestinal tube is usually placed in the stomach and allowed to advance through peristalsis through the pyloric sphincter (may take up to 24 hours).
- Test pH of aspirate when tube has advanced to marked point to confirm placement in the intestine. Check position by radiograph. Tape in place when confirmed.

involves local anesthesia, passage of an endoscope into the stomach, a small incision or stab wound through the skin of the abdomen, pushing a cannula through the small incision, insertion of a guide wire or suture material through the cannula, and introduction and placement of the PEG tube through one of several methods (Fig. 41-6 illustrates a PEG tube in place in the stomach). Use of a PEG tube or other type of gastrostomy tube requires an intact, functional gastrointestinal tract. In long-term feeding situations in which gastric problems exist, the jejunostomy is an alternate method through which nutrition can be delivered. These tubes may be inserted surgically or through

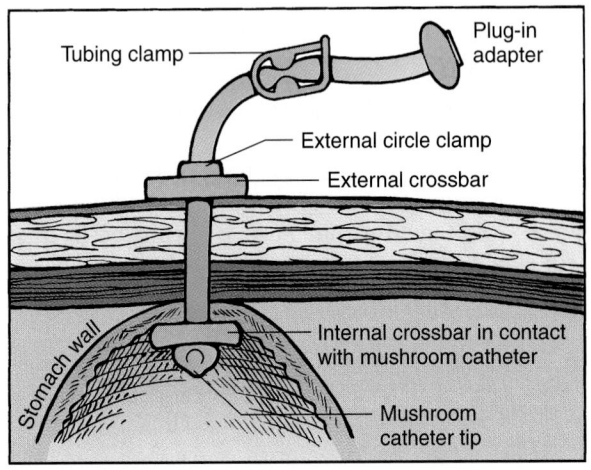

Figure 41-6
Percutaneous endoscopic gastrostomy tube in place in the stomach. (Smeltzer, S. C., & Bare, B. G. [2000]. *Brunner and Suddarth's textbook of medical surgical nursing* [9th ed.]. Philadelphia: Lippincott, Williams & Wilkins.)

a laparoscopy. Gastrostomy or jejunostomy tubes are not easily dislodged.

For patients who are active yet require long-term continuous or intermittent feedings, a low-profile gastrostomy device (LPGD) may be an option. Children are also excellent candidates for LPGDs. The external apparatus is minimal and consists of a button or skin disk that is stable, less irritating to the skin, and has no external tubing. Additional advantages include the fact that it can be immersed in water and is less likely to migrate or become dislodged (Hall, 1997).

Confirming Placement of Tubes

After the initial insertion of a feeding tube, before beginning a feeding or instilling liquids, and at regular intervals during continuous feedings, the placement of a nasogastric or nasointestinal tube must be verified (see the accompanying Research in Nursing box). A misplaced feeding tube in the lungs or pulmonary tissue places the patient at risk for aspiration. It is estimated that about 5% of feeding tube insertions are inadvertently placed in the respiratory tract (Metheny, Smith, Wehrle, Wiersema, & Clark, 1998b). Radiographic examination is the standard procedure to ver-

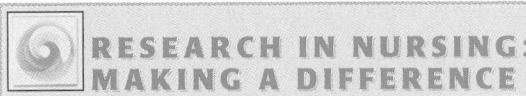

RESEARCH IN NURSING: MAKING A DIFFERENCE

Using pH and Bilirubin Concentration to Predict Feeding Tube Placement

Proper insertion of a feeding tube through the nasal route is imperative, and nurses have the responsibility to always check tube placement before initiating a tube feeding or irrigating a tube. Lethal complications can result if a tube has migrated to or been accidentally misplaced in the respiratory tract. Although still commonly used, the auscultatory method to check tube placement is considered unreliable. Testing the pH of fluid aspirated from the tube has proved moderately reliable in distinguishing between gastric and respiratory or gastric and intestinal placement. Because respiratory and intestinal aspirates usually have a pH value greater than 6, it still can remain unclear whether a tube is located in the respiratory tree or in the intestines. Chest radiographs conclusively confirm correct tube placement, but research may identify a reliable bedside method.

Related Research
Metheny, N., Stewart, B., Smith, L., Yan, H., Diebold, M., & Clouse, R. (1999). pH and concentration of bilirubin in feeding tube aspirates as predictors of tube placement. *Nursing Research, 48*(4), 189–197.
Bilirubin results from the breakdown of hemoglobin in the red blood cells. It is excreted through bile into

the duodenum. It is not typically found in gastric fluid and is only rarely found in fluid from the respiratory tract. This study measured the concentration of bilirubin and pH level in aspirate from newly inserted small-bore feeding tubes within 5 minutes of radiographs taken to confirm tube location. The samples were obtained during a 3-year period from 437 acutely ill adult patients who had small-bore feeding tubes recently placed. The combination of measurement of pH and bilirubin levels correctly identified all cases in which respiratory placement had occurred, 75% of the tubes located in the intestines, and more than 60% of the gastric tubes.

Relevance to Nursing Practice
Results of this nursing research study indicate that testing pH and bilirubin content has the potential to reduce the number of radiographs required to exclude respiratory placement, assuming that aspirate can be obtained from the tube. This could also result in a significant reduction in healthcare costs. At this point, pH can be measured easily at the bedside, but bilirubin determination is a laboratory function. This research team is currently involved in developing a bedside method to measure bilirubin.

ify initial placement of a feeding tube (Loan, Magnuson, & Williams, 1998; Metheny, Wehrle, Wiersema, & Clark, 1998a). This is especially a priority when a small-bore tube has been used or when patients are at high risk for aspiration. Because radiographs expose the patient to radiation, must be interpreted by a physician, and may be inaccessible, other methods are also used to check tube placement. These include aspirating gastric contents and measuring the pH of the aspirate (refer to the accompanying box for guidelines for measuring gastric pH). After radiographic examination, measurement of pH is the recommended method for determining correct placement of a feeding tube. Some clinicians remain reluctant to abandon the auscultatory method of checking tube placement (injecting 10 to 30 cc of air into the tube while listening with stethoscope placed over the epigastrium for a "whooshing" sound). This procedure has been proved unreliable and may result in tragic consequences if used as the sole indicator of tube placement. Refer to the accompanying box, Through the Eyes of a Student, for a student nurse's experience with checking tube placement.

Small-bore tubes offer greater resistance during aspiration than larger feeding tubes. Because they are less rigid, they may be more likely to collapse when negative pressure is applied during aspiration. More than likely, the difficulty is a result of a blocked tube or the fact that the ports on the tip of the tube are not positioned in fluid. Research by clinicians has demonstrated that aspiration is easier in small-bore tubes if there are multiple ports rather than a single port. Several attempts may be necessary to aspirate gastric contents. If repeated instillations of 30 mL of air and repositioning prove ineffective, tube placement should be checked by radiograph, or the tube should be removed and reinserted after checking with the physician (Metheny et al., 1998a and 1998b).

Checking placement of a gastrostomy or jejunostomy tube requires regular comparisons (according to agency policy) of the tube length to the measurement (inches or centimeters) that was documented after insertion. An indelible marker can be used to identify the exit point of the tube from the abdomen (O'Brien et al., 1999).

Administering the Feeding to the Patient

Feeding Schedule

Based on the patient's physical, medical, and nutritional condition, the nutritionist usually makes recommendations concerning the feeding pattern or schedule. *Continuous feedings* allow gradual introduction of the formula into the gastrointestinal tract, promoting maximal absorption. They require use of an enteral feeding pump, which limits the patient's mobility and increases cost. Feedings into the intestine are always continuous to avoid triggering the dumping syndrome. Continuous feeding into the stomach is controversial because of the risk for reflux and aspiration.

Intermittent feedings are delivered at regular intervals using a gravity drip or a feeding pump to introduce the formula gradually over a set period of time. Bolus intermittent feedings, whereby a syringe is used to deliver the formula quickly into the stomach, may place the patient at risk for aspiration or cause distention. They are usually not recommended but may be used in long-term situations if tolerated by the patient. Another option is *cyclic feeding.* This involves administering continuous feeding for a portion of the 24-hour period. The usual routine is to feed the patient for 12 to 16 hours, most often overnight. Cyclic feeding allows the patient to attempt eating regular meals during the day, if this is possible, and makes ambulation and activity easier. The basic method for administering a tube feeding is outlined in Procedure 41-2.

Feeding Formulas

The nutritional composition of tube feedings depends on the feeding route, the patient's ability to digest and absorb nutrients, and his or her nutrient and fluid requirements. Other considerations include the availability and cost of the formula, medical conditions that require diet modifications, food intolerance, and allergies. The typical feeding formula has the following caloric breakdown: 16% protein, 54% carbohydrate, and 30% fat (Dudek, 1997). Protein is the most critical component; the patient's needs will determine the complexity of the protein that is required. Many enteral feeding formulas are available. In addition to being nutritionally balanced, formulas may be high in calories, contain fiber, contain additional protein, or be especially formulated for patients with respiratory, renal, or other health problems. Detailed information on their composition and caloric value (most formulas contain 1 cal/mL, although 2 cal/mL concentrations are available) can be obtained from the product label.

Enteral Feeding Pumps

An enteral feeding pump regulates the amount of feeding solution that is delivered to the patient. The newer pumps are user friendly, have built-in safeguards that protect the patient from risk for complications, and can be used in both institutions and the home. Safety features include automatic tube flush, cassettes that prevent free-flow of formula, safety tips that prevent accidental attachment to an intravenous setup, and various audible and visible alarms (Jones & Guenter, 1997; Krupp & Heximer, 1998). Most pumps can operate for up to 8 hours on battery, but manufacturers recommend that whenever the patient is seated or resting for a period of time, the pump should be plugged into an electrical outlet for recharging.

Nursing Considerations With Tube Feeding

Agency protocols may differ and should be followed, but nursing actions that contribute to successful tube feedings include the following.

Promote Patient Safety

- Check tube placement (for technique for testing gastric pH, see the box earlier in this section). The practice of

(*text continues on page 1115*)

Guidelines for Nursing Care

Measuring pH of Gastric Fluids

- Allow 1-hour interval after patient has received medication or completed an intermittent feeding before testing pH of gastric fluid. If feeding is continuous, plan pH testing at a time when feeding can be withheld.
- Irrigate tube with 30 mL of warm water after medications or feeding.
- Insert 30 mL of air into tube before aspirating GI contents.
- Withdraw small amount (5–10 mL) of gastric secretions.
- If unable to obtain specimen, reposition the patient and flush tube again with 30 mL of air. It may be necessary to retry several times, especially if a small-bore feeding tube is in place.
- Place drop of gastric secretions onto pH test paper or place small amount in plastic cup and dip the pH paper into it. Within 30 seconds, compare the color on the paper with the chart supplied by the manufacturer. (A pH meter and color chart are also an option.)
- Document results in the patient's chart. The following are indications of placement:

pH

- Stomach: pH 0–4.0 (If patient is taking an acid-inhibiting agent [eg, Zantac], the range may be 4.0–6.0)
- Intestines: pH 7.0 or higher
- Respiratory tract: pH 6.0 or higher

Color of Aspirate

- Stomach: grassy green, tan, off-white, bloody, or brown
- Intestines: medium to deep golden yellow (may be greenish-brown if stained with bile)
- Respiratory tract: off-white and tinged with mucus

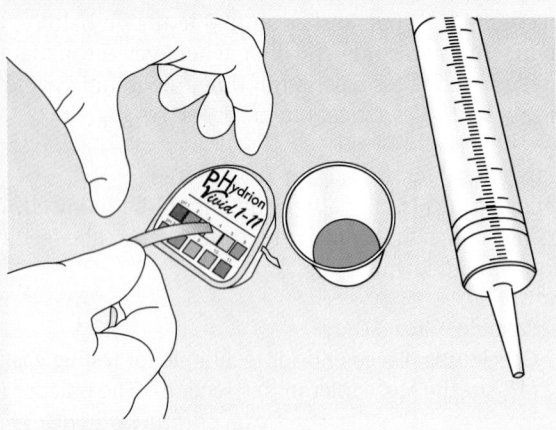

Through the Eyes of a Student

She looked lost in that big hospital bed, so thin and frail. Her hair was as white as her pillowcase and blankets, and her skin looked almost transparent. And then I saw it. Snaking under her blankets into her belly was the feeding tube surrounded by thick, green, smelly discharge.

During preconference my instructor had told me that I needed to check residual every 2 hours to monitor her absorption rate. The first time, with my instructor standing beside me like my guardian angel (or my patient's guardian angel, I'm not sure which), the procedure naturally went off without a hitch. I could do this, I thought, feeling more confident.

Because my patient had chronic diarrhea as well as skin breakdown at her sacrum, the next 2 hours flew by in a whirlwind of bathing. But now the time had come. This is it, I thought. I'm on my own for the second residual check. And, again, I breathed a sigh of relief when the procedure was completed with no problems.

As the day progressed, I got myself a little behind schedule because I was determined to remove the hardened crusts from underneath her nails. Before I knew it, I got the message from another student that it was postconference time. Oh no! I didn't do my last residual check yet. Quickly, I emptied the basin I was using on her fingernails and grabbed the plunger. I reached into my pocket for my hemostat to clamp off the line and the next thing I saw was Jevity squirting all over the bed, my patient, the clean Chux and me! I had cut the line instead of clamping it!

I quickly pinched both ends to stop the Jevity from squirting and frantically called for help. While waiting for rescue, I checked on my patient's response, not knowing how she was going to react. Thankfully, she was sound asleep, soothed by her recent nail massage. It seemed like forever before my instructor rushed in. With my eyes filling up, I attempted to explain that I had grabbed the scissors from my pocket instead of the hemostat. Guardian angel that she was (I think she was both of ours), my instructor calmly and efficiently proceeded to attach both ends of the tube together with the use of an adapter.

Many lessons were learned that day, such as don't attempt a procedure in haste, and have all your supplies readily at hand. But the one thing I'll never, ever forget is that the scissors are the crooked ones!

—Eileen Cooper
Delaware County Community College, Media, PA

PROCEDURE 41-2

Administering a Tube Feeding

Equipment

Tube feeding at room temperature
Stethoscope
Feeding bag or prefilled tube
    feeding set
Alcohol preps

Clamp (Hoffman or butterfly)
Disposable pad or towel
Sterile water for irrigation
Asepto or Toomey syringe

Rubber band
Enteral feeding pump (if ordered)
IV pole
Disposable gloves

Action	Rationale
1. Explain procedure to patient. Use stethoscope to assess bowel sounds.	This facilitates cooperation and provides reassurance for patient. Presence of bowel sounds indicates functional GI tract.
2. Assemble equipment. Check amount, concentration, type, and frequency of tube feeding on patient's chart. Check expiration date of formula.	This provides for organized approach to task. Ensures that correct feeding will be administered. Outdated formula may be contaminated.
3. Wash your hands. Don disposable gloves.	Handwashing deters the spread of microorganisms. Gloves protect from exposure to blood or body fluids.
4. Position patient with head of bed elevated at least 30 degrees or as near normal position for eating as possible.	This position minimizes possibility of aspiration into trachea.
5. Unpin tube from patient's gown and check to see that the nasogastric tube is properly located in the stomach, as described in Procedure 42-1, Action 14.	Even when initially positioned correctly, a nasogastric tube left in place can become dislodged between feedings. The instillation of water or nourishment could lead to serious respiratory problems if a gastric tube is in the trachea or a bronchus, rather than in the stomach.
6. Aspirate all gastric contents with a syringe and measure. Return immediately through tube, saving small amount to measure gastric pH. Flush tube with 30 mL of sterile water for irrigation. Proceed with feeding if amount of residual does not exceed policy of agency or physician's guideline. Disconnect syringe from tubing.	This indicates gastric emptying time. A residual of more than 100 mL or more than 10% to 20% above the hourly feeding rate must be reported to physician. Fluid should be returned to stomach so as not to cause any fluid or electrolyte losses.
7. Measure pH of aspirated gastric fluid.	Gastric contents have a pH of 0 to 4.0; intestinal secretions have a pH of 7.0 or higher.

For Intermittent Feedings

Action	Rationale
8. When using a feeding bag (open system):	
a. Hang bag on IV pole and adjust to about 12 inches above the stomach. Clamp tubing.	Formula displaces air in the tubing.
b. Cleanse top of feeding container with alcohol before opening it. Pour formula into feeding bag and allow solution to run through tubing. Close clamp.	Cleansing container top with alcohol minimizes risk for contaminants entering feeding bag. Formula displaces air in tubing.
c. Attach feeding setup to feeding tube, open clamp, and regulate drip according to physician's order or allow feeding to run in over 30 minutes.	Introducing the formula at a slow, regular rate allows the stomach to accommodate to the feeding and decreases gastrointestinal distress.

(continued)

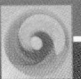

PROCEDURE 41-2

Administering a Tube Feeding (Continued)

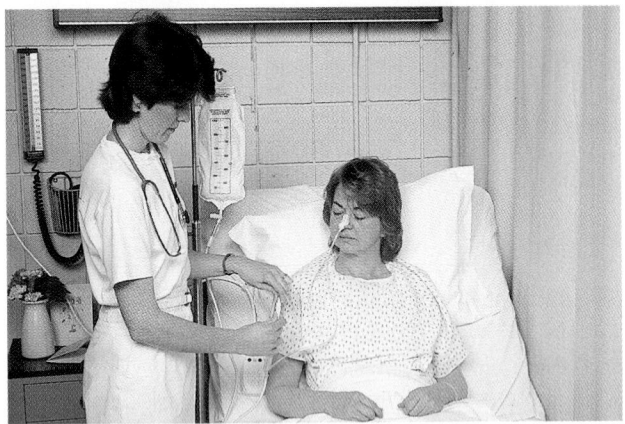

Action 7c: Attaching feeding-bag tubing to tube.

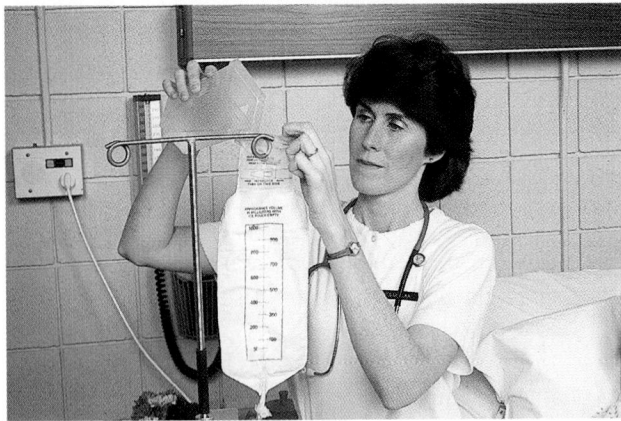

Action 7d: Adding water to rinse feeding tube.

d. Add 30 to 60 mL (1–2 oz) of sterile water for irrigation to feeding bag when feeding is almost completed and allow it to run through tube.

Water rinses the feeding from the tube and helps to keep it patent.

e. Clamp the tubing immediately after water has been instilled. Disconnect from tube. Clamp tube and cover end with sterile gauze secured with a rubber band or apply cap.

Clamping the tube prevents air from entering the stomach. Cover on end of tube deters entry of microorganisms and protects patient and linens from fluid leakage from tube.

9. When using prefilled tube feeding set-up (closed system):

   a. Remove screw-on cap and attach administration set-up with drip chamber and tubing. Hang set on IV pole and adjust to about 12 inches above the stomach. Clamp tubing and squeeze drip chamber to fill one third to one half of capacity. Release clamp and run formula through tubing. Close clamp.

   Formula displaces air in tubing.

   b. Follow Actions 8c, 8d, and 8e. Feeding pump may be used with tube feeding set-up to regulate drip.

10. When using a feeding pump:

    a. Close flow-regulator clamp on tubing and fill feeding bag with prescribed formula. The amount used depends on agency policy. Place label on container.

    Feeding intolerance is less likely to occur with smaller volumes. Hanging smaller amounts of feeding also reduces risk for bacteria growth and contamination of feeding at room temperature.

    b. Hang feeding container on IV pole and allow solution to flow through tubing.

    This prevents air from being forced into the stomach or intestines.

    c. Connect to feeding pump following manufacturer's directions. Set rate.

    Smaller volume of feeding is infused continuously and is more easily tolerated by patient.

    d. Check residual every 4 to 8 hours.

    Checking verifies placement of the tube and proper absorption of the feeding.

(*continued*)

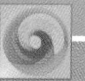

PROCEDURE 41-2

Administering a Tube Feeding (Continued)

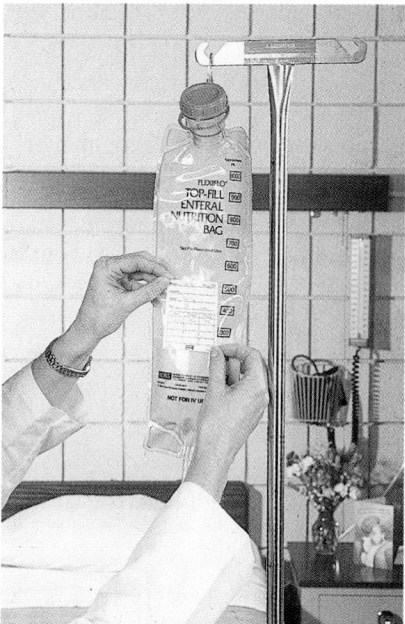

Action 10a: Placing label on container. (Photo © B. Proud.)

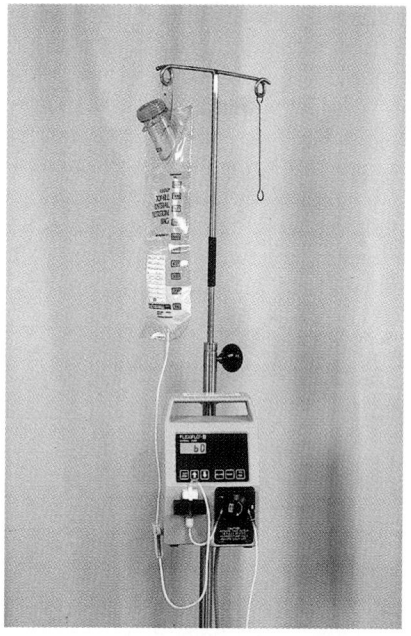

Action 10c: Feeding pump with feeding.

11. Observe patient's response during and after tube feeding.

12. Have patient remain in upright position for at least 30 minutes to 1 hour after feeding.

13. Wash and clean equipment or replace according to agency policy. Remove gloves and wash your hands.

14. Record type and amount of feeding and patient's response. Monitor blood glucose, if ordered by physician.

Pain may indicate stomach distention, which may lead to vomiting.

This position minimizes risk for backflow and discourages aspiration, if any vomiting should occur.

This prevents contamination and deters spread of microorganisms.

This provides accurate documentation of procedure. Many feedings contain high amounts of carbohydrates.

adding food dye or coloring to the tube feeding as a means of detecting aspirated fluid is not recommended (Dudek, 1997). Blue food coloring may be added to the tube feeding, particularly if the patient has an endotracheal tube, to detect the presence of aspirate in pulmonary secretions. The coloring may be contaminated with bacteria because it usually sits by the bedside, can cause diarrhea because it contains sorbitol, and can interfere with guaiac testing of stool. It is safer to test pulmonary secretions with a glucose dipstick. Unless blood is present in pulmonary secretions, they usually do not contain any glucose.

- Check *residual* (feeding remaining in the stomach) before each feeding or every 4 to 6 hours during a continuous feeding. Record residuals on flow sheet

or progress notes. Check agency procedure, but a residual of more than 100 mL or more than 10% to 20% above the hourly rate for the feeding may indicate that the feeding should be interrupted or delayed for 30 minutes to 1 hour. Some experts now recommend that the patient's pattern of residual is more important than the amount. Many patients can tolerate amounts in excess of 300 mL without experiencing any complications (Loan et al., 1998).

- Assess for bowel sounds at least once per shift to check for the presence of peristalsis and a functional intestinal tract. Experts, however, have recently come to the conclusion that it is not uncommon for acutely ill patients to have delayed or absent gastric emptying; therefore, delaying enteral feedings based on the absence of bowel sounds may place a patient at risk for malnutrition. Gastric distention or pain may be a better indicator of how well a patient is tolerating a tube feeding (Loan et al., 1998).

- Prevent contamination during enteral feedings by maintaining the integrity of the feeding system and using proper technique. Loan and colleagues (1998) state that a *closed system* reduces the opportunity for bacterial contamination. A closed system consists of a sterile, prefilled, ready-to-hang container, whereas an *open system* exists when formula from a can or bottle is added to a feeding setup. The expiration date of formula should always be checked; hands should be washed before touching the equipment; all equipment should be labeled with the patient's name, date, and

time the feeding was hung; sterile water should be used for flushing the tube; and disconnected tubing should be capped or covered. A reusable feeding system is usually cleansed with soap and hot water every 24 hours, whereas a disposable feeding apparatus is usually replaced every 24 hours.

Monitor Patient for Presence of Complications

A summary of common complications and preventive nursing measures is given in the accompanying Guidelines for Nursing Care box.

- Prevent the tube from becoming clogged or obstructed. Common causes of clogged enteral tubes include aspirated stomach contents, residue from

---

Guidelines for Nursing Care
Preventing Complications in Enteral Feeding

Potential Complications for Aspiration

- Use appropriate measures to check tube placement.
- Elevate head of bed at least 30 degrees during feeding and for 1 hour afterward.
- Give small, frequent feedings.
- Avoid oversedation of patient.

Potential Complications for Clogged Tube

- Flush tube before and after feeding, every 4 hours during continuous feeding, and after withdrawing aspirate.
- Instill 30 mL of water with 50-mL syringe.

Potential Complications for Nasal Erosion With Nasogastric or Nasointestinal Tubes

- Check nostrils every shift for signs of pressure.
- Clean and moisten nares every 4 to 8 hours.

Potential Complication for Diarrhea

- Start feeding at slow rate.
- Prevent contamination in both open and closed systems:
  - Change delivery set every 12 to 24 hours according to agency policy.
  - Refrigerate opened cans of formula and discard after 24 hours.
  - Limit hang time to 8 hours when using open system.
- Use aseptic technique for patients who are immunosuppressed or acutely ill.
- Assess for fecal impaction.

Potential for Other GI Symptoms (Nausea, Vomiting, Distention)

- Check residual prior to intermittent feedings and every 4 hours during continuous feedings.

- Avoid oversedating client (delays gastric emptying).

Potential Complication for Unplanned Extubation

- Anchor tube adequately with tape.
- Check on patient frequently.
- Measure external length of tubing at regular intervals.

Potential Complication for Gastrostomy or Jejunostomy: "Buried Bumper" Syndrome (bumper or retaining disc presses too tightly against abdominal wall)

- Notify physician for complaints of bloating, abdominal discomfort, or signs of tube malfunction or bleeding.

Potential Complication for Stoma Infection

- Clean skin every shift with soap and warm water. Dry thoroughly.
- Use topical antibiotics as ordered.
- Assess for signs of infection.
- Request consult with wound care specialist.

Potential Complication for Refeeding Syndrome (electrolyte and metabolic disorder that can occur when a nutritionally depleted patient is fed enterally or parenterally)

- Monitor for muscle weakness that can progress to respiratory failure (due to decreased phosphorus in the cells).
- Assess for potassium depletion.
- Administer phosphorus and potassium supplements as ordered by physician (Belcaster, 1997).

medications, feeding flow rate of less than 50 mL/h, infrequent or inadequate addition of water to the system, and using a tube with a small lumen (Dudek, 1997). Flush tube with 30 to 50 mL of water before and after each feeding or introduction of medications, at least every 4 hours during a continuous feeding, and after aspirating a tube for gastric contents. Use of a feeding pump helps to prevent clogging. If an occlusion occurs, fill a large piston syringe with warm water and use a gentle push-and-pull motion. Carbonated beverages have not proved effective in unclogging a feeding tube (Kohn-Keeth, 2000).

Provide Comfort Measures

- Administer oral hygiene frequently to prevent drying of tissues and to relieve thirst. Offer the patient the opportunity to rinse the mouth with warm water and mouthwash solution frequently. Lubricate the lips generously.
- Keep the nares clean, especially around the tube where secretions tend to accumulate. Using a lubricant after cleaning the nares is recommended.
- Help control local irritation from the tube in the throat. Analgesic throat lozenges or anesthetic sprays may be effective.
- Encourage the patient, if able, to verbalize concerns about tube feeding and presence of tube. A visit from another person who has learned to cope with this alternate feeding method may prove helpful.

Provide Instruction

- Provide health teaching to the patient and caregivers if enteral feedings will continue in the home.
- Individualized instructions should be provided in written form as a reference for the patient and caregivers.
- Include information about the administration of feedings, operation of the pump, formula, instructions regarding rate and how to check for tube placement.
- Review care of the tube insertion site and possible complications that need to be reported.
- Discuss proper preparation, cleaning, and disposal of equipment.
- Provide emergency telephone numbers, including the number for the home healthcare agency and the physician.
- Arrangements should be made for a visit from the home health nurse as soon as possible after discharge (Dudek, 1997; O'Brien et al., 1999).

Removing the Tube

The tube must be removed as carefully as it is inserted to provide as much comfort as possible to the patient. Oral hygiene follows removal of the tube. This is especially important to remove disagreeable tastes and odors and should be done thoroughly when the tube has been in the intestinal tract and in contact with intestinal contents. Directions for removing the nasogastric tube are given in Procedure 41-3.

Using Nasoenteric Tubes for Decompression

In addition to providing enteral feedings, nasogastric tubes can be used for other purposes. They may be inserted to decompress or drain the stomach of fluid and air, allowing it to rest, or before or after surgery, to promote healing. Nasogastric tubes may also be used to monitor gastrointestinal bleeding and prevent intestinal obstruction. Single- and double-lumen tubes (the lumen is the inner open space) are available. A single-lumen Levin tube lacks a venting system, and mucosal damage can occur when suction is applied continuously. Double-lumen sump tubes are a tube within a tube (eg, the Salem sump tube). One lumen empties the stomach, and the second lumen provides for a continuous flow of air. The airflow lumen controls suction by preventing the drainage lumen from pulling stomach mucosa into the tube's eyes and irritating the stomach lining. Suction can be continuous rather than intermittent, as is required when a single-lumen tube is used. Nasogastric tubes used for decompression require irrigation with 30 to 60 mL of normal saline solution (0.9% sodium chloride) to compensate for electrolytes that are lost in the gastric fluids removed by suction (McConnell, 1994). This is different from tubes used for feeding purposes, which are cleared before and after use with sterile water or tap water according to the physician's order. Procedure 41-4 outlines techniques for irrigating a nasogastric tube that is being used for decompression.

Providing Parenteral Nutrition

Patients who have nonfunctional gastrointestinal tracts, who are comatose, or who cannot consume a nutritionally adequate diet enterally (eg, patients undergoing aggressive cancer therapy and those recovering from extensive burns, surgery, sepsis, or multiple fractures) may require parenteral nutrition. **Total parenteral nutrition (TPN)** bypasses the gastrointestinal tract for patients who are unable to take fluid orally and meets the patient's nutritional needs by way of nutrient-filled solutions administered intravenously through a central line, usually the subclavian or internal jugular veins. *Hyperalimentation* is another term used synonymously with parenteral nutrition.

TPN therapy is costly, requires constant monitoring, and has the potential for causing infectious, metabolic, and mechanical complications. It should be used only when enteral intake is inadequate or contraindicated and should be gradually discontinued as soon as possible. *Partial parenteral nutrition or peripheral parenteral nutrition* (PPN) is prescribed for patients who have an inadequate intake of oral feedings but require supplementation of nutrients through a peripheral vein. Isotonic solutions may be delivered peripherally (PPN), whereas hypertonic solutions must be administered through a central vein (TPN).

Identifying Patients Who Need Parenteral Nutrition

Assessment of serum albumin level is the best indicator of a patient in need of TPN. Patients whose levels are 2.5 g/dL or less are at severe risk for malnutrition. TPN contains the three primary components necessary to maintain nutrition: proteins, carbohydrates, and fats.

PROCEDURE 41-3

Removing a Nasogastric Tube

Equipment

Tissues
Bath towel or disposable pad
Disposable plastic bag

50-mL syringe (optional)
Normal saline solution for irrigation
(optional)

Disposable gloves

Action	Rationale
1. Check physician's order for removal of nasogastric tube.	This ensures correct implementation of physician's order.
2. Explain procedure to patient and assist to semi-Fowler's position.	Explanation facilitates patient cooperation. Sitting position decreases risk of aspiration, if vomiting should occur.
3. Gather equipment.	This provides for organized approach to task.
4. Wash your hands. Don clean disposable gloves.	Handwashing deters the spread of microorganisms. Gloves protect hands from contact with abdominal secretions.
5. Place towel or disposable pad across patient's chest. Give tissues to patient.	Precautions protect patient from contact with gastric secretions. Tissues are necessary if patient wants to blow his or her nose when tube is removed.
6. Discontinue suction and separate tube from suction. Unpin tube from patient's gown and carefully remove adhesive tape from patient's nose.	Disconnecting tube allows for its unrestricted removal.
7. Attach syringe and flush with 10 mL normal saline solution or clear with 30 to 50 cc of air (optional).	Air or saline solution clears the tube of feeding or debris.
8. Instruct patient to take a deep breath and hold it.	This prevents accidental aspiration of gastric secretions in tube.
9. Clamp tube with fingers by doubling tube on itself. Quickly and carefully remove tube while patient holds breath.	Careful removal minimizes trauma and discomfort for patient. Clamping prevents drainage of gastric contents in tube.
10. Place tube in disposable plastic bag. Remove gloves and place in bag.	This prevents contamination with microorganisms.
11. Offer mouth care to patient and facial tissue to blow nose.	Provides for comfort.
12. Measure nasogastric drainage. Remove all equipment and dispose according to agency policy. Wash your hands.	Measuring nasogastric drainage provides for accurate recording of output. Proper disposal deters spread of microorganisms.
13. Record removal of tube, patient's response, and measurement of drainage. Continue to monitor patient for 2–4 hours after tube removal for gastric distention, nausea, or vomiting.	Facilitates documentation and provides for comprehensive care.

Additional components of parenteral nutrition include electrolytes, vitamins, and trace elements. Medications such as insulin (because TPN contains large concentrations of glucose) and heparin (to prevent formation of a blood clot on the tip of the catheter) may also added to the solution. The concentration of glucose in TPN is usually about 25%, yielding a hypertonic solution that, because of its concentration, must be delivered through a central vein. Fat or lipid emulsions and the dextrose add caloric value that the body needs to meet energy requirements. TPN can be given for extended periods of time (up to 3 months) through a peripherally inserted central catheter (PICC; refer to Chap. 45 for additional discussion of PICCs). PPN solutions provide fewer calories and supplement a patient's inadequate oral intake. This solution usually contains 10% glucose, which is suitable for

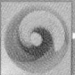

PROCEDURE 41-4

Irrigating a Nasogastric Tube Connected to Suction

Equipment

Nasogastric tube connected to continuous or intermittent suction
Irrigation set (Asepto or Toomey syringe and container for irrigating solution)

Normal saline solution (0.9% sodium chloride solution) for irrigation
Stethoscope

Disposable pad or bath towel
Clamp
Disposable gloves

Action	Rationale
1. Check physician's order for irrigation. Explain procedure to patient.	This clarifies schedule and irrigating solution. An explanation encourages patient cooperation and reduces apprehension.
2. Gather necessary equipment. Check expiration dates on irrigating saline solution and irrigation set.	This provides for organized approach to task. Agency policy dictates safe interval for reuse of equipment.
3. Wash your hands.	Handwashing deters the spread of microorganisms.
4. Assist patient to semi-Fowler's position, unless this is contraindicated.	This position minimizes risk for aspiration.
5. Check placement of nasogastric tube (refer to Procedure 41-1, Action 14).	
6. Pour irrigating solution into container. Draw up 30 mL of saline solution (or amount ordered by physician) into syringe.	This delivers measured amount of irrigant through tube. Saline solution compensates for electrolytes lost through nasogastric drainage.
7. Clamp suction tubing near connection site. Disconnect tube from suction apparatus and lay on disposable pad or towel or hold both tubes upright in nondominant hand.	This protects patient from leakage of nasogastric drainage.
8. Place tip of syringe in tube. If Salem sump or double-lumen tube is used, make sure that syringe tip is placed in drainage port and not in air vent. Hold syringe upright and gently insert the irrigant (or allow solution to flow in by gravity if agency or physician indicates). Do not force solution into tube.	Position of syringe prevents entry of air into stomach. Gentle insertion of saline solution (or gravity insertion) is less traumatic to gastric mucosa.

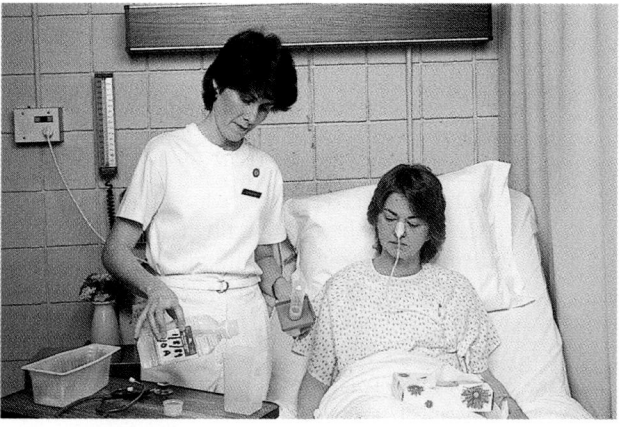

Action 7: Preparing irrigant.

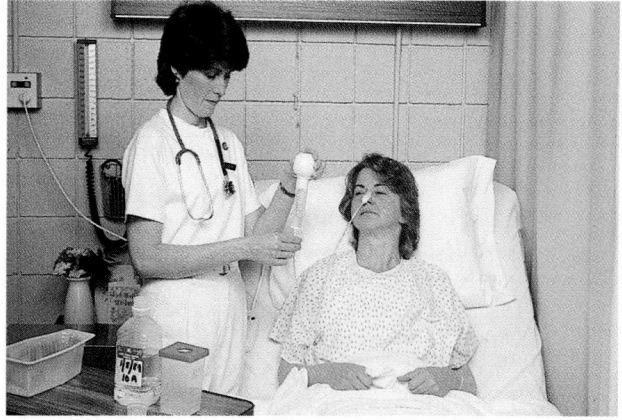

Action 8: Introducing irrigant into tube.

(continued)

9. If unable to irrigate tube, reposition patient and attempt irrigation again. Check with physician if repeated attempts to irrigate tube fail.	Tube may be positioned against gastric mucosa, making it difficult to irrigate.
10. Withdraw or aspirate fluid into syringe. If no return, inject 20 cc of air and aspirate again.	Injection of air may reposition the end of tube.
11. Reconnect tube to suction. Observe movement of solution or drainage.	Observation determines patency of tube and correct operation of suction apparatus.
12. Measure and record amount and description of irrigant and returned solution.	Irrigant placed in tube is considered intake; solution returned is recorded as output.
13. Rinse equipment if it will be reused.	This promotes cleanliness and prepares equipment for next irrigation.
14. Wash your hands.	Handwashing deters the spread of microorganisms.
15. Record irrigation procedure, description of drainage, and patient's response.	This facilitates documentation of procedure and provides for comprehensive care.

administration into a peripheral vessel. The accompanying Guidelines for Nursing Care box lists nursing guidelines for monitoring administration of parenteral nutrition.

Although the benefits of parenteral nutrition are extensive, return to oral or enteral nutrition is recommended as soon as possible. This lessens the risk for sepsis and prevents wasting and deterioration of the gastrointestinal tract. Prevention of potential complications associated with total parenteral nutrition requires vigilance and careful monitoring by the nurse. They include the following (Phipps, Sands, & Marek, et al., 1999):

- Insertion problems, such as pneumothorax, air embolism, and thromboembolism
- Infection
- Metabolic alterations, such as hyperglycemia or hypoglycemia when infusion is discontinued or interrupted (see Procedure 41-5, Monitoring the Blood Glucose Level)
- Fluid, electrolyte, and acid–base imbalances

Guidelines for Nursing Care

Monitoring Administration of Parenteral Nutrition

- Check that catheter lumen used for administration of parenteral nutrition is labeled to indicate this.
- Use a pump to administer infusion of parenteral nutrition.
- If administration of parenteral nutrition is interrupted, administer a 5% to 10% dextrose solution to prevent hypoglycemia.
- Discard unused parenteral nutrition solution within 24 hours of starting its administration.
- Check vital signs every 4 hours to monitor for development of infection or sepsis.
- Monitor blood glucose levels every 6 hours. (Procedure 41-5 explains the technique for monitoring serum glucose levels.)

- Use aseptic technique when changing solution, tubing, filter, or dressings according to agency policy. Most infection control practitioners recommend changing infusion administration sets every 24 hours. Dressings should be changed at least every 24 hours or according to agency protocol.
- Check that all connections are securely taped, catheter is clamped before opening the system, and insertion site is covered with an air-occlusive or transparent polyurethane dressing to prevent an air embolism.
- Compare the patient's daily weight to fluid intake and output. Total weight gain should not be greater than 3 lb per week.
- Assess serum protein and electrolyte levels for signs of imbalance.

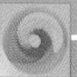

PROCEDURE 41-5

Monitoring the Blood Glucose Level

Equipment

Blood glucose meter   Sterile lancet   Alcohol swab or soap and water
Testing strips   Cotton balls   Disposable gloves

Action	Rationale
1. Check physician's order for monitoring schedule.	This confirms times for checking blood glucose.
2. Gather equipment.	This provides an organized approach to the task.
3. Explain procedure to patient.	Explanation encourages patient cooperation.
4. Wash hands. Don disposable gloves.	Handwashing deters the spread of microorganisms. Gloves protect from exposure to blood or body fluids.
5. Prepare lancet.	Aseptic technique maintains sterility.
6. Remove test strip from the vial and recap container immediately. Turn monitor on and check that code number on strip matches the code number on the monitor screen.	Immediate recapping protects strips from exposure to light and discoloration. Matching code numbers on the strip and glucose monitor ensure that machine is calibrated correctly.
7. Massage side of finger for adult (or heel for child) toward puncture site.	Massage encourages blood flow to the area.

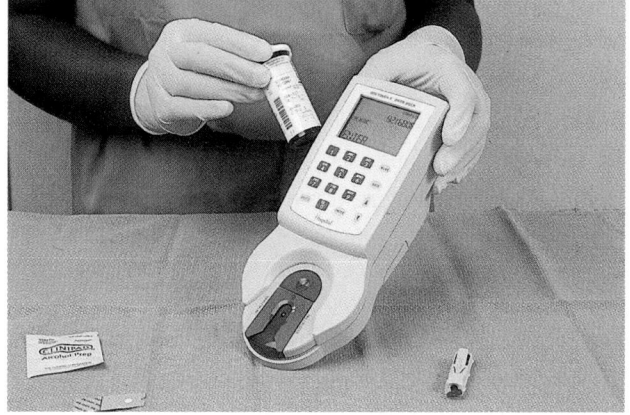

Action 6: Comparing the code number on the strip to the code number on the monitor screen.

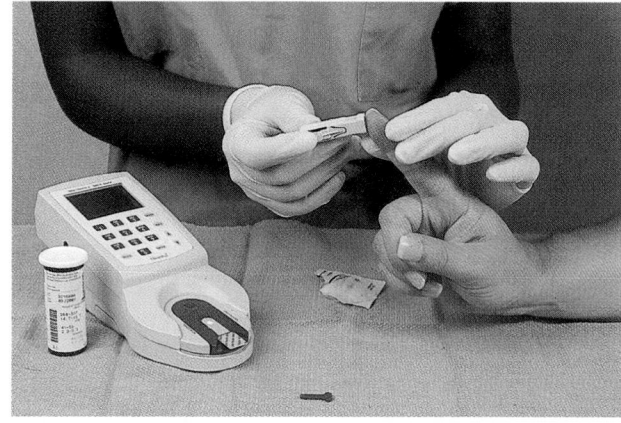

Action 9: Using the lancet to prick the skin.

8. Have patient wash hands with soap and warm water or cleanse area with alcohol. Dry thoroughly.	Washing with soap and water or alcohol cleanses the puncture site. Warm water also helps to cause vasodilation.
9. Hold lancet perpendicular to skin and prick site with the lancet.	Holding lancet in proper position facilitates proper skin penetration.
10. Wipe away first drop of blood with cotton ball if recommended by manufacturer of monitor.	Some feel first drop of blood may be contaminated by serum or cleansing product and produce an inaccurate reading.
11. Lightly squeeze or milk the puncture site until a hanging drop of blood has formed (check instructions for monitor).	Large droplet facilitates accurate test results.

(continued)

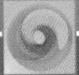

PROCEDURE 41-5

Monitoring the Blood Glucose Level (Continued)

12. Gently touch drop of blood to pad on test strip without smearing it.

13. Insert strip into the meter according to directions for that specific device. Some devices require that the drop of blood is applied to a test strip that has already been inserted in the monitor.

Smearing blood on strip may result in inaccurate test results.

Correctly inserted strip allows meter to read blood glucose level accurately.

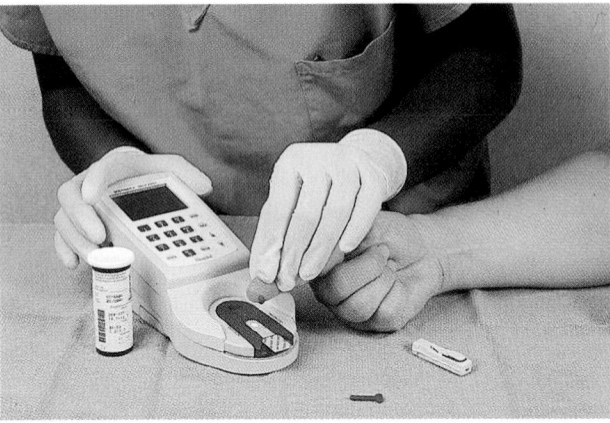

Action 12: Preparing to place a drop of blood on the strip.

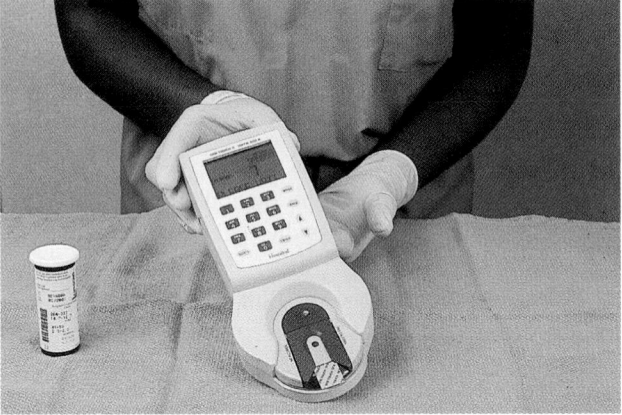

Action 14: Awaiting test results while the timer counts down.

14. Press timer if directed by manufacturer.

15. Apply pressure to puncture site.

16. Read blood glucose results and document appropriately at bedside. Inform patient of test result.

17. Turn meter off, dispose of supplies appropriately, and place lancet in sharps container.

18. Remove gloves and wash hands.

19. Record blood glucose on chart or medication record.

Timing produces accurate results.

Pressure causes hemostasis.

Timing when awaiting results depends on type of meter.

Proper disposal prevents exposure to blood and accidental needle sticks.

Handwashing prevents the spread of microorganisms.

This facilitates documentation of procedure and provides for comprehensive care.

Many patients, however, require long-term parenteral nutrition and continue this therapy in the home. Individuals with acquired immunodeficiency syndrome (AIDS), advanced cancer, difficulty swallowing, or chronic bowel problems are candidates for this type of nutritional support. Nurses are involved in educating the patient and caregiver about the techniques and responsibilities associated with parenteral nutrition, providing technical and psycho-

logical support, and documenting the assessments that allow parenteral nutrition to be continued in the home.

EVALUATING

The effectiveness of the plan of care is evaluated as the last step in the nursing care process. On an ongoing basis, the nurse should accomplish the following:

- Evaluate the patient's progress toward meeting nutritional goals
- Evaluate the patient's tolerance and adherence to the diet, when appropriate
- Assess the patient's level of understanding of the diet and the need for further diet instruction or reinforcement

- Communicate findings to other members of the healthcare team
- Revise the plan of care, as needed, or terminate nursing care

See the accompanying Applying Learning to Practice: Patient Care Study and Nursing Plan of Care boxes.

APPLYING LEARNING TO PRACTICE

Patient Care Study

Susan Oakland, a 21-year-old student, was seen at the prenatal clinic for her first pregnancy at 5 weeks' gestation. On her next visit, 4 weeks later, she complained of nausea and vomiting and had lost 3 lb (1.4 kg).

Assessment Findings

A comprehensive nutritional assessment revealed the following data:

ANTHROPOMETRIC DATA

Usual body weight: 112 lb (50.8 kg)
Weight at 9 weeks' gestation 109 lb (49.4 kg)
Height: 5 feet 5 inches (165.1 cm)
Ideal body weight: 125 lb (56.7 kg; range is 113 to 137 lb [51.3 to 62.1 kg])
Expected weight gain for 9 weeks' gestation: 1 to 2 lb (0.45 to 0.9 kg)

BIOCHEMICAL DATA

Laboratory data revealed low hemoglobin level and hematocrit.

MEDICAL AND SOCIOECONOMIC DATA

- Patient complains of nausea and vomiting, which begin in the morning and continue until midafternoon. Her appetite is poor. She also states, "I'm always tired."
- Patient and her husband are first-semester graduate students; their source of income is graduate assistantships, and their food budget is limited.
- Patient states that she did not intend to become pregnant, but both she and her husband are excited about becoming parents. She plans to take a leave of absence from school for one semester when the baby is born; she wants to breastfeed.

CLINICAL DATA

Patient appears pale. No other abnormal physical findings were noted.

DIETARY DATA

- Patient's 24-hour recall revealed an inadequate intake from the milk group and a marginal intake from the grain and meat groups. She skips breakfast because of a hurried schedule, which is now complicated by nausea; lunch comprises soup, salad, and fruit; dinner usually comprises chicken; cooked vegetables; pasta, rice, or potatoes; and fruit. Patient dislikes red meat and eats it only once or twice a month. She also dislikes milk and substitutes sugar-free soft drinks and water. Before becoming pregnant, she drank five or six cups of black coffee a day, but now she avoids it. Her snacks usually consist of fresh fruit and vegetables.
- Patient is very weight conscious; she periodically crash diets to maintain her weight at 112 lb (50.8 kg).
- Patient does not take vitamins, medications, or drugs; she drinks socially.
- Nutritional problems and contributing factors include the following:
  - Inadequate intake of milk and calories contributed to by nausea and vomiting, dislike for milk, limited food budget, weight consciousness
  - Poor iron intake contributed to by lack of good sources of iron in her diet, no supplemental iron intake
  - Meal-skipping contributed to by nausea and vomiting, hurried schedule
  - Underweight or weight loss contributed to by weight consciousness, nausea, and vomiting

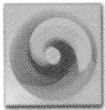

NURSING PLAN OF CARE
for Susan Oakland

Nursing Diagnosis

Altered Nutrition: Less than Body Requirements related to increased requirements imposed by pregnancy, nausea and vomiting, weight consciousness, hurried schedule, food dislikes as manifested by: reports of anorexia, fatigue, 3-lb weight loss in 4 weeks' time, pale color, and low hemoglobin and hematocrit values.

Expected Outcome

By the next monthly assessment, 6/26/01, the patient will:
* Eat three or more small meals a day

Nursing Interventions	Rationale	Evaluative Statement
Determine how the patient's schedule may be altered to allow time for meals. Encourage the patient to have easy-to-eat foods available for quick snacks, like cartons of yogurt, cheese and crackers, muffins, and fresh fruit.	Patient complained that her current schedule prevents regular meals. Easy-to-eat foods may be more acceptable and can be nutritionally comparable to traditional meals.	6/26/01 Goal met. Patient eats three meals daily. Tries snacking on easy-to-eat foods when possible. *Recommendation:* Encourage more snacking to increase overall food intake. *L. Swift, RN*
Advise the patient that nausea may be lessened by avoiding periods of hunger, and that later in the pregnancy, avoiding hunger will help ensure a steady supply of nutrients to the fetus.	Low blood glucose may contribute to nausea early in pregnancy; later in pregnancy, low blood glucose and resultant ketosis may be harmful to the fetus.	

Expected Outcome

By the next monthly assessment, 6/26/01, the patient will:
* Eat dry crackers, bread sticks, or dry cereal 30 minutes before rising

Nursing Interventions	Rationale	Evaluative Statement
Advise the patient to eat a source of dry carbohydrates before getting up in the morning.	Eating dry carbohydrates 30 minutes before rising helps avoid nausea.	6/26/01 Goal met. Patient eats dry crackers every morning 30 minutes before getting out of bed. Reports that it prevents morning nausea. *L. Swift, RN*

Expected Outcome

By the next monthly assessment, 6/26/01, the patient will:
* Drink water between meals

Nursing Interventions	Rationale	Evaluative Statement
Advise the patient to avoid fluid with meals. Recommend fluids be consumed 1 hour before or 2 hours after eating.	Fluid with meals may contribute to nausea.	6/26/01 Goal met. Patient avoids liquids with meals. Nausea is occurring less frequently throughout the day. *L. Swift, RN*

(continued)

NURSING PLAN OF CARE (Continued)
for Susan Oakland

Expected Outcome

By the next monthly assessment, 6/26/01, the patient will:
- Avoid diet soft drinks

Nursing Interventions	Rationale	Evaluative Statement
Advise the patient to avoid diet soft drinks. Recommend acceptable nutritional alternatives to the patient.	Saccharin and aspartame have not been proved safe for the fetus.	6/26/01 Goal partially met. Patient reports that she drinks two or three cans of diet soft drinks a week at school to relieve thirst because nothing else is available. *Recommendation:* Encourage the patient to bring something to drink during the day from home, such as frozen drink boxes of 100% fruit juice, which will thaw at room temperature, or an insulated container of ice water or milk flavored with vanilla (dislikes plain milk). *L. Swift, RN*

Expected Outcome

By the next monthly assessment, 6/26/01, the patient will:
- Eat the recommended number of servings from each food group as suggested by the daily food guide for pregnancy

Nursing Interventions	Rationale	Evaluative Statement
Provide the patient with a daily food guide for pregnancy, and explain the rationale for the increased recommendations. Investigate acceptable alternatives for red meat and milk, which the patient normally does not consume.	Because this is the patient's first pregnancy, she is not aware of the recommendations for eating during pregnancy. Although no one particular food is essential during pregnancy, red meat is essential during pregnancy and an excellent source of iron, and milk is an excellent source of calcium, two minerals important for the developing fetus. If the patient is not provided with nutritionally equivalent alternatives, her diet may not be optimal, even if she consumes the recommended number of servings from the meat and milk groups (ie, patient may not be getting as much iron as she can from her diet if she relies on fish, cheese, and white-meat poultry to satisfy the meat group recommendations).	6/26/01 Goal partially met. Patient's intake is improved: intake from the grain and meat groups is adequate instead of marginal. However, the patient still has difficulty consuming enough items from the milk group. *Recommendation:* Continue encouraging the patient to consume more items from the milk group, such as cheese, yogurt, and pudding. Will advise the patient to add skim milk powder whenever possible to fortify home-cooked and home-baked products. Will recommend that the patient increase her intake of non-dairy sources of calcium, such as broccoli, spinach, and greens. *L. Swift, RN*

(continued)

NURSING PLAN OF CARE (Continued)
for Susan Oakland

Expected Outcome	By the next monthly assessment, 6/26/01, the patient will: • Gain 1 to 2 lb

Nursing Interventions	Rationale	Evaluative Statement
Advise the patient on the recommended rate and amount of weight gain. Stress the importance of quality weight gain.	Patient needs to understand that a 25- to 35-lb gradual weight gain is considered optimal for fetal development, and results in little gain in maternal fat tissue. However, because the fetus and maternal tissues require nutrients along with calories, it is essential that the weight gain comes from eating nutrient-dense calories instead of empty calories.	6/26/01 Goal met. Noting a relief from nausea and an increase in the number of daily meals, the patient gained 2 lb. *L. Swift, RN*

Expected Outcome	By the next monthly assessment, the patient will: • Take prenatal vitamins as prescribed by the physician

Nursing Interventions	Rationale	Evaluative Statement
Advise the patient to take the supplement as prescribed and that the supplements are not a substitute for an adequate diet.	Supplements are intended to be used in conjunction with an optimal diet, not in place of one, because they do not provide optimal amounts of all required nutrients. Because the requirements for folic acid and iron during pregnancy are usually not met through diet alone, supplements of these two nutrients in particular are necessary.	6/26/01 Goal met. Patient reports taking supplement as prescribed. No adverse effects noted. *Recommendation:* Will continue to monitor patient's tolerance of supplement. Will continue to implement plan and reassess at next monthly appointment, 7/28/01. *L. Swift, RN*
Advise the patient that the iron content in the supplements may cause constipation and the stools to become black.	Common adverse effects of large iron doses are constipation and black stools.	

Sample Documentation	5/22/01 Nursing

Mrs. Oakland was seen for routine prenatal checkup at 9 weeks' gestation. Assessment findings reveal that the patient is underweight, has lost 3 lb (1.4 kg) in the past 4 weeks, is experiencing nausea and vomiting, has a deficient hemoglobin and hematocrit, and is fatigued. Other contributing factors include weight consciousness, hurried schedule, and food dislikes. Discussion centered on maintaining good dietary habits, improving overall intake and meal patterns to meet the demands of pregnancy and subsequent lactation, initiating dietary changes aimed at avoiding nausea and vomiting, and increasing iron intake. See plan of care. Patient's progress will be evaluated at the next monthly visit, 6/26/01.

L. Swift, RN

Learning Outcomes

After completing this chapter, the learner should be able to accomplish the following:

1. Define the key terms used in the chapter.

anorexia	nutrition
anthropometric	obesity
basal metabolism	percutaneous endoscopic
calorie	gastrostomy tube (PEG)
carbohydrate	protein
cholesterol	recommended dietary
enteral nutrition	allowance (RDA)
lipid	total parenteral
minerals	nutrition (TPN)
nasogastric (NG) tube	triglycerides
nasointestinal (NI) tube	vitamins
nutrient	

2. List the six classes of nutrients and explain the significance of each.
3. Evaluate a diet using the Food Guide Pyramid.
4. Identify risk factors for poor nutritional status.
5. Describe nutritional implications of growth and development throughout the life cycle.
6. Discuss the components of a nutritional assessment.
7. Develop nursing diagnoses that correctly identify nutritional problems that may be treated by independent nursing interventions.
8. Describe nursing interventions to help patients achieve their nutritional goals.
9. Plan, implement, and evaluate nursing care related to selected nursing diagnoses that involve nutritional problems.
10. Differentiate between enteral and parenteral nutrition.

Critical Thinking Exercises

1. Prepare a diet for an economically disadvantaged family consisting of a single working mother and three children, ages 3 to 14 years, taking into consideration the family's culture (specify a minority culture in your locale) and yearly income (below poverty level).
2. Prepare a 1-day menu that meets the recommended daily allowance of essential nutrients for the following patients:

   - An obese teenager
   - A child vegetarian
   - An executive with high blood pressure who dines out frequently with clients
   - A woman running a minimum of 12 miles daily as she trains for a marathon

Study Questions

1. The most concentrated source of energy in the body is
   a. protein
   b. carbohydrates
   c. fat
   d. macrominerals
2. The Food Guide Pyramid that is a replacement for the food group wheel
   a. puts meat and dairy products at the peak
   b. gives equal emphasis to all food groups
   c. focuses on wellness and the role that food plays in the prevention of chronic diseases
   d. focuses on deficiencies in our diet
3. Which laboratory test result indicates that a patient is at risk for poor nutritional status?
   a. decreased serum albumin level
   b. increased lymphocyte count
   c. decreased blood urea nitrogen level
   d. increased platelet count
4. Mr. Yow is refusing to eat. What nursing action may stimulate his appetite?
   a. administer pain medication after meals
   b. encourage food from home when possible
   c. schedule his respiratory therapy before each meal
   d. reinforce the importance of his eating exactly what is delivered to him
5. Mrs. James has progressed to a full liquid diet. The nurse expects to see what items on her tray?
   a. apple juice and bouillon
   b. water ice and ginger ale
   c. puréed beef and cream of broccoli soup
   d. custard and a glass of milk
6. Parenteral nutrition provides nutrients to the patient by way of the
   a. gastrostomy tube
   b. intravenous route
   c. nasointestinal route
   d. jejunostomy tube
7. The nurse completing anthropometric measurements for a patient collects the following information
   a. height and weight
   b. serum hemoglobin and hematocrit levels
   c. diet history
   d. intake and output
8. The nurse and Mrs. Young discuss a weight reduction plan. The nurse teaches Mrs. Young that 1 lb of body fat is equal to about
   a. 1500 cal
   b. 2400 cal
   c. 3500 cal
   d. 5000 cal

9. Mr. White has been admitted to the alcoholic referral unit in the local hospital. Nutritionally, he will most commonly be prone to
   a. vitamin B malnutrition
   b. obesity
   c. dehydration
   d. vitamin C deficiency

10. A patient has a nasogastric tube inserted for feeding purposes. Using the stomach as a reservoir for food is advantageous in preventing what complication?
   a. dumping syndrome
   b. duodenal ulcers
   c. hyperglycemia
   d. gastric ulcers

11. Intermittent suction is used in the patient with a single-lumen nasogastric tube for the purpose of
   a. draining the stomach more effectively
   b. preventing electrolyte losses
   c. helping to prevent dumping syndrome
   d. helping to prevent the tube from suctioning the mucosa

12. Mr. Lang is receiving continuous tube feedings through a nasogastric tube. The nurse checks the tube's placement once a shift because

a. the physician ordered it to be done
b. the tube could be misplaced in the ileum
c. the tube should be in the esophagus for feeding
d. the tube can become dislodged and enter the trachea

13. Saline solution is used to irrigate a nasogastric tube used for decompression. The rationale for this is
   a. irrigating with water is a contaminated procedure
   b. saline solution is a hypertonic solution
   c. saline solution replaces electrolytes lost through nasogastric suction
   d. saline solution is less irritating to the gastric mucosa

14. Gorging followed by purging with self-induced vomiting describes the disorder of
   a. anorexia
   b. morbid obesity
   c. bulimia
   d. cachexia

15. Protein helps to regulate fluid balance by
   a. oncotic pressure
   b. hydrostatic pressure
   c. secretion of antidiuretic hormone
   d. retention of sodium

Answers With Rationale

1. The correct response is *c*. Fat provides 9 cal for every gram compared with 4 cal/g of protein and carbohydrates. Macrominerals are regulatory nutrients, not energy nutrients.

2. The correct response is *c*. The focus of the Food Guide Pyramid is on wellness and prevention of nutritionally related diseases. Fats are at the peak of the pyramid, whereas the greatest focus is on grains and cereals as the basic food group.

3. The correct response is *a*. A decreased serum protein level places a patient at nutritional risk. The other test results do not represent a nutritional risk.

4. The correct response is *b*. Food from home that the patient enjoys may stimulate him to eat. Pain medication should be given before meals, respiratory therapy should be scheduled after meals, and telling the patient what he must eat is no guarantee that he will comply.

5. The correct response is *d*. Custard and milk are items found in a full liquid diet. Apple juice, bouillon, water ice, and ginger ale are clear liquids, and puréed beef and cream of broccoli soup are more likely to be found in a soft diet.

6. The correct response is *b*. Parenteral nutrition is given intravenously. Gastrostomy tube, nasointestinal route, and jejunostomy tube are routes for enteral feedings.

7. The correct response is *a*. Intake and output measurements indicate fluid balance, hemoglobin and

hematocrit are biochemical data, and a diet history is used to complete dietary data.

8. The correct response is *c*. One pound of body fat is equal to about 3500 cal.

9. The correct response is *a*. The need for B vitamins is increased in alcoholics because they are used to metabolize alcohol.

10. The correct response is *a*. When the stomach is used as a reservoir, the formula is released at a controlled rate, preventing the occurrence of the dumping syndrome.

11. The correct response is *d*. Intermittent suction prevents damage to the mucosa of the stomach, and that is the primary purpose for using it with a single-lumen tube.

12. The correct response is *d*. Checking tube placement verifies that the tube is in the stomach and has not slipped into the trachea. The nurse's concern is to prevent aspiration of the feeding, leading to severe respiratory problems.

13. The correct response is *c*. Saline solution reduces loss of electrolytes through nasogastric suction and is, therefore, the irrigant of choice.

14. The correct response is *c*. Bulimia is the only eating disorder mentioned that involves the cycle of gorging and purging.

15. The correct response is *a*. Serum proteins are responsible for maintaining oncotic pressure, which exerts a "pull" pressure.

Bibliography

Belcaster, A. (1997). Helping your patients avoid refeeding syndrome. *Nursing, 27*(9), 32hn8.

Bliss, D., & Lehmann, S. (1999). Tube feeding: Immune-boosting formulas. *RN, 62*(8), 26–28.

Bliss, D., & Lehmann, S. (1999). Tube feeding: Administration tips. *RN, 62*(8), 29–32.

Bloom, A. (1998). *Tips for your fingertips.* Alexandria, VA: American Diabetes Association.

Cason, K. (1998). Maintaining nutrition during drug therapy. *Nursing, 28*(9), 54–55.

Cerrato, P. (1997). Vitamins and minerals. *RN, 60*(11), 52–55.

Cerrato, P. (1999). When food is the culprit. *RN, 62*(6), 52–58.

Cobb, M. (1997). Improving your patient's nutritional status. *Nursing, 27*(6), 32hn4–32hn6.

Dudek, S. (1997). *Nutrition handbook for nursing practice,* (3rd ed.). Philadelphia: Lippincott-Raven.

Fischbach, F. (1996). *A manual of laboratory and diagnostic tests,* (5th ed.). Philadelphia: Lippincott-Raven.

Gallagher, S. (1999). Tailoring care for obese patients. *RN, 62*(5), 43–48.

Hall, J. (1997). Learning about low-profile gastrostomy devices. *Nursing, 27*(6), 62–63.

Jones, S., & Guenter, P. (1997). Automatic flush feeding pumps. *Nursing, 27*(2), 56–58.

Kayser-Jones, J., & Pengilly, K. (1999). Dysphagia among nursing home residents. *Geriatric nursing, 20*(2), 77–82.

Kohn-Keeth, C. (2000). How to keep feeding tubes flowing freely. *Nursing, 30*(1), 58–59.

Krupp, K., & Heximer, B. (1998). Going with the flow: How to prevent feeding tubes from clogging. *Nursing, 28*(4), 54–55.

Liebman, B. (1998). 3 Vitamins and a Mineral: What to take. *Nutrition Action Health Letter, 25*(4), 3–7.

Liebman, B., & Wootan, M. (1999). Trans fat. *Nutrition Action Health Letter, 26*(5), 9–11.

Liebman, B. (1999). Ten tips for staying lean. *Nutrition Action Health Letter, 26*(6), 3–7.

Loan, T., Kearney, P., Magnuson, B., & Williams, S. (1997). Enteral feeding in the home environment. *Home Healthcare Nurse, 15*(8), 531–536.

Loan, T., Magnuson, B. & Williams, S. (1998). Debunking six myths about enteral feeding. *Nursing, 28*(8), 43–48.

Lyman, B., & Marquardt, P. (1997). Nutrition screening tool for home care patients. *Home Healthcare Nurse, 15*(12), 835–841.

McCloskey, J., & Bulechek, J. (1996). *Nursing interventions classification (NIC)* (2nd ed.). St. Louis: C. V. Mosby.

McConnell, M. (1994). Managing a nasoenteric decompression tube. *Nursing, 24*(3), 18.

McConnell, M. (1997). Inserting a nasogastric tube. *Nursing, 27*(1), 72.

McConnell, M. (1997). How to determine gastric pH. *Nursing, 27*(8), 26.

McConnell, M. (1998). Administering parenteral nutrition. *Nursing, 28*(7), 18.

Metheny, N., Wehrle, A., Wiersema, L., & Clark, J. (1998a). Testing feeding tube placement: Auscultation vs. pH method. *American Journal of Nursing, 98*(5), 37–42.

Metheny, N., Smith, L., Wehrle, M., Wiersema, L., & Clark, J. (1998b). pH, color, and feeding tubes. *RN, 61*(1), 25–27.

North American Nursing Diagnosis Association. (1999). *NANDA nursing diagnoses: Definitions & classification, 1999–2000.* Philadelphia: Author.

O'Brien, B., Davis, S., & Erwin-Toth, P. (1999). G-tube site care: A practical guide. *RN, 62*(2), 52–56.

Peckenpaugh, N., & Poleman, C. (1999). *Nutrition essentials and diet therapy* (8th ed.). Philadelphia: W. B. Saunders.

Phipps, W., Sands, J., & Marek, J. (1999). *Medical-surgical nursing: Concepts & clinical practice* (6th ed.). St. Louis: C. V. Mosby.

Purnell, L., & Paulanka, B. (1998). *Transcultural health care.* Philadelphia: F. A. Davis.

Russell, R., Rasmussen, H., & Lichtenstein, A. (1999). Modified food guide pyramid for people over seventy years of age. *Journal of Nutrition, 129*(3), 751–753.

Selekman, J. (1998). Sensitivity toward those who are obese. *American Journal of Nursing, 98*(5), 16RR–16WW.

Williams, S. (1999). *Essentials of nutrition and diet therapy,* (7th ed.). St. Louis: C. V. Mosby.

Yen, P. (1997). Tube feeding safety. *Geriatric nursing, 18*(1), 40–41.

Chapter 42
Urinary Elimination

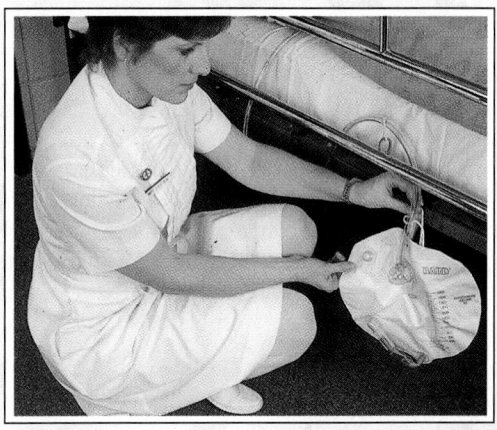

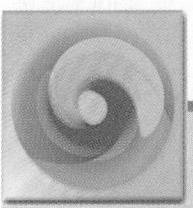

**Thinking Critically About
Nursing's Blended Skills**

Before reading this chapter, think about the types of skills you will need to address the following challenges related to urinary elimination.

- You've been monitoring Jewel's urinary output since the delivery of her healthy twins and are growing concerned. Her bladder is palpably full and distended but she has been unable to void on her own.

- You have been instructed to do hourly urine outputs on a patient in the intensive care unit who is at risk for renal shutdown. Your last hourly measurement was 42 mL. The patient has a Foley catheter.

- Mrs. Fleming asks you (a home healthcare nurse) if she should talk with her husband's doctor about getting him a Foley catheter. "Ever since he came back from the hospital this last time, he seems unable to use the urinal. He dribbles constantly and I can't keep up with the sheets. He had a catheter in the hospital."

- You are asked to collect surprise urine specimens from all hospital employees in your unit. Narcotic drugs have been missing, and management is hoping to identify the potential thief by detecting the missing drugs in some employee's urine.

What cognitive, technical, interpersonal, and ethical/legal skills do you think you will need to meet the needs of the patients described above?

Elimination from the urinary tract helps to rid the body of waste products and materials that exceed bodily needs. A properly functioning urinary system is essential to the body's physical well-being, to life itself, and to a person's general sense of well-being. Nurses assisting a patient with urination or intervening to resolve health problems related to urination need many specialized abilities.

This chapter describes the physiology of the urinary system and the many factors that affect urination. A practical guide to assessing urinary elimination is included along with detailed information on specific assessment measures, such as monitoring fluid intake, collecting urine specimens, testing urine, and assisting with other diagnostic procedures. Analysis of urinary assessment data may lead to identifying one or more nursing diagnoses or, when reported to the physician, to the early detection of a medical problem. Expected patient outcomes are established when planning care, for which specific nursing strategies are presented. The concluding patient care study illustrates how the nurse's knowledge of the urinary system and urinary pathology combines with specific nursing interventions to resolve urinary problems successfully.

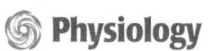 Physiology

Kidneys and Ureters

The kidneys are located on either side of the vertebral column behind the peritoneum, in the posterior portion of the abdominal cavity. One of the more significant functions of the kidneys is to help maintain the composition and volume of body fluids. They filter and excrete blood constituents that are not needed and retain those that are. The body's total blood volume passes through the kidneys for waste removal about every half hour. Despite varying kinds and amounts of food and fluids ingested, body fluids remain relatively stable if the kidneys are functioning properly. Urine, the waste product excreted by the kidneys, contains organic, inorganic, and liquid wastes.

The nephron is the basic structural and functional unit of the kidneys. There are about 1 million nephrons in each kidney. Nephrons remove the end products of metabolism, such as urea, creatinine, and uric acid, from the blood plasma and form urine. Each nephron is a complicated system of arterioles, capillaries, and tubules. Fluid balance is also maintained and regulated by the nephrons by means of selective reabsorption and secretion processes. Urine from the nephrons empties into the pelvis of each kidney. From each kidney, urine is transported by rhythmic peristalsis through the ureters to the urinary bladder. The ureters enter the bladder obliquely, and a fold of membrane in the bladder closes the entrance to the ureters so that urine is not forced up the ureters to the kidneys when pressure exists in the bladder. Figure 42-1 shows the male and female urinary systems and the position of the kidneys and ureters in the abdomen.

Bladder

The urinary bladder is a smooth muscle sac that serves as a reservoir for urine. There are three layers of muscle tissue in the bladder: the inner longitudinal layer, the middle circular layer, and the outer longitudinal layer. These three layers are called the *detrusor muscle*. At the base of the bladder, the middle circular layer of muscle tissue forms the internal, or involuntary, sphincter, which guards the

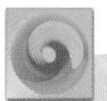

COGNITIVE SKILLS

- Knowledge of the anatomy and physiology of the urinary system and variables that influence urination
- Knowledge of how to promote normal urination; facilitate use of the toilet, bedpan, urinal, and commode; perform catheterizations; and assist with urinary diversions
- Knowledge of how to use the nursing process to identify and care for patients with diagnoses associated with urinary problems

TECHNICAL SKILLS

- Ability to use the equipment and protocols necessary to diagnose and treat urinary problems

INTERPERSONAL SKILLS

- Strong people skills to establish trusting relationships with each of these patients
- Special interpersonal competence to determine how best to meet the need to identify the source of the missing narcotics

ETHICAL/LEGAL SKILLS

- First and foremost a strong sense of accountability for the health and well-being of these individuals; a commitment to getting them the help they need to achieve their health goals—within the scope of your nursing responsibilities and available resources
- A willingness to hold colleagues accountable for safe and good-quality practice
- A knowledge of the ethical and legal principles surrounding drug testing in the workplace

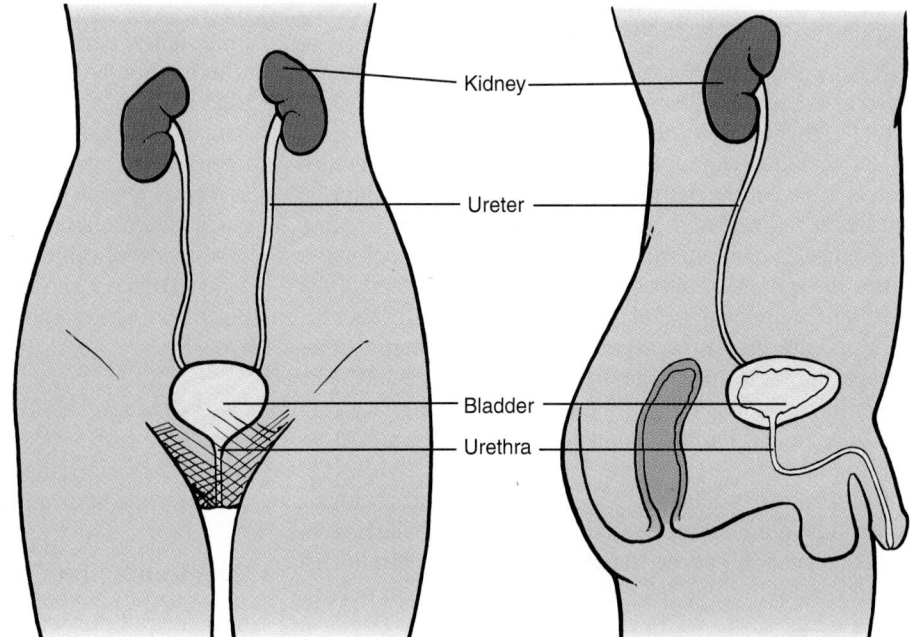

Figure 42-1
Frontal view of the female urinary tract (*left*) and lateral view of the male urinary tract (*right*).

opening between the urinary bladder and the urethra. The urethra conveys urine from the bladder to the exterior of the body.

The urinary bladder muscle is innervated by the autonomic nervous system. The sympathetic system carries inhibitory impulses to the bladder and motor impulses to the internal sphincter. These impulses cause the detrusor muscle to relax and the internal sphincter to constrict, retaining urine in the bladder. The parasympathetic system carries motor impulses to the bladder and inhibitory impulses to the internal sphincter. These impulses cause the detrusor muscle to contract and the sphincter to relax. The male and female urinary bladders are shown in Figure 42-1.

The bladder normally contains urine under very little pressure, and as the volume of urine increases, the pressure increases only slightly. The bladder wall adapts to pressure, apparently because of the muscle tissue in the bladder, and this makes it possible for urine to continue to enter the bladder from the ureters against low pressure. When the pressure becomes sufficient to stimulate nerves, called *stretch receptors,* in the bladder wall, the person feels a desire to empty the bladder.

Urethra

The urethra's function is to convey urine from the bladder to the exterior. The anatomy of the urethra differs in males and females. The male urethra functions in both the excretory system and the reproductive system. It is about $5\frac{1}{2}$ to $6\frac{1}{4}$ inches (13.7 to 16.2 cm) long and consists of three parts: the prostatic, the membranous, and the cavernous portions (Fig. 42-2). The external urethral sphincter consists of striated muscle and is located just beyond the prostatic portion of the urethra. The external sphincter is under voluntary control.

The female urethra is about $1\frac{1}{2}$ to $2\frac{1}{2}$ inches (3.7 to 6.2 cm) long. The external, or voluntary, sphincter is located about midurethra. No portion of the female urethra is external to the body, as in the male, although the muscle at the meatus is usually called the *external sphincter.*

Act of Micturition

The process of emptying the bladder is known as **micturition,** *voiding,* or *urination.* The nerve centers for micturition are situated in the brain and the spinal cord. Voiding

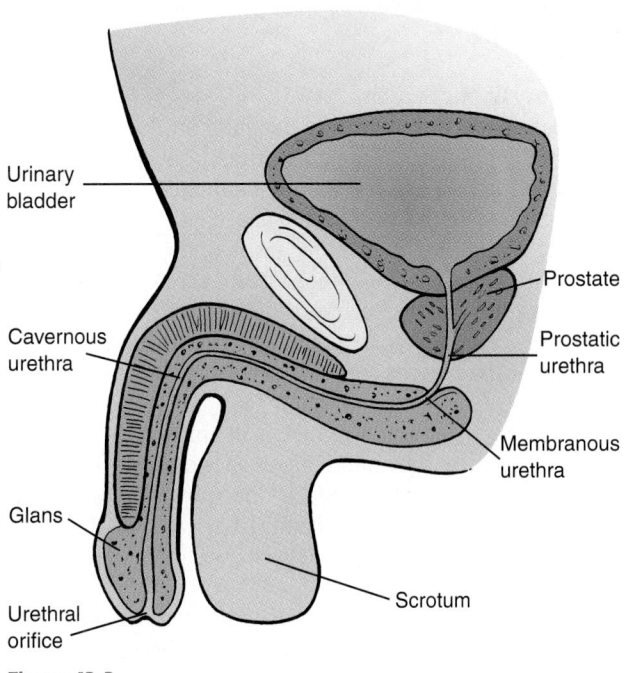

Figure 42-2
Parts of the male urethra.

is largely an involuntary reflex act, but its control can be learned.

After the stretch receptors in the bladder are stimulated as the urine collects, the person feels a desire to void. Usually, this occurs when about 100 to 200 mL for a child or 200 to 300 mL for an adult has collected. When micturition is initiated, the detrusor muscle contracts, the internal sphincter relaxes, and urine enters the posterior urethra. The muscles of the perineum and the external sphincter relax, the muscle of the abdominal wall contracts slightly, the diaphragm lowers, and micturition occurs. During micturition, the pressure within the bladder is many times greater than it is during the time the bladder is filling. The act of micturition is normally painless. The voluntary control of voiding is limited to initiating, restraining, and interrupting the act.

Restraint of voiding is thought to occur subconsciously when the volume of urine in the bladder is small. If voiding is delayed, however, the bladder continues to fill. Discomfort may then be felt when undue distention occurs, and the urgency to void becomes paramount.

Sometimes, increased abdominal pressure, such as occurs during coughing and sneezing, forces an involuntary escape of urine, especially in females, because the urethra is shorter. Any involuntary loss of urine that causes a problem is referred to as **urinary incontinence**. Strong psychological factors, such as marked fear, also may result in involuntary urination. In certain conditions, it may be difficult for a person to relax the restraining muscles sufficiently to void, such as when a shy or embarrassed person needs to give a urine specimen.

When the higher nerve centers develop after infancy, the voluntary control of micturition develops also. Until that time, voiding is purely a reflex action. People whose bladders are no longer controlled by the brain because of injury or disease also void by reflex only. This is called *autonomic bladder*.

Frequency of Micturition

The **frequency** of micturition depends on the amount of urine being produced. The more urine produced, the more often voiding is necessary. Except when fluid intake is very large, most healthy people do not void during normal sleeping hours. The first voided urine of the day is usually more concentrated than other urine excreted during the day. Because the first urine of the day is not fresh, but rather an accumulation of a number of hours of kidney output, this urine may or may not be used as a specimen for certain tests.

Some people normally void small amounts at frequent intervals because they habitually respond to the first early urge to void. This habit usually does not mean anything and is not necessarily an indication of disease. On the other hand, if this pattern occurs as a change in urination routine, it may indicate illness.

Other people have habits of infrequent voiding. For example, some people go 8 to 12 waking hours or longer without urinating. A habitual low fluid intake or a decrease in the sensation of thirst associated with aging may be the reason. The inaccessibility of toilet facilities owing to

travel, work circumstances, or illness, as well as limitations in mobility, can also lead to infrequent urination. People who habitually urinate infrequently develop more urinary tract infections and kidney disorders than those who urinate at least every 3 to 4 hours. The reason for this is believed to be stagnation of urine in the bladder, which serves as a good medium for bacterial growth. Newly occurring infrequent voiding can also indicate a decreased production of urine caused by a kidney or circulatory disorder. **Urinary retention** occurs when urine is produced normally but not appropriately excreted from the bladder.

Factors Affecting Micturition

Numerous factors affect the amount and quality of urine produced by the body and the manner in which it is excreted.

Developmental Considerations

Infants are born without voluntary control of micturition and with little ability to concentrate urine. An infant's urine is usually very light in color and without odor. At about 6 weeks of age, the infant's nephrons are able to control reabsorption of fluids in the tubules and effectively concentrate urine. Most children develop urinary control between the ages of 2 and 5 years. Daytime control precedes nighttime control, and girls generally develop control earlier than boys. Older children and adults control urination voluntarily and seldom wake to void at night because their kidneys are able to concentrate urine and produce less urine at night as a result of decreased renal blood flow.

Toilet Training

Most children begin to control urination voluntarily at 18 to 24 months of age. Toilet training should not begin until the child is able to (1) hold urine for 1 to 2 hours, (2) recognize the feeling of bladder fullness, and (3) communicate the need to void and control urination until seated on the toilet. The child's desire to gain control is also important. Wanting to be like a parent or older sibling often provides adequate motivation. Lifelong attitudes toward urination, the body, and cleanliness may develop during the time of toilet training. Involuntary urination that occurs after an age when continence should be present is termed **enuresis.**

Toilet training is taught a variety of ways in different cultural patterns. Initiation of toilet training begins in some cultures before the child is 1 year old but in others may not be considered until the child is near 5 years of age. Nurses must recognize cultural influences on this parenting responsibility while promoting flexibility. It is always reassuring for parents to hear that any regression of toileting skills that occurs during a child's hospitalization is not unexpected and is usually short-lived.

Aging

Physiologic changes that accompany normal aging may affect urination in older adults:

- Diminished ability of the kidneys to concentrate urine may result in nocturia.

- Decreased bladder muscle tone may reduce the capacity of the bladder to hold urine and increase frequency.
- Decreased bladder contractility may lead to urine retention and stasis, which increase the likelihood of urinary tract infection.
- Neuromuscular problems, degenerative joint problems, alterations in thought processes, and weakness may interfere with voluntary control and the ability to reach a toilet in time.

Individuals who view themselves as old, powerless, and neglected may cease to value voluntary control over urination and simply find toileting too much bother no matter what the setting. Incontinence is often the result.

Food and Fluid

When the body is functioning well, the kidneys help the body maintain a careful balance of fluid intake and output, which should be about equal. When the body is dehydrated, the kidneys reabsorb fluid, and the urine produced is more concentrated and decreased in amount. Conversely, with fluid overload, the kidneys excrete a large quantity of dilute urine.

Caffeine-containing beverages (cola, coffee, and tea) have a diuretic effect and increase urine production. Alcohol produces the same effect by inhibiting the release of antidiuretic hormone. Foods high in water may increase urine production. Foods and beverages with high sodium content cause sodium and water reabsorption and retention, thereby decreasing urine formation. As well, certain foods may affect the odor of the urine (asparagus, onions) or its color (beets). The accompanying Applying Learning to Practice boxes include a checklist for the nurse (Nurse as Role Model) and suggested behaviors to maintain healthy urinary elimination patterns (Promoting Health).

Psychological Variables

Many individual, family, and sociocultural variables influence a person's normal voiding habits. For some people, voiding is a personal and private act—something one does not talk about. Needing assistance with a bedpan or urinal thus provokes great embarrassment and anxiety, especially when the bedpan is offered by a nurse of the opposite sex. For others, voiding is a natural act that does not cause embarrassment, and these people readily excuse themselves to void whenever the urge presents.

Many people who experience stress void smaller amounts of urine at more frequent intervals. Stress can also interfere with the ability to relax the perineal muscles and the external urethral sphincter. When this happens, the person may feel an urge to void, but emptying the bladder completely becomes difficult or impossible.

Activity and Muscle Tone

Among the many benefits of regular exercise are increased metabolism and optimal urine production and elimination. During prolonged periods of immobility, decreased bladder and sphincter tone can result in poor urinary control and urinary stasis. People with indwelling urinary catheters lose bladder tone because the bladder muscle is not being stretched by the bladder filling with urine. Other causes of decreased muscle tone include childbearing, menopausal muscle atrophy, and damage to muscles from trauma.

Pathologic Conditions

Certain renal or urologic problems can affect both the quantity and the quality of urine produced. Diseases associated with renal problems include congenital urinary tract abnormalities, polycystic kidney disease, urinary tract infection, urinary calculi (kidney stones), hypertension, diabetes mellitus, gout, and certain connective tissue disorders.

Diseases that reduce physical activity or lead to generalized weakness, such as arthritis, Parkinson's disease, and degenerative joint disease, may interfere with toileting. Cognitive deficits and certain psychiatric problems can interfere with a person's ability or desire to control urination voluntarily. Fever and diaphoresis (profuse perspiration) result in the kidney's conservation of body fluids. Urine production is decreased, and the urine is highly concentrated. Other pathologic conditions, such as congestive heart failure, may lead to fluid retention and decreased urine output.

APPLYING LEARNING TO PRACTICE

The Nurse as Role Model: Urinary Elimination

Before intervening to help patients develop healthy urinary elimination patterns, it is important for nurses to assess the adequacy of their own urinary elimination habits and patterns. If you are unable to meet the following goals, you may want to take the time now to revise your own health practices, so that you will be an effective role model for patients. Your elimination habits should include the following:

- Empty the bladder completely at regular intervals.
- Respond to the urge to void (ie, do not routinely postpone voiding because of being too busy)
- Drink 8 to 10 glasses of water daily.
- Respond to changes in urinary characteristics (or frequency) by seeking their cause and getting medical assistance when necessary.

APPLYING LEARNING TO PRACTICE

Promoting Health

Urine Elimination

Use the assessment checklist to determine how well you are meeting your need for urine elimination. Then develop a prescription for self-care by choosing appropriate behaviors from the list of suggestions.

ASSESSMENT CHECKLIST

almost always	sometimes	almost never	
☐	☐	☐	1. I urinate at regular intervals throughout the day.
☐	☐	☐	2. I have an adequate fluid intake.
☐	☐	☐	3. I limit my sodium intake.
☐	☐	☐	4. My urine volume remains relatively constant.

SELF-CARE BEHAVIORS

1. Maintain a normal voiding pattern and volume.
2. Respond as soon as possible to the urge to void.
3. Drink 8 to 10 glasses of water daily.
4. Avoid foods that contain excess sodium.
5. Monitor use of caffeine, alcohol, or medication schedules that promote voiding and may interfere with sleep.
6. Seek medical assistance for any change in the characteristics of urine or presence of pain on urination.

Medications

Medications have numerous effects on urine production and elimination. Of gravest concern are the many prescription and nonprescription drugs known to be nephrotoxic (capable of causing kidney damage). Abuse of analgesics, such as aspirin, can cause nephrotoxicity; some antibiotics, such as kanamycin, can be nephrotoxic.

Diuretics (water pills), which commonly are used in the treatment of hypertension and other disorders, prevent the reabsorption of water and certain electrolytes in the tubules. Depending on their strength, they cause moderate to severe increases in production and excretion of dilute urine. *Cholinergic* medications stimulate contraction of the detrusor muscle and produce urination. Some *analgesics* and *tranquilizers* that suppress the central nervous system interfere with urination by diminishing the effectiveness of the neural reflex.

Certain drugs cause urine to change color, including the following:

- Anticoagulants may cause **hematuria** (blood in the urine) or red color
- Diuretics can lighten urine color to pale yellow.
- Pyridium (a urinary tract analgesic) can cause orange or orange-red urine.
- Elavil (an antidepressant) or B-complex vitamins can cause urine that is green or blue-green.
- Levodopa (antiparkinsonian drug) or injectable iron compounds can lead to brown or black urine.

The Nursing Process

ASSESSING

A comprehensive nursing assessment of the functioning of a patient's urinary system includes the following:

- Collection of data about the patient's voiding patterns, habits, and difficulties and a history of current or past urinary problems
- Physical examination of the kidneys, bladder, and urethral meatus; assessment of skin integrity and hydration; and examination of the urine
- Correlation of these findings with the results of diagnostic tests and procedures for examining the urine and the urinary tract

Nursing History

In the initial nursing history, the nurse questions the patient (or caregiver) about his or her usual voiding habits and any current or past voiding difficulties. Terminology should be used that the patient understands. Elements of a urinary elimination history that should be incorporated into the initial nursing assessment are listed in the accompanying Focused Assessment Guide.

With infants and young children, it is important to assess whether the child has achieved bladder control and whether a toileting schedule has been established. The nursing history and plan also should note the words the child uses to indicate the need to void.

With older adults, decreased bladder tone may be a problem, and the nursing history should note any problems, how the person normally handles these problems, and the nurse's judgment of the adequacy of the solution.

People with limited or no bladder control and those with urinary diversions usually have well-established routines for emptying the bladder. *Urinary diversions* involve surgical creation of an alternate route for excretion of urine and are discussed later in the chapter. The procedures and equipment the patient uses should be assessed to make sure they follow accepted guidelines and do not predispose the person to infection or other risk. Any special routine, equipment, or supplies the patient uses for urinary elimination should be noted in both the history and the nursing plan of care.

FOCUSED ASSESSMENT GUIDE

Urinary Elimination

Factors to Assess	Questions and Approaches
Usual patterns of urinary elimination	How often do you urinate (pass your water) during the day?
	Do you awaken at night to empty your bladder?
	How would you describe your urine?
Recent changes in urinary elimination	Have you noticed any changes in your usual voiding patterns (frequency, amount, force of stream, difficulty, comfort)?
	Do you ever leak urine (eg, on your way to the bathroom or when you sneeze or cough)?
	Do you ever notice that your undergarments are wet or damp?
Aids to elimination	Is there anything you do that helps you to urinate?
Present or past occurrence of voiding difficulties (nature of problem, onset, frequency, causes, severity, symptoms, intervention attempted, and results)	Tell me about any problems you are having now when you urinate (urgency, pain or burning, difficulty starting or stopping stream, dribbling, incontinence).
	If there is a problem, describe what you feel like before you urinate and while you are urinating.
	Have you had any urinary problems in the past (any history or urinary tract infections, kidney or bladder disease or problems)?
	Do you use any type of absorbent pad or product to protect your clothes?
Presence of artificial orifices (normal routine, history of problems)	Tell me about your usual routine with your ureterostomy.

When a patient reports a problem with voiding, its duration, severity, and precipitating factors should be explored. (See the accompanying box for terms used to describe such problems.) Also noted are the patient's perception of the problem and the adequacy of the patient's self-care behaviors.

Physical Assessment

The physical assessment of urinary functioning includes an examination of the kidneys, urinary bladder, urethral meatus, skin, and urine.

Kidneys

The kidneys are normally well protected by considerable fat and connective tissue and are difficult to palpate. The right kidney is at the level of the 12th rib, lower than the left kidney. The right kidney can sometimes be palpated if it is pushed down by the diaphragm when the patient inhales. The nurse stands to the right of the supine patient and places the left hand under the patient's flank while the right hand palpates the abdominal wall. This technique requires deep palpation and should be practiced only under supervision. The left kidney is palpated similarly. The contour and size of the kidneys are noted, as is any tenderness or lumps.

The examination of the kidneys includes checking for *costovertebral tenderness*. The costovertebral angle is

formed by the 12th rib and the spine. When the kidneys are inflamed, the patient feels pain when this angle is percussed. The nurse places one palm flat over the costovertebral angle and strikes the back of this hand with the other fist.

Bladder

The bladder is normally positioned below the symphysis pubis and cannot be palpated or percussed when empty. When the bladder is distended, it rises above the symphysis pubis and may reach to just below the umbilicus (Fig. 42-3). Before palpating the bladder, the nurse should ask the patient when he or she voided last. The nurse then observes the lower abdominal wall, noting any swelling, and palpates this area for tenderness, also noting the smoothness and roundness of the bladder. The height of the edge of the bladder above the symphysis pubis may be measured, and the bladder may also be percussed. A full bladder produces a dull sound.

Urethral Orifice

The urethral orifice is inspected for any signs of inflammation, discharge, or foul odor. In females, the urethral meatus is a pink, slitlike opening below the clitoris and above the vaginal orifice. Female patients should be in the dorsal recumbent position with the inner labia retracted for good visualization of the meatus. In males, the meatus is at the tip of the penis. If the male patient is uncircumcised, the

Terms Used to Describe Additional Urinary Problems

Anuria: Technically, no urine voided; 24-hour urine output is less than 100 mL; synonyms are complete *kidney shutdown* or *renal failure*

Dysuria: Difficulty in voiding; may or may not be associated with pain; a feeling of warm local irritation occurring during voiding is called *burning*

Frequency: Increased incidence of voiding

Glycosuria: Presence of sugar in the urine; if due to an unusually large intake of sugar or to marked emotional disturbances and is temporary, there is little cause for alarm

Nocturia: Frequency of urination during the night

Oliguria: Scanty or greatly diminished amount of urine voided in a given time; 24-hour urine output is 100 to 400 mL

Orthostatic albuminuria: Presence of albumin in urine that is voided after periods of standing, walking, or running; phenomenon of the circulatory system and not necessarily a symptom of kidney disorders

Pneumaturia: Passage of urine containing gas

Polyuria: Excessive output of urine (diuresis)

Proteinuria: Albumin in the urine; indication of kidney disease

Pyuria: Pus in the urine; urine appears cloudy

Suppression: Stoppage of urine production; normally the adult kidneys produce urine continuously at the rate of 60 to 120 mL/h

Urgency: Strong desire to void

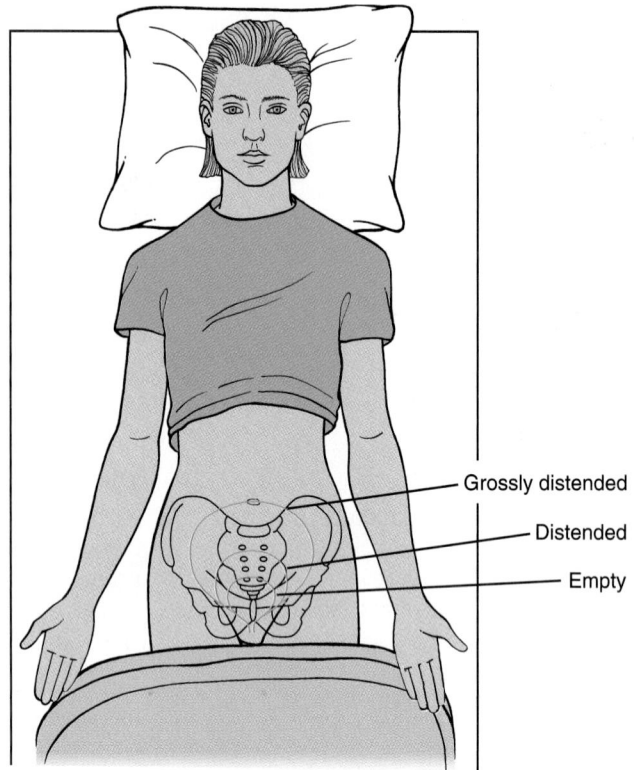

Figure 42-3
Position of bladder when empty and distended.

— Grossly distended

— Distended

— Empty

such as protein, blood, glucose, ketone bodies, and bacteria. The normal characteristics of urine are detailed in Table 42-1.

Assessment Measures

In addition to the nursing history and physical examination, the nurse gathers data about urinary elimination through the following assessment measures: measuring urine output, collecting urine specimens, determining the presence of abnormal constituents in the urine, and assisting with diagnostic procedures. These are discussed in the following sections.

Measuring Urine Output

Measuring the patient's intake and output is an important nursing responsibility. Accuracy of the total fluid intake and output from all sources is essential for planning the patient's nursing and medical care. The measurement of intake and output is described further in Chapter 45. Gloves are required when handling urine to protect the nurse from possible exposure to pathogenic microorganisms or blood that may be present in the urine.

The Voiding Patient

The procedure for measuring the urine output of a patient who is voiding is as follows:

foreskin may need to be retracted for visualization of the meatus.

Skin Integrity and Hydration

Because problems with urinary functioning may result in disturbances in hydration and excretion of body wastes, the skin should be carefully assessed for color, texture, turgor, and the excretion of any wastes. The integrity of the skin in the perineal area is also assessed. Problems with incontinence may result in severe excoriation.

Urine

Whenever a patient's urine is handled, it should be assessed for color, odor, clarity, and the presence of any sediment. Abnormalities should be noted. In select patients, the pH and specific gravity of the urine are monitored, and the urine is checked for abnormal constituents

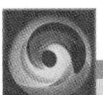

Table 42-1
Characteristics of Urine

Characteristic	Normal Findings	Special Considerations
Color	A freshly voided specimen is pale yellow, straw-colored, or amber, depending on its concentration.	Urine is darker than normal when it is scanty and concentrated. Urine is lighter than normal when it is excessive and diluted. Certain drugs, such as cascara, L-dopa, and sulfonamides, alter the color or urine.
Odor	Normal urine smell is aromatic. As urine stands, it often develops an ammonia odor because of bacterial action.	Some foods cause urine to have a characteristic odor; for example, asparagus causes urine to have a strong, musty odor. Urine high in glucose content has a sweet odor. Urine that is heavily infected has a fetid odor.
Turbidity	Fresh urine should be clear or translucent; as urine stands and cools, it becomes cloudy.	Cloudiness observed in freshly voided urine is abnormal and may be due to the presence of red blood cells, white blood cells, bacteria, vaginal discharge, sperm, or prostatic fluid.
pH	The normal pH is about 6.0, with a range of 4.6 to 8. (Urine alkalinity or acidity may be promoted through diet to inhibit bacterial growth or urinary stone development or to facilitate the therapeutic activity of certain medications.) Urine becomes alkaline on standing when carbon dioxide diffuses into the air.	A high-protein diet causes urine to become excessively acid. Certain foods tend to produce alkaline urine, such as citrus fruits, dairy products, and vegetables, especially legumes. Certain foods tend to produce acidic urine, for example, meat and cranberry juice. Certain drugs influence the acidity or alkalinity of urine; for example, ammonium chloride produces acidic urine, and potassium citrate and sodium bicarbonate produce alkaline urine.
Specific gravity	This is a measure of the concentration of dissolved solids in the urine. The normal range is 1.010 to 1.025.	Concentrated urine will have a higher than normal specific gravity, and diluted urine will have a lower than normal specific gravity. In the absence of kidney disease, a high specific gravity usually indicates dehydration and a low specific gravity indicates overhydration.
Constituents	*Organic* constituents of urine include urea, uric acid, creatinine, hippuric acid, indican, urene pigments, and undetermined nitrogen. *Inorganic* constituents are ammonia, sodium, chloride, traces of iron, phosphorus, sulfur, potassium, and calcium.	*Abnormal constituents* of urine include blood, pus, albumin, glucose, ketone bodies, casts, gross bacteria, and bile.

1. Ask the patient to void into a bedpan or urinal, either in bed or in the bathroom. Urinary devices used to collect or measure urine are shown in Figure 42-4.
2. Pour the urine from the bedpan or urinal into the appropriate measuring device provided by the agency. The devices are calibrated in milliliters.
3. Place the calibrated container on a flat surface, such as a shelf, for an accurate reading. Note the amount of urine voided, read at eye level, and record it on the appropriate form. Figure 42-5 shows a form commonly used for recording urine output. The form is usually kept at the patient's bedside. The total amount voided during each shift and 24-hour period is recorded on the patient's permanent record.
4. Do *not* discard the urine if a specimen is required. Otherwise, the urine is discarded in the toilet.
5. Tell patients who are ambulatory when their urine output is to be measured and recorded, so that they do not use the bathroom without measuring output. A specimen hat can be placed under the toilet seat to collect and measure voided urine (see Fig. 42-4). Patients who are willing and able

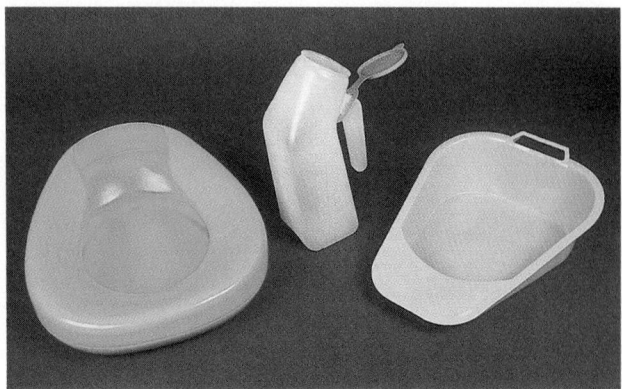

Bedpan and fracture pan: containers used to collect urine from nonambulatory patients.
Urinal: container used to collect urine from nonambulatory male patients

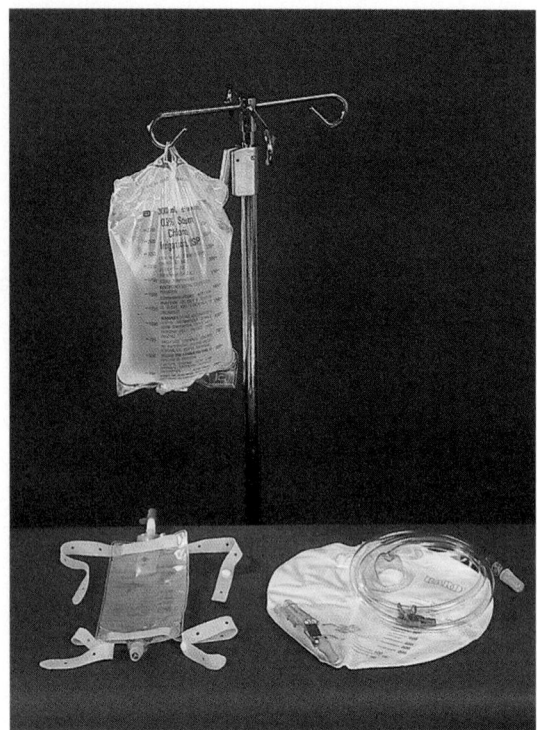

Bladder irrigation fluid for continuous bladder irrigation.
Small urine collection bag for use by ambulatory patients.
Large urine collection bag

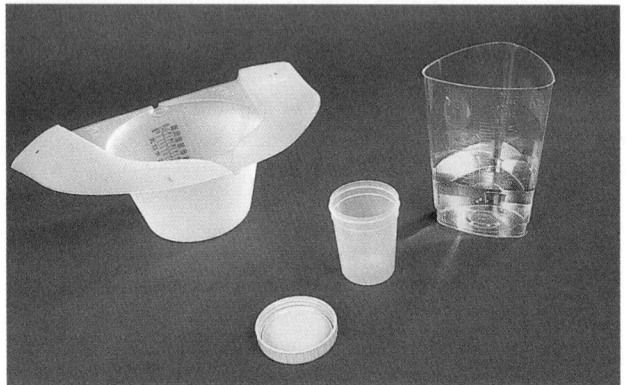

Specimen hat: container that is placed anteriorly on the toilet, underneath the seat. Used to collect urine.
Specimen cup: container that holds urine
Calibrated measuring device: makes possible the recording of an accurate urine output

Figure 42-4
Devices for collecting and measuring urine.

can be taught to measure and record their own output.

The Patient With an Indwelling Catheter

When a patient has an indwelling catheter, the procedure for measuring urine output is as follows:

1. Wear clean gloves.
2. Place a calibrated measuring device beneath the collection bag at the bedside.
3. Place the drainage spout from the collection bag above, but not touching, the calibrated measuring device, and open the clamp.
4. Allow the urine to flow from the collection bag into the measuring device.
5. Reclamp the drainage tube, wipe the spout of the tube with an alcohol pad, and replace the tube into the slot on the drainage bag. Then proceed with measurement as described above.

Catheterized patients who are acutely ill may require hourly measurements of urine. This is facilitated by using a special collection bag with a built-in calibrated measuring chamber. After the nurse assesses and records the amount of urine produced hourly, the measuring chamber is tilted so that this urine flows into the general collection bag. The measuring chamber is then empty and ready to collect the next hour's urine.

Collecting Urine Specimens

Nurses have specific responsibilities for diagnostic tests pertinent to urinary elimination. They routinely collect clean and sterile urine specimens, measure specific gravity of urine, and assess urine for abnormal constituents.

Routine Urinalysis

The collection of urine specimens for urinalysis is a nursing responsibility. A sterile urine specimen is not re-

Intake and Output Chart

7:00 AM _11-18-01_ to 7:00 AM _11-19-01_

	Intake					Output						
	Oral	I.V.		Blood	Other	Comments	Urine	Stool	Gastric tube	Drainage tubes	Vomitus	Other	Comments
7-8	250					Force fluids to 1100cc/shift	300						
8-9													
9-10	120												
10-11	60												
11-12	100						250						
12-1	300												
1-2	240												
2-3	100						200						
8 hr Tot	1170						750						voiding s̄ discomfort
3-4													
4-5													
5-6													
6-7													
7-8													
8-9													
9-10													
10-11													
8 hr Tot													
11-12													
12-1													
1-2													
2-3													
3-4													
4-5													
5-6													
6-7													
8 hr Tot													
24 hr Tot													

Total intake   **Total output**

Figure 42-5
An example of a form commonly used for recording intake and output.

quired for a routine urinalysis. Urine is collected by having the patient void into a clean bedpan, urinal, or receptacle in the toilet bowl. Care is taken to avoid contamination with feces. If a woman is menstruating at the time when a urine sample is obtained, this is noted on the laboratory slip because red blood cells may appear in the urine. If voiding into a bedpan or collection device on the toilet, patients are instructed not to place toilet tissue into the urine because this makes analysis more difficult. Using aseptic technique, the nurse pours the urine into an appropriate container; labels it with the patient's name, date, and time of collection; packages it appropriately; and sends it to the laboratory for examination. Urine should not be left standing at room temperature for a long period before being sent to the laboratory because this may alter both the appearance and chemistry of the urine.

Specimens From Infants and Children. Plastic disposable collection bags are available for infants and young children who have not achieved voluntary bladder control (Fig. 42-6). The manufacturer's instructions should be followed and care taken when applying and removing the bag to avoid irritating the sensitive perineal skin.

Clean-Catch or Midstream Specimen. A clean-catch specimen of urine is required in some situations. Most health agencies specify that a clean-catch specimen be collected during midstream. This means that the patient voids a little urine, which is discarded; the specimen is then collected during midstream in a sterile specimen container, and the last urine in the bladder is also discarded. The first voided urine helps to flush away any organisms near the meatus because the urinalysis findings may be inaccurate if these organisms enter the specimen. As well, it is generally thought that urine voided at midstream is most characteristic of the urine the body is producing. A clean-catch midstream specimen from a male is sterile. A female may be catheterized if a sterile specimen is required. (Catheterization is discussed later in this chapter.)

A patient who can carry out the technique properly may collect his or her own clean-catch midstream urine specimen and often prefers to do so. The nurse provides the appropriate equipment and instructions for the proce-

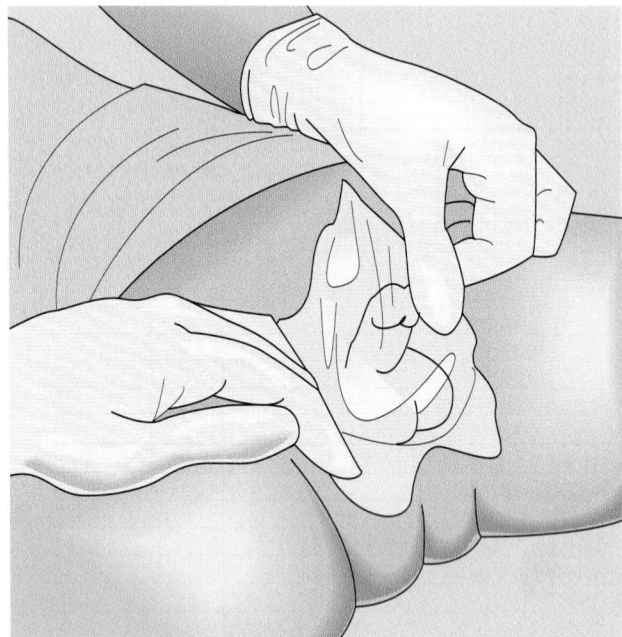

Figure 42-6
Disposable plastic urine collection device for infants.

dure. Refer to the accompanying Guidelines for Nursing Care for techniques for obtaining a clean-catch midstream urine specimen.

Sterile Specimen From an Indwelling Catheter. Sterile urine specimens may be obtained by catheterizing the patient's bladder (see Procedures 42-2 and 42-3 later in this chapter) or by taking the specimen from an indwelling catheter already in place.

When it is necessary to collect a urine specimen from a patient with an indwelling catheter, it should be done from the catheter itself using the special port for specimens. A specimen from the collecting receptacle (drainage bag) may not be fresh urine and could result in an inaccurate analysis. Sterile technique must be observed.

The size of the syringe for the specimen depends on the specific laboratory test. A urine culture requires about 3 mL, whereas routine urinalysis requires at least 10 mL of urine. A sterile 21- to 25-gauge needle, an antiseptic swab, a specimen container, and possibly a clamp are necessary equipment. Wearing gloves protects the nurse from any accidental contact with the specimen.

If urine is not present in the tube, it may be necessary to clamp the tube below the collection port briefly (not to exceed 30 minutes) to allow urine to accumulate. Most catheters have a self-sealing area designed for a needle puncture. It is unsafe to puncture a Silastic or plastic catheter because leakage will probably occur. Clean the entry port with an antiseptic swab, and carefully insert the sterile needle into the catheter. Aspirate urine into the syringe, remove the syringe, release the clamp if one was used, and transfer the specimen into the appropriate container. The uncapped needle and syringe should be placed in the "sharps" container, and the spec-

Guidelines for Nursing Care

Collecting a Clean-Catch or Midstream Urine Specimen

Female

- Wear clean gloves.
- Clean the area at the meatus with soap and water.
- Have patient void about 30 mL, and discard this urine.
- Position the sterile specimen container near, but not touching, the meatus, and ask the patient to void forcibly if she is lying down to prevent urine from dribbling across the perineum.
- Stop collecting urine before the patient empties the bladder. Allow patient to continue voiding into a bedpan or the commode and discard this urine.
- Use a sterilized bedpan to collect the midstream specimen if the patient has difficulty voiding into the container, and then transfer the urine into the sterile specimen container.
- Label the specimen container, package it appropriately, and send the specimen to the laboratory.

Male

- Wear clean gloves.
- Retract the foreskin to expose the glans penis in the uncircumcised male patient.
- Clean the area of the external meatus with soap and water.
- Have the patient void about 30 mL, and discard this urine.
- Have the patient void directly into the sterile container.
- Stop collecting urine before the patient empties his bladder. Allow the patient to void the remaining urine in his bladder and discard it.
- Return the foreskin to its normal position in an uncircumcised patient to prevent swelling and irritation of the glans penis.
- Use a sterile urinal to collect the midstream specimen if the patient has difficulty voiding into the container, and then transfer the urine into the sterile specimen container.
- Label the specimen container appropriately, and send the specimen to the laboratory.

imen is then packaged and transported according to agency policy.

Figure 42-7 demonstrates removal of urine from an indwelling catheter.

Collecting 24-Hour Urine Specimens. For some laboratory studies, 24-hour specimens are required. It is crucial that the patient and the entire nursing team understand the importance of collecting *all* the urine voided in a 24-hour period. A sign posted on the patient's bathroom door is a helpful reminder not to discard urine. The collection is initiated at a specific time (which is recorded) by asking the patient to empty his or her bladder. This urine is discarded. All urine voided for the next 24 hours is collected.

Depending on the type of examination, the urine from each voiding may be kept in a separately marked container and the time of each voiding recorded, or all voidings may be collected in a common receptacle. The laboratory should specify whether a preservative is used to retard decomposition and whether the specimens are refrigerated or kept on ice. Many laboratories have a transport service to pick up specimens from a patient's home and return them to the laboratory within the appropriate time frame.

Determining Abnormal Constituents in the Urine

In some situations, the nurse may perform tests on urine specimens, especially when specimens are being tested repeatedly for known abnormalities, when screening tests are being used, or when laboratory facilities are not readily available. For example, a nurse may test urine for the presence of glucose, protein, bilirubin, and blood. The results of the test are recorded on the patient's record. Many commercially prepared diagnostic kits are available for such tests and can be used in the home or the healthcare facility. Although these tests are economical and fast, laboratory analysis is recommended when precise results are needed.

Most diagnostic kits contain all needed equipment and the appropriate reagent, a substance used in a chemical reaction to detect another substance. Reagents are available in tablets, fluids, impregnated paper, and plastic strips with a special coating. When the reagent contacts the urine, a chemical reaction occurs that causes a color change. This color is then compared with an accompanying chart that describes the significance of the color.

The precise directions for the amount of the specimen, the time allowance for the chemical reaction, and the interpretation of the color vary with the manufacturer. Therefore, it is important to follow the directions accompanying the diagnostic kit exactly.

Determining Specific Gravity

The specific gravity of urine is determined with an instrument called a urinometer or *hydrometer*. The urinometer has a calibrated scale for the measurement of specific gravity. Urine is placed in a cylindrical container, and the urinometer is inserted with a gentle twisting motion to prevent it from touching the bottom or side of the container. The reading on a urinometer should be made at eye level at the bottom of the meniscus formed by the urine (Fig. 42-8). The density of the urine floats the urinometer. If the urine is concentrated, the urinometer is buoyed up high, registering high on the measurement scale. If the urine is diluted, the urinometer floats lower in the urine with a low specific gravity reading.

Assisting With Diagnostic Procedures

Various diagnostic procedures, typically performed in a hospital operating room or outpatient facility, are used to study the urinary system. Nurses are responsible for preparing the patient and giving appropriate aftercare. Explaining the procedure helps reduce the patient's anxieties. Common diagnostic procedures include urodynamics studies, cystoscopy, intravenous pyelogram, retrograde pyelogram, computed tomography (CT) scans, and ultrasound examination. The

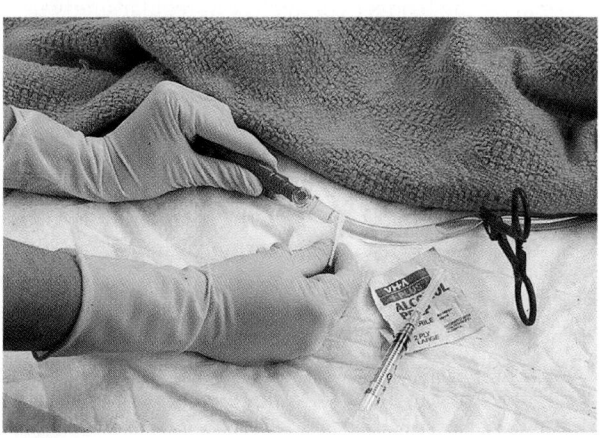
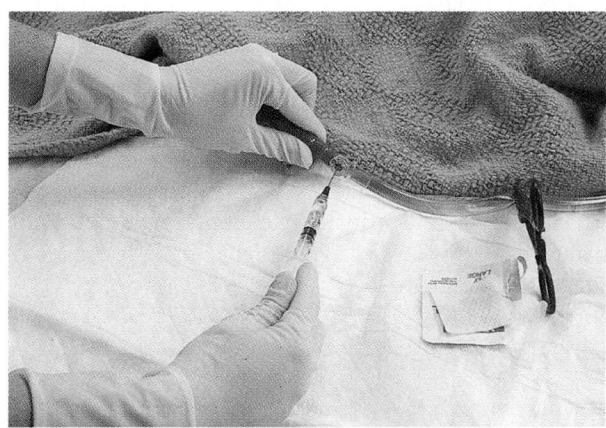

Figure 42-7
The nurse is obtaining a urine specimen from a patient using an indwelling catheter. (**A**) She first uses a swab moistened with an antiseptic to clean the area where she will introduce a sterile needle. (**B**) She then inserts the needle and withdraws a specimen of urine. Body substance precautions require that gloves be used when contact with urine is probable. (Photos © B. Proud.)

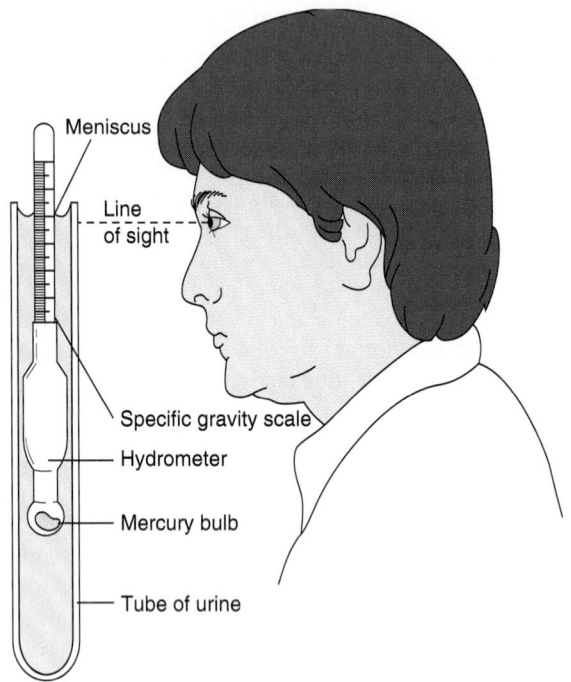

Figure 42-8
To determine specific gravity, the urinometer should be read at eye level at the base of the meniscus formed by the urine.

preparation and aftercare of the patient for each of these procedures are described in Table 42-2.

DIAGNOSING

The data the nurse collects about the patient's urinary functioning may lead to one or more nursing diagnoses. Some data are appropriately reported to the physician and may contribute to the physician's identification of a medical diagnosis. Nurses must identify significant urinary findings, record these appropriately, and report them to the proper people.

Urinary Functioning as the Problem

Nursing diagnoses that specifically address problems in urinary functioning include problems of incontinence, pattern alteration, and urinary retention. Sample defining characteristics for these diagnoses appear in the accompanying box.

Urinary Functioning as the Etiology

Difficulty with urination or changes in normal voiding patterns may affect other areas of human functioning. Examples of nursing diagnoses related to urinary problems include the following:

Anxiety related to incontinence, diagnostic procedures
Caregiver Role Strain related to incontinence of family member

Risk for Infection related to indwelling urinary catheter
Impaired Skin Integrity (Actual, Risk for) related to incontinence
Knowledge Deficit related to any existing or new urinary disease or disorder, lack of information about personal hygiene
Noncompliance With Medication Regimen related to misunderstanding the need to finish all doses of medication for urinary tract infection
Pain related to bladder spasms, dysuria, urinary retention, cancer of the bladder, diagnostic procedures
Self-Esteem Disturbance related to urinary incontinence, urinary diversion
Sexual Dysfunction related to urinary incontinence, urinary diversion
Sleep Pattern Disturbance related to nocturia
Toileting Self-Care Deficit related to parent's lack of knowledge or motivation to toilet train child, neuromuscular impairment or musculoskeletal disorders, immobility, trauma or surgical procedures, confusion, disorientation

The nurse's challenge is to identify correctly human responses to alterations in urinary elimination that pose specific health problems for the patient and his or her family.

PLANNING: EXPECTED OUTCOMES

When the patient is ambulatory and not experiencing difficulties with the urinary system, normal voiding is usually not a problem. Trauma or illness, however, may result in the patient's need for nursing assistance with voiding. Nursing interventions should support planned patient goals. The patient will achieve the following:

- Produce urine output about equal to fluid intake
- Maintain fluid and electrolyte balance
- Empty the bladder completely at regular intervals
- Report ease of voiding
- Maintain skin integrity

IMPLEMENTING

Any alteration in urinary elimination invariably invokes anxiety and fear in people. Nursing interventions focus on maintaining and promoting normal urinary patterns regardless of the healthcare setting, improving or curing urinary incontinence, preventing potential problems associated with bladder catheterization, and assisting with care of urinary diversions. Nurses can assist the patient and family to achieve desirable outcomes for their urination needs.

Promoting Normal Urination

Maintaining Normal Voiding Habits
If the patient's voiding habits are adequate, the nurse provides care or teaches the patient to maintain these habits

Table 42-2
Common Diagnostic Procedures Used to Study the Urinary Tract

Preparation	Aftercare
Urodynamic Studies: A group of tests that measure how urine flows, is stored, and is eliminated in the lower urinary tract	
There are usually no fluid or food restrictions before the test.	Drink 8 to 10 glasses of water in the 24 hours after the test.
Bladder should be full before the test.	Teach patient the signs and symptoms of a urinary tract infection.
Inform the patient that a catheter will be inserted during the test.	
Cystoscopy: The direct visual examination of the bladder, ureteral orifices, and urethra with a cystoscope	
The patient is allowed liquids on the morning of the examination.	Tissue swelling, dysuria, and hematuria may occur owing to trauma from the procedure.
Sedation and analgesics are usually prescribed before the procedure.	Encourage a generous fluid intake, and observe and measure urine output for at least 24 hours.
A signed consent form is required for the procedure.	Observe the patient for urinary retention and for signs of infection; nosocomial infection after a cystoscopy is common.
The procedure is ordinarily painless.	
Intravenous Pyelography (excretory urography): The radiographic examination of the kidney and ureter after a contrast material is injected intravenously	
No fluids or food are given for at least 12 hours before the examination so that contrast material will concentrate in the urinary system. Elderly, debilitated, or young patients may not tolerate this dehydration, and compromises may need to be made.	Fluids and food may be given immediately after the examination.
	Observe the patient for signs of a reaction to the contrast material, such as a rash, nausea, and hives.
A laxative the evening before the examination and an enema the morning of the examination are given so that stool and gas do not interfere with visualization.	
The patient should void before the examination.	
Retrograde Pyelography: The radiographic examination of the kidney and ureters after a contrast material is injected into the renal pelvis through the ureter	
No fluids or food are given after midnight before the examination.	Foods and fluids may be given, but if anesthesia has been used, this is delayed for several hours.
A laxative the evening before the examination and an enema the morning of the examination are given so that stool and gas do not interfere with visualization.	Check the vital signs regularly if anesthesia has been used.
The patient should void before the examination.	Observe the patient for signs of a reaction to the contrast material, such as a rash, nausea, and hives.
A signed consent form is recommended for the procedure.	Ureteral catheters may be in place and should be connected to drainage receptacles so that the amount and character of drainage from each catheter can be noted.
Ultrasonography: A noninvasive procedure that involves the use of ultrasound to produce an image or photograph of an organ or tissue	
A signed consent form is required.	No special care is required after the test.
Food and fluids are restricted for 8–12 hours before an abdominal ultrasound.	Inform patient that results are usually available 1–2 days after the study.
The patient should not smoke or chew gum before the procedure to prevent swallowing air.	
The procedure is painless.	

(continued)

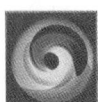

Table 42-2 (Continued)

Preparation	Aftercare
Computed Tomography (CT Scanning): A noninvasive radiographic procedure whereby a body part can be scanned from different angles with an x-ray beam and a computer that calculates varying tissue densities and records a cross-sectional image on paper	
A consent form should be signed.	Observe for a delayed reaction to the contrast dye (skin rash, urticaria, headache, vomiting). An oral antihistamine may be given for mild reactions.
The patient is usually NPO for 8 hours before the test if a contrast dye is used.	
Check for any history of allergic reaction or hypersensitivity to shellfish, iodine, or any contrast dyes.	Be supportive to patient and family. Test can be frightening.
All metal objects need to be removed before the test.	Instruct patient to resume usual diet and activity unless otherwise indicated.
Medications may usually be taken until 2 hours before the test.	
Renal Biopsy: Invasive procedure that involves obtaining a small piece of renal tissue for microscopic examination. Tissue sample may be obtained by needle and syringe through a skin puncture or small incision, during an open surgical procedure during which a wedge of tissue is removed, or through a cystoscope during which a brush is used to obtain a tissue fragment.	
Coagulation studies and hematocrit must be obtained.	Instruct patient to lie quietly for 4 hours.
Baseline vital signs must be obtained.	Monitor urine for hematuria during the first 24 hours. Collect each voided specimen in a separate cup labeled with the time.
Food and fluid are withheld before the procedure.	
A signed consent form is required.	Monitor vital signs and dressing for any indication of shock or bleeding.
Sedation may be necessary, depending on the type of procedure.	Instruct patient to avoid strenuous activities or heavy lifting for several days and to report any flank pain, hematuria, or dizziness.

to ensure comfort and satisfactory urine output. Attention to the following variables is helpful:

Schedule: Some patients report voiding on demand in no apparent pattern. Others have inflexible patterns that have developed over the years and become anxious if these are interrupted. Some patients need assistance voiding and may experience urgency. Nursing actions should support the patient's usual voiding pattern as much as possible.

Privacy: Many adults and children cannot void in the presence of another person. Unless the patient is extremely weak and requires assistance, privacy should be offered in the healthcare facility and in the home.

Position: Helping patients assume their usual voiding position may be all that is necessary to resolve an inability to void. Some male patients cannot use a urinal while lying down or sitting; the nurse should encourage them to void while standing at the bedside unless this is contraindicated. Similarly, some female patients cannot void easily on a bedpan but respond favorably with a bedside commode.

Hygiene: Patients who are confined to bed find it difficult to perform their usual genital hygiene. Careful cleansing of the perineal and genital areas is needed for patient comfort and to prevent infection. This is easily accomplished for patients on bed rest by using a bedpan and then pouring warm soapy water over the perineal area followed by clear water. Families providing care for ill members at home may be taught this technique.

Because many people customarily wash their hands after toileting, patients confined to bed should be offered a moistened towelette or soap and water to wipe their hands after the nurse removes the bedpan. Specific recommendations for urinary elimination problems that affect older adults are listed in the accompanying box, Focus on the Older Adult.

Promoting Fluid Intake

Many people routinely drink less fluid than is optimal to promote healthy urinary functioning. Adults with no disease-related fluid restrictions should drink 2000 to 2400 mL (8 to 10 8-ounce glasses) of fluid daily. A common misperception is that drinking this much fluid causes water retention and contributes to weight gain. If a good proportion of the daily fluid intake is water, the kidneys and urinary structures are well flushed and waste products are removed, including potentially harmful bacteria. Fluid intake

Nursing Diagnoses for Common Problems

Urinary Elimination

Problem	*Related Factors*	*Sample Defining Characteristics*
Altered Urinary Elimination	Enuresis (maturational)	Parents report 6-year-old son wets bed three or four times a week.
	Dysuria	Small bladder capacity, less than 300 mL
		"It hurts when I pass my water."
		Urinalysis reveals hematuria and proteinuria.
Functional Urinary Incontinence	Altered environment	"I don't know why Johnny started wetting since he's been hospitalized. He has been toilet trained for 6 months now."
	Sensory, cognitive, or mobility deficits	"When I remember to take mother to the toilet she urinates fine. But if I don't remember, I find her wet."
Reflex Urinary Incontinence	Neurologic impairment	Patient with spinal cord lesion reports no awareness of bladder filling, no urge to void or feelings of bladder fullness, involuntary loss of urine at somewhat regular intervals.
Stress Incontinence	Age-related degenerative changes	Obese mother of four reports involuntary dribbling of urine with coughs, sneezes, hearty laughter.
	High intraabdominal pressure	Patient "too busy to void" during day reports involuntary leakage of urine with sudden movement, cough, and so on.
	Incompetent bladder outlet	
	Overdistention between voidings	
	Weak pelvic muscles and structural supports	
Total Incontinence	Neurologic impairment	Constant flow of urine at unpredictable times without distention or uninhibited bladder contractions.
	Trauma or disease affecting spinal cord nerves	Nocturia
Urge Incontinence	Decreased bladder capacity	"I can never make it to the bathroom in time."
	Bladder spasms	Urgency, frequency, nocturia, bladder contracture or spasm
	Increased intake of caffeine or alcohol	
	Increased urine concentration	
	Overdistention of bladder	
Urinary Retention	High urethral pressure caused by weak detrusor	Elderly man diagnosed with benign prostatic hypertrophy complains of inability to urinate despite feeling bladder is full.
	Inhibition of reflex arc	Woman 6 hours after delivery has had no urine output since labor; 800 mL IV fluids infused; fundus of uterus is displaced to the right by a full bladder.
	Strong sphincter	
	Blockage	

should be monitored for potentially harmful excesses of caffeine-containing beverages, high-sodium beverages, such as diet sodas, and high-sugar beverages.

Fresh water, juices, and fluids of preference should be made available to patients confined to bed. Confused patients and children may need to be reminded to drink. Fluid restrictions may be ordered by the physician for patients with certain diseases. For others, forced fluids (above-average intake of fluids) are prescribed. This needs to be incorporated in the plan of care and explained to the patient.

Focus on the Older Adult

Nursing Strategies for Urinary Elimination Problems Affecting Older Adults

Nocturia, Frequency, and Urgency

- Ensure easy access to the bathroom or commode.
- Discourage fluid intake at bedtime.
- Discourage alcohol use before bedtime.
- Evaluate medication regimen and schedule, particularly diuretics and drugs that produce sedation or confusion.
- Use a night light.
- Use clothing that is easily removed for voiding.
- Keep assistive ambulatory devices (walkers, canes, etc.) readily available.
- Provide call bell if assistance is necessary.
- Evaluate gait and ability to ambulate safely.
- Assess for urinary tract infection.

Incontinence

- Maintain a fluid intake of 1500 to 2000 mL/day.
- Discourage use of alcohol, NutraSweet, and caffeine.
- Provide easy access to the bathroom.
- Assess factors that influence voiding.
- Use assistive devices when necessary (raised toilet seat, grab bars, walker).
- Use collection devices when necessary (urinal or bed pan).
- Ensure safety when ambulating (eg, skid-proof slippers).
- Encourage use of whole, unprocessed, coarse wheat bran to prevent constipation and fecal impaction.
- Perform Kegel exercises several times daily.
- Encourage participation in a bladder retraining program.
- Consider insertion of an indwelling catheter as the *last resort.*

Urinary Tract Infections

- Maintain a liberal fluid intake
- Encourage shower instead of tub bath to decrease opportunity for bacteria in bath water to enter urethra.
- Void at frequent intervals.
- Void immediately after sexual intercourse.
- Assess for signs of urinary tract infection (may be nonspecific in elderly patient).
- Use dipstick (Microstix) if recommended to monitor bacteria count in urine.
- Continue antimicrobial therapy as ordered.

Strengthening Muscle Tone

Strengthening perineal and abdominal muscle tone can facilitate voluntary control of urination and significantly reduce or eliminate problems with stress incontinence. Weakening of the pelvic floor muscles is a common cause of urinary incontinence. **Kegel exercises**, which are pelvic muscle exercises, target the inner muscles that lie under and support the bladder. These muscles can be toned, strengthened, and actually made larger by a regular routine of tightening and relaxing them. Often, patients have difficulty determining which muscles to exercise. These are the same muscles that you contract to stop urinating midstream or to control defecation. Patients are instructed to contract the pelvic floor muscles for 10 seconds and to relax them for 10 seconds. Kegel exercises should be performed without involving the muscles in the abdomen, inner thigh, and buttocks. When the patient is familiar with these sensations, he or she should perform these exercises 30 to 80 times a day for at least 6 weeks and possibly longer, depending on the response (Loughrey, 1999). The exercises can be done anywhere, and patients should be assisted to incorporate them into their daily activities. Kegel exercises can also be combined with biofeedback therapy. The auditory and visual cues from biofeedback help the patient isolate and hold the pelvic floor muscles correctly (Sasso, 1998).

Stimulating Urination and Resolving Urinary Retention

When urinary retention occurs, the bladder continues to fill and may distend to hold 3000 to 4000 mL of urine. Retention is often temporary, such as occurs commonly after surgery involving the lower abdomen, pelvis, bladder, or urethra, especially if ambulation is delayed or fluid intake is minimal. Any mechanical obstruction, such as swelling at the meatus, which often occurs after childbirth, or an enlarged prostate in men, may cause retention. Many people experience **hesitancy**—a delay or difficulty in initiating voiding. Routinely delaying urination may result in difficulty initiating a stream; therefore, the nurse should assist the patient to void when he or she first feels the urge to void. This problem may be resolved through additional measures that can be used by the nurse in the healthcare facility or caregivers at home (see the standardized Nursing Interventions Classification [NIC] listing.)

Occasionally, a physician may request the patient to perform *Credé's maneuver,* which is a manual bladder compression used to stimulate urination by creating a sensation of bladder fullness and relaxing the urethral sphincter. The patient is taught to place both hands flat on the abdomen, between the umbilicus and the symphysis pubis, with fingers pointing downward. The patient applies pressure over the bladder while holding the abdomen tight and holding his or her breath. This maneuver should be performed only in cases of bladder flaccidity when the patient is not expected to regain voluntary control. It usually requires a physician's order.

Using the Nursing Interventions Classification (NIC)

Urinary Retention Care

- Provide privacy for elimination.
- Use the power of suggestion by running water or flushing the toilet.
- Stimulate the reflex bladder by applying cold to the abdomen, stroking the inner thigh, or running water.
- Provide enough time for bladder emptying (10 min).
- Use spirits of wintergreen in bedpan or urinal.
- Monitor degree of bladder distention by palpation and percussion.
- Assist with toileting at regular intervals, as appropriate.

From McClosky, J., & Bulechek, G. (2000). *Nursing interventions classification (NIC)* (3rd ed.) (p. 692). St. Louis: C.V. Mosby. A full listing of nursing activities for each nursing intervention can be found in this book.

Assisting With Toileting

Toilet

Even when the patient can use the bathroom toilet, the nurse may be responsible for noting any abnormalities of elimination. In some instances, patients may need to be taught to report abnormalities to the nurse and instructed not to flush the toilet until the nurse checks the urine. In other instances, when the urine volume is to be calculated, the patient may need to urinate in a bedpan or some other receptacle placed in the toilet so that the urine can be measured before it is discarded. Although many patients can easily be taught to measure their urine output, the nurse should observe the urine at least once during a work shift and more frequently if warranted.

Weak patients should be assisted to the bathroom. Someone should remain in attendance if there is any danger of the patient's falling. Bathrooms should not be locked, and a signal bell should be within easy reach so that the patient can summon help easily if he or she feels weak and needs assistance. A hand rail near the toilet is helpful.

Commode

Commodes can be used for patients who can get out of bed but are unable to use the bathroom toilet. Commodes are chairs, straight-back chairs, or wheelchairs with open seats under which there is a shelf or a holder on which a bedpan is placed. The commode can be placed adjacent to the bed, and the patient can be assisted to it with minimal exertion.

Bedpan and Urinal

Male patients confined to bed usually use the urinal for voiding and the bedpan for defecation; female patients use the bedpan for both. The bedpan and the urinal are difficult for patients to use and embarrassing to many. Privacy is important to almost all patients when they use a bedpan or urinal.

A special bedpan called a *fracture bedpan* is frequently used by people with fractures of the femur or lower spine. Smaller and flatter than the ordinary bedpan, it is helpful for patients who cannot easily raise themselves onto the regular bedpan. Very thin or elderly patients often find it easier and more comfortable to use the fracture bedpan.

Figure 42-4 shows types of bedpans and urinals, and Procedure 42-1 shows how to help a patient use a bedpan or urinal.

Preventing Urinary Tract Infections

Urinary tract infections (UTIs) account for more than 7 million physician office visits and more than 1 million hospital admissions yearly in the United States (Marchiondo, 1998). Because their urethra is shorter and in close proximity to the vagina and rectum, women are especially vulnerable. UTIs can affect both the upper (kidneys and ureters) and lower (bladder and urethra) urinary tract. *Escherichia coli*, bacteria commonly found in the gastrointestinal tract, are the most common causal organism (Stockert, 1999).

Risk Factors

Those at greatest risk for a UTI include the following:

- Sexually active women—during intercourse, perineal bacteria can migrate into the urethra and bladder; as well, the spermicide used with a diaphragm decreases the amount of normally protective vaginal flora.
- Postmenopausal women—urinary stasis, which is common at this age, provides an optimal environment for bacteria to multiply; decreased estrogen contributes to loss of protective vaginal flora.
- Individuals with an indwelling urinary catheter in place—about one half of all patients with an indwelling catheter become infected within 1 week after its insertion.
- Individuals with diabetes mellitus—bacteria proliferate more easily in urine when glucose is present.
- Elderly people—the physiologic changes associated with aging (listed earlier in the chapter) predispose older people to development of UTI (Marchiondo, 1998; Stockert, 1999).

Diagnostic Evaluation

In addition to the nursing history and physical examination, laboratory findings can identify the presence of UTI. Clinicians believe that the presence of bacteria in a clean-catch midstream or sterile urine specimen, accompanied by symptoms (eg, dysuria, urinary frequency or urgency, or cloudy urine with a foul odor), indicates UTI. Red blood cells may be present in the urine.

PROCEDURE 42-1

Offering and Removing a Bedpan or Urinal

Equipment

Bedpan or urinal
Toilet tissue

Handwashing supplies
Disposable gloves

Cover for bedpan or urinal (use
Chux or disposable cover if
others not available)

Action	Rationale
1. Bring the bedpan or urinal and equipment to bedside. Don disposable gloves.	Having equipment on hand saves time by avoiding unnecessary trips to the storage area. Gloves protect against exposure to blood and body substances.
2. Warm the bedpan, if it is made of metal, by rinsing it with warm water.	A cold bedpan feels uncomfortable and may make it difficult for the patient to void. Plastic bedpans do not require warming.
3. Place an adjustable bed in the high position.	Having the bed in the high position reduces strain on the nurse's back while assisting the patient onto the bedpan.
4. Place the bedpan or urinal on the chair next to the bed or on the foot of the bed. Fold the top linen back just enough to allow for placement of bedpan or urinal.	Folding back the linen in this manner prevents unnecessary exposure while still allowing the nurse to place the bedpan or urinal.
5. If the patient needs assistance to move onto the bedpan, have him or her bend the knees and rest some of his or her weight on the heels. Lift the patient by placing one hand under the lower back, and slip the bedpan into place with the other hand.	The patient uses less energy as the nurse assists by lifting him or her onto the bedpan. The nurse uses less energy when the patient can assist by placing some of his or her weight on the heels.

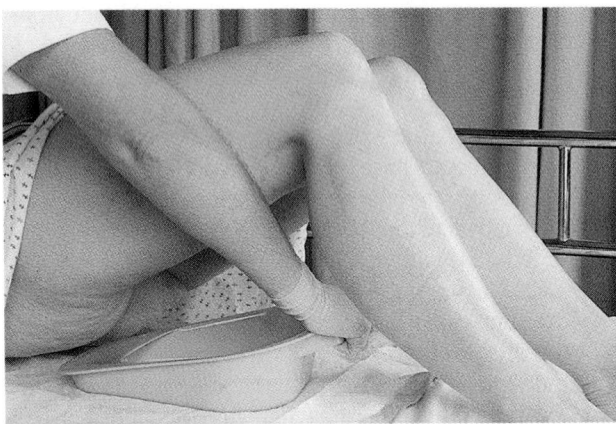

Action 5: Placing a fracture pan under buttocks.

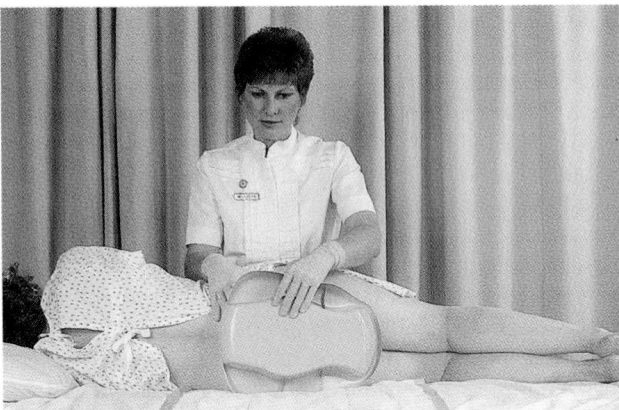

Action 6: Placing bedpan against buttocks while patient is on his side.
(PHOTOS © B. PROUD.)

6. If the patient is helpless, two people may be required to lift him or her onto the bedpan. Or, the patient may be placed on his or her side, the bedpan is placed against the buttocks, and the patient is rolled back onto the bedpan, as shown.

Having two people lift a helpless patient causes less strain on the nurse's back. Rolling the patient takes less energy than lifting the patient onto a bedpan.

(continued)

Offering and Removing a Bedpan or Urinal (Continued)

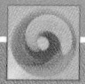

7. When the bedpan is in the proper place, the patient's buttocks rest on the rounded shelf of the bedpan, as shown. For male patients, the urinal is properly placed between slightly spread legs with the penis positioned in it and with the urinal resting on the bed.

Having the bedpan or urinal in the proper place prevents spilling contents onto the bed and prevents injury to the skin from a misplaced bedpan.

8. If permitted, raise the head of the bed as near to the sitting position as tolerated.

This position makes it easier for the patient to void or defecate, avoids strain on the patient's back, and allows gravity to aid in elimination.

9. Place call device and toilet tissue within easy reach. Leave the patient if it is safe to do so. Use side rails appropriately.

Falls can be prevented when the patient does not have to reach for items he or she needs. Side rails are an additional safety precaution. Leaving patient alone, if possible, promotes self-esteem and respects privacy.

10. Remove the bedpan in the same manner in which it was offered, being careful to hold it steady. If necessary to assist the patient, don disposable gloves, wrap tissue around the hand several times, and wipe the patient clean, using one stroke from the pubic area toward the anal area. Discard tissue, and use more until the patient is clean. Place the patient on his or her side, and spread the buttocks to clean the anal area. Cover bedpan.

Holding the pan steady prevents spilling its contents. Cleaning an area from front to back minimizes fecal contamination of the vagina and urinary meatus. Cleaning the patient after he or she has used the bedpan prevents offensive odors and irritation to the skin.

11. Do not place toilet tissue in the bedpan if a specimen is required. Have a receptacle handy for discarding the tissue.

Toilet tissue mixed with a specimen makes laboratory examination more difficult and interferes with accurate output measurement.

12. Offer the patient supplies to wash and dry his or her hands, assisting as necessary.

Washing hands after using the bedpan or urinal helps prevent the spread of organisms.

13. Empty and clean the bedpan and urinal. Wash your hands. Record according to agency procedure.

Provides adequate documentation. Handwashing helps prevent the spread of organisms.

Nursing Considerations   If it is difficult to slide patient onto the bedpan, powder may be used on the resting surfaces of the pan to eliminate friction. Powder should not be used if a specimen is required because contamination could result.

Treatment

Various protocols are used to treat UTI. A short-course antibiotic regimen (3 to 5 days) usually eradicates UTI of the lower urinary tract, whereas longer antimicrobial therapy is required for upper tract infections. A single large dose of an oral antibiotic is the newest approach to treatment of acute UTI and effectively eliminates the bacteria 80% of the time (Stockert, 1999).

By educating patients, nurses can significantly help prevent UTI recurrence. When risk factors have been identified, the nurse can teach the patient about measures that promote health and decrease the severity and incidence of UTIs. Nursing education focuses on teaching patients the following measures:

- Drink 8 to 10 8-ounce glasses of water daily.
- Observe the urine for color, amount, odor, and frequency. Report any sign of infection to healthcare provider.
- Dry the perineal area after urination or defecation from the front to the back, or from the urethra toward the rectum.
- Drink two glasses of water before and after sexual intercourse and void immediately after intercourse.
- Take showers rather than baths.
- Wear underwear with a cotton crotch, and avoid clothing that is tight and restrictive on the lower half of the body.

- Drink 2 to 3 glasses of cranberry or blueberry juice daily because this acidifies the urine and makes it more difficult for bacteria to adhere to the bladder wall (Jackson & Hicks, 1997). Regular intake of vitamin C appears to have a similar effect.
- Use an estrogen vaginal cream if postmenopausal and prone to UTIs.

Nursing interventions for a patient with an indwelling catheter are discussed later in the chapter.

Caring for an Incontinent Patient

Urinary incontinence, the inability to retain urine in the bladder, is widely underreported and underdiagnosed. It is a common but treatable health problem that is not, as widely believed, an inevitable result of growing old or bearing children. Many people self-manage this life-altering condition for many years before seeking assistance from a healthcare provider. Conservatively, as many as 35% of the American population older than 60 years of age and 50% of people who live in extended-care facilities or receive home care are incontinent (Agency for Health Care Policy and Research [AHCPR], 1996; Loughrey, 1999). Urinary incontinence is the leading cause of placement of older adults in long-term care facilities (Scura & Whipple, 1997). Although urinary incontinence is more prevalent in older women, 10% to 25% of women between the ages of 15 and 65 years report this condition (Johnson, 2000). Twice as many women as men are incontinent, and healthcare costs related to managing incontinent episodes are staggering.

The annual cost of incontinence care in the United States is estimated at $16.4 billion annually, with more than $1.5 billion spent for adult diapers (Scura & Whipple, 1997; Johnson, 2000). As the numbers of elderly increase, the cost of managing urinary incontinence will continue to escalate. The AHCPR, in its 1996 guideline on urinary incontinence in adults, recognized the role of nurses as healthcare professionals in delivering quality care and ensuring long-term improvement, thus reducing the cost and personal suffering caused by urinary incontinence.

As the statistics indicate, urinary incontinence is a special problem for older adults who may experience decreasing control over micturition and who may find it more difficult to reach a toilet in time to void because of mobility problems or dexterity problems in undressing. The discomfort, odor, and embarrassment of urine-soaked clothing can greatly diminish a person's self-concept and cause the individual to feel like a social outcast. Age-related changes do affect urinary function, but urinary incontinence can be treated, and individualized interventions can help the patient lead a normal life. Of those who seek treatment, 80% are either cured or their symptoms notably improved. Advertisements for adult disposable undergarments have increased public awareness about urinary incontinence, but they fail to mention possible treatment strategies. Refer to the box on Developing Critical Thinking Skills.

Types of Urinary Incontinence

The AHCPR guidelines (1996) recognized four major types of urinary incontinence: stress, urge, mixed, and overflow, and three minor classes: functional, transient, and unconscious incontinence. **Stress incontinence** occurs when there is an involuntary loss of urine related to an increase in intraabdominal pressure during coughing, sneezing, laughing, or other physical activities. Childbirth, menopause, obesity, or straining from chronic constipation can also result in urine loss. The leakage usually does not occur when the person is supine. **Urge incontinence** is the involuntary loss of urine associated with an abrupt and strong desire to void (urgency). It is usually associated with instability or involuntary contractions of the detrusor muscle that may or may not be associated with a neurologic disorder. A diagnosis of **mixed incontinence** indicates that symptoms of urge and stress incontinence are present, although one type may predominate. With **overflow incontinence**, the involuntary loss of urine is associated with overdistention and overflow of the bladder. The signal to empty the bladder may be underactive or absent, the bladder fills, and dribbling occurs. It may be due to a secondary effect of some drugs, fecal impaction, or neurologic conditions. **Functional incontinence** is urine loss caused by factors outside the lower urinary tract, such as chronic impairments of physical or cognitive functioning. A temporary reversible loss of bladder control, known as *transient incontinence*, may result from UTI or certain medications, such as diuretics. *Unconscious incontinence* is common in paraplegic patients and patients with multisystem failure (AHCPR, 1996).

Diagnostic Evaluation

In addition to the assessment strategies mentioned earlier in the chapter, physical examination and specific diagnostic tests aid in identifying urinary incontinence. The nurse examines the patient's abdomen for a distended bladder, any masses, or tenderness. Pelvic and rectal examinations can determine muscle and sphincter tone and detect any irregularities. Measurement of the **postvoid residual** (PVR) urine can be accomplished by the traditional method of catheterization or use of a portable ultrasound device that scans the bladder. A *bladder scan* can be performed at the bedside, poses no risk for infection, and is a safer alternative. Results are most accurate when the patient is in the supine position during the scanning. Both indicate the amount of urine remaining in the bladder immediately after the completion of urination. A PVR less than 50 mL is adequate, a volume greater than 200 mL is considered inadequate bladder emptying, and results between these two numbers indicate the need for further evaluation. If a bladder scan measures the urine volume at greater than 300 mL, catheterization should be performed to relieve distention. A voiding record or diary provides information about the frequency, timing, and amount of voiding (see the Research in Nursing box).

Developing Critical Thinking Skills

Situation

You have been assigned to care for an 80-year-old patient who was admitted with a recurrent leg ulcer and is due to be discharged the following day. Her nursing notes indicate that she has had two or three episodes of urinary incontinence every day while in the hospital and her plan of care states "use adult diapers." You go into the room to answer Mrs. Bartowski's call bell and help her into the bathroom. She is wearing an adult diaper, and a half-used package of diapers is on the chair. After voiding 150 mL of urine, she tearfully begs, "Please don't put that diaper back on me; I'm not a child." According to her chart, Mrs. Bartowski is mentally alert, lives at home with her daughter who visits frequently, and appears able to identify her need to urinate. You're aware that there are effective alternative therapies to resolve or minimize urinary incontinence rather than relying on absorbent products. However, the nurses have obviously made a decision to use diapers in this situation. You prefer to leave the diaper off, try some other measures, and, possibly, discuss this with her daughter; but as a student nurse you are only here for 2 days. You want to be a patient advocate and do the right thing. What should you do?

1. **Identify Goal of Thinking**

   Determine whether it is more important to replace the diaper against the patient's wishes or leave it off and discuss the possibility of using behavioral strategies with the staff.

2. **Assess Adequacy of Knowledge**

   Pertinent circumstances: Mrs. Bartowski is alert and oriented and obviously upset that diapers are being used. She has used her call light when she feels the urge to urinate, but incontinent episodes have also been documented. The nursing staff have decided that diapers are appropriate for this patient. Her daughter, with whom she lives, appears supportive and attentive. Discharge is scheduled for tomorrow.

   Prerequisite knowledge: Before you decide what to do in this situation, you need to discuss your options with your instructor. Of primary importance is whether the patient and her daughter are interested in pursuing alternatives. They can also provide invaluable information about her elimination pattern at home. The physician must be consulted to determine the etiology of the incontinence and validate that her urinary tract is intact and functioning adequately. You will also need to review the various treatment options for incontinence because these will have to be communicated to the patient and her daughter before discharge.

   Room for error/time constraints: Absorbent products can provide a sense of security and are widely used for incontinence. There is, however, an 80% chance that continence can be restored once incontinence is assessed, recognized, and addressed. Early dependence on absorbent products can remove motivation to seek treatment and promote acceptance of the condition. The treatment options should be discussed with Mrs. Bartowski and her daughter before discharge tomorrow.

3. **Address Potential Problems**

   Continuing to use absorbent products offers a temporary solution to the problem. They protect the patient from embarrassment and provide a sense of security, although they do nothing to prevent incontinent episodes. Using behavioral techniques to control incontinence will require health teaching before discharge and a long-term commitment to follow-up in the home.

4. **Consult Helpful Resources**

   The patient's motivation to restore continence is your most valuable resource. The primary nurse or case manager, the physician, and your instructor can also help you sort through your priorities in this situation. The AHCPR Guideline on Urinary Incontinence in Adults reflects the latest research and recommends use of behavioral techniques first to treat incontinence.

5. **Critique Judgment/Decision**

   If you decide to reapply a diaper against the patient's wishes, you may, in fact, be supporting the myth that incontinence is inevitable and untreatable. Long-term use of absorbent products can place the patient at risk for skin breakdown and a urinary tract infection if used improperly. You decide to leave the diaper off and establish regular intervals for voiding for the 2 days you will be caring for Mrs. Bartowski. In this short time, you hope to demonstrate to the patient, her daughter, and the staff that it is possible for Mrs. Bartowski to maintain a pattern of continence. Because she will most likely be discharged tomorrow, you also discuss the possibility of referral to home care or a continence expert who will instruct, support, and follow through with the necessary components of care. When you discuss your situation at postconference, your clinical group supports your decision.

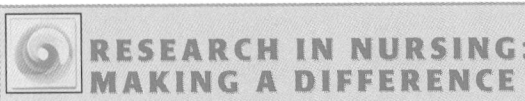

RESEARCH IN NURSING: MAKING A DIFFERENCE

Assisting Older Adults to Manage Urinary Incontinence

Urinary incontinence is an embarrassing, potentially disabling, and costly health problem that affects people of all ages. It is particularly disabling for older adults and is the most common reason older adults are relocated to long-term care facilities. Rather than being viewed as an inevitable outcome of aging for which there is no effective treatment, urinary incontinence can be cured or substantially alleviated with appropriate treatment options. Careful assessment and evaluation of an individual's voiding amounts and pattern can significantly affect the choice of interventions that will have a beneficial effect on the episodes of urinary incontinence.

Related Research

Pfister, S. (1999). Bladder diaries and voiding patterns in older adults. *Journal of Gerontological Nursing*, 25(3), 36–41.
All participants in this descriptive study lived in retirement settings and agreed to record fluid intake, the occurrence and timing of voluntary voiding, and involuntary urine leakage episodes in a diary. Information was collected over a 3-day period by 51 residents who averaged 67 years of age. Eight-eight percent were women, and 82% of the participants reported episodes of urinary incontinence. Nurses reviewed the data recorded in the bladder diary at a follow-up meeting and discussed treatment options based on individual concerns. Possible interventions included fluid and dietary modifications, behavioral management techniques such as Kegel exercises, and other medical or surgical options for bladder control. The bladder diary was viewed as a helpful assessment tool that clearly demonstrated factors that affected urinary elimination and provided a basis for approaches that result in regaining or improving urinary incontinence.

Relevance to Nursing Practice

The cause of urinary incontinence must be considered as nurses strive to identify the most successful and clinically realistic methods of significantly improving urinary incontinence. After careful assessment, home healthcare nurses can assist older patients to manage urinary leakage problems effectively in their home setting. Informing patients of therapeutic options helps them to maintain self-esteem and self-respect and live life to the fullest.

Treatment

Many patients incorrectly believe that surgery is the only treatment option for urinary incontinence. Surgical intervention is considered only if behavioral and pharmacologic measures prove ineffective. The most recent AHCPR guideline (1996) recommends using the least invasive treatment measures first. Nursing skills and creativity can help patients become continent again. The accompanying box summarizes the recommended treatment regimen for urinary incontinence.

Patients frequently turn to absorbent products for protection when they are incontinent of urine if they have not had this condition properly diagnosed and treated. When used improperly, such products may cause skin breakdown and place the patient at risk for UTI. Many types of products are available, including adult diapers, liners, pads, pant systems, and drip collectors. Long-term use of these products is not recommended according to AHCPR guideline until the following factors have been considered and discussed with a healthcare provider:

- Functional disability of the patient
- Type and severity of incontinence
- Gender
- Availability of caregivers
- Failure with previous treatment programs
- Patient preference

Through careful assessment and planned interventions, the nurse can restore a patient's continence and help postpone a caregiver's decision to place a family member in a costly healthcare facility. Environmental factors are of paramount importance and require careful assessment. It may be necessary to provide equipment that gives the person better access to toileting facilities (eg, walker, cane, wheelchair, Velcro closings on clothing). Dietary habits, such as excess caffeine intake or insufficient fluid intake, indicate the need for nutritional health teaching. Caffeine and concentrated urine irritate the bladder and may contribute to incontinence. The home setting, particularly, is ideally suited for the use of noninvasive, low-risk behavioral interventions, which are the first line of therapy. Nurses can identify patients who are incontinent and use these techniques or refer them to nurse or physician continence experts in the community. All nurses caring for older adults need to be familiar with education about urinary incontinence.

Catheterizing the Patient's Bladder

Urinary catheterization is the introduction of a catheter through the urethra into the bladder for the purpose of withdrawing urine. A *catheter* is a tube for injecting or removing fluids. Catheterization is considered the most common cause of nosocomial infections, that is, infections

Treatment Options for Urinary Incontinence

Behavioral Techniques

- Bladder training—a substantial retraining effort consisting of education, scheduled voiding, and positive reinforcement that requires resisting the sensation of urgency, postponing voiding, and urinating according to a timetable.
- Habit training—a program that focuses on voiding at regular intervals with an attempt to match the schedule to the person's natural elimination pattern.
- Pelvic muscle exercises—Kegel exercises that strengthen the voluntary periurethral and pelvic muscles. Biofeedback is an effective adjunct to Kegel exercises.

Pharmacologic Treatment

- This depends on the type of incontinence and involves a drug regimen for detrusor over-activity (urge incontinence) or drugs to improve urethral sphincter insufficiency (stress incontinence).
- Estrogen preparations or the vaginal ring that releases estrogen may be effective for post-menopausal women.

Prosthetic Supports for the Bladder Neck
External Barriers

- These adhere to the urethral opening to stop urine leakage but must be removed prior to voiding.

Urethral Inserts

- Devices that fit into the urethra; an inflated balloon keeps it in place and blocks the flow of urine.

Surgical Intervention

- Used as a last resort. The type of surgery depends on the etiology of the incontinence.

Adapted from Sasso, K. (1998). New treatment options for stress incontinence. *RN, 61*(9), 36–39.

acquired in a hospital. Whenever possible, catheterization should be avoided. When deemed necessary, it should be performed with careful technique.

Types of Catheters

If a catheter is to remain in place for continuous drainage, an **indwelling urethral catheter** is used. Indwelling catheters are also called *retention* and *Foley catheters*. The indwelling urethral catheter is designed so that it does not slip out of the bladder. These catheters are used for the gradual decompression of an overdistended bladder, for intermittent bladder drainage and irrigation, and for continuous bladder drainage.

An indwelling catheter uses a balloon that is inflated to retain it in place after the catheter is inserted into the bladder. Several types of indwelling catheters are available, but the principles on which they operate are similar.

The indwelling catheter has more than one lumen or open tube within the catheter. In a double-lumen catheter, one lumen is connected directly with the balloon, which is distended with sterile water, and the other is the lumen through which the urine drains. The triple-lumen catheter provides an additional lumen for the instillation of irrigating solution. Figure 42-9 shows a triple-lumen, a double-lumen, and a straight catheter.

Intermittent catheters, or *straight catheters*, are used to drain the bladder for shorter periods (5 to 10 minutes). Patients can be taught to insert and remove intermittent catheters themselves. Intermittent catheters are discussed later in this section.

A **suprapubic catheter** is occasionally used for continuous drainage. This type of catheter is surgically inserted through a small incision above the pubic area (Fig. 42-10). Suprapubic bladder drainage diverts urine from the urethra when injury, stricture, prostatic obstruction, or gynecologic or abdominal surgery have compromised the flow of urine through the urethra. Care of the patient with a suprapubic catheter is more appropriately discussed in clinical texts.

When a patient has a urinary tract obstruction and is not a candidate for surgery, a *urologic stent* may be inserted. The stent may be temporary (when placed in the ureters) or permanent (when positioned in the urethra). Temporary stents are usually made of a pliable material, such as radiopaque silicone, whereas permanent stents must be stronger and typically are made of a flexible metal mesh. They are inserted during a cystoscopic procedure, and in most cases, the patient receives only a local anesthetic and sedation. Urologic stents relieve urinary obstructions and provide a path for the flow of urine. Major nursing responsibilities include assessment, measurement, and documentation of urinary output. The nurse should never irrigate a blocked stent (Phipps, Sands, & Marek, 1999). Patients with a urologic stent must be instructed to notify the physician *immediately* if the urine becomes bright red in color, severe pain occurs, the drainage pattern changes, or there is any sign of infection. The patient should also be encouraged to wear a medical alert bracelet at all times.

Facts About the Lower Urinary Tract System

The following basic facts about the lower urinary tract system should be considered when catheterization is planned:

- The bladder is normally a sterile cavity.
- The external opening to the urethra can never be sterilized.
- The bladder has defense mechanisms. It empties itself of urine regularly and maintains an acidic environment, which has antibacterial advantages. These

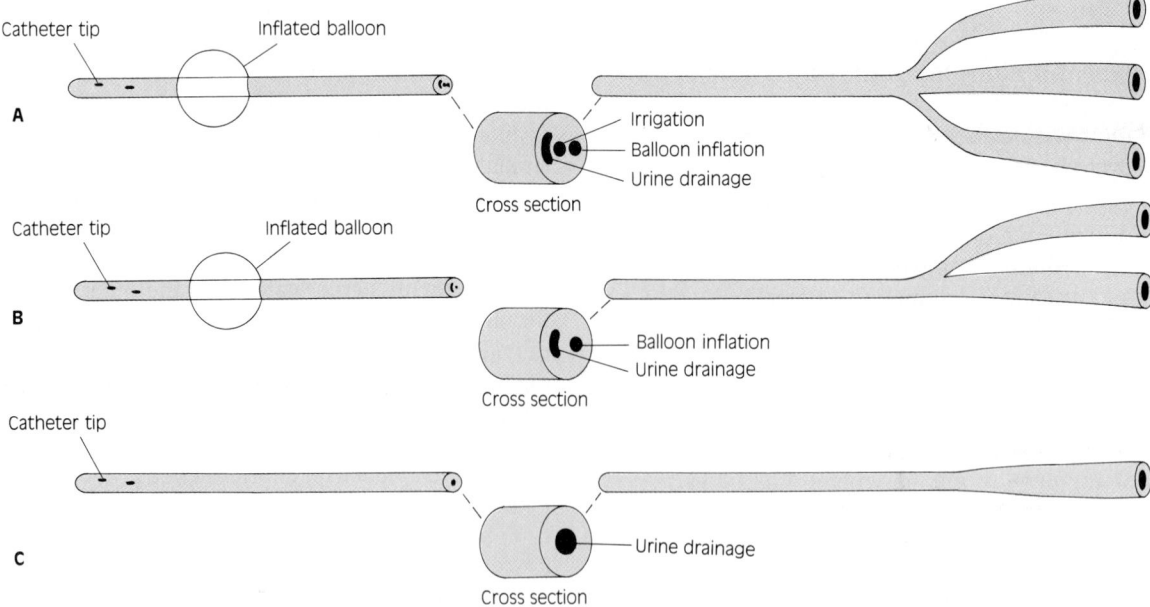

Figure 42-9
(**A**) Triple-lumen indwelling catheter. (**B**) Double-lumen indwelling catheter. (**C**) Straight catheter.

help to maintain a sterile bladder under normal circumstances and also help in clearing an infection if it occurs.

- Pathogens introduced into the bladder can ascend the ureters and cause bladder and kidney infection.

- A healthy bladder is not as susceptible to infection as an injured one. A state of lowered resistance, present in many diseases and stressful situations, predisposes the patient to urinary infection.

Reasons for Catheterization

Following are common reasons for a urinary catheterization:

- To relieve urinary retention
- To obtain a sterile urine specimen from a woman
- To measure the amount of PVR urine in the bladder. The patient is first asked to void and is then catheterized to determine how much urine stays in the bladder after normal voiding.
- To obtain a urine specimen when a specimen cannot be secured satisfactorily by other means. Examples include collecting an uncontaminated specimen from a woman who is menstruating or from an incontinent patient.
- To empty the bladder before, during, or after surgery and before certain diagnostic examinations

Hazards of Catheterization

The hazards of introducing an instrument or a catheter into the bladder are sepsis and trauma. The male urethra is especially vulnerable to injury because of its length. An object forced through a stricture or an irregular opening from the wrong angle can seriously damage the urethra. Although the female urethra is shorter than the male urethra, it is also susceptible to damage if a catheter is forced through it. The mucous membrane lining the urethra is delicate and easily damaged by the friction resulting from the insertion of a catheter. Bacteria can enter the bladder when the catheter is inserted. When the catheter

Figure 42-10
A suprapubic catheter positioned in the bladder. (From Smeltzer S., & Bare B. [2000]. *Brunner & Suddarth's textbook of medical surgical nursing* [9th ed.]. Philadelphia: Lippincott Williams & Wilkins.)

is left in place, the organisms may move up the catheter lumen or the space between the catheter and the urethral wall. This asymptomatic condition in which bacteria is present in the urine is known as *bacteriuria.* Most patients with an indwelling catheter in place for more than 4 weeks develop bacteriuria (Sienty & Dawson, 1999; Evans, 1999).

Intermittent catheterization may be necessary for patients with spinal cord injuries or other neurologic conditions. It may be done by the patient or a caregiver in the home. Although the risk for UTI is always present, most research supports the use of clean rather than sterile technique in this environment. The procedure for self-catheterization is essentially the same as that used by the nurse to catheterize a patient. A female patient may initially use a mirror to locate the meatus but eventually can learn to insert the catheter using just touch. Self-catheterization is recommended at regular intervals to prevent overdistention of the bladder and decreased blood flow through the wall of the bladder (Smeltzer & Bare, 2000).

Equipment

The equipment used for catheterization is usually pre-packaged in a sterile, disposable tray. Most kits already contain a standard-sized catheter. The trays used for catheterizing male and female patients are the same. Catheters are graded on the French (F) scale according to lumen size. For long-term use for an adult, a 12F to 14F catheter with a 5- to 10-mL balloon is commonly used. Smaller catheters usually are not necessary, and a smaller sized lumen would be so small that it would increase the time necessary for emptying the bladder. Larger catheters distend the urethra and increase the discomfort of the procedure. Size 8F or 10F catheters are commonly used for children.

Patient Preparation

Before the catheterization, the patient should be given an adequate explanation about the procedure and the reason for it. A catheter being inserted produces a sensation of pressure and some discomfort, and this should be explained to the patient. In addition, the patient should be assured that measures will be taken to avoid exposure and embarrassment. The more relaxed the patient is, the easier it is to insert the catheter.

The most common position for the patient is the dorsal recumbent, preferably on a solid surface such as a firm mattress or a treatment table. Catheterizing a patient in a bed with a soft mattress, especially a female patient, is not as satisfactory because the patient's pelvic surfaces are not firmly supported and visualization of the meatus is difficult. Also, the patient may sink into the bed, causing the bladder to be lower than the outlet of the catheter. If the patient is in bed, supporting the buttocks on a firm cushion is helpful.

The Sims, or lateral, position is an alternate position for female patients. This position may allow better visualization and be more comfortable for the patient, especially if hip and knee movements are difficult. The smaller area of exposure is also less stressful for the patient. The patient may lie on either side, depending on which position is easiest for the nurse and best for the patient's comfort. The patient's buttocks are placed near the edge of the bed with her shoulders at the opposite edge and her knees drawn toward her chest. The nurse lifts the upper buttock and labia to expose the urinary meatus. This position is shown in Figure 42-11.

Procedure

Catheterization of the urinary bladder in female and male patients is described in Procedures 42-2 and 42-3. Tech-

(*text continues on page 1162*)

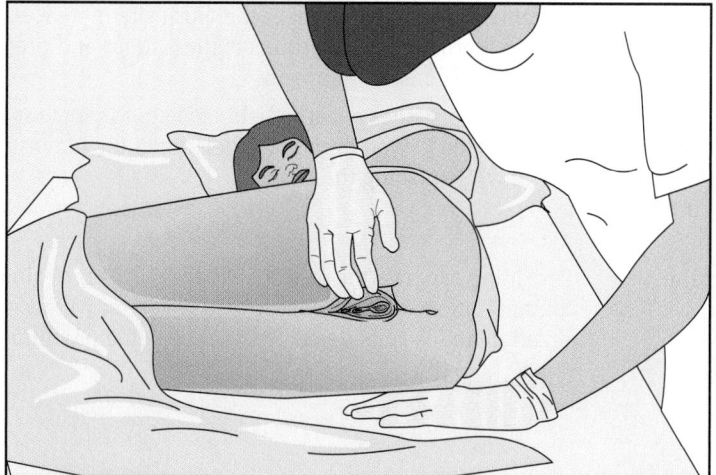
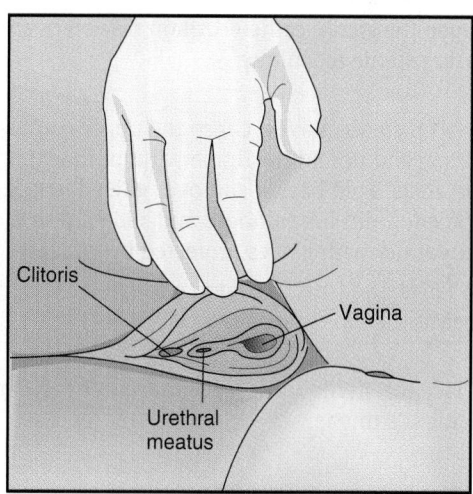

Figure 42-11
Demonstration of the side-lying position (*left*) and of how to expose the urinary meatus when catheterizing a female patient in the side-lying position (*right*).

PROCEDURE 42-2

Catheterizing the Female Urinary Bladder (Straight and Indwelling)

Equipment

Sterile catheterization kit that
   contains:
   Sterile gloves
   Sterile drapes (one of which is
     fenestrated)
   Antiseptic solution
   Lubricant
   Cotton balls or gauze squares

Forceps
Straight or indwelling catheter
   (size must be appropriate for
   patient)
Prefilled syringe
Basin (base of kit usually serves
   as this)
Specimen container

Flashlight or lamp
Urine collection bag and drainage
   tubing (may be connected to
   sterile indwelling catheter if a
   closed drainage system is used)
Velcro leg strap or tape
Disposal bag
Waterproof pad or Chux

Action	Rationale
1. Assemble equipment. Wash your hands. Explain the procedure and its purpose to the patient.	Organization facilitates performance of the task. Hand-washing deters spread of microorganisms. An explanation encourages patient cooperation and reduces apprehension.
2. Provide for good light. Artificial light is recommended (use of a flashlight requires an assistant to hold and position it).	Good lighting is necessary to see the meatus clearly.
3. Provide for privacy by closing the curtains or door.	The procedure may be embarrassing for the patient.
4. Assist the patient to the dorsal recumbent position with the knees flexed and the feet about 2 feet apart and drape the patient. Or, if preferable, the patient can be placed in the side-lying position as shown in Figure 42-11. Slide the waterproof drape under the patient.	Good visualization of the meatus is important. Embarrassment, chilliness, and feeling tense can interfere with introducing the catheter. The patient's comfort will promote relaxation. The drape will protect bed linens from moisture.
5. Clean the genital and perineal area with warm soap and water. Rinse and dry. Wash your hands again.	Clean technique decreases the possibility of introducing organisms into the bladder.
6. Prepare urine drainage setup if indwelling catheter is to be inserted and separate urine collection system is used. Secure to bed frame according to manufacturer's directions.	This facilitates connection of the catheter to the drainage system and provides for easy access.
7. Open the sterile catheterization tray on overbed table using sterile technique.	Placement of equipment near the work site increases efficiency. Sterile technique protects the patient and prevents the spread of microorganisms.
8. Put on sterile gloves. Grasp the upper corners of the drape and unfold the drape without touching unsterile areas. Fold back a cuff over gloved hands. Ask the patient to lift her buttocks and slide the sterile drape under her with gloves protected by cuff.	The drape provides a sterile field close to the meatus. Covering the gloved hands will help keep the gloves sterile while placing the drape.
9. A fenestrated sterile drape may be placed over the perineal area, exposing the labia.	The drape expands the sterile field and protects against contamination. Use of a fenestrated drape may limit visualization and is considered optional by some practitioners.
10. Place the sterile tray on the drape between the patient's thighs.	This provides easy access to supplies.

(continued)

Catheterizing the Female Urinary Bladder (Continued)

11. Open all supplies:
    a. *If the catheter is to be indwelling,* test the catheter balloon. Remove the protective cap on the tip of the syringe and attach the syringe prefilled with sterile water to injection port. Inject appropriate amount of fluid. If the balloon inflates properly, withdraw fluid and leave the syringe attached to the port.

    A balloon that does not inflate or that leaks needs to be replaced before insertion in the patient.

    b. Pour antiseptic solution over cotton balls or gauze. Open the specimen container if specimen is to be obtained.

    It is necessary to open all supplies and prepare for the procedure while both hands are sterile.

    c. Lubricate 1 to 2 inches of the catheter tip.

    Lubrication facilitates the insertion of the catheter and reduces trauma to the tissues.

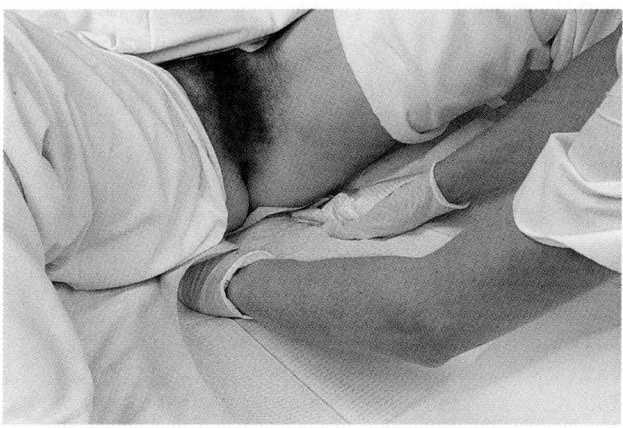

Action 8: Keeping sterile gloves protected while positioning drape under patient.

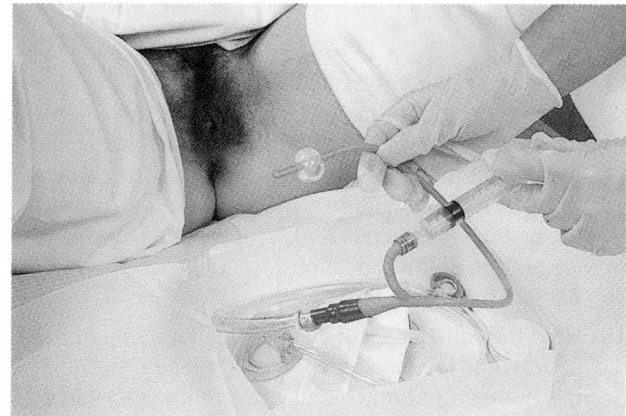

Action 11a: Testing the balloon.

12. With the thumb and one finger of your nondominant hand, spread the labia and identify the meatus, as shown in figure. Be prepared to maintain separation of the labia with one hand until urine is flowing well and continuously.

    Smoothing the area immediately surrounding the meatus helps to make it visible. Allowing the labia to drop back into position may contaminate the area around the meatus, as well as the catheter. Your nondominant hand is now contaminated.

13. Using cotton balls held with forceps, clean both labial folds and then directly over the meatus. Move the cotton ball from above the meatus down toward the rectum. Discard each cotton ball after one downward stroke.

    Moving from an area where there is likely to be less contamination to an area where there is more contamination helps prevent the spread of organisms. Cleaning the meatus last helps reduce the possibility of introducing organisms into the bladder.

14. With the uncontaminated gloved hand, place the drainage end of the catheter in the receptacle. *For insertion of an indwelling catheter* that is preattached to sterile tubing and drainage container (closed drainage system), position the catheter and setup within easy reach on the sterile field.

    This facilitates drainage of urine and minimizes risk of contaminating sterile equipment.

(continued)

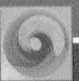

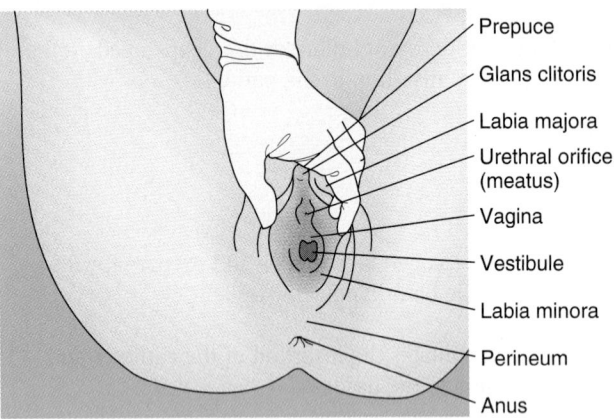

Action 12: Spreading the labia with nondominant band to identify the meatus.

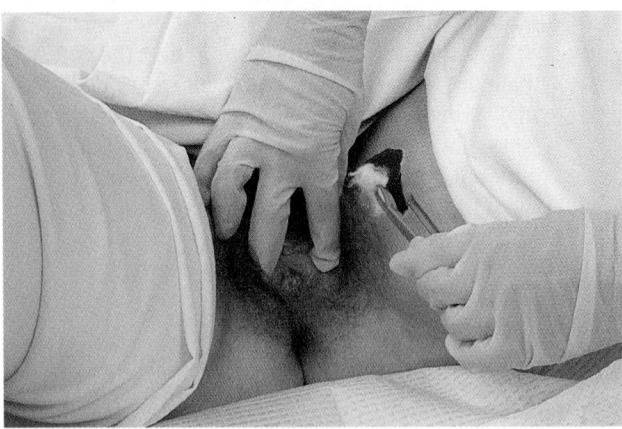

Action 13: Preparing to clean the labial folds.

15. Insert the catheter tip into the meatus 5 to 7.5 cm (2–3 in) or until urine flows. Do not use force to push the catheter through the urethra into the bladder. Ask the patient to breathe deeply, and rotate the catheter gently if slight resistance is met as the catheter reaches the external sphincter. *For an indwelling catheter, once urine drains, advance the catheter another 2.5 to 5.0 cm (1–2 in).*

16. Hold the catheter securely with the nondominant hand while the bladder empties. Collect a specimen if required. Continue drainage according to agency policy.

17. Remove the catheter smoothly and slowly if a straight catheterization was ordered.

18. *If the catheter is to be indwelling:*
    a. Inflate the balloon according to the manufacturer's recommendations. Inject the entire volume supplied in the prefilled syringe.
    b. Tug gently on the catheter after the balloon is inflated to feel resistance.
    c. Attach the catheter to the drainage system if necessary.
    d. Secure to the upper thigh with a Velcro leg strap or tape. Leave some slack in the catheter to allow for leg movement.
    e. Check that the drainage tubing is not kinked and that movement of side rails does not interfere with catheter or drainage bag.

The female urethra is about 3.7 to 6.2 cm (1½–2½ in) long. Applying force on the catheter is likely to injure mucous membranes. The sphincter relaxes, and the catheter can enter the bladder easily when the patient relaxes. Advancing an indwelling catheter an additional 1.3 to 2.5 cm (½ to 1 in) ensures placement in the bladder and facilitates inflation of the balloon without damaging the urethra.

Withdrawing and reinserting the catheter increases the chances of contaminating it. In general, no more than 750 mL of urine should be removed at one time. Pelvic floor blood vessels may become engorged from the sudden release of pressure leading to possible hypotensive episode.

This causes less discomfort to the patient.

The balloon anchors the catheter in place in the bladder. Sterile water is used to inflate the balloon as a precaution in case the balloon ruptures.
Improper inflation can cause patient discomfort and malpositioning of catheter.
Closed drainage system minimizes the risk for organisms being introduced into the bladder.
Proper attachment prevents trauma to the urethra and meatus from tension on the tubing.

This facilitates drainage of urine and prevents the backflow of urine.

(continued)

Catheterizing the Female Urinary Bladder (Continued)

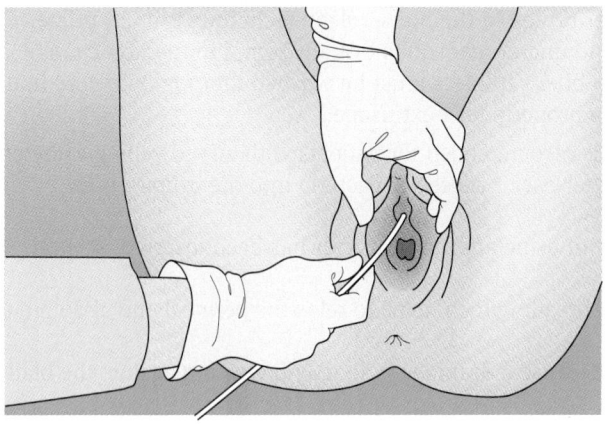

Action 15: Inserting the tip of the catheter into the meatus, using the uncontaminated gloved band.

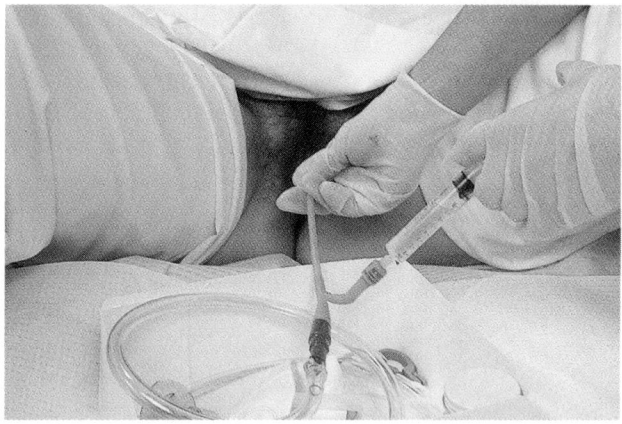

Action 18a: Injecting sterile water to inflate balloon.

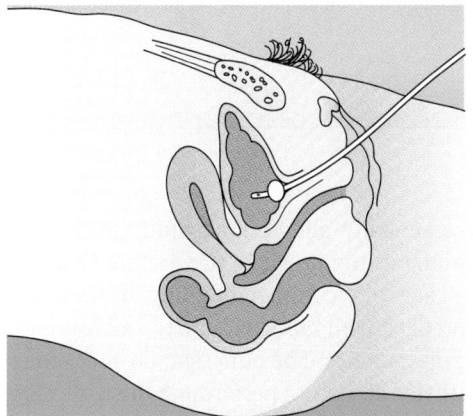

Action 18b: Tugging gently on catheter after balloon is in place to feel resistance.

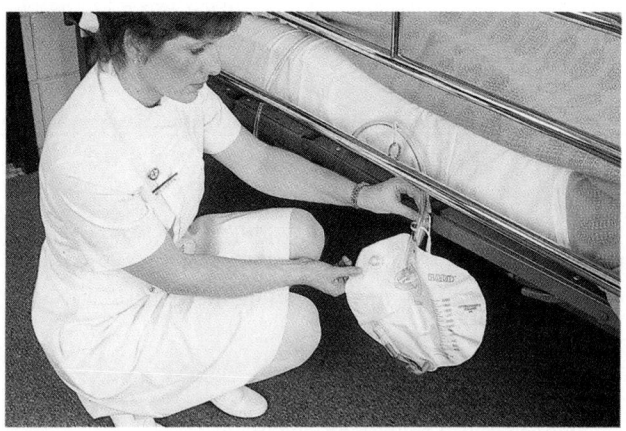

Action 18e: Checking position of drainage setup.

19. Remove the equipment and make the patient comfortable in bed. Clean and dry the perineal area, if necessary. Care for the equipment according to agency policy. Send the urine specimen to the laboratory promptly or refrigerate it.

Urine kept at room temperature may cause organisms, if present, to grow and distort laboratory findings.

20. Wash your hands.

Handwashing deters the spread of microorganisms.

21. Record the time of the catheterization, the amount of urine removed, a description of the urine, the patient's reaction to the procedure, and your name.

A careful record is important for planning the patient's care.

(continued)

Catheterizing the Female Urinary Bladder (Continued)

Home Care Considerations	If self-catheterization must be performed in the home, clean technique is appropriate. The bladder's natural resistance to microorganisms normally found in the home make sterile technique unnecessary. Rubber catheters must be washed thoroughly before boiling for 20 minutes. Dry and store properly for next usage.
	A shower rather than a tub bath is recommended for patients with an indwelling catheter. Sitting in the bathtub may allow for easier access of bacteria into the urinary tract.
Special Considerations	If there is not an immediate flow of urine after the catheter has been inserted, several measures may prove helpful:

- Have the patient take a deep breath, which helps to relax the perineal and abdominal muscles.
- Rotate the catheter slightly because a drainage hole may be resting against the bladder wall.
- Raise the head of the patient's bed to increase pressure in the bladder area.
- Placed a gloved finger in the vagina to feel digitally for the position of the catheter through the anterior vaginal wall.
- Temporarily leave a catheter that has inadvertently been placed in the vagina in place as a guide while the nurse regloves and inserts another sterile catheter directly above it into the urinary meatus.

niques of surgical asepsis are extraordinarily important to help prevent urinary tract infection. See the box, Through the Eyes of a Student, for a student's experience with catheterization.

Indwelling Catheters

Inserting and Connecting to the Drainage System

The nurse inserts the indwelling catheter and cares for the patient. The procedure for inserting an indwelling catheter is similar to that for inserting a straight single-lumen catheter, with a few differences. An inflated balloon holds the indwelling catheter in position in the bladder. The prefilled syringe included in the catheter kit contains the amount of sterile water needed to inflate the balloon to the desired spherical shape. If the nurse were to inject only 5 mL into a catheter into a 5 mL balloon, some solution would remain in the tubing leading to the balloon, and the partially inflated balloon could cause irritation and erosion to the mucosa in the bladder. Usually, 7 to 10 mL of fluid is necessary to inflate a 5-mL balloon completely. If a patient complains of pain immediately after the catheter is inflated, it is allowed to empty, and the catheter is replaced with another one; the balloon was probably in the urethra and caused discomfort because of the distention of the urethra.

The technique of applying lubricant on the catheter before inserting it in a male patient is no longer practiced. Lubricant applied externally to the catheter remains at the

meatus, essentially allowing an unlubricated catheter to cause trauma to the lining of the urethra. Instead, Procedure 42-3, step 8, recommends gently inserting the tip of a syringe prefilled with lubricant into the male urethra before inserting the catheter. The nurse should check the contents of the catheter kit before performing the male catheterization procedure to ensure that it contains a prefilled syringe of lubricant rather than a single packet of lubricant (Gerard & Sueppel, 1997).

The indwelling catheter is connected to a drainage and collection system that must be properly positioned and secured to minimize the risk for infection. The following technique is used to complete the closed urinary drainage system:

- Check to see that the patient is not lying on the drainage tubing and compressing it.
- Keep the catheter drainage bag below the level of the bladder at all times.
- Keep the drainage bag off the floor at all times to reduce the risk of infection. The floor is grossly contaminated!
- Check that all connections are secure and that no leakage is occurring.

An indwelling catheter must be properly secured to prevent injury or friction (see Procedures 42-2 and 42-3 for appropriate methods).

Catheterizing the Male Urinary Bladder (Straight and Indwelling)

Equipment

Sterile catheterization kit that
    contains:
    Sterile gloves
    Sterile drapes (one of which is
      fenestrated)
    Antiseptic solution
    Lubricant in 10 mL syringe
    Cotton balls or gauze squares

Forceps
Straight or indwelling catheter
Prefilled syringe
Basin (base of kit usually serves
    as this)
Specimen container
Flashlight or lamp

Urine collection bag and drainage
    tubing (may be connected to
    sterile indwelling catheter if a
    closed drainage system is used)
Velcro leg strap or tape
Disposal bag
Waterproof pad or Chux

Action	Rationale
1. Assemble equipment and follow actions 1 through 3 for female catheterization in Procedure 42-2.	
2. Position the patient on his back with the thighs slightly apart. Drape the patient so that only the area around the penis is exposed.	This prevents unnecessary exposure.
3. Follow actions 5 to 7 for female catheterization in Procedure 42-2.	

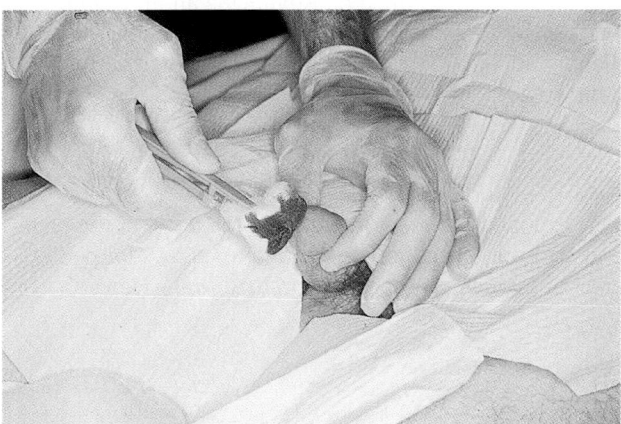

Action 3: Cleaning area of the meatus.

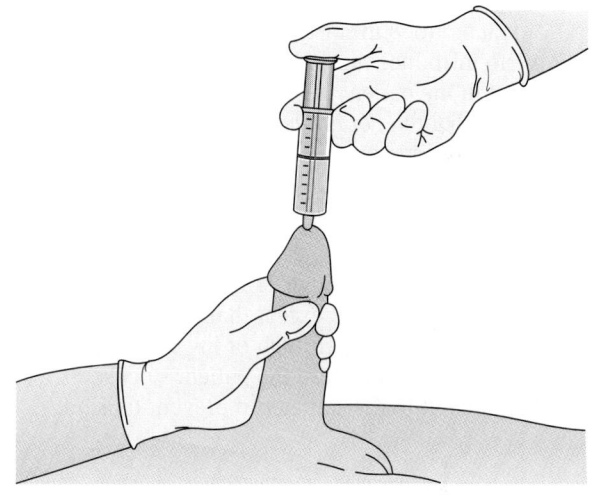

Action 8: Instillation of lubrication before male catheterization.

Action	Rationale
4. Put on sterile gloves. Open the sterile drape and place on the patient's thighs. Place the fenestrated drape with the opening over the penis.	This maintains a sterile working area.
5. Place the catheter set on or next to the patient's legs on the sterile drape.	The sterile setup should be arranged so that the nurse's back is not turned to it, nor should it be out of the nurse's range of vision.
6. Open all supplies:	
a. *If the catheter is to be indwelling,* test the catheter balloon. Remove the protective cap on the tip of the syringe and attach the syringe prefilled with sterile water to the injection port. Inject appropriate amount of fluid. If balloon inflates properly, withdraw fluid and leave syringe attached to port.	A balloon that does not inflate or that leaks must be replaced before insertion in the patient.
b. Pour antiseptic solution over cotton balls or gauze. Open the specimen container if specimen is to be obtained.	It is necessary to open all supplies and prepare for the procedure while both hands are sterile.
c. Remove the cap from the syringe prefilled with lubricant.	

(continued)

PROCEDURE 42-3

Catheterizing the Male Urinary Bladder (Continued)

7. Lift the penis with your nondominant hand, which is then considered contaminated. Retract the foreskin in the uncircumcised male patient. Clean the area at the meatus with a cotton ball held with a forceps. Use a circular motion, moving from the meatus toward the base of the penis for three cleansings.

The hand touching the penis becomes contaminated. Cleansing the area around the meatus and under the foreskin in the uncircumcised male patient helps prevent infection. Moving from the meatus toward the base of the penis prevents bringing organisms to the meatus.

8. Hold the penis with slight upward tension and perpendicular to the patient's body. Gently insert the tip of the syringe with lubricant into the urethra and instill the 10 mL of lubricant.

The lubricant causes the urethra to distend slightly and facilitates passage of the catheter without traumatizing the lining of the urethra.

9. Ask the patient to bear down as if voiding. With your dominant hand, place the drainage end of the catheter in the receptacle. *For insertion of an indwelling catheter* that is preattached to sterile tubing and a drainage container (closed drainage system), position the catheter and setup within easy reach on the sterile field.

Bearing down eases the passage of the catheter through the urethra.

10. Insert the tip into the meatus. Advance the catheter 15 to 20 cm (6–8 in) or until urine flows. Do not use force to introduce the catheter. If the catheter resists entry, ask the patient to breathe deeply and rotate the catheter slightly. *For an indwelling catheter,* once urine drains, advance the catheter to the bifurcation of the catheter. Once the balloon is inflated, the catheter may be gently pulled back into place. Lower the penis.

The male urethra is about 20 cm long. Deep breaths or slight twisting of the catheter may ease the catheter past resistance at the sphincters. Advancing an indwelling catheter to the bifurcation ensures its placement in the bladder and facilitates inflation of the balloon without damaging the urethra.

11. Follow Actions 16 through 21 for female catheterization in Procedure 42-2 except that the catheter may be secured to the upper thigh or lower abdomen with the penis directed toward the patient's chest. Slack should be left in the catheter to prevent tension.

This is done to prevent irritation at the angle of the penis and scrotum. Slack left in the catheter allows for penile erection, which can occur naturally during sleep.

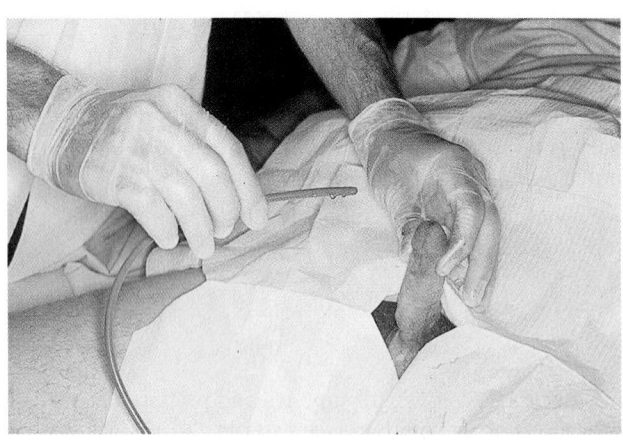

Action 9: Preparing to insert the catheter.

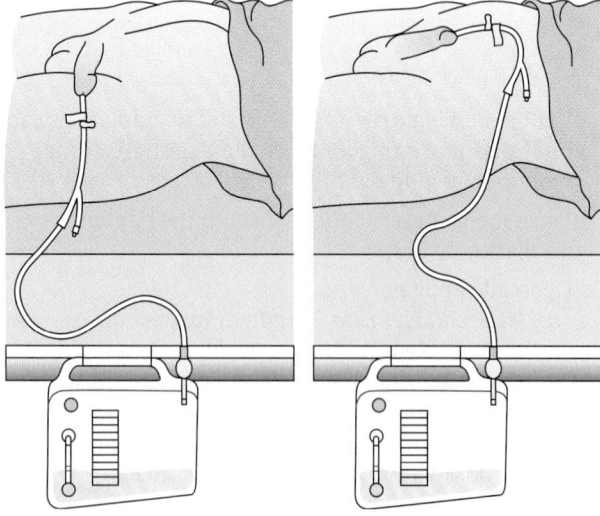

Action 11: Secure the catheter to the upper thigh or lower abdomen, allowing slack to prevent tension.

Through the Eyes of a Student

Remembering my first hospital experiences, I would have to say that doing my first catheterization was the scariest. I was working with a nurse on the maternity floor. Our patient had not voided in more than 8 hours and seemed to be in great discomfort. We palpated her abdomen to see if her bladder was distended, and it was. Because she didn't have an urge to void, we decided to straight cath her to lessen her discomfort. The nurse I was working with turned and handed me the kit. She said, "You know what to do, right?" Automatically I replied, "Sure."

My heart began to race. Of course I knew the procedure, but I never actually did it on a real person. Not only was I nervous about doing the procedure, but I also didn't want to make her labor more painful. The nurse, out of courtesy, asked the patient if she minded if I did the procedure. Thank God the patient had a soft side for a beginner. Smiling, she looked at me and said, "You know what you're doing, right?" Again I said, "Sure." I began setting up to begin my mission. To my amazement, I really did remember how to prepare for a catheterization. I even was amazed that my sterile procedure wasn't bad for the first time. When it was time to insert the catheter, I took a deep breath. Thankfully, it went in nice and smooth, and I reached the bladder in seconds. The urine began flowing through rapidly. It seemed like it would never stop. Amazingly, it filled the container. I removed the catheter, cleaned up, and let out my breath.

In summary, I was glad that I had the experience to do a catheterization. The nurse told me that I did a good job, which made me feel good. Also, my patient thanked me for relieving some of her discomfort and gave me a reassuring smile. As I look back now, it wasn't as bad as I had myself believed it would be. Even though it's invasive to the patient, sometimes it's necessary. I want to do everything I can to help my patients. Now, I look at all my new adventures as helping my patients feel better.

—ALYSIA PAXSON,
HOLY FAMILY COLLEGE, PHILADELPHIA

Irrigating the Indwelling Catheter or Bladder

The flushing of a tube, canal, or area with solution is called *irrigation*. The purpose of catheter irrigation is to restore or maintain its patency. A bladder irrigation rinses out the bladder and can also instill medication that acts directly on the bladder wall. Procedure 42-4 describes how to irrigate an indwelling catheter using the closed system.

Continuous or frequent irrigations may be ordered when blood clots or other debris threaten to block the catheter. In the past, an open procedure was done routinely for almost all indwelling catheters, but because this is another means of introducing pathogens, it is now recommended that the closed system be used. Natural irrigation of the catheter through increased fluid intake by the patient is preferred.

Preferably, the patient who needs frequent irrigation so that the catheter and tubing remain patent will have a triple-lumen catheter using continuous irrigation. Procedure 42-5 describes continuous bladder irrigation, and Figure 42-12 illustrates this system.

Caring for Patients With an Indwelling Catheter

Following are nursing measures used to care for patients with an indwelling catheter:

- Wash hands before and after caring for a patient with an indwelling catheter and wear gloves to protect against possible exposure to blood and body substances.
- Clean the perineal area thoroughly, especially around the meatus, daily and after each bowel movement.
- Cleanse the catheter by cleaning gently from the meatus outward.
- Use mild soap and water or a perineal cleanser to clean the perineal area; rinse the area well. Do not use powders and lotions after cleaning.
- Make sure that the patient maintains a generous fluid intake. This helps prevent infection and irrigates the catheter naturally by increasing urine output.
- Encourage the patient to be up and about, as ordered.
- Note the volume and character of urine, and record observations carefully. The urine can be observed through the drainage tubing and in the collecting container. The usual procedure is to note and record the amount of urine on the patient's intake-and-output record every 8 hours. The collecting container is calibrated, but the volume markings are only approximations. The urine should be emptied into a graduated container that is accurately calibrated for correct determination of output.
- Do not open the drainage system to obtain urine specimens or to measure urine. If the tubing becomes disconnected, wipe the ends of both tubes with antiseptic solution before reconnecting them. When emptying the drainage bag, make sure the drainage spout does not touch a contaminated surface.
- Teach the patient the importance of personal hygiene, especially the importance of careful clean-

PROCEDURE 42-4

Irrigating the Catheter Using the Closed System

Equipment

Sterile basin or container
Gauze squares or cotton balls with
  disinfectant or alcohol swabs
Waterproof drape

30- to 50-mL syringe with 18- or 19-
  gauge needle
Sterile irrigating solution (at room
  temperature or warmed to body
  temperature)

Bath blanket
Disposable gloves

Action	Rationale
1. Assemble equipment. Wash your hands. Explain the procedure and its purpose to the patient.	Organization facilitates performance of task. Handwashing deters spread of microorganisms. An explanation encourages patient cooperation and reduces apprehension.
2. Provide for privacy by closing the curtains or door and draping the patient with the bath blanket.	The procedure may be embarrassing for the patient.
3. Assist the patient to a comfortable position and expose the aspiration port on the catheter setup. Place the waterproof drape under the catheter and aspiration port.	This provides for adequate visualization. The drape protects the patient and the bed from leakage.
4. Open the sterile supplies. Pour sterile solution into the sterile basin. Aspirate irrigant (30 to 50 mL) into the sterile syringe and attach the capped sterile needle. Don gloves.	This prevents the spread of microorganisms and contact with blood or body substances.
5. Disinfect the aspiration port with alcohol swabs or gauze square with antiseptic solution.	This prevents the spread of microorganisms.
6. Clamp or fold the catheter tubing distal to the aspiration port.	This directs the irrigating solution into the bladder.
7. Remove the cap and insert the needle into the port. Gently instill solution into the catheter.	Gentle irrigation prevents damage to the lining of the bladder.
8. Remove the needle from the port. Unclamp the tubing and allow irrigant and urine to drain. Repeat the procedure as necessary.	Gravity aids drainage of urine and irrigant from the bladder.
9. Assess the patient's response to the procedure and the quality and amount of drainage. Document on the patient's chart.	This provides accurate documentation of the procedure.
10. Record the amount of irrigant used on the intake and output record. Subtract this from the urine output when totaled.	Subtracting irrigant total from drainage in urine collection bag provides accurate recording of urine output.
11. Remove equipment and discard uncapped needle and syringe in appropriate receptacle. Remove gloves and wash your hands. Make patient comfortable.	Handwashing deters the spread of microorganisms. Proper disposal of needle prevents the nurse accidentally puncturing self.

ing after having a bowel movement and thorough, frequent handwashing.
- Promptly report any signs of infection. These include a burning sensation and irritation at the meatus, cloudy urine, a strong odor to the urine, an elevated temperature, and chills.

- Help keep the urine acidic because acidity retards bacterial growth. As mentioned earlier, plain water in increased amounts, cranberry juice, and ascorbic acid are helpful for acidifying urine.
- Help the patient take a tub or shower bath when permitted. The catheter should be clamped

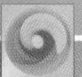

PROCEDURE 42-5

Giving a Continuous Bladder Irrigation

Equipment

Sterile irrigating solution (at room temperature or warmed to body temperature), usually 200-mL bags

Sterile tubing with drip chamber and clamp for connection to irrigating solution
IV pole
Three-way Foley catheter in place in patient's bladder

Foley drainage setup (tubing and collection bag)
Bath blanket
Disposable gloves

Action	Rationale
1. Explain the procedure and its purpose to the patient.	An explanation encourages patient cooperation and reduces apprehension.
2. Assemble the equipment.	Organization facilitates performance of tasks.
3. Wash your hands.	Handwashing deters the spread of microorganisms.
4. Provide for privacy by closing the curtains or door and draping the patient with the bath blanket.	The procedure may be embarrassing for the patient.
5. Prepare the sterile irrigation bag for use as directed by the manufacturer. Secure the clamp and attach the sterile tubing with drip chamber to the container. Hang the bag on IV pole 2½ to 3 feet above the level of the patient's bladder. Release the clamp and remove the protective cover on the end of the tubing without contaminating it. Allow the solution to flush the tubing and remove air. Reclamp.	Irrigation solution continuously bathes the lining of the bladder and keeps the catheter patent. Flushing the tubing before irrigation clears air from the tubing that might cause bladder distention.
6. Using sterile technique, attach the irrigation tubing to the irrigation port of the three-way Foley catheter. If a closed system is used, tubing may already be connected to the irrigation port on the catheter.	Sterile technique prevents the spread of microorganisms into the bladder.

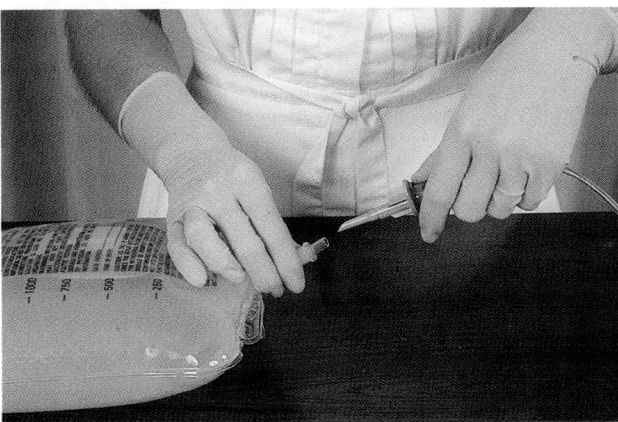

Action 5: Inserting spike into container of irrigating solution.

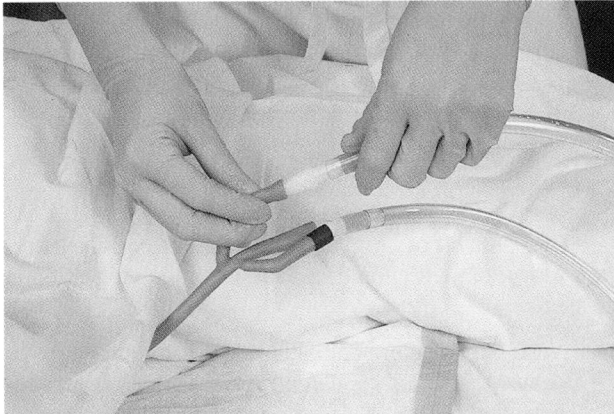

Action 6: Attaching irrigation tubing to irrigation port of three-way Foley catheter using sterile technique.

7. Release the clamp on the irrigation tubing and regulate the flow according to the physician's order.	This allows for continual gentle irrigation without causing discomfort to the patient.

(continued)

8. As irrigation is completed, clamp the tubing. Do not allow the drip chamber to empty. Disconnect the empty bag and attach a full irrigation bag. Continue as ordered by the physician.

9. Assess the patient's response to the procedure and the quality and amount of drainage. Document on the patient's chart.

10. Record the amount of irrigant used on the intake and output record. Don gloves and empty the drainage collection bag as each new container is hung and record.

11. Wash your hands.

This eliminates the need to separate tubing from the catheter and clear air from the tubing. Opening the drainage system provides access for introduction of microorganisms.

This provides accurate documentation of the procedure.

This ensures accurate recording of urine output. Gloves protect against exposure to blood, body substances, and microorganisms.

Handwashing deters the spread of microorganisms.

---

temporarily if the collecting container is higher than the bladder at any time. In a tub, with the catheter clamped, the container can be hung over the side of the tub. Care should be taken so that the catheter does not remain clamped after the bath. In a shower, the catheter can be attached to a smaller urinary drainage bag that can be secured to the patient's leg, in which case clamping the tube is usually unnecessary.

- Plan to change indwelling catheters only as necessary. If rolling the drainage tubing between the hands frees the tubing of sandy particles, it is time to change the catheter. The interval between catheter changes varies and should be individualized for the patient. The less often a catheter is changed, the lower the likelihood of an infection developing.

Removing the Indwelling Catheter

The removal of an indwelling catheter and the aftercare of the patient should include the following nursing measures:

- Wash hands before and after and wear gloves.
- *Be sure the balloon is deflated before attempting to remove the catheter.* This is done by inserting a syringe into the balloon valve and aspirating the fluid used to inflate the balloon. Always verify the size of the balloon, which is printed either on the catheter or documented in the chart, so that you know how much fluid to remove before proceeding. Do *not* cut the tubing with scissors.
- Ask the patient to take several deep breaths to relax while gently removing the catheter. Wrap

the catheter in a towel or disposable, waterproof drape.
- Clean the perineal area after the catheter is removed.
- See to it that the patient's fluid intake is generous, and record the patient's intake as well as time and amount of output for at least 24 hours or according to agency policy. Instruct the patient to void into the bedpan or urinal.
- Inform the patient that it may take a little while for the bladder to reestablish voluntary control and that an accident now is not unusual.
- Tell the patient that there may be a slight burning sensation the one or two times the patient voids after the catheter is removed.
- Observe the urine carefully for any abnormalities.
- Record and report any unusual signs, such as discomfort, a burning sensation when voiding, bleeding, or changes in vital signs, especially the patient's temperature. Be alert to any signs of infection, and report them promptly.

Clinicians are currently investigating this standard technique for catheter removal. Some believe that a totally deflated, wrinkled balloon may sometimes cause urethral trauma. A recommendation to wait 30 to 60 seconds after deflating the balloon and then to instill 0.5 to 1 mL of water into the balloon before removing it is a subject of present research. The hypothesis is that the addition of this small amount of fluid creates a smoother surface (Evans, 1999).

Teaching the Patient

Patients who have an indwelling catheter should be taught how the system functions and how they can assist with

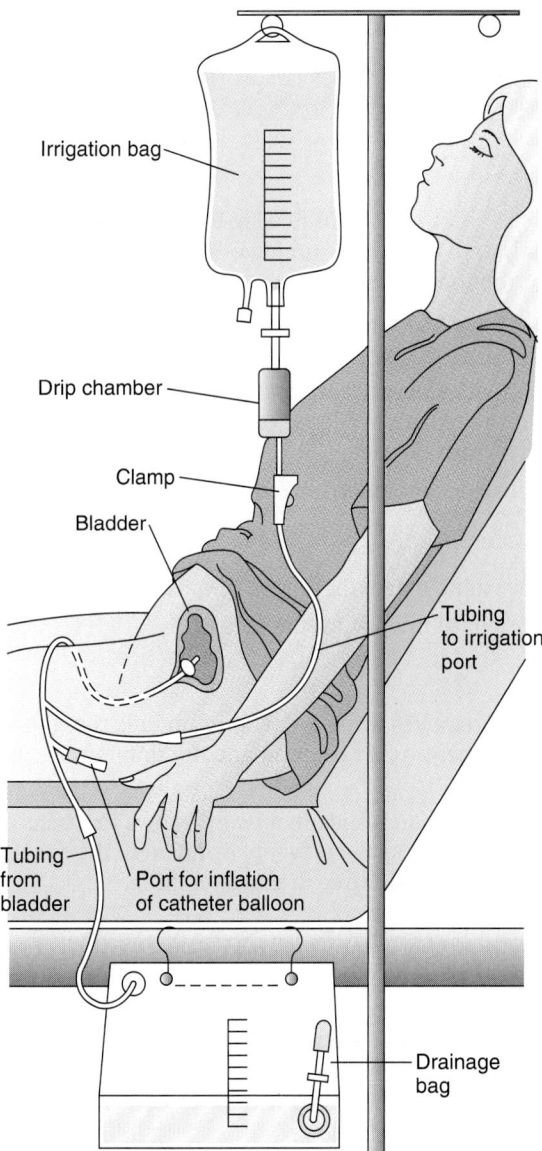

Figure 42-12
A continuous bladder irrigation (CBI) set up.

their care. Teaching points include keeping the tubing free of kinks, maintaining a constant downward flow of the urine, maintaining an adequate fluid intake, and promptly reporting any unusual symptoms.

An ambulatory patient can connect the indwelling catheter to a smaller drainage bag that can be secured to the lower leg. Instructions for patients who use this apparatus include the following:

- Empty the leg bag at regular intervals. A full drainage bag may cause reflux of urine into the bladder or may pull away from its attachment on the leg.
- Wash hands before and after emptying the leg bag. Use an antiseptic solution to cleanse the connections.

- Disinfect the leg bag at regular intervals with a chlorine solution consisting of 2 ounces bleach mixed with 5 ounces water (Evans, 1999).

Applying a Condom Catheter

When voluntary control of urination is not possible for male patients, an alternative to an indwelling catheter is the **condom catheter.** This soft, pliable device made of plastic or rubberized material is applied externally to the penis. It is connected to tubing and a leg bag during the day and a drainage bag at night and thus allows the patient to be dressed and to participate in activities without problem. Steps for applying a condom catheter are described in Procedure 42-6.

Nursing care includes vigilant skin care to prevent excoriation. The condom should be removed daily and the penis washed with soap and water, carefully dried, and inspected for irritation. The manufacturer's instructions for applying the condom should be followed because there are several variations. In all cases, care must be taken to fasten the condom securely enough to prevent leakage, yet not so tightly as to constrict the blood vessels in the area. Self-adhesive condom catheters are also available. The tip of the tubing should be kept 1 to 2 inches (2.5 to 5 cm) beyond the tip of the penis to prevent irritation to the sensitive glans. Maintaining free urinary drainage is another nursing priority, to prevent tubing from becoming kinked. To prevent urine from excoriating the glans, the tubing that collects urine from the condom should be positioned to draw urine away from the penis.

Assisting With Urinary Diversions

Obstructions or tumors in the urinary tract may require some patients to have the urinary flow diverted surgically. An **ileal conduit** is a surgical diversion of the ureters to the ileum rather than the bladder. This separated section of the small intestine is then brought to the abdominal wall, where urine is excreted through a stoma, a surgically created opening on the body surface. Figure 42-13 shows how the ureters are diverted in an ileal conduit. Such diversions are usually permanent, and the patient wears an external appliance to collect the urine because elimination of the urine from the stoma cannot be voluntarily controlled.

Patients with an ileal conduit must adapt to an altered body image and usually need assistance in coping. The time required for adaptation varies, and the adjustment can often be assisted with the support of family, friends, nurses, physicians, and people with a similar health problem. Most of all, the patient needs to understand that an active, useful life is compatible with a urinary diversion.

Another option is a *continent urostomy* (eg, the Kock continent ileal reservoir). This is a surgical alternative that creates an internal reservoir that holds urine using a sec-

PROCEDURE 42-6

Applying a Condom Catheter

Equipment

Condom sheath in appropriate size
Basin of warm water and soap
Washcloth and towel

Bath blanket
Disposable gloves (optional)
Elastic strip or Velcro strap (optional)

Reusable leg bag with drainage
tubing or urinary drainage setup

Action	Rationale
1. Explain the procedure to the patient. Ask if the patient is aware of any allergy to latex.	This provides reassurance and promotes patient cooperation. If the patient is allergic to latex, a latex-free condom catheter must be used.
2. Assemble the equipment. Prepare urinary drainage setup or reusable leg bag for attachment to the condom sheath.	This provides for an organized approach to the task.
3. Wash your hands.	Handwashing deters the spread of microorganisms.
4. Assist the patient to the supine position. Close the curtain or door. Use the bath blanket and sheet to expose only the patient's genital area.	This provides privacy for the patient.
5. Don disposable gloves. Wash the genital area with soap and water, rinse, and dry thoroughly.	Washing removes urine, secretions, and microorganisms. The penis must be clean and dry to minimize skin irritation.
6. Roll the condom sheath outward onto itself. Grasp the penis firmly with your nondominant hand. Apply the condom sheath by rolling it onto the penis with your dominant hand. Leave 2.5- to 5-cm (1 to 2-inch) space between the tip of the penis and the end of the condom sheath.	Rolling the condom sheath outward allows for easier application. The space prevents irritation to the tip of the penis and allows for free drainage of urine.
7. Apply the elastic or Velcro strap in a snug but not tight manner. Do not allow the elastic or Velcro to come in contact with the skin.	The elastic or Velcro strap should secure the condom sheath but not interfere with blood circulation to the penis.

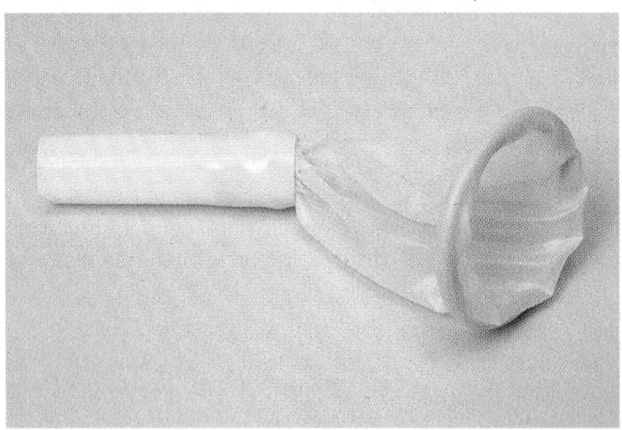

Condom sheath.

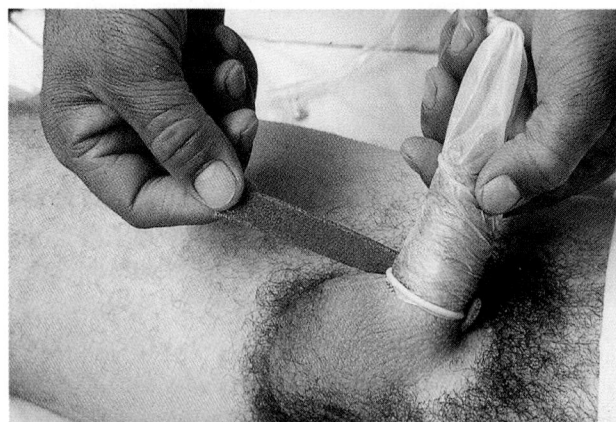

Action 7: Application of a Velcro strap at the base of the condom sheath.

(*continued*)

8. Connect the condom sheath to the drainage setup. Avoid kinking or twisting of the drainage tubing.

9. Remove the equipment. Place the patient in a comfortable, safe position. Wash your hands.

10. Assess the patient's response and record observations on the patient's chart.

The collection device keeps the patient dry. Kinked tubing encourages backflow of urine.

This provides a safe, comfortable setting for the patient. Handwashing deters the spread of microorganisms.

This provides accurate documentation and observation of urine output.

---

tion of the intestines. The external stoma or outlet must be catheterized at regular intervals to drain urine that has collected in this reservoir.

Appliances to Collect Urine

With a urinary diversion, the external appliance to collect the urine is typically a soft rubber or plastic pouch that is either reusable or disposable. The upper part of the pouch has a firm faceplate several inches in diameter that has an opening the size of the stoma. Some faceplates are detachable from the pouch. The plate surface is firmly secured around the stoma opening with a moisture-proof adherent

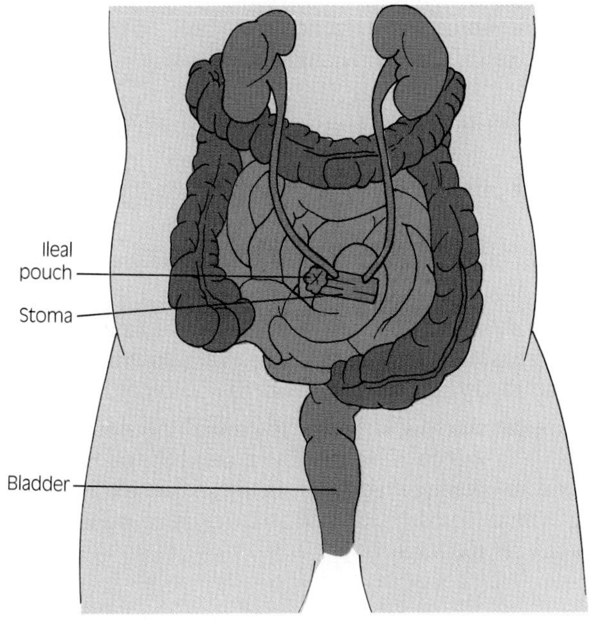

Figure 42-13
Location of an ileal conduit. The ureters are brought to the ileum of the small intestine and a stoma is made where the urine is excreted. (Redrawn after Types of Ostomies. Copyright 1979. Hollister Inc. All rights reserved.)

so that no urine leakage occurs. Many patients also wear an elasticized belt around the waist for added support. The lower end of the pouch may have a drainage valve, which is used for emptying the pouch.

The pouch should be emptied before it becomes heavy with the weight of urine and causes the seal to loosen. For most people, this means emptying the appliance several times a day. Urine-collection receptacles designed to be placed under the bed can be used at night.

Changing the Urinary Appliance

The frequency of changing the appliance depends on the type being used. The appliance should be changed after a time of low fluid intake, such as in the early morning. Urine production is less at this time, which makes changing the appliance easier. Procedure 42-7 describes how to change an appliance worn over an ileal conduit.

Teaching the Patient

Nursing care includes patient education for the achievement of optimal self-care. As the patient assumes responsibility for self-care, he or she should be taught to make the necessary observations, to be aware of indications of problems, and to recognize when to seek assistance. For these goals to be met, the patient needs to be able to do the following:

- Explain the reason for the urinary diversion and the rationale for treatment
- Demonstrate self-care behaviors that effectively manage the diversion
- Describe follow-up care and existing support resources
- Report where supplies may be obtained in the community
- Verbalize related fears and concerns
- Demonstrate a positive body image

The assistance of an enterostomal therapist can help the patient achieve these outcomes. As well, the patient

PROCEDURE 42-7

Changing a Stoma Appliance on an Ileal Conduit

Equipment

Basin with warm water, soap, towel, washcloth or cotton balls
Graduated container
Skin protectant or barrier

Sterile 2 × 2 gauze squares
Ostomy bag cut to the correct stomal size (with adhesive-backed faceplate, if available)

Ostomy belt (optional)
Adhesive cement (optional for reusable pouches)
Disposable gloves

Action	Rationale
1. Explain the procedure and encourage the patient to observe or participate if possible. Provide for privacy.	Observing or assisting with procedure encourages self-acceptance.
2. Assemble the equipment.	Organization facilitates performance of task.
3. Wash your hands and don disposable gloves.	Handwashing deters the spread of microorganisms. Gloves protect the nurse from blood, body substances, and microorganisms.
4. Have the patient sit or stand if able to assist with procedure or assume supine position in bed.	These positions result in less abdominal folds and facilitate removal and application of the device.
5. Empty the pouch being worn into the graduated container (before removing if it is reusable and not attached to straight drainage).	Having the pouch empty before handling it reduces the likelihood of spilling the excretions. The physician may have ordered recording of intake and output.
6. Gently remove the pouch faceplate from the skin.	The seal between the surface of the faceplate and the skin must be broken before the faceplate can be removed. Harsh handling of the appliance can damage the skin and impair the development of a secure seal in the future.
7. Discard the pouch appropriately if disposable, or wash reusable pouch in lukewarm soap and water and allow to air dry.	Thorough cleaning and airing of the appliance reduce odor and deterioration. For aesthetic and infection-control purposes, used appliances should be discarded appropriately.
8. Clean the skin around the stoma with soap and water or a commercial cleaner using a washcloth or cotton balls. Make sure you remove all of old adhesive from the skin.	Cleaning the skin removes excretions and old adhesive and skin protectant. Excretions or a buildup of other substances can irritate and damage the skin.
9. Gently pat dry. Make sure the skin around the stoma is thoroughly dry. Assess the stoma and the condition of the surrounding skin.	Careful drying prevents trauma to the skin and stoma. An intact, properly applied urinary collection device protects skin integrity. Any change in the color and size of the stoma may indicate circulatory problems.
10. Place a gauze square or two over the stoma opening.	Continuous drainage must be absorbed to keep the skin dry during the appliance change.
11. Apply a skin protectant to a 5-cm (2-in) radius around the stoma, and allow it to dry completely, which takes about 30 seconds.	The skin needs protection from the excoriating effect of the excretion and appliance adhesive. Allowing the protectant to dry completely enhances its effectiveness.
12. If necessary, enlarge the size of the faceplate opening to fit the stoma.	The appliance should fit snugly around the stoma, with only $\frac{1}{16}$ to $\frac{1}{8}$ inch of skin visible around the opening. A faceplate opening that is too small can cause trauma to the stoma. Exposed skin will be irritated by urine if the opening is too large.

(continued)

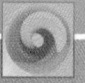

PROCEDURE 42-7

Changing a Stoma Appliance on an Ileal Conduit (Continued)

13. Apply adhesive to the faceplate or remove the protective covering from the disposable faceplate, carefully position the appliance, and press it in place, moving from the center outward. Remove the gauze squares from the stoma before applying the pouch.

The appliance is effective only if it is properly positioned and securely adhered. Commercial deodorants may be used if odor is a problem.

14. Secure the optional belt to the appliance and around the patient.

An elasticized belt helps support the appliance for some people.

15. Remove or discard the equipment and assess the patient's response to the procedure. Wash your hands and remove gloves.

The patient's response may indicate acceptance of the ostomy as well as the need for health teaching. Hand-washing deters the spread of microorganisms.

16. Record the appearance of the stoma and the surrounding skin as well as the patient's reaction to the procedure.

A careful record is important for planning the patient's care.

---

may be referred to the United Ostomy Association for further information and helpful periodicals. Detailed discussion of other aspects of caring for a patient with a urinary diversion can be found in clinical texts.

EVALUATING

The nurse evaluates the effectiveness of a plan of care to promote healthy urinary functioning by checking whether the patient has met the individualized patient goals specified in the plan. Nursing care is considered effective if the patient expresses satisfaction with the regular voiding pattern and is able to achieve the following:

- Produce a sufficient quantity of urine to maintain fluid, electrolyte, and acid–base balance
- Empty the bladder completely at regular intervals without discomfort
- Develop a plan to modify any factors that contribute to current urinary problems or that might adversely affect urinary functioning in the future
- Correct unhealthy urinary habits, such as delaying voiding, drinking insufficient fluids, or abusing diuretics

See the accompanying Applying Learning to Practice and Nursing Plan of Care boxes.

APPLYING LEARNING TO PRACTICE

Patient Care Study

Mrs. Jaspers is an alert, 83-year-old woman whose husband of 59 years died 6 months ago. Although Mrs. Jaspers was adamant about wanting to live independently in her own home, arthritis severely restricted her movement and ability to manage. After a hospitalization for pneumonia, she was transferred to a nursing home 1 month ago. The admitting medical diagnoses included hypertension, osteoarthritis, and depression. A comprehensive nursing assessment of Mrs. Jaspers performed 1 month after her admission to the nursing home included the following notations:

- Continent of urine on admission
- At present, incontinent of urine one or two times a day; often found wet in the morning; states it is "too much bother to get into the bathroom"
- Sits in chair in room unless encouraged and assisted to walk, although capable of independent ambulation with care; progressive muscle atrophy and joint stiffness
- No identifiable pathology underlying incontinence
- Medications include a diuretic for hypertension and a tricyclic antidepressant
- Reddened skin in the perineal area

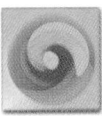

NURSING PLAN OF CARE
for Mrs. Jaspers

Nursing Diagnosis

Functional Urinary Incontinence related to difficult transition to nursing home and mobility deficit as manifested by incontinence of urine one or two times a day; feeling toileting is too much bother; mobility deficits secondary to osteoarthritis; taking a diuretic and antidepressant.

Expected Outcome

By the next monthly assessment, 5/1/01, the patient will:
* Verbalize the importance of getting to bathroom or toilet when she first feels the need to void.

Nursing Interventions	Rationale	Evaluative Statement
Assess the value the patient attaches to voluntary control of urination and urinary continence; counsel appropriately.	Unless the patient is committed to the plan of care, goal achievement is impossible.	5/1/01 Goal partially met. Patient has commented on the importance of regular toileting but still finds this "too much trouble" some days.
Teach the importance of complete bladder emptying at regular intervals and the harmful effects of ignoring the urge to void.	Patient understanding of the causes and harmful effects of urinary incontinence may motivate desire for reestablishment of voluntary control.	*Revision:* Reinforce value. *D. Mora, RN*
Assess patient's normal voiding habits at home and assist her to reestablish these. Initial reminders to toilet herself may be necessary.	Respect for the patient's normal voiding schedule and patterns communicates nursing's sincere concern for the individual and encourages patient achievement of goals.	

Expected Outcome

By the next monthly assessment, 5/1/01, the patient will:
* Demonstrate the ability to walk independently to the bathroom (using cane) to toilet herself.

Nursing Interventions	Rationale	Evaluative Statement
Assess the patient's ability to toilet herself independently. Work consistently with her to increase activity tolerance: encourage short walks throughout the day to increase mobility.	One response to experiencing the multiple losses associated with aging is to surrender all control and become increasingly dependent. Non–pathology-based incontinence is less likely to occur if the daily living of the person keeps her more mobile, flexible, oriented, and motivated. An older person who seeks to take control and has a positive self-image is more continent.	5/1/01 Goal met. Patient can safely walk to bathroom using cane and toilet herself when she wants to. *D. Mora, RN*
Refer patient to occupational therapy for assistance with diagnosis and treatment if necessary.		
Communicate clearly that the patient is expected to use the toilet to urinate. Refrain from using incontinent briefs or pads. Talk with family about patient's having sufficient undergarments to allow changes as needed until control is reestablished.	The specialized skills of the occupational therapist may facilitate relearning toileting skills. Understanding that the staff *expects* continence and is committed to working with the patient to achieve it is a powerful patient motivator.	

(continued)

NURSING PLAN OF CARE (Continued)
for Mrs. Jaspers

Nursing Interventions	Rationale	Evaluative Statement
Assess patient's motivation and ability to be clean, dry, and comfortable.	Patient may not understand how easily skin irritation can occur and danger of pressure ulcers.	5/1/01 Goal not met. Patient repeatedly neglects AM perineal care.
Teach perineal hygiene.	Keeping the perineal area clean and dry promotes intact skin around the urinary meatus and the perineal area. Proper hygiene measures also decrease the possibility of bacteria or organisms migrating into the bladder.	*Revision:* Reteach both the importance and procedure of perineal care. Assess each AM. *D. Mora, RN*

Expected Outcome	By the next monthly assessment, 5/1/01, the patient will: • Decrease urinary incontinent episodes to less than three or four per week

Nursing Interventions	Rationale	Evaluative Statement
Communicate to patient that the nurses *care* about her reestablishing urinary continence and believe she can do this. Use verbal reinforcement to reward "dry" days.	A common feeling of recently institutionalized elderly people is *abandonment* and the sense that no one cares; response: "Why should I?" Communicating that the patient's progress toward goal achievement is valued by the nurses is an excellent encouragement to continue progress.	5/1/01 Goal met. Patient in last week was completely dry for 4 of 7 days. Recorded four incontinent episodes. *D. Mora, RN*
Chart incontinent episodes and monitor progress; discuss this with patient.	This records progress with incontinent episodes and provides positive reinforcement.	

Nursing Diagnosis	Impaired Skin Integrity related to functional urinary incontinence as manifested by reddened perineal area (skin still intact)
Expected Outcome	By the next monthly assessment, 5/1/01, the patient will: • Demonstrate healing of reddened perineal area

Nursing Interventions	Rationale	Evaluative Statement
Assess skin for breakdown each AM and PM and after each incontinent episode.	Perineal care is often neglected or assigned to the least trained personnel in care settings. Skin irritation not detected and treated early may progress to serious pressure ulcers.	5/1/01 Goal partially met. Perineal area is less inflamed. *Revision:* Continue to monitor perineal hygiene. No need for protective ointment. *D. Mora, RN*
Teach the patient the importance of washing this area carefully with soap and water each AM and after incontinent episodes. Teach the importance of always cleaning and wiping the perineum from front to back to prevent autoinfection. Until incontinent episodes are eliminated, a protective waterproof ointment may be indicated.	The woman who is doing self-care may neglect it entirely or use incorrect technique.	

(continued)

NURSING PLAN OF CARE (Continued)
for Mrs. Jaspers

Nursing Interventions	Rationale	Evaluative Statement
Cotton underwear should be worn. Nylon pantyhose, girdles, tight-fitting pants should be avoided.	Nylon products tend to hold moisture and may minimize airflow to the perineal area.	

Sample Documentation

4/3/01   Nursing

This AM, after an incontinent episode, Mrs. Jaspers began to talk about how hard it is to get adjusted to living here, and commented, "I feel like just giving up." We talked about the importance of being as independent as possible and the dangers of becoming passively dependent. Nursing teaching and counseling included values of independently adhering to usual toileting schedule and importance of perineal hygiene. Two hours later, after lunch, Mrs. Jaspers walked to bathroom and toileted herself. Progress with urinary incontinence will continue to be monitored. Ability definitely present but encouragement needed.

D. Mora, RN

Learning Outcomes

After completing this chapter, the learner should be able to accomplish the following:

1. Define the key terms used in the chapter.

condom catheter	mixed incontinence
enuresis	nocturia
frequency	oliguria
functional incontinence	overflow incontinence
hematuria	postvoid residual (PVR)
hesitancy	stress incontinence
ileal conduit	suprapubic catheter
indwelling urethral catheter	urge incontinence
	urgency
Kegel exercises	urinary incontinence
micturition	urinary retention

2. Describe the physiology of the urinary system.
3. Identify variables that influence urination.
4. Assess urinary elimination, using appropriate interview questions and physical assessment skills.
5. Perform the following assessment measures: measure urine output, collect urine specimens, determine the presence of select abnormal urine constituents, determine urine specific gravity, and assist with diagnostic tests and procedures.
6. Develop nursing diagnoses that correctly identify urinary problems amenable to nursing therapy.
7. Demonstrate how to promote normal urination; facilitate use of the toilet, bedpan, urinal, and commode; perform catheterizations; and assist with urinary diversions.
8. Describe nursing interventions that can be used to manage urinary incontinence effectively.
9. Describe nursing interventions that can prevent the development of urinary tract infections.
10. Plan, implement, and evaluate nursing care related to selected nursing diagnoses associated with urinary problems.

Critical Thinking Exercises

1. The daughter of an older patient who is about to be discharged to the daughter's home requests that a catheter be inserted in her mother to make home care easier. The mother knows when she needs to void but needs assistance to get into the bathroom. How do you respond to the daughter's request?
2. If you noted the following when assessing a patient, what would you do?
   - A 6-year-old refuses to give a urine sample.
   - Frank blood appears in urine of a patient who has no history of urinary problems.
   - When you ask for a urine sample, a teenager asks, "This won't reveal drugs, will it?"
   - A young woman complains of painful urination with burning.
   - An older man reports frequency and pain when voiding.

Study Questions

1. The nurse collects a urine specimen for routine urinalysis from a patient. She is aware that
   a. a sterile specimen is required
   b. standing at room temperature for a prolonged period may alter the urine chemistry
   c. the external meatus should be cleaned with antiseptic soap and water before voiding
   d. a clean-catch midstream specimen is required

2. Which statement would be correct to teach the patient in regard to healthy urinary functioning?
   a. Drinking more than 2000 mL of fluid per day will cause fluid retention.
   b. The healthy adult should drink four to six 8-ounce glasses of water per day.
   c. Because of greater thirst sensitivity, children will drink required amounts of fluid without being reminded.
   d. Caffeine-containing beverages should be monitored to prevent excess intake.

3. When a person has a fever or diaphoresis, the urine output will be which of the following?
   a. decreased and highly concentrated
   b. decreased and highly dilute
   c. increased and concentrated
   d. increased and dilute

4. The physician has ordered an indwelling catheter inserted in a hospitalized male patient. The nurse is aware that
   a. the male urethra is more vulnerable to injury during insertion
   b. normally a clean technique is required
   c. the catheter is inserted 2 to 3 inches into the meatus
   d. smaller catheters are usually necessary because of the size of the urethra

5. Nursing care for a patient with an indwelling catheter includes
   a. irrigation of the catheter with 30 mL of normal saline solution every 4 hours
   b. disconnecting and reconnecting the drainage system quickly to obtain a urine specimen
   c. encouraging a generous fluid intake if permitted
   d. informing the patient that burning and irritation at the meatus are normal and should subside within a few days

6. After surgery, Ms. Young is having difficulty voiding. Which nursing action will cause increased difficulty with voiding rather than stimulation of voiding?
   a. pouring warm water over Ms. Young's fingers
   b. having Ms. Young ignore the urge to void until her bladder is full
   c. using a warm bedpan when Ms. Young feels the urge to void
   d. stroking Ms. Young's leg or thigh

7. Mr. Cheng is hospitalized and has developed a urinary tract infection. He is 80 years old, has an indwelling catheter in place, and has diabetes mellitus. Which factor is most likely the cause of his UTI?
   a. the close proximity of the male genitalia to the rectum
   b. decreased immunity
   c. a high urine glucose level
   d. the indwelling urinary catheter

8. The inability to void although the kidneys are producing urine and it enters the bladder is known as
   a. urgency
   b. retention
   c. oliguria
   d. dysuria

9. Mrs. D'Ambrosia, an alert, ambulatory, older nursing home resident, voids frequently and has difficulty making it to the bathroom on time. As the nurse plans her care, she is aware that
   a. incontinence is to be expected in a woman Mrs. D'Ambrosia's age
   b. 1 of every 10 nursing home residents is incontinent
   c. Kegel exercises at regular intervals throughout the day may be helpful
   d. an indwelling catheter should be inserted as soon as possible

10. The priority treatment option for Mrs. D'Ambrosia would most likely involve
    a. behavioral techniques
    b. pharmacologic measures
    c. surgical intervention
    d. use of absorbent products

11. A patient taking Pyridium (a urinary tract analgesic) should be cautioned that her urine color may change to
    a. pale yellow
    b. green
    c. orange-red
    d. brown

12. Mr. Bales is 60 years old and alert. He is timid and reluctant to talk about his urinary retention problem. Which part of this plan could create stress for Mr. Bales and possibly increase his inability to urinate?
    a. assisting him in assuming his normal voiding position
    b. pulling curtains around him to provide privacy during voiding
    c. staying with him while voiding
    d. offering the urinal on a regular schedule

13. Which of the following is a nursing priority when caring for a male patient with a condom catheter?
    a. preventing the tubing from kinking to maintain free urinary drainage
    b. not removing the catheter for any reason
    c. fastening the condom securely to prevent the possibility of leakage

d. maintaining bed rest at all times to prevent the catheter from slipping off

14. If you read the nursing diagnosis, Altered Urinary Elimination related to maturational enuresis, you would recognize that your patient is which of the following?
    a. an adult older than 65 years of age who is incontinent
    b. a child older than 4 years of age who has involuntary urination
    c. a 12-month-old child who has involuntary urination

d. a patient with neurologic damage resulting in bladder dysfunction

15. Data must be collected to evaluate the effectiveness of a plan to reduce urinary incontinence in an older adult patient. Of the data below, which is least necessary for the evaluation process?
    a. the incontinence pattern
    b. state of physical mobility
    c. medications being taken
    d. age of the patient

Answers With Rationale

1. The correct response is *b.* For a routine urinalysis, a clean specimen is adequate. The external meatus does not need to be cleaned with an antiseptic, as is required for a clean-catch midstream specimen.

2. The correct response is *d.* Caffeine intake should be limited because it is irritating to the bladder mucosa. It is recommended that a healthy adult drink 8 to 10 8-ounce glasses of fluid daily. Unless a disease process is present, this will not cause fluid retention. Children frequently need to be reminded to drink fluids.

3. The correct response is *a.* Fever and diaphoresis cause the kidneys to conserve body fluids. Thus, the urine is concentrated and decreased in amount.

4. The correct response is *a.* Because of its length, the male urethra is more prone to injury and requires that the catheter be inserted 6 to 8 inches or until urine flows. This procedure requires surgical asepsis to prevent introducing bacteria into the urinary tract. Larger catheters are used for male catheterization.

5. The correct response is *c.* A generous fluid intake promotes healthy urinary tract functioning. Irrigation may introduce bacteria into the urinary tract and is not routinely ordered. The drainage system should never be disconnected to obtain a specimen because this may provide the opportunity for bacteria to enter the urinary tract. Burning and irritation may indicate that an infection is present and should never be disregarded.

6. The correct response is *b.* Ignoring the urge to void makes urination even more difficult and should be avoided. The other activities are all recommended nursing activities to promote voiding.

7. The correct response is *d.* Most UTIs in hospitalized patients are caused by the presence of an indwelling catheter. Additional, although less significant, causes of UTI include a decrease in immunity common in elderly people and the presence of glucose in the urine, as seen with diabetes.

8. The correct response is *b.* Urgency is a strong desire to void. Oliguria is scanty or greatly diminished amount of urine voided in a given time. Dysuria is difficulty urinating.

9. The correct response is *c.* Kegel exercises may help a patient regain better control of the micturition process. Incontinence is not a normal consequence of aging, and at least half of nursing home residents may be incontinent. An indwelling catheter is the last choice of treatment.

10. The correct response is *a.* The least invasive interventions should be attempted first. Pharmacologic and surgical interventions are not recommended until behavioral techniques have been attempted. Using absorbent products may remove motivation from the patient and caregiver to seek evaluation and treatment of the incontinence. They should be used only after careful evaluation by a healthcare provider.

11. The correct response is *c.* Pyridium is noted for turning the urine orange-red, and the patient needs to be aware of this.

12. The correct response is *c.* Mr. Bales will be embarrassed if the nurse remains with him as he attempts to void and is more likely to have difficulty voiding.

13. The correct response is *a.* The catheter should be removed daily to prevent skin excoriation and should not be fastened too tightly, or restriction of blood vessels in the area is likely. Confining a patient to bed rest increases the risk for other hazards related to immobility.

14. The correct response is *b.* Maturational enuresis is involuntary urination after an age when continence should be present. A 12-month-old child is not expected to be continent, and incontinence and neurologic damage are not maturational problems.

15. The correct response is *d.* Incontinence is not a natural consequence of the aging process. All the other factors are necessary information for the plan of care.

Bibliography

Agency for Health Care Policy and Research, Public Health Service, Urinary Incontinence Guideline Panel (1996). *Urinary incontinence in adults: Acute and chronic management.* Clinical Practice Guideline No. 2, 1996 update. AHCPR Pub. No. 96-0684. Rockville, MD: U. S. Department of Health and Human Services.

Bradway, C., Hernly, S., & the NICHE faculty. (1998). Urinary incontinence in older adults admitted to acute care. *Geriatric Nursing, 19*(2), 98–101.

Evans, E. (1999). Indwelling catheter care: Dispelling the misconceptions. *Geriatric Nursing, 20*(2), 85–88.

Fischbach, F. (1996). *A manual of laboratory and diagnostic tests* (5th ed.). Philadelphia: Lippincott-Raven.

Gerard, L., & Sueppel, C. (1997). Lubrication technique for male catheterization. *Urologic Nursing, 17*(4), 156–158.

Gray, M. (2000). Urinary retention: Management in the acute care setting. *American Journal of Nursing, 100*(7), 40–47.

Haus, E. (1998). Urinary tract infections in the homebound elderly. *Home Healthcare Nurse, 16*(5), 323–327.

Jackson, B., & Hicks, L. (1997). Effect of cranberry juice on urinary pH in older adults. *Home Healthcare Nurse, 15*(3), 199–202.

Jirovec, M., Wyman, J., & Wells, T. (1998). Addressing urinary incontinence with educational continence-care competencies. *Image—The Journal of Nursing Scholarship, 30*(4), 375–378.

Johnson, S. (2000). From incontinence to confidence. *American Journal of Nursing, 100*(2), 69–75.

Kirton, C. (1997). Assessing for bladder distension. *Nursing, 27*(4), 64.

Loughrey, L. (1999). Taking a sensitive approach to urinary incontinence. *Nursing, 29*(5), 60–61.

Luft, J., & Vriheas-Nichols, A. (1998). Identifying the risk factors for developing incontinence: Can we modify individual risk? *Geriatric Nursing, 19*(2), 66–70.

Lyons, S., & Specht, J. (2000). Prompted voiding protocol for individuals with urinary incontinence. *Journal of Gerontological Nursing, 26*(6), 5–13.

Marchiondo, K. (1998). A new look at urinary tract infection. *American Journal of Nursing, 98*(3), 34–39.

McCloskey, J., & Bulechek, J. (1996). *Nursing interventions classification (NIC)* (2nd ed.). St. Louis: C. V. Mosby.

McConnell, E. (1997). Maintaining a closed urinary drainage system. *Nursing, 27*(10), 22.

North American Nursing Diagnosis Association. (1999). *NANDA nursing diagnoses: Definitions & classification, 1999–2000.* Philadelphia: Author.

Phipps, W., Sands, J., & Marek, J. (1999). *Medical-surgical nursing: Concepts & clinical practice* (6th ed.). St. Louis: C. V. Mosby.

Sasso, K. (1998). New treatment options for stress incontinence. *RN, 61*(9), 36–39.

Scura, K., & Whipple, B. (1997). How to provide better care for the postmenopausal woman. *American Journal of Nursing, 97*(4), 36–43.

Sienty, M., & Dawson, N. (1999). Preventing urosepsis from indwelling urinary catheters. *American Journal of Nursing, 99*(1), 24C–24H.

Smeltzer, S., & Bare, B. (2000). *Brunner & Suddarth's textbook of medical-surgical nursing* (9th ed.). Philadelphia: Lippincott Williams & Wilkins.

Smith, D. (1999). Gauging bladder volume. *Nursing, 29*(12), 52–53.

Stockert, P. (1999). Getting UTI patients back on track. *RN, 62*(3), 49–52.

Weber, E., McDowell, J., Engberg, S., Brodak, I., & Donovan, N. (1998). Protocol for indwelling bladder catheter removal in the homebound older adult. *Home Healthcare Nurse, 16*(9), 603–609.

Chapter 43
Bowel Elimination

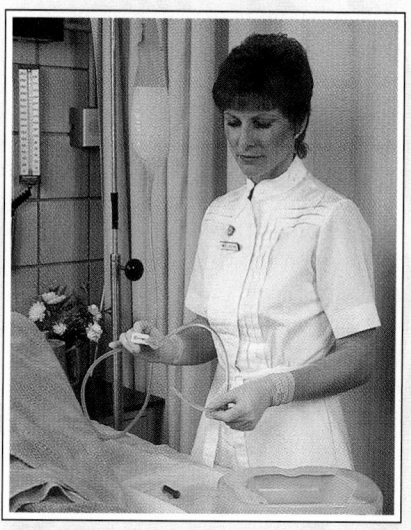

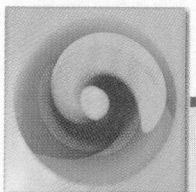

Thinking Critically About
Nursing's Blended Skills

Before reading this chapter, think about the types of skills you will need to care for patients with bowel elimination problems.

- Baby boy Seth has had no stool recorded since his birth 30 hours ago. When you reexamine Seth, you realize he has no anus and that this was not detected in the newborn physical.

- Sally, a college junior with Crohn's disease, has frequent episodes of diarrhea. "It's so embarrassing. Sometimes, I don't make it fast enough to the bathroom. If I have one more accident in a public place, I think I'll die. Somedays, I think I should never go out in public again."

- Mr. Cobbs, newly diagnosed with cancer, was taking Tylenol with codeine for pain. He said no one warned him about constipation or told him how to prevent it. He became so impacted that he had to be hospitalized. This is day seven of his hospitalization, and he is still not moving his bowels normally. He tells you, "I didn't know anything could hurt so bad. I'll take my chances with the cancer pain in the future, rather than take more pain meds and have this happen again."

- Mrs. Fisher reports during her health history that she frequently notices blood when she wipes herself after a bowel movement. "It's just hemorrhoids, right? Nothing to worry about?"

What cognitive, technical, interpersonal, and ethical/legal skills do you think you will need to meet effectively the needs of the patients described above?

limination of the waste products of digestion is a natural process critical for human functioning. Patients differ widely in their expectations about bowel elimination, their usual pattern of defecation, and the ease with which they speak of bowel problems. Although most people have experienced minor acute bouts of diarrhea or constipation, some patients experience severe or chronic bowel elimination alterations that affect their fluid and electrolyte balance, hydration, nutritional status, skin integrity, comfort, and self-concept. Because many patients experience illnesses that affect bowel elimination or are undergoing diagnostic testing and pharmacologic or surgical treatments that affect functioning, nurses need to be knowledgeable for both preventing and treating bowel problems.

This chapter discusses the physiology of bowel elimination and the multiple factors that influence this process. A practical guide for assessing bowel elimination is presented that includes a description of nursing responsibilities related to diagnostic studies of the gastrointestinal tract. Numerous examples of nursing diagnoses are included.

The chapter describes goals for both the nurse and the patient and nursing strategies to meet those goals. The concluding patient care study illustrates how the nurse uses specific nursing interventions and caring to resolve bowel elimination problems successfully.

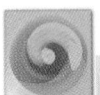 Anatomy and Physiology

The anatomy of the gastrointestinal tract is shown in Figure 43-1.

Large Intestine

The large intestine, the primary organ of bowel elimination, is the lower, or distal, part of the alimentary tract. It extends from the ileocecal valve to the anus. Waste products of digestion, called **chyme**, move from the small intestine to the large intestine. About 1500 mL of chyme is processed daily by the large intestine, and most is absorbed in the proximal portion of the colon, except for about 100 mL of fluid that is eliminated in the feces. Functions of the large intestine include the completion of absorption, the manufacture of certain vitamins, the formation of feces, and the expulsion of feces from the body.

The large intestine in adults is about 1.5 m long (about 59 inches), but variations in length are normal. The width of the colon varies. At its narrowest point, the colon is about 2.5 cm (1 inch) wide; at its widest point, it is about 7.5 cm (3 inches). Its diameter decreases from the cecum to the anus.

The connection between the ileum of the small intestine and the large intestine is the ileocecal, or ileocolic, valve. This valve normally prevents contents from entering the large intestine prematurely and prevents waste products from returning to the small intestine.

Waste contents pass through the ileocecal valve and enter the cecum, the first part of the large intestine. It is situated on the right side of the body, and to it is attached the vermiform process, or appendix. When waste products enter the large intestine, the contents are liquid or watery. While passing through the large intestine, most water is absorbed. About 800 to 1000 mL of liquid is absorbed daily by the intestinal tract, allowing for the formed, semisolid consistency of the normal stool. When

COGNITIVE SKILLS

- Knowledge of the anatomy and physiology of bowel elimination and variables that influence bowel elimination

- Knowledge of how to promote regular bowel habits; use cathartics, laxatives, and antidiarrheals; empty the colon of feces; design and implement bowel training programs; and use comfort measures to ease defecation

- Knowledge of how to use the nursing process to identify and care for patients with diagnoses associated with bowel problems

TECHNICAL SKILLS

- Ability to use the equipment and protocols necessary to diagnose and treat bowel problems

INTERPERSONAL SKILLS

- Strong people skills to establish trusting relationships with each of these patients

- Special interpersonal competence to help Sally, Mr. Cobbs, and Mrs. Fisher to initiate new self-care behaviors

ETHICAL/LEGAL SKILLS

- First and foremost, a strong sense of accountability for the health and well-being of these individuals; a commitment to getting them the help they need to achieve their health goals—within the scope of your nursing responsibilities and available resources

- A willingness to hold colleagues accountable for safe and good-quality practice

- Knowledge of your legal responsibilities within the scope of your nursing responsibilities

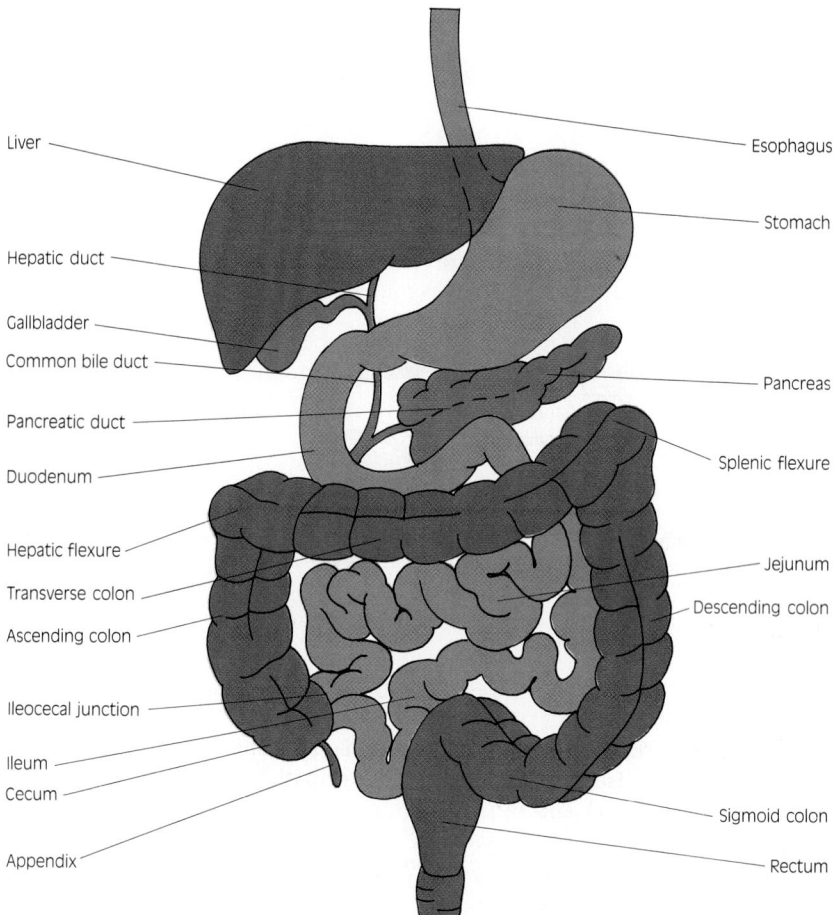

Figure 43-1
Organs of the gastrointestinal system.

Labels (top to bottom, left side): Liver, Hepatic duct, Gallbladder, Common bile duct, Pancreatic duct, Duodenum, Hepatic flexure, Transverse colon, Ascending colon, Ileocecal junction, Ileum, Cecum, Appendix

Labels (right side): Esophagus, Stomach, Pancreas, Splenic flexure, Jejunum, Descending colon, Sigmoid colon, Rectum

absorption does not occur properly, such as when the waste products pass through the large intestine at a rapid rate, the stool is soft and watery. If the stool remains in the colon too long, or if too much water is absorbed, the stool becomes dry and hard.

From the cecum, the digestive contents enter the colon, which has several segments. The ascending colon extends from the cecum upward toward the liver, where it turns to cross the abdomen. This turn is called the hepatic flexure. The transverse colon crosses the abdomen from right to left. The turn from the transverse colon to the descending colon is called the splenic flexure. The descending colon passes down the left side of the body, from the splenic flexure to the sigmoid, or pelvic, colon. When the waste products reach the distal end of the colon, they are called **feces**, and when excreted, feces are called **stool**.

The sigmoid colon contains feces ready for excretion and empties into the rectum, the last part of the large intestine. The rectum is about 12 cm (about 5 inches) long, 2.5 cm (1 inch) of which is the anal canal. Three transverse folds of tissue are normally present in the rectum. These folds may help to hold the fecal material in the rectum temporarily. There are also vertical folds, each of which contains an artery and a vein. Abnormally distended veins in this area are called **hemorrhoids**.

The rectum is empty except immediately before and during defecation. Feces are excreted from the rectum through the anal canal and the anus, which is about 1 to 1.5 inches (2.5 to 3.8 cm) long.

The muscles of the colon are innervated by the autonomic nervous system. The parasympathetic system stimulates movement, and the sympathetic system inhibits movement. Contractions of the circular and longitudinal muscles of the intestine (**peristalsis**) occur every 3 to 12 minutes to move waste products continually along the length of the intestine (Fig. 43-2). Mass peristaltic sweeps occur one to four times each 24-hour period in most people, propelling the fecal mass forward. This movement is different from the frequent peristaltic rushes that occur in the small intestine. Mass peristalsis often occurs after food has been ingested, accounting for the urge to defecate that often occurs after meals. Timing nursing interventions to evacuate bowel contents with this natural urge to defecate is helpful. One third to one half of ingested food waste is normally excreted in the stool within 24 hours, and the remainder within the next 24 to 48 hours.

Anal Canal and Anus

The internal sphincter in the anal canal and the external sphincter at the anus control the discharge of feces and intestinal gas, or **flatus**. The internal sphincter consists of involuntary smooth muscle tissue. The innervation of the

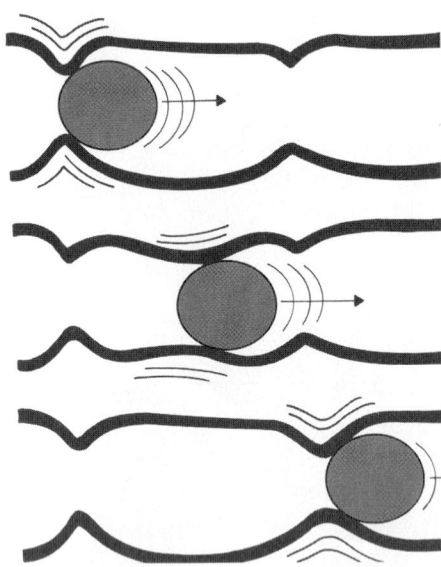

Figure 43-2
Peristaltic movements in the intestine.

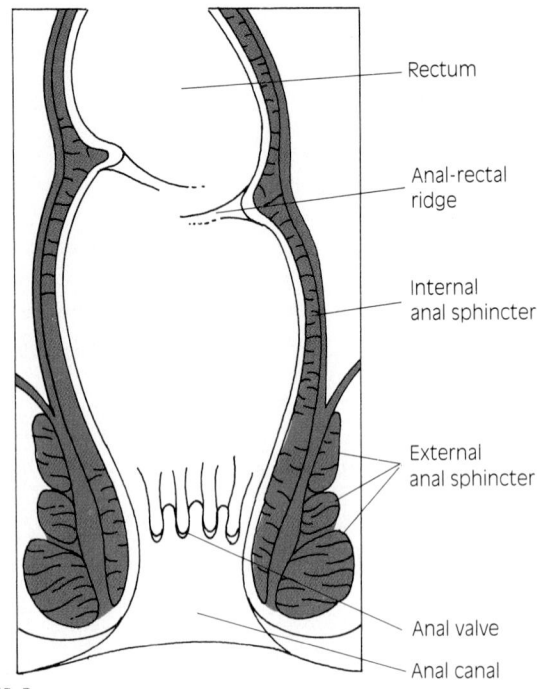

Figure 43-3
Interior view of the rectum and anal canal.

internal sphincter occurs through the autonomic nervous system. Motor impulses are carried by the sympathetic system (thoracolumbar) and inhibitory impulses by the parasympathetic system (craniosacral). These two divisions of the autonomic nervous system function antagonistically in a dynamic equilibrium.

The external sphincter at the anus has striated muscle tissue and is under voluntary control. The levator ani muscle reinforces the action of the external sphincter and is controlled voluntarily. Interference with the normal functioning of elimination from the intestines can occur in health as during illness. Elimination can be affected by the amount and quality of fluid or food intake, the level of activity, and emotional states.

Figure 43-3 shows these structures.

Act of Defecation

Defecation, often called a **bowel movement**, is the emptying of the large intestine. Two centers govern the reflex to defecate, one in the medulla and a subsidiary one in the spinal cord. When parasympathetic stimulation occurs, the internal anal sphincter relaxes, and the colon contracts. The defecation reflex is stimulated chiefly by the fecal mass in the rectum. When the rectum is distended, the intrarectal pressure rises, the defecation reflex is stimulated by the muscle stretch, and the urge to eliminate occurs. The external anal sphincter is constricted or relaxed at will. If the urge to defecate is ignored, defecation often can be delayed voluntarily.

During the act of defecation, several additional muscles aid the process. Voluntary contraction of the muscles of the abdominal wall, fixing of the diaphragm, and closing of the glottis increase intraabdominal pressure up to four or five times the normal pressure, aiding in expelling feces. This technique, termed the **Valsalva maneuver**, may be contraindicated in people with cardiovascular problems and other illnesses. When an individual bears down to defecate, the increased pressures in the abdominal and thoracic cavities result in a decreased blood flow to the atria and ventricles, thus temporarily lowering cardiac output. Once bearing down ceases, the pressure is lessened, and a larger than normal amount of blood returns to the heart and may dangerously elevate blood pressure in an already hypertensive individual (Smeltzer & Bare, 2000). Simultaneously, the muscles on the pelvic floor contract and aid in expulsion of the fecal mass.

Defecation is eased by flexing the thigh muscles, which increases abdominal pressure, and by the sitting position, which increases downward pressure on the rectum.

The act of defecation is usually painless. If the bowels move at regular intervals and the stools are formed and soft, functional problems of frequency of elimination seldom occur. Nurses find that many people show concern if they do not have a daily bowel movement, but a normal frequency of bowel movements cannot be stated arbitrarily. Although many adults pass one stool each day, other healthy people have more frequent or less frequent bowel movements. Some people have a bowel movement two or three times a week; others, two or three times a day.

◉ Factors Affecting Bowel Elimination

Developmental Considerations

Age affects what a person eats and the body's ability to digest nutrients and eliminate wastes. There is a marked difference between the stools of an infant and those of an older person. Because patients are often reluctant to discuss their bowel habits and stool characteristics, nurses need to be familiar with bowel concerns pertinent to each developmental group.

Infant

The stool characteristics depend on whether the infant is being fed breast milk or formula. Breastfed babies have more frequent, yellow to golden stools of salvelike consistency. With formula or cow's milk feedings, the stools vary from yellow to brown, are firmer, and have a stronger fecal odor because of the decomposition of protein. Both stools may have curds and mucus. Infants have no voluntary control over bowel elimination.

The number of stools infants pass varies greatly. It can vary from two to four stools daily (breastfed infant) or one to two daily (bottle-fed infant) to one stool daily at 1 year of age. Parents may mistake the infant's liquid stool for diarrhea. Loose stools may be related to overfeeding or too much corn syrup in formula. True diarrhea, however, requires evaluation. If constipation occurs, dietary manipulation is the initial treatment, and consistent use of suppositories and laxatives should be discouraged. Infants with persistent constipation should be evaluated for structural defects.

Toddler

Between the ages of 18 and 24 months, the nerve fibers innervating the anal sphincter become fully developed, and voluntary control of defecation becomes possible. Voluntary defecation requires intact muscular, sensory, and nervous structures. Successful bowel training includes an awareness by the toddler of the need to defecate, the ability to communicate this need, the wish to please the significant person involved in bowel training, and praise and reinforcement for the toddler's successful behavior. Daytime bowel control is normally attained by 30 months.

Parents need to understand that physiologic maturity is the first priority for successful bowel training. A child should never be punished or shamed for elimination accidents or for a lack of readiness to become toilet-trained. As well, toddlers who are toilet-trained often regress when hospitalized and experience soiling. Scolding or acting disgusted only reinforces this behavior, and the only constructive approach is to seek out the underlying cause.

Child, Adolescent, and Adult

From childhood into adulthood, defecation patterns vary in quantity, frequency, and rhythmicity. Many people at these ages may not understand the significance of changes in bowel habits or may worry needlessly about normal stool characteristics or bowel habits. It is important to emphasize that use of over-the-counter laxatives and enemas can have serious consequences and that any problems prompting such use need to be evaluated.

Older Adult

Constipation is often a chronic problem for older adults. Diarrhea, fecal impaction, or fecal incontinence can also result from physiologic or lifestyle changes (see the accompanying box for factors related to bowel elimination problems in older adults). *metamucil - better lax b/c veg based*
mineral oil - worst - coats large int &↓
absorb'd manufacture Vit E, C, D, K

Daily Patterns

Most people have individual regular patterns of bowel elimination involving frequency, timing considerations, position, and place. Changes in any of these may upset a person's routine and lead to constipation. For example, many people defecate after breakfast, when the gastrocolic and duodenocolic reflexes cause mass propulsive movements in the large intestine. If this urge to defecate is ignored because the person finds the time inconvenient, the feces remain in the rectum until the defecation reflex is again initiated. Meanwhile, water continues to be absorbed from the unexpelled feces, which makes stool dry, hard, and painful to pass.

The position most people assume for defecation is squatting or sitting slightly forward with the thighs flexed. In this position, increased pressure is placed on the abdomen as well as downward pressure on the rectum; both facilitate defecation. It is difficult to obtain the same results when seated on a bedpan, and embarrassment may further inhibit defecation.

For many people, defecation is a private affair experienced easily only in the comfort of one's own bathroom. Defecation in a shared hospital room with only a curtain separating one from a roommate or other people may be difficult.

Food and Fluid *20-30ccs per Kg of body weight*

Both the type and the amount of foods eaten and the amount of fluids ingested affect elimination. Healthy elimination is facilitated by a high-fiber diet and a daily fluid intake of 2000 to 3000 mL. High-fiber foods increase the bulk in fecal material. Bulkier feces place more pressure on the intestinal wall, which serves as a stimulus for peristalsis, moving the feces more quickly. When fecal material moves quickly through the intestine, there is less time for water to be reabsorbed, and the resultant stool is soft and easily passed. There is also less time for toxins to be absorbed from feces by the colon. Many believe that such toxins play an important role in colon cancer.

People digest and tolerate different foods differently. This variation is determined in part by one's culture. When traveling to a different country, eating native foods may result in severe indigestion and elimination problems; differences in water may also affect elimination when traveling.

Focus on the Older Adult

Older adults frequently experience problems with bowel elimination. These can be due to a variety of causes and can have serious implications for the elderly patient.

Bowel Elimination Problem	Related Factors and Implications
• Chronic constipation	Can be caused by: Decreased gastrointestinal motility Effect of medications (eg, antacids, opioids, antihypertensives) Decreased fluid intake Less active lifestyle Inadequate fiber intake Incomplete emptying of the bowel Can lead to laxative abuse
• Diarrhea	Can be caused by: Laxative abuse Effect of medications/tube feedings Can lead to life-threatening dehydration and electrolyte imbalance
• Fecal impaction	Can result from chronic constipation May be preceded by oozing of liquid feces—often mistaken for diarrhea
• Fecal incontinence	Can be caused by: Decreased muscle tone Alteration in nervous system innervation to rectum Altered cognition

People who lack the enzyme lactase, which helps to break down the simple sugar lactose found in milk and milk products, cannot digest milk; this is called lactose intolerance. Food intolerance may result in diarrhea, gaseous distention, and cramping.

In addition to high-fiber, bulk-producing foods, other foods that influence bowel elimination include the following:

Constipating foods: processed cheese, lean meat, eggs, and pasta
Foods with laxative effect: certain fruits and vegetables (eg, prunes), bran, chocolate, spicy foods, alcohol, and coffee
Gas-producing foods: onions, cabbage, beans, cauliflower

Activity and Muscle Tone

Regular exercise improves gastrointestinal motility and muscle tone, whereas inactivity decreases both. Adequate tone in the abdominal muscles, the diaphragm, and the perineal muscles is essential for ease of defecation. Patients on prolonged bed rest are prime candidates for constipation.

Lifestyle

Many individual, family, and sociocultural variables influence a person's usual elimination habits. The long-term effects of bowel training may result in a person's (1) acceptance of bowel elimination as a normal life process, (2) preoccupation with bowel elimination, or (3) feeling that bowel elimination is a "dirty" process. Rituals associated with bowel elimination, cleanliness considerations, the language used to talk about bowel elimination or reluctance to discuss it, individual responses to involuntary passage of flatus (gas), and so on vary widely among different people. A person's daily schedule, occupation, and leisure activities may contribute to a habit of defecating at regular times or to an irregular pattern (see the accompanying Applying Learning to Practice boxes).

Psychological Variables

Emotional stress affects the body in many ways. In some people, anxiety seems to have a direct effect on gastrointestinal motility, and diarrhea accompanies periods of high anxiety. In the fight-or-flight response, when the body mobilizes itself for intense action, blood is shunted away from the stomach and intestines, and gastrointestinal motility slows. Chronic worriers and certain personality types who tend to hold on to problems and negative feelings may experience frequent constipation.

Pathologic Conditions

Numerous pathologic processes may change a person's usual bowel elimination. When a patient reports that his or her stool has become narrower or ribbon-like, it is

APPLYING LEARNING TO PRACTICE

The Nurse as Role Model: Bowel Elimination

Before intervening to help patients develop healthy bowel elimination patterns, it is important for nurses to assess the adequacy of their own bowel elimination habits and patterns. If you are unable to meet the following goals, you may want to take the time now to revise your own health practices, so that you will be an effective role model for patients. Use the assessment checklist to see how well you are meeting bowel elimination needs. The nurse:

- Has a regular bowel elimination pattern without discomfort

- Responds to the urge to defecate
- Includes in each day's nutritional intake sufficient high-fiber foods and fluid to promote peristalsis and reduce stool retention
- Identifies many ways to increase fiber and fluid in different types of diets
- Exercises vigorously for 30 to 45 minutes three or four times a week
- Responds to changes in stool characteristics (or frequency) by seeking their cause and getting medical assistance when necessary

important for the nurse to consider the possibility of a tumor in the colon forming an obstruction to normal stool passage and to report this finding to the physician. Similarly, if a parent reports that a child's stools are frequent, bulky, greasy, and foul smelling, one possible explanation is cystic fibrosis; this would need to be ruled out if other clinical manifestations are present. Changes in stool characteristics or frequency may be one of the first clinical manifestations of a disease, and their evaluation may lead to the diagnosis of the disease.

Pathologic conditions that may result in diarrhea include diverticulitis, infection, malabsorption syndromes, neoplastic diseases, diabetic neuropathy, hyperthyroidism, and uremia. Conditions that predispose to constipation include diseases within the colon or rectum, injury to or degeneration of the spinal cord, and megacolon. Conditions that traumatize the stomach or intestines or that interfere with normal digestion may change the color, contents, odor, and appearance of the stool, mak-

ing stool assessment an important diagnostic task for nursing.

Outbreaks of food poisoning can result in severe gastrointestinal symptoms, including diarrhea. Infections caused by *Escherichia coli* are particularly dangerous for young children and older adults. They can progress quickly to life-threatening hematologic and renal complications (Sheff, 1999). Severe abdominal cramping followed by watery or bloody diarrhea may signal the presence of an infection from this microbe, and a stool sample may confirm it. Treatment is supportive, and these patients require careful monitoring and attentive nursing care.

Medications

Medications are available to either promote peristalsis (cathartics and laxatives) or inhibit peristalsis (antidiarrheal medications). These are discussed later in the chapter.

APPLYING LEARNING TO PRACTICE

Promoting Health

Bowel Elimination

Use the assessment checklist to determine how well you are meeting your need for bowel elimination. Then develop a prescription for self-care by choosing appropriate behaviors from the list of suggestions.

ASSESSMENT CHECKLIST

almost always | sometimes | almost never
1. I have a regular bowel elimination pattern, satisfactory to support comfort and activities of daily living.
2. I eat a diet high in fiber.
3. I exercise regularly.
4. I have an adequate intake of fluids.

SELF-CARE BEHAVIORS

1. Accept individual patterns of defecation as normal.
2. Eat a balanced diet, including high-fiber foods, such as fruits, vegetables, and nuts.
3. Follow a regular exercise program with 30 to 45 minutes of activity three to four times a week.
4. Do not ignore the urge to defecate.
5. Establish a routine, if needed (1 hour after meals is usually best).
6. Avoid prolonged use of over-the-counter medications or enemas to treat constipation.

Other types of medications may affect bowel elimination and stool characteristics. Opioids, antacids containing aluminum, and anticholinergic medications may all cause constipation by decreasing gastrointestinal motility. Many medications can cause diarrhea as a side effect. Twenty percent of the time, antibiotic use causes diarrhea (Abrams, 1998). The use of antidiarrheal drugs in this situation is not recommended because this would further prolong the exposure of the intestinal mucosa to the irritating effect of the antibiotics or toxins. The diarrhea may be severe enough to warrant cessation of the drug.

Medications may also influence the appearance of the stool, for a variety of reasons. Any drug with the potential to cause gastrointestinal bleeding (eg, anticoagulants, aspirin products) may result in the stool appearing pink to red to black. Iron salts result in a black stool from the oxidation of iron. Antacids may cause a white discoloration or speckling in the stool. Antibiotics may cause a green-gray color because of impaired digestion.

Pepto Bismol & iron turn stool black

Diagnostic Tests

Patients may need to fast for diagnostic studies, and all patients need a clear explanation about the nature and purpose of tests. The stress of hospitalization and waiting for the results of the study, combined with changes in food intake, can severely alter a patient's usual elimination patterns. Bowel cleansing by use of cathartics or enemas is a prerequisite for certain diagnostic studies of the gastrointestinal tract (see Table 43-2 later in this chapter).

Surgery and Anesthesia

Direct manipulation of the bowel during abdominal surgery inhibits peristalsis, causing a condition termed paralytic ileus. This temporary stoppage of peristalsis normally lasts 24 to 48 hours, and during this time, food and fluids are withheld. If this condition persists, it may cause distention and symptoms of acute obstruction and may require surgical intervention. Inhaled general anesthetic agents also inhibit peristalsis by blocking the parasympathetic impulses to the intestinal musculature. Local and regional anesthetics have little effect on peristalsis.

The Nursing Process

ASSESSING

Nursing History

Because many patients are reluctant to initiate a conversation about their bowel status, nurses should include pertinent bowel elimination questions in each comprehensive nursing history (see the accompanying Focused Assessment Guide).

If the patient is experiencing any disturbance in bowel elimination, a more detailed assessment is conducted with attention directed to those factors described earlier that may influence bowel elimination.

Patients who are critically ill or who have impaired cognition may be incapable of reporting their bowel status accurately. In this case, nurses need to record the patient's daily bowel status to be alert to impending problems. While making daily rounds, nurses can ask patients who give reliable answers, "Did you move your bowels yesterday or today?" and chart the response. If the patient cannot provide this information, the nurse who is assisting with bowel elimination records the daily stools.

Physical Assessment

Assessment of bowel elimination includes physical assessment of the abdomen, anus, and rectum (discussed in Chap. 25). Described below are examination techniques that may be helpful when assessing the functioning of the gastrointestinal tract.

Abdomen

The sequence for abdominal assessment proceeds from inspection, auscultation, and percussion to palpation. Auscultation is done before palpation because palpation may disturb normal peristalsis and bowel motility (Kirton, 1997). The patient is comfortably positioned in the supine position with the abdomen exposed, the chest and pubic area draped, and the knees slightly flexed. The bladder should be emptied.

Inspection

The nurse first observes the contour of the abdomen, noting any masses or areas of distention. Peristalsis is usually not visible except in very thin patients. When an intestinal obstruction is present, the visible waves of peristalsis to the point of the obstruction may be observed on the abdomen.

Auscultation

The nurse uses a warmed stethoscope to listen for bowel sounds in a systematic, clockwise manner in all abdominal quadrants. If the patient has a nasogastric tube in place, it should be disconnected from suction during this assessment to allow for accurate interpretation of sounds. The timing of the patient's most recent meal or a bladder that has not been emptied may also affect the examination. The frequency and character of bowel sounds are noted. Bowel sounds are audible clicks and gurgles produced by the movement of air and flatus in the gastrointestinal tract. They are usually high pitched, gurgling, and soft. Their frequency may range from 5 to 30 bowel sounds per minute, depending on the rate of peristalsis (Weber & Kelley, 1998). Of significance are absent or infrequent bowel sounds, indicating hypoperistalsis or paralytic ileus (no decision should be made until the nurse has listened for 5 minutes), or abnormally intense and frequent bowel sounds (borborygmus), indicating hyperperistalsis. Bowel sounds are usually described as being audible, hyperactive, hypoactive, or inaudible.

FOCUSED ASSESSMENT GUIDE

Bowel Elimination

Factors to Assess	Questions and Approaches
Usual patterns of bowel elimination	How often do you move your bowels?
	Any special time of the day?
	What does your stool look like:
	• Frequency
	• Time of day
	• Description of usual stool characteristics (amount, consistency, shape, color, odor)
Aids to elimination	Do you use anything to help move your bowels?
	• Natural aids (liquids, food)
	• Pharmacologic aids (laxatives)
	• Enemas
Recent changes in bowel elimination	Have you noticed any changes in your stool recently?
	Have you noticed any blood in your stool?
	Have you noted a difference in the appearance of your stool (narrowing, presence of mucus)?
Problems with bowel elimination	Are your bowels causing you any problem now?
	• Nature of disturbance
	• Onset and frequency
	• Causes (*physical:* food and fluid intake, exercise status, history of surgery or illnesses influencing GI tract; *psychosocial; medicine related*)
	• Severity
	• Symptoms
	• Interventions attempted and results
Presence of artificial orifices	What is your usual routine with your colostomy or ileostomy?
	Do you have any problems with it?

Percussion

The nurse next percusses all quadrants of the abdomen in a systematic, clockwise manner to identify any masses, fluid, or air in the abdomen. A resonant sound or tympany is expected over the abdomen and stomach because these are hollow organs. With practice, the nurse can distinguish normal resonance from the hyperresonance that occurs when excess flatus is trapped in the intestines. An intestinal obstruction sounds dull on percussion. Areas of increased dullness may be caused by fluid, a mass, or a tumor.

Palpation

Both light and deep palpation in each quadrant are next performed by a skilled nurse, noting muscular resistance, tenderness, enlargement of organs, and masses. The beginning nurse quickly learns the feel of a distended abdomen. If the patient is in pain, medication should be administered before proceeding with the palpation.

Anus and Rectum

The nurse's skill level determines the extent of the rectal examination. A superficial examination is performed each

time a nurse washes a patient's anal area or assists with bowel evacuation. The patient is most often positioned in left Sims' position.

Inspection and Palpation

The nurse first examines the anal area for cracks, nodules, distended veins (hemorrhoids), masses, or polyps. A fecal mass may be observed distending the anus. A gloved, lubricated finger is inserted through the anus into the rectum to assess sphincter tone and smoothness of the mucosal lining and to note the presence of any masses, polyps, hardened stool, bleeding, or abnormal discharge. The perineal area is also inspected for areas of skin irritation or breakdown secondary to diarrhea or fecal incontinence.

Stool Characteristics

Nurses are responsible for observing and recording information about the patient's stool. Table 43-1 describes the characteristics of a normal stool along with special considerations when observing a stool. Anything unusual should be reported and recorded. Passing little or no gas or unusual amounts should also be recorded and reported.

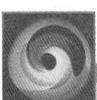

Table 43-1
The Stool: Normal Characteristics and Special Considerations for Observation

Characteristic	Normal Finding	Special Considerations for Observation
Volume	Variable	The volume of the stool depends on the amount the person eats and the nature of the diet. For example, a diet high in roughage produces more feces than a soft, bland diet.
		Consistently large diarrheal stools suggest a disorder in the small bowel or proximal colon; small, frequent stools with urgency to pass them suggest a disorder of the left colon or rectum.
Color	Infant: Yellow Adult: Brown	The brown color of the stool is due to stercobilin, a bile pigment derivative. The rapid rate of peristalsis in the infant causes the stool to be yellow.
		The color of the stool is influenced by diet. For example, the stool will be almost black if the person eats red meat and dark green vegetables, such as spinach. The stool will be light brown if the diet is high in milk and milk products and low in meat.
		The absence of bile may cause the stool to appear white or clay-colored.
		Certain drugs influence the color of the stool. For example, iron salts cause the stool to be black. Antacids cause it to be whitish.
		Bleeding high in the intestinal tract causes a stool to be black owing to the digestion of the blood. Bleeding low in the intestinal tract results in fresh blood in the stool.
		The stool darkens with standing.
Odor	Pungent; may be affected by foods ingested	The characteristic odor of the stool is due to indole and skatole, caused by putrefaction and fermentation in the lower intestinal tract.
		The odor of the stool is influenced by its pH value, which normally is neutral or slightly alkaline.
		Excessive putrefaction causes a strong odor.
		The presence of blood in the stool causes a unique odor.
Consistency	Soft, semisolid, and formed	The consistency of the stool is influenced by fluid and food intake and gastric motility. The less time stool spends in the intestine (or the shorter the intestine), the more liquid the stool. Many pathologic conditions influence consistency.
Shape	Formed stool is usually about 1 inch (2.5 cm) in diameter and has the tubular shape of the colon, but may be larger or smaller, depending on the condition of the colon.	A gastrointestinal obstruction may result in a narrow, pencil-shaped stool. Rapid peristalsis thins the stool. Increased time spent in the large intestine may result in a hard, marblelike fecal mass.
Constituents	Waste residues of digestion: bile, intestinal secretions, shedded epithelial cells, bacteria, and inorganic material (chiefly calcium and phosphates); seeds, meat fibers, and fat may be present in small amounts	Internal bleeding, infection, inflammation, and other pathologic conditions may result in abnormal constituents. These include blood, pus, excessive fat, parasites, ova, and mucus.
		Foreign bodies also may be found in the stool.

The frequency with which the patient has bowel movements is noted and recorded. Frequency is recorded as I, II, III, or i, ii, iii, to indicate the number of bowel movements in a given period of time. The frequency of the patient's bowel movements, as well as specific information about the amount and characteristics of stool, is usually appropriately recorded on a bedside flow sheet. Any additional unusual observations are described in the nurses' notes on the patient's permanent record. When auxiliary personnel or the patient assumes this responsibility, the nurse should check at regular intervals to see that it is being done correctly.

Warning Signs of Colon Cancer

- Change in the bowel elimination pattern
- Blood in the stools
- Rectal or abdominal pain
- Change in the character of the stool
- Sensation of incomplete emptying after bowel movement

Ideally, populations at high risk for bowel elimination problems are identified before problems occur, and such problems are prevented or minimized through vigilant nursing care. The nurse must also be aware of the clinical manifestations of colon cancer because early detection significantly improves survival statistics (see the accompanying box, Warning Signs of Colon Cancer). When assessing bowel function, the nurse needs a thorough knowledge of the factors that affect defecation.

Assisting With Diagnostic Studies

The nurse is often responsible for caring for patients with elimination problems who are undergoing diagnostic testing. Following are specific guidelines for nursing's role in stool collection and direct and indirect visualization studies.

Stool Collection

The nurse is responsible for obtaining the specimen according to agency procedure, labeling the specimen, and ensuring that the specimen is transported to the laboratory in a timely manner. The institution's policy and procedure manual or laboratory manual determine specifics regarding the amount of stool needed, the time frame during which stool is to be collected, and the type of specimen container to use.

Medical aseptic techniques are imperative. Disposable gloves should be worn when any contact or handling of a stool specimen is likely. Handwashing before and after glove use is essential. Care must also be taken not to contaminate the outside of the specimen container with stool. Specimens should be packaged, labeled, and transported to the laboratory according to agency policy in a manner that guarantees that there is no leakage of the specimen.

Specific instructions the nurse needs to give the patient when collecting a stool specimen may include the following:

- Void first because the laboratory study may be inaccurate if the stool contains urine.
- Use a clean or sterile bedpan or the bedside commode, depending on the specific specimen required.
- Defecate into the required container rather than the toilet bowl because the analysis results may be affected by the water in the bowl.
- Do not place toilet tissue in the bedpan or specimen container because contents in the paper may influence laboratory results.

- Notify the nurse when the specimen is available, so that it may be collected and transported to the laboratory in the required manner.

To place a specimen in a laboratory container, the nurse should put on gloves and use two clean tongue blades. Usually, 1 inch (2.5 cm) of formed stool or 15 to 30 mL of liquid stool is sufficient. If portions of the stool include visible blood, mucus, or pus, include these with the specimen. The specimen should also be free of any barium and enema solution. Because a fresh specimen produces the most accurate results, the specimen should be sent to the laboratory immediately. If this is not possible, it should be refrigerated, unless contraindicated.

To test the stool for pH or blood, use a commercial tape, dipstick, or solution according to the manufacturer's directions. **Occult blood** in the stool—that is, blood that is hidden in the specimen or cannot be seen on gross examination—can be detected with simple screening tests. Certain conditions, such as ulcer disease, inflammatory bowel disorders, and colon cancer, place the patient at high risk for intestinal bleeding. The color of the stool may reflect the source of the bleeding. Generally, black stools reflect a reaction between hemoglobin and gastric acid and indicate upper gastrointestinal bleeding (eg, peptic ulcer). Lower gastrointestinal bleeding (eg, hemorrhoids) may produce bright red blood in the stool. Certain foods and medications can also cause a black or reddish colored stool.

Tests for occult blood in the stool may be performed quickly by nurses within an institution or by patients at home. These simple tests use reagent substances to detect the presence of the enzyme peroxidase in the hemoglobin molecule. A diet high in red meat, chicken, fish, or other food substances, such as horseradish, raw fruits, and raw vegetables, and certain medications (eg, salicylate intake of more than 325 mg daily, steroids, iron preparations, and anticoagulants) may result in a false-positive reading (American College of Physicians, 1997). The ingestion of vitamin C can produce false-negative results even if bleeding is present. For home testing, recommendations usually include the following:

- Before the stool testing, restricting the types of food (for 3 days) and drugs (for 7 days) that may alter test results
- Postponing the test if a women has her menstrual period until 3 days after it has ceased
- Delaying the test if bleeding hemorrhoids or hematuria are present
- Recommending that a person who is color-blind to the color blue not attempt to interpret the test results (Dammel, 1997)

In clinical settings, these restrictions are usually not practical. The Hematest and guaiac test are chemical tests used to determine occult blood in the stool. The accompanying box, Guidelines for Nursing Care, gives additional nursing considerations for fecal occult blood testing, and Figure 43-4 demonstrates the procedure for a Hemoccult test.

Guidelines for Nursing Care

Testing for Fecal Occult Blood

- Instruct the patient about food and drug restrictions for at least 2 to 3 days before the test, if they apply.
- Review manufacturer's directions for collecting the specimen. Equipment may include a specimen card, collection tissues, or test paper.
- Avoid mixing the specimen with urine or water.
- Inform the patient that multiple or serial specimens are usually collected from different bowel movements to verify results.
- Collect the amount recommended for the particular test (usually only a small amount is required).
- Wear gloves and wash hands thoroughly if collecting a specimen from a bedpan, commode, or plastic receptacle.
- Use tongue blades to transfer the stool to the test tape or folder.
- Follow instructions based on type of test. Hemoccult slide test requires placing 2 drops of developer solution on the back side of the specimen paper. The tablet test directions include placing 2 to 3 drops of tap water on the tablet, which is centered on the stool specimen.
- Document the test results according to agency policy. *A blue color is a positive result and needs to be reported.*
- Inform the patient of the test results.

Timed Specimens

Consider the first stool passed by the patient as the start of the collection period. Collect a specimen of *every* stool passed within the designated period (the test may require saving the entire stool passed or only a sample). Follow instructions for sending stools to the laboratory.

Pinworms

Use clear cellophane tape for collecting a specimen for pinworms (frosted tape makes examination difficult). The tape is pressed against the anal opening, removed immediately, and then placed on a slide. Collect this specimen in the morning, immediately after the patient awakens and before the patient has a bowel movement or bath. Pinworms tend to come to the anal area during the night to deposit eggs and retreat into the anal canal during the day. They are visible to the naked eye if the buttocks are spread and the anus is visualized while the child is asleep. Pinworm eggs can usually be detected on the tape under a microscope. For accurate results, this test may need to be repeated on consecutive days.

Direct Visualization Studies

Endoscopy is the direct visualization of the lining of a hollow body organ using a fiber optic endoscope, which is a long, flexible tube containing glass fibers that transmits light into the organ and returns an image that can be viewed. Pincers may be inserted through the tube to obtain a biopsy tissue sample. An endoscope enables the physician to view the integrity of the mucosa, blood vessels, and specific organ parts and is helpful for diagnosing inflammatory, ulcerative, and infectious diseases; benign and malignant neoplasms; and other lesions of the esophageal, gastric, and intestinal mucosa. Endoscopic studies include the following:

Esophagogastroduodenoscopy: visual examination of the lining of the esophagus, the stomach, and the upper duodenum with a flexible, fiber optic endoscope

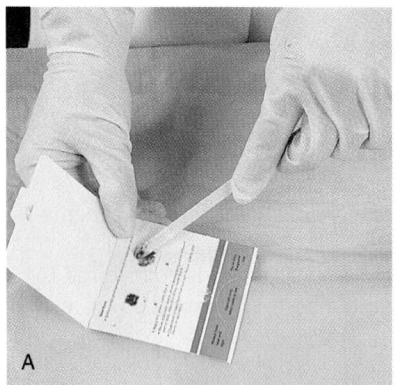
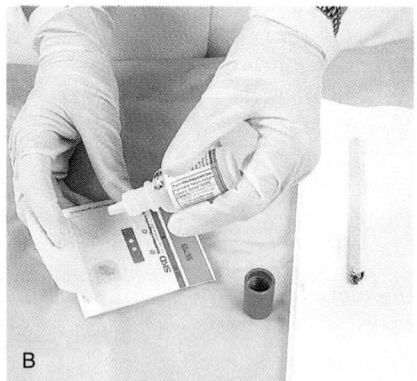
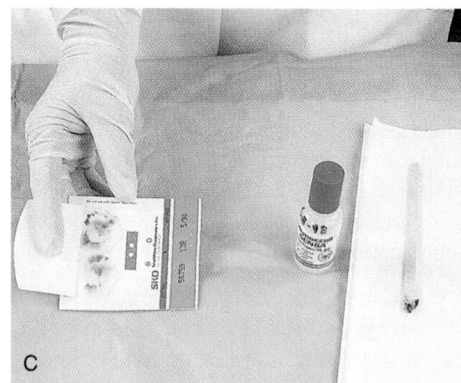

Figure 43-4
Testing a stool specimen for occult blood. (**A**) Applying a stool specimen to the test paper; (**B**) adding developing solution to the back side of the paper according to directions; (**C**) *blue coloration* indicating positive results. (Copyright © B. Proud.)

Colonoscopy: visual examination of the lining of the large intestine with a flexible, fiber optic endoscope

Sigmoidoscopy: visual examination of the lining of the distal sigmoid colon, the rectum, and the anal canal using either a flexible or rigid instrument. The tube has an attached light source and is equipped to allow biopsy. The rigid sigmoidoscope may be more uncomfortable for the patient, especially one who is not relaxed.

Nursing responsibilities before and after these studies are described in Table 43-2.

Indirect Visualization Studies

Indirect visualization of the gastrointestinal tract is commonly achieved through radiography. The passage of x-rays through the patient creates a radiograph or film depicting body structures. This technique is useful for detecting obstructions, strictures, inflammatory disease, tumors, ulcers, and other lesions and for diagnosing hiatal hernia and other structural changes in the gastrointestinal tract. Use of a radiopaque contrast medium, such as barium sulfate, accentuates the body structures being visualized. In the *upper gastrointestinal examination* and *small bowel series*, the patient drinks the barium sulfate like a milk shake, which coats the esophagus, stomach, and small intestine to be better visualized. In the *barium enema* or *lower gastrointestinal examination*, barium sulfate is instilled into the large intestine through a rectal tube inserted through the anus. Fluoroscopy projects consecutive x-ray images onto a screen for continuous observation of the flow of the barium. The specific nursing responsibilities are included in Table 43-2.

Scheduling Diagnostic Studies

Because nurses are commonly involved in the scheduling of diagnostic studies when a patient is to undergo multiple studies, guidelines for scheduling studies of the gastrointestinal tract are important:

1. The following is a logical sequence when more than one test is required for accurate diagnosis:

   Fecal occult blood tests: to detect gastrointestinal bleeding

   Barium studies: to visualize gastrointestinal structures and reveal any inflammation, ulcers, tumors, strictures, or other lesions

   Endoscopic examinations: to visualize an abnormality, locate a source of bleeding, and if necessary, provide biopsy tissue samples

2. A barium enema and routine radiography should precede an upper gastrointestinal series because retained barium from an upper gastrointestinal series could take several days to pass through the gastrointestinal tract and cloud anatomic detail on the barium enema studies.

3. Noninvasive procedures usually take precedence over invasive procedures, such as endoscopic studies, when sufficient diagnostic data can be obtained. (In some instances, endoscopic studies may be done before barium studies to ensure visualization.)

DIAGNOSING

Bowel Elimination as the Problem

When the analysis of assessment data points to a bowel elimination problem that can be prevented or resolved by independent nursing intervention, a nursing diagnosis is developed. If alterations in bowel elimination require new self-care behaviors (eg, colostomy management), Knowledge Deficit may be an appropriate nursing diagnosis. Examples of specific causes and defining characteristics for common alterations in bowel elimination are listed in the accompanying box.

Bowel Elimination as the Etiology

Problems of bowel elimination may also affect other areas of human functioning. In the nursing diagnoses that follow, problems of bowel elimination are the etiology for other problems:

Altered Growth and Development related to parents' misconceptions about bowel and bladder training

Altered Nutrition: Less Than Body Requirements related to loss of appetite from flatulence or impaction

Anxiety related to lack of voluntary control of fecal elimination and significant others' response to ostomy

Body Image Disturbance related to ostomy, need to wear disposable adult briefs

Fluid Volume Deficit related to prolonged diarrhea

Impaired Skin Integrity related to prolonged diarrhea, fecal incontinence

Ineffective Individual Coping related to inability to accept permanent ostomy

Knowledge Deficit: Bowel Training related to no previous experience

Pain related to intestinal distention, prolonged constipation or impaction, fecal incontinence, hemorrhoids

Self-Care Deficit: Toileting, related to mobility deficit, weakness, confusion

Self-Esteem Disturbance related to need for assistance with toileting, fecal incontinence

Sexual Dysfunction related to perceived change in body image, lack of interest, loss of self-esteem

PLANNING: EXPECTED OUTCOMES

Nursing measures for patients without specific bowel elimination problems are directed toward the patient's achievement of the following goals. The patient will achieve the following:

- Have a soft, formed bowel movement every 1 to 3 days without discomfort

(*text continues on page 1196*)

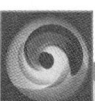

Table 43-2
Common Diagnostic Procedures Used to Study the Gastrointestinal Tract

Preparation	Aftercare

Esophagogastroduodenoscopy: Allows visual examination of the esophagus, stomach, and upper duodenum by means of a long, flexible, fiberoptic-lighted scope

Preparation	Aftercare
A signed consent form is required for this procedure.	Withhold food and fluids until the gag reflex returns.
Fasting is required 6 to 12 hours before the test (check agency policy).	Check vital signs according to the protocol.
Dentures need to be removed before the test.	Observe for signs of perforation: pain, persistent difficulty swallowing, vomiting blood, or black, tarry stools.
Remind the patient that he will be awake but sedated and that a local anesthetic will be sprayed into the mouth and throat to depress the gag reflex.	Explain to the patient that it is normal to sense throat soreness and hoarseness for several days; saline gargles and lozenges may be helpful.

Colonoscopy: Allows visual examination of the rectum, colon, and distal small bowel using a long, flexible, fiberoptic-lighted scope.

Preparation	Aftercare
Ensure that an informed consent is signed. Preparation prior to test may involve: • Clear liquid diet (24–48 h before test) • 2 day bowel preparation—strong cathartic and Dulcolax on day 1 and enema the day of the test, *or* • 1 day bowel preparation—ingestion of a gallon of bowel cleanser such as GoLytely in a short period of time Sedation will be given before the test.	May experience flatulence or gas pains because air was used to distend the intestines for better visibility. Usual diet may be resumed once patient recovers from the sedation. Check vital signs according to agency protocol. Observe for signs of bowel perforation: rectal bleeding, abdominal pain and distention, fever, malaise.

Sigmoidoscopy: Allows visual examination of the distal sigmoid colon, the rectum, and the anal canal through a flexible or rigid sigmoidoscope.

Preparation	Aftercare
Obtain an informed consent for this procedure. Preparation usually consists of light meal before the test and two Fleet enemas. Sedation is not usually required.	May experience flatulence or gas pains because air was used to distend the intestines for better visibility. Observe for signs of bowel perforation. If biopsy was performed, patient should be informed that slight rectal bleeding may occur.

Upper Gastrointestinal (UGI) and Small Bowel Series: Fluoroscopic examination of the esophagus, stomach, and small intestine after ingestion of barium sulfate.

Preparation	Aftercare
Ensure that an informed consent is signed. Keep patient NPO after midnight the day of the test. Inform patient that a chalky-tasting barium contrast mixture will be given to drink before the test.	A posttest cathartic (eg, Milk of Magnesia) is usually prescribed to prevent fecal impaction from barium sulfate that has hardened. Explain that the barium may lighten the color of stools for the next several days. After the barium is expelled, the stool color will return to normal.

Barium Enema: A series of radiographs that examine the large intestine after rectal instillation of barium sulfate

Preparation	Aftercare
An informed consent must be signed. Preparation may consist of dietary modifications, increased fluid intake, a cathartic, NPO after midnight, and enemas until clear before the test. Review the patient's history for any history of ulcerative colitis or active GI bleeding that would prohibit the use of the standard bowel preparation.	Encourage fluids to prevent dehydration. Inform the patient that the barium may lighten the color of the stools. A cathartic may be prescribed. Encourage rest because the bowel preparation and the test exhaust many patients.

Adapted from Fischbach, F. (1998). *A manual of laboratory diagnostic tests* (6th ed.). Philadelphia: Lippincott Williams & Wilkins; and Pagana, K., & Pagana, T. (1998). *Manual of diagnostic and laboratory Tests*. St. Louis: C. V. Mosby.

Nursing Diagnoses for Common Problems

Bowel Elimination

Problem	*Related Factors*	*Sample Defining Characteristics*
Constipation	• Decreased fiber in diet • Decreased fluid intake • Inactivity • Delaying defecation when urge is present • Abuse of laxatives • Use of constipating medications (antacids, narcotic analgesics [opioids], anticholinergics) • Change in routine • Pain associated with defecation	• "I feel bloated and know I have to move my bowels but I can't." • "Whenever I'm constipated I feel lethargic and lose my appetite." • Reports straining during defecation with little result • Passes small "marbles" of dry, hard stool • Decreased frequency • Decreased frequency of bowel sounds or changes in abdominal growling • Straining often results in small amount of bleeding from swollen external hemorrhoids • Reports feeling rectal fullness or pressure in rectum • Headache
Risk for constipation	• Habitually ignores urge to defecate • Inactivity • Decreased fiber in diet • Inadequate fluid intake • Use of pharmacologic agents that can result in constipation (iron, opioids, anticholinergics) • Stress, confusion	• "I'm in such a rush in the morning that I never take time to go to the bathroom." • Reports straining during defecation • Passes small, hard, dry stool • Reports feeling bloated
Perceived constipation	• Culture • Family health beliefs • Faulty appraisal • Impaired thought processes	• Expectation of daily bowel movement with resulting abuse of laxatives, enemas, suppositories • Expected passage of stool at the same time every day
Diarrhea	• Food intolerance (coarse, greasy, or spicy foods) • Food or drug allergies • Abuse of laxatives • Alteration in normal bacterial flora of the intestine (antibiotic therapy) • Emotional stress • Intestinal infection • Colon disease and other diseases • Surgical alterations	• Loose liquid stools, increased frequency • Urgency with soiling • Reports of abdominal pain and cramping • Increased frequency of bowel sounds
Bowel incontinence	• Gross constipation with impaction and subsequent overflow • Organic changes in neural innervation of the rectum • Local causes (inflammation, cancer of rectum, prolapsed anus, semifluid stool) • Extreme debilitation • Cognitive impairment	• Involuntary passage of stool (stool characteristics vary) • "I'm sorry, I couldn't get into the bathroom (or onto the bedpan) quickly enough." • "It came so fast I couldn't hold it back." • History of constipation with sudden development of oozing diarrhea stool

- Explain the relation between bowel elimination and dietary fiber, fluid intake, and exercise
- Relate the importance of seeking medical evaluation if changes in stool color or consistency persist

IMPLEMENTING

Promoting Regular Bowel Habits

Regular bowel habits can be promoted in both well and ill patients by attention to timing, positioning, privacy, nutrition, and exercise.

Timing

Once the nurse knows when a patient usually experiences the urge to defecate (often about an hour after meals when mass colonic peristalsis occurs), the nurse offers whatever assistance is needed to help the patient to the bathroom, commode, or bedpan at this time. Nursing care or treatments should not be scheduled during this time. Because many patients feel uncomfortable about requesting time for elimination, the nurse should communicate to all patients the importance of heeding this natural urge, explaining that postponing it only results in constipation and other problems.

Positioning

The squatting position best facilitates defecation, but most patients routinely use a sitting position while leaning a bit forward. Most patients who are able to use the bedside commode or bathroom toilet have little difficulty assuming this position, although they may need support. An elevated toilet seat may be ordered for patients with orthopedic problems who cannot lower themselves to a toilet seat.

Patients who need to use a bedpan in bed benefit from having the head of the bed elevated 30 degrees, unless this is contraindicated. This eliminates the hyperextension of the back that occurs when a patient who is lying flat attempts to lift his or her hips onto the pan. After the head of the bed is elevated, the patient raises the hips by bending the knees, digging in the heels, and lifting the hips upward. An overhead trapeze may be helpful for patients with weak lower extremities. The head of the bed should not be raised more than 45 degrees because this makes it harder to lift the hips straight up. Positioning a patient with a bedpan is described in Procedure 42-1 in Chapter 42. Many patients on bed rest appreciate having moistened hand wipes at the bedside to substitute for handwashing after toileting. Bedpans should be emptied, cleaned, and returned to the patient's bedside stand promptly.

Privacy

Because most people consider elimination a private act, nurses must respect the patient's need to be alone while defecating, unless the patient's weakness makes this impossible. Bedside drapes should be pulled around a patient using a bedside commode or bedpan. Well patients who cannot defecate in a public restroom or strange environment may need assistance in developing a workable schedule of defecation that makes use of private toilet facilities.

Nutrition

Patients with elimination problems may need a dietary analysis to determine which foods and fluids are contributing to their problem and which may help in its treatment. General dietary recommendations to promote regular defecation include a fluid intake of 2000 to 3000 mL and a high-fiber intake. Water is recommended as the fluid of choice because other fluids (ie, coffee, tea, and juice) may have a diuretic effect (Benton et al., 1997). Increasing fiber intake without sufficient fluid intake can result in severe gastrointestinal problems, including fecal impaction. Specific recommendations are discussed in the next section.

Exercise

Regular exercise improves gastrointestinal motility and aids in defecation. Well patients should be encouraged to exercise regularly three to five times a week. Ill patients should be ambulated as soon as possible and should be instructed about how inactivity can lead to constipation, distention, and impaction. Bedside exercises may be helpful for immobilized patients.

Patients with weak abdominal and perineal muscles who are using a bedpan may be helped by the following exercises:

Abdominal setting: The patient, lying in a supine position, tightens and holds the abdominal muscles for 6 seconds and then relaxes them. This should be repeated several times each waking hour.

Thigh strengthening: The thigh muscles are flexed and contracted by slowly bringing the knees up to the chest one at a time and then lowering them to the bed. This also should be performed several times for each knee each waking hour.

Preventing and Treating Constipation

Constipation is the passage of dry, hard stools. Decreased gastric motility slows the passage of feces through the large intestine, resulting in increased fluid absorption from the fecal mass, causing dry, hard stool. Straining often accompanies defecation. Some people may be constipated and yet have a daily bowel movement, whereas others who regularly defecate no more than three times a week are not constipated. Individuals at high-risk for constipation include (1) patients on bed rest who take constipating medications (opioids, anticholinergics), (2) patients with reduced fluids or bulk in their diet, (3) depressed people, and (4) patients with central nervous system disease or local lesions that cause pain.

Teaching About Nutrition

The nurse's promotion of healthy behaviors can assist the patient and family to achieve mutually desirable outcomes for preventing constipation. Strategies for health teaching include those that have been previously discussed as well as specific nutritional recommendations to increase high-fiber foods (fruits, vegetables, whole-grain cereals and bread) and fluid intake (water, fruit juices, especially prune juice, and hot liquids). Bran and fluids are more effective than medications for reducing constipation (Stewart, 1998).

Teaching About Cathartics and Laxatives

Cathartics and **laxatives** are drugs that induce emptying of the intestinal tract. Although these terms are sometimes used interchangeably, cathartics exert a stronger effect on the intestines than laxatives. Some of these drugs, such as castor oil, cascara, senna, phenolphthalein, and bisacodyl (Dulcolax), act chemically by stimulating peristalsis. Others, such as magnesium sulfate and psyllium hydrophilic mucilloid (Metamucil), act by increasing the intestinal bulk, which promotes additional mechanical stimulation on the intestine. Still others, such as mineral oil and dioctyl sodium sulfosuccinate (Colace), soften the fecal material. Another frequently used laxative is milk of magnesia. It has antacid properties in small dosages and laxative properties when taken in larger doses. Table 43-3 summarizes the types of laxatives.

Laxatives have their rightful place in healthcare. They are necessary at times for people whose activity is limited or whose food intake is poor. They are also used for emptying the intestinal tract in preparation for surgical or diagnostic exploration. Their occasional use is not harmful for most people, but all efforts should be taken to prevent a person from becoming dependent on them. Because many laxatives are available as nonprescription drugs, and because modern advertising promotes their use, many people take them frequently on their own initiative, whether they need them or not.

Some people are aware that because of their chemical action, laxatives should not be taken when there is abdominal pain because an intestinal pathologic condition could be harmed by the increased peristalsis. Although many people take laxatives because they believe they are constipated, most are unaware that habitual use of laxatives is the most common cause of chronic constipation.

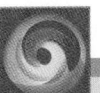

Table 43-3
Classification of Laxatives

Type	Action	Advantages	Caution
Bulk-forming (eg, Metamucil)	Psyllium, grain, or synthetic product that causes stool to absorb water and swell, thus stimulating peristalsis	Usually acts within 24 hours	May interfere with absorption of calcium and iron and certain drugs Should not be given to bedridden patients or those with intestinal strictures May be expensive
Emollient/stool softener (eg, Colace)	Agents with detergent activity that allow water and fat to penetrate and lubricate the stool	Recommended for those who must avoid straining	Lubricant component of drug may interfere with absorption of fat-soluble vitamins
Lubricant (eg, mineral oil)	Lubricant absorbed from intestinal tract and softens stool, making it easier to pass	Usually effective within 8 hours	May interfere with absorption of fat-soluble vitamins Aspiration of drug may result in a lipid pneumonia
Stimulant (eg, Dulcolax)	Promotes peristalsis by irritating the intestinal mucosa or stimulating nerve endings in intestinal wall	Works more quickly than bulking agents	Most abused laxatives on the market Causes lazy bowel syndrome May affect absorption of vitamin D and calcium Not recommended for elderly patients because of prolonged action Alters electrolyte transport
Saline-osmotic (eg, Fleet)	Draws water into intestine and stimulates peristalsis	Use when rapid cleansing desired	Should not be used by elderly people Can produce dehydration Not recommended in patients with kidney disease or heart failure

Nurses are often in a position to help patients who abuse laxatives. Breaking the physical and psychological habit of using laxatives is not easy for a person who has come to depend on them. It often requires much patience, support, and teaching by the nurse. The person also frequently needs to be helped with diet, fluid intake, activity, and regularity of habits (see the accompanying Research in Nursing box).

Preventing and Treating Diarrhea

Diarrhea is the passage of excessively liquid, unformed stools. Frequent bowel movements do not necessarily mean that diarrhea is present, although patients with diarrhea usually pass stools more frequently. Diarrhea is often associated with intestinal cramps. Nausea and vomiting may occur, along with blood in the stools. Diarrhea occurs protectively when its cause is irritants in the intestinal tract. Large amounts of fluids and electrolytes may be lost relatively quickly through diarrhea, however. This is especially true with infants and young children; if neglected, such loss may easily place a youngster's life in jeopardy. If oral intake is possible, cold fluids and rich foods, especially sweets, should be avoided.

Additional nursing measures include the following:

- Answer the patient's call bell immediately or ensure that a bedpan or commode is within easy reach. Diarrhea can be embarrassing, and the patient needs to know that the nurse is there to help.
- Whenever possible, remove the cause of the diarrhea. Discontinuation of medications that cause diarrhea usually results in a return to normal defecation within 1 to 3 days.
- If there is any indication of an impaction, a rectal examination should be performed before using antidiarrheal medications.
- Give special care to the region around the anus, where skin irritation is common. Keep the area clean and dry. Use skin creams, ointments, or powders as necessary.
- After the diarrhea stops, it is important to promote a return to normal bowel flora. Fermented dairy products, such as buttermilk or yogurt, aid this process.

Teaching About Nutrition

An initial precaution is to ensure that food is safe for consumption and prepared and stored properly. Food poison-

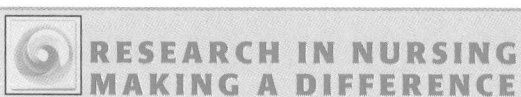

RESEARCH IN NURSING: MAKING A DIFFERENCE

Managing Chronic Constipation in Long-Term Care Residents

Changes in bowel elimination patterns are distressing to patients and caregivers. Laxatives, enemas, and manual removal of fecal impactions are commonly prescribed to alleviate constipation in long-term care residents. In addition to being unpleasant for the resident, they are also costly and require additional nursing assistance. Nursing interventions that can help to alleviate the hopelessness and stress associated with constipation promote the emotional as well as the physical well-being of an individual. The results of previous studies supported the use of bran to treat constipation, but controlled research is necessary to define an effective bran protocol and decrease reliance on pharmacologic and invasive measures.

Related Research
Howard, L., West, D., & Ossip-Klein, D. (2000). Chronic constipation management for institutionalized older adults. *Geriatric Nursing*, 21(2), 78–82.
The subjects in this study were 12 male residents of a Veterans Administration Medical Center who had chronic constipation (two or fewer stools per week) and regularly used laxatives or enemas. They were paired into groups of two: one resident in the control group continued with the usual treatments and medications, and the other participated in the bran-treatment regi-

men. During a 4-month period, as the amount of bran was gradually increased to a maximal dose of 6 tablespoons per day, laxative use was significantly reduced in the bran-treatment group. At the conclusion of this study, oral laxatives were totally discontinued for this test group, and the use of other bowel medication was reduced by 80%. Nurses also reported a decrease in patient discomfort with bowel elimination in the bran-treatment group. The control group did not experience any change in bowel habits or their medication and treatment regimen.

Relevance to Nursing Practice
This study verified that a simple dietary measure, over time, can have a dramatic effect on bowel elimination. Bran that is added slowly to the diet usually has minimal adverse effects and results in positive outcomes. Additional investigations will be necessary to compare the bran protocol with other treatment measures for constipation. The amount of bran and the length of time it is used merit additional study. Problems in bowel elimination are commonly identified and treated by nurses, and the nurse can play an essential role in helping a vulnerable population to regain control of this body function and maintain their dignity.

ing and the diarrhea that frequently accompanies it can be prevented by these common measures (Cerrato, 1999):

- Never purchase food with damaged packaging. Items that require refrigeration should be taken home immediately.
- Raw eggs in any form should not be used because of the danger of infection with the *Salmonella* bacillus. When cooking eggs, use only fresh ones purchased within 3 to 5 weeks and kept refrigerated.
- Ground meat should not be eaten uncooked. When cooked, it should not have a pink center when cut or drain pink juices. Avoid placing cooked meat on platters or cutting boards or using knives previously used for uncooked meat.
- Seafood should not be eaten raw and should not be used if it has a strong, unpleasant odor.
- Vegetables and fruit should be thoroughly cleaned before eating.
- Refrigerate leftovers within 2 hours of eating them.

Additional measures for preventing or treating diarrhea include avoiding highly spiced foods and foods with laxative effects such as raw fruits and vegetables. Encourage foods with low-fiber content. Replace lost fluids and electrolytes with weak tea, water, bouillon, clear soup, and gelatin; if diarrhea is severe, intravenous therapy may be needed.

Teaching About Antidiarrheal Medication

Antidiarrheal medications are usually reserved for treatment of chronic diarrhea and are not recommended initially for acute episodes of diarrhea. Acute diarrhea may result from a viral or bacterial infection, reactions to medications, or alterations in diet and is characterized by its sudden onset and a duration of several hours to several days. The duration of chronic diarrhea (more than 3 to 4 weeks) and the many possible causative agents (secondary disease states, surgery, laxative and alcohol abuse, and radiation and chemotherapeutic agents) usually necessitate pharmacologic intervention along with fluid and electrolyte replacement. Whatever the type of diarrhea, every effort should be made to identify and eliminate its underlying cause. The most effective nonspecific antidiarrheal medications are the opiates (eg, opium tincture [paregoric]) and related opiate derivatives (eg, loperamide [Imodium]), which act systemically to reduce intestinal hypermotility and slow peristalsis.

Eisenhauer and coauthors (1998) review basic characteristics of various antidiarrheal agents:

- The opiates are effective but have the potential for serious adverse effects. These drugs should not be used with infectious diarrhea because they decrease intestinal motility and may result in additional exposure of the intestinal mucosal to the causative agent. Commonly prescribed agents in this group include Lomotil and Imodium.
- Some antidiarrheal medications may cause drowsiness, and patients need to be cautioned about the hazards of driving or performing certain tasks when using these drugs.

- Kaolin-pectin preparations (Kaopectate) are available as over-the-counter medications, but their effectiveness for diarrhea is questionable. They may absorb nutrients and other antidiarrheal agents if given with them.
- Bismuth subsalicylate (Pepto-Bismol) has proved effective because it also has antisecretory, antimicrobial, and antiinflammatory effects. It is used to prevent traveler's diarrhea.

The nurse should focus on eliminating the cause of the diarrhea and replacing lost fluid as well as treating the symptoms. Some commercial products, such as Gatorade, may prove helpful. Pillitteri (1999) suggests the BRAT routine (*b*ananas, *r*ice cereal, *a*pplesauce, and *t*oast) as the protocol for a bland diet while replacing fluids and electrolytes during acute episodes of diarrhea in children. Oral rehydration therapy for adults is cost-effective and replaces fluid loss. It is particularly important that a fluid balance be maintained in older patients.

Decreasing Flatulence

Excessive formation of gases in the stomach or intestines is known as **flatulence**. When the gas is not expelled but accumulates in the intestinal tract, the condition is referred to as *intestinal distention* or *tympanites*. Gas-producing foods, such as beans, cabbage, onions, cauliflower, and beer, often predispose a person to flatulence and distention. Avoiding these foods may be helpful for people with ostomies who are concerned about odor.

In addition to avoiding irritating foods, other nursing interventions are helpful in decreasing flatus. Having the patient move about in bed and walk promotes peristalsis and the escape of flatus. Reclining after meals should be avoided.

A rectal tube may also be used to help gas escape if ambulation proves ineffective. The tube helps to stimulate peristalsis and provides a passageway for the escape of flatus. The procedure for inserting a rectal tube is as follows:

1. Use a 22 to 34 French tube for adults, smaller sizes for children.
2. Position the patient on his or her side, and drape the patient properly when preparing to insert a rectal tube.
3. Lubricate the rectal tube to reduce irritation to mucous membranes when inserting it.
4. Separate the buttocks well so that the anus is in plain view, and introduce the rectal tube beyond the anal canal into the rectum for about 10 cm (about 4 inches). It may be inserted a bit further if it is noted that no flatus is being removed.
5. Secure a dressing or waterproof pad to the end of the rectal tube, or place the end of the tube in a specimen container or urinal placed between the patient's legs. These techniques allow any discharge that empties through the rectal tube to be caught.
6. Leave the rectal tube in place for a short period—no longer than about 20 minutes; the tube no longer acts as a stimulant for peristalsis if left in place longer. If distention is not relieved, use the rectal tube intermittently every 2 to 3 hours, as necessary.

7. Have the patient assume various positions to help move flatus along the intestinal tract toward the anus. Gas is lighter than fluids and solids, and it will rise. Positions that help gas rise include lying on the abdomen, assuming the knee–chest position, and positioning the upper part of the body over the edge of the bed while the lower part rests across the bed. Do not use these positions if they are contraindicated or unsafe for the patient.

8. Confer with the physician if these measures bring no relief. An enema, a suppository, or a medication may be prescribed to help bring relief.

Emptying the Colon of Feces

Several methods are used to help promote elimination of feces: enemas, suppositories, oral intestinal lavage, and digital removal of stool.

Enemas

An **enema** is the introduction of a solution into the large intestine, usually for the purpose of removing feces. The instilled solution distends the intestine, may irritate intestinal mucosa, and thus increases peristalsis.

Types of Enemas

Enemas are classified as cleansing, retention, or return-flow enemas.

Cleansing Enemas. Cleansing enemas are given to remove feces from the colon. They are used for four common purposes:

- To relieve constipation or fecal impaction
- To prevent involuntary escape of fecal material during surgical procedures
- To promote visualization of the intestinal tract by radiographic or instrument examination
- To help establish regular bowel function during a bowel training program

The most common types of solutions used for cleansing enemas are tap water, normal saline solution, soap solution, and hypertonic solution. These are described in Table 43-4. Hypotonic (tap water) and isotonic (normal saline solution) enemas are large-volume enemas that result in rapid colonic emptying. The large volumes of solution (adults, 500 to 1000 mL; infants, 150 to 250 mL) may present a danger to patients with weakened intestinal walls. These solutions often require special preparation and equipment. Hypertonic solution preparations are available commercially and are administered in smaller volumes (adult, 70 to 130 mL). These solutions draw water into the colon, which stimulates the defecation reflex. They may be contraindicated in patients for whom sodium retention is a problem.

Retention Enemas. Retention enemas are retained in the bowel for a prolonged period for different reasons.

Oil-retention enemas: lubricate the stool and intestinal mucosa, making defecation easier. About 150 to 200 mL of solution is administered to adults.

Carminative enemas: help to expel flatus from the rectum and provide relief from gaseous distention. Common solutions include the milk-and-molasses enema (equal parts) and the MGW enema (30 mL of magnesium sulfate, 60 mL of glycerin, and 90 mL of warm water).

Medicated enema: used to administer medications that are absorbed through the rectal mucosa

Anthelmintic enemas: administered to destroy intestinal parasites

Nutritive enemas: administer fluids and nutrition rectally

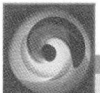

Table 43-4
Commonly Used Enema Solutions

Solution	Amount	Action	Time to Take Effect	Adverse Effects
Tap water (hypotonic)	500–1000 mL	Distends intestine, increases peristalsis, softens stool	15 min	Fluid and electrolyte imbalance, water intoxication
Normal saline (isotonic)	500–1000 mL	Distends intestine, increases peristalsis, softens stool	15 min	Fluid and electrolyte imbalance, sodium retention
Soap	500–1000 mL (concentrate at 3–5 mL/1000 mL)	Distends intestine, irritates intestinal mucosa, softens stool	10–15 min	Rectal mucosa irritation or damage
Hypertonic	70–130 mL	Distends intestine, irritates intestinal mucosa	5–10 min	Sodium retention
Oil (mineral, olive, or cottonseed oil)	150–200 mL	Lubricates stool and intestinal mucosa	30 min	

Return-Flow Enemas. *Return-flow,* or *Harris flush,* enemas are occasionally prescribed to expel flatus. For an adult, 100 to 200 mL of a solution is instilled into the rectum and sigmoid colon, and then the solution container is lowered so that the solution flows back into the container. This process is repeated five or six times, and the alternating flow of solution stimulates peristalsis and aids in the expelling of flatus. The procedure is terminated when abdominal distention is relieved. If the return solution becomes thick with feces, it is replaced by fresh solution.

Equipment

Commercially prepared enema kits include a flexible bottle containing hypertonic solution with an attached prelubricated firm tip about 5 to 7.5 cm (2 to 3 inches) long. Its ease of use makes it particularly convenient in the home. Patients can readily administer their own enema in many instances.

For tap water, saline solution, or soap solution enema, a container, rubber or plastic tubing with side openings near its distal end, a tubing clamp, lubricant, and the solution are necessary. Although the commercially prepared equipment is sterile and reusable equipment is sterilized between patients in a health agency, the procedure for administering an enema requires clean or medical asepsis technique, not sterile technique. Disposable gloves protect the caregiver from exposure to blood, body substances, and microorganisms.

Patient Preparation

Because enemas are a common procedure, some patients already understand why they are used and how they are administered. Patients who have not previously experienced an enema need an explanation of its purpose, what they can expect, and how they can participate. The procedure offers an excellent opportunity for health teaching because many people are not familiar with the functioning of the intestinal tract. Failure to provide explanations and protect privacy may result in the patient finding the procedure disagreeable.

A reclining position during the enema is recommended, but a patient with a respiratory disorder may need the head of the bed elevated slightly. Results are usually ineffective if the enema is given in Fowler's position because the solution remains in the rectum and expulsion occurs rapidly with minimal cleansing effect.

Some patients think the solution is to be expelled as soon as possible. When the solution is to be retained, care should be taken to have the patient understand this.

Administering an Enema Using a Large Volume of Solution

The procedure for administering a cleansing enema using either a large volume of solution or a commercially prepared solution is described in Procedure 43-1.

Administering an Enema Using a Hypertonic Solution

Administering a cleansing enema using a hypertonic solution differs from the procedure described in Procedure 43-1 in the following ways:

- The equipment is included in the commercially prepared set. The only additional equipment needed is the bedpan for a bedridden patient and a disposable waterproof pad to protect bed linens.
- It is unnecessary to warm the hypertonic solution. Administer it at room temperature, and warm it only if it is very cold.
- The side-lying position is usually used. The knee–chest position helps to distribute the solution throughout the lower intestinal tract and is recommended if the patient can assume it. Additional lubrication of the rectal tips is recommended, even though they are prelubricated.
- The solution is forced into the rectum by applying gentle pressure on the collapsible solution container. It should take 1 to 2 minutes to administer the enema.
- The hypertonic enema solution (Fleet enema) should be administered cautiously to a patient with hemorrhoids. The rigid tip may tear fragile rectal mucosa that is enlarged and inflamed, causing pain, torn rectal tissue, and necrosis. A rectal examination and generous lubrication are recommended before inserting the enema tip.

Administering an Oil-Retention Enema

The procedure for giving an oil enema differs from that of giving a cleansing enema in the following respects:

- A small rectal tube is used. The small size helps to reduce intestinal contractions so that the patient can retain the oil more easily. Oil enemas are available in commercial kits similar to those for hypertonic solution enemas. The kits contain a small rectal tube.
- Oil is given at body temperature to minimize muscle contractions caused by a warmer or cooler solution.
- The patient should be instructed to retain the oil for at least 30 minutes for best cleansing results.

Rectal Suppositories

A **suppository** is a conical or oval solid substance shaped for easy insertion into a body cavity and designed to melt at body temperature. Various rectal suppositories are available. Some are fecal softeners, others have direct action on the nerve endings in the rectal mucosa, and some liberate carbon dioxide when moistened. Fecal softeners are useful when the stool is very hard; substances that stimulate the rectal nerves are helpful for people with weak muscle tone or poor innervation. The carbon dioxide suppositories liberate about 200 mL of gas, which causes distention, causing stimulation and elimination impulses (see the accompanying Guidelines for Nursing Care box).

Oral Intestinal Lavage

An oral solution, such as GoLYTELY or Colyte, can be used to cleanse the intestine of feces. This solution is prescribed by the physician and can be administered before diagnostic (*text continues on page 1204*)

PROCEDURE 43-1

Administering a Cleansing Enema

Equipment

Disposable enema set
Water-soluble lubricant
Solution as ordered by physician:
  Temperature:
    For adult—105°–110F (40°–43°C)
    For children—100°F (37.7°C)
  Amount: Will vary, depending on
    type of solution, age of the
person, and the patient's ability to retain the solution. Average cleansing enema for an adult may range from 750 to 1000 mL.
Necessary additives (soap, salt, and so forth)
Bath thermometer
Waterproof pad
Bath blanket
Bedpan and toilet tissue
IV pole
Disposable gloves
Paper towel
Washcloth, soap, and towel or Handi-wipes

Action	Rationale
1. Assemble the necessary equipment. Warm solution in amount ordered, and check temperature with a bath thermometer if available. If tap water is used, adjust temperature as it flows from faucet.	Organization facilitates performance of task. If bath thermometer is not available, warm to room temperature or slightly higher, and test on inner wrist.
2. Explain the procedure to the patient and plan where he or she will defecate. Have a bedpan, commode, or nearby bathroom ready for his use.	The patient is better able to relax and cooperate if he or she is familiar with the procedure and knows everything is in readiness when the urge to defecate is felt. Defecation usually occurs within 5 to 15 minutes.
3. Wash your hands.	Handwashing deters the spread of microorganisms.
4. Add enema solution to container. Release the clamp and allow fluid to progress through tube before reclamping.	This causes any air to be expelled from the tubing. Although allowing air to enter the intestine is not harmful, it may further distend the intestine.
5. Position waterproof pad under the patient.	This protects bed linen.
6. Provide for patient's privacy. Position and drape the patient on the left side (Sims' position) with anus exposed or on the back, as dictated by patient comfort and condition.	The patient's comfort and warmth help him or her relax. The exact position of the reclining person has not been found to alter results of an enema significantly.
7. Put on disposable gloves.	This protects the nurse from microorganisms in the feces.
8. Elevate the solution so that it is 45 cm (18 inches) above the level of the patient's anus. Plan to give the solution slowly over a period of 5 to 10 minutes. The container may be hung on an IV pole or held in the nurse's hands at the proper height.	Gravity forces the solution to enter the intestine. The amount of pressure determines the rate of flow and pressure exerted on the intestinal wall. Giving the solution too quickly causes rapid distention and pressure in the intestine, resulting in too rapid expulsion of the solution, poor defecation, or damage to the mucous membrane.
9. Generously lubricate the end of the rectal tube for 5 to 7 cm (2–3 inches). A disposable enema set may have a prelubricated rectal tube.	This facilitates passage of the rectal tube through the anal sphincter and prevents injury to the mucosa.
10. Lift the buttock to expose the anus. Slowly and gently insert the rectal tube 7 to 10 cm (3–4 inches). Direct it at an angle pointing toward the umbilicus.	Good visualization of the anus helps prevent injury to tissues. The anal canal is about 2.5 to 5 cm (1–2 inches) in length. The tube should be inserted past the internal sphincter. Further insertion may damage intestinal mucous membrane. The suggested angle follows the normal intestinal contour. Slow insertion of the tube minimizes spasms of the intestinal wall and sphincters.

(continued)

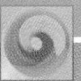

PROCEDURE 43-1

Administering a Cleansing Enema (Continued)

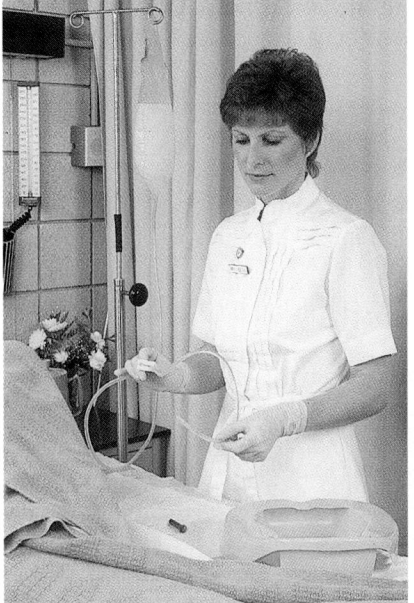

Action 8: Preparing to administer the enema.

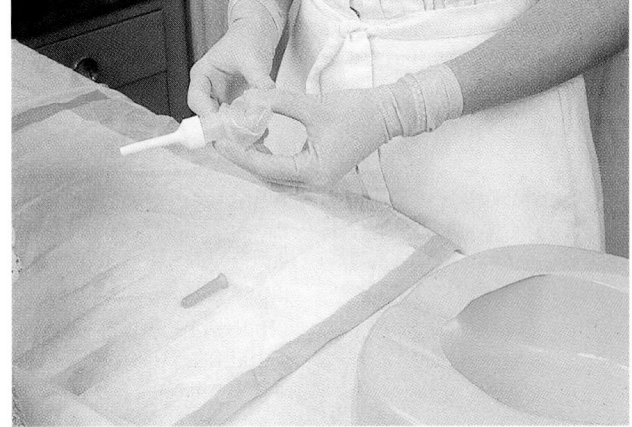

Action 12: Technique for compressing Fleet enema container.

11. If the tube meets resistance while inserting it, permit a small amount of solution to enter, withdraw the tube slightly and then continue to insert it. Do not force entry of the tube. Ask the patient to take several deep breaths.

Resistance may be due to spasms of the intestine or failure of the internal sphincter to open. The solution may help to reduce spasms and relax the sphincter, thus making continued insertion of the tube safe. Forcing a tube may injure the intestinal wall. Taking deep breaths helps relax the anal sphincter.

12. Introduce the solution slowly over a period of 5 to 10 minutes. Hold tubing all the time that solution is being instilled. Commercial preparations may be administered by compressing container with hands, according to package directions (see photo).

Introducing the solution slowly helps prevent rapid distention of the intestine and a desire to defecate.

13. Clamp the tubing or lower the container if the patient has the desire to defecate or cramping occurs. Patient also may be instructed to take small, fast breaths or to pant.

These techniques help relax muscles and prevent the expulsion of the solution prematurely.

14. After solution has been given, clamp the tubing and remove the tube. Have paper towel ready to receive tube as it is withdrawn. Have the patient retain the solution until the urge to defecate becomes strong, usually in about 5 to 15 minutes.

This amount of time usually allows muscle contractions to become sufficient to produce good results.

15. Remove disposable gloves from inside out and discard.

This protects the nurse from contact with any microorganisms.

16. When the patient has a strong urge to defecate, place him or her in a sitting position on a bedpan or assist to a commode or to the bathroom.

The sitting position is most natural and facilitates the act of defecation.

(continued)

17. Record the character of the stool and the patient's reaction to the enema. Remind the patient not to flush commode before nurse inspects results of enema.	The nurse needs to observe and record the results. Additional enemas may be necessary if physician has ordered enemas "until clear."
18. Assist patient if necessary with cleaning of anal area. Offer washcloth, soap, and water to wash patient's hands.	Deters spread of microorganisms.
19. Leave the patient clean and comfortable. Care for the equipment properly.	There is abundant growth of bacteria in the intestine, which can be spread to others when equipment is not properly cared for.
20. Wash your hands.	Handwashing deters the spread of microorganisms.

Age Considerations	Infirm or elderly patients who are unable to retain the enema solution should receive the enema while on the bedpan in the supine position. For comfort, the head of the bed can be elevated 30 degrees if necessary and pillows used appropriately. Disposable gloves protect the hands as the enema is being expelled.
	Modify amount of solution according to client's ability to tolerate procedure and size of patient.
Home Care Considerations	Give enema in area that is as close to bathroom as possible. If using bedpan or commode, have it readily accessible.
	Inform patient about availability of commercially prepared solutions and equipment.
Special Considerations	The limit for "enemas until clear" is usually three. Check with the physician before continuing with additional enemas because fluid and electrolyte imbalance can occur.

tests that require a clear bowel for visualization purposes or as a "bowel prep" before intestinal surgery. Evacuation of feces usually begins within 1 hour after the first glass and is completed within 4 to 6 hours. As with an enema, a clear return indicates that the bowel preparation is complete. A clear diet for 24 hours before taking this solution lessens the time needed for completion of the bowel prep, but potassium replacement may be required before surgery because of the limited potassium in a clear diet. The solution has a slightly salty taste and is easier to tolerate if it is cold and consumed quickly. Older patients require careful assessment because they are more prone to electrolyte imbalances (Abrams, 1998).

Digital Removal of Stool

Fecal impaction is prolonged retention or an accumulation of fecal material that forms a hardened mass in the rectum. Fecal impaction often prevents the passage of normal stools. Small amounts of fluid may go around the impacted mass, and liquid fecal seepage with no passage of normal feces is a symptom of an impaction.

If a patient with a fecal impaction cannot expel the fecal mass voluntarily, and oil and cleansing enemas fail to break up the mass, the impaction must be broken up manually. A physician's order is required. This procedure may cause great discomfort to the patient as well as irritation of the rectal mucosa and bleeding. Digital removal of a fecal mass can stimulate the vagus nerve, resulting in a slowed heart rate. If this occurs, the procedure should be terminated immediately and the physician notified. The following technique is recommended:

1. Have a second person assist with the procedure. The second person can assure and comfort the patient while the first person works to break up the mass.
2. Place the patient in a side-lying position.
3. Place a bedpan on the bed for removed feces to be deposited into it.
4. Drape the patient to preserve privacy yet provide easy access.
5. Use clean gloves for the procedure because the intestinal tract is not sterile.

Guidelines for Nursing

Inserting a Rectal Suppository

- Use a glove for protection while inserting the suppository.
- Have the patient lie on either side, and pie-fold top linens over him or her.
- Lubricate the suppository and fingertips to reduce irritation on intestinal mucosa while inserting the suppository.
- Separate the buttocks and then have the patient relax by breathing through the mouth while the suppository is inserted.
- Introduce the suppository well beyond the internal sphincter (4 inches for adults and 2 inches for children and infants) so that the suppository is in the rectum, where its effect is desired.
- Avoid embedding the suppository in the fecal mass. Correct placement when there is stool in the rectum is between the stool and the rectal mucosa.
- Be sure the patient understands that he or she is to retain the suppository, usually for 30 to 45 minutes after insertion.

- Encourage the patient to walk about if ambulatory; this often helps promote peristalsis.

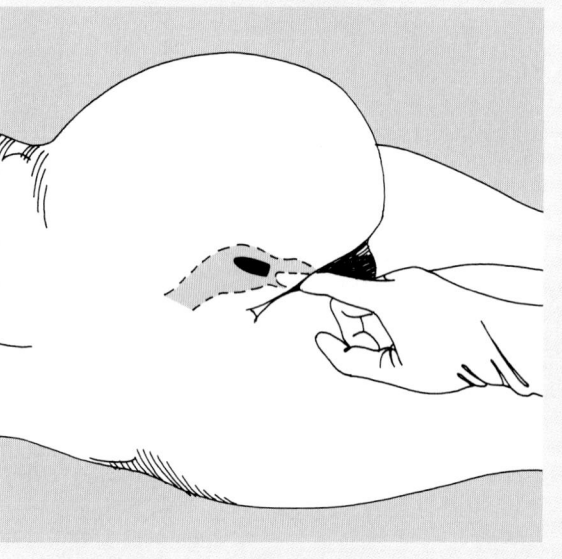

6. Lubricate the forefinger generously to reduce irritating the rectum, and insert the finger *gently* into the anal canal. The presence of the finger added to the mass tends to cause discomfort for the patient if the work is not done slowly and gently.
7. Work the finger around and into the hardened mass to break it up and then remove pieces of it. Instruct the patient to bear down, if possible, while extracting feces to ease in removal.
8. Remove the impaction at intervals if it is severe. This helps to avoid discomfort as well as irritation, which can injure intestinal mucosa.
9. Use an oil-retention enema if necessary. The enema may be given before attempts are made to break up and remove the impaction digitally, or it may be ordered after digital attempts fail. A cleansing enema is often ordered after an oil-retention enema.

Figure 43-5 demonstrates the procedure for removal of fecal impaction. Many patients find that a sitz bath or tub bath after this procedure soothes the irritated perineal area.

Managing Bowel Incontinence

Bowel incontinence is the inability of the anal sphincter to control the discharge of fecal and gaseous material. The cause of incontinence is usually an organic disease, resulting either in a mechanical condition that hinders the proper functioning of the anal sphincter or an impairment in the nerve supply to the anal sphincter. Mental illness may also cause a patient to be indifferent to the passage of stool. Although bowel incontinence is seldom a threat to life, incontinent patients suffer embarrassment, may become emotionally disturbed, and pose a challenge for nurses because of the risk for skin breakdown.

Nursing interventions that are helpful for a patient who suffers from bowel incontinence are as follows:

- Note when incontinence is most likely to occur, and place the patient on a bedpan at those times. If there is no pattern, offer a bedpan at regular intervals, such as every few hours.
- Keep the skin clean and dry by using proper hygienic measures. Pressure ulcers may develop when such measures are overlooked.
- Change bed linens and clothing as necessary to avoid odor, skin irritation, and embarrassment. Disposable bed pads and moisture-proof undergarments can be considered but should not be used until other measures have been attempted.
- Confer with the physician about using a suppository or a daily cleansing enema. These measures empty the lower colon regularly and often help to decrease incontinence. Bowel training programs may be helpful.

Rectal Indwelling Catheter

In many healthcare agencies, the rectal indwelling catheter has been used for patients with uncontrollable diarrhea. Relatively little research supports the safety of this procedure. Some nurses claim that the rectal indwelling catheter

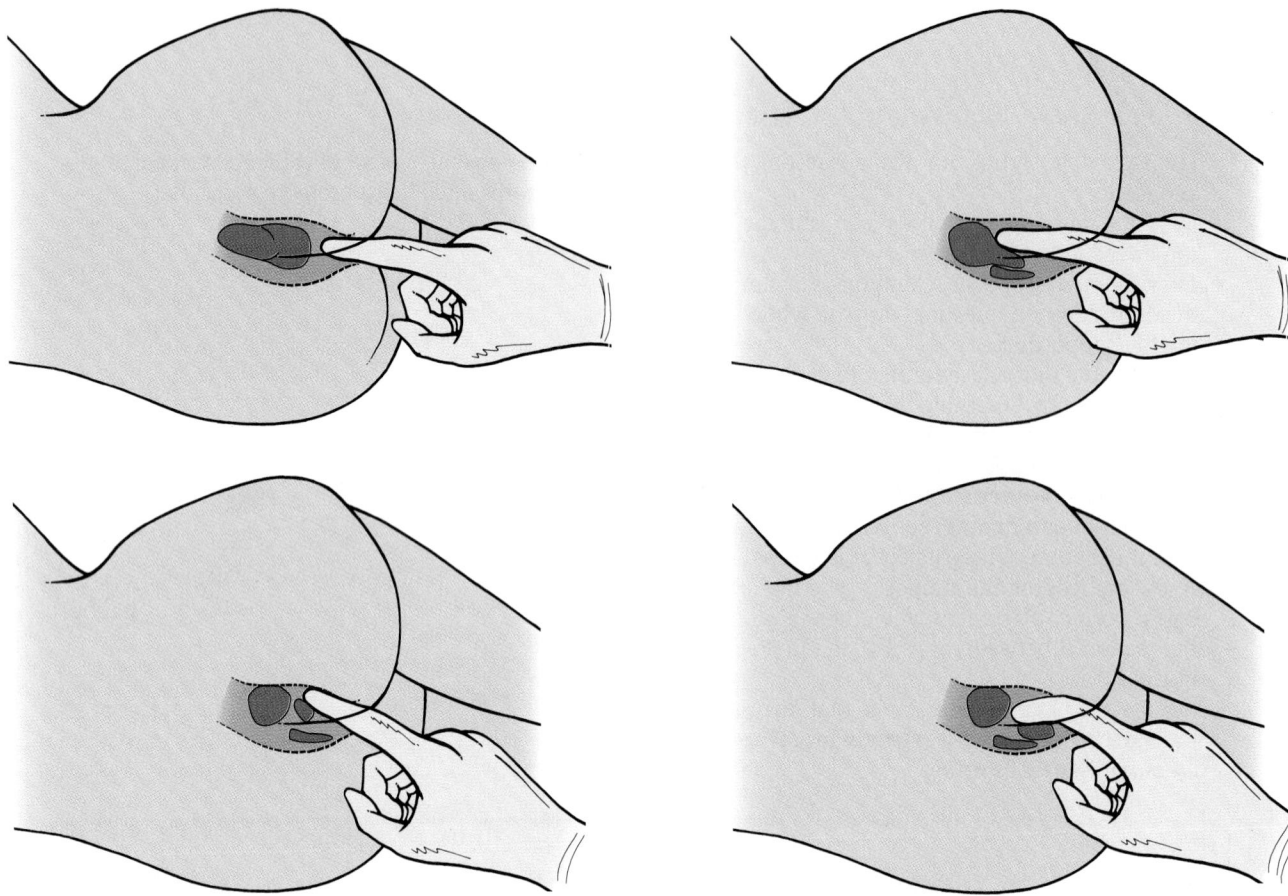

Figure 43-5
Digital removal of fecal impaction. *Step 1:* Inserting the gloved, lubricated finger into the fecal mass. *Step 2:* Using the finger to break up some of the hardened mass. *Step 3:* Breaking off a section of the impaction. *Step 4:* Removing a section of the impaction.

stimulates sensory nerve fibers in the rectum, thus increasing peristalsis and worsening the diarrhea. Others are concerned about the danger of rectal perforation and the development of mucosal necrosis. Most experts agree that indwelling rectal catheters should not be used to manage large volumes of diarrhea.

Fecal Incontinence Pouch

An alternative measure to protect perianal skin from repeated episodes of fecal incontinence is the fecal incontinence pouch. This device can be secured around the anal opening and attached to gravity drainage, allowing liquid stool to accumulate in a collection bag. It is best applied before the perianal area becomes excoriated, but a skin barrier is effective if this has already occurred.

Nursing responsibilities include careful regular assessment and documentation of the perianal skin condition and attentive management of the drainage system. The pouch should be changed at least every 72 hours, or sooner if it is not intact or leakage has occurred. Family members may need explanation and support to understand the benefits of this system.

Designing and Implementing Bowel Training Programs

Patients with a history of chronic constipation and impaction and those who are incontinent of stool may benefit from a **bowel training program**. The purpose of this program is to manipulate factors within the person's control (food and fluid intake, exercise, time for defecation) to produce the elimination of a soft, formed stool at regular intervals without laxative support. This effort to regain bowel control may be initiated in the healthcare setting or the patient's home. Steps in a bowel training program are described in the accompanying Nursing Interventions Classification box of standardized interventions. When the patient has established a pattern of regular defecation, continue to offer assistance with toileting at the successful time but discontinue use of the suppository if one was used.

Using the Nursing Interventions Classification (NIC)

Bowel Training

- Plan bowel program with patient and appropriate others.
- Instruct patient about which foods are high in bulk.
- Ensure adequate fluid intake.
- Initiate an uninterrupted, consistent time for defecation.
- Ensure privacy.
- Administer suppository, as appropriate.
- Evaluate bowel status regularly.
- Modify bowel program, as needed.

From McClosky, J., & Bulechek, G. [2000]. *Nursing interventions classification [NIC]* [3rd ed.] [p. 190]. St. Louis: C. V. Mosby. A full listing of nursing activities for each nursing intervention can be found in this book.

Meeting Needs of Patients With Bowel Diversions

Sometimes, surgical procedures are required to create an opening into the abdominal wall for fecal elimination. The intestinal mucosa is brought out to the abdominal wall, and a **stoma** is formed by suturing the mucosa to the skin. The word **ostomy** is a general term for an opening into the body; it is usually used to refer to an opening created for the excretion of body wastes. An **ileostomy** allows liquid fecal content from the ileum of the small intestine to be eliminated through the stoma. A **colostomy** permits formed feces from the colon to exit through the stoma. Figure 43-6 shows the location of an ileostomy and variously placed colostomies.

A *continent ileostomy* is an alternative to the traditional surgical procedure. An internal pouch is created that the patient accesses through a nipple-like valve constructed from the ileum on the abdominal wall. An advantage is that the patient is not required to wear an external collection device, but because the value malfunctions frequently, this procedure has limited use at this time. Another surgical alternative that does not involve an external stoma is the creation of an *ileoanal reservoir*. The terminal ileum is sutured directly to the anus, a pouch is created, and the patient is able to control expulsion of feces through the intact anal sphincter (Fig. 43-7). This procedure also has complications, and candidates are carefully selected for this surgery.

An ileostomy or colostomy may be either temporary or permanent. Temporary ostomies are performed to allow the intestine to repair itself after inflammatory disease, some types of intestinal surgery, or injury. Permanent ostomies are performed for debilitating intestinal diseases or cancer of the colon or rectum. Clinical texts further discuss the pathophysiologic conditions for which ostomies are required.

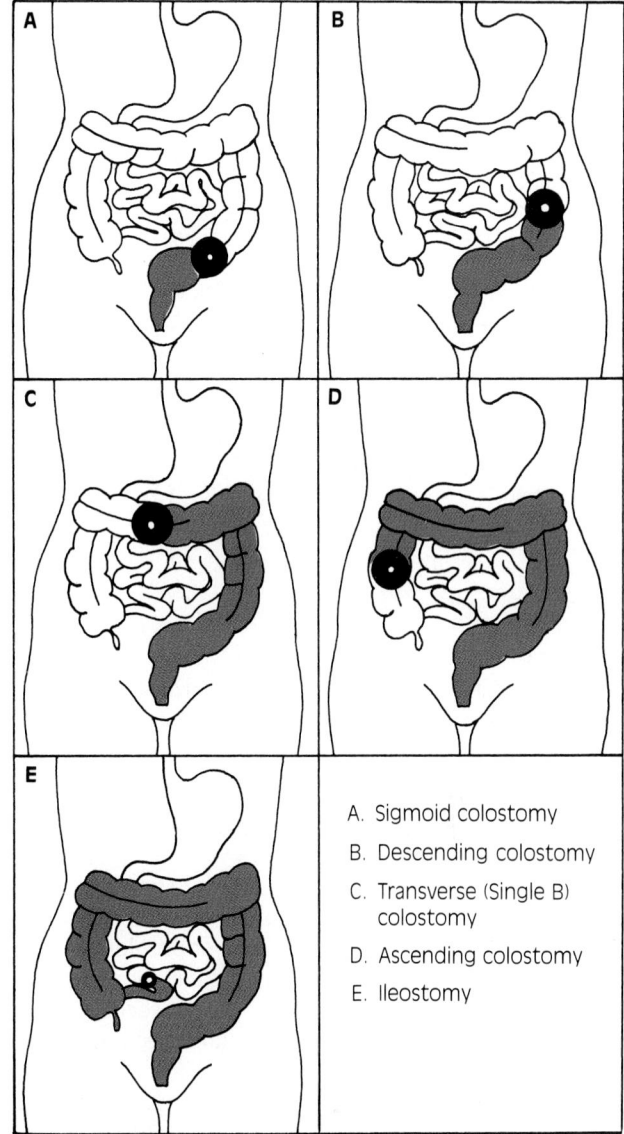

A. Sigmoid colostomy
B. Descending colostomy
C. Transverse (Single B) colostomy
D. Ascending colostomy
E. Ileostomy

Figure 43-6
(**A–D**) Location of various colostomies, and (**E**) the location of an ileostomy. The *shaded portions* represent the sections of the bowel that have been removed or are currently inactive.

Colostomy and Ileostomy Care

The patient with an ostomy needs physical and psychological support both preoperatively and postoperatively. This support can come from the patient's significant others as well as from members of the health team and from people who have had similar experiences. The ostomy requires specific physical care for which the nurse is initially responsible. The following guidelines help to promote the ostomy patient's physical and psychological comfort:

- Keep the patient as free of odors as possible. The application of a temporary appliance after surgery or during the time of the first dressing change postoperatively can eliminate much of the fecal odor

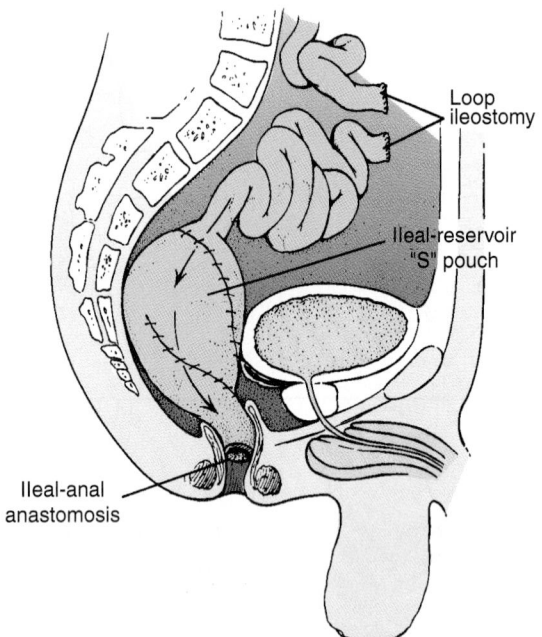

Figure 43-7
Ileoanal reservoir. (From Smeltzer, S. C. & Bare, B. G (2000). *Brunner & Suddarth's textbook of medical-surgical nursing* (9th ed.). Philadelphia: Lippincott Williams & Wilkins.)

from a bulky dressing. The ostomy appliance should be emptied frequently.

- Check the patient's stoma regularly. The color should be dark pink to red and moist. A pale-colored stoma may indicate anemia, and a dark or purple-blue stoma may reflect compromised circulation or ischemia (Bradley & Pupiales, 1997). Bleeding around the stoma and its stem should be minimal.

The physician should be notified promptly if bleeding persists or is excessive or if color changes occur in the stoma. The size of the stoma stabilizes within 6 to 8 weeks. Most stomas protrude $\frac{1}{2}$ to 1 inch from the abdominal surface and may initially appear swollen and edematous. After 6 weeks, the edema has usually subsided. If an abdominal dressing is in place, it should also be checked frequently for drainage and bleeding. Figure 43-8 compares varieties of stomal appearance.

- Keep the skin around the stoma site (peristomal area) clean and dry. If care is not taken to protect the skin around the stoma, irritation or infection may occur. A leaking appliance frequently causes skin erosion.
- Measure the patient's fluid intake and output. Check the ostomy appliance for the quality and quantity of discharge. Intake and output should be recorded every 4 hours for the first 3 days after surgery. If the patient's output decreases while intake remains stable, the condition should be reported promptly.
- Explain each aspect of care to the patient and explain what his or her role will be when he or she begins self-care. Patient teaching is one of the most important aspects of colostomy care and should include family members when appropriate.
- Encourage the patient to participate in care and to look at the ostomy. Patients normally experience emotional depression during the early postoperative period. The nurse can help the patient to cope by listening, explaining, and being available and supportive. A visit from a representative of the local ostomy support group may be helpful. Patients usually begin to accept their altered body image when they are willing to look at the stoma, make neutral or positive statements concerning the ostomy, and express interest in learning self-care.

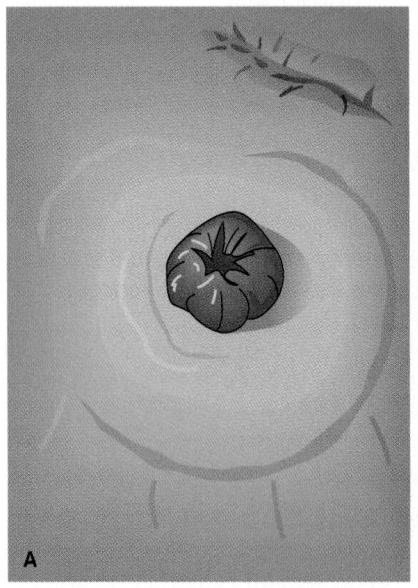
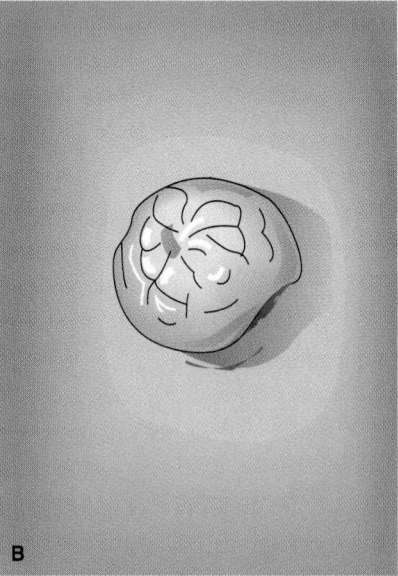
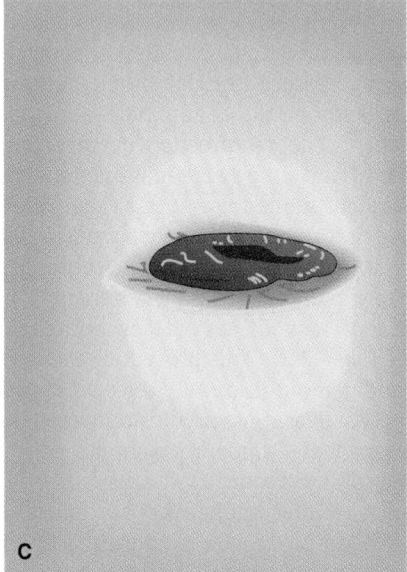

Figure 43-8
Comparison of stomal appearance. (**A**) Normal-appearing stoma is bright red, moist, and perfectly round. (**B**) A pale stoma indicates severe anemia. (**C**) Eroded skin around the area may lead to a flush stoma.

Changing the Ostomy Appliance

The ostomy appliance should protect the skin, collect the fecal discharge, and control odor. For the first few days after surgery, most patients wear an open-ended *appliance* or *pouch* that allows for drainage of fecal material without removing the appliance. The *skin barrier* has an adhesive that also protects the surrounding skin from the stoma output (O'Brien, 1999). Appliances are either one-piece (barrier already attached to the pouch) or two-piece (separate pouch that fastens to the barrier). Appliances can be either drainable or closed. It is unusual to see any output from a colostomy until normal peristalsis returns (2 to 5 days). An ileostomy drains within 24 to 48 hours because of the liquid contents in the small intestine. A pouch that can be drained should be emptied when it is one-third full and replaced every 3 to 7 days. Nondrainable pouches require removal and changing when they are half full. The drainable pouch is cleansed by rinsing the inside with tepid water and wiping the lower 2 inches of the pouch with tissue to remove any fecal material. Types of ostomy equipment are illustrated in Figure 43-9 and include the following:

- Various types of one-piece and two-piece pouches (drainable and nondrainable)
- Skin-barrier rings that surround the stoma and protect the peristomal skin
- Clamps that securely close drainable pouches

Changing or emptying an ostomy appliance is shown in Procedure 43-2.

Colostomy Irrigation

Ileostomies are not irrigated because the fecal content of the ileum is liquid and cannot be controlled. Irrigations may be used to help promote regular evacuation of some colostomies, typically those in the lower right portion of the colon. Various factors, such as the site of the colostomy in the colon and the patient's and physician's preferences, determine whether a colostomy is irrigated.

If an irrigation is to be done, the nurse should familiarize the patient with the technique to be used. The nurse should explain the procedure, demonstrate the equipment, and explain how the return fluid can be directed into a bedpan, commode, or toilet bowl. It may also be helpful to have a family member learn the irrigation techniques in case there are times when the patient cannot do the irrigation. The procedure for irrigating a colostomy is similar to that for administering an enema, except that the irrigating catheter is inserted into the abdominal stoma instead of into the anus. A commercially obtained irrigation set usually has all the equipment needed and comes with explicit directions.

In many health agencies, ostomy care, colostomy irrigations, and patient teaching are done by specially trained enterostomal therapists.

Long-Term Ostomy Care

The patient can live an active and useful life with an ostomy. He or she should be aware of community resources available for assistance, such as home healthcare nurses, special clinics, and ostomy support groups. The patient should be encouraged to seek medical follow-up care on a regular basis.

(*text continues on page 1212*)

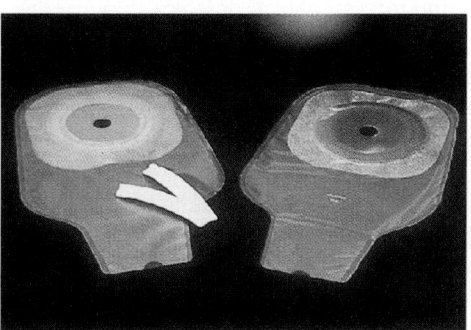

One-piece pouch

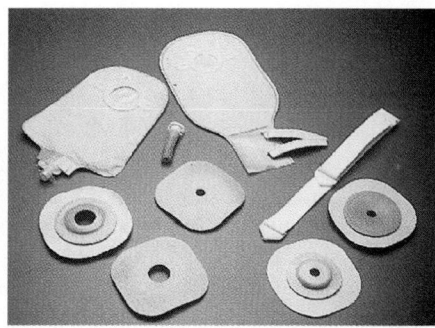

Two-piece pouch

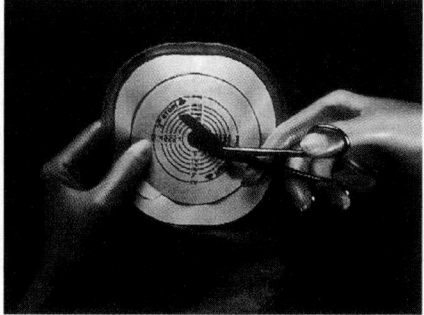

Cut-to-fit pouch

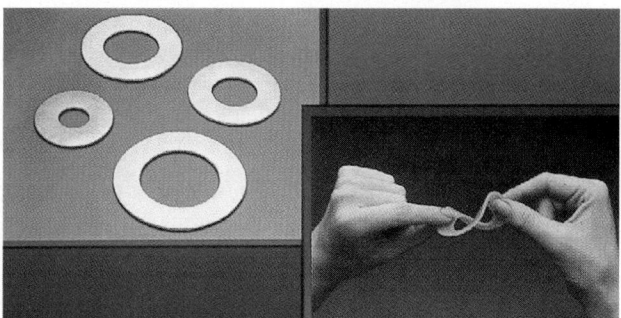

Skin-barrier rings

Figure 43-9
Examples of ostomy pouches, closures, and skin barriers. This equipment comes in various models and sizes. Convex pouches, belts, and other devices to prevent leaks and irritation are also available.

PROCEDURE 43-2

Changing or Emptying an Ostomy Appliance

Equipment

Clean ostomy appliance
Closure clamp
Stoma measuring guide
Scissors
Toilet tissue
Cleansing products (warm water,
    mild soap [optional], washcloth,
    and towel)

Adhesive solvent (optional)
Plastic bag
Toilet or bedpan
Water or special solution to clean
    pouch

Gauze pad
Disposable gloves
Disposable pad (optional)
Skin barrier (optional)
Deodorant for pouch (optional)

Action	Rationale
1. Assemble the necessary equipment	Organization facilitates performance of the task.
2. Explain the procedure to the patient.	The patient is better able to cooperate and learn the technique when he or she is aware of the procedure.
3. Wash your hands and don disposable gloves.	Handwashing deters the spread of microorganisms. Gloves protect the nurse from exposure to blood or microorganisms in the feces.
4. Provide for patient's privacy. Assist to a comfortable sitting or lying position in bed or a standing or sitting position in the bathroom.	Either position should allow the patient to view the procedure in preparation for learning to apply it independently. Lying flat or sitting upright facilitates smooth application of the appliance.

To Change the Pouch

Action	Rationale
5. Empty the partially filled appliance into a bedpan if it is a drainable pouch.	Emptying the contents before removal of the pouch prevents accidental spillage of fecal material. Pouches that are too full can detach or leak.
6. Slowly remove the appliance beginning at the top while keeping the abdominal skin taut. If any resistance is felt, use warm water or the adhesive solvent to facilitate removal. Discard the disposable pouch in the plastic bag.	Careful removal protects the underlying skin from damage and minimizes discomfort for the patient. Solvent is rarely necessary to ease removal of the pouch.
7. Use toilet tissue to remove any excess stool from the stoma. Cover stoma with a gauze pad. Gently wash and pat dry the peristomal skin. Mild soap or a cleansing agent may be used according to agency policy.	Soap may not be recommended because it may be irritating to the peristomal skin. Toilet tissue, used gently, will not damage the stoma. The gauze absorbs any drainage from the stoma while the skin is being prepared.
8. Assess the appearance of the peristomal skin and stoma. A moist, reddish-pink stoma is considered normal.	Any change in normal appearance may indicate either anemia (pale stoma) or altered circulation (bluish purple color), and the physician should be notified.
9. Apply the skin barrier and appliance together (wafer or disc style): • Select size for stoma opening by using the measurement guide. • Trace same size circle on the back and center of the skin barrier. • Use scissors to cut an opening ¼- to ⅛-inch larger than stoma.	Placing both the skin barrier disc and the appliance together over the stoma makes application easier for the patient. The opening is cut slightly larger to prevent irritation to the stoma as peristalsis occurs. Smooth application of the pouch prevents escape of odor and feces. The warmth from the nurse's hands facilitates a tight seal.

(continued)

PROCEDURE 43-2

Changing or Emptying an Ostomy Appliance (Continued)

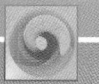

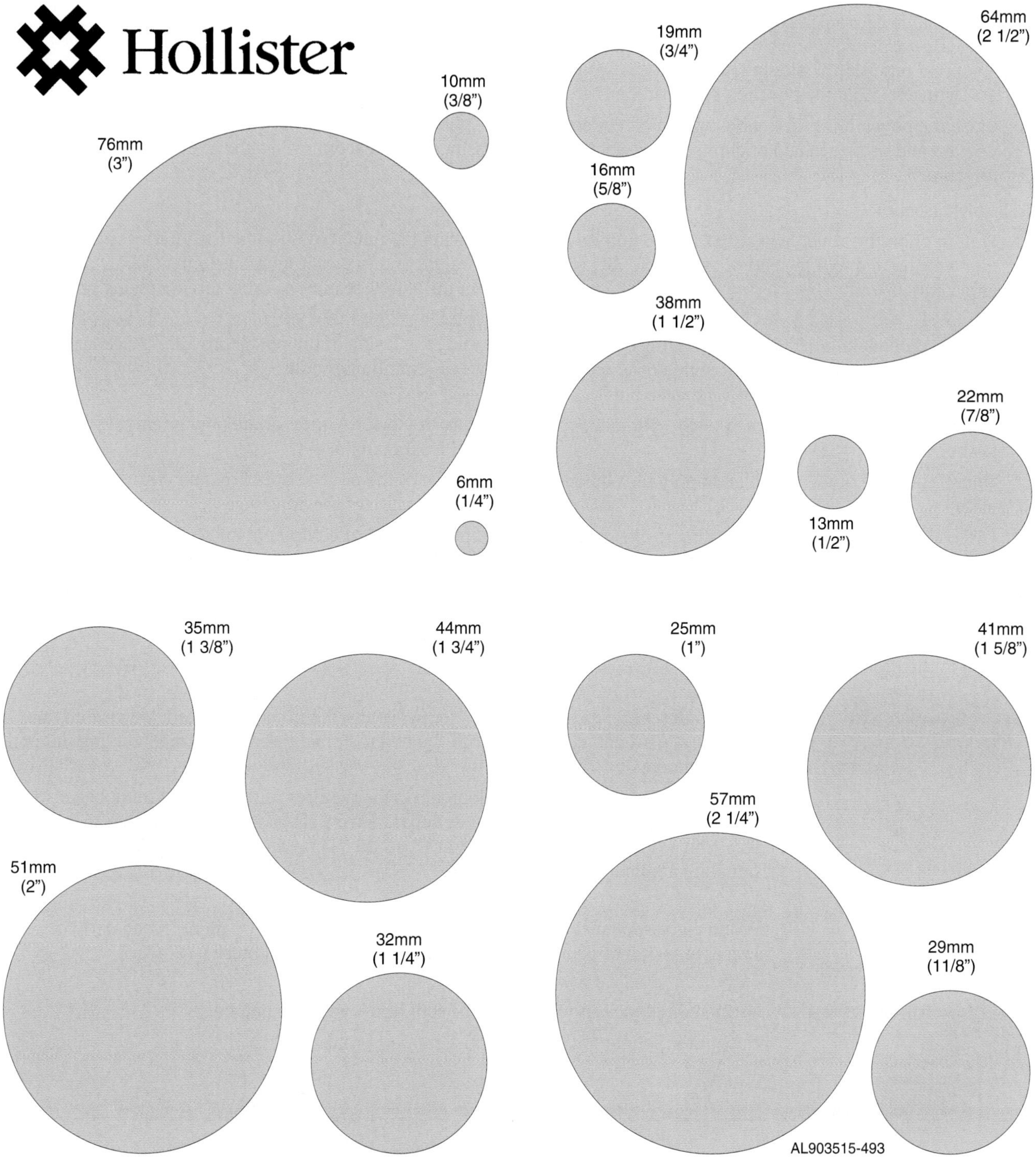

Hollister
76mm
(3")
10mm
(3/8")
6mm
(1/4")
19mm
(3/4")
16mm
(5/8")
38mm
(1 1/2")
64mm
(2 1/2")
13mm
(1/2")
22mm
(7/8")
35mm
(1 3/8")
44mm
(1 3/4")
51mm
(2")
32mm
(1 1/4")
25mm
(1")
41mm
(1 5/8")
57mm
(2 1/4")
29mm
(11/8")
AL903515-493

(continued)

- Remove the backing to expose sticky side.
- Remove gauze pad covering stoma.
- Ease barrier and pouch over the stoma and gently press onto skin while smoothing out creases or wrinkles. Hold the pouch in place for 5 minutes.

10. Close the pouch if it is drainable by folding the end upward and using a clamp or clip (see manufacturer's directions).

A tightly sealed appliance will not leak and cause embarrassment and discomfort for the patient.

To Empty the Pouch

11. Plan to drain the pouch when it is ⅓ to ½ full. Remove clamp and fold the end of the pouch upward like a cuff.

Allowing the pouch to fill more than half-way increases its weight and makes it more likely to separate or loosen from the skin. Creating a cuff before emptying prevents additional soilage and odor.

12. Empty contents into bedpan or toilet. Rinse pouch with tepid water or water mixed with a drop of mouthwash administered with a squeeze bottle.

Rinsing the inside of the pouch provides a cleaner appearance and minimizes odor.

13. Wipe the lower 2 inches of the pouch with toilet tissue.

Drying the lower section of the pouch removes any additional fecal material.

14. Uncuff the edge of the pouch and apply the clip or clamp.

The edge of the pouch should remain clean. The clamp secures closure of the appliance.

15. Dispose of used equipment according to agency policy. Remove gloves and wash hands.

Proper disposal of equipment and handwashing prevent contamination from microorganisms.

16. Document appearance of stoma, condition of peristomal skin, characteristics of drainage (amount, color, consistency, unusual odor), and patient's reaction to the procedure.

Careful documentation facilitates continuity of care.

Special Considerations	Many different types of appliances are available; the nurse should always read manufacturer's instructions or check with the enterostomal therapist before handling unfamiliar equipment.
	Flatus may cause a pouch to balloon out. This requires immediate attention because if flatus is not released, the pouch may separate from the skin barrier, causing seepage of fecal contents or release of fecal odor. Open the clamp and release the flatus. Never puncture a hole in the appliance.
Age Considerations	A one-piece appliance makes application easier for an older patient, particularly if impaired vision or compromised mobility from arthritis is present.
Home Care Considerations	Written directions should always be sent home with the patient.
	Encourage patient to participate in a support group.

Ostomy patients are encouraged initially to avoid foods high in fiber content (eg, foods with skins, seeds, and shells) as well as any other foods that cause diarrhea or excessive amounts of flatus (Table 43-5). By gradually adding new foods, the ostomy patient can build up to a normal diet. Foods that are bothersome should be avoided. The patient should be instructed to drink at least two quarts of fluids, preferably water, daily.

Health teaching about medication use is frequently overlooked for ostomy patients. Some medications may

Table 43-5
Nutritional Impact on Ostomies

Foods that should be eaten in moderation for a person who has a *colostomy* or *ileostomy*:

- Foods that may increase odor

Asparagus	Eggs
Broccoli	Fish
Brussel sprouts	Garlic
Cabbage	Onions
Cauliflower	Some spices

- Foods and beverages that may increase gas

Beans	Cauliflower
Beer	Corn
Broccoli	Cucumbers
Brussel sprouts	Mushrooms
Cabbage	Peas
Carbonated beverages	Spinach

- Foods and beverages that may thicken stools

Applesauce	Peanut butter (creamy,
Bananas	not chunky)
Buttermilk	Pretzels
Cheese	Rice
Marshmallows	Tapioca pudding
Milk (boiled)	Toast
Noodles (any type)	Yogurt

- Foods and beverages that may cause loose stools

Beer or other alcohol	Green beans
Broccoli	Prunes or prune juice
Fresh fruits	Spicy foods
(except bananas)	Spinach
Grape juice	

Foods that are high in fiber and can cause blockages that may not easily pass through the stoma in the person with an *ileostomy*:

- Foods that are high in fiber

Celery	Meats with casings
Chinese vegetables	(sausage, weiners,
Coconut	bologna)
Cole slaw (raw cabbage)	Mushrooms
Corn	Nuts
Dried Fruits	Popcorn
Foods with nondigestible	
peels (apples, potatoes,	
grapes)	

From *Managing your colostomy* and *Managing your ileostomy* (1997). Illinois: Hollister Incorporated.

discolor the stool and cause unusual odors, some may cause constipation, and some may not dissolve or be absorbed completely because the small bowel is where most absorption occurs. Ostomy patients should use liquid, chewable, or injectable forms rather than long-acting, enteric-coated, or sustained-release medications. Laxatives and enemas are dangerous because they may cause severe fluid and electrolyte imbalance.

Patients with ostomies should also be taught various methods of odor control. The chlorophyll content in dark green vegetables helps to deodorize the feces when these vegetables are included in the diet, and buttermilk, cranberry juice, and yogurt can also effectively prevent odor (Bradley & Pupiales, 1997). The enterostomal therapist can help with the selection of odor-control strategies.

Some patients can achieve control over fecal elimination from a colostomy by regular irrigations and by habitual emptying of the colon at a certain time each day. Few patients with an ileostomy gain any degree of control of excretion and seldom may dispense with the use of an appliance, except for short periods.

The ostomy patient can resume normal activity, including work. Direct physical contact sports and heavy lifting should be avoided. The patient can go swimming and need only wear gauze or a large adhesive bandage over the stoma. Whenever travel is required, the patient should carry a 1- to 2-day supply of equipment in a carry-on bag in case checked luggage is lost.

Providing Comfort Measures

Comfort measures related to defecation include working with the patient to develop a bowel elimination routine that results in the easy passage of a soft, formed stool; being attentive to perineal hygiene and the maintenance of skin integrity; and using warm moist heat (sitz bath or tub bath) to soothe the perineal area. Additional nonsurgical treatment options include the following (Smeltzer & Bare, 2000):

- A high-residue diet that includes fruit and bran
- Use of a laxative that absorbs water as it passes through the intestines and softens the stool
- Ointments or astringents (witch hazel)
- Suppositories that contain anesthetics
- Bed rest

EVALUATING

The nurse evaluates the effectiveness of the plan of care to promote regular bowel elimination by checking to see if the patient has met the individualized patient goals specified in the plan. Nursing care is considered effective if the patient expresses satisfaction with his or her regular pattern of defecation and the ability to pass a soft, formed stool comfortably without the use of medications or laxatives. The plan of care is most successful when the patient is able to accomplish the following:

- Verbalize the relationships among bowel elimination and nutrition, fluid intake, exercise, and stress management
- Develop a plan to modify any factors that contribute to current bowel problems or that might adversely affect bowel functioning in the future.

See the accompanying Applying Learning to Practice: Patient Care Study and Nursing Plan of Care boxes.

(text continues on page 1216)

APPLYING LEARNING TO PRACTICE

Patient Care Study

Jeremy Green, 4 years of age, height 45 inches (114.3 cm), weight 36 lb (16.3 kg), was placed in day care when his mother returned to work 6 months ago. He presents at the hospital with a diagnosis of viral gastroenteritis. A comprehensive nursing assessment included the following notations:

- Admitted with complaints of diarrhea beginning 3 days ago
- Seen today by pediatrician who recommended admission and work-up to exclude causes other than viral
- Mother reports liquid stools (no observable blood, pus, or mucus) six to seven times daily beginning 3 days ago with amounts of "one to two cups."

- Urgency results in soiling of pants.
- Child has sipped boiled skim milk and cola and eaten a small amount of broth and a few pretzels but has no appetite.
- Complained of nausea and vomited twice 3 days ago
- Child is pale and eyes are sunken.
- Skin is warm and dry with decreased turgor, dry mucous membranes.
- Hyperactive bowel sounds
- Height, 45 inches; weight, 36 lb; temperature, 99.8°F (rectally); pulse, 88 beats/min; respiratory rate, 18 breaths/min
- Mother reported several other children in same day care center are out sick with diarrhea

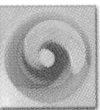

NURSING PLAN OF CARE
for Jeremy Green

Nursing Diagnosis	Diarrhea related to unknown cause (possibly viral, rule out malabsorption of lactose and other causes) as manifested by passage of liquid stools (1–2 cups) for 3 days; urgency with fecal soiling; anorexia, nausea, vomiting twice on day 1; signs of dehydration: decreased skin turgor, dry mucous membranes, sunken eyeballs
Expected Outcome	At the time of discharge, the patient will: • Voluntarily pass a formed stool of usual consistency (experience less or no diarrhea)

Nursing Interventions	Rationale	Evaluative Statement
Assess and chart frequency and amount of diarrhea, stool characteristics, precipitating factors, and accompanying manifestations (gastrointestinal symptoms, hyperactive bowel sounds).	This assists in identifying the cause of the diarrhea.	5/8/01 Goal partially met. No recurrence of liquid stools for 24 hours. *Revision:* Continue to monitor. *D. Lentsky, RN*

Expected Outcome	At the time of discharge, the patient will: • Exhibit decreased bowel sounds (8–10/min)

Nursing Interventions	Rationale	Evaluative Statement
Work collaboratively with the physician to identify the cause of the diarrhea. Obtain stool specimens and send to laboratory.	Correct treatment depends on identification of the cause of the diarrhea. Viral diarrhea is usually self-limiting and lasts 24 to 72 hours. Prolonged diarrhea after acute viral illness may be from temporary malabsorption of lactose or other simple sugars.	5/8/01 Goal met. Bowel sounds are normal. *D. Lentsky, RN*

(continued)

Nursing Interventions	Rationale	Evaluative Statement
Instruct Jeremy and his parents (if they want to participate in care) on correct enteric precautions for handling stool.	Prevents transmissions of infectious diarrhea to others.	
Increase frequency and length of rest periods and discourage strenuous activity.	Exercise and activity stimulate peristalsis.	
Administer prescribed antidiarrheal medication and observe for adverse effects.	Antidiarrheal medications may cause drowsiness and dizziness.	

Expected Outcome	At the time of discharge, the patient will:
	• Demonstrate signs of fluid and electrolyte balance: (1) improved skin turgor, (2) moist mucous membranes, and (3) normal eyeballs

Nursing Interventions	Rationale	Evaluative Statement
Continue to assess hydration status and be alert to signs of electrolyte imbalance.	Reestablishing normal fluid and electrolyte balance by replacing ongoing fluid losses and providing maintenance fluids is a priority for the child with severe and prolonged diarrhea. Diarrhea stools contain large amounts of water and often are relatively low in sodium and high in potassium.	5/8/01 Goal partially met. Skin turgor improved, eyeballs normal, mucous membranes still dry. *Revision:* Continue to encourage PO fluids. Enjoys clear chicken broth and half-strength gelatin products. *D. Lentsky, RN*
Administer prescribed intravenous therapy and clear liquids—note patient response as new fluids and foods are added to the diet.	There is no ideal oral replacement fluid. Some may cause diarrhea or provide inappropriate amounts of electrolytes.	
Chart daily weight.	Daily weights are the most accurate indicator of fluid balance.	
Monitor intake and output. Note concentration of urine.	Urine becomes more concentrated when a person is dehydrated.	

Expected Outcome	At the time of discharge, the patient will:
	• Demonstrate signs of improved nutritional status: (1) eats low-fiber diet without abdominal cramping, nausea, or vomiting; and (2) maintains or increases admission weight

Nursing Interventions	Rationale	Evaluative Statement
Discontinue milk products and solid foods. Until the diarrhea resolves, offer a combination of clear liquids (half-strength apple juice or gelatin products; commercial products: Lytren, Pedialyte, 5% glucose water): 30 mL/hr for first 8 hours, then 60 to 90 mL every 1 to 2 hours if number of stools lessens.	If one fluid is used exclusively, inappropriate amounts of electrolytes may be provided. Commercial preparations tend to be expensive. Objective is to provide the necessary water, electrolytes, and minimal calories in a milk-free and solid-free diet—until the diarrhea resolves.	5/8/01 Goal met. Tolerating rice cereal and bananas. Gained 1 lb since admission. *D. Lentsky, RN*

(continued)

Nursing Interventions	Rationale	Evaluative Statement
As gastrointestinal symptoms subside, advance to other liquids and solids (bananas, applesauce, and rice cereal solidify stool)—milk should be the last liquid added.	Adding new fluids and foods slowly enables intolerances to be quickly detected.	

Expected Outcome

At the time of discharge, the patient will:
- Show no signs of skin breakdown in the perianal area

Nursing Interventions	Rationale	Evaluative Statement
Assess the perianal area after each passage of stool and note any irritation.	Perianal irritation is a common problem with severe diarrhea. The goal of treatment is prevention.	5/8/01 Goal partially met. Small area of excoriation remains around anus. Continue plan. *D. Lentsky, RN*
Wash and dry the area carefully after each episode of diarrhea and apply protective ointment (as ordered or per agency protocol).	Keeping the skin clean and dry and protected with a waterproof ointment or skin barrier may prevent breakdown.	

Sample Documentation

5/7/01 Nursing

Liquid stools have decreased to two in the past 24 hours. Negative report on stool culture. Normal bowel sounds auscultated in all four quadrants. Skin turgor normal and mucous membranes pink in color with moist appearance. Urine clear and light amber in color. Has gained 1 lb since admission. Jeremy stated this AM, "My stomach doesn't hurt so much anymore." Rice cereal and bananas will be added to diet tomorrow. Milk and milk products will be last items added to diet. Parents instructed to monitor child for manifestations of lactose intolerance.

D. Lentsky, RN

Learning Outcomes

After completing this chapter, the learner should be able to accomplish the following:

1. Define the key terms used in the chapter.

bowel movement	flatus
bowel training program	hemorrhoids
cathartic	ileostomy
chyme	incontinence (bowel)
colostomy	laxative
constipation	occult blood
diarrhea	ostomy
endoscopy	peristalsis
enema	stoma
fecal impaction	stool
feces	suppository
flatulence	Valsalva maneuver

2. Describe the physiology of bowel elimination.
3. Identify variables that influence bowel elimination.
4. Assess bowel elimination using appropriate interview questions and physical assessment skills.
5. Assist with the following diagnostic measures: stool collection for laboratory analysis and direct and indirect visualization studies of the gastrointestinal tract.
6. Develop nursing diagnoses that correctly identify bowel elimination problems amenable to nursing therapy.
7. Demonstrate how to (1) promote regular bowel habits (timing, positioning, privacy, nutrition, exercise); (2) use cathartics, laxatives, and antidiarrheals; (3) empty the colon of feces (enemas, rectal suppositories, rectal catheters, digital removal of stool); (4) design and implement bowel training programs; and (5) use comfort measures to ease defecation.
8. Describe nursing care for a patient with an ostomy.
9. Plan, implement, and evaluate nursing care related to select nursing diagnoses that involve bowel problems.

Critical Thinking Exercises

1. If you noticed the following when assessing a patient, what would you do?
   - Patient has frank blood in stool.
   - Parent reports that child's stool is unusually foul-smelling and greasy.
   - Patient's stool is ribbon-like.
   - Patient receiving cancer pain medication reports chronic constipation.
   - Teenager reports frequent episodes of diarrhea that leave her weak and dehydrated.

2. A 52-year-old man presents with acute stomach pain and altered bowel elimination: diarrhea. Role-play with another student the interview you would use to assess his bowel elimination status. Identify variables that make you, as either the nurse or patient, uncomfortable talking about elimination. Discuss how you can best address your discomfort.

Study Questions

1. The nurse encourages Mr. Brown to avoid foods that have a laxative effect. He is instructed to avoid
   a. cheese
   b. alcohol
   c. eggs
   d. pasta

2. Which of the following is a true statement about the effects of medication on bowel elimination?
   a. Diarrhea occurs with antibiotic use about 20% of the time.
   b. Anticoagulants cause a white discoloration of the stool.
   c. Narcotic analgesics increase gastrointestinal motility.
   d. Iron salts impair digestion and cause a green stool.

3. Mr. Jones has a fecal impaction. The nurse correctly administers an oil-retention enema by
   a. administering a large volume of solution (500 to 1000 mL)
   b. mixing milk and molasses in equal parts for an enema
   c. instructing the patient to retain the enema for at least 30 minutes
   d. following the return-flow or Harris flush procedure

4. As the nurse prepares to assist Mrs. Perez with her newly created ileostomy, she is aware that
   a. an appliance will not be required on a continual basis
   b. the size of the stoma stabilizes within 2 weeks
   c. irrigation is necessary for regulation
   d. fecal drainage will be liquid

5. The class of laxative that acts by causing stool to absorb water and swell is
   a. bulk forming
   b. emollient
   c. lubricant
   d. stimulant

6. Mr. Toney is nervous about a colonoscopy scheduled for tomorrow. The nurse describes the test by explaining that

   a. it allows visual examination of the esophagus and stomach
   b. it allows visual examination of the large intestine
   c. it is a radiographic examination of the large intestine
   d. it is a fluoroscopic examination of the small intestine

7. A bowel training program includes
   a. a diet that is low in bulk
   b. decreasing fluid intake to 1000 mL
   c. administering an enema once a day to stimulate peristalsis
   d. allowing ample time for evacuation

8. Your patient complains of excessive flatulence. Which food, if eaten regularly, may be responsible for this?
   a. meat
   b. cauliflower
   c. potatoes
   d. ice cream

9. The barium enema should be done before the upper gastrointestinal series because of which of the following?
   a. Retained barium may cloud the colon.
   b. Barium can cause lower gastrointestinal bleeding.
   c. The physician orders are in that sequence.
   d. Barium is absorbed readily in the lower intestine.

10. Nurses should recommend to their patients the avoidance of habitual use of laxatives. Which of the following is the rationale for this?
    a. They will cause a fecal impaction.
    b. They will cause chronic constipation.
    c. They change the pH of the gastrointestinal tract.
    d. They inhibit the intestinal enzymes.

11. Which of the following is the physiology behind a hypertonic solution enema?
    a. bowel mucosa irritation
    b. diffusion of water out of colon
    c. osmosis of water into colon
    d. softening of fecal contents

12. Which of the following is the rationale for discouraging use of rectal Foley catheters?
    a. decrease peristalsis

b. require a physician's order
c. cause rectal necrosis
d. prevent the liquid stool from draining

13. During removal of a fecal impaction, which of the following could occur because of vagal stimulation?
    a. bradycardia
    b. atelectasis
    c. tachycardia
    d. cardiac tamponade

14. Which of the following would be a common nursing diagnosis for the patient with an ileostomy?

a. Body Image Disturbance
b. Constipation
c. Altered Growth and Development
d. Fluid Volume Excess

15. Your patient who is experiencing flatulence would be helped if he were placed in which of the following positions?
    a. Trendelenburg position
    b. knee–chest position
    c. semi-Fowler's position
    d. Fowler's position

Answers With Rationale

1. The correct response is *b*. All the foods listed except alcohol have a constipating effect.

2. The correct response is *a*. Anticoagulants may result in the stool having a pink to red to black appearance, whereas iron salts also cause a black stool. Narcotic analgesics decrease gastric motility.

3. The correct response is *c*. The usual amount of solution administered with a retention enema is 150 to 200 mL for an adult. The milk-and-molasses mixture is a carminative enema that helps to expel flatus, as does the Harris flush procedure.

4. The correct response is *d*. An appliance is usually required on a continual basis because the fecal drainage is liquid. Stoma size usually stabilizes within 4 to 6 weeks, and irrigation is not necessary because fecal matter is liquid.

5. The correct response is *a*. Emollients lubricate the stool; lubricants soften the stool, making it easier to pass; and stimulants promote peristalsis by irritating the intestinal mucosa or stimulating nerve endings in the intestinal wall.

6. The correct response is *b*. An esophagogastroduodenoscopy allows visual examination of the esophagus and stomach. The radiographic examination of the large intestine is a barium enema, and a fluoroscopic examination of the small intestine is an upper gastrointestinal series.

7. The correct response is *d*. For a bowel training program to be effective, the patient must have ample time for evacuation (usually 20 to 30 minutes). Fluid intake is increased to 2500 to 3000 mL; food high in bulk is recommended as part of the program; and a daily enema is not administered in a bowel training program. A cathartic suppository may be used 30 minutes before the patient's usual defecation time to stimulate peristalsis.

8. The correct response is *b*. Cauliflower is a gas-producing food that results in flatulence.

9. The correct response is *a*. The barium enema should always precede the upper gastrointestinal series because retained barium from the latter may take several days to pass through the gastrointestinal tract and may cloud anatomic detail on the barium enema studies.

10. The correct response is *b*. Habitual use of laxatives is the most common cause of chronic constipation.

11. The correct response is *c*. Hypertonic solutions draw water into the colon by osmosis, thus stimulating the defecation reflex. Oil solutions soften fecal contents, and soap solutions distend the intestine and irritate the bowel mucosa.

12. The correct response is *c*. Concern for mucosal necrosis is one of the main reasons that the use of rectal Foley catheters is discouraged. Nurses also feel that the catheter stimulates sensory nerve fibers in the rectum, thus worsening diarrhea. The catheter allows liquid feces to drain, and the necessity of obtaining a physician's order is not a factor in determining the safety of the rectal catheter.

13. The correct response is *a*. Removing a fecal impaction manually may result in stimulation of the vagal nerve and a resulting bradycardia.

14. The correct response is *a*. Constipation cannot occur with an ileostomy because the drainage is liquid. Growth and development are not affected by the formation of an ileostomy. Fluid volume excess is unlikely to occur because the drainage is liquid and probably continual.

15. The correct response is *b*. Because gas rises, the knee–chest position facilitates the passage of flatus.

Bibliography

Abrams, A. (1998). *Clinical drug therapy* (5th ed.). Philadelphia: Lippincott Williams & Wilkins.

American College of Physicians. (1997). Suggested techniques for fecal occult blood testing and interpretation in colo-rectal cancer screening. *Annals of Internal Medicine, 126*(5), 808.

Benton, J., O'Hara, P., Chen, H., Harper, D., & Johnston, S. (1997). Changing bowel hygiene practice successfully: A program to reduce laxative use in a chronic care hospital. *Geriatric Nursing, 18*(1), 12–17.

Bradley, M., & Pupiales, M. (1997). Essential elements of ostomy care. *American Journal of Nursing, 97*(7), 38–45.

Cerrato, P. (1999). When food is the culprit. *RN, 62*(6), 52–58.

Dammel, T. (1997). Fecal occult-blood testing. *Nursing, 27*(7), 44–45.

Dunne, D. (1997). Common questions about ileoanal reservoirs. *American Journal of Nursing, 97*(11), 67–75.

Eisenhauer, L., Nichols, L., Spencer, R., & Bergan, F. (1998). *Clinical pharmacology and nursing management* (5th ed.). Philadelphia: Lippincott Williams & Wilkins.

Fischbach, F. (1998). *A manual of laboratory diagnostic tests* (6th ed.). Philadelphia: Lippincott Williams & Wilkins.

Fries, C. (1999). Managing an ostomy. *Nursing, 29*(8), 26.

Kirton, C. (1997). Assessing bowel sounds. *Nursing, 27*(3), 64.

Mackenzie, D. (1999). When *E. coli* turns deadly. *RN, 62*(7), 28–31.

McClosky. J., & Bulechek, J. (1996). *Nursing interventions classification (NIC)* (2nd ed.). St. Louis: C. V. Mosby.

North American Nursing Diagnosis Association. (1999). *NANDA nursing diagnosis: Definitions & classification, 1999–2000.* Philadelphia: Author.

O'Brien, B. (1999). Coming of age with an ostomy. *American Journal of Nursing, 99*(9), 71–75.

Pagana, K., & Pagana, T. (1998). *Manual of diagnostic and laboratory tests.* St. Louis: C. V. Mosby.

Phipps, W., Sands, J., & Marek, J. (1999). *Medical-surgical nursing: Concepts & clinical practice* (6th ed.). St. Louis: C. V. Mosby.

Pillitteri, A. (1999). *Maternal and child health nursing* (3rd ed.). Philadelphia: Lippincott Williams & Wilkins.

Sheff, B. (1999). Microbe of the month: *Escherichia coli (E. coli)* 0157.H7. *Nursing, 29*(5), 25.

Smeltzer, S., & Bare, B. (2000). *Brunner and Suddarth's textbook of medical–surgical nursing* (9th ed.). Philadelphia: Lippincott Williams & Wilkins.

Stewart, K. (1998). Helping your patient contend with constipation. *Nursing, 28*(6), 32hn24–32hn26.

Tolch, M. (1997). 4 Steps to teaching ostomy care. *Nursing, 27*(6), 32hn9–32hn10.

Weber, J., & Kelley, J. (1998). *Health assessment in nursing.* Philadelphia: Lippincott Williams & Wilkins.

Chapter 44
Oxygenation

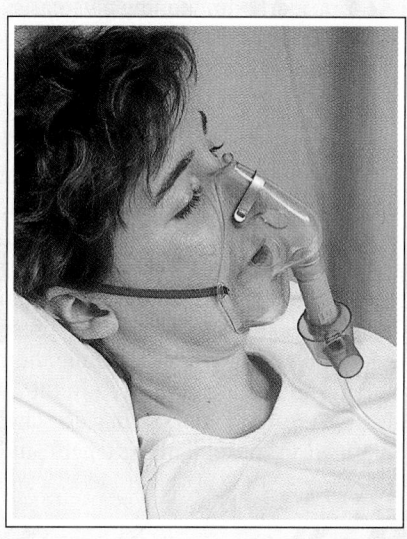

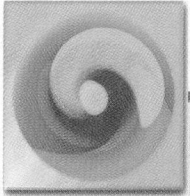

**Thinking Critically About
Nursing's Blended Skills**

Before reading this chapter, think about the types of skills you will need to nurse people effectively with respiratory problems.

- Jeremy, a 2-year old, is brought to the emergency room gasping for breath. His parents are frantic. You suspect an acute asthma attack and immediately work to protect his airway.

- Jim is in the medical intensive care unit on a ventilator. Efforts are being made to wean him from the ventilator, but he has been unable to breathe on his own for any length of time. He has written notes asking you to "let him go" the next time he fails to be weaned.

- Wheeling a resident into the dining room, you observe another resident choking and clutching her throat. She seems unable to speak or cough.

- You are invited to speak with local high school students about the dangers of smoking.

- Laura reports during her health history that she and her husband visit an "oxygen bar" several times a week. "We sit back in recliners, they hook us up to an oxygen tank, and I can feel my stress melting away. It seems to clear my head and renews my energy. I recommend it for anyone."

What cognitive, technical, interpersonal, and ethical/legal skills do you think you will need to meet the needs of the patients described above?

ost people take respiratory functioning for granted, but adequate respiratory functioning is necessary for life. Living cells require oxygen. The air passages must remain patent (open) for oxygen to enter the system. Any condition that interferes with normal functioning must be minimized or eliminated to prevent pulmonary distress, which could lead to death.

Normal functioning depends on essentially three factors:

- The integrity of the airway system to transport air to and from the lungs
- A properly functioning alveolar system in the lungs to oxygenate venous blood and to remove carbon dioxide from the blood
- A properly functioning cardiovascular system to carry nutrients and wastes to and from body cells

This chapter describes the respiratory system's physiology and general purpose as well as general factors affecting respiratory functioning. Practical suggestions for performing a comprehensive respiratory assessment are included. Sample interview questions for both a general and focused respiratory history are presented, along with a description of the nursing examination. Laboratory and radiology studies are addressed in the assessment. After analyzing the data, nurses decide whether the respiratory data lead to a problem statement, indicate another prob-

lem, or are the possible cause of a problem. Numerous examples of nursing diagnoses are given. Expected patient outcomes and specific nursing strategies for implementation are described. The concluding patient care study illustrates how, with knowledge of respiratory functioning and skilled nursing interventions, the nurse resolves respiratory problems successfully.

Physiology of Respiration

Knowing the basic anatomy and physiology of the respiratory system helps nurses understand assessment findings and the rationale for nursing interventions.

The Respiratory System

The airway is a pathway for the transport and exchange of oxygen and carbon dioxide. The upper airway is composed of the nose, pharynx, larynx, and epiglottis. Its main function is to warm, filter, and humidify inspired air. The lower airway, known as the tracheobronchial tree, includes the trachea, right and left mainstem bronchi, segmental bronchi, and terminal bronchioles. Its major functions are conduction of air, mucociliary clearance, and production of pulmonary surfactant. *Cilia*, which are microscopic hairlike projections, propel sheets of mucus toward the upper

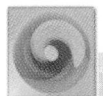

COGNITIVE SKILLS

- Knowledge of respiratory physiology and the variables that affect respiratory function
- Knowledge about how to use the nursing process to identify and care for patients with respiratory problems
- Knowledge of how to teach young people about the dangers related to smoking and to motivate healthy lifestyles
- Knowledge about new health beliefs and practices, such as "oxygen bars"

TECHNICAL SKILLS

- Ability to use the equipment and protocols necessary to diagnose and treat respiratory problems
- Competence in particular skills, such as Heimlich maneuver and ventilatory assistance

INTERPERSONAL SKILLS

- Strong people skills to establish trusting relationships with Jeremy and his parents, Jim, and the other patients

- Special interpersonal competence to help high school students value making the lifestyle changes necessary to improve their health and respiratory functioning
- A good working relationship with colleagues to make sure that all of the above patients receive excellent care

ETHICAL/LEGAL SKILLS

- First and foremost, a strong sense of accountability for the health and well-being of these individuals; a commitment to getting them the help they need to achieve their health goals—within the scope of your nursing responsibilities and available resources
- A willingness to hold colleagues accountable for safe and good-quality practice
- Knowledge of the ethical and legal principles that guide decision making about withholding and withdrawing life-sustaining medical treatment (ventilator)

airway so that the mucus can be removed (by coughing) after it has trapped cells, particles, and infectious debris. Fluid is necessary for the production of watery mucus normally present in the respiratory tract and for ciliary action. This covering of mucus also protects the underlying tissues from irritation and infection. A few milliliters of fluid between the pleural surfaces allows the lungs to move easily along the chest wall as they expand and contract. Without this fluid, filling and emptying of the lungs are difficult. *Surfactant*, a detergent-like phospholipid, reduces surface tension of the fluid lining the alveoli. When surfactant production is reduced, the lung becomes stiff, and the alveoli collapse.

The main organs of respiration, the lungs, are located within the thoracic cavity (Fig. 44-1). The right lung has three lobes, and the left has two lobes. Each lobe is further subdivided into segments or lobules. The right lung has 10 bronchopulmonary segments; the left has 8. The lungs extend from the base at the level of the diaphragm to the apex (top), which is above the first rib. The heart lies between the right and left lung. The lungs are composed of elastic tissue that can stretch or recoil. Normally, the elastic fibers are partially stretched at all times, partially filling the thoracic cavity. The actual lung is composed of **alveoli**, small air sacs at the end of the terminal bronchioles (Fig. 44-2). These structures are the site of gas exchange. The average adult has more than 300 million alveoli.

The *pleurae* are two-layered membranes: the visceral pleura covers the lungs, and the parietal pleura lines the

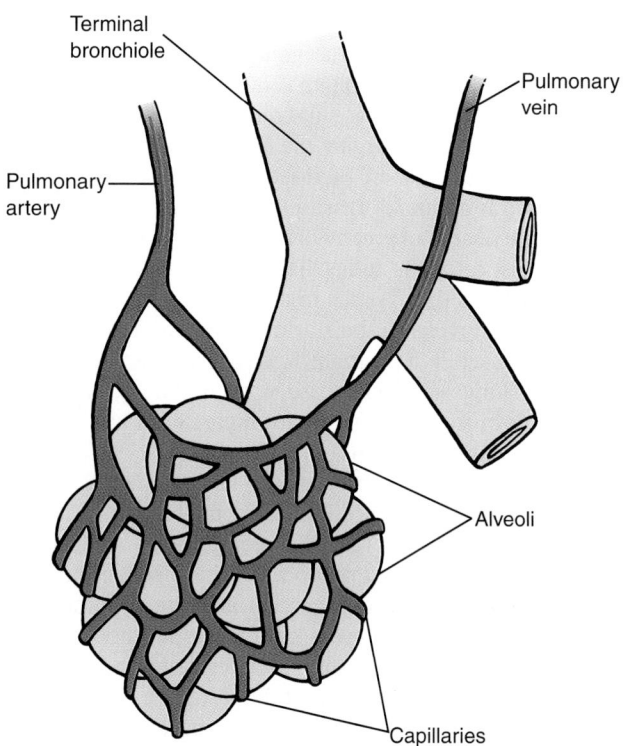

Figure 44-2
Alveoli and the intrapulmonary system where gas exchange occurs. The terminal bronchioles lead into the alveoli. Air in the alveoli and blood in the capillaries are separated by only a very thin partition, which is readily crossed by diffusing gases. The pulmonary artery carries unoxygenated blood to the capillaries, and the pulmonary veins return oxygenated blood to the left side of the heart.

thoracic cavity. These two are continuous with each other and form a closed sac. There is normally a potential space between them, not an actual space. Pleural fluid between the membranes acts as a lubricant and as an adhesive agent to hold the lungs in an expanded position. Pressure within the pleural space (intrapleural pressure) is always subatmospheric (a negative pressure). This constant intrapleural negative pressure is essential for normal ventilation.

Pulmonary Ventilation

Ventilation is the movement of air into and out of the lungs. The process of ventilation has two phases: inspiration (inhalation) and expiration (exhalation). **Inspiration,** the active phase, involves movement of muscles and the thorax to bring air into the lungs. **Expiration**, the passive phase, is the movement of air out of the lungs. The diaphragm and the intercostal muscles are responsible for normal inspiration and expiration.

Immediately before inspiration, the air pressure in the lungs is equal to that of the surrounding atmospheric pressure. According to *Boyle's law,* the volume of a gas at a constant temperature varies inversely with the pressure. This means that less pressure in the lungs facilitates the movement of more air into the lungs. The pressure within the lungs (intrapulmonic pressure) decreases as the volume of

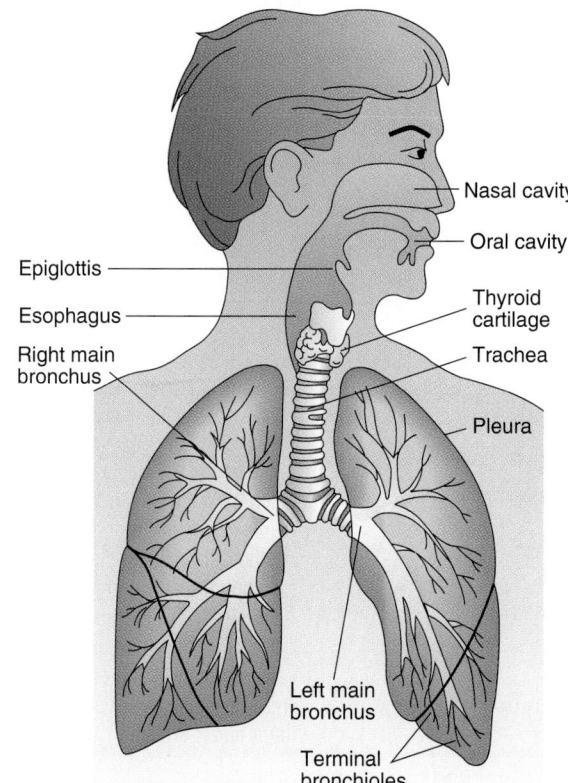

Figure 44-1
The organs of the respiratory tract.

the lungs increases. During inspiration, the following events occur: the diaphragm contracts and descends, lengthening the thoracic cavity; the external intercostal muscles contract, lifting the ribs upward and outward; and the sternum is pushed forward, enlarging the chest from front to back. This combination of an increased lung volume and decreased intrapulmonic pressure allows atmospheric air to move from an area of greater pressure (outside air) into the lesser pressure of the lungs. The relaxation, or recoil, of these structures then results in expiration. The diaphragm relaxes and moves up, the ribs move down, and the sternum drops back into position. This causes a decreased volume in the lungs and an increase in intrapulmonic pressure, and the air in the lungs moves from greater to lesser pressure and is expired (Fig. 44-3).

The accessory muscles of the abdomen, neck, and back are used to maintain respiratory movements at times when breathing is difficult. The condition of the body's musculature can affect the process of respiration. For example, when the respiratory center is depressed and pulmonary congestion is present, normal respiratory effort is compromised. The accessory muscles help to maintain movement of air into and out of the lungs.

The compliance of lung tissue also affects lung volume. *Lung compliance* refers to the stretchability of the lungs, the ease with which lungs can be inflated. Porth (1998) compares the varying changes in lung pressure and resulting lung compliance to differences in blowing up a new, noncompliant balloon versus one that was previously inflated. A stiff, noncompliant lung (like a new balloon) requires a greater inspiratory effort to inflate it. Emphysema, a chronic lung condition, and the normal changes associated with aging are examples of conditions that result in decreased elasticity in lung tissue, which decreases compliance. Surfactant increases the ease of inflation or lung compliance. Without surfactant, lung inflation would be very difficult.

Any impediment or obstruction that air meets as it moves through the airway is known as *airway resistance*. There is less airway resistance during inspiration than ex-

piration because the size of the airway opening is increased. Obstruction in any part of the normal passageways impedes respiration. Obstruction can be caused by a foreign substance, such as a piece of food, a coin, or a toy or by liquids, as in the case of a drowning victim. Obstruction can also result from tissues or secretions within the body (eg, excessive or thickened secretions, tumor growths, or edema in the respiratory tract). A decrease in the size of air passages resulting from constriction or to poor sitting, standing, and lying positions can also impede respiration.

Alveolar Gas Exchange

Respiration occurs at the terminal alveolar capillary system, where there is an exchange of gases between the air and blood (Fig. 44-4). The dense network of capillaries in the respiratory portion of the lungs and the thin alveolar walls facilitate gas exchange. *Diffusion* refers to the movement of oxygen and carbon dioxide between the air (in the alveoli) and the blood (in the capillaries). The appropriate gas moves passively from an area of higher concentration to an area of lesser concentration. The greater pressure of oxygen in the alveoli causes the oxygen to move into the capillaries containing unoxygenated venous blood. Likewise, the carbon dioxide in the returning venous blood exerts a greater pressure than the carbon dioxide in the air in the alveoli. The carbon dioxide diffuses across into the alveoli and is expired.

Diffusion of gases in the lung is influenced by four factors. Any change in the surface area available for diffusion negatively affects diffusion (eg, removal of a lung or the presence of a disease that destroys lung tissue). Incomplete lung expansion or lung collapse, known as **atelectasis**, prevents the pressure changes and the exchange of gas by diffusion in the lungs. Atelectatic areas of the lung cannot fulfill a function of respiration. Examples of conditions that predispose a patient to atelectasis include obstructions of the airway by foreign bodies, mucus, constricted airways, external compression by tumors or enlarged blood vessels,

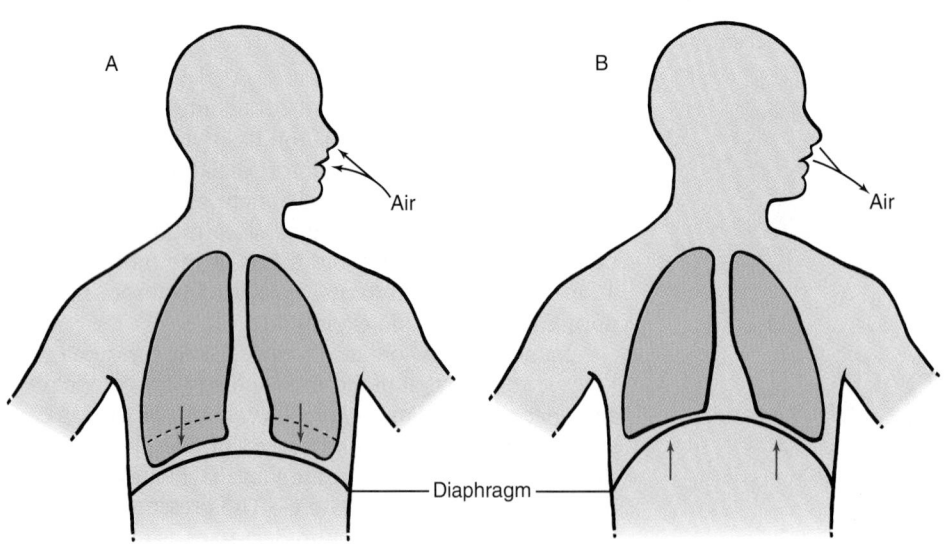

Figure 44-3
Movement of the diaphragm in ventilation. With inspiration (**A**), the diaphragm contracts and descends, the thoracic cavity lengthens, intrapulmonic pressure decreases, and air rushes in. With expiration (**B**), the diaphragm relaxes and moves upward, intrapulmonic pressure increases, and air moves out of the lungs and is expired.

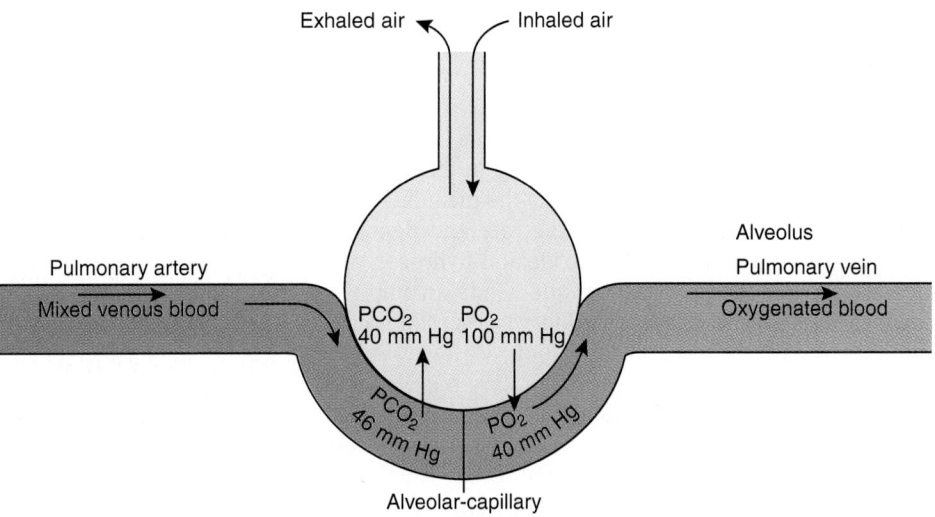

Figure 44-4
Gas exchange in the alveolus. The greater pressure of the oxygen in the air inhaled into the alveoli causes the oxygen to move into the capillaries, which contain unoxygenated blood. The carbon dioxide in the returning venous blood moves from the capillaries (area of greater concentration) into the alveoli (area of lesser concentration).

and immobility. Any disease or condition that results in thickening of the alveolar–capillary membrane (eg, pneumonia or pulmonary edema) makes diffusion more difficult. The *partial pressure*, or pressure resulting from any gas in a mixture depending on its concentration, can also affect diffusion. If environmental oxygen is reduced (eg, at higher altitudes and in the presence of toxic fumes), less is available for diffusion. When oxygen is administered therapeutically, the increased amount available results in greater diffusion across capillary membranes. Finally, the solubility and molecular weight of the gas are factors in diffusion; carbon dioxide has greater solubility in the respiratory membranes and diffuses more rapidly than oxygen.

This oxygenated capillary blood passes through tissue in the process called **perfusion**. The amount of blood flow through the lungs is a factor in the amount of oxygen and other gases that are exchanged. The amount of blood present in any given area of lung tissue depends partially on whether the person is sitting, standing, or lying down. Perfusion is greater in dependent areas. The perfusion of lung tissue also depends on the person's activity level. Greater activity results in increased cellular oxygen need and cardiac output and, consequently, in increased blood return to the lungs. In addition, perfusion depends on an adequate blood supply and proper cardiovascular functioning to carry oxygen and carbon dioxide to and from the lungs. Cardiovascular function is discussed in relation to vital signs in Chapter 24.

Transport of Respiratory Gases

Oxygen and carbon dioxide must move through the alveoli and be carried to and from body cells by the blood. Oxygen is carried two ways in the body. It is dissolved in plasma, but because oxygen is insoluble in liquids, little oxygen is carried in this way. The hemoglobin in red blood cells has a strong affinity for oxygen, and therefore most oxygen (97%) is carried in the body by red blood cells in the form of oxyhemoglobin. Hemoglobin also carries carbon dioxide easily. Any abnormality in the alveoli or in the blood's constituents affects internal respiration. (the exchange of oxygen and carbon dioxide between the circulating blood and the tissue cells). A decrease in cardiac output (eg, caused by hemorrhage or loss of blood) means a reduction in the amount of circulating blood that is available to deliver oxygen to the tissues. Any decrease in the amount of red blood cells or erythrocytes results in insufficient hemoglobin available to transport oxygen. Anemia occurs when the hemoglobin content of the blood is inadequate to meet the body's oxygen demands. Exercise can have a positive effect on the transport of oxygen because the heart pumps more effectively and cells are better able to utilize oxygen.

If a problem exists in any part of the respiratory process, **hypoxia**, the condition in which an inadequate amount of oxygen is available to cells, may occur. The most common symptoms of hypoxia are *dyspnea* (difficulty breathing), an elevated blood pressure with a small pulse pressure, increased respiratory and pulse rates, paleness, and cyanosis. Anxiety and restlessness are also common signs of hypoxia. Hypoxia is often caused by **hypoventilation**, a decreased rate or depth of air movement into the lungs. The effects of chronic hypoxia can be detected in all body systems and include altered thought processes, headaches, chest pain, enlarged heart, clubbing of the fingers and toes, anorexia, constipation, decreased urinary output, decreased libido, weakness of extremity muscles, and muscle pain. At the other extreme is **hyperventilation**, which is an increased rate and depth of ventilation above the body's normal metabolic requirements. This is discussed in more detail in the later Diagnosing section.

Control of Respirations

The medulla in the brain stem immediately above the spinal cord is the respiratory center. It is stimulated by an increased concentration of carbon dioxide and hydrogen ions and, to a lesser degree, by the decreased amount of oxygen in the arterial blood. Chemoreceptors in the aortic arch and carotid bodies are also sensitive to the same arterial blood gas levels and can activate the medulla. Stimulation of the medulla increases the rate and depth of ventilation to blow off carbon dioxide and hydrogen and increase oxygen levels. The medulla sends an impulse down the spinal cord to the respiratory muscles to stimulate a contraction leading to inhalation. If the system is intact, the diaphragm, the major respiratory muscle, contracts and descends into the abdomen. The thoracic cavity enlarges. The lungs expand in response to pressure changes in the intrapleural space and lungs. Inhalation ceases when the atmospheric air pressure and pulmonary air pressure are equal. Exhalation occurs, and the lungs return to their resting position.

Developmental Variations

Birth necessitates many adaptations by a newborn. The most obvious of these changes occur in the lungs, which are transformed from fluid-filled structures to air-filled organs. The normal infant's chest is small, the airways are short, and aspiration is a potential problem. The respiratory rate is more rapid in infants than at any other age (Table 44-1). As the alveoli increase in number and size, adequate oxygenation is accomplished at lower respiratory rates. Respiratory rates stabilize in young adulthood.

Respiratory activity is primarily abdominal in infants. The infant's chest wall is so thin and has so little musculature that the ribs, sternum, and xiphoid process are easily seen. Infants have a rounded chest wall in which the anteroposterior diameter (ie, the measurement from the front to back of the thorax) equals the transverse diameter. Occasional fine crackles at the end of deep inspiration (a sound that occurs when air moves through airways that contain fluids) heard on auscultation of the infant's thorax are normal.

In preschool-aged and school-aged children, some subcutaneous fat is deposited on the chest wall, making landmarks less prominent than in infants. Muscular development is also more noticeable. The ratio of transverse diameter to anteroposterior diameter reaches the adult configuration of 1:2 by the age 6 years. The preschool child's eustachian tubes, bronchi, and bronchioles are elongated and less angular, and therefore the average number of routine colds and infections decreases until they enter school and are exposed more frequently to pathogens. As well, young children usually have not had the opportunity to develop antibodies for the variety of viruses and bacteria they encounter. Good handwashing techniques and tissue etiquette are practices to be encouraged. Most children at this age experience colds or upper respiratory infections, but some have more serious problems of otitis media, bronchitis, and pneumonia. By the end of late childhood and during adulthood, the immune system is sufficiently seasoned to protect the person from most infections.

Specific physical changes occur in older people that are unrelated to any pathology. Bony landmarks are more prominent because of the loss of subcutaneous fat. Kyphosis (curvature of the spine) contributes to the older person's appearance of leaning forward. Barrel chest deformity (see Fig. 25-31 in Chap. 25) may result in an increased anteroposterior diameter; in the absence of any abnormal findings in the physical examination, this is known as senile emphysema. The tissues and airways of

Table 44-1
Respiratory Variations in the Life Cycle

	Infant (Birth–1 year)	Early Childhood (1–5 years)	Late Childhood (6–12 years)	Aged Adult (65+ years)
Respiratory rate	30–60 breaths/min	20–40 breaths/min	15–25 breaths/min	16–20 breaths/min
Respiratory pattern	Abdominal breathing, irregular in rate and depth	Abdominal breathing, irregular	Thoracic breathing, regular	Thoracic, regular
Chest wall	Thin, little muscle, ribs and sternum easily seen	Same as infant's but with more subcutaneous fat	Further subcutaneous fat deposited, structures less prominent	Thin, structures prominent
Breath sounds	Loud, harsh crackles at end of deep inspiration	Loud, harsh expiration longer than inspiration	Clear inspiration is longer than expiration	Clear
Shape of thorax	Round	Elliptical	Elliptical	Barrel shaped or elliptical

the respiratory tract (including alveoli) become more rigid with age. The power of respiratory and abdominal muscles is reduced, and therefore the diaphragm moves less efficiently. These alterations increase the risk for disease, especially pneumonia.

Factors Affecting Respiratory Functioning

A variety of factors affect adequate respiratory functioning. Six important factors are described in the following sections.

Levels of Health

People with renal or cardiac disorders often have compromised respiratory functioning because of fluid overload. People with chronic illnesses often have muscle wasting and poor muscle tone, including muscles of the respiratory system. Anemia results in diminished carbon dioxide exchange resulting from the decreased amount of hemoglobin.

Development

Developmental variations were described earlier. Physical changes such as scoliosis (curvature of the spine) influence breathing patterns and may cause air trapping. There is a statistically significant correlation between obesity and chronic bronchitis. Obese people are often short of breath during activity and thus often participate less in exercise. The alveoli at the base of the lungs are rarely stimulated to expand fully.

Opioids

Opioids are chemical agents that depress the medullary respiratory center such that the rate and depth of respirations decrease. This occurs especially with the use of morphine and meperidine (Demerol). The nurse must be alert to the potential for respiratory arrest when administering any narcotic or sedative.

Lifestyle

Sedentary activity patterns do not encourage the expansion of alveoli and the development of pulmonary exercise patterns (deep breathing). People who exercise routinely (eg, aerobics, walking, swimming) three to six times per week can better respond to stressors to respiratory health. Cigarette smoking (active or passive) is a major contributor to lung disease and respiratory distress (refer to the accompanying Applying Learning to Practice boxes).

Environment

It is impossible to pinpoint all the effects of air pollution, but researchers have demonstrated a statistically high correlation between air pollution and cancer and lung diseases. For example, occupational exposure to asbestos, silica, or coal dust can lead to chronic pulmonary disease. A person with adequate respiratory functioning who is exposed to air pollution experiences stinging of eyes and nasal passages, coughing, choking, headache, and dizziness. People who have experienced an alteration in respiratory functioning in the past often cannot continue self-care activities in a polluted environment.

Psychological Health

Individuals responding to stress may sigh excessively or have a hyperventilation breathing pattern. Generalized anxiety has been shown to cause enough bronchospasm to produce an episode of bronchial asthma. Those experiencing an alteration in respiratory functioning often develop some anxiety as a result.

The Nursing Process

ASSESSING

The patient's health history is an essential component for assessing respiratory functioning. Either the patient or a family member or significant other can provide information. The

---

APPLYING LEARNING TO PRACTICE

The Nurse as Role Model: Oxygenation

Nurses working with patients to initiate changes in health habits that affect respiration must also examine themselves as a factor in the success of the plan. Patients view nurses as role models for achieving healthy lifestyles. Nurses dealing with stresses from professional and personal aspects of their own lives sometimes channel their energies into destructive behaviors. If the nurse wishes to encourage optimal respiratory functioning, he or she must demonstrate behaviors that support a healthy lifestyle. With this goal in mind, the nurse will do the following:

- Maintain adequate fluid intake and proper nutrition.
- Use deep-breathing exercises.
- Evaluate his or her own use of nicotine.
- Incorporate a plan to reduce smoking and then stop smoking on a specific target date.
- Reduce activity patterns (ie, rest at home) in the presence of infection.
- Create a pollution-reduced environment by avoiding use of strong perfumes, aftershaves, or other scents.
- Arrange to have a tuberculin test (PPD) done annually.
- Schedule three or four periods of exercise per week.

APPLYING LEARNING TO PRACTICE

Promoting Health

Oxygenation

Use the assessment checklist to determine how well you are meeting oxygenation needs. Then develop a prescription for self-care by choosing appropriate behaviors from the list of suggestions.

ASSESSMENT CHECKLIST

almost always / sometimes / almost never

- [ ] [ ] [ ] 1. I breathe easily, without discomfort and without feeling short of breath.
- [ ] [ ] [ ] 2. I exercise regularly.
- [ ] [ ] [ ] 3. I maintain normal weight for my height and body frame.
- [ ] [ ] [ ] 4. I live in an environment free of pollution.
- [ ] [ ] [ ] 5. I avoid substances (tobacco, chemicals) that cause respiratory problems.

SELF-CARE BEHAVIORS

1. Follow a regular exercise program with 30 to 45 minutes of moderate activity three or four times a week.
2. Maintain normal body weight.
3. Obtain medical evaluation for chest pain, problems with breathing, chronic cough with sputum or blood.
4. Avoid smoking cigarettes, cigars, or pipes.
5. Avoid chemical substances that cause respiratory depression.
6. Maintain a pollution-free environment (as much as possible).
7. Support federal and community efforts to keep the air free of pollution.
8. Avoid exposure to second-hand smoke (from another's cigarette) when possible.

nursing examination combined with laboratory findings can provide information to identify a patient's strengths, the nature of the problem, its course, related signs and symptoms, and its onset, frequency, and effects on activities of daily living. The nurse decides, based on these findings, what problems can be treated independently by nursing. Other problems are referred to a physician for decisions on treatment.

Nursing History

The nursing history, an important clinical tool in the early steps of the nursing process, always includes a respiratory component. The information gained provides data about why the patient needs nursing care and what kind of care is required to maintain a sufficient intake of air. Interview questions help identify current or potential health deviations, patient actions for meeting respiratory needs and the effects of such actions, contributing factors, the use of any aids to improve the intake of air, and effects on the patient's current lifestyle and relationships with others.

Before starting the interview, the nurse ascertains that the patient and family members are comfortable. If the patient is in any respiratory distress, appropriate actions should be initiated to relieve symptoms. Family members or others may help answer questions. The nurse can expand this initial database when the patient is able to provide more information. If no emergency interventions are necessary for the patient's clinical condition, a comprehensive history can be obtained.

When a health deviation is noted during the data collection, the nurse needs to collect as much descriptive information as possible, including whether the problem evolved suddenly or slowly. Sample questions are given in the accompanying Focused Assessment Guide.

Physical Assessment

The basic examination of the lungs and respiratory status is discussed in Chapter 25. The nurse proceeds in a well-organized manner through a sequence of inspection, palpation, percussion, and auscultation.

Inspection

Observation of the chest normally shows that the contour is slightly convex with no sternal depression. The antero-posterior diameter should be less than the transverse diameter. Any abnormalities in thoracic structure should be described or sketched (see Fig. 25-30 in Chap. 25 for examples). The contour of the intercostal spaces should be flat or depressed. Movement of the chest should be symmetric. The skin over the thorax should be warm and dry and even in color, with no cyanosis or pallor. Note any scars, the origin of which should be recorded in the history under previous surgery or accidents. Observe the respiratory rate and rhythm for 1 full minute. Normally, respirations are quiet and nonlabored. Any flaring of nostrils, intercostal restriction, tachypnea, or bradypnea suggests a health deviation that necessitates further evaluation. Abnormal breathing patterns are shown in Figure 25-35 in Chapter 25.

The nurse must always be alert for common clinical manifestations that may indicate an airway emergency. Specific disease processes and conditions leading to acute respiratory failure, as well as specific clinical manifestations, are discussed in medical–surgical nursing textbooks.

FOCUSED ASSESSMENT GUIDE

Respiration

Factors to Assess	Questions and Approaches
Usual patterns of respiration	How would you describe your breathing patterns?
	Do you have allergies?
	Do you smoke?
	Do you live with a smoker or are there smokers or other pollutants in your workplace?
Recent changes	Have you noticed any changes in your breathing pattern (out of breath, cough, pain)?
	Do you have chest pain?
Cough	How much and how often do you cough?
	Is the cough related to the time of day or any activity?
	What is it like (dry, bubbly, hoarse)?
	Do you have a history of allergies?
	Do you ever wheeze?
	Are you exposed to dust? Fumes?
	Where do you work? What kind of work?
	How are you treating the cough?
Sputum	Do you ever cough up and spit out mucus?
	How much do you spit out and do you associate it with anything (time of day, environment)?
	What color is it? Is it ever blood tinged?
	What is its odor?
Chest pain	On a scale of 0 to 5 (5 being very painful), how severe is the pain?
	Where is the pain?
	Is the pain worse with inspiration? Expiration? Cough?
	Does the pain radiate?
	What measures are you using to relieve the pain?
Dyspnea	Is it constant or remittent or related to any activity?
	How do different positions affect it?
	How does it affect your daily activities?
	Is any part of your body bluish during the breathing problem?
	What do you do during and after the breathing attack?
	Have you ever been told that you have asthma? Emphysema? Tuberculosis? Heart disease?
	Do you think the problem is getting worse or staying the same?
Fever	Have you had pneumonia recently?
	Do you have any contact with people who have tuberculosis?
	Do you have night sweats?
	Are others in your household well or ill?
	Have you traveled anywhere recently?
	What medications are you using?
	Have you been exposed to any pollutants?
Fatigue	Have you noticed you feel more tired lately?
	Are you getting your normal amount of sleep at night?
	Has your sleep at night been affected by any difficulty breathing?
	Do you become easily fatigued when you climb stairs?
	Has your pattern of daily activity changed lately?

Palpation

The trachea should be equidistant from each clavicle. Skin temperature should be the same as the rest of the body. Respiratory excursion is measured by placing one's hand on the patient's posterior thorax at the 10th rib, with both thumbs almost touching the vertebrae. While the patient takes a few deep breaths, the nurse's thumbs should move 5 to 8 cm symmetrically at maximal inspiration (see Fig. 25-37 in Chap. 25). To assess *tactile fremitus* (the capacity to feel sound on the chest wall), the nurse should place his or her palm surface to the patient's chest wall, avoiding bony areas (eg, scapulae); the nurse should detect equal vibrations as the patient says some multisyllable word (eg, "ninety-nine"). Bilaterally equal mild fremitus should be detected, with the greatest intensity noted at the anterior and posterior base of the neck and along the trachea and large bronchi. Increased fremitus occurs in patients with pneumonia because solid tissue conducts sound well. Conversely, patients with chronic obstructive pulmonary disease (COPD) have decreased fremitus because air does not conduct sound as well. The presence or absence of crepitation, masses, edema, or tenderness should be noted.

Percussion

Percussion is performed posteriorly as the patient pulls shoulders forward; the examination proceeds down the patient's back, comparing one side to the other. The anterior and lateral thorax can be examined with the patient in a supine position. The nurse must listen to the intensity and quality of each sound as the chest wall and underlying structures are percussed. Resonance, a loud, hollow, low-pitched sound, is heard over normal lungs. Emphysematous lungs produce a loud, low, booming sound called hyperresonance. A flat sound is detected over bone or heavy muscle. A dull sound with medium pitch and intensity is percussed on the liver (fifth intercostal space at the right midclavicular line). Tympany is a high-pitched, loud, drumlike sound produced over the stomach. Dullness over the lung field occurs when fluid or solid tissue replaces normal lung tissue in the pleural space; this finding requires further investigation.

Auscultation

The nurse moves from apex to base with the stethoscope, comparing one side with the other side. Normal breath sounds are of three types: *vesicular* (low pitch, soft expiration, and heard over most of lung); *bronchial* (high pitch and longer and heard over the trachea); and *bronchovesicular* (medium pitch and medium expiration and heard over the upper anterior chest and intercostal area; see Fig. 25-34 in Chap. 25). The patient should breathe through an open mouth slowly. Nasal breathing produces false abnormal breath sounds. Hyperventilation may cause syncope and patient distress. If any abnormal breath sound is detected, the nurse should instruct the patient to cough and should auscultate again for at least two breaths. It is imperative with any abnormal sound to record location, change in breath sounds after coughing, and phase of respiration (eg, expiration).

Adventitious, or abnormal, lung sounds are categorized as either crackles (formerly called rales) or wheezes. **Crackles** are discontinuous (intermittent) sounds that occur when air moves through airways that contain fluid. They are produced by a delayed reopening of deflated airways. Crackles can be further classified as fine, medium, or coarse. Fine crackles, which are high-pitched sounds similar to static that are heard toward the end of inspiration or early expiration, indicate congestion in small air passages and alveoli. Rubbing strands of hair between your fingers creates a sound similar to fine crackles. Medium crackles are louder and may sound moist, whereas coarse crackles are somewhat louder, bubbly noises heard during inspiration and possibly expiration and not cleared by coughing. They result when air passes through fluid in the larger airways and indicate increasing pulmonary congestion. They are usually first detected in the lung bases, usually cannot be cleared with coughing, and may be auscultated in a patient with pneumonia. **Wheezes** are continuous sounds heard on expiration and sometimes on inspiration. They originate as air passes through airways constricted by swelling, secretions, or tumors. They can be further classified as *sibilant wheezes* (formerly called wheezes) or *sonorous wheezes* (formerly known as rhonchi). Sibilant wheezes originate in smaller airways and are high pitched and whistling, whereas sonorous wheezes can be heard over larger airways and sound like a snore (Smeltzer & Bare, 2000). They are often heard in patients with asthma or emphysema. A *pleural friction rub* is a continuous, dry grating sound caused by inflammation of pleural surfaces. It is more often heard on inspiration than expiration, is unaltered by coughing, and resembles the sound made by rubbing two leather surfaces together.

Common Methods to Assess Respiratory Functioning

Diagnostic Procedures

In addition to the nursing history and physical examination, the laboratory and radiologic tests described in Table 44-2 provide further assessment data that can aid in the formation of nursing diagnoses. The following tests are not distinctive for a particular disease but reflect how well the respiratory system is functioning.

Pulmonary Function Studies

Pulmonary function studies are routinely done to evaluate pulmonary status and detect abnormalities. They include spirometry studies that measure lung capacity, volumes, and flow rates while the patient inhales deeply and exhales forcefully into a **spirometer**, an instrument that measures these volumes and airflow. Individuals with chronic lung disease are usually exhausted after these tests. Drugs affecting the respiratory tract, such as bronchodilators, are withheld before the examination so that test results reflect the patient's present status. Pulmonary

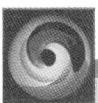

Table 44-2
Common Diagnostic Procedures Used to Assess Respiratory Functioning

Preparation	Aftercare

Arterial blood gas and pH analysis examine arterial blood to determine the pressure exerted by oxygen and carbon dioxide in the blood and the blood pH. This test measures the adequacy of oxygenation, ventilation, and perfusion. Normal results are: pH (7.35–7.45), PCO_2 (35–45 mm Hg), PO_2 (80–100 mm Hg), and HCO_3 (22–26 mEq/L).

Preparation	Aftercare
• Explain to the patient that this test requires an arterial puncture and collection of a blood specimen. • The radial, brachial, or femoral arteries are usually the sites of choice.	• The arterial specimen is immediately placed on ice and taken to the laboratory. • Apply pressure for 3–5 minutes and watch for evidence of bleeding. If patient is taking anticoagulants, pressure must be applied for a longer interval.

A **cytologic study** involves a microscopic examination of sputum and the cells it contains. It is done primarily to detect cells that may be malignant, to determine organisms causing infection, and to identify blood or pus in the sputum.

Preparation	Aftercare
• Collect the specimen, if possible, in the morning before breakfast. The test usually involves 3 successive days of sputum collection. About 1 teaspoon of sputum is needed for a specimen. • Instruct the patient that saliva is not a satisfactory specimen. • Patient should take a deep breath and then expel the air with a deep cough. • Expectorate the specimen into a sterile specimen container that contains 50% alcohol. • Close the container with a tight-fitting lid.	• Advise the patient to inform the nurse when the specimen has been obtained. • Label and package the specimen and send it to the laboratory as soon as possible.

Endoscopic studies involve direct visualization of a body cavity. A *bronchoscope* is used to examine the larynx, bronchi, and trachea. Bronchoscopy is used to view lesions, obtain a biopsy, improve drainage, remove foreign substances, and drain abscesses.

Preparation	Aftercare
• Obtain an informed consent. • The patient should be NPO for 4–8 hours before the test. • An analgesic, sedative, and/or anticholinergic may be administered before the test. • Local anesthetic is sprayed into the throat.	• Withhold food and fluids until the gag reflex returns. • Check vital signs according to the protocol. • Observe carefully for signs of respiratory impairment. Emergency resuscitation equipment should be available. • Warm saline gargles may relieve throat irritation once the gag reflex has returned.

Skin tests determine antigen–antibody reactions. In intradermal tests, antigens (to which the patient may have previously been exposed) are injected into the superficial layer of the skin with a needle and syringe to evaluate immune response.

Preparation	Aftercare
• Check patient's history for hypersensitivity to any of the test antigens. If positive, notify the physician before performing test. • Cleanse the test area with alcohol and allow it to dry.	• Instruct the patient to have the test results read at the appropriate time. • After reading the results, document the reaction, noting the amount of erythema or induration. Record the test, time, date, method, and site of administration on the patient record.

Radiography is an x-ray examination of the lungs and the thoracic cavity. Radiographic examinations of the lungs are done to help diagnose pulmonary diseases and to determine the progress or development of disease.

Preparation	Aftercare
• Instruct patient to remove clothing to the waist and put on gown. All metal jewelry should be removed. • The patient will be required to take a deep breath and hold it during the radiograph.	• No special care is required after chest radiograph.

Lung scan is the recording on a photographic plate of the emissions of radioactive waves from a substance injected into a vein as it circulates through the lung. A *perfusion scan* (Q scan) is done to measure integrity of pulmonary blood vessels and evaluate blood flow abnormalities (eg, pulmonary emboli). A *ventilation scan* (V scan) is done to detect ventilation abnormalities (especially in patients with emphysema). Both scans used together provide greater and more accurate diagnostic information than either test used solely.

Preparation	Aftercare
• Obtain an informed consent if required by agency. • Explain that no fasting is required. • Patient should be told to remove jewelry from the chest area.	• No special care is required after the lung scan. • Reassure patient that no radiation precautions are necessary.

(Adapted from Fischbach, F. [2000]. *A manual of laboratory diagnostic tests* [6th ed.]. Philadelphia: Lippincott Williams & Wilkins; and Pagana, K., & Pagana, T. [1998]. *Manual of diagnostic and laboratory tests*. St. Louis: C. V. Mosby.)

function tests measure the following lung volumes and capacities:

- *Tidal volume (TV):* the amount of air inspired and expired in a normal respiration. Normal is 500 mL.
- *Inspiratory reserve volume (IRV):* the amount of air that can be inspired beyond tidal volume. Normal is 3100 mL.
- *Expiratory reserve volume (ERV):* the amount of air that can be exhaled beyond tidal volume. Normal is 1200 mL.
- *Residual volume (RV):* the amount of air remaining in the lungs after a maximal expiration. Normal is 1200 mL.
- *Vital capacity (VC):* the maximal amount of air that can be exhaled after a maximal inhalation. Normal is 4800 mL.
- *Inspiratory capacity (IC):* the largest amount of air that can be inhaled after a normal quiet exhalation. Normal is 3600 mL.
- *Functional residual volume (FRV):* equal to the expiratory reserve volume plus the residual volume. Normal is 2400 mL.
- *Total lung capacity (TLC):* the sum of the TV, IRV, ERV, and RV. Normal is 6000 mL.

Pulse Oximetry

Pulse oximetry is a noninvasive technique that measures the oxygen saturation (SaO_2) of arterial blood. Pulse oximetry is useful for monitoring people on oxygen, those at risk for hypoxia, and postoperative patients. It effectively records trends in oxygen saturation. It is not a replacement for arterial blood gas analysis but can be used as an adjunct diagnostic test. It is important to be aware of the patient's hemoglobin level before evaluating oxygen saturation because the test measures only the percentage of oxygen carried by the available hemoglobin. Even a patient with a low hemoglobin could appear to have a normal SaO_2 because most of that hemoglobin is saturated yet may not have enough oxygen to meet body needs. A range of 95% to 100% is considered normal oxygen saturation (SaO_2); values less than 85% indicate that oxygenation to the tissues is inadequate. Figure 44-5 demonstrates a nurse using a pulse oximetry unit, and Procedure 44-1 outlines nursing responsibilities when using a pulse oximetry unit.

Thoracentesis

Thoracentesis is the procedure of entering the pleural cavity and aspirating fluid. The pleural cavity is a potential cavity because it is normally not distended with fluid or air. The physician usually performs thoracentesis at the bedside with the nurse assisting. The patient is required to sign a permit for this procedure. A thoracentesis may be performed to obtain and analyze a specimen for diagnostic purposes or to remove fluid that has accumulated in the pleural cavity and is causing respiratory difficulty and discomfort. Because the cavity being entered is sterile, surgical asepsis is required. Body substance precautions are used.

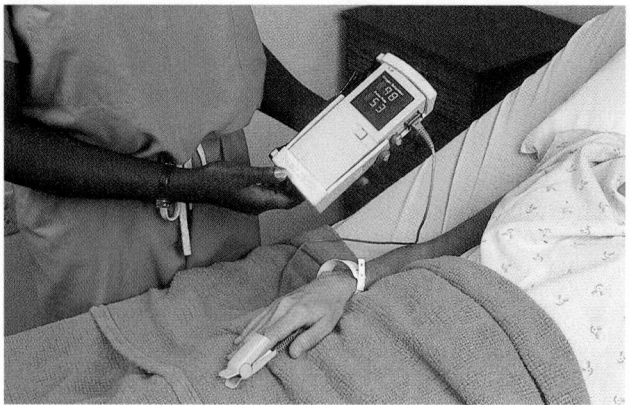

Figure 44-5
Portable pulse oximetry unit, used to measure oxygen saturation (SaO_2) of arterial blood. (Copyright © B. Proud.)

Procedure. One way to remove fluid or air from the pleural cavity is to aspirate it with a syringe. Another method for removing fluid is to drain the fluid into a bottle in which a partial vacuum has been created. A small plastic catheter may be threaded through the needle, allowing the needle to be withdrawn. This catheter reduces the possibility of puncturing the lung. When this method is used, the tubing connecting the needle and the bottle should be sterile. It is convenient to use a calibrated bottle for the drainage to determine the amount of fluid removed. The upper limit is usually 1000 mL.

The skin is prepared over the area where the physician indicates the needle will be inserted. The exact location depends on the area in which fluid is present and where the physician can best aspirate it. After a local anesthetic is administered, the needle is inserted between the ribs through the intercostal muscles and fascia and into the pleura. After the procedure, the needle or plastic catheter is removed, and a small sterile dressing is placed over the entry site.

Nursing Responsibilities. The nurse is responsible for the collection of baseline data before the examination. The patient is instructed not to cough or breathe deeply during the procedure. It is imperative that the patient remain as still as possible to diminish the risk for accidental injury to the lung. Pain medication should be administered before the test if requested.

This procedure is usually carried out when the patient is sitting on a chair or on the edge of the bed with the legs supported and the arms folded and resting on a pillow on the bedside table. Figure 44-6 shows this position. If unable to sit up, the patient may lie on the unaffected side with the hand of the affected side raised above the shoulder (McConnell, 1997).

During the procedure, the nurse observes the patient for reactions. The patient's color, pulse, and respiratory rates are observed, and any deviation from the norm is reported to the physician immediately. Fainting, nausea, and vomiting may occur. After the procedure, the patient should be observed for changes in respirations. If a large amount of fluid is removed, respirations are usually eased. Any medications that the patient is currently taking, particularly antibiotics, should be indicated on the laboratory

PROCEDURE 44-1

Using a Pulse Oximeter

Equipment

Pulse oximeter
Nail polish remover (if necessary)

Action	Rationale
1. Explain procedure to patient.	An explanation relieves anxiety and facilitates patient cooperation.
2. Wash your hands.	Handwashing deters the spread of microorganisms.

3. Select an adequate site for application of the sensor:
  a. Use the patient's index, middle, or ring finger.
  b. Check the proximal pulse and capillary refill at the pulse closest to the site.
  c. If circulation at site is inadequate, the ear lobe or bridge of nose may be considered.
  d. Use a toe only if lower extremity circulation is not compromised.
	Inadequate circulation can interfere with the SaO_2 reading.
	
	Brisk capillary refill and a strong pulse indicate that circulation to the site is adequate.
	These alternate sites are highly vascular alternatives.
	
	Peripheral vascular disease is common in lower extremities.

4. Use the proper equipment:
  a. If one finger is too large for the probe, use a smaller one. A pediatric probe may be used for a small adult.
  b. Use probes appropriate for patient's age and size.
  c. Check if patient is allergic to adhesive. A non-adhesive finger clip or reflectance sensor is available.
	Inaccurate readings can result if probe or sensor is not attached correctly.
	
	A reaction may occur if patient is allergic to adhesive substance.

5. Prepare the monitoring site:
  a. Cleanse the selected area and allow it to dry.
  b. Remove nail polish and artificial nails after checking manufacturer's instructions.
	Skin oils, dirt, or grime on site; polish; and artificial nails can interfere with the passage of light waves.

6. Apply the probe securely to the skin. Make sure that the light-emitting sensor and the light-receiving sensor are aligned opposite each other (not necessary to check if placed on the forehead or bridge of the nose).	Secure attachments and proper alignment of the markings for the light-emitting and light-receiving sensor promote satisfactory operation of the equipment and accurate recording of the SaO_2.
7. Connect the sensor probe to the pulse oximeter and check operation of the equipment (presence of audible beep and fluctuation of bar of light or waveform on the face of the oximeter).	Audible beep represents the arterial pulse, and fluctuating waveform indicates strength of the pulse. A weak signal will produce an inaccurate recording of the SaO_2.
8. Set the alarms on the pulse oximeter. Check manufacturer's alarm limits for high and low pulse rate settings.	Alarm provides additional safeguard for patient and signals when high or low limits have been surpassed.
9. Check oxygen saturation at regular intervals as ordered by physician and necessitated by alarms. Monitor patient's hemoglobin level.	Monitoring SaO_2 provides ongoing assessment of patient's condition. A low hemoglobin level may be satisfactorily saturated yet not be adequate to meet a patient's oxygen needs.
10. Remove sensor on a regular basis and check for skin irritation or signs of pressure (every 2 hr for spring-tension sensor or every 4 hr for adhesive finger or toe sensor).	Prolonged pressure may lead to tissue necrosis and adhesive sensor may cause skin irritation.

(continued)

PROCEDURE 44-1

Using a Pulse Oximeter (Continued)

11. Evaluate any malfunctions or problems with equipment.

    a. For absent or weak signal, check the patient's vital signs and condition. If satisfactory, check connections and circulation to site.

    Hypotension makes an accurate recording difficult. Equipment (restraint, BP cuff) may compromise circulation to site and cause venous blood to pulsate, giving an inaccurate reading.

    b. For inaccurate reading, check prescribed medications and history of circulatory disorders. Try device on a healthy person to see if problem is equipment related or patient related.

    Drugs that cause vasoconstriction interfere with accurate recording of oxygen saturation.

    c. If bright light (sunlight or fluorescent light) is suspected of causing equipment malfunction, cover probe with a dry washcloth.

    Bright light can interfere with operation of light sensors and cause unreliable report.

12. Document and report SaO_2 appropriately.

    Ensures continuity of care and ongoing assessment record.

Home Care Consideration   Portable units are available for use in the home or an outpatient setting.

---

slip that accompanies the specimen. If the lung is punctured inadvertently, respiratory distress becomes acute. If blood appears in the sputum or the patient has severe coughing, the physician should be notified promptly. A chest radiograph is usually done after the procedure to verify the absence of complications.

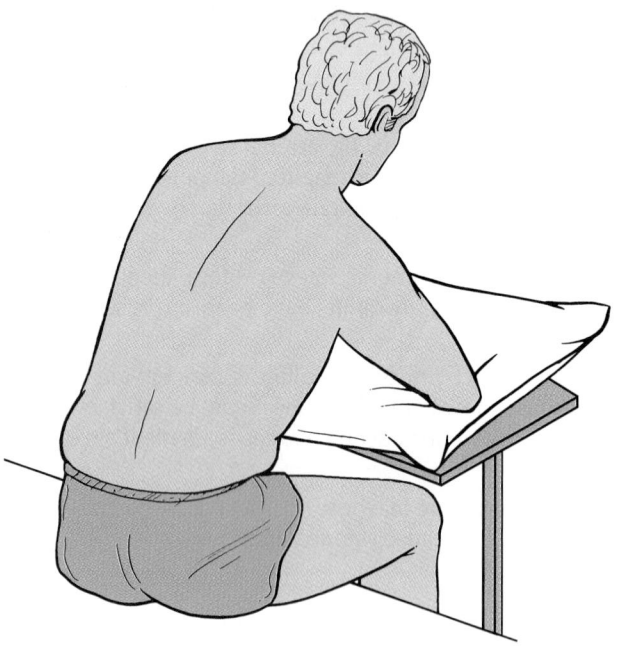

Figure 44-6
Position of the patient for thoracentesis.

DIAGNOSING

Alterations in Respiratory Function as the Problem

After the assessment is completed and the data are examined, the nurse concludes either that there is no problem at this time or that there is an actual or potential respiratory problem that is amenable to independent or interdependent nursing action. Nursing diagnoses indicating alterations in respiratory function are as follows:

Ineffective Airway Clearance
Ineffective Breathing Pattern
Impaired Gas Exchange

Common etiologies for these diagnoses include an inability to maintain proper position, pain or fear of pain, viscous secretions, fatigue, decreased level of consciousness, lack of knowledge, smoking, allergy, mechanical obstruction, medications, and decreased elasticity of the lungs.

Examples of these diagnoses, etiologic factors, and defining characteristics are given in the accompanying box.

Alterations in Respiratory Function as the Etiology

An alteration in respiratory functioning may affect other areas of human functioning. Other nursing diagnoses resulting from alterations in respiratory functioning include the following:

Activity Intolerance related to shortness of breath
Anxiety related to feeling of suffocation

Nursing Diagnoses for Common Problems

Respiration

Problem	Related Factors	Sample Defining Characteristics
Ineffective Airway Clearance	Thick yellow secretions, fever, fatigue, dehydration, poor nutrition	"I never feel as though I am getting enough air." Seventy-year-old man with a 20-year history of COPD, recent development of pneumonia. He is pale with circumoral cyanosis. His respiratory rate is 40 breaths/min and shallow. Rhonchi are auscultated bilaterally. He does not sit quietly in chair or on bed. He cannot walk length of room without coughing episode, which produces little sputum.
Impaired Gas Exchange	Smokes one pack per day; works with asbestos in auto factory; has had a cold for 7 days	Cyanotic 50-year-old man. Using pursed-lip breathing while sitting on emergency room stretcher. Sitting hunched forward with overbed table supporting arms. Altered blood gases show respiratory acidosis. Admits to shortness of breath, nausea, and ankle edema for 1 week.
Ineffective Breathing Pattern	Anxious about results of cardiac catheterization and possible cardiac surgery	Hyperventilating, tachypneic (40 minutes). "I have a tingling feeling in my fingers."

Pain related to pleural inflammation

Impaired Verbal Communication related to endotracheal intubation

Ineffective Individual Coping related to frequent hospitalization resulting from acute symptoms of COPD

Diversional Activity Deficit related to loss of ability to perform specific activities because of shortness of breath

Fatigue related to impaired oxygen transport system

Fear related to disabling respiratory illness

Dysfunctional Grieving related to loss of normal respiratory functioning

Altered Health Maintenance related to smoking

Noncompliance With (eg, Performance of Daily Respiratory Exercises) related to side effects of therapy

Altered Nutrition: Less Than Body Requirements, related to difficulty breathing

Altered Oral Mucous Membrane related to presence of endotracheal tube

Powerlessness related to inability for self-care because of COPD

Self-Esteem Disturbance related to loss of normal respiratory function

Sleep Pattern Disturbance related to orthopnea and bronchodilators

Social Isolation related to inability to walk to usual "people places"

Risk for Suffocation related to child playing with a plastic bag

Risk for Aspiration related to reduced level of consciousness

Important Distinctions

Each nursing statement identifies a patient problem and suggests expected patient outcomes. The etiology of the problem directs nursing interventions. The nurse, in analyzing the assessment data, must determine whether the alteration in respiratory functioning:

- Is the problem
- Is contributing to a different problem
- Is a sign or symptom of a problem

Altered respiratory functioning can fit into all three categories. Consider, for example, how ineffective airway clearance in a 17-year-old asthmatic baseball player who is waiting to hear from the college of his choice plays a role in three different nursing diagnoses:

Ineffective Airway Clearance related to pollen exposure, exercise, and stress of waiting to hear about college applications

The airway clearance is the problem statement. Nursing interventions are directed to reducing exposure to pollens, specific stressors, and timing or degree of exercise. The outcome is that the patient will achieve effective airway clearance.

Activity Intolerance related to ineffective airway clearance during and after baseball games, fatigue, and stress

Here, the activity intolerance is the problem statement, and ineffective airway clearance is just one of the many factors contributing to the problem. All the nursing interventions are directed to improving airway clearance, combating fatigue, and coping with stress.

> Ineffective Individual Coping related to stress of career choices and stress of performance during baseball games as demonstrated by recent increase in episodes of asthmatic attacks

In this case, the ineffective airway clearance is a symptom of the patient's real problem—ineffective coping. Nursing interventions are directed to reducing stressors. When the patient is able to improve his use of coping skills, the expected outcome is that the number of asthma attacks will decrease.

Each nursing diagnosis is unique to the situation, and the etiology varies with each patient. The nurse, with the patient, decides which problem is the priority. With creativity and patience, the nurse develops a nursing diagnosis that clearly directs nursing interventions and expected outcomes. However, there may also be interventions initiated by another member of the healthcare team for the nurse to follow (eg, a prescription for administering medications), which are a dependent aspect of nursing practice. Interdependent nursing actions involve problems the nurse and other healthcare team members collaborate to treat (eg, nurses monitoring side effects of prescribed medications).

PLANNING: EXPECTED OUTCOMES

Whenever nurses care for patients with an alteration in respiratory functioning, nursing measures support the following general expected outcomes. The patient will achieve the following:

* Demonstrate improved gas exchange in his or her lungs by an absence of cyanosis or chest pain
* Relate the causative factors, if known, and demonstrate an adaptive method of coping with these factors
* Preserve pulmonary function by maintaining an optimal level of activity
* Demonstrate self-care behaviors that provide relief from symptoms and prevent further pulmonary problems

When the patient's physical, psychosocial, and spiritual dimensions contribute to alterations in respiratory function, individualized expected outcomes are developed with the patient's input. For example: "By March 15, the patient will be able to walk up one flight of steps at home without dyspnea."

IMPLEMENTING

Teaching About Pollution-Free Environments

A pollution-free environment is particularly important for individuals with respiratory problems. The nurse needs to teach the patient to assess the environment and make adjustments, whenever possible, to factors that impair respiratory functioning. The patient must actively plan to prevent exposure to pollutants. This might involve a job change, use of protective equipment, requesting enforcement of existing laws by government agencies, or subcontracting jobs. Dusting and vacuuming the office and home must be done minimally twice per week. In some situations, the patient may wear a mask to prevent some symptoms of respiratory distress. Exposure to industrial or occupational hazards (eg, paint, varnish, gaseous fumes, and asbestos) must be restricted.

In the United States, fine pollutants that pose a hazard to health are monitored closely. These include carbon monoxide, sulfur dioxide, total suspended particulates, ozone, and nitrogen dioxide. On days when pollutant levels are significantly elevated, morbidity and mortality rates among people with preexisting pulmonary disease are greatly increased. Thus, on those days when pollution alerts are announced, the nurse instructs patients with an alteration in respiratory function to reduce activities, stay indoors, and use an air conditioner, electronic air cleaner, or air filter. If pollen alters the patient's respiratory function, the same principles apply.

Cigarette smoking is the most important risk factor in pulmonary disease. The inhalation of cigarette smoke increases airway resistance, reduces ciliary action, increases mucus production, causes thickening of the alveolar–capillary membrane, and causes bronchial walls to thicken and lose their elasticity. These effects occur in both smokers and nonsmokers (children and adults) who live with smokers. Habitual smokers usually have great difficulty quitting or reducing their smoking and need much encouragement. The American Lung Association and the American Heart Association offer many free educational materials to aid and support patients who are trying to stop smoking. Their addresses and phone numbers are listed in local telephone directories. Nurses are in a prime position to present accurate information regarding the negative effects of smoking and to encourage the decision to stop smoking or never to start smoking (see the Research in Nursing box, p. 1265).

Establishing a Trusting Nurse–Patient Relationship

Most people with altered respiratory functioning experience anxiety as a result of their symptoms and the actual or potential loss of independence. Oxygen deficits, particularly in older people, negatively affect all aspects of their daily living. The accompanying box focuses on oxygen problems and nursing education strategies for the older adult.

The nurse needs to create an environment that is likely to reduce anxiety. Immediate discomfort should be treated. Using effective listening skills and accurate observation helps validate the nurse's caring attitude. Nurses must seek to understand patients' life experiences and habits without prejudging them. Patients often bring a fear of stigma into a professional relationship (especially with detrimental health habits), and this impedes the use of nursing interventions. Patients who believe nurses are genuinely concerned about them and their family are more willing to work toward achieving mutually desirable outcomes.

Focus on the Older Adult

Physiologic Changes and Nursing Strategies for Oxygen Problems Affecting Older Adults

Decreased Gas Exchange and Increased Work of Breathing

Physiologic Changes

- Decreased elastic recoil of the lungs
- Expiration requires use of accessory muscles.
- Fewer functional capillaries and more fibrous tissue in alveoli
- Decreased skeletal muscle strength in thorax
- Reduction in vital capacity and increase in residual volume

Nursing Strategies

- Encourage rest periods as necessary.
- Teach stair-climbing techniques.
- Encourage cessation or moderation of smoking.
- Teach breathing exercises.
- Remind about avoiding air pollutants.
- Caution about effect of extreme weather conditions.
- Instruct to avoid narcotics and sleeping pills.
- Discuss home management with patient and family.
- Teach avoidance of infection and preventive measures (ie, flu vaccination).
- Use pillows as necessary to sleep.

Decreased Ventilation and Ineffective Cough

Physiologic Changes

- Less air exchange; more secretions remain in lungs
- Drier mucous membranes
- Altered pain sensation
- Different norms for body temperature; fever may be atypical
- Greater risk for aspiration due to slower gastric motility
- Impaired mobility and inactivity, effects of medication

Nursing Strategies

- Encourage increased fluid intake, especially water, as allowed.
- Use cool-mist humidifier.
- Encourage attendance at pulmonary exercise rehabilitation program.
- Discourage use of over-the-counter medications.
- Teach how to splint thorax and cough effectively.
- Instruct in use of supplemental oxygen.
- Teach avoidance of milk products if they are troublesome

Promoting Proper Breathing

Breathing exercises are designed to help patients achieve more efficient and controlled ventilations, to decrease the work of breathing, and to correct respiratory defects. The accompanying Nursing Interventions Classification box focuses on nursing interventions that maximize oxygen and carbon dioxide exchange in the lungs.

Deep Breathing

Habits of breathing that are not conducive to maximal respiratory functioning are common in both well and ill people. Some people develop a pattern of shallow breathing or walk with a posture that makes the chest wall appear to be caved in. Ill people, for any number of reasons, may limit their respiratory efforts. Hypoventilation occurs when a decreased amount of air enters and leaves the lungs. Deep-breathing exercises to produce hyperventilation are often used to overcome hypoventilation.

The nurse instructs the patient to make each breath deep enough to move the bottom ribs. Unless the patient has a nasal condition that prohibits or prevents normal breathing, the patient should start slow, deep ventilations nasally and expire slowly through the mouth. Breathing through the nose warms, filters, and humidifies the air. The patient's respiratory status, motivation, and general clinical condition dictate the timing of this exercise, done hourly while awake or four times daily.

Using Incentive Spirometry

In incentive spirometry, the patient takes a deep breath and observes the results of his or her efforts registered on the spirometry equipment while sustaining that maximal inspiration. Incentive spirometry keeps the alveoli from collapsing so that gas exchange can occur and secretions can be cleared and expectorated (Lezon, 1999). Instructions are necessary before the patient uses incentive spirometry equipment, and the nurse should validate patients' correct use of this equipment in both healthcare and home environments. This intervention offers immediate positive reinforcement to the patient for his or her breathing efforts. See the accompanying Guidelines for Nursing Care for additional suggestions when teaching patients to use this device.

Abdominal or Diaphragmatic Breathing

Many people with COPD have a tendency to breathe in a shallow, rapid, and exhausting pattern. This type of upper chest breathing can be changed to diaphragmatic breathing, reducing the rate, increasing the tidal volume, and reducing the functional residual capacity. The patient is

Using the Nursing Interventions Classification (NIC)

Ventilation Assistance

- Maintain a patent airway
- Auscultate breath sounds, noting areas of decreased or absent ventilation, and presence of adventitious sounds
- Initiate and maintain supplemental oxygen, as prescribed
- Administer appropriate pain medication to prevent hypoventilation
- Ambulate three to four times per day, as appropriate
- Monitor respiratory and oxygenation status
- Administer medications (eg, bronchodilators and inhalers) that promote airway patency and gas exchange
- Teach pursed-lip breathing techniques, as appropriate
- Teach breathing techniques as appropriate
- Initiate a program of respiratory muscle strength and/or endurance training, as appropriate

(From McClosky, J., & Bulechek, G. [2000]. *Nursing interventions classification [NIC]* [3rd ed.]. [p. 697]. St. Louis: C. V. Mosby. A full listing of nursing activities for each nursing intervention can be found in this book.)

instructed to place one hand on the stomach and the other on the middle of the chest. The patient then should breathe in slowly through the nose, letting the abdomen protrude as far as it will go. Next, he or she should breathe out through pursed lips while contracting the abdominal muscles while one hand presses inward and upward on the abdomen. These steps should be repeated for 1 minute followed by rest for 2 minutes. The patient should practice this breathing pattern several times during the day. Eventually it will become automatic.

Pursed-Lip Breathing

Patients who experience dyspnea and feelings of panic can often gain control of their respiration by using pursed-lip breathing. This exercise trains the muscles to prolong exhalation, increasing airway pressure during expiration and reducing the amount of airway trapping and resistance. To do this, the patient inhales through the nose while counting to three and exhales slowly and evenly against pursed lips while tightening the abdominal muscles. During exhalation, the patient counts to seven. To purse the lips, the patient should position the lips as though he or she were sucking through a straw or whistling. When walking, the patient should inhale while taking two steps and then exhale through pursed lips while taking the next four steps, and then repeat the cycle. Before teaching these techniques, the nurse should practice them alone and then with a partner.

Managing Chest Tubes

Patients who develop fluid (*pleural effusion*), blood (*hemothorax*), or air (*pneumothorax*) in the pleural space require the assistance of a chest tube to drain these substances and allow the compressed lung to reexpand. A chest tube is a

---

Guidelines for Nursing Care

Using an Incentive Spirometer

- Assist patient to upright position if possible.
- Remove dentures if they fit poorly.
- Demonstrate how to steady device with one hand and hold mouthpiece with other hand.
- Instruct the patient to exhale normally and then place lips securely around mouthpiece.
- Instruct patient not to breathe through his or her nose. Use a nose clip if necessary.
- Instruct the patient to inhale slowly and as deeply as possible through the mouthpiece.
- Tell patient to hold breath and count to three. Check position of gauge to determine progress and level attained.
- Instruct patient to remove lips from mouthpiece and exhale normally.
- Tell patient to complete breathing exercises about 10 times every hour if possible. Rest in between breaths as necessary.

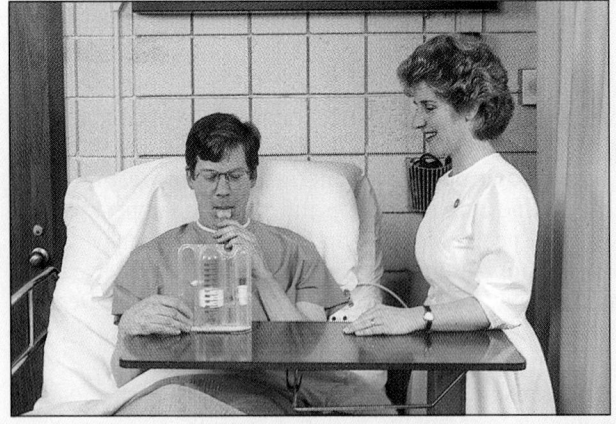

firm plastic tube with drainage holes in the proximal end that is placed in the pleural space, secured with a suture and tape, covered with an air-tight dressing, and attached to a drainage system that may or may not include suction. Other components of the system may include an air seal to prevent air from reentering the chest once it has escaped and a suction control chamber that protects against excess suction pressure in the pleural cavity (Pettinicchi, 1998). Most healthcare agencies use molded plastic, three-compartment disposable chest drainage units in place of the one-, two-, or three-bottle system formerly used. Placement of the chest tube in the chest cavity is determined by the type of drainage. To drain air, the tube is placed higher in the chest, whereas a lower tube is used for fluids, which settle at the base of the lung.

Nursing responsibilities include assisting with insertion and removal of a chest tube and, once the tube is in place, monitoring the patient's respiratory status and vital signs, checking the dressing, and maintaining the patency and integrity of the drainage system. Figure 44-7 illustrates a chest drainage system, and the accompanying Guidelines for Nursing Care list guidelines for monitoring a patient with a chest tube.

Promoting and Controlling Coughing

The presence of excessive fluids or secretions in an organ or body tissue is called *congestion*, and a person with secretions or fluid in the lungs is said to have congested lungs. If the cough is dry, the patient is said to be congested with a *nonproductive cough*. If the cough produces respiratory tract secretions, the patient is referred to as being congested

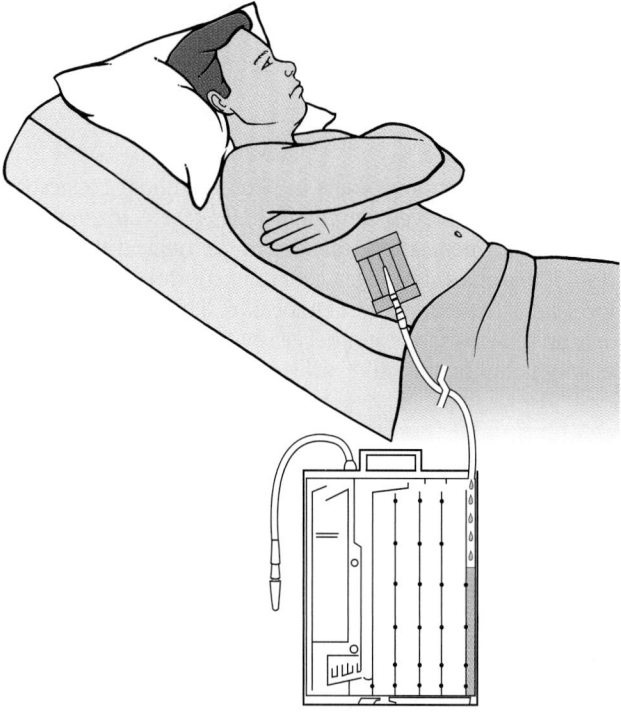

Figure 44-7
A chest drainage system attached to a patient.

Guidelines for Nursing Care
Monitoring a Patient With a Chest Tube

- Assess the patient's respiratory status, vital signs, and breath sounds. Monitor for any indication of change in respiratory status.
- Observe the dressing around the chest tube insertion site and ensure that it is occlusive. All connections should also be securely taped.
- Check that the drainage tube has no dependent loops or kinks. The drainage collection device must be positioned below the tube insertion site to facilitate drainage.
- Check that two padded Kelly clamps are available and secured at the bedside. If the drainage unit requires changing, one clamp is positioned 1½ to 2½ inches from the insertion site, and the second clamp is placed 1 inch down from the first one until the unit has been switched. The physician may order a chest tube clamped before its removal to observe the patient's tolerance when it is discontinued or the chest tube may be clamped to assess for an air leak.
- *Never* clamp the tube if the patient leaves the unit for a test or moves away from the bed. Disconnect the suction tubing from the drainage system, allowing the unit to continue to collect drainage by gravity.
- Avoid milking or stripping the tube to promote drainage. This creates excessive negative pressure that can damage delicate lung tissue.
- Assess the suction control chamber if suction is in use. If it is not at the appropriate level (fluid can evaporate), water must be added to ensure that suction is adequate. Gentle bubbling in the suction chamber indicates that suction is being applied to assist drainage.
- Assist the patient to remain in high-Fowler's position (if hemothorax is present) or semi-Fowler's position (for pneumothorax) for improved drainage or evacuation.
- Measure drainage output at the end of each shift by marking the level on the container or placing a small piece of tape at the drainage level to indicate date and time. Drainage is never emptied from the collection chamber. Document color and consistency of drainage. Drainage exceeding 100 mL/hr or a change in drainage to a bright red color that indicates fresh bleeding requires immediate notification of the physician.

with a *productive cough*. Thick respiratory secretions are sometimes called *phlegm*. A patient who is coughing with no congestion or secretions produced is described as being noncongested with a nonproductive cough.

Cough Mechanism

The cough mechanism (Fig. 44-8) consists of an initial irritation; a deep inspiration; a quick, tight closure of the glottis together with a forceful contraction of the expiratory intercostal muscles; and an upward push of the diaphragm. This causes an explosive movement of air from the lower to the upper respiratory tract. To be effective, a cough should have enough muscle contraction to force air to be expelled and to propel a liquid or a solid on its way out of the respiratory tract. Coughing is most effective when the patient is sitting upright with feet flat on the floor. A cough is a cleaning mechanism of the body. It is a means of helping to keep the airway clear of secretions and other debris.

Voluntary Coughing

When a cough does not occur as a result of reflex stimulation of the cough-sensitive areas, it can be induced voluntarily. Teaching the patient to cough voluntarily is an important aspect of preoperative and postoperative care. Although the teaching of deep breathing and coughing is relatively easy, experience has shown that it is difficult to motivate patients to follow through and perform coughing on their own. Frequent reminders throughout the day are necessary for many patients. A specific schedule for coughing on the nursing plan of care is advised. Coughing early in the morning after rising removes phlegm that accumulated during the night. Coughing before meals improves the taste of food and oxygenation. At bedtime, coughing removes any buildup of phlegm and improves sleep patterns. For a patient who is unable to cough voluntarily, manual stimulation over the trachea and prolonged exhalation can be helpful. If neither of these methods is successful, mechanical endotracheal suctioning with a catheter is used sometimes.

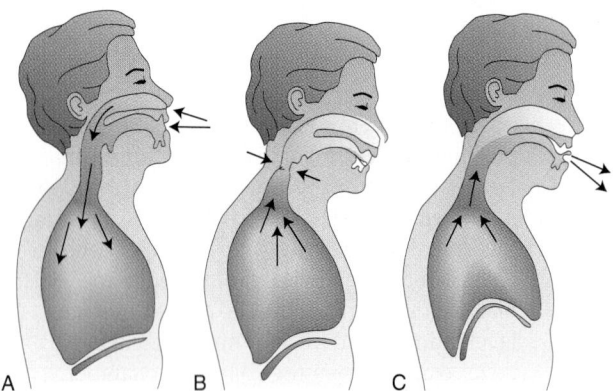

Figure 44-8

(**A**) A cough begins with a deep inspiration, distending the trachea and hyperinflating the lungs. (**B**) After inspiration, the glottis closes while intercostal and abdominal muscles contract forcibly. (**C**) When intrathoracic pressure reaches a high level, the glottis opens slightly, and the diaphragm is pushed up, producing an explosive movement of air.

Involuntary Coughing

Involuntary coughing often accompanies respiratory tract infections and irritations. It helps clear the airway if it is productive, but it is fatiguing and irritating when it is nonproductive. Medication may control involuntary coughing. Observation of the patient's breathing and coughing characteristics is necessary to determine the appropriate type of medication.

Cough Suppressants

Suppressants are drugs that depress a body function, in this case, the cough reflex. Codeine, which is present in many cough preparations, is generally considered the preferred cough suppressant ingredient. However, codeine can be addictive. Because of possible abuse, many states require a physician's prescription for its use. Drowsiness (also common with antihistamines) is a side effect of its use. Therefore, it may not be safe to use codeine when the person must remain alert, such as when driving a car.

An irritating nonproductive cough in people without congestion may be appropriately treated with suppressants. Inappropriate suppression of the cough in a person with respiratory congestion can result in harmful retention of the secretions.

Expectorants

Expectorants are drugs that facilitate the removal of respiratory tract secretions by reducing the secretion viscosity. Patients with extremely tenacious secretions may need the secretions liquefied for their cough to be effective. In that way, the nonproductive cough of a person with lung congestion can become productive. An expectorant used by a person who does not have congestion is inappropriate. Guaifenesin is widely used as an expectorant in cough preparations (eg, Robitussin). Adequate fluid intake and air humidification are considered effective expectorants by some authorities.

Lozenges

Mild, nonproductive coughs in people without congestion can often be relieved by cough lozenges. A lozenge is a small, solid medication intended to be held in the mouth until it dissolves. Lozenges generally control coughs by the local anesthetic effect of benzocaine. The local anesthetic acts on sensory and motor nerves by controlling the primary irritation and by inhibiting afferent and efferent impulses.

Teaching About Cough Preparations

Because cough preparations are so readily available and people who purchase them are usually eager for relief, consumers sometimes take excessive amounts of more than one type. The nurse can offer health teaching about the appropriate choice of expectorants and suppressants. Also, the nurse should teach patients about other misuses of cough mixtures. For example, cough syrups with a high sugar or alcohol content can disturb the metabolic balance of people with diabetes mellitus. Preparations containing antihistamines have an anticholinergic action, which can cause serious problems for people with glaucoma or cause urinary retention in men with prostate enlargement. Other cough preparations can be detrimental to people with hypertension or with thyroid or cardiac diseases. In addition, prolonged use of self-prescribed cough preparations can conceal more serious health problems.

Promoting Comfort

Positioning
Helping an incapacitated patient assume a position that allows free movement of the diaphragm and expansion of the chest wall promotes ease of respiration. For example, sitting in a slumped position, which permits the abdominal contents to push upward on the diaphragm, results in less lung expansion during inspiration. People with dyspnea and orthopnea are most comfortable in high Fowler's position because accessory muscles can then be used easily to promote respiration. Recent research has demonstrated that turning patients who are acutely ill with pulmonary disease into the prone position on a regular basis promotes oxygenation. This position allows posterior dependent sections of the lungs to be better ventilated and perfused (Dirkes & Dickinson, 1998). A partially prone position appears to be sufficient and allows access to invasive lines and airway access.

Maintaining Adequate Fluid Intake
Secretions can be kept thin by asking the patient to drink 2 to 3 quarts (1.9 to 2.9 L) of clear fluids daily. The patient's fluid intake should be increased to the maximum that his or her health state can tolerate. Special attention needs to be given to the fluid intake of patients who have an elevated temperature, who are breathing through the mouth, who are coughing, or who are losing excessive body fluids in other ways. If there is an incidence of right side heart failure, fluid intake should not exceed 1½ quarts (1.4 L) daily. Milk products (milk, ice cream, yogurt, cheese, and so forth) thicken secretions and congestion and should be avoided. Clear fluids include water, tea, coffee, apple juice, broths, fruit ices, and flavored gelatin.

Providing Humidified Air
When air humidity is low, artificial means for humidifying inspired air may be helpful. The inspiration of dry air removes normal moisture in the respiratory passages that is essential for protection from irritation and infection. Room humidifiers may be helpful for some patients. Electric vaporizers that produce steam or cool mist are also useful. Neither device has been demonstrated to have greater therapeutic value than the other. A cool-mist vaporizer does not present dangers with burns because it does not generate heat or hot water. However, it can be a medium for pathogen growth if inadequately cleaned. The steam vaporizer does not present this problem.

Percussing
Cupping is the manual percussion of lung areas to loosen pulmonary secretions so that they can be expectorated with greater ease. Percussion by cupping uses the hand

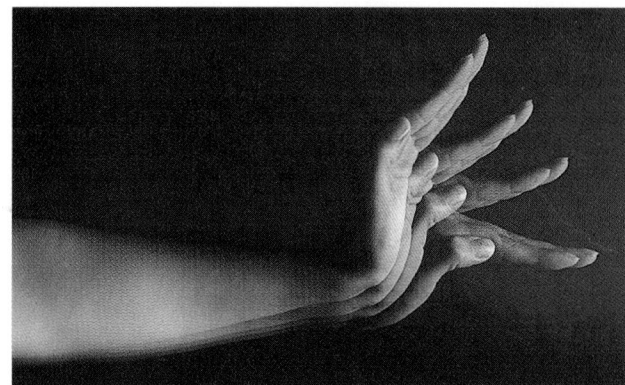

Figure 44-9
The cupping position and action of the hand on manual percussion of the lung area. (Copyright © B. Proud.)

held in a rigid, dome-shaped position (Fig. 44-9), striking rhythmically over the lobes of the lungs to be drained. The patient should be supine or prone and should not experience any pain. Cupping is never done on bare skin or performed below the ribs or over the spine or breasts because of the danger of tissue damage. Percussion may be done for 30 to 60 seconds over an area several times a day, or for up to 3 to 5 minutes for patients with tenacious secretions. The patient may learn to percuss anterior surfaces of his or her chest wall, or family members can be taught to percuss posterior surfaces. Also, mechanical devices are available for percussion on the chest wall.

Vibrating
Vibration involves the nurse's rhythmic contraction and relaxation of his or her arm and shoulder muscles while holding the hands flat on the patient's chest wall as the patient exhales. The purpose is to help loosen respiratory secretions so that they can be expectorated with ease. Vibration (at a rate of about 200 per minute) can be done for several minutes several times a day but should never be done over the patient's breasts, spine, sternum, and lower rib cage. Vibration (Fig. 44-10) can also be taught to family members or accomplished using a mechanical device.

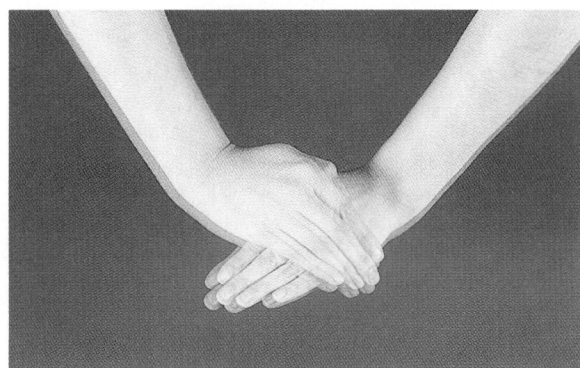

Figure 44-10
The position and action of the hands necessary to use vibration to loosen respiratory secretions in the lungs. (Copyright © B. Proud.)

Providing Postural Drainage

In *postural drainage*, gravity is used to drain secretions from the lungs. The patient is positioned in a way that promotes the drainage of secretions from smaller pulmonary branches into larger ones, where they can be removed by drainage or coughing (Fig. 44-11). Postural drainage is often preceded by vibration, percussion, or both. Postural drainage is carried out as follows:

1. Have tissues and an emesis basin close at hand for the patient to use when coughing and expectorating secretions.
2. Place the patient in an appropriate position to promote drainage from the lobes of the lungs, as follows:

   Use high Fowler's position to drain the apical sections of the upper lobes of the lungs.

   Place the patient in a lying position, half on the abdomen and half on the side, right and left, to drain the posterior sections of the upper lobes of the lungs.

   Place the patient lying on the left side with a pillow under the chest wall to drain the right lobe of the lung.

   Place the patient in Trendelenburg's position to drain the lower lobes of the lungs.

3. Carry out postural drainage two to four times a day for 20 to 30 minutes. Discontinue the drainage if the patient begins to feel weak or faint.
4. Delay postural drainage for 1 to 2 hours after meals to avoid vomiting.

Maintaining Good Nutrition

People who are working hard at breathing often do not have energy for eating. Nutritional status is assessed by measuring the patient's height, weight, upper arm circumference, serum protein levels, and nitrogen balance. Special attention and deliberate planning should be directed to adequate intake of proteins, vitamins, and minerals. Six small meals should be distributed over the course of the day instead of the usual three larger meals. Nutritional in-

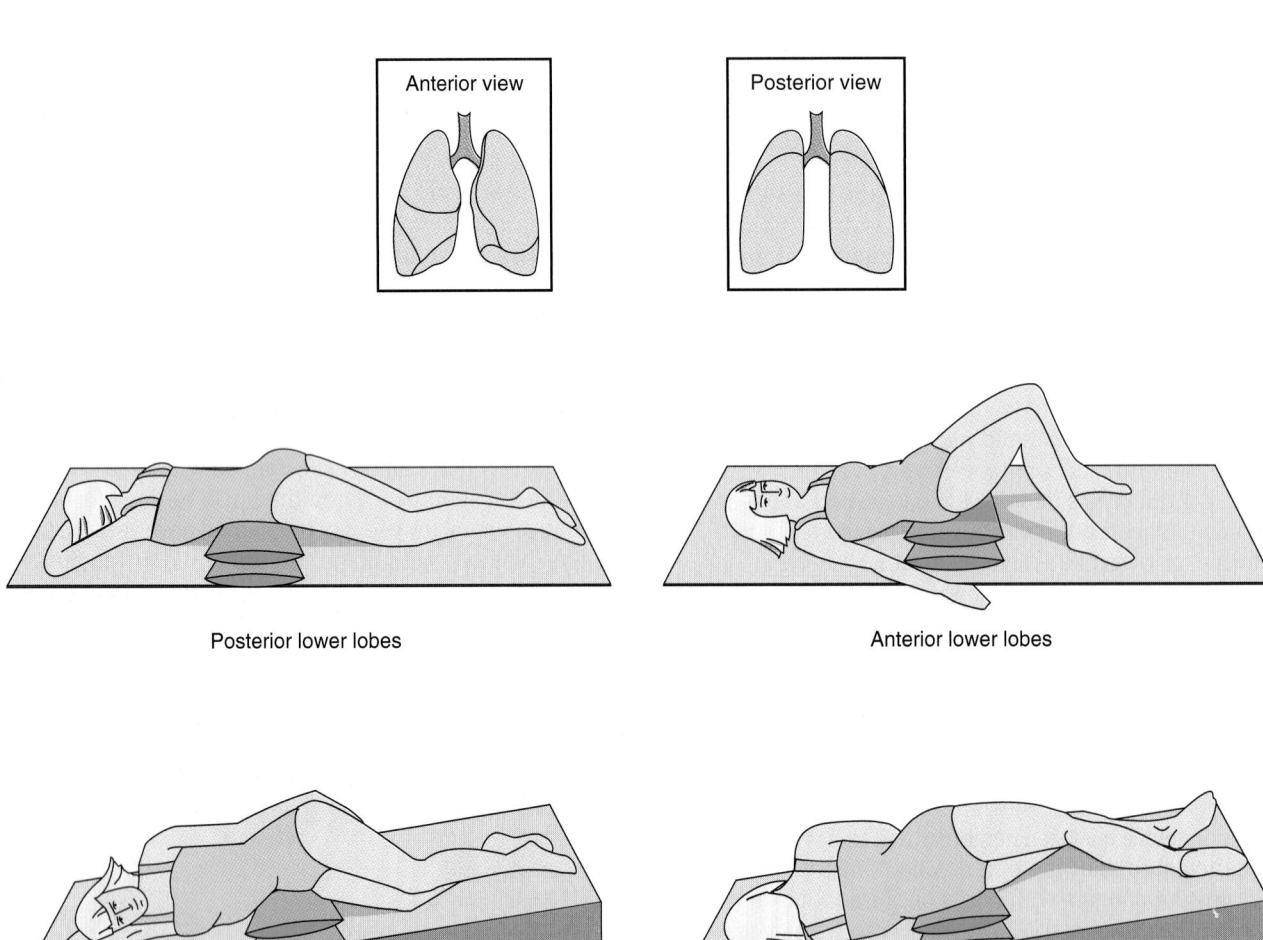

Anterior view

Posterior view

Posterior lower lobes

Anterior lower lobes

Left lower lobe

Right lower lobe

Figure 44-11
Postural drainage. Shown are four positions that use the force of gravity to assist the drainage of secretions from the smaller bronchial airways into the main bronchi and trachea so the patient is able to cough them up.

take can be improved by providing frequent oral hygiene and rest periods before eating. Meals should be arranged 1 to 2 hours after breathing treatments and exercises.

In patients who have COPD or are ventilator dependent, it is important to provide nutrients in the proper balance to reduce production of CO_2 (from metabolism). Fat metabolism produces the least amount of CO_2, and carbohydrate metabolism produces the most. Thus, nonprotein calories in the diet should be equally divided between fat and carbohydrates for these types of patients. Some healthcare facilities call this type of diet a COPD or respiratory diet (Grodner, Anderson, & DeYoung, 2000).

Meeting Respiratory Needs With Medications

Although treating patients with medications is a dependent nursing intervention, monitoring the patient's response and side effects to medication is an independent nursing action. Table 44-3 shows some common medications for respiratory functioning, their side effects, and nursing implications. Patients and caregivers need a reminder that caffeine may potentiate the side effects of drugs commonly used to dilate bronchial airways.

Using Nebulizers

Patients use nebulizers to disperse fine particles of medication into the deeper passages of the respiratory tract where absorption occurs. Inhaled medications may be administered to open narrowed airways (**bronchodilators**), to liquefy or loosen thick secretions (mucolytic agents), or to reduce inflammation in airways (corticosteroids). A *metered-dose inhaler* (MDI) delivers a controlled dose of medication with each compression of the canister, whereas a *small-volume nebulizer* is used until all the medication in the nebulizer cup has been inhaled. Patients need instruction on how to use inhalers and nebulizers effectively and safely (Gazarian, 1997). Overuse may result in serious side effects and eventual ineffectiveness of the medication. Nurses need to be aware of the common mistakes that patients make when using an MDI. They include the following:

- Failing to shake the canister
- Holding the inhaler upside down
- Inhaling through the nose rather than the mouth
- Inhaling too rapidly
- Stopping the inhalation when the cold propellant is felt in the throat
- Failing to hold their breath after inhalation
- Inhaling two sprays with one breath

For some patients, a spacing or extender device is necessary to aid delivery of medication by the inhalation route. Using an MDI requires that the patient activate the device while continuing to inhale. Young children and older patients are candidates for the addition of a spacer if inhalation therapy is prescribed. The spacer acts as a reservoir. When the MDI is compressed, the medication is deposited in the reservoir of the spacer, and the patient then inhales the medication from the spacer device. This makes administration less complicated and the dose more predictable. To ensure

correct use, slow, deep inspirations are still necessary. To prevent inhaling too quickly, some spacers are equipped with a whistle device that sounds if inhalation is too rapid. A spacer is also recommended for patients using steroid inhalers because it reduces the risk for an oral fungal infection. The accompanying Guidelines for Nursing Care provide information to instruct patients in the proper use of MDIs and small-volume nebulizers. Package inserts with the medication also reinforce correct technique for using inhalers.

A microchip-based inhaler has been developed that determines when the patient is breathing at an ideal rate to deliver a metered dose of asthma medication. This device (eg, SmartMist) delivers a standard dose with a high degree of precision. Several companies are working on similar pulmonary drug-delivery systems.

Providing Supplemental Oxygen

The amount of oxygen the patient uses for inspiration can be increased by providing a supplemental supply. This is called oxygen therapy and is usually prescribed by the physician. Oxygen therapy can frighten patients. Explanations from the nurse regarding procedures and purpose help reduce this fear. Patients should be encouraged to discuss their anxieties. If oxygen is given in an emergency, explanations concurrent with administration are appropriate.

Sources of Oxygen

Therapeutic oxygen is supplied from a wall outlet or a portable cylinder. The wall outlet source can be prepared for use quickly. The oxygen is supplied from a central source in the agency through a pipeline, usually at 50 to 60 pounds per square inch (psi) of pressure. A specially designed flowmeter is attached to the outlet (see Procedure 44-2 later for an illustration of a flowmeter). A valve regulates the oxygen flow.

Oxygen can also be dispersed under pressure from steel cylinders or tanks. The tank is delivered with a protective cap to prevent accidental damage of the cylinder outlet. When a standard, large-sized cylinder is full, its contents are under more than 2000 psi of pressure. The force through an accidentally partially opened outlet could cause the tank to take off like an uncontrolled, dangerous missile. Smaller cylinders are available for emergency and ambulatory settings. The principles and precautions are the same for all size cylinders.

To release oxygen safely and at the desired rate, a regulator is used. The regulator has two gauges. The one nearest the tank shows the pressure or amount of oxygen in the tank. The other gauge indicates the number of liters per minute of oxygen being released.

The oxygen cylinder and the regulator must be handled cautiously. The oxygen cylinder should be transported carefully, preferably strapped onto a wheeled carrier to avoid possible falling and breaking of the outlet. The cylinder should be stabilized securely in a properly fitting stand.

Because dust or other particles that may be present in the outlet of the tank could be forced in the regulator,

(*text continues on page 1246*)

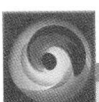

Table 44-3
Medications Used to Improve Respiratory Functioning

Medication	Activity	Route	Side Effects	Nursing Implications
Epinephrine	Relaxes muscles that line bronchi and bronchioles	IV, SQ	Tremors, anxiety, insomnia, headache, palpitations, elevated blood pressure, vomiting	Position patient upright to prevent aspiration if vomiting occurs. Monitor heart rate, respirations, breath sounds, and blood pressure every 15 minutes. May repeat medication within 15 minutes with an order.
Isoproterenol (Isuprel)	Bronchodilator	Inhaler	Same as with epinephrine but milder	Monitor heart rate. Demonstrate proper use of inhaler. Warn patient not to exceed prescribed frequency of doses.
Metaproterenol (Alupent)	Bronchodilator	PO, inhalation	Same as with epinephrine	Same as with epinephrine
Theophylline (aminophylline)	Bronchodilator	PO, IV, rectally	Nausea, vomiting, rapid heart rate, diuresis, irritability, vertigo, convulsions, nervousness, irritability	Monitor vital signs closely. Force fluids as clinical status allows. Monitor serum theophylline levels, especially if patient does not respond to drug or severe side effects develop.
Corticosteroids (ACTH, prednisone, dexamethasone)	Reduces inflammation	PO, IV	Fluid retention, hypertension, mood swings, weight gain, gastritis, hyperglycemia, insomnia	Reduce sodium intake. Make patient and family aware of potential for labile emotions. Weigh daily in morning. Monitor blood pressure and blood sugar. Warn patient to follow administration directions accurately. Instruct patient about correct use of inhaler.
Antihistamines	Blocks histamine and relieves congestion of an allergic origin	PO	Drowsiness, anorexia, constipation, dry mouth, blurred vision, urinary retention	Warn patient to use only with physician's advice in presence of bronchial asthma. Do not mix with alcohol, tranquilizers, or sedatives. Patient should avoid driving or using machinery. Observe patients for prolonged bleeding if they are using warfarin anticoagulants.
Cromolyn sodium (Intal)	Prevents the release of histamines, serotonin, prostaglandin by the mast cell in an antigen–antibody reaction in asthma	Inhaler	Cough	Remind patient this is used to prevent asthma attacks, not to treat acute episodes. This drug contains lactose and will cause diarrhea in lactose-deficient patients. Inform patient that this is effective only if taken routinely (two to four times per day).

IV, intravenous; SQ, subcutaneous; PO, oral.

Guidelines for Nursing Care

Using a Nebulizer Device

- Assess the patient's ability to manage a metered-dose inhaler or small-volume nebulizer.
- Explain, demonstrate, and encourage the patient to manipulate the inhaler or nebulizer apparatus.
- Encourage the patient to wash hands thoroughly before using device.

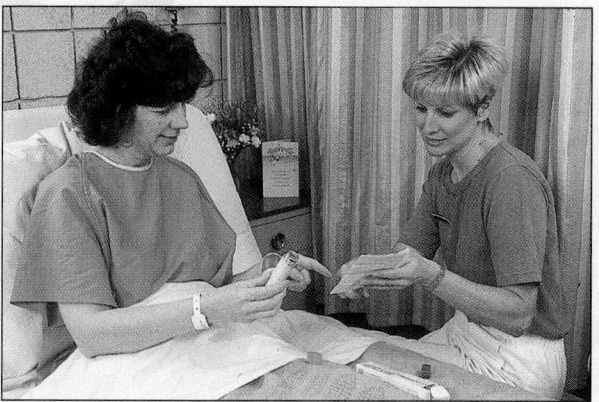

Teaching a patient about the inhaler.

Using a metered-dose inhaler with an extender.

The Metered-Dose Inhaler

- Remove the mouthpiece cover and shake inhaler well.
- Follow caregiver's or manufacturer's recommendations for placement of the mouthpiece. Two methods are possible:
  - Hold the inhaler 1–2 inches in front of open mouth; or
  - Place mouthpiece into mouth grasping securely with teeth and lips (an MDI coupled with a spacer or extender is always placed in the mouth)
- Take a deep breath and exhale.
- Inhale slowly and deeply through the mouth. Press down on the medication canister while continuing to inhale a full breath (when using a spacer or extender, depress the canister about one fourth or one third through the inspiration).
- Hold your breath for 5 to 10 seconds or as long as possible.
- Exhale slowly through pursed lips.
- If another puff is prescribed, wait 1 to 5 minutes before the next inhalation.
- If desired, gargle with tap water and blow nose into a tissue to remove any remaining trace of medication.
- Use mild soap and water to clean the mouthpiece, rinse it, and let it dry before replacing it.
- Follow physician's order regarding frequency of inhaler use.

Special Considerations

- Teach patients how to tell when their inhaler is empty. They can either count the number of times they have used the inhaler (usually about 200 sprays per container) or separate the canister from the plastic holder and place it in a bowl of water. When full, it sinks; when empty, it floats.

Home Considerations

- Once a week, MDI mouthpiece, spacer or extender, or nebulizer parts should be soaked in a vinegar solution (1 pint of water to 2 oz. of vinegar) for 20 minutes. Rinse with clean water and allow to air dry.

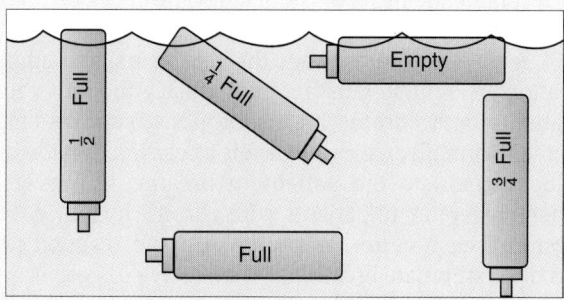

(*continued*)

Guidelines for Nursing Care (Continued)

The Small-Volume Nebulizer

- Remove the nebulizer cup from the device, open it, and place it on a flat working surface.
- Place premeasured unit dose medication in the bottom section of the cup or use a dropper to place concentrated dose of medication in cup and add prescribed fluid to dilute it.
- Screw the top portion of nebulizer cup back in place and attach the cup to the nebulizer.
- Attach one end of tubing to the stem on the bottom of the nebulizer cuff and the other end to the air compressor or oxygen source (if valve to control airflow is not available, a Y tube can be added to the tubing so that one branch of the Y tube connects to the nebulizer cup and the other branch is left open).
- Turn on the air compressor or oxygen.
- Check that a fine medication mist is produced by opening valve or placing thumb over open branch of Y tube.
- Place mouthpiece into mouth and grasp securely with teeth and lips.
- Inhale slowly through the mouth (a nose clip may be necessary if patient is also breathing through the nose).
- Hold each breath for 5 to 10 seconds or as long as possible before exhaling.
- Continue this inhalation technique until all medication in the nebulizer cup has been aerosolized (usually about 15 minutes).
- If desired, gargle with tap water after using nebulizer.
- Rinse the equipment in warm water and allow to air dry on a clean towel.

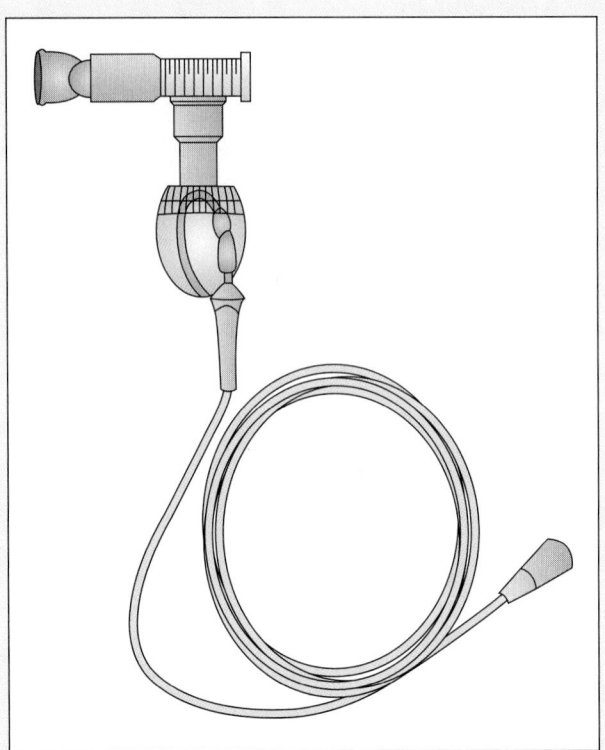

Small-volume nebulizer.

the tank is primed with two hands before the regulator is attached. The handle of the tank is turned slightly counterclockwise. This releases a small amount of oxygen and flushes out the outlet. The cylinder is closed again by turning the handle clockwise. The force with which the oxygen is released from this opening causes a loud, hissing sound that startles most people. Thus, patients and visitors need to be prepared for the noise with an appropriate explanation. It is recommended that tanks be primed away from the bedside. The accompanying Guidelines for Nursing Care give additional suggestions for transporting a patient with a portable oxygen tank.

Oxygen Flow Rate

The flow rate of oxygen, measured in liters per minute, regulates the amount of oxygen available to the patient. The rate varies depending on the condition of the patient and the route of administration of the oxygen. The flow rate does not necessarily reflect the oxygen concentration actually inspired by the patient because there is leaking and mixing with atmospheric air. More precise doses are usually prescribed in terms of percentage of inspired oxygen. To regulate oxygen concentration accurately, analysis of samples of the air mixture the patient is actually inhaling is recommended every 4 hours. Several types of commercial oxygen analyzers are available.

A physician prescribes the rate of oxygen administration. The nurse must monitor closely the flow rate for patients with chronic lung conditions, such as emphysema. Normally, excessive levels of carbon dioxide in the blood stimulate the patient to breathe. However, the chemoreceptors of patients with chronic lung disease become insensitive to carbon dioxide and respond to hypoxia to stimulate breathing. If excessive oxygen is given, the stimulus to breathe is removed, and the patient may stop breathing completely. Most patients with chronic

Guidelines for Nursing Care

Transporting a Patient With a Portable Oxygen Cylinder

Before the Transfer:

- Check that the oxygen cylinder contains oxygen.
- Check that additional oxygen source is available where patient is being transferred.
- Check amount of oxygen in cylinder (place cylinder key or wrench on valve stem and turn fully counterclockwise until needle on gauge indicates amount of available oxygen; turn the key back a half turn; use cylinder only if gauge indicates more than 500 psi).
- Connect oxygen tubing or humidifier bottle with tubing to the flowmeter adapter and attach other end to patient's oxygen cannula.
- Adjust the flow-control dial to the prescribed setting.
- Ensure that the cylinder is secured in holder before transporting patient (it is a dangerous practice to place the cylinder between the patient's legs or next to the patient during transfer because injury to the patient may result).
- Place coiled tubing under pillow or attach to linen or patient's gown.

After the Transfer:

- Attach patient to wall oxygen.
- Turn off the oxygen flow from the cylinder by turning the cylinder key clockwise until it is tight.
- Remove any excess oxygen in the pressure gauge by "bleeding" it. Turn the flow-control dial back on until hissing sound stops and needle on gauge has fallen to zero. Turn flow-control dial off.

(From Mathews, P. [1995]. Safely delivering a breath of fresh air. *Nursing, 25*[5], 66–69.)

---

lung disease can tolerate oxygen with a nasal cannula at 2 L/min, but arterial blood gas analysis should be monitored closely.

Humidifying Oxygen

The benefits of humidifying oxygen before delivering it to the patient by way of a nasal cannula are controversial. Research shows that with very-low-flow oxygen (2 L/min or less) delivered by nasal cannula, humidification is unnecessary. Because oxygen dries and dehydrates the respiratory mucous membranes, humidifying devices are commonly used for delivery of oxygen at higher flow rates. These supply 20% to 40% humidity. Distilled or sterile water is commonly used to humidify oxygen.

Precautions for Oxygen Administration

Oxygen, which constitutes 20% of normal air, is a tasteless, odorless, colorless gas. It supports combustion. To prevent fires and injuries, the following precautions must be taken:

- Avoid open flames in the patient's room.
- Place NO SMOKING signs in conspicuous places in the patient's room or home. Instruct the patient and visitors about the hazard of smoking when oxygen is in use.
- Check to see that electric equipment used in the room, such as electric bell cords, razors, radios, and suctioning equipment, is in good working order and emits no sparks.

- Avoid wearing and using synthetic fabrics that build up static electricity.
- Avoid using oils in the area. Oil can ignite spontaneously in the presence of oxygen.

Oxygen Administration

Oxygen can be administered by nasal cannula, nasal catheter, transtracheal catheter, simple mask, partial rebreather mask, nonrebreather mask, Venturi mask, and tent. Table 44-4 compares oxygen delivery systems.

Nasal Cannula

A **nasal cannula**, also called nasal prongs, is probably the most commonly used aid to breathing. The cannula is a disposable, plastic device with two protruding prongs for insertion into the nostrils; the cannula is connected to an oxygen source with a humidifier and flowmeter. The cannula does not impede eating or speaking and is easily used in the home. Disadvantages of this system are that it can easily be dislodged and can cause dryness of the nasal mucosa. Procedure 44-2 describes oxygen administration by nasal cannula.

Nasal Catheter

A nasal, or oropharyngeal, catheter is another efficient means for administering oxygen, but it is infrequently used because it is uncomfortable for the patient and may cause trauma to respiratory mucous membranes. It is inserted into the throat through one nostril and must be changed to the other nostril every 8 hours. Gastric distention often occurs because the gas flow can be misdirected into the stomach.

Face Masks

Disposable and reusable face masks are available in plastic or rubber. The mask should be fitted carefully to the patient's face to avoid leakage of oxygen. It should be comfortably snug but not tight against the patient's face. The most commonly used types of masks include the simple face mask, the partial rebreather mask, the nonrebreather mask, and the Venturi mask. Procedure 44-3 describes the actions and rationales for steps in using face masks.

The *simple oxygen mask* connects to oxygen tubing, a humidifier, and a flowmeter, just as the nasal cannula does. This mask has vents on its sides that allow room air to leak in at many places, thereby diluting the source oxygen, and exhaled carbon dioxide to escape (see Table 44-4). Often, it is used when an increased delivery of oxygen is needed for short periods (eg, less than 12 hours). The mask should fit closely to the face to deliver this higher concentration of oxygen effectively. Patients may have difficulty keeping the mask in position over the nose and mouth, and because of this pressure and the presence of moisture, skin

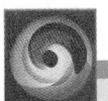

Table 44-4
Oxygen Delivery Systems

Method	Amount Delivered FiO$_2$ (Fraction Inspired Oxygen)	Priority Nursing Interventions
Nasal cannula	*Low Flow* 1 L/min = 24% 2 L/min = 28% 3 L/min = 32% 4 L/min = 36% 5 L/min = 40% 6 L/min = 44%	Check frequently that both prongs are in patient's nares. Never deliver more than 2–3 L/min to patient with chronic lung disease.
Simple mask	*Low Flow* 6–10 L/min = 35%–60% (5 L/min is minimum setting)	Monitor patient frequently to check placement of the mask. Support patient if claustrophobia is a concern. Secure physician's order to replace mask with nasal cannula during meal time.
Partial rebreather mask	*Low Flow* 6–15 L/min = 70%–90%	Set flow rate so that mask remains two thirds full during inspiration. Keep reservoir bag free of twists or kinks.
Nonrebreather mask	*Low Flow* 6–15 L/min = 60%–100%	Maintain flow rate so reservoir bag collapses only slightly during inspiration. Check that valves and rubber flaps are functioning properly (open during expiration and closed during inhalation). Monitor SaO$_2$ with pulse oximeter.
Venturi mask	*High Flow* 4–10 L/min = 24%–55%	Requires careful monitoring to verify FiO$_2$ at flow rate ordered. Check that air intake valves are not blocked.

PROCEDURE 44-2

Administering Oxygen by Nasal Cannula

Equipment

Flowmeter connected to oxygen supply

Humidifier with sterile distilled water (optional with low-flow system)

Nasal cannula and tubing
Gauze to pad tubing over ears (optional)

Action	Rationale
1. Explain procedure to patient and review safety precautions necessary when oxygen is in use. Place NO SMOKING signs in appropriate areas.	Oxygen supports combustion.
2. Wash your hands.	Handwashing deters the spread of microorganisms.
3. Connect the nasal cannula to the oxygen setup with humidification, if one is in use. Adjust the flow rate as ordered by physician (see photo). Check that oxygen is flowing out of prongs.	Oxygen forced through a water reservoir is humidified before it is delivered to the patient, thus preventing dehydration of the mucous membranes. Recent research has questioned the necessity of humidification with low-flow oxygen delivery by way of cannula.

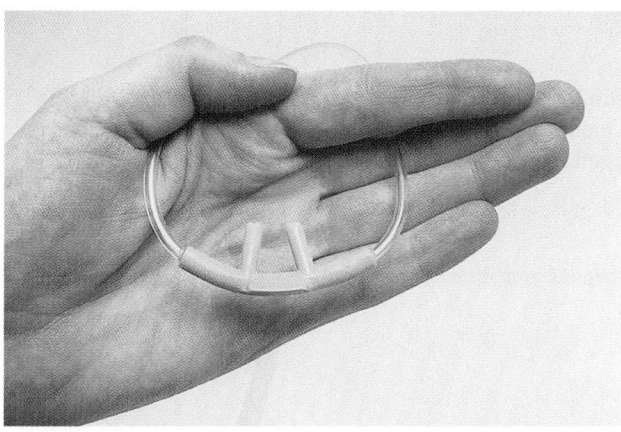

Nasal cannula.

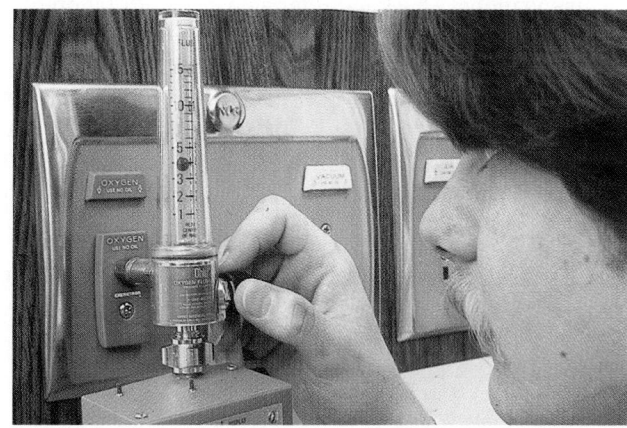

Action 3: Adjusting flow rate.

Action	Rationale
4. Place the prongs in the patient's nostrils (see photo). Adjust according to type of equipment. 　a. Over and behind each ear with adjuster comfortably under chin; *or* 　b. Around the patient's head	Correct placement of the prongs and fastener facilitates oxygen administration and comfort for the patient.
5. Use gauze pads at ear beneath the tubing as necessary.	Pads reduce irritation and pressure and protect the skin.
6. Encourage patient to breathe through his or her nose with mouth closed.	Provides for optimal delivery of oxygen to patient.
7. Wash your hands.	Handwashing deters the spread of microorganisms.
8. Assess and chart patient's response to therapy.	Patient's respirations, color, breathing pattern, and chest movements indicate effectiveness of oxygen therapy.

(continued)

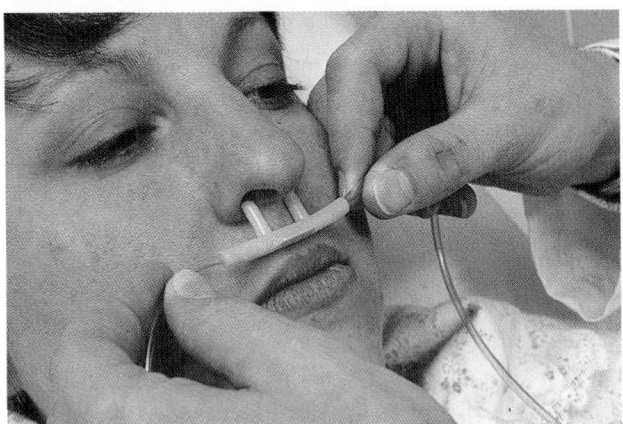

Action 4: Placing cannula prongs in nostrils.

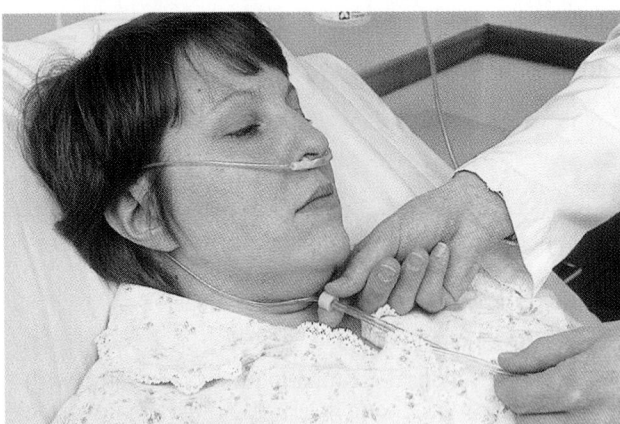

Action 4: Adjusting for comfort.

9. Remove and clean the cannula and assess nares at least every 8 hours or according to agency recommendations. Check nares for evidence of irritation or bleeding.

The continued presence of the cannula causes irritation and dryness of the mucous membranes. Lubricant counteracts the drying effects of oxygen.

Home Care Considerations   Patients may require oxygen administration to continue in the home setting. Portable oxygen concentrators are used most frequently. Caregivers require instruction concerning safety precautions with oxygen use and an understanding of the rationale for the specific liter flow of oxygen.

---

breakdown is a possibility. It is difficult to eat or talk with the mask in place.

The *partial rebreather mask* is equipped with a reservoir bag for the collection of the first part of the patient's exhaled air. The remaining exhaled air exits through vents. The air in the reservoir is mixed with 100% oxygen for the next inhalation. The patient thus rebreathes about one third of the expired air from the reservoir bag. This type of mask permits the conservation of oxygen. An additional advantage is that the patient can inhale room air through openings in the mask if the oxygen supply is briefly interrupted. The disadvantages are those of any mask: eating and talking are difficult, a tight seal is required, and there is the potential for skin breakdown. The reservoir bag should deflate slightly with inspiration. If it deflates completely, the flow rate should be increased until only a slight deflation is noted.

The *nonrebreather mask* provides the highest concentration of oxygen with a mask to a spontaneously breathing patient. It is similar to the partial rebreather mask except two one-way valves prevent rebreathing exhaled air. The reservoir bag is filled with oxygen that enters the mask on

inspiration. A malfunction could possibly cause CO_2 buildup and suffocation. Exhaled air escapes through side vents. This mask can also be used to administer other gases.

The *Venturi mask* gets its name from the Venturi effect, which allows the mask to deliver the most precise concentrations of oxygen. This mask has a large tube with an oxygen inlet. As the tube narrows, the pressure drops, causing air to be sucked in through side ports. These ports are adjusted according to the prescription for oxygen concentration. It is a nursing responsibility to make sure the ports are always open. If these are occluded by linens, clothing, or a patient rolling on the mask, the oxygen delivered might be at an unsafe concentration.

Oxygen Tent

Oxygen also can be administered by way of a tent—a light, portable structure made of clear plastic and attached to a motor-driven unit. The motor helps to circulate and cool the air in the tent. The cooling device functions like an electric refrigeration unit. A thermostat in the unit keeps the tent at the temperature considered most comfortable for the patient. The tent fits over the top part of the bed so

PROCEDURE 44-3

Administering Oxygen by Mask

Equipment

Flowmeter connected to oxygen
   supply

Humidifier with sterile distilled water
Face mask specified by physician

Gauze to pad elastic band (optional)

Action	Rationale
1. Explain procedure to patient and review safety precautions necessary when oxygen is in use. Place No Smoking signs in appropriate areas.	Oxygen supports combustion. Explanation alleviates anxiety.
2. Wash your hands.	Handwashing deters the spread of microorganisms.
3. Attach the face mask to the oxygen setup with humidification. Start the flow of oxygen at the specified rate. For a mask with a reservoir, allow O_2 to fill the bag before placing the mask over the patient's nose and mouth.	Oxygen forced through a water reservoir is humidified before it is delivered to the patient, thus preventing dehydration of the mucous membranes. A reservoir bag must be inflated with oxygen because the bag is the source of oxygen supply for the patient.
4. Position the face mask over the patient's nose and mouth. Adjust it with the elastic strap so that the mask fits snugly but comfortably on the face.	A loose or poorly fitting mask will result in oxygen loss and decreased therapeutic value. Masks may cause feeling of suffocation, and patient needs frequent attention and reassurance.
5. Use gauze pads to reduce irritation to the patient's ears and scalp.	Pads reduce irritation and pressure and protect the skin.
6. Wash your hands.	Handwashing deters the spread of microorganisms.
7. Remove the mask and dry the skin every 2 to 3 hours if the oxygen is running continuously. Do not powder around the mask.	The tight-fitting mask and moisture from condensation can irritate the skin on the face. There is danger of inhaling powder if it is placed on the mask.
8. Assess and chart patient's response to therapy.	Patient's respiratory rate and pattern, color, and so forth indicate effectiveness of oxygen therapy.

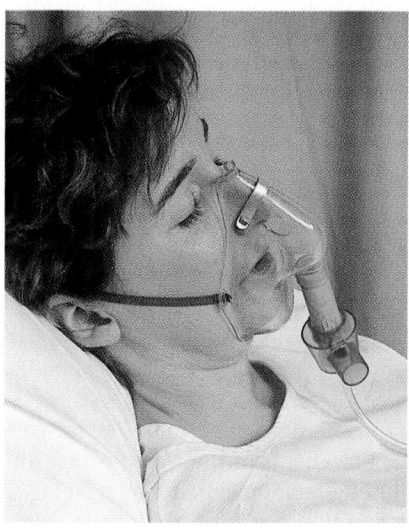

Venturi mask. (Photos © Ken Kasper.)

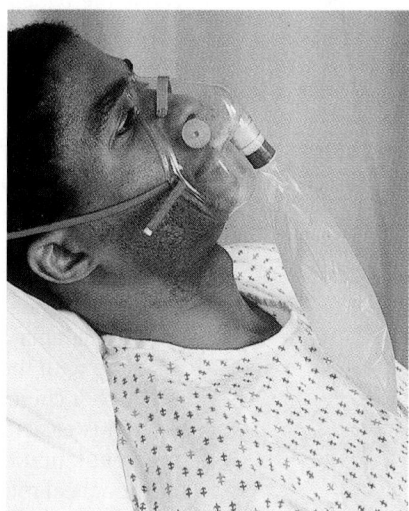

Nonrebreather mask.

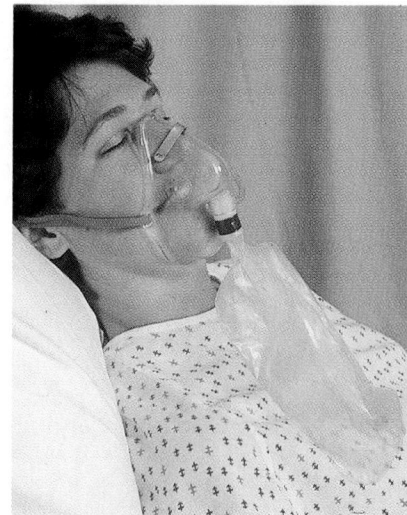

Partial rebreather mask.

that the patient's head and thorax are inside. It has side openings through which nursing care can be administered. It is commonly used with children who need a cool and highly humidified airflow (eg, children with pneumonia). The tent does not allow the maintenance of a satisfactory or precise oxygen concentration and thus is rarely used except for children.

Oxygen Therapy in the Home

Oxygen concentrators rather than cylinders are used more commonly in the home setting. They are portable, cost-effective, and easy to use but cannot deliver oxygen flow at greater than 4 liters (FiO_2 of about 36%).

Patients using continuous supplemental oxygen therapy in the home have another alternative—*transtracheal oxygen delivery*. A small catheter is inserted into the trachea under local anesthesia. Patients usually report improved mobility, comfort, appearance, and lower cost with this delivery system. A transtracheal catheter does not interfere with talking, eating, or drinking and delivers oxygen throughout the respiratory cycle rather than just at inspiration. This system does require that the patient or family assume responsibility for daily catheter care. A transtracheal oxygen setup is illustrated in Figure 44-12.

Patients using oxygen at home need instruction regarding safety precautions. The following items must be reviewed and stressed (Rice, 1995):

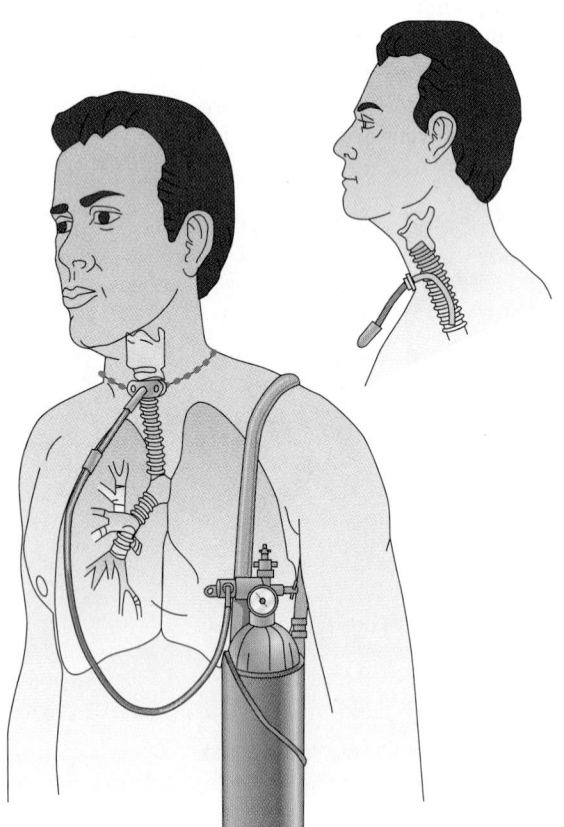

Figure 44-12
A transtracheal oxygen setup.

- No smoking or open flames are allowed within 10 feet of the oxygen source. Remind visitors of the restriction on smoking.
- Do not use electrical equipment near the oxygen administration setup (eg, space heaters).
- Remove oxygen when patient uses an electric razor.
- Use caution with gas or electric appliances when patient is receiving oxygen therapy.
- Follow the physician's prescription for the oxygen flow rate (using too little or too much oxygen can prove life-threatening).
- Secure the oxygen tank in a holder and away from direct sunlight or heat.
- Allow adequate airflow around the oxygen concentrator (avoid placing concentrator flush against wall).
- Ground oxygen concentrators.
- Have the physician's and nurse's telephone numbers readily available.
- Review with the patient the directions for reaching the oxygen equipment vendor and the reasons for contacting vendor.
- Discuss the signs and symptoms that indicate the need to call for emergency assistance or visit the local emergency room.

Using Artificial Airways

Oropharyngeal and Nasopharyngeal Airways

An *oropharyngeal* or *nasopharyngeal airway* is a semicircular tube of plastic or rubber inserted into the back of the pharynx through the mouth or nose in a spontaneously breathing patient. It is used to keep the tongue clear of the airway and to permit suctioning of secretions. It is often used for postoperative patients until they regain consciousness. It is important to not use tape to hold it in place because the patient should be able to expel the airway once he or she becomes alert. Refer to the accompanying Guidelines for Nursing Care for an illustration and techniques to use when inserting an oropharyngeal airway.

Endotracheal Tube

An **endotracheal tube** is a polyvinylchloride airway that is inserted through the nose or the mouth into the trachea using a laryngoscope as a guide. It is used to administer oxygen by mechanical ventilator, to suction secretions easily, or to bypass upper airway obstructions (eg, tongue or tracheal edema). Although uncomfortable and easy to manipulate with the tongue, orotracheal insertion is often the method of choice, especially in an emergency, because insertion is easier and a larger-sized tube can be used making ventilation easier. Placement of the tube through the nasotracheal route, although tolerated better by patients, is more difficult and requires the use of a narrower tube. Most commonly, a cuffed endotracheal tube is used that prevents air leakage and bronchial aspiration of foreign material, while allowing more precise control of oxygen and mechanical ventilation (Fig. 44-13). Careful monitoring of endotracheal cuff pressure decreases the risk for tracheal necrosis. The smallest amount of air that results in

Guidelines for Nursing Care

Inserting an Oropharyngeal Airway

- Use an airway that is the correct size (size 4 or 5 is appropriate for the average adult).
- Explain what you are doing to the patient even though the patient appears unconscious.
- Wash your hands and don gloves (if patient is coughing, wear mask and goggles or face shield).
- Remove dentures if they are present.
- Position patient on his or her back with neck hyperextended (unless this is inappropriate).
- Open patient's mouth by using your thumb and index finger to gently pry teeth apart.
- Insert the airway with the curved tip pointing up toward the roof of the mouth.
- Slide the airway across the tongue to the back of the mouth.
- Rotate the airway 180 degrees as it passes the uvula (a flashlight can confirm the position of the airway with the curve fitting over the tongue).
- Ensure adequate ventilation by auscultating breath sounds.
- Position patient on his or her side when airway is in place.
- Remove airway for a brief period every 4 hours. Provide mouth care and rinse airway before reinserting it.

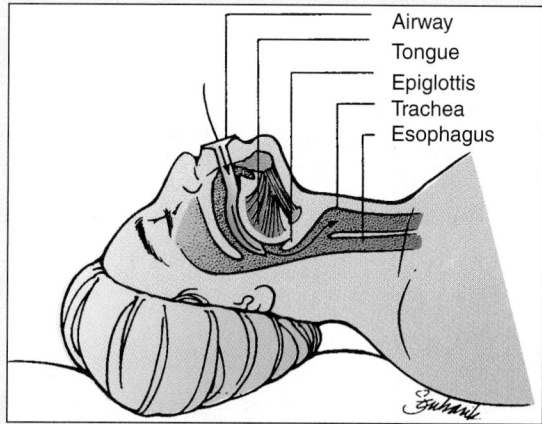

Airway — Tongue — Epiglottis — Trachea — Esophagus

Airway in place in a patient after anesthesia. Airway allows air to pass over the tongue and into the pharynx. (Reprinted with permission from Smeltzer, S. C., & Bare, B. G. [2000]. *Brunner & Suddarth's textbook of medical-surgical nursing* [9th ed.]. Philadelphia: Lippincott Williams & Wilkins, p. 350.)

---

an airtight seal between the trachea and the tube is desirable and less likely to result in complications.

Tracheostomy

A *tracheostomy* is an artificial opening made into the trachea. The curved **tracheostomy tube** inserted into this opening is made of semiflexible plastic, rigid plastic, or metal and comes in multiple sizes with varied angles. A tracheostomy tube consists of an outer cannula or main shaft, the inner cannula, and an obturator. An obturator guides the direction of the outer cannula and is inserted into the tube during placement. It is removed once the outer cannula of the tube is in place (Fig. 44-14). Many tubes also have inner cannulas, which may or may not be disposable. The outer cannula remains in place in the trachea, and the inner cannula is removed for cleaning or replaced with a new one. A tube with an inner cannula is necessary when patients have excessive secretions or have difficulty clearing their secretions and may also be recommended for a patient discharged with a tracheostomy tube in place. The condition and needs of the patient determine the selection of either a metal or plastic tracheostomy tube. Although metal tubes are more cost-effective for long-term use, only plastic tubes have an adapter at the neckplate that permits connection to respiratory therapy equipment (eg, an oxygen delivery system, Ambu bag, or mechanical ventilator). A *fenestrated* tracheostomy tube has one large or several small openings or windows on its outer curve, has an inner cannula, and can be cuffed or cuffless. When the patient is

being mechanically ventilated, the inner cannula is in place blocking the small openings. After the patient is no longer connected to the ventilator, the inner cannula can be removed, the cuff deflated, and the tube plugged, allowing the patient to speak. Because the tube has these openings, it is not recommended for use if a patient has a history of aspiration (Phipps, Sands, & Marek, 1999).

Tracheostomy tubes may be either cuffed or cuffless (see Fig. 44-14). The inflated cuff seals the opening around the tube against air leakage, prevents aspiration, and permits mechanical ventilation. Newer tracheal cuffs are low pressure, do not require deflating for short intervals every few hours, and can be maintained at lower than tracheal capillary pressure. A cuffed tube should be deflated before oral feeding unless the patient is at high risk for aspiration. If left cuffed, the balloon can cause pressure that extends through the trachea and onto the esophagus, possibly impeding swallowing.

A tracheostomy tube is inserted for a variety of reasons (eg, to replace an endotracheal tube, to provide a method to mechanically ventilate the patient, to bypass an upper airway obstruction, or to remove tracheobronchial secretions). It is inserted in the operating room or intensive care unit under sterile conditions using local anesthesia. The tracheostomy tube is held in place by twill tapes or a Velcro strip fastened around the patient's neck. Usually, a sterile, square gauze pad that has been precut by the manufacturer is placed between the skin and outer wings of the tube before the tube is tied. This tracheostomy dressing

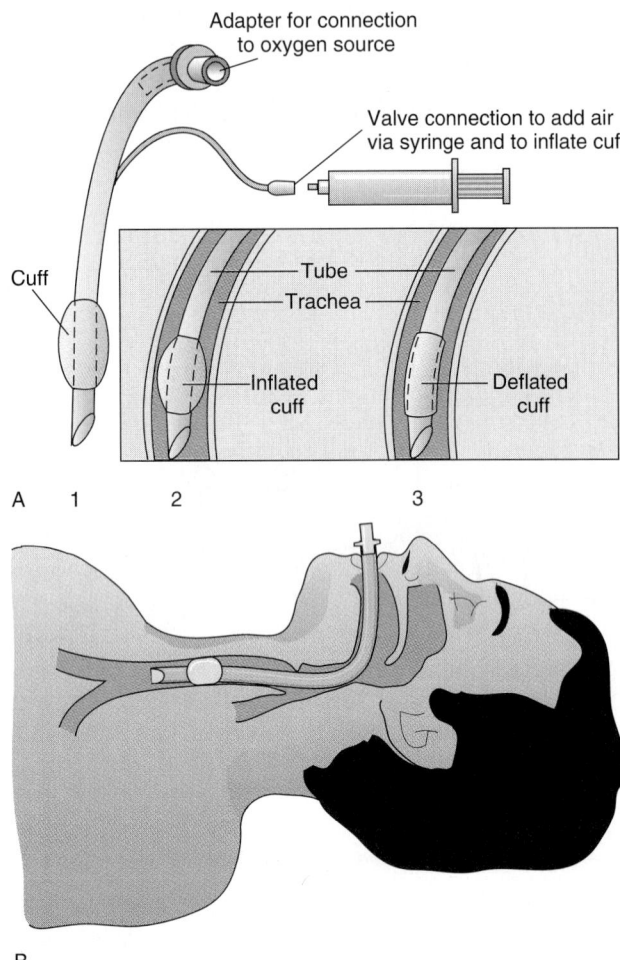

Figure 44-13
Endotracheal tube. **(A)** (1) Parts of a cuffed endotracheal tube, (2) tube in place with the cuff inflated, (3) tube in place with the cuff deflated. **(B)** Endotracheal tube in place.

must be kept dry to prevent infection and skin irritation. The tracheostomy can be temporary or permanent.

Nursing responsibilities may include regularly checking cuff pressure, although some tubes have a pressure-release valve that prevents pressure from increasing to damaging levels. Also, because the tracheostomy tube bypasses the natural humidifying and heating mechanisms in the nose and mouth, the oxygen must be heated and humidified to prevent secretions from becoming dry.

The tracheostomy tube must remain free from foreign objects and nonsterile materials. Cotton balls, loose threads from dressings, needles, and other small objects must be kept away from the opening. Suctioning to remove secretions is performed using the sterile technique described in Chapter 27. The frequency of suctioning varies with the amount of secretions present, but it should be done often enough to keep ventilation effective and as effortless as possible.

A tracheotomized patient is unable to speak. The patient's care should include consideration of his or her impaired ability to communicate. Communication tools (eg, writing board, letters, vocabulary cards) should be kept close at hand along with the call light or bell. To prevent anxiety, this patient requires reassurance and frequent explanations and anticipation of needs.

Suctioning

If the patient is unable to remove secretions with coughing after the application of artificial airways, secretions can be aspirated with a suctioning device (Procedure 44-4). Suctioning irritates the mucosa and removes oxygen from the respiratory tract, possibly causing *hypoxemia* (insufficient oxygen in the blood). Thus, the patient must be hyperoxygenated before suctioning. Tracheal suctioning may be performed by passing a sterile catheter through the mouth
(*text continues on page 1257*)

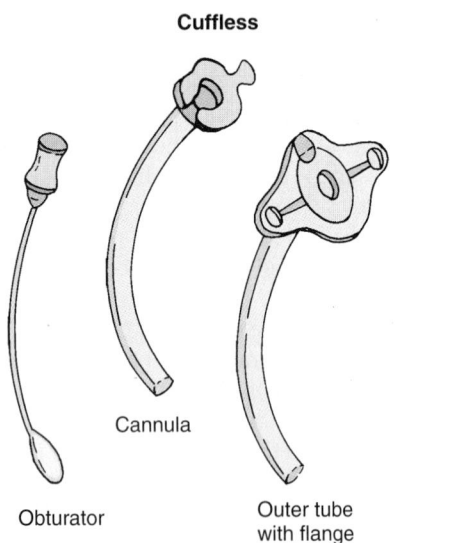

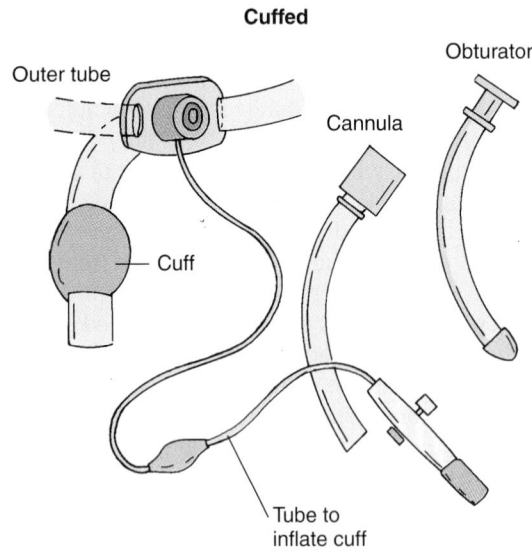

Figure 44-14
Two types of tracheostomy sets—cuffless and cuffed.

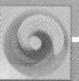

PROCEDURE 44-4

Suctioning the Nasopharyngeal and Oropharyngeal Areas

Equipment

Portable or wall suction unit with tubing

Sterile suction catheter with Y port

Sterile water or saline

Sterile disposable container

Sterile gloves

Towel or waterproof pad

Action	Rationale
1. Determine the need for suctioning. Administer pain medication before suctioning to postoperative patient.	Suctioning should be done only when secretions have accumulated or adventitious breath sounds are audible. This minimizes trauma to airway mucosa. Suctioning stimulates coughing, which is painful for patients with surgical incisions.
2. Explain procedure to patient.	This provides reassurance and promotes cooperation.
3. Assemble equipment.	This provides for organized approach.
4. Wash your hands.	Handwashing deters spread of microorganisms.
5. Adjust bed to comfortable working position. Lower side rail closer to you. Place the patient in a semi-Fowler's position if conscious. An unconscious patient should be placed in the lateral position facing you.	Having the patient in a sitting position helps him or her to cough and makes breathing easier. Gravity also facilitates the insertion of the catheter. Lateral position prevents the airway from becoming obstructed and promotes drainage of secretions.
6. Place towel or waterproof pad across patient's chest.	This protects bed linens.

7. Turn suction to appropriate pressure:
 a. Wall unit
   Adult: 100 to 120 mm Hg
   Child: 95 to 110 mm Hg
   Infant: 50 to 95 mm Hg
 b. Portable unit
   Adult: 10 to 15 mm Hg
   Child: 5 to 10 mm Hg
   Infant: 2 to 5 mm Hg
	Negative pressure must be at a safe level or pneumothorax may occur.

8. Open sterile suction package. Set up sterile container, touching only the outside surface, and pour sterile saline or water into it.	Sterile normal saline or water is used to lubricate the outside of the catheter, thus minimizing irritation of mucosa as it is being introduced.
9. Don sterile gloves. The dominant hand that will handle the catheter must remain sterile, while the nondominant hand is considered clean rather than sterile.	Handling the sterile catheter with a hand wearing a sterile glove helps prevent introducing organisms into the respiratory tract and the clean glove protects the nurse from microorganisms.
10. With sterile gloved hand, pick up sterile catheter and connect to suction tubing that is held with unsterile hand.	Sterilization can be maintained.
11. Moisten the catheter by dipping it into the container of sterile saline (see photo). Occlude Y tube to check suction.	Lubricating the inside of the catheter with saline helps move secretions in the catheter.
12. Estimate the distance from the ear lobe to the nostril, and place thumb and forefinger of gloved hand at that point on the catheter.	Ensures that catheter remains in pharynx rather than trachea.

(continued)

PROCEDURE 44-4

Suctioning the Nasopharyngeal and Oropharyngeal Areas (Continued)

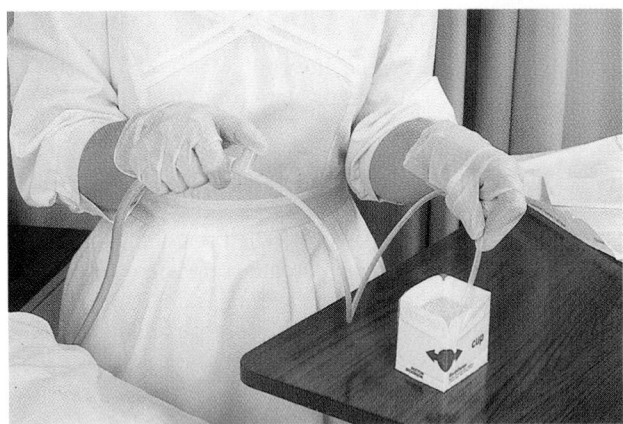

Action 11: Moisten the catheter by dipping it into the sterile saline container and occlude Y tube to check suction.

13. Gently insert the catheter with the suction off by leaving the vent on the Y connector open (see photo). Slip the catheter gently along the floor of an unobstructed nostril toward the trachea to suction the nasopharynx. Or, insert the catheter along the side of the mouth toward the trachea to suction the oropharynx. Never apply suction as the catheter is introduced.

Using suction while inserting the catheter can cause trauma to the mucosa and removes oxygen from the respiratory tract. Coughing is induced when the trachea is touched. This helps the patient raise secretions.

14. Apply suction by occluding the suctioning port with your thumb and gently rotate the catheter as it is being withdrawn (see photo). Do not allow the suctioning to continue for more than 10 to 15 seconds at a time.

Turning the catheter as it is withdrawn helps clean all surfaces of the respiratory passageways. Suctioning the patient for longer than 10 to 15 seconds robs the respiratory tract of oxygen, which may result in hypoxia.

15. Flush the catheter with saline and repeat suctioning as needed and according to patient's toleration of procedure.

Flushing cleans and clears catheter and lubricates it for next insertion.

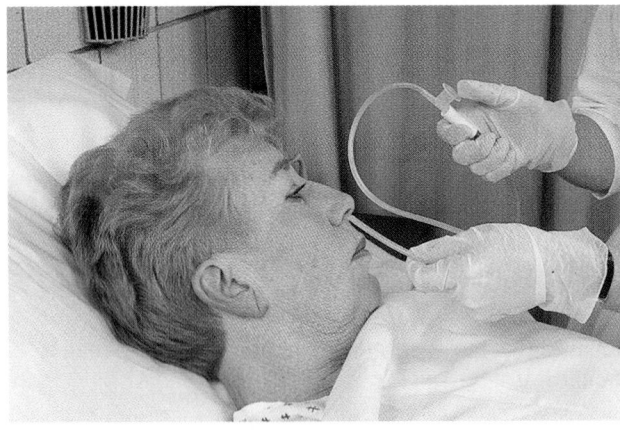

Action 13: Inserting the catheter.

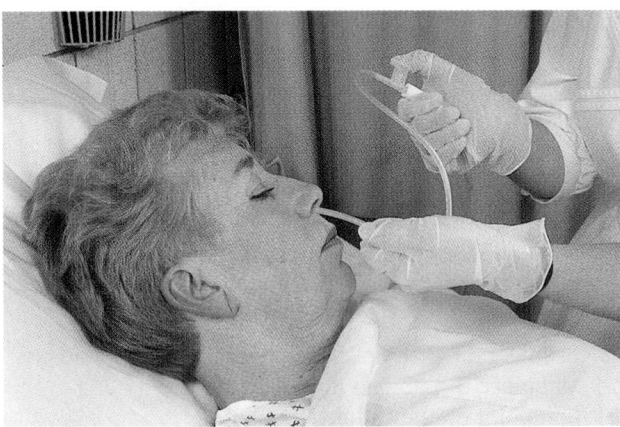

Action 14: Occluding port and rotating catheter while withdrawing.

(continued)

PROCEDURE 44-4

Suctioning the Nasopharyngeal and Oropharyngeal Areas (Continued)

16. Allow at least 20- to 30-second interval if additional suctioning is needed. The nares should be alternated when repeated suctioning is required. Do not force catheter through the nares. Encourage patient to cough and deep breathe between suctionings.

Normal breathing between suctioning helps compensate for any hypoxia induced by the previous suctioning.

17. When suctioning is completed, remove gloves inside out and dispose of gloves, catheter, and container with solution in proper receptacle. Wash your hands.

Handwashing prevents transmission of microorganisms.

18. Use auscultation to listen to chest and breathing sounds to assess the effectiveness of suctioning (see photo).

Listening to chest and breathing sounds helps determine whether the respiratory passageways are clear of secretions.

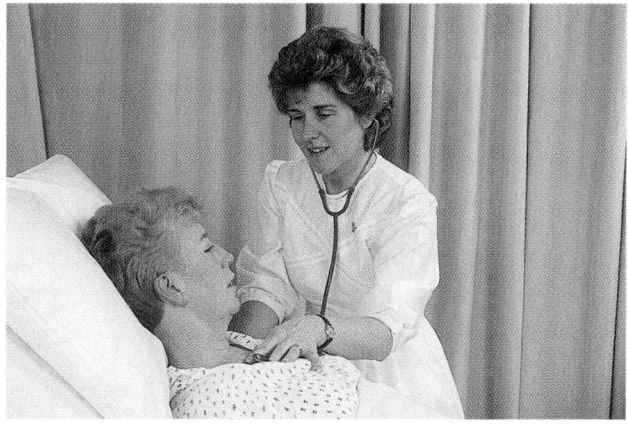

Action 18: Assessing effectiveness of suctioning. (Photos © 1992 B. Proud.)

19. Record the time of suctioning and the nature and amount of secretions. Also note the character of the patient's respirations before and after the suctioning.

Records of nursing measures used help assess, evaluate, and coordinate care.

20. Offer oral hygiene after suctionings.

Respiratory secretions that are allowed to accumulate in the mouth are irritating to mucous membranes and unpleasant for the patient.

(orotracheal), through the nose (nasotracheal), through an endotracheal tube, or through a tracheostomy tube. Procedure 44-5 describes suctioning a tracheostomy. When performed correctly, suctioning provides comfort by relieving respiratory distress. It is normally painless; however, a postoperative or trauma patient should receive analgesic medication before suctioning because the cough reflex will be stimulated. When performed incorrectly, it can increase anxiety and pain and cause respiratory arrest. Possible complications include infection, cardiac arrhythmias, hypoxia, mucosa trauma, and death. The suctioning catheter should be small enough not to occlude the airway being suctioned but large enough to remove secretions. Carroll

(1998) recommends that the outer diameter of the suction catheter should be half the inner diameter of the endotracheal or tracheostomy tube. Several sizes of soft, plastic, clear catheters are available.

Previously, it was common practice to instill a small amount of normal saline into the airway during the suctioning procedure to help liquefy secretions. This is no longer recommended for routine suctioning because research identified that the addition of liquid into the airway further reduces oxygenation, has no effect on thinning secretions, and may dislodge bacteria adhered to the tube and flush it into the lungs (Carroll, 1998; Galvin & Cusano, 1998).

PROCEDURE 44-5

Suctioning the Tracheostomy

Equipment

Portable or wall suction device with connecting tubing
Sterile suction kit containing the following or gather separately:
    Sterile suction catheter of appropriate size with Y port

Infants: 6–8 F
Children: 8–10 F
Adults: 12–16 F
Sterile container
Sterile glove
Sterile normal saline

Clean towel or sterile drape (optional)
Goggles (or glasses) and mask
Gown (optional)
Resuscitation bag connected to 100% oxygen

Action	Rationale
1. Explain procedure to patient and reassure him or her that you will interrupt procedure if the patient indicates respiratory difficulty. Administer pain medication before suctioning to postoperative patient.	Explanation facilitates cooperation and provides reassurance for patient. Any procedure that compromises respiration is frightening for the patient. Suctioning stimulates coughing, which is painful for patients with surgical incisions.
2. Gather equipment and provide privacy for patient.	This provides for organized approach to task.
3. Wash your hands.	Handwashing deters spread of microorganisms.
4. Assist the patient to a semi-Fowler's or Fowler's position if conscious. An unconscious patient should be placed in the lateral position facing you.	Sitting position helps patient to cough and breathe more easily. This position also uses gravity to aid in the insertion of catheter. Lateral position prevents the airway from becoming obstructed and promotes drainage of secretions.

5. Turn suction to appropriate pressure:
  a. Wall unit
     Adult: 100 to 120 mm Hg
     Child: 95 to 110 mm Hg
     Infant: 50 mm Hg
  b. Portable unit
     Adult: 10 to 15 mm Hg
     Child: 5 to 10 mm Hg
     Infant: 2 to 5 mm Hg
	Negative pressure must be at safe level or damage to tracheal mucosa may occur.

6. Place clean towel, if being used, across patient's chest. Don goggles, mask, and gown, if necessary.	Towel protects patient and bed linens. Wearing protective equipment prevents contamination of the caregiver's mucous membranes.
7. Open sterile kit or set up equipment, and prepare to suction: a. Place sterile drape, if available, across patient's chest.	Drape protects patient and bed linens.
b. Open sterile container (see photo) and place on bedside table or overbed table without contaminating inner surface. Pour sterile saline into it.	This maintains sterile setup.
c. Hyperoxygenate patient using manual resuscitation bag or sigh mechanism on mechanical ventilator.	This prevents hypoxemia that can occur during suctioning.
d. Don sterile gloves or one sterile glove on dominant hand and clean glove on nondominant hand.	Gloves maintain sterility of procedure and protect the nurse from microorganisms.
e. Connect sterile suction catheter to suction tubing that is held with unsterile gloved hand (see photo).	Sterile technique helps prevent introduction of organisms into the respiratory tract.

(continued)

PROCEDURE 44-5

Suctioning the Tracheostomy (Continued)

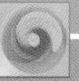

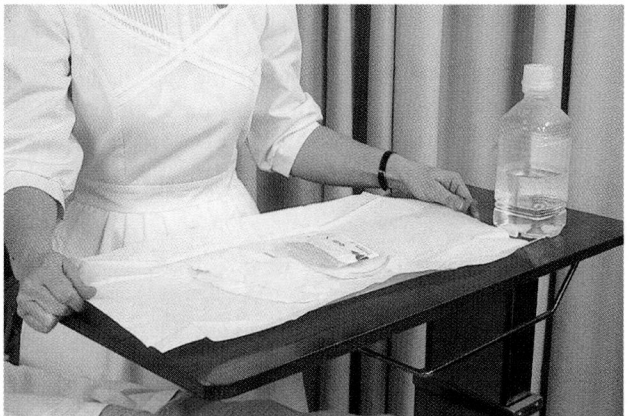

Action 7: Opening the sterile kit.

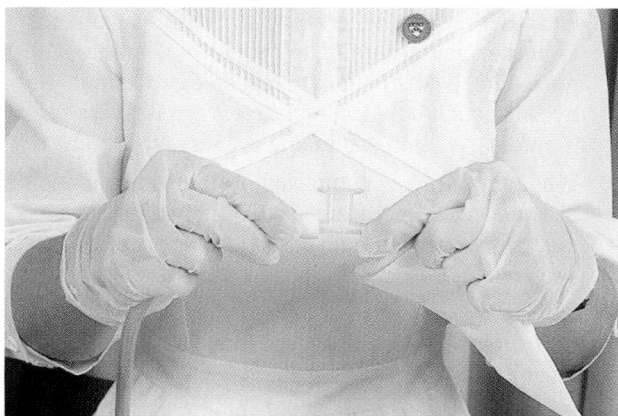

Action 7e: Connecting catheter to the suction tube.

8. Moisten the catheter by dipping it into the container of sterile saline unless it is one of the newer silicone catheters that do not require lubrication.

9. Remove oxygen delivery setup with unsterile gloved hand if it is still in place.

10. Using sterile gloved hand, gently and quickly insert catheter into the trachea (see photo). Advance about 10 to 12.5 cm (4 to 5 inches) or until patient coughs. *Do not occlude Y port when inserting catheter.*

Lubricating the inside of catheter with saline helps move secretions in the catheter. Silicone catheters do not require lubrication.

This exposes tracheostomy tube.

Using suction when inserting catheter can cause trauma to mucosa and removes oxygen from the respiratory tract.

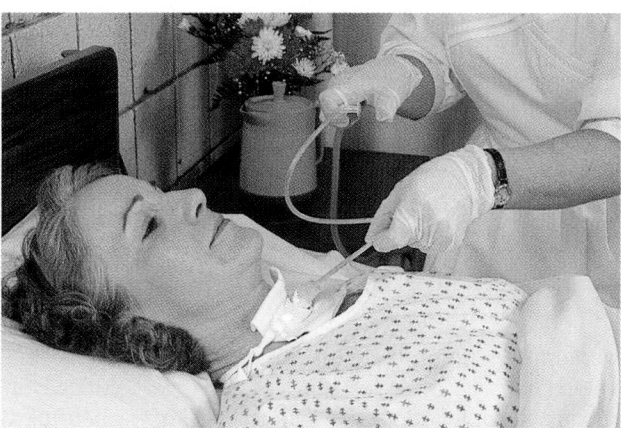

Action 10: Inserting the catheter with the Y port open.

11. Apply intermittent suction by occluding Y port with thumb of unsterile gloved hand. Gently rotate catheter with thumb and index finger of sterile gloved hand as catheter is being withdrawn. Do not allow suctioning to continue for more than 10 seconds. Hyperventilate 3 to 5 times between suctionings or encourage patient to cough and deep breathe between suctionings.

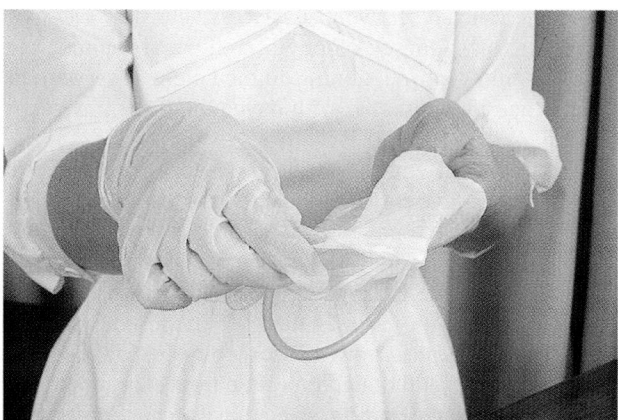

Action 13: Removing glove over the catheter. (Photos © B. Proud.)

Turning the catheter while withdrawing it helps clean surfaces of respiratory tract and prevents injury to tracheal mucosa. Suctioning for longer than 10 seconds may result in hypoxia. Hyperventilation reoxygenates the lungs.

(continued)

PROCEDURE 44-5

Suctioning the Tracheostomy (Continued)

12. Flush the catheter with saline and repeat suctioning as needed and according to patient's toleration of procedure. Allow patient to rest at least 1 minute between suctionings, and replace oxygen delivery setup if necessary. Limit suctioning events to three times.

Flushing cleans and clears catheter and lubricates it for next insertion. Allowing time interval and replacing oxygen delivery setup helps compensate for hypoxia induced by the previous suctioning. Irritation from multiple suctionings results in an increased amount of secretions.

13. When procedure is completed, turn off suction and disconnect catheter from suction tubing. Remove gloves inside out and dispose of gloves, catheter, and container with solution in proper receptacle (see photo). Wash hands.

This prevents transmission of microorganisms.

14. Adjust patient's position. Auscultate chest to evaluate breath sounds.

Auscultation helps determine whether respiratory passageways are cleared of secretions.

15. Record the time of suctioning and the nature and amount of secretions. Also note the character of patient's respirations before and after suctioning.

This provides accurate documentation and provides for comprehensive care.

16. Offer oral hygiene.

Respiratory secretions that accumulate are irritating to mucous membranes and unpleasant for the patient.

The nurse should wear gloves on both hands, goggles, mask, and gown if necessary for protection from microorganisms. The patient's color and heart rate and the color, amount, and consistency of secretions should be monitored continuously. If cyanosis, excessively slow or rapid heart rate, or suddenly bloody secretions are noted, the nurse should stop suctioning immediately. The patient should then be ventilated with oxygen and the physician notified.

For a patient with an artificial airway on continuous mechanical ventilation, a closed airway suction system reduces the risk that a patient will become hypoxemic or develop an infection. The catheter (Fig. 44-15), encased in a plastic sleeve, remains connected to the patient's airway or ventilator tubing for up to 24 hours. This closed system is cost-effective because only one catheter is used daily and the caregiver has additional protection from exposure to the patient's secretions. Some systems have an access valve, a safety feature that completely closes off access between the suction catheter, and the endotracheal tube (Carroll, 1998; Galvin & Cusano, 1998).

Providing Tracheostomy Care

In addition to suctioning the tracheostomy, the nurse is responsible for either cleaning a nondisposable inner cannula or replacing a disposable one. The inner cannula requires cleaning or replacement to prevent accumulation of secretions that can interfere with respiration and occlude the airway. Because soiled tracheostomy dressings place the patient at risk for development of skin breakdown and

infection, the nurse regularly changes dressings and ties. Non–cotton-filled gauze dressings are used to prevent aspiration of foreign bodies (eg, lint or cotton fibers) into the trachea. Care must be exercised when changing the tracheostomy ties to prevent accidental extubation or expulsion of the tube. It is recommended either that an assistant holds the tube in place during the change or that the soiled tie is left in place until a clean one is securely attached. Agency policy determines specific procedures and schedules; however, a newly inserted tracheostomy may require attention every 1 to 2 hours. Procedure 44-6 outlines the care of a patient's tracheostomy.

Assisting Ventilation

Mechanical ventilators are used to assist or completely control ventilation. These machines are used with critically ill patients in conjunction with endotracheal or tracheostomy tubes in acute care facilities, extended care settings, and the home. Mechanical ventilation improves oxygenation and ventilation and supports the patient's breathing function during emergency or acute care episodes as well as in some long-term situations. Many types of ventilators are available, and the nurse must address both physical and psychological concerns of the patient and family. The nurse has responsibility for evaluating the patient's response to ventilation therapy, using safe practices and techniques, and monitoring the patient carefully for complications. (Clinical texts and literature discuss the use of mechanical ventilators in great detail.)

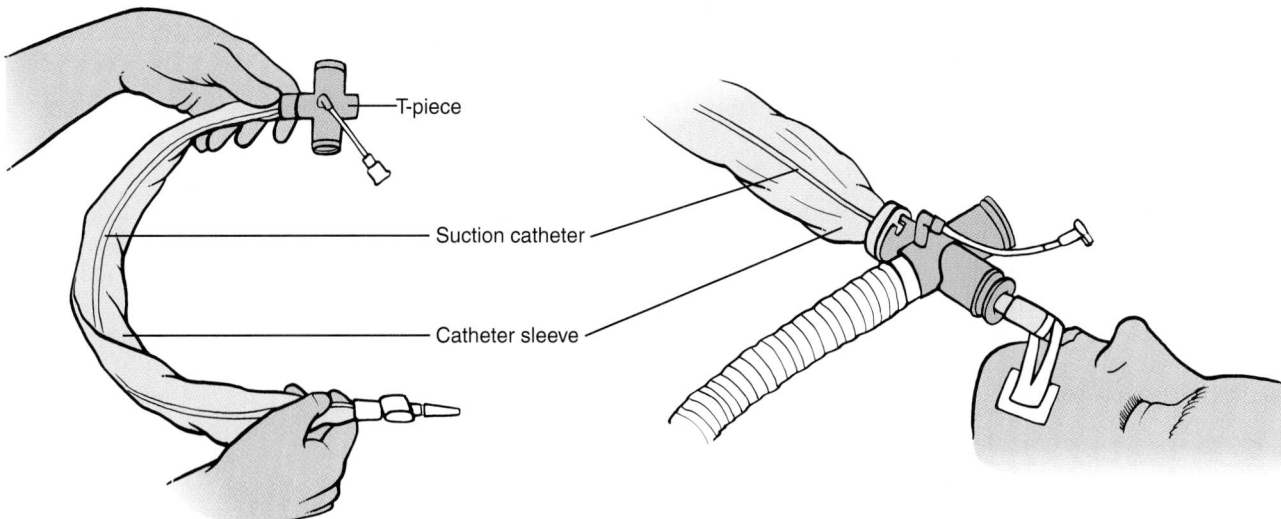

Figure 44-15
Closed airway suction system. **(A)** Closed tracheal suction system. **(B)** Closed system connected by a T piece to the endotracheal tube and ventilator.

Another mechanical device used to assist ventilation is *intermittent positive-pressure breathing* (IPPB). This is a method of providing a specific amount of air, oxygen, and aerosolized medication under increased pressure to the respiratory tract. The patient receiving IPPB inhales the aerosol therapy through a mouthpiece or face mask. IPPB forces deeper inspiration by positive-pressure inhalation and then permits passive exhalation. The amount of pressure varies with each patient. It is now recognized as an alternative therapy when the patient is unable or unwilling to make the effort to ventilate his or her lungs. Conservative methods should be attempted first, such as deep breathing and coughing exercises, percussion, vibration, and postural drainage.

In emergency situations, the manual resuscitation bag (or Ambu bag) can be used to assist ventilation in patients whose respirations have ceased. With the patient's head tilted back, jaw pulled forward, and airway cleared, the mask is held tightly over the patient's nose and mouth. The operator's other hand compresses the bag at a rate that approximates normal respiratory rate (eg, 16 to 20 breaths/min in adults). The one-way valve in the mask allows exhaled air to escape. Artificial ventilation can be sustained until spontaneous breathing starts, until other mechanical assistance is available, or until death is confirmed. The bag is self-inflating.

Clearing an Obstructed Airway

Foreign-body obstruction of the airway usually occurs during eating. In adults, meat is the most common cause. In children, any variety of foods or objects can obstruct the upper airway. A semiconscious or unconscious patient can develop airway obstruction because the tongue covers the pharynx as it falls back, causing an obstruction. The tongue is the most common cause of airway obstruction.

Foreign bodies can cause either partial airway obstruction or complete airway obstruction. In partial airway obstruction with good air exchange, the patient can cough forcefully. This person should be allowed and encouraged to cough and breathe spontaneously. At this time, the nurse should not interfere with the patient's efforts to expel the object. Good air exchange can progress to poor air exchange, indicated by a weak, ineffective cough, high-pitched noises while inhaling, increased breathing difficulties, and cyanosis. This situation should be managed the same way as complete airway obstruction.

With a complete airway obstruction, the victim is unable to speak or cough. The patient may demonstrate the universal distress signal (ie, clutching his or her throat with both hands). Immediate action is necessary, or the patient will become unconscious as the brain becomes hypoxic. After complete airway obstruction has been determined, the Heimlich maneuver (abdominal thrusts) should be performed. The American Heart Association has developed and continually updates its protocols for cardiopulmonary resuscitation and obstructed airways.

Administering Cardiopulmonary Resuscitation

Cardiopulmonary resuscitation (CPR) is the combination of mouth-to-mouth breathing, which supplies oxygen to the lungs, and chest compressions, which circulate blood. It is often described in terms of the ABCs of basic life support:

Airway: Tip the head and check for breathing. The respiratory tract must be opened so that air can enter.
Breathing: If the victim does not start to breathe spontaneously after the airway is opened, give two breaths lasting 1.5 to 2 seconds.
Circulation: Check the pulse. If the victim has no pulse, artificial circulation must be started with compressions.

(*text continues on page 1264*)

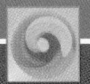

PROCEDURE 44-6

Providing Tracheostomy Care

Equipment

Disposable gloves	Sterile cotton-tipped applicators	Commercially prepared tracheostomy
Sterile gloves	Sterile cleaning solutions:	dressing or sterile non–cotton-
Goggles or face shield (optional)	Hydrogen peroxide	filled 4 × 4 gauze pad, additional
Sterile tracheostomy cleaning kit	Normal saline solutions	sterile gauze pad
(if available) *or*	Replacement inner cannula	Tracheostomy ties (twill tape or
Sterile basins (2)	(if available)	Velcro)
Sterile brush/pipe cleaners	Sterile suction catheter and	Scissors
	glove set	Plastic disposal bag

Action	Rationale
1. Explain procedure to patient.	Explanation facilitates cooperation and provides reassurance for patient.
2. If tracheostomy tube has just been suctioned, remove soiled dressing from around tube and discard with gloves when they are removed.	Suctioning prevents secretions from accumulating in inner cannula and occluding airway.
3. Wash your hands and open necessary supplies.	Handwashing deters spread of microorganisms.

Cleaning a Nondisposable Inner Cannula

Action	Rationale
4. Prepare supplies before cleaning inner cannula:	
a. Open tracheostomy care kit and separate basins touching only the edges. If kit is not available, open two sterile basins.	Basins are sterile receptacles for cleaning solutions.
b. Fill one basin ½ in (1.25 cm) deep with hydrogen peroxide.	Hydrogen peroxide facilitates removal of dry, encrusted secretions.
c. Fill other basin ½ in (1.25 cm) deep with saline.	Saline rinses and removes hydrogen peroxide and lubricates the outer surface of the inner cannula for easier reinsertion.
d. Open sterile brush or pipe cleaners if they are not already available in a cleaning kit. Open additional sterile gauze pad.	Sterile brush or pipe cleaner provides friction to clean inner surface of cannula.
5. Don disposable gloves.	Gloves protect from exposure to blood and body substances.
6. Remove the oxygen source if one is present. Rotate the lock on the inner cannula in a counterclockwise motion to release it.	Releasing the lock permits removal of the inner cannula.
7. Gently remove the inner cannula and carefully drop it in the basin with hydrogen peroxide. Remove gloves and discard.	Soaking in hydrogen peroxide loosens dry, hardened secretions.
8. Clean the inner cannula:	
a. Don sterile gloves.	Sterile gloves maintain surgical asepsis.
b. Remove inner cannula from soaking solution. Moisten brush or pipe cleaners in saline and insert into tube, using back-and-forth motion.	Movement of brush creates friction and aids in removal of accumulated secretions.
c. Agitate cannula in saline solution. Remove and tap against inner surface of basin.	Saline rinses inner cannula. Tapping tube against basin removes excess saline in inner tube.
d. Place on sterile gauze pad.	Maintains sterility and frees both hands for suctioning.
9. Suction the outer cannula using sterile technique.	Removes any remaining secretions.

(continued)

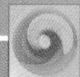

PROCEDURE 44-6

Providing Tracheostomy Care (Continued)

10. Replace inner cannula into outer cannula. Turn lock clockwise and check that inner cannula is secure. Reapply oxygen source if needed.

Clockwise motion secures inner cannula in place.

Replacing a Disposable Inner Cannula

11. Release lock. Gently remove inner cannula and place in disposal bag. Discard gloves and don sterile ones to insert new cannula. Replace with appropriately sized new cannula. Engage lock on inner cannula.

Disposable cannulas, although more costly, ensure that airway is clean and patent.

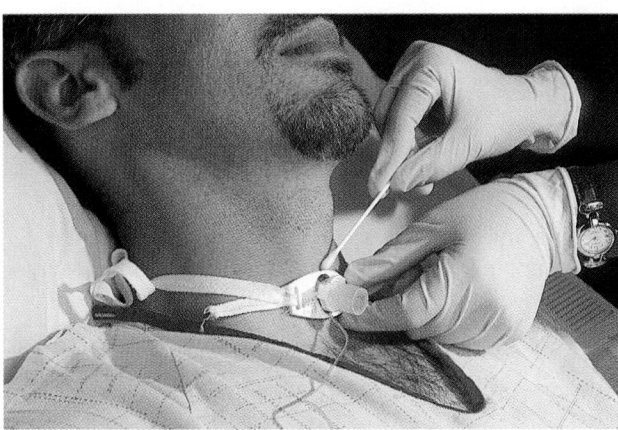

Action 12: Cleaning underneath the faceplate.

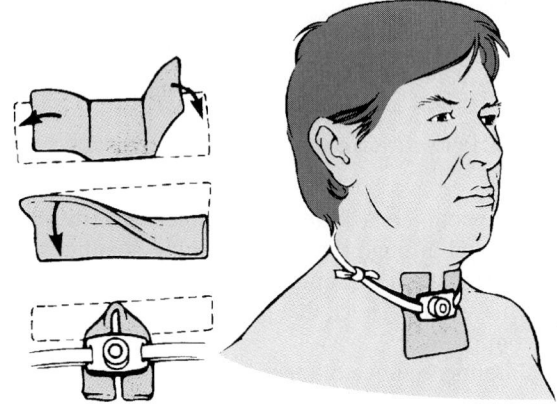

Action 15: Folding gauze square or placing commercially prepared dressing under faceplate of tracheostomy tube.

Applying Clean Dressing and Tape

12. Dip cotton-tipped applicator in saline and clean stoma under faceplate (see photo). Use each applicator only once, moving from stoma site outward.

Saline is nonirritating to tissue. Cleansing from stoma outward and using each applicator only once promotes aseptic technique.

13. Apply hydrogen peroxide to area around stoma, faceplate, and outer cannula if secretions prove difficult to remove. Rinse area with saline.

Hydrogen peroxide may cause tissue damage and needs to be removed from skin and surrounding area.

14. Pat skin gently with dry 4 × 4 gauze.

Gauze removes excess moisture.

15. Slide commercially prepared tracheostomy dressing or prefolded non–cotton-filled 4 × 4 dressing under faceplate (see drawing).

Lint or fiber from cotton-filled gauze pad can be aspirated into the trachea and cause irritation.

16. Change the tracheostomy tape:
    a. Leave soiled tape in place until new one is applied.
    b. Cut piece of tape that is twice the neck circumference plus 4 in (10 cm). Trim ends of tape on the diagonal.
    c. Insert one end of tape through faceplate opening alongside old tape. Pull through until both ends are even.

Ensures that tracheostomy will not be expelled if patient coughs or moves.
Provides for secure attachment with knot in front at neckplate. Diagonal cut facilitates insertion of tape into openings on faceplate.
Provides attachment for one side of faceplate.

(continued)

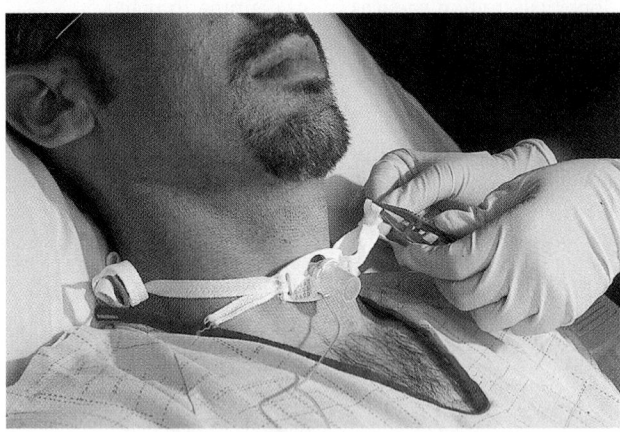

Action 16d: Inserting the tracheostomy tape through the opening and pulling through. (Photos © B. Proud.)

d. Slide both tapes under patient's neck and insert one end through remaining opening on other side of faceplate. Pull snugly and tie ends in double square knot. Check that patient can flex neck comfortably.	A secure tape prevents accidental expulsion of the tracheostomy tube. Neck flexion that is comfortable assures that tape will not compromise circulation to the area.
e. Carefully remove old tape. Reapply oxygen source if necessary.	New tape provides for secure attachment.
17. Remove gloves and discard. Wash hands. Assess the patient's respirations. Document assessments and completion of procedure.	Assessment and accurate documentation provide for comprehensive care.

Home Care Considerations   The patient and home caregiver are given instructions on how to perform tracheostomy care. The nurse observes the return demonstration and provides feedback. Clean rather than sterile technique can be used in the home setting. Sterile saline can be made by mixing 1 teaspoon of table salt in 1 quart of water and boiling for 15 minutes. The solution is cooled and stored in a clean, dry container. Saline is discarded at the end of each day to prevent growth of bacteria. If the patient is performing self-care, the nurse recommends the use of a mirror to view the steps in the procedure.

CPR should be started in any situation in which either breathing alone or breathing and heart beat are absent. The brain is sensitive to hypoxia and will sustain irreversible damage after 4 to 6 minutes of no oxygen. The faster that CPR is initiated, the greater the chance of survival (see the accompanying Research in Nursing box).

At regular intervals, the American Heart Association revises the CPR protocols. Blood and body substance precautions should be followed even though contact with a patient's blood or body fluids may not occur during CPR. Occupational Safety and Health Administration (OSHA) standards require healthcare facilities to provide an ample supply of ventilation masks along with other protective barriers for staff to use during resuscitation efforts.

The automated external defibrillator (AED) has also proved effective in reducing deaths attributed to cardiac arrest. This computer-based device is easy to use and designed to deliver a shock quickly to the heart muscle to interrupt ventricular fibrillation, the most common initial rhythm occurring in cardiac arrest. The AED has the ability to analyze the heart's rhythm, direct the operator to deliver a shock when appropriate or deliver one automatically, and then reanalyze the rhythm to determine whether it has returned to normal (Fig. 44-16). In healthcare facilities in

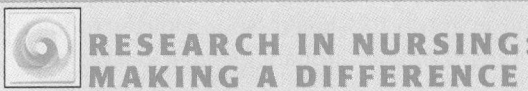

RESEARCH IN NURSING: MAKING A DIFFERENCE

Evaluating a *Breathe Easy!* Smoking-Cessation Program for Adolescents

Annual deaths related to smoking-related diseases total almost 500,000 in the Unites States. There also is a significant economic impact related to smoking when medical expenses and lost productivity are calculated. Smoking cessation programs have helped to gradually decrease tobacco use among adults, but the increase in cigarette smoking among youth is alarming. It is imperative that healthcare providers initiate successful prevention and smoking-cessation programs for this adolescent population. Programs using a passive instructional approach have proved less effective for young people than those programs that include peer and social reinforcement approaches.

Related Research
Higgs, P., & Edwards, D. (2000). Evaluation of a self-directed smoking prevention and cessation program. *Pediatric Nursing, 26*(2), 150–153.
This study evaluated the effectiveness of the *Breathe Easy!* smoking and prevention program for adolescents. Because this age group traditionally has not responded to lectures from adults emphasizing behaviors they should avoid, an interactive experience was developed. Adult instructors acted as facilitators for small peer group discussions. The student interactions focused on acquiring social skills to resist pressure to smoke and accepting the consequences of personal choices. Young people at a summer youth program at

four different sites participated in the study. Subjects at two of the sites participated in the *Breathe Easy!* intervention, while the control groups were not exposed to the antismoking group experiences. Surveys were administered to all groups at the start of the summer youth program and at 1- or 6-month intervals during the program. Results of this study indicated a significant difference in smoking behaviors in the intervention group surveyed at 6 months, with the prevalence of smoking dropping from 18.7% to 8.9%. There was no significant difference between 1-month survey results for the experimental group and the control group.

Relevance to Nursing Practice
Healthcare providers, particularly nurses, can help adolescents to make positive changes in their smoking behaviors and overall health status. Because they are recognized as credible resources, healthcare providers need to become actively involved in interactions that focus on prevention or cessation of smoking in this target population. Innovative and interactive approaches that address this growing health concern and also consider the ethnic, racial, and socioeconomic background of the students will prove more effective. These types of programs also have the additional positive outcome of promoting personal responsibility for one's own health behaviors.

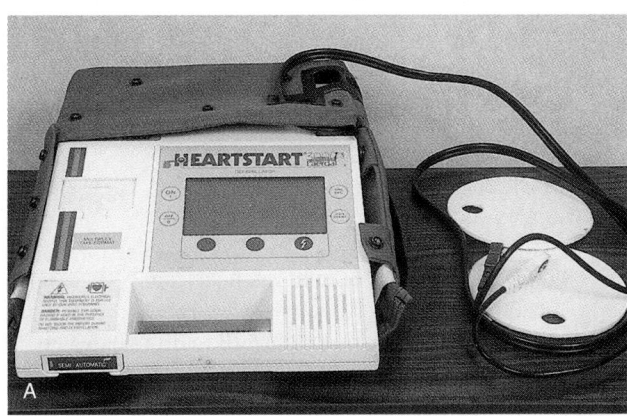

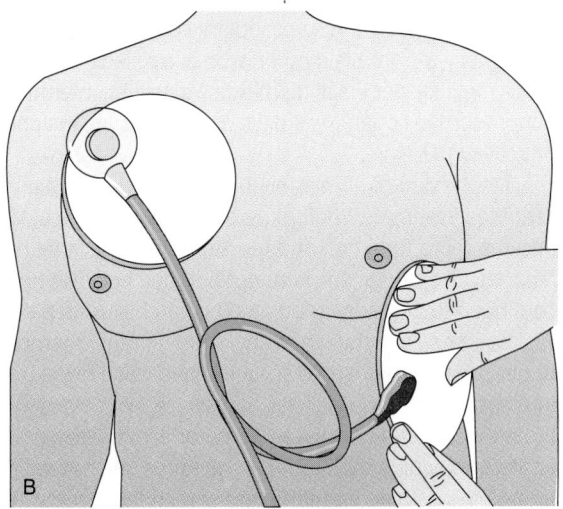

Figure 44-16
Placement of the automated external defibrillator (AED). (**A**) AED device. (**B**) Place the AED pad attached to the red cable connector to the left of the heart apex. To help remember where to place the pads, think "white right, red ribs." (Placement of both electrode pads is the same as it is for manual defibrillation or cardioversion.) (Photograph copyright © B. Proud.)

which defibrillation equipment is readily available, using the AED takes priority over CPR unless the AED is not immediately available (Mancini & Kaye, 1999). Despite recommendations of the American Heart Association, many hospitals have not established AED response programs, and AED use is still most often initiated by ACLS teams. In the community, more than half of states permit healthcare workers who are not emergency medical technicians to use AEDs, and six states allow lay responders to use them. In many cases, reducing deaths from cardiac arrest appears to depend on early delivery of AED.

Most professional organizations recommend and support widespread efforts to teach CPR to lay people and all health professionals. Mannequins for practice can be obtained from the American Heart Association, the American Red Cross, and health agencies. It is a nurse's professional responsibility to maintain proficiency in CPR skills. This necessitates periodic practice with mannequins

(adult and infant). CPR should be administered quickly and accurately, without hesitation, when cardiac arrests occurs.

EVALUATING

Evaluation is an ongoing and deliberate part of the nursing process that involves the nurse, patient, family, and other healthcare team members. It compares the patient's health status with previously defined expected outcomes and examines the patient's projected progress in meeting those outcomes. Everyone involved in the evaluation process needs to identify effective interventions and reasons for any failures in achieving these expected outcomes. Adjustments in the nursing plan of care are then made accordingly.

See the accompanying Applying Learning to Practice: Patient Care Study and Nursing Plan of Care boxes.

APPLYING LEARNING TO PRACTICE

Patient Care Study

Freddie is a 1-year-old, alert, well-developed child who has been a patient on the pediatric unit for 3 days with status asthmaticus. He has had two other hospitalizations for acute asthma, during which he responded quickly to intravenous and inhalation bronchodilators. During this hospitalization, either his mother, a teacher, or his father, a psychologist, has stayed with him. Other relatives are caring for Freddie's 9-year-old sister and 5-year-old brother.

Freddie interacts happily with staff as long as a parent is within sight. Gross and fine motor coordination are appropriate for his age. His vocabulary consists of 25 words. The history is from his mother, who is a reliable source. He has had a clear nasal discharge with slight, intermittent, nonproductive cough for 3 days with no change in appetite or activity pattern.

On the day of admission, he attended the daycare center as usual. After being there for 3 hours, his cough became more frequent, and his respirations became more labored. The caregivers were not alarmed because he continued to eat, drink, nap, and play in his usual pattern. His mother states that when she arrived in the afternoon to pick up the boys, she discovered him to be using his intercostal and neck muscles excessively with every breath. His respirations were 50 breaths/min, labored, and accompanied by a grunt. By the time she arrived home, he was pale and fitful and was crying weakly. Respirations were 60 breaths/min, and peripheral cyanosis was noted. The pediatrician advised lung evaluation in the emergency department. While there, three subcutaneous injections of epinephrine were administered 5 min-

utes apart. The child did not respond satisfactorily, so he was admitted for intravenous aminophylline and steroid administration.

In addition to a history of asthma, Freddie is allergic to eggs and peanuts and has eczema on his face, arms, legs, and upper back. His current medications include metaproterenol sulfate (Alupent) every 8 hours; a topical steroid (Lidex Cream); and a multivitamin and mineral supplement (Poly-Vi-Sol drops). No one in the family smokes. The caregivers at the daycare center smoke outside the building. The daycare center is clean and had the rugs shampooed the night before this child's illness. This child had no sputum production or fever. Immunizations are current. A comprehensive assessment revealed the following findings:

Respiratory rate, 44 breaths/min
Irregular rhythm
Excessive use of accessory muscles
Nonproductive, frequent cough
Gurgles and expiratory wheezes noted
Pale, no cyanosis
Blood pressure, 100/60 mm Hg; heart rate,
  120 beats/min
Restless child who naps for only 20 to 30 minutes at
  intervals day and night
Arterial blood gases: normal values
Chest radiograph: normal
Poor appetite, vomiting one or two times
Up early in morning
Sweat test: negative for cystic fibrosis

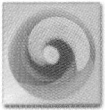

NURSING PLAN OF CARE
for Freddie

Nursing Diagnosis	Ineffective Airway Clearance related to exposure to allergens, viral infection, broncho-spasm, overproduction of mucus as manifested by: nonproductive frequent cough, presence of gurgles (rhonchi) and expiratory wheeze, restlessness, interrupted sleep.
Expected Outcome	By 12/5/01, the patient will: • Have rare episodes of coughing and no vomiting

Nursing Interventions	Rationale	Evaluative Statement
Hold meals until inhalation treatments are done.	Bronchodilators stimulate coughing and often cause vomiting if given after meals.	12/4/01 Goal met. Freddie has not vomited in 2 days and has 2-hour intervals between coughing episodes.
Avoid milk products.	Milk accelerates the production of mucus.	*Mary Jones, RN*
Offer clear juices every 3 hours in a bottle or cup.	Clear liquids help to liquefy secretions and prevent dehydration.	
Perform percussion during morning and evening bath.	Percussion loosens pulmonary secretions so that they are more easily expectorated.	

Expected Outcome	By 12/5/01, the patient's parents will: • Remove dust-collecting toys

Nursing Interventions	Rationale	Evaluative Statement
Give parents allergy pamphlets from American Lung Association.	Adequate information reinforces instruction given by healthcare providers.	12/2/01 Goal met. Parents removed furry toys from hospital room.
Review with both parents methods to reduce exposure to possible allergens at home.	Constant exposure to allergens (dust, mold, mildew, and so forth) and irritants (perfume, smog, cleaners, and so forth) produces bronchospasm and stimulates copious mucus production. Medications are most effective when allergens are removed.	*Mary Jones, RN*
Encourage parents to examine daycare environment. Explore options with them.	Environment in daycare may contain allergens. The least irritating setting is desirable.	

Sample Documentation	12/1/01 Nursing
	Family and staff conference to discuss Freddie's respiratory disturbance initiated by primary nurse's concern. Present were Freddie's mother; MJ (primary nurse); TK (clinical coordinator); TR (head of respiratory department); and MM and LQ (staff nurses). Primary nurse presented findings from assessment and nursing examination. Discussion centered on strategies to control airway edema and reduce wheezes, reduce coughing episodes and control vomiting, and prevent further bronchospasms and edema resulting from exposure to allergens in environment. See plan of care. Patient progress will be evaluated in 4 days during nursing grand rounds, 12/5/01. *Mary Jones, RN*

Learning Outcomes

After completing this chapter, the learner should be able to accomplish the following:

1. Define the key terms used in the chapter.

alveoli	inspiration
atelectasis	nasal cannula
bronchodilator	perfusion
crackles	pulse oximetry
endotracheal tube	spirometer
expiration	thoracentesis
hyperventilation	tracheostomy tube
hypoventilation	ventilation
hypoxia	wheezes

2. Describe the principles of respiratory physiology.

3. Describe age-related differences that influence the care of patients with respiratory problems.
4. Identify factors that influence respiratory function.
5. Perform a comprehensive respiratory assessment using appropriate interview questions and physical assessment skills.
6. Develop nursing diagnoses that correctly identify problems that may be treated by independent nursing interventions.
7. Describe nursing strategies to promote adequate respiratory functioning, identifying their rationale.
8. Plan, implement, and evaluate nursing care related to select nursing diagnoses involving respiratory problems.

Critical Thinking Exercises

1. Using the Focused Assessment Guide earlier in this chapter, work with a partner to assess the respiratory functioning of the following patients. Discuss ways in which you would modify your assessment to meet the specific needs of individual patients.
   - A 6-year-old who presents with asthma and is experiencing difficulty breathing
   - A 12-year-old who is brought to emergency room after use of inhalants ("huffing")
   - An adult dying of cancer who is receiving increasing doses of narcotics, which depress respiratory functioning

   - A hospitalized young adult with a 24-pack/year history of smoking who is noted to have a persistent, hacking cough
2. A postoperative patient who is at high risk for pulmonary complications because of a long history of smoking refuses to use the incentive spirometer or to cooperate with instructions to deep breathe. How would you respond to this patient? Discuss with other students what nursing response is most likely to secure his cooperation in necessary self-care measures.

Study Questions

1. A patient has a fractured rib and is breathing less often and with less depth because of the pain. This is best described as
   a. fremitus
   b. hyperventilation
   c. pleural friction rub
   d. hypoventilation
2. When auscultating Mr. Chang's breath sounds, the nurse detects a continuous sound heard on expiration. She assesses this as
   a. crackles or rales
   b. wheezes
   c. bronchial sounds
   d. pleural friction rub
3. Air that develops in the pleural space is referred to as
   a. pneumothorax
   b. pleural effusion
   c. hemothorax
   d. atelectasis
4. When planning care for a patient with chronic lung disease who is receiving oxygen through a nasal cannula, the nurse expects that

   a. the oxygen must always be humidified
   b. the rate will be 2 L/min or less
   c. arterial blood gases must be drawn every 4 hours to determine flow rate
   d. the rate will be 6 L/min or more
5. The highest concentration of oxygen is provided by the
   a. partial rebreather mask
   b. nonrebreather mask
   c. simple mask
   d. Venturi mask
6. Which of the following is a correct statement about pulse oximetry measurement?
   a. A range of 95% to 98% is considered normal oxygen saturation.
   b. Oximetry measurement measures oxygen saturation of venous blood.
   c. Fasting is required for 12 hours before the test.
   d. Pulse oximetry is a replacement for arterial blood gas analysis.
7. The nurse correctly performs oropharyngeal suctioning on a patient by

a. using clean technique

b. applying suction as the catheter is introduced

c. flushing the catheter with saline between catheter insertions

d. limiting suctioning to 25- to 30-second intervals at one time

8. Effective use of a metered-dose inhaler requires that the patient

a. breathe in through the nose

b. inhale two sprays with one breath

c. hold his or her breath after inspiration for 5 to 10 seconds

d. exhale quickly through an open mouth

9. Mr. Parks has chronic obstructive pulmonary disease. The nurse has taught him pursed-lip breathing that helps him by

a. increasing carbon dioxide, which stimulates breathing

b. teaching him to prolong inspiration and shorten expiration

c. helping liquefy his secretions

d. decreasing the amount of air trapping and resistance

10. A patient has suddenly had a cardiac arrest. What is the critical time that the nurse must keep in mind before irreversible brain damage occurs?

a. 1 to 3 minutes

b. 2 to 4 minutes

c. 4 to 6 minutes

d. 8 to 10 minutes

11. David White is in the hospital with a medical diagnosis of viral pneumonia. He is receiving oxygen through a simple face mask. Why must the mask fit snugly over the patient's face?

a. It prevents mask movement and consequent skin breakdown.

b. It helps the patient feel secure.

c. It maintains carbon dioxide retention.

d. It aids in maintaining expected oxygen delivery.

12. When suctioning her patient through a tracheostomy tube, the nurse was careful not to occlude the Y port when inserting the suction catheter because it would

a. prevent suctioning from occurring

b. cause trauma to the tracheal mucosa

c. break the sterile technique

d. suction out all the carbon dioxide

13. The nurse follows safe technique when using a portable oxygen cylinder by

a. checking the amount of oxygen in the cylinder before using it

b. using a cylinder for a patient transfer that indicates available oxygen is 500 psi

c. placing the oxygen cylinder on the stretcher next to the patient

d. discontinuing the oxygen flow by turning the cylinder key counterclockwise until it is tight

14. Which of the following blood gas values are considered within the normal range?

a. pH, 7.25 to 7.35; $PaCO_2$, 25 to 35 mm Hg; PaO_2, 50 to 100 mm Hg

b. pH, 7.35 to 7.45; $PaCO_2$, 45 to 50 mm Hg; PaO_2, 90 to 100 mm Hg

c. pH, 7.35 to 7.45; $PaCO_2$, 35 to 45 mm Hg; PaO_2, 80 to 100 mm Hg

d. pH, 7.30 to 7.40; $PaCO_2$, 30 to 45 mm Hg; PaO_2, 70 to 100 mm Hg

15. Abdominal breathing at 30 to 60 breaths/min with an irregular pattern of rate and depth would closely describe the breathing patterns of what age group?

a. aged adult

b. infant

c. early childhood

d. late childhood

Answers With Rationale

1. The correct response is *d*. Hypoventilation is a decreased rate or depth of air movement into the lungs. Hyperventilation is an increased rate and depth of ventilation, whereas fremitus is the vibration of the chest wall that can be palpated. A pleural friction rub is a dry grating sound caused by inflammation of pleural surfaces.

2. The correct response is *b*. Crackles are not described as squeaky, and the pleural friction rub is a dry, grating sound. Bronchial breath sounds are normal sounds heard over the trachea.

3. The correct response is *a*. Fluid in the pleural space is referred to as a pleural effusion, and blood in the pleural space is called hemothorax. Atelectasis is an incomplete expansion or collapse of the lungs.

4. The correct response is *b*. A rate higher than 2 L/min may destroy the hypoxic drive that stimulates respirations in the medulla in a patient with chronic lung

disease. Oxygen delivered at low rates does not necessarily have to be humidified, and arterial blood gases are not required at regular intervals to determine flow rate.

5. The correct response is *b*. The nonrebreather mask provides the highest concentration of oxygen to a spontaneously breathing patient.

6. The correct response is *a*. Pulse oximetry measures oxygen saturation levels of arterial blood, fasting is not required before the test, and pulse oximetry is an adjunct therapy, not a replacement for arterial blood gas analysis.

7. The correct response is *c*. The nurse should use sterile technique and should not apply suction as the catheter is being introduced; suctioning should be limited to 10- to 15-second intervals to avoid causing hypoxia.

8. The correct response is *c*. Holding one's breath for 5 to 10 seconds after inspiration of the medication

allows the drug to reach the alveoli. Correct technique for using an MDI includes breathing in through the mouth so that all the medication is properly delivered to the lungs, using one spray of medication for each breath to receive the correct dose, and exhaling slowly through pursed lips to minimize airway trapping and resistance.

9. The correct response is *d*. Pursed-lip breathing prolongs expiration, increases airway pressure, and loosens the amount of airway trapping and resistance. Doing pursed-lip breathing correctly diminishes carbon dioxide retention.

10. The correct response is *c*. After 4 to 6 minutes without oxygen, irreversible brain damage can occur.

11. The correct response is *d*. A snug-fitting mask is necessary to deliver expected rates of oxygen. A simple face mask does not trap carbon dioxide or cause retention.

12. The correct response is *b*. Occluding the Y port causes suction and may traumatize the tracheal mucosa if applied when the catheter is inserted.

13. The correct response is *a*. The cylinder must always be checked before use to ensure that enough oxygen is available for the patient. It is unsafe to use a cylinder that reads 500 psi or less because not enough oxygen remains for a patient transfer. A cylinder that is not secured properly may result in injury to the patient. Oxygen flow is discontinued by turning the valve clockwise until it is tight.

14. The correct response is *c*. These are the normal arterial blood gas ranges for pH, carbon dioxide, and oxygen.

15. The correct response is *b*. Respirations in the infant are more rapid and have not stabilized. As alveoli increase in number and size, the respiratory rate is lower.

Bibliography

Carroll, P. (1998). Closing in on safer suctioning. *RN, 61*(5), 22–26.

Carroll, P. (1999). Evolutions/revolutions: Respiratory monitoring. *RN, 62*(5), 68–77.

Dirkes, S. E., & Dickinson, S. (1998). Common questions about prone positioning for ARDs. *American Journal of Nursing, 98*(6), 16JJ–16PP.

Eliopoulis, C. (1997). *Gerontological nursing* (4th ed.). Philadelphia: Lippincott-Raven.

Fischbach, F. (2000). *A manual of laboratory tests* (6th ed.). Philadelphia: Lippincott Williams & Wilkins.

Gallauresi, B. (1998). Pulse oximeters: Monitor your patient closely to avoid serious injuries. *Nursing, 28*(9), 31.

Galvin, W., & Cusano, A. (1998). Making a clean sweep: Using a closed tracheal suction system. *Nursing, 28*(6), 50–51.

Gazarian, P. (1997). The direct route for asthma therapy. *Nursing, 27*(10), 52–54.

Grodner, M., Anderson, S., & DeYoung, S. (2000). *Foundations and clinical applications of nutrition: A nursing approach* (2nd ed.). St. Louis: C. V. Mosby.

Lazzara, D. (1999). Shocking facts about semiautomatic defibrillation. *Nursing, 29*(4), 55–57.

Lezon, K. (1998). Code blue: Defibrillate. *Nursing, 28*(4), 58–60.

Lezon, K. (1999). Teaching incentive spirometry. *Nursing, 29*(1), 60–61.

Mancini, M., & Kaye, W. (1998). Learning the latest about AEDs. *Nursing, 28*(9), 32hn10–32hn11.

Mancini, M., & Kaye, W. (1999). AEDs: Changing the way you respond to cardiac arrest. *American Journal of Nursing, 99*(5), 26–30.

Mathews, P. (1995). Safely delivering a breath of fresh air. *Nursing, 25*(5), 66–69.

McCloskey, J., & Bulechek, J. (1996). *Nursing Interventions Classification (NIC)* (2nd ed.). St. Louis: C. V. Mosby.

McConnell, E. (1997a). Your role in thoracentesis. *Nursing, 27*(3), 76.

McConnell, E. (1997b). Administering oxygen by mask. *Nursing, 27*(9), 26.

McConnell, E. (1999). Performing pulse oximetry. *Nursing, 29*(11), 17.

McConnell, E. (2000). Suctioning a tracheostomy tube, *Nursing, 30*(1), 80.

North American Nursing Diagnosis Association. (1999). *NANDA nursing diagnoses: Definitions and classification, 1999–2000*. Philadelphia: Author.

Owen, A. (1998), Respiratory assessment revisited. *Nursing, 28*(4), 48–49.

Pagana, K., & Pagana, T. (1998). *Manual of diagnostic and laboratory tests*. St. Louis: C. V. Mosby.

Pettinicchi, T. (1998). Trouble shooting chest tubes. *Nursing, 28*(3), 58–59.

Phipps, W., Sands, J. & Marek, J. (1999). *Medical-surgical nursing: Concepts & clinical practice* (6th ed.). Philadelphia: Lippincott Williams & Wilkins.

Porth, C. (1998). *Pathophysiology: Concepts of altered health states* (5th ed.). Philadelphia: Lippincott Williams & Wilkins.

Rice, R. (1995). *Home health nursing procedures*. St. Louis: C. V. Mosby.

Rokosky, J. (1997). Misuse of metered-dose inhalers: Helping patients get it right. *Home Healthcare Nurse, 15*(1), 13–21.

Shortall, S., & Perkins, L. (1999). Interpreting the ins and outs of pulmonary function tests. *Nursing, 29*(12), 41–47.

Smeltzer, S., & Bare, B. (2000). *Brunner and Suddarth's textbook of medical–surgical nursing* (9th ed.). Philadelphia: Lippincott Williams & Wilkins.

Tamburri, L. (1998). How to handle an airway emergency. *Nursing, 28*(12), 32hn2–32hn6.

Chapter 45
Fluid, Electrolyte, and Acid–Base Balance

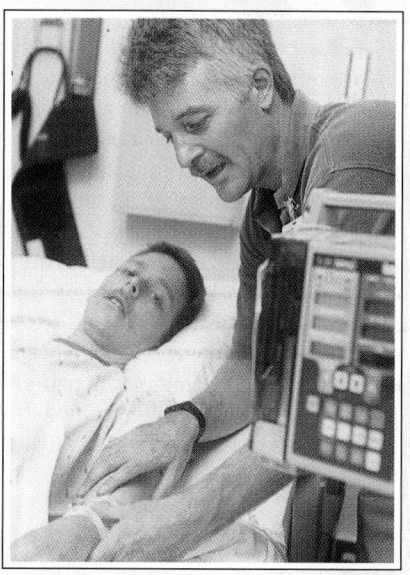

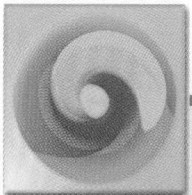

**Thinking Critically About
Nursing's Blended Skills**

Before reading this chapter, think about the types of skills you will need to care for patients with fluid, electrolyte, or acid–base disturbances.

- A number of students report to the student health center with what appears to be a gastrointestinal virus. Nausea, vomiting, and diarrhea have resulted in generalized weakness, dehydration, and electrolyte imbalance.

- You receive a patient helicoptered out of the Grand Canyon experiencing heat exhaustion and dehydration.

- Physical examination findings in a patient, including a bounding pulse, distended neck veins, and crackles and wheezes in the lungs, make you suspect fluid volume excess. Rechecking the intravenous fluids your patient has been receiving, you detect an administration error that resulted in overhydration.

- Ten-year-old Billy requires surgery that may result in life-threatening blood loss and the need for blood transfusions. His parents, who are Jehovah's witnesses, refuse to consent to the administration of blood products. You are asked to speak to them.

- When you conduct a drug history with an elderly woman you are visiting at home you learn that she is unknowingly taking twice the prescribed dose of her diuretic. You suspect serious alterations in her electrolytes.

What cognitive, technical, interpersonal, and ethical/legal skills do you think you will need to meet effectively the needs of the patients described above?

Between 50% and 60% of the human body by weight is water. Because fluid is the main constituent of the body, the body's fluid balance is very important. Body fluids contain other dissolved substances in the form of electrolytes, gases, and nonelectrolytes. The balance, or homeostasis, of water and dissolved substances is maintained through functions of almost every organ of the body. Nurses routinely care for patients with serious and even life-threatening fluid, electrolyte, and acid–base disturbances. One of nursing's most important roles is the prevention of these disturbances in high-risk populations, such as infants, older people, and patients with cardiac and renal disorders.

This chapter discusses the principles of fluid, electrolyte, and acid–base balance and common disturbances. Sample interview questions for performing a fluid balance assessment are included along with information on specific physical assessment measures and laboratory studies. Numerous examples of nursing diagnoses are provided. Expected outcomes and specific nursing interventions to promote fluid and electrolyte balance are described. These interventions include modifying dietary and fluid intake; administering medications; and assisting with intravenous (IV) therapy, blood replacement, and total parenteral nutrition (TPN). The concluding patient care study illustrates how nurses combine their knowledge of fluid, electrolyte, and acid–base balance with skilled nursing interventions and caring to resolve alterations in health status and improve patient outcome.

Physiology

Body Fluids

As the primary body fluid, water is the most important nutrient of life. Although life can be sustained for many days without food, humans can survive for only a few days without water. Following are the primary functions of water in the body:

- Provides a medium for transporting nutrients to cells and wastes from cells and for transporting substances such as hormones, enzymes, blood platelets, and red and white blood cells
- Facilitates cellular metabolism and proper cellular chemical functioning
- Acts as a solvent for electrolytes and nonelectrolytes
- Helps maintain normal body temperature
- Facilitates digestion and promotes elimination
- Acts as a tissue lubricant

Body Fluid Compartments

Fluids are located in two main compartments, or spaces, in the body—the *intracellular fluid* (ICF) and *extracellu-*

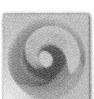

COGNITIVE SKILLS

- Knowledge of the functions, regulation, sources, and losses of body fluids, electrolytes, and acid–base balance
- Knowledge of how to use the nursing process to identify and care for patients at risk for problems related to fluid, electrolyte, and acid–base balance
- Knowledge of specific variables that may influence fluid, electrolyte, and acid–base balance (eg, Jehovah's Witnesses beliefs about not receiving blood or blood products)

TECHNICAL SKILLS

- Ability to use the nursing process to identify and treat patients at risk for fluid, electrolyte, and acid–base problems
- Competence in particular skills, such as intravenous therapy, blood replacement, and total parenteral nutrition

INTERPERSONAL SKILLS

- Strong people skills to establish trusting relationships with each of the patients described

above, especially in the case of the Jehovah's Witnesses parents

- A good working relationship with colleagues, which will be essential to the unit's taking ownership of an error in the administration of intravenous fluids

ETHICAL/LEGAL SKILLS

- First and foremost, a strong sense of accountability for the health and well-being of these individuals; a commitment to getting them the help they need to achieve their health goals—within the scope of your nursing responsibilities and available resources
- A willingness to hold colleagues accountable for safe and good-quality practice; knowledge of how to report and document an error in the administration of intravenous fluids
- Knowledge of your legal responsibilities when caring for the patients described above

lar fluid (ECF). ICF is the fluid within cells. It constitutes about 40% of an adult's body weight, or 70% of the total-body water. ECF is all the fluid outside the cells. It constitutes about 20% of an adult's body weight, or 30% of total-body water (Metheny, 2000). ECF includes intravascular and interstitial fluids. *Intravascular fluid,* or plasma, is the liquid constituent of blood (ie, fluid found within the vascular system). *Interstitial fluid* is the fluid that surrounds tissue cells and includes lymph. The term *total-body water* or fluid refers to the total amount of water in the body expressed as a percentage of body weight. Figure 45-1 illustrates the components of total-body fluid; Figure 45-2 shows body fluid distribution on the microscopic level.

Variations in Fluid Content

In a healthy person, total-body water constitutes about 50% to 60% of the body's weight, depending on such factors as the person's age, lean body mass, and sex. Table 45-1 illustrates age-related differences in total-body water and in the various water compartments of the body. An infant has considerably more body fluid and ECF than an adult. Because ECF is more easily lost from the body than ICF, infants are more prone to fluid volume deficits.

Total-body water also differs by sex and the person's amount of fat cells. Because fat cells contain little water and lean tissue is rich in water, the more obese the person, the smaller the percentage of total body water compared with body weight. Because females tend to have proportionally more body fat than males, they also have less body fluid than males. Similarly, the decreasing percentage of body fluid in older people is related to an increase in fat cells.

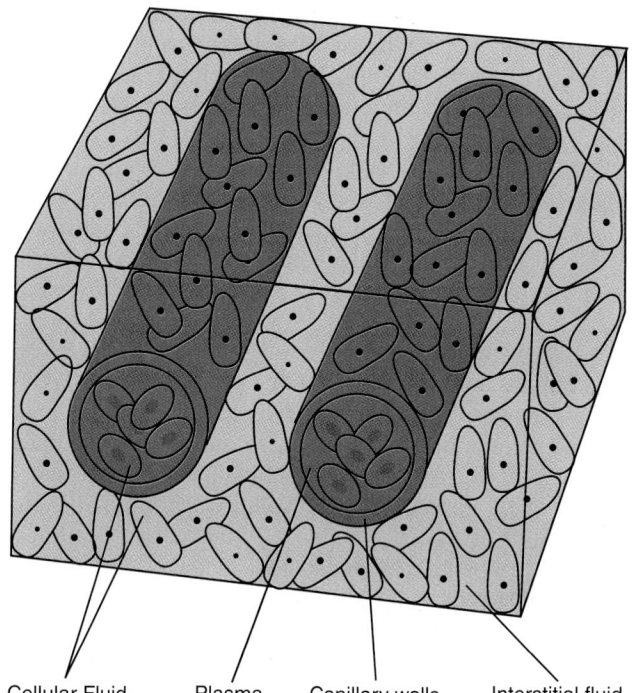

Cellular Fluid   Plasma   Capillary walls   Interstitial fluid

Figure 45-2
Microscopic visualization of body fluid distribution.

Electrolytes

Certain compounds dissociate in solution or separate into simpler molecules to form ions. An **ion** is an atom or molecule carrying an electric charge. Substances capable of breaking into electrically charged ions when dissolved in a solution are called **electrolytes**. Some ions develop a positive charge and are called **cations**. Others develop a negative charge and are called **anions**. These charges are the basis of chemical interactions in the body necessary for metabolism and other functions.

Molecules in the body's chemical compounds that remain intact are called nonelectrolytes. In the human body,

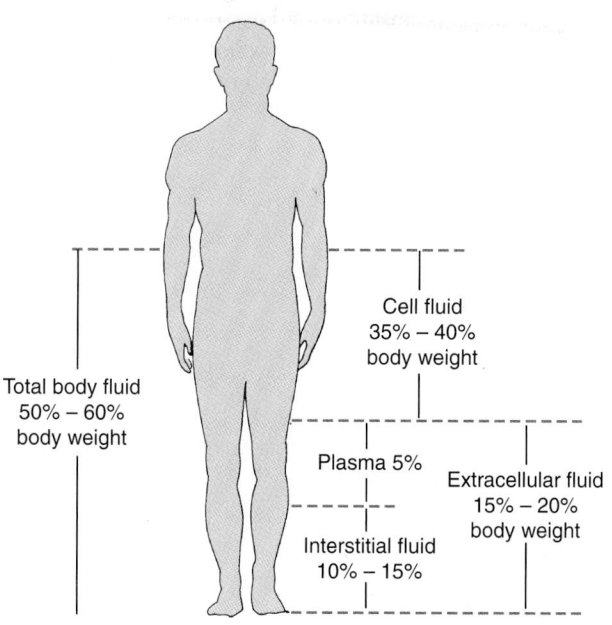

Cell fluid
35% – 40%
body weight

Total body fluid
50% – 60%
body weight

Plasma 5%

Extracellular fluid
15% – 20%
body weight

Interstitial fluid
10% – 15%

Figure 45-1
Total body fluid represents 50% to 60% of body weight of a normal adult.

Table 45-1
Water as a Percentage of Body Weight

Water Compartment	Infant (%)	Adult (%) Man	Adult (%) Woman	Elderly Person (%)
Extracellular				
Intravascular	4	4	5	5
Interstitial	25	11	10	15
Intracellular	48	45	35	25
Total-body water	77	60	50	45

for example, urea and glucose are nonelectrolytes. **Solvents** are liquids that hold a substance in solution; **solutes** are substances that are dissolved in a solution. Water is the primary solvent in the body. The solutes are electrolytes and nonelectrolytes.

Fluids in various compartments of the body differ in their constituents. For example, ICF has higher concentrations of certain electrolytes than ECF. Figure 45-3 illustrates differences in the electrolyte composition of body fluids according to the compartments in which the fluids are found.

Measurement of Electrolytes

Electrolytes are measured in terms of their chemical combining power, or chemical activity. The milliequivalent (mEq) is the unit of measure that describes the chemical activity of electrolytes. One milliequivalent of either a cation or an anion is chemically equivalent to the activity of 1 mg of hydrogen. Therefore, 1 mEq of any cation is equivalent to 1 mEq of any anion.

For the body to be in homeostasis, the total cations in the body are normally equal to the total anions. In healthy people, the milliequivalents per liter for electrolytes in the body vary within a relatively narrow range. When electrolytes are not in normal balance, the person is in a state of risk for alterations in health.

Regulation of Electrolytes

Electrolytes regulate water distribution, regulate acid–base balance, and maintain a balanced degree of neuromuscular excitability (Porth, 1998). There are many different electrolytes in the body. The following sections describe the most prevalent ones. Electrolyte disturbances are discussed later in the chapter.

Sodium (Na+)

Sodium is the chief electrolyte of ECF. It moves easily between intravascular and interstitial spaces and moves across cell membranes by active transport. Many chemical reactions in the body are influenced by sodium, particularly in nervous tissue cells and muscle tissue cells.

Functions
- Controls and regulates the volume of body fluids
- Maintains water balance throughout the body
- Is the primary regulator of ECF volume
- Influences ICF volume
- Participates in the generation and transmission of nerve impulses
- Is an essential electrolyte in the sodium–potassium pump

Sources and Losses
- The average daily requirements for sodium are not known precisely, but the Daily Value cited on the Nutrition Facts label is 2400 mg, which is about 1 teaspoon of salt. The RDA for sodium for adults is about 500 mg, or 0.5 g (Dudek, 1997).
- Sodium is found in many foods and is typically present in large amounts, particularly in bacon, ham, sausage, catsup, mustard, relish, processed cheese, canned vegetables, bread, cereal, and salted snack foods. It is found in table salt (sodium chloride), which is about 46% sodium. Sodium excesses are eliminated primarily by the kidneys; small amounts are lost in feces and perspiration.

Regulation
- Sodium is normally maintained in the body within a relatively narrow range, and deviations quickly result in a serious health problem.
- Salt intake affects sodium concentrations.
- Sodium is conserved through reabsorption in the kidneys, a process stimulated by aldosterone.
- The normal extracellular concentration of sodium is 135 to 145 mEq/L (mmol/L).

Potassium (K+) +charge

Potassium is the major cation of ICF. Potassium and sodium work reciprocally. For example, an excessive intake of sodium results in an excretion of potassium, and vice versa.

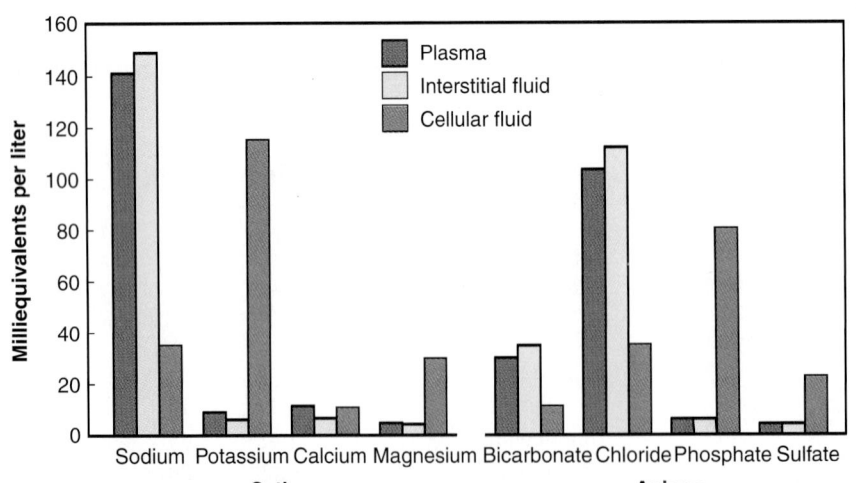

Figure 45-3
Electrolyte composition of body fluids according to compartment.

Functions

- Is the chief regulator of cellular enzyme activity and cellular water content
- Plays a vital role in such processes as the transmission of electric impulses, particularly in nerve, heart, skeletal, intestinal, and lung tissue; protein and carbohydrate metabolism; and cellular building
- Assists in regulation of acid–base balance by cellular exchange with H^+

Sources/Losses

- The average daily requirements for potassium are not known precisely, but an intake of 50 to 100 mEq daily maintains K^+ balance.
- A well-balanced diet contains adequate quantities of potassium. Leading food sources include bananas, peaches, kiwi, figs, dates, apricots, oranges, prunes, melons, raisins, broccoli, and potatoes. Meat and dairy products also provide adequate amounts of potassium.
- Potassium is excreted primarily by the kidneys. The kidneys have no effective method of conserving potassium. Therefore, deficits develop readily if potassium is excreted in excess without being replaced simultaneously.
- Gastrointestinal (GI) secretions contain potassium in large quantities. Some is also found in perspiration and saliva.

Regulation

- Cellular K^+ is conserved by the sodium pump (described later in the chapter) when Na^+ is excluded.
- The kidneys conserve K^+ when cellular K^+ is decreased.
- Aldosterone secretion triggers K^+ excretion in urine.
- The normal range for serum potassium is 3.5 to 5 mEq/L.

Calcium (Ca^{2+})

Calcium is the most abundant electrolyte in the body. Up to 99% of the total amount of calcium in the body is found in bones and teeth in ionized form. There is a close link between concentrations of calcium and phosphorus.

Functions

- Is necessary for nerve impulse transmission and blood clotting
- Is a catalyst for muscle contraction
- Is needed for vitamin B_{12} absorption and for its use by body cells
- Acts as a catalyst for many cell chemical activities
- Is necessary for strong bones and teeth
- Determines the thickness and strength of cell membranes

Sources/Losses

- The average daily requirement for calcium is about 1 g for adults. Higher amounts according to body weight are required for children and pregnant and lactating women. Older adults, particularly post-menopausal women not taking estrogen and men

older than 65 years of age, are urged to consume 1500 mg/day (Dudek, 1997).
- It is found in milk, cheese, and dried beans. Some calcium is present in meats and vegetables.
- The use of calcium is stimulated by vitamin D. The most active form of vitamin D (calcitriol) promotes calcium absorption and limits calcium excretion when levels are inadequate.
- It leaves bones and teeth to maintain normal blood calcium levels, if necessary.
- It is excreted in urine, feces, bile, digestive secretions, and perspiration.

Regulation

- When ECF calcium levels decrease, the parathyroid glands increase the secretion of parathyroid hormone (PTH), which acts on bones to increase the release of calcium into the blood and acts on the kidney tubules and the intestinal mucosa to increase the reabsorption of calcium from the kidneys and the intestine.
- A high serum phosphate concentration decreases the serum calcium level; a low serum phosphate concentration increases serum calcium.
- Calcitonin, a hormone secreted by the thyroid gland, has an effect on calcium opposite that of PTH. Increases in calcitonin reduce serum calcium concentration primarily by opposing osteoclast bone resorption.

Magnesium (Mg^{2+})

Most of the cation magnesium is found within body cells. It is present in heart, bone, nerve, and muscle tissues. Magnesium is the second most important cation in the ICF.

Functions

- Is important for the metabolism of carbohydrates and proteins
- Is important for many vital reactions involving enzymes
- Is necessary for protein and DNA synthesis, DNA and RNA transcription, and translation of RNA
- Maintains normal intracellular levels of potassium
- Helps maintain electric activity in nervous tissue membranes and muscle membranes

Sources and Losses

- The average daily adult requirement for magnesium is about 18 to 30 mEq; children require larger amounts.
- Magnesium is found in most foods but especially in vegetables, nuts, fish, whole grains, peas, and beans.

Regulation

- Magnesium is absorbed by the intestines and excreted by the kidneys.
- Plasma concentrations of magnesium range from 1.3 to 2.1 mEq/L, with about one third of that amount bound to plasma proteins.

Chloride (Cl^-)

Chloride, the chief extracellular anion, is found in blood, interstitial fluid, and lymph and in minute amounts in ICF.

Functions

- Acts with sodium to maintain the osmotic pressure of the blood
- Plays a role in the body's acid–base balance
- Has important buffering action when oxygen and carbon dioxide exchange in red blood cells
- Is essential for the production of hydrochloric acid in gastric juices

Sources/Losses

- The average daily requirements of chloride are unknown.
- It is found in foods high in sodium, dairy products, and meat.

Regulation

- It is normally paired with sodium and is excreted and conserved with sodium by the kidneys.
- Chloride deficits lead to potassium deficits, and vice versa.
- Normal serum chloride levels range from 95 to 105 mEq/L (mmol/L).

Bicarbonate (HCO_3^-)

The bicarbonate molecule is an anion. It is the major chemical base buffer within the body and is found in both ECF and ICF.

Function

- Is essential for acid–base balance; bicarbonate and carbonic acid constitute the body's primary buffer system

Regulation

- Bicarbonate levels are regulated primarily by the kidneys.
- Bicarbonate is readily available as a result of carbon dioxide formation during metabolism.
- Normal bicarbonate levels range between 25 and 29 mEq/L (mmol/L).

Phosphate (PO_4^-)

The phosphate ion is the major anion in body cells. It is a buffer anion in both ICF and ECF.

Functions

- Helps maintain the body's acid–base balance
- Is involved in important chemical reactions in the body; for example, phosphorus is necessary for many B vitamins to be effective, helps promote nerve and muscle action, and plays a role in carbohydrate metabolism
- Is important for cell division and for the transmission of hereditary traits

Sources/Losses

- The average daily requirements for phosphorus are similar to those for calcium.
- It is found in most foods but especially in beef, pork, and dried peas and beans.
- It is metabolized in the same manner as calcium.

Regulation

- Phosphate is regulated by PTH and by activated vitamin D.
- Calcium and phosphate are inversely proportional; an increase in one results in a decrease in the other.
- The normal range of phosphate is 2.5 to 4.5 mEq/L (mmol/L).

Additional Electrolytes

The anion sulfate is found primarily within cells and is associated with cellular protein. Excesses are excreted by the kidneys. The organic acid anions normally have an intermediary role in cell metabolism. A major anion is lactic acid. The protein anion functions in the process of diffusion to move substances to and from the capillaries. Plasma proteins include albumin, globulin, and fibrinogen.

Other electrolytes are required for proper cell functioning but are found only in traces in the body. One example is chromium. A well-balanced diet ordinarily ensures an adequate supply of required trace substances in the body.

Fluid and Electrolyte Movement

The ECF takes nourishment to each body cell and receives each cell's waste products. These exchanges, which normally result in fluid balance and homeostasis, are essential to life. The most common routes for transporting materials to and from intracellular compartments are osmosis, diffusion, active transport, and filtration, described in the following sections.

Osmosis

The membranes of cells are semipermeable. This makes it possible for water, a pure solvent, to be transported through cell walls. **Osmosis** is the major method of transporting body fluids. Water shifts, and thus balance depends heavily on this route of transport.

Through the process of osmosis, the solvent water passes from an area of lesser solute concentration to an area of greater solute concentration until equilibrium is established. As a result, the volume of the more concentrated solution increases, and the volume of the weaker solution decreases. The greater the difference in the concentration of the two solutions on each side of a semipermeable membrane, the greater the osmotic pressure or drawing power of water.

The concentration of particles in a solution, or its pulling power, is referred to as the **osmolarity** of a solution. A solution that has about the same concentration of particles, or osmolarity, as plasma (between 275 and 295 mOsm/L) is considered an *isotonic* solution. An isotonic fluid remains in the intravascular compartment without any net flow across the semipermeable membrane. In contrast, a *hypertonic* solution has a greater osmolarity than plasma (more than 295 mOsm/L), whereas a *hypotonic* solution has less osmolarity than plasma (less than 275 mOsm/L). Because a hypertonic solution has a greater concentration of particles in solution, water moves out of the cells and into the intravascular compartment in which the fluid is hypertonic, causing the cells to shrink. A hypotonic solution in the intravascular space, with a lower osmolarity, moves out of the intravascular space into intracellular fluid, causing cells to swell and possibly burst (Young, 1998). Figure 45-4 illustrates the process of osmosis.

Diffusion

Diffusion is the tendency of solutes to move freely throughout a solvent. The solute moves from an area of higher concentration to an area of lower concentration (ie, "downhill") until equilibrium is established. Gases also move by diffusion. Oxygen and carbon dioxide exchange in the lung's alveoli and capillaries occurs by diffusion.

Active Transport

Active transport is a process that requires energy for the movement of substances through a cell membrane from an area of lesser concentration to an area of higher concentration. Adenosine triphosphate released from a cell makes it possible for certain substances to acquire energy needed to pass through the cell membrane. Although this process is not entirely understood, the energy requirements for active transport are affected by characteristics of the cell membrane, specific enzymes, and concentrations of ions. This process explains the so-called pump mechanism. If diffusion can be called "coasting downhill," active trans-

port can be called "pumping uphill." Substances believed to use active transport are amino acids; glucose (in certain places only, such as in the kidneys and intestines); and ions of sodium, chloride, potassium, hydrogen, phosphate, calcium, and magnesium.

Filtration

Filtration is the passage of fluid through a permeable membrane. Passage is from an area of high pressure to one of lower pressure.

Certain substances, such as plasma proteins, which have high molecular weights, exert **colloid osmotic pressure,** or **oncotic pressure,** on permeable membranes in the body. **Hydrostatic pressure** is a force exerted by a fluid against the container wall. Blood hydrostatic pressure is the pressure of plasma and blood cells in the capillaries: it depends primarily on arterial blood pressure on the arteriolar side of capillaries, and on venous blood pressure on the venular side of capillaries. *Filtration pressure* is the difference between colloid osmotic pressure and blood hydrostatic pressure.

These pressures are important in understanding how fluid leaves arterioles, enters the interstitial compartment, and eventually returns to the venules. The filtration pressure is positive in the arterioles, helping to force or filter fluids into interstitial spaces; it is negative in the venules and thus helps fluid enter the venules. This is illustrated in Figure 45-5. Filtration is also involved in the proper functioning of the glomeruli of the kidneys.

Fluid Balance

The desirable amount of fluid intake and loss in adults ranges from 1500 to 3500 mL each 24 hours, with most people averaging 2500 mL per day. Although these figures are helpful guidelines, the individual's balance between actual intake and loss must be considered when assessing nursing needs. A person's intake should normally be approximately balanced by output or fluid loss. A general rule is that in healthy adults, the output of urine normally approximates the ingestion of liquids; and the water from food and oxidation is balanced by the water loss through the feces, the skin, and the respiratory process. The intake–output balance may not always occur in a single 24-hour period but should normally be achieved within 2 to 3 days.

Fluid Sources

Water for the body derives from several sources, including ingested liquids, food, and metabolism.

Ingested Liquids

This source makes up the largest amount of water normally taken into the body. Fluid intake is primarily regulated by the thirst mechanism. Located within the hypothalamus, the thirst control center is stimulated by intracellular dehydration and decreased blood volume.

Water in Food

This is the second largest source of water for the body. The amount ingested depends on the diet. For example,

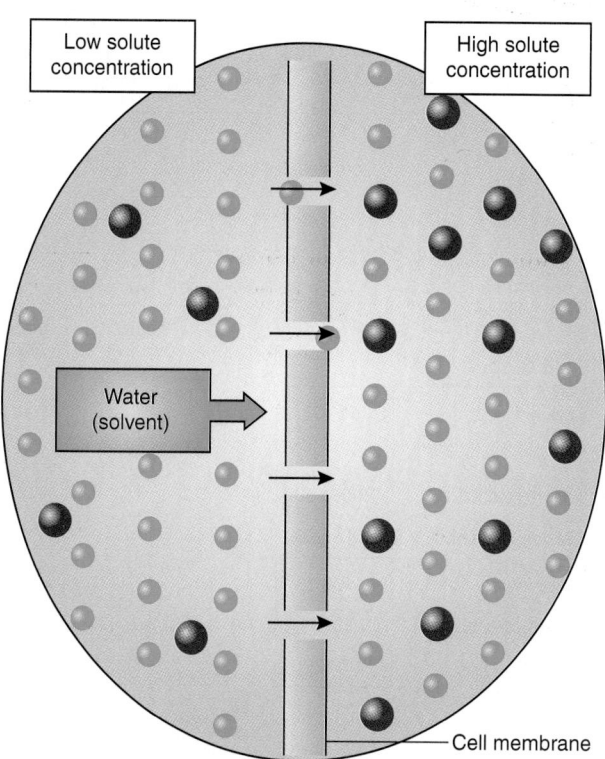

Figure 45-4
Body fluids are transported through cell membranes through the process of osmosis. Water, a solvent, moves from an area of lesser solute concentration to one of greater solute concentration, until equilibrium is established.

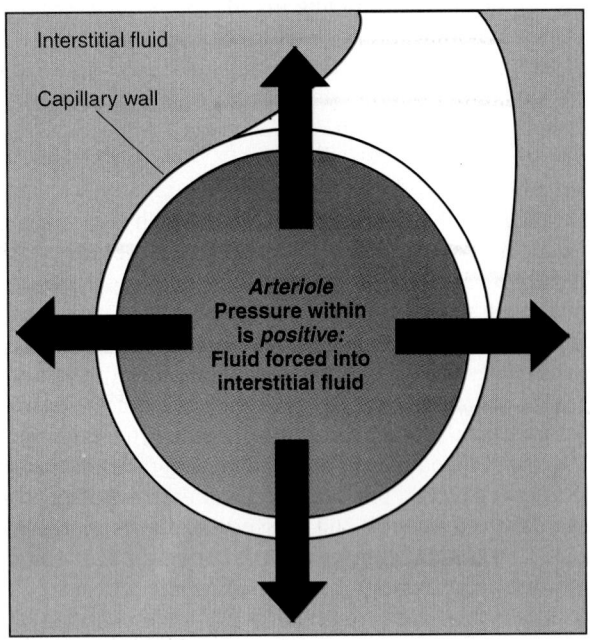

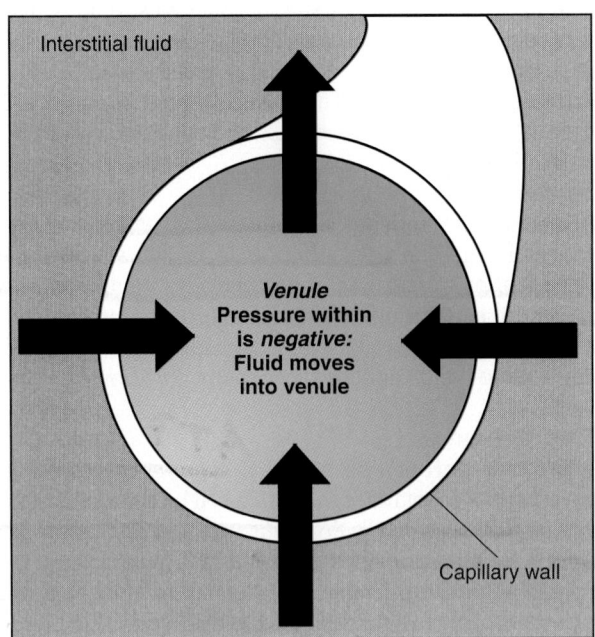

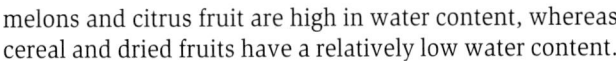

Figure 45-5
Filtration.

melons and citrus fruit are high in water content, whereas cereal and dried fruits have a relatively low water content.

Water From Metabolic Oxidation

Water is an end product of the oxidation that occurs during the metabolism of food substances. This source also varies among different types of nutrients. A person whose diet is high in fat has a proportionately greater amount of water resulting from metabolic processes than a person whose diet is high in protein.

Fluid Losses

Water is lost from the body through the kidneys as urine, through the intestinal tract in feces, and through the skin as perspiration. Water is also lost as *insensible water loss*, which is imperceptible. For example, an invisible amount of water is lost from the skin constantly through evaporation. Insensible loss from the lungs is moisture exhaled in breaths. Water losses vary according to the person and the circumstances.

Figure 45-6 illustrates fluid intake and output balance in healthy adults. Deviations from normal ranges for a balanced water intake and output should alert the nurse to potential imbalances. The accompanying Applying Learning to Practice boxes reflect on self-care behaviors vital for maintaining a healthy fluid and electrolyte balance.

Homeostatic Mechanisms

Fluid homeostasis normally functions automatically and effectively. Almost every organ and system in the body helps in some way to maintain fluid homeostasis. The following sections describe the primary organs of homeostasis. Their functions are highlighted in Table 45-2. Fluid balance is threatened when any organ fails to function properly.

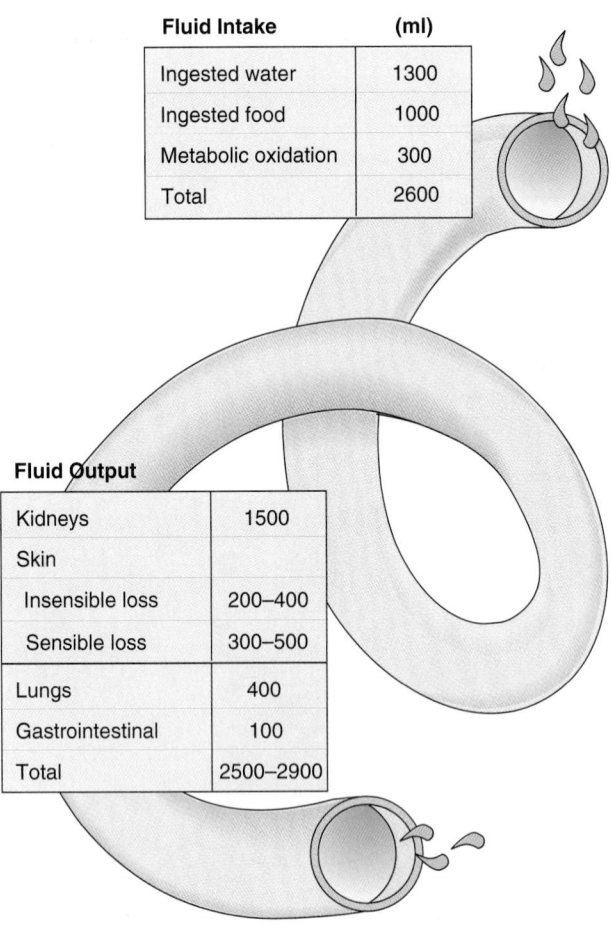

Fluid Intake	(ml)
Ingested water	1300
Ingested food	1000
Metabolic oxidation	300
Total	2600

Fluid Output	
Kidneys	1500
Skin	
Insensible loss	200–400
Sensible loss	300–500
Lungs	400
Gastrointestinal	100
Total	2500–2900

Figure 45-6
In health, fluid intake and fluid losses are about equal. The amounts indicated are average adult daily fluid sources and losses.

APPLYING LEARNING TO PRACTICE

The Nurse as Role Model: Fluid, Electrolyte, and Acid–Base Balance

Nurses wishing to be a role model of self-care behaviors that promote fluid, electrolyte, and acid–base balance should meet the following goals. The nurse will:

- Daily ingest the quantity and type of fluids (to include six to eight glasses of water) that promote healthy hydration and urinary functioning
- Evaluate use of fad diets, diuretics, laxatives, and alcohol, identifying potential risks to health
- Identify situations of high risk for fluid and electrolyte imbalance and intervene appropriately

Kidneys   *filter*

The kidneys are frequently referred to as the master chemists of the body. They normally ~~filter~~ 170 L of plasma daily in the adult while excreting only 1.5 L of urine. They selectively retain electrolytes and water and excrete wastes and excesses. Renal failure results in serious fluid and electrolyte problems.

Cardiovascular System   *circulation*

The cardiovascular system is responsible for ~~pumping and carrying nutrients~~ and water throughout the body.

Lungs

The lungs ~~regulate oxygen and carbon dioxide~~ levels of the blood. The regulation of the carbon dioxide level is especially crucial in maintaining acid–base balance; this is explained later in this chapter.

Adrenal Glands   *regulates metabolic rate*

The adrenal glands secrete aldosterone, a hormone that helps the body conserve sodium. ~~The hormone also helps save chloride and water and causes potassium to be excreted.~~

Thyroid Gland

Thyroxine, released by the thyroid gland, increases blood flow in the body. This in turn ~~increases renal circulation,~~ which results in increased glomerular filtration and urinary output.

Parathyroid Glands

The parathyroid glands secrete parathyroid hormone, which regulates the level of ~~calcium~~ in ECF.

Gastrointestinal Tract

The GI tract ~~absorbs water and nutrients~~ that enter the body through this route. *absorbs vit A, D, E, K*

APPLYING LEARNING TO PRACTICE

Promoting health

Fluid and Electrolyte Balance

Use the assessment checklist to determine how well you are meeting fluid and electrolyte needs. Then develop a prescription for self-care by choosing appropriate behaviors from the list of suggestions.

ASSESSMENT CHECKLIST

(columns: almost always / sometimes / almost never)

- ☐ ☐ ☐ 1. I drink six to eight glasses of water every day.
- ☐ ☐ ☐ 2. I am aware of early signs of dehydration or fluid retention.
- ☐ ☐ ☐ 3. I limit sugar, alcohol, and caffeine in my diet.
- ☐ ☐ ☐ 4. I am alert for any sudden variations in my weight.
- ☐ ☐ ☐ 5. I am aware of fluid and electrolyte imbalances that may be associated with intake of certain medications.
- ☐ ☐ ☐ 6. I diet sensibly when I need to lose weight.

SELF-CARE BEHAVIORS

1. Consume about 1½ quarts of water daily.
2. Maintain normal body weight.
3. Avoid consuming excess amounts of products high in salt, sugar, and caffeine.
4. Limit alcohol intake because of its diuretic effect.
5. Obtain medical evaluation for any ongoing indications of fluid imbalance.
6. Monitor side effects of medications, especially diuresis and diarrhea.

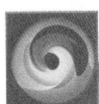

Table 45-2
Homeostatic Mechanisms That Maintain the Composition and Volume of Body Fluid Within Narrow Limits of Normal

Organs of Homeostasis	Functions
Kidneys	• Regulate extracellular fluid (ECF) volume and osmolality by selective retention and excretion of body fluids • Regulate electrolyte levels in the ECF by selective retention of needed substances and excretion of unneeded substances • Regulate pH of ECF by excretion or retention of hydrogen ions • Excrete metabolic wastes (primarily acids) and toxic substances
Heart and blood vessels	• Circulate blood through the kidneys under sufficient pressure for urine to form (pumping action of the heart) • React to hypovolemia by stimulating fluid retention (stretch receptors in the atria and blood vessels)

Lungs	• Eliminate about 13,000 mEq of hydrogen ions (H^+) daily, as opposed to only 40 to 80 mEq excreted daily by the kidneys
	• Act promptly to correct metabolic acid–base disturbances; regulate H^+ concentration (pH) by controlling the level of carbon dioxide (CO_2) in the extracellular fluid as follows:
	  1. Metabolic alkalosis causes compensatory hypoventilation, resulting in CO_2 retention (increases acidity of the extracellular fluid).
	  2. Metabolic acidosis causes compensatory hyperventilation, resulting in CO_2 excretion (decreases acidity of the extracellular fluid).
	• Remove approximately 300 mL of water daily through exhalation (insensible water loss) in the normal adult

Adrenal glands	• Regulate blood volume and sodium and potassium balance by secreting aldosterone, a mineral corticoid secreted by the adrenal cortex
	  1. The primary regulator of aldosterone appears to be angiotensin II, which is produced by the renin–angiotensin system. A decrease in blood volume triggers this system and increases aldosterone secretion, which causes sodium retention (and thus water retention) and potassium loss.
	  2. Decreased secretion of aldosterone causes sodium and water loss and potassium retention.
	• Cortisol, another adrenocortical hormone, has only a fraction of the potency of aldosterone.
	• However, secretion of cortisol in large quantities can produce sodium and water retention and potassium deficit.

Pituitary gland	• Stores and releases the antidiuretic hormone (ADH), which makes the body retain water; functions of ADH include:
	  1. Maintains osmotic pressure of the cells by controlling renal water retention or excretion
	    a. When osmotic pressure of the ECF is greater than that of the cells (as in hypernatremia—excess sodium—or hyperglycemia), ADH secretion is increased, causing renal retention of water.
	    b. When osmotic pressure of the ECF is less than that of the cells (as in hyponatremia), ADH secretion is decreased, causing renal excretion of water.
	  2. Controls blood volume (less influential than aldosterone)
	    a. When blood volume is decreased, an increased secretion of ADH results in water conservation.
	    b. When blood volume is increased, a decreased secretion of ADH results in water loss.

Parathyroid glands	• Regulate calcium (Ca^{2+}) and phosphate (HPO_4^{2-}) balance by means of parathyroid hormone (PTH); PTH influences bone reabsorption, calcium absorption from the intestines, and calcium reabsorption from the renal tubules.
	  1. Increased secretion of PTH causes:
	    a. Elevated serum calcium concentration
	    b. Lowered serum phosphate concentration
	  2. Conversely, decreased secretion of PTH causes:
	    a. Lowered serum calcium concentration
	    b. Elevated serum phosphate concentration

(Data from Metheny, N. M. [2000]. *Fluid and electrolyte balance* [4th ed.]. Philadelphia: Lippincott-Raven.)

Nervous System

The nervous system acts as a switchboard and inhibits and stimulates mechanisms that influence fluid balance. It functions chiefly as the regulator of sodium and water intake and excretion. The thirst center is located in the hypothalamus. The posterior lobe of the pituitary gland stores antidiuretic hormone (ADH), a hormone manufactured in the hypothalamus. Neurons called *osmoreceptors* are sensitive to changes in the concentration of ECF and send appropriate impulses to the pituitary to release ADH or inhibit its release.

Acid–Base Balance

Body fluids must maintain an acid–base balance to sustain health and life. Acidity or alkalinity of a solution is determined by its concentration of hydrogen ions (H^-). An **acid** is a substance containing hydrogen ions that can be liberated or released. An *alkali*, or **base**, is a substance that can accept or trap hydrogen ions. The following equations illustrate:

An acid releases hydrogen, as follows:

$$H_2CO_3 \rightarrow H^+ + HCO_3-$$

Carbonic acid   releases hydrogen ion to form   bicarbonate base

A base traps hydrogen, as follows:

$$HCO_3- + H^+ \rightarrow H_2CO_3$$

Bicarbonate base   traps hydrogen ion to form   carbonic acid

An acid that is strong dissociates (separates) completely in solution and releases all of its hydrogen ions, whereas a weak acid releases only a small number. A base that binds or accepts hydrogen ions easily is considered a strong base, whereas one that accepts hydrogen ions less readily is considered weak.

The unit of measure used to describe acid–base balance is **pH**, which is an expression of hydrogen ion concentration and the resulting acidity or alkalinity of a substance. The pH scale ranges from 1 to 14. A neutral solution measures 7; an example is pure water. Because pH is based on a negative logarithm, as the hydrogen ions increase and a solution becomes more acid, the pH becomes less than 7. When the concentration of hydrogen ions in a solution is reduced or accepted by another substance, the solution is alkaline, and the pH is greater than 7. Gastric secretions that are strongly acidic have an approximate pH of 1 to 1.3, whereas strongly alkaline pancreatic secretions have an approximate pH of 10.

Normal blood plasma is slightly alkaline and has a normal pH range of 7.35 to 7.45. When the blood plasma pH exceeds the normal pH range in either direction, the person develops signs and symptoms of illness, and if the condition goes on unabated, death results. **Acidosis** is the condition characterized by an excess of hydrogen ions in ECF in which the pH falls below 7.35. **Alkalosis** occurs when there is a lack of hydrogen ions and the pH exceeds 7.45. Figure 45-7 illustrates normal pH, acidosis, and alkalosis and shows the points at which death typically occurs.

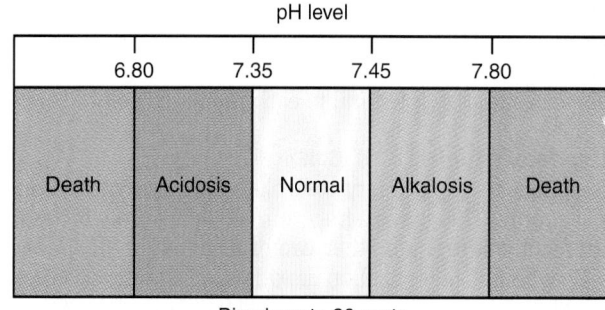

Figure 45-7

Acid–base balance. Note that *acidosis* is used to describe the condition when the pH falls below 7.35, and *alkalosis* describes a pH above 7.45. When the normal pH is exceeded in either direction, death can occur.

The narrow range of normal pH is achieved through three major homeostatic regulators of hydrogen ions: (1) buffer systems, (2) respiratory mechanisms, and (3) renal mechanisms. A **buffer** is a substance that prevents body fluids from becoming overly acidic or alkaline. The body has three buffer systems: (1) the carbonic acid–sodium bicarbonate buffer system, (2) the phosphate buffer system, and (3) the protein buffer system, as described in the following sections.

Buffer Systems

Carbonic Acid–Sodium Bicarbonate Buffer System

The most important buffer system of the body is the carbonic acid–sodium bicarbonate system. This system buffers up to 90% of the H^- of ECF. Horne and Derrico (1999) refer to buffers as "chemical sponges." They either act like a base and bind or soak up free hydrogen ions or act like an acid and release hydrogen ions when too few are present in a solution. Buffers attempt to bring a body fluid as close as possible to the pH of normal body fluid (7.35 to 7.45).

The ratio of carbonic acid (H_2CO_3), the most common acid in human body fluid, to the body's most common base, bicarbonate (HCO_3-), is important for acid–base balance. Normal ECF has a ratio of 20 parts bicarbonate to 1 part carbonic acid. The exact quantities are unimportant for acid–base balance as long as they remain in a 20:1 ratio. Carbonic acid and bicarbonate must be carefully controlled to maintain this ratio; if either is increased or decreased, the 20:1 ratio is no longer in effect.

Phosphate Buffer System

This chemical buffer system is active in intracellular fluids and converts alkaline sodium phosphate (Na_2HPO_4), a weak base, to acid–sodium phosphate (NaH_2PO_4) in the kidneys.

Protein Buffer System

The third buffer system is a mixture of plasma proteins and the globin portion of hemoglobin in red blood cells. Because plasma proteins and hemoglobin possess chemical groups that can combine with or liberate hydrogen ions, they tend to minimize changes in pH and serve as excellent buffering agents over a wide range of pH values. For example, excess hydrogen ions in the blood cross over the plasma membrane of red blood cells and bind to the hemoglobin molecules that are plentiful in each red blood cell.

Respiratory Control of H⁻ Balance

The lungs are the primary controller of the body's carbonic acid supply. They have a huge surface area from which CO_2 can readily diffuse, and they can bring about rapid changes in H⁻ when needed. Carbon dioxide is constantly produced by cellular metabolism (carbonic acid [H_2CO_3] yields CO_2 and H_2O) and is excreted by exhalation. When the amount of CO_2 in the blood increases, the sensitive respiratory center in the medulla is stimulated and increases the rate and depth of respirations to eliminate more CO_2. As more CO_2 is exhaled, the H_2CO_3 level in the blood decreases, and the pH of the blood becomes more alkaline. When the blood level of CO_2 decreases, the respiratory center decreases the rate and depth of respirations to retain the CO_2 so that carbonic acid can be formed and the delicate balance maintained. This total respiratory process occurs almost as rapidly as the buffering action in the carbonic acid–sodium bicarbonate system.

Renal Control of H⁻ Balance

The concentration of bicarbonate in the plasma is regulated by the kidneys. Essentially, the kidneys excrete or retain hydrogen ions and form or excrete bicarbonate ions in response to the pH of the blood. In the presence of acidosis, the kidneys excrete hydrogen ions and form and conserve bicarbonate ions, thus raising the pH to the normal range. If alkalosis is present, the kidneys retain hydrogen ions and excrete bicarbonate ions in an effort to return to a balanced state.

Acid–base regulation by the kidneys occurs more slowly than by the carbonic acid–sodium bicarbonate system or by respiratory regulation. It may take up to 3 days for a normal fluid pH to be restored by the kidneys. The pH of urine varies, depending on the ions that are being excreted, but generally it is between 4.5 and 8.2.

⊚ Disturbances in Fluid, Electrolyte, and Acid–Base Balance

Nurses commonly encounter disturbances in fluid, electrolyte, and acid–base balance while caring for acutely or chronically ill patients. Although many of these disturbances are interrelated and may occur together, they are described here separately for learning purposes.

Fluid Imbalances

Fluid imbalances occur when the body's compensatory mechanisms are unable to maintain a homeostatic state. Fluid imbalances involve either the volume or distribution of water or electrolytes.

Fluid Volume Deficit

Fluid volume deficit can be caused by a deficiency in the amount of both water and electrolytes in the ECF when the water and electrolyte proportions remain near normal. The state is commonly known as *hypovolemia*. Both os-

motic and hydrostatic pressure changes force the interstitial fluid into the intravascular space. As the interstitial space is depleted, its fluid becomes hypertonic, and cellular fluid is then drawn into the interstitial space, leaving cells without adequate fluid to function properly.

The term dehydration is sometimes used as a synonym for hypovolemia, but this is technically inaccurate. *Dehydration* refers only to a decreased volume of water, but water is not decreased without electrolyte changes also. The term *hydration* refers to the union of a substance with water and is often used to indicate that there is normal water volume in the body.

Fluid volume deficits result from the loss of body fluids, especially if fluid intake is simultaneously decreased. Table 45-7 later in the chapter summarizes fluid volume deficits, common assessments, and general nursing interventions.

Young children, elderly people, and people who are ill are especially at risk for hypovolemia. A weight loss of 5% in adults and 10% in infants can occur rapidly. A 5% weight loss is considered to be pronounced fluid deficit, and an 8% loss or more is considered severe. A 15% weight loss caused by fluid deficiency usually threatens life.

Third-space fluid shift refers to a distributional shift of body fluids into potential body spaces such as the pleural, peritoneal, pericardial, or joint cavities; the bowel; or the interstitial space (plasma-to-interstitial shift). Once trapped in these spaces, the fluid is not easily exchanged with ECF. With third-space fluid shift, a deficit in ECF volume occurs. The fluid has not been lost but is trapped in another body space for a period of time and is essentially unavailable for use. A third-space shift may occur as a result of a severe burn, a bowel obstruction, or pancreatitis. Decreased body weight does not occur as it does with an ECF volume deficit (vomiting or diarrhea), nor can the fluid loss be measured (Metheny, 2000). Treatment is directed toward correction of the cause of the third-space shift, or third-spacing, as it is also commonly called.

Fluid Volume Excess

Excessive retention of water and sodium in ECF in near-normal proportions results in a condition termed *fluid volume excess*. It is also called *hypervolemia.* The term overhydration is commonly used as a synonym for hypervolemia, but strictly speaking, this is inaccurate. *Overhydration* refers only to above-normal amounts of water in extracellular spaces. Common causes are malfunction of the kidneys, causing an inability to excrete the excesses, and failure of the heart to function as a pump, resulting in accumulation of fluid in the lungs and dependent parts of the body. When water is retained in excessive amounts, so is sodium.

Because of the increased extracellular osmotic pressure from the retained sodium, fluid is pulled from the cells to equalize the tonicity. By the time the intracellular and extracellular spaces are isotonic to each other, an excess of both water and sodium is in the ECF, whereas the cells are nearly depleted. The excessive ECF may accumulate in tissue spaces; this is known as *edema*. Edema can be observed around the eyes, fingers, ankles, and sacral space (Fig. 45-8) and can also accumulate in or around body organs. It may result in a weight gain in excess of 5%. When

1+ Pitting Edema

- Slight indentation (2mm)
- Normal contours
- Associated with interstitial fluid volume 30% above normal

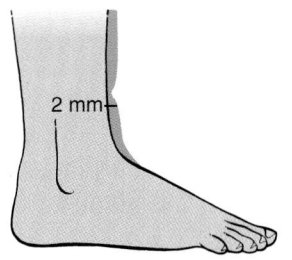

2+ Pitting Edema

- Deeper pit after pressing (4mm)
- Lasts longer than 1+
- Fairly normal contour

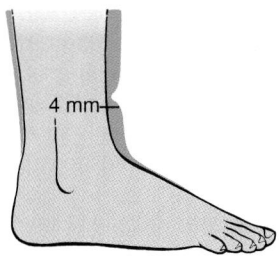

3+ Pitting Edema

- Deep pit (6mm)
- Remains several seconds after pressing
- Skin swelling obvious by general inspection

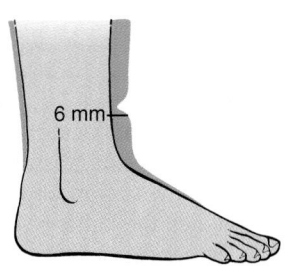

4+ Pitting Edema

- Deep pit (8mm)
- Remains for a prolonged time after pressing, possibly minutes
- Frank swelling

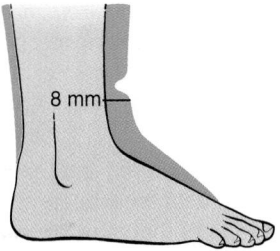

Brawny Edema   *a brawt on a grill- fluid seeps out*

- Fluid can no longer be displaced secondary to excessive interstitial fluid accumulation
- No pitting
- Tissue palpates as firm or hard
- Skin surface shiny, warm, moist

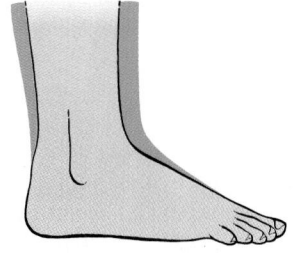

Figure 45-8
System for grading edema.

the excess fluid remains in the intravascular space, the concentration of solids in the blood is decreased.

Interstitial-to-plasma shift is the movement of fluid from the space surrounding the cells to the blood. This shift, also called hypervolemia, is a compensatory response to volume or osmotic pressure changes of the intravascular fluid. Although the body attempts to maintain normal balance in all fluid spaces, the intravascular fluid is usually protected at the expense of interstitial fluid and ICF.

Electrolyte Imbalances

When patients present with deficits or excesses of sodium, potassium, calcium, magnesium, or phosphate, careful nursing assessment depends on an understanding of the effects of these imbalances.

Hyponatremia and Hypernatremia

Hyponatremia refers to a sodium deficit in ECF caused by a loss of sodium or a gain of water. Osmotic pressure changes result in ECF moving into the cells. When this occurs, prints from the examiner's fingers tend to remain on the patient's skin over the sternum when pressure is applied with the fingers. The phenomenon results from tissue plasticity as fluid moves into cells in excess amounts.

Hypernatremia refers to a surplus of sodium in ECF that can result from excess water loss or an overall excess of sodium. Because of the increased extracellular osmotic pressure, fluids move from the cells, leaving them without sufficient fluid.

Hypokalemia and Hyperkalemia

Hypokalemia refers to a potassium deficit in ECF. When the extracellular potassium level falls, potassium moves from the cell, creating an intracellular potassium deficiency. Sodium and hydrogen ions are then retained by the cells to maintain isotonic fluids. These electrolyte shifts influence normal cellular functioning, the pH of ECF, and the functions of most body systems. Skeletal muscles are generally the first to demonstrate a potassium deficiency. Typical signs of hypokalemia include muscle weakness and leg cramps. *Hyperkalemia* refers to an excess of potassium in ECF. Although this condition occurs less frequently than hypokalemia, it can be hazardous. The transmission of stimuli through heart muscle is slowed or prevented, and cardiac arrest eventually occurs if hyperkalemia is not corrected.

Hypocalcemia and Hypercalcemia

Hypocalcemia refers to a calcium deficit in ECF. If the condition is prolonged, calcium is taken from the bones. This results in *osteomalacia*, which is characterized by soft and pliable bones. Common signs of hypocalcemia include numbness and tingling of fingers, muscle cramps, and tetany. *Hypercalcemia* refers to an excess of calcium in ECF. Hypercalcemia is an emergency situation because the condition often leads to cardiac arrest.

Hypomagnesemia and Hypermagnesemia

Hypomagnesemia refers to a magnesium deficit. The body's potassium level also drops because the kidneys tend to excrete more potassium when magnesium supplies are poor. As a result, hypomagnesemia and hypokalemia often occur together. *Hypermagnesemia* refers to a magnesium excess. It can occur especially in end-stage renal failure when the kidneys fail to excrete magnesium and excessive amounts are administered therapeutically.

Hypophosphatemia and Hyperphosphatemia

Hypophosphatemia refers to a below-normal serum concentration of inorganic phosphorus. Although this may indicate phosphorus deficiency, multiple factors may lower serum phosphate levels while total-body phosphorus stores are normal. *Hyperphosphatemia* refers to above-normal serum concentrations of inorganic phosphorus.

Acid–Base Imbalances

Arterial blood gases (ABGs) are laboratory tests commonly used in the assessment and treatment of acid–base imbalances. Results from venous blood, in contrast, are only specific for the particular extremity or area where the blood was sampled and do not provide information on how well the lungs are oxygenating the blood. The pH of plasma indicates balance or impending acidosis or alkalosis. In addition, a study of the blood's oxygen and carbon dioxide gases is important. The partial pressures (indicated by "P") of these gases, or their tensions, are determined by the use of a nomogram, which reflects the chemical and physical activities of the two gases. The partial pressure of carbon dioxide is abbreviated $PaCO_2$; for oxygen, it is PaO_2. The "a" indicates an arterial specimen. When the PaO_2 is low, hemoglobin carries less than normal amounts of oxygen; when the PaO_2 is high, the hemoglobin carries more oxygen. Oxygen saturation readings (SaO_2) reveal the percentage of oxygen in the blood that combines with hemoglobin. The $PaCO_2$ is influenced almost entirely by respiratory activity. When the $PaCO_2$ is low, carbonic acid leaves the body in excessive amounts; when the $PaCO_2$ is high, there are excessive amounts of carbonic acid in the body. Laboratory levels for ABGs are listed in Table 45-3.

Acid–base imbalances occur when the carbonic acid or bicarbonate levels become disproportionate. When there is a single primary cause, these disturbances are known as respiratory acidosis or alkalosis and metabolic acidosis or alkalosis, which are described in the sections that follow. These disturbances are a result of an upset in acid–base balance, as follows:

- A respiratory disturbance alters the carbonic acid portion:

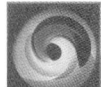

Table 45-3
Acid–Base Parameters for Arterial Blood Gas Studies

	Normal	Acid	Base
pH	7.35–7.45	<7.35	>7.45
$PaCO_2$	35–45	>45	<35
HCO_3^-	22–26	<22	>26

- Respiratory acidosis and alkalosis are the results of respiratory disturbances.
- Compensation for a respiratory disturbance occurs when the kidneys attempt to restore balance by either conserving or excreting more bicarbonate.
- A metabolic disturbance alters the bicarbonate portion:
  - Metabolic acidosis and alkalosis are almost entirely the result of metabolic processes.
  - The primary organs for compensation with a metabolic disorder are the lungs, which either try to conserve or excrete more carbon dioxide (available in weakly ionized carbonic acid).
  - Although compensation is the body's natural attempt to restore balance, correction may also be required. Correction involves using nursing and medical interventions to promote a return to homeostasis (eg, pharmacologic agents or mechanical ventilation).

Complicated clinical situations may occur when respiratory and metabolic imbalances coexist.

Respiratory Acidosis

Respiratory acidosis is a primary excess of carbonic acid in ECF. Any decrease in alveolar ventilation that results in retention of carbon dioxide can cause respiratory acidosis. Because the lungs are the source of the problem, they are unable to participate in compensation. As the carbonic acid content increases, the kidneys attempt to retain more bicarbonate and increase their hydrogen excretion. Thus:

$$\text{Respiratory acidosis} = \text{high } PaCO_2 \text{ because of} \\ \text{alveolar hypoventilation}$$

Respiratory Alkalosis

Respiratory alkalosis is a primary deficit of carbonic acid in ECF. It is the result of increased alveolar ventilation and the consequent decrease in carbon dioxide. An increase in respiratory rate and depth causes the carbon dioxide loss because the carbon dioxide is excreted faster than normal.

Because of the deficit of carbon dioxide, which is a respiratory stimulant sensed in the medulla of the brain, depression or cessation of respirations eventually can occur. Because the lungs are the source of the problem, they are unable to participate in compensation. Therefore, the kidneys attempt to alleviate the imbalance by increasing the bicarbonate excretion and by retaining more hydrogen. Thus:

Respiratory alkalosis = low $PaCO_2$ because of alveolar hyperventilation

Metabolic Acidosis

Metabolic acidosis is a proportionate deficit of bicarbonate in ECF. The deficit can occur as the result of an increase in acid components or an excessive loss of bicarbonate. The lungs attempt to increase the carbon dioxide excretion by increasing the rate and depth of respirations. The kidneys attempt to compensate by retaining bicarbonate and by excreting more hydrogen. If the body is unable to achieve normal balance, the person may lose consciousness as metabolic acidosis increases, and death eventually results. Thus:

Metabolic acidosis = low bicarbonate. Nonvolatile acid is present to use up HCO_3- in disproportionate amounts, or HCO_3- is lost in similar amounts

Metabolic Alkalosis

Metabolic alkalosis is a primary excess of bicarbonate in ECF. This may be the result of excessive acid losses or increased base ingestion or retention. The body attempts to compensate by retaining carbon dioxide. The respirations become slow and shallow, and periods of no breathing may occur. The kidneys attempt to excrete potassium and sodium with the excessive bicarbonate, and retain hydrogen in carbonic acid. Thus:

Metabolic alkalosis = high bicarbonate. Nonvolatile acid is lost and is not using up HCO_3- or HCO_3- is gained in disproportionate amounts

The Nursing Process

ASSESSING

The pathophysiology underlying acute and chronic illness, trauma, and certain therapeutic interventions may place a patient at high risk for fluid, electrolyte, and acid–base imbalances. Such imbalances can seriously compromise the patient's health status and may prove life-threatening. The nursing assessment is directed toward the following:

- Identifying patients at high risk for fluid, electrolyte, and acid–base imbalance
- Determining that a specific imbalance is present and identifying the nature of the imbalance along with its severity, etiology, and defining characteristics
- Determining the effectiveness of the plan of care

Important assessment parameters include the nursing history and nursing examination, a record of fluid intake and output, daily weights, and laboratory studies.

Nursing History

A comprehensive nursing history includes questions related to the patient's fluid, electrolyte, and acid–base balance. The accompanying Focused Assessment Guide includes interview questions helpful in identifying the patient's usual pattern of fluid intake and elimination and the patient's evaluation of his or her hydration status and awareness of particular problems. Interview questions are also directed toward identifying patients at high risk for imbalances. Risk factors include the following:

- The pathophysiology underlying acute and chronic illnesses (eg, diabetes mellitus, congestive heart failure, renal failure)
- Abnormal losses of body fluids (eg, prolonged or severe vomiting or diarrhea, draining wounds, fistulas). Table 45-4 lists imbalances that result from loss of specific body fluids.
- Burns
- Trauma
- Therapies that may disrupt fluid and electrolyte balance (eg, medications such as diuretics and steroids, treatments such as IV therapy and TPN)

Physical Assessment

Metheny (2000) recommends that the nurse pay attention to certain parameters when assessing a patient's fluid and electrolyte status:

- Comparison of total intake and output of fluids
- Urine volume and concentration
- Skin and tongue turgor
- Degree of moisture in oral cavity
- Body weight
- Thirst
- Tearing and salivation
- Appearance and temperature of skin
- Facial appearance
- Edema
- Vital signs
- Neck and hand vein filling
- Results of hemodynamic monitoring (eg, central venous pressure [CVP] and pulmonary artery pressure [PAP])
- Neuromuscular irritability

When an imbalance of particular electrolytes is suspected, the nurse needs to understand that the associated assessment is vital. Table 45-5 presents select nursing considerations for each of these parameters, findings in a healthy adult, and significant findings.

Measuring Fluid Intake and Output

When either the physician or nurse orders that a patient's fluid intake and output be continuously measured, the patient, family, and all caregivers should be alert to the

(*text continues on page 1291*)

FOCUSED ASSESSMENT GUIDE

Fluid, Electrolyte, and Acid–Base Balance

Factors to Assess	Questions and Approaches
Usual patterns of fluid intake	Describe the amount and types of fluids you usually drink in a 24-hour period. Have there been any recent changes?
Usual pattern of fluid elimination	Describe your usual voiding/urination habits.
	Any recent changes in frequency or amount?
	Is your body losing fluids in any other major way? • Vomiting • Diarrhea • Excessive perspiration • Fistula
Patient's evaluation of hydration status	Do you think there is an approximate balance between your fluid intake and output?
	Have you noticed any signs that your body is experiencing too much or too little hydration (difficulty breathing, edema, dry skin and mucous membranes, thirst)?
History of disease process	Is there any history of disease process or injury that might disrupt fluid and electrolyte balance (eg, diabetes mellitus, cancer, burns)?
Medication history	Do you take any medications or treatments that might disrupt fluid and electrolyte balance (eg, steroids, diuretics, total parenteral nutrition, dialysis)?
Fluid, electrolyte, and acid–base imbalances and contributing factors	Are you aware of any other fluid balance problems you may be experiencing? • Nature • Onset of problem and frequency • Causes • Severity • Symptoms • Intervention attempted and results

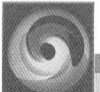

Table 45-4
Imbalances Resulting From Loss of Specific Body Fluid

Fluid Lost	Imbalances Likely to Occur	Fluid Lost	Imbalances Likely to Occur
Gastric juice	Extracellular fluid volume deficit Metabolic alkalosis Sodium deficit Potassium deficit	Pancreatic juice	Metabolic acidosis Sodium deficit Calcium deficit Extracellular fluid volume deficit
	Tetany (if metabolic alkalosis is present)	Sensible perspiration	Extracellular fluid volume deficit Sodium deficit
	Ketosis of starvation Magnesium deficit	Insensible water loss	Water deficit (dehydration) Sodium excess
Intestinal juice	Extracellular fluid volume deficit Metabolic acidosis Sodium deficit Potassium deficit	Wound exudate	Protein deficit Sodium deficit Extracellular fluid volume deficit
Bile	Sodium deficit Metabolic acidosis	Ascites	Protein deficit Sodium deficit Plasma-to-interstitial fluid shift Extracellular fluid volume deficit

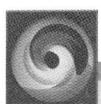

Table 45-5
Parameters to Be Considered in Clinical Assessment for Fluid, Electrolyte, and Acid–Base Balance

Assessment Parameters	Nursing Considerations	Findings in Healthy Adult	Significant Findings
Comparison of total intake and output of fluids	• Records may be initiated by the nurse for any patient with a real or potential water or electrolyte problem. • Intake should include all fluids taken into the body. • Output should include urine, vomitus, diarrhea, drainage from fistulas, and drainage from suction apparatus. Perspiration and drainage from lesions should be noted and estimated. Prolonged hyperventilation should also be noted because it is an important route of water vapor loss.	• Fluid intake about equals fluid output—when averaged over 2 or 3 days. • Range of 1500 to 3500 mL fluid intake and loss; 2000 mL is average adult intake and loss per day. • Output of urine normally approximates the ingestion of liquids; water from food and oxidation is balanced by the water loss through feces, the skin, and the respiratory process.	• When the total intake is substantially less than the total output, the patient is in danger of fluid volume deficit. • When the total intake is substantially more than the total output, the patient is in danger of fluid volume excess.

Urine volume and concentration	• Measure all fluid loses according to routes.
	• Use a device calibrated for small volumes of urine when hourly urine volumes need to be measured.
	• Account for factors that can alter urinary output:
	  1. Amount of fluid intake
	  2. Losses from skin, lungs, and GI tract
	  3. Amount of waste products for excretions
	  4. Renal concentrating ability
	  5. Blood volume
	  6. Hormonal influences (primarily aldosterone and ADH)
		• Normal urinary output is about 1 mL/kg of body weight per hour (for the average adult: 1500 mL/24 hr, which is equivalent to about 40 to 80 mL/hr).
		• Stress may diminish the 24-hour urine volume in the adult to 750 to 1000 mL (or 30 to 50 mL/hr) because of increased aldosterone and ADH secretion.
		• The range of specific gravity is from 1.003 to 1.035. Urine osmolality ranges between 500 mOsm and 800 mOsm/kg (mmol/kg).
			• A low urine volume with a high specific gravity indicates fluid volume deficit.
			• A low urine volume with a low specific gravity indicates renal disease.
			• A high urine volume suggests fluid volume excess.
			• Urine volume is increased in conditions with high solute loads, such as diabetes mellitus.
			• Hypovolemia causes decreased renal perfusion and thus oliguria; hypervolemia causes increased urinary volume if the kidneys are functioning normally.

Body weight	• Because of the common inaccuracies in recording intake and output, body weight is believed to be a more accurate indicator of fluid gained and lost.
	• Guidelines for weighing patients:
	  1. Use the same scale each time.
	  2. Measure weight at the same time each day: in the morning before breakfast and after voiding.
	  3. Be sure the patient is wearing the same or similar clothing (clothing should be dry).
		• A patient's dry weight should remain relatively stable.	• Rapid variations in weight closely reflect changes in body fluid volume.
			• A rapid loss of body weight occurs when the total fluid intake is less than the total fluid output.
			  1. Rapid loss of 2% total body weight (TBW) indicates mild fluid volume deficit.
			  2. Rapid loss of 5% TBW indicates moderate fluid volume deficit.
			  3. Rapid loss of 8% or more of TBW indicates severe fluid volume deficit.

(continued)

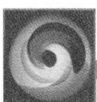

Table 45-5 (Continued)

Assessment Parameters	Nursing Considerations	Findings in Healthy Adult	Significant Findings

	4. If the patient is unable to stand on a small, portable scale, use a bed scale.
	• A patient may have a severe fluid volume deficit even though body weight is essentially unchanged when there is a third-space loss of body fluid.
			• A rapid gain of body weight occurs when the total fluid intake is greater than the total fluid output.
			  1. Rapid gain of 2% TBW indicates mild fluid volume excess.
			  2. Rapid gain of 5% TBW indicates moderate fluid volume excess.
			  3. Rapid gain of 8% or more of TBW indicates severe fluid volume excess.
			• A rapid gain or loss of 1 kg (2.2 lb) of body weight is about equal to the gain or loss of 1 L of fluid.

Skin turgor (elasticity)	• Pinch the patient's skin over the sternum, inner aspect of the thighs, or forehead. • Some prefer to test skin turgor in children over the abdominal area and on the medial aspect of the thighs. • Skin turgor can vary with age, nutritional state, and even race and complexion.	• Pinched skin immediately falls back to its normal position when released. • Reduced skin turgor is common in older patients (those more than 55 to 60 years of age) because of a primary decrease in skin elasticity.	• In a person with a fluid volume deficit, the skin flattens more slowly after the pinch is released; the skin may remain elevated for many seconds. • Severe malnutrition, particularly in infants, can cause depressed skin turgor even in the absence of fluid depletion.
Tongue turgor	• Unlike skin turgor, tongue turgor is not affected appreciably by age and thus is a useful assessment for all age groups. (In an arid climate, this may not be a reliable parameter.)	• Tongue has one longitudinal furrow.	• In the person with fluid volume deficit, there are additional longitudinal furrows and the tongue is smaller. • Sodium excess causes the tongue to look red and swollen.
Moisture and oral cavity	• A dry mouth may be the result of fluid volume deficit or of mouth breathing. (Exposure to an arid climate may result in a dry mouth.)	• Mucous membranes in oral cavity are moist.	• Dryness of the membrane where the cheek and gum meet indicates fluid volume deficit. • Dry sticky mucous membranes are noted in sodium excess. (The oral cavity feels like flypaper.)
Tearing and salivation		• Tearing and salivation decrease normally with age.	• The absence of tearing and salivation in a child is a sign of fluid volume deficit; it becomes obvious with a fluid loss of 5% of TBW.
Appearance of skin and skin temperature			• Metabolic acidosis can cause warm, flushed skin (due to peripheral vasodilation).
Facial appearance			• A person with a severe fluid volume deficit has a pinched and drawn facial expression.

(continued)

Table 45-5 (Continued)

Assessment Parameters	Nursing Considerations	Findings in Healthy Adult	Significant Findings
			• A fluid volume deficit of 10% of body weight causes decreased intraocular pressure, causing the eyes to appear sunken and to feel soft to the touch.
Edema (excessive accumulation of interstitial fluid)	• Pitting edema (see Fig. 45-8) • Measurement of an extremity or body part with a millimeter tape, in the same area each day, is a more exact method of measurement. • An excess of interstitial fluid may accumulate predominantly in the lower extremities of ambulatory patients and in the presacral region of bedridden patients. • The presence of periorbital (around the eyes) edema or pedal edema should prompt one to look for edema in other parts of the body.	• No edema	• Clinically edema is not usually apparent in the adult until the retention of 5 to 10 lb of excess fluid occurs. • Pitting edema is not evident until at least a 10% increase in weight has occurred. • Formation of edema may be localized (as in thrombophlebitis) or generalized (as in heart failure, cirrhosis of liver, or nephrotic syndrome). Edema of congestive heart failure, liver cirrhosis, or nephrotic syndrome is the result of sodium retention.
Body temperature	• Because fever increases the loss of body fluids, it is important that temperature elevations be detected early and appropriate interventions be taken. • Body temperature and other vital signs should be assessed at the nurse's discretion.	• Baseline temperature: diurnal variations	• There is an elevation of body temperature in hypernatremia (dehydration) probably related to lack of available fluid for sweating. • There is a decrease in body temperature in fluid volume deficit, when uncomplicated by infection. • Fever increases the loss of body fluids. • A temperature elevation between 101°F (38.3°C) and 103°F (39.4°C) increases the 24-hour fluid requirement by at least 500 mL, and a temperature above 103°F increases it by at least 1000 mL.
Pulse		• Baseline pulse rate, rhythm, and volume	• Tachycardia is usually the earliest sign of the decreased vascular volume associated with fluid volume deficit. • Irregular pulse rates also occur with potassium imbalances and magnesium deficit. • Pulse volume is decreased in fluid volume deficit and increased in fluid volume excess.

b/c insensible losses from resp & sweat

(continued)

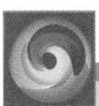

Table 45-5 (Continued)

Assessment Parameters	Nursing Considerations	Findings in Healthy Adult	Significant Findings
Respirations		• Baseline respiratory rate, rhythm, and qualities	• Deep, ~~rapid respirations~~ may be a compensatory mechanism for metabolic acidosis or a primary disorder causing respiratory alkalosis. • Slow, shallow respirations may be a compensatory mechanism for metabolic alkalosis or a primary disorder causing respiratory acidosis. • Moist crackles, in the absence of cardiopulmonary disease, indicate fluid volume excess.
~~Blood pressure~~	• Whenever a fluid imbalance is suspected, check the ~~patient's blood pressure while he or she is lying down, sitting, and standing.~~	• Baseline blood pressure	• A fall in systolic pressure greater than 15 mm Hg from the lying to the sitting or standing position (postural hypotension) usually indicates fluid volume deficit.

Neck veins and central venous pressure (CVP)	• The jugular veins provide a built-in manometer for following changes in CVP.
	• To estimate CVP, the nurse:
	  1. Positions the patient in a semi-Fowler's position (head of bed elevated to a 30- to 45-degree angle), keeping the neck straight
	  2. Removes any of the patient's clothing that could constrict the neck or upper chest
	  3. Provides adequate lighting to visualize effectively the external jugular veins on each side of the neck
	  4. Measures the levels to which the veins are distended on the neck or above the level of the manubrium
	• More accurate assessments of blood volume are obtained by measuring CVP by hemodynamic monitoring.
		• Normally, when the patient is supine, the external jugular veins fill to the anterior border of the sternocleidomastoid muscle. With the patient positioned sitting at a 45-degree angle, the venous distentions normally should not extend higher than 2 cm above the sternal angle.
		• Pressure in the right atrium is usually 0 to 4 cm H_2O; pressure in the vena cava is about 4 to 11 cm H_2O.
			• A low CVP may indicate:
			  1. Decreased blood volume
			  2. Drug-induced vasodilation (causing pooling of blood in peripheral veins)
			• A high CVP may indicate:
			  1. Increased blood volume
			  2. Heart failure
			  3. Vasoconstriction

Neuromuscular irritability	• When imbalances in calcium, magnesium, and sodium are suspected it is important to assess patients for increased or decreased neuromuscular irritability.		

Handwritten annotations: "body's straining to keep up" (top right); "distended when ↑FV" (left, next to CVP); "↑ deep tendon reflexes" (center, near Neuromuscular irritability)

(continued)

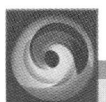

Table 45-5 (Continued)

Assessment Parameters	Nursing Considerations	Findings in Healthy Adult	Significant Findings
	• To test for *Chvostek's sign*, the facial nerve should be percussed about 2 cm anterior to the ear lobe.	• Negative response	• Patients with hypocalcemia or hypomagnesemia respond positively with a unilateral twitching of the facial muscles, including the eyelid and lips.
	• To test for *Trousseau's sign*, place a blood pressure cuff on the arm and inflate above systolic pressure for 3 minutes.	• Negative response	• A positive response is the development of carpal spasm.
	• A deep tendon reflex is elicited by briskly tapping a partially stretched tendon with a rubber percussion hammer, preferably over the tendon insertion of the muscle.	• The response in the prospective muscle is a sudden contraction (2+).	• Deep tendon reflexes may be hyperactive in the presence of hypocalcemia, hypomagnesemia, hypernatremia, and alkalosis.
	• The muscle being tested should be slightly stretched, and the patient should be relaxed.		• Deep tendon reflexes may be hypoactive in the presence of hypercalcemia, hypermagnesemia, hyponatremia, hypokalemia, and acidosis.

	• Reflexes usually graded on a 0 to 4+ scale
	    0 = no response
	    1+ = somewhat diminished, but present
	    2+ = normal
	    3+ = brisker than average and possibly but not necessarily indicative of disease
	    4+ = hyperactive		

Behavior Sensation Fatigue level	• Because these changes are often vague, they are best evaluated in context with specific imbalances.		

(Data from Metheny, N. M. [2000]. *Fluid and electrolyte balance* [4th ed.]. Philadelphia: Lippincott-Raven.)

need to measure all fluids entering and leaving the body. The patient's condition dictates the strictness of these intake and output measurements. Adherence to the guidelines in the accompanying box helps eliminate common errors in measuring fluid intake and output.

Daily Weights

Because there are numerous sources of inaccuracies in fluid intake and output measurement, the record of a patient's daily weight may more accurately depict fluid balance status.

Laboratory Studies

Laboratory tests are helpful in determining whether fluid, electrolyte, and acid–base balance exist. As a safety precaution and in compliance with Centers for Disease Control

and Prevention guidelines, nurses must apply a "biohazard" label to all blood specimens collected from patients at home. The specimen should be transported to the laboratory as soon as possible or refrigerated if a delay of more than 1 hour is expected. Standard tests include the following (tables of normal values are given in Appendix B):

Complete Blood Count

This basic screening test determines the total number of red blood cells and values for hemoglobin and hematocrit. Significant values include the following:

• *Increased hematocrit values:* found in severe dehydration and shock (when hemoconcentration rises considerably)

got good blood – just not enough of it.

Guidelines for Nursing Care
Measuring Fluid Intake and Output

As soon as measured intake and output is ordered for the patient, the patient and family are instructed that the nurse needs a record of all fluids entering the body and all fluid output. A simple explanation of why this is being done is offered as well as specific instructions as to how the patient can help to keep his or her record accurate. Some patients may need to be reminded during nursing rounds each morning that this measurement will continue.

The patient's plan of care and nursing Kardex are used to communicate to nursing personnel the need to measure fluid intake and output. A sign posted in the patient's room and bedside form for recording intake and output are helpful reminders for both the patient and nurses.

The Patient's Fluid Intake Includes the Following:

- All fluids and foods that are liquid at room temperature (ice cream, gelatin dessert [Jell-O], and so forth)

  Use the agency's designation of specific volumes for common food containers (eg, juice glass = 90 mL; milk carton = 240 mL). Remind the patient that sips of water or other fluids in between meals need to be recorded; small, disposable calibrated cups at the bedside facilitate accurate measurement. Remember that liquid medications or water taken with pills may significantly increase the fluid intake of some patients.
- All parenteral fluids

- Other fluids taken into the body: subcutaneous fluids, fluids instilled into drainage tubes, enema solutions

The Patient's Fluid Output Includes the Following:

- Urine; vomitus; diarrhea; drainage from fistulas, wounds, and ulcers; and drainage from suctioning devices. Calibrated measuring devices should be readily available for accurate measurement. Disposable, calibrated urine collection containers that fit under the toilet seat are available for ambulatory patients. Urine or liquid feces in diapers or bed clothes, vomitus on clothing or bed linens, wound drainage saturating dressings, and so forth, need to be estimated.
- Heavy perspiration should be noted on the output record, especially when the patient's clothing or bed linens are soaked.
- Hyperventilation (water vapor loss) should also be noted on the output record. Record rate and depth of respirations.

Both intake and output should be measured whenever possible, rather than estimated. Output measurement is described in chapter 42. Failure to record intake or output when it is measured may result in its being forgotten.

Intake and output totals are generally recorded for each 8-hour shift and totaled each 24 hours. At varying intervals throughout the shift, the alert patient should be questioned about his or her intake and output.

- *Decreased hematocrit values:* found with acute, massive blood loss and with hemolytic reaction after transfusion of incompatible blood
- *Increased levels of hemoglobin:* found in hemoconcentration of the blood
- *Decreased levels of hemoglobin:* found with anemia states, severe hemorrhage, and after a hemolytic reaction

Serum Electrolytes

This screening test determines plasma levels of certain electrolytes. Commonly determined are plasma levels of sodium, potassium, chloride, and bicarbonate ions.

Urine pH and Specific Gravity

Both the urine pH and specific gravity may be obtained by dipstick measurement using a fresh voided specimen or through laboratory analysis. Specific gravity is a measure of the urine's concentration. The range depends on the patient's state of hydration and varies with urine volume and

the load of solutes to be excreted. Normal values range from 1.003 to 1.035 (concentrated urine—1.025 to 1.030 or more; dilute urine—1.001 to 1.010).

Arterial Blood Gases

ABGs are obtained to determine the adequacy of oxygenation and ventilation and to assess acid–base status. See the earlier Table 45-3 for the primary laboratory values used to determine acid–base balance. Additional ABG values exist but are not included in this simple interpretation of acid–base imbalances. Partial pressure of oxygen ($PaCO_2$) and oxygen saturation (SaO_2) results also directly reflect the adequacy of oxygenation and ventilation. The following are necessary steps to take when interpreting blood gases:

1. Determine whether the pH is alkalotic or acidotic.
2. Check for the cause of the change in pH. Is it respiratory ($PaCO_2$) or metabolic (HCO_3^-)? In respiratory acid–base imbalances, the pH and $PaCO_2$ values are inversely abnormal (move in opposite directions):

Respiratory acidosis:
  $\downarrow$ pH   < 7.35 $\uparrow$ PaCO$_2$ Normal HCO$_3$–
Respiratory alkalosis:
  $\uparrow$ pH   > 7.45 $\downarrow$ PaCO$_2$ Normal HCO$_3$–

In metabolic acid–base imbalances, the pH and HCO$_3$ values are both high or both low:

Metabolic acidosis:
  $\downarrow$ pH   < 7.35 $\downarrow$ HCO$_3$–   Normal PaCO$_2$
Metabolic alkalosis:
  $\uparrow$ pH   > 7.45 $\uparrow$ HCO$_3$–   Normal PaCO$_2$

3. Determine whether the body is compensating for the pH change. When the problem is respiratory, the renal system attempts to compensate either by increasing or by decreasing HCO$_3$–. In contrast, the respiratory system compensates for a metabolic acid–base imbalance by regulating CO$_2$ levels. When compensation occurs, the PaCO$_2$ and the HCO$_3$– will always point in the same direction. The focus of compensation efforts is to return the pH to the normal range:

Respiratory acidosis:
  $\downarrow$ pH   < 7.35 $\uparrow$ PaCO$_2$ $\uparrow$ HCO$_3$–
  (compensation attempt)
Respiratory alkalosis:
  $\uparrow$ pH   > 7.45 $\downarrow$ PaCO$_2$ $\downarrow$ HCO$_3$–
  (compensation attempt)
Metabolic acidosis:
  $\downarrow$ pH   < 7.35 $\downarrow$ HCO$_3$– $\downarrow$ PaCO$_2$
  (compensation attempt)
Metabolic alkalosis:
  $\uparrow$ pH   > 7.45 $\uparrow$ HCO$_3$– $\uparrow$ PaCO$_2$
  (compensation attempt)

4. Look at the total picture and determine whether compensation has occurred. Compensation is classified as follows:
   Absent if:
   pH abnormal
   One component abnormal
   Second component within normal range
   Partial if:
   pH abnormal
   One component abnormal
   Second component beginning to change
   Complete if:
   pH within normal range
   One component abnormal
   Second changed to move pH within normal range

Table 45-6 lists assessments and nursing interventions related to these acid–base disturbances.

Fluid and Electrolyte Disturbances as the Problem

When assessment data point to fluid and electrolyte problems amenable to nursing therapy, they receive one of three diagnostic labels:

Fluid Volume Excess
Fluid Volume Deficit
Risk for Fluid Volume Deficit

Excess fluid volume may result from greatly increased fluid intake or, more frequently, from decreased excretion such as occurs in progressive renal disease and with certain cancers. Fluid volume deficits may result from decreased intake; increased excretion of fluids; fluid shifts; and the special need for fluids and electrolytes in situations involving strenuous exercise, extreme heat or dryness, and conditions (eg, fever) that increase the metabolic rate. The accompanying box presents contributing factors and defining characteristics for these diagnoses.

The nurse's analysis of assessment data may also lead to the diagnosis of specific electrolyte or acid–base disturbances that are collaborative problems because they require joint intervention by nursing and medicine.

Fluid and Electrolyte Disturbances as the Etiology

Disturbances in fluid, electrolyte, and acid–base balance may affect many other areas of human functioning. Sample diagnoses follow:

  Activity Intolerance related to imbalance between oxygen supply and demand
  Ineffective Breathing Pattern related to compensatory mechanism by lungs (hypoventilation or hyperventilation)
  Decreased Cardiac Output related to decreased blood volume, shock
  Risk for Injury related to neuromuscular irritability, cardiac arrhythmia
  Knowledge Deficit: Harmful Effects of Abuses of Dieting, Alcohol, Diuretics, Laxatives, and Enemas related to no previous experience
  Altered Oral Mucous Membrane related to dehydration
  Impaired Skin Integrity related to dehydration, edema
  Altered Thought Processes related to cerebral edema, mental confusion or disorientation, convulsions
  Altered Tissue Perfusion: [specify type] related to decreased cardiac output
  Altered Urinary Elimination related to decreased kidney perfusion secondary to decreased plasma volume

Nursing care supports the following expected outcomes. The healthy adult patient will achieve the following:

• Maintain an approximate balance between fluid intake and fluid output (average about 2500 mL fluid intake and output over 3 days)
• Maintain a urine specific gravity within normal range (1.010 to 1.025)

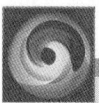

Table 45-6
Acid–Base Disturbances

Risk Factors	Assessments	Nursing Interventions
Respiratory Acidosis (Carbonic Acid Excess)		
Acute respiratory disease:	Acute respiratory acidosis	Treatment is directed at improving
Pulmonary edema	Mental cloudiness	ventilation:
Aspiration of a foreign body	Dizziness	Pharmacologic measures
Atelectasis	Muscular twitching	Pulmonary hygiene measures
Overdose of sedative or	Unconsciousness	Adequate hydration
anesthetic	ABGs	Supplemental oxygen
Cardiac arrest	pH <7.35	Mechanical ventilation may be neces-
Chronic respiratory disease:	$PaCO_2$ >45 mm Hg (primary)	sary to correct disorder but must be
Emphysema	HCO_3- normal or only slightly elevated	used cautiously to decrease $PaCO_2$
Bronchial asthma	Chronic respiratory acidosis	slowly.
Cystic fibrosis	Weakness	
Inadequate mechanical	Dull headache	
ventilation	ABGs	
CNS depression	pH <7.35 or low N	
Neuromuscular disease	$PaCO_2$ >45 mm Hg (primary)	
	HCO_3- >26 mEq/L (compensatory)	
Respiratory Alkalosis (Carbonic Acid Deficit)		
Extreme anxiety (most common	Lightheadedness	If anxiety is the cause, the patient
cause)	Inability to concentrate	should be encouraged to breathe
Hypoxemia	Hyperventilation syndrome	more slowly (causes accumulation of
High fever	Tinnitus	CO_2) or breathe into a closed system
Early sepsis	Palpitations	(paper bag). Sedative may also be
Excessive ventilation by	Sweating	necessary in extreme anxiety.
mechanical ventilator	Dry mouth	Treatment of other causes is directed
CNS lesion involving the	Tremulousness	at correcting the underlying problem.
respiratory center	Convulsions and loss of consciousness	
Thyrotoxicosis	ABGs	
	pH >7.45	
	$PaCO_2$ <35 mm Hg (primary)	
	HCO_3- <22 mEq/L (compensatory)	
Metabolic Acidosis (Base Bicarbonate Deficit)		
Diarrhea	Headache	Treatment is directed toward correct-
Intestinal fistulas	Confusion	ing the metabolic deficit. If the cause
Ureterosigmoidostomy	Drowsiness	of the problem is excessive intake of
Hyperalimentation	Increased respiratory rate and depth	chloride, treatment obviously focuses
Excessive intake of acids, such	Nausea and vomiting	on eliminating the source. When nec-
as salicylates	Peripheral vasodilation	essary, bicarbonate is administered.
Diabetic ketoacidosis	ABGs	
Renal failure	pH <7.35	
Starvational ketoacidosis	HCO_3- <22 mEq/L (primary)	
	$PaCO_2$ <35 mm Hg	
	Hyperkalemia frequently present	
Metabolic Alkalosis (Base Bicarbonate Excess)		
Vomiting or gastric suction	Dizziness	Treatment is aimed at reversal of the
Hypokalemia	Tingling of fingers and toes	underlying disorder. Sufficient chlo-
Potassium-wasting diuretics	Hypertonic muscles	ride must be supplied for the kidney
Alkali ingestion (bicarbonate-	Depressed respirations (compensatory)	to absorb sodium with chloride (al-
containing antacids)	ABGs	lowing the excretion of excess bicar-
Renal loss of H^+ (eg, from steroid	pH >7.45	bonate). Treatment also includes
or diuretic use)	HCO_3- >26 mEq/L (primary)	administration of NaCl fluids to re-
	$PaCO_2$ >45 mm Hg (compensatory)	store normal fluid volume.
	Hypokalemia may be present	

(Adapted from Metheney, N. [2000]. *Fluid and electrolyte balance* [4th ed.]. Philadelphia: Lippincott-Raven.)

Nursing Diagnoses for Common Problems

Fluid and Electrolyte Balance

Problem	Related Factors	Sample Defining Characteristics
Fluid Volume Excess	Pathophysiologic factors: renal failure, decreased cardiac output, liver disease, abnormal fluid accumulations, hormonal problems	• "I've noticed that my wedding ring is tight . . . also my clothes don't fit as well as they used to. I guess I've gained some weight." • Reports dyspnea with exertion, feeling weak and fatigued • Pitting edema in feet, ankles, lower legs • Taut, shiny skin • Jugular venous distention
	Situational factors: excessive IV infusion	• Bounding pulse, increased from baseline • Shallow, rapid respirations, rales • Increased blood pressure
	Nutritional factors: excessive sodium intake, low protein intake	• 10-lb (4.5-kg) weight gain over past month • Fluid intake greater than output • "Sometimes I can't catch my breath and I feel like my heart is pounding away." • "I feel bloated."
Fluid Volume Deficit; Risk for Fluid Volume Deficit	Decreased fluid intake: imposed fluid restrictions, inability to obtain or swallow fluids (debilitation, oral pain), depression	• "After I got the flu I got so weak I couldn't get out of bed. . . . I think I was out of it for a couple of days." • Increased pulse and respirations • Dry oral mucosa, cracked lips, furrowed tongue • Scanty urine output
	Abnormal fluid loss: vomiting; diarrhea; abnormal drainage; excessive use of laxative, enemas, diuretics; blood loss; diaphoresis; burns	• "I'm thirsty all the time." • "I've been vomiting and I have diarrhea—several times a day." • Weight loss: 5 lb (2–3 kg) • Urine is concentrated (specific gravity, 1.035). • Fluid output greater than fluid intake • Neck veins collapsed when lying flat • Decreased skin turgor
	Increased need for fluids: strenuous exercise, extreme heat or dryness, fever (increased metabolic rate)	• Skin is warm to touch, moist, and flushed • Increased temperature, pulse, respirations • Decreased blood pressure

• Practice self-care behaviors to promote fluid, electrolyte, and acid–base balance; maintain adequate intake of fluid and electrolytes; respond appropriately to the body's signals of impending fluid, electrolyte, or acid–base imbalance

When an imbalance exists, the patient will achieve the following:

• Relate relief of symptoms (specify) after implementation of treatment regimen (eg, 1 month after decreasing sodium intake patient reports 4 lb [1.8 kg] weight loss)

IMPLEMENTING

Nursing interventions to prevent or correct fluid, electrolyte, and acid–base imbalances include dietary modification,

modification of fluid intake, medication administration, IV therapy, blood and blood products replacement, and TPN.

Preventing Fluid Imbalances

An adequate fluid intake and a well-balanced, nutritious diet with appropriate adjustments throughout the life cycle are essential to promote fluid balance. Table 45-7 lists the risk factors, related assessments, and specific nursing interventions for fluid volume disturbances. Following are general measures the nurse needs to consider to help prevent fluid imbalances:

• Be familiar with common events in life that lead to fluid imbalances, and observe the patient carefully. Infants are particularly vulnerable to fluid imbalances

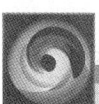

(handwritten note): every 2.2 lbs = 1 liter of H₂O gained or lost.

Table 45-7
Fluid Volume Disturbances

Risk Factors	Assessments	Nursing Interventions
Fluid Volume Deficit (Hypovolemia)		
GI: Vomiting, diarrhea, suction, fistulas	Thirst	Assess for presence or worsening of FVD
Hemorrhage	Weight loss over short period	Administer oral fluids if indicated
Excessive sweating	Weakness, fatigue, anorexia	If patient unable to eat and drink, TPN or tube feedings may be ordered
Skin trauma, burns, draining wounds	Dry mucous membranes	Monitor patient's response to fluid intake, either oral or parenteral
Third-space fluid shifts *burns*	Poor skin and tongue turgor	Be alert for signs of fluid overload
Excessive laxative or diuretic use	Sunken eyes	Provide appropriate skin care
Polyuria from renal disease or diuretics	Flat neck veins	
Hyperglycemia	Urine output <30 mL/hr	
Change in mental status (unable to gain access to fluids, depression, confusion)	Postural hypotension *orthostatic hypotension*	
	Weak, rapid pulse	
	↑Urine specific gravity *Concentration*	
	↑Hematocrit	
	↑BUN	
	↑Serum sodium	
	Altered sensorium	
Fluid Volume Excess (Hypervolemia)		
Compromised regulatory mechanisms: renal failure, CHF, cirrhosis of liver, Cushing's syndrome	Weight gain over short period *5-10 lbs*	Assess for presence or worsening of FVE
GI irrigation with hypotonic fluid	Peripheral edema (may be pitting)	Encourage adherence to sodium-restricted and fluid-restricted diet, if ordered
Excess IV fluids with sodium	Increased BP	Avoid OTC drugs or check with physician or pharmacist about sodium content
Corticosteroid therapy	Shortness of breath	Encourage rest periods
Excessive ingestion of sodium-containing substances in diet or sodium-containing medications	Crackles and wheezes in lungs	Monitor patient's response to diuretics
	Full, bounding pulse	Teach self-monitoring of weight and intake and output
	Neck vein distention	Attentive skin care
	Polyuria if renal function is normal	
	Ascites, pleural effusion	
	Pulmonary edema *if bad enough*	
	↓BUN (due to plasma dilution)	
	↓Hematocrit	
	↓Serum sodium	
	↓Urine specific gravity	

GI, gastrointestinal; BUN, blood urea nitrogen; FVD, fluid volume deficit; TPN, total parenteral nutrition; CHF, congestive heart failure; IV, intravenous; BP, blood pressure; FVE, fluid volume excess; OTC, over-the-counter.

because body water accounts for a greater percentage of their weight, and fluid fluctuations are more common. Loss of fluid because of an illness can cause serious and life-threatening problems in infants.

- Note the patient's present fluid and food intake, and learn what his or her previous eating and drinking patterns have been. Learn whether the patient has been using a fad diet, which may lead to imbalances.
- Note whether the patient experiences excessive thirst or little or no thirst. Thirst is a subjective sensation and an important factor determining water intake

and, eventually, output through the kidneys. Thirst is poorly understood, although both psychological and physiologic factors appear to be involved.

- Be aware of excessive losses of fluids from the body, and attempt to prevent losses when possible. Vomiting, pronounced perspiration, diarrhea, draining wounds, and excessive urinary output, for example, may cause excessive losses.
- Consider ways in which the patient's medical regimen may lead to fluid and electrolyte imbalances. For example, diuretics that stimulate urine formation

may increase the elimination of potassium. If food supplements high in potassium are not included in the diet or if drug therapy is not started, hypokalemia often follows (Table 45-8 describes nursing interventions for specific electrolyte disturbances).

- Learn whether the patient has been "treating" himself or herself in some way that may threaten fluid balance. Common practices that threaten fluid balance include the indiscriminate use of enemas, laxatives, antacids, and over-the-counter drugs to promote urination.
- Consider conditions with destructive effects on the body as threats to fluid balance. Examples include immobilization, trauma, burns, surgical procedures, and exposure to toxic agents.
- Teach patients to observe for fluid imbalances and to report them promptly. Examples include rapid weight gains and losses; swollen fingers, feet, and ankles; puffy eyelids; muscle weakness; change in skin sensations; and scanty or profuse urine production.
- Help patients and their families understand the significance of maintaining fluid balance and preventing imbalances.
- Be aware that normal physiologic changes associated with aging affect elder patients' ability to maintain fluid balance. Dehydration is a common fluid and electrolyte disorder in this population. The accompanying box, Focus on the Older Adult, suggests specific nursing strategies to prevent and correct fluid and electrolyte imbalances.

Developing a Dietary Plan

Simple dietary changes may help to resolve fluid and electrolyte disturbances. After doing a nutritional assessment to identify actual or potential imbalances and food preferences, the nurse can initiate teaching. When developing the nutritional plan, it is important to involve both the patient and the person who prepares the patient's meals. The plan should include foods that help to resolve the fluid or electrolyte imbalance and that are acceptable to the patient. For example, for fluid volume deficit, increase foods with high water content (eg, citrus fruit, melons, celery); for hypokalemia, increase foods with high potassium content (eg, bananas, citrus fruits, apricots, melons, broccoli, potatoes); for hypernatremia, avoid foods high in sodium (eg, processed cheese, lunch meats, canned soups and vegetables, salted snack foods) and eliminate use of table salt.

When given a list of foods, the patient should be able to identify those that can be eaten freely or moderately as well as those that should be avoided. Both the patient and person responsible for the patient's food preparation should be able to describe a 24-hour diet plan compatible with the recommended modifications.

Modifying Fluid Intake

Depending on the nature of the fluid or electrolyte imbalance, a patient's fluids may need to be increased, decreased, or modified in terms of types of fluids ingested. The nurse is responsible for the following:

- Identifying the appropriate fluid modification (with certain illnesses; the physician may order fluid directives (eg, "Restrict fluids to 1000 mL/d")
- Determining whether the patient understands the rationale for the fluid modification, is motivated to follow the modification, and is capable of adhering to the plan (eg, a bedridden patient who needs to increase fluid intake cannot do this independently)
- Developing and implementing a plan of care based on the preceding information. For example, three patients with the same tendency to retain fluids may need different nursing care. One has never learned that the high-sodium beverages she frequently drinks are contributing to her problem; one teaching session may be sufficient to resolve her fluid imbalance. A second patient has a history of poor self-care behaviors. Intelligent and the recipient of much health education in the past, this patient has no need for further teaching. Nursing time is best invested in counseling and exploring why the patient fails to value his health sufficiently to follow the treatment regimen. Until the patient values the proposed fluid modification, compliance will probably be poor. The third patient is a frail older woman with pneumonia and a history of congestive heart failure who depends on the nursing staff for care. Her fluid intake will be determined by the fluids offered her by the nursing staff. This patient's fluid retention may also be affected by diuretic medication, which places her at risk for fluid deficits and potassium imbalances.

Increasing Fluids

An above-average intake of fluids is prescribed for certain patients. The usual order reads, "Force fluids," and indicates the amount of fluid the patient is to have in each 24-hour period. The plan of care should specify the amount of fluid to be ingested in 24 hours (for hospitalized patients, shift totals are helpful [eg, 7 to 3, 1200 mL; 3 to 11, 900 mL; 11 to 7, 300 mL]) and the patient's food preferences. Fluids should be chosen that best provide the calories and electrolytes needed by the patient.

Several techniques are recommended to help the patient take more than average amounts of fluids:

- Explain to the patient in understandable terms the specific goal of taking the daily amount of fluid prescribed. This promotes motivation and is more meaningful than simply telling the patient to increase fluid intake.
- Mutually establish short-term goals with the patient. Examples include a glass of water every hour, a particular beverage by the time a television program is finished, or a pitcher of water by lunch. Most patients try to reach goals that they help to set, even when they do not feel thirsty.
- Plan to offer a proportionately larger amount of fluid during the early hours of the patient's waking day. The patient can usually take fluids relatively easily after having few or no fluids during sleeping hours.

(text continues on page 1300)

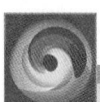

Table 45-8
Electrolyte Disturbances

Risk Factors	Assessments	Nursing Interventions
Hyponatremia		

Loss of sodium, as in:
  Loss of GI fluids
  Use of diuretics
  Adrenal insufficiency
Gains of water, as in:
  Excessive administration of D₅W
Disease states associated with SIADH (a form of hyponatremia)
Pharmacologic agents that may impair water excretion
	Anorexia
	Nausea and vomiting
	Lethargy
	Confusion
	Muscle cramps
	Fingerprinting over sternum
	Muscular twitching
	Seizures
	Coma
	Serum Na below 135 mEq/L
	Urine specific gravity <1.010
		Monitor fluid losses and gains
		Monitor for presence of GI and CNS symptoms
		Monitor serum Na levels
		Check urine specific gravity
		If able to eat, encourage foods and fluids with high sodium content
		Be aware of sodium content of common IV fluids
		Avoid giving large water supplements to patients receiving isotonic tube feedings

Hypernatremia		

Water deprivation
Increased sensible and insensible water loss
Ingestion of large amount of salt
Excessive parenteral administration of sodium-containing solutions
Profuse sweating
Diabetes insipidus
	Thirst
	Elevated body temperature
	Tongue dry and swollen, sticky mucous membranes, _furrowed tongue_
	Severe hypernatremia
	  Disorientation
	  Hallucinations
	  Lethargy when undisturbed
	  Irritable and hyperactive
	  Focal or grand mal seizures
	  Coma
	Serum Na above 145 mEq/L
	Urine specific gravity >1.015
		Monitor fluid losses and gains _ask 24 hr I&O_
		Observe for excessive intake of high sodium foods
		Monitor sodium content of prescriptions and OTC drugs
		Monitor for changes in behavior such as restlessness, lethargy, and disorientation
		Look for excessive thirst and elevated body temperature
		Monitor serum Na levels
		Check urine specific gravity
		Give sufficient water with tube feedings to keep serum Na and BUN at normal limits

Hypokalemia		

Diarrhea _due to ↓K (from Lasics?)_
Vomiting or gastric suction
Potassium-wasting diuretics
Steroid administration and certain antibiotics
Poor intake as in anorexia nervosa, alcoholism, potassium-free parenteral fluids
Polyuria
	Fatigue
	Anorexia, nausea, and vomiting
	Muscle weakness
	Decreased bowel motility
	Cardiac arrhythmias
	Increased sensitivity to digitalis
	Polyuria, nocturia, dilute urine _↑urine output_
	Postural hypotension
	Serum K below 3.5 mEq/L
	ECG changes
	Paresthesias or tender muscles
		Monitor for occurrence of hypokalemia
		Assess digitalized patients at risk for hypokalemia, which potentiates the action of digitalis
		Prevent hypokalemia by:
		  Encouraging extra K intake if possible
		  Educating about abuse of laxatives and diuretics
		Administer oral K supplements if ordered
		Be knowledgeable about danger of IV potassium administration

Hyperkalemia		

Decreased potassium excretion:
  Oliguric renal failure
  Potassium-sparing diuretics
  Hypoaldosteronism
High potassium intake, especially in presence of renal insufficiency
	Vague muscle weakness
	Cardiac arrhythmias
	Paresthesias of face, tongue, feet, and hands
	Flaccid muscle paralysis
		Monitor for hyperkalemia, which is life-threatening
		Prevent hyperkalemia by:
		  Following rules for safe administration of K

(continued)

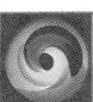

Table 45-8 (Continued)

Risk Factors	Assessments	Nursing Interventions
Shift of potassium out of cells (acidosis, tissue trauma, malignant cell lysis)	GI symptoms such as nausea, intermittent intestinal colic, or diarrhea may occur Serum K above 5.0 mEq/L	Avoiding giving patients with renal insufficiency K-saving diuretics, K supplements, or salt substitutes Cautioning about foods high in potassium content
Hypocalcemia		
Surgical hypoparathyroidism Malabsorption Vitamin D deficiency Acute pancreatitis Excessive administration of citrated blood Alkalotic states	Trousseau's and Chvostek's signs Numbness and tingling of fingers and toes Mental changes Convulsions *tetney* Spasm of laryngeal muscles ECG changes Cramps in muscles of extremities Total serum calcium <8.5 mg/dL	Take seizure precautions when hypocalcemia is severe Monitor condition of airway Take safety precautions if confusion is present Educate people at risk for osteoporosis about need for dietary calcium intake Discuss calcium-losing aspects of nicotine and alcohol use
Hypercalcemia		
Hyperparathyroidism Malignant neoplastic disease Prolonged immobilization Large doses of vitamin D Overuse of calcium supplements Thiazide diuretics	Muscular weakness Tiredness, lethargy Constipation Anorexia, nausea, and vomiting Decreased memory and attention span Polyuria and polydipsia Renal stones Neurotic behavior Cardiac arrest Serum calcium >10.5 mg/dL	Increase mobilization when feasible Encourage sufficient oral intake Discourage excessive consumption of milk products Encourage bulk in the diet Take safety precautions if confusion is present Be alert for signs of digitalis toxicity in hypercalcemic patients Force fluids to prevent formation of renal stones
Hypomagnesemia		

Chronic alcoholism
Intestinal malabsorption
Diarrhea
Nasogastric suction
Drugs
  Thiazide diuretics
  Aminoglycoside antibiotics
  Excessive doses of vitamin D
  Citrate preservative in blood
	Neuromuscular irritability
	  Increased reflexes
	  Coarse tremors
	  Convulsions
	Cardiac manifestations
	  Tachyarrhythmias
	  Increased susceptibility to digitalis toxicity
	Mental changes
	  Disorientation
	  Mood changes
	Serum magnesium <1.3 mEq/L
		Assess for magnesium deficit because it predisposes patient to digitalis toxicity
		Take seizure precautions if necessary
		Monitor condition of airway because laryngeal stridor can occur
		Educate patient if abuse of diuretics or laxatives is a problem
		Educate about intake of foods rich in magnesium

Hypermagnesemia		
Renal failure Adrenal insufficiency Excessive magnesium administration during treatment of eclampsia	Early sign is serum magnesium level of 3 to 5 mEq/L Flushing and sense of skin warmth	If hypermagnesemia is present, be alert for low BP and shallow respirations, lethargy, drowsiness, and coma

(continued)

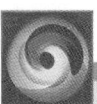

Table 45-8 (Continued)

Risk Factors	Assessments	Nursing Interventions
Hemodialysis with hard water or dialysate high in magnesium content	Hypotension Depressed respirations Drowsiness, hypoactive reflexes, and muscular weakness Cardiac abnormalities	Do not give magnesium-containing medications to patient with renal failure or compromised renal function Be cautious of OTC drugs
Hypophosphatemia		
Glucose administration Refeeding after starvation Hyperalimentation Alcohol withdrawal Diabetic ketoacidosis Respiratory alkalosis	Cardiomyopathy Acute respiratory failure Seizures Decreased tissue oxygenation Joint stiffness Serum phosphate <2.5 mg/dL	Be aware that severely hypophosphatemic patients are at greater risk for infection Administer IV phosphate products cautiously Introduce hyperalimentation cautiously in patients who are malnourished Monitor for diarrhea when taking oral supplements Sudden increase in serum phosphate level can cause hypocalcemia
Hyperphosphatemia		
Renal failure Chemotherapy Large intake of milk Excessive intake of phosphate-containing laxatives (Fleet phosphosoda) Large vitamin D intake Hyperthyroidism	Short-term consequences: Symptoms of tetany, such as tingling of the fingertips and around the mouth, numbness, and muscle spasms Long-term consequences: Precipitation of calcium phosphate in nonosseous sites, such as the kidneys, joints, arteries, skin, or cornea. Serum phosphate above 4.5 mg/dL	Monitor for signs of tetany Be aware that soft tissue calcification can be a long-term complication of chronically elevated serum phosphate levels Instruct patients that use of phosphate-containing laxatives can result in hyperphosphatemia. Avoid foods high in phosphorus content

SIADH, syndrome of inappropriate antidiuretic hormone; ECG, electrocardiographic; CNS, central nervous system.
(Adapted from Metheny, N. [2000]. *Fluid and electrolyte balance* [4th ed.]. Philadelphia: Lippincott-Raven.)

- Try to avoid making it necessary to offer large amounts of fluid before sleep. This helps prevent the patient's rest from being disturbed by a need to urinate.
- Encourage as wide a variety of liquids as possible to make larger intake more interesting and palatable. If patients dislike taking fluids (a common problem with children) or have swallowing difficulties, offering a gelatin dessert (Jell-O), flavored frozen water (Popsicles), water ice, and so forth may meet with more success.
- Keep fluids readily available for the patient. Take care to avoid a situation in which patients are unable to secure their own fluids left with an unfilled water pitcher, an empty glass, a full pitcher out of reach, or a pitcher too heavy to lift.
- Serve fluids at the appropriate temperature. For example, the patient is likely to drink more when some liquids are iced and cold, and coffee and tea when they are hot but not hot enough to cause a burn.
- Use attractive, clean, and easily handled cups and glasses, a practice that helps to encourage the patient's desire to take fluids.
- Have the patient help keep a record of his or her intake when possible. This often serves as a motivating factor to increase fluid intake.
- Provide support, understanding, and encouragement because forcing fluid intake for the person experiencing no thirst can be uncomfortable.

Increasing the fluid intake of patients is among the most common nursing care objective. Often, creativity and considerable patience by the nurse and family are necessary to reach desired goals (see the accompanying Research in Nursing box). Fluids may also be replaced through nasogastric, gastrostomy, or jejunostomy tubes, and any irrigations of these tubes should also be included in the fluid balance summary (see Chap. 41).

Focus on the Older Adult

Nursing Strategies for Ensuring Fluid Balance in Older Adults

Decrease in Total Body Weight

- Ensure that oral intake is at least 1500 mL for 24 hours.
- Assess for signs of dehydration or fluid retention.
- Assess 24-hour intake and output for consistency and balance.
- Teach family to notify physician when persistent diarrhea or vomiting occur.
- Assess skin turgor and mucous membranes.
- Be aware of schedule for diagnostic tests (and associated dietary and fluid restrictions).
- Assess medication history for drugs that have a diuretic action or require additional fluid intake.

Altered Sense of Thirst

- Offer fluids at regular intervals.
- Replace fluids as necessary either orally or IV.
- Investigate individual fluid preferences.
- Provide assistance or assistive devices for encouraging fluid intake.

Loss of Nephrons and Decreased Renal Blood Flow

- Record output accurately.
- Note appearance and specific gravity of urine.
- Check laboratory values for abnormal levels.

Restricting Fluids

Restricting the patient's fluid intake is sometimes necessary. The usual order reads "Restrict fluids" and indicates the amount of fluid the patient is to have in each 24-hour period.

Several techniques are recommended to help patients restrict their intake of fluids:

- Explain to the patient in understandable terms the specific goal of taking the daily amount of fluid prescribed.
- Discuss with the patient the time intervals at which fluids will be served. Usually, it is best to offer fluids between meals because food often helps to relieve some feelings of thirst.
- Mutually establish short-term or interim goals for offering small amounts of fluids at 1- or 2-hour intervals when this seems helpful and when the patient can cooperate.
- Serve ice chips instead of water from time to time. When they melt, the water is about one half of its volume when frozen and helps to quench thirst.

- Use small glasses or cups so that the container appears to contain more fluid than it actually does. Large containers partially full make the amount of fluid seem smaller than it actually is.
- Provide oral hygiene at regular intervals so that the patient's mouth remains clean. Lubricate the lips and mucous membranes as indicated.
- Allow cooperative patients to rinse their mouth with water without swallowing the fluid and exceeding the intake limit.
- Avoid offering patients dry, salty, or sweet foods and fluids, because they tend to increase thirst.
- Avoid offering patients hard candy or gum. Formerly they were thought to relieve thirst by stimulating salivation, as the sugar content increases oral tonicity and temporarily draws fluids to the mouth membranes. After about 15 to 30 minutes, however, the membranes are even drier than before. Sugarless gum may be offered to some patients.
- Divert patients' attention from thirst by involving them in activities to the degree that they can participate.
- Keep fluids not intended for the patient out of sight.
- Have the patient help keep the intake record when possible. This may serve as a motivating factor to limit fluid intake.
- Provide understanding, support, and encouragement because limiting fluid intake is uncomfortable for a thirsty person.

Administering Medications

Patients with fluid, electrolyte, and acid–base imbalances are often prescribed medications as part of the therapeutic regimen. Nurses need to be knowledgeable about the therapeutic effects of mineral–electrolyte preparations and diuretics as well as alert for adverse effects of other medications, such as steroids and hormone replacements.

Mineral–Electrolyte Preparations

Mineral–electrolyte preparations are frequently prescribed to correct electrolyte imbalances. Nursing responsibilities include the following:

- Accurately administering the medications, following manufacturer's guidelines (eg, dilute potassium supplements to disguise the unpleasant taste and decrease gastric irritation; monitor ABGs for increased pH after each 50 to 100 mEq of sodium bicarbonate to avoid overtreatment and metabolic alkalosis)
- Knowing and evaluating the intended therapeutic effect (eg, with magnesium sulfate, look for decreased restlessness and irritability, decreased muscle tremors, and control of convulsions)
- Assessing for adverse effects (eg, with sodium chloride injection, observe for hypernatremia and circulatory overload)

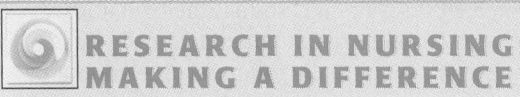

RESEARCH IN NURSING: MAKING A DIFFERENCE

Identifying the Adequacy of Water Intake in an Elderly Population

Monitoring and maintaining fluid balance in patients is a major component of nursing care. The older population is particularly at risk for life-threatening imbalances; however, research is limited that documents the water intake of elderly patients and the factors that are associated with this imbalance. Studies have consistently reported that water intake is inadequate but have been unable to document significant association between environmental factors. Nurses need an awareness of associated causative factors to initiate effective measures to prevent dehydration in this vulnerable population.

Related Research
Gaspar, P. (1999). Water intake of nursing home residents. *Journal of Gerontological Nursing, 25*(4), 23–29.
This study was conducted in several urban nursing homes and included 99 subjects. To participate in the study, the residents were 70 years or older, not receiving tube feedings, and not on a fluid restriction. Researchers collected data regarding water intake during two 24-hour periods and recorded all food and fluid offered and ingested on the Intake/

Situational Modifier Sheet. Examples of situational modifiers included level of assistance, swallowing ability, occurrence of drooling, availability of fluids, and who initiated the ingestion. The mean water intake, including water from food and fluids, was 1968 mL per day, or 76% of the required intake for this age group with a range from 597 mL to 2998 mL. Results indicated that the older residents were more likely to have inadequate intake and fewer ingestion sessions per day. Also, impaired speech, difficulty feeding self, and drooling were associated significantly with inadequate water intake.

Relevance to Nursing Practice
Nurses working in long-term care settings need to focus on development of a protocol for the assessment, prevention, and treatment of inadequate water intake in residents. Scheduling more opportunities for fluid intake is especially important because the thirst sensation is diminished in this at-risk population. Nurses need to target their interventions to problem-solve and address other factors identified in this study, ensuring that fluid needs of long-term care residents are met.

- Knowing the risks associated with administration of IV potassium—*never* give potassium IV push and carefully monitor the infusion rate for IV KCl solutions (maximum rate should be 20 mEq/h). An error can result in a sudden and fatal hyperkalemia (Lilley & Guanci, 1997).
- Assessing for drug interactions (eg, drugs that increase the effects of minerals and electrolytes include acidifying agents, alkalinizing agents, cation exchange resin, iron salts, and potassium salts)
- Teaching patients appropriate self-care behaviors

Diuretics

Diuretics are drugs that increase renal excretion of water, sodium, and other electrolytes. Although helpful in treating patients with fluid volume excess, they increase the risk for dehydration and serious electrolyte deficiencies. Patients need careful monitoring (eg, check urine output and serum K level) and education while on diuretic therapy.

Administering Intravenous Therapy

A relatively common form of therapy for handling fluid disturbances is the use of various solutions infused intravenously. IV therapy is delivered annually to millions of patients in homes and hospitals. The physician is respon-

sible for prescribing the kind and amount of solution to be used. The nurse is responsible for initiating, monitoring, and discontinuing the therapy. The accompanying box lists a selection of standardized nursing interventions related to IV therapy.

As with other therapeutic agents, the nurse should understand the patient's need for IV therapy, the type of solution being used, its desired effect, and untoward reactions that may occur. The contents of selected IV solutions are listed along with comments about their use in Table 45-9.

Equipment

Sterile technique must be observed when puncturing a vein. Disposable infusion tubing and needles are used to help eliminate many possible sources of contamination and to reduce the cost of equipment aftercare.

Equipment varies according to the manufacturer. Nurses are responsible for being familiar with the equipment used in their agency or home settings. Typically, most solutions for infusions are dispensed in 1-L or 500-mL flexible or rigid plastic containers. Plastic bags collapse under atmospheric pressure as the solution enters the patient's vein and do not require air to replace fluid flowing from the container. Small 50- and 100-mL solution bags are available to administer intermittent IV medications (such as antibiotics given by IV piggyback).

Using the Nursing Interventions Classification (NIC)

Intravenous (IV) Therapy

- Maintain strict aseptic technique
- Examine the solution for type, amount, expiration date, character of the solution, and lack of damage to container
- Select and prepare an IV infusion pump, as indicated
- Administer IV fluids at room temperature
- Monitor for IV patency before administration of IV medication
- Maintain occlusive dressing
- Flush intravenous lines between administration of incompatible solutions

(From McClosky, J., & Bulechek, G. [2000]. *Nursing interventions classification [NIC]* [3rd ed.] [p. 409]. St. Louis: C. V. Mosby. A full listing of nursing activities for each nursing intervention can be found in this book.)

Many options are available for the IV tubing that is attached to the solution container. A basic administration set is illustrated in Figure 45-9. A spike or piercing pin is inserted into the container, usually with a twisting motion. The rate of flow is manually controlled by a clamp or constricting device on the tubing. A device called a drip meter or drip chamber connects the solution bottle and tubing and permits the number of drops per minute of solution to be determined.

A variety of needles and catheters are commonly used for IV infusions. IV catheters are plastic tubes that have been mounted on a needle or are threaded through a needle for insertion. Once inserted, the needle is withdrawn and the flexible catheter remains in the vein. The over-the-needle catheter is easy to insert and stable, and its placement is easily detected with radiography. Infiltration is rare with this device. Single- or double-winged infusion needles (butterflies) are short-beveled, thin-walled needles with plastic flaps. They are used in pediatric settings and when short-term therapy is expected. Butterfly or scalp vein needles are not flexible and, thus, more likely to infiltrate. Other equipment necessary to start an IV infusion is listed in Procedure 45-1.

The nurse is the healthcare provider most at risk for a needlestick injury. Many devices are available that minimize the potential for injury and promote safety when connecting, accessing, or disposing of IV equipment. Needleless systems and needle-housing systems in which the needle is recessed and protected are becoming increasingly common. Refer to Chapters 27 and 28 for additional information about these protective measures.

Vascular Access Devices

Multiple vascular access devices are available for delivery of solutions and medications into a vein. The length of time the infusion therapy is needed, the type of medication or product that will be delivered intravenously, and the patient's individualized needs determine which option is used. The nursing care depends on the type of device.

Short or Midline Peripheral Catheters

When infusion therapy will be brief, a short or midline peripheral catheter may be ordered by the physician. The smallest-gauge device is usually selected to minimize trauma to the vein, and a dextrose solution that is 10% or less may be administered by this route. The optimal site for a midline catheter is the basilic vein in the arm, which is larger in diameter, provides for improved hemodilution, and allows short-term or intermittent infusions of irritating drugs.

Central Venous Access Devices

A *central venous access device* (CVAD) is usually introduced into the subclavian or internal jugular vein and passed to the superior vena cava just above the right atrium. CVADs are now an integral component of patient care in acute, ambulatory, and subacute care settings as well as in the home and long-term care facilities. They provide access for a variety of IV fluids, medications, blood products, and nutritional solutions and allow a means for hemodynamic monitoring. All CVADs require radiographic confirmation of position. The patient's diagnosis, the type of care that is required, and other factors such as limited venous access, irritating drugs, patient request, or the need for long-term intermittent infusions determine the type of CVAD used. Types of CVAD include the following:

- Peripherally inserted central catheters (PICCs)
- Nontunneled percutaneous central venous catheters
- Tunneled central venous catheters
- Implanted ports

PICCs are a type of central venous access that can be introduced into a peripheral vein (usually the basilic or cephalic veins), ideally above or below the antecubital space, and advanced as far as the superior vena cava (Fig. 45-10). Both the Intravenous Nurses Society and the National Association of Vascular Access networks agree that complications are less prevalent when the PICC tip rests in the superior vena cava (Hadaway, 1999). Radiographic verification is always required before use. PICCs may have single or dual lumens, and specially trained registered nurses or physicians insert these catheters. PICCs are used extensively in the home for IV therapy and have become an increasingly popular venous access device in acute care settings. Indications for use of PICCs include administration of IV antibiotics for an extended period (2 to 6 weeks), infusion of parenteral nutrition, chemotherapy, continuous narcotic infusions, blood components, other specific medications (eg, vasopressors, anticoagulants), and long-term rehydration (Macklin, 1997). Advantages of this type of IV access include the ability for a PICC to be inserted at the bedside, a decreased risk for pneumothorax because of peripheral insertion, cost-effectiveness, and adequate hemodilution for medications. Nursing responsibilities include sterile dressing changes per agency schedule and protocol, routine heparin or saline flushes to maintain patency, and careful observation for any complications of PICC therapy, such as

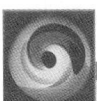

Table 45-9
Selected IV Solutions

Solution	Comments
Isotonic Solutions	
5% dextrose in water (D_5W)	Supplies about 170 cal/L and contains 50 g of glucose
	Should not be used in excessive volumes because it does not contain any sodium, thus the fluid dilutes the amount of sodium in the serum. Brain swelling, or *hyponatremic encephalopathy*, can develop rapidly and cause death unless it is promptly recognized and treated.
0.9% NaCl (normal saline)	Not desirable as routine maintenance solution because it provides only Na^+ and Cl^-, which are provided in excessive amounts.
	May be used to expand temporarily the extracellular compartment if circulatory insufficiency is a problem; also used to treat diabetic ketoacidosis.
Lactated Ringer's solution	A roughly isotonic solution that contains multiple electrolytes in about the same concentrations as found in plasma (note that this solution is lacking in Mg and PO_4)
	Used in the treatment of hypovolemia, burns, and fluid lost as bile or diarrhea
	Useful in treating mild metabolic acidosis
Hypotonic Solutions	
0.33% NaCl (⅓-strength saline)	A hypotonic solution that provides Na^+, Cl^-, and free water Na^+ and Cl^- allows kidneys to select and retain needed amounts
	Free water desirable as aid to kidneys in elimination of solutes
0.45% NaCl (½-strength saline)	A hypotonic solution that provides Na^+, Cl^- and free water
	Often used to treat hypernatremia (because this solution contains a small amount of Na^+, it dilutes the plasma sodium while not allowing it to drop too rapidly)
Hypertonic Solutions	
5% dextrose in 0.45% NaCl	A common hypertonic solution used to treat hypovolemia; used to maintain fluid intake
10% dextrose in water ($D_{10}W$)	Supplies 340 cal/L
	Used for peripheral parenteral nutrition (PPN)
5% dextrose in 0.9% NaCl (normal saline)	Replaces nutrients and electrolytes
	Can temporarily be used to treat hypovolemia if plasma expander is not available

(Data from Metheny, N. M. [2000]. *Fluid and electrolyte balance* [4th ed.]. Philadelphia: Lippincott-Raven; and Young, J. [1998]. A closer look at IV fluids. *Nursing, 28*[10], 52–55.)

phlebitis, cellulitis, infiltration, and infection or sepsis. The accompanying box provides additional information related to nursing care for patients with a PICC.

Nontunneled percutaneous central venous catheters (Fig. 45-11) have a shorter dwell time (3 to 10 days) and are introduced through the skin into the jugular, subclavian, or femoral veins and sutured into place. The catheter tip rests in the superior vena cava. They may be inserted at the bedside or in outpatient settings. This type of central venous catheter has a high risk for complications, particularly infection.

A *tunneled central venous catheter* is intended for long-term use and is placed through a small incision into the jugular or subclavian vein and tunneled in subcutaneous tissue under the skin (usually the midchest area) for 3 to 6 inches to its exit site. It is initially sutured into place, but after 7 to 14 days, the sutures are removed. Subcutaneous tissue attaches to a Dacron polyester cuff around the catheter, helping to stabilize the catheter and minimize the risk for infection.

Another type of long-term CVAD is an *implanted port*. The catheter tip is placed in the subclavian or jugular vein, but the proximal end or port is usually implanted in a subcutaneous pocket of the upper chest wall, and no external parts of the system are visible. Implanted ports placed in the antecubital area of the arm are referred to as peripheral

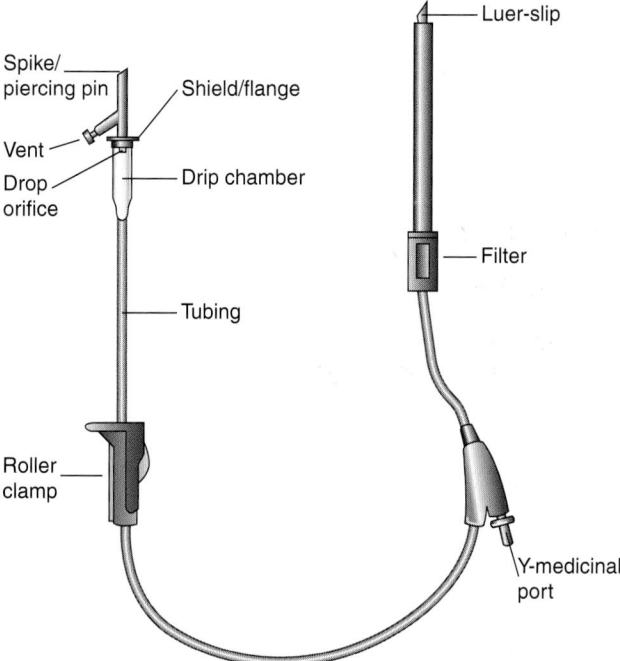

Figure 45-9
Basic administration set for intravenous therapy.

access system ports. Implanted ports were initially used for chemotherapy but are also used for any patient requiring long-term intermittent infusions. A special angled noncoring needle is inserted through the skin and rubber septum and into the port reservoir (Fig. 45-12). Implanted ports require minimal care, but the discomfort of accessing the port may be a disadvantage for some patients.

Nursing responsibilities with central venous catheters include using sterile technique, changing the dressing according to agency policy, carefully assessing for any sign of infection, changing injection caps on the lumens, and flushing with a prescribed solution (usually saline and heparin) to prevent clotting and blockage of the lumen. Many agencies have a policy to discard the injection cap once it is removed (eg, when blood is drawn) and replace it with a sterile cap because contaminated caps have been implicated as a cause of systemic infections. Nurses have many opportunities for health teaching about medical and surgical asepsis and meticulous skin care as they care for patients with central venous access devices.

Site Selection
The suitability of particular veins for IV infusions varies with individual circumstances. Selection should be determined after considering the following factors.

Accessibility of a Vein
- Determine the most desirable accessible vein. The lower cephalic vein, accessory cephalic vein, and basilic vein are good sites for infusion. The superficial veins on the dorsal aspect of the hand can also be used successfully for some people. Figure 45-13 illustrates common infusion sites on the arm and

hand. Either arm may be used for IV therapy. If the patient is right-handed and both arms appear equally usable, usually the left arm is selected to free the right arm for the patient's use.
- Determine accessibility based on the patient's condition. For example, a person with severe burns on both forearms does not have vessels available in these areas or a patient with a history of axillary node dissection should not have venipunctures in the affected arm.
- Do not use the antecubital veins for long-term infusions. They are not a good choice for infusion because flexion of the patient's arm can displace the IV catheter over time. These vessels are satisfactory for blood withdrawal or for small amounts of IV medication administration.
- Do not use veins in the leg, unless other sites are inaccessible, because of the danger of stagnation of peripheral circulation and possible serious complications.
- Do not use veins in surgical areas. For example, infusions in the arm should not be given on the same side as recent extensive breast surgery, because of vascular disturbances in the area, or in an arm with a dialysis access device (eg, fistula or shunt).
- Select scalp veins for infants because of their accessibility and because of relative ease of preventing dislocation of the needle.

Condition of the Vein
- Determine the condition of the vein. Thin-walled and scarred veins, especially in some older patients, make continued infusion a problem. Experience helps the nurse acquire skill in palpating veins to determine their general condition.

Type of Fluid to Be Infused
- Select a vein appropriate for the solution. Hypertonic solutions, those containing irritating medications, those administered at a rapid rate, and those with a high viscosity should be given in a large vein to minimize vessel trauma and to facilitate the rate of flow.
- Advise the patient that some medications administered intravenously in a peripheral vein may cause irritation and pain (eg, potassium chloride and certain antibiotics) and that the patient should tell the nurse if this occurs.

Anticipated Duration of Infusion
- Select a site where restriction in movement is kept to a minimum if this is a consideration.
- Change peripheral venous catheter sites every 48 to 72 hours, if possible, starting with sites as distal as possible and moving in a proximal direction on the alternate arms.

Other
- Select the catheter with the smallest gauge and shortest possible length that will maintain the ordered infusion. Insert it into the largest vein available (Angeles, 1997).
- Select a site that is naturally splinted by bone, such as the back of the hand or the forearm.

(*text continues on page 1309*)

PROCEDURE 45-1

Starting an Intravenous Infusion

Equipment

IV solution
IV infusion set
IV tubing
IV catheter (over-the-needle,
    angiocath) or butterfly needle
Tourniquet
Cleansing swabs (alcohol,
    povidone-iodine)

Towel or disposable pad
Gauze or transparent dressing
    (according to agency policy)
Time tape or label (for IV container)
Site protector or tube-shaped elastic
    netting (optional)

Nonallergenic tape
Electronic infusion device
    (if ordered)
Armboard, if needed
Disposable gloves
IV pole

Action	Rationale
1. Gather all equipment and bring to bedside. Check IV solution and medication additives with physician's order.	Having equipment available saves time and facilitates accomplishment of task. Ensures that patient receives the correct IV solution and medication as ordered by physician.
2. Explain procedure to patient.	Explanation allays client's anxiety.
3. Wash your hands.	Handwashing deters the spread of microorganisms.
4. Prepare IV solution and tubing:	
a. Maintain aseptic technique when opening sterile packages and IV solution	This prevents spread of microorganisms.
b. Clamp tubing, uncap spike, and insert into entry site on bag as manufacturer directs.	This punctures the seal in the IV bag.
c. Squeeze drip chamber and allow it to fill at least half way.	Suction effect causes fluid to move into drip chamber. Also prevents air from moving down the tubing.

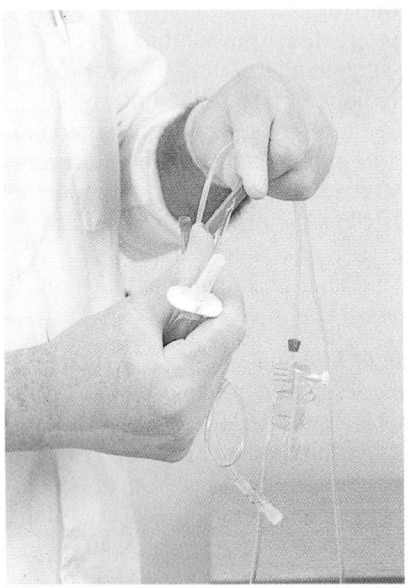

Action 4b: Clamping tubing.

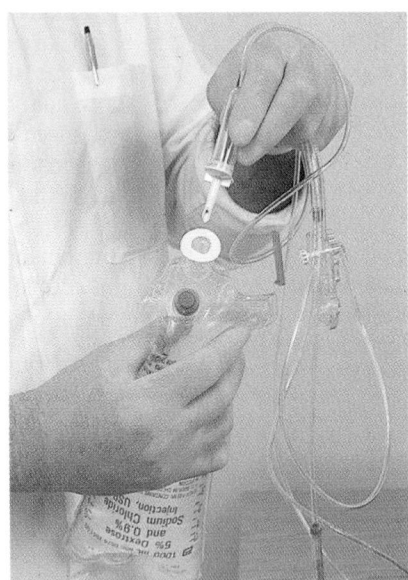

Action 4b: Inserting spike.

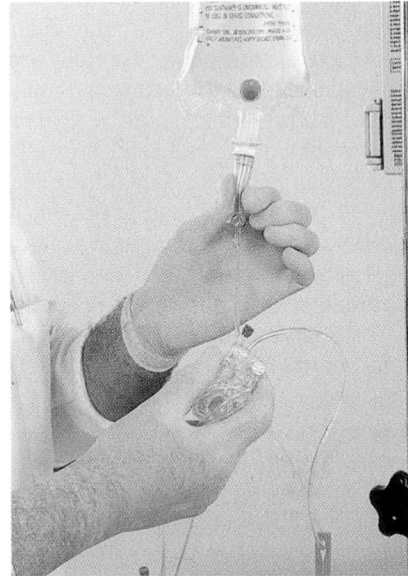

Action 4c: Squeezing drip chamber.

(continued)

Starting an Intravenous Infusion (Continued)

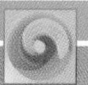

d. Remove cap at end of tubing, release clamp, and allow fluid to move through tubing. Allow fluid to flow until all air bubbles have disappeared. Close clamp and recap end of tubing, maintaining sterility of setup.	This removes air from tubing that can, in larger amounts, act as an air embolus.
e. If an electronic device is to be used, follow manufacturer's instructions for inserting tubing and setting infusion rate.	This ensures correct flow rate and proper use of equipment.
f. Apply label if medication was added to container (pharmacy may have added medication and applied label).	This provides for administration of correct solution with prescribed medication or additive.
g. Place time-tape on container.	This permits immediate evaluation of IV according to schedule.
5. Have the patient in a low Fowler's position in bed. Place protective towel or pad under patient's arm.	The supine position permits either arm to be used and allows for good body alignment. The low Fowler's position is usually most comfortable for the patient.
6. Select an appropriate site and palpate accessible veins.	The selection of an appropriate site decreases discomfort for the patient and possible damage to body tissues.
7. If the site is hairy and agency policy permits, clip a 2-inch area around the intended site of entry.	It is difficult to clean the site of entry in the presence of hair because hair can harbor microorganisms.
8. Apply a tourniquet 5 to 6 inches above the venipuncture site to obstruct venous blood flow and distend the vein. Direct the ends of the tourniquet away from the site of entry. Check to be sure that the radial pulse is still present.	Interrupting the blood flow to the heart causes the vein to distend. Interruption of the arterial flow impedes venous filling. Distended veins are easy to see, palpate, and enter. The end of the tourniquet could contaminate the area of injection if directed toward the site of entry.
9. Ask the patient to open and close his or her fist. Observe and palpate for a suitable vein. Try the following techniques if a vein cannot be felt: a. Release the tourniquet and have the patient lower his or her arm below the level of the heart to fill the veins. Reapply tourniquet and gently tap over the intended vein to help distend it. b. Remove tourniquet and place warm moist compresses over the intended vein for 10 to 15 minutes.	Contraction of the muscles of the forearm forces blood into the veins, thereby distending them further. Lowering the arm below the level of the heart, tapping the vein, and applying warmth help distend veins by filling them with blood.
10. Don clean gloves.	Care must be used when handling any blood or body fluids to prevent transmission of HIV and other blood-borne infections.
11. Cleanse the entry site with an antiseptic solution (alcohol swab) followed by antimicrobial solution (povidone-iodine) according to agency policy. Use a circular motion to move from the center outward for several inches.	Cleansing that begins at the site of entry and moves outward in a circular motion carries organisms away from the site of entry. Organisms on the skin can be introduced into the tissues or the bloodstream with the needle.
12. Use the nondominant hand, placed about 1 inch or 2 inches below entry site, to hold the skin taut against the vein. Avoid touching the prepared site.	Pressure on the vein and surrounding tissues helps prevent movement of the vein as the needle or catheter is being inserted. The needle entry site and catheter must remain free of contamination from unsterile hands.

(continued)

PROCEDURE 45-1

Starting an Intravenous Infusion (Continued)

13. Enter the skin gently with the catheter held by the hub in the dominant hand, bevel side up, at a 10- to 30-degree angle. The catheter may be inserted from directly over the vein or the side of the vein. While following the course of the vein, advance the needle or catheter into the vein. A sensation of "give" can be felt when the needle enters the vein.

This allows needle or catheter to enter the vein with minimal trauma and deters passage of the needle through the vein.

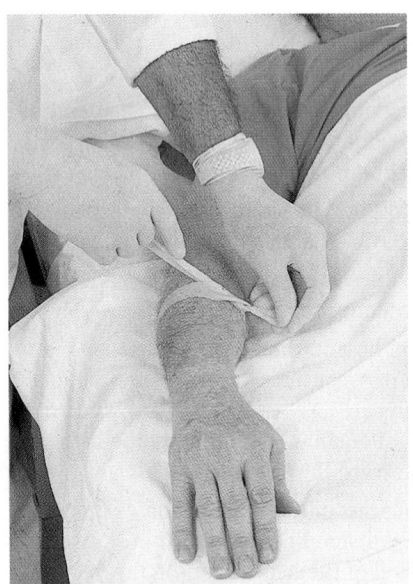

Action 8: Applying tourniquet.

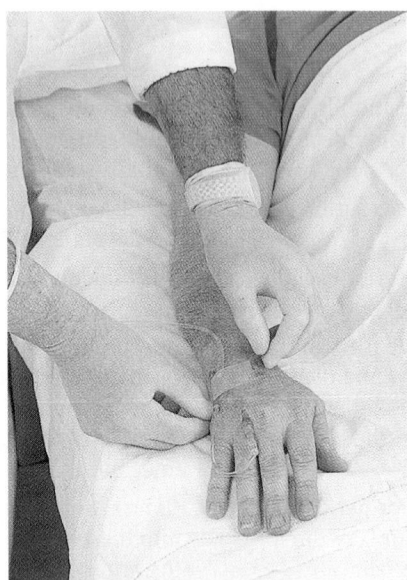

Action 18: Looping and anchoring tubing.

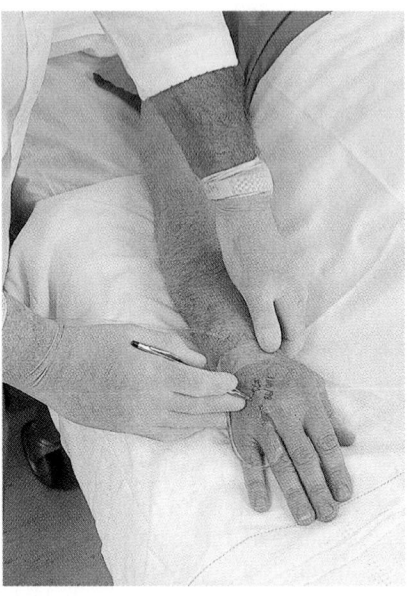

Action 19: Marking pertinent information on tape.
(Photos © B. Proud.)

14. When blood returns through the lumen of the needle or the flashback chamber of the catheter, advance either device ⅛ to ¼ inch farther into the vein. A catheter needs to be advanced until the hub is at the venipuncture site, but the exact technique depends on the type of device used.

The tourniquet causes increased venous pressure resulting in automatic backflow. Having the catheter placed well into the vein helps to prevent dislodgement.

15. Release the tourniquet. Quickly remove protective cap from the IV tubing and attach the tubing to the catheter or needle. Stabilize the catheter or needle with nondominant hand.

Bleeding is minimized and patency of the vein is maintained if the connection is made smoothly between the catheter and tubing.

16. Start the flow of solution promptly by releasing the clamp on the tubing. Examine the tissue around the entry site for signs of infiltration.

Blood clots readily if intravenous flow is not maintained. If catheter accidentally slips out of vein, solution will accumulate and infiltrate into surrounding tissue.

(continued)

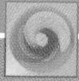

PROCEDURE 45-1

Starting an Intravenous Infusion (Continued)

17. Secure the catheter with narrow nonallergenic tape (½ inch) placed sticky side up under the hub and crossed over the top of the hub.

18. Place sterile dressing over venipuncture site. Agency policy may direct nurse to use gauze dressing or transparent dressing. Apply tape to dressing if necessary. Loop the tubing near the site of entry, and anchor to dressing.

19. Mark the date, time, site and type and size of the catheter used for the infusion on the tape anchoring the tubing.

20. Anchor arm to an armboard for support if necessary or apply a site protector or tube-shaped mesh netting over the insertion site.

21. Adjust the rate of solution flow according to the amount prescribed or follow manufacturer's directions for adjusting flow rate on infusion pump.

22. Remove all equipment and dispose in proper manner. Remove gloves and wash hands.

23. Document the procedure and patient's response. Chart time, site, device used, and solution.

24. Return to check flow rate and observe for infiltration 30 minutes after starting infusion.

The smooth structure of the vein does not offer resistance to the movement of the catheter. The weight of the tubing is sufficient to pull it out of the vein if it is not well anchored. Nonallergenic tape is less likely to tear fragile skin.

Transparent dressing allows easy visualization of site but may place patient at increased risk for infection. Gauze dressing absorbs drainage and may have a decreased infection rate. Discussion continues about effectiveness of types of dressings.

Personnel working with the infusion will know what type of device is being used, the site, and when it was inserted. Protects patient and IV site from infection.

An armboard or site protectors help to prevent change in the position of the catheter in the vein.

The physician prescribes the rate of flow.

Handwashing deters the spread of microorganisms.

This provides accurate documentation and ensures continuity of care.

This documents patient's response to infusion.

Age Considerations

- *Older adults:* Avoid vigorous friction at the insertion site and using too much alcohol. Both can traumatize fragile skin and veins in the elderly (Roth, 1997).
- Experienced nurses may elect to omit use of a tourniquet on individuals with prominent but especially fragile veins. This decreases trauma to the vessel.
- *Children:* Hand insertion sites should not be the first choice for children because nerve endings are very close to the surface of the skin and it is more painful. Research indicates that peripheral IVs should not remain in place longer than 6 days for children or the risk for infection increases. Adults have a 2- to 3-day limit because they are at risk for developing phlebitis, which is rarely seen in children (Frey, 1998).

- Select a site distal to the heart and move proximally, as necessary, to find an appropriate injection site.
- Select a site while moving toward the heart away from a damaged vein.

Starting an Intravenous Infusion

Before the infusion is started, a final check should be made of the solution to ensure that it is clear and contains no particles or precipitates. This check is especially important when substances have been added to the solution because

some additives create precipitates. Commercially available in-line filters help reduce the risk for contamination by filtering the solution immediately before it enters the patient's vein. Filters are routinely recommended for any patient receiving long-term IV therapy, TPN, or IV chemotherapy.

Some adults and young children have a fear of needles, and it may be advisable to use a product that eases the discomfort of venipuncture. One such system (eg, Numby Stuff) uses a mild electrical current to apply local analgesia to the skin. The analgesic takes effect in 10 minutes.

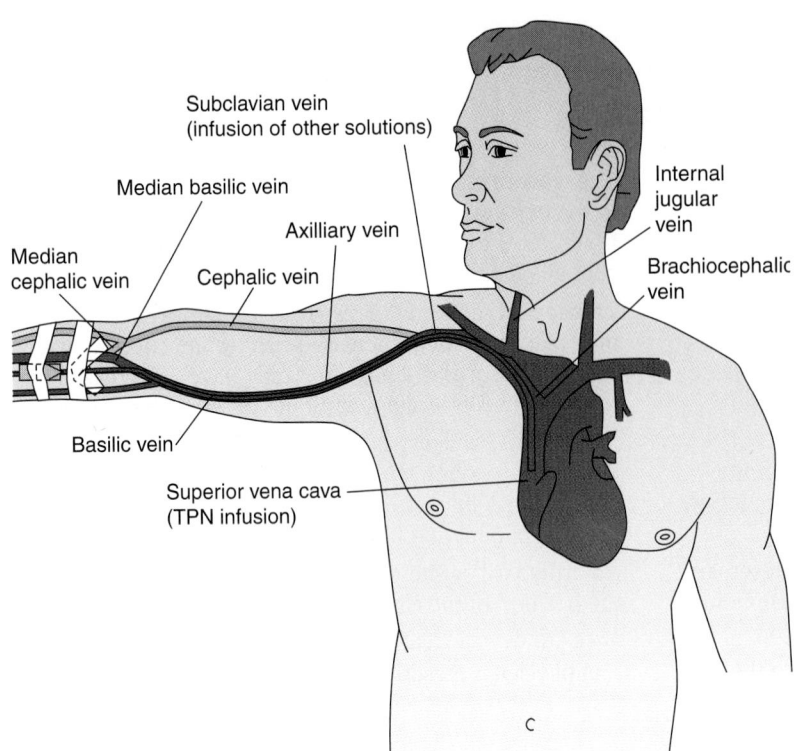

Figure 45-10
Placement of peripherally inserted central catheter (PICC).

Lidocaine (Emla) cream also numbs the skin, but it requires as much as 60 minutes to become effective. A subcutaneous injection of local anesthetic would likely also be rejected by a patient with a fear of needles.

Techniques for starting an IV infusion are described in Procedure 45-1.

Regulating and Monitoring

The nurse is responsible for maintaining the proper flow rate while ensuring the comfort and safety of the patient. The physician prescribes the amount of solution to be infused within a specified period. The rate is then determined on the basis of the amount of solution to be infused over 1 hour. This is called the drip rate.

The drop factor, or drops per milliliter of solution, is determined by the size of the opening in the infusion apparatus. It varies among different products from different companies. Most health agencies use the products of a single company. The most common drop factors are macrodrop systems (10, 15, 20 drops per mL), a microdrip or pediatric setup (60 drops per mL), and a blood administration set (10 drops per mL). Sixty drops per milliliter is used most often when small fluid volumes are important, such as with infants and small children. A buretrol or volume-control device can also be used to reduce the risk for fluid overload or medication overdose. A method for determining flow rate is described in the accompanying Guidelines for Nursing Care.

A time tape can be placed on the container of solution to provide a quick reference for the nurse to monitor the rate at which the solution is entering the patient. The tape gives an hourly indication of where the fluid level should be, based on the nurse's calculation of the drip rate.

Many factors can alter the rate of flow of an IV infusion, such as the height of the container in relation to the patient, the patient's blood pressure, the patient's position, the patency of the IV catheter, infiltration, and any knot or kink in the tubing. The nurse periodically checks the infusion every hour and determines quickly by glancing at the time tape whether the solution is being infused at the proper hourly rate. If it is not, the nurse again regulates the flow. Because the patient's movements, disturbances of the regulation mechanism, or change in the height of the infusion bottle or bed can alter the flow rate, even after it is regulated, the nurse needs to continue to check on the infusion at regular intervals. It has been reported that standard IV administration sets lose up to one half of their initial flow rate during the first hour of infusion because of tubing flexibility; therefore, the rate needs adjustment.

Maintenance of the flow rate is important because of the implications for the patient's fluid balance. Too slow a flow may result in a fluid volume deficit because the input is not balancing fluid lost, or in delaying the restoration of the balance. Infusing IV fluid too rapidly can overtax the body's capacities to adjust to the increase in the water volume or the electrolytes it contains and lead to fluid volume excess. Allowing an infusion to get behind schedule and then increasing the rate to catch up might seriously insult the patient's compensatory mechanisms and jeopardize the patient's well-being.

Electronic infusion control devices limit the amount of fluid to be infused at any one time and, in some healthcare facilities, are used to regulate all IV infusions. They can automatically regulate the flow rate at preset limits and notify the nurse by an alarm system when air is in the tubing, the flow is obstructed, the solution level of the

Guidelines for Nursing Care

Caring for a Client With a PICC

Maintenance

Always check agency policy for specific guidelines.

- Use sterile technique when changing dressings (24 hours after insertion and once a week thereafter). Also change dressing if soiled or loose.
- When accessing port or changing dressing, many agencies require nurse and patient to wear a mask.
- Keep external portion of catheter coiled under dressing.
- Change catheter caps every 3 to 7 days on frequency of access and agency policy. Many agencies have a policy to replace caps once they have been removed (eg, when blood is drawn).
- Flush: Using a 10-mL syringe, flush *open-ended catheter* with heparin solution after intermittent use or every 12 hours if catheter is not currently in use. Using a 10-mL syringe, flush a *close-ended catheter* with saline after each intermittent use or once a week if not in use. After withdrawing a blood specimen, flush PICC with 20 mL of normal saline and follow with a final flush of heparin solution.
- Avoid blood pressure measurement in the involved arm.
- Document:
    Appearance of site
    Length of external part of catheter
    Dates of dressing and cap change
    Flushing frequency and routine
    Any problems

Client Instruction

- Demonstrate procedures, care, and maintenance of PICC catheter as well as potential complications.
- Provide simple, written instructions for patient/caregiver at home. Instruct concerning reasons to notify nurse or doctor.
- Emphasize that there are minimal activity restrictions.
- Instruct to protect insertion site when showering or bathing.
- Advise to wear a Medic-Alert tag if use is long-term.
- Instruct to have repair kit on hand at home.
- Avoid strenuous physical activity that may cause displacement of the catheter.

(From Sansivero, G. [1997]. Maintaining a PICC line: What you should know. *Nursing, 27*[4], 14.)

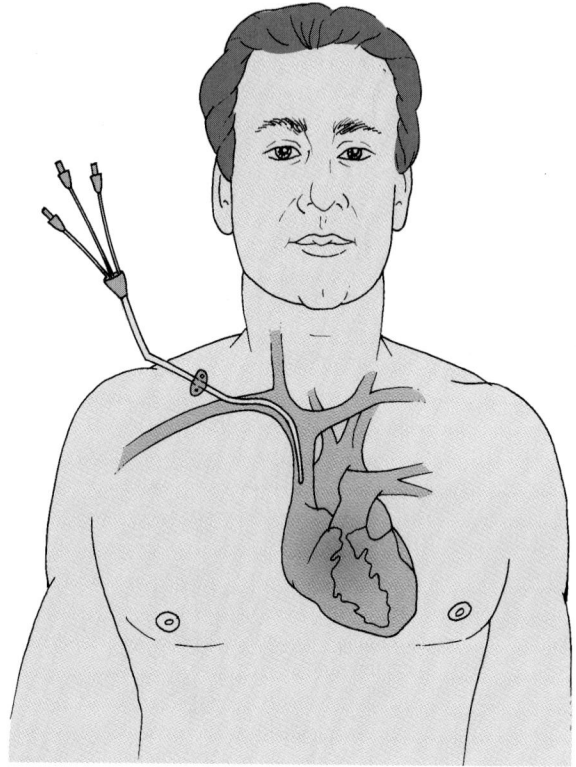

Figure 45-11
Placement of triple-lumen nontunneled percutaneous central venous catheter.

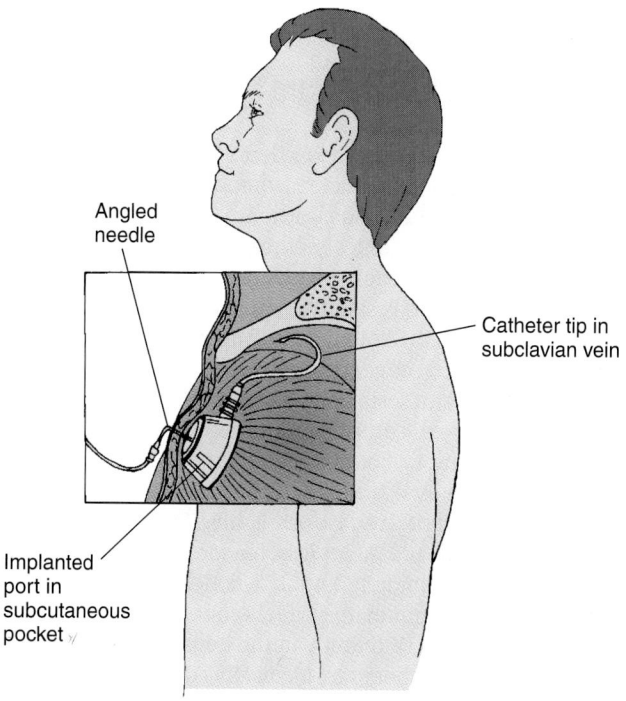

Figure 45-12
Placement of an implanted port with the tip in the subclavian vein. Angled needle is inserted through skin and rubber septum into port.

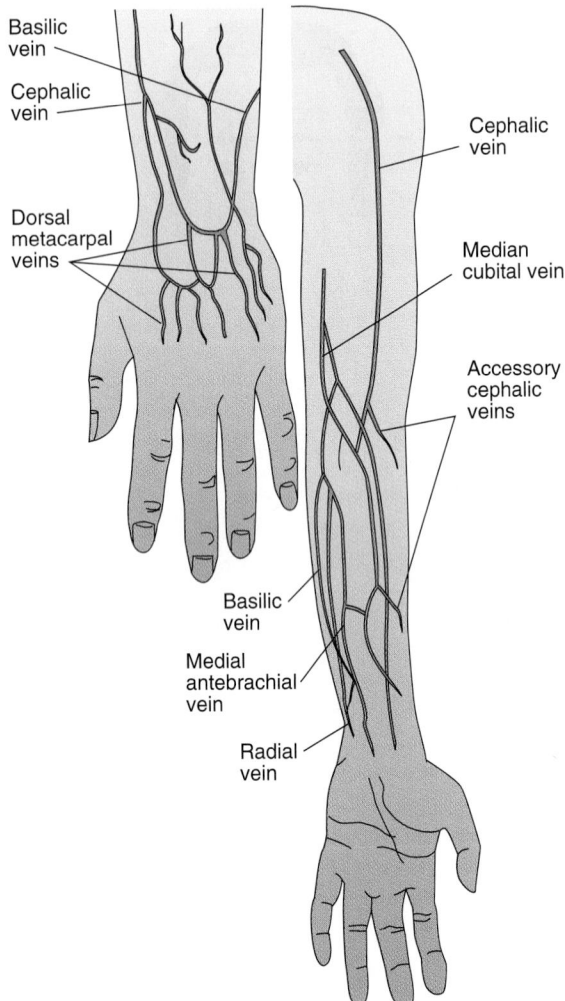

Basilic vein

Cephalic vein

Dorsal metacarpal veins

Cephalic vein

Median cubital vein

Accessory cephalic veins

Basilic vein

Medial antebrachial vein

Radial vein

Figure 45-13
Infusion sites on the ventral and dorsal aspects of the lower arm and hand.

bottle or bag is getting low, or there is increased pressure in the system such as occurs when an IV infiltrates and fluid flows into the tissues. Either a pump or controller may be used, but many healthcare facilities use pumps because their accuracy is greater, they deliver fluids against gravity or resistance, and there are fewer IV-related problems (Skokal, 1997). Pumps totally control the delivery rate by exerting positive pressure based on preset limits when resistance develops. Controllers do not rely on pressure to control solution flow but rather rely on the height of the IV container in relation to the IV site to affect flow rate over time.

Syringe pumps are also available. They deliver small amounts of fluid, 100 mL or less, and are particularly useful with infants and children. Portable models are also available and are useful in ambulatory and home settings. Candidates for infusion pump IV therapy in the home should meet certain criteria. They should be medically stable, have a full- or part-time caregiver, have access to a telephone, and have a refrigerator available for storage of prefilled medication cassettes. Patients can receive insulin infusions, pain medication, antibiotic therapy, cancer chemotherapy, or TPN

Guidelines for Nursing Care
Regulating IV Flow Rate

- Check physician's order for IV solution.
- Check patency of IV line and needle.
- Verify drop factor (number of drops in 1 mL) of the equipment in use.
- Calculate the flow rate:
  a. *Standard formula*

$$gtt/min = \frac{volume\ (mL) \times drop\ factor\ (gtt/mL)}{time\ (in\ minutes)}$$

EXAMPLE—Administer 1000 mL D$_5$W over 10 hours (set delivers 60 gtt/1 mL).

$$gtt/min = \frac{1000\ mL \times 60}{600\ (60\ min \times 10\ h)}$$

$$= \frac{60,000}{600}$$

$$= 100\ gtt/min$$

  b. *Short formula using milliliters per hour*

$$gtt/min = \frac{milliliters\ per\ hour \times drop\ factor\ (gtt/mL)}{time\ (60\ min)}$$

EXAMPLE—Administer 1000 mL D$_5$W over 10 hours (set delivers 60 gtt/1 mL).

Find milliliters per hour by dividing 1000 mL by 10 hours:

$$\frac{1000}{10} = 100\ mL/hr$$

$$gtt/min = \frac{100\ mL \times 60}{60\ min}$$

$$= \frac{6,000}{600}$$

$$= 100\ gtt/min$$

- Count drops per minute in drip chamber (number of gtt/15-sec interval × 4 = gtt/min). Hold watch beside drip chamber.
- Adjust IV clamp as needed and recount drops per minute.
- Mark IV container according to agency policy and manufacturer's recommendations. Use a time tape or label to measure amount to be infused at timed intervals.
- Monitor IV flow rate at frequent intervals. Document patient's response to infusion at prescribed rate.

through portable infusion pumps at home. Procedure 45-3 later in this chapter illustrates an infusion pump.

Changing Solutions and Tubing

If more than one bottle of solution is ordered for the patient, the nurse attaches the additional bottles, using the method determined in the agency. Some IV equipment is designed to simplify the procedure by making it possible to attach additional bottles with a tandem-like arrangement. Because infusions are often continued after the responsibility for a patient's care changes from one nurse to another, it is a good practice to agree on one common method for managing infusions. Without such uniformity, serious errors can occur, or valuable time is lost in checking and rechecking. One method for changing the solution and tubing is presented in Procedure 45-2.

Caring for the Infusion Site

Scrupulous care of the infusion site is needed to help control contamination and to help prevent the introduction of microorganisms into the bloodstream. Catheter contamination can occur from the following sources (Masoorli, 1997b):

- Hands of the caregiver
- Skin bacteria that contaminate the catheter during insertion
- Disconnection of the tubing or injection cap from the catheter hub, allowing bacteria to enter the closed system or multiple-lumen catheters
- Poor insertion technique
- An IV solution that becomes contaminated when solutions are changed, a medication is added, or the solution is allowed to infuse for too long a period

Regular dressing changes and tubing replacements are important means of preventing infection. Gauze and transparent membrane dressings are used most commonly to protect the insertion site. Transparent dressings (eg, Tegaderm or OpSite IV) allow easy inspection of the IV site, permit moisture to evaporate that accumulates under the dressing, and help to secure the catheter. Additional IV securement systems include plastic shields and adhesive anchors. Hard plastic shields that are ventilated and secured with tape are often used in pediatric settings. Adhesive anchors eliminate the need for tape but are more costly and use strong adhesives (Hanchett, 1999). Agency policy generally determines the type of dressing and the intervals for dressing change. The Intravenous Nurses Society recommends an IV dressing change every 48 hours, whereas the Centers for Disease Control and Prevention suggest changing them every 48 to 72 hours. All guidelines state that any dressing that is damp, loosened, or soiled should be changed immediately. Procedures 45-3 and 45-4 explain how to monitor an IV site and how to change an IV dressing.

A controversial aspect of the care of the insertion site concerns irrigation of the needle. An irrigation is sometimes used when the needle begins to clog with blood and the patient does not have other good sites for starting another infusion. *The procedure should not be used unless agency policy recommends it.*

Complications

The patient can be an important source of information regarding the possibility of complications associated with IV therapy. If the patient is uncomfortable, the nurse should check to see that the infusion is entering the vein as intended, that the flow rate is not too rapid, and that the patient's position is satisfactory. Anxiety over the implications of an infusion can also cause discomfort for the patient.

Local complications, such as infiltration, phlebitis, and thrombophlebitis, occur more frequently than systemic complications. Systemic complications (eg, fluid overload, embolus, sepsis), however, are more serious and may be life-threatening. Table 45-10 defines these complications, noting common causes, signs and symptoms, and pertinent nursing considerations.

Capping a Primary Line for Intermittent Use

When a continuous IV is no longer necessary, the primary IV line can be capped and converted to a heparin lock or another needleless system, which provides venous access for intermittent or emergency medications. A heparin or saline lock consists of a plastic tube with a sealed injection port on the end that is connected to an indwelling catheter. Blunt cannula systems and other needleless adapters are also commonly used in healthcare facilities to cap a primary line. Periodic injection with heparin or saline according to agency policy is required to keep the catheter patent. Procedure 45-5 describes this technique.

Discontinuing the Infusion

When the amount of solution the physician has ordered has been infused or when the insertion site shows signs of local complications, the nurse assumes responsibility for discontinuing the infusion. If the catheter is to be removed, the tubing is clamped, and the adhesive strips and sterile dressing are removed. The catheter is withdrawn in line with the vein, and pressure is immediately applied to the site. A dry sterile gauze pad is preferable to an alcohol preparation to apply pressure to the site because alcohol tends to burn and does not stop blood flow from the puncture wound. If the patient can do so, he or she may be asked to hold the pressure for a minute or more.

Nurses also have responsibility for removing a PICC line. Specific protocols must be followed to prevent breaking or fracture of the catheter. Guidelines for removal of a PICC are as follows:

- Wear clean gloves. If a culture of the catheter tip is ordered, sterile gloves are required for removal of the PICC.
- Place the patient in supine position with the arm straight and have the insertion site below heart level (to prevent the risk for an air embolus).
- Remove the dressing carefully and clip and remove any sutures if they are present.
- Remove the catheter slowly. Two methods are suggested:
  - Grasp the catheter close to the insertion site and slowly ease the catheter out, 1 inch at a time,

(*text continues on page 1317*)

PROCEDURE 45-2

Changing IV Solution and Tubing

Equipment

For solution change:
IV solution as ordered
by physician

For tubing change:
Administration set
Sterile gauze
Timing tape or label

Sterile dressings and antiseptic
solutions (according to agency
recommendations)
Disposable gloves

Action	Rationale
1. Gather all equipment and bring to bedside. Check IV solution and medication additives with physician's order.	Having equipment available saves time and facilitates accomplishment of task. Ensures that patient receives the correct IV solution and medication as ordered by physician.
2. Explain procedure to patient.	Explanation allays patient's anxiety.
3. Wash your hands.	Handwashing deters the spread of microorganisms.

To Change IV Solution

Action	Rationale
4. Carefully remove protective cover from new solution container and expose entry site.	This maintains sterility of IV solution.
5. Close clamp on tubing.	Clamping stops the flow of IV fluid during change of solution.
6. Lift container off IV pole and invert it. Quickly remove the spike from the old IV container, being careful not to contaminate it.	This maintains sterility of IV setup.
7. Steady new container and insert spike. Hang on IV pole.	This allows for uninterrupted flow of new solution.
8. Reopen clamp on tubing and adjust flow.	Opening clamp regulates flow rate into drip chamber.
9. Label container according to agency policy. Record on intake and output record and document on chart according to agency policy. Discard used equipment in proper manner. Wash your hands.	This ensures accurate continuation and administration of correct IV solution. Handwashing deters the spread of microorganisms.

To Change IV Tubing and Solution

Action	Rationale
10. Follow actions 1 through 4.	This maintains sterility of IV setup. Once clamp is closed, the bag can be spiked without loss of solution.
11. Open the administration set and close clamp on new tubing. Remove protective covering from infusion spike. Using sterile technique, insert into new container.	
12. Hang IV container on pole and squeeze drip chamber to fill at least halfway.	Gravity and suction effect cause fluid to move into drip chamber.
13. Remove cap at end of tubing, release clamp, and allow fluid to move through tubing until all air bubbles have disappeared. Close clamp and recap end of tubing maintaining sterility of setup.	This removes air from tubing that can, in larger amounts, act as an air embolus.
14. Loosen tape at IV insertion site. Don clean gloves. Carefully remove dressing and tape.	Care must be used when blood contact is possible. This prevents transmission of HIV and other blood-borne infections. Removing dressing provides access to needle hub necessary for tubing change.

(continued)

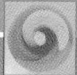

PROCEDURE 45-2

Changing IV Solution and Tubing (Continued)

15. Place sterile gauze square under needle hub.

Gauze absorbs any leakage when tubing is disconnected from needle.

16. Place new IV tubing close to patient's IV site and slightly loosen protective cap.

This facilitates removal of cap and attachment to needle hub.

17. Clamp the old IV tubing. Steady the needle hub with nondominant hand until change is completed. Remove tubing with dominant hand using a twisting motion. A short closed tubing set with an injection port and closure clamp between the needle or angiocath hub and the tubing may also be used.

This stabilizes needle and prevents inadvertently dislodging it. The use of a short closed tubing set reduces risk for blood exposure.

18. Set old tubing aside. While maintaining sterility, carefully remove cap and insert sterile end of tubing into the needle hub. Twist to secure it. Remove soiled gloves.

This maintains sterility of IV setup.

19. Open the clamp.

Opening clamp allows solution to flow to patient.

20. Reapply sterile dressing to site according to agency protocol (see Procedure 45-4).

This deters entry of microorganisms at site.

21. Regulate the IV flow according to physician's order.

This ensures that patient receives IV solution at the prescribed rate.

22. Attach to IV tubing tape or label (see photo) that states date, time, and your initials. Label container and record procedure (see photo) according to agency policy. Discard used equipment in proper manner and wash hands.

This documents IV tubing change. Handwashing deters the spread of microorganisms.

23. Record patient's response to IV infusion.

This ensures accurate documentation of patient's response.

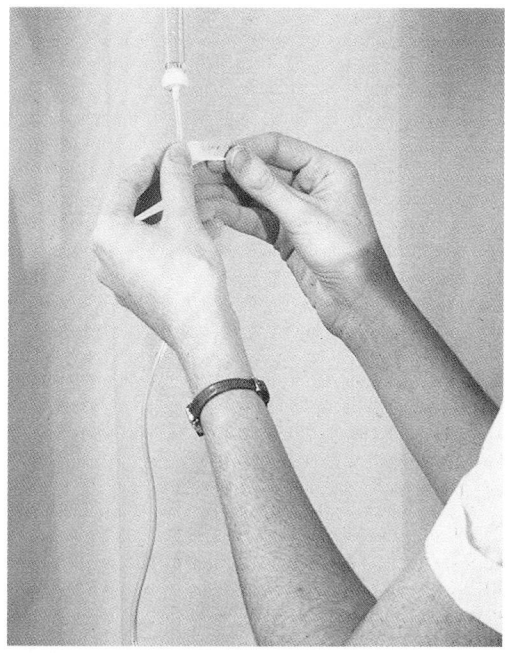

Action 22: Labeling IV tubing.

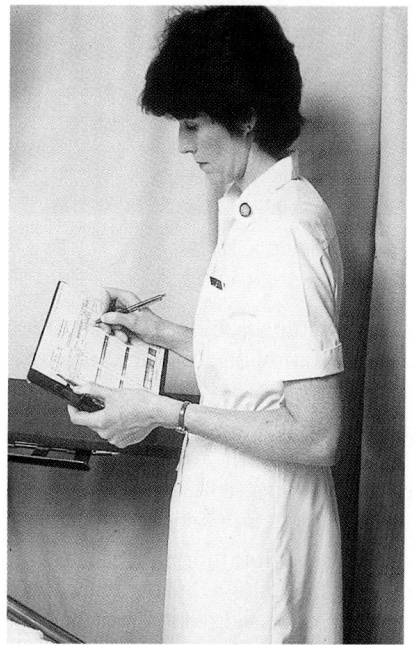

Action 23: Recording patient's response to infusion.

PROCEDURE 45-3

Monitoring an IV Site and Infusion

Action	Rationale
1. Monitor IV infusion several times a shift. More frequent checks may be necessary if medication is being infused:	This promotes safe administration of IV fluids and medication. Too rapid administration of medications can result in the development of speed shock.
a. Check physician's order for IV solution.	This ensures that correct solution is being given at the correct rate and in the proper sequence with the correct medications.
b. Check drip chamber and time drops (see photo) if IV is not regulated by an infusion control device.	This ensures that flow rate is correct.
c. Check tubing for anything that might interfere with flow. Be sure that clamp is in the open position. Observe dressing for leakage of IV solution.	Any kink or pressure on tubing may interfere with flow. Leakage may occur at connection of tubing with hub of needle or catheter and allow for loss of IV solution.

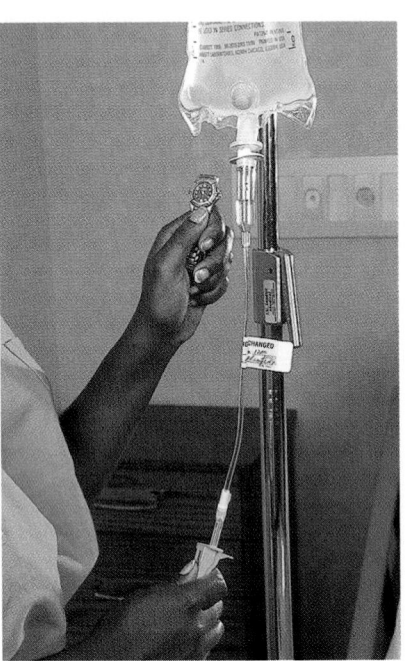

Action 1b: Timing the drops.

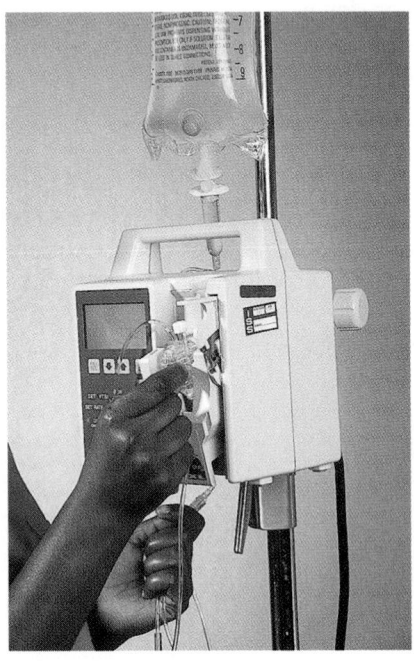

Action 1d: Setting up the pump.

Action	Rationale
d. Observe settings, alarm, and indicator lights on infusion control device if one is being used (see photo).	Observation ensures that infusion control device is functioning and that alarm is in ON position.
2. Inspect site for swelling, pain, coolness, or pallor at site of insertion, which may indicate infiltration of IV. This necessitates removing IV and restarting at another site.	Catheter may become dislodged from vein, and IV solution may flow into subcutaneous tissue.
3. Inspect site (see photo) for redness, swelling, heat, and pain at the IV site, which may indicate phlebitis is present. IV will need to be discontinued and restarted at another site. Notify physician if you suspect that phlebitis may have occurred.	Chemical irritation or mechanical trauma cause injury to the vein and can lead to the development of phlebitis.

(continued)

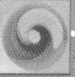

PROCEDURE 45-3

Monitoring an IV Site and Infusion (Continued)

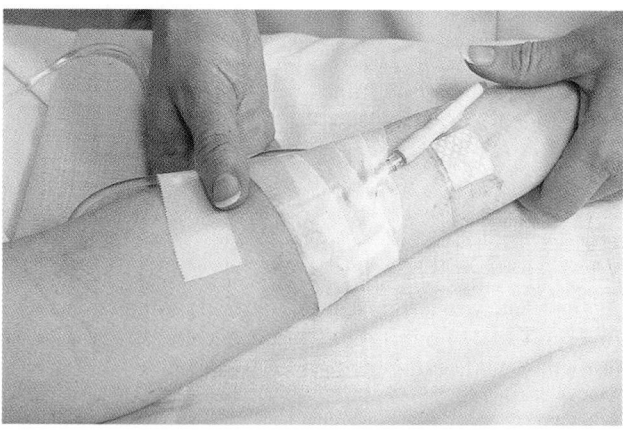

Action 3: Checking inflammation surrounding infusion site. (PHOTOS © B. PROUD.)

4. Check for local or systemic manifestations that indicate an infection is present at the site. IV will be discontinued and physician notified. Be careful not to disconnect IV tubing when putting on patient's hospital gown.

Poor aseptic technique may allow bacteria to enter the needle or catheter insertion site or tubing connection.

5. Be alert for additional complications of IV therapy.
   a. Circulatory overload can result in signs of cardiac failure and pulmonary edema. Monitor intake and output during IV therapy.
   b. Bleeding at the site is most likely to occur when the IV is discontinued.

Infusing too much IV solution results in an increased volume of circulating fluid.

Bleeding may be caused by anticoagulant medication.

6. If possible, instruct patient to call for assistance if any discomfort is noted at site, solution container is nearly empty, or flow has changed in any way.

This facilitates cooperation of patient and safe administration of IV solution.

7. Document IV infusion, any complications of therapy, and patient's reaction to therapy.

This provides accurate documentation and ensures continuity of care.

---

keeping it parallel to the skin. Continue removing 1-inch segments using a smooth and regular motion (Macklin, 2000).
- Slowly remove the catheter with a hand-over-hand technique. Removal may take up to 2 minutes.
- Apply pressure to the site and place a small sterile dressing.
- Measure the catheter and compare it with the length listed in the chart when it was inserted. This ensures that the entire catheter was removed.
- Document the procedure in the chart (Sansivero, 1997; Masoorli, 1998).

After the infusion has been discontinued, record the date and time the infusion was completed, the kind and amount of solution infused, the name of the person discontinuing the infusion, and symptoms of any adverse reactions.

Teaching About Home Infusion

Many patients return to their home from a healthcare facility with IV infusions. Portable infusion pumps and the availability of home care nurses have made this an acceptable alternative. After a patient has been identified as a candidate for home infusion therapy, the nurse needs to begin assessment and education to ensure a successful outcome. The patient and any caregivers must be able to perform necessary skills independently before discharge from the healthcare facility.

(*text continues on page 1320*)

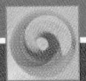

PROCEDURE 45-4

Changing an IV Dressing

Equipment

Sterile gauze (2 × 2 or 4 × 4) or
   transparent occlusive dressing
Povidone-iodine (Betadine) swabs
Adhesive remover (optional)

Alcohol swabs
Tape
Clean gloves

Towel or disposable pad
Masks for nurse and patient
   (optional)

Action	Rationale
Peripheral	
1. Assess patient's need for dressing change.	Agency policy determines interval for dressing change (every 24 to 72 hours). The presence of moisture or a nonadhering dressing increases risk for bacterial contamination at the site.
2. Gather equipment and bring to bedside. Place towel or disposable pad under extremity.	Having equipment available saves time and facilitates the performance of the task.
3. Explain procedure to patient.	Explanation allays patient's anxiety.
4. Wash your hands. Don clean gloves.	Handwashing deters the spread of microorganisms. Gloves prevent transmission of HIV and other blood-borne infections.
5. Carefully remove old dressing but leave tape that anchors IV needle or catheter in place. Discard in proper manner.	This prevents dislodging of IV needle or catheter.
6. Assess IV site for presence of inflammation or infiltration. Discontinue and relocate the IV if noted.	Inflammation or infiltration causes trauma to tissues and necessitates removal of the IV needle or catheter.
7. Loosen tape and gently remove, being careful to steady catheter with one hand. Use adhesive remover if necessary.	Tape stabilizes needle and prevents inadvertently dislodging it.
8. Cleanse the entry site with an alcohol swab using a circular motion moving from the center outward. Allow to dry. Follow with povidone-iodine swab using the same process.	Cleaning in a circular motion while moving outward carries organisms away from the entry site. Use of antiseptic solutions reduces the number of microorganisms on the skin surface.
9. Reapply tape strip to needle or catheter at entry site.	Tape anchors needle or catheter to prevent dislodgement.
10. Apply sterile gauze or transparent polyurethane dressing over entry site. Remove gloves and dispose of properly.	Dressing protects site and deters contamination with microorganisms.
11. Secure IV tubing with additional tape if necessary. Label dressing with date, time of change, and initials. Check that IV flow is accurate and system is patent.	Label documents IV dressing change.
Central Venous Access Device	
12. Follow Actions 1–5.	
13. Remove gloves and wash hands thoroughly. If agency requires, nurse and patient should put on a mask. Open dressing kit using sterile technique.	Unclean hands and improper technique are potential sources for infecting a central venous access device. Most facilities have all sterile dressing supplies gathered in a single unit.
14. Put on sterile gloves.	Maintains surgical asepsis.

(continued)

Changing an IV Dressing (Continued)

15. Using the alcohol swabs, move in a circular fashion from the insertion site outward (1½- to 2-inch area). Allow to dry.

16. Follow alcohol cleansing with povidone-iodine swabs using the same technique. Allow to dry.

The alcohol kills *Staphylococcus aureus* and *epidermis,* which are the most common causes of central line infections (Masoorli, 1997).

Povidone-iodine kills fungi that are responsible for 25% of central line infections (Masoorli, 1997c).

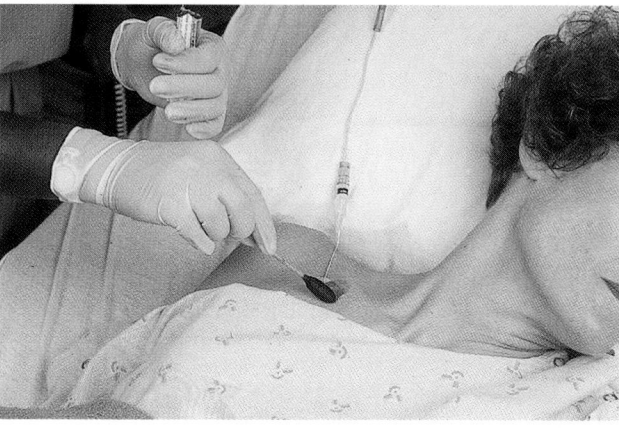

Action 16: Cleaning with povidone-iodine swabs.

17. Reapply sterile dressing or securement device according to agency policy. Secure tubing or lumens to prevent tugging on insertion site.

Prevents contamination of the IV catheter and protects insertion site.

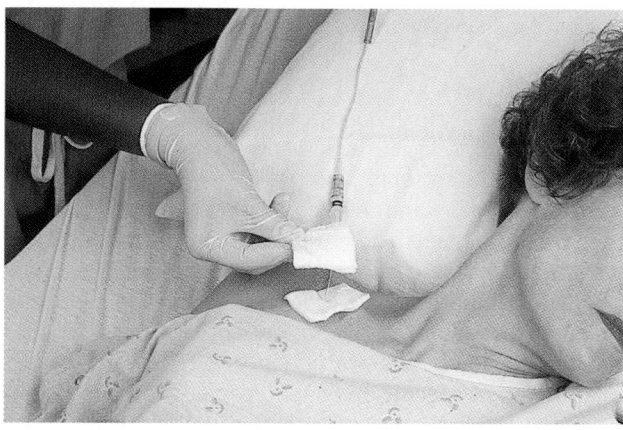

Action 17: Applying a sterile dressing.

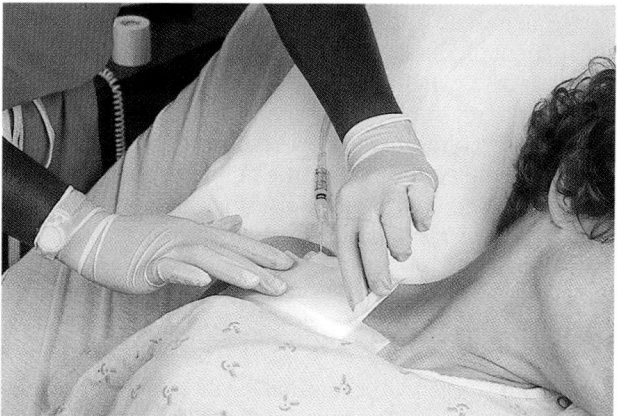

Action 17: Securing the dressing with tape.

18. Note date, time of dressing change, size of catheter, and initials on tape or dressing.

Documents that dressing change occurred.

(continued)

PROCEDURE 45-4

Changing an IV Dressing (Continued)

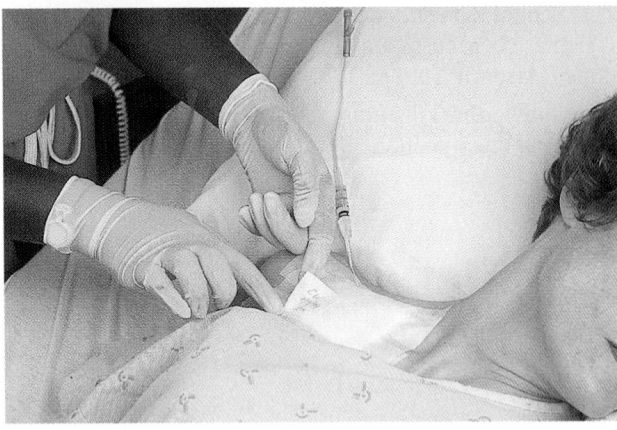

Action 18: Labeling the dressing.

19. Discard equipment properly and wash hands.

20. Record patient's response to dressing change and observation of site.

Handwashing protects against spread of microorganisms.

This provides accurate documentation and ensures continuity of care.

Important points to be addressed include proper handwashing technique, handling all equipment, performing dressing changes, assessing for indications of infection or other complications, and maintaining the supplies necessary to continue home infusion. The nurse ensures that the patient understands the physician's orders and is familiar with when and how to contact the physician or nurses if questions or concerns arise. Before initiating this therapy, the nurse and the infusion service consider the home environment, the ability of the patient or caregiver to maintain the IV infusion, and any other potential considerations necessary to promote a smooth transition.

Replacing Blood and Blood Products

A *blood transfusion* is the infusion of whole blood or a blood component such as plasma, red blood cells, or platelets into the patient's venous circulation. Whole blood is infrequently used because the various components can be easily separated and used for replacement therapy. The person receiving the blood is the *recipient*. The person giving the blood is the *donor*. Steps in administering blood transfusions are described in Procedure 45-6.

Typing and Cross-Matching

Before blood can be given to a patient, it must be determined that the blood of the donor is compatible with the patient. If incompatible, clumping and hemolysis of the recipient's blood cells result, and death can occur. The laboratory examination to determine a person's blood type is called *typing*. The process of determining compatibility between blood specimens is *cross-matching*.

Blood Types

The four main blood groups in the ABO system of blood typing are A, B, AB, and O. Some groups are further broken down into subgroups.

Blood type is an inherited trait and is determined by the type of antigens and antibodies present in the blood. An *antigen* is a substance that causes the formation of antibodies. An *antibody* is a protein substance developed in the body in response to the presence of an antigen that has entered the body. An *agglutinin* is an antibody that causes a clumping of specific antigens. People who have type A blood have an A antigen in their red blood cells; those with type B blood have B antigens in their cells; those in the AB group have both A and B antigens; and people with type O blood have neither A nor B antigens in their red blood cells. People in each blood group have the agglutinins to the red blood cell antigens that they lack. Group A people have the agglutinin for B; group AB people have no agglutinins for A and B, whereas group O people have both A and B agglutinins in their blood serum. If a person with type O blood were transfused with blood from a person *(text continues on page 1325)*

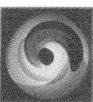

Table 45-10
Complications Associated With Intravenous Infusions

Complication/Cause	Signs and Symptoms	Nursing Considerations

Infiltration: the escape of fluid into the subcutaneous tissue
  Dislodged needle
  Penetrated vessel wall
	Swelling, pallor, coldness, or pain around the infusion site; significant decrease in the flow rate	Check the infusion site several times per shift for symptoms.
		Discontinue the infusion if symptoms occur.
		Restart the infusion at a different site.
		Limit the movement of the extremity with the IV.

Sepsis: microorganisms invade the bloodstream through the catheter insertion site
  Poor insertion technique
  Multilumen catheters
  Long-term catheter insertion
  Frequent dressing changes
	Red and tender insertion site
	Fever, malaise, other vital sign changes
		Assess catheter site daily.
		Notify physician immediately if any signs of infection.
		Follow agency protocol for culture of drainage.
		Use scrupulous aseptic technique when starting an infusion.

Phlebitis: an inflammation of a vein
  Mechanical trauma from needle or catheter
  Chemical trauma from solution
  Septic (due to contamination)
	Local, acute tenderness; redness, warmth, and slight edema of the vein above the insertion site	Discontinue the infusion immediately.
		Apply warm, moist compresses to the affected site.
		Avoid further use of the vein.
		Restart the infusion in another vein.

Thrombus: a blood clot Tissue trauma from needle or catheter	Symptoms similar to phlebitis IV fluid flow may cease if clot obstructs needle	Stop the infusion immediately. Apply warm compresses as ordered by the physician. Restart the IV at another site. *Do not rub or massage the affected area.*
Speed shock: the body's reaction to a substance that is injected into the circulatory system too rapidly Too rapid a rate of fluid infusion into circulation	Pounding headache, fainting, rapid pulse rate, apprehension, chills, back pains, and dyspnea	If symptoms develop, discontinue the infusion immediately. Report symptoms of speed shock to the physician immediately. Monitor vital signs if symptoms develop. Use the proper IV tubing. A microdrip (60 gtt/mL) should be used on all pediatric patients. Carefully monitor the rate of fluid flow. Check the rate frequently for accuracy. A time tape is useful for this purpose.
Fluid overload: the condition caused when too large a volume of fluid infuses into the circulatory system Too large a volume of fluid infused into circulation	Engorged neck veins, increased blood pressure, and difficulty in breathing (dyspnea)	If symptoms develop, slow the rate of infusion. Notify the physician immediately. Monitor vital signs. Carefully monitor the rate of fluid flow. Check the rate frequently for accuracy.
Air embolus: air in the circulatory system Break in the IV system above the heart level allowing air in the circulatory system as a bolus	Respiratory distress Increased heart rate Cyanosis Decreased blood pressure Change in level of consciousness	Pinch off catheter or secure system to prevent entry of air. Place patient on left side in Trendelenburg position. Call for immediate assistance. Monitor vital signs and pulse oximetry.

Capping a Primary Line for Intermittent Use

Equipment

Lock device
Clean gloves
4 × 4 gauze pad

Normal saline or heparin flush
  prepared in a syringe (1–3 mL)
  according to agency policy

Alcohol wipe
Tape
Extension tubing (optional)

Action	Rationale
1. Gather equipment and verify physician's order. Fill lock and extension tubing with normal saline or heparin flush. Recap syringe for use in number 10.	Having equipment available saves time and facilitates the task; ensures that the procedure has been ordered by the physician. Flush maintains patency of lock and tubing.
2. Explain the procedure to the patient.	Explanation allays the patient's anxiety.
3. Wash your hands.	Handwashing deters the spread of microorganisms.
4. Assess the IV site.	Complications such as infiltration or phlebitis necessitate discontinuation of the IV infusion at that site.
5. Clamp off primary line.	Protects patient and nurse from inadvertent blood loss when IV and tubing are disconnected.
6. Don clean gloves.	Gloves protect the nurse from contact with the patient's blood.
7. Place gauze 4 × 4 sponge underneath IV connection hub between IV catheter and tubing.	Gauze absorbs any blood leakage when IV and tubing are disconnected.
8. Stabilize hub of IV catheter with nondominant hand. Use dominant hand to quickly twist and disconnect IV tubing from the catheter, discard it, and attach prefilled lock device or needleless cap to hub without contaminating the tips of the catheter and lock. Extension tubing may also be attached.	This maintains sterility of IV setup.

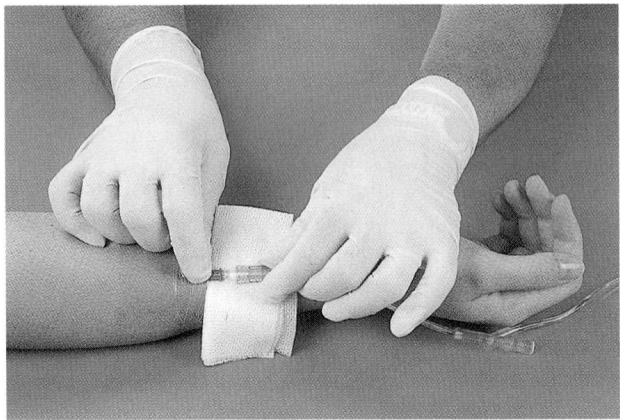

Action 8: Disconnecting tubing from an IV catheter.

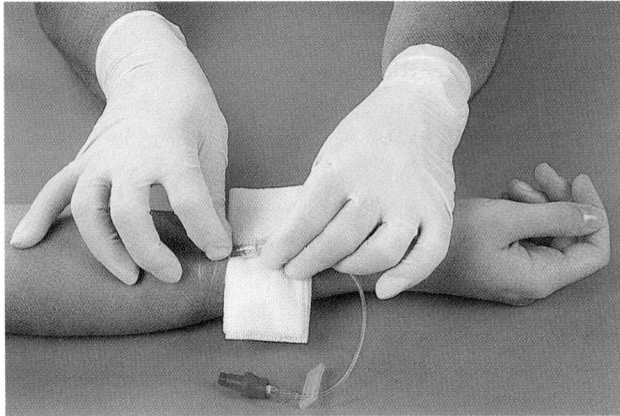

Action 8: Attaching a lock device with extension tubing to the IV catheter hub.

Action	Rationale
9. Cleanse cap with an alcohol wipe.	Cleansing removes surface bacteria at the heparin lock entry site.
10. Insert the syringe with blunt cannula or standard syringe and gently flush catheter with saline or heparin flush as per agency policy. Remove syringe carefully.	This maintains patency of the IV access line. Clinical evidence has demonstrated that a saline flush is as effective as heparin for peripheral IVs and avoids the adverse effects of heparin, is less expensive, and prevents drug incompatibilities.
11. Tape lock or cap securely in place.	Tape secures the lock and IV in place.
12. Chart on IV administration record or medication Kardex per institutional policy.	Accurate documentation is necessary to prevent error.

Administering a Blood Transfusion

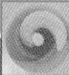

Equipment

Blood product
Blood administration set (tubing
    with in-line filter and Y for saline
    administration)

0.9% Normal saline
IV pole
Intravenous catheter (20 gauge or
    larger)

Disposable gloves
Tape

Action	Rationale
1. Determine whether patient knows reason for transfusion. Ask if the patient has had a transfusion or a transfusion reaction in the past.	This directs teaching before beginning transfusion.
2. Explain procedure to patient. Check for signed consent for transfusion if required by agency. Advise patient to report any chills, itching, rash, or unusual symptoms.	Explanation provides reassurance and facilitates cooperation. Prompt reporting of any reaction to transfusion necessitates stopping immediately.
3. Wash your hands and put on clean gloves.	Handwashing deters the spread of microorganisms. Gloves protect against accidental exposure to the patient's blood.
4. Hang container of 0.9% normal saline with blood administration set to initiate IV infusion and follow administration of blood.	Dextrose may lead to clumping of red blood cells and hemolysis. Filter in blood administration set removes particulate material formed during storage of blood.

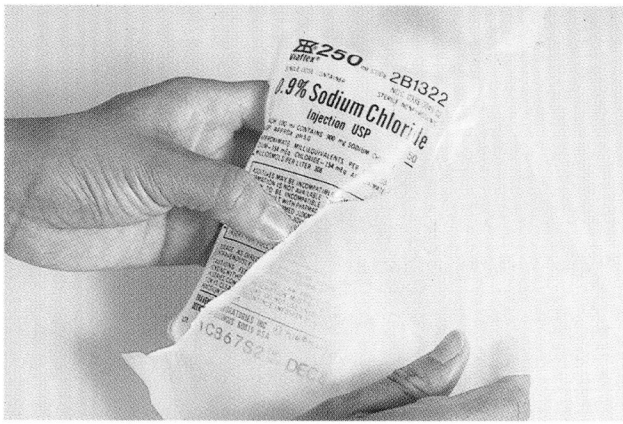

Normal saline container.

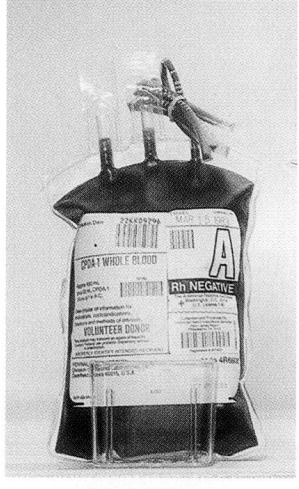

Unit of packed red blood cells.

Action	Rationale
5. Start intravenous with #18 or #19 catheter if not already present (see Procedure 45-1). Keep IV open by starting flow of normal saline.	Large-bore needle or catheter is necessary for infusion of blood products. The lumen must be large enough not to cause damage to red blood cells.
6. Obtain blood product from blood bank according to agency policy.	Blood must be stored in refrigerated unit at carefully controlled temperature (4°C).

7. Complete identification and checks as required by agency:
  a. Identification number
  b. Blood group and type
  c. Expiration date
 	
  d. Patient's name
  e. Inspect blood for clots
	Some agencies require two registered nurses to verify information:
	  Verifies that unit numbers match
	  Verifies that ABO group and Rh type are the same
	  Safe storage of blood is limited to 35 days before red blood cells begin to deteriorate.
	  Never administer blood to a patient without a name band. If clots are present, blood should be returned to blood bank.

(continued)

PROCEDURE 45-6

Administering a Blood Transfusion (Continued)

8. Take baseline set of vital signs before beginning transfusion.

9. Start infusion of the blood product:
   a. Prime in-line filter with blood.
   b. Start administration slowly (no more than 25–50 mL for the first 15 minutes). Stay with the patient for the first 5–15 minutes of transfusion.

   c. Check vital signs at least every 15 minutes for the first half hour after the start of the transfusion and then every half hour or hour after the transfusion depending on agency policy.

Any change in vital signs during the transfusion may indicate a reaction.

Priming is necessary if blood is to flow properly. Transfusion reactions typically occur during this period, and a slow rate will minimize the volume of red blood cells infused. If there have been no adverse effects during this time, the infusion rate is increased.
If complications occur, they can be observed, and the blood can be stopped immediately.

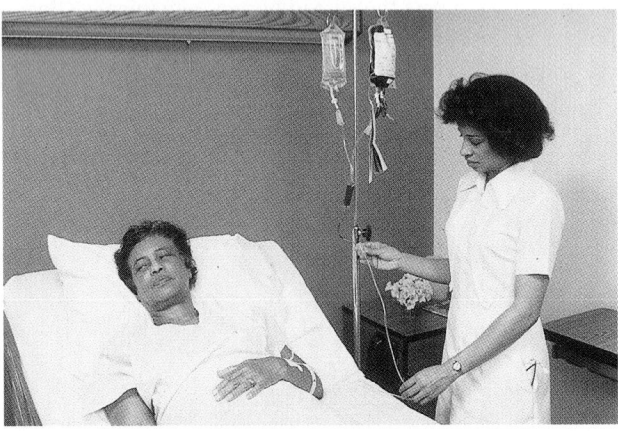

Action 9a: Priming the in-line filter.

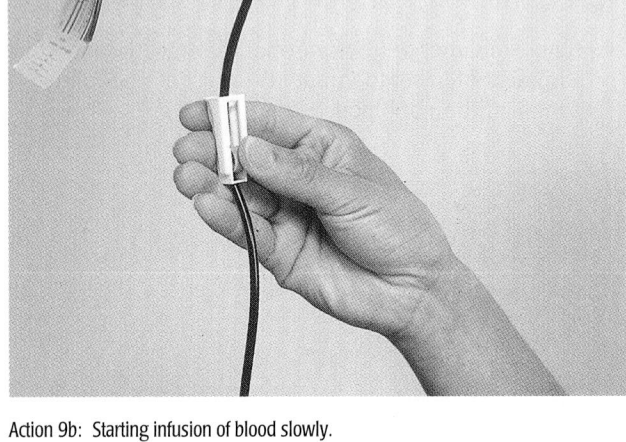

Action 9b: Starting infusion of blood slowly.

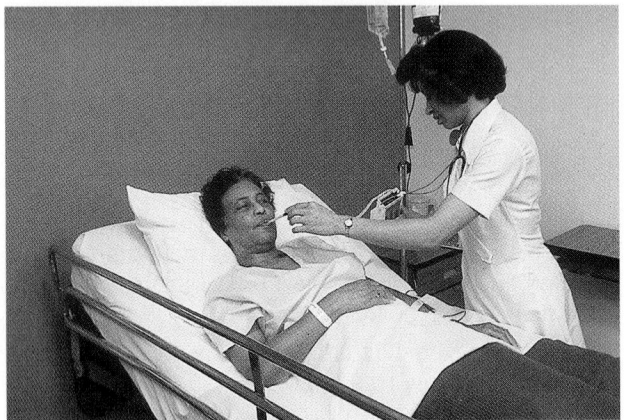

Action 9c: Checking temperature with electronic thermometer.

   d. Observe patient for flushing, dyspnea, itching, hives, or rash.
   e. Use a blood warming device, if indicated, especially with rapid transfusions through a CVP catheter.

These symptoms may be early indication of a transfusion reaction.
Rapid administration of cold blood can result in cardiac arrhythmias.

(*continued*)

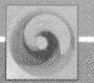

Administering a Blood Transfusion (Continued)

10. Maintain the prescribed flow rate as ordered or as deemed appropriate by the patient's overall condition, keeping in mind the outer limits for safe administration. Assess frequently for transfusion reaction. Stop blood transfusion and allow saline to flow if you suspect a reaction. Notify physician and blood bank.

    Rate must be carefully controlled, and patient's reaction must be monitored on a frequent basis.

11. When transfusion is complete, infuse 0.9% normal saline.

    Saline prevents hemolysis of red blood cells and clears remainder of blood in IV line.

12. Record administration of blood and patient's reaction as ordered by agency. Return blood transfusion bag to blood bank according to agency policy.

    This provides for accurate documentation of patient's response to blood transfusion.

Special Considerations   Electronic infusion devices may be used to maintain prescribed rate but must be specifically designed for use with blood transfusions.

Home Care Administrations   Home care agencies evaluate patients who are candidates for a blood transfusion at home. Home transfusion is not appropriate for patients who are actively bleeding, require more than 4 hours for the transfusion, or recently had a reaction to a blood transfusion. Written consent must be obtained from the patient and the physician. The nurse transports the blood product to the patient's home in a special cooler. The nurse and patient's caregiver check serial number and other identification information together.

---

with either group A or group B blood, there would be destruction of the recipient's red blood cells because his or her anti-A or anti-B agglutinins would react with the A or B antigens in the donor's red blood cells. This example shows why group AB people are often called universal recipients (because people in this blood group have no agglutinins for either A or B antigens) and group O people are often called universal donors (because they have neither A nor B antigens).

Rh Factor

The Rh factor is an inherited antigen in human blood. There are five antigens in the Rh system, but the one designated D is of first concern. A person whose blood contains a D antigen is called Rh positive; an Rh-negative person lacks D. It is important that an Rh-negative person receive blood from another Rh-negative person. If Rh-positive blood is injected into an Rh-negative person, the recipient develops anti-Rh agglutinins. Subsequent transfusion with Rh-positive blood may cause serious reactions with clumping and hemolysis of red blood cells.

Selection of Blood Donors

Blood donors must be selected with care. Not only must the donor's blood be accurately typed, but it is also important to determine that the donor is free from diseases. The

blood will be tested for human immunodeficiency virus (HIV), hepatitis B virus (HBV), and other viruses that can be transmitted to the recipient. Blood donated from people who have allergies or those with a history of a chronic disease, such as tuberculosis, certain types of cancer, and hemophilia, is usually not used. As a further precaution, some blood banks do not accept blood from a donor who has been immunized recently because of a possible allergic reaction to the blood by a recipient.

The donor is examined carefully at the time of donation and receives specific information about eligibility as well as a confidential method to allow or disallow the distribution of the donated blood. Prospective donors are questioned about high-risk behaviors, such as unsafe sex, IV drug abuse, and the presence of any of the signs and symptoms of acquired immunodeficiency syndrome (AIDS). Individuals may give blood only if their blood count, temperature, pulse, respiration, and blood pressure are within normal range. *There is no way that donors may contract HIV or any other disease by giving blood.*

Some patients who know in advance that they will need blood can give their own blood (*autologous transfusion*). Autotransfusion eliminates the danger of transmitting cross-infection from donor to recipient and decreases the risk for complications from mismatched blood but requires advance planning (the blood must be donated 5 weeks before the surgery). This practice is growing in popularity. A patient's own blood can also be salvaged during surgery or collected from tubes and drains to allow for autologous transfusions.

Blood Extracts

Whole blood is rarely used unless blood loss has been massive. With current technology, whole blood can be easily separated into its components, and patients receive only the blood product they need. For example, a patient may need red blood cells but not the blood plasma and its constituents. Red blood cells in concentrated form, called packed red blood cells, may be used in the following situations:

- Patient with anemia suffering with a low red blood cell count
- Patient with cardiovascular failure, with a need to increase blood volume and red blood cells while avoiding cardiovascular overload
- Patient with gastrointestinal bleeding, with a need to maintain adequate hemoglobin levels without increasing blood pressure, which would likely lead to more bleeding

In other situations, only plasma is required, such as when plasma protein or the blood's clotting factor is low. Fresh-frozen plasma is particularly useful in emergencies for immediate restoration of fluid because serum transfusion presents no compatibility problems and time need not be lost seeking donors and matching blood. It is also an excellent blood-volume expander when time is of essence, for example, in a patient who is severely burned and losing plasma rapidly from burn areas. Components of plasma that are used therapeutically include human albumin (used for hypovolemic shock, albuminemia, liver failure); cryoprecipitates (used for bleeding due to hemophilia or disseminated intravascular coagulation); and gamma globulins—the antibody-containing part of plasma (used for gamma globulin deficiencies).

Platelet infusion is indicated for the treatment or prevention of bleeding associated with deficiencies in the number or function of a patient's platelets. The demand for platelets has noticeably risen during the past several decades, and specialized products and preparation methods have been developed to reduce the risk for complications and improve the patient's response to platelet therapy.

Initiating the Transfusion

The procedure for starting a blood transfusion (see Procedure 45-6) is basically the same as for an IV solution. If possible, larger veins should be selected because a catheter no smaller than 20 gauge should be used. This size is necessary because of the viscosity of blood. Vital signs should be taken and recorded just before starting the transfusion. If the patient's temperature is 100°F (37.8°C) or higher, the physician should be notified. Blood that has not been used within 30 minutes after its arrival from the blood bank must be returned, and blood that has been infusing for more than 4 hours must be discontinued to prevent the risk for bacterial contamination.

Transfusion Reactions

When preparing and administering the transfusion, the nurse should take every precaution to prevent the occurrence of a transfusion reaction through scrupulous technique. Table 45-11 describes potential transfusion reactions that can be serious.

Giving Total Parenteral Nutrition

Hypertonic solutions consisting of dextrose, amino acids, and select electrolytes and minerals may be infused using a central vein by TPN. This is frequently performed in cases of malnutrition. This procedure and related nursing responsibilities are described in Chapter 41.

EVALUATING

When evaluating the effectiveness of the plan of care aimed at promoting healthy fluid, electrolyte, and acid–base balance, nurses pay attention to the following parameters:

- Are the patient's drinking and eating patterns supplying the needed fluid and electrolytes? Are food and fluid likes and dislikes interfering with the implementation of the care plan? Is the patient having any difficulties with oral fluids, tube feedings, IV therapy, or TPN?
- Is the patient's urine output about equal to the fluid intake? Does the patient void at least once each shift (except when sleeping)? Do urine characteristics (color, odor, specific gravity) indicate healthy functioning of the kidneys and excretion of fluids?
- Are abnormal sources of fluid loss (vomiting, diarrhea, draining wounds, fistula, and so forth) responding to treatment? Are these fluid losses effectively being replaced by the designated therapy? Are the signs of fluid volume deficit improving?
- Do the patient's weight and record of fluid intake and output indicate fluid balance?
- Are the signs and symptoms that initially manifested the fluid, electrolyte, or acid–base imbalances absent or improved? Has therapy led to any troublesome new signs or symptoms?
- Is the patient now able to practice self-care behaviors to maintain fluid, electrolyte, and acid–base balance? Can the patient describe appropriate responses to potential future problems?

This evaluation should be ongoing as the plan of care is implemented. As the patient achieves the expected outcomes, these should be noted and reinforced. Before nursing care is terminated, the patient and family should be able to independently promote fluid, electrolyte, and acid–base balance.

See the accompanying Applying Learning to Practice: Patient Care Study and Nursing Plan of Care boxes.

(*text continues on page 1329*)

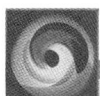

Table 45-11
Transfusion Reactions

Reaction	Signs and Symptoms	Nursing Activity
Allergic reaction: allergy to transfused blood	Hives, itching Anaphylaxis	• Stop transfusion immediately and keep vein open with normal saline. • Notify physician stat. • Administer antihistamine parenterally as necessary.
Febrile reaction: fever develops during infusion	Fever and chills Headache Malaise	• Stop transfusion immediately and keep vein open with normal saline. • Notify physician. • Treat symptoms.
Hemolytic transfusion reaction: incompatibility of blood product	Immediate onset Facial flushing Fever, chills Headache Low back pain Shock	• Stop infusion immediately and keep vein open with normal saline. • Notify physician stat. • Obtain blood samples from site. • Obtain first voided urine. • Treat shock if present. • Send unit, tubing, and filter to lab. • Draw blood sample for serologic testing and send urine specimen to the lab.
Circulatory overload: too much blood administered	Dyspnea Dry cough Pulmonary edema	• Slow or stop infusion. • Monitor vital signs. • Notify physician. • Place in upright position with feet dependent.
Bacterial reaction: bacteria present in blood	Fever Hypertension Dry, flushed skin Abdominal pain	• Stop infusion immediately. • Obtain culture of patient's blood and return blood bag to lab. • Monitor vital signs. • Notify physician. • Administer antibiotics stat.

APPLYING LEARNING TO PRACTICE

Patient Care Study

Gerry Stein is a 22-year-old Jewish man who is a senior in the premed program at a large state university. Although his grades were poor his first year in college, he currently is an honors student and plans to take the MCAT examination in 2 weeks. His overwhelming ambition is to be accepted into a prestigious medical school and to become a psychiatrist. He presents at the campus health clinic with the following assessment findings:

- History of problems with diarrhea since his junior year in high school; self-treatment with kaolin and pectin (Kaopectate) and limiting his food and fluid intake; believes diarrhea is stress related; no medical evaluation to date

- Has had two or three loose bowel movements per day for the past week with urgency and occasional incontinence; believes this is related to anxiety about performance on MCAT and his need for good grades; always thirsty but afraid to drink much; urine output is decreased, and he noted that urine is darker in color and has a stronger odor

Nursing examination: temperature, 99.8°F (37.6°C); pulse, 92 beats/min; respirations, 18 breaths/min; blood pressure, 100/60 mm Hg; skin and mucous membranes are pale and dry; weight is 4 lb less than usual (current weight, 170 lb)

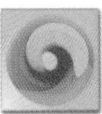

NURSING PLAN OF CARE
for Mr. Stein

Nursing Diagnosis

Fluid Volume Deficit related to prolonged diarrhea and decreased fluid intake secondary to stress management as evidenced by 4-lb weight loss, dry skin and mucous membranes, and report of decreased urine output and concentrated urine

Expected Outcome

By next week's visit, 3/24/01, the patient will:
- Describe two effective means he has used to cope with stress

Nursing Interventions	Rationale	Evaluative Statement
Explore with the patient (1) what he finds most stressing at present, (2) the control he believes he has over these stressors, and (3) the adequacy of his past and present stress management strategies.	Assisting the patient to eliminate and reduce stress where possible and learn to cope better with unavoidable stress (identify and eliminate causative factors) is critical in controlling stress-related diarrhea.	3/24/01 Goal not met. Patient reports little progress in coping with stress. With MCATs 1 week away, he feels more tense than ever before. Reports no time to explore stress management techniques.
Assess for other factors contributing to diarrhea and fluid volume deficit.	Diarrhea may have a functional basis.	*Revision:* Goal is appropriate. Encourage visit to counseling center if not before MCATs then as soon as possible afterward.
Teach relation between stress and bouts of diarrhea.	Stress may result in increased intestinal mobility.	*C. Ryan, RN*
Refer to counseling center on campus for assistance with stress management.	Professional assistance may facilitate identification and management of stressful situation.	

Expected Outcome

By the next week's visit, 3/24/01, the patient will:
- Report that his diarrhea is eliminated or decreased to one or two episodes per day

Nursing Interventions	Rationale	Evaluative Statement
Teach patient to link causative factors with diarrhea and to note anything that brings relief or assists in establishment of usual pattern of defecation.	Being able to make these connections helps patient to assume charge of own condition and to reinforce preventive strategies and successful relief measures.	3/24/01 Goal met. Patient reports diarrhea decreased to one or two episodes per day.
Make sure patient understands diet: chemically and mechanically nonirritating diet high in calories, protein, and minerals; exclude foods such as cocoa, chocolate, alcohol, cold or carbonated beverages, citrus juices; try frequent, small meals.	Some patients fear eating because it stimulates the gastrocolic reflex and may result in a stool. Eating the proper diet actually reduces bowel irritation and decreases peristalsis.	*Recommendation:* Advise patient that it is important to keep appointment with gastroenterologist because relief may only be temporary.
Teach patient proper use of prescribed medications.	Loperamide hydrochloride controls diarrhea, and methylcellulose increases consistency of stool.	*C. Ryan, RN*

(continued)

NURSING PLAN OF CARE (Continued)
for Mr. Stein

Expected Outcome

By next week's visit, 3/24/01, the patient will:
- Demonstrate improved fluid and electrolyte balance as evidenced by (1) maintenance of present weight (170 lb), (2) moist mucous membranes, and (3) report of increased urinary output

Nursing Interventions	Rationale	Evaluative Statement
Explore with patient workable plan for oral replacement of fluids. Have patient note which calorie- and electrolyte- (sodium and potassium) rich fluids he can tolerate. Increase fluid intake to maintain a normal urine specific gravity. Instruct patient to weigh himself every other day and to note changes in the volume or appearance of his urine. Teach patient defining characteristics of electrolyte imbalances associated with prolonged diarrhea—hyponatremia and hypokalemia.	Collaboration with patient to determine acceptable sources of fluid intake may allay his fear that fluid intake causes diarrheal episodes. Increased fluid intake is necessary to compensate for excessive loss in diarrhea and to reestablish fluid balance. All other things being equal, weight loss is a good indicator of continued fluid volume deficit. Other signs include decreased urinary output and high specific gravity. Excreted stool pulls electrolytes with it, especially sodium and potassium.	3/24/01 Goal partially met. Patient reports diarrhea decreased to once or twice a day. Two days there was no diarrhea. Weight, 169 lb. Mucous membranes are moist. Urine output is increased. *C. Ryan, RN*

Sample Documentation

3/24/01, nursing

Mr. Stein returned to the clinic reporting that his diarrhea is decreased to one to two episodes per day and that he has an appointment with a gastroenterologist. He believes that modifying his diet, increasing rest periods, and medications (loperamide hydrochloride to control diarrhea and methylcellulose to increase the consistency of stool) were of great help. He still does not know how he can reduce his stress level. Nursing examination revealed temperature, 98.9°F (37.1°C); pulse, 88 beats/min; respirations, 18 breaths/min; blood pressure, 110/60 mm Hg; weight, 169 lb; skin and mucous membranes less dry than on previous visit. States he has not noted much change in urine output but possibly less concentrated.

C. Ryan, RN

Learning Outcomes

After completing this chapter, the learner should be able to accomplish the following:

1. Define the key terms used in the chapter.

acid	electrolyte
acidosis	filtration
active transport	hydrostatic pressure
alkalosis	ion
anion	oncotic pressure
base	osmolarity
buffer	osmosis
cation	pH
colloid osmotic pressure	solute
diffusion	solvent

2. Describe the location and functions of body fluids and factors that affect variations in fluid compartments.
3. Describe the functions, regulation, sources, and losses of the main electrolytes of the body.
4. Explain the principles of osmosis, diffusion, active transport, and filtration.
5. Describe how thirst and the organs of homeostasis (kidneys, heart and blood vessels, lungs, adrenal glands, pituitary gland, and parathyroid glands) function to maintain fluid homeostasis.
6. Describe the role of buffer systems and respiratory and renal mechanisms in achieving and maintaining acid–base balance.

7. Identify the etiologies, defining characteristics, and treatment modalities for common fluid, electrolyte, and acid–base disturbances.
8. Perform a fluid, electrolyte, and acid–base balance assessment.
9. Describe the role of dietary modification, modification of fluid intake, medication administration, IV therapy, blood replacement, and TPN in resolving fluid, electrolyte, and acid–base imbalances.
10. Plan, implement, and evaluate nursing care related to select nursing diagnoses involving fluid, electrolyte, and acid–base imbalances.

Critical Thinking Exercises

1. Using Table 45-5 earlier in this chapter, which describes parameters to be considered in clinical assessment for fluid, electrolyte, and acid–base balance, assess a healthy individual and then a patient whose fluid and electrolyte or acid–base balance is altered. Compare and contrast your findings.

2. Review the record of a patient who has been receiving IV fluids over a period of 3 or more days. Note the daily intake and output records, pertinent laboratory values, and clinical behaviors, and make a judgment about the patient's fluid, electrolyte, and acid–base balance. What factors complicate a hospitalized patient's usual ability to remain in balance?

Study Questions

1. Plasma, the liquid constituent of blood, is correctly identified as
    a. interstitial fluid
    b. intravascular fluid
    c. intracellular fluid
    d. 40% of total body fluid
2. Potassium functions as
    a. the chief electrolyte of extracellular fluid
    b. the most abundant electrolyte in the body
    c. the major cation of intracellular fluid
    d. the chief extracellular anion
3. The movement of the solvent water from an area of lesser solute concentration to an area of greater solute concentration until equilibrium is established is known as
    a. osmosis
    b. diffusion
    c. active transport
    d. filtration
4. The most accurate indication of fluid balance status is
    a. intake and output
    b. skin turgor
    c. complete blood count
    d. daily weight
5. After assessing the following arterial blood gas values (pH, 7.30; $PaCO_2$, 32; HCO_3^-, 14), the nurse correctly identifies
    a. respiratory acidosis
    b. respiratory alkalosis
    c. metabolic acidosis
    d. metabolic alkalosis
6. Mrs. Podralski, a patient in the hospital, has been encouraged to increase her fluid intake. The nurse can best facilitate this by

    a. explaining the mechanisms involved in transporting fluids to and from intracellular compartments
    b. keeping fluids readily available for the patient
    c. emphasizing the long-term goal of increasing fluids when she returns home
    d. planning to offer most daily fluids in the evening
7. As the nurse prepares to assist the physician with insertion of a nontunneled percutaneous central venous catheter, she is aware that
    a. this catheter usually remains in place for 2 to 3 months
    b. the catheter is introduced by way of the basilic or cephalic veins in the antecubital space
    c. nursing responsibility includes accessing the catheter with an angled needle
    d. a chest radiograph is required to confirm placement
8. The nurse alertly assesses the acid–base balance of a patient because she is aware that the patient will be unable to control effectively his carbonic acid supply. This is most likely a patient with badly damaged
    a. kidneys
    b. lungs
    c. adrenal glands
    d. blood vessels
9. Having the patient focus on breathing more slowly would be the most helpful intervention for the problem of
    a. respiratory acidosis (carbonic acid excess)
    b. respiratory alkalosis (carbonic acid deficit)
    c. metabolic acidosis (base bicarbonate deficit)
    d. metabolic alkalosis (base bicarbonate excess)
10. Which of the following is the most common etiologic factor related to the nursing diagnosis of fluid volume excess?

a. increased need for fluids secondary to fever
b. abnormal fluid loss from vomiting
c. excessive IV infusion
d. decreased fluid intake secondary to depression

11. When the nurse evaluates for complications of IV therapy, which of the following is evidence that the IV has infiltrated?
    a. In the past hour, only 50 mL of fluid has infused.
    b. The insertion site is red, hot, and swollen.
    c. The patient's temperature has risen to 101°F (38.3° C).
    d. The site is pale, cool, swollen, and painful.

12. For a patient at risk for hyperkalemia, it is important to teach the patient to avoid certain foods. Included in the foods to avoid would be
    a. carrots and squash
    b. canned soups and potato chips
    c. bananas, apricots, broccoli
    d. whole grain cereals

13. Your patient has multiple injuries after an automobile accident, and you are to start IV therapy. His right arm is in a cast. Which site would you choose for venipuncture?
    a. left antecubital
    b. dorsal aspect of either foot
    c. right hand
    d. left forearm

14. For patients who are receiving IV therapy, the nurse should
    a. change the IV catheter and entry site daily
    b. change the tubing every 8 hours
    c. increase the rate to catch up if the correct amount has not been infused at the end of the shift
    d. monitor the flow rate at least every hour

15. While a patient is receiving blood, the nurse should evaluate for a transfusion reaction
    a. 15 minutes after the infusion is started
    b. after the blood is all infused
    c. every hour
    d. every 15 minutes

Answers With Rationale

1. The correct response is *b*. Intravascular fluid or plasma is extracellular fluid and composes 5% of total-body fluid.

2. The correct response is *c*. Sodium is the chief electrolyte of extracellular fluid, calcium is the most abundant electrolyte in the body, and chloride is the chief extracellular anion.

3. The correct response is *a*. Gases move around by diffusion. Active transport is a process that requires energy for the movement of substances through a cell membrane from an area of lesser to higher concentration. Filtration is the passage of fluids through a permeable membrane from an area of high pressure to one of low pressure.

4. The correct response is *d*. Intake and output are not always as accurate and may involve a subjective component. Measurement of skin turgor is subjective, and the complete blood count does not necessarily reflect fluid balance.

5. The correct response is *c*. Metabolic acidosis equals low bicarbonate. Acidosis equals low pH. Decreased $PaCO_2$ represents a respiratory compensatory attempt.

6. The correct response is *b*. Explanation of the fluid transportation mechanisms is inappropriate and does not focus on the immediate problem of increasing fluid intake. Meeting short-term goals provides further reinforcement, and additional fluids should be taken earlier in the day.

7. The correct response is *d*. Nontunneled percutaneous central venous catheters remain in place for 3 to 7 days, are introduced into the subclavian or internal jugular vein, and are never accessed through an angled needle (used with an implanted port).

8. The correct response is *b*. The lungs are the primary controller of the body's carbonic acid supply.

9. The correct response is *b*. Breathing more slowly causes accumulation of carbon dioxide to reverse carbonic acid deficit.

10. The correct response is *c*. The other alternatives are related to fluid volume deficit.

11. The correct response is *d*. A decrease in flow rate may indicate an infiltration but is not as significant as the other signs of a pale, cool, swollen, and painful site. Phlebitis is an inflammatory process and results in redness, warmth, and possibly a temperature elevation.

12. The correct response is *c*. Hyperkalemia is an elevated serum potassium level; bananas, apricots, and broccoli are foods high in potassium and should be avoided in this situation.

13. The correct response is *d*. Based on the condition of the right arm, this is not a choice. The left forearm is preferable to the antecubital space of the left arm or the lower extremities.

14. The correct response is *d*. The IV catheter and entry site should be changed every 48 to 72 hours in most circumstances. The tubing is changed according to agency policy but not at the frequency of every 8 hours. Increasing the rate may lead to fluid overload.

15. The correct response is *d*. The nurse should closely observe a patient for the first 15 minutes and then check the patient thereafter every 15 minutes while he or she is receiving the blood transfusion.

Bibliography

Angeles, T. (1997). How to prevent phlebitis. *Nursing, 27*(1), 26.

Barbone, M. (1999). A tip of the cap to intermittent infusions. *Nursing, 29*(2), 53–54.

Bennett, J. (2000). Dehydration: Hazards and benefits. *Geriatric Nursing, 21*(2), 84–87.

Castiglione, V. (2000). Hyperkalemia. *American Journal of Nursing, 100*(1), 55–56.

Dudek, S. (1997). *Nutrition handbook for nursing practice* (3rd ed.). Philadelphia: Lippincott-Raven.

Ellenberger, A. (1999). Starting an IV line. *Nursing, 29*(3), 56–59.

Faries, J. (1998). Easing the discomfort of venipuncture. *Nursing, 28*(3), 30.

Fischbach, F. (1998). *A manual of laboratory tests* (6th ed.). Philadelphia: Lippincott Williams & Wilkins.

Fitzpatrick, L., & Fitzpatrick, T. (1997). Blood transfusion: Keeping your patient safe. *Nursing, 27*(8), 34–41.

Frey, A. (1997). Tips for pediatric IV insertion. *Nursing, 27*(9), 32.

Frey, A. (1998). When a child needs peripheral IV therapy. *Nursing, 28*(4), 18.

Goldy, D. (1998). Circulatory overload secondary to blood transfusion. *American Journal of Nursing, 98*(7), 33.

Hadaway, L. (1999). Choosing the right vascular access device, part I. *Nursing, 29*(2), 18.

Hadaway, L. (1999). Choosing the right vascular access device, part II. *Nursing, 29*(7), 28.

Hadaway, L. (1999). IV infiltration. *Nursing, 29*(9), 41–47.

Hanchett, M. (1999). Choosing an intravenous securement system. *Home Healthcare Nurse, 17*(4), 239–244.

Horne, C., & Derrico, D. (1999). Mastering ABGs: The art of arterial blood measurement. *American Journal of Nursing, 99*(8), 26–32.

Johndrow, P. (1999). Phlebotomy techniques in the home. *Home Healthcare Nurse, 17*(4), 247–251.

Jones, R. (1998). Managing a venous air embolism. *Nursing, 28*(10), 25.

Kokotis, K. (1998). Preventing chemical phlebitis. *Nursing, 28*(11), 41–46.

Larouere, E. (1999). The art of accessing an implanted port. *Nursing, 29*(5), 56–58.

Larouere, E. (1999). Deaccessing an implanted port. *Nursing, 29*(6), 60–61.

Lilley, L., & Guanci, R. (1997). Persistent potassium problems. *American Journal of Nursing, 97*(6), 14.

Macklin, D. (1997). How to manage PICCs. *American Journal of Nursing, 97*(9), 27.

Macklin, D. (2000). Removing PICC. *American Journal of Nursing, 100*(1), 52–54.

Masoorli, S. (1997a). Central lines: Controversies in care. *Nursing, 27*(3), 72.

Masoorli, S. (1997b). How to prevent IV catheter contamination. *Nursing, 27*(6), 60.

Masoorli, S. (1997c). Managing complications of central venous access devices. *Nursing, 27*(8), 59–63.

Masoorli, S. (1998). Removing a PICC: Proceed with caution. *Nursing, 28*(3), 56–57.

Masoorli, S. (1999). Air embolism. *RN, 62*(11), 32–34.

Masoorli, S., Angeles, T., & Barbone, M. (1998). Danger points: How to prevent nerve injuries from venipuncture. *Nursing, 28*(9), 35–39.

McCloskey, J., & Bulechek, J. (1996). *Nursing interventions classification (NIC)* (2nd ed.). St. Louis: C. V. Mosby.

McConnell, E. (1997). Safely administering a blood transfusion. *Nursing, 27*(6), 30.

Metheny, N. (2000). *Fluid and electrolyte balance: Nursing considerations* (4th ed.). Philadelphia: Lippincott-Raven.

Metheny, N. (1997). Focusing on the dangers of D$_5$W. *Nursing, 27*(10), 55–59.

Millam, D., & Hadaway, L. (2000). On the road to successful IV starts. *Nursing, 30*(4), 34–38.

Millam, D., & Hadaway, L. (2000). From container to cannula: Trends in I.V. therapy. *Nursing, 30*(4), 39–48.

North American Nursing Diagnosis Association. (1999). *NANDA nursing diagnoses: Definitions and classification, 1999–2000.* Philadelphia: Author.

Phipps, W., Sands, J., & Marek, J. (1999). *Medical-surgical nursing: Concepts and clinical practice* (6th ed.). St. Louis: C. V. Mosby.

Porth, C. (1998). *Pathophysiology: Concepts of altered health states* (5th ed.). Philadelphia: Lippincott Williams & Wilkins.

Powers, F. (1999). Your elderly patient needs IV therapy: Can you keep her safe? *Nursing, 29*(7), 54–55.

Rice, R. (1995). *Handbook of home health nursing procedures.* St. Louis: C. V. Mosby.

Robb, W. (1998). Searching for an ideal blood substitute. *RN, 61*(8), 26–29.

Roth, D. (1997). Venipuncture tips for geriatric patients. *Nursing, 27*(10), 69.

Sansivero, G. (1997a). Maintaining a PICC line: What you should know. *Nursing, 27*(4), 14.

Sansivero, G. (1997b). How to withdraw a PICC. *Nursing, 27*(12), 25.

Satarawala, R. (2000). Confronting the legal perils of IV therapy. *Nursing, 30*(8), 44–48.

Skokal, W. (1997). Infusion pump update. *RN, 60*(10), 35–38.

Smeltzer, S., & Bare, B. (2000). *Brunner and Suddarth's textbook of medical–surgical nursing* (9th ed.). Philadelphia: Lippincott Williams & Wilkins.

Tasota, F., & Wesmiller, S. (1998). Balancing act: Keeping blood pH in equilibrium. *Nursing, 28*(12), 34–40.

Wise, M. (1997). Understanding needle-free access devices. *Nursing, 27*(7), 32.

Wong, F. (1999). A new approach to ABG interpretation. *American Journal of Nursing, 99*(8), 34–36.

Young, J. (1998). A closer look at IV fluids. *Nursing, 28*(10), 52–55.

Appendix A
Equivalents

METRIC UNITS

The metric system, developed by the French, uses the *meter* as the basic unit. The metric system is a decimal system, with prefixes that designate the various multiples or divisibles of 10. The most commonly used prefixes in medicine are:

Milli, which means one one-thousandth (0.001)
Centi, which means one one-hundredth (0.01)
Kilo, which means one thousand (1000)

These prefixes may be affixed to any of the three basic units of measurements, which are

Meter (m), the unit of length
Gram (g), the unit of weight
Liter (L), the unit of volume

Therefore

1 millimeter (mm) = 0.001 m
1 milligram (mg) = 0.001 g
1 milliliter (mL) = 0.001 L
1 kilometer (km) = 1000 m
1 kilogram (kg) = 1000 g
1 kiloliter (kl) = 1000 L

Length

The meter (a little longer than a yard) and the kilometer (about 0.6 mile) seldom are used in medicine or nursing. The commonly used measure of length is 1 centimeter (cm) = 0.01 m = about 0.4 inch.

Volume

The most frequently used measures of volume are the *liter* and the *milliliter*. Some useful equivalents to know are

1000 milliliters (mL) = 1 liter (L)
1000 cubic centimeters (cc) = 1 liter (L)
1 milliliter (mL) = 1 cc

Weight

The gram designates the weight of 1 mL of distilled water at 4°C. The most frequently used units of weight are

1,000,000 micrograms (mcg or µg) = 1 gram (g)
1000 micrograms (mcg) = 1 milligram (mg)
1000 milligrams (mg) = 1 gram (g)
1000 grams (g) = 1 kilogram (kg) = 2.2 pounds (lb)

Metric Units and Their Household Equivalents

Household measurement is inaccurate, with wide variations in the size of teaspoons, teacups, and so forth. The generally accepted household measures are:

60 drops (gtt) = 1 teaspoon (tsp or t)
3 tsp = 1 tablespoon (Tbs or T)
12 Tbs = 1 teacup
16 Tbs = 1 glass (or a standard measuring cup)

APOTHECARY UNITS

In the apothecary system

The unit of weight is the *grain.*
The unit of volume is the *minim.*

Of the many units of measure in the apothecary system, you should know the following units, abbreviations, and equivalents.

Weight

60 grains (gr) = 1 dram (dr or ʒ)
8 drams (dr or ʒ) = 1 ounce (oz or ℥)

Volume

60 minims (min) = 1 fluid dram (fl dr or fʒ)
8 fl dr = 1 fluid ounce (fl oz or f℥)
16 fl oz = 1 pint (pt)

Table A-1
Metric and Household Equivalents

Metric Unit	Household Unit
5 mL	1 tsp
15 mL	1 Tbs
180 mL	1 full teacup
240 mL	1 full glass

2 pt = 1 quart (qt)
4 qt = 1 gallon (gal)

In the apothecary system, when the symbol or abbreviation is used, the quantity is written in lowercase Roman numerals and follows the symbol. Arabic numerals are used, however, in preference to large Roman numerals. For example

5 gr = gr v
8 dr = ʒ viii

The quantity one-half may be indicated by the symbol ss.

1¹/₂ gr = gr iss
7¹/₂ gr = gr viiss

Other fractional parts are expressed as common fractions, for example, gr ¹/₂₅₀, gr ¹/₁₀.
When pint, quart, and gallon are written, the quantity is expressed in Arabic numerals, (eg, 1¹/₂ pints or 7¹/₂ quarts).

Table A-2
Most Commonly Used Approximate Equivalents*

Metric	Apothecary	Household
0.06 g	gr i	
0.06 mL	min i	1 drop
1.0 g	gr xv	
1.0 mL	min xv	¹/₅ tsp
5 mL	(1 dr) ʒ i	1 tsp
15 mL	(¹/₂ oz) ʒ ss	1 Tbs
30 mL	(1 oz) ʒ i	2 Tbs
500 mL	(16 oz) ʒ 16	1 pt
1000 mL	(32 oz) ʒ 32	1 qt

* There are many discrepancies among these approximate equivalents. For example, 30 mL is the accepted equivalent for 1 oz (29.57 mL is the exact equivalent). Such discrepancies are inevitable when two systems are used whose equivalents are not exact. If the discrepancies are within a 10% margin of error, they usually are acceptable in pharmacology.

Apothecary Units and Their Household Equivalents

1 drop = 1 minim (m i)
1 tsp = 1 dr (ʒ i)
1 Tbs = ¹/₂ oz (ʒ ss)
2 Tbs = 1 oz (ʒ i)
1 teacup = 6 oz (ʒ vi)
1 glass or measuring cup = 8 oz (ʒ viii)
2 measuring cups = 1 pt

Appendix B
Normal Adult Laboratory Values*

COMMONLY USED ABBREVIATIONS

kg = kilogram
g = gram
mg = milligram
µg = microgram
µµg = micromicrogram
ng = nanogram
mEq = milliequivalent
L = liter
dl = 100 milliliters
mL = milliliter

cu mm (mm3) = cubic millimeter
nM = nanomolar
mIU = milliInternational Unit
pg = picogram
mm = millimeter
µ = micron or micrometer
mm Hg = millimeters of mercury
mU = milliunit
µU = microunit
IU = International Unit

* Laboratory values may vary according to techniques used in different laboratories.

Table B-1
Hematologic Values—Reference Ranges

Determination	Conventional	SI
Coagulation Factors		
Factor I (fibrinogen)	0.15–0.35 g/100 mL	4.0–10.0 µmol/L
Factor II (prothrombin)	60%–140%	0.60–1.40 µmol/L
Factor V (accelerator globulin)	60%–140%	0.60–1.40 µmol/L
Factors VII to X (proconvertin to Stuart factor)	70%–130%	0.70–1.30 µmol/L
Factor X (Stuart factor)	60%–140%	0.70–1.30 µmol/L
Factor VIII (antihemophilic globulin)	50%–200%	0.50–2.0 µmol/L
Factor IX (plasma thromboplastic cofactor)	60%–140%	0.60–1.40 µmol/L
Factor XI (plasma thromboplastic antecedent)	60%–140%	0.60–1.40 µmol/L
Factor XII (Hageman factor)	60%–140%	0.60–1.40 µmol/L
Coagulation Screening Tests		
Bleeding time (Simplate)	2–8 min	180–540 sec
Prothrombin time	9.5–12 sec	Less than 2 sec from control
Partial thromboplastin time (activated)	20–45 sec	25–37 sec
Whole blood clot lysis	No clot lysis in 24 hr	0/day

(continued)

Table B-1 (Continued)

Determination	Conventional	SI
Fibrinolytic Studies		
Euglobin lysis	No lysis in 2 hr	0 (in 2 hr)
Thrombin time		Control +5 sec
Complete Blood Count		
Hematocrit	Male: 42%–50%	Male: 0.42–0.52
	Female: 40%–48%	Female: 0.37–0.48
Hemoglobin	Male: 13–18 g/dL	Male: 8.1–11.2 mmol/L
	Female: 12–16 g/dL	Female: 7.4–9.9 mmol/L
Leukocyte count	5000–10,000/mm^3	4.3–10.8×10^9/L
Erythrocyte count	4.2 million–5.9 million/mm^3	4.2–5.9×10^{12}/L
Mean corpuscular volume (MCV)	80–94 μm^3	80–94 fl
Mean corpuscular hemoglobin (MCH)	27–32 pg	1.7–2.0 fmol
Mean corpuscular hemoglobin concentration (MCHC)	33%–38%	19–22.8 mmol/L
Erythrocyte sedimentation rate (Zeta Centrifuge)	41%–54%	Male: 1–13 mm/h
		Female: 1–20 mm/h
Erythrocyte Enzymes		
Glucose-6-phosphate dehydrogenase	5–15 U/g Hb	5–15 U/g
Pyruvate kinase	13–17 U/g Hb	13–17 U/g
Ferritin (serum)	Females: 5–100 ng/mL	
	Males: 10–270 ng/mL	
Folic acid, RIA	4–16 ng/mL	
Haptoglobin	50–250 mg/dL	1.0 g–3.0 g/L
Hemoglobin Studies		
Electrophoresis for A$_2$ hemoglobin	1.5%–3.5%	0.015–0.035
Hemoglobin, met- and sulf-	0	0
Serum hemoglobin	2–3 mg/100 mL	1.2–1.9 μmol/L
Lupus erythematosus (LE) preparation		
Heparin as anticoagulant	0	0
Defibrinated blood	0	0
Muramidase	Serum, 3–7 μg/mL	3–7 mg/L
	Urine, 0–2 μg/mL	0–2 mg/L
Osmotic fragility of erythrocyte	Increased if hemolysis occurs in over 0.5% NaCl; decreased if hemolysis is incomplete in 0.3% NaCl	
Peroxide hemolysis	Less than 10%	< 0.10
Platelet count	100,000–400,000/mm^3	150–350×10^9/L
Platelet Function Tests		
Clot retraction	50%–100%/2 hr	0.50–1.00/2 hr
Platelet aggregation	Full response to ADP, epinephrine and collagen	1.0
Platelet factor 3	33–57 sec	33–57 sec
Reticulocyte count	0.5%–1.5% red cells	0.005–0.15
Vitamin B$_{12}$	90–280 pg/mL (borderline: 70–90)	66–207 pmol/L (borderline: 52–66)

Table B-2
Blood, Plasma or Serum Values—Reference Ranges

Determination	Conventional	SI
Acetoacetate plus acetone	0.3–2.0 mg/dL	3–20 mg/L
Aldolase	1.3–8.2 mU/mL	12–75 nmol sec^{-1}/L
Alpha amino nitrogen	3.0–5.5 mg/100 mL	2.1–3.9 mmol/L
Ammonia	80–110 µg/100 mL	47–65 µmol/L
Ascorbic acid	0.4–1.5 mg/100 mL	23–85 µmol/L
Bilirubin (van den Bergh test)	1 minute: 0.4 mg/100 mL	Up to 7 µmol/L
	Direct: 0.1–0.2 mg/dL	Up to 17 µmol/L
	Total: 1.0 mg/100 mL	
	Indirect: 0.1–1.0 mg/dL	
Blood volume	8.5%–9.0% of body weight in kg	80–85 mL/kg
	Toxic level: 17 mEq/L	
Bromsulphalein (BSP)	Less than 5% retention 45 min after 5 mg/kg IV	< 0.05 L
Calcium	8.5–10.5 mg/100 mL	2.1–2.5 mmol/L
Carbon dioxide content	24 mEq–32 mEq/L	24–30 mmol/L
Carcinoembryonic antigen (CEA)	0.25 mg/mL	0–2.5 µg/L
Carotenoids	0.8–4.0 µg/mL	1.5–7.4 µmol/L
Ceruloplasmin	27–37 mg/100 mL	1.8–2.4 µmol/L
Chloride	95–105 mEq/L	100–106 mmol/L
Cholesterol	< 200 mg/dL	
Cholinesterase (pseudocholinesterase)	0.5 pH U or more/hr	0.5 arb unit or more
	0.7 pH U or more/hr for packed cells	
Copper	Total: 100–200 µg/100 mL	16–31 µmol/L
Creatine phosphokinase (CPK)	Female: 50–250 mU/mL	0.08–0.58 µmol sec^{-1}/L
	Male: 50–325 mU/mL	
Creatinine	0.7–1.4 mg/100 mL	60–130 µmol/L
Ethanol	0.3%–0.4%, marked intoxication;	65–87 mmol/L
	0.4%–0.5%, alcoholic stupor;	87–109 mmol/L
	0.5% or over, alcoholic coma	> 109 mmol/L
Glucose	Fasting: 60–110 mg/100 mL	3.9–5.6 mmol/L
Iron	65–170 µg/100 mL (higher in males)	9.0–26.9 µmol/L
Iron-binding capacity	250–410 µg/100 mL	44.8–73.4 µmol/L
Lactic acid	0.6–1.8 mEq/L	0.6–1.8 mmol/L
Lactic dehydrogenase isoenzymes	100–225 mU/mL	1.00–2.00 µmol sec^{-1}/L
Lead	50 µg/100 mL or less	Up to 2.4 µmol/L
Lipase	2 U/mL or less	Up to 2 arb units
Lipids, total	400–1000 mg/dL	3.10–5.69 mmol/L
Magnesium	0.33–2.4 mEq/L	0.8–1.3 mmol/L
5′ Nucleotidase	0.3–3.2 Bodansky U	30–290 nmol sec^{-1}/L
Osmolality	280–300 mOsm/kg water	285–295 mmol/kg
Oxygen saturation (arterial)	95%–100%	0.96–1.00 L
P$_{CO_2}$	35–45 mm Hg	4.7–6.0 kPg
pH	7.35–7.45	Same
P$_{O_2}$	95–100 mm Hg (dependent on age while breathing room air)	10.0–13.3 kPa
	Above 500 mm Hg while on 100% O_2	
Phenylalanine	0–2 mg/100 mL	0–120 µmol/L

(*continued*)

Table B-2 (Continued)

Determination	Conventional	SI
Phosphorus (inorganic)	3.0–4.5 mg/100 mL	1.0–1.5 mmol/L
Potassium	3.8–5.0 mEq/L	3.5–5.0 mmol/L
Primidone (Mysoline)	Therapeutic level, 4–12 µg/mL	18–55 µmol/L
Protein, total	6.0–8.0 g/100 mL	60–84 g/L
Albumin	3.5–5.0 g/100 mL	33–50 g/L
Globulin	1.5–3.0 g/100 mL	23–35 g/L
Electrophoresis	% of total protein	% of total protein
Albumin	3.3–5.0 g/dL	0.52–0.68
Globulin		
Alpha$_1$	0.2–0.4 g/dL	0.042–0.072
Alpha$_2$	0.6–1.0 g/dL	0.068–0.12
Beta	0.6–1.2 g/dL	0.093–0.15
Gamma	0.7–1.5 g/dL	0.13–0.23
	0.3–0.7 mg/dL	0–0.11 mmol/L
Sodium	135–145 mEq/L	135–145 mmol/L
Sulfate	0.5–1.5 mg/100 mL	0.05–1.2 mmol/L
Transaminase (SGOT) (aspartate aminotransferase)	7–40 U/mL	0.08–0.32 µmol sec^{-1}/L
Urea nitrogen (BUN)	10–20 mg/100 mL	2.9–8.9 mmol/L
Uric acid	2.5–8.0 mg/100 mL	0.13–0.42 mmol/L
Vitamin A	50–220 µg/dL	0.5–2.1 µmol/L

Table B-3
Urine Values—Reference Ranges

Determination	Conventional	SI
Acetone plus acetoacetate (quantitative)	0	0 mg/L
Alpha amino nitrogen	64–199 mg/day; not over 1.5% of total nitrogen	4.6–14.2 mmol/day
Amylase	35–260 U/mL	24–76 arb units
Calcium	150 mg/day or less	3.8 mmol/day or less
Catecholamines	Epinephrine, 10%–40%	< 55 nmol/day
	Norepinephrine, 60%–90%	< 590 nmol/day
Copper	20–70 µg/day	0–1.6 µmol/day
Coproporphyrin	50–300 µg/day	80–380 nmol/day
Creatine	0–200 mg/24 hr	< 0.75 mmol/day
Cystine or cysteine	0	0
Follicle-stimulating hormone		
Follicular phase	5–20 IU/day	Same
Midcycle	15–60 IU/day	
Luteal phase	5–15 IU/day	
Menopausal	50–100 IU/day	
Men	5–25 IU/day	

(continued)

Table B-3 (Continued)

Determination	Conventional			SI		
Hemoglobin and myoglobin	0					
5-Hydroxyindole acetic acid	2–9 mg/day (women lower than men)			10–45 µmol/day		
Phenolsulfonphthalein (PSP)	At least 25% excreted by 15 min; 40% by 30 min; 60% by 120 min			0.25 L		
Phosphorus (inorganic)	Varies with intake; average 1 g/day			32 mmol/day		
Porphobilinogen	0			0		
Protein, quantitative	< 150 mg/24 hr			< 0.15 g/day		
Steroids						
17-Ketosteroids (per day)	Age (yr)	Male (mg)	Female (mg)	Male (µmol/day)	Female (µmol/day)	
	10	1–4	1–4	3–14	3–14	
	20	6–21	4–16	21–73	14–56	
	30	8–26	4–14	28–90	14–49	
	50	5–18	3–9	17–62	10–31	
	70	2–10	1–7	7–35	3–24	
17-Hydroxysteroids	3–8 mg/day (women lower than men)			8–22 µmol/day as hydrocortisone		
Sugar						
Quantitative glucose	0			0 mmol/L		
Identification of reducing substances						
Fructose	0			0 mmol/L		
Pentose	0			0 mmol/L		
Titratable acidity	20–40 mEq/day			20–40 mmol/day		
Urobilinogen	< 0.25 mg/dL			To 1.0 arb unit		
Uroporphyrin	Up to 50 µg in 24 hr			0 nmol/day		
Vanilmandelic acid (VMA)	0.7–6.8 mg/24 hr			Up to 45 µmol/day		

Table B-4
Cerebrospinal Fluid Values—Reference Ranges

Determination	Conventional	SI
Bilirubin	0	0 µmol/L
Chloride	100–130 mEq/L	
Albumin	15.5–32.0 mg/dL	0.295 g/L 6 2 SD (0.11–0.48)
IgG	0–6.6 mg/dL	0.043 g/L 6 2 SD (0–0.086)
Glucose	50–75 mg/100 mL (30%–50% less than blood)	2.8–4.2 mmol/L
Pressure (initial)	70–180 mm H_2O	70–80 arb units
Protein		
Lumbar	15–45 mg/100 mL	0.15–0.45 g/L
Cisternal	15–25 mg/100 mL	0.15–0.25 g/L
Ventricular	5–15 mg/100 mL	0.05–0.15 g/L

Table B-5
Special Endocrine Tests—Reference Ranges

Steroid Hormones

Aldosterone	Excretion: 5–19 µg/24 hr	14–53 nmol/day
Fasting, at rest, 210 mEq sodium diet	Supine: 48 ± 29 pg/mL	133 ± 80 pmol/L
	Upright: (2h) 65 ± 23 pg/mL	180 ± 64 pmol/L
Fasting, at rest, 110 mEq sodium diet	Supine: 107 ± 45 pg/mL	279 ± 125 pmol/L
	Upright: (2h) 239 ± 123 pg/mL	663 ± 341 pmol/L
Fasting, at rest, 10 mEq sodium diet	Supine: 175 ± 75 pg/mL	485 ± 208 pmol/L
	Upright: (2h) 532 ± 228 pg/mL	1476 ± 632 pmol/L

Steroid Hormones

Cortisol		
Fasting	8 AM: 5–25 µg/100 mL	0.14–0.69 µmol/L
At rest	8 PM: below 10 µg/100 mL	0–0.28 µmol/L
20 U ACTH	4-hour ACTH test: 30–45 µg/100 mL	0.83–1.24 µmol/L
Dexamethasone at midnight	Overnight suppression test: below 5 µg/100 mL	< 0.14 nmol/L
	Excretion: 20–70 µg/24 hr	55–193 nmol/day
11-Deoxycortisol	Responsive: over 7.5 µg/100 mL (after metrapone)	> 0.22 µmol/L
Testosterone	Adult male: 300–1100 ng/100 mL	10.4–38.1 nmol/L
	Adolescent male: over 100 ng/100 mL	> 3.5 nmol/L
	Females: 25–90 ng/100 mL	0.87–3.12 nmol/L
Unbound testosterone	Adult male: 3.06–24.0 ng/100 mL	106–832 pmol/L
	Adult female: 0.09–1.28 ng/100 mL	3.1–44.4 pmol/L

Polypeptide Hormones

Adrenocorticotrophin (ACTH)	15–70 pg/mL	3.3–15.4 pmol/L
Calcitonin	Undetectable in normals	0
	> 100 pg/mL in medullary carcinoma	> 29.3 pmol/L
Growth hormone		
Fasting, at rest	Below 5 ng/mL	< 233 pmol/L
After exercise	Children: over 10 ng/mL	> 465 pmol/L
	Male: below 5 ng/mL	< 233 pmol/L
	Female: up to 30 ng/mL	0–1395 pmol/L
After glucose	Male: below 5 ng/mL	< 233 pmol/L
	Female: below 10 mg/mL	0–465 pmol/L
Insulin		
Fasting	6–26 µU/mL	43–187 pmol/L
During hypoglycemia	Below 20 µU/mL	< 144 pmol/L
After glucose	Up to 150 µU/mL	0–1078 pmol/L
Luteinizing hormone	Male: 6–18 mU/mL	6–18 U/L
Preovulatory or postovulatory	Female: 5–22 mU/mL	5–22 U/L
Midcycle peak	30–250 mU/mL	30–250 U/L
Parathyroid hormone	< 10 µl equiv/mL	< 10 mL equiv/L
Prolactin	2–15 ng/mL	0.08–6.0 nmol/L
Renin activity		
Normal diet	Supine: 1.1 ± 0.8 ng/mL/hr	0.9 ± 0.6 nmol/L/hr
	Upright: 1.9 ± 1.7 ng/mL/hr	1.5 ± 1.3 nmol/L/hr

(continued)

Table B-5 (Continued)

Low-sodium diet	Supine: 2.7 ± 1.8 ng/mL/hr	2.1 ± 1.4 nmol/L/hr
	Upright: 6.6 ± 2.5 ng/mL/hr	5.1 ± 1.9 nmol/L/hr
High-sodium diet	Diuretics: 10.0 ± 3.7 ng/mL/hr	7.7 ± 2.9 nmol/L/hr

Thyroid Hormones

Thyroid-stimulating hormone (TSH)	0.5–3.5 µU/mL	0.5–3.5 mU/L
Thyroxine-binding globulin capacity	15–25 µg T_4/100 mL	193–322 mU/L
Total triiodothyronine by radioimmunoassay (T_3)	70–190 ng/100 mL	1.08–2.92 nmol/L
Total thyroxine (T_4) by RIA	4–12 µg/100 mL	52–154 nmol/L
T_3 resin uptake	25%–35%	0.25–0.35
Free thyroxine index (FT_4I)	1–4 ng/100 mL	12.8–51.2 pmol/L

Glossary

A

Abduction: lateral movement of the body part away from the midline of the body

Absorption: process by which drugs are transferred from the site of entry into the body to the bloodstream

Accommodation: (1) ability to adjust the eye to see at various distances; (2) process by which intellectual acts are changed to handle increasingly complex information

Accreditation: process by which an educational program is evaluated and then recognized as having met certain predetermined standards of education

Acid: substance containing a hydrogen ion that can be liberated or released

Acidosis: condition characterized by a proportionate excess of hydrogen ions in the extracellular fluid, in which the pH falls below 7.35

Acquired immunodeficiency syndrome (AIDS): fatal condition in which the body's immune system is rendered ineffective as a result of infection by the retrovirus HIV

Active exercise: joint movement activated by the person

Active euthanasia: someone other than the patient commits an action with the intent to end the patient's life, for example, injecting him or her with a lethal dose

Active immunity: antibodies against harmful effects of microorganisms or toxins that are self-produced

Active transport: movement of ions or molecules across cell membranes, usually against a pressure gradient and with the expenditure of metabolic energy

Acute illness: rapidly occurring illness that runs its course, allowing the person to return to his or her previous level of functioning

Acute pain: episode of pain that lasts for seconds to less than 6 months

Adaptation: adjustment of living to other living things and environmental conditions

Addictive: substance to which a person develops a psychological and physiologic dependency

Adduction: movement of a body part toward the midline of the body

Adolescence: the period of time between childhood and adulthood; a time of rapid physical change, reproductive maturity, and emotional development

Advance directive: written directive that allows people to state in advance what their choices for healthcare would be if certain circumstances should develop

Adventitious breath sounds: abnormal breath sound heard over the lungs

Advocacy: protection and support of another's rights

Aerobic bacteria: bacteria that require oxygen to live and grow

Aerobic exercise: exercise that promotes cardiovascular fitness; it increases blood flow, heart rate, and the metabolic demand for oxygen over a period of time

Afebrile: a condition in which the body temperature is not elevated

Affective learning: changes in attitudes, values, and feelings

Ageism: attitudes that stereotype the older adult on the basis of chronologic age

Agency for Health Care Policy and Research (AHCPR): a group of multidisciplinary experts who utilize research as well as a broad range of input from professional and consumer organizations and individuals to develop clinical practice guidelines; established by the Omnibus Budget Reconciliation Act of 1989

Agnostic: person who holds that nothing can be known about the existence of a god

Albuminuria: albumin in the urine; indication of kidney disease

Alkali: substance that can accept or trap a hydrogen ion; synonym for base

Alkalosis: condition, characterized by a proportionate lack of hydrogen ions in the extracellular fluid concentration, in which the pH exceeds 7.45

Alopecia: baldness

Alternative care: general term used to identify various methods of nonhospital healthcare, including residential housing, day care, respite care, hospice, and extended-care facilities

Alveoli: small air sacs at the end of the terminal bronchioles that are the site of gas exchange

Alzheimer's disease: type of dementia in which discrete patches of brain tissue degenerate; this devastating disease eventually affects all body systems

Ambulatory care: healthcare settings located in areas that are convenient for people to walk into and receive care; may be provided in hospitals, clinics, or centers

Amino acid: basic building blocks used to manufacture protein and the end products of protein digestion

Ampule: glass flask containing a single dose of medication for parenteral administration

Anaerobic bacteria: bacteria that can live without oxygen

Anaerobic exercise: exercise in which the supply of oxygen is less than the demand created by contracting muscles; oxygen debt results

Analgesic drug: pharmaceutical agent used to relieve pain

Anaphylactic reaction: severe reaction occurring immediately after exposure to a drug; characterized by respiratory distress and vascular collapse

Anion: ion that carries a negative electric charge

Ankylosis: fixation or immobilization of a joint

Anorexia: lack or loss of appetite for food

Anorexia nervosa: eating disorder characterized by the denial of appetite and bizarre eating habits

Anoxia: absence of oxygen

Antagonistic effect: combined effect of two or more drugs that produces less than the effect of each drug alone

Anthropometric: measurements of the body and body parts

Antibacterial: agent that kills bacteria or suppresses their growth

Antibody: immunoglobin produced by the body in response to a specific antigen

Antigen: foreign material capable of inducing a specific immune response

Antimicrobial: antibacterial agent that kills bacteria or suppresses their growth

Antipyretic: agent that reduces fever

Antiseptic: substance that inhibits the growth of bacteria

Anuria: technically, no urine voided; 24-hour urine output is less than 100 mL; synonyms are *complete kidney shutdown* and *renal failure*

Anxiety: vague sense of impending doom or apprehension precipitated by new and unknown experiences

Apnea: absence of breathing

Arousal: condition in which the cortical area of the brain receives and responds appropriately to stimuli

Ascites: accumulation of fluid in the peritoneal cavity

Asepsis: absence of disease-producing microorganisms; being free of infection

Asphyxiation: stoppage of breathing or the lack of air reaching the lungs; synonym for suffocation

Assault: threat or an attempt to make bodily contact with another person without that person's permission

Assertiveness: ability to stand up for oneself and others using open, honest, and direct communication

Assessing: systematic and continuous collection, validation, and communication of patient data

Assimilation: process by which a person interprets information to fit the current level of cognition

Assisted suicide: the act of making a means of suicide (eg, providing pills or a weapon) available to a patient with knowledge of his or her intention; in assisted suicide, someone makes the means of death available but does not act as the direct agent of death

Atelectasis: incomplete expansion or collapse of a part of the lungs

Atheist: person who denies the existence of a god

Atrophy: decrease in the size of a body structure

Attachment: active, affectionate, reciprocal relationship between two persons

Attitude: feeling or emotion, generally including a positive or negative judgment toward people, objects, or ideas

Auditory: pertaining to hearing

Auscultation: listening for sounds within the body

Authoritative knowledge: knowledge that comes from an expert and is accepted as truth based on a perceived level of expertise

Autocratic leadership: leadership style in which the leader assumes complete control over the decisions and activities of the group

Autonomy: self-determination; being independent and self-governing

B

Bacteria: the most significant and most commonly observed infection-causing agents

Bacteriuria: an asymptomatic condition that occurs when bacteria enter the bladder during catheterization or when organisms migrate up the catheter lumen or the urethra into the bladder

Bandage: piece of gauze or other material used to cover a wound

Basal metabolism: amount of energy required to carry out involuntary activities of the body at rest

Base: substance that can accept or trap a hydrogen ion; synonym for alkali

Base of support: foundation that provides stability for an object

Basic human needs: something essential to the health and survival of humans; common to all people

Battery: assault that is carried out

Beliefs: special class of intellectual attitudes based primarily on faith as opposed to fact

Beneficence: principle of doing good

Bereavement: state of grieving or going through the grief process

Bilateral: pertaining to two sides of the body

Binder: type of bandage, usually designed to fit a large body area

Biologic gender: the term used to denote chromosomal sexual development: male (XY) or female (XX)

Biopsy: removal of a piece of tissue for microscopic examination

Bisexuality: having sexual feelings for people of both sexes

Blended family: two single-parent families joined together to form a new family unit

Blood pressure: force of blood against arterial walls

Body image: how a person experiences his or her body

Body language: nonverbal communication

Body mechanics: efficient use of the body as a machine and as a means of locomotion

Body substance isolation (BSI): type of isolation that considers all body substances as potentially infective regardless of a person's diagnosis

Bolus: single injection of a concentrated solution administered intravenously

Bonding: a process of initial fusing of the mother and infant that occurs most often in the first few hours after birth and is necessary for later attachment

Bowel movement: emptying of the intestinal tract; synonym for defecation

Bowel training program: program that manipulates factors within a person's control (timing of defecation, exercise, diet) to produce a regular pattern of comfortable defecation without medication or enemas

Bradycardia: slow heart rate

Bradypnea: abnormally slow rate of breathing

Bronchial sounds: those heard over the trachea; high in pitch and intensity with expiration being longer than inspiration

Bronchodilator: medication that relaxes contractions of smooth muscles of the bronchioles

Bronchoscopy: visual examination of the trachea and bronchi

Bronchovesicular: normal breath sounds heard over the upper anterior chest and intercostal area

Bruit: unusual sound, usually abnormal, heard in auscultation

Buffer: substance that prevents body fluid from becoming overly acid or alkaline

Bulimia: eating disorder characterized by episodes of gorging followed by purging; often occurs in conjunction with anorexia nervosa

Burnout: behaviors exhibited as the result of prolonged occupational stress

C

Calorie: measure of heat, or energy; kilocalorie, commonly referred to as a calorie, defined as the amount of heat required to raise 1 kg of water 1°C

Carbohydrate: organic compounds (commonly known as sugars and starches) that are composed of carbon, hydrogen, and oxygen; the most abundant and least expensive source of calories in the diet worldwide

Cardiac output: volume of blood pumped from the left ventricle per minute

Cardinal signs: body temperature, pulse and respiratory rates, and blood pressure; synonym for vital signs

Caregiver burden: stress responses experienced during prolonged periods of home care by family caregivers

Caries: cavitation of the teeth

Case management: the process of coordinating an individual's healthcare for the purpose of maximizing positive outcomes and containing costs

Cathartic: medication that strongly increases gastrointestinal motility and promotes defecation

Catheter: tube for injecting or removing fluids

Cation: ion that carries a positive electric charge

Center of gravity: point at which the mass of an object is centered

Centers for Disease Control (CDC): U.S. government agency whose responsibilities include investigation, identification, prevention, and control of disease

Central venous catheter: venous access device usually introduced into the subclavian or internal jugular veins and passed to the superior vena cava just above the right atrium

Certification: process by which a person who has met certain criteria established by a non-governmental association is granted recognition

Ceruminal gland: gland found in the external auditory canal that secretes a substance called cerumen

Change: process of transforming, altering, or modifying something

Change agent: person who purposefully and systematically implements change

Change of shift report: communication method used by nurses completing care for a patient to transmit patient information to nurses about to assume responsibility for continuing care; may be exchanged verbally in a meeting or audiotaped

Channel: a term used in communication theory to denote the medium selected to convey the message; the channel may target any of the receiver's senses

Charting by exception: shorthand method for documenting patient data that is based on well-defined standards of practice; only exceptions to these standards are documented in narrative notes

Chemical name: precise description of a drug's chemical composition

Cheyne-Stokes respirations: gradual increase and then gradual decrease in depth of respirations followed by a period of apnea

Child abuse: intentional, nonaccidental physical or mental abuse of a child by a parent or other caregiver

Cholesterol: fat-like substance found only in animal tissues; it is important for cell membrane structure, a precursor of steroid hormones, and a constituent of bile; high serum cholesterol levels are a risk factor in the development of atherosclerosis

Chronic illness: irreversible illness that causes permanent physical impairment and requires long-term healthcare

Chronic pain: episode of pain that lasts for 6 months or longer; may be intermittent or continuous

Chyme: semifluid state that food is in when it leaves the stomach

Circadian rhythm: rhythm that completes a full cycle every 24 hours; synonym for *diurnal rhythm*

Circumduction: moving the distal part of the limb to trace a complete circle while the proximal end of the bone remains fixed

Civil law: rule that regulates relationships among people; synonym for *private law*

Clinical pathway/critical path: case management tools used to communicate the standardized, interdisciplinary plan of care for a particular group of patients; care guidelines and outcomes are specified for each day of the patient's stay

Clubbing: rounding and swelling of nailbeds

Cognition: cerebral functioning; process of perceiving and understanding one's world

Cognitive competency: enables nurses to reason about the nature of things sufficiently to "make sense" of their world and to conceptually grasp what is necessary to achieve valued goals

Cognitive learning: storing and recalling of new knowledge in the brain

Coitus: sexual activity in which the penis is placed in the vagina; synonym for *sexual intercourse*

Colic: acute abdominal pain caused by spasmodic contractions of the intestine during the first 3 months of life

Collaborative problem: actual or potential health problem that may occur from complications of disease, diagnostic studies, or the treatment regimen; the nurse works together with other members of the healthcare team toward its resolution

Colloid osmotic pressure: pressure exerted by plasma proteins on permeable membranes in the body; synonym for *oncotic pressure*

Colon: section of the large intestine from the cecum to the rectum

Colostomy: an opening into the colon that permits feces from the colon to exit through the stoma

Comfort measures only: an order written to indicate that the goal of treatment is a comfortable, dignified death and that further life-sustaining measures are no longer indicated

Common law: law resulting from court decisions that is then followed when other cases involving similar circumstances and facts arise; common law is as binding as civil law

Communication: process of sharing information; process of generating and transmitting meanings

Community-based healthcare: healthcare that is provided to people who live within a defined geographic region or who have common needs; designed to meet the needs of people as they move between and among healthcare settings

Complaint: legal statement of the plaintiff's claim; once filed, it initiates legal proceedings

Compliance: act of completing what is expected of one

Computerized nursing care plan: plan of patient care developed by computer software programs that enable the nurse to call up screens listing causes, goals, and related nursing interventions for nursing diagnoses and medical diagnoses

Concept: abstract images that are formed as impressions from the environment and organized into symbols of reality

Conceptual framework/model: set of concepts, along with the statements that arrange the concepts into an understandable pattern

Concurrent audit: evaluation of nursing care and patient outcomes conducted while the patient is receiving care; may use direct observation of nursing care, patient interview, and chart review

Condom catheter: tube for draining urine; it connects a device applied externally to the penis to a collection bag

Confidentiality: respecting privileged information

Congestion: presence of excessive fluids or secretions in an organ or body tissue

Constipation: passage of dry, hard, fecal material

Consultation: a process in which two or more individuals with varying degrees of experience and expertise deliberate about a problem and its solution

Consumer: the person who uses healthcare services (the patient)

Continuity of care: coordination of services provided to patients before they enter a healthcare setting, during the time they are in the setting, and after they leave the setting

Continuum: graduated scale

Contraception: prevention of conception or pregnancy; also used to describe methods used for birth control

Contractual agreement: pact made between two persons for the achievement of mutually set goals

Contracture: permanent contraction state of a muscle

Convalescent period: stage of an infection that represents recovery from the infection

Coping mechanism: patterns of behavior used to neutralize, deny, or counteract anxiety

Counseling: giving guidance, assisting with problem solving

Crackles: fine crackling sounds made as air moves through wet secretions in the lungs

Credentialing: general term that refers to ways in which professional competence is maintained

Crime: offense against people or property; the act is considered to be against the government, referred to in a lawsuit as "the people," and the accused is prosecuted by the state

Crisis: (1) point at which body temperature drops rapidly to normal; (2) occurs when coping and defense mechanisms are no longer effective, resulting in high levels of anxiety, disorganized behavior, and the inability to function normally

Crisis intervention: five-step problem-solving technique to promote adaptation and improve future coping

Criteria: specified behavior; for example, the measurable criteria in a patient goal specifies how the patient must perform the desired behavior

Critical thinking: thought that is disciplined, comprehensive, based on intellectual standards, and, as a result, well-reasoned; a systematic way to form and shape one's thinking that functions purposefully and exactingly

Crossmatching: act of determining the compatibility of two blood specimens

Cue: significant data that is helpful in making decisions

Cultural assimilation: process that occurs when a minority group, living as part of a dominant group within a culture, loses the cultural characteristics that made it different

Cultural blindness: the process of ignoring differences in people and proceeding as though the differences do not exist

Cultural care deprivation: a lack of culturally assistive, supportive, or facilitative acts in the healthcare setting

Cultural imposition: tendency of some to impose their beliefs, practices, and values on another culture because they believe that their ideas are superior to those of another person or group

Culture: sum total of human behavior or social characteristics peculiar to a specific group and passed from generation to generation or from one to another within the group

Culture shock: those feelings, usually negative, a person experiences when placed in a different culture

Cumulative effect: occurs when the body cannot metabolize a drug before additional doses are administered

Cutaneous pain: superficial pain usually involving the skin or subcutaneous tissue

Cyanosis: bluish coloring of the skin and mucous membranes

Cystoscopy: direct visual examination of the bladder, ureteral orifices, and urethra with a cystoscope

Cytologic study: study of cells and fluids from the body

D

Data: information

Data base: all the pertinent patient information that enables a comprehensive and effective plan of care to be designed and implemented for the patient

Data cluster: grouping of patient data or cues that points to the existence of a patient health problem

Day-care center: centers that provide care for infants, children, elderly people, and people with special healthcare needs

Death: termination of life and its related clinical signs

Débridement: cleaning away of devitalized tissue and foreign matter from a wound; can be accomplished by various methods

Deductive reasoning: a cognitive process in which one examines a general idea and then considers specific actions or ideas

Defamation: wrongs of slander and libel; making derogatory remarks about one person or another

Defecation: emptying of the intestinal tract; synonym for *bowel movement*

Defense mechanisms: forms of self-deception; unconscious process the self uses to protect itself from anxiety or threats to self-esteem

Dehiscence: separation of the layers of a surgical wound; may be partial, superficial, or a complete disruption of the surgical wound

Dehydration: decreased water volume

Delta sleep: deep sleep, occurring during stage III and especially stage IV in NREM sleep

Dementia: organic impairment of intellectual functioning, gradually leading to interference with social or occupational functioning, memory, and often personality integration

Democratic leadership: leadership style characterized by a sense of equality between the leader and followers

Deontologic: ethical system in which actions are right or wrong independent of the consequences they produce

Dependent action: nursing action carried out at the instruction or order of an authorized healthcare professional other than a nurse; synonym for *physician-initiated or physician-prescribed intervention*

Dermis: underlying portion of the skin

Development: increase in the complexity of function and progression to skill advancement

Development theory: theory to describe the orderly and predictable process of the growth and development of humans, individualized by social, biologic, and environmental factors

Developmental crisis: predictable patterns of behavior and change occurring throughout the lifespan

Developmental delay: measure of development that lags behind the normal range for a given age

Developmental task: successful achievement of psychomotor, psychosocial, or cognitive skills at certain periods in life; failure to obtain the developmental task can lead to unhappiness and difficulty with later tasks

Diagnosis (nursing): analysis of patient data to identify patient strengths and health problems that independent nursing intervention can prevent or resolve

Diagnosis related groups (DRGs): classification of patients by major medical diagnosis for the purpose of standardizing healthcare costs (see *prospective payment*)

Diarrhea: passage of liquid and unformed stools

Diastolic pressure: least amount of pressure exerted on arterial walls, which occurs when the heart is at rest between ventricular contractions

Dietary Guidelines: recommendations for choosing a healthy diet made by the U.S. Department of Agriculture and the U.S. Department of Health and Human Services

Diffuse pain: pain that covers a large area

Diffusion: tendency of solutes to move freely throughout a solvent from an area of higher concentration to an area of lower concentration until equilibrium is established

Direct transfusion: infusion of blood while it is being taken from the donor

Discharge planning: systematic process of preparing the patient to leave the healthcare facility and for maintaining continuity of care

Discharge summary: description of where the patient stands in relation to problems identified in the record at discharge; documents any special teaching or counseling the patient received, including referrals

Discipline: specific and unique body of knowledge that uses existing and new knowledge to creatively solve problems and meet human needs within ever-changing boundaries

Disease: pathologic change in the structure or function of the body or mind

Distribution: movement of drugs by the circulatory system to the site of action

Documentation: written, legal record of all pertinent interventions with the patient—assessments, diagnoses, plans, interventions, and evaluations

Dominant group: group within a culture that has the authority to control the value system and determine the rewards of the system; usually the largest group in a society

Donor: person who donates blood to be given to another person

Do-not-hospitalize: an order specifying that a patient, usually one who is terminally ill and anticipating death, not be admitted to the hospital in the event of a worsening of condition

Do-not-resuscitate: An order specifying that there be no attempt to resuscitate a patient in the event of cardiopulmonary arrest

Dressing: protective covering placed over a wound

Drug: substance that modifies body functions when taken into the living organism; synonym for *medication*

Drug allergy: hypersensitivity caused by previous exposure to a medication; may occur immediately or be delayed; manifestations range from mild to severe

Drug tolerance: tendency of the body to become accustomed to a drug over time; larger doses are required to produce the desired effects

Dysrhythmia: an abnormal cardiac rhythm; synonym for *arrhythmia*

Dysuria: difficulty in voiding; may or may not be associated with pain; a feeling of warm local irritation occurring during voiding is called *burning*

E

Ecchymosis: collection of blood in subcutaneous tissues that causes a purplish discoloration

Edema: accumulation of fluid in extracellular spaces

Elective surgery: surgery that is recommended but can be omitted or delayed without catastrophe

Electrocardiogram (ECG; EKG): graphic record produced by the electrocardiograph

Electroencephalograph: instrument that measures and records electric impulses of the brain

Electrolyte: substance capable of breaking into ions and developing an electric charge when dissolved in solution

Electromyograph (EMG): instrument that records muscle tone

Electrooculogram: recording of the electric current or potential produced by eye movements

Embolism: blocking of an artery by a blood clot or by other foreign matter brought to the site by the blood flow

Embolus: foreign body or air in the circulatory system; plural form is *emboli*

Emergency surgery: surgery that must be performed immediately to save the person's life or a body organ

Empathy: intellectually identifying with the way another person feels

Endogenous: infection in which the causative organism comes from microbial life the person himself or herself harbors

Endorphins: morphine-like substances released by the body that appear to alter the perception of pain

Endoscopy: direct visualization of hollow organs of the body using an endoscope or flexible, lighted tube

Endotracheal tube: polyvinyl-chloride airway that is inserted through the nose or the mouth into the trachea using a laryngoscope as a guide

Enema: introduction of solution into the lower intestinal tract

Enkephalins: opioids that are widespread throughout the brain and dorsal horn of the spinal cord and are believed to reduce pain sensation by inhibiting the release of substance P

Enteral nutrition: alternate form of feeding that involves passing a tube into the gastrointestinal tract to allow instillation of the appropriate formula

Entry phase: the phase of the home visit in which the nurse develops rapport with the patient and family members, mutually determines outcomes, makes assessments, plans and implements prescribed care, and provides teaching

Enuresis: involuntary urination; most often used to refer to a child who involuntarily urinates during the night

Epidermis: a superficial portion of the skin

Epidural analgesia: means of providing pain relief with an opioid injection delivered by way of a catheter inserted in the midlumbar region into the epidural space

Epithelialization: stage of wound healing in which epithelial cells move across the surface of a wound; tissue color ranges from the color of "ground glass" to pink

Erection: condition that results when erectile tissue of the penis fills with blood as a result of stimulation

Erogenous zones: areas of the body that produce sexual desire and arousal when stimulated

Erythema: redness of the skin

Eschar: a thick, leathery scab or dry crust that is necrotic and must be removed for adequate pressure ulcer staging to occur

Ethical/legal competencies: enable nurses to live life in a manner that is consistent with their personal moral code and role responsibilities

Ethics: system dealing with standards of character and behavior related to what is right and wrong

Ethnicity: sense of identification that a cultural group collectively has; the sharing of common and unique cultural and social beliefs and behavior patterns, including language and dialect, religious practices, literature, folklore, music, political interests, food preferences, and employment patterns

Ethnocentrism: judgment of other people based on the standards and practices of one's own culture

Euphoria: unrealistic sense of well-being

Eupnea: normal respirations

Euthanasia: mercy killing; the deliberate termination of the life of a person

Evaluating: measurement of the extent to which the patient has achieved the goals specified in the plan of care; factors that positively or negatively influence goal achievement are identified, and the plan of care is terminated or revised

Evisceration: protrusion of viscera through an incisional area

Excretion: removal of a drug from the body

Exercise: active exertion of muscles involving the contraction and relaxation of muscle groups

Exogenous: infection in which the causative organism is acquired from outside the host

Expected outcome: the specific, measurable criteria used to evaluate whether the patient goal has been met

Expectorant: drug that facilitates the removal of respiratory secretions

Expert witness: nurse who explains to the judge and jury what happened based on the patient's record and who offers an opinion as to whether the nursing care met acceptable standards of practice

Expiration: act of breathing out; synonym is *exhalation*

Extended-care facility: type of care given after hospitalization of acute illness; includes residential care and intermediate or skilled nursing home care

Extended family: nuclear family and other related people

Extracellular fluid (ECF): fluid outside the cells; includes intravascular and interstitial fluids

Exudate: fluid that accumulates in a wound; may contain serum, cellular debris, bacteria, and white blood cells

F

Fact witness: nurse who has knowledge of the actual incident prompting a legal case; bases testimony on firsthand knowledge of the incident not on assumptions

Failure to thrive (FTT): physical and developmental retardation of infants or children resulting from physical or emotional neglect

Faith: (1) spiritual dimensions of a person's life regardless of religious affiliation; (2) confident belief in something for which there is no proof or material evidence

Family: any group of two or more people who live together and are emotionally involved with each other

Febrile: a condition in which the body temperature is elevated

Fasting state: abstinence from food and fluids

Fecal impaction: collection in the rectum of hardened feces that cannot be passed

Feces: intestinal waste products

Feedback: verbal and nonverbal evidence that the message is received and understood

Felony: (1) crime punishable by imprisonment in a state or federal penitentiary for more than 1 year; (2) crime of greater offense than a misdemeanor

Fever: elevation above the upper limit of normal body temperature; synonym for *pyrexia*

Fiber: all dietary plant material that is not digestible by gastrointestinal tract, enzymes, and secretions

Fidelity: keeping promises and commitments made to others

Fight-or-flight response: the body prepares itself against threat, to either resist (fight) or evade (flight) the danger

Filtration: passage of a fluid through a permeable membrane whose spaces do not allow certain solutes to pass; passage is from an area of higher pressure to one of lower pressure

Flaccidity: decreased muscle tone; synonym for *hypotonicity*

Flatulence: excessive formation of gases in the gastrointestinal tract

Flatus: intestinal gas

Flexibility: ability to use a muscle through its entire range of motion

Flexion: state of being bent

Flowsheets: graphic record of abbreviated aspects of patient's condition (eg, vital signs, routine aspects of care)

Fluid balance: state in which water and its solutes in the body are in normal proportions and concentrations and are in appropriate body compartments

Fluid imbalance: state in which water and its solutes in the body are in improper proportions and concentrations or are improperly located in body compartments

Fluid volume deficit: deficiency in the amount of both water and electrolytes in extracellular fluid; water and electrolyte proportions remain near normal

Fluid volume excess: excessive retention of water and sodium in extracellular fluid in near-normal proportions

Flushing: red appearance of the skin

Focus charting: a documentation system that replaces the problem list with a focus column that incorporates many aspects of a patient and patient care; the focus may be a patient strength or a problem or need; the narrative portion of focus charting uses the data (D), action (A), response (R) format

Foley catheter: indwelling or retention catheter that remains in place to drain urine

Footdrop: complication resulting from extended plantar flexion

Formal teaching: planned teaching based on learner objectives

Frail-old: term for people over age 75; the fastest-growing segment of the population

Fraud: willful and purposeful misrepresentation that could cause, or has caused, loss or harm to people or property

Fremitus: vibration of the chest wall that can be palpated during the physical examination

Frequency: increased incidence of voiding

Friction: occurs when two surfaces rub against each other; the resulting injury resembles an abrasion and can also damage superficial blood vessels directly under the skin

Friction rub: crackling sounds heard in the chest cavity caused by inflamed pleura rubbing against the chest wall

Functional health: level of health defined by one's ability to carry out usual and desired daily activities

Functional incontinence: state in which a person experiences an involuntary, unpredictable passage of urine

Fungi: plant-like organisms (molds and yeasts) that also can cause infection

G

Gate control theory: theory that explains that excitatory pain stimuli carried by small-diameter nerve fibers can be blocked by inhibiting signals carried by large-diameter nerve fibers

Gender identity: the inner sense a person has of being male or female, which may be the same as or different from biologic gender; synonym is *sexual identity*

Gender role behavior: the behavior a person conveys about being male or female, which may or may not be the same as biologic gender or gender identity (Pilliteri, 1995)

General adaptation syndrome (GAS): biochemical model of stress describing the body's general response to stress

General anesthesia: anesthetic drugs that produce narcosis, relaxation of skeletal muscles, and reduced or absent reflex action

Generic name: name assigned by the manufacturer who first develops a drug; it is often derived from the chemical name

Gerontologic nursing: nursing specialty concerned with the care of both the well and the ill older adult

Gerontology: study of all aspects of the aging process and their consequences

Gingivitis: inflammation of the gingivae or gums

Glycosuria: presence of sugar in the urine; if due to an unusually large intake of sugar or to marked emotional disturbances and is temporary, there is little cause for alarm

Good Samaritan law: law that holds certain health practitioners blameless when undertaking to aid a person in an emergency

Gram-negative bacteria: bacteria with chemically more complex cell walls that can be decolorized by alcohol

Gram-positive bacteria: bacteria with a thick cell wall that resists decolorization (loss of color) and are stained violet

Granulation tissue: new tissue that is pink/red in color and composed of fibroblasts and small blood vessels that fill an open wound when it starts to heal

Graphic sheet: a form used to record specific patient variables

Grief: emotional response to loss. *Dysfunctional grief:* distorted or abnormal grief response, including *inhibited grief* (suppression of grief reaction) and *unresolved grief* (lengthy or denied grief reaction). *Abbreviated grief:* short but genuine grief reaction. *Anticipatory grief:* grief reaction before actual loss.

Ground: conducting connection between a source of electricity and the earth

Group dynamics: study of a group's characteristics and ways of functioning

Gurgles: continuous musical sounds that are audible in expiration or inspiration, or both; formerly called *rhonchi*

Gustatory: pertaining to taste

H

Halitosis: offensive breath

Health: state of optimal functioning or well-being

Health-belief model: what people believe to be true about themselves in relation to health

Health maintenance organization (HMO): broad term encompassing various healthcare delivery systems that use group practice and provide an incentive to use a prepaid comprehensive healthcare system

Health problem: condition related to health requiring intervention if disease or illness is to be prevented or resolved and coping and wellness are to be promoted

Helping relationship: interaction that sets the climate of movement of the participants toward common goals

Hematuria: blood in the urine; if present in large enough quantities, urine may be bright red or reddish brown

Hemolysis: process of freeing a red blood cell of its hemoglobin by destruction of the cell membrane

Hemoptysis: sputum containing blood

Hemorrhage: excessive blood loss due to the escape of blood from blood vessels

Hemorrhoids: abnormally distended rectal veins

Heparin lock: intravenous needle or catheter with an injection pad attached at the end

Hesitancy: delay or difficulty in initiating voiding

Heterosexuality: having sexual feelings for a person of the opposite sex

Hierarchy of needs: as defined by Maslow, certain needs are more basic than others; a person strives to at least minimally meet certain needs before attending to others

High-level wellness: functioning to one's maximum potential while maintaining balance and purposeful direction in the environment

Holistic healthcare: healthcare that takes into account the whole person interacting in the environment

Home health agency: agency, eligible to receive federal funds, that provides home-based care; may be independent, hospital operated, or health department managed

Home healthcare: healthcare services provided in a patient's home

Homeostasis: various physiologic and psychological mechanisms respond to changes in the internal and external environment to maintain a balanced state

Homosexuality: having sexual feelings for a person of the same sex

Hospice: a type of end-of-life care for persons who are terminally ill, characterized by the following: (1) patients are kept as free of pain as possible so that they may die comfortably and with dignity; (2) patients receive continuity of care, are not abandoned, and do not lose personal identity; (3) patients retain as much control as possible over decisions regarding their care and are allowed to refuse further life-prolonging technologic interventions; and (4) patients are viewed as individuals with personal fears, thoughts, feelings, values, and hopes

Hospitals: acute-care settings that provide various healthcare services, such as emergency care, in-patient care, surgery, diagnostic tests, and patient education

Host: animal or person on or within which microorganisms live

Hydration: union of a substance with water; term often is used as the opposite of dehydration, in which case it means that there is normal intracellular and extracellular water volume

Hydrometer: instrument used to determine the specific gravity of urine

Hydrostatic pressure: force exerted by a fluid against the container wall

Hypercalcemia: excess of calcium in the extracellular fluid

Hyperkalemia: excess of potassium in the extracellular fluid

Hypermagnesemia: excess of magnesium in the extracellular fluid

Hypernatremia: excess of sodium in the extracellular fluid

Hyperphosphatemia: above normal serum concentration of inorganic phosphorus

Hyperpyrexia: high fever, above 41°C (105.8°F)

Hypersomnia: condition characterized by excessive sleeping, especially daytime sleeping

Hypertension: blood pressure elevated above the upper limit of normal

Hypertonic: having a greater concentration than the solution with which it is being compared

Hyperventilation: condition in which there is more than the normal amount of air entering and leaving lungs

Hypervolemia: excess of plasma

Hypnotic: pharmaceutical agent used to induce sleep

Hypocalcemia: insufficient amount of calcium in the extracellular fluid

Hypokalemia: insufficient amount of potassium in the extracellular fluid

Hypomagnesemia: insufficient amount of magnesium in the extracellular fluid

Hyponatremia: insufficient amount of sodium in the extracellular fluid

Hypophosphatemia: below normal serum concentration of inorganic phosphorus

Hypoproteinemia: insufficient amount of protein substances in the extracellular fluid

Hypotension: blood pressure below the lower limit of normal

Hypotonic: having a lesser concentration than the solution with which it is being compared

Hypoventilation: a decreased rate or depth of air movement into the lungs

Hypovolemia: deficiency of plasma

Hypovolemic shock: shock due to a decrease in blood volume

Hypoxemia: deficient oxygenation of blood

Hypoxia: inadequate amount of oxygen available to the cells

I

Iatrogenic infection: infection that occurs as a result of a treatment or diagnostic procedure

Ideal self: self a person would like to be or thinks he or she should be; includes aspirations, moral ideas, and values

Idiosyncratic effect: unusual, unexpected response to a drug that may manifest itself by overresponse, underresponse, or response different from the expected outcome

Ileal conduit: urinary diversion in which the ureters are connected to the ileum with a stoma created on the abdominal wall

Ileostomy: allows fecal content from the ileum to be eliminated through the stoma

Illness: abnormal process in which any aspect of the person's functioning is altered (in comparison to the previous condition of health)

Immunization: process of rendering a person immune or resistant to particular antigenic agents or bacteria

Implementing: carrying out the plan of care

Impotence: condition in which a man is unable to attain or maintain an erection to such an extent that he cannot have satisfactory sexual intercourse; synonym for *erectile failure*

Incentive spirometer: equipment to help maximize lung inflation

Incident report: documentation that describes any injury or potential for injury suffered by a patient in a healthcare agency

Incision: wound made with a sharp, cutting instrument

Incontinence: inability to voluntarily control the discharge of urine or feces

Independent action: (1) nursing action carried out at the instruction or order of a nurse; (2) actions within the legal scope of nursing's independent domain; synonym for *nurse-initiated* or *nurse-prescribed intervention*

Inductive reasoning: a cognitive process in which one identifies a specific idea or action and then makes conclusions about general ideas

Indwelling urethral catheter: catheter that remains in place for continuous urine drainage; synonym for *Foley catheter*

Infancy: period from 1 month to 1 year of age

Infection: disease state resulting from pathogens in or on the body

Infiltration: escape of fluid into subcutaneous tissue

Inflammatory response: localized response of the body to injury or infection; protective mechanism that eliminates invading pathogens and allows for tissue repair to occur

Informal teaching: unplanned teaching sessions dealing with the patient's immediate learning needs and concerns

Informed consent: knowledgeable, voluntary permission obtained from a patient to perform a specific test or procedure

Inhalation: (1) act of breathing in; synonym for inspiration; (2) administration of a drug in solution by way of the respiratory tract

Injection: introduction of medication into the body by a syringe attached to a needle

Inpatient: person who enters a healthcare setting for a stay ranging from 24 hours to many years

Insomnia: difficulty in falling asleep, intermittent sleep, or early awakening from sleep

Inspection: purposeful and systematic observation

Inspiration: act of breathing in; synonym is *inhalation*

Integument: skin

Integumentary system: skin and its appendages (ie, hair, glands in the skin, and nails)

Interdependent action: nursing action performed by the nurse in collaboration with other members of the healthcare team

Intermittent fever: body temperature that alternates between fever and normal or subnormal temperature

Intermittent pulse: normal pulse rhythm broken by periods of irregular rhythm

Interpersonal competency: skills that enable a nurse to establish and maintain caring relationships that facilitate the achievement of valued goals while simultaneously affirming the worth of participants in the relationship

Interstitial fluid: fluid between the cells

Interview: planned communication for a specific purpose (eg, data collection)

Interviewing techniques: communication skills specifically designed to gather and validate information

Intracellular fluid (ICF): fluid within the cell; synonym for *cellular fluid*

Intractable pain: severe pain that is extremely resistant to relief measures

Intradermal injection: injection placed just below the epidermis

Intramuscular injection: an injection into deep muscle tissue, usually of the buttock, thigh, or upper arm

Intraoperative phase: period lasting from admission to the operating room area to transfer to the postanesthesia recovery area after surgery is completed

Intravascular fluid: fluid within the vascular system; synonym for *plasma*

Intravenous infusion: injection of relatively large quantities of solution into a vein

Intravenous route: injection of a solution into the vein

Intuitive problem solving: direct understanding of a situation based on a background of experience, knowledge, and skill that makes expert decision making possible

Ion: atom or molecule carrying an electric charge in solution

Irrigation: flushing of a tube, canal, or area with solution

Ischemia: deficiency of blood in a particular area

Isokinetic exercise: exercise involving muscle contractions with resistance varying at a constant rate

Isolation: protective procedure designed to prevent the transmission of specific microorganisms; also called *protective aseptic techniques* and *barrier techniques*

Isometric exercise: exercise in which muscle tension occurs without a significant change in muscle length

Isotonic: (1) having about the same concentration as the solution with which it is being compared; (2) exercise in which muscles shorten (contract) and move

J

Jaundice: yellow appearance of the skin

Justice: process that distributes benefits, risks, and costs fairly

K

Kardex nursing care plan: trade name for a care plan documentation system that encompasses (1) prescriptions for nursing care related to activities of daily living; (2) nursing diagnoses and related patient goals and nursing orders; and (3) the nursing care related to diagnostic measures and the medical regimen

Kegel exercises: repetitious contraction and relaxation of the pubococcygeal muscle to improve vaginal tone and urinary continence

Kinesthesia: awareness of positioning of body parts and body movement

Korotkoff sounds: series of sounds that correspond to changes in blood flow through an artery as pressure is released

Kussmaul's respiration breathing: an extreme rate and depth of breathing

L

Laissez-faire leadership: leadership style in which the leader relinquishes all power to the group

Language: prescribed way of using words; a means to express thoughts and feelings

Law: rule of conduct established and enforced by the government of a society

Lawsuit: legal action in a court of law

Laxative: drug used to induce emptying of the intestinal tract

Leadership: ability to direct or motivate others toward the achievement of predetermined goals

Learning: increasing one's knowledge; having one's behavior changed in a measurable way as a result of an experience

Liability: legal responsibility for one's acts (and failure to act); includes responsibility for financial restitution of harms resulting from negligent acts

Licensure: to be given a license to practice nursing in a state or province after successfully meeting requirements

Life review/reminiscence: universal phenomenon identified by Butler as a review of one's life through one's recollections

Line of gravity: vertical line that passes through the center of gravity

Lipid: group name for fatty substances, including fats, oils, waxes, and related compounds

Literacy: ability to read and write

Litigation: process of lawsuit

Living will: advance directive specifying the medical care a person would want or refuse should he or she lack the capacity to consent to or refuse treatment himself or herself

Local adaptation syndrome (LAS): localized response of the body to stress, precipitated by trauma or pathology

Localized symptoms: symptoms that are limited or restricted to a discrete area

Long-term care: facilities for long-term care provide healthcare and help with activities of daily living for people of any age who are physically or mentally unable to independently care for themselves

Loss: inaccessibility or change in a valued person, object, or situation. *Actual loss:* loss tangible to both the person sustaining the loss and to others. *Perceived loss:* loss tangi-

ble only to the person sustaining it. *Physical loss:* loss of life, limb, an object, person, pet, or job. *Psychological loss:* loss that affects a person's self-image. *Anticipatory loss:* loss behaviors displayed before the actual loss occurs

Love and belonging needs: understanding and acceptance of others in giving and receiving love

M

Macromineral: mineral that is needed by the body in amount greater than 100 mg/day

Macronutrient: essential nutrient that supplies energy and builds tissue, such as carbohydrate, fat, and protein

Macroshock: electric current passing through a relatively large area of a person

Malpractice: act of negligence as applied to a professional person such as a physician, nurse, or dentist

Managed care: an organized, high-quality; cost-effective system of healthcare that influences the selection and use of healthcare services of a population

Management: process of directing others toward goal achievement

Masturbation: self-stimulation for sexual satisfaction

Medicaid: Title XIX (Social Security Act, 1965) to make healthcare available to those people with less than the minimum income who do not qualify for Medicare

Medical asepsis: practices designed to reduce the number and transfer of pathogens; synonym for *clean technique*

Medical diagnosis: statement about a specific disease process using terminology from a well-developed classification system accepted by the medical profession

Medicare: Title XVIII (Social Security Act, 1965) to provide a measure of health coverage to all Social Security recipients

Medication: substance that modifies body functions when taken into the living organisms; synonym for *drug*

Medication record: record documenting all medications administered to the patient, the nurse administering the drugs, and sometimes the reason the drug was administered and its effectiveness

Menarche: initiation of the menstrual cycle

Meniscus: curved surface at the top of a column of liquid in a tube

Menopause: decrease of cyclic hormonal production and cessation of menses in females, usually between ages 45 and 60 years

Menstruation: a cycle of about 20 days during which the female body prepares for the presence of a fertilized ovum

Mentorship: relationship in which an experienced person (the mentor) advises and assists a less experienced person

Message: term used in communication theory to denote the actual physical product of the source or encoder (eg, a speech, interview, phone conversation, chart)

Metabolic acidosis: proportionate deficiency of bicarbonate ions in the extracellular fluid

Metabolic alkalosis: proportionate excess of bicarbonate ions in the extracellular fluid

Metabolism: (1) chemical changes in the body by which energy is provided; (2) breakdown of a drug to an inactive form; also referred to as *biotransformation*

Micromineral: mineral or trace element that is needed by the body in an amount less than 100 mg/day

Micronutrient: vitamin or mineral needed in much smaller amount to regulate and control body processes

Microshock: electric current passing through a relatively small area of a person, usually part of the heart

Micturition: process of emptying the bladder; urination; voiding

Middle adult: the adult between the ages of 40 and 60 years; also called *middle adulthood*

Midlife crisis: realization that the halfway point in life has been reached and youthful goals may not have been achieved

Minerals: inorganic elements found in nature

Minority group: group having some physical or cultural characteristic that identifies the people within the group as different from the dominant culture

Misdemeanor: crime of lesser offense than a felony and punishable by fines, imprisonment (usually for less than 1 year) or both

Morals: like ethics, concerned with what constitutes right action; more informal and personal than the term ethics

Mourning: period during which a person learns to accept grief

N

Narcolepsy: condition characterized by an uncontrolled desire to sleep

Narrative: descriptive record of the patient's condition; includes patient's response to interventions by health professionals and patient's progress toward goal achievement

Nasal cannula: disposable, plastic device that delivers oxygen with two protruding prongs for insertion into the nostrils

Nasogastric tube: a tube inserted through the nose and into the stomach

Nasointestinal tube: a tube inserted through the nose and into the upper portion of the small intestine

National Medical Care: healthcare services in Canada, funded by taxes and provided to every Canadian citizen

Necrosis: death of cells

Negative reinforcement: an ineffective teaching strategy that uses criticism or punishment

Negativism: negative verbalizations and behaviors

Negligence: performing an act that a reasonably prudent person under similar circumstances would not do, or failing to perform an act that a reasonably prudent person under similar circumstances would do

Neonate: period from birth to 1 month of age

Neuromodulator: endogenous opioid chemical regulators that appear to have analgesic activity and alter pain perception

Neurotransmitters: substances that either excite or inhibit target nerve cells

Nociceptors: pain receptors

Nocturia: frequency of urination during the night

Nocturnal myoclonus: condition characterized by marked muscle contraction that results in the jerking of one or both legs during sleep

Noncompliance: nonadherence to a therapeutic recommendation

Nonmaleficence: principle of avoiding evil

Nonproductive cough: forceful expiratory effort without production of mucus; also called a *dry cough*

Nonverbal communication: exchange of information without the use of words

Normal flora: microorganisms that normally inhabit various body sites and are part of the body's natural defense system

Nosocomial infection: hospital-acquired infection

NREM: non–rapid eye movement that characterizes four stages of sleep

Nuclear family: family unit, family of marriage, parenthood, or procreation, and their immediate children

Nurse practice act: law established to regulate nursing practice

Nursing: profession focusing on the holistic person receiving healthcare services and providing a unique contribution to the prevention of illness and maintenance of health

Nursing actions: any action performed by a nurse to assist patients to meet health goals: promote wellness, prevent disease or illness, restore health, facilitate coping with altered functioning

Nursing audit: method of evaluating the outcomes of nursing care or the process by which these outcomes are achieved using a review of patient records

Nursing care conference: formal meeting of nurses to discuss some aspect of patient's care

Nursing care rounds: procedure in which a group of nurses visit patients individually at bedside to gather information that helps to plan and evaluate nursing care

Nursing diagnosis: actual or potential health problem that independent nursing intervention can prevent or resolve. *Actual problem* is present. *Possible problem* may be present, but more data are needed to confirm or disconfirm the problem. *Potential problem* may occur; defining characteristics are present as risk factors

Nursing history: assessment of the patient by interview to identify the patient's health status, strengths, health problems, health risks, and need for nursing

Nursing order: prescribes the nursing care to be given to assist patients to meet health goals

Nursing plan of care: written guide to direct the efforts of the nursing team as they work with patients to meet health goals; specifies prioritized nursing diagnoses, patient goals, and nursing orders

Nursing process: five-step systematic method for giving patient care; involves assessing, diagnosing, planning, implementing, and evaluating

Nutrient: specific biochemical substance used by the body for growth, development, activity, reproduction, lactation, health maintenance, and recovery from illness or injury

Nutrition: study of the nutrients and how they are handled by the body, as well as the impact of human behavior and environment on the process of nourishment

O

Obesity: weight greater than 20% above ideal body weight

Objective data: information perceptible to the senses; may be verified by another person

Observation: conscious and deliberate use of the five senses to gather data

Occult blood: blood present in such minute quantities that it cannot be detected with the unassisted eye

Occupational Safety and Health Administration (OSHA): government agency that establishes minimum health and safety standards for workers

Official name: name by which a drug is identified in official publications

Old-old: term used to describe older adults over age 75; sometimes referred to as frail-old

Older adult: after middle age; refers to adults over age of 65

Olfactory: pertaining to smell

Oliguria: scanty or greatly diminished amount of urine voided in a given time; 24-hour urine output is 100 to 400 mL

Oncotic pressure: pressure exerted by plasma proteins on permeable membranes in the body; synonym for *colloid osmotic pressure*

Opioid: more correct term for narcotic analgesics, since these drugs act by binding to opiate receptor sites in the central nervous system

Opportunist: bacteria that may potentially be harmful

Organism: a living being

Orgasm: apex of sexual activity in which rhythmic contractions of the genital organs and many other physiologic changes occur

Orthopnea: type of dyspnea in which breathing is easier when the patient sits or stands

Orthostatic hypotension: temporary fall in blood pressure associated with assuming an upright position; synonym for *postural hypotension*

Osmolarity: the concentration of particles in a solution, or a solution's pulling power

Osmosis: passage of a solvent through a semipermeable membrane from an area of lesser concentration to an area of greater concentration until equilibrium is established

Osmotic pressure: drawing power for water or the attraction for water exerted by solute particles

Osteoporosis: condition characterized by loss of calcium from bone tissue

Ostomy: general term referring to an artificial opening; usually used to refer to an opening created for the excretion of body wastes

Outcome: end product of nursing care; patient outcomes are measurable changes in patient behavior or state of health

Outpatient: a person who requires healthcare services but does not need to stay in an institution for those services

Overflow incontinence: the involuntary loss of urine associated with overdistention and overflow of the bladder

Ovulation: discharge of ovum from the female ovary at about the midpoint of each menstrual cycle

Ovum: female reproductive cell, often called an *egg*

P

Pain: sensation of physical or mental suffering or hurt that usually causes distress or agony to the one experiencing it

Pain threshold: amount of stimulation required before a person experiences the sensation of pain

Pain tolerance: point beyond which a person is no longer willing to endure pain (ie, pain of greater duration or intensity)

Pallor: paleness of the skin

Palpation: method of examining by feeling a part with the fingers or hand

Palpitation: perception of one's own heartbeat

Paracentesis: withdrawal of fluid from a body cavity, usually from the abdominal cavity

Parasomnia: patterns of waking behavior that appear during sleep (eg, sleep walking, sleep talking, nocturnal erections)

Paralytic ileus: paralysis of intestinal peristalsis

Paraplegia: paralysis of the legs

Parenteral: outside of intestines or alimentary canal; popularly used to refer to injection routes

Paresthesia: numbness and tingling

Passive exercise: manual or mechanical means of moving the joints

Paternalism: an action that is based on what a parent would do

Pathogen: disease-producing microorganism

Patient: the person receiving care

Patient-controlled analgesia (PCA): method of controlling pain that involves an infusion pump that holds a vial of an intravenous analgesic that the patient controls and self-administers in small doses

Patient goal: statement describing an expected patient outcome

Patient record: a compilation of a patient's health information; the patient record is the only permanent legal document that details the nurse's interactions with the patient

Pediculosis: infestation with lice

Perception: conscious process of organizing and interpreting data from the senses into meaningful information

Percussion: the act of striking one object against another for the purpose of producing a sound; used to assess the location, shape, size, and density of body tissues

Percutaneous endoscopic gastrostomy tube (PEG): a surgically or laparoscopically placed gastrostomy tube

Perfusion: passing of fluid through body tissue

Perioperative nursing: wide variety of nursing activities carried out before, during, and after surgery

Peripheral resistance: restraint to blood flow created by arteriole walls in a partial state of contraction

Peripherally inserted central catheter (PICC): a type of venous access device that can be introduced into a peripheral vein and advanced as far as the superior vena cava

Peristalsis: involuntary, progressive wave-like movement of the musculature of the gastrointestinal tract

Personal identity: an individual's conscious sense of who he or she is

Personal space: external environment surrounding a person that is regarded as being part of that person

Petechiae: small, purplish hemorrhagic spots on the skin that do not blanch with applied pressure

pH: expression of hydrogen ion concentration and resulting acidity of a substance

Phagocytosis: engulfing of microorganisms, foreign particles, or other cells by phagocytes

Phantom pain: sensation of pain without demonstrable physiologic or pathologic substance; commonly observed after the amputation of a limb

Pharmacology: study of actions of chemicals on living organisms

Phlebitis: inflammation of a vein

Phlegm: thick, respiratory secretions

Physical assessment: systematic examination of the patient for objective data to better define the patient's condition and help the nurse in planning care; usually performed in a head-to-toe format

Physiologic needs: need for oxygen, food, water, temperature, elimination, sexuality, activity, and rest; these needs have the highest priority and are essential for survival

PIE charting: a documentation system that is unique in that it does not develop a separate care plan; the care plan is incorporated into the progress notes in which problems are identified by number, worked up using the problem (P), intervention (I), evaluation (E) format, and evaluated each shift

Piggyback infusion: intermittent intravenous administration of medications through a primary intravenous line with the additive container positioned higher than the primary intravenous solution

Placebo: Latin word meaning "I shall please"; an inactive substance that gives satisfaction to the person using it

Plaintiff: person or government bringing a lawsuit against another

Planning: establishment of patient goals to prevent, reduce, or resolve the problems identified in the nursing diagnoses and determination of related nursing interventions

Plaque: transparent, adhesive coating on teeth consisting of mucin, carbohydrate, and bacteria

Plasma: liquid constituent of blood; synonym for *intravascular fluid*

Pneumonia: inflammation or infection of the lungs

Podiatrist: one who treats foot disorders; synonym for *chiropodist*

Polyp: tumor on a stem that bleeds easily and may become malignant

Polysomnography: sleep study consisting of an electroencephalographic recording of the stages of sleep and any episodes of apnea, continuous monitoring of arterial oxygen saturation, and an electrocardiographic recording to detect any cardiac dysrhythmias

Polyuria: excessive output of urine (diuresis)

Positive reinforcement: affirmation of the efforts of patients

Postoperative: period lasting from admission to the postanesthesia recovery area through recovery and convalescence

Postural hypotension: temporary fall in blood pressure associated with assuming an upright position; synonym for *orthostatic hypotension*

Post-void residual (PVR): urine that remains in the bladder after the act of micturition; a synonym for *residual urine*

Power: ability to influence others to achieve a desired effect

Preceptorship: process by which an experienced person facilitates an orientee's introduction to new responsibilities by way of teaching and guidance

Precordium: anterior surface of the chest wall overlying the heart and its related structures

Pre-entry phase: the phase of the home visit in which the nurse collects information about the patient's healthcare needs, gathers needed supplies, and evaluates safety factors

Preferred provider organization (PPO): any arrangement whereby patients are channeled to specific organizations as providers of health plans

Premenstrual (tension) syndrome (PMS): menstrual cycle–related distress; occurs a few days before the onset of menstruation

Preoperative: period lasting from the decision that surgery is necessary until the patient is transferred to the operating room area

Presbycusis: age-related hearing loss in which there is decreased ability to distinguish higher frequencies

Presbyopia: condition of aging in which decreased elasticity of the eye lens hinders accommodation to close vision

Preschooler: period from ages 3 to 6 years

Prescription: used by physician to convey medication plans for a patient

Pressure ulcer: any lesion caused by unrelieved pressure that results in damage to underlying tissue

Primary healthcare: essential healthcare based on practical, scientifically sound, and socially acceptable methods and technology, made universally accessible through the community's full participation and at a cost the community can afford

Primary preventive care: care directed toward health promotion and specific protection against illness

Principle-based approach: an approach to bioethics that offers specific action guides

Problem-oriented record (POR): documentation system organized according to the person's specific health problems; includes data base, problem list, plan of care, and progress notes

Process: series of actions, changes, or functions to bring about a result

Productive cough: cough that produces respiratory tract secretions

Professionalism: a way of being/commitment to secure the interests and welfare of those entrusted to one's care

Progress notes: any of a variety of methods of notes that relate how a patient is progressing toward expected outcomes

Protein: vital component of every living cell; composed of carbon, hydrogen, oxygen, and nitrogen

Proteinuria: albumin in the urine; indication of kidney disease

Protocol: written plan that details the nursing activities to be executed in specific situations

Psychogenic pain: pain for which no physical cause can be identified

Psychomotor learning: acquisition of physical skills

Psychosomatic disorder: physiologic alterations and illness believed to be due to psychological influences

Puberty: period during which primary and secondary sexual characteristics develop and the capability of sexual reproduction is attained

Public health agencies: local, state, provincial, or federal agencies that provide public health services to members of communities

Pulse: wave produced in the wall of an artery with each beat of the heart

Pulse deficit: difference between the apical and radial pulse rates

Pulse oximetry: noninvasive technique that measures the oxygen saturation (SaO₂) of arterial blood

Pulse pressure: difference between systolic and diastolic pressures

Purulent: containing pus

Pyorrhea: extensive inflammation of the gums and alveolar tissues; synonym for *periodontitis*

Pyrexia: elevation above the upper limit of normal body temperature; synonym for *fever*

Pyuria: pus in the urine; urine appears cloudy

Q

Quality assurance program: ongoing evaluation program designed and implemented to secure the excellence of healthcare; may involve an assessment of structure, process, and outcome standards

Quality improvement: the commitment and approach used to continuously improve every process in every part of an organization, with the intent of meeting and exceeding customer expectations and outcomes (also known as continuous quality improvement [CQI] or total quality management [TQM])

R

Race: division of human beings based on distinct physical characteristics

Radiography: examination by x-ray film

Range of motion: complete extent of movement of which a joint is normally capable

Rape: sexual violation of a person by someone who uses force, threats, and abuse

Rapid eye movement sleep: stage that constitutes 20% to 25% of a person's nightly sleep; person is difficult to arouse during this stage

Rapport: feeling of mutual trust experienced by people in a satisfactory relationship

Reactive hyperemia: the body's flooding of an area with blood after it has suffered from poor circulation for a period; the occurrence of a blanchable reddening of the skin when pressure is removed

Reality orientation: method of care used to promote awareness of reality in confused or disoriented patients

Receiver (decoder): term used in communication theory that specifies the person or object to which the message is directed

Reception: process of receiving data about the internal or external environment through the senses

Recommended dietary allowance (RDA): recommendations for average daily amounts of essential nutrients that healthy population groups should consume over time

Referral: process of sending or guiding someone to another source for assistance

Referred pain: pain in an area removed from that in which stimulation has its origin

Reflex pain response: automatic response of the central nervous system to the stimulus of pain

Regional anesthesia: anesthetic drug is injected or applied topically to inhibit transmission of sensory stimuli

Regression: behavior that is more characteristic of an earlier age

Rehabilitation: process of restoring a person's highest level of possible wellness and returning that person's ability to live and work as normally as possible after a disabling illness or injury

Rehabilitation centers: centers specializing in services for patients requiring physical or emotional rehabilitation and for treatment of any type of drug dependency

Relationship: interaction of people over time

Religion: organized system of beliefs about a higher power; often includes set forms of worship, spiritual practices, and codes of conduct

REM: rapid eye movement that characterizes the dream state of sleep

Report: oral, written, or computer-based communication of patient data with the purpose of informing others

Repression: exclusion of an anxiety-producing event from conscious awareness

Reservoir: natural habitat for the growth and multiplication of microorganisms

Residual urine: urine that remains in the bladder after the act of micturition

Respiration: act of breathing and using oxygen in body cells

Respiratory acidosis: proportionate excess of carbonic acid in the extracellular fluid

Respiratory alkalosis: proportionate deficiency of carbonic acid in the extracellular fluid

Rest: condition in which the body is in a decreased state of activity with the consequent feeling of being refreshed

Restraint: device used to limit movement or immobilize a client

Retention: inability to void although urine is produced by the kidneys and enters the bladder; excessive storage of urine in the bladder

Retention sutures: sutures used to provide extra support in wounds in obese patients or in wounds with increased risk of dehiscence

Reticular activating system: network of neurons in the core of the brain stem with ascending and descending tracts to other areas of the brain that monitors and regulates incoming sensory stimuli and level of arousal

Retrospective audit: evaluation of nursing care and patient outcomes after the patient has been discharged (may use postdischarge questionnaires, patient interviews, or chart review)

Risk factor: something that increases a person's chance for illness or injury

Role performance: ability to successfully execute societal expectations regarding role-specific behaviors

S

Safety and security needs: person's need to be protected from actual or potential harm and to have freedom from fear

Sanguineous: containing or mixed with blood

Scar: connective tissue that fills a wound area

School-age: period from ages 6 to 12 years

Scientific knowledge: knowledge arrived at by applying scientific methods

Scientific problem solving: systematic problem-solving process that involves (1) problem identification, (2) data collection, (3) hypothesis formulation, (4) plan of action, (5) hypothesis testing, (6) interpretation of results, and (7) evaluation resulting in conclusion or revision of the study

Scrub nurse: nurse who assists the surgeon during surgery, maintaining surgical asepsis while draping, handling instruments, and handling supplies

Scultetus binder: type of bandage with multiple tails; synonym for *many-tailed binder*

Sebaceous gland: gland found in the skin that secretes an oily substance called sebum

Secondary preventive care: care directed to health maintenance for patients experiencing health problems or to prevention of complications or disabilities

Self-actualization needs: need to reach one's potential through full development of one's unique capabilities; highest level need

Self-concept: mental image or picture of self; includes body image, subjective self, ideal self, and social self

Self-esteem: person's perception of his or her total being, including self-worth and body image

Self-esteem needs: need to feel good about oneself and to believe others hold one in high regard

Semantics: study of the meaning of words

Semen: seminal plasma containing sperm

Semipermeable membrane: selectively permeable membrane that allows water to pass through it but is either impermeable or selectively permeable to solutes

Sensoristasis: arousal state of the reticular activating system; general drive state

Sensory deficit: impaired or absent functioning of one or more senses

Sensory deprivation: condition resulting from decreased sensory input or input that is monotonous, unpatterned, or meaningless

Sensory overload: condition resulting from excessive sensory input to which the brain is unable to meaningfully respond

Sensory/perceptual alteration: disturbance in the body's ability to receive or process data from its internal or external environment. NANDA-approved nursing diagnosis

Separation anxiety: condition that occurs when a child is afraid of being sent away from caregivers who are loved and provide security

Serous: resembling blood serum; clear and watery in appearance

Set point: level at which the hypothalamus attempts to maintain body temperature

Sexual dysfunction: condition that prevents a person or couple from engaging in or obtaining satisfaction from sexual activity

Sexual harassment: unwelcome verbal or physical advance or sexually explicit statement (eg, leers, pats, grabs, jokes, requests for dates, and even rape) that interferes with one's ability to do one's job by making one feel humiliated, intimidated, or uncomfortable

Sexuality: degree to which a person exhibits and experiences maleness and femaleness physically, emotionally, and mentally

Sexually transmitted disease: a disease that spreads from one person to another through intimate sexual contact

Shearing force: force created when layers of tissue move on one another

Shock: body's reaction to acute peripheral circulatory failure due to an abnormality of circulatory control or to a loss of circulating fluid

Situational crisis: change that results when a person faces an event or situation that causes a disruption in his life

Sitz bath: special type of bath that applies heated water to the pelvic or rectal area

Skin sutures: used to approximate wound tissues and skin; may be silk, synthetic, wire, or metal staples

Skin tests: tests to determine antigen–antibody reaction

Sleep: state of altered consciousness throughout which varying degrees of stimuli preclude wakefulness

Sleep apnea: periods of no breathing during sleep that may last from 15 seconds to 2 minutes

Sleep cycle: passage through the four states of NREM sleep (I, II, III, IV), then reversal (IV, III, II), and finally, instead of reentering stage I and awakening, entering REM sleep and returning to stage II

Sleep deprivation: a decrease in the amount, consistency, and quality of sleep; results from decreased REM or NREM sleep

SOAP format: method of charting narrative progress notes; organizes data according to subjective information (S), objective information (O), assessment (A), and plan (P)

Social isolation: sense of aloneness because of decreasing relationships with others, resulting from attitudinal, geographic, financial, or illness-related factors

Social self: way a person believes that others see him or her

Solute: substance dissolved in a solution

Solvent: liquid holding a substance in solution

Somatic pain: pain originating in structures in the body's external wall

Somnambulism: sleep walking

Sordes: accumulation of mucus and crust formation on the teeth and around the lips

Source (encoder): term used in communication theory to specify the one who prepares and sends a message to the receiver

Source-oriented record: documentation system in which each healthcare group records data on its own separate form

Spasticity: increased muscle tone

Sperm: male reproductive cell; synonym for spermatozoan

Spermicide: chemical agent used to destroy sperm

Sphincter: circular muscle that constricts a passage or closes a natural orifice

Spiritual distress: nursing diagnosis describing an alteration in spiritual health (eg, spiritual pain, alienation, anxiety, guilt, anger, loss, despair)

Spiritual need: lack of anything necessary for spiritual health (eg, meaning and purpose, love and relatedness, forgiveness)

Spirituality: anything that pertains to a person's relationship with a nonmaterial life force or higher power

Spirometer: instrument used to measure lung capacities and volumes; one type is used to encourage deep breathing (incentive spirometry)

Standard: acceptable, expected, level of performance established by authority, custom, or consent

Standardized plan of care: prepared plan of care that identifies the nursing diagnoses, patient goals, and related nursing orders common to a specific population (eg, normal neonates) or problem

Standard Precautions: new CDC precautions used in the care of all patients regardless of their diagnosis or possible infection status; this category combines universal and body substance precautions

Standing order: document that details the nursing care to be implemented in specific nursing situations, frequently when a physician is not present; may expand scope of nursing responsibilities

Statutory law: law enacted by a legislative body

Stereognosis: the sense that perceives the solidity of objects, their size, shape, and texture

Stereotyping: assigning characteristics to a group of people without considering specific individuality

Sterilization: (1) the process by which all microorganisms, including spores, are destroyed; (2) surgical procedure performed to render a person infertile

Stertorous breathing: noisy respirations

Stimulus: agent, act, or other influence capable of initiating a response by the nervous system

Stoma: artificial opening for waste excretion located on the body surface

Stool: excreted feces

Strength (muscle): ability of the muscle to move actively against resistance

Stress: condition in which the human system responds to change in its normal balanced state

Stress incontinence: state in which the person experiences a loss of urine of less than 50 mL that occurs with increased abdominal pressure

Stressor: anything causing a person to experience stress; change in the balanced state

Stridor: harsh, high-pitched sound usually heard on inspiration when upper airways become narrowed

Subculture: group of people with different interests or goals than the primary culture

Subcutaneous injection: injection into the subcutaneous tissue that lies between the epidermis and the muscle

Subjective data (symptoms, covert data): information perceived only by the affected person

Subjective self: how one sees oneself; who one thinks one is

Sublingual: area in the mouth under the tongue

Sudden infant death syndrome (SIDS): sudden death of any infant or young child without demonstrated cause

Sundowning syndrome: describes a phenomenon when a person habitually becomes confused or disoriented with darkness

Suppository: oval- or cone-shaped substance that is inserted into a body cavity and that melts at body temperature

Suprapubic catheter: catheter inserted into the bladder through a small abdominal incision above the pubic area

Surgical asepsis: practices that render and keep objects and areas free from microorganisms; synonym for *sterile technique*

Susceptibility: degree of resistance of a host to a pathogen

Symptom: abnormality indicative of illness as experienced by the patient; synonym for *subjective data*

Synergistic effect: combined effect of two or more drugs is greater than the effect of each drug alone

Systemic symptoms: symptoms manifested throughout the entire body

Systolic pressure: highest point of pressure on arterial walls when the ventricles contract

T

Tachycardia: rapid heart rate

Tachypnea: abnormally rapid rate of breathing

Tactile: pertaining to touch

Tartar: hard deposit on the teeth near the gum line formed by plaque buildup and dead bacteria

Teaching: planned method or series of methods used to help someone learn

Technical competencies: skills that enable a nurse to skillfully manipulate equipment in a manner conducive to achieving a desired goal

Temperament: person's style of approaching people, situations, or events

Temperature: refers to the hotness or coldness of a substance

Terminal illness: illness from which there is no reasonable expectation of recovery or cure

Terminal wean: the withdrawal of life-sustaining therapy with the understanding that death may result, generally after a decision is made that the therapy in question is medically futile or disproportionately burdensome

Tertiary preventive care: care directed at helping rehabilitate patients and restore them to a maximum level of functioning after an illness

Therapeutic touch: an alternative therapy that involves using one's hands to consciously direct an energy exchange from the practitioner to the patient to facilitate healing or pain relief

Third-space fluid shift: distributional shift and trapping of body fluids into body spaces such as the pleural, peritoneal, or pericardial, or into the interstitial space (plasma-to-interstitial shift)

Thoracentesis: aspiration of fluid or air from the pleural space

Thrill: abnormal tremor accompanying a vascular or cardiac murmur felt on palpation

Thrombophlebitis: inflammation in a vein associated with thrombus formation

Thrombus: blood clot; plural is *thrombi*

Toddler: period from ages 1 to 3 years

Tonus: normal, partially steady state of muscle contraction

Topical application: application of a substance directly to a body site

Tort: wrong committed by a person against another person or his property

Total body water (TBW): total amount of water in the body, expressed as a percentage of body weight. The term total body fluid also is used; fluids usually are considered to include water and electrolytes

Total parenteral nutrition (TPN): nutritional therapy that bypasses the gastrointestinal tract for patients who are unable to take food orally; meets the patient's nutritional needs by way of nutrient-filled solutions administered intravenously through a central vein

Trace elements: minerals found in the body in quantities less than 5 g and needed in only small amounts (18 mg or less)

Tracheostomy tube: curved tube inserted into an artificial opening made into the trachea that comes with varied angles and in multiple sizes

Trade name: drug name selected and trademarked by the company selling the drug to market the drug; also called *brand name* or *proprietary name*

Traditional family: composed of a husband, wife, and their children, who live together in one house

Traditional knowledge: knowledge passed down from generation to generation

Transcultural nursing: providing nursing care that is planned and implemented in a way that is sensitive to the needs of individuals, families, and groups representing the diverse cultural populations within our society

Transformational leadership: type of leadership in which the person creates revolutionary change and commits to the personal and professional growth of self and others

Transmission-based precautions: new CDC precautions used in patients known or suspected to be infected with pathogens that can be transmitted by airborne, droplet, or contact routes; used in addition to Standard Precautions

Trauma: injury

Tremor: involuntary muscular movements

Trial: hearing of evidence in a legal case before a judge (and jury) with the intent of reaching a decision or verdict

Triglycerides: predominant form of fat in food and the major storage form of fat in the body; composed of one glyceride molecule and three fatty acids

Turgor: tension of a cell determined by its hydration

Typing: determining a person's blood type

U

Unilateral: affecting or occurring on one side only

Universal precautions: isolation system that considers blood, body fluids containing blood, semen, and vaginal secretions of all patients as potentially infective

Urge incontinence: state in which a person experiences involuntary passage of urine that occurs soon after a strong sense of urgency to void

Urgency: strong desire to void

Urinary retention: inability to void although urine is produced by the kidneys and enters the bladder; excessive storage of urine in the bladder

Urination: process of emptying the bladder; micturition; voiding

Utilitarianism: ethical theory that states that those acts that produce the greatest overall balance of good for the greatest number of people are right

V

Validation: act of confirming or verifying

Valsalva maneuver: forcible exhalation against a closed glottis, resulting in increased intrathoracic pressure

Value system: organization of values ranked along a continuum of importance

Values: set of beliefs that are meaningful in life and that influence relationships with others

Values clarification: process by which people come to understand their own values and value system

Variables: factors in a research study

Variance charting: documentation method in case management that records unexpected events, the cause for the event, actions taken in response to the event, and discharge planning when appropriate

Varicosity: swollen, twisted vein

Ventilation: exchange of gases

Veracity: truth telling

Verbal communication: exchange of information using words

Vesicular breath sounds: normal sound of respirations heard on auscultation over peripheral lung areas

Vial: glass bottle with self-sealing stopper through which medication is removed; may be single or multiple dose

Virulence: ability to produce disease

Virus: smallest of all microorganisms that can be seen only by using an electron microscope

Visceral: pertaining to inner organs

Visceral pain: pain originating in the internal organs in the thorax, cranium, or abdomen

Visual: pertaining to sight

Vital signs: body temperature, pulse and respiratory rates, and blood pressure; synonym for *cardinal signs*

Vitamins: organic substances needed by the body in small amounts to help regulate body processes; are susceptible to oxidation and destruction

Voiding: process of emptying the bladder; also called *micturition* or *urination*

Voluntary agencies: community agencies that are often funded by private donations, grants, or fund-raising and that provide a wide variety of direct services and education

W

Wellness: an active process in which an individual progresses toward the maximum possible potential, regardless of his or her current state of health

Wellness diagnosis: clinical judgment about an individual, family, or community in transition from a specific level of wellness to a higher level of wellness

Wheeze: a continuous, high-pitched squeak or musical sound made as air moves through narrowed or partially obstructed airway passages

Whistleblowing: term generally used to refer to employees who report their employers' violation of the law to appropriate law enforcement agencies outside the employers' facilities

Wound: injury that results in a disruption in the normal continuity of a body structure

X

X-ray: high-energy electromagnetic wave capable of penetrating solid matter and acting on photographic film; synonym for *roentgen ray*

Yin-yang: energy forces in Chinese teaching that must be in balance for good health; expression of strong emotions results in disharmony and imbalance between these forces

Young adult: the adult between the ages of 20 and 40 years; also called *early adulthood*

Z

Z-track: zigzag technique used to administer medications intramuscularly

Photo Credits

Chapter and Unit Openers

© Kathy Sloane: Chapters 1, 7, 8, 26, 30, 31, 40

© Gates Rhodes, courtesy of the School of Nursing, University of Pennsylvania: Chapter 2

© David Wagner/Phototake: Chapter 3

Courtesy of Nursing Spectrum: Units IV, V, and VI
    Children's Seashore House: Unit VII
    Daniel Hagan/Mercy Catholic Memorial Center: Chapter 14
    Linda Hadly, Montgomery ICU: Unit II
    Einrosia Photography, Shore Memorial Hospital: Chapter 4

© Mark Roberts/Custom Medical Stock Photo: Chapter 6

© Steve Rubin/Johns Hopkins School of Nursing: Chapters 9, 15

© Ed Eckstein/Phototake: Chapters 10, 13, 36

© Johns Hopkins School of Nursing: Chapters 11, 20, 23, 33

© Rick Lance/Phototake: Chapters 12, 21

© Yoav Levy/Phototake: Chapters 17, 28

© Mike McGovern, Johns Hopkins School of Nursing: Chapters 19, 45

© Eric Kamp/Phototake: Chapter 22

© B. Proud: Chapter 27, Unit VIII

Courtesy of Linda Hadley/Montgomery ICU: Chapter 29

Courtesy of John Harkins: Chapter 34

Courtesy of Ed Woods: Chapter 35

Courtesy of Brett Ainsworth: Chapters 37, 39, Unit III

© Richard T. Nowitz/Phototake: Chapter 38

© Mauritius, GMBH/Phototake: Chapter 41

© Ken Kasper: Chapter 44

Courtesy of Bill Rowe/Rockford Health System: Unit I

INDEX

Expand Your Learning Power... with the
Study Guide...
that Brings the
Fundamentals of Nursing to Life!

STUDY GUIDE
to accompany
Fundamentals of
NURSING
The Art & Science of Nursing Care
FOURTH EDITION

Carol Taylor   Priscilla LeMone
Carol Lillis   Marilee LeBon

Study Guide to Accompany Fundamentals of Nursing:

The Art and Science of Nursing Care
Fourth Edition

Carol Taylor, CSFN, RN, PhD, MSN,
Carol Lillis, RN, MSN and
Priscilla LeMone, RN, DSN, FAAN
Marilee Lebon, Journalist

Developing a learning strategy that
consistently boosts your understanding
and improves your test scores can seem
like a challenge. With this superior *Study Guide*
as your learning partner, you'll be sure to retain
and integrate all the essential material from
Fundamentals of Nursing, Fourth Edition.

This knowledge-builder provides...
- Hundreds of incisive questions that review
  vital information from each area of the
  parent text.

- Correct and incorrect responses that help
  you evaluate comprehension, reinforce
  key nursing concepts, and identify areas
  needing further study.

- Easy-to-follow format that helps you learn
  the sound foundation needed to meet
  future LPN/LVN challenges.

*Make this Study Guide part of
your successful learning strategy!*

AVAILABLE AT YOUR HEALTH
SCIENCE BOOK STORE
OR CALL TOLL FREE
1-800-638-3030

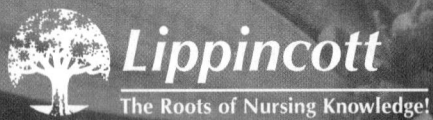

Lippincott
The Roots of Nursing Knowledge!

G322-00   CO/GD